Cancer of the Thoracic Cavity

From

Cancer

Principles & Practice of Oncology

10th edition

Cancer of the Thoracic Cavity

From
Cancer
Principles & Practice of Oncology
10th edition

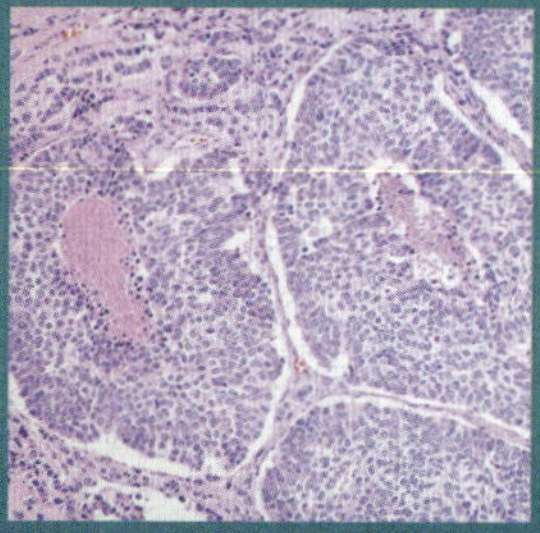
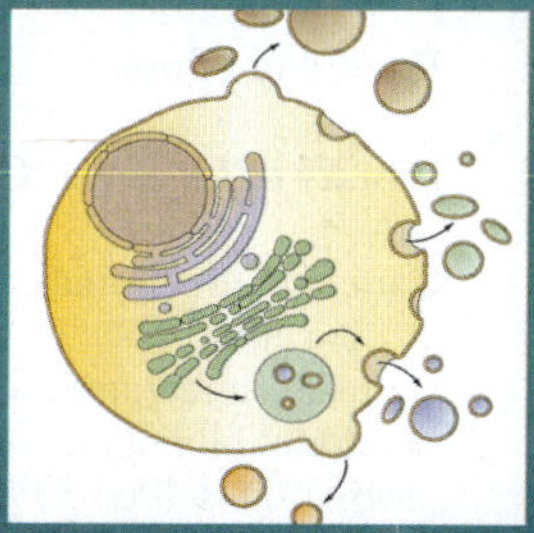
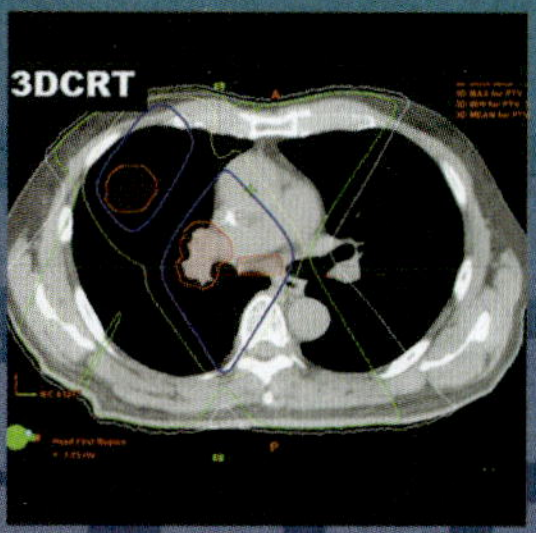

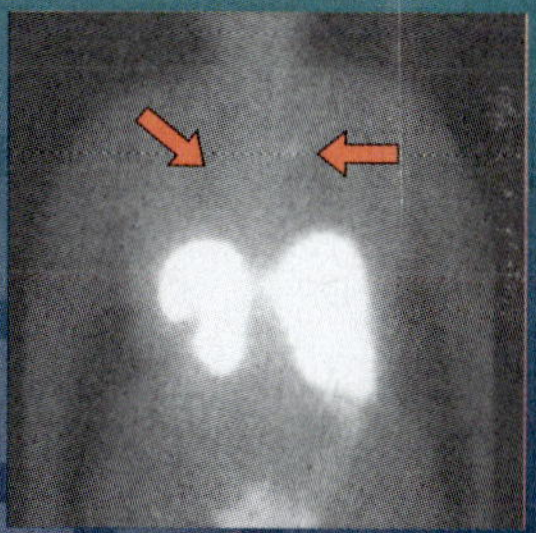

Vincent T. DeVita, Jr., MD
Amy & Joseph Perella Professor of Medicine
Yale Comprehensive Cancer Center and Smilow
Cancer Hospital at Yale-New Haven
Professor of Epidemiology and Public Health
Yale University School of Public Health
New Haven, Connecticut

Theodore S. Lawrence, MD, PhD
Isadore Lampe Professor and Chair
Department of Radiation Oncology
University of Michigan
Ann Arbor, Michigan

Steven A. Rosenberg, MD, PhD
Chief, Surgery Branch, National Cancer Institute, National Institutes of Health
Professor of Surgery, Uniformed Services University of the Health Sciences
School of Medicine
Bethesda, Maryland
Professor of Surgery
George Washington University School of Medicine
Washington, DC

Wolters Kluwer
Philadelphia • Baltimore • New York • London
Buenos Aires • Hong Kong • Sydney • Tokyo

Acquisitions Editor: Julie Goolsby
Senior Product Development Editor: Emilie Moyer
Editorial Assistant: Brian Convery
Production Project Manager: David Orzechowski
Marketing Manager: Stephanie Kindlick
Senior Designer: Stephen Druding
Illustration Coordinator: Jennifer Clements
Illustrator: Jason McAlexander, Electronic Publishing Services, Inc.
Manufacturing Coordinator: Beth Welsh
Prepress Vendor: Absolute Service, Inc.
Prepress Vendor Project Manager: Harold Medina

9 8 7 6 5 4 3 2 1

Printed in China

Library of Congress Cataloging-in-Publication Data

Cancer of the thoracic cavity / editors, Vincent T. DeVita, Jr., Theodore S. Lawrence, Steven A. Rosenberg.
p. ; cm.
"From Cancer: principles & practice of oncology, 10th edition."
Includes bibliographical references and index.
ISBN 978-1-4963-3395-7 (alk. paper)
I. DeVita, Vincent T., Jr., 1935- , editor. II. Lawrence, Theodore S., editor. III. Rosenberg, Steven A., editor. IV. Devita, Hellman and Rosenberg's cancer. 10th ed. Abridgement of (expression):
[DNLM: 1. Thoracic Neoplasms. WF 970]
RC280.C5
616.99'494–dc23

2015031786

LWW.com

CONTRIBUTORS

Gregory P. Adams, PhD
Associate Professor, Developmental Therapeutics Program
Director of Biological Research and Therapeutics
Fox Chase Cancer Center
Philadelphia, Pennsylvania

Bharat B. Aggarwal, PhD
Professor of Cancer Research
Professor of Cancer Medicine (Biochemistry)
Chief, Cytokine Research Laboratory
Department of Experimental Therapeutics
The University of Texas MD Anderson Cancer Center
Houston, Texas

Shirin Arastu-Kapur, PhD
Associate Director
Biology at Onyx Pharmaceuticals
South San Francisco, California

Luiz Henrique de Lima Araujo, MD, MSc
Postdoctoral Researcher
James Cancer Center
The Ohio State University Medical Center
Columbus, Ohio

Alan Ashworth, FRS
Professor and Chief Executive
The Institute of Cancer Research
London, United Kingdom

Sharyn D. Baker, PharmD, PhD
Associate Member
Pharmaceutical Sciences Department
St. Jude Children's Research Hospital
Memphis, Tennessee

Alberto Bardelli, MD
Laboratory of Molecular Genetics
Institute for Cancer Research and Treatment
University of Torino Medical School
Candiolo, Italy

Susan E. Bates, MD
Head, Molecular Therapeutics Section
Developmental Therapeutics Branch
Center for Cancer Research
National Cancer Institute
Bethesda, Maryland

Stephen B. Baylin, MD
Professor of Oncology
Professor of Medicine
Johns Hopkins University School of Medicine
Deputy Director of the Cancer Center
Baltimore, Maryland

Andrew Berchuck, MD
Professor and Director
Gynecologic Oncology Program
Division of Gynecologic Oncology
Department of Obstetrics and Gynecology
Duke Cancer Institute
Duke University Medical Center
Durham, North Carolina

Leslie Bernstein, MS, PhD
Professor and Director
Division of Cancer Etiology
Department of Population Sciences
Beckman Research Institute
City of Hope Dean for Faculty Affairs
City of Hope National Medical Center and the Beckman Research Institute
Duarte, California

Bryan L. Betz, PhD
Assistant Professor
Department of Pathology
University of Michigan
Technical Director
Molecular Diagnostics Laboratory
University of Michigan Health System
Ann Arbor, Michigan

Lawrence H. Boise, PhD
Professor
Winship Cancer Institute of Emory University
Departments of Hematology/Medical Oncology and Cell Biology
Emory School of Medicine
Atlanta, Georgia

Danielle C. Bonadies, MS, CGC
Director, Cancer Genetics Division
Gene Counsel, LLC
New Haven, Connecticut

Hossein Borghaei, MS, DO
Associate Professor
Chief, Thoracic Medical Oncology
Fox Chase Cancer Center
Philadelphia, Pennsylvania

Otis W. Brawley, MD, FACP
Chief Medical Officer
American Cancer Society, Inc.
Atlanta, Georgia

Dean E. Brenner, MD
Kutsche Family Professor of Internal Medicine
Professor of Pharmacology
University of Michigan Comprehensive Cancer Center
Ann Arbor, Michigan

Christopher B. Buck, PhD
Investigator
Head, Tumor Virus Molecular Biology Section
Laboratory of Cellular Oncology
Center for Cancer Research
National Cancer Institute
Bethesda, Maryland

Tim E. Byers, MD, MPH
Associate Dean for Public Health Practice
Colorado School of Public Health
Associate Director for Cancer Prevention and Control
University of Colorado Cancer Center
Aurora, Colorado

A. Hilary Calvert
Professor
Gynecologic Oncology
University College Hospitals (UCLH)
London, United Kingdom

Robert B. Cameron, MD
Professor, Cardiothoracic Surgery and Surgical Oncology
David Geffen School of Medicine
University of California, Los Angeles
Chief, Thoracic Surgery
West Los Angeles Virginia Medical Center
Los Angeles, California

David P. Carbone, MD, PhD
Barbara J. Bonner Chair in Lung Cancer Research
Professor of Medicine
Director, James Thoracic Center
James Cancer Center
The Ohio State University Medical Center
Columbus, Ohio

Michele Carbone, MD, PhD
Director
University of Hawaii Cancer Center
Professor, Department of Pathology
John A. Burns School of Medicine
Honolulu, Hawaii

Cindy H. Chau, PharmD, PhD
Scientist
Medical Oncology Branch
Center for Cancer Research
National Cancer Institute
National Institutes of Health
Bethesda, Maryland

Edward Chu, MD
Professor of Medicine and Pharmacology & Chemical Biology
Chief, Division of Hematology-Oncology
Deputy Director, University of Pittsburgh Cancer Institute
University of Pittsburgh School of Medicine
Pittsburgh, Pennsylvania

Jessica Clague, PhD, MPH
Assistant Research Professor
Division of Cancer Etiology
Department of Population Sciences
Beckman Research Institute
City of Hope National Medical Center
Duarte, California

M. Sitki Copur, MD, FACP
Medical Director of Oncology
Saint Francis Cancer Treatment Center
Grand Island, Nebraska
Professor, Department of Medicine
Division of Hematology Oncology
Adjunct Faculty
University of Nebraska Medical Center
Omaha, Nebraska

Roy H. Decker, MD, PhD
Associate Professor
Department of Therapeutic Radiology
Yale University School of Medicine
New Haven, Connecticut

Marcello Deraco, MD
Peritoneal Surface Malignancies
Department of Surgery-Colorectal Unit
Fondazione IRCCS
Instituto Nazionale dei Tumori
Milano, Italy
Professor Postgraduation on Digestive Surgery
Tor Vergata University
Roma, Italy

Hari A. Deshpande, MD
Associate Professor of Medicine
Yale University School of Medicine
Section of Medical Oncology
Yale New Haven Hospital
New Haven, Connecticut

Frank C. Detterbeck, MD
Professor and Chief
Section of Thoracic Surgery
Yale University School of Medicine
New Haven, Connecticut

Khanh T. Do, MD
Senior Clinical Fellow
Division of Cancer Treatment and Diagnosis
National Cancer Institute
National Institutes of Health
Bethesda, Maryland

James H. Doroshow, MD
Director, Division of Cancer Treatment and Diagnosis
Deputy Director for Clinical and Translational Research
National Cancer Institute
National Institutes of Health
Bethesda, Maryland

Dominique M. Elias, MD, PhD
Professor, Department of Surgical Oncology
Villejuif, France

Charles Erlichman, MD
Professor, Department of Oncology
Deputy Director, Clinical Research
Peter and Frances Georgeson Professor of Gastroenterology Cancer Research
Mayo Clinic
Rochester, Minnesota

Steven A. Feldman, PhD
Staff Scientist
Director, Surgery Branch
Vector Production Facility
National Cancer Institute
Bethesda, Maryland

William Douglas Figg, Sr., PharmD, MBA
Senior Investigator and Head of the Clinical Pharmacology Program
Clinical Director, Center for Cancer Research
Head of the Molecular Pharmacology Section
Medical Oncology Branch
Center for Cancer Research
National Cancer Institute
National Institutes of Health
Bethesda, Maryland

Antonio Tito Fojo, MD, PhD
Medical Oncology Branch and Affiliates
Head, Experimental Therapeutics Section
Senior Investigator
Center for Cancer Research
National Cancer Institute
Bethesda, Maryland

Larissa V. Furtado, MD
Assistant Professor
Department of Pathology
Assistant Director
Division of Genomics and Molecular Pathology
University of Chicago
Chicago, Illinois

Sheryl G. A. Gabram-Mendola, MD, MBA, FACS
Surgeon-in-Chief
Grady Memorial Hospital
Emory University School of Medicine
Deputy Director
Georgia Cancer Center for Excellence
Director, AVON Comprehensive Breast Center at Grady
Director, High Risk Assessment Program
Winship Cancer Institute of Emory University
Georgia Cancer Coalition Distinguished Cancer Scholar
Atlanta, Georgia

Jared J. Gartner, DO
Biologist, National Cancer Institute
Surgery Branch
National Institute of Health
Bethesda, Maryland

Scott Nicholas Gettinger, MD
Associate Professor of Medicine
Thoracic Oncology Program
Developmental Therapeutics
Yale Cancer Center
New Haven, Connecticut

Olivier Glehen, MD, PhD
Professor Lyon 1 University
Chief, Division of General Surgery
Hospices Civils de Lyon
Department of General and Oncologic Surgery
Centre Hospitalier Lyon Sud
Pierre-Bénite, France

Matthew P. Goetz, MD
Associate Professor of Pharmacology
Associate Professor of Oncology
Mayo Clinic
Rochester, Minnesota

Sarah B. Goldberg, MD, MPH
Assistant Professor of Internal Medicine
Medical Oncology
Yale Cancer Center
Yale University School of Medicine
New Haven, Connecticut

Steven D. Gore, MD
Yale University School of Medicine
New Haven, Connecticut

Ellen R. Gritz, PhD
Professor and Chair
Department of Behavioral Science
The University of Texas MD Anderson Cancer Center
Houston, Texas

José G. Guillem, MD, MPH
Department of Surgery
Memorial Sloan-Kettering Cancer Center
New York, New York

Douglas Hanahan, PhD
Director
Swiss Institute for Experimental Cancer Research (ISREC)
Lausanne, Switzerland

Lyndsay N. Harris, MD, FRCP(C)
Diana Hyland Chair in Breast Cancer
Director, Breast Cancer Program
Seidman Cancer Center
University Hospitals Case Medical Center
Professor of Medicine
Division of Hematology and Oncology
Case Western Reserve University
Cleveland, Ohio

C. William Helm, MBBChir, FRCS
Northern Gynaecological Oncology Center
Queen Elizabeth Hospital, Gateshead
Tyne and Wear, United Kingdom

James G. Herman, MD
Johns Hopkins University
Baltimore, Maryland

Jay L. Hess, MD, PhD
Professor, Department of Pathology
Carl V. Weller Professor and Chair
Professor, Department of Internal Medicine
University of Michigan Health System
Ann Arbor, Michigan

Christopher J. Hoimes, DO
Assistant Professor
UH Case Medical Center
Department of Medicine-Hematology and Oncology
Cleveland, Ohio

Leora Horn, MD, MSc
Associate Professor, Department of Medicine
Vanderbilt University Medical Center
Nashville, Tennessee

Vanessa W. Hui, MD
Department of Surgery
Memorial Sloan-Kettering Cancer Center
New York, New York

Christopher J. Kirk, MD
Vice President of Research
Onyx Pharmaceuticals, Inc.
South San Francisco, California

James N. Kochenderfer, MD
Investigator, Experimental Transplantation and Immunology Branch
National Cancer Institute
National Institutes of Health
Bethesda, Maryland

Manish Kohli, MD
Associate Professor of Oncology
Department of Oncology
College of Medicine
Mayo Clinic
Joint Appointment, Department of Urology
Mayo Clinic
Rochester, Minnesota

Mark G. Kris, MD
Professor of Medicine
Weill Cornell Medical College
Attending Physician, Thoracic Oncology Service
Memorial Sloan-Kettering Cancer Center
New York, New York

Lee M. Krug, MD
Associate Attending Physician
Department of Medicine
Memorial Sloan-Kettering Cancer Center
Associate Professor of Medicine
Weill Medical College of Cornell University
New York, New York

Shivaani Kummar, MD, FACP
Head, Early Clinical Trials Development
Office of the Director
Division of Cancer Treatment and Diagnosis
National Cancer Institute
Bethesda, Maryland

Theodore S. Lawrence, MD, PhD
Isadore Lampe Professor and Chair
Department of Radiation Oncology
University of Michigan Health System
Ann Arbor, Michigan

Percy P. Lee, MD
Associate Professor of Radiation Oncology
Chief, Thoracic Radiation Oncology
Chief, Gastrointestinal Radiation Oncology
Director, Stereotactic Body Radiation Oncology Program
David Geffen School of Medicine at University of California, Los Angeles
University of California Los Angeles Jonsson Comprehensive Cancer Center
Los Angeles, California

Rogerio C. Lilenbaum, MD
Chief Medical Officer of Smilow Cancer Hospital
Thoracic Oncology Program
Yale University School of Medicine
New Haven, Connecticut

Scott M. Lippman, MD
Director, Senior Associate Dean, & Associate Vice Chancellor
Cancer Research and Care
Chugai Pharmaceutical Chair
Professor of Medicine
University of California, San Diego
Moores Cancer Center
La Jolla, California

Mats Ljungman, PhD
Professor, Departments of Radiation Oncology and Environmental Health Sciences
Translational Oncology Program
University of Michigan Medical School
Ann Arbor, Michigan

Patrick J. Loehrer, Sr, MD
H. H. Gregg Professor of Oncology
Director, Indiana University Melvin and Bren Simon Cancer Center
Associate Dean for Cancer Research
Indiana University School of Medicine
Indianapolis, Indiana

Carlos López-Otin, PhD
Professor, Department of Biochemistry and Molecular Biology
Universidad de Oviedo
Principality of Asturias, Spain

Charles L. Loprinzi, MD
Regis Professor of Breast Cancer Research
Department of Oncology
Mayo Clinic
Rochester, Minnesota

Yani Lu, PhD
Assistant Research Professor
Division of Cancer Etiology
Department of Population Science
Beckman Research Institute of the City of Hope
Duarte, California

Xiaomei Ma, PhD
Associate Professor, Department of Chronic Disease Epidemiology
Yale University School of Public Health
New Haven, Connecticut

Ellen T. Matloff, MS, CGC
President & CEO
Gene Counsel, LLC
New Haven, Connecticut

Susan T. Mayne, PhD
C.-E.A. Winslow Professor of Epidemiology
Chair, Department of Chronic Disease Epidemiology
Yale University School of Public Health
Associate Director for Population Sciences
Yale Cancer Center
New Haven, Connecticut

Howard L. McLeod, PharmD
Medical Director, DeBartolo Family Personalized Medicine Institute
Senior Member, Division of Population Sciences
H. Lee Moffitt Cancer Center
Tampa, Florida

Karin B. Michels, ScD, PhD
Associate Professor
Obstetrician/Gynecologist
Epidemiology Center
Department of Obstetrics, Gynecology and Reproductive Biology
Brigham and Women's Hospital
Harvard Medical School
Boston, Massachusetts

Jeffrey F. Moley, MD
Chief, Section of Endocrine and Oncologic Surgery
Professor of Surgery
Washington University School of Medicine
St. Louis, Missouri

Meredith A. Morgan, PhD
Research Assistant Professor
Department of Radiation Oncology
University of Michigan
Ann Arbor, Michigan

Patrick Nana-Sinkam, MD
Associate Professor, Department of Internal Medicine
Division of Pulmonary, Allergy, Critical Care and Sleep Medicine
The Ohio State University
Columbus, Ohio

Jeffrey A. Norton, MD
Professor, Department of Surgery
Chief, Section of Surgical Oncology and Division of General Surgery
Department of Surgery
Stanford University Hospital
Stanford, California

Richard J. O'Connor, PhD
Associate Member, Department of Health Behavior
Division of Cancer Prevention and Population Sciences
Roswell Park Cancer Institute
Buffalo, New York

Peter J. O'Dwyer, MD
Professor of Medicine
Abramson Cancer Center
University of Pennsylvania
Philadelphia, Pennsylvania

Gregory A. Otterson, MD
Professor, Department of Internal Medicine
Division of Medical Oncology
Director, Hematology/Oncology Fellowship Program
The Ohio State University Comprehensive Cancer Center
Columbus, Ohio

Howard L. Parnes, MD
Chief
Prostate and Urologic Cancer Research Group
Division of Cancer Prevention
National Cancer Institute
Rockville, Maryland

Harvey I. Pass, MD
Stephen E. Banner Professor of Thoracic Oncology
Vice-Chairman, Research Department of Cardiothoracic Surgery
Director, General Thoracic Surgery
New York University Langone Medical Center
New York, New York

Giao Q. Phan, MD, FACS
Associate Professor
Division of Surgical Oncology
Massey Cancer Center
Virginia Commonwealth University
Richmond, Virginia

M. Catherine Pietanza, MD
Thoracic Oncology
Memorial Sloan-Kettering Cancer Center
New York, New York

Yves Pommier, MD, PhD
Chief, Laboratory of Molecular Pharmacology
Head, DNA Topoisomerase/Integrase Group
Center for Cancer Research
National Cancer Institute
Bethesda, Maryland

Sahdeo Prasad, PhD
Cytokine Research Laboratory
Department of Experimental Therapeutics
The University of Texas MD Anderson Cancer Center
Houston, Texas

Lee Ratner, MD, PhD
Professor Departments of Medicine and Molecular Microbiology
Co-Director, Medical & Molecular Oncology
Washington University School of Medicine
Barnes-Jewish Hospital
St. Louis, Missouri

Paul F. Robbins, PhD
National Institutes of Health
Bethesda, Maryland

Matthew K. Robinson, PhD
Assistant Professor, Developmental Therapeutics Program
Fox Chase Cancer Center
Philadelphia, Pennsylvania

Steven A. Rosenberg, MD, PhD
Chief, Surgery Branch, National Cancer Institute, National Institutes of Health
Professor of Surgery, Uniformed Services University of the Health Sciences
School of Medicine
Bethesda, Maryland
Professor of Surgery
George Washington University School of Medicine
Washington, District of Columbia

Kenneth E. Rosenzweig, MD
Professor, Department of Radiation Oncology
Icahn School of Medicine at Mount Sinai
Chair, Department of Radiation Oncology
Mount Sinai Health System
New York, New York

Charles M. Rudin, MD, PhD
Chief, Thoracic Oncology Service
Memorial Sloan-Kettering Cancer Center
New York, New York

M. Wasif Saif, MD, MBBS
Director, Gastrointestinal Oncology Program
Leader, Experimental Therapeutics Program
Tufts Medical Center
Tufts University School of Medicine
Boston, Massachusetts

Yardena Samuels, PhD
Knell Family Professorial Chair
Department of Molecular Cell Biology
Weizmann Institute of Science
Rehovot, Israel

Charles L. Sawyers, MD
Investigator, Howard Hughes Medical Institute
Chair, Human Oncology and Pathogenesis Program
Memorial Sloan-Kettering Cancer Center
New York, New York

Peter G. Shields, MD
Deputy Director, Comprehensive Cancer Center
Professor, College of Medicine
James Cancer Hospital
The Ohio State University
Columbus, Ohio

Alex Sparreboom, PhD
Associate Member, Department of Pharmaceutical Sciences
St. Jude Children's Research Hospital
Memphis, Tennessee

Paul H. Sugarbaker, MD, FACS, FRCS
Medical Director, Center for Gastrointestinal Malignancies
Chief, Program in Peritoneal Surface Oncology
MedStar Washington Hospital Center
Washington, District of Columbia

Irene M. Tamí-Maury, DMD, DrPH, MSc
The University of Texas MD Anderson Cancer Center
Houston, Texas

Lynn Tanoue, MD
Professor of Internal Medicine
Medical Director
Yale Cancer Center
Thoracic Oncology Program
Yale University School of Medicine
New Haven, Connecticut

Randall K. Ten Haken, PhD, FAAPM, FInstP, FASTRO, FACR
Professor, Associate Chair, and Physics Division Director
Department of Radiation Oncology
University of Michigan Medical School
Ann Arbor, Michigan

Kenneth D. Tew, PhD, DSc
Chairman and John C. West Chair in Cancer Research
Cell and Molecular Pharmacology
Medical University of South Carolina
Charleston, South Carolina

Benjamin A. Toll, PhD
Associate Professor of Psychiatry
Yale University School of Medicine
Yale Comprehensive Cancer Center
Program Director, Smoking Cessation Service
Smilow Cancer Hospital at Yale-New Haven
New Haven, Connecticut

William D. Travis, MD
Professor of Pathology
Weill Medical College of Cornell University
Memorial Sloan-Kettering Cancer Center
New York, New York

Brian B. Tuch, PhD
Associate Director, Translational Genomics
Onyx Pharmaceuticals
South San Francisco, California

Vic J. Verwaal, MD, PhD
The Netherlands Cancer Institute
Amsterdam, The Netherlands

Christine M. Walko, PharmD, BCOP
Clinical Pharmacogenetic Scientist
DeBartolo Family Personalized Medicine Institute
Applied Clinical Scientist, Division of Population Science
H. Lee Moffitt Cancer Center and Research Institute
Tampa, Florida

Graham W. Warren, MD, PhD
Associate Professor
Vice Chair for Research in Radiation Oncology
Department of Radiation Oncology
Department of Cell and Molecular Pharmacology
Hollings Cancer Center
Medical University of South Carolina
Charleston, South Carolina

Robert A. Weinberg, PhD
Member, Whitehead Institute for Biomedical Research
Department of Biology
Massachusetts Institute of Technology
Director, Ludwig Center for Molecular Oncology
Whitehead Institute for Biomedical Research
Cambridge, Massachusetts

Louis M. Weiner, MD
Director, Lombardi Comprehensive Cancer Center
Professor and Chair, Department of Oncology
Francis L. and Charlotte G. Gragnani Chair
Georgetown University Medical Center
Washington, District of Columbia

Walter C. Willett, MD, DrPH
Professor and Chair, Department of Nutrition
Harvard School of Public Health
Boston, Massachusetts

Terence M. Williams, MD, PhD
Assistant Professor, Department of Radiation Oncology
The Ohio State University
Arthur G. James and Richard Solove Research Institute
Columbus, Ohio

Abraham J. Wu, MD
Assistant Attending Physician
Department of Radiation Oncology
Memorial Sloan-Kettering Cancer Center
New York, New York

Herbert Yu, MD, PhD
Professor and Director
Cancer Epidemiology Program
Associate Director for Population Sciences and Cancer Control
University of Hawaii Cancer Center
Adjunct Professor, Department of Chronic Disease Epidemiology
Yale School of Public Health
Honolulu, Hawaii

Stuart H. Yuspa, MD
Chief, Laboratory of Cancer Biology and Genetics
Center for Cancer Research
National Cancer Institute
Bethesda, Maryland

CONTENTS

PART IV

Cancer Prevention and Screening

PART V

Cancer of the Thoracic Cavity

PART I

Principles of Oncology

1 The Cancer Genome

Yardena Samuels, Alberto Bardelli, Jared J. Gartner, and Carlos López-Otin

INTRODUCTION

There is a broad consensus that cancer is, in essence, a genetic disease, and that accumulation of molecular alterations in the genome of somatic cells is the basis of cancer progression (Fig. 1.1).[1] In the past 10 years, the availability of the human genome sequence and progress in DNA sequencing technologies has dramatically improved knowledge of this disease. These new insights are transforming the field of oncology at multiple levels:

1. The genomic maps are redesigning the tumor taxonomy by moving it from a histologic- to a genetic-based level.
2. The success of cancer drugs designed to target the molecular alterations underlying tumorigenesis has proven that somatic genetic alterations are legitimate targets for therapy.
3. Tumor genotyping is helping clinicians individualize treatments by matching patients with the best treatment for their tumors.
4. Tumor-specific DNA alterations represent highly sensitive biomarkers for disease detection and monitoring.
5. Finally, the ongoing analyses of multiple cancer genomes will identify additional targets, whose pharmacologic exploitation will undoubtedly result in new therapeutic approaches.

This chapter will review the progress that has been made in understanding the genetic basis of sporadic cancers. An emphasis will be placed on an introduction to novel integrated genomic approaches that allow a comprehensive and systematic evaluation of genetic alterations that occur during the progression of cancer. Using these powerful tools, cancer research, diagnosis, and treatment are poised for a transformation in the next years.

CANCER GENES AND THEIR MUTATIONS

Cancer genes are broadly grouped into oncogenes and tumor suppressor genes. Using a classical analogy, oncogenes can be compared to a car accelerator, so that a mutation in an oncogene would be the equivalent of having the accelerator continuously pressed.[2] Tumor suppressor genes, in contrast, act as brakes,[2] so that when they are not mutated, they function to inhibit tumorigenesis. Oncogene and tumor suppressor genes may be classified by the nature of their somatic mutations in tumors. Mutations in oncogenes typically occur at specific hotspots, often affecting the same codon or clustered at neighboring codons in different tumors.[1] Furthermore, mutations in oncogenes are almost always missense, and the mutations usually affect only one allele, making them heterozygous. In contrast, tumor suppressor genes are usually mutated throughout the gene; a large number of the mutations may truncate the encoded protein and generally affect both alleles, causing loss of heterozygosity (LOH). Major types of somatic mutations present in malignant tumors include nucleotide substitutions, small insertions and deletions (*indels*), chromosomal rearrangements, and copy number alterations.

IDENTIFICATION OF CANCER GENES

The completion of the Human Genome Project marked a new era in biomedical sciences.[3] Knowledge of the sequence and organization of the human genome now allows for the systematic analysis of the genetic alterations underlying the origin and evolution of tumors. Before elucidation of the human genome, several cancer genes, such as *KRAS*, *TP53*, and *APC*, were successfully discovered using approaches based on an oncovirus analysis, linkage studies, LOH, and cytogenetics.[4,5] The first curated version of the Human Genome Project was released in 2004,[3] and provided a sequence-based map of the normal human genome. This information, together with the construction of the HapMap, which contains single nucleotide polymorphisms (SNP), and the underlying genomic structure of natural human genomic variation,[6,7] allowed an extraordinary throughput in cataloging somatic mutations in cancer. These projects now offer an unprecedented opportunity: the identification of all the genetic changes associated with a human cancer. For the first time, this ambitious goal is within reach of the scientific community. Already, a number of studies have demonstrated the usefulness of strategies aimed at the systematic identification of somatic mutations associated with cancer progression. Notably, the Human Genome Project, the HapMap project, as well as the candidate and family gene approaches (described in the following paragraphs), utilized capillary-based DNA sequencing (first-generation sequencing, also known as Sanger sequencing).[8] Figure 1.2 clearly illustrates the developments in the search of cancer genes, its increased pace, as well as the most relevant findings in this field.

Cancer Gene Discovery by Sequencing Candidate Gene Families

The availability of the human genome sequence provides new opportunities to comprehensively search for somatic mutations in cancer on a larger scale than previously possible. Progress in the field has been closely linked to improvements in the throughput of DNA analysis and in the continuous reduction in sequencing costs. What follows are some of the achievements in this research area, as well as how they affected knowledge of the cancer genome.

A seminal work in the field was the systematic mutational profiling of the genes involved in the RAS-RAF pathway in multiple tumors. This candidate gene approach led to the discovery that *BRAF* is frequently mutated in melanomas and is mutated at a lower frequency in other tumor types.[9] Follow-up studies quickly revealed that mutations in *BRAF* are mutually exclusive with alterations in *KRAS*,[9,10] genetically emphasizing that these genes function in the same pathway, a concept that had been previously demonstrated in lower organisms such as *Caenorhabditis elegans* and *Drosophila melanogaster*.[11,12]

In 2003, the identification of cancer genes shifted from a candidate gene approach to the mutational analyses of gene families. The first gene families to be completely sequenced were those that

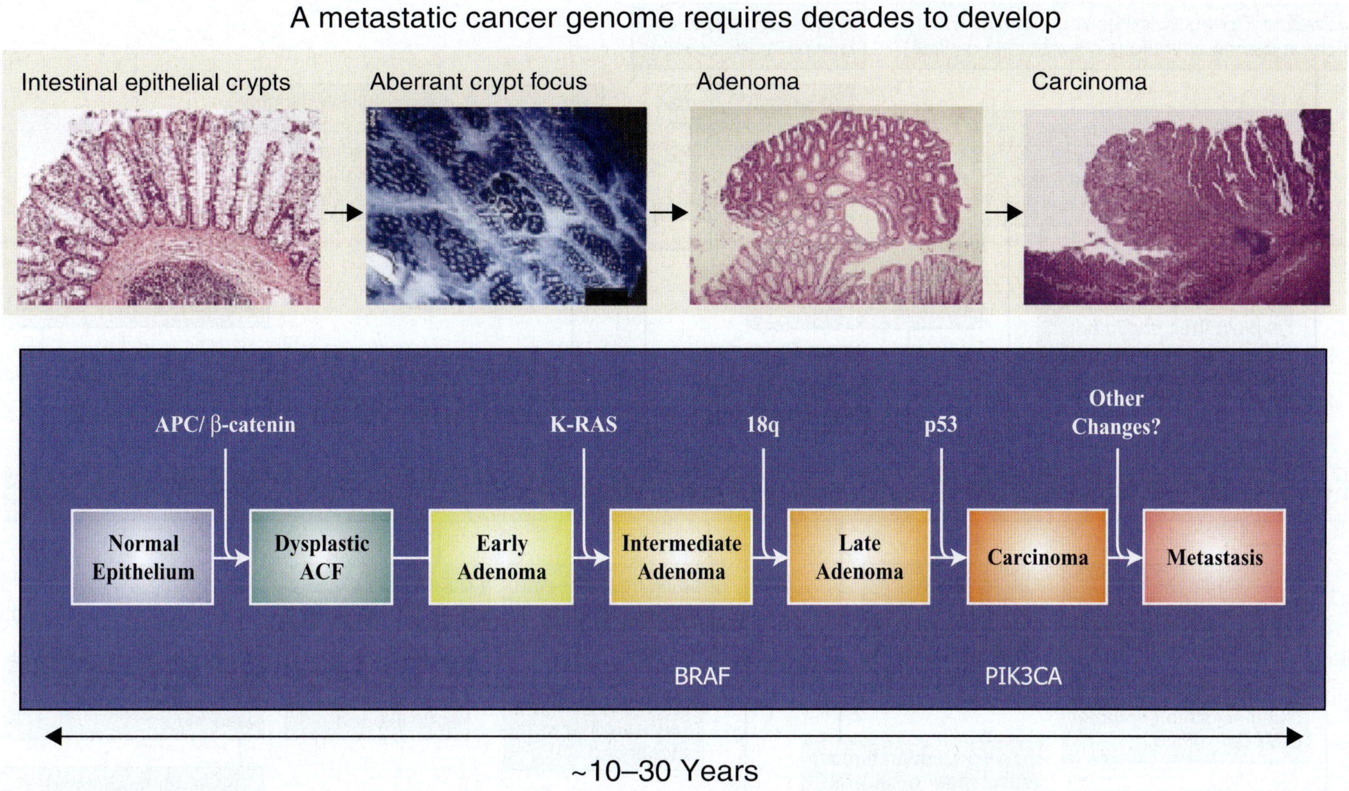

Figure 1.1 Schematic representation of the genomic and histopathologic steps associated with tumor progression: from the occurrence of the initiating mutation in the founder cell to metastasis formation. It has been convincingly shown that the genomic landscape of solid tumors such as that of pancreatic and colorectal tumors requires the accumulation of many genetic events, a process that requires decades to complete. This timeline offers an incredible window of opportunity for the early detection, which is often associated with an excellent prognosis, of this disease.

involved protein[13,14] and lipid phosphorylation.[15] The rationale for initially focusing on these gene families was threefold:

- The corresponding proteins were already known at that time to play a pivotal role in the signaling and proliferation of normal and cancerous cells.
- Multiple members of the protein kinases family had already been linked to tumorigenesis.
- Kinases are clearly amenable to pharmacologic inhibition, making them attractive drug targets.

The mutational analysis of all the tyrosine-kinase domains in colorectal cancers revealed that 30% of cases had a mutation in at least one tyrosine-kinase gene, and overall mutations were identified in eight different kinases, most of which had not previously been linked to cancer.[13] An additional mutational analysis of the coding exons of 518 protein kinase genes in 210 diverse human cancers, including breast, lung, gastric, ovarian, renal, and acute lymphoblastic leukemia, identified approximately 120 mutated genes that probably contribute to oncogenesis.[14] Because kinase activity is attenuated by enzymes that remove phosphate groups called phosphatases, the rational next step in these studies was to perform a mutation analysis of the protein tyrosine phosphatases. A mutational investigation of this family in colorectal cancer identified that 25% of cases had mutations in six different phosphatase genes (*PTPRF*, *PTPRG*, *PTPRT*, *PTPN3*, *PTPN13*, or *PTPN14*).[16] A combined analysis of the protein tyrosine kinases and the protein tyrosine phosphatases showed that 50% of colorectal cancers had mutations in a tyrosine-kinase gene, a protein tyrosine phosphatase gene, or both, further emphasizing the pivotal role of protein phosphorylation in neoplastic progression. Many of the identified genes had previously been linked to human cancer, thus validating the unbiased comprehensive mutation profiling. These landmark studies led to additional gene family surveys.

The phosphatidylinositol 3 kinase (*PI3K*) gene family, which also plays a role in proliferation, adhesion, survival, and motility, was also comprehensively investigated.[17] Sequencing of the exons encoding the kinase domain of all 16 members belonging to this family pinpointed *PIK3CA* as the only gene to harbor somatic mutations. When the entire coding region was analyzed, *PIK3CA* was found to be somatically mutated in 32% of colorectal cancers. At that time, the *PIK3CA* gene was certainly not a newcomer in the cancer arena, because it had previously been shown to be involved in cell transformation and metastasis.[17] Strikingly, its staggeringly high mutation frequency was discovered only through systematic sequencing of the corresponding gene family.[15] Subsequent analysis of *PIK3CA* in other tumor types identified somatic mutations in this gene in additional cancer types, including 36% of hepatocellular carcinomas, 36% of endometrial carcinomas, 25% of breast carcinomas, 15% of anaplastic oligodendrogliomas, 5% of medulloblastomas and anaplastic astrocytomas, and 27% of glioblastomas.[18–22] It is known that *PIK3CA* is one of the two (the other being *KRAS*) most commonly mutated oncogenes in human cancers. Further investigation of the *PI3K* pathway in colorectal cancer showed that 40% of tumors had genetic alterations in one of the *PI3K* pathway genes, emphasizing the central role of this pathway in colorectal cancer pathogenesis.[23]

Although most cancer genome studies of large gene families have focused on the kinome, recent analyses have revealed that members of other families highly represented in the human genome are also a target of mutational events in cancer. This is the case of proteases, a complex group of enzymes consisting of at least 569 components that constitute the so-called human degradome.[24] Proteases exhibit an elaborate interplay with kinases and

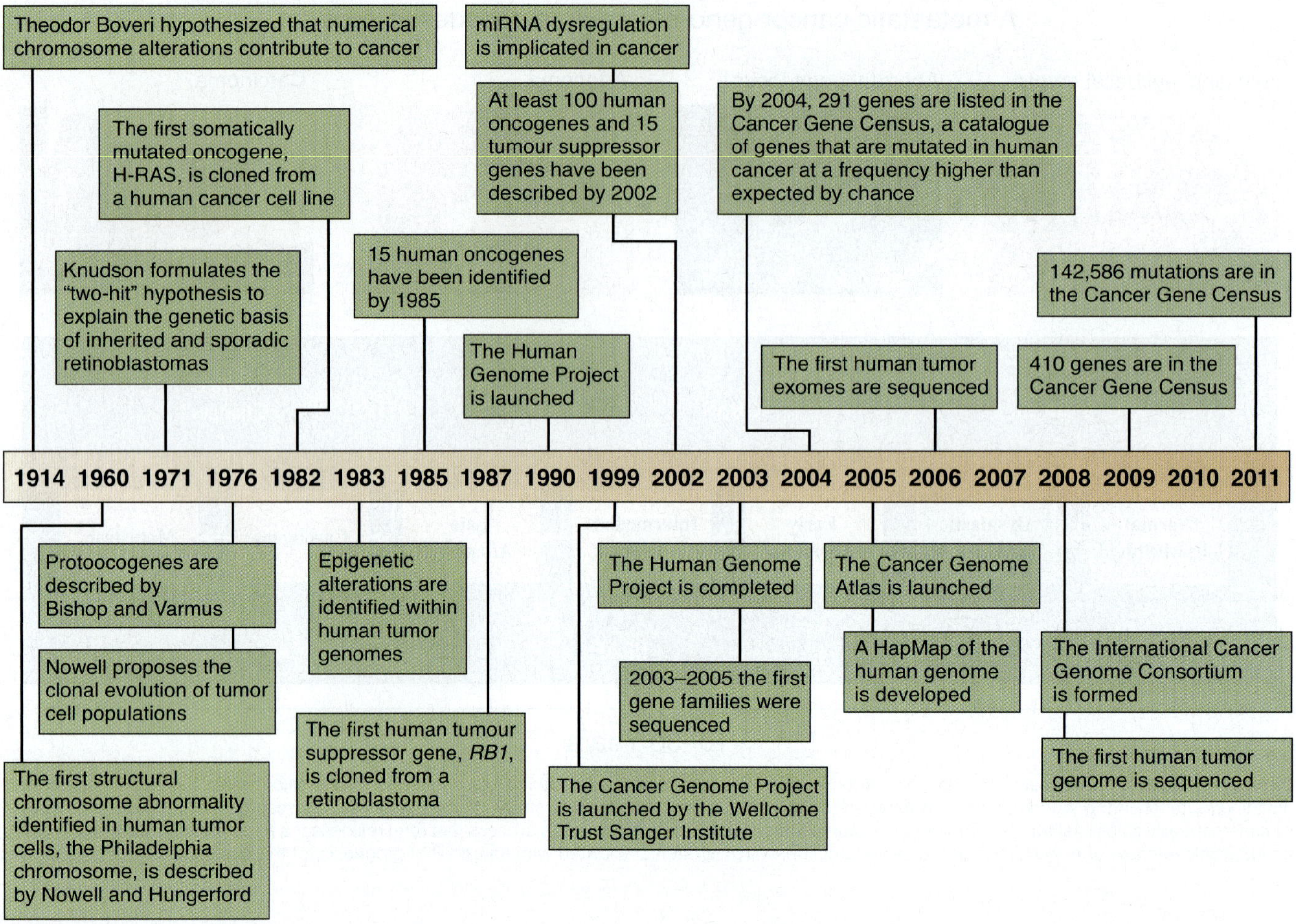

Figure 1.2 Timeline of seminal hypotheses, research discoveries, and research initiatives that have led to an improved understanding of the genetic etiology of human tumorigenesis within the past century. The consensus cancer gene data were obtained from the Wellcome Trust Sanger Institute Cancer Genome Project Web site (http://www.sanger.ac.uk/genetics/CGP). (Redrawn from Bell DW. Our changing view of the genomic landscape of cancer. *J Pathol* 2010;220:231–243.)

have traditionally been associated with cancer progression because of their ability to degrade extracellular matrices, thus facilitating tumor invasion and metastasis.[25,26] However, recent studies have shown that these enzymes hydrolyze a wide variety of substrates and influence many different steps of cancer, including early stages of tumor evolution.[27] These functional studies have also revealed that beyond their initial recognition as prometastatic enzymes, they play dual roles in cancer, as assessed by the identification of a growing number of tumor-suppressive proteases.[28]

These findings emphasized the possibility that mutational activation or inactivation of protease genes occurs in cancer. A systematic analysis of genetic alterations in breast and colorectal cancers revealed that proteases from different catalytic classes were somatically mutated in cancer.[29] These results prompted the mutational analysis of entire protease families such as matrix metalloproteinases (MMP), a disintegrin and metalloproteinase (ADAM), and ADAMs with thrombospondin domains (ADAMTS) in different tumors. These studies led to the identification of protease genes frequently mutated in cancer, such as *MMP8*, which is mutated and functionally inactivated in 6.3% of human melanomas.[30,31]

The mutational status of caspases has also been extensively analyzed in different tumors because these proteases play a fundamental role in the execution of apoptosis, one of the hallmarks of cancer.[32] These studies demonstrated that *CASP8* is deleted in neuroblastomas and inactivated by somatic mutations in a variety of human malignancies, including head and neck, colorectal, lung, and gastric carcinomas.[33–35] Other large protease families whose components are often mutated in cancer are the deubiquitinating enzymes (DUB), which catalyze the removal of ubiquitin and ubiquitin-like modifiers of their target proteins.[36] Some DUBs were initially identified as oncogenic proteins, but further work has shown that other deubiquitinases, such as CYLD, A20, and BAP1, are tumor suppressors inactivated in cancer. *CYLD* is mutated in patients with familial cylindromatosis, a disease characterized by the formation of multiple tumors of skin appendages.[37] A20 is a DUB family member encoded by the *TNFAIP3* gene, which is mutated in a large number of Hodgkin lymphomas and primary mediastinal B-cell lymphomas.[38–41] Finally, the *BAP1* gene, encoding an ubiquitin C-terminal hydrolase, is frequently mutated in metastasizing uveal melanomas[42] and in other human malignancies, such as mesothelioma and renal cell carcinoma.[43]

Mutational Analysis of Exomes Using Sanger Sequencing

Although the gene family approach for the identification of cancer genes has proven extremely valuable, it still is a candidate approach and thus biased in its nature. The next step forward in the mutational profiling of cancer has been the sequencing of exomes, which is the entire coding portion of the human genome (18,000 protein-encoding genes). The exomes of many different tumors—including breast, colorectal, pancreatic, and ovarian clear cell carcinomas; glioblastoma multiforme; and medulloblastoma—have been analyzed using Sanger sequencing. For the first time, these large-scale analyses allowed researchers to describe and understand the genetic complexity of human cancers.[29,44–48] The declared goals of these exome studies were to provide methods for exomewide mutational analyses in human tumors, to characterize their spectrum and quantity of somatic mutations, and, finally, to discover new genes involved in tumorigenesis as well as novel pathways that have a role in these tumors. In these studies, sequencing data were complemented with gene expression and copy number analyses, thus providing a comprehensive view of the genetic complexity of human tumors.[45–48] A number of conclusions can be drawn from these analyses, including the following:

- Cancer genomes have an average of 30 to 100 somatic alterations per tumor in coding regions, which was a higher number than previously thought. Although the alterations included point mutations, small insertions, deletions, or amplifications, the great majority of the mutations observed were single-base substitutions.[45,46]
- Even within a single cancer type, there is a significant intertumor heterogeneity. This means that multiple mutational patterns (encompassing different mutant genes) are present in tumors that cannot be distinguished based on histologic analysis. The concept that individual tumors have a unique genetic milieu is highly relevant for personalized medicine, a concept that will be further discussed.
- The spectrum and nucleotide contexts of mutations differ between different tumor types. For example, over 50% of mutations in colorectal cancer were C:G to T:A transitions, and 10% were C:G to G:C transversions. In contrast, in breast cancers, only 35% of the mutations were C:G to T:A transitions, and 29% were C:G to G:C transversions. Knowledge of mutation spectra is vital because it allows insight into the mechanisms underlying mutagenesis and repair in the various cancers investigated.
- A considerably larger number of genes that had not been previously reported to be involved in cancer were found to play a role in the disease.
- Solid tumors arising in children, such as medulloblastomas, harbor on average 5 to 10 times less gene alterations compared to a typical adult solid tumor. These pediatric tumors also harbor fewer amplifications and homozygous deletions within coding genes compared to adult solid tumors.

Importantly, to deal with the large amount of data generated in these genomic projects, it was necessary to develop new statistical and bioinformatic tools. Furthermore, an examination of the overall distribution of the identified mutations allowed for the development of a novel view of cancer genome landscapes and a novel definition of cancer genes. These new concepts in the understanding of cancer genetics are further discussed in the following paragraphs. The compiled conclusions derived from these analyses have led to a paradigm shift in the understanding of cancer genetics.

A clear indication of the power of the unbiased nature of the whole exome surveys was revealed by the discovery of recurrent mutations in the active site of *IDH1*, a gene with no known link to gliomas, in 12% of tumors analyzed.[46] Because malignant gliomas are the most common and lethal tumors of the central nervous system, and because glioblastoma multiforme (GBM; World Health Organization grade IV astrocytoma) is the most biologically aggressive subtype, the unveiling of *IDH1* as a novel GBM gene is extremely significant. Importantly, mutations of *IDH1* predominantly occurred in younger patients and were associated with a better prognosis.[49] Follow-up studies showed that mutations of *IDH1* occur early in glioma progression; the R132 somatic mutation is harbored by the majority (greater than 70%) of grades II and III astrocytomas and oligodendrogliomas, as well as in secondary GBMs that develop from these lower grade lesions.[49–55] In contrast, less than 10% of primary GBMs harbor these alterations. Furthermore, analysis of the associated *IDH2* revealed recurrent somatic mutations in the R172 residue, which is the exact analog of the frequently mutated R132 residue of *IDH1*. These mutations occur mostly in a mutually exclusive manner with *IDH1* mutations,[49,51] suggesting that they have equivalent phenotypic effects. Subsequently, *IDH1* mutations have been reported in additional cancer types, including hematologic neoplasias.[56–58]

Next-Generation Sequencing and Cancer Genome Analysis

In 1977, the introduction of the Sanger method for DNA sequencing with chain-terminating inhibitors transformed biomedical research.[8] Over the past 30 years, this first-generation technology has been universally used for elucidating the nucleotide sequence of DNA molecules. However, the launching of new large-scale projects, including those implicating whole-genome sequencing of cancer samples, has made necessary the development of new methods that are widely known as next-generation sequencing technologies.[59–61] These approaches have significantly lowered the cost and the time required to determine the sequence of the 3×10^9 nucleotides present in the human genome. Moreover, they have a series of advantages over Sanger sequencing, which are of special interest for the analysis of cancer genomes.[62] First, next-generation sequencing approaches are more sensitive than Sanger methods and can detect somatic mutations even when they are present in only a subset of tumor cells.[63] Moreover, these new sequencing strategies are quantitative and can be used to simultaneously determine both nucleotide sequence and copy number variations.[64] They can also be coupled to other procedures such as those involving paired-end reads, allowing for the identification of multiple structural alterations, such as insertions, deletions, and rearrangements, that commonly occur in cancer genomes.[63] Nonetheless, next-generation sequencing still presents some limitations that are mainly derived from the relatively high error rate in the short reads generated during the sequencing process. In addition, these short reads make the task of de novo assembly of the generated sequences and the mapping of the reads to a reference genome extremely complex. To overcome some of these current limitations, deep coverage of each analyzed genome is required and a careful validation of the identified variants must be performed, typically using Sanger sequencing. As a consequence, there is a substantial increase in both the cost of the process and in the time of analysis. Therefore, it can be concluded that whole-genome sequencing of cancer samples is already a feasible task, but not yet a routine process. Further technical improvements will be required before the task of decoding the entire genome of any malignant tumor of any cancer patient can be applied to clinical practice.

The number of next-generation sequencing platforms has substantially grown over the past few years and currently includes technologies from Roche/454, Illumina/Solexa, Life/APG's SOLiD3, Helicos BioSciences/HeliScope, and Pacific Biosciences/PacBio RS.[61] Noteworthy also are the recent introduction of the Polonator G.007 instrument, an open source platform with freely available software and protocols; the Ion Torrent's semiconductor sequencer; as well as those involving self-assembling DNA nanoballs or nanopore technologies.[65–67] These new machines are driving the field toward the era of third-generation sequencing, which brings enormous clinical interest because it can substantially increase the speed and accuracy of analyses at reduced costs and can facilitate the possibility of single-molecule sequencing of human genomes. A comparison of next-generation sequencing platforms is shown in Table 1.1. These various platforms differ in the method utilized for template preparation and in the nucleotide sequencing and imaging strategy, which finally result in their different performance. Ultimately, the most suitable approach depends on the specific genome sequencing projects.[61]

Current methods of template preparation first involve randomly shearing genomic DNA into smaller fragments, from which

TABLE 1.1

Comparative Analysis of Next-Generation Sequencing Platforms

Platform	Library/Template Preparation	Sequencing Method	Average Read-Length (Bases)	Run Time (Days)	Gb Per Run	Instrument Cost (U.S.$)	Comments
Roche 454 GS FLX	Fragment, mate-pair Emulsion PCR	Pyrosequencing	400	0.35	0.45	500,000	Fast run times High reagent cost
Illumina HiSeq 2000	Fragment, mate-pair Solid phase	Reversible terminator	100–125	8 (mate-pair run)	150–200	540,000	Most widely used platform Low multiplexing capability
Life/APG's SOLiD 5500xl	Fragment, mate-pair Emulsion PCR	Cleavable probe, sequencing by ligation	35–75	7 (mate-pair run)	180–300	595,000	Inherent error correction Long run times
Helicos BioSciences HeliScope	Fragment, mate-pair Single molecule	Reversible terminator	32	8 (fragment run)	37	999,000	Nonbias template representation Expensive, high error rates
Pacific Biosciences PacBio RS	Fragment Single molecule	Real-time sequencing	1,000	1	0.075	NA	Greatest potential for long reads Highest error rates
Polonator G.007	Mate pair Emulsion PCR	Noncleavable probe, sequencing by ligation	26	5 (mate-pair run)	12	170,000	Least expensive platform Shortest read lengths

NA, not available.
Data represent an update of information provided in Metzker ML. Sequencing technologies—the next generation. *Nat Rev Genet* 2010;11:31–46.

a library of either fragment templates or mate-pair templates are generated. Then, clonally amplified templates from single DNA molecules are prepared by either emulsion polymerase chain reaction (PCR) or solid-phase amplification.[68,69] Alternatively, it is possible to prepare single-molecule templates through methods that require less starting material and that do not involve PCR amplification reactions, which can be the source of artifactual mutations.[70] Once prepared, templates are attached to a solid surface in spatially separated sites, allowing thousands to billions of nucleotide sequencing reactions to be performed simultaneously.

The sequencing methods currently used by the different next-generation sequencing platforms are diverse and have been classified into four groups: cyclic reversible termination, single-nucleotide addition, real-time sequencing, and sequencing by ligation (Fig. 1.3).[61,71] These sequencing strategies are coupled with different imaging methods, including those based on measuring bioluminescent signals or involving four-color imaging of single molecular events. Finally, the extraordinary amount of data released from these nucleotide sequencing platforms is stored, assembled, and analyzed using powerful bioinformatic tools that have been developed in parallel with next-generation sequencing technologies.[72]

Next-generation sequencing approaches represent the newest entry into the cancer genome decoding arena and have already been applied to cancer analyses. The first research group to apply these methodologies to whole cancer genomes was that of Ley et al.,[73] who reported in 2008 the sequencing of the entire genome of a patient with acute myeloid leukemia (AML) and its comparison with the normal tissue from the same patient, using the Illumina/Solexa platform. As further described, this work allowed for the identification of point mutations and structural alterations of putative oncogenic relevance in AML and represented proof of principle of the relevance of next-generation sequencing for cancer research.

Whole-Genome Analysis Utilizing Second-Generation Sequencing

The sequence of the first whole cancer genome was reported in 2008, where AML and normal skin from the same patient were described.[73] Numerous additional whole genomes, together with the corresponding normal genomes of patients with a variety of malignant tumors, have been reported since then.[56,63,74–86]

The first available whole genome of a cytogenetically normal AML subtype M1 (AML-M1) revealed eight genes with novel mutations along with another 500 to 1,000 additional mutations found in noncoding regions of the genome. Most of the identified genes had not been previously associated with cancer. However, validation of the detected mutations did not identify novel recurring mutations in AML.[73] Concomitantly, with the expansion in the use of next-generation sequencers, many other whole genomes from a number of cancer types started to be evaluated in a similar manner (Fig. 1.4).[87]

In contrast to the first AML whole genome, the second did observe a recurrent mutation in *IDH1*, encoding isocitrate dehydrogenase.[56] Follow-up studies extended this finding and reported that mutations in *IDH1* and the related gene *IDH2* occur at a 20% to 30% frequency in AML patients and are associated with a poor prognosis in some subgroups of patients.[79,80,88] A good example illustrating the high pace at which second-generation technologies and their accompanying analytical tools are found is demonstrated by the following finding derived from a reanalysis of the first AML whole genome. Thus, when improvements in sequencing

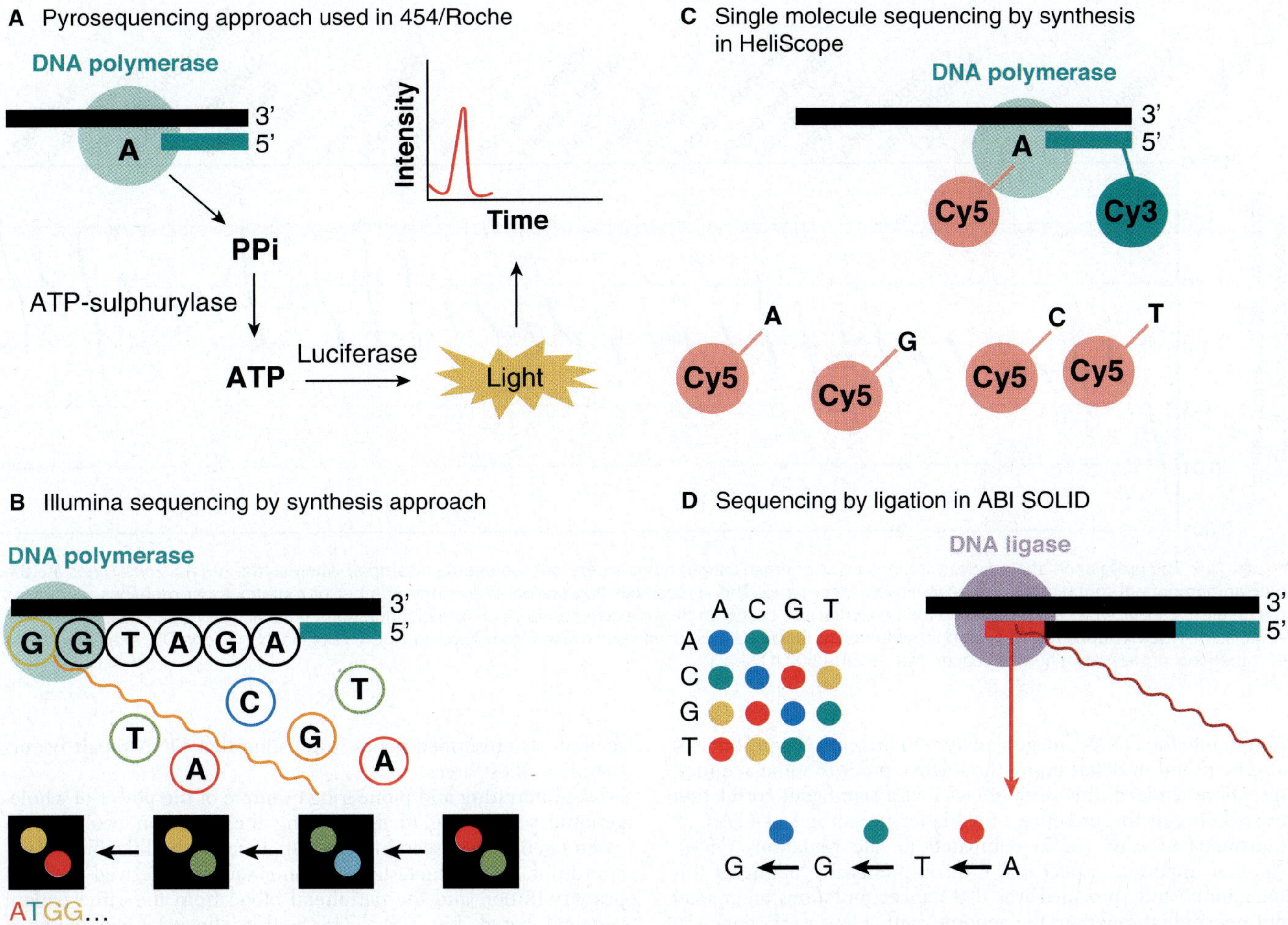

Figure 1.3 Advances in sequencing chemistry implemented in next-generation sequencers. **(A)** The pyrosequencing approach implemented in 454/Roche sequencing technology detects incorporated nucleotides by chemiluminescence resulting from PPi release. **(B)** The Illumina method utilizes sequencing by synthesis in the presence of fluorescently labeled nucleotide analogs that serve as reversible reaction terminators. **(C)** The single-molecule sequencing by synthesis approach detects template extension using Cy3 and Cy5 labels attached to the sequencing primer and the incoming nucleotides, respectively. **(D)** The SOLiD method sequences templates by sequential ligation of labeled degenerate probes. Two-base encoding implemented in the SOLiD instrument allows for probing each nucleotide position twice. (From Morozova O, Hirst M, Marra MA. Applications of new sequencing technologies for transcriptome analysis. *Annu Rev Genomics Hum Genet* 2009;10:135–151.)

techniques were available, the first AML whole genome (described previously), which identified no recurring mutations and had a 91.2% diploid coverage, was reevaluated by deeper sequence coverage, yielding 99.6% diploid coverage of the genome. This improvement, together with more advanced mutation calling algorithms, allowed for the discovery of several nonsynonymous mutations that had not been identified in the initial sequencing. This included a frameshift mutation in the DNA methyltransferase gene *DNMT3A*. Validation of *DNMT3A* in 280 additional de novo AML patients to define recurring mutations led to the significant discovery that a total of 22.1% of AML cases had mutations in *DNMT3A* that were predicted to affect translation. The median overall survival among patients with *DNMT3A* mutations was significantly shorter than that among patients without such mutations (12.3 months versus 41.1 months; $p < 0.001$).

Shortly after this study, complete sequences of a series of cancer genomes, together with matched normal genomes of the same patients, were reported.[56,78,83,84] These works opened the way to more ambitious initiatives, including those involving large international consortia, aimed at decoding the genome of malignant tumors from thousands of cancer patients. Thus, over the last 2 years, many whole genomes of different human malignancies have been made available.[74–76]

In addition to direct applications of next-generation sequencing technologies for the mutational analysis of cancer genomes, these methods have an additional range of applications in cancer research. Thus, genome sequencing efforts have begun to elucidate the genomic changes that accompany metastasis evolution through a comparative analysis of primary and metastatic lesions from breast and pancreatic cancer patients.[77,81,82,85] Likewise, massively parallel sequencing has been used to analyze the evolution of a tongue adenocarcinoma in response to selection by targeted kinase inhibitors.[89] Detailed information of several of these whole genome projects is found in the following paragraph.

The first solid cancer to undergo whole-genome sequencing was a malignant melanoma that was compared to a lymphoblastoid cell line from the same individual.[83] Impressively, a total of 33,345 somatic base substitutions were identified, with 187 nonsynonymous substitutions in protein-coding sequences, at least one order of magnitude higher than any other cancer type. Most somatic base substitutions were C:G > T:A transitions, and of the 510 dinucleotide substitutions, 360 were CC.TT/GG.AA changes, which is consistent with ultraviolet light exposure mutation signatures previously reported in melanoma.[14] Such results from the most comprehensive catalog of somatic mutations not only provide

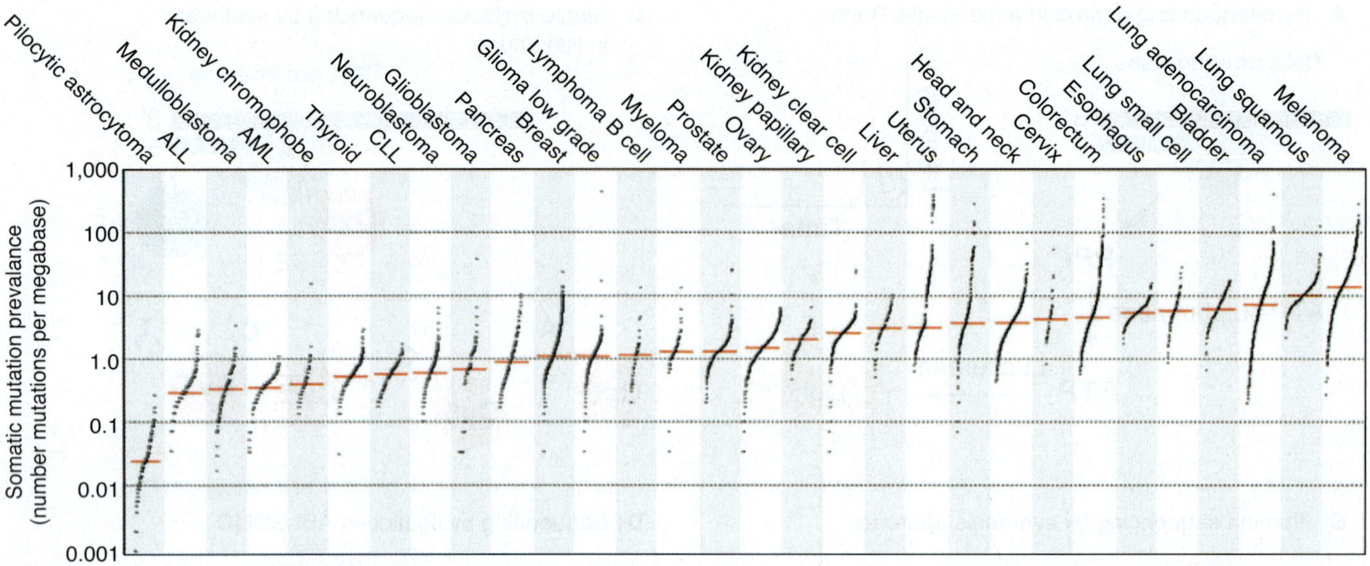

Figure 1.4 The prevalence of somatic mutations across human cancer types. Every *dot* represents a sample, whereas the *red horizontal lines* are the median numbers of mutations in the respective cancer types. The vertical axis (log scaled) shows the number of mutations per megabase, whereas the different cancer types are ordered on the horizontal axis based on their median numbers of somatic mutations. ALL, acute lymphoblastic leukemia; AML, acute myeloid leukemia; CLL, chronic lymphocytic leukemia. (Used with permission from Alexandrov LB, Nik-Zainal S, Wedge DC, et al. Signatures of mutational processes in human cancer. *Nature* 2013;500:415–421.)

insight into the DNA damage signature in this cancer type, but can also be useful in determining the relative order of some acquired mutations. Indeed, this study shows that a significant correlation exists between the presence of a higher proportion of C.A/G.T transitions in early (82%) compared to late mutations (53%). Another important aspect that the comprehensive nature of this melanoma study provided was that cancer mutations are spread out unevenly throughout the genome, with a lower prevalence in regions of transcribed genes, suggesting that DNA repair occurs mainly in these areas.

An interesting and pioneering example of the power of whole-genome sequencing in deciphering the mutation evolution in carcinogenesis was seen in a study in which a basallike breast cancer tumor, a brain metastasis, a tumor xenograft derived from the primary tumor, and the peripheral blood from the same patient were compared (Fig. 1.5).[85] This analysis showed a wide range of

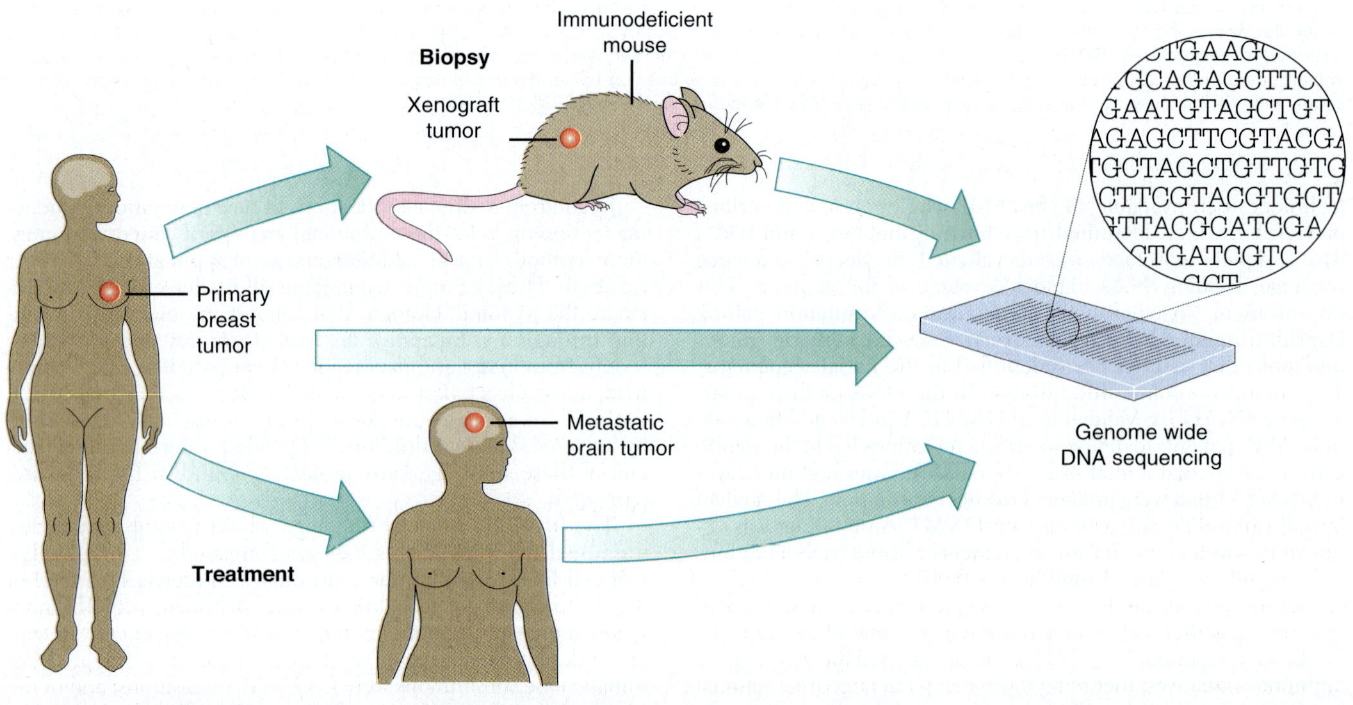

Figure 1.5 Covering all the bases in metastatic assessment. Ding et al.[85] performed a genomewide analysis on three tumor samples: a patient's primary breast tumor; her metastatic brain tumor, which formed despite therapy; and a xenograft tumor in a mouse, originating from the patient's breast tumor. They find that the primary tumor differs from the metastatic and xenograft tumors mainly in the prevalence of genomic mutations. (With permission from Gray J. Cancer: genomics of metastasis. *Nature* 2010;464:989–990.)

mutant allele frequencies in the primary tumor, which was narrowed in the metastasis and xenograft samples. This suggested that the primary tumor was significantly more heterogeneous in its cell populations compared to its matched metastasis and xenograft samples because these underwent selection processes whether during metastasis or transplantation. The clear overlap in mutation incidence between the metastatic and xenograft cases suggests that xenografts undergo similar selection as metastatic lesions and, therefore, are a reliable source for genomic analyses. The main conclusion of this whole-genome study was that, although metastatic tumors harbor an increased number of genetic alterations, the majority of the alterations found in the primary tumor are preserved. Interestingly, single-cell genome sequencing of a breast primary tumour and its liver metastasis indicated that a single clonal expansion formed the primary tumor and seeded the metastasis.[90] Further studies have confirmed and extended these findings to metastatic tumors from different types, including renal and pancreatic carcinomas.[91]

The importance of performing whole-genome sequencing has also been emphasized by the recent identification of somatic mutations in regulatory regions, which can also elicit tumorigenesis. In a study reviewing the noncoding mutations in 19 melanoma whole-genome samples, two recurrent mutations in 17 of the 19 cases studied within the *telomerase reverse transcriptase* (*TERT*) promoter region were revealed.[92] When these two mutations were investigated in an extension of 51 additional tumors and their matched normal tissues, it was observed that 33 tumors harbored one of the mutations and that the mutations occurred in a mutually exclusive manner. These two mutations generate an identical 11 bp nucleotide stretch that contains the consensus binding site for E-twenty-six (ETS) transcription factors. When cloned into a luciferase reporter assay system, it was shown that these mutations conferred a two- to fourfold increase in transcriptional activity of this promoter in five melanoma cell lines. Although this alteration is much more frequent in melanoma, it is also present in other cancer types because 16% of the cancers listed in the Cancer Cell Line Encyclopedia harbor one of the two *TERT* mutations. In combination, these *TERT* mutations are seen in a greater frequency than *BRAF*- and *NRAS*-activating mutations. They occur in a mutually exclusive manner and in regions that do not show a large background mutation rate, all suggesting that these mutations are important driver events contributing to oncogenesis. Further supporting this was another recent study that identified these same two mutations in the germ line of familial melanoma patients.[93]

As the *TERT* promoter mutation discovery shows, regions of the genome that do not code for proteins are just as vital in our understanding of the biology behind tumor development and progression. Another class of non–protein-coding regions in the genome are the noncoding RNAs. One class of noncoding RNAs are microRNAs (miRNA). Discovered 20 years ago, miRNAs are known to be expressed in a tissue or developmentally specific manner and their expression can influence cellular growth and differentiation along with cancer-related pathways such as apoptosis or stress response. miRNAs do this through either overexpression, leading to the targeting and downregulation of tumor suppressor genes, or inversely through their own downregulation, leading to increased expression of their target oncogene. miRNAs have been extensively studied in cancer and their functional effects have been noted in a wide variety of cancers like glioma[94] and breast cancer,[95] to name just a few.

Another class of noncoding RNAs (ncRNA) are the long noncoding RNAs (lncRNA). These RNAs are typically greater than 200 bp and can range up to 100 kb in size. They are transcribed by RNA polymerase II and can undergo splicing and polyadenylation. Although much less extensively studied when compared to miRNAs for their role in cancer, lncRNAs are beginning to come under much more scrutiny. A recent study of the steroid receptor RNA activator (SRA) revealed two transcripts, a lncRNA (SRA) and a translated transcript (steroid receptor RNA activator protein [SRAP]), that coexist within breast cancer cells. However, their expression varies within breast cancer cell lines with different phenotypes. It was shown that in a more invasive breast cancer line, higher relative levels of the noncoding transcript were seen.[96] Because this ncRNA acts as part of a ribonucleoprotein complex that is recruited to the promoter region of regulatory genes, it has been hypothesized that this shift in balance between both noncoding and coding transcripts may be associated with growth advantages. When this balance was shifted in vitro, it led to a large increase in transcripts associated with invasion and migration. The results of this study highlight the importance of the investigation into the roles of ncRNA in tumor development or progression and confirm again that the study of coding variants is not sufficient in determining the full genomic spectrum of cancer.

It must be also noted that the recent analysis of whole genomes of many different human tumors has provided additional insights into cancer evolution. Thus, it has been demonstrated that multiple mutational processes are operative during cancer development and progression, each of which has the capacity to leave its particular mutational signature on the genome. A remarkable and innovative study in this regard was aimed at the generation of the entire catalog of somatic mutations in 21 breast carcinomas and the identification of the mutational signatures of the underlying processes. This analysis revealed the occurrence of multiple, distinct single- and double-nucleotide substitution signatures. Moreover, it was reported that breast carcinomas harboring *BRCA1* or *BRCA2* mutations showed a characteristic combination of substitution mutation signatures and a particular profile of genomic deletions. An additional contribution of this analysis was the identification of a distinctive phenomenon of localized hypermutation, which has been termed *kataegis*, and which has also subsequently been observed in other malignancies distinct from breast carcinomas.[87]

Whole-genome sequencing of human carcinomas has also allowed for the ability to characterize other massive genomic alterations, termed *chromothripsis* and *chromoplexy*, occurring across different cancer subtypes.[97] Chromothripsis implies a massive genomic rearrangement acquired in a one-step catastrophic event during cancer development and has been detected in about 2% to 3% of all tumors, but is present at high frequency in some particular cases, such as bone cancers.[98] Chromoplexy has been originally described in prostate cancer and involves many DNA translocations and deletions that arise in a highly interdependent manner and result in the coordinate disruption of multiple cancer genes.[99] These newly described phenomena represent powerful strategies of rapid genome evolution, which may play essential roles during carcinogenesis.

Whole-Exome Analysis Utilizing Second-Generation Sequencing

Another application of second-generation sequencing involves utilizing nucleic acid "baits" to capture regions of interest in the total pool of nucleic acids. These could either be DNA, as described previously,[100,101] or RNA.[102] Indeed, most areas of interest in the genome can be targeted, including exons and ncRNAs. Despite inefficiencies in the exome-targeting process—including the uneven capture efficiency across exons, which results in not all exons being sequenced, and the occurrence of some off-target hybridization events—the higher coverage of the exome makes it highly suitable for mutation discovery in cancer samples.

Over the last few years, thousands of cancer samples have been subjected to whole-exome sequencing. These studies, combined with data from whole-genome sequencing, have provided an unprecedented level of information about the mutational landscape of the most frequent human malignancies.[74–76] In addition, whole-exome sequencing has been used to identify the somatic mutations characteristic of both rare tumors and those that are prevalent in certain geographical regions.[76]

Overall, these studies have provided very valuable information about mutation rates and spectra across cancer types and subtypes.[87,103,104] Remarkably, the variation in mutational frequency between different tumors is extraordinary, with hematologic and pediatric cancers showing the lowest mutation rates (0.001 per Mb of DNA), and melanoma and lung cancers presenting the highest mutational burden (more than 400 per Mb). Whole-exome sequencing has also contributed to the identification of novel cancer genes that had not been previously described to be causally implicated in the carcinogenesis process. These genes belong to different functional categories, including signal transduction, RNA maturation, metabolic regulation, epigenetics, chromatin remodeling, and protein homeostasis.[74] Finally, a combination of data from whole-exome and whole-genome sequencing has allowed for the identification of the signatures of mutational processes operating in different cancer types.[87] Thus, an analysis of a dataset of about 5 million mutations from over 7,000 cancers from 30 different types has allowed for the extraction of more than 20 distinct mutational signatures. Some of them, such as those derived from the activity of APOBEC cytidine deaminases, are present in most cancer types, whereas others are characteristic of specific tumors. Known signatures associated with age, smoking, ultraviolet (UV) light exposure, and DNA repair defects have been also identified in this work, but many of the detected mutational signatures are of cryptic origin. These findings demonstrate the impressive diversity of mutational processes underlying cancer development and may have enormous implications for the future understanding of cancer biology, prevention, and treatment.

SOMATIC ALTERATION CLASSES DETECTED BY CANCER GENOME ANALYSIS

Whole-genome sequencing of cancer genomes has an enormous potential to detect all major types of somatic mutations present in malignant tumors. This large repertoire of genomic abnormalities includes single nucleotide changes, small insertions and deletions, large chromosomal reorganizations, and copy number variations (Fig. 1.6).

Nucleotide substitutions are the most frequent somatic mutations detected in malignant tumors, although there is a substantial variability in the mutational frequency among different cancers.[60] On average, human malignancies have one nucleotide change per million bases, but melanomas reach mutational rates 10-fold higher, and tumors with mutator phenotype caused by DNA mismatch repair deficiencies may accumulate tens of mutations per million nucleotides. By contrast, tumors of hematopoietic origin have less than one base substitution per million. Several bioinformatic tools and pipelines have been developed to efficiently detect somatic nucleotide substitutions through comparison of the genomic information obtained from paired normal and tumor samples from the same patient. Likewise, there are a number of publicly available computational methods to predict the functional relevance of the identified mutations in cancer specimens.[60] Most of these bioinformatic tools exclusively deal with nucleotide changes in protein coding regions and evaluate the putative structural or functional effect of an amino acid substitution in a determined protein, thus obviating changes in other genomic regions, which can also be of crucial interest in cancer. In any case, current computational methods used in this regard are far from being optimal, and experimental validation is finally required to assess the functional relevance of nucleotide substitutions found in cancer genomes.

For years, the main focus of cancer genome analyses has been on identifying coding mutations that cause a change in the amino acid sequence of a gene. The rationale behind this is quite sound because any mutation that creates a novel protein or truncates an essential protein has the potential to drastically change the cellular environment. Examples of this have been shown earlier in the chapter with *BRAF* and *KRAS* along with many others. With the advancements in next-generation sequencing, larger studies are able to be conducted. These studies give the power to detect mutations occurring in the cancer genome at a lower frequency. Interesting to note is that these studies are leading to the discovery that recurrent synonymous mutations occur in cancer. Previously believed to be merely neutral mutations that maintain no functional role in tumorigenesis, these mutations were largely ignored, but a recent study shows[105] that simply dismissing these mutations as silent may be premature.

In a review of only 29 melanoma exomes and genomes, 16 recurring synonymous mutations were discovered. When these mutations were screened in additional samples, a synonymous mutation in the gene *BCL2L12* was discovered in 12 out of 285 total samples. The observed frequency of this recurrent mutation is greater than expected by chance, suggesting that it has undergone some type of selective pressure during tumor development.[105] Noting that *BCL2L12* had previously been linked to tumorigenesis, the mutation was further evaluated for its functional effect, with the finding that it led to an abrogation of the effect of a miRNA, leading to the deregulated expression of *BCL2L12*. BCL2L12 is a negative regulator of the gene p53, which functions by binding and inhibiting apoptosis in glioma.[106] Accordingly, the dysregulation observed in *BCL2L12* led to a reduction in p53 target gene expression.

Small insertions and deletions (*indels*) represent a second category of somatic mutations that can be discovered by whole-genome sequencing of cancer specimens. These mutations are about 10-fold less frequent than nucleotide substitutions, but may also have an obvious impact in cancer progression. Accordingly, specific bioinformatic tools have been created to detect these *indels* in the context of the large amount of information generated by whole-genome sequencing projects.[107]

The systematic identification of large chromosomal rearrangements in cancer genomes represents one of the most successful applications of next-generation sequencing methodologies. Previous strategies in this regard had mainly been based on the utilization of cytogenetic methods for the identification of recurrent translocations in hematopoietic tumors. More recently, a combination of bioinformatics and functional methods has allowed for the finding of recurrent translocations in solid epithelial tumors such as *TMPRSS2–ERG* in prostate cancer and *EML4–ALK* in non–small-cell lung cancer.[108,109] Now, by using a next-generation sequencing analysis of genomes and transcriptomes, it is possible to systematically search for both intrachromosomal and interchromosomal rearrangements occurring in cancer specimens. These studies have already proven their usefulness for cancer research through the discovery of recurrent translocations involving genes of the *RAF* kinase pathway in prostate and gastric cancers and in melanomas.[110] Likewise, massively parallel paired-end genome and transcriptome sequencing has already been used to detect new gene fusions in cancer and to catalog all major structural rearrangements present in some tumors and cancer cell lines.[63,111–113] The ongoing cancer genome projects involving thousands of tumor samples will likely lead to the detection of many other chromosomal rearrangements of relevance in specific subsets of cancers. It is also remarkable that whole-genome sequencing may also facilitate the identification of other types of genomic alterations, including rearrangements of repetitive elements, such as active retrotransposons, or insertions of foreign gene sequences, such as viral genomes, which can contribute to cancer development. Indeed, a next-generation sequencing analysis of the transcriptome of Merkel cell carcinoma samples has revealed the clonal integration within the tumor genome of a previously unknown polyomavirus likely implicated in the pathogenesis of this rare but aggressive skin cancer.[114]

Finally, next-generation sequencing approaches have also demonstrated their feasibility to analyze the pattern of copy number

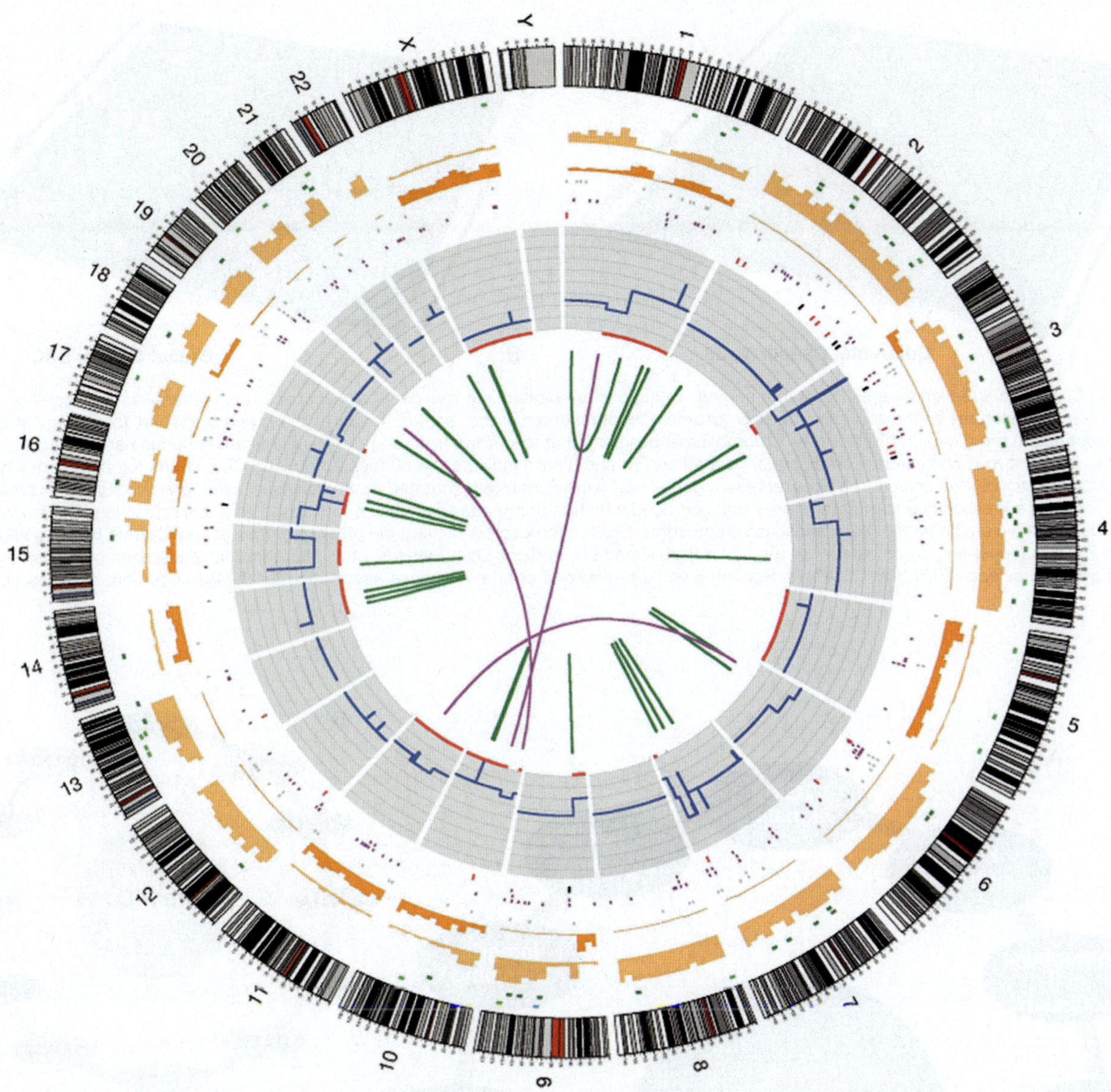

Figure 1.6 The catalog of somatic mutations in COLO-829. Chromosome ideograms are shown around the *outer ring* and are oriented pter–qter in a clockwise direction with centromeres indicated in *red*. Other tracks contain somatic alterations (*from outside to inside*): validated insertions *(light green rectangles)*; validated deletions *(dark green rectangles)*; heterozygous *(light orange bars)*, and homozygous *(dark orange bars)* substitutions shown by density per 10 megabases; coding substitutions *(colored squares: silent in gray, missense in purple, nonsense in red, and splice site in black)*; copy number *(blue lines)*; regions of loss of heterozygosity (LOH) *(red lines)*; validated intrachromosomal rearrangements *(green lines)*; validated interchromosomal rearrangements *(purple lines)*. (From Pleasance ED, Cheetham RK, Stephens PJ, et al. A comprehensive catalogue of somatic mutations from a human cancer genome. *Nature* 2010;463:191–196.)

alterations in cancer, because they allow researchers to count the number of reads in both tumor and normal samples at any given genomic region and then to evaluate the tumor-to-normal copy number ratio at this particular region. These new methods offer some advantages when compared with those based on microarrays, including much better resolution, precise definition of the involved breakpoints, and absence of saturation, which facilitates the accurate estimation of high copy number levels occurring in some genomic loci of malignant tumors.[60]

PATHWAY-ORIENTED MODELS OF CANCER GENOME ANALYSIS

Genomewide mutational analyses suggest that the mutational landscape of cancer is made up of a handful of genes that are mutated in a high fraction of tumors, otherwise known as *mountains*, and most mutated genes are altered at relatively low frequencies, otherwise known as *hills* (Fig. 1.7).[29] The mountains probably give a high selective advantage to the mutated cell, and the hills might provide a lower advantage, making it hard to distinguish them from passenger mutations. Because the hills differ between cancer types, it seems that the cancer genome is more complex and heterogeneous than anticipated. Although highly heterogeneous, bioinformatic studies suggest that the mountains and hills can be grouped into sets of pathways and biologic processes. Some of these pathways are affected by mutations in a few pathway members and others by numerous members. For example, pathway analyses have allowed for the stratification of mutated genes in pancreatic adenocarcinomas to 12 core pathways that have at least one member mutated in 67% to 100% of the tumors analyzed (Fig. 1.8).[45] These core pathways deviated to some that harbored one single highly mutated gene,

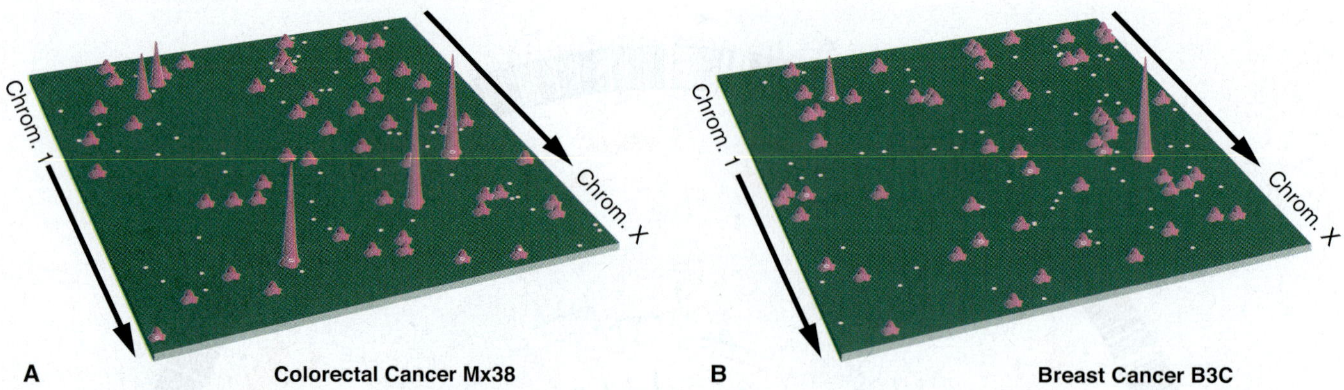

Figure 1.7 Cancer genome landscapes. Nonsilent somatic mutations are plotted in a two-dimensional space representing chromosomal positions of RefSeq genes. The telomere of the short arm of chromosome 1 is represented in the rear left corner of the *green plane* and ascending chromosomal positions continue in the direction of the arrow. Chromosomal positions that follow the front edge of the plane are continued at the back edge of the plane of the adjacent row, and chromosomes are appended end to end. Peaks indicate the 60 highest ranking CAN genes for each tumor type, with peak heights reflecting CaMP scores. The *dots* represent genes that were somatically mutated in the individual colorectal (Mx38) **(A)** or breast tumor (B3C) **(B)**. The *dots* corresponding to mutated genes that coincided with hills or mountains are black with white rims; the remaining *dots* are white with red rims. The mountain on the right of both landscapes represents *TP53* (chromosome 17), and the other mountain shared by both breast and colorectal cancers is *PIK3CA* (upper left, chromosome 3). (Redrawn from Wood LD, Parsons DW, Jones S, et al. The genomic landscapes of human breast and colorectal cancers. *Science* 2007;318:1108–1113. Reprinted with permission from the American Association for the Advancement of Science).

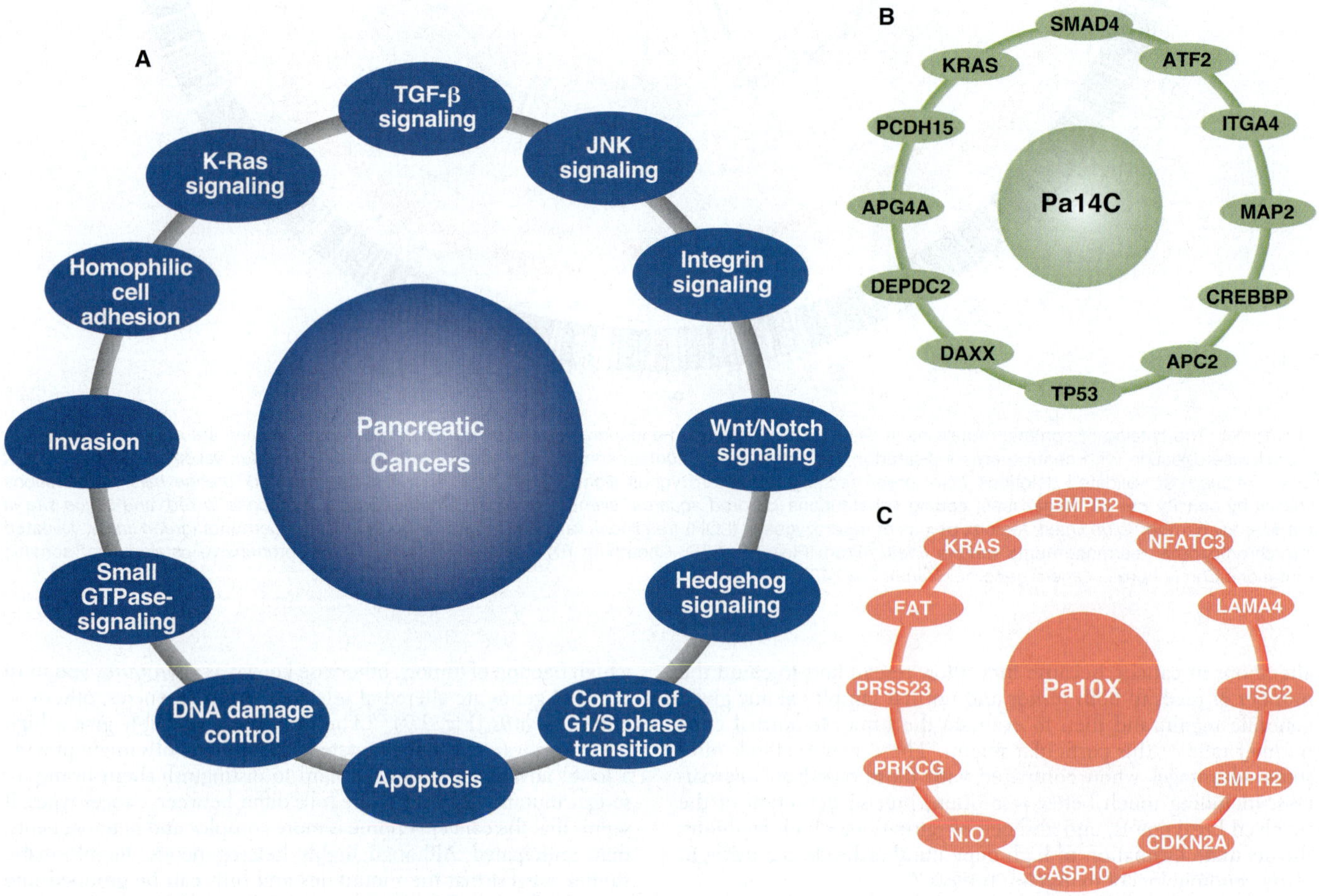

Figure 1.8 Signaling pathways and processes. **(A)** The 12 pathways and processes whose component genes were genetically altered in most pancreatic cancers. **(B,C)** Two pancreatic cancers (Pa14C and Pa10X) and the specific genes that are mutated in them. The positions around the circles in **(B)** and **(C)** correspond to the pathways and processes in **(A)**. Several pathway components overlapped, as illustrated by the BMPR2 mutation that presumably disrupted both the SMAD4 and Hedgehog signaling pathways in Pa10X. Additionally, not all 12 processes and pathways were altered in every pancreatic cancer, as exemplified by the fact that no mutations known to affect DNA damage control were observed in Pa10X. NO, not observed. (Redrawn from Jones S, Zhang X, Parsons DW, et al. Core signaling pathways in human pancreatic cancers revealed by global genomic analyses. *Science* 2008;321:1801–1806. Reprinted with permission from the American Association for the Advancement of Science).

such as in *KRAS* in the G1/S cell cycle transition pathway and pathways where a few mutated genes were found, such as the transforming growth factor (TGF-β) signaling pathway. Finally, there were pathways in which many different genes were mutated, such as invasion regulation molecules, cell adhesion molecules, and integrin signaling. Importantly, independent of how many genes in the same pathway are affected, if they are found to occur in a mutually exclusive fashion in a single tumor, they most likely give the same selective pressure for clonal expansion.

The idea of genetically analyzing pathways rather than individual genes has been applied previously, revealing the concept of mutual exclusivity. Mutual exclusivity has been shown elegantly in the case of *KRAS* and *BRAF*, where a *KRAS*-mutated cancer generally does not also harbor a *BRAF* mutation, because *KRAS* is upstream of *BRAF* in the same pathway.[9] A similar concept was applied for *PIK3CA* and *PTEN*, where both mutations do not usually occur in the same tumor.[23]

With the ever expanding amounts of genetic information being gathered, the ability to search for common pathways being affected in cancer is increasing. One new pathway that is beginning to emerge is the glutamate-signaling pathway. Glutamate dysregulation has been implicated in a number of cancers. In a study of pancreatic duct adenocarcinoma (PDAC), it was seen that glutamate levels were significantly higher in the tissue of individuals with chronic pancreatitis (CP) and PDAC when compared to normal pancreas tissue.[115] It was also observed that the increased glutamate levels led to proinvasion and antiapoptotic signaling through the activation of AMPA receptors.

Also in this regard, and through the use of whole-exome sequencing, it has been recently shown that the glutamate receptor gene *GRIN2A* is highly mutated in melanoma. The finding that many of these mutations are nonsense has suggested that *GRIN2A* is a novel tumor suppressor. Additional genes in the glutamate pathway have also found mutated in melanomas.[116] Pathway analyses and statistical testing on the whole-exome data have also revealed the glutamate signaling pathway to be dysregulated. These results have been further corroborated in another study reporting mutations in the metabotropic glutamate receptor GRM3[117,118] in melanoma. A functional analysis of mutations found in *GRM3* in melanoma tumor samples has shown an increased activation of MEK1/2 kinase, increased migration, and anchorage-independent growth.[117]

Passenger and Driver Mutations

By the time a cancer is diagnosed, it is comprised of billions of cells carrying DNA abnormalities, some of which have a functional role in malignant proliferation; however, many genetic lesions acquired along the way have no functional role in tumorigenesis.[14] The emerging landscapes of cancer genomes include thousands of genes that were not previously linked to tumorigenesis but are found to be somatically mutated. Many of these changes are likely to be *passengers*, or neutral, in that they have no functional effects on the growth of the tumor.[14] Only a small fraction of the genetic alterations are expected to drive cancer evolution by giving cells a selective advantage over their neighbors. Passenger mutations occur incidentally in a cell that later or in parallel develops a *driver* mutation, but are not ultimately pathogenic.[119] Although neutral, cataloging passengers mutations is important because they incorporate the signatures of the previous exposures the cancer cell underwent as well as DNA repair defects the cancer cell has. In many cases, the passenger and driver mutations occur at similar frequencies and the identification of drivers versus the passenger is of utmost relevance and remains a pressing challenge in cancer genetics.[120–122] This goal will eventually be achieved through a combination of genetic and functional approaches, some of which are listed as follows.

The most reliable indicator that a gene was selected for and therefore is highly likely to be pathogenic is the identification of recurrent mutations, whether at the same exact amino acid position or in neighboring amino acid positions in different patients. More than that, if somatic alterations in the same gene occur very frequently (mountains in the tumor genome landscape), these can be confidently classified as drivers. For example, cancer alleles that are identified in multiple patients and different tumors types, such as those found in *KRAS*, *TP53*, *PTEN*, and *PIK3CA*, are clearly selected for during tumorigenesis.

However, most genes discovered thus far are mutated in a relatively small fraction of tumors (hills), and it has been clearly shown that genes that are mutated in less than 1% of patients can still act as *drivers*.[123] The systematic sequencing of newly identified putative cancer genes in the vast number of specimens from cancer patients will help in this regard. However, even if examining large numbers of samples can provide helpful information to classify drivers versus passengers, this approach alone is limited by the marked variation in mutation frequency among individual tumors and individual genes. The statistical test utilized in this case calculates the probability that the number of mutations in a given gene reflects a mutation frequency that is greater than expected from the nonfunctional background mutation rate,[29,124] which is different between different cancer types. These analyses incorporate the number of somatic alterations observed, the number of tumors studied, and the number of nucleotides that were successfully sequenced and analyzed.

Another approach often used to distinguish driver from passenger mutations exploits the statistical analysis of synonymous versus nonsynonymous changes.[125] In contrast to nonsynonymous mutations, synonymous mutations do not alter the protein sequence. Therefore, they do not usually apply a growth advantage and would not be expected to be selected during tumorigenesis. This strategy works by comparing the observed-to-expected ratio of synonymous with that of nonsynonymous mutation. An increased proportion of nonsynonymous mutations from the expected 2:1 ratio implies selection pressure during tumorigenesis.

Other approaches are based on the concept that driver mutations may have characteristics similar to those causing Mendelian disease when inherited in the germ line and may be identifiable by constraints on tolerated amino acid residues at the mutated positions. In contrast, passenger mutations may have characteristics more similar to those of nonsynonymous SNPs with high minor allele frequencies. Based on these premises, supervised machine learning methods have been used to predict which missense mutations are drivers.[126] Additional approaches to decipher drivers from passengers include the identification of mutations that affect locations that have previously been shown to be cancer causing in protein members of the same gene family. Enrichment for mutations in evolutionarily conserved residues are analyzed by algorithms, such as SIFT (sorting intolerant from tolerant (SIFT),[127] which estimates the effects of the different mutations identified.

Probably the most conclusive methods to identify driver mutations will be rigorous functional studies using biochemical assays as well as model organisms or cultured cells, using knockout and knockin of individual cancer alleles.[128] Unfortunately, these methods are not well suited to the analysis of the hundreds of gene candidates that arise from every large-scale cancer genome project. In conclusion, it is fair to say that sequencing cancer genomes is only the beginning of a journey that will ultimately be completed when the thousands of the newly discovered alleles are annotated as being the drivers of this disease. A summary of the various next-generation applications and approaches for their analysis is summarized in Figure 1.9 and Table 1.2.

NETWORKS OF CANCER GENOME PROJECTS

The repertoire of oncogenic mutations is extremely heterogeneous, suggesting that it would be difficult for independent cancer genome initiatives to address the generation of comprehensive

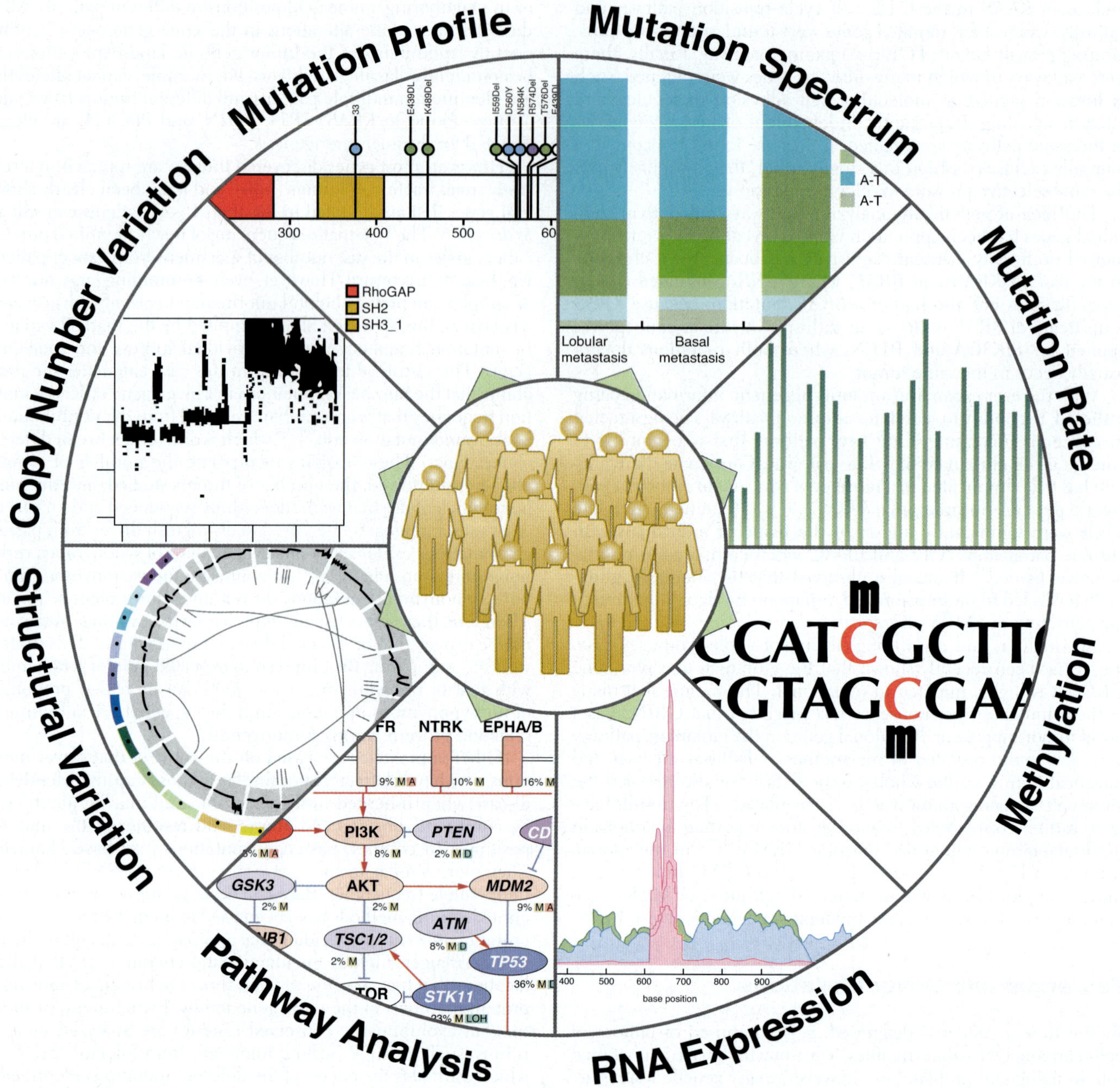

Figure 1.9 Landscape of cancer genomics analyses. NGS data will be generated for hundreds of tumors from all major cancer types in the near future. The integrated analysis of DNA, RNA, and methylation sequencing data will help elucidate all relevant genetic changes in cancers. (Used with permission from Ding L, Wendl MC, Koboldt DC, et al. Analysis of next-generation genomic data in cancer: accomplishments and challenges. *Hum Mol Genet* 2010;19:R188–R196.)

catalogs of mutations in the wide spectrum of human malignancies. Accordingly, there have been different efforts to coordinate the cancer genome sequencing projects being carried out around the world, including The Cancer Genome Atlas (TCGA) and the International Cancer Genome Consortium (ICGC). Moreover, there are other initiatives that are more focused on specific tumors, such as that led by scientists at St. Jude Children's Research Hospital in Memphis, and Washington University, which aims at sequencing multiple pediatric cancer genomes.[129]

TCGA began in 2006 in the United States as a comprehensive program in cancer genomics supported by the U.S. National Institutes of Health (NIH). The initial project focused on three tumors: GBM, serous cystadenocarcinoma of the ovary, and lung squamous carcinoma. These studies have already generated novel and interesting information regarding genes mutated in these malignancies.[134] On the basis of these positive results, the NIH announced an expansion of the TCGA program with the aim to produce genomic data sets for at least 20 to 25 cancers during the next few years.

The ICGC was formed in 2008 to coordinate the generation of comprehensive catalogs of genomic abnormalities in tumors from 50 different cancer types or subtypes that are of clinical and societal importance across the world.[130] The project aims to perform systematic studies of over 25,000 cancer genomes at the genomic level and integrate this information with epigenomic and transcriptomic studies of the same cases as well as with clinical features of patients. At present, there are a total of 69 committed projects involving at least 16 different countries coordinated by

TABLE 1.2

Computational Tools and Databases Useful for Cancer Genome Analyses

Category	Tool/Database	URL
Alignment	Maq[a]	http://maq.sourceforge.net
	Burrows-Wheeler Aligner (BWA)[b]	http://bio-bwa.sourceforge.net
Mutation calling	SNVMix[c]	http://www.bcgsc.ca/platform/bioinfo/software/SNVMix
	SAMtools[d]	http://samtools.sourceforge.net
	VarScan[e]	http://varscan.sourceforge.net
	MuTect[f]	http://www.broadinstitute.org/cancer/cga/mutect
Indel calling	Pindel[g]	http://gmt.genome.wustl.edu/pindel/current/
Copy number analysis	CBS[h]	http://www.bioconductor.org
	SegSeq[i]	http://www.broadinstitute.org/cgi-bin/cancer/publications/pub_paper.cgi?mode=view&paper_id=182
Functional effect	SIFT[j]	http://sift.jcvi.org/
	PolyPhen-2[k]	http://genetics.bwh.harvard.edu/pph2
Visualization	CIRCOS[l]	http://mkweb.bcgsc.ca/circos
	Integrative Genomics Viewer (IGV)[m]	http://www.broadinstitute.org/igv
Repository	Catalogue of Somatic Mutations in Cancer (COSMIC)[n]	http://www.sanger.ac.uk/genetics/CGP/cosmic
	Cancer Genome Project (CGP)[o]	http://www.sanger.ac.uk/genetics/CGP
	dbSNP[p]	http://www.ncbi.nlm.nih.gov/SNP
	Gene Ranker[q]	http://cbio.mskcc.org/tcga-generanker/

[a] Li H, Durbin R. Fast and accurate short read alignment with Burrows–Wheeler transform. *Bioinformatics* 2009;25:1754–1760.
[b] Li H, Durbin R. Fast and accurate long-read alignment with Burrows–Wheeler transform. *Bioinformatics* 2010;26:589–595.
[c] Goya R, Sun MG, Morin RD, et al. SNVMix: predicting single nucleotide variants from next-generation sequencing of tumors. *Bioinformatics* 2010;26:730–736.
[d] Li H, Handsaker B, Wysoker A, et al. The Sequence Alignment/Map format and SAMtools. *Bioinformatics* 2009;25:2078–2079.
[e] Koboldt DC, Chen K, Wylie T, et al. VarScan: variant detection in massively parallel sequencing of individual and pooled samples. *Bioinformatics* 2009;25:2283–2285.
[f] Cibulski K, Lawrence MS, Carter SL, et al. Sensitive detection of somatic point mutations in impure and heterogeneous cancer samples. *Nat Biotechnol* 2013;31:213–219.
[g] Ye K, Schulz MH, Long Q, et al. Pindel: a pattern growth approach to detect break points of large deletions and medium sized insertions from paired-end short reads. *Bioinformatics* 2009;25:2865–2871.
[h] Venkatraman ES, Olshen AB. A faster circular binary segmentation algorithm for the analysis of array CGH data. *Bioinformatics* 2007;23:657–663.
[i] Chiang DY, Getz G, Jaffe DB, et al. High-resolution mapping of copy-number alterations with massively parallel sequencing. *Nature Methods* 2009;6:99–103.
[j] Ng PC, Henikoff S. Predicting deleterious amino acid substitutions. *Genome Res* 2001;11:863–874.
[k] Idzhubei IA, Schmidt S, Peshkin L, et al. A method and server for predicting damaging missense mutations. *Nature Methods* 2010;7:248–249.
[l] Krzywinski M, Schein J, Birol I, et al. Circos: an information aesthetic for comparative genomics. *Genome Res* 2009;19:1639–1645.
[m] Robinson JT, Thorvaldsdóttir H, Winckler W, et al. Integrative Genomics Viewer. *Nat Biotechnol* 2011;29:24–26.
[n] Forbes SA, Bhamra S, Dawson E, et al. The catalogue of somatic mutations in cancer (COSMIC). *Curr Protoc Hum Genet* 2008;Chapter 10:Unit 10.11.
[o] Futreal PA, Coin L, Marshall M, et al. A census of human cancer genes. *Nat Rev Cancer* 2004;4:177–183.
[p] Sherry ST, Ward MH, Kholodov M, et al. dbSNP: The NCBI Database of genetic variation. *Nucleic Acids Res* 2001,29.308–311.
[q] The Cancer Genome Atlas Research Network. Comprehensive genomic characterization defines human glioblastoma genes and core pathways. *Nature* 2008;455:1061–1068.
Based on Meyerson M, Stacey G, Getz G. Advances in understanding cancer genomes through second generation sequencing. *Nature Rev Genet* 2010;11: 685–696, Table 2.

the ICGC. All of these projects deal with at least 500 samples per cancer type from cancers affecting a variety of human organs and tissues, including blood, the brain, the breast, the esophagus, the kidneys, the liver, the oral cavity, the ovaries, the pancreas, the prostate, the skin, and the stomach.[130]

All of these coordinated projects have already provided new insights into the catalog of genes mutated in cancer and have unveiled specific signatures of the mutagenic mechanisms, including carcinogen exposures or DNA-repair defects, implicated in the development of different malignant tumors.[83,84,87,131] Furthermore, these cancer genome studies have also contributed to define clinically relevant subtypes of tumors for prognosis and therapeutic management, and in some cases have identified new targets and strategies for cancer treatment.[74–76] The rapid technological advances in DNA sequencing will likely drop the costs of sequencing cancer genomes to a small fraction of the current price and will allow researchers to overcome some of the current limitations of these global sequencing efforts. Hopefully, worldwide coordination of cancer genome projects, including Pan-Cancer initiative, with those involving large-scale, functional analyses of genes in both cellular and animal models will likely provide us with the most comprehensive collection of information generated to date about the causes and molecular mechanisms of cancer.

THE GENOMIC LANDSCAPE OF CANCERS

Examining the overall distribution of the identified mutations redefined the cancer genome landscapes whereby the *mountains* are the handful of commonly mutated genes and the *hills* represent the vast majority of genes that are infrequently mutated.

One of the most striking features of the tumor genomic landscape is that it involves different sets of cancer genes that are mutated in a tissue-specific fashion.[132,133] To continue with the analogy, the scenery is very different if we observe a colorectal, a lung, or a breast tumor. This indicates that mutations in specific genes cause tumors at specific sites, or are associated with specific stages of development, cell differentiation, or tumorigenesis, despite many of those genes being expressed in various fetal and adult tissues. Moreover, different types of tumors follow specific genetic pathways in terms of the combination of genetic alterations that it must acquire. For example, no cancer outside the bowel has been shown to follow the classic genetic pathway of colorectal tumorigenesis. Additionally, *KRAS* mutations are almost always present in pancreatic cancers but are very rare or absent in breast cancers. Similarly, *BRAF* mutations are present in 60% of melanomas, but are very infrequent in lung cancers.[1] Another intriguing feature is that alterations in ubiquitous housekeeping genes, such as those involved in DNA repair or energy production, occur only in particular types of tumors.

In addition to tissue specificity, the genomic landscape of tumors can also be associated with gender and hormonal status. For example, *HER2* amplification and *PIK3C2A* mutations, two genetic alterations associated with breast cancer development, are correlated with the estrogen-receptor hormonal status.[134] The molecular basis for the occurrence of cancer mutations in tissue- and gender-specific profiles is still largely unknown. Organ-specific expression profiles and cell-specific neoplastic transformation requirements are often mentioned as possible causes for this phenomenon. Identifying tissue and gender cancer mutations patterns is relevant because it may allow for the definition of individualized therapeutic avenues.

INTEGRATIVE ANALYSIS OF CANCER GENOMICS

The implementation of novel high-throughput technologies is generating an extraordinary amount of information on cancer samples in many different ways other than those derived from whole-exome or whole-genome sequencing. Accordingly, there is a growing need to integrate genomic, epigenomic, transcriptomic, and proteomic landscapes from tumor samples, and then linking this integrated information with clinical outcomes of cancer patients. There are some examples of human malignancies in which this integrative approach has been already performed, such as for AML, glioblastoma, medulloblastoma, and renal cell, colorectal, ovarian, endometrial, prostate, and breast carcinomas.[135–142] In these cases, the integration of whole-exome and whole-genome sequencing with studies involving genomic DNA copy number arrays, DNA methylation, transcriptomic arrays, miRNA sequencing, and proteomic profiling has contributed to improving the molecular classification of complex and heterogeneous tumors. These integrative molecular analyses have also provided new insights into the mechanisms disrupted in each particular cancer type or subtype and have facilitated the association of genomic information with distinct clinical parameters of cancer patients and the discovery of novel therapeutic targets.[143] Also in this regard, there has been significant progress in the definition of the mechanisms by which the cancer genome and epigenome influence each other and cooperate to facilitate malignant transformation.[144,145] Thus, many tumor-suppressor genes are inactivated by either mutation or epigenetic silencing, and in some cases such as colorectal carcinomas, both mechanisms work coordinately to create a permissive environment for oncogenic transformation.[146] Moreover, mutations in epigenetic regulators such as DNA methyl transferases, chromatin remodelers, histones, and histone modifiers, are very frequent events in many tumors, including hepatocellular carcinomas, renal carcinomas leukemias, lymphomas, glioblastomas, and medulloblastomas. These genetic alterations of epigenetic modulators cause widespread transcriptomic changes, thereby amplifying the initial effect of the mutational event at the cancer genome level.[145]

The recent availability of different platforms for integrative cancer genome analyses will be very helpful in enabling the classification, biologic characterization, and personalized clinical management of human cancers (Table 1.3).[144,147]

THE CANCER GENOME AND THE NEW TAXONOMY OF TUMORS

Deciphering the cancer genome has already impacted clinical practice at multiple levels. On the one hand, it allowed for the identification of new cancer genes such as *IDH1*, a gene involved in glioma, which was discovered recently (see previous), and on the other hand, it is redesigning the taxonomy of tumors.

Until the genomic revolution, tumors had been classified based on two criteria: their localization (site of occurrence) and their appearance (histology). These criteria are also currently used as primary determinants of prognosis and to establish the best treatments. For many decades, it has been known that patients with histologically similar tumors have different clinical outcomes. Furthermore, tumors that cannot be distinguished based on an histologic analysis can respond very differently to identical therapies.[148]

It is becoming increasingly clear that the frequency and distribution of mutations affecting cancer genes can be used to redefine the histology-based taxonomy of a given tumor type. Lung and colorectal tumors represent paradigmatic examples. Genomic analyses led to the identification of activating mutations in the receptor tyrosine kinase *EGFR* in lung adenocarcinomas.[149] The occurrence of *EGFR* mutations molecularly defines a subtype of non–small-cell lung cancers (NSCLC) that occur mainly in nonsmoking women, that tend to have a distinctly enhanced prognosis, and that typically respond to epidermal growth factor receptor (EGFR)-targeted therapies.[150–152] Similarly, the recent discovery of the *EML4-ALK* fusion identifies yet another subset of NSCLC that is clearly distinct from those that harbor *EGFR* mutations, that have distinct epidemiologic and biologic features, and that respond to ALK inhibitors.[109,153]

The second example is colorectal cancers (CRC), the tumor type for which the genomic landscape has been refined with the highest accuracy. CRCs can be clearly categorized according to the mutational profile of the genes involved in the *KRAS* pathway (Fig. 1.10). It is now known that *KRAS* mutations occur in approximately 40% of CRCs. Another subtype of CRC (approximately 10%) harbors mutations in *BRAF*, the immediate downstream effectors of *KRAS*.[10]

In CRCs and other tumor types, *KRAS* and *BRAF* mutations are known to be mutually exclusive. The mutual exclusivity pattern indicates that these genes operate in the same signaling pathway. Large epidemiologic studies have shown that the prognosis of tumors harboring wild-type *KRAS/BRAF* genes is distinct, and typically more favorable, than that of the mutated ones.[154,155] Of note, *KRAS* and *BRAF* mutations have been recently shown to impair responsiveness to the anti-EGFR monoclonal antibodies therapies in CRC patients.[156–158] Clearly distinct subgroups can be genetically identified in both NSCLCs and CRCs with respect to prognosis and response to therapy. It is likely that as soon as the genomic landscapes of other tumor types are defined, molecular subgroups like those described previously will also become defined.

Genotyping tumor tissue in search of somatic genetic alterations for *actionable* information has become routine practice in clinical oncology. The genetic profile of solid tumors is currently obtained from surgical or biopsy specimens. As the techniques

TABLE 1.3

Useful Information for the Description and Management of Cancer

Bioinformatic Tool or Webservices	Database Used	Webservice or Tool	Upload of Data Possible	Gene Search	Chromosomal Region Search	mRNA Expression	SNV	CNV	Methylation	miRNA Expression	Protein	Pathways
cBioPortal for Cancer Genomics	TCGA	Webservice	—	✓	—	✓	✓	✓	—	—	✓	✓
PARADIGM, Broad GDAC Firehose	TCGA	Webservice	✓	✓	—	✓	✓	✓	✓	—	—	✓
WashU Epigenome Browser	ENCODE	Webservice	✓	✓	✓	✓	✓	✓	✓	—	—	✓
UCSC Cancer Genomics Browser	UCSC	Webservice	✓	✓	✓	✓	✓	✓	✓	✓	—	—
The Cancer Genome Workbench	TCGA	Webservice	—	✓	✓	✓	✓	✓	✓	—	—	—
EpiExplorer	ENCODE and ROADMAP	Webservice	✓	✓	✓	✓	✓	✓	✓	—	—	—
EpiGRAPH	ENCODE	Webservice	✓	✓	✓	✓	✓	✓	✓	—	—	—
Catalogue of Somatic Mutations in Cancer (COSMIC)	TCGA and ICGC	Webservice	—	✓	—	—	✓	✓	—	—	—	—
PCmtl, MAGIA, miRvar, CoMeTa, etc.*	GEO and TCGA	Webservice	✓	✓	—	✓	—	—	—	✓	—	✓
ICGC	ICGC	Webservice	—	✓	—	✓	✓	✓	—	—	—	—
Genomatix	User defined	Tool	—	✓	—	✓	✓	✓	✓	—	—	✓
Caleydo	TCGA	Tool	—	✓	✓	✓	✓	✓	✓	✓	—	✓
Integrative Genomics Viewer (IGV)	ENCODE	Tool	—	✓	✓	✓	✓	✓	✓	—	—	—
iCluster and iCluster Plus	User defined	Tool	—	✓	—	✓	—	✓	—	—	—	—

* Web Site with links for integrated analysis of microRNA and mRNA expression.
CNV, copy-number variation; ENCODE, Encyclopedia of DNA Elements; ICGC, the International Cancer Genome Consortium; GDAC, Genomic Data Analysis Center; GEO, Gene Expression Omnibus; miRNA, microRNA; SNV, single-nucleotide variation; TCGA, The Cancer Genome Atlas; USCS, University of California, Santa Cruz;
Based on Plass C, Pfister SM, Lindroth AM, et al. Mutations in regulators of the epigenome and their connections to global chromatin patterns in cancer. *Nat Rev Genet* 2013;14:765–780, Table 1.

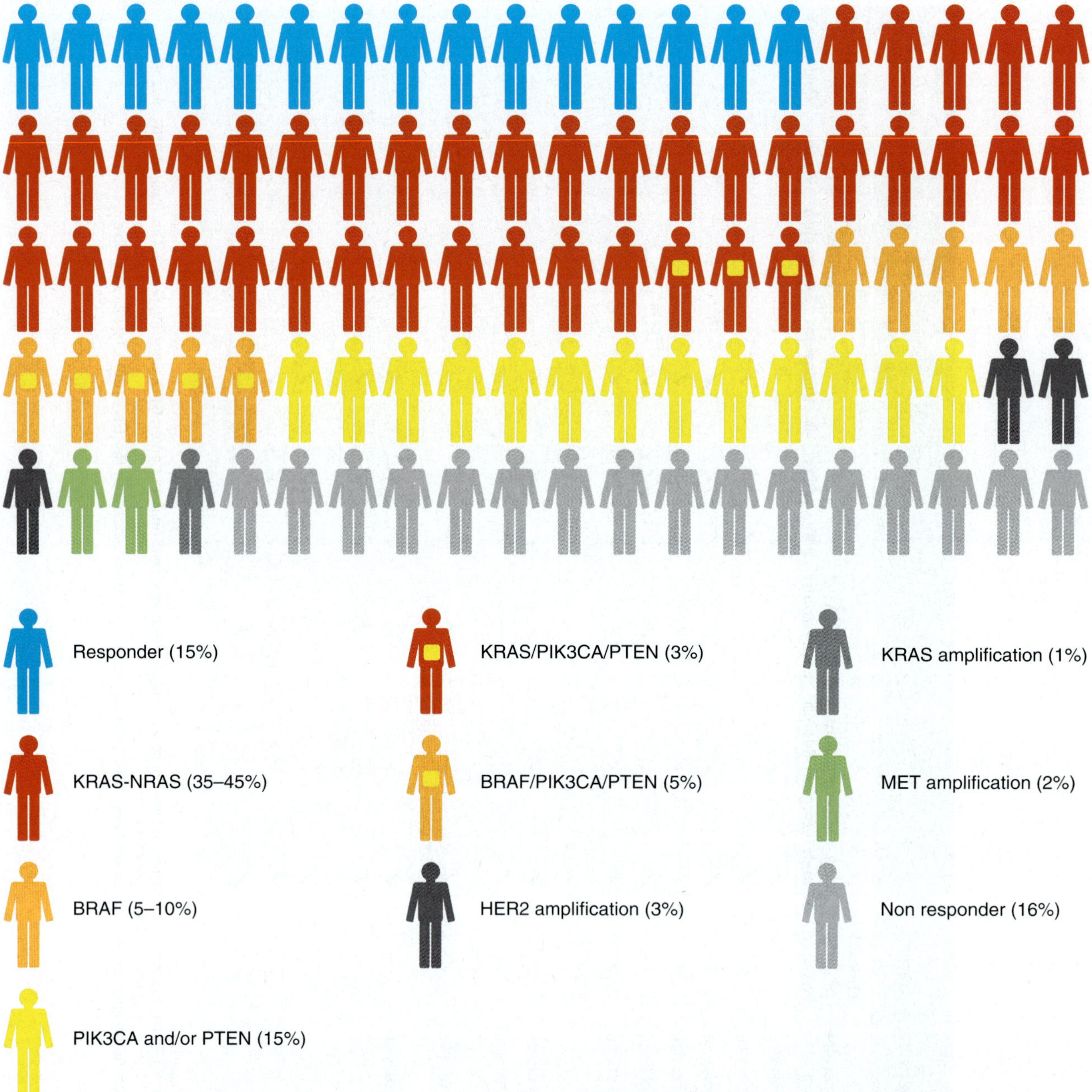
Responder (15%)
KRAS/PIK3CA/PTEN (3%)
KRAS amplification (1%)
KRAS-NRAS (35–45%)
BRAF/PIK3CA/PTEN (5%)
MET amplification (2%)
BRAF (5–10%)
HER2 amplification (3%)
Non responder (16%)
PIK3CA and/or PTEN (15%)

Figure 1.10 Graphic representation of a cohort of 100 patients with colorectal cancer treated with cetuximab or panitumumab. The genetic milieu of individual tumors and their impacts on the clinical response are listed. *KRAS, BRAF,* and *PIK3CA* somatic mutations as well as loss of PTEN protein expression are indicated according to different color codes. Molecular alterations mutually exclusive or coexisting in individual tumors are indicated using different color variants. The relative frequencies at which the molecular alterations occur in colorectal cancers are described. (Redrawn from Bardelli A, Siena S. Molecular mechanisms of resistance to cetuximab and panitumumab in colorectal cancer. *J Clin Oncol* 2010;28:1254–1261.)

that have enabled us to analyze tumor tissues become ever more sophisticated, we have realized the limitations of this approach. As previously discussed, cancers are heterogeneous, with different areas of the same tumor showing different genetic profiles (i.e., intratumoral heterogeneity); likewise, heterogeneity exists between metastases within the same patient (i.e., intermetastatic heterogeneity).[159] A tissue section (or a biopsy) from one part of a solitary tumor will miss the molecular intratumoral as well as intermetastatic heterogeneity. To capture tumor heterogeneity, techniques that are capable of interrogating the genetic landscapes of the overall disease in a single patient are needed.

In 1948, the publication of a manuscript describing the presence of cell-free circulating DNA (cfDNA) in the blood of humans offered—probably without realizing it—unprecedented opportunities in this area.[160] Only recently, the full potential of this seminal discovery has been appreciated. Several groups have reported that the analysis of circulating tumor DNA can, in principle, provide the same genetic information obtained from tumor tissue.[161] The levels of cfDNA are typically higher in cancer patients than healthy individuals, indicating that it is possible to screen for the presence of disease through a simple blood test. Furthermore, the specific detection of tumor-derived cfDNA has been shown to correlate with tumor burden, which changes in response to treatment or surgery.[162–164]

Although the detection of ctDNA has remarkable potential, it is also challenging for several reasons. The first is the need to discriminate DNA released from tumor cells (ctDNA) from circulating *normal* DNA. Discerning ctDNA from normal cfDNA is aided by the fact that tumor DNA is defined by the presence of mutations. These somatic mutations, commonly single base pair substitutions, are present only in the genomes of cancer cells or precancerous cells and are present in the DNA of normal cells of the same individual. Accordingly, ctDNA offers exquisite specificity as a biomarker. Unfortunately, cfDNA derived from tumor cells often represents a very small fraction (<1%) of the total cfDNA, thus limiting the applicability of the approach. The development and refinement of next-generation sequencing strategies as well as recently developed digital PCR techniques have made it possible to define rare mutant variants in complex mixtures of DNA. Using these approaches, it is possible to detect point mutations, rearrangements, and gene copy number changes in individual genes starting from a few milliliters of plasma.[165] Very recently, several groups have opened a new frontier by showing that exome analyses can also be performed from circulating DNA extracted from the blood of cancer patients.[166]

The detection of tumor-specific genetic alterations in patients' blood (often referred to as *liquid biopsies*) has several applications in the field of oncology, which are summarized as follows. Analyses of cfDNA can be used to genotype tumors when a tissue sample is not available or is difficult to obtain. Circulating tumor DNA fragments contain the identical genetic defects as the tumor themselves, thus the blood can reveal tumor point mutations (*EGFR, KRAS, BRAF, PIK3CA*), rearrangements (e.g., *EML4-ALK*), as well as tumor amplifications (*MET*).[167–169] *Liquid biopsies* may also be useful in monitoring tumor burden—a central aspect in the management of patients with cancer that is typically assessed with imaging. In this regard, several investigational studies have shown that ctDNA can be a surrogate for tumor burden and that, much like viral load changes (e.g., HIV viral load), levels of ctDNA correspond with clinical course. Another application of ctDNA is the detection of minimal residual disease following surgery or therapy with curative intent.[163] Finally, *liquid biopsies* can be used to monitor the genomic drift (clonal evolution) of tumors upon treatment.[166] In this setting, the analysis of ctDNA in plasma samples obtained pretreatment, during, and posttreatment can lead to an understanding of the mechanisms of primary and, especially, acquired resistance to therapies.[170,171]

Importantly, the advances in sequencing technologies have made the idea of personalized treatment of cancer a reality, which is most evident in the field of adoptive cell therapy (ACT). Although already a treatment in use, the ability to use a patient's autologous tumor-infiltrating lymphocytes (TIL) is in position to benefit greatly from advances in sequencing technologies. A recent study demonstrated this when whole-exome data, along with a major histocompatibility complex (MHC)-binding algorithm, were utilized to identify candidate tumor epitopes that are recognized by the patients' TILs.[172] This study should allow for future work in which the information obtained from the direct sequencing of a patient's tumor can quickly be used to generate tumor-reactive T cells that can then be used for a personalized treatment.

In conclusion, the taxonomy of tumors is being rewritten using the presence of genetic lesions as major criteria. Genome-based information will improve the diagnosis and will be used to determine personalized therapeutic regimens based on the genetic landscape of individual tumors.

CANCER GENOMICS AND DRUG RESISTANCE

Cancer genomics has dramatically impacted disease management, because its application is helping researchers determine which patients are likely to benefit from which drug. As discussed in great detail in Chapter 22, good examples for such treatment include targeted therapy using imatinib for chronic myeloid leukemia (CML) patients and the use of gefitinib and erlotinib for NSCLC patients.

The key to the successful development and application of anticancer agents is a better understanding of the effect of the therapeutic regimens and of resistance mechanisms that may develop. In most tumor types, a fraction of patients' tumors are refractory to therapies (intrinsic resistance). Even if an initial response to therapies is obtained, the vast majority of tumors subsequently become refractory (i.e., acquired resistance), and patients eventually succumb to disease progression. Therefore, secondary resistance should be regarded as a key obstacle to treatment progress. The analysis of the cancer genome represents a powerful tool both for the identification of chemotherapeutic signatures as well as to understand resistance mechanisms to therapeutic agents. Examples for each of these are described as follows.

An important application of systematic sequencing experiments is the identification of the effects of chemotherapy on the cancer genome. For example, gliomas that recur after temozolomide treatment have been shown to harbor large numbers of mutations with a signature typical of a DNA alkylating agent.[173,174] Because these alterations were detected using Sanger sequencing, which as described previously has limited sensitivity, the data suggested that the detected alterations were clonal. The model that unfolds from this study indicates that although temozolomide has limited efficacy, almost all of the cells in a glioma respond to the drug. However, a single cell that was resistant to the chemotherapy proliferated and formed a cell clone. Later genomic analyses of the cell clone allowed for the identification of the underlying mutated resistance genes.[173,174]

Single-molecule–targeted therapy is almost always followed by acquired drug resistance.[175–177] Genomic analyses can be successfully exploited to decipher resistance mechanisms to such inhibitors. A few paradigmatic examples are presented as follows, which will be discussed extensively in other chapters. Despite the effectiveness of gefitinib and erlotinib in EGFR mutant cases of NSCLC,[178] drug resistance develops within 6 to 12 months after the initiation of therapy. The underlying reason for this resistance was identified as a secondary mutation in *EGFR* exon 20, T790M, which is detectable in 50% of patients who relapse.[179–181] Importantly, some studies have shown the mutation to be present before the patient was treated with the drug,[182,183] suggesting that exposure to the drug selected for these cells.[184] Because the drug-resistant *EGFR* mutation is structurally analogous to the mutated gatekeeper residue T315I in BCR-ABL, T670I in c-Kit, and L1196M in EML4-ALK, which have been shown previously to confer resistance to imatinib and other kinase inhibitors,[176,185,186] this mechanism of resistance represents a general problem that needs to be overcome.

A recent elegant study, which also represents the use of genomics in understanding drug-resistance mechanisms, focused on the inhibition of activating *BRAF* (V600E) mutations, which occur in 7% of human malignancies and in 60% of melanomas.[9] Clinical trials using PLX4032, a novel class I RAF-selective inhibitor, showed an 80% antitumor response rate in melanoma patients with *BRAF* (V600E) mutations; however, cases of drug resistance were observed.[187] The use of microarray and sequencing technologies showed that, in this case, the resistance was not due to secondary mutations in *BRAF*, but due rather to either upregulation of *PDGFRB* or *NRAS* mutations.[188]

It was, however, the introduction of two anti-EGFR monoclonal antibodies, cetuximab and panitumumab, for the treatment of metastatic colorectal cancer, that provided the largest body of knowledge on the relationship between tumors' genotypes and the response to targeted therapies. The initial clinical analysis

PRINCIPLES OF ONCOLOGY

pointed out that only a fraction of metastatic CRC patients benefited from this novel treatment. Different from the NSCLC paradigm, it was found that EGFR mutations do not play a major role in the response. On the contrary, from the initial retrospective analysis, it became clear that somatic *KRAS* mutations, thought to be present in 35% to 45% of metastatic colorectal cancers, are important negative predictors of efficacy in patients who are given panitumumab or cetuximab.[156–158] Among tumors carrying wild-type *KRAS*, mutations of *BRAF* or *PIK3CA*, or a loss of phosphatase and tensin homolog (PTEN) expression may also predict resistance to EGFR-targeted monoclonal antibodies, although the latter biomarkers require further validation before they can be incorporated into clinical practice. From these few examples, it is clear that a future, deeper genomic understanding of targeted drug resistance is crucial to the effective development of additional as well as alternative therapies to overcome this resistance.

PERSPECTIVES OF CANCER GENOME ANALYSIS

The completion of the human genome project has marked a new beginning in biomedical sciences. Because human cancer is a genetic disease, the field of oncology has been one of the first to be impacted by this historic revolution. Knowledge of the sequence and organization of the human genome allows for the systematic analysis of the genetic alterations underlying the origin and evolution of tumors. High-throughput mutational profiling of common tumors, including lung, skin, breast, and colorectal cancers, and the application of next-generation sequencing to whole genome, whole exome, and whole transcriptome of cancer samples has allowed substantial advances in the understanding of this disease by facilitating the detection of all main types of somatic cancer genome alterations. These have also led to historical results, such as the identification of genetic alterations that are likely to be the major drivers of these diseases.

However, the genetic landscape of cancers is by no means complete, and what has been learned so far has raised new and exciting questions that must be addressed. There are still important technical challenges for the detection of somatic mutations.[60] Clinical tumor samples often contain large amounts of nonmalignant cells, which makes the identification of mutations in cancer genomes more challenging when compared with similar analyses of peripheral blood samples for germ-line genome studies. Moreover, the genomic instability inherent to cancer development and progression largely increases the complexity and diversity of genomic alterations of malignant tumors, making it necessary to distinguish between driver and passenger mutations. Likewise, the fact that malignant tumors are genetically heterogeneous and contain several clones simultaneously growing within the same tumor mass raises additional questions regarding the quality of the information currently derived from cancer genomes. Hopefully, in the near future, advances in third-generation sequencing technologies will make it feasible to obtain high-quality sequence data of a genome isolated from a single cell, an aspect of crucial relevance for cancer research.

One of the next imperatives is the definition of the oncogenomic profile of all tumor types. In particular, the less common—although not less lethal—ones are still largely mysterious to scientists and untreatable to clinicians. For some of these diseases, few new therapeutically amenable molecular targets have been discovered in the past years. For example, the identification of drugable genetic lesions associated with pancreatic and ovarian cancers could help define new therapeutic strategies for these aggressive diseases. To achieve this, detailed oncogenomic maps of the corresponding tumors must be drafted. The latter will hopefully be completed in the coming years, thanks to the systematic cancer genome projects that are presently being performed.

Even in the case of common cancers, a lot of genomic profiling efforts still lay ahead. For example, in a significant fraction of breast and lung tumors, the mutations that are likely to be drivers have not yet been found. This is not surprising considering that even in these tumor types only a limited number of samples have been systematically analyzed so far. Therefore, low incidence mutations that could represent potentially key therapeutic targets in a subset of tumors might have escaped detection. Consequently, the scaling up of the mutational profiling to large numbers of specimens for each tumor type is warranted.

Finally, understanding the cellular properties imparted by the hundreds of recently discovered cancer alleles is another area that must be developed. As a matter of fact, compared to the genomic discovery stage, the functional validation of putative novel cancer alleles, despite their potential clinical relevance, is substantially lagging behind. To achieve this, high-throughput functional studies in model systems that accurately recapitulate the genetic alterations found in human cancer must be developed.

To conclude, the eventual goal of profiling the cancer genome is not only to further understand the molecular basis of the disease, but also to discover novel diagnostic and drug targets. One might anticipate that the most immediate application of these new technologies will be noninvasive strategies for early cancer detection. Considering that oncogenic mutations are present only in cancer cells, screening for tumor-derived mutant DNA in patients' blood holds great potential and will progressively substitute current biomarkers, which have poor sensitivity and lack specificity.[171] Further improvements in next-generation sequencing technologies are likely to reduce their cost as well as make these analyses more facile in the future. Once this happens, most cancer patients will undergo in-depth genomic analyses as part of their initial evaluation and throughout their treatment. This will offer more precise diagnostic and prognostic information, which will affect treatment decisions. Although many challenges remain, the information gained from next-generation sequencing platforms is laying a foundation for personalized medicine, in which patients are managed with therapies that are tailored to the specific gene mutations found in their tumors. Ultimately, these should lead to therapeutic successes similar to the ones attained for CML patients with imatinib,[189,190] melanoma patients with PLX4032,[187] and NSCLC patients with gefitinib and erlotinib.[178] Clearly, this is the absolute goal for all of this work.

ACKNOWLEDGMENTS

This work was supported by the Intramural Research Programs of the National Human Genome Research Institute, National Institutes of Health, USA, YS is supported by the Henry Chanoch Krenter Institute for Biomedical Imaging and Genomics, Louis and Fannie Tolz Collaborative Research Project, Dukler Fund for Cancer Research, De Benedetti Foundation-Cherasco 1547, Peter and Patricia Gruber Awards, Gideon Hamburger, Israel, Estate of Alice Schwarz-Gardos, Estate of John Hunter and the Knell Family. YS is supported by the Israel Science Foundation grant numbers 1604/13 and 877/13 and the ERC (StG-335377). A.B. is supported by the European Communityís Seventh Framework Programme under grant agreement no. 259015 COLTHERES, Associazione Italiana per la Ricerca sul Cancro (AIRC) IG grant no. 12812 and Fondazione Piemontese per la Ricerca sul Cancro–ONLUS. C.L-O. is an Investigator of the Botin Foundation supported by grants from Ministerio de Economía y Competitividad-Spain and Instituto de Salud Carlos III (RTICC), Spain.

REFERENCES

1. Vogelstein B, Kinzler KW. Cancer genes and the pathways they control. *Nat Med* 2004;10:789–799.
2. Kinzler KW, Vogelstein B. Lessons from hereditary colon cancer. *Cell* 1996; 87:159–170.
3. International Human Genome Sequencing Consortium. Finishing the euchromatic sequence of the human genome. *Nature* 2004;431:931–945.
4. Stehelin D, Varmus HE, Bishop JM, et al. DNA related to the transforming gene(s) of avian sarcoma viruses is present in normal avian DNA. *Nature* 1976;260:170–173.
5. Rous P. Transmission of a malignant new growth by means of a cell-free filtrate. *J Am Med Assoc* 1911;56:198.
6. International HapMap Consortium. The International HapMap Project. *Nature* 2003;426:89–96.
7. International HapMap Consortium. A haplotype map of the human genome. *Nature* 2005;437:1299–1320.
8. Sanger F, Nicklen S, Coulson AR. DNA sequencing with chain-terminating inhibitors. *Proc Natl Acad Sci U S A* 1977;74:5463–5467.
9. Davies H, Bignell GR, Cox C, et al. Mutations of the BRAF gene in human cancer. *Nature* 2002;417:949–954.
10. Rajagopalan H, Bardelli A, Lengauer C, et al. Tumorigenesis: RAF/RAS oncogenes and mismatch-repair status. *Nature* 2002;418:934.
11. Moodie SA, Wolfman A. The 3Rs of life: Ras, Raf and growth regulation. *Trends Genet* 1994;10:44–48.
12. Hafen E, Dickson B, Brunner D, et al. Genetic dissection of signal transduction mediated by the sevenless receptor tyrosine kinase in Drosophila. *Prog Neurobiol* 1994;42:287–292.
13. Bardelli A, Parsons DW, Silliman N, et al. Mutational analysis of the tyrosine kinome in colorectal cancers. *Science* 2003;300:949.
14. Greenman C, Stephens P, Smith R, et al. Patterns of somatic mutation in human cancer genomes. *Nature* 2007;446:153–158.
15. Samuels Y, Wang Z, Bardelli A, et al. High frequency of mutations of the PIK3CA gene in human cancers. *Science* 2004;304:554.
16. Wang Z, Shen D, Parsons DW, et al. Mutational analysis of the tyrosine phosphatome in colorectal cancers. *Science* 2004;304:1164–1166.
17. Vivanco I, Sawyers CL. The phosphatidylinositol 3-Kinase AKT pathway in human cancer. *Nat Rev Cancer* 2002;2:489–501.
18. Broderick DK, Di C, Parrett TJ, et al. Mutations of PIK3CA in anaplastic oligodendrogliomas, high-grade astrocytomas, and medulloblastomas. *Cancer Res* 2004;64:5048–5050.
19. Lee JW, Soung YH, Kim SY, et al. PIK3CA gene is frequently mutated in breast carcinomas and hepatocellular carcinomas. *Oncogene* 2005;24:1477–1480.
20. Bachman KE, Argani P, Samuels Y, et al. The PIK3CA gene is mutated with high frequency in human breast cancers. *Cancer Biol Ther* 2004;3: 772–775.
21. Oda K, Stokoe D, Taketani Y, et al. High frequency of coexistent mutations of PIK3CA and PTEN genes in endometrial carcinoma. *Cancer Res* 2005;65:10669–10673.
22. Samuels Y, Waldman T. Oncogenic mutations of PIK3CA in human cancers. *Curr Top Microbiol Immunol* 2010;2:21–42.
23. Parsons DW, Wang TL, Samuels Y, et al. Colorectal cancer: mutations in a signalling pathway. *Nature* 2005;436:792.
24. Lopez-Otin C, Overall CM. Protease degradomics: a new challenge for proteomics. *Nat Rev Mol Cell Biol* 2002;3:509–519.
25. Liotta LA, Tryggvason K, Garbisa S, et al. Metastatic potential correlates with enzymatic degradation of basement membrane collagen. *Nature* 1980;284: 67–68.
26. Lopez-Otin C, Hunter T. The regulatory crosstalk between kinases and proteases in cancer. *Nat Rev Cancer* 2010;10:278–292.
27. Egeblad M, Werb Z. New functions for the matrix metalloproteinases in cancer progression. *Nat Rev Cancer* 2002;2:161–174.
28. Lopez-Otin C, Matrisian LM. Emerging roles of proteases in tumour suppression. *Nat Rev Cancer* 2007;7:800–808.
29. Wood LD, Parsons DW, Jones S, et al. The genomic landscapes of human breast and colorectal cancers. *Science* 2007;318:1108–1113.
30. Palavalli LH, Prickett TD, Wunderluch JR, et al. Analysis of the matrix metalloproteinase family reveals that MMP8 is often mutated in melanoma. *Nat Genet* 2009;41:518–520.
31. Lopez-Otin C, Palavalli LH, Samuels Y. Protective roles of matrix metalloproteinases: from mouse models to human cancer. *Cell Cycle* 2009;8:3657–3662.
32. Hanahan D, Weinberg RA. The hallmarks of cancer. *Cell* 2000;100:57–70.
33. Teitz T, Wei T, Valentine MB, et al. Caspase 8 is deleted or silenced preferentially in childhood neuroblastomas with amplification of MYCN. *Nat Med* 2000;6:529–535.
34. Mandruzzato S, Brasseur F, Andry G, et al. A CASP-8 mutation recognized by cytolytic T lymphocytes on a human head and neck carcinoma. *J Exp Med* 1997;186:785–793.
35. Soung YH, Lee JW, Kim SY, et al. CASPASE-8 gene is inactivated by somatic mutations in gastric carcinomas. *Cancer Res* 2005;65:815–821.
36. Fraile JM, Quesada V, Rodríguez D, et al. Deubiquitinases in cancer: new functions and therapeutic options. *Oncogene* 2012;31:2373–2388.
37. Bignell GR, Warren W, Seal S, et al. Identification of the familial cylindromatosis tumour-suppressor gene. *Nat Genet* 2000;25:160–165.
38. Schmitz R, Hansmann ML, Bohle V, et al. TNFAIP3 (A20) is a tumor suppressor gene in Hodgkin lymphoma and primary mediastinal B cell lymphoma. *J Exp Med* 2009;206:981–989.
39. Compagno M, Lim WK, Grunn A, et al. Mutations of multiple genes cause deregulation of NF-kappaB in diffuse large B-cell lymphoma. *Nature* 2009;459:717–721.
40. Kato M, Sanada M, Kato I, et al. Frequent inactivation of A20 in B-cell lymphomas. *Nature* 2009;459:712–716.
41. Novak U, Rinaldi A, Kwee I, et al. The NF-kappa B negative regulator TNFAIP3 (A20) is inactivated by somatic mutations and genomic deletions in marginal zone lymphomas. *Blood* 2009;113: 4918–4921.
42. Harbour JW, Onken MD, Roberson ED, et al. Frequent mutation of BAP1 in metastasizing uveal melanomas. *Science* 2010;330:1410–1413.
43. Carbone M, Yang H, Pass HI, et al. BAP1 and cancer. *Nat Rev Cancer* 2013; 13:153–159.
44. Sjöblom T, Jones S, Wood LD, et al. The consensus coding sequences of human breast and colorectal cancers. *Science* 2006;314:268–274.
45. Jones S, Zhang X, Parsons DW, et al. Core signaling pathways in human pancreatic cancers revealed by global genomic analyses. *Science* 2008;321:1801–1806.
46. Parsons DW, Jones S, Zhang X, et al. An integrated genomic analysis of human glioblastoma multiforme. *Science* 2008;321:1807–1812.
47. Jones S, Wang TL, Shih leM, et al. Frequent mutations of chromatin remodeling gene ARID1A in ovarian clear cell carcinoma. *Science* 2010;330:228–231.
48. Parsons DW, Li M, Zhang X, et al. The genetic landscape of the childhood cancer medulloblastoma. *Science* 2011;331:435–439.
49. Yan H, Parsons DW, Jin G, et al. IDH1 and IDH2 mutations in gliomas. *N Engl J Med* 2009;360:765–773.
50. Bleeker FE, Lamba S, Leenstra S, et al. IDH1 mutations at residue p.R132 (IDH1(R132)) occur frequently in high-grade gliomas but not in other solid tumors. *Hum Mutat* 2009;30:7–11.
51. Hartmann C, Meyer J, Balss J, et al. Type and frequency of IDH1 and IDH2 mutations are related to astrocytic and oligodendroglial differentiation and age: a study of 1,010 diffuse gliomas. *Acta Neuropathol* 2009;118:469–474.
52. Hayden JT, Frühwald MC, Hasselblatt M, et al. Frequent IDH1 mutations in supratentorial primitive neuroectodermal tumors (sPNET) of adults but not children. *Cell Cycle* 2009;8:1806–1807.
53. Ichimura K, Pearson DM, Kocialkowski S, et al. IDH1 mutations are present in the majority of common adult gliomas but rare in primary glioblastomas. *Neuro Oncol* 2009;11:341–347.
54. Kang MR, Kim MS, Oh JE, et al. Mutational analysis of IDH1 codon 132 in glioblastomas and other common cancers. *Int J Cancer* 2009;125:353–355.
55. Watanabe T, Nobusawa S, Kleihues P, et al. IDH1 mutations are early events in the development of astrocytomas and oligodendrogliomas. *Am J Pathol* 2009;174:1149–1153.
56. Mardis ER, Ding L, Dooling DJ, et al. Recurring mutations found by sequencing an acute myeloid leukemia genome. *N Engl J Med* 2009;361:1058–1066.
57. Green A, Beer P. Somatic mutations of IDH1 and IDH2 in the leukemic transformation of myeloproliferative neoplasms. *N Engl J Med* 2010;362:369–370.
58. Gross S, Cairns RA, Minden Md, et al. Cancer-associated metabolite 2-hydroxyglutarate accumulates in acute myelogenous leukemia with isocitrate dehydrogenase 1 and 2 mutations. *J Exp Med* 2010;207:339–344.
59. Mardis ER, Wilson RK. Cancer genome sequencing: a review. *Hum Mol Genet* 2009;18:R163–R168.
60. Meyerson M, Gabriel S, Getz G. Advances in understanding cancer genomes through second generation sequencing. *Nat Rev Genet* 2010;11:685–696
61. Metzker ML. Sequencing technologies - the next generation. *Nat Rev Genet* 2010;11:31–46.
62. Bell DW. Our changing view of the genomic landscape of cancer. *J Pathol* 2010;220:231–243.
63. Campbell PJ, Pleasance ED, Stephens PJ, et al. Subclonal phylogenetic structures in cancer revealed by ultra-deep sequencing. *Proc Natl Acad Sci U S A* 2008;105:13081–13086.
64. Kidd JM, Cooper GM, Donahue WF, et al. Mapping and sequencing of structural variation from eight human genomes. *Nature* 2008;453:56–64.
65. Drmanac R, Sparks AB, Callow MJ, et al. Human genome sequencing using unchained base reads on self-assembling DNA nanoarrays. *Science* 2010; 327:78–81.
66. Clarke J, Wu HC, Jayasinghe L, et al. Continuous base identification for single-molecule nanopore DNA sequencing. *Nat Nanotechnol* 2009;4:265–270.
67. Schadt EE, Turner S, Kasarskis A. A window into third-generation sequencing. *Hum Mol Genet* 2010;19:R227–R240.
68. Dressman D, Yan H, Traverso G, et al. Transforming single DNA molecules into fluorescent magnetic particles for detection and enumeration of genetic variations. *Proc Natl Acad Sci U S A* 2003;100:8817–8822.
69. Fedurco M, Romieu A, Williams S, et al. BTA, a novel reagent for DNA attachment on glass and efficient generation of solid-phase amplified DNA colonies. *Nucleic Acids Res* 2006;34:e22.
70. Harris TD, Buzby PR, Babcock H, et al. Single-molecule DNA sequencing of a viral genome. *Science* 2008;320:106–109.
71. Morozova O, Hirst M, Marra MA. Applications of new sequencing technologies for transcriptome analysis. *Annu Rev Genomics Hum Genet* 2009;10: 135–151.

PRINCIPLES OF ONCOLOGY

72. Pop M, Salzberg SL. Bioinformatics challenges of new sequencing technology. *Trends Genet* 2008;24:142–149.
73. Ley TJ, Mardis ER, Ding L, et al. DNA sequencing of a cytogenetically normal acute myeloid leukaemia genome. *Nature* 2008;456:66–72.
74. Garraway LA, Lander ES. Lessons from the cancer genome. *Cell* 2013;15: 17–37.
75. Vogelstein B, Papadopoulos N, Velculescu VE, et al. Cancer genome landscapes. *Science* 2013;339:1546–1558.
76. Watson IR, Takahashi K, Futreal PA, et al. Emerging patterns of somatic mutations in cancer. *Nat Rev Genet* 2013;14:703–718.
77. Campbell PJ, Yachida S, Mudie LJ, et al. The patterns and dynamics of genomic instability in metastatic pancreatic cancer. *Nature* 2010;467:1109–1113.
78. Lee W, Jiang Z, Liu J, et al. The mutation spectrum revealed by paired genome sequences from a lung cancer patient. *Nature* 2010;465:473–477.
79. Marcucci G, Maharry K, Wu YZ, et al. IDH1 and IDH2 gene mutations identify novel molecular subsets within de novo cytogenetically normal acute myeloid leukemia: a Cancer and Leukemia Group B study. *J Clin Oncol* 2010;28:2348–2355.
80. Paschka P, Schlenk RF, Gaidzik VI, et al. IDH1 and IDH2 mutations are frequent genetic alterations in acute myeloid leukemia and confer adverse prognosis in cytogenetically normal acute myeloid leukemia with NPM1 mutation without FLT3 internal tandem duplication. *J Clin Oncol* 2010;28:3636–3643.
81. Shah SP, Morin Rd, Khattra J, et al. Mutational evolution in a lobular breast tumour profiled at single nucleotide resolution. *Nature* 2009;461:809–813.
82. Yachida S, Jones S, Bozic I, et al. Distant metastasis occurs late during the genetic evolution of pancreatic cancer. *Nature* 2010;467:1114–1117.
83. Pleasance ED, Cheetham RK, Stephens PJ, et al. A comprehensive catalogue of somatic mutations from a human cancer genome. *Nature* 2010;463:191–196.
84. Pleasance ED, Stephens PJ, O'Meara S, et al. A small-cell lung cancer genome with complex signatures of tobacco exposure. *Nature* 2010;463:184–190.
85. Ding L, Ellis MJ, Li S, et al. Genome remodelling in a basal-like breast cancer metastasis and xenograft. *Nature* 2010;464:999–1005.
86. Ley TJ, Ding L, Walter MJ, et al. DNMT3A mutations in acute myeloid leukemia. *N Engl J Med* 2010;363:2424–2433.
87. Alexandrov LB, Nik-Zainal S, Wedge DC, et al. Signatures of mutational processes in human cancer. *Nature* 2013;500:415–421.
88. Ward PS, Patel J, Wise DR, et al. The common feature of leukemia-associated IDH1 and IDH2 mutations is a neomorphic enzyme activity converting alpha-ketoglutarate to 2-hydroxyglutarate. *Cancer Cell* 2010;17:225–234.
89. Jones SJ, Laskin J, Lu YY, et al. Evolution of an adenocarcinoma in response to selection by targeted kinase inhibitors. *Genome Biol* 2010;11:R82.
90. Navin N, Kendall J, Troge J, et al. Tumour evolution inferred by single-cell sequencing. *Nature* 2011;472:90–94.
91. Vanharanta S, Massague J. Origins of metastatic traits. *Cancer Cell* 2013; 24:410–421.
92. Huang FW, Hodis E, Xu MJ, et al. Highly recurrent TERT promoter mutations in human melanoma. *Science* 2013;339:957–959.
93. Horn S, Figl A, Rachakonda PS, et al. TERT promoter mutations in familial and sporadic melanoma. *Science* 2013;339:959–961.
94. Ying Z, Li Y, Wu J, et al. Loss of miR-204 expression enhances glioma migration and stem cell-like phenotype. *Cancer Res* 2013;73:990–999.
95. Liang YJ, Wang QY, Zhou CX, et al. MiR-124 targets Slug to regulate epithelial-mesenchymal transition and metastasis of breast cancer. *Carcinogenesis* 2013;34:713–722.
96. Cooper C, Guo J, Yan Y, et al. Increasing the relative expression of endogenous non-coding Steroid Receptor RNA Activator (SRA) in human breast cancer cells using modified oligonucleotides. *Nucleic Acids Res* 2009;37:4518–4531.
97. Stephens PJ, Greenman CD, Fu B, et al. Massive genomic rearrangement acquired in a single catastrophic event during cancer development. *Cell* 2011; 144:27–40.
98. Korbel JO, Campbell PJ. Criteria for inference of chromothripsis in cancer genomes. *Cell* 2013;152:1226–1236.
99. Baca SC, Prandi D, Lawrence MS, et al. Punctuated evolution of prostate cancer genomes. *Cell* 2013;153:666–677.
100. Turner EH, Lee C, Ng SB, et al. Massively parallel exon capture and library-free resequencing across 16 genomes. *Nat Methods* 2009;6:315–316.
101. Gnirke A, Melnikov A, Maguire J, et al. Solution hybrid selection with ultra-long oligonucleotides for massively parallel targeted sequencing. *Nat Biotechnol* 2009;27:182–189.
102. Levin JZ, Berger MF, Adiconis X, et al. Targeted next-generation sequencing of a cancer transcriptome enhances detection of sequence variants and novel fusion transcripts. *Genome Biol* 2009;10:R115.
103. Lawrence MS, Stojanov P, Polak P, et al. Mutational heterogeneity in cancer and the search for new cancer-associated genes. *Nature* 2013;499:214–218.
104. Kandoth C, McLellan MD, Vandin F, et al. Mutational landscape and significance across 12 major cancer types. *Nature* 2013;502:333–339.
105. Gartner JJ, Parker SC, Prickett TD, et al. Whole-genome sequencing identifies a recurrent functional synonymous mutation in melanoma. *Proc Natl Acad Sci U S A* 2013;110:13481–13486.
106. Stegh AH, Brennan C, Mahoney JA, et al. Glioma oncoprotein Bcl2L12 inhibits the p53 tumor suppressor. *Genes Dev* 2010;24:2194–2204.
107. Mullaney JM, Mills RE, Pittard WS, et al. Small insertions and deletions (INDELs) in human genomes. *Hum Mol Genet* 2010;19:R131–R136.
108. Tomlins SA, Rhodes DR, Perner S, et al. Recurrent fusion of TMPRSS2 and ETS transcription factor genes in prostate cancer. *Science* 2005;310:644–648.
109. Soda M, Choi YL, Enomoto M, et al. Identification of the transforming EML4-ALK fusion gene in non-small-cell lung cancer. *Nature* 2007;448:561–566.
110. Palanisamy N, Ateeq B, Kalyana-Sundaram S, et al. Rearrangements of the RAF kinase pathway in prostate cancer, gastric cancer and melanoma. *Nat Med* 2010;16:793–798.
111. Leary RJ, Kinde I, Diehl F, et al. Development of personalized tumor biomarkers using massively parallel sequencing. *Sci Transl Med* 2010;2:20ra14.
112. Maher CA, Kumar-Sinha C, Cao X, et al. Transcriptome sequencing to detect gene fusions in cancer. *Nature* 2009;458:97–101.
113. Stephens PJ, McBride DJ, Lin ML, et al. Complex landscapes of somatic rearrangement in human breast cancer genomes. *Nature* 2009;462:1005–1010.
114. Feng H, Shuda M, Chang Y, et al. Clonal integration of a polyomavirus in human Merkel cell carcinoma. *Science* 2008;319:1096–1100.
115. Herner A, Sauliunaite D, Michalski CW, et al. Glutamate increases pancreatic cancer cell invasion and migration via AMPA receptor activation and Kras-MAPK signaling. *Int J Cancer* 2011;129:2349–2359.
116. Wei X, Walia V, Lin JC, et al. Exome sequencing identifies GRIN2A as frequently mutated in melanoma. *Nat Genet* 2011;43:442–446.
117. Prickett TD, Wei X, Cardenas-Navia I, et al. Exon capture analysis of G protein-coupled receptors identifies activating mutations in GRM3 in melanoma. *Nat Genet* 2011;43:1119–1126.
118. Krauthammer M, Kong Y, Ha BH, et al. Exome sequencing identifies recurrent somatic RAC1 mutations in melanoma. *Nat Genet* 2012;44:1006–1014.
119. Davies H, Hunter C, Smith R, et al. Somatic mutations of the protein kinase gene family in human lung cancer. *Cancer Res* 2005;65:7591–7595.
120. Bozic I, Antal T, Ohtsuki H, et al. Accumulation of driver and passenger mutations during tumor progression. *Proc Natl Acad Sci U S A* 2010;107:18545–18550.
121. Parmigiani G, Boca S, Lin J, et al. Design and analysis issues in genome-wide somatic mutation studies of cancer. *Genomics* 2009;93:17–21.
122. Kaminker JS, Zhang Y, Waugh A, et al. Distinguishing cancer-associated missense mutations from common polymorphisms. *Cancer Res* 2007;67:465–473.
123. Futreal PA. Backseat drivers take the wheel. *Cancer Cell* 2007;12:493–494.
124. Greenman C, Wooster R, Futreal PA, et al. Statistical analysis of pathogenicity of somatic mutations in cancer. *Genetics* 2006;173:2187–2198.
125. Baudot A, Real FX, Izarzugaza JM, et al. From cancer genomes to cancer models: bridging the gaps. *EMBO Rep* 2009;10:359–366.
126. Carter H, Chen S, Isik L, et al. Cancer-specific high-throughput annotation of somatic mutations: computational prediction of driver missense mutations. *Cancer Res* 2009;69:6660–6667.
127. Ng PC, Henikoff S. SIFT: Predicting amino acid changes that affect protein function. *Nucleic Acids Res* 2003;31:3812–3814.
128. Kohli M, Rago C, Lengauer C, et al. Facile methods for generating human somatic cell gene knockouts using recombinant adeno-associated viruses. *Nucleic Acids Res* 2004;32:e3.
129. Downing JR, Wilson RK, Zhang J, et al. The Pediatric Cancer Genome Project. *Nat Genet* 2012;44:619–622.
130. Hudson TJ, Anderson W, Artez A, et al. International network of cancer genome projects. *Nature* 2010;464:993–998.
131. Bignell GR, Greenman CD, Davies H, et al. Signatures of mutation and selection in the cancer genome. *Nature* 2010;463:893–898.
132. Sieber OM, Tomlinson SR, Tomlinson IP. Tissue, cell and stage specificity of (epi)mutations in cancers. *Nat Rev Cancer* 2005;5:649–655.
133. Benvenuti S, Frattini M, Arena S, et al. PIK3CA cancer mutations display gender and tissue specificity patterns. *Hum Mutat* 2008;29:284–288.
134. Karakas B, Bachman KE, Park BH. Mutation of the PIK3CA oncogene in human cancers. *Br J Cancer* 2006;94:455–459.
135. Brennan CW, Werhaak RG, McKenna A, et al. The somatic genomic landscape of glioblastoma. *Cell* 2013;155:462–477.
136. Cancer Genome Atlas Network. Comprehensive molecular characterization of human colon and rectal cancer. *Nature* 2012;487:330–337.
137. Cancer Genome Atlas Network. Comprehensive molecular portraits of human breast tumours. *Nature* 2012;490:61–70.
138. Cancer Genome Atlas Research Network. Integrated genomic analyses of ovarian carcinoma. *Nature* 2011;474:609–615.
139. Cancer Genome Atlas Research Network. Comprehensive molecular characterization of clear cell renal cell carcinoma. *Nature* 2013;499:43–49.
140. Cancer Genome Atlas Research Network. Integrated genomic characterization of endometrial carcinoma. *Nature* 2013;497:67–73.
141. Weischenfeldt J, Simon R, Feuerbach L, et al. Integrative genomic analyses reveal an androgen-driven somatic alteration landscape in early-onset prostate cancer. *Cancer Cell* 2013;23:159–170.
142. Cancer Genome Atlas Research Network. Genomic and epigenomic landscapes of adult de novo acute myeloid leukemia. *N Engl J Med* 2013;368:2059–2074.
143. Dawson SJ, Rueda OM, Aparicio S, et al. A new genome-driven integrated classification of breast cancer and its implications. *EMBO J* 2013;32:617–628.
144. Plass C, Pfister SM, Lindroth AM, et al. Mutations in regulators of the epigenome and their connections to global chromatin patterns in cancer. *Nat Rev Genet* 2013;14:765–780.
145. Shen H, Laird PW. Interplay between the cancer genome and epigenome. *Cell* 2013;153:38–55.
146. Yamamoto E, Suzuki H, Yamano HO, et al. Molecular dissection of premalignant colorectal lesions reveals early onset of the CpG island methylator phenotype. *Am J Pathol* 2012;181:1847–1861.
147. Gao J, Aksoy BA, Dogrusoz U, et al. Integrative analysis of complex cancer genomics and clinical profiles using the cBioPortal. *Sci Signal* 2013;6:pl1.

148. Bleeker FE, Bardelli A. Genomic landscapes of cancers: prospects for targeted therapies. *Pharmacogenomics* 2007;8:1629–1633.
149. Paez JG, Jänne PA, Lee JC, et al. EGFR mutations in lung cancer: correlation with clinical response to gefitinib therapy. *Science* 2004;304:1497–1500.
150. Ciardiello F, Tortora G. EGFR antagonists in cancer treatment. *N Engl J Med* 2008;358:1160–1174.
151. Janku F, Stewart DJ, Kurzrock R. Targeted therapy in non-small-cell lung cancer—is it becoming a reality? *Nat Rev Clin Oncol* 2010;7:401–414.
152. Pao W, Chmielecki J. Rational, biologically based treatment of EGFR-mutant non-small-cell lung cancer. *Nat Rev Cancer* 2010;10:760–774.
153. Gerber DE, Minna JD. ALK inhibition for non-small cell lung cancer: from discovery to therapy in record time. *Cancer Cell* 2010;18:548–551.
154. Andreyev HJ, Norman AR, Cunningham D, et al. Kirsten ras mutations in patients with colorectal cancer: the multicenter "RASCAL" study. *J Natl Cancer Inst* 1998;90:675–684.
155. Roth AD, Tejpar S, Delorenzi M, et al. Prognostic role of KRAS and BRAF in stage II and III resected colon cancer: results of the translational study on the PETACC-3, EORTC 40993, SAKK 60-00 trial. *J Clin Oncol* 2010;28:466–474.
156. Bardelli A, Siena S. Molecular mechanisms of resistance to cetuximab and panitumumab in colorectal cancer. *J Clin Oncol* 2010;28:1254–1261.
157. Siena S, Sartore-Bianchi A, Di Nicolantonio F, et al. Biomarkers predicting clinical outcome of epidermal growth factor receptor-targeted therapy in metastatic colorectal cancer. *J Natl Cancer Inst* 2009;101:1308–1324.
158. Tejpar S, Bertagnolli M, Bosman F, et al. Prognostic and predictive biomarkers in resected colon cancer: current status and future perspectives for integrating genomics into biomarker discovery. *Oncologist* 2010;15:390–404.
159. Gerlinger M, Rowan AJ, Horswell S, et al. Intratumor heterogeneity and branched evolution revealed by multiregion sequencing. *N Engl J Med* 2012;366:883–892.
160. Mandel P, Metais P. [Not Available]. *C R Seances Soc Biol Fil* 1948;142: 241–243.
161. Crowley E, Di Nicolantonio F, Loupakis F, et al. Liquid biopsy: monitoring cancer-genetics in the blood. *Nat Rev Clin Oncol* 2013;10:472–484.
162. Diehl F, Li M, Dressman D, et al. Detection and quantification of mutations in the plasma of patients with colorectal tumors. *Proc Natl Acad Sci U S A* 2005;102:16368–16373.
163. Diehl F, Schmidt K, Choti MA, et al. Circulating mutant DNA to assess tumor dynamics. *Nat Med* 2008;14:985–990.
164. Frattini M, Gallino G, Signoroni S, et al. Quantitative and qualitative characterization of plasma DNA identifies primary and recurrent colorectal cancer. *Cancer Lett* 2008;263:170–181.
165. Chan KC, Jiang P, Zheng YW, et al. Cancer genome scanning in plasma: detection of tumor-associated copy number aberrations, single-nucleotide variants, and tumoral heterogeneity by massively parallel sequencing. *Clin Chem* 2013;59:211–224.
166. Murtaza M, Dawson SJ, Tsui DW, et al. Non-invasive analysis of acquired resistance to cancer therapy by sequencing of plasma DNA. *Nature* 2013;497: 108–112.
167. Bardelli A, Corso S, Bertotti A, et al. Amplification of the MET receptor drives resistance to anti-EGFR therapies in colorectal cancer. *Cancer Discov* 2013;3:658–673.
168. Higgins MJ, Jelovac D, Barnathan E, et al. Detection of tumor PIK3CA status in metastatic breast cancer using peripheral blood. *Clin Cancer Res* 2012;18:3462–3469.
169. Leary RJ, Sausen M, Kinde I, et al. Detection of chromosomal alterations in the circulation of cancer patients with whole-genome sequencing. *Sci Transl Med* 2012;4:162ra154.
170. Misale S, Yaeger R, Hobor S, et al. Emergence of KRAS mutations and acquired resistance to anti-EGFR therapy in colorectal cancer. *Nature* 2012;486:532–536.
171. Diaz LA Jr, Williams RT, Wu J, et al. The molecular evolution of acquired resistance to targeted EGFR blockade in colorectal cancers. *Nature* 2012;486:537–540.
172. Robbins PF, Lu YC, El-Gamil M, et al. Mining exomic sequencing data to identify mutated antigens recognized by adoptively transferred tumor-reactive T cells. *Nat Med* 2013;19:747–752.
173. Hunter C, Smith R, Cahill DP, et al. A hypermutation phenotype and somatic MSH6 mutations in recurrent human malignant gliomas after alkylator chemotherapy. *Cancer Res* 2006;66:3987–3991.
174. Cahill DP, Levine KK, Betensky RA, et al. Loss of the mismatch repair protein MSH6 in human glioblastomas is associated with tumor progression during temozolomide treatment. *Clin Cancer Res* 2007;13:2038–2045.
175. Engelman JA, Zejnullahu K, Mitsudomi T, et al. MET amplification leads to gefitinib resistance in lung cancer by activating ERBB3 signaling. *Science* 2007;316:1039–1043.
176. Gorre ME, Mohmmed M, Ellwood K, et al. Clinical resistance to STI-571 cancer therapy caused by BCR-ABL gene mutation or amplification. *Science* 2001;293:876–880.
177. Heinrich MC, Corless CL, Blanke CD, et al. Molecular correlates of imatinib resistance in gastrointestinal stromal tumors. *J Clin Oncol* 2006;24:4764–4774.
178. Shepherd FA, Rodrigues Pereira J, Ciuleanu T, et al. Erlotinib in previously treated non-small-cell lung cancer. *N Engl J Med* 2005;353:123–132.
179. Kobayashi S, Boggon TJ, Dayaram T, et al. EGFR mutation and resistance of non-small-cell lung cancer to gefitinib. *N Engl J Med* 2005;352:786–792.
180. Kwak EL, Sordella R, Bell DW, et al. Irreversible inhibitors of the EGF receptor may circumvent acquired resistance to gefitinib. *Proc Natl Acad Sci U S A* 2005;102:7665–7670.
181. Pao W, Miller VA, Politi KA, et al. Acquired resistance of lung adenocarcinomas to gefitinib or erlotinib is associated with a second mutation in the EGFR kinase domain. *PLoS Med* 2005;2:e73.
182. Shih JY, Gow CH, Yang PC. EGFR mutation conferring primary resistance to gefitinib in non-small-cell lung cancer. *N Engl J Med* 2005;353:207–208.
183. Bell DW, Gore I, Okimoto Ra, et al. Inherited susceptibility to lung cancer may be associated with the T790M drug resistance mutation in EGFR. *Nat Genet* 2005;37:1315–1316.
184. Inukai M, Toyooka S, Ito S, et al. Presence of epidermal growth factor receptor gene T790M mutation as a minor clone in non-small cell lung cancer. *Cancer Res* 2006;66:7854–7858.
185. Daub H, Specht K, Ullrich A. Strategies to overcome resistance to targeted protein kinase inhibitors. *Nat Rev Drug Discov* 2004;3:1001–1010.
186. Choi YL, Soda M, Yamashita Y, et al. EML4-ALK mutations in lung cancer that confer resistance to ALK inhibitors. *N Engl J Med* 2010;363:1734–1739.
187. Flaherty KT, Puzanov I, Kim KB, et al. Inhibition of mutated, activated BRAF in metastatic melanoma. *N Engl J Med* 2010;363:809–819.
188. Nazarian R, Shi H, Wang Q, et al. Melanomas acquire resistance to B-RAF(V600E) inhibition by RTK or N-RAS upregulation. *Nature* 2010;468:973–977.
189. Pompetti F, Spadano A, Sau A, et al. Long-term remission in BCR/ABL-positive AML-M6 patient treated with Imatinib Mesylate. *Leuk Res* 2007;31:563–567.
190. Druker BJ, Builhot F, O'Brien SG, et al. Five-year follow-up of patients receiving imatinib for chronic myeloid leukemia. *N Engl J Med* 2006;355:2408–2417.

2 Hallmarks of Cancer: An Organizing Principle for Cancer Medicine

Douglas Hanahan and Robert A. Weinberg

INTRODUCTION

The hallmarks of cancer comprise eight biologic capabilities acquired by incipient cancer cells during the multistep development of human tumors. The hallmarks constitute an organizing principle for rationalizing the complexities of neoplastic disease. They include sustaining proliferative signaling, evading growth suppressors, resisting cell death, enabling replicative immortality, inducing angiogenesis, activating invasion and metastasis, reprogramming energy metabolism, and evading immune destruction. Facilitating the acquisition of these hallmark capabilities are genome instability, which enables mutational alteration of hallmark-enabling genes, and immune inflammation, which fosters the acquisition of multiple hallmark functions. In addition to cancer cells, tumors exhibit another dimension of complexity: They contain a repertoire of recruited, ostensibly normal cells that contribute to the acquisition of hallmark traits by creating the *tumor microenvironment*. Recognition of the widespread applicability of these concepts will increasingly influence the development of new means to treat human cancer.

At the beginning of the new millennium, we proposed that six *hallmarks of cancer* embody an organizing principle that provides a logical framework for understanding the remarkable diversity of neoplastic diseases.[1] Implicit in our discussion was the notion that, as normal cells evolve progressively to a neoplastic state, they acquire a succession of these hallmark capabilities, and that the multistep process of human tumor pathogenesis can be rationalized by the need of incipient cancer cells to acquire the diverse traits that in aggregate enable them to become tumorigenic and, ultimately, malignant.

We noted as an ancillary proposition that tumors are more than insular masses of proliferating cancer cells. Instead, they are complex tissues composed of multiple distinct types of neoplastic and normal cells that participate in heterotypic interactions with one another. We depicted the recruited normal cells, which form tumor-associated stroma, as active participants in tumorigenesis rather than passive bystanders; as such, these stromal cells contribute to the development and expression of certain hallmark capabilities. This notion has been solidified and extended during the intervening period, and it is now clear that the biology of tumors can no longer be understood simply by enumerating the traits of the cancer cells, but instead must encompass the contributions of the *tumor microenvironment* to tumorigenesis. In 2011, we revisited the original hallmarks, adding two new ones to the roster, and expanded on the functional roles and contributions made by recruited stromal cells to tumor biology.[2] Herein we reiterate and further refine the hallmarks-of-cancer perspectives we presented in 2000 and 2011, with the goal of informing students of cancer medicine about the concept and its potential utility for understanding the pathogenesis of human cancer, and the potential relevance of this concept to the development of more effective treatments for this disease.

HALLMARK CAPABILITIES, IN ESSENCE

The eight hallmarks of cancer—distinct and complementary capabilities that enable tumor growth and metastatic dissemination—continue to provide a solid foundation for understanding the biology of cancer (Fig. 2.1). The sections that follow summarize the essence of each hallmark, providing insights into their regulation and functional manifestations.

Sustaining Proliferative Signaling

Arguably, the most fundamental trait of cancer cells involves their ability to sustain chronic proliferation. Normal tissues carefully control the production and release of growth-promoting signals that instruct entry of cells into and progression through the growth-and-division cycle, thereby ensuring proper control of cell number and thus maintenance of normal tissue architecture and function. Cancer cells, by deregulating these signals, become masters of their own destinies. The enabling signals are conveyed in large part by growth factors that bind cell-surface receptors, typically containing intracellular tyrosine kinase domains. The latter proceed to emit signals via branched intracellular signaling pathways that regulate progression through the cell cycle as well as cell growth (that is, increase in cell size); often, these signals influence yet other cell-biologic properties, such as cell survival and energy metabolism.

Remarkably, the precise identities and sources of the proliferative signals operating within normal tissues remain poorly understood. Moreover, we still know relatively little about the mechanisms controlling the release of these mitogenic signals. In part, the study of these mechanisms is complicated by the fact that the growth factor signals controlling cell number and position within normal tissues are thought to be transmitted in a temporally and spatially regulated fashion from one cell to its neighbors; such paracrine signaling is difficult to access experimentally. In addition, the bioavailability of growth factors is regulated by their sequestration in the pericellular space and associated extracellular matrix. Moreover, the actions of these extracellular mitogenic proteins is further controlled by a complex network of proteases, sulfatases, and possibly other enzymes that liberate and activate these factors, apparently in a highly specific and localized fashion.

The mitogenic signaling operating in cancer cells is, in contrast, far better understood.[3–6] Cancer cells can acquire the capability to sustain proliferative signaling in a number of alternative ways: They may produce growth factor ligands themselves, to which they can then respond via the coexpression of cognate receptors, resulting in autocrine proliferative stimulation. Alternatively, cancer cells may send signals to stimulate normal cells within the supporting tumor-associated stroma; the stromal cells then reciprocate by supplying the cancer cells with various growth factors.[7,8] Mitogenic signaling can also be deregulated by elevating the levels of receptor proteins displayed at the cancer cell

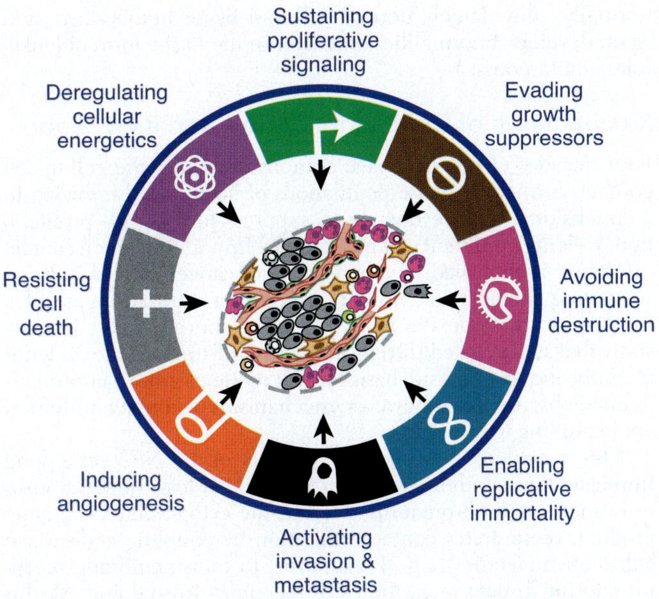

Figure 2.1 The hallmarks of cancer. Eight functional capabilities—the hallmarks of cancer—are thought to be acquired by developing cancers in the course of the multistep carcinogenesis that leads to most forms of human cancer. The order in which these hallmark capabilities are acquired and the relative balance and importance of their contributions to malignant disease appears to vary across the spectrum of human cancers. (Adapted from Hanahan D, Weinberg R. The hallmarks of cancer. *Cell* 2000;100:57–70; Hanahan D, Weinberg RA. Hallmarks of cancer: the next generation. *Cell* 2011;144:646–674.)

surface, rendering such cells hyperresponsive to otherwise limiting amounts of growth factor ligands; the same outcome can result from structural alterations in the receptor molecules that facilitate ligand-independent firing.

Independence from externally supplied growth factors may also derive from the constitutive activation of components of intracellular signaling cascades operating downstream of these receptors within cancer cells. These intracellular alterations obviate the need to stimulate cell proliferation pathways by ligand-mediated activation of cell-surface receptors. Of note, because a number of distinct downstream signaling pathways radiate from ligand-stimulated receptors, the activation of one or another of these downstream branches (e.g., the pathway responding to the Ras signal transducer) may only provide a subset of the regulatory instructions transmitted by a ligand-activated receptor.

Somatic Mutations Activate Additional Downstream Pathways

DNA sequencing analyses of cancer cell genomes have revealed somatic mutations in certain human tumors that predict constitutive activation of the signaling circuits, cited previously, that are normally triggered by activated growth factor receptors. The past 3 decades have witnessed the identification in tens of thousands of human tumors of mutant, oncogenic alleles of the *RAS* proto-oncogenes, most of which have sustained point mutations in the 12th codon, which results in RAS proteins that are constitutively active in downstream signaling. Thus, more than 90% of pancreatic adenocarcinomas carry mutant K-*RAS* alleles. More recently, the repertoire of frequently mutated genes has been expanded to include those encoding the downstream effectors of the RAS proteins. For example, we now know that ~40% of human melanomas contain activating mutations affecting the structure of the B-RAF protein, resulting in constitutive signaling through the RAF to the mitogen-activated protein (MAP)–kinase pathway.[9] Similarly, mutations in the catalytic subunit of phosphoinositide 3-kinase (PI3K) isoforms are being detected in an array of tumor types; these mutations typically serve to hyperactivate the PI3K signaling pathway, causing in turn, excess signaling through the crucial Akt/PKB signal transducer.[10,11] The advantages to tumor cells of activating upstream (receptor) versus downstream (transducer) signaling remain obscure, as does the functional impact of cross-talk between the multiple branched pathways radiating from individual growth factor receptors.

Disruptions of Negative-Feedback Mechanisms that Attenuate Proliferative Signaling

Recent observations have also highlighted the importance of negative-feedback loops that normally operate to dampen various types of signaling and thereby ensure homeostatic regulation of the flux of signals coursing through the intracellular circuitry.[12–15] Defects in these negative-feedback mechanisms are capable of enhancing proliferative signaling. The prototype of this type of regulation involves the RAS oncoprotein. The oncogenic effects of mutant RAS proteins do not result from a hyperactivation of its downstream signaling powers; instead, the oncogenic mutations affecting *RAS* genes impair the intrinsic GTPase activity of RAS that normally serves to turn its activity off, ensuring that active signal transmission (e.g., from upstream growth factor receptors) is transient; as such, oncogenic RAS mutations disrupt an autoregulatory negative-feedback mechanism, without which RAS generates chronic proliferative signals.

Analogous negative-feedback mechanisms operate at multiple nodes within the proliferative signaling circuitry. A prominent example involves phosphatase and tensin homolog (PTEN), which counteracts PI3K by degrading its product, phosphatidylinositol 3,4,5-phosphate (PIP_3). Loss-of-function mutations in PTEN amplify PI3K signaling and promote tumorigenesis in a variety of experimental models of cancer; in human tumors, PTEN expression is often lost by the methylation of DNA at specific sites associated with the promoter of the *PTEN* gene, resulting in the shutdown of its transcription.[10,11]

Yet another example involves the mammalian target of rapamycin (mTOR) kinase, a key coordinator of cell growth and metabolism that lies both upstream and downstream of the PI3K pathway. In the circuitry of some cancer cells, mTOR activation results, via negative feedback, in the inhibition of PI3K signaling. Accordingly, when mTOR is pharmacologically inhibited in such cancer cells (e.g., by the drug rapamycin), the associated loss of negative feedback results in increased activity of PI3K and its effector, the Akt/PKB kinase, thereby blunting the antiproliferative effects of mTOR inhibition.[16,17] It is likely that compromised negative feedback loops in this and other signaling pathways will prove to be widespread among human cancer cells, serving as important means by which cancer cells acquire the capability of signaling chronically through these pathways. Moreover, disruption of such normally self-attenuating signaling can contribute to the development of adaptive resistance toward therapeutic drugs targeting mitogenic signaling.

Excessive Proliferative Signaling Can Trigger Cell Senescence

Early studies of oncogene action encouraged the notion that ever-increasing expression of such genes and the signals released by their protein products would result in proportionately increased cancer cell proliferation and, thus, tumor growth. More recent research has undermined this notion, in that it is now apparent that excessively elevated signaling by oncoproteins, such as RAS, MYC, and RAF, can provoke counteracting (protective) responses from cells, such as induction of cell death; alternatively, cancer cells expressing high levels of these oncoproteins may be forced to enter into the nonproliferative but viable state called senescence. These responses contrast with those seen in cells expressing lower levels of these proteins, which permit cells to avoid senescence or cell death and, thus, proliferate.[18–21]

Cells with morphologic features of senescence, including enlarged cytoplasm, the absence of proliferation markers, and the expression of the senescence-induced β-galactosidase enzyme, are abundant in the tissues of mice whose genomes have been reengineered to cause overexpression of certain oncogenes[19,20]; such senescent cells are also prevalent in some cases of human melanoma.[22]

These ostensibly paradoxical responses seem to reflect intrinsic cellular defense mechanisms designed to eliminate cells experiencing excessive levels of certain types of mitogenic signaling. Accordingly, the intensity of oncogenic signaling observed in naturally arising cancer cells may represent compromises between maximal mitogenic stimulation and avoidance of these anti-proliferative defenses. Alternatively, some cancer cells may adapt to high levels of oncogenic signaling by disabling their senescence- or apoptosis-inducing circuitry.

Evading Growth Suppressors

In addition to the hallmark capability of inducing and sustaining positively acting growth-stimulatory signals, cancer cells must also circumvent powerful programs that negatively regulate cell proliferation; many of these programs depend on the actions of tumor suppressor genes. Dozens of tumor suppressors that operate in various ways to limit cell proliferation or survival have been discovered through their inactivation in one or another form of animal or human cancer; many of these genes have been validated as bona fide tumor suppressors through gain- or loss-of-function experiments in mice. The two prototypical tumor suppressor genes encode the retinoblastoma (RB)-associated and TP53 proteins; they operate as central control nodes within two key, complementary cellular regulatory circuits that govern the decisions of cells to proliferate, or alternatively, to activate growth arrest, senescence, or the cell-suicide program known as apoptosis.

The RB protein integrates signals from diverse extracellular and intracellular sources and, in response, decides whether or not a cell should proceed through its growth-and-division cycle.[23–25] Cancer cells with defects in the RB pathway function are thus missing the services of a critical gatekeeper of cell-cycle progression whose absence permits persistent cell proliferation. Whereas RB transduces growth-inhibitory signals that largely originate outside of the cell, TP53 receives inputs from stress and abnormality sensors that function within the cell's intracellular operating systems. For example, if the degree of damage to a cell's genome is excessive, or if the levels of nucleotide pools, growth-promoting signals, glucose, or oxygenation are insufficient, TP53 can call a halt to further cell-cycle progression until these conditions have been normalized. Alternatively, in the face of alarm signals indicating overwhelming or irreparable damage to such cellular systems, TP53 can trigger apoptosis. Of note, the alternative effects of activated TP53 are complex and highly context dependent, varying by cell type as well as by the severity and persistence of conditions of cell-physiologic stress and genomic damage.

Although the two canonical suppressors of proliferation—TP53 and RB—have preeminent importance in regulating cell proliferation, various lines of evidence indicate that each operates as part of a larger network that is wired for functional redundancy. For example, chimeric mice populated throughout their bodies with individual cells lacking a functional *Rb* gene are surprisingly free of proliferative abnormalities, despite the expectation that a loss of RB function should result in unimpeded advance through the cell division cycle by these cells and their lineal descendants; some of the resulting clusters of *Rb*-null cells should, by all rights, progress to neoplasia. Instead, the *Rb*-null cells in such chimeric mice have been found to participate in relatively normal tissue morphogenesis throughout the body; the only neoplasia observed is of pituitary tumors developing late in life.[26] Similarly, *TP53*-null mice develop normally, show largely normal cell and tissue homeostasis, and again develop abnormalities only later in life in the form of leukemias and sarcomas.[27]

Mechanisms of Contact Inhibition and Its Evasion

Four decades of research have demonstrated that the cell-to-cell contacts formed by dense populations of normal cells growing in 2-dimensional culture operate to suppress further cell proliferation, yielding confluent cell monolayers. Importantly, such *contact inhibition* is abolished in various types of cancer cells in culture, suggesting that contact inhibition is an in vitro surrogate of a mechanism that operates in vivo to ensure normal tissue homeostasis that is abrogated during the course of tumorigenesis. Until recently, the mechanistic basis for this mode of growth control remained obscure. Now, however, mechanisms of contact inhibition are beginning to emerge.[28]

One mechanism involves the product of the *NF2* gene, long implicated as a tumor suppressor because its loss triggers a form of human neurofibromatosis. Merlin, the cytoplasmic *NF2* gene product, orchestrates contact inhibition by coupling cell-surface adhesion molecules (e.g., E-cadherin) to transmembrane receptor tyrosine kinases (e.g., the EGF receptor). In so doing, Merlin strengthens the adhesiveness of cadherin-mediated cell-to-cell attachments. Additionally, by sequestering such growth factor receptors, Merlin limits their ability to efficiently emit mitogenic signals.[28–31]

Corruption of the TGF-β Pathway Promotes Malignancy

Transforming growth factor beta (TGF-β is best known for its antiproliferative effects on epithelial cells. The responses of carcinoma cells to TGF-β's proliferation–suppressive effects is now appreciated to be far more elaborate than a simple shutdown of its signaling circuitry.[32–35] In normal cells, exposure to TGF-β blocks their progression through the G1 phase of the cell cycle. In many late-stage tumors, however, TGF-β signaling is redirected away from suppressing cell proliferation and is found instead to activate a cellular program, termed the epithelial-to-mesenchymal transition (EMT), which confers on cancer cells multiple traits associated with high-grade malignancy, as will be discussed in further detail.

Resisting Cell Death

The ability to activate the normally latent apoptotic cell-death program appears to be associated with most types of normal cells throughout the body. Its actions in many if not all multicellular organisms seems to reflect the need to eliminate aberrant cells whose continued presence would otherwise threaten organismic integrity. This rationale explains why cancer cells often, if not invariably, inactivate or attenuate this program during their development.[21,36–38]

Elucidation of the detailed design of the signaling circuitry governing the apoptotic program has revealed how apoptosis is triggered in response to various physiologic stresses that cancer cells experience either during the course of tumorigenesis or as a result of anticancer therapy. Notable among the apoptosis-inducing stresses are signaling imbalances resulting from elevated levels of oncogene signaling and from DNA damage. The regulators of the apoptotic response are divided into two major circuits, one receiving and processing extracellular death-inducing signals (the extrinsic apoptotic program, involving for example the Fas ligand/Fas receptor), and the other sensing and integrating a variety of signals of intracellular origin (the intrinsic program). Each of these circuits culminates in the activation of a normally latent protease (caspase 8 or 9, respectively), which proceeds to initiate a cascade of proteolysis involving effector caspases that are responsible for the execution phase of apoptosis. During this final phase, an apoptotic cell is progressively disassembled and then consumed, both by its neighbors and by professional phagocytic cells. Currently, the intrinsic apoptotic program is more widely implicated as a barrier to cancer pathogenesis.

The molecular machinery that conveys signals between the apoptotic regulators and effectors is controlled by counterbalancing pro- and antiapoptotic members of the Bcl-2 family of regulatory proteins.[36,37] The archetype, Bcl-2, along with its closest relatives (Bcl-XL, Bcl-W, Mcl-1, A1) are inhibitors of apoptosis, acting in large part by binding to and thereby suppressing two proapoptotic triggering proteins (Bax and Bak); the latter are embedded in the mitochondrial outer membrane. When relieved of inhibition by their antiapoptotic relatives, Bax and Bax disrupt the integrity of the outer mitochondrial membrane, causing the release into the cytosol of proapoptotic signaling proteins, the most important of which is cytochrome C. When the normally sequestered cytochrome C is released, it activates a cascade of cytosolic caspase proteases that proceed to fragment multiple cellular structures, thereby executing the apoptotic death program.[37,39]

Several abnormality sensors have been identified that play key roles in triggering apoptosis.[21,37] Most notable is a DNA damage sensor that acts through the TP53 tumor suppressor[40]; TP53 induces apoptosis by upregulating expression of the proapoptotic, Bcl-2-related Noxa and Puma proteins, doing so in response to substantial levels of DNA breaks and other chromosomal abnormalities. Alternatively, insufficient survival factor signaling (e.g., inadequate levels of interleukin (IL)-3 in lymphocytes or of insulinlike growth factors 1/2 [IGF1/2] in epithelial cells) can elicit apoptosis through another proapoptotic Bcl-2–related protein called Bim. Yet another condition triggering apoptosis involves hyperactive signaling by certain oncoproteins, such as Myc, which acts in part via Bim and other Bcl-2–related proteins.[18,21,40]

Tumor cells evolve a variety of strategies to limit or circumvent apoptosis. Most common is the loss of TP53 tumor suppressor function, which eliminates this critical damage sensor from the apoptosis-inducing circuitry. Alternatively, tumors may achieve similar ends by increasing the expression of antiapoptotic regulators (Bcl-2, Bcl-XL) or of survival signals (IGF1/2), by downregulating proapoptotic Bcl-2–related factors (Bax, Bim, Puma), or by short-circuiting the extrinsic ligand-induced death pathway. The multiplicity of apoptosis-avoiding mechanisms presumably reflects the diversity of apoptosis-inducing signals that cancer cell populations encounter during their evolution from the normal to the neoplastic state.

Autophagy Mediates Both Tumor Cell Survival and Death

Autophagy represents an important cell-physiologic response that, like apoptosis, normally operates at low, basal levels in cells but can be strongly induced in certain states of cellular stress, the most obvious of which is nutrient deficiency.[41–43] The autophagic program enables cells to break down cellular organelles, such as ribosomes and mitochondria, allowing the resulting catabolites to be recycled and thus used for biosynthesis and energy metabolism. As part of this program, intracellular vesicles (termed autophagosomes) envelope the cellular organelles destined for degradation; the resulting vesicles then fuse with lysosomes in which degradation occurs. In this fashion, low–molecular-weight metabolites are generated that support survival in the stressed, nutrient-limited environments experienced by many cancer cells. When acting in this fashion, autophagy favors cancer cell survival.

However, the autophagy program intersects in more complex ways with the life and death of cancer cells. Like apoptosis, the autophagy machinery has both regulatory and effector components.[41–43] Among the latter are proteins that mediate autophagosome formation and delivery to lysosomes. Of note, recent research has revealed intersections between the regulatory circuits governing autophagy, apoptosis, and cellular homeostasis. For example, the signaling pathway involving PI3K, AKT, and mTOR, which is stimulated by survival signals to block apoptosis, similarly inhibits autophagy; when survival signals are insufficient, the PI3K signaling pathway is downregulated, with the result that autophagy and/or apoptosis may be induced.[41,42,44,45]

Another interconnection between these two programs resides in the Beclin-1 protein, which has been shown by genetic studies to be necessary for the induction of autophagy.[41–44] Beclin-1 is a member of the Bcl-2 family of apoptotic regulatory proteins, and its BH3 domain allows it to bind the Bcl-2/Bcl-XL proteins. Stress sensor–coupled BH3-containing proteins (e.g. Bim, Noxa) can displace Beclin-1 from its association with Bcl-2/Bcl-XL, enabling the liberated Beclin-1 to trigger autophagy, much as they can release proapoptotic Bax and Bak to trigger apoptosis. Hence, stress-transducing Bcl-2–related proteins can induce apoptosis and/or autophagy depending on the physiologic state of the cell.

Genetically altered mice bearing inactivated alleles of the *Beclin-1* gene or of certain other components of the autophagy machinery exhibit increased susceptibility to cancer.[42,46] These results suggest that the induction of autophagy can serve as a barrier to tumorigenesis that may operate independently of or in concert with apoptosis. For example, excessive activation of the autophagy program may cause cells to devour too many of their own critical organelles, such that cell growth and division are crippled. Accordingly, autophagy may represent yet another barrier that needs to be circumvented by incipient cancer cells during multistep tumor development.[41,46]

Perhaps paradoxically, nutrient starvation, radiotherapy, and certain cytotoxic drugs can induce elevated levels of autophagy that apparently protect cancer cells.[45–48] Moreover, severely stressed cancer cells have been shown to shrink via autophagy to a state of reversible dormancy.[46,49] This particular survival response may enable the persistence and eventual regrowth of some late-stage tumors following treatment with potent anticancer agents. Together, observations like these indicate that autophagy can have dichotomous effects on tumor cells and, thus, tumor progression.[46,47] An important agenda for future research will involve clarifying the genetic and cell-physiologic conditions that determine when and how autophagy enables cancer cells to survive or, alternatively, causes them to die.

Necrosis Has Proinflammatory and Tumor-Promoting Potential

In contrast to apoptosis, in which a dying cell contracts into an almost invisible corpse that is soon consumed by its neighbors, necrotic cells become bloated and explode, releasing their contents into the local tissue microenvironment. A body of evidence has shown that cell death by necrosis, like apoptosis, is an organized process under genetic control, rather than being a random and undirected process.[50–52]

Importantly, necrotic cell death releases proinflammatory signals into the surrounding tissue microenvironment, in contrast to apoptosis, which does not. As a consequence, necrotic cells can recruit inflammatory cells of the immune system,[51,53,54] whose dedicated function is to survey the extent of tissue damage and remove associated necrotic debris. In the context of neoplasia, however, multiple lines of evidence indicate that immune inflammatory cells can be actively tumor-promoting by fostering angiogenesis, cancer cell proliferation, and invasiveness (discussed in subsequent sections). Additionally, necrotic cells can release bioactive regulatory factors, such as IL1α, which can directly stimulate neighboring viable cells to proliferate, with the potential, once again, to facilitate neoplastic progression.[53] Consequently, necrotic cell death, while seemingly beneficial in counterbalancing cancer-associated hyperproliferation, may ultimately do more damage to the patient than good.

Enabling Replicative Immortality

Cancer cells require unlimited replicative potential in order to generate macroscopic tumors. This capability stands in marked contrast to the behavior of the cells in most normal cell lineages in the body, which are only able to pass through a limited number of successive cell growth-and-division cycles. This limitation has been associated with two distinct barriers to proliferation: *replicative senescence*, a typically irreversible entrance into a nonproliferative but viable state, and *crisis*, which involves cell death. Accordingly, when cells are propagated in culture, repeated cycles of cell division lead first to induction of replicative senescence and then, for those cells that succeed in circumventing this barrier, to the crisis phase, in which the great majority of cells in the population die. On rare occasion, cells emerge from a population in crisis and exhibit unlimited replicative potential. This transition has been termed immortalization, a trait that most established cell lines possess by virtue of their ability to proliferate in culture without evidence of either senescence or crisis.

Multiple lines of evidence indicate that telomeres protecting the ends of chromosomes are centrally involved in the capability for unlimited proliferation.[55–58] The telomere-associated DNA, composed of multiple tandem hexanucleotide repeats, shortens progressively in the chromosomes of nonimmortalized cells propagated in culture, eventually losing the ability to protect the ends of chromosomal DNA from end-to-end fusions; such aberrant fusions generate unstable dicentric chromosomes, whose resolution during the anaphase of mitosis results in a scrambling of karyotype and entrance into crisis that threatens cell viability. Accordingly, the length of telomeric DNA in a cell dictates how many successive cell generations its progeny can pass through before telomeres are largely eroded and have consequently lost their protective functions.

Telomerase, the specialized DNA polymerase that adds telomere repeat segments to the ends of telomeric DNA, is almost absent in nonimmortalized cells but is expressed at functionally significant levels in the great majority (~90%) of spontaneously immortalized cells, including human cancer cells. By extending telomeric DNA, telomerase is able to counter the progressive telomere erosion that would otherwise occur in its absence. The presence of telomerase activity, either in spontaneously immortalized cells or in the context of cells engineered to express the enzyme, is correlated with a resistance to induction of both senescence and crisis/apoptosis; conversely, the suppression of telomerase activity leads to telomere shortening and to activation of one or the other of these proliferative barriers.

The two barriers to proliferation—replicative senescence and crisis/apoptosis—have been rationalized as crucial anticancer defenses that are hardwired into our cells and are deployed to impede the outgrowth of clones of preneoplastic and, frankly, neoplastic cells. According to this thinking, most incipient neoplasias exhaust their endowment of replicative doublings and are stopped in their tracks by either of these barriers. The eventual immortalization of rare variant cells that proceed to form tumors has been attributed to their ability to maintain telomeric DNA at lengths sufficient to avoid triggering either senescence or apoptosis, which is achieved most commonly by upregulating the expression of telomerase or, less frequently, via an alternative recombination-based (ALT) telomere maintenance mechanism.[59] Hence, telomere shortening has come to be viewed as a clocking device that determines the limited replicative potential of normal cells and, thus, one that must be overcome by cancer cells.

Reassessing Replicative Senescence

The senescent state induced by oncogenes, as described previously, is remarkably similar to that induced when cells are explanted from living tissue and introduced into culture, the latter being the replicative senescence just discussed. Importantly, the concept of replication-induced senescence as a general barrier requires refinement and reformulation. Recent experiments have revealed that the induction of senescence in certain cultured cells can be delayed and possibly eliminated by the use of improved cell culture conditions, suggesting that recently explanted primary cells may be intrinsically able to proliferate unimpeded in culture up the point of crisis and the associated induction of apoptosis triggered by critically shortened telomeres.[60–63] This result indicates that telomere shortening does not necessarily induce senescence prior to crisis. Additional insight comes from experiments in mice engineered to lack telomerase; this work has revealed that shortening telomeres can shunt premalignant cells into a senescent state that contributes (along with apoptosis) to attenuated tumorigenesis in mice genetically destined to develop particular forms of cancer.[58] Such telomerase-null mice with highly eroded telomeres exhibit multiorgan dysfunction and abnormalities that provide evidence of both senescence and apoptosis, perhaps similar to the senescence and apoptosis observed in cell culture.[58,64] Thus, depending on the cellular context, the proliferative barrier of telomere shortening can be manifested by the induction of senescence and/or apoptosis.

Delayed Activation of Telomerase May Both Limit and Foster Neoplastic Progression

There is now evidence that clones of incipient cancer cells in spontaneously arising tumors experience telomere loss-induced crisis relatively early during the course of multistep tumor progression due to their inability to express significant levels of telomerase. Thus, extensively eroded telomeres have been documented in premalignant growths through the use of fluorescence in situ hybridization (FISH), which has also revealed the end-to-end chromosomal fusions that signal telomere failure and crisis.[65,66] These results suggest that such incipient cancer cells have passed through a substantial number of successive telomere-shortening cell divisions during their evolution from fully normal cells of origin. Accordingly, the development of some human neoplasias may be aborted by telomere-induced crisis long before they have progressed to become macroscopic, frankly neoplastic growths.

A quite different situation is observed in cells that have lost the TP53-mediated surveillance of genomic integrity and, thereafter, experience critically eroded telomeres. The loss of the TP53 DNA damage sensor can enable such cells to avoid apoptosis that would otherwise be triggered by the DNA damage resulting from dysfunctional telomeres. Instead, such cells lacking TP53 continue to divide, suffering repeated cycles of interchromosomal fusion and subsequent breakage at mitosis. Such breakage-fusion-bridge (BFB) cycles result in deletions and amplifications of chromosomal segments, evidently serving to mutagenize the genome, thereby facilitating the generation and subsequent clonal selection of cancer cells that have acquired mutant oncogenes and tumor suppressor genes.[58,67] One infers, however, that the clones of cancer cells that survive this telomere collapse must eventually acquire the ability to stabilize and thus protect their telomeres via the activation of telomerase or the ALT mechanism noted previously.

These considerations present an interesting dichotomy: Although dysfunctional telomeres are an evident barrier to chronic proliferation, they can also facilitate the genomic instability that generates hallmark-enabling mutations, as will be discussed further. Both mechanisms may be at play in certain forms of carcinogenesis in the form of transitory telomere deficiency prior to telomere stabilization. Circumstantial support for this concept of transient telomere deficiency in facilitating malignant progression has come from comparative analyses of premalignant and malignant lesions in the human breast.[68,69] The premalignant lesions did not express significant levels of telomerase and were marked by telomere shortening and chromosomal aberrations. In contrast, overt carcinomas exhibited telomerase expression concordantly with the reconstruction of longer telomeres and the fixation of the aberrant karyotypes that would seem to have been acquired after telomere failure but before the acquisition of telomerase activity. When portrayed in this way, the delayed acquisition of telomerase function serves to generate tumor-promoting mutations, whereas its subsequent expression stabilizes the mutant genome and confers the unlimited replicative capacity that cancer cells require in order to generate clinically apparent tumors.

Inducing Angiogenesis

Like normal tissues, tumors require sustenance in the form of nutrients and oxygen as well as an ability to evacuate metabolic wastes and carbon dioxide. The tumor-associated neovasculature, generated by the process of angiogenesis, addresses these needs. During embryogenesis, the development of the vasculature involves the birth of new endothelial cells and their assembly into tubes (vasculogenesis) in addition to the sprouting (angiogenesis) of new vessels from existing ones. Following this morphogenesis, the normal vasculature becomes largely quiescent. In the adult, as part of physiologic processes such as wound healing and female reproductive cycling, angiogenesis is turned on, but only transiently. In contrast, during tumor progression, an *angiogenic switch* is almost always activated and remains on, causing normally quiescent vasculature to continually sprout new vessels that help sustain expanding neoplastic growths.[70]

A compelling body of evidence indicates that the angiogenic switch is governed by countervailing factors that either induce or oppose angiogenesis.[71,72] Some of these angiogenic regulators are signaling proteins that bind to stimulatory or inhibitory cell-surface receptors displayed by vascular endothelial cells. The well-known prototypes of angiogenesis inducers and inhibitors are vascular endothelial growth factor-A (VEGF-A) and thrombospondin-1 (Tsp-1), respectively.

The VEGF-A gene encodes ligands that are involved in orchestrating new blood vessel growth during embryonic and postnatal development, in the survival of endothelial cells in already-formed vessels, and in certain physiologic and pathologic situations in the adult. VEGF signaling via three receptor tyrosine kinases (VEGFR1–3) is regulated at multiple levels, reflecting this complexity of purpose. VEGF gene expression can be upregulated both by hypoxia and by oncogene signaling.[73–75] Additionally, VEGF ligands can be sequestered in the extracellular matrix in latent forms that are subject to release and activation by extracellular matrix-degrading proteases (e.g., matrix metallopeptidase 9 [MMP-9]).[76] In addition, other proangiogenic proteins, such as members of the fibroblast growth factor (FGF) family, have been implicated in sustaining tumor angiogenesis.[71] TSP-1, a key counterbalance in the angiogenic switch, also binds transmembrane receptors displayed by endothelial cells and thereby triggers suppressive signals that can counteract proangiogenic stimuli.[77]

The blood vessels produced within tumors by an unbalanced mix of proangiogenic signals are typically aberrant: Tumor neovasculature is marked by precocious capillary sprouting, convoluted and excessive vessel branching, distorted and enlarged vessels, erratic blood flow, microhemorrhaging, leaking of plasma into the tissue parenchyma, and abnormal levels of endothelial cell proliferation and apoptosis.[78,79]

Angiogenesis is induced surprisingly early during the multistage development of invasive cancers both in animal models and in humans. Histologic analyses of premalignant, noninvasive lesions, including dysplasias and in situ carcinomas arising in a variety of organs, have revealed the early tripping of the angiogenic switch.[70,80] Historically, angiogenesis was envisioned to be important only when rapidly growing macroscopic tumors had formed, but more recent data indicate that angiogenesis also contributes to the microscopic premalignant phase of neoplastic progression, further cementing its status as an integral hallmark of cancer.

Gradations of the Angiogenic Switch

Once angiogenesis has been activated, tumors exhibit diverse patterns of neovascularization. Some tumors, including highly aggressive types such as pancreatic ductal adenocarcinomas, are hypovascularized and replete with stromal deserts that are largely avascular and indeed may even be actively antiangiogenic.[81] In contrast, many other tumors, including human renal and pancreatic neuroendocrine carcinomas, are highly angiogenic and, consequently, densely vascularized.[82,83]

Collectively, such observations suggest an initial tripping of the angiogenic switch during tumor development, which is followed by a variable intensity of ongoing neovascularization, the latter being controlled by a complex biologic rheostat that involves both the cancer cells and the associated stromal microenvironment.[71,72] Of note, the switching mechanisms can vary, even though the net result is a common inductive signal (e.g., VEGF). In some tumors, dominant oncogenes operating within tumor cells, such as *Ras* and *Myc*, can upregulate the expression of angiogenic factors, whereas in others, such inductive signals are produced indirectly by immune inflammatory cells, as will be discussed.

Endogenous Angiogenesis Inhibitors Present Natural Barriers to Tumor Angiogenesis

A variety of secreted proteins have been reported to have the capability to help shut off normally transitory angiogenesis, including thrombospondin-1 (TSP-1), fragments of plasmin (angiostatin) and type 18 collagen (endostatin), along with another dozen candidate antiangiogenic proteins.[77,84–88] Most are proteins, and many are derived by proteolytic cleavage of structural proteins that are not themselves angiogenic regulators.

A number of these endogenous inhibitors of angiogenesis can be detected in the circulation of normal mice and humans. Genes that encode several endogenous angiogenesis inhibitors have been deleted from the mouse germ line without untoward developmental or physiologic effects; however, the growth of autochthonous and implanted tumors is enhanced as a consequence.[84,85,88] By contrast, if the circulating levels of an endogenous inhibitor are genetically increased (e.g., via overexpression in transgenic mice or in xenotransplanted tumors), tumor growth is impaired.[85,88] Interestingly, wound healing and fat deposition are impaired or accelerated by elevated or ablated expression of such genes.[89,90] The data suggest that, under normal conditions, endogenous angiogenesis inhibitors serve as physiologic regulators modulating the transitory angiogenesis that occurs during tissue remodeling and wound healing; they may also act as intrinsic barriers to the induction and/or persistence of angiogenesis by incipient neoplasias.

Pericytes Are Important Components of the Tumor Neovasculature

Pericytes have long been known as supporting cells that are closely apposed to the outer surfaces of the endothelial tubes in normal tissue vasculature, where they provide important mechanical and physiologic support to the endothelial cells. Microscopic studies conducted in recent years have revealed that pericytes are associated, albeit loosely, with the neovasculature of most, if not all, tumors.[91–93] More importantly, mechanistic studies (discussed subsequently) have revealed that pericyte coverage is important for the maintenance of a functional tumor neovasculature.

A Variety of Bone Marrow-Derived Cells Contribute to Tumor Angiogenesis

It is now clear that a repertoire of cell types originating in the bone marrow play crucial roles in pathologic angiogenesis.[94–97] These include cells of the innate immune system—notably, macrophages, neutrophils, mast cells, and myeloid progenitors—that assemble at the margins of such lesions or infiltrate deeply within them; the tumor-associated inflammatory cells can help to trip the angiogenic switch in quiescent tissue and sustain ongoing angiogenesis associated with tumor growth. In addition, they can help protect the vasculature from the effects of drugs targeting endothelial cell signaling.[98] Moreover, several types of bone marrow–derived *vascular progenitor cells* have been observed to have migrated into neoplastic lesions and become intercalated into the existing neovasculature, where they assumed the roles of either pericytes or endothelial cells.[92,99,100]

Activating Invasion and Metastasis

The multistep process of invasion and metastasis has been schematized as a sequence of discrete steps, often termed the invasion–metastasis cascade.[101,102] This depiction portrays a succession of cell-biologic changes, beginning with local invasion, then intravasation by cancer cells into nearby blood and lymphatic vessels, transit of cancer cells through the lymphatic and hematogenous systems, followed by the escape of cancer cells from the lumina of such vessels into the parenchyma of distant tissues (extravasation), the formation of small nests of cancer cells (micrometastases), and finally, the growth of micrometastatic lesions into macroscopic tumors, this last step being termed *colonization*. These steps have largely been studied in the context of carcinoma pathogenesis. Indeed, when viewed through the prism of the invasion–metastasis cascade, the diverse tumors of this class appear to behave in similar ways.

During the malignant progression of carcinomas, the neoplastic cells typically develop alterations in their shape as well as their attachment to other cells and to the extracellular matrix (ECM). The best-characterized alteration involves the loss by carcinoma cells of E-cadherin, a key epithelial cell-to-cell adhesion molecule. By forming adherens junctions between adjacent epithelial cells, E-cadherin helps to assemble epithelial cell sheets and to maintain the quiescence of the cells within these sheets. Moreover, increased expression of E-cadherin has been well established as an antagonist of invasion and metastasis, whereas a reduction of its expression is known to potentiate these behaviors. The frequently observed downregulation and occasional mutational inactivation of the E-cadherin–encoding gene, *CDH1*, in human carcinomas provides strong support for its role as a key suppressor of the invasion–metastasis hallmark capability.[103,104]

Notably, the expression of genes encoding other cell-to-cell and cell-to-ECM adhesion molecules is also significantly altered in the cells of many highly aggressive carcinomas, with those favoring cytostasis typically being downregulated. Conversely, adhesion molecules normally associated with the cell migrations that occur during embryogenesis and inflammation are often upregulated. For example, N-cadherin, which is normally expressed in migrating neurons and mesenchymal cells during organogenesis, is upregulated in many invasive carcinoma cells, replacing the previously expressed E-cadherin.[104]

Research into the capability for invasion and metastasis has accelerated dramatically over the past decade as powerful new research tools, and refined experimental models have become available. Although still an emerging field replete with major unanswered questions, significant progress has been made in delineating important features of this complex hallmark capability. An admittedly incomplete representation of these advances is highlighted as follows.

The Epithelial-to-Mesenchymal Transition Program Broadly Regulates Invasion and Metastasis

A developmental regulatory program, termed the EMT, has become implicated as a prominent means by which neoplastic epithelial cells can acquire the abilities to invade, resist apoptosis, and disseminate.[105–110] By co-opting a process involved in various steps of embryonic morphogenesis and wound healing, carcinoma cells can concomitantly acquire multiple attributes that enable invasion and metastasis. This multifaceted EMT program can be activated transiently or stably, and to differing degrees, by carcinoma cells during the course of invasion and metastasis.

A set of pleiotropically acting transcriptional factors (TF), including Snail, Slug, Twist, and Zeb1/2, orchestrate the EMT and related migratory processes during embryogenesis; most were initially identified by developmental genetics. These transcriptional regulators are expressed in various combinations in a number of malignant tumor types. Some of these EMT-TFs have been shown in experimental models of carcinoma formation to be causally important for programming invasion; others have been found to elicit metastasis when experimentally expressed in primary tumor cells.[105,111–114] Included among the cell-biologic traits evoked by these EMT-TFs are loss of adherens junctions and associated conversion from a polygonal/epithelial to a spindly/fibroblastic morphology, concomitant with expression of secreted matrix-degrading enzymes, increased motility, and heightened resistance to apoptosis, which are implicated in the processes of invasion and metastasis. Several of these transcription factors can directly repress E-cadherin gene expression, thereby releasing neoplastic epithelial cells from this key suppressor of motility and invasiveness.[115]

The available data suggest that EMT-TFs regulate one another as well as overlapping sets of target genes. Results from developmental genetics indicate that contextual signals received from neighboring cells in the embryo are involved in triggering expression of these transcription factors in cells that are destined to pass through an EMT[111]; in an analogous fashion, heterotypic interactions of cancer cells with adjacent tumor-associated stromal cells have been shown to induce expression of the malignant cell phenotypes that are known to be choreographed by one or more of these EMT-TFs.[116,117] Moreover, cancer cells at the invasive margins of certain carcinomas can be seen to have undergone an EMT, suggesting that these cancer cells are subject to microenvironmental stimuli distinct from those received by cancer cells located in the cores of these lesions.[118] Although the evidence is still incomplete, it would appear that EMT-TFs are able to orchestrate most steps of the invasion–metastasis cascade, except perhaps the final step of colonization, which involves adaptation of cells originating in one tissue to the microenvironment of a foreign, potentially inhospitable tissue.

We still know rather little about the various manifestations and temporal stability of the mesenchymal state produced by an EMT. Indeed, it seems increasingly likely that many human carcinoma cells only experience a *partial EMT*, in which they acquire mesenchymal markers while retaining many preexisting epithelial ones. Although the expression of EMT-TFs has been observed in certain nonepithelial tumor types, such as sarcomas and neuroectodermal tumors, their roles in programming malignant traits in these tumors are presently poorly documented. Additionally, it remains to be determined whether aggressive carcinoma cells invariably acquire their malignant capabilities through activation of components of the EMT program, or whether alternative regulatory programs can also enable expression of these traits.

Heterotypic Contributions of Stromal Cells to Invasion and Metastasis

As mentioned previously, cross-talk between cancer cells and cell types of the neoplastic stroma is involved in the acquired capabilities of invasiveness and metastasis.[94,119–121] For example, mesenchymal stem cells (MSC) present in the tumor stroma have been found to secrete CCL5/RANTES in response to signals released by cancer cells; CCL5 then acts reciprocally on the cancer cells to stimulate invasive behavior.[122] In other work, carcinoma cells secreting IL-1 have been shown to induce MSCs to synthesize a spectrum of other cytokines that proceed thereafter to promote activation of the EMT program in the carcinoma cells; these effectors include IL-6, IL-8, growth-regulated oncogene alpha (GRO-α), and prostaglandin E2.[123]

Macrophages at the tumor periphery can foster local invasion by supplying matrix-degrading enzymes such as metalloproteinases and cysteine cathepsin proteases[76,120,124,125]; in one model system, the invasion-promoting macrophages are activated by IL-4 produced by the cancer cells.[126] And in an experimental model of metastatic breast cancer, tumor-associated macrophages (TAM) supply epidermal growth factor (EGF) to breast cancer cells, while the cancer cells reciprocally stimulate the macrophages with colony stimulating factor 1 (CSF-1). Their concerted interactions facilitate intravasation into the circulatory system and metastatic dissemination of the cancer cells.[94,127]

Observations like these indicate that the phenotypes of high-grade malignancy do not arise in a strictly cell-autonomous manner, and that their manifestation cannot be understood solely through analyses of signaling occurring within tumor cells. One important implication of the EMT model, still untested, is that the ability of carcinoma cells in primary tumors to negotiate most of the steps of the invasion–metastasis cascade may be acquired in certain tumors without the requirement that these cells undergo additional mutations beyond those that were needed for primary tumor formation.

Plasticity in the Invasive Growth Program

The role of contextual signals in inducing an invasive growth capability (often via an EMT) implies the possibility of reversibility, in that cancer cells that have disseminated from a primary tumor to more distant tissue sites may no longer benefit from the activated stroma and the EMT-inducing signals that they experienced while residing in the primary tumor. In the absence of ongoing exposure to these signals, carcinoma cells may revert in their new tissue environment to a noninvasive state. Thus, carcinoma cells that underwent an EMT during initial invasion and metastatic dissemination may reverse this metamorphosis, doing so via a mesenchymal-to-epithelial transition (MET). This plasticity may result in the formation of new tumor colonies of carcinoma cells exhibiting an organization and histopathology similar to those created by carcinoma cells in the primary tumor that never experienced an EMT.[128]

Distinct Forms of Invasion May Underlie Different Cancer Types

The EMT program regulates a particular type of invasiveness that has been termed *mesenchymal*. In addition, two other distinct modes of invasion have been identified and implicated in cancer cell invasion.[129,130] *Collective invasion* involves phalanxes of cancer cells advancing en masse into adjacent tissues and is characteristic of, for example, squamous cell carcinomas. Interestingly, such cancers are rarely metastatic, suggesting that this form of invasion lacks certain functional attributes that facilitate metastasis. Less clear is the prevalence of an *amoeboid* form of invasion,[131,132] in which individual cancer cells show morphologic plasticity, enabling them to slither through existing interstices in the ECM rather than clearing a path for themselves, as occurs in both the mesenchymal and collective forms of invasion. It is presently unresolved whether cancer cells participating in the collective and amoeboid forms of invasion employ components of the EMT program, or whether entirely different cell-biologic programs are responsible for choreographing these alternative invasion programs.

Another emerging concept, noted previously, involves the facilitation of cancer cell invasion by inflammatory cells that assemble at the boundaries of tumors, producing the ECM-degrading enzymes and other factors that enable invasive growth.[76,94,120,133] These functions may obviate the need of invading cancer cells to produce these proteins through activation of EMT programs. Thus, rather than synthesizing these proteases themselves, cancer cells may secrete chemoattractants that recruit proinvasive inflammatory cells; the latter then proceed to produce matrix-degrading enzymes that enable invasive growth.

The Daunting Complexity of Metastatic Colonization

Metastasis can be broken down into two major phases: the physical dissemination of cancer cells from the primary tumor to distant tissues, and the adaptation of these cells to foreign tissue microenvironments that results in successful colonization (i.e., the growth of micrometastases into macroscopic tumors). The multiple steps of dissemination would seem to lie within the purview of the EMT and similarly acting migratory programs. Colonization, however, is not strictly coupled with physical dissemination, as evidenced by the presence in many patients of myriad micrometastases that have disseminated but never progress to form macroscopic metastatic tumors.[101,102,134–136]

In some types of cancer, the primary tumor may release systemic suppressor factors that render such micrometastases dormant, as revealed clinically by explosive metastatic growth soon after resection of the primary growth.[87,137] In others, however, such as breast cancer and melanoma, macroscopic metastases may erupt decades after a primary tumor has been surgically removed or pharmacologically destroyed. These metastatic tumor growths evidently reflect dormant micrometastases that have solved, after much trial and error, the complex problem of adaptation to foreign tissue microenvironments, allowing subsequent tissue colonization.[135,136,138] Implicit here is the notion that most disseminated cancer cells are likely to be poorly adapted, at least initially, to the microenvironment of the tissue in which they have landed. Accordingly, each type of disseminated cancer cell may need to develop its own set of ad hoc solutions to the problem of thriving in the microenvironment of one or another foreign tissue.[139]

One can infer from such natural histories that micrometastases may lack certain hallmark capabilities necessary for vigorous growth, such as the ability to activate angiogenesis. Indeed, the inability of certain experimentally generated dormant micrometastases to form macroscopic tumors has been ascribed to their failure to activate tumor angiogenesis.[135,140] Additionally, recent experiments have shown that nutrient starvation can induce intense autophagy that causes cancer cells to shrink and adopt a state of reversible dormancy. Such cells may exit this state and resume active growth and proliferation when permitted by changes in tissue microenvironment, such as increased availability of nutrients, inflammation from causes such as infection or wound healing, or other local abnormalities.[49,141] Other mechanisms of micrometastatic dormancy may involve antigrowth signals embedded in normal tissue ECM[138] and tumor-suppressing actions of the immune system.[135,142]

Metastatic dissemination has long been depicted as the last step in multistep primary tumor progression; indeed, for many tumors, that is likely the case, as illustrated by recent genome sequencing studies that provide genetic evidence for clonal evolution of pancreatic ductal adenocarcinoma to a metastatic stage.[143–145] Importantly, however, recent results have revealed that some cancer cells can disseminate remarkably early, dispersing from apparently noninvasive premalignant lesions in both mice and humans.[146,147] Additionally, micrometastases can be spawned from primary tumors that are not obviously invasive but possess a neovasculature lacking in luminal integrity.[148] Although cancer cells can clearly disseminate from such preneoplastic lesions and seed the bone marrow and other tissues, their capability to colonize these sites and develop into pathologically significant macrometastases remains unproven. At present, we view this early metastatic dissemination as a demonstrable phenomenon in mice and humans, the clinical significance of which is yet to be established.

Having developed such a tissue-specific colonizing ability, the cells in metastatic colonies may proceed to disseminate further, not only to new sites in the body, but also back to the primary tumors in which their ancestors arose. Accordingly, tissue-specific colonization programs that are evident among certain cells within a primary tumor may originate not from classical tumor progression occurring entirely within the primary lesion, but instead from immigrants that have returned home.[149] Such reseeding is consistent with the aforementioned studies of human pancreatic cancer metastasis.[143–145] Stated differently, the phenotypes and underlying gene expression programs in focal subpopulations of cancer cells within primary tumors may reflect, in part, the reverse migration of their distant metastatic progeny.

Implicit in this *self-seeding* process is another notion: The supportive stroma that arises in a primary tumor and contributes to its acquisition of malignant traits provides a hospitable site for reseeding and colonization by circulating cancer cells released from metastatic lesions.

Clarifying the regulatory programs that enable metastatic colonization represents an important agenda for future research. Substantial progress is being made, for example, in defining sets of genes (*metastatic signatures*) that correlate with and appear to facilitate the establishment of macroscopic metastases in specific tissues.[139,146,150–152] Importantly, metastatic colonization almost certainly requires the establishment of a permissive tumor microenvironment composed of critical stromal support cells. For these reasons, the process of colonization is likely to encompass a large number of cell-biologic programs that are, in aggregate, considerably more complex and diverse than the preceding steps of metastatic dissemination that allow carcinoma cells to depart from primary tumors to sites of lodging and extravasation throughout the body.

Reprogramming Energy Metabolism

The chronic and often uncontrolled cell proliferation that represents the essence of neoplastic disease involves not only deregulated control of cell proliferation but also corresponding adjustments of energy metabolism in order to fuel cell growth and division. Under aerobic conditions, normal cells process glucose, first to pyruvate via glycolysis in the cytosol and thereafter via oxidative phosphorylation to carbon dioxide in the mitochondria. Under anaerobic conditions, glycolysis is favored and relatively little pyruvate is dispatched to the oxygen-consuming mitochondria. Otto Warburg first observed an anomalous characteristic of cancer cell energy metabolism[153–155]: Even in the presence of oxygen, cancer cells can reprogram their glucose metabolism, and thus their energy production, leading to a state that has been termed *aerobic glycolysis*.

The existence of this metabolic specialization operating in cancer cells has been substantiated in the ensuing decades. A key signature of aerobic glycolysis is upregulation of glucose transporters, notably GLUT1, which substantially increases glucose import into the cytoplasm.[156–158] Indeed, markedly increased uptake and utilization of glucose has been documented in many human tumor types, most readily by noninvasively visualizing glucose uptake using positron-emission tomography (PET) with a radiolabeled analog of glucose (^{18}F-fluorodeoxyglucose [FDG]) as a reporter.

Glycolytic fueling has been shown to be associated with activated oncogenes (e.g., *RAS*, *MYC*) and mutant tumor suppressors (e.g., *TP53*),[18,156,157,159] whose alterations in tumor cells have been selected primarily for their benefits in conferring the hallmark capabilities of cell proliferation, subversion of cytostatic controls, and attenuation of apoptosis. This reliance on glycolysis can be further accentuated under the hypoxic conditions that operate within many tumors: The hypoxia response system acts pleiotropically to upregulate glucose transporters and multiple enzymes of the glycolytic pathway.[156,157,160] Thus, both the Ras oncoprotein and hypoxia can independently increase the levels of the HIF1α and HIF2α hypoxia-response transcription factors, which in turn upregulate glycolysis.[160–162]

The reprogramming of energy metabolism is seemingly counterintuitive, in that cancer cells must compensate for the ~18-fold lower efficiency of ATP production afforded by glycolysis relative to mitochondrial oxidative phosphorylation. According to one long-forgotten[163] and a recently revived and refined hypothesis,[164] increased glycolysis allows the diversion of glycolytic intermediates into various biosynthetic pathways, including those generating nucleosides and amino acids. In turn, this facilitates the biosynthesis of the macromolecules and organelles required for assembling new cells. Moreover, Warburg-like metabolism seems to be present in many rapidly dividing embryonic tissues, once again suggesting a role in supporting the large-scale biosynthetic programs that are required for active cell proliferation.

Interestingly, some tumors have been found to contain two subpopulations of cancer cells that differ in their energy-generating pathways. One subpopulation consists of glucose-dependent (Warburg-effect) cells that secrete lactate, whereas cells of the second subpopulation preferentially import and utilize the lactate produced by their neighbors as their main energy source, employing part of the citric acid cycle to do so.[165–168] These two populations evidently function symbiotically: The hypoxic cancer cells depend on glucose for fuel and secrete lactate as waste, which is imported and preferentially used as fuel by their better oxygenated brethren. Although this provocative mode of intratumoral symbiosis has yet to be generalized, the cooperation between lactate-secreting and lactate-utilizing cells to fuel tumor growth is in fact not an invention of tumors, but rather again reflects the co-opting of a normal physiologic mechanism, in this case one operative in muscle[165,167,168] and the brain.[169] Additionally, it is becoming apparent that oxygenation, ranging from normoxia to hypoxia, is not necessarily static in tumors, but instead fluctuates temporally and regionally,[170] likely as a result of the instability and chaotic organization of the tumor-associated neovasculature.

Finally, the notion of the Warburg effect needs to be refined for most if not all tumors exhibiting aerobic glycolysis. The effect does not involve a switching off oxidative phosphorylation concurrent with activation of glycolysis, the latter then serving as the sole source of energy. Rather, cancer cells become highly adaptive, utilizing both mitochondrial oxidative phosphorylation and glycolysis in varying proportions to generate fuel (ATP) and biosynthetic precursors needed for chronic cell proliferation. Finally, this capability for reprograming energy metabolism, dubbed to be an *emerging hallmark* in 2011,[2] is clearly intertwined with the hallmarks conveying deregulated proliferative signals and evasion of growth suppressors, as discussed earlier. As such, its status as a discrete, independently acquired hallmark remains unclear, despite growing appreciation of its importance as a crucial component of the neoplastic growth state.

Evading Immune Destruction

The eighth hallmark reflects the role played by the immune system in antagonizing the formation and progression of tumors. A longstanding theory of immune surveillance posited that cells and tissues are constantly monitored by an ever alert immune system, and that such immune surveillance is responsible for recognizing and eliminating the vast majority of incipient cancer cells and, thus, nascent tumors.[171,172] According to this logic, clinical detectable cancers have somehow managed to avoid detection by the various arms of the immune system, or have been able to limit the extent of immunologic killing, thereby evading eradication.

The role of defective immunologic monitoring of tumors would seem to be validated by the striking increases of certain cancers in immune-compromised individuals.[173] However, the great majority of these are virus-induced cancers, suggesting that much of the control of this class of cancers normally depends on reducing viral burden in infected individuals, in part through eliminating virus-infected cells. These observations, therefore, shed little light on the possible role of the immune system in limiting formation of the >80% of tumors of nonviral etiology. In recent years, however, an increasing body of evidence, both from genetically engineered mice and from clinical epidemiology, suggests that the immune system operates as a significant barrier to tumor formation and progression, at least in some forms of non–virus-induced cancer.[174–177]

When mice genetically engineered to be deficient for various components of the immune system were assessed for the development of carcinogen-induced tumors, it was observed that tumors arose more frequently and/or grew more rapidly in the immunodeficient mice relative to immune-competent controls. In particular, deficiencies in the development or function of either $CD8^+$ cytotoxic T lymphocytes (CTL), $CD4^+$ T_H1 helper T cells, or natural killer (NK) cells, each led to demonstrable increases in tumor incidence. Moreover, mice with combined immunodeficiencies in both T cells and NK cells were even more susceptible to cancer development. The results indicated that, at least in certain experimental models, both the innate and adaptive cellular arms of the immune system are able to contribute significantly to immune surveillance and, thus, tumor eradication.[142,178]

In addition, transplantation experiments have shown that cancer cells that originally arose in immunodeficient mice are often inefficient at initiating secondary tumors in syngeneic immunocompetent hosts, whereas cancer cells from tumors arising in immunocompetent mice are equally efficient at initiating transplanted tumors in both types of hosts.[142,178] Such behavior has been interpreted as follows: Highly immunogenic cancer cell clones are routinely eliminated in immunocompetent hosts—a process that has been referred to as *immunoediting*—leaving behind only weakly immunogenic variants to grow and generate solid tumors. Such weakly immunogenic cells can thereafter successfully colonize both immunodeficient and immunocompetent hosts. Conversely, when arising in immunodeficient hosts, the immunogenic cancer cells are not selectively depleted and can, instead, prosper along with their weakly immunogenic counterparts. When cells from such nonedited tumors are serially transplanted into syngeneic recipients, the immunogenic cancer cells are rejected when they confront, for the first time, the competent immune systems of their secondary hosts.[179] (Unanswered in these particular experiments is the question of whether the chemical carcinogens used to induce such tumors are prone to generate cancer cells that are especially immunogenic.)

Clinical epidemiology also increasingly supports the existence of antitumoral immune responses in some forms of human cancer.[180–182] For example, patients with colon and ovarian tumors that are heavily infiltrated with CTLs and NK cells have a better prognosis than those who lack such abundant killer lymphocytes.[176,177,182,183] The case for other cancers is suggestive but less compelling and is the subject of ongoing investigation. Additionally, some immunosuppressed organ transplant recipients have been observed to develop donor-derived cancers, suggesting that in ostensibly tumor-free organ donors, the cancer cells were held in check in a dormant state by a functional immune system,[184] only to launch into proliferative expansion once these *passenger cells* in the transplanted organ found themselves in immunocompromised patients who lack the physiologically important capabilities to mount immune responses that would otherwise hold latent cancer cells in check or eradicate them.

Still, the epidemiology of chronically immunosuppressed patients does not indicate significantly increased incidences of the major forms of nonviral human cancers, as noted previously. This might be taken as an argument against the importance of immune surveillance as an effective barrier to tumorigenesis and tumor progression. We note, however, that HIV and pharmacologically immunosuppressed patients are predominantly immunodeficient in the T- and B-cell compartments and thus do not present with the multicomponent immunologic deficiencies that have been produced in the genetically engineered mutant mice lacking both NK cells and CTLs. This leaves open the possibility that such patients still have residual capability for mounting an anticancer immunologic defense that is mediated by NK and other innate immune cells.

In truth, the previous discussions of cancer immunology simplify tumor–host immunologic interactions, because highly immunogenic cancer cells may well succeed in evading immune destruction by disabling components of the immune system that have been dispatched to eliminate them. For example, cancer cells may paralyze infiltrating CTLs and NK cells by secreting TGF-β or other immunosuppressive factors.[32,185,186] Alternatively, cancer cells may express immunosuppressive cell-surface ligands, such as PD-L1, that prevent activation of the cytotoxic mechanisms of the CTLs. These PD-L1 molecules serve as ligands for the PD-1 receptors displayed by the CTLs, together exemplifying a system of *checkpoint* ligands and receptors that serve to constrain immune responses in order to avoid autoimmunity.[187–189] Yet other localized immunosuppressive mechanisms operate through the recruitment of inflammatory cells that can actively suppress CTL activity, including regulatory T cells (Tregs) and myeloid-derived suppressor cells (MDSC).[174,190–193]

In summary, these eight hallmarks each contribute qualitatively distinct capabilities that seem integral to most lethal forms of human cancer. Certainly, the balance and relative importance of their respective contributions to disease pathogenesis will vary among cancer types, and some hallmarks may be absent or of minor importance in some cases. Still, there is reason to postulate their generality and, thus, their applicability to understanding the biology of human cancer. Next, we turn to the question of how these capabilities are acquired during the multistep pathways through which cancers develop, focusing on two facilitators that are commonly involved.

TWO UBIQUITOUS CHARACTERISTICS FACILITATE THE ACQUISITION OF HALLMARK CAPABILITIES

We have defined the hallmarks of cancer as acquired functional capabilities that allow cancer cells to survive, proliferate, and disseminate. Their acquisition is made possible by two *enabling characteristics* (Fig. 2.2). Most prominent is the development of genomic instability in cancer cells, which generates random mutations, including chromosomal rearrangements, among which are rare genetic changes that can orchestrate individual hallmark capabilities. A second enabling characteristic involves the inflammatory state of premalignant and frankly malignant lesions. A variety of cells of the innate and adaptive immune system infiltrate neoplasias, some of which serve to promote tumor progression through various means.

An Enabling Characteristic: Genome Instability and Mutation

Acquisition of the multiple hallmarks enumerated previously depends in large part on a succession of alterations in the genomes of neoplastic cells. Basically, certain mutant genotypes can confer selective advantage to particular subclones among proliferating nests of incipient cancer cells, enabling their outgrowth and eventual dominance in a local tissue environment. Accordingly, multistep tumor progression can be portrayed as a succession of clonal expansions, most of which are triggered by the chance acquisition of an enabling mutation.

Indeed, it is apparent that virtually every human cancer cell genome carries mutant alleles of one or several growth-regulating genes, underscoring the central importance of these genetic alterations in driving malignant progression.[194] Still, we note that many heritable phenotypes—including, notably, inactivation of tumor suppressor genes—can be acquired through epigenetic

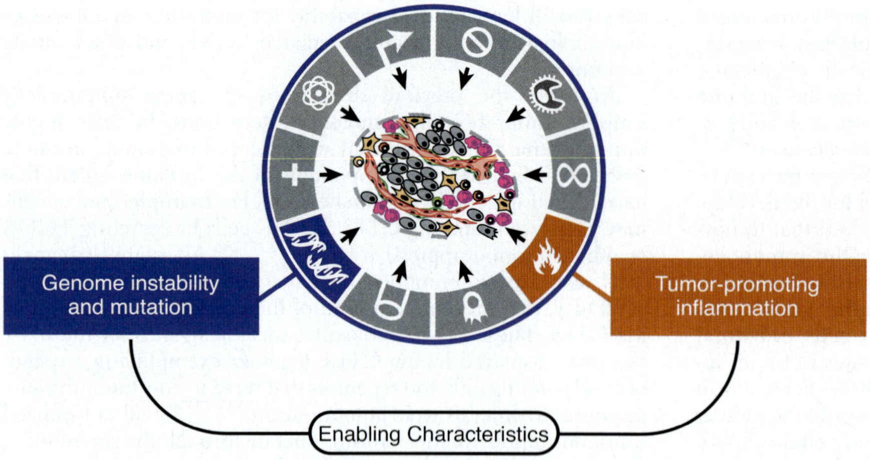

Figure 2.2 Enabling characteristics. Two ostensibly generic characteristics of cancer cells and the neoplasias they create are involved in the acquisition of the hallmark capabilities. First and foremost, the impairment of genome maintenance systems in aberrantly proliferating cancer cells enables the generation of mutations in genes that contribute to multiple hallmarks. Secondarily, neoplasias invariably attract cells of the innate immune system that are programmed to heal wounds and fight infections; these cells, including macrophages, neutrophils, and partially differentiated myeloid cells, can contribute functionally to acquisition of many of the hallmark capabilities. (Adapted from Hanahan D, Weinberg RA. Hallmarks of cancer: the next generation. *Cell* 2011;144:646–674.)

mechanisms, such as DNA methylation and histone modifications.[195–198] Thus, many clonal expansions may also be triggered by heritable nonmutational changes affecting the regulation of gene expression. At present, the relative importance of genetic versus heritable epigenetic alterations to the various clonal expansions remains unclear, and likely, varies broadly amongst the catalog of human cancer types.

The extraordinary ability of genome maintenance systems to detect and resolve defects in the DNA ensures that rates of spontaneous mutation in normal cells of the body are typically very low, both in quiescent cells and during cell division. The genomes of most cancer cells, by contrast, are replete with these alterations, reflecting loss of genomic integrity with concomitantly increased rates of mutation. This heightened mutability appears to accelerate the generation of variant cells, facilitating the selection of those cells whose advantageous phenotypes enable their clonal expansion.[199,200] This mutability is achieved through increased sensitivity to mutagenic agents, through a breakdown in one or several components of the genomic maintenance machinery, or both. In addition, the accumulation of mutations can be accelerated by aberrations that compromise the surveillance systems that normally monitor genomic integrity and force such genetically damaged cells into either quiescence, senescence, or apoptosis.[201–203] The role of TP53 is central here, leading to its being called the *guardian of the genome*.[204]

A diverse array of defects affecting various components of the DNA-maintenance machinery, referred to as the *caretakers* of the genome,[205] have been documented. The catalog of defects in these caretaker genes includes those whose products are involved in (1) detecting DNA damage and activating the repair machinery, (2) directly repairing damaged DNA, and (3) inactivating or intercepting mutagenic molecules before they have damaged the DNA.[199,201,202,206–208] From a genetic perspective, these caretaker genes behave much like tumor suppressor genes, in that their functions are often lost during the course of tumor progression, with such losses being achieved either through inactivating mutations or via epigenetic repression. Mutant copies of many of these caretaker genes have been introduced into the mouse germ line, resulting, not unexpectedly, in increased cancer incidence, thus supporting their involvement in human cancer development.[209]

In addition, research over the past decade has revealed another major source of tumor-associated genomic instability. As described earlier, the loss of telomeric DNA in many tumors generates karyotypic instability and associated amplification and deletion of chromosomal segments.[58] When viewed in this light, telomerase is more than an enabler of the hallmark capability for unlimited replicative potential. It must also be added to the list of critical caretakers responsible for maintaining genome integrity.

Advances in the molecular–genetic analysis of cancer cell genomes have provided the most compelling demonstrations of function-altering mutations and of ongoing genomic instability during tumor progression. One type of analysis—comparative genomic hybridization (CGH)—documents the gains and losses of gene copy number across the cell genome. In many tumors, the pervasive genomic aberrations revealed by CGH provide clear evidence for loss of control of genome integrity. Importantly, the recurrence of specific aberrations (both amplifications and deletions) at particular locations in the genome indicates that such sites are likely to harbor genes whose alteration favors neoplastic progression.[210]

More recently, with the advent of efficient and economical DNA sequencing technologies, higher resolution analyses of cancer cell genomes have become possible. Early studies are revealing distinctive patterns of DNA mutations in different tumor types (see: http://cancergenome.nih.gov/). In the not-too-distant future, the sequencing of entire cancer cell genomes promises to clarify the importance of ostensibly random mutations scattered across cancer cell genomes.[194] Thus, the use of whole genome resequencing offers the prospect of revealing recurrent genetic alterations (i.e., those found in multiple independently arising tumors) that in aggregate represent only minor proportions of the tumors of a given type. The recurrence of such mutations, despite their infrequency, may provide clues about the regulatory pathways playing causal roles in the pathogenesis of the tumors under study.

These surveys of cancer cell genomes have shown that the specifics of genome alteration vary dramatically between different tumor types. Nonetheless, the large number of already documented genome maintenance and repair defects, together with abundant evidence of widespread destabilization of gene copy number and nucleotide sequence, persuade us that instability of the genome is inherent to the cancer cells forming virtually all types of human tumors. This leads, in turn, to the conclusion that the defects in genome maintenance and repair are selectively advantageous and, therefore, instrumental for tumor progression, if only because they accelerate the rate at which evolving premalignant cells can accumulate favorable genotypes. As such, genome instability is clearly an *enabling characteristic* that is causally associated with the acquisition of hallmark capabilities.

An Enabling Characteristic: Tumor-Promoting Inflammation

Among the cells recruited to the stroma of carcinomas are a variety of cell types of the immune system that mediate various inflammatory functions. Pathologists have long recognized that some (but not all) tumors are densely infiltrated by cells of both the innate and adaptive arms of the immune system, thereby mirroring inflammatory conditions arising in nonneoplastic tissues.[211] With the advent of better markers for accurately identifying the distinct cell types of the immune system, it is now clear that virtually every neoplastic lesion contains immune cells present at densities ranging from subtle infiltrations detectable only with cell type–specific antibodies to gross inflammations that are apparent even by standard histochemical staining techniques.[183] Historically, such immune responses were largely thought to reflect an attempt by the immune system to eradicate tumors, and indeed, there is increasing evidence for antitumoral responses to many tumor types with an attendant pressure on the tumor to evade immune destruction,[174,176,177,183] as discussed earlier.

By 2000, however, there were also clues that tumor-associated inflammatory responses can have the unanticipated effect of facilitating multiple steps of tumor progression, thereby helping incipient neoplasias to acquire hallmark capabilities. In the ensuing years, research on the intersections between inflammation and cancer pathogenesis has blossomed, producing abundant and compelling demonstrations of the functionally important tumor-promoting effects that immune cells—largely of the innate immune system—have on neoplastic progression.[19,53,94,174,212,213] Inflammatory cells can contribute to multiple hallmark capabilities by supplying signaling molecules to the tumor microenvironment, including growth factors that sustain proliferative signaling; survival factors that limit cell death; proangiogenic factors; extracellular matrix-modifying enzymes that facilitate angiogenesis, invasion, and metastasis; and inductive signals that lead to activation of EMT and other hallmark-promoting programs.[53,94,116,212,213]

Importantly, localized inflammation is often apparent at the earliest stages of neoplastic progression and is demonstrably capable of fostering the development of incipient neoplasias into full-blown cancers.[94,214] Additionally, inflammatory cells can release chemicals—notably, reactive oxygen species—that are actively mutagenic for nearby cancer cells, thus accelerating their genetic evolution toward states of heightened malignancy.[53] As such, inflammation by selective cell types of the immune system is demonstrably an *enabling characteristic* for its contributions to the acquisition of hallmark capabilities. The cells responsible for this enabling characteristic are described in the following section.

THE CONSTITUENT CELL TYPES OF THE TUMOR MICROENVIRONMENT

Over the past 2 decades, tumors have increasingly been recognized as tissues whose complexity approaches and may even exceed that of normal healthy tissues. This realization contrasts starkly with the earlier, reductionist view of a tumor as nothing more than a collection of relatively homogeneous cancer cells, whose entire biology could be understood by elucidating the cell-autonomous properties of these cells (Fig. 2.3A). Rather, assemblages of diverse cell types associated with malignant lesions are increasingly documented to be functionally important for the manifestation of symptomatic disease (Fig. 2.3B). When viewed from this perspective, the biology of a tumor can only be fully understood by studying the individual specialized cell types within it. We enumerate as follows a set of accessory cell types recruited directly or indirectly by neoplastic cells into tumors, where they contribute in important ways to the biology of many tumors, and we discuss the regulatory mechanisms that control their individual and collective functions. Most of these observations stem from the study of carcinomas, in which the neoplastic epithelial cells constitute a compartment (the parenchyma) that is clearly distinct from the mesenchymal cells forming the tumor-associated stroma.

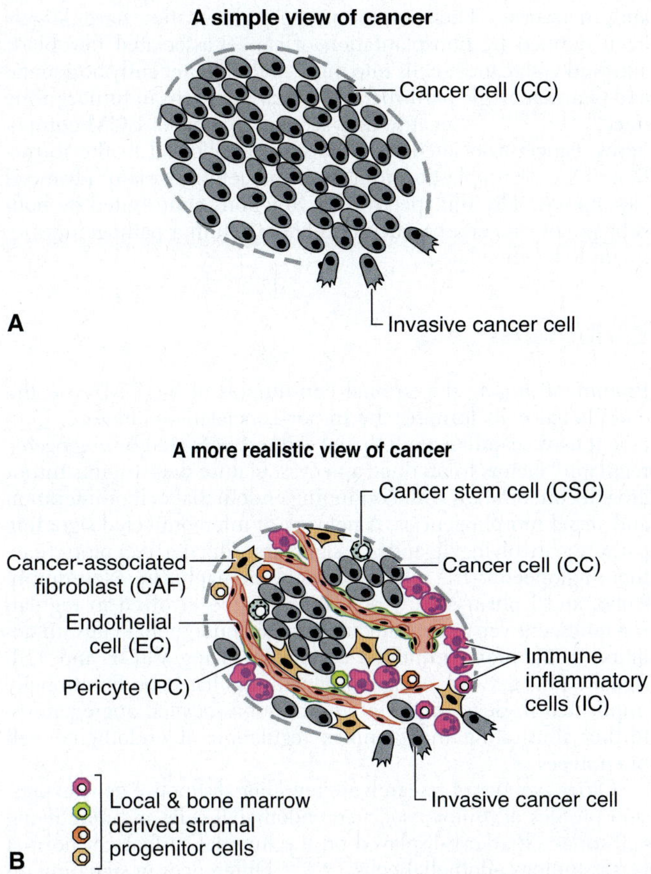

Figure 2.3 Tumors as outlaw organs. Research aimed at understanding the biology of tumors has historically focused on the cancer cells, which constitute the drivers of neoplastic disease. This view of tumors as nothing more than masses of cancer cells **(A)** ignores an important reality, that cancer cells recruit and corrupt a variety of normal cell types that form the tumor-associated stroma. Once formed, the stroma acts reciprocally on the cancer cells, affecting almost all of the traits that define the neoplastic behavior of the tumor as a whole **(B)**. The assemblage of heterogeneous populations of cancer cells and stromal cells is often referred to as the tumor microenvironment (TME). (Adapted from Hanahan D, Weinberg R. The hallmarks of cancer. *Cell* 2000;100:57–70; Hanahan D, Weinberg RA. Hallmarks of cancer: the next generation. *Cell* 2011;144:646–674.)

Cancer-Associated Fibroblasts

Fibroblasts are found in various proportions across the spectrum of carcinomas, in many cases constituting the preponderant cell population of the tumor stroma. The term *cancer-associated fibroblasts* (CAFs) subsumes at least two distinct cell types: (1) cells with similarities to the fibroblasts that create the structural foundation supporting most normal epithelial tissues, and (2) myofibroblasts, whose biologic roles and properties differ markedly from those of the widely distributed tissue-derived fibroblasts. Myofibroblasts are identifiable by their expression of α-smooth muscle actin (αSMA). They are rare in most healthy epithelial tissues, although certain tissues, such as the liver and pancreas, contain appreciable numbers of αSMA-expressing cells. Myofibroblasts transiently increase in abundance in wounds and are also found in sites of chronic inflammation. Although beneficial to tissue repair, myofibroblasts are problematic in chronic inflammation, in that they contribute to the pathologic fibrosis observed in tissues such as the lung, kidney, and liver.

Recruited myofibroblasts and variants of normal tissue-derived fibroblastic cells have been demonstrated to enhance tumor phenotypes, notably cancer cell proliferation, angiogenesis, invasion, and metastasis. Their tumor-promoting activities have largely been defined by transplantation of cancer-associated fibroblasts admixed with cancer cells into mice, and more recently by genetic and pharmacologic perturbation of their functions in tumor-prone mice.[8,121,133,215–219] Because they secrete a variety of ECM components, cancer-associated fibroblasts are implicated in the formation of the desmoplastic stroma that characterizes many advanced carcinomas. The full spectrum of functions contributed by both subtypes of cancer-associated fibroblasts to tumor pathogenesis remains to be elucidated.

Endothelial Cells

Prominent among the stromal constituents of the TME are the endothelial cells forming the tumor-associated vasculature. Quiescent tissue capillary endothelial cells are activated by *angiogenic* regulatory factors to produce a neovasculature that sustains tumor growth concomitant with continuing endothelial cell proliferation and vessel morphogenesis. A network of interconnected signaling pathways involving ligands of signal-transducing receptors (e.g., the Angiopoeitin-1/2, Notch ligands, Semaphorin, Neuropilin, Robo, and Ephrin-A/B) is now known to be involved in regulating quiescent versus activated angiogenic endothelial cells, in addition to the aforementioned counterbalancing VEGF and TSP signals. This network of signaling pathways has been functionally implicated in developmental and tumor-associated angiogenesis, further illustrating the complex regulation of endothelial cell phenotypes.[220–224]

Other avenues of research are revealing distinctive gene expression profiles of tumor-associated endothelial cells and identifying cell-surface markers displayed on the luminal surfaces of normal versus tumor endothelial cells.[78,225,226] Differences in signaling, in transcriptome profiles, and in vascular *ZIP codes* will likely prove to be important for understanding the conversion of normal endothelial cells into tumor-associated endothelial cells. Such knowledge may lead, in turn, to opportunities to develop novel therapies that exploit these differences in order to selectively target tumor-associated endothelial cells. Additionally, the activated (*angiogenic*) tumor vasculature has been revealed as a barrier to efficient intravasation and a functional suppressor of cytotoxic T cells,[227] and thus, tumor endothelial cells can contribute to the hallmark capability for evading immune destruction. As such, another emerging concept is to normalize rather than ablate them, so as to improve immunotherapy[190] as well as delivery of chemotherapy.[228]

Closely related to the endothelial cells of the circulatory system are those forming lymphatic vessels.[229] Their role in the tumor-associated stroma, specifically in supporting tumor growth, is poorly understood. Indeed, because of high interstitial pressure within solid tumors, intratumoral lymphatic vessels are typically collapsed and nonfunctional; in contrast, however, there are often functional, actively growing (*lymphangiogenic*) lymphatic vessels at the periphery of tumors and in the adjacent normal tissues that cancer cells invade. These associated lymphatics likely serve as channels for the seeding of metastatic cells in the draining lymph nodes that are commonly observed in a number of cancer types. Recent results that are yet to be generalized suggest an alternative role for the activated (i.e., lymphangiogenic) lymphatic endothelial cells associated with tumors, not in supporting tumor growth like the blood vessels, but in inducing (via VEGF-C–mediated signaling) a lymphatic tissue microenvironment that suppresses immune responses ordinarily marshaled from the draining lymph nodes.[230] As such, the real value to a tumor from activating the signaling circuit involving the ligand VEGF-C and its receptor VEGFR3 may be to facilitate the evasion of antitumor immunity by abrogating the otherwise immunostimulatory functions of draining lymphatic vessels and lymph nodes, with the collateral effect of inducing lymphatic endothelial cells to form the new lymphatic vessels that are commonly detected in association with tumors.

Pericytes

Pericytes represent a specialized mesenchymal cell type that are closely related to smooth muscle cells, with fingerlike projections that wrap around the endothelial tubing of blood vessels. In normal tissues, pericytes are known to provide paracrine support signals to the quiescent endothelium. For example, Ang-1 secreted by pericytes conveys antiproliferative stabilizing signals that are received by the Tie2 receptors expressed on the surface of endothelial cells. Some pericytes also produce low levels of VEGF that serve a trophic function in endothelial homeostasis.[93,231] Pericytes also collaborate with the endothelial cells to synthesize the vascular basement membrane that anchors both pericytes and endothelial cells and helps vessel walls to withstand the hydrostatic pressure created by the blood.

Genetic and pharmacologic perturbation of the recruitment and association of pericytes has demonstrated the functional importance of these cells in supporting the tumor endothelium.[93,217,231] For example, the pharmacologic inhibition of signaling through the platelet-derived growth factor (PDGF) receptor expressed by tumor pericytes and bone marrow–derived pericyte progenitors results in reduced pericyte coverage of tumor vessels, which in turn destabilizes vascular integrity and function.[91,217,231] Interestingly, and in contrast, the pericytes of normal vessels are not prone to such pharmacologic disruption, providing another example of the differences in the regulation of normal quiescent and tumor vasculature. An intriguing hypothesis, still to be fully substantiated, is that tumors with poor pericyte coverage of their vasculature may be more prone to permit cancer cell intravasation into the circulatory system, thereby enabling subsequent hematogenous dissemination.[91,148]

Immune Inflammatory Cells

Infiltrating cells of the immune system are increasingly accepted to be generic constituents of tumors. These inflammatory cells operate in conflicting ways: Both tumor-antagonizing and tumor-promoting leukocytes can be found in various proportions in most, if not all, neoplastic lesions. Evidence began to accumulate in the late 1990s that the infiltration of neoplastic tissues by cells of the immune system serves, perhaps counterintuitively, to promote tumor progression. Such work traced its conceptual roots back to the observed association of tumor formation with sites of chronic inflammation. Indeed, this led some to liken tumors to "wounds that do not heal."[211,232] In the course of normal wound healing and the resolution of infections, immune inflammatory cells appear transiently and then disappear, in contrast to their persistence in sites of chronic inflammation, where their presence has been associated with a variety of tissue pathologies, including fibrosis, aberrant angiogenesis, and as mentioned, neoplasia.[53,233]

We now know that immune cells play diverse and critical roles in fostering tumorigenesis. The roster of tumor-promoting inflammatory cells includes macrophage subtypes, mast cells, and neutrophils, as well as T and B lymphocytes.[96,97,119,133,212,234,235] Studies of these cells are yielding a growing list of tumor-promoting signaling molecules that they release, which include the tumor growth factor EGF, the angiogenic growth factors VEGF-A/-C, other proangiogenic factors such as FGF2, plus chemokines and cytokines that amplify the inflammatory state. In addition, these cells may produce proangiogenic and/or proinvasive matrix-degrading enzymes, including MMP-9 and other MMPs, cysteine cathepsin proteases, and heparanase.[94,96] Consistent with the expression of these diverse signals, tumor-infiltrating inflammatory cells have been shown to induce and help sustain tumor angiogenesis, to stimulate cancer cell proliferation, to facilitate tissue invasion, and to support the metastatic dissemination and seeding of cancer cells.[94,96,97,119,120,234–237]

In addition to fully differentiated immune cells present in tumor stroma, a variety of partially differentiated myeloid progenitors have been identified in tumors.[96] Such cells represent intermediaries between circulating cells of bone marrow origin and the differentiated immune cells typically found in normal and inflamed tissues. Importantly, these progenitors, like their more differentiated derivatives, have demonstrable tumor-promoting activity. Of particular interest, a class of tumor-infiltrating myeloid cells has been shown to suppress CTL and NK cell activity, having been identified as MDSCs that function to block the attack on tumors by the adaptive (i.e., CTL) and innate (i.e., NK) arms of the immune system.[94,133,193] Hence, recruitment of certain myeloid cells may be doubly beneficial for the developing tumor, by directly promoting angiogenesis and tumor progression, while at the same time affording a means of evading immune destruction.

These conflicting roles of the immune system in confronting tumors would seem to reflect similar situations that arise routinely in normal tissues. Thus, the immune system detects and targets infectious agents through cells of the adaptive immune response. Cells of the innate immune system, in contrast, are involved in wound healing and in clearing dead cells and cellular debris. The balance between the conflicting immune responses within particular tumor types (and indeed in individual patients' tumors) is likely to prove critical in determining the characteristics of tumor growth and the stepwise progression to stages of heightened aggressiveness (i.e., invasion and metastasis). Moreover, there is increasing evidence supporting the proposition that this balance can be modulated for therapeutic purposes in order to redirect or reprogram the immune response to focus its functional capabilities on destroying tumors.[133,238,239]

Stem and Progenitor Cells of the Tumor Stroma

The various stromal cell types that constitute the tumor microenvironment may be recruited from adjacent normal tissue—the most obvious reservoir of such cell types. However, in recent years, bone marrow (BM) has increasingly been implicated as a key source of tumor-associated stromal cells.[99,100,240–243] Thus, mesenchymal stem and progenitor cells can be recruited into tumors from BM, where they may subsequently differentiate into the various well-characterized stromal cell types. Some of these recent arrivals may also persist in an undifferentiated or partially differentiated state, exhibiting functions that their more differentiated progeny lack.

The BM origins of stromal cell types have been demonstrated using tumor-bearing mice in which the BM cells (and thus their disseminated progeny) have been selectively labeled with reporters such as green fluorescent protein (GFP). Although immune inflammatory cells have been long known to derive from BM, more recently progenitors of endothelial cells, pericytes, and several subtypes of cancer-associated fibroblasts have also been shown to originate from BM in various mouse models of cancer.[100,240–243] The prevalence and functional importance of endothelial progenitors for tumor angiogenesis is, however, currently unresolved.[99,242] Taken together, these various lines of evidence indicate that tumor-associated stromal cells may be supplied to growing tumors by the proliferation of preexisting stromal cells or via recruitment of BM-derived stem/progenitor cells.

In summary, it is evident that virtually all cancers, including even the *liquid tumors* of hematopoietic malignancies, depend not only on neoplastic cells for their pathogenic effects, but also on diverse cell types recruited from local and distant tissue sources to assemble specialized, supporting tumor microenvironments. Importantly, the composition of stromal cell types supporting a particular cancer evidently varies considerably from one tumor type to another; even within a particular type, the patterns and abundance can be informative about malignant grade and prognosis. The inescapable conclusion is that cancer cells are not fully autonomous, and rather depend to various degrees on stromal cells of the tumor microenvironment, which can contribute functionally to seven of the eight hallmarks of cancer (Fig. 2.4).

Heterotypic Signaling Orchestrates the Cells of the Tumor Microenvironment

Every cell in our bodies is governed by an elaborate intracellular signaling circuit—in effect, its own microcomputer. In cancer cells, key subcircuits in this integrated circuit are reprogrammed so as to activate and sustain hallmark capabilities. These changes are induced by mutations in the cells' genomes, by epigenetic alterations affecting gene expression, and by the receipt of a diverse array of signals from the tumor microenvironment. Figure 2.5A illustrates some of the circuits that are reprogrammed to enable cancer cells to proliferate chronically, to avoid proliferative brakes and cell death, and to become invasive and metastatic. Similarly, the intracellular integrated circuits that regulate the actions of stromal cells are also evidently reprogrammed. Current evidence suggests that stromal cell reprogramming is primarily affected by extracellular cues and epigenetic alterations in gene expression, rather than gene mutation.

Given the alterations in the signaling within both neoplastic cells and their stromal neighbors, a tumor can be depicted as a network of interconnected (cellular) microcomputers. This dictates that a complete elucidation of a particular tumor's biology will require far more than an elucidation of the aberrantly functioning integrated circuits within its neoplastic cells. Accordingly, the rapidly growing catalog of the function-enabling genetic mutations within cancer cell genomes[194] provides only one dimension to this problem. A reasonably complete, graphical depiction of the network of microenvironmental signaling interactions remains far beyond our reach, because the great majority of signaling molecules and their circuitry are still to be identified. Instead, we provide a hint of such interactions in Figure 2.5B. These few well-established examples are intended to exemplify a signaling network of remarkable complexity that is of critical importance to tumor pathogenesis.

Coevolution of the Tumor Microenvironment During Carcinogenesis

The tumor microenvironment described previously is not static during multistage tumor development and progression, thus creating another dimension of complexity. Rather, the abundance and functional contributions of the stromal cells populating neoplastic lesions will likely vary during progression in two respects. First, as the neoplastic cells evolve, there will be a parallel coevolution occurring in the stroma, as indicated by the shifting composition of stroma-associated cell types. Second, as cancer cells enter into different locations, they encounter distinct stromal microenvironments. Thus, the microenvironment in the interior of a primary tumor will likely be distinct both from locally invasive breakout lesions and from the one encountered by disseminated cells in distant organs (Fig. 2.6A). This dictates that the observed histopathologic progression of a tumor reflects underlying changes in heterotypic signaling between tumor parenchyma and stroma.

We envision back-and-forth reciprocal interactions between the neoplastic cells and the supporting stromal cells that change during the course of multistep tumor development and progression, as depicted in Figure 2.6B. Thus, incipient neoplasias begin the interplay by recruiting and activating stromal cell types that assemble into an initial preneoplastic stroma, which in turn responds reciprocally by enhancing the neoplastic phenotypes of the nearby cancer cells. The cancer cells, in response, may then undergo further genetic evolution, causing them to feed signals back to the stroma. Ultimately, signals originating in the stroma of primary tumors enable cancer cells to invade normal adjacent tissues and disseminate, seeding distant tissues and, with low efficiency, metastatic colonies (see Fig. 2.6B).

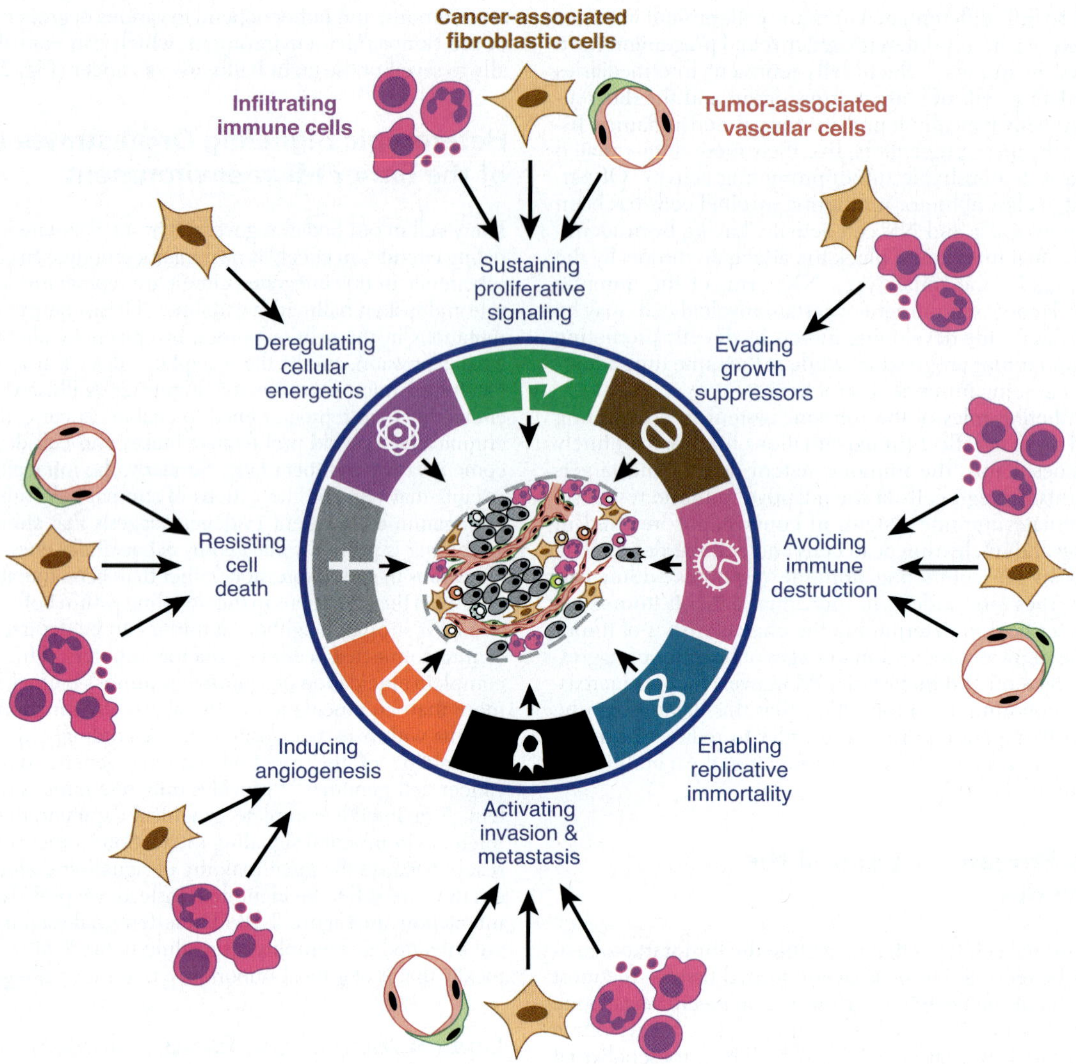

Figure 2.4 Diverse contributions of stromal cells to the hallmarks of cancer. Of the eight hallmark capabilities acquired by cancer cells, seven depend on contributions by stromal cells forming the tumor microenvironment.[2,213] The stromal cells can be divided into three general classes: infiltrating immune cells, cancer-associated fibroblastic cells, and tumor-associated vascular cells. The association of these corrupted cell types with the acquisition of individual hallmark capabilities has been documented through a variety of experimental approaches that are often supported by descriptive studies in human cancers. The relative importance of each of these stromal cell classes to a particular hallmark varies according to tumor type and stage of progression. (Adapted from Hanahan D, Coussens LM. Accessories to the crime: functions of cells recruited to the tumor microenvironment. *Cancer Cell* 2012;21:309–322.)

The circulating cancer cells that are released from primary tumors leave a microenvironment supported by this coevolved stroma. Upon landing in a distant organ, however, disseminated cancer cells must find a means to grow in a quite different tissue microenvironment. In some cases, newly seeded cancer cells must survive and expand in naïve, fully normal tissue microenvironments. In other cases, the newly encountered tissue microenvironments may already be supportive of such disseminated cancer cells, having been preconditioned prior to their arrival. Such permissive sites have been referred to as *premetastatic niches*.[146,244,245] These supportive niches may already preexist in distant tissues for various physiologic reasons,[101] including the actions of circulating factors dispatched systemically by primary tumors.[245]

The fact that signaling interactions between cancer cells and their supporting stroma are likely to evolve during the course of multistage primary tumor development and metastatic colonization clearly complicates the goal of fully elucidating the mechanisms of cancer pathogenesis. For example, this complexity poses challenges to systems biologists seeking to chart the crucial regulatory networks that orchestrate malignant progression, because much of the critical signaling is not intrinsic to cancer cells and instead operates through the interactions that these cells establish with their neighbors.

Cancer Cells, Cancer Stem Cells, and Intratumoral Heterogeneity

Cancer cells are the foundation of the disease. They initiate neoplastic development and drive tumor progression forward, having acquired the oncogenic and tumor suppressor mutations that define cancer as a genetic disease. Traditionally, the cancer cells within tumors have been portrayed as reasonably homogeneous cell populations until relatively late in the course of tumor progression, when hyperproliferation combined with increased genetic instability spawn genetically distinct clonal subpopulations. Reflecting such clonal heterogeneity, many human tumors are histopathologically diverse, containing regions demarcated by various

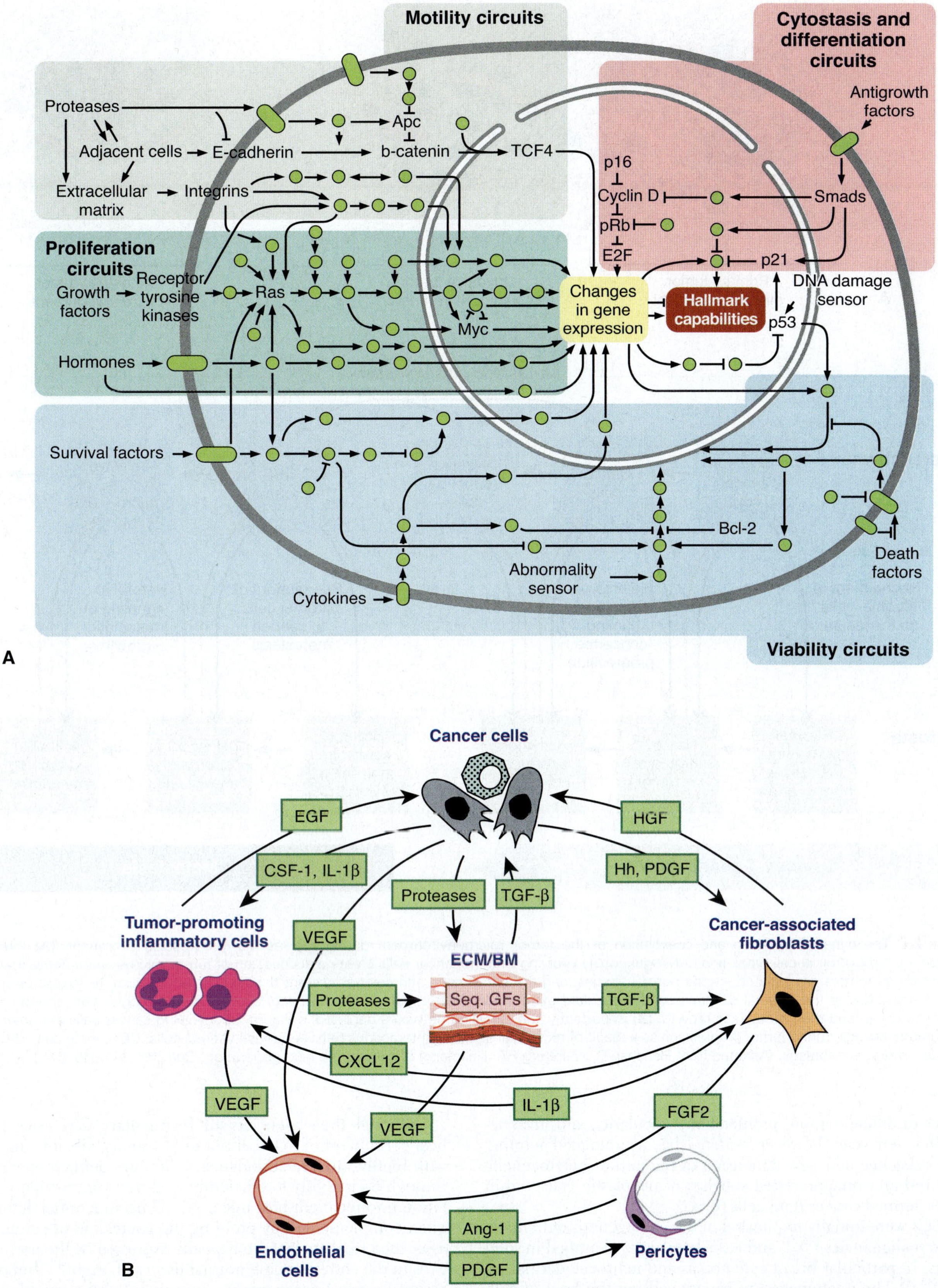

Figure 2.5 Reprogramming intracellular circuits and cell-to-cell signaling pathways dictates tumor inception and progression. An elaborate integrated circuit operating within normal cells is reprogrammed to regulate the hallmark capabilities acquired by cancer cells **(A)** and by associated stromal cells. Separate subcircuits, depicted here in differently colored fields, are specialized to orchestrate distinct capabilities. At one level, this depiction is simplistic, because there is considerable cross-talk between such subcircuits. More broadly, the integrated circuits operating inside cancer cells and stromal cells are interconnected via a complex network of signals transmitted by the various cells in the tumor microenvironment (in some cases via the extracellular matrix *[ECM]* and basement membranes *[BM]* they synthesize), of which a few signals are exemplified **(B).** HGF, hepatocyte growth factor for the cMet receptor; Hh, hedgehog ligand for the Patched (PTCH) receptor; Seq. GF, growth factors sequested in the ECM/BM. (Adapted from Hanahan D, Weinberg RA. Hallmarks of cancer: the next generation. *Cell* 2011;144:646–674.)

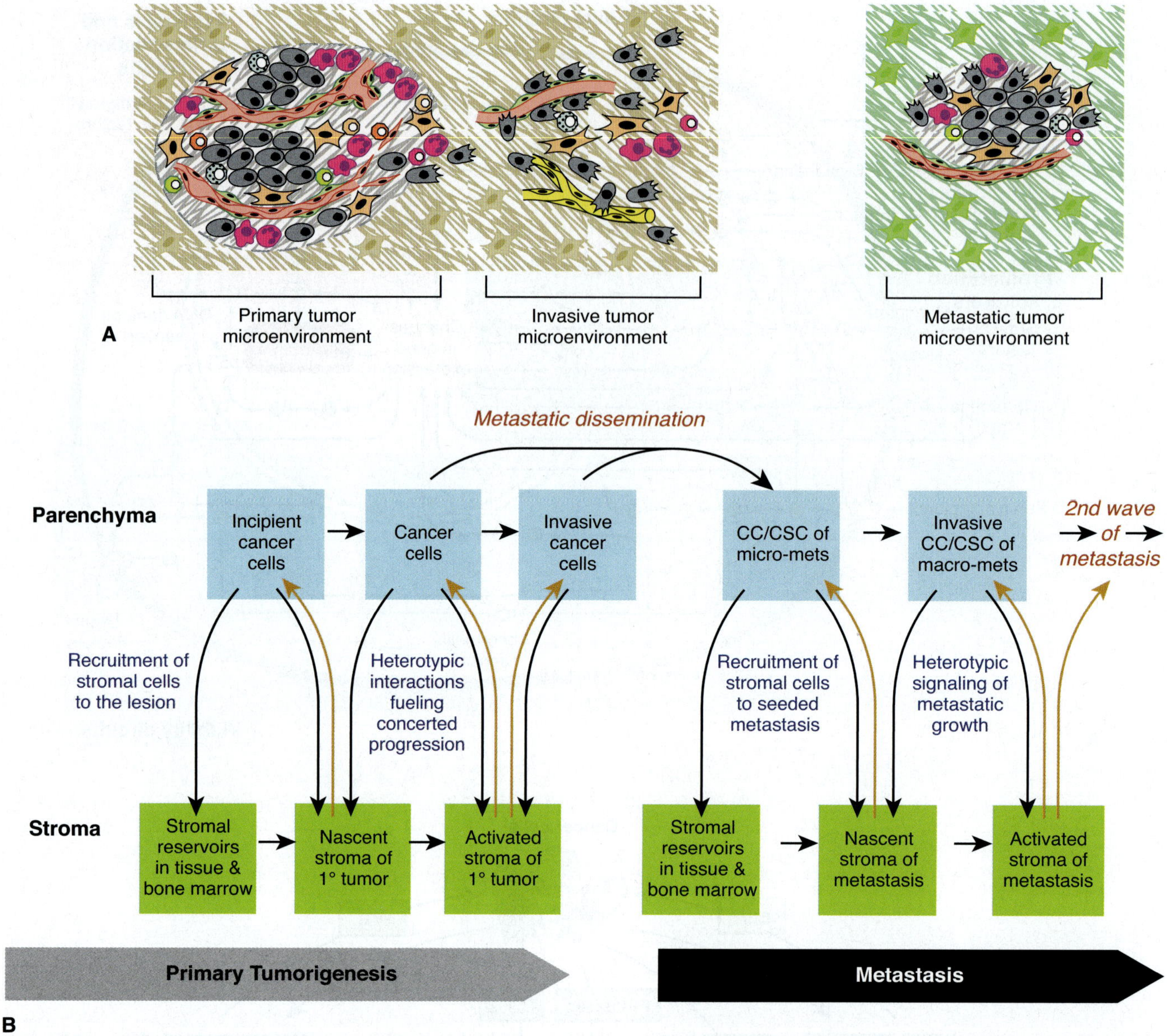

Figure 2.6 The dynamic variation and coevolution of the tumor microenvironment during the lesional progression of cancer. **(A)** Interactions between multiple stromal cell types and heterogeneously evolving mutant cancer cells create a succession of tumor microenvironments that change dynamically as tumors are initiated, invade normal tissues, and thereafter seed and colonize distant tissues. The abundance, histologic organization, and characteristics of the stromal cell types and associated extracellular matrix *(hatched background)* evolves during progression, thereby enabling primary, invasive, and then metastatic growth. **(B)** Importantly, the signaling networks depicted in Figure 2.5 involving cancer cells and their stromal collaborators change during tumor progression as a result of reciprocal signaling interactions between these various cells. CC, cancer cell; CSC, cancer stem cell; mets, metastases. (Adapted from Hanahan D, Weinberg RA. Hallmarks of cancer: the next generation. *Cell* 2011;144:646–674.)

degrees of differentiation, proliferation, vascularity, and invasiveness. In recent years, however, evidence has accumulated pointing to the existence of a new dimension of intratumor heterogeneity and a hitherto unappreciated subclass of neoplastic cells within tumors, termed cancer stem cells (CSC).

CSCs were initially implicated in the pathogenesis of hematopoietic malignancies,[246,247] and years later, were identified in solid tumors, in particular breast carcinomas and neuroectodermal tumors.[248,249] The fractionation of cancer cells on the basis of cell-surface markers has yielded subpopulations of neoplastic cells with a greatly enhanced ability, relative to the corresponding majority populations of non-CSCs, to seed new tumors upon implantation in immunodeficient mice. These, often rare, tumor-initiating cells have proven to share transcriptional profiles with certain normal tissue stem cells, thus justifying their designation as stemlike.

Although the evidence is still fragmentary, CSCs may prove to be a constituent of many, if not most tumors, albeit being present with highly variable abundance. CSCs are defined operationally through their ability to efficiently seed new tumors upon implantation into recipient host mice.[250–253] This functional definition is often complemented by profiling the expression of certain CSC-associated markers that are typically expressed by the normal stem cells in the corresponding normal tissues of origin.[249] Importantly, recent in vivo lineage-tracing experiments have provided an additional functional test of CSCs by demonstrating their ability to spawn large numbers of progeny, including non-CSCs within tumors.[250] At the same time, these experiments have provided the most compelling evidence to date that CSCs exist, and that they can be defined functionally through tests that do not depend on the implantation of tumor cells into appropriate mouse hosts.

The origins of CSCs within a solid tumor have not been clarified and, indeed, may well vary from one tumor type to another.[250,251,254] In some tumors, normal tissue stem cells may serve as the cells of origin that undergo oncogenic transformation to yield CSCs; in others, partially differentiated transit-amplifying cells, also termed progenitor cells, may suffer the initial oncogenic transformation, thereafter assuming more stemlike characters. Once primary tumors have formed, the CSCs, like their normal counterparts, may self-renew as well as spawn more differentiated derivatives. In the case of neoplastic CSCs, these descendant cells form the great bulk of many tumors and thus are responsible for creating many tumor-associated phenotypes. It remains to be established whether multiple distinct classes of increasingly neoplastic stem cells form during the inception and subsequent multistep progression of tumors, ultimately yielding the CSCs that have been described in fully developed cancers.

Recent research has interrelated the acquisition of CSC traits with the EMT transdifferentiation program discussed previously.[250,255] The induction of this program in certain model systems can induce many of the defining features of stem cells, including self-renewal ability and the antigenic phenotypes associated with both normal and cancer stem cells. This concordance suggests that the EMT program may not only enable cancer cells to physically disseminate from primary tumors, but can also confer on such cells the self-renewal capability that is crucial to their subsequent role as founders of new neoplastic colonies at sites of dissemination.[256] If generalized, this connection raises an important corollary hypothesis: The heterotypic signals that trigger an EMT, such as those released by an activated, inflammatory stroma, may also be important in creating and maintaining CSCs.

An increasing number of human tumors are reported to contain subpopulations with the properties of CSCs, as defined operationally through their efficient tumor-initiating capabilities upon xenotransplantation into mice. Nevertheless, the importance of CSCs as a distinct phenotypic subclass of neoplastic cells remains a matter of debate, as does their oft cited rarity within tumors.[254,257–259] Indeed, it is plausible that the phenotypic plasticity operating within tumors may produce bidirectional interconversion between CSCs and non-CSCs, resulting in dynamic variation in the relative abundance of CSCs.[250,260] Such plasticity could complicate a definitive measurement of their characteristic abundance. Analogous plasticity is already implicated in the EMT program, which can be engaged reversibly.[261]

These complexities notwithstanding, it is already evident that this new dimension of tumor heterogeneity holds important implications for successful cancer therapies. Increasing evidence in a variety of tumor types suggests that cells exhibiting the properties of CSCs are more resistant to various commonly used chemotherapeutic treatments.[255,262,263] Their persistence following initial treatment may help to explain the almost inevitable disease recurrence occurring after apparently successful debulking of human solid tumors by radiation and various forms of chemotherapy. Moreover, CSCs may well prove to underlie certain forms of tumor dormancy, whereby latent cancer cells persist for years or even decades after initial surgical resection or radio/chemotherapy, only to suddenly erupt and generate life-threatening disease. Hence, CSCs represent a double threat in that they are more resistant to therapeutic killing, and at the same time, are endowed with the ability to regenerate a tumor once therapy has been halted.

This phenotypic plasticity implicit in the CSC state may also enable the formation of functionally distinct subpopulations within a tumor that support overall tumor growth in various ways. Thus, an EMT can convert epithelial carcinoma cells into mesenchymal, fibroblast-like cancer cells that may well assume the duties of CAFs in some tumors (e.g., pancreatic ductal adenocarcinoma).[264] Intriguingly, several recent reports that have yet to be thoroughly validated in terms of generality, functional importance, or prevalence have documented the ability of glioblastoma cells (or possibly their associated CSC subpopulations) to transdifferentiate into endothelial-like cells that can substitute for bona fide host-derived endothelial cells in forming a tumor-associated neovasculature.[265–267] These examples suggest that certain tumors may induce some of their own cancer cells to undergo various types of metamorphoses in order to generate stromal cell types needed to support tumor growth and progression, rather than relying on recruited host cells to provide the requisite hallmark-enabling functions.

Another form of phenotypic variability resides in the genetic heterogeneity of cancer cells within a tumor. Genomewide sequencing of cancer cells microdissected from different sectors of the same tumor[145] has revealed striking intratumoral genetic heterogeneity. Some of this genetic diversity may be reflected in the long recognized histologic heterogeneity within individual human tumors. Thus, genetic diversification may produce subpopulations of cancer cells that contribute distinct and complementary capabilities, which then accrue to the common benefit of overall tumor growth, progression, and resistance to therapy, as described earlier. Alternatively, such heterogeneity may simply reflect the genetic chaos that arises as tumor cell genomes become increasingly destabilized.

THERAPEUTIC TARGETING OF THE HALLMARKS OF CANCER

We do not attempt here to enumerate the myriad therapies that are currently under development or have been introduced of late into the clinic. Instead, we consider how the description of hallmark principles is likely to inform therapeutic development at present and may increasingly do so in the future. Thus, the rapidly growing armamentarium of therapeutics directed against specific molecular targets can be categorized according to their respective effects on one or more hallmark capabilities, as illustrated in the examples presented in Figure 2.7. Indeed, the observed efficacy of these drugs represents, in each case, a validation of a particular capability: If a capability is truly critical to the biology of tumors, then its inhibition should impair tumor growth and progression.

Unfortunately, however, the clinical responses elicited by these targeted therapies have generally been transitory, being followed all too often by relapse. One interpretation, which is supported by growing experimental evidence, is that each of the core hallmark capabilities is regulated by a set of partially redundant signaling pathways. Consequently, a targeted therapeutic agent inhibiting one key pathway in a tumor may not completely eliminate a hallmark capability, allowing some cancer cells to survive with residual function until they or their progeny eventually adapt to the selective pressure imposed by the initially applied therapy. Such adaptation can reestablish the expression of the functional capability, permitting renewed tumor growth and clinical relapse. Because the number of parallel signaling pathways supporting a given hallmark must be limited, it may become possible to therapeutically cotarget all of these supporting pathways, thereby preventing the development of adaptive resistance.

Another dimension of the plasticity of tumors under therapeutic attack is illustrated by the unanticipated responses to antiangiogenic therapy, in which cancer cells reduce their dependence on this hallmark capability by increasing their dependence on another. Thus, many observers anticipated that potent inhibition of angiogenesis would starve tumors of vital nutrients and oxygen, forcing them into dormancy and possibly leading to their dissolution.[86,87,268] Instead, the clinical responses to antiangiogenic therapies have been found to be transitory, followed by relapse, implicating adaptive or evasive resistance mechanisms.[220,269–271] One such mechanism of evasive resistance, observed in certain preclinical models of antiangiogenic therapy, involves reduced dependence on continuing angiogenesis by increasing the activity of two other capabilities: invasiveness and metastasis.[269–271] By invading nearby and distant tissues, initially hypoxic cancer cells gain access to normal,

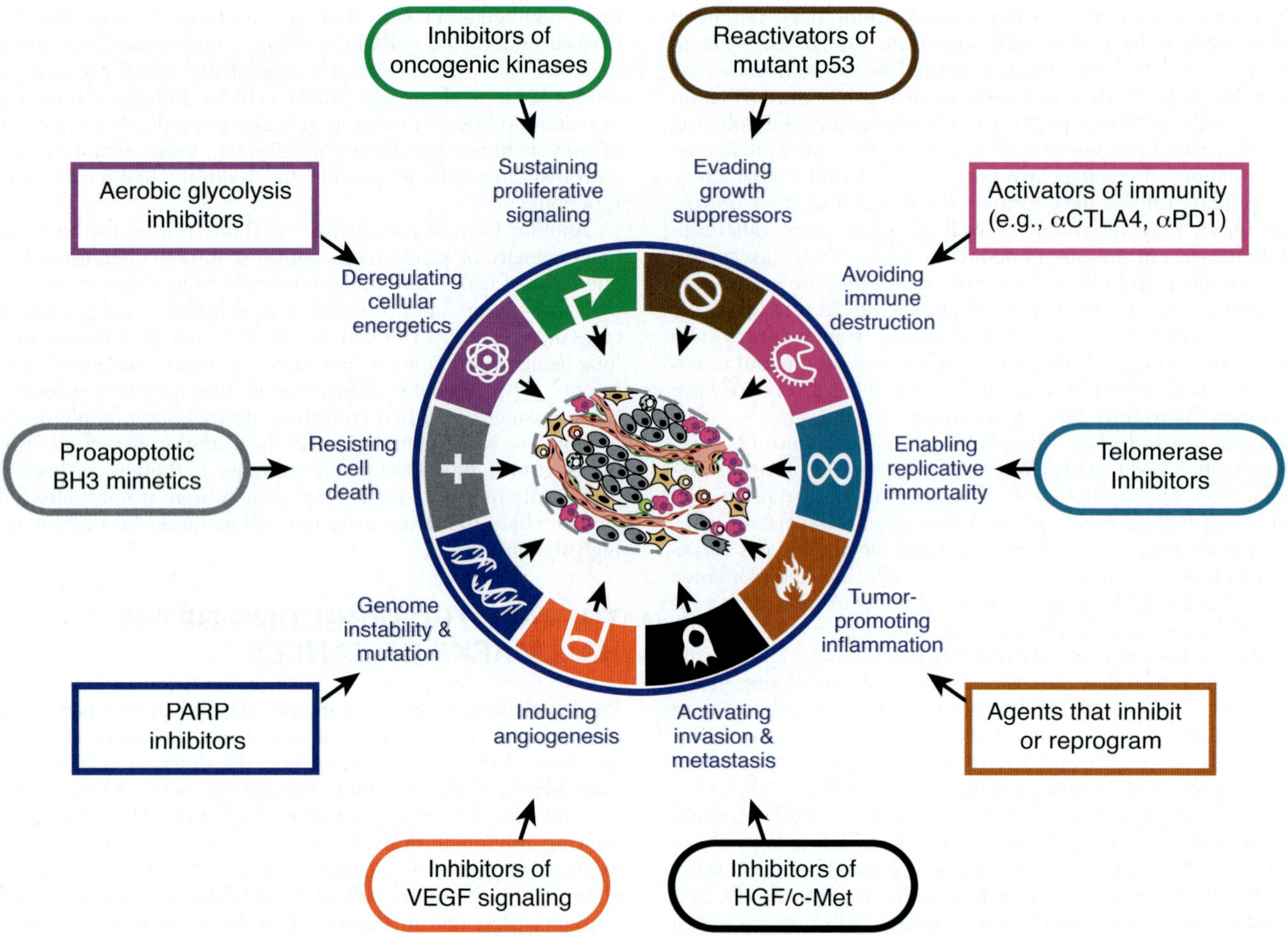

Figure 2.7 Therapeutic targeting of the hallmarks of cancer. Drugs that interfere with each of the hallmark capabilities and hallmark-enabling processes have been developed and are in preclinical and/or clinical testing, and in some cases, approved for use in treating certain forms of human cancer. A focus on antagonizing specific hallmark capabilities is likely to yield insights into developing novel, highly effective therapeutic strategies. PARP, poly ADP ribose polymerase. (Adapted from Hanahan D, Weinberg RA. Hallmarks of cancer: the next generation. *Cell* 2011;144:646–674.)

preexisting tissue vasculature. The initial clinical validation of this adaptive/evasive resistance is apparent in the increased invasion and local metastasis seen when human glioblastomas are treated with antiangiogenic therapies.[272–274] The applicability of this lesson to other human cancers has yet to be established.

Analogous adaptive shifts in dependence on other hallmark traits may also limit the efficacy of analogous hallmark-targeting therapies. For example, the deployment of apoptosis-inducing drugs may induce cancer cells to hyperactivate mitogenic signaling, enabling them to compensate for the initial attrition triggered by such treatments. Such considerations suggest that drug development and the design of treatment protocols will benefit from incorporating the concepts of functionally discrete hallmark capabilities and of the multiple biochemical pathways involved in supporting each of them. For these reasons, we envisage that attacking multiple hallmark capabilities with hallmark-targeting drugs (see Fig. 2.7), in carefully considered combinations, sequences, and temporal regimens,[275] will result in increasingly effective therapies that produce more durable clinical responses.

CONCLUSION AND A VISION FOR THE FUTURE

Looking ahead, we envision significant advances in our understanding of invasion and metastasis during the coming decade. Similarly, the role of altered energy metabolism in malignant growth will be elucidated, including a resolution of whether this metabolic reprogramming is a discrete capability separable from the core hallmark of chronically sustained proliferation. We are excited about the new frontier of immunotherapy, which will be empowered to leverage detailed knowledge about the regulation of immune responses in order to develop pharmacologic tools that can modulate them therapeutically for the purpose of effectively and sustainably attacking tumors and, most importantly, their metastases.

Other areas are currently in rapid flux. In recent years, elaborate molecular mechanisms controlling transcription through chromatin modifications have been uncovered, and there are clues that specific shifts in chromatin configuration occur during the acquisition of certain hallmark capabilities.[195,196] Functionally significant epigenetic alterations seem likely to be factors not only in the cancer cells, but also in the altered cells of the tumor-associated stroma. At present, it is unclear whether an elucidation of these epigenetic mechanisms will materially change our overall understanding of the means by which hallmark capabilities are acquired, or simply add additional detail to the regulatory circuitry that is already known to govern them.

Similarly, the discovery of hundreds of distinct regulatory microRNAs has already led to profound changes in our understanding of the molecular control mechanisms that operate in health and disease. By now, dozens of microRNAs have been implicated in various tumor phenotypes.[276,277] Still, these only scratch the surface of the true complexity, because the functions of hundreds of microRNAs known to be present in our cells and to be altered in expression levels in different forms of cancer remain total mysteries. Here again, we are unclear whether future progress will cause fundamental shifts in our understanding of the pathogenic mechanisms of cancer, or only add detail to the elaborate regulatory circuits that have already been mapped out.

Finally, the existing diagrams of heterotypic interactions between the multiple distinct cell types that collaborate to produce malignant tumors are still rudimentary. We anticipate that, in another decade, the signaling pathways describing the intercommunication between these various cell types within tumors will be charted in far greater detail and clarity, eclipsing our current knowledge. And, as before,[1,2] we continue to foresee cancer research as an increasingly logical science, in which myriad phenotypic complexities are manifestations of an underlying organizing principle.

ACKNOWLEDGMENT

This chapter is modified from Hanahan D, Weinberg RA. Hallmarks of cancer: the next generation. *Cell* 2011;144(5):646–674.

REFERENCES

1. Hanahan D, Weinberg R. The hallmarks of cancer. *Cell* 2000;100:57–70.
2. Hanahan D, Weinberg RA. Hallmarks of cancer: the next generation. *Cell* 2011;144:646–674.
3. Lemmon MA, Schlessinger J. Cell signaling by receptor tyrosine kinases. *Cell* 2010;141:1117–1134.
4. Witsch E, Sela M, Yarden Y. Roles for growth factors in cancer progression. *Physiology* 2010;25:85–101.
5. Hynes NE, MacDonald G. ErbB receptors and signaling pathways in cancer. *Curr Opin Cell Biol* 2009;21:177–184.
6. Perona T. Cell signalling: growth factors and tyrosine kinase receptors. *Clin Transl Oncol* 2006;8:77–82.
7. Franco OE, Shaw AK, Strand DW, et al. Cancer associated fibroblasts in cancer pathogenesis. *Semin Cell Dev Biol* 2010;21:33–39.
8. Bhowmick NA, Neilson EG, Moses HL. Stromal fibroblasts in cancer initiation and progression. *Nature* 2004;432:332–337.
9. Davies MA, Samuels Y. Analysis of the genome to personalize therapy for melanoma. *Oncogene* 2010;29:5545–5555.
10. Jiang BH, Liu LZ. PI3K/PTEN signaling in angiogenesis and tumorigenesis. *Adv Cancer Res* 2009;102:19–65.
11. Yuan TL, Cantley LC. PI3K pathway alterations in cancer: variations on a theme. *Oncogene* 2008;27:5497–5510.
12. Wertz IE, Dixit VM. Regulation of death receptor signaling by the ubiquitin system. *Cell Death Differ* 2010;17:14–24.
13. Cabrita MA, Christofori G. Sprouty proteins, masterminds of receptor tyrosine kinase signaling. *Angiogenesis* 2008;11:53–62.
14. Amit I, Citri A, Shay T, et al. A module of negative feedback regulators defines growth factor signaling. *Nature Genet* 2007;39:503–512.
15. Mosesson Y, Mills GB, Yarden Y. Derailed endocytosis: an emerging feature of cancer. *Nat Rev Cancer* 2008;8:835–850.
16. Sudarsanam S, Johnson DE. Functional consequences of mTOR inhibition. *Curr Opin Drug Discov Devel* 2010;13:31–40.
17. O'Reilly KE, Rojo F, She QB, et al. mTOR inhibition induces upstream receptor tyrosine kinase signaling and activates Akt. *Cancer Res* 2006;66:1500–1508.
18. Dang CV. MYC on the path to cancer. *Cell* 2012;149:22–35.
19. Collado M, Serrano M. Senescence in tumours: evidence from mice and humans. *Nat Rev Cancer* 2010;10:51–57.
20. Evan GI, d'Adda di Fagagna F. Cellular senescence: hot or what? *Curr Opin Genet Dev* 2009;19:25–31.
21. Lowe SW, Cepero E, Evan G. Intrinsic tumour suppression. *Nature* 2004;432:307–315.
22. Mooi WJ, Peeper DS. Oncogene-induced cell senescence—halting on the road to cancer. *N Engl J Med* 2006;355:1037–1046.
23. Burkhart DL, Sage J. Cellular mechanisms of tumour suppression by the retinoblastoma gene. *Nat Rev Cancer* 2008;8:671–682.
24. Deshpande A, Sicinski P, Hinds PW. Cyclins and cdks in development and cancer: a perspective. *Oncogene* 2005;24:2909–2915.
25. Sherr CJ, McCormick F. The RB and p53 pathways in cancer. *Cancer Cell* 2002;2:103–112.
26. Lipinski MM, Jacks T. The retinoblastoma gene family in differentiation and development. *Oncogene* 1999;18:7873–7882.
27. Ghebranious N, Donehower LA. Mouse models in tumor suppression. *Oncogene* 1998;17: 3385–3400.
28. McClatchey AI, Yap AS. Contact inhibition (of proliferation) redux. *Curr Opin Cell Biol* 2012;24:685–694.
29. Curto M, Cole BK, Lallemand D, et al. Contact-dependent inhibition of EGFR signaling by Nf2/Merlin. *J Cell Biol* 2007;177:893–903.
30. Okada T, Lopez-Lago M, Giancotti FG. Merlin/NF-2 mediates contact inhibition of growth by suppressing recruitment of Rac to the plasma membrane. *J Cell Biol* 2005;171:361–371.
31. Stamenkovic I, Yu Q. Merlin, a "magic" linker between the extracellular cues and intracellular signaling pathways that regulate cell motility, proliferation, and survival. *Curr Protein Pept Sci* 2010;11:471–484.
32. Pickup M, Novitskiv S, Moses HL. The roles of TGFβ in the tumour microenvironment. *Nat Rev Cancer* 2013;13:788–799.
33. Ikushima H, Miyazono K. TGFbeta signalling: a complex web in cancer progression. *Nat Rev Cancer* 2010;10:415–424.
34. Massagué J. TGF-beta in cancer. *Cell* 2008;134:215–230.
35. Bierie B, Moses HL. Tumour microenvironment: TGF-beta: the molecular Jekyll and Hyde of cancer. *Nat Rev Cancer* 2006;6:506–520.
36. Strasser A, Cory S, Adams JM. Deciphering the rules of programmed cell death to improve therapy of cancer and other diseases. *EMBO J* 2011;30:3667–3683.
37. Adams JM, Cory S. The Bcl-2 apoptotic switch in cancer development and therapy. *Oncogene* 2007;26:1324–1337.
38. Evan G, Littlewood T. A matter of life and cell death. *Science* 2004;281:1317–1322.
39. Willis SN, Adams JM. Life in the balance: how BH3-only proteins induce apoptosis. *Curr Opin Cell Biol* 2005;17:617–625.
40. Junttila MR, Evan GI. p53 — a jack of all trades but master of none. *Nat Rev Cancer* 2009;9:821–829.
41. White E. Deconvoluting the context-dependent role for autophagy in cancer. *Nat Rev Cancer* 2012;12:401–410.
42. Levine B, Kroemer G. Autophagy in the pathogenesis of disease. *Cell* 2008;132:27–42.
43. Mizushima N. Autophagy: process and function. *Genes Dev* 2007;21:2861–2873.
44. Sinha S, Levine B. The autophagy effector Beclin 1: a novel BH3-only protein. *Oncogene* 2008;27:S137–S148.
45. Mathew R, Karantza-Wadsworth V, White E. Role of autophagy in cancer. *Nat Rev Cancer* 2007;7:961–967.
46. White E, DiPaola RS. The double-edged sword of autophagy modulation in cancer. *Clin Cancer Res* 2009;15:5308–5316.
47. Apel A, Zentgraf H, Büchler MW, et al. Autophagy—A double-edged sword in oncology. *Int J Cancer* 2009;125:991–995.
48. Amaravadi RK, Thompson CB. The roles of therapy-induced autophagy and necrosis in cancer treatment. *Clin Cancer Res* 2007;13:7271–7279.
49. Lu Z, Luo RZ, Lu Y, et al. The tumor suppressor gene ARHI regulates autophagy and tumor dormancy in human ovarian cancer cells. *J Clin Invest* 2008;118:3917–3929.
50. Vanden Berghe T, Linkermann A, Jouan-Lanhouet S, et al. Regulated necrosis: the expanding network of non-apoptotic cell death pathways. *Nat Rev Mol Cell Biol* 2014;15:135–147.
51. Galluzzi L, Kroemer G. Necroptosis: a specialized pathway of programmed necrosis. *Cell* 2008;135:1161–1163.
52. Zong WX, Thompson CB. Necrotic death as a cell fate. *Genes Dev* 2006;20:1–15.
53. Grivennikov SI, Greten FR, Karin M. Immunity, inflammation, and cancer. *Cell* 2010;140:883–899.
54. White E, Karp C, Strohecker AM, et al. Role of autophagy in suppression of inflammation and cancer. *Curr Opin Cell Biol* 2010;22:212–217.
55. Blasco MA. Telomeres and human disease: ageing, cancer and beyond. *Nat Rev Genet* 2005;6:611–622.
56. Shay JW, Wright WE. Hayflick, his limit, and cellular ageing. *Nat Rev Mol Cell Biol* 2000;1:72–76.
57. Shay JW, Wright WE. Telomeres and telomerase in cancer. *Sem Cancer Biol* 2011;21:349–353.
58. Artandi SE, DePinho RA. Telomeres and telomerase in cancer. *Carcinogenesis* 2010;31:9–18.
59. Cesare AJ, Reddel RR. Alternative lengthening of telomeres: models, mechanisms and implications. *Nat Rev Genet* 2010;11:319–330.
60. Ince TA, Richardson AL, Bell GW, et al. Transformation of different human breast epithelial cell types leads to distinct tumor phenotypes. *Cancer Cell* 2007;12:160–170.
61. Passos JF, Saretzki G, von Zglinicki T. DNA damage in telomeres and mitochondria during cellular senescence: is there a connection? *Nucleic Acids Res* 2007;35:7505–7513.
62. Zhang H, Herbert BS, Pan KH, et al. Disparate effects of telomere attrition on gene expression during replicative senescence of human mammary epithelial cells cultured under different conditions. *Oncogene* 2004;23:6193–6198.
63. Sherr CJ, DePinho RA. Cellular senescence: mitotic clock or culture shock? *Cell* 2000;102:407–410.
64. Feldser DM, Greider CW. Short telomeres limit tumor progression in vivo by inducing senescence. *Cancer Cell* 2007;11:461–469.
65. Kawai T, Hiroi S, Nakanishi K, et al. Telomere length and telomerase expression in atypical adenomatous hyperplasia and small bronchioloalveolar carcinoma of the lung. *Am J Clin Pathol* 2007;127:254–262.

66. Hansel DE, Meeker AK, Hicks J. Telomere length variation in biliary tract metaplasia, dysplasia, and carcinoma. *Mod Pathol* 2006;19:772–779.
67. Artandi SE, DePinho RA. Mice without telomerase: what can they teach us about human cancer? *Nature Med* 2000;6:852–855.
68. Raynaud CM, Hernandez J, Llorca FP, et al. DNA damage repair and telomere length in normal breast, preneoplastic lesions, and invasive cancer. *Am J Clin Oncol* 2010;33:341–345.
69. Chin K, de Solorzano CO, Knowles D, et al. In situ analyses of genome instability in breast cancer. *Nature Genet* 2004;36:984–988.
70. Hanahan D, Folkman J. Patterns and emerging mechanisms of the angiogenic switch during tumorigenesis. *Cell* 1996;86:353–364.
71. Baeriswyl V, Christofori G. The angiogenic switch in carcinogenesis. *Semin Cancer Biol* 2009;19:329–337.
72. Bergers G, Benjamin LE. Tumorigenesis and the angiogenic switch. *Nat Rev Cancer* 2003;3:401–410.
73. Ferrara N. Vascular endothelial growth factor. *Arterioscler Thromb Vasc Biol* 2009;29:789–791.
74. Mac Gabhann F, Popel AS. Systems biology of vascular endothelial growth factors. *Microcirculation* 2008;15:715–738.
75. Carmeliet P. VEGF as a key mediator of angiogenesis in cancer. *Oncology* 2005;69:4–10.
76. Kessenbrock K, Plaks V, Werb Z. Matrix metalloproteinases: regulators of the tumor microenvironment. *Cell* 2010;141:52–67.
77. Kazerounian S, Yee KO, Lawler J. Thrombospondins in cancer. *Cell Mol Life Sci* 2008;65:700–712.
78. Nagy JA, Chang SH, Shih SC, et al. Heterogeneity of the tumor vasculature. *Semin Thromb Hemost* 2010;36:321–331.
79. Baluk P, Hashizume H, McDonald DM. Cellular abnormalities of blood vessels as targets in cancer. *Curr Opin Genet Dev* 2005;15:102–111.
80. Raica M, Cimpean AM, Ribatti D. Angiogenesis in pre-malignant conditions. *Eur J Cancer* 2009;45:1924–1934.
81. Olive KP, Jacobetz MA, Davidson CJ, et al. Inhibition of Hedgehog signaling enhances delivery of chemotherapy in a mouse model of pancreatic cancer. *Science* 2009;324:1457–1461.
82. Zee YK, O'Connor JP, Parker GJ, et al. Imaging angiogenesis of genitourinary tumors. *Nat Rev Urol* 2010;7:69–82.
83. Turner HE, Harris AL, Melmed S, et al. Angiogenesis in endocrine tumors. *Endocr Rev* 2003;24:600–632.
84. Xie L, Duncan MB, Pahler J, et al. Counterbalancing angiogenic regulatory factors control the rate of cancer progression and survival in a stage-specific manner. *Proc Natl Acad Sci U S A* 2011;108:9939–9944.
85. Ribatti D. Endogenous inhibitors of angiogenesis: a historical review. *Leuk Res* 2009;33:638–644.
86. Folkman J. Angiogenesis. *Annu Rev Med* 2006;57:1–18.
87. Folkman J. Role of angiogenesis in tumor growth and metastasis. *Semin Oncol* 2002;29:15–18.
88. Nyberg P, Xie L, Kalluri R. Endogenous inhibitors of angiogenesis. *Cancer Res* 2005;65:3967–3979.
89. Cao Y. Adipose tissue angiogenesis as a therapeutic target for obesity and metabolic diseases. *Nat Rev Drug Discov* 2010;9:107–115.
90. Seppinen L, Sormunen R, Soini Y, et al. Lack of collagen XVIII accelerates cutaneous wound healing, while overexpression of its endostatin domain leads to delayed healing. *Matrix Biol* 2008;27:535–546.
91. Raza A, Franklin MJ, Dudek AZ. Pericytes and vessel maturation during tumor angiogenesis and metastasis. *Am J Hematol* 2010;85:593–598.
92. Kovacic JC, Boehm M. Resident vascular progenitor cells: an emerging role for non-terminally differentiated vessel-resident cells in vascular biology. *Stem Cell Res* 2009;2:2–15.
93. Bergers G, Song S. The role of pericytes in blood-vessel formation and maintenance. *Neuro Oncol* 2005;7:452–464.
94. Qian BZ, Pollard JW. Macrophage diversity enhances tumor progression and metastasis. *Cell* 2010;141:39–51.
95. Zumsteg A, Christofori G. Corrupt policemen: inflammatory cells promote tumor angiogenesis. *Curr Opin Oncol* 2009;21:60–70.
96. Murdoch C, Muthana M, Coffelt SB, et al. The role of myeloid cells in the promotion of tumour angiogenesis. *Nat Rev Cancer* 2008;8:618–631.
97. De Palma M, Murdoch C, Venneri MA, et al. Tie2-expressing monocytes: regulation of tumor angiogenesis and therapeutic implications. *Trends Immunol* 2007;28:519–524.
98. Ferrara N. Pathways mediating VEGF-independent tumor angiogenesis. *Cytokine Growth Factor Rev* 2010;21:21–26.
99. Patenaude A, Parker J, Karsan A. Involvement of endothelial progenitor cells in tumor vascularization. *Microvasc Res* 2010;79:217–223.
100. Lamagna C, Bergers G. The bone marrow constitutes a reservoir of pericyte progenitors. *J Leukoc Biol* 2006;80:677–681.
101. Talmadge JE, Fidler IJ. AACR centennial series: the biology of cancer metastasis: historical perspective. *Cancer Res* 2010;70:5649–5669.
102. Fidler IJ. The pathogenesis of cancer metastasis: the "seed and soil" hypothesis revisited. *Nat Rev Cancer* 2003;3:453–458.
103. Berx G, van Roy F. Involvement of members of the cadherin superfamily in cancer. *Cold Spring Harb Perspect Biol* 2009;1:a003129.
104. Cavallaro U, Christofori G. Cell adhesion and signaling by cadherins and Ig-CAMs in cancer. *Nat Rev Cancer* 2004;4:118–132.
105. De Craene B, Berx G. Regulatory networks defining EMT during cancer initiation and progression. *Nat Rev Cancer* 2013;13:97–110.
106. Klymkowsky MW, Savagner P. Epithelial-mesenchymal transition: a cancer researcher's conceptual friend and foe. *Am J Pathol* 2009;174:1588–1592.
107. Polyak K, Weinberg RA. Transitions between epithelial and mesenchymal states: acquisition of malignant and stem cell traits. *Nat Rev Cancer* 2009;9:265–273.
108. Thiery JP, Acloque H, Huang RY, et al. Epithelial-mesenchymal transitions in development and disease. *Cell* 2009;139:871–890.
109. Yilmaz M, Christofori G. EMT, the cytoskeleton, and cancer cell invasion. *Cancer Metastasis Rev* 2009;28:15–33.
110. Barrallo-Gimeno A, Nieto MA. The Snail genes as inducers of cell movement and survival: implications in development and cancer. *Development* 2005;132:3151–3161.
111. Micalizzi DS, Farabaugh SM, Ford HL. Epithelial-mesenchymal transition in cancer: parallels between normal development and tumor progression. *J Mammary Gland Biol Neoplasia* 2010;15:117–134.
112. Taube JH, Herschkowitz JI, Komurov K, et al. Core epithelial-to-mesenchymal transition interactome gene-expression signature is associated with claudin-low and metaplastic breast cancer subtypes. *Proc Natl Acad Sci U S A* 2010; 107:15449–15454.
113. Schmalhofer O, Brabletz S, Brabletz T. E-cadherin, beta-catenin, and ZEB1 in malignant progression of cancer. *Cancer Metastasis Rev* 2009;28:151–166.
114. Yang J, Weinberg RA. Epithelial-mesenchymal transition: at the crossroads of development and tumor metastasis. *Develop Cell* 2008;14:818–829.
115. Peinado H, Marin F, Cubillo E, et al. Snail and E47 repressors of E-cadherin induce distinct invasive and angiogenic properties in vivo. *J Cell Sci* 2004;117: 2827–2839.
116. Karnoub AE, Weinberg RA. Chemokine networks and breast cancer metastasis. *Breast Dis* 2006;26:75–85.
117. Brabletz T, Jung A, Reu S, et al. Variable beta-catenin expression in colorectal cancers indicates tumor progression driven by the tumor environment. *Proc Natl Acad Sci U S A* 2001;98:10356–10361.
118. Hlubek F, Brabletz T, Budczies J, et al. Heterogeneous expression of Wnt/beta-catenin target genes within colorectal cancer. *Int J Cancer* 2007;121: 1941–1948.
119. Egeblad M, Nakasone ES, Werb Z. Tumors as organs: complex tissues that interface with the entire organism. *Dev Cell* 2010;18:884–901.
120. Joyce JA, Pollard JW. Microenvironmental regulation of metastasis. *Nat Rev Cancer* 2009;9:239–252.
121. Kalluri R, Zeisberg M. Fibroblasts in cancer. *Nat Rev Cancer* 2006;6: 392–401.
122. Karnoub AE, Dash AB, Vo AP, et al. Mesenchymal stem cells within tumour stroma promote breast cancer metastasis. *Nature* 2007;449:557–563.
123. Li HJ, Reinhart F, Herschman HR, et al. Cancer-stimulated mesenchymal stem cells create a carcinoma stem cell niche via prostaglandin E2 signaling. *Cancer Discov* 2012;2:840–855.
124. Palermo C, Joyce JA. Cysteine cathepsin proteases as pharmacological targets in cancer. *Trends Pharmacol Sci* 2008;29:22–28.
125. Mohamed MM, Sloane BF. Cysteine cathepsins: multifunctional enzymes in cancer. *Nat Rev Cancer* 2006;6:764–775.
126. Gocheva V, Wang HW, Gadea BB, et al. IL-4 induces cathepsin protease activity in tumor-associated macrophages to promote cancer growth and invasion. *Genes Dev* 2010;24:241–255.
127. Wyckoff JB, Wang Y, Lin EY, et al. Direct visualization of macrophage-assisted tumor cell intravasation in mammary tumors. *Cancer Res* 2007;67: 2649–2656.
128. Hugo H, Ackland ML, Blick T, et al. Epithelial-mesenchymal and mesenchymal-epithelial transitions in carcinoma progression. *J Cell Physiol* 2007;213:374–383.
129. Friedl P, Wolf K. Plasticity of cell migration: a multiscale tuning model. *J Cell Biol* 2009;188:11–19.
130. Friedl P, Wolf K. Tube travel: the role of proteases in individual and collective cancer cell invasion. *Cancer Res* 2008;68:7247–7249.
131. Madsen CD, Sahai E. Cancer dissemination—lessons from leukocytes. *Dev Cell* 2010;19:13–26.
132. Sabeh F, Shimizu-Hirota R, Weiss SJ. Protease-dependent versus-independent cancer cell invasion programs: three-dimensional amoeboid movement revisited. *J Cell Biol* 2009;185:11–19.
133. Quail DF, Joyce JA. Microenvironmental regulation of tumor progression and metastasis. *Nat Med* 2013;19:1423–1437.
134. McGowan PM, Kirstein JM, Chambers AF. Micrometastatic disease and metastatic outgrowth: clinical issues and experimental approaches. *Future Oncol* 2009;5:1083–1098.
135. Aguirre-Ghiso JA. Models, mechanisms and clinical evidence for cancer dormancy. *Nat Rev Cancer* 2007;7:834–846.
136. Townson JL, Chambers AF. Dormancy of solitary metastatic cells. *Cell Cycle* 2006;5:1744–1750.
137. Demicheli R, Retsky MW, Hrushesky WJ, et al. The effects of surgery on tumor growth: a century of investigations. *Ann Oncol* 2008;19:1821–1828.
138. Barkan D, Green JE, Chambers AF. Extracellular matrix: a gatekeeper in the transition from dormancy to metastatic growth. *Eur J Cancer* 2010;46: 1181–1188.
139. Gupta GP, Minn AJ, Kang,Y, et al. Identifying site-specific metastasis genes and functions. *Cold Spring Harb Symp Quant Biol* 2005;70:149–158.
140. Naumov GN, Folkman J, Straume O, et al. Tumor-vascular interactions and tumor dormancy. *APMIS* 2008;116:569–585.

141. Kenific CM, Thorburn A, Debnath J. Autophagy and metastasis: another double-edged sword. *Curr Opin Cell Biol* 2010;22:241–245.
142. Teng MW, Swann JB, Koebel CM, et al. Immune-mediated dormancy: an equilibrium with cancer. *J Leukoc Biol* 2008;84:988–993.
143. Campbell PJ, Yachida S, Mudie LJ, et al. The patterns and dynamics of genomic instability in metastatic pancreatic cancer. *Nature* 2010;467:1109–1113.
144. Luebeck EG. Cancer: genomic evolution of metastasis. *Nature* 2010;467: 1053–1055.
145. Yachida S, Jones S, Bozic I, et al. Distant metastasis occurs late during the genetic evolution of pancreatic cancer. *Nature* 2010;467:1114–1117.
146. Coghlin C, Murray GI. Current and emerging concepts in tumour metastasis. *J Pathol* 2010;222:1–15.
147. Klein CA. Parallel progression of primary tumours and metastases. *Nat Rev Cancer* 2009;9:302–312.
148. Gerhardt H, Semb H. Pericytes: gatekeepers in tumour cell metastasis? *J Mol Med* 2008;86:135–144.
149. Kim MY, Oskarsson T, Acharyya S, et al. Tumor self-seeding by circulating cancer cells. *Cell* 2009;139:1315–1326.
150. Bos PD, Zhang XH, Nadal C, et al. Genes that mediate breast cancer metastasis to the brain. *Nature* 2009;459:1005–1009.
151. Olson P, Lu J, Zhang H, et al. MicroRNA dynamics in the stages of tumorigenesis correlate with hallmark capabilities of cancer. *Genes Dev* 2009;23: 2152–2165.
152. Nguyen DX, Bos PD, Massagué J. Metastasis: from dissemination to organ-specific colonization. *Nat Rev Cancer* 2009;9:274–284.
153. Warburg OH. *The Metabolism of Tumours: Investigations from the Kaiser Wilhelm Institute for Biology, Berlin-Dahlem.* London, UK: Arnold Constable; 1930.
154. Warburg O. On the origin of cancer cells. *Science* 1956;123:309–314.
155. Warburg O. On respiratory impairment in cancer cells. *Science* 1956;124: 269–270.
156. Jones RG, Thompson CB. Tumor suppressors and cell metabolism: a recipe for cancer growth. *Genes Dev* 2009;23:537–548.
157. DeBerardinis RJ, Lum JJ, Hatzivassiliou G, et al. The biology of cancer: metabolic reprogramming fuels cell growth and proliferation. *Cell Metab* 2008;7:11–20.
158. Hsu PP, Sabatini DM. Cancer cell metabolism: Warburg and beyond. *Cell* 2008;134:703–707.
159. Ward PS, Thompson CB. Metabolic reprogramming: a cancer hallmark even warburg did not anticipate. *Cancer Cell* 2012;21:297–308.
160. Semenza GL. HIF-1: upstream and downstream of cancer metabolism. *Curr Opin Genet Dev* 2010;20:51–56.
161. Semenza GL. Defining the role of hypoxia-inducible factor 1 in cancer biology and therapeutics. *Oncogene* 2010;29:625–634.
162. Kroemer G, Pouyssegur J. Tumor cell metabolism: cancer's Achilles' heel. *Cancer Cell* 2008;13:472–482.
163. Potter V. The biochemical approach to the cancer problem. *Fed Proc* 1958; 17:691–697.
164. Vander Heiden MG, Cantley LC, Thompson CB. Understanding the Warburg effect: the metabolic requirements of cell proliferation. *Science* 2009; 324:1029–1033.
165. Semenza GL. Tumor metabolism: cancer cells give and take lactate. *J Clin Invest* 2008;118:3835–3837.
166. Nakajima EC, Van Houten B. Metabolic symbiosis in cancer: refocusing the Warburg lens. *Mol Carcinog* 2013;52:329–337.
167. Kennedy KM, Dewhirst MW. Tumor metabolism of lactate: the influence and therapeutic potential for MCT and CD147 regulation. *Future Oncol* 2010;6:127–148.
168. Feron O. Pyruvate into lactate and back: from the Warburg effect to symbiotic energy fuel exchange in cancer cells. *Radiother Oncol* 2009;92:329–333.
169. Magistretti PJ. Neuron-glia metabolic coupling and plasticity. *J Exp Biol* 2006;209:2304–2311.
170. Hardee ME, Dewhirst MW, Agarwal N, et al. Novel imaging provides new insights into mechanisms of oxygen transport in tumors. *Curr Mol Med* 2009;9:435–441.
171. Burnet FM. The concept of immunological surveillance. *Prog Exp Tumor Res* 1970;13:1–27.
172. Thomas L. On immuosurveillance in human cancer. *Yale J Biol Med* 1982;55:329–333.
173. Vajdic CM, van Leeuwen MT. Cancer incidence and risk factors after solid organ transplantation. *Int J Cancer* 2009;125:1747–1754.
174. Elinav E, Nowarski R, Thaiss CA, et al. Inflammation-induced cancer: crosstalk between tumours, immune cells and microorganisms. *Nat Rev Cancer* 2013;13:759–771.
175. Swann JB, Smyth MJ. Immune surveillance of tumors. *J Clin Invest* 2007;117: 1137–1146.
176. Fridman WH, Mlecnik B, Bindea G, et al. Immunosurveillance in human non-viral cancers. *Curr Opin Immunol* 2011;23:272–278.
177. Galon J, Angell HK, Bedognetti D, et al. The continuum of cancer immunosurveillance: prognostic, predictive, and mechanistic signatures. *Immunity* 2013;39:11–26.
178. Kim R, Emi M, Tanabe K. Cancer immunoediting from immune surveillance to immune escape. *Immunology* 2007;121:1–14.
179. Smyth MJ, Dunn GP, Schreiber RD. Cancer immunosurveillance and immune-editing: the roles of immunity in suppressing tumor development and shaping tumor immunogenicity. *Adv Immunol* 2006;90:1–50.
180. Bindea G, Mlecnik B, Fridman WH, et al. Natural immunity to cancer in humans. *Curr Opin Immunol* 2010;22:215–222.
181. Ferrone C, Dranoff G. Dual roles for immunity in gastrointestinal cancers. *J Clin Oncol* 2010;28:4045–4051.
182. Nelson BH. The impact of T-cell immunity on ovarian cancer outcomes. *Immunol Rev* 2008;222:101–116.
183. Pagès F, Galon J, Dieu-Nosjean MC, et al. Immune infiltration in human tumors: a prognostic factor that should not be ignored. *Oncogene* 2010;29: 1093–1102.
184. Strauss DC, Thomas JM. Transmission of donor melanoma by organ transplantation. *Lancet Oncol* 2010;11:790–796.
185. Yang L, Pang Y, Moses HL. TGF-beta and immune cells: an important regulatory axis in the tumor microenvironment and progression. *Trends Immunol* 2010;31:220 –227.
186. Shields JD, Kourtis IC, Tomei AA, et al. Induction of lymphoidlike stroma and immune escape by tumors that express the chemokine CCL21. *Science* 2010;328:749–752.
187. Korman AJ, Peggs KS, Allison J. Checkpoint blockade in cancer immunotherapy. *Adv Immunol* 2006;90:297–339.
188. Fife BT, Pauken KE, Eagar TN, et al. Interactions between programmed death-1 and programmed death ligand-1 promote tolerance by blocking the T cell receptor-induced stop signal. *Nat Immunol* 2009;10:1185–1192.
189. Pardoll DM. The blockade of immune checkpoints in cancer immunotherapy. *Nat Rev Cancer* 2012;12:252–264.
190. Motz GT, Coukos G. Deciphering and reversing tumor immune suppression. *Immunity* 2013;39:61–73.
191. Gabrilovich DI, Nagaraj S. Myeloid-derived suppressor cells as regulators of the immune system. *Nat Rev Immunol* 2009;9:162–174.
192. Mougiakakos D, Choudhury A, Lladser A, et al. Regulatory T cells in cancer. *Adv Cancer Res* 2010;107:57–117.
193. Ostrand-Rosenberg S, Sinha P. Myeloid-derived suppressor cells: linking inflammation and cancer. *J Immunol* 2009;182:4499–4506.
194. Garraway LA, Lander ES. Lessons from the cancer genome. *Cell* 2013;153: 17–37.
195. You JS, Jones PA. Cancer genetics and epigenetics: two sides of the same coin? *Cancer Cell* 2012;22:9–20.
196. Berdasco M, Esteller M. Aberrant epigenetic landscape in cancer: how cellular identity goes awry. *Dev Cell* 2010;19:698–711.
197. Esteller M. Cancer epigenomics: DNA methylomes and histone-modification maps. *Nat Rev Genet* 2007;8:286–298.
198. Jones PA, Baylin SB. The epigenomics of cancer. *Cell* 2007;128:683–692.
199. Negrini S, Gorgoulis VG, Halazoneitis TD. Genomic instability—an evolving hallmark of cancer. *Nat Rev Mol Cell Bio* 2010;11:220–228.
200. Loeb LA. A mutator phenotype in cancer. *Cancer Res* 2001;61:3230–3239.
201. Jackson SP, Bartek J. The DNA-damage response in human biology and disease. *Nature* 2009;461:1071–1078.
202. Kastan MB. DNA damage responses: mechanisms and roles in human disease. *Mol Cancer Res* 2008;6:517–524.
203. Sigal A, Rotter V. Oncogenic mutations of the p53 tumor suppressor: the demons of the guardian of the genome. *Cancer Res* 2000;60:6788–6793.
204. Lane DP. Cancer. p53, guardian of the genome. *Nature* 1992;358:15–16.
205. Kinzler KW, Vogelstein B. Cancer-susceptibility genes. Gatekeepers and caretakers. *Nature* 1997;386:761–763.
206. Ciccia A, Elledge SJ. The DNA damage response: making it safe to play with knives. *Mol Cell* 2010;40:179–204.
207. Harper JW, Elledge SJ. The DNA damage response: ten years after. *Mol Cell* 2007;28:739–745.
208. Friedberg EC, Aguilera A, Gellert M, et al. DNA repair: from molecular mechanism to human disease. *DNA Repair (Amst)* 2006;5:986–996.
209. Barnes DE, Lindahl T. Repair and genetic consequences of endogenous DNA base damage in mammalian cells. *Annu Rev Genet* 2004;38:445–476.
210. Korkola J, Gray JW. Breast cancer genomes—form and function. *Curr Opin Genet Dev* 2010;20:4–14.
211. Dvorak HF. Tumors: wounds that do not heal. Similarities between tumor stroma generation and wound healing. *N Engl J Med* 1986;315:1650–1659.
212. De Nardo DG, Andreu P, Coussens LM. Interactions between lymphocytes and myeloid cells regulate pro- versus anti-tumor immunity. *Cancer Metastasis Rev* 2010;29:309–316.
213. Hanahan D, Coussens LM. Accessories to the crime: functions of cells recruited to the tumor microenvironment. *Cancer Cell* 2012;21:309–322.
214. de Visser KE, Eichten A, Coussens LM. Paradoxical roles of the immune system during cancer development. *Nat Rev Cancer* 2006;6:24–37.
215. Servais C, Erez N. From sentinel cells to inflammatory culprits: cancer-associated fibroblasts in tumour-related inflammation. *J Pathol* 2013;229: 198–207.
216. Dirat B, Bochet L, Escourrou G, et al. Unraveling the obesity and breast cancer links: a role for cancer-associated adipocytes? *Endocr Dev* 2010;19:45–52.
217. Pietras K, Ostman A. Hallmarks of cancer: interactions with the tumor stroma. *Exp Cell Res* 2010;316:1324–1331.
218. Räsänen K, Vaheri A. Activation of fibroblasts in cancer stroma. *Exp Cell Res* 2010;316:2713–2722.
219. Shimoda M, Mellody KT, Orimo A. Carcinoma-associated fibroblasts are a rate-limiting determinant for tumour progression. *Sem Cell Dev Biol* 2010;21:19–25.
220. Welti J, Loges S, Dimmeler S, et al. Recent molecular discoveries in angiogenesis and antiangiogenic therapies in cancer. *J Clin Invest* 2013;123:3190–3200.

221. Pasquale EB. Eph receptors and ephrins in cancer: bidirectional signalling and beyond. *Nat Rev Cancer* 2010;10:165–180.
222. Ahmed Z, Bicknell R. Angiogenic signalling pathways. *Methods Mol Biol* 2009;467:3–24.
223. Dejana E, Orsenigo F, Molendini C, et al. Organization and signaling of endothelial cell-to-cell junctions in various regions of the blood and lymphatic vascular trees. *Cell Tissue Res* 2009;335:17–25.
224. Carmeliet P, Jain RK. Angiogenesis in cancer and other diseases. *Nature* 2000;407:249–257.
225. Ruoslahti E, Bhatia SN, Sailor MJ. Targeting of drugs and nanoparticles to tumors. *J Cell Biol* 2010;188:759–768.
226. Ruoslahti E. Specialization of tumour vasculature. *Nat Rev Cancer* 2002;2: 83–90.
227. Motz GT, Coukos G. The parallel lives of angiogenesis and immunosuppression: cancer and other tales. *Nat Rev Immunol* 2011;11:702–711.
228. Carmeliet P, Jain RK. Principles and mechanisms of vessel normalization for cancer and other angiogenic diseases. *Nat Rev Drug Discov* 2011;10: 417–427.
229. Tammela T, Alitalo K. Lymphangiogenesis: Molecular mechanisms and future promise. *Cell* 2010;140:460–476.
230. Card CM, Yu SS, Swartz MA. Emerging roles of lymphatic endothelium in regulating adaptive immunity. *J Clin Invest* 2014;124:943–952.
231. Gaengel K, Genové G, Armulik A, et al. Endothelial-mural cell signaling in vascular development and angiogenesis. *Arterioscler Thromb Vasc Biol* 2009;29:630–638.
232. Schäfer M, Werner S. Cancer as an overhealing wound: an old hypothesis revisited. *Nat Rev Mol Cell Biol* 2008;9:628–638.
233. Karin M, Lawrence T, Nizet V. Innate immunity gone awry: linking microbial infections to chronic inflammation and cancer. *Cell* 2006;124:823–835.
234. Coffeldt SB, Lewis CE, Naldini L, et al. Elusive identities and overlapping phenotypes of proangiogenic myeloid cells in tumors. *Am J Pathol* 2010;176: 1564–1576.
235. Johansson M, Denardo DG, Coussens LM. Polarized immune responses differentially regulate cancer development. *Immunol Rev* 2008;222:145–154.
236. Mantovani A. Molecular pathways linking inflammation and cancer. *Curr Mol Med* 2010;10:369–373.
237. Mantovani A, Allavena P, Sica A, et al. Cancer-related inflammation. *Nature* 2008;454:436–444
238. DeNardo DG, Brennan DJ, Rexhepaj E, et al. Leukocyte complexity predicts breast cancer survival and functionally regulates response to chemotherapy. *Cancer Discov* 2011;1:54–67.
239. De Palma M, Coukos G, Hanahan D. A new twist on radiation oncology: low-dose irradiation elicits immunostimulatory macrophages that unlock barriers to tumor immunotherapy. *Cancer Cell* 2013;24:559–561.
240. Koh BI, Kang Y. The pro-metastatic role of bone marrow-derived cells: a focus on MSCs and regulatory T cells. *EMBO Rep* 2012;13:412–422.
241. Bergfeld SA, DeClerck YA. Bone marrow-derived mesenchymal stem cells and the tumor microenvironment. *Cancer Metastasis Rev* 2010;29:249–261.
242. Fang S, Salven P. Stem cells in tumor angiogenesis. *J Mol Cell Cardiol* 2011;50:290–295.
243. Giaccia AJ, Schipani E. Role of carcinoma-associated fibroblasts and hypoxia in tumor progression. *Curr Top Microbiol Immunol* 2010;345:31–45.
244. Labelle M, Hynes RO. The initial hours of metastasis: the importance of cooperative host-tumor cell interactions during hematogenous dissemination. *Cancer Discov* 2012;2:1091–1099.
245. Peinado H, Lavothskin S, Lyden D. The secreted factors responsible for pre-metastatic niche formation: old sayings and new thoughts. *Semin Cancer Biol* 2011;21:139–146.
246. Reya T, Morrison SJ, Clarke MF, et al. Stem cells, cancer, and cancer stem cells. *Nature* 2001;414:105–111.
247. Bonnet D, Dick JE. Human acute myeloid leukemia is organized as a hierarchy that originates from a primitive hematopoietic cell. *Nature Med* 1997;3: 730–737.
248. Gilbertson RJ, Rich JN. Making a tumour's bed: glioblastoma stem cells and the vascular niche. *Nat Rev Cancer* 2007;7:733–736.
249. al-Hajj M, Wicha M, Benito-Hernandez A, et al. Prospective identification of tumorigenic breast cancer cells. *Proc Natl Acad Sci U S A* 2003;100:3983–3988.
250. Beck B, Blanpain C. Unravelling cancer stem cell potential. *Nat Rev Cancer* 2013;13:727–738.
251. Magee JA, Piskounova E, Morrison SJ. Cancer stem cells: impact, heterogeneity, and uncertainty. *Cancer Cell* 2012;21:283–296.
252. Cho RW, Clarke MF. Recent advances in cancer stem cells. *Curr Opin Genet Devel* 2008;18:1–6.
253. Lobo NA, Shimono Y, Qian D, et al. The biology of cancer stem cells. *Annu Rev Cell Dev Biol* 2007;23:675–699.
254. Meacham CE, Morrison SJ. Tumour heterogeneity and cancer cell plasticity. *Nature* 2013;501:328–337.
255. Singh A, Settleman J. EMT, cancer stem cells and drug resistance: an emerging axis of evil in the war on cancer. *Oncogene* 2010;29:4741–4751.
256. Brabletz T, Jung A, Spaderna S, et al. Opinion: migrating cancer stem cells – an integrated concept of malignant tumor progression. *Nat Rev Cancer* 2005;5:744–749.
257. Boiko AD, Razorenova OV, van de Rijn M, et al. Human melanoma-initiating cells express neural crest nerve growth factor receptor CD271. *Nature* 2010;466:133–137.
258. Gupta P, Chaffer CL, Weinberg RA. Cancer stem cells: mirage or reality? *Nature Med* 2009;15:1010–1012.
259. Quintana E, Shackleton M, Sabel MS, et al. Efficient tumour formation by single human melanoma cells. *Nature* 2008;456:593–598.
260. Chaffer CL, Brueckmann I, Scheel C, et al. Normal and neoplastic nonstem cells can spontaneously convert to stem-like state. *Proc Natl Acad Sci U S A* 2011;108:7950–7955.
261. Thiery JP, Sleeman JR. Complex networks orchestrate epithelial-mesenchymal transitions. *Nat Rev Mol Cell Biol* 2006;7:131–142.
262. Creighton CJ, Li X, Landis M, et al. Residual breast cancers after conventional therapy display mesenchymal as well as tumor-initiating features. *Proc Natl Acad Sci U S A* 2009;106:13820–13825.
263. Buck E, Eyzaguirre A, Barr S, et al. Loss of homotypic cell adhesion by epithelial-mesenchymal transition or mutation limits sensitivity to epidermal growth factor receptor inhibition. *Mol Cancer Therap* 2007;6:532–541.
264. Rhim AD, Mirek ET, Aiello NM, et al. EMT and dissemination precede pancreatic tumor formation. *Cell* 2012;148:349–361.
265. Soda Y, Marumoto T, Friedmann-Morvinski D, et al. Transdifferentiation of glioblastoma cells into vascular endothelial cells. *Proc Natl Acad Sci U S A* 2011;108:4274–4280.
266. El Hallani S, Boisselier B, Peglion F, et al. A new alternative mechanism in glioblastoma vascularization: tubular vasculogenic mimicry. *Brain* 2010;133: 973–982.
267. Wang R, Chadalavada K, Wilshire J, et al. Glioblastoma stem-like cells give rise to tumour endothelium. *Nature* 2010;468:829–833.
268. Folkman J, Kalluri R. Cancer without disease. *Nature* 2004;427:787.
269. Azam F, Mehta S, Harris AL. Mechanisms of resistance to antiangiogenesis therapy. *Eur J Cancer* 2010;46:1323–1332.
270. Ebos JM, Lee CR, Kerbel RS. Tumor and host-mediated pathways of resistance and disease progression in response to antiangiogenic therapy. *Clin Cancer Res* 2009;15:5020–5025.
271. Bergers G, Hanahan D. Modes of resistance to anti-angiogenic therapy. *Nat Rev Cancer* 2008;8:592–603.
272. Ellis LM, Reardon DA. Cancer: the nuances of therapy. *Nature* 2009;458: 290–292.
273. Norden AD, Drappatz J, Wen PY. Antiangiogenic therapies for high-grade glioma. *Nat Rev Neurol* 2009;5:610–620.
274. Verhoeff JJ, van Tellingen O, Claes A, et al. Concerns about anti-angiogenic treatment in patients with glioblastoma multiforme. *BMC Cancer* 2009; 9:444.
275. Hanahan D. Rethinking the war on cancer. *Lancet* 2014;383:558–563.
276. Pencheva N, Tavazoie SF. Control of metastatic progression by microRNA regulatory networks. *Nat Cell Biol* 2013;15:546–554.
277. Garzon R, Marcucci G, Croce CM. Targeting microRNAs in cancer: rationale, strategies and challenges. *Nat Rev Drug Discov* 2010;9:775–789.

3 Molecular Methods in Cancer

Larissa V. Furtado, Jay L. Hess, and Bryan L. Betz

APPLICATIONS OF MOLECULAR DIAGNOSTICS IN ONCOLOGY

Molecular diagnostics is increasingly impacting a number of areas of cancer care delivery including diagnosis, prognosis, in predicting response to particular therapies, and in minimal residual disease monitoring. Each of these depends on detection or measurement of one or more disease-specific molecular biomarkers representing abnormalities in genetic or epigenetic pathways controlling cellular proliferation, differentiation, or cell death (Table 3.1). In addition, molecular diagnostics is beginning to play a role in predicting host metabolism of drugs—for example, in predicting fast versus slow thiopurine metabolizers using polymorphisms in the thiopurine methyltransferase (TPMT) allele and in use in dosing patients with thiopurine drugs.[1] Molecular diagnostics has also had a major impact on assessing an engraftment after bone marrow transplantation and in tissue typing for bone marrow and solid organ transplantation.

The ideal cancer biomarker is only associated with the disease and not the normal state. The utility of the biomarker largely depends on what the clinical effect the biomarker predicts for, how large the effect is, and how strong the evidence is for the effect. For clinical application, biomarkers need a high level of *analytic validity*, *clinical validity*, and *clinical utility*. Analytic validity refers to the ability of the overall testing process to accurately detect and, in many cases, measure the biomarker. Clinical validity is the ability of a biomarker to predict a particular disease behavior or response to therapy. Clinical utility, arguably the most difficult to assess, addresses whether the information available from the biomarker is actually beneficial for patient care.

Biomarkers can take many forms including *chromosomal translocations* and *other chromosomal rearrangements*, *gene amplification*, *copy number variation*, *point mutations*, *single nucleotide polymorphisms*, *changes in gene expression* (including micro RNAs), and *epigenetic alterations*. Most biomarkers in widespread use represent either gain of function or loss of function alterations in key signaling pathways. Those that occur early and at a high frequency in tumors tend to be *driver mutations*, whose function is important for the cancer cell's proliferation and/or survival. These are particularly useful as biomarkers because they often represent important therapeutic targets. However, cancer cells accumulate many genetic alterations, called *passenger mutations*, which tend to occur at a lower frequency overall and in a subset of a heterogeneous population of tumor cells that may contribute to the cancer phenotype but are not absolutely essential.[2] Distinguishing passenger from driver mutations using various functional assays has become a major focus of translational research in cancer. The same biomarker may have utility in a variety of settings. For example, the detection of the *BCR-ABL1* translocation, pathognomonic for chronic myelogenous leukemia (CML), is used for establishing the diagnosis, for the selection of therapy, and for monitoring for minimal residual disease during and after therapy.

Some of the most heavily used genetic biomarkers in cancer, particularly in hematologic malignancies, are *chromosomal translocations*. For certain diseases such as CML, detection of the *BCR-ABL1* translocation or in Burkitt lymphoma the immunoglobulin gene-*MYC* translocation is required, according to current World Health Organization (WHO) guidelines, to make the diagnosis. Identification of translocations is important in the diagnosis and subtyping of acute leukemias (e.g., detection of *PML-RARA* and variant translocations in acute promyelocytic leukemia) and is also extremely important for the diagnosis of sarcomas such as Ewing sarcoma. The discovery of chromosomal translocations, such as the *TMPRSS-ETS* in prostate cancer and *ALK* translocations in non–small-cell lung cancer, portends an importance of detecting translocations in solid tumors.[3] Chromosomal translocations, especially for hematologic malignancies, have been traditionally detected by classical karyotyping. This approach has limitations; in particular, it requires viable, dividing cells, which are often not readily available from solid tumor biopsies. In addition, a significant proportion of chromosomal translocations are not detectable by conventional karyotyping. For example, 5% to 10% of CML cases lack detectable t(9;22) by G banding. Such "cryptic" translocations require other approaches for detection, which are to be discussed, including *fluorescent in situ hybridization (FISH)*, *polymerase chain reaction (PCR)*, as well as *nucleic acid sequencing-based methods*.

In certain settings, it can be helpful to detect if a population of cells is clonal. For example, in some lymphoid infiltrates, the cells are well differentiated and it can be difficult to determine whether these represent a reactive or neoplastic infiltrate. If dispersed, cells are available and these could be analyzed by flow cytometer to detect whether a monotypic population expressing either immunoglobulin kappa or lambda light chains is present. In theory, immunohistochemical staining (IHC) for immunoglobulin light chains could be used to assess clonality; however, in practice this is done with more sensitivity using RNA in situ hybridization for immunoglobulin kappa and lambda light chain transcripts. The most sensitive way to detect clonality in a B-cell population is to analyze the size of the break point cluster region that arises as a result of VDJ recombination by *PCR*. Reactive B cells will show a distribution in the size of the VDJ recombination for the *IGH* or *IGK* or *IGL*, whereas clonal cells will show a predominant band that represents the size of the VDJ region of the dominant clone. Similarly, sometimes it can be difficult to distinguish neoplastic from reactive T-cell infiltrates. Given the large number of T-cell antigen receptors, it is not as simple to detect clonality by IHC or flow cytometry in T-cell proliferations. One approach is to use aberrant loss of T-cell antigen expression to aid in the diagnosis of T-cell neoplasms. Another is to detect clonal rearrangement of the VDJ region of the T-cell receptor gamma (*TCRγ*) gene, which can be done by PCR on both fresh and formalin-fixed paraffin-embedded (FFPE) tissue.

Gene amplification is another important mechanism in cancer that has been found to have high utility in a subset of cancers. *MYCN* amplification occurs in approximately 40% of undifferentiated or poorly differentiated neuroblastoma subtypes,[4,5] either appearing as double minute chromosomes or homogeneously

TABLE 3.1

Genomic Alterations as Putative Predictive Biomarkers for Cancer Therapy

Genes	Pathways	Aberration Type	Disease Examples	Putative or Proven Drugs
PIK3CA,[51,52] *PIK3R1*,[53] *PIK3R2*, *AKT1*, *AKT2*, and *AKT3*[54,55]	Phosphoinositide 3-kinase (PI3K)	Mutation or amplification	Breast, colorectal, and endometrial cancer	■ PI3K inhibitors ■ AKT inhibitors
PTEN[56]	PI3K	Deletion	Numerous cancers	■ PI3K inhibitors
MTOR,[57] *TSC1*,[58] and *TSC2*[59]	mTOR	Mutation	Tuberous sclerosis and bladder cancer	■ mTOR inhibitors
RAS family (*HRAS*, *NRAS*, *KRAS*), *BRAF*,[60] and *MEK1*	RAS–MEK	Mutation, rearrangement, or amplification	Numerous cancers, including melanoma and prostate cancers	■ RAF inhibitors ■ MEK inhibitors ■ PI3K inhibitors
Fibroblast growth factor receptor 1 (*FGFR1*), *FGFR2*, *FGFR3*, *FGFR4*[36]	FGFR	Mutation, amplification, or rearrangement	Myeloma, sarcoma, and bladder, breast, ovarian, lung, endometrial, and myeloid cancers	■ FGFR inhibitors ■ FGFR antibodies
Epidermal growth factor receptor (*EGFR*)	EGFR	Mutation, deletion, or amplification	Lung and gastrointestinal cancer	■ EGFR inhibitors ■ EGFR antibodies
ERBB2[61]	ERBB2	Amplification or mutation	Breast, bladder, gastric, and lung cancers	■ ERBB2 inhibitors ■ ERBB2 antibodies
SMO[62,63] and *PTCH1*[64]	Hedgehog	Mutation	Basal cell carcinoma	■ Hedgehog inhibitor
MET[65]	MET	Amplification or mutation	Bladder, gastric, and renal cancers	■ MET inhibitors ■ MET antibodies
JAK1, *JAK2*, *JAK3*,[66] *STAT1*, *STAT3*	JAK–STAT	Mutation or rearrangement	Leukemia and lymphoma	■ JAK–STAT inhibitors ■ STAT decoys
Discoidin domain-containing receptor 2 (*DDR2*)	RTK	Mutation	Lung cancer	■ Some tyrosine kinase inhibitors
Erythropoietin receptor (*EPOR*)	JAK–STAT	Rearrangement	Leukemia	■ JAK–STAT inhibitors
Interleukin-7 receptor (*IL-7R*)	JAK–STAT	Mutation	Leukemia	■ JAK–STAT inhibitors
Cyclin-dependent kinases (*CDKs*[67]; *CDK4*, *CDK6*, *CDK8*), *CDKN2A*, and cyclin D1 (*CCND1*)	CDK	Amplification, mutation, deletion, or rearrangement	Sarcoma, colorectal cancer, melanoma, and lymphoma	■ CDK inhibitors
ABL1	ABL	Rearrangement	Leukemia	■ ABL inhibitors
Retinoic acid receptor-α (*RARA*)	RARα	Rearrangement	Leukemia	■ All-trans retinoic acid
Aurora kinase A (*AURKA*)[68]	Aurora kinases	Amplification	Prostate and breast cancers	■ Aurora kinase inhibitors
Androgen receptor (*AR*)[69]	Androgen	Mutation, amplification, or splice variant	Prostate cancer	■ Androgen synthesis inhibitors ■ Androgen receptor inhibitors
FLT3[70]	FLT3	Mutation or deletion	Leukemia	■ FLT3 inhibitors
MET	MET–HGF	Mutation or amplification	Lung and gastric cancers	■ MET inhibitors
Myeloproliferative leukemia (*MPL*)	THPO, JAK–STAT	Mutation	Myeloproliferative neoplasms	■ JAK–STAT inhibitors
MDM2[71]	MDM2	Amplification	Sarcoma and adrenal carcinomas	■ MDM2 antagonist
KIT[72]	KIT	Mutation	GIST, mastocytosis, and leukemia	■ KIT inhibitors
PDGFRA and *PDGFRB*	PDGFR	Deletion, rearrangement, or amplification	Hematologic cancer, GIST, sarcoma, and brain cancer	■ PDGFR inhibitors
Anaplastic lymphoma kinase (*ALK*)[9,37,73,74]	ALK	Rearrangement or mutation	Lung cancer and neuroblastoma	■ ALK inhibitors

(continued)

TABLE 3.1

Genomic Alterations as Putative Predictive Biomarkers for Cancer Therapy *(continued)*

Genes	Pathways	Aberration Type	Disease Examples	Putative or Proven Drugs
RET	RET	Rearrangement or mutation	Lung and thyroid cancers	■ RET inhibitors
ROS1[75]	ROS1	Rearrangement	Lung cancer and cholangiocarcinoma	■ ROS1 inhibitors
NOTCH1 and *NOTCH2*	Notch	Rearrangement or mutation	Leukemia and breast cancer	■ Notch signalling pathway inhibitors

PIK3CA, PI3K catalytic subunit-α; *PIK3R1*, PI3K regulatory subunit 1; *PI3K*, phosphoinositide 3-kinase; *AKT*, v-akt murine thymoma viral oncogene homolog; *PTEN*, phosphatase and tensin homolog; mTOR, mechanistic target of rapamycin; *TSC1*, tuberous sclerosis 1 protein; RAS–MEK, rat sarcoma; *MEK*, MAPK/ERK (mitogen-activated protein kinase/extracellular signal-regulated kinase) kinase; RAF, v-raf murine sarcoma viral oncogene homolog; *ERBB2*, also known as *HER2*; *SMO*, smoothened homolog; *PTCH1*, patched homolog; *MET*, hepatocyte growth factor receptor; *JAK*, Janus kinase; *THPO*, thrombopoietin; *STAT*, signal transducer and activator of transcription; RTK, receptor tyrosine kinase; *CDKN2A*, cyclin-dependent kinase inhibitor 2A; ABL, Abelson murine leukemia viral oncogene homolog 1; *FLT3*, FMS-like tyrosine kinase 3; *HGF*, hepatocyte growth factor; *MDM2*, mouse double minute 2; *KIT*, v-kit Hardy-Zuckerman 4 feline sarcoma viral oncogene homolog; GIST, gastrointestinal stromal tumor; PDGFR, platelet-derived growth factor receptor; *ROS1*, v-ros avian UR2 sarcoma virus oncogene homolog.

PRINCIPLES OF ONCOLOGY

staining regions. *MYCN* amplification is a very strong predictor of poor outcomes, particularly in patients with localized (stage 1 or stage 2) disease or in infants with stage 4S metastatic disease, where fewer than half of patients survive beyond 5 years.[6]

Use of *other chromosome abnormalities* has been largely limited to the diagnosis and prognostication of hematologic disorders. Roughly half of all myelodysplastic disorders show cytogenetically detectable chromosomal abnormalities, such as monosomy 5 or 7, partial chromosomal loss (5q-, 7q-), or complex chromosomal abnormalities. Certain abnormalities in isolation (e.g., 5q-) have a favorable prognosis, whereas many others (e.g., "complex" karyotypes with three or more abnormalities) carry a worse prognosis. Differences in ploidy have proven to be useful predictors in pediatric acute lymphocytic leukemia (ALL), with hyperdiploid cases (>50 chromosomes) showing a distinctly more favorable course compared with hypodiploid or near diploid cases.[7] Overall, DNA ploidy can be assessed by flow cytometry. Specific chromosomal copy number alterations can be detected by *conventional karyotyping, array hybridization methods*, or *FISH*.

Copy number variation (CNV) represents the most common type of structural chromosomal alteration. Regions affected by CNVs range from approximately 1 kilobase to several megabases that are either amplified or deleted. It is estimated that about 0.4% of the genomes of healthy individuals differ in copy number.[8] CNVs resulting in deletion of genes such as *BRCA1*, *BRCA2*, *APC*, mismatch repair genes, and *TP53* have been implicated in a wide range of highly penetrant cancers.[9,10] CNVs can be detected by a variety of means including *FISH*, *comparative or array genomic hybridization*, or *virtual karyotyping* using *single nucleotide polymorphism (SNP) arrays*. Increasingly, CNV is detected using *next-generation sequencing*.

Large-scale sequencing of tumors has identified many *mutations* that are of potential prognostic and therapeutic significance. As will be discussed further, a wide range of strategies is available for the detection of point mutations (Fig. 3.1). It is important to

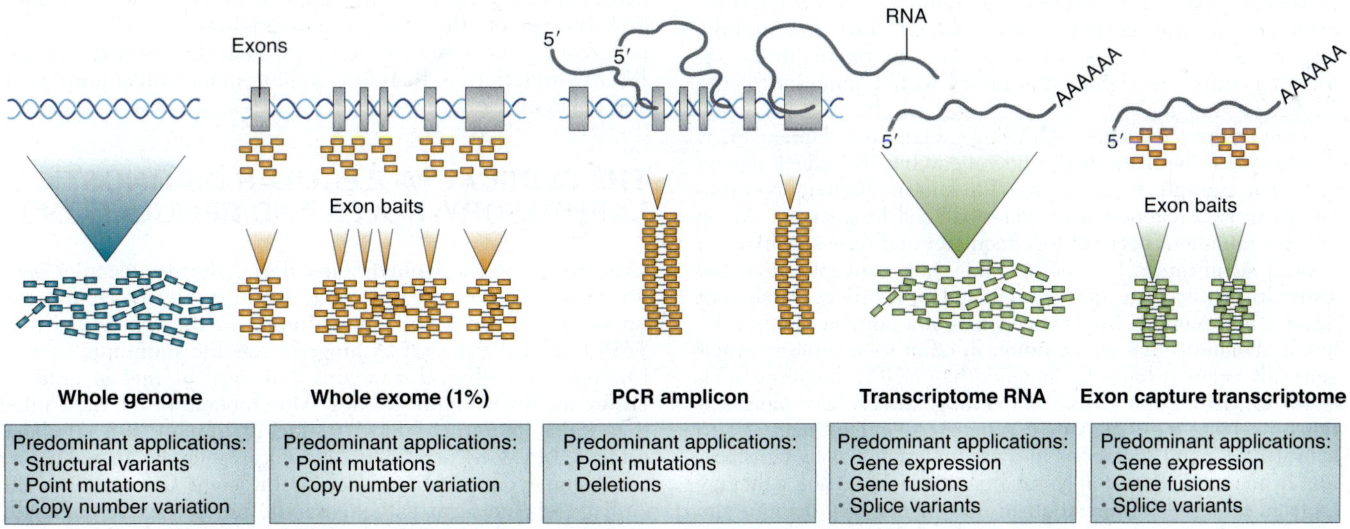

Figure 3.1 Strategies for the detection of mutations, translocations, and other structural genomic abnormalities in cancer. Whole genome sequencing, which involves determining the entire sequence of both introns and exons, is not only the most comprehensive, but also the most laborious and expensive approach. Exome sequencing uses *baits* to capture either the entire exome (roughly 20,000 genes [about 1% of the genome]) or else a subset of genes of interest. Amplicon-based sequencing uses PCR or other amplification techniques to amplify targets of interest for sequencing. Transcriptome sequencing, also known as RNAseq, is based on sequencing expressed RNA and can be used to detect not only mutations, but also translocations, other structural abnormalities, as well as differences in expression levels. This can be combined with exome capture techniques for a higher sensitivity analysis of genes of particular interest. (Reprinted by permission from Macmillan Publishers Limited: Nature Reviews Drug Discovery, Simon, R. and Rowchodhury, S. 12:358–369, 2013, ©2013.)

recognize that many nucleotide variations occur at any given allele in populations. Formally, the term *polymorphism* is used to describe genetic differences present in ≥1% of the human population, whereas *mutation* describes less frequent differences. However, in practice, *polymorphism* is often used to describe a nonpathogenic genetic change, and mutation a deleterious change, regardless of their frequencies.

Mutations can be classified according to their effect in the structure of a gene. The most common of these disease-associated alterations are single nucleotide substitutions (point mutations); however, many deletions, insertions, gene rearrangements, gene amplification, and copy number variations have been identified that have clinical significance. Point mutations may affect promoters, splicing sites, or coding regions. Coding region mutations can be classified into three kinds, depending on the impact on the codon: *missense mutation*, a nucleotide change leads to the substitution of an amino acid to another; *nonsense mutation*, a nucleotide substitution causes premature termination of codons with protein truncation; and *silent mutation*, a nucleotide change does not change the coded amino acid.

Loss of function mutations, either through point mutations or deletions in tumor suppression genes such as *APC* and *TP53*, are the most common mutations in cancers. Tumor suppression genes require two-hit (biallelic) mutations that inactivate both copies of the gene in order to allow tumorigenesis to occur. The first hit is usually an inherited or somatic point mutation, and the second hit is assumed to be an acquired deletion mutation that deletes the second copy of the tumor suppression gene. Promoter methylation of tumor suppressor genes is an alternative route to tumorigenesis that, to date, has not been commonly employed for molecular diagnostics.

Oncogenes originate from the deregulation of genes that normally encode for proteins associated with cell growth, differentiation, apoptosis, and signal transduction (proto-oncogenes, [e.g., *BRAF* and *KRAS*]). Proto-oncogenes generally require only one gain of function or activating mutation to become oncogenic. Common mutation types that result in proto-oncogene activation include point mutations, gene amplifications, and chromosomal translocations. One example is mutations in the epidermal growth factor receptor (*EGFR*) that occur in lung cancer, which are almost exclusively seen in nonmucinous bronchoalveolar carcinomas. Somatic mutations of *EGFR* constitutively activate the receptor tyrosine kinase (TK). Importantly, responsiveness of tumors harboring these mutations to the inhibitor gefitinib is highly coordinated with a mutation of the EGFR TK domain.[11,12]

One of the challenges with using mutations as biomarkers is that there can be many nucleotide alterations that affect a given gene. For example, there are over 100 known different point mutations in *EGFR* reported in non–small-cell lung cancer. Many of these mutations occur at low frequency and have an unknown clinical significance.[13,14] Another important concept is that the same driver oncogene may be mutated in a variety of different tumors. For example, lung cancers harbor a number of other different alterations that are common in other solid tumors, which generally occur at lower frequencies than *EGFR* mutations such as *KRAS*, *BRAF*, and *HER2*. Some lung cancers have translocations involving the *ALK* kinase gene. *ALK*, interestingly, is also activated by point mutations in a neuroblastoma as by translocation in anaplastic large cell lymphoma (Fig. 3.2). Hence, a therapy targeted to a genetic alteration in one cancer may demonstrate efficacy in other cancers.

The detection of mutations is also important in the evaluation of chemotherapy resistance. Roughly a third of CML patients are resistant to the frontline ABL1 kinase inhibitor imatinib, either at the time of initial treatment or, more commonly, secondarily. In cases of primary failure or secondary failure, over 100 different *ABL1* mutations have been identified, including particularly common ones such as T315I and P loop mutations. While some

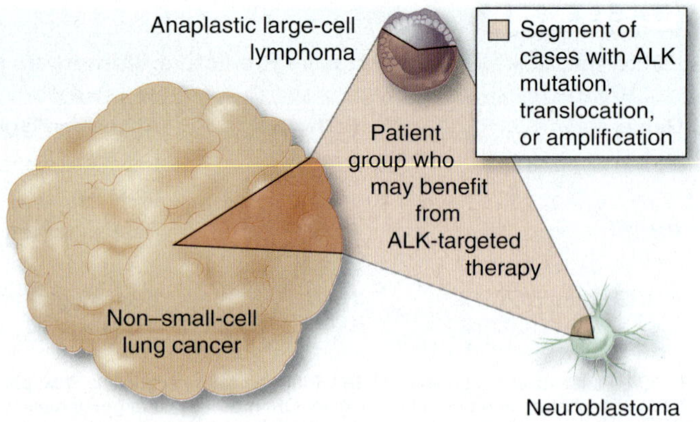

Figure 3.2 Activating genomic alterations occur in a variety of tumor types. *ALK* translocations, mutations, and amplifications occur in non–small-cell lung cancer, neuroblastomas, and in anaplastic large cell lymphomas. Such recurrent alterations in cancer, together with effective inhibitors of these pathways, are transforming oncologic therapies from organ-specific to pathway-specific interventions and are driving the use of molecular diagnostics in a wider range of tumor types. (Modified from McDermott, U. and Settleman, J. *J Clin Oncol* 2009;27:5650–5659.)

mutations, such as Y253H, respond to second generation TK inhibitors (TKI), others, such as the T315I mutation, are noteworthy because they confer resistance not only to imatinib, but also to nilotinib and dasatinib.

Mutations are also used as important predictive biomarkers (Table 3.1). Two of the most notable examples are the use of the *BRCA1* and *BRCA2* mutation analysis for women with a strong family history of breast cancer. Over 200 mutations (loss of function point mutations, small deletions, or insertions) occur in *BRCA* genes, which are distributed across the genes necessitating full sequencing for their detection. The overall prevalence of these occur in about 0.1% of the general population.[15,16] The lifetime risk of breast cancer for women carrying *BRCA1* mutations is in the range of 47% to 66%, whereas for *BRCA2* mutations, it is in the range of 40% to 57%.[17,18] In addition, the risk of other tumors including ovarian, fallopian, and pancreatic cancer is also increased. Detection of *BRCA1* and *BRCA2* mutations is, therefore, important for cancer prevention and risk reduction.

THE CLINICAL MOLECULAR DIAGNOSTICS LABORATORY: RULES AND REGULATIONS

Laboratories in the United States that perform molecular diagnostic testing are categorized as high-complexity laboratories under the Clinical Laboratory Improvement Amendments of 1988 (CLIA).[19] The CLIA program sets the minimum administrative and technical standards that must be met in order to ensure quality laboratory testing. Most laboratories in the United States that perform clinical testing in humans are regulated under CLIA. CLIA-certified laboratories must be accredited by professional organizations such as the Joint Commission, the College of American Pathologists, or another agency officially approved by the Centers for Medicare & Medicaid Services (CMS), and must comply with CLIA standards and guidelines for quality assurance. Although the regulation of laboratory services is in the U.S. Food and Drug Administration's (FDA) jurisdiction, the FDA has historically exercised enforcement discretion. Therefore, FDA approval is not currently required for clinical implementation of molecular tests as long as other regulations are met.[20,21]

SPECIMEN REQUIREMENTS FOR MOLECULAR DIAGNOSTICS

Samples typically received for molecular oncology testing include blood, bone marrow aspirates and biopsies, fluids, organ-specific fresh tissues in saline or tissue culture media such as Roswell Park Memorial Institute (RPMI), FFPE tissues, and cytology cell blocks. Molecular tests can be ordered electronically or through written requisition forms, but never through verbal requests only. All samples submitted for molecular testing need to be appropriately identified. Sample type, quantity, and specimen handling and transport requirements should conform to the laboratory's stated requirements in order to ensure valid test results.

Blood and bone marrow samples should be drawn into anticoagulated tubes. The preferred anticoagulant for most molecular assays is ethylenediaminetetraacetic acid (EDTA; lavender). Other acceptable collection tubes include ACD (yellow) solutions A and B. Heparinized tubes are not preferred for most molecular tests because heparin inhibits the polymerase enzyme utilized in PCR, which may lead to assay failure. Blood and bone marrow samples can be transported at ambient temperature. Blood samples should never be frozen prior to separation of cellular elements because this causes hemolysis, which interferes with DNA amplification. Fluids should be transported on ice. Tissues should be frozen (preferred method) as soon as possible and sent on dry ice to minimize degradation. Fresh tissues in RPMI should be sent on ice or cold packs. Cells should be kept frozen and sent on dry ice; DNA samples can be sent at ambient temperature or on ice.

For FFPE tissue blocks, typical collection and handling procedures include cutting 4 to 6 microtome sections of 10-micron thickness each on uncoated slides, air-drying unstained sections at room temperature, and staining one of the slides with hematoxylin and eosin (H&E). A board-certified pathologist reviews the H&E slides to ensure the tissue block contains a sufficient quantity of neoplastic tumor cells, and circles an area on the H&E slide that will be used as a template to guide macrodissection or microdissection of the adjacent, unstained slides. The pathologist also provides an estimate of the percentage of neoplastic cells in the area that will be tested, which should exceed the established limit of detection (LOD) of the assay.

MOLECULAR DIAGNOSTICS TESTING PROCESS

The workflow of a molecular test begins with receipt and accessioning of the specimen in the clinical molecular diagnostics laboratory followed by extraction of the nucleic acid (DNA or RNA), test setup, detection of analyte (e.g., PCR products), data analysis, and result reporting to the patient medical record (Fig. 3.3).

An extraction of intact, moderately high-quality DNA is essential for molecular assays. For DNA extraction, the preferred age for blood, bone marrow, and fluid samples is less than 5 days; for frozen or fixed tissue, it is indefinite; and for fresh tissue, it is overnight. Although there is no age limit for the use of a fixed and embedded tissue specimen for analysis, older specimens may yield a lower quantity and quality of DNA. Because RNA is significantly more labile than DNA, the preferred age for blood and bone marrow is less than 48 hours (from time of collection). Tissue samples intended for an RNA analysis should be promptly processed in fresh state, snap frozen, or preserved with RNA stabilizing agents for transport.

Dedicated areas, equipment, and materials are designated for various stages of DNA and RNA extraction procedures. DNA and RNA isolation can be done by manual or automated methods. Currently, most clinical laboratories employ commercial protocols based on liquid- or solid-phase extractions. Nucleated cells are isolated from biological samples prior to nucleic acid extraction.

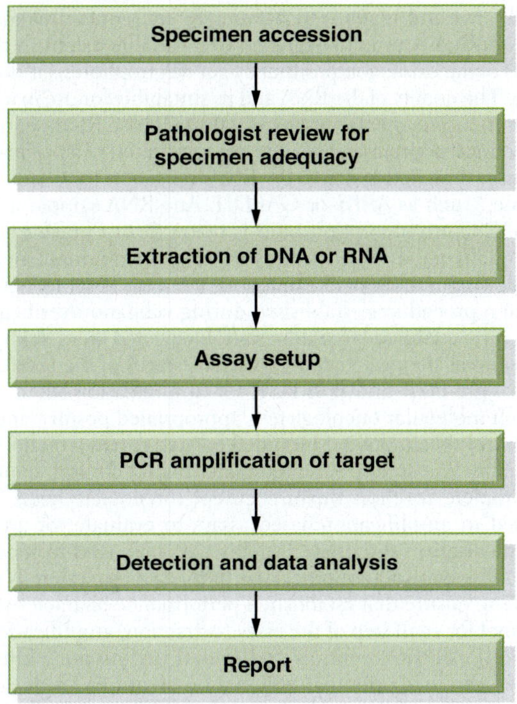

Figure 3.3 Simplified workflow of clinical molecular diagnostic testing.

White blood cells (WBC) can be isolated from blood and bone marrow samples by different methods. One method involves lysing the red blood cells with an ammonium chloride solution, which yields the total WBC population and other nucleated cells present. Another method involves a gradient preparation with a Ficoll solution, which yields the mononuclear cell population only. Sections of FFPE tissue blocks are prepared for DNA extraction by first removing the paraffin and disrupting the cell membranes with proteinase K digestion. Fresh and frozen tissues also undergo proteinase K digestion prior to nucleic acid extraction. DNA isolation protocols consist of several steps, including cell lysis, DNA purification by salting out the proteins and other debris (nonorganic method), or by solvent extractions of the proteins with phenol and chloroform solutions (organic method). The DNA is then precipitated out of the solution with isopropanol or ethanol. The pellet is washed with 70% to 80% ethanol and then solubilized in buffer, such as Tris-EDTA solution. Proteinase K can be added to assist in the disruption and to prevent nonspecific degradation of the DNA. RNase is sometimes added to eliminate contaminating RNA. The DNA yield is quantitated spectrophotometrically, and the DNA sample integrity is visually checked, if necessary, on an agarose gel followed by ethidium bromide staining. Intact DNA appears as a high–molecular-weight single band, whereas degraded DNA is identified as a smear of variably sized fragments. After extraction, the DNA is stored at 4°C prior to use in a PCR assay, and is then stored at −70°C after completion of the assay. Because the DNA extracted from formalin-fixed tissue is degraded to a variable extent, an analysis of the extraction product by gel electrophoresis is not informative. Yield and integrity of the extracted DNA is best assessed by an amplification control to ensure that the quality and quantity of input DNA is adequate to yield a valid result.

RNA isolation steps are similar to the ones described previously for DNA extraction. However, RNA is inherently less stable than DNA due to its single-strand conformation and susceptibility to degradation by RNase, which is ubiquitous in the environment. To ensure preservation of target RNA, special precautions are required, including the use of diethylpyrocarbonate (DEPC) water in all reagents used in RNA procedures, and special decontamination of work area and pipettes to prevent RNase contamination. The extracted RNA is usually degraded to a variable extent so that the analysis of the extraction product by gel electrophoresis is not informative. The quality of the RNA and its suitability for use in a reverse transcriptase polymerase chain reaction (RT-PCR)–based assay is assessed most appropriately by the demonstration of a positive result in an assay designed to detect the RNA transcripts for a "housekeeping gene," such as *ABL1* or *GAPDH*. Any RNA sample in which the 260/280-nm absorption ratio is below 1.9 or greater than 2.0 may contain contaminants and must be cleaned prior to analysis.

Following nucleic acid extraction, the assay is set up according to written procedures established during validation/verification of the assay by qualified laboratory staff. Dedicated areas, equipment, and materials are designated for various stages of the test (e.g., extraction, pre-PCR and post-PCR for amplification-based assays). For each molecular oncology test, appropriated positive and negative control specimens are included to each run as a matter of routine quality assessment. A no template (blank) control, containing the complete reaction mixture except for nucleic acids, is also included in amplification-based assays to evaluate for amplicon contamination in the assay reagents that may lead to inaccurate results. The controls are processed in the same manner as patient samples to ensure that established performance characteristics are being met for each step of the assay (extraction, amplification, and detection). All assay controls and overall performance of the run must be examined prior to interpretation of sample results. Following acceptance of the controls, results are electronically entered into reports. The final report is reviewed and signed by the laboratory director or a qualified designee who meets the same qualifications as the director, as defined by CLIA (see previous).

TECHNOLOGIES

Several traditional and emerging techniques are currently available for mutation detection in cancer (Table 3.2). In the era of personalized medicine, molecular oncology assays are rapidly moving from a mutational analysis of single genes toward a multigene panel analysis. As the number of "actionable" mutations such as *ALK*, *EGFR*, *BRAF*, and others increase, the use of next-generation sequencing platforms is expected to become much more widespread. Both traditional and emerging testing approaches have advantages and disadvantages that need to be balanced before a test platform is implemented into practice.

An important consideration when adding a new oncology test in the clinical laboratory menu is to define the intended use of the assay (e.g., diagnosis, prognosis, prediction of therapy response). The clinical utility of the assay, appropriate types of specimens, the spectrum of possible mutations that can be found in the genomic region of interest, and available methods for testing should also be determined. The laboratory director and ordering physicians should also discuss the estimated test volume, optimal reporting format, and required turnaround time for the proposed new test.[21–23]

Polymerase Chain Reaction

Polymerase chain reaction (PCR)[24,25] is widely used in all molecular diagnostics laboratories for the rapid amplification of targeted DNA sequences. The reaction includes the specimen template DNA, forward and reverse primers (18 to 24 oligonucleotides long), Taq DNA polymerase, and each of the four nucleotides bases (dATP, dTTP, dCTP, dGTP). During PCR, selected genomic sequences undergo repetitive temperature cycling (sequential heat and cooling) that allows for *denaturation* of double-stranded DNA template, *annealing* of the primers to the targeted complementary sequences on the template, and *extension* of new strands of DNA by Taq polymerase from nucleotides, using the primers as the starting point. Each cycle doubles the copy number of PCR templates for the next round of polymerase activity, resulting in an exponential amplification of the selected target sequence. The PCR products (amplicons) are detected by electrophoresis or in real-time systems simultaneously to the amplification reaction (see real-time PCR, which follows).

PCR is specifically designed to work on DNA templates because the Taq polymerase does not recognize RNA as a starting material. Nonetheless, PCR can be adapted to RNA testing by including a reverse transcription step to convert a RNA sequence into its cognate cDNA sequence before the PCR reaction is performed (see reverse-transcription PCR, which follows). Multiplex PCR reactions can also be designed with multiple primers for simultaneous amplification of multiple genomic targets. PCR is a highly sensitive and specific technique that can be employed in different capacities for the detection of point mutations, small deletions, insertions and duplications, as well as gene rearrangements and clonality assessment. Limits of detection can reach 0.1% mutant allele or lower, which is important for the detection of somatic mutations in oncology because tumor specimens are usually composed of a mixture of tumor and normal cells. Reverse transcription PCR can also be used for the relative quantification of target RNA in minimal residual disease testing, such as *BCR-ABL1* transcripts in CML. Another advantage of PCR is its ability to amplify small amounts of low quality FFPE-derived DNA. However, applications of PCR can be limited because it cannot amplify across large or highly repetitive genomic regions. Also, the PCR reaction can be inhibited by heparin or melanin if present in the extracted DNA, which may lead to assay failure. Finally, the risk of false positives due to specimen or amplicon contamination is an important issue when using PCR-based techniques; therefore, stringent laboratory procedures, as described previously, are used to minimize contamination. With the exception of hybridization assays, such as fluorescence in situ hybridization and genomic microarrays, PCR is the necessary initial step in all current molecular oncology assays.

Targeted Mutation Analysis Methods

Real-Time PCR (q-PCR)

In real-time PCR (q-PCR), the polymerase chain reaction is performed with a PCR reporter that is usually a fluorescent double-stranded DNA binding dye or a fluorescent reporter probe. The intensity of the fluorescence produced at each amplification cycle is monitored in real time, and both quantification and detection of targeted sequences is accomplished in the reaction tube as the PCR amplification proceeds.

The intensity of the fluorescent signal for a given DNA fragment (wild type or mutant) is correlated with its quantity, based on the PCR cycle in which the fluorescence rises above the background (crossing threshold [Ct] or crossing point [Cp]).[26] The Ct value can be used for qualitative or quantitative analysis. Qualitative assays use the Ct as a cutoff for determining "presence" or "absence" of a given target in the reaction. A qualitative analysis by q-PCR is particularly useful for a targeted detection of point mutations that are located in mutational hotspots. Examples include the *JAK2* V617F mutation, which is located within exon 14, and is found in several myeloproliferative neoplasms (polycythemia vera, essential thrombocythemia, and primary myelofibrosis),[27] and the *BRAF* V600E,[28] which is located within exon 15, and is found in various cancer types including melanomas and thyroid and lung cancers.

For a quantitative analysis, the Ct of standards with known template concentration is used to generate a standard curve to which Ct values of unknown samples are compared. The concentration of the unknown samples is then extrapolated from values from the standard curve. The quantity of amplicons produced in a PCR reaction is proportional to the prevalence of the targeted sequence;

TABLE 3.2

Molecular Methods in Oncology

Method	Advantages	Disadvantages	Analytic Sensitivity	Examples of Applications in Oncology
Real-time PCR (q-PCR) Allele-specific PCR (AS-PCR) Reverse transcriptase PCR (RT-PCR)	Flexible platforms that permit detection of a variety of conserved hotspot mutations including nucleotide substitutions, small length mutations (deletions, insertions), and translocations High sensitivity is beneficial for residual disease testing and specimens with limited tumor content Adaptable to quantitative assays	Detects only specific targeted mutations/ chromosomal translocations Not suitable for variable mutations May not determine the exact change in nucleotide sequence	Very high	*KRAS, BRAF,* and *EGFR* mutations in solid tumors *JAK2* V617F and *MPL* mutations in myeloproliferative neoplasms *KIT* D816V mutation in systemic mastocytosis and AML Quantitation of *BCR-ABL1* and *PML-RARA* transcripts for residual disease monitoring in CML and APL, respectively
Fragment analysis	Detects small to medium insertions and deletions Detects variable insertions and deletions regardless of specific alteration Provides semiquantitative information regarding mutation level	Does not determine the exact change in nucleotide sequence Does not detect single nucleotide substitution mutations Limited multiplex capability	High	*NPM1* insertion mutations in AML *FLT3* internal tandem duplications in AML *JAK2* exon 12 insertions and deletions in PV *EGFR* exon 19 deletions in NSCLC
FISH	Detects chromosomal translocation, gene amplification, and deletion Morphology of tumor is preserved, allowing for a more accurate interpretation of heterogeneous samples	High cost Unable to detect small insertions and deletions Limited multiplex capability Does not determine the exact breakpoint and change in nucleotide sequence	High	*IGH/BCL2* translocation detection in follicular lymphoma and in a subset of diffuse large B-cell lymphoma *ALK* translocation in NSCLC *EWSR1* translocation in soft tissue tumors *HER2* amplification in breast cancer 1p/19q deletion in oligodendroglioma
High-resolution melting (HRM) curve analysis	Qualitative detection of variable single nucleotide substitutions and small insertions and deletions	Does not determine the exact mutation Result interpretation may require testing via an alternate technology Limited multiplex capability	Medium	*KRAS* and *BRAF* mutations in solid tumors *JAK2* exon 12 mutations in PV
Sanger sequencing	Detects variable single nucleotide substitutions and small insertions and deletions Provides semiquantitative information about mutation level Current gold standard for mutation detection	Low throughput Low analytic sensitivity limits application in specimens with low tumor burden Does not detect copy number changes or large (>500 bp) insertions and deletions	Low	*KIT* mutations in GIST and melanoma *CEBPA* mutations in AML *EGFR* mutations in NSCLC
Pyrosequencing	Higher analytical sensitivity than Sanger sequencing Detects variable single nucleotide substitutions and small insertions and deletions Provides quantitative information about mutation level	Short read lengths limit analysis to mutational hotspots Low throughput	Medium	*KRAS* and *BRAF* mutations in solid tumors
Single nucleotide extension assay (SNaPshot)	Simultaneous detection of targeted nucleotide substitution mutations Multiplex capability	Detects only targeted mutations	High	Small gene panels (3–10) for melanoma, NSCLC, breast cancer, and metastatic colorectal cancer

(continued)

TABLE 3.2

Molecular Methods in Oncology *(continued)*

Method	Advantages	Disadvantages	Analytic Sensitivity	Examples of Applications in Oncology
Next-generation sequencing (NGS)	Quantitative detection of variable single nucleotide substitutions, small insertions and deletions, chromosomal translocations, and gene copy number variations Highly multiplexed High throughput	Requires costly investment in instrumentation and bioinformatics Technology is rapidly evolving Higher error rates for insertion and deletion mutations Limited ability to sequence GC-rich regions	High	Small to large gene panels (3–500) for solid tumor and hematologic malignancies
Genomic microarray	Simultaneous detection of copy number variation and LOH (SNP array)	Limited application to FFPE tissue Does not detect balanced translocations May not detect low-level mutant allele burden	Medium	Analysis of recurrent copy number variation and LOH in chronic lymphocytic leukemia and myeloproliferative neoplasms

AML, acute myelogenous leukemia; CML, chronic myelogenous leukemia; APL, acute promyelocytic leukemia; PV, polycythemia vera; NSCLC, non–small-cell lung carcinoma; GIST, gastrointestinal stromal tumor; GC, guanine-cytosine; LOH, loss of heterozygosity; FFPE, formalin-fixed paraffin-embedded.

therefore, samples with a higher template concentration reaches the Ct at earlier PCR cycles than one with a low concentration of the amplified target. Quantitative q-PCR has high analytical sensitivity for the detection of low mutant allele burden. For that reason, this method has been widely utilized for monitoring minimal residual disease.

Allele-Specific PCR

Allele-specific PCR (AS-PCR) is a variant of conventional PCR. The method is based on the principle that Taq polymerase is incapable of catalyzing chain elongation in the presence of a mismatch between the 3′ end of the primer and the template DNA. Selective amplification by AS-PCR is achieved by designing a forward primer that matches the mutant sequence at the 3′ end primer. A second mismatch within the primer can be introduced at the adjacent -1 or -2 position to decrease the efficiency of mismatched amplification products. This will minimize the chance of amplifying and, therefore, detecting the wild-type target. AS-PCR is usually performed as two PCR reactions: one employing a forward primer specific for the mutant sequence, the other using a forward primer specific for the correspondent wild-type sequence. In this case, a common reverse primer is used for both reactions. Following amplification, the PCR products are detected by electrophoresis (capillary or agarose gel) or in q-PCR systems. The detection of adequate PCR product in the wild-type amplification reaction is important to control for adequate specimen quality and quantity, particularly when the specimen is negative in the mutation-specific PCR reaction.

AS-PCR is particularly useful for the detection of targeted point mutations. Multiplex AS-PCR reactions can be designed for the simultaneous detection of multiple mutations by including several mutation-specific primers. The method has high analytical sensitivity and specificity and can be easily deployed in most clinical laboratories. However, an important limitation is that this approach will not detect mutations other than those for which specific primers are designed. Therefore, it is utilized for highly recurrent mutations that occur at specific locations within genes, rather than for the detection of variable mutations that may occur throughout a gene.

Examples of AS-PCR applications in oncology include the detection of *JAK2* V617F and *MPL* mutations in myeloproliferative neoplasms (primary myelofibrosis, essential thrombocythemia, and/or polycythemia vera),[29] the *BRAF* V600E mutation,[30] and *KIT* D816V mutations in cases of systemic mastocytosis and in acute myelogenous leukemia (AML).

Reverse Transcriptase PCR

RT-PCR is utilized for the detection and quantification of RNA transcripts. The first step for all amplification-based assays that use RNA as a starting material is reverse transcription of RNA into cDNA, because RNA is not a suitable substrate for Taq polymerase. In RT-PCR, RNA is isolated and reverse transcribed into cDNA by using a reverse transcriptase enzyme and one of the following: (1) random hexamer primers, which anneal randomly to RNA and reverse transcribe all RNA in the cell; (2) oligo dT primers, which anneal to the polyA tail of mRNA and reverse transcribe only mRNA; or (3) gene-specific primers that reverse transcribe only the target of interest. PCR is subsequently performed on the cDNA with forward and reverse primers specific to the gene(s) of interest. The RT-PCR products may then be analyzed by capillary electrophoresis or in real-time systems as in a standard PCR reaction.

RT-PCR is commonly used for detecting gene fusions during translocation analysis because breakpoints frequently occur within the intron of each partner gene and the precise intronic breakpoint locations may be variable. This variability complicates the design of primers used in DNA-based PCR assays. RT-PCR tests are advantageous because mature mRNA has intronic sequence spliced out, allowing for simplified primer design within the affected exon of each partner gene. In this setting, RT-PCR is useful in tests where both translocation partners are recurrent and only one or a few exons are involved in each partner gene. For instance, 95% of acute promyelocytic leukemia (APL) cases harbor the reciprocal t(15;17) chromosomal translocation and these breakpoints always occur within intron 2 of the *RARA* gene. By contrast, three distinct chromosome 15 breakpoints are involved, all occurring within the *PML* gene: intron 6, exon 6, and intron 3. Because the breakpoints in the two genes are recurrent, most of the reported *PML-RARA* fusions can be detected by targeting these three transcript isoforms.

RT-PCR is the method of choice when high sensitivity is required to detect gene translocations. For example, *PML-RARA*

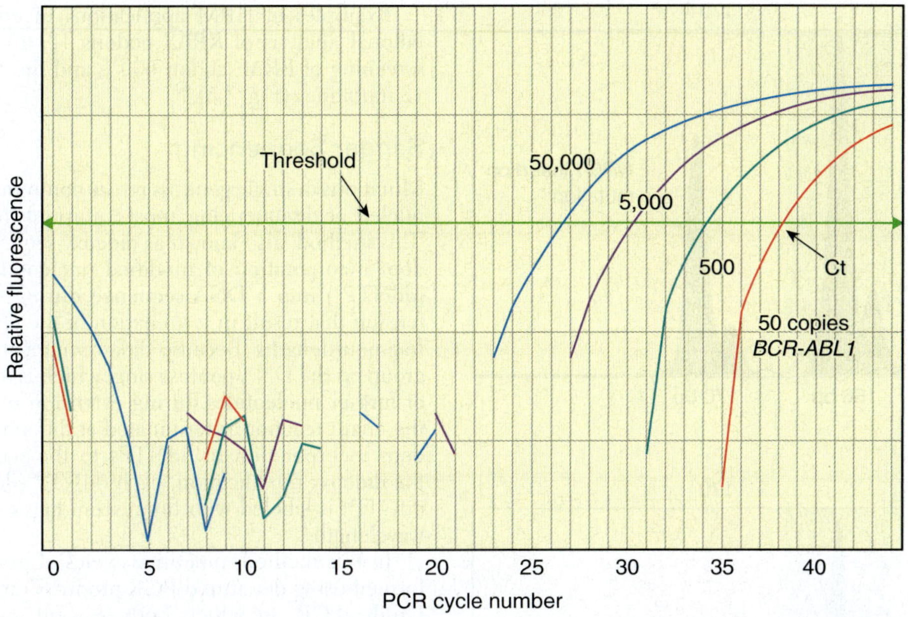

Figure 3.4 Reverse transcriptase PCR (RT-PCR) is a sensitive means to detect *BCR-ABL1* fusion transcripts in CML. RT-PCR can be combined with real-time PCR (q-PCR) to quantitate *BCR-ABL1* transcripts across four to six log range levels. Amplification products are detected during each PCR cycle using a fluorescent probe specific to the PCR product. The accumulated fluorescence in log(10) value is plotted against the number of PCR cycles. For a given specimen, the PCR cycle number is measured when the increase in fluorescence is exponential and exceeds a threshold. This point is called the Ct, which is inversely proportional to the amount of PCR target in the specimen (i.e., lower Ct values indicate a greater amount of target). Calibration standards of known quantity are used in standard curves to calculate the amount of target in a tested specimen. These are shown in the chart as different colored plots. Note that PCR increases the amount of amplification product by a factor of two with each PCR cycle. Therefore, specimens that produce a Ct value that is one cycle lower are expected to have a twofold higher concentration of target. Specimens that differ in target concentration by a factor of 10 (as shown) are expected to have a Ct value 3.3 cycles apart ($2^{3.3} = 10$).

transcript detection by RT-PCR can detect this fusion transcript down to 1 tumor cell in the background of 100,000 normal cells. Detecting low levels of fusion transcript can reveal relapse after consolidation and guide further treatment.[31] RT-PCR can also be used to quantitate the amount of expression of a gene. One major application of RT-PCR in this setting includes quantitative detection of *BCR-ABL1* fusion transcript for prognostication and minimal residual disease testing in CML (Fig. 3.4). In this setting, a three log decrease in *BCR-ABL1* levels is associated with an improved outcome.[32,33]

Fragment Analysis

A fragment analysis is a PCR amplicon-sizing technique that is relevant for the detection of small- to medium-length–affecting mutations (deletions, insertions, and duplications). This is typically performed by capillary electrophoresis, which is capable of resolving length mutations from approximately 1 to 500 base pairs in size.

Fragment analysis represents a practical strategy because it enables comprehensive detection of a wide variety of possible length mutations and has high analytic sensitivity. Further, it can provide semiquantitative information regarding the relative amount of mutated alleles. Limitations of this approach include the inability to objectively quantitate mutant allele burdens, the inability to determine the exact change in nucleotide sequence, and the inability to detect non–length-affecting mutations such as substitution mutations.

Examples of fragment analysis applications in oncology include the detection of *NPM1* insertion mutations (Fig. 3.5),[34] *EGFR* exon 19 deletions, *FLT3* internal tandem duplications, and *JAK2* exon 12 mutations.[35]

High-Resolution Melting Curve Analysis

A high-resolution melting (HRM) curve analysis is a mutation screening method that allows for the detection of DNA sequence variations based on specific sequence-related melting profiles of PCR products.[36] Because the melting property of DNA duplexes is dependent on the biophysical and chemical properties of the nucleotide sequences, mutant and wild-type DNA sequences can be differentiated from one another based on their melting characteristics.

An HRM analysis is preceded by a PCR. The reaction employs a pair of gene-specific forward and reverse primers, template DNA, and a reporter that can either be a double-stranded DNA binding dye or a fluorescent reporter probe. Following the last cycle of the PCR, the amplification products undergo a cooling step that generates homoduplexes (double-stranded molecules with perfect complementarity between alleles) and heteroduplexes (double-stranded molecules with sequence mismatch between alleles) followed by a heating step that denatures (i.e., melts) the double-stranded products. Heteroduplexes (mutant DNA) produce a melting profile different from that of wild-type samples (homoduplexes). In most cases, the reaction is performed in a q-PCR system that allows for an analysis of amplification and

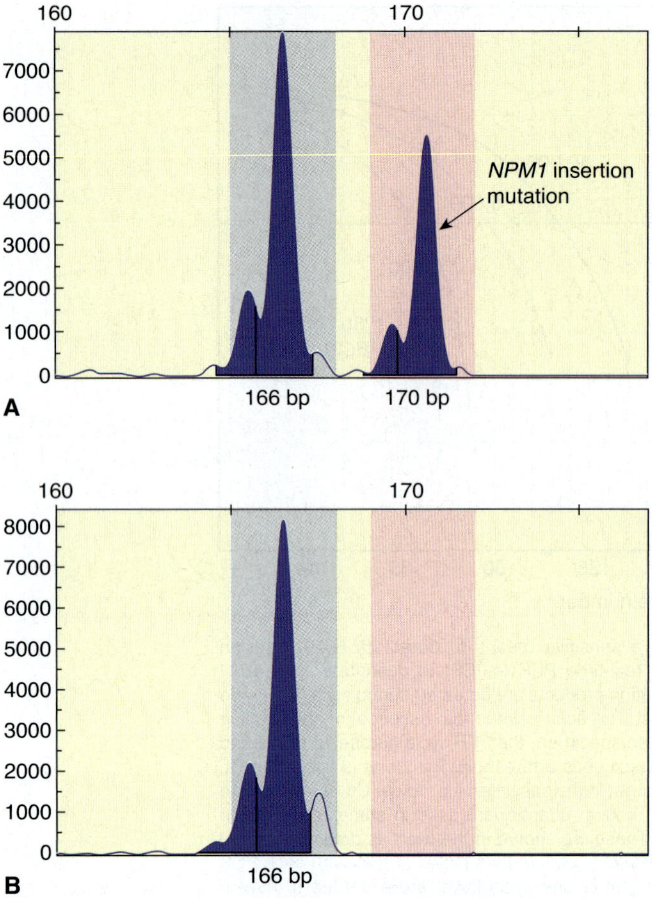

Figure 3.5 Fragment analysis. *NPM1* mutations are important prognostic markers in acute myeloid leukemia. Virtually all *NPM1* mutations result in a four nucleotide insertion within exon 12. Detection of these mutations can be accomplished by PCR utilizing primers that flank the mutation region. The amplification products are sized using capillary electrophoresis. A mutation is indicated by a PCR fragment that is 4 bp larger than the wild-type fragment. Mutation positive **(A)** and negative **(B)** cases are shown.

melting data in a close-tube format, thereby minimizing the risk of amplicon contamination.

An HRM analysis is useful for the qualitative detection of variable point mutations and small length-affecting mutations that occur within mutational hotspot regions. This method has high analytical sensitivity and can detect mutations even in a small fraction of alleles in a background of wild-type DNA. However, this assay does not characterize the specific sequence alteration in the mutant allele and may be challenging to interpret, especially for cases with mutation levels that approach the detection limit of the assay. Samples with a lower abundance of mutant alleles, and consequently a decreased fraction of heteroduplexes that produced fluorescence decay during the melting analysis, usually produce a melting curve that may not differ significantly from that of wild-type samples. Likewise, the detection of duplication mutations may be hampered by the similarity between the mutant and the duplicated wild-type genome sequences, which may produce only subtle differences in the melting behavior of the DNA duplexes, especially for samples with low mutant allele burden. Therefore, both the mutant sequence and the allelic burden play in the ability of an HRM analysis to detect mutations.[37] Poor quality and impurity of genomic DNA may also lower the sensitivity of an HRM analysis.[38] In instances of patients with a low mutant allelic burden, equivocal mutations identified by this approach may not be confirmable by an alternate method such as Sanger sequencing.

Examples of HRM applications in oncology include a mutational analysis of *KRAS* codons 12, 13, and 61[39]; a mutation screening of *BRAF* codon 600[39]; and the detection of *JAK2* exon 12 mutations (Fig. 3.6).[40]

Sanger Sequencing

Mutations in single gene assays are commonly analyzed by targeted nucleic acid sequencing, most commonly by Sanger sequencing.[41] This method, also known as dideoxy sequencing, is based on random incorporation of modified nucleotides (dideoxynucleotides [ddNTP]) into a DNA sequence during rounds of template extension that result in termination of the chain reaction at various fragment lengths. Because dideoxynucleotides lack a 3′ hydroxyl group on the DNA pentose ring, which is required for the addition of further nucleotides during extension of the new DNA strand, the chain reaction is terminated at different lengths with the random incorporation of ddNTPs to the sequence. In addition to the dideoxy modification, each ddNTP (ddATP, ddTTP, ddCTP, ddGTP) is labeled with fluorescent tags of different fluorescence wavelengths.

In this method, repetitive cycles of primer extension are performed using denatured PCR products (amplicons) as templates. Unlike PCR, in which both forward and reverse primers are added to the same reaction, in Sanger sequencing, the forward and reverse reactions are performed separately. Bidirectional sequencing is performed to ensure that the entire region of interest

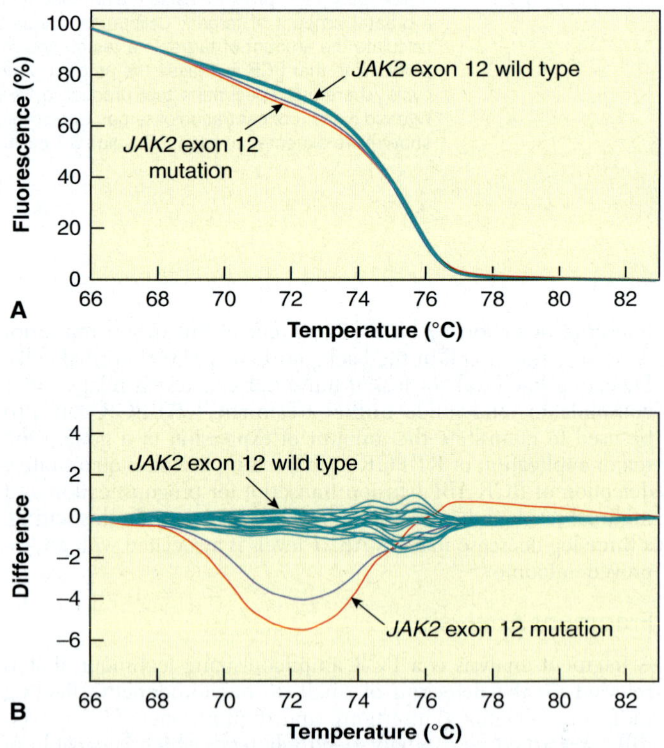

Figure 3.6 High resolution melting (HRM) curve analysis. An HRM analysis can be an efficient screening method for detecting a variety of mutations that may cluster in one or more hotspot regions, such as occurs with *JAK2* exon 12 mutations in polycythemia vera. PCR is utilized to amplify the target region in the presence of a fluorescent double-stranded DNA-binding dye. Following PCR, the product is gradually melted, and the emitted fluorescence is measured. **(A)** Plotting fluorescence versus temperature generates a melt curve characteristic of each amplicon. The presence of a mutation alters the melt profile due to mismatched double-stranded heteroduplexes of mutant and wild-type fragments. **(B)** A difference plot in which sample curves are subtracted from a wild-type control can accentuate the different melt profiles.

for each analysis is visualized adequately to produce unequivocal sequence readout. The sequencing products of increasing size are resolved by capillary electrophoresis, and the DNA sequence is determined by detection of the fluorescently labeled nucleotide sequences.

Sanger sequencing has the ability to detect a wide variety of nucleotide alterations in the DNA, including point mutations, deletions, insertions, and duplications. This technique is especially useful when mutations are scattered across the entire gene, when genes have not been sufficiently studied to determine mutational hot spots, or when it is relevant to determine the exact change in DNA sequence. Sanger sequencing can also provide semiquantitative information about mutation levels in a sample based on the evaluation of average peak drop values from forward and reverse mutant peaks on sequence chromatograms. Limitations of this approach include low throughput and limited diagnostic sensitivity. In general, heterozygous mutations at allelic levels lower than 20% may be difficult to detect by Sanger sequencing. This may be particularly problematic when testing for somatic mutations in oncogenes, such as *JAK2* exon 12 in polycythemia vera, which may occur at low levels.[35]

Examples of Sanger sequencing applications in oncology include the detection of *KIT* mutations for gastrointestinal stromal tumors (GIST) and melanomas that arise from mucosal membranes and acral skin, *EGFR* mutations for non–small-cell lung cancers, and *KRAS* mutations for colorectal and lung carcinomas (Fig. 3.7).

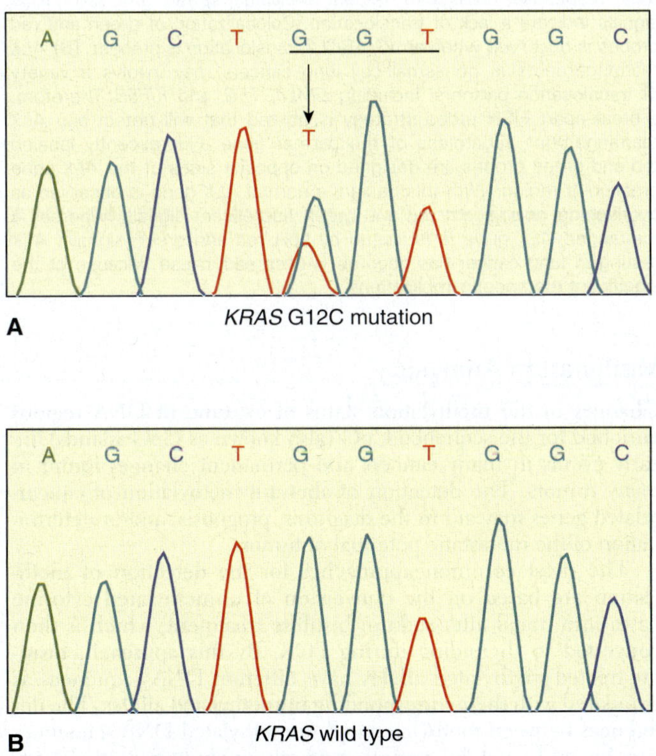

Figure 3.7 Sanger sequencing. *KRAS* mutation testing requires a technology like Sanger sequencing, which can detect the diverse variety of mutations that span multiple nucleotide sites. Overlapping peaks in the DNA sequence chromatogram indicate the presence of a mutation. The top panel **(A)** displays a G to T nucleotide substitution in codon 12. This results in a GGT to TGT codon change, leading to a glycine to cysteine (G12C) amino acid substitution. Activating mutations in *KRAS* such as G12C are associated with resistance to epidermal growth factor receptor (EGFR) targeted therapies in colon cancer. The bottom panel **(B)** displays a wild-type *KRAS* sequence.

Pyrosequencing

Pyrosequencing, also known as *sequencing by synthesis*, is based on the real-time detection of pyrophosphate release by nucleotide incorporation during DNA synthesis.[42] In the pyrosequencing reaction, as nucleotides are added to the nucleic acid chain by polymerase, pyrophosphate molecules are released and subsequently converted to ATP by ATP sulfurylase. Light is produced by an ATP-driven luciferase reaction via oxidation of a luciferin molecule. The amount of light produced is proportional to the number of incorporated nucleotides in the sequence. When a nucleotide is not incorporated into the reaction, no pyrophosphate is released and the unused nucleotide is degraded by apyrase. Light is converted into peaks in a charge-coupled device (CCD) camera. Individual dNTP nucleotides are sequentially added to the reaction, and the sequence of nucleotides that produce chemiluminescent signals allow the template sequence to be determined. Mutations appear as new peaks in the pyrogram sequence or variations of the expected peak heights.[43]

Pyrosequencing is particularly useful for the detection of point mutations and insertion/deletion mutations that occur at short stretches in mutational hotspots. This method has higher analytical sensitivity than Sanger sequencing and can provide quantitative information about mutation levels in a sample. Pyrosequencing can also be used for the detection and quantification of gene-specific DNA methylation and gene copy number assessments. A microfluidic pyrosequencing platform is available for massive parallel sequencing. However, this method is not well suited for detecting mutations that are scattered across the entire gene because pyrosequencing read lengths are limited to ~100 to 250 base pairs.[43]

Examples of pyrosequencing applications in oncology include the mutational analysis of *BRAF* (codon 600),[44,45] *KRAS* (codons 12, 13, 61),[45] *NRAS* (codon 61),[45] and the methylation analysis of *MGMT* in glioblastoma multiforme.[46,47]

Single Nucleotide Extension Assay (SNaPshot®)

The single nucleotide extension assay is a variant of dideoxy sequencing. This method consists of a single base extension of an unlabeled primer that anneals one base upstream to the relevant mutation with fluorophore-labeled dideoxynucleotides (ddNTP). Multiplexed reactions can be designed with multiple primers of differing lengths for simultaneous amplification of multiple genomic targets.[48] Mutations are identified based on amplicon size and fluorophore color via capillary electrophoresis. When a mutation is present, an alternative dideoxynucleotide triphosphate is incorporated, resulting in a different colored peak with a different amplicon length than the expected wild-type one.

The single nucleotide extension assay is particularly useful for the simultaneous detection of recurrent point mutations. Clinically, it has been employed for analyses of mutational hotspots in multiple genes involved in melanomas, non–small-cell lung cancers, breast cancers, and metastatic colorectal cancers.[49] The assay has higher analytical sensitivity than Sanger sequencing and can detect low-level mutations in FFPE-derived DNA, making it advantageous for biopsy specimens with limited tumor involvement. This assay, however, can only detect mutations that are immediately adjacent to the 3′ to the end of the primer.

Fluorescence In Situ Hybridization

FISH allows for the visualization of specific chromosome nucleic acid sequences within a cellular preparation. This method involves the annealing of a large single-stranded fluorophore-labeled oligonucleotide probe to complementary DNA target sequences within a tissue or cell preparation. The hybridization of the probe at the specific DNA region within a nucleus is visible by direct detection using fluorescence microscopy.

FISH can be used for the quantitative assessment of gene amplification or deletion and for the qualitative evaluation of gene rearrangements. Many oncologic FISH assays employ two probe types: *locus specific probes*, which are complementary to the gene of interest, and *centromeric probes*, which hybridize to the alpha-satellite regions near the centromere of a specific chromosome and help in the enumeration of the number of copies of that chromosome.

For the quantitative assessment of gene amplification, a locus-specific probe and a centromeric probe are labeled with two different fluorophores. The signals generated by each of these probes are counted and a ratio of the targeted gene to the chromosome copy number is calculated. The amount of signal produced by the locus-specific probe is proportional to the number of copies of the targeted gene in a cell. This type of gene amplification assay can be used for the detection of *HER2* gene amplification as an adjunct to existing clinical and pathologic information as an aid in the assessment of stage II, node-positive breast cancer patients for whom Herceptin treatment is being considered. It can also be used for an assessment of *MYCN* amplification in neuroblastoma.

For the detection of deletion mutations, dual-probe hybridization is usually performed using locus-specific probes. For instance, for the detection of 1p/19q codeletion in oligodendrogliomas, locus-specific probe sets for 1p36 and 19q13, and 1q25 and 19p13 (control) are used. The frequencies of signal patterns for each of these loci are evaluated. A signal pattern with 1p and 19q signals that are less than control signals is consistent with deletion of these loci.

Gene rearrangements/chromosomal translocations in hematologic or solid malignancies can be tested using locus-specific dual-fusion or break-apart probes. Dual-color, dual-fusion translocation assays employ two probes that are located in two separate genes involved in a specific rearrangement. Each gene probe is labeled in a different color. This design detects translocations by the juxtaposition of both probe signals. Dual-color, dual-fusion translocation assays are very specific for detecting a selected translocation. But, it can only be used for detecting translocations that involve consistent partners, where both partners are known. Alternate translocations with different fusion partners are not detected by this approach. Examples of application of dual-fusion probes in oncology include for the detection of the *IGH-BCL2* translocation that occurs in most follicular lymphomas and a subset of diffuse large B-cell lymphomas (Fig. 3.8) and for the detection of *IGH-CCND1* rearrangements in mantle cell lymphomas.

In break-apart FISH assays, both dual-colored probes flank the breakpoint region in a single gene that represents the constant partner in the translocation. By this approach, rearranged alleles show two split signals, whereas normal alleles show fusion signals. This design is particularly useful for genes that fuse with multiple translocation partners (e.g., *EWSR1* gene, which may undergo rearrangement with multiple partner genes, including *FLI1*, *ERG*, *ETV1*, *FEV*, and *E1AF* in Ewing sarcoma/primitive neuroectodermal tumor [PNET]; *WT1* in desmoplastic small round cell tumors; *CHN* in extraskeletal myxoid chondrosarcoma; and *ATF1* in clear cell sarcoma and angiomatoid fibrous histiocytoma).[50] The disadvantage of this approach is that break-apart FISH does not allow for the identification of the "unknown" partner in the translocation.

FISH has the advantage of being applicable to a variety of specimen types, including FFPE tissue. Because probes are hybridized to tissue in situ, the tumor morphology is preserved, which allows for an interpretation of the assay even in the context of heterogeneous samples. However, FISH is a targeted approach that will only detect specific alterations. Because most probes are large (e.g., >100 kb), small deletions or insertions will not be detected. In addition, poor tissue fixation, fixation artifacts, nuclear truncation on tissue slides, and nuclear overlaps are potential pitfalls of this technique that may hamper interpretation. Some intrachromosomal rearrangements (e.g., *RET-PTC* and *EML4-ALK*) may be challenging to interpret by FISH due to subtle rearrangements of the probe signals on the same chromosome arm.

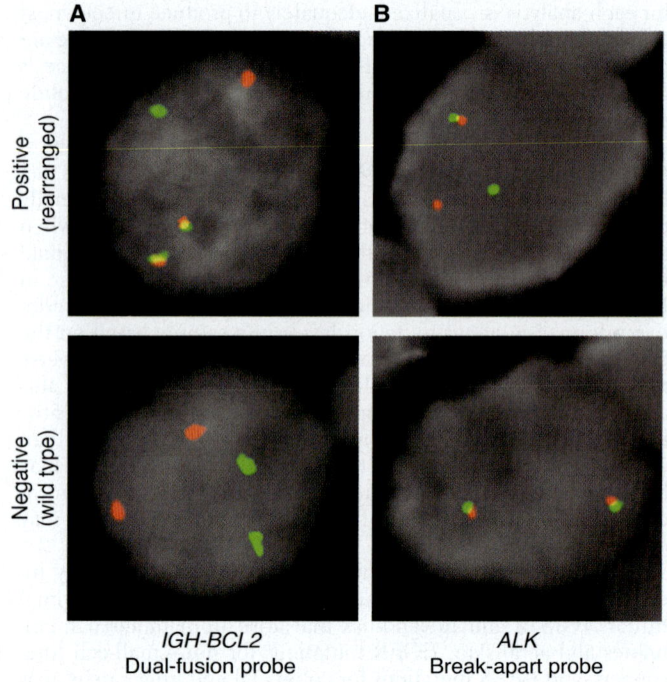

Figure 3.8 Fluorescence in situ hybridization (FISH). **(A)** Recurrent chromosomal translocations such as *IGH-BCL2* (occurring in B-cell lymphomas) can be effectively detected with a dual-fusion probe strategy. This design utilizes a green probe specific to the *IGH* locus and a red probe specific to the *BCL2* gene, with each probe spanning their respective breakpoint region. Individual green and red probe signals indicate a lack of translocation. Colocalization of green and red probes is observed when an *IGH-BCL2* translocation is present. **(B)** *ALK* rearrangements in non–small-cell lung cancers may involve a variety of translocation partners, including *EML4*, *TFG*, and *KIF5B*. Therefore, a break-apart FISH probe strategy is utilized that will detect any *ALK* rearrangement, regardless of the partner gene. Fluorescently labeled red and green probes are designed on opposite sides of the *ALK* gene breakpoint region. With this design, a normal *ALK* gene is observed as overlapping or adjacent red and green fluorescent signals, whereas a rearranged *ALK* gene is indicated by split red and green signals. *ALK* testing in lung cancer has become widespread in use because of the significant therapeutic implications.

Methylation Analysis

Changes in the methylation status of cytosine in DNA regions enriched for the sequence CpG (also known as CpG islands) are early events in many cancers and permanent changes found in many tumors. The detection of aberrant methylation of cancer-related genes may aid in the diagnosis, prognosis, and/or determination of the metastatic potential of tumors.

The most common approaches for the detection of methylation are based on the conversion of unmethylated cytosine bases into uracil after sodium bisulfite treatment, which is then converted to thymidine during PCR. By this approach, bisulfite-treated methylated alleles have different DNA sequences as compared with their corresponding unmethylated alleles. The differences between methylated and unmethylated DNA sequences can be evaluated by several methods, including methylation-sensitive restriction enzyme analysis, methylation-specific PCR, semiquantitative q-PCR, Sanger sequencing, pyrosequencing, and next-generation sequencing.

The methylation status of oncogenic genes can also be assessed by methylation-sensitive multiplex ligation-dependent probe amplification (MS-MLPA) assay.[51,52] MS-MLPA is a variant of multiplex PCR in which oligonucleotide probes hybridized to the targeted DNA samples are directly amplified using one pair of universal primers. This method is not based on bisulfite conversion of unmethylated cytosine bases into uracil. Instead, the target sequences detected by MS-MLPA probes contain a restriction site recognized by methylation-sensitive endonucleases. A probe amplification product will only be obtained if the CpG site is methylated because digested probes cannot be amplified during PCR. The level of methylation is determined by resolving PCR products by capillary electrophoresis and calculating the normalized ratio of each target probe peak area in both digested and undigested specimens. The ratio corresponds to the percentage of methylation present in the specimen.

Examples of applications of methylation analysis in oncology include an analysis of *MLH1* promoter hypermethylation in microsatellite unstable sporadic colorectal carcinomas, an analysis of *MGMT* promoter methylation status in glioblastoma multiforme patients treated with alkylating chemotherapy, and *SEPT9* promoter methylation in DNA derived from blood plasma in colorectal cancer patients.[53]

Microsatellite Instability Analysis

Microsatellites are short, tandem-repeated DNA sequences with repeating units of one to six base pairs in length. Microsatellites are distributed throughout the human genome, and individual repeat loci often vary in length from one individual to another. Microsatellite instability (MSI) is the change in length of a microsatellite allele due to either insertion or deletion of repeating units and a failure of the DNA mismatch repair (MMR) system to repair these replication errors. This genomic instability arises in a variety of human neoplasms where tumor cells have a decreased ability to faithfully replicate DNA. MSI is particularly associated with colorectal cancer, where 15% to 20% of sporadic tumors show MSI, in contrast to the more common chromosomal instability (CIN) phenotype, with MSI status being an independent prognostic indicator. MSI analysis is also clinically useful in identifying patients at increased risk of hereditary nonpolyposis colorectal cancer (HNPCC)/Lynch syndrome, where a germline mutation of an MMR gene causes a familial predisposition to colorectal cancer. MSI analysis alone is not sufficient to make a diagnosis of a germline MMR mutation given the high rate of sporadic MSI-positive colorectal tumors, but a positive result is an indication for follow-up genetic testing and counseling.

In an MSI analysis, DNA is extracted from tumor tissue and the corresponding adjacent normal mucosa. The DNA is subjected to multiplex PCR using fluorescent-labeled primers for coamplification of five mononucleotide repeat markers for MSI determination and two pentanucleotide markers for confirming tumor/normal sample identity. The resulting PCR fragments are separated and detected using capillary electrophoresis. Allelic profiles of normal versus tumor tissues are compared, and MSI is scored as the presence of novel microsatellite lengths in tumor DNA compared to normal DNA. Instability in two or more out of five mononucleotide microsatellite markers in tumor DNA compared to normal DNA is defined as MSI-H (high). MSI-L (low) is defined as instability in one out of five mononucleotide markers in tumor DNA compared to normal DNA. Tumors with no instability (zero out of five altered mononucleotide markers) are defined as microsatellite stable (MSS).[54,55]

Loss of Heterozygosity Analysis

Loss of heterozygosity (LOH) is a common event in cancer that usually occurs due to deletion of a chromosome segment and results in a loss of one copy of an allele. LOH is a common occurrence in tumor suppressor genes and may contribute to tumorigenesis when the second allele is subsequently inactivated by a second "hit" due to mutation or deletion.

LOH studies are used to identify genomic imbalance in tumors, indicating possible sites of tumor suppressor gene (TSG) deletion. LOH studies can be done by multiplex PCR analysis of microsatellites (short tandem repeats [STRs]), FISH, and genomic microarrays). By PCR, microsatellites located in the vicinity of a tumor suppressor gene are used as surrogate markers for the presence of the gene of interest. DNA is extracted from tumor tissue and corresponding adjacent normal mucosa. The DNA is subjected to multiplex PCR using fluorescent-labeled STR primers. Peak height ratio of informative (nonhomozygous) alleles at each locus is calculated from both normal and tumor tissues. LOH is defined as the decrease in peak height of one of the two alleles, relative to the allele peak heights of the normal sample.

An example of applications of LOH studies in oncology include an analysis of 1p/19q loss in oligodendrogliomas, and an analysis of 1p loss in parathyroid carcinomas.

Whole Genome Analysis Methods

Next-Generation Sequencing

Next-generation sequencing (NGS), also known as massive parallel sequencing or deep sequencing, is an emerging technology that has revolutionized the speed, throughput, and cost of sequencing and has facilitated the discovery of clinically relevant genetic biomarkers for diagnosis, prognosis, and personalized therapeutics. By way of this technology, multiple genes or the entire exome or genome can be interrogated simultaneously in multiple parallel reactions instead of a single-gene basis as in Sanger sequencing or pyrosequencing. Currently, the most common NGS approach for cancer testing in the clinical setting employs targeted sequencing of specific genes and mutation hotspot regions. This targeted approach increases sensitivity for the detection of low-level mutations by increasing the depth of sequence coverage.

Presently, there are numerous NGS platforms that employ different sequencing technologies. A comprehensive review and comparison of NGS platforms is beyond the scope of this chapter and has been reviewed elsewhere.[56,57] A generalized clinical workflow is shown (Fig. 3.9). Frequently, multiple DNA samples are individually barcoded and pooled together to leverage platform throughput. Pooled libraries are prepared and enriched, and single DNA molecules are arrayed in solid surfaces, glass slides, or beads and sequenced in situ using reversible DNA chain terminators or iterative cycles of oligonucleotide ligation. NGS signal outputs are based on luminescence, fluorescence, or changes in ion concentration. Robust bioinformatics pipelines are required for an alignment of reads to a reference genome sequence, variant calling, variant annotation, and to assist with result reporting.[58]

NGS can be used for the detection of single nucleotide variants, small insertions and deletions, translocations, inversions, alternative splicing, and copy number variations given sufficient depth of genomic DNA sequence (Fig. 3.10). Technical limitations of this technique include difficulty in sequencing guanine-cytosine (GC)–rich genomic regions, and erroneous sequencing of homologous DNA regions (e.g., pseudogenes) that may confound interpretation.

Examples of applications of NGS in oncology include small targeted panels (3 to 50 genes) for non–small-cell lung cancers, melanomas, colon cancers, and acute myeloid leukemias.[57,59–62] Larger panels (50 to 500 genes) are increasingly being utilized, particularly in both clinical trials and research.

Massively parallel sequencing of RNA (RNA-Seq) can be used for determining sequence variants, alternative splicing, gene rearrangements, and allelic expression of mutant transcripts. To date, this technique has been used primarily for discovery rather than clinical applications, but it is likely to play an increasing role in clinical diagnostics as the technology improves. For transcriptome sequencing, the RNA must first be converted to cDNA, which is then fragmented and entered into library construction. After sequencing, reads are aligned to a reference genome, compared with known transcript sequences, or assembled de novo

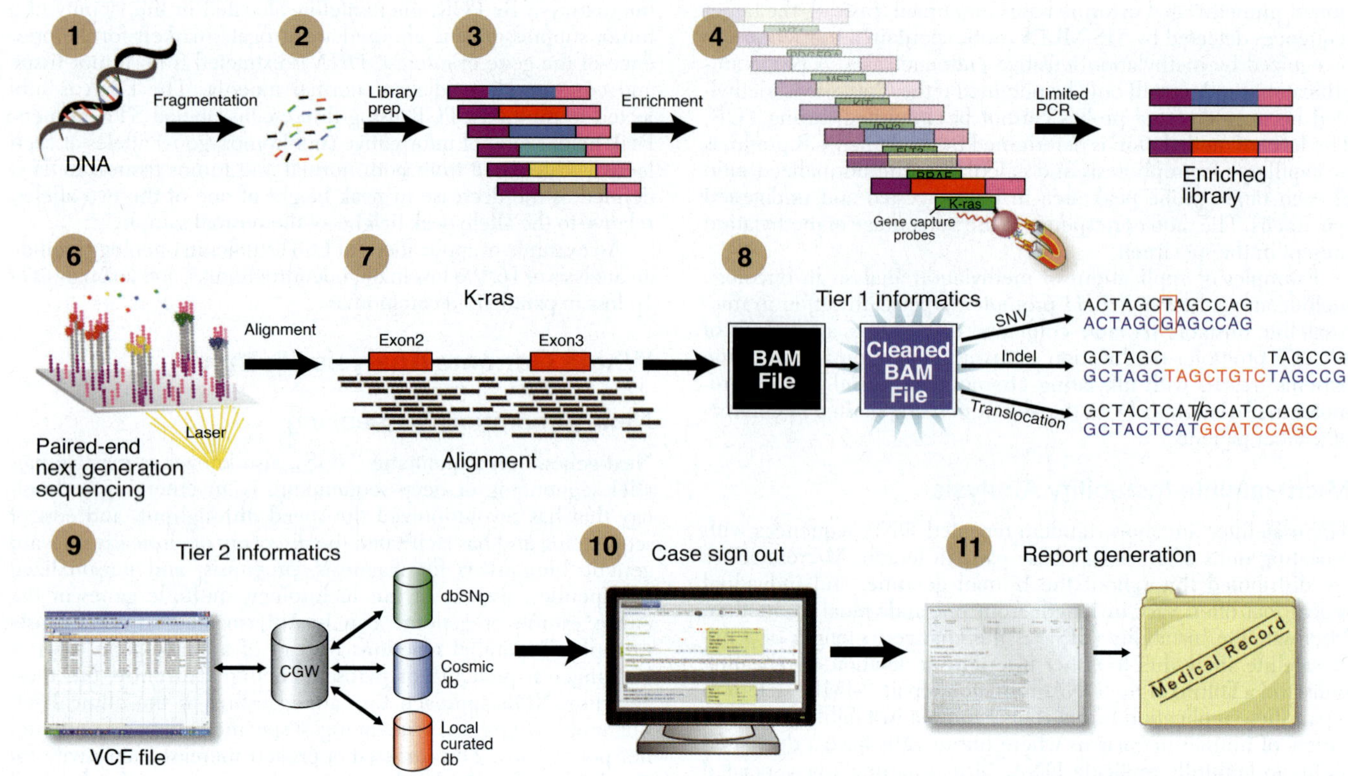

Figure 3.9 Next-generation sequencing (NGS) workflow in a clinical laboratory. Targeted-panel sequencing offers tremendous promise for cancer diagnostics due to the massive improvement in throughput, speed, and cost. NGS is a complex, multiday process that requires significant infrastructure and expertise to deploy in a clinical setting. The process begins with genomic DNA extraction, which is fragmented and to which linkers are ligated. In this targeted gene panel–based example, the sequencing libraries are enriched for the target genes, which are subjected to a limited PCR prior to sequencing. Sequence reads are mapped to a reference genome and subjected to several bioinformatics tools to provide variant calling results and variant annotation. Clinical interpretation and case sign out is performed by a physician with expertise in molecular pathology. BAM, Binary Sequence Alignment/Map; SNV, Single Nucleotide Variant; VCF, Variant Call Format; CGW, Clinical Genomicist Workstation; dbSNP, The Single Nucleotide Polymorphism Database. (Used with permission from Shashikant Kulkarni PhD and Eric Duncavage MD.)

to construct a genome-scale transcription map. Expression levels are determined from the total number of sequence reads that map to the exons of a particular gene, normalized by the length of exons that can be uniquely mapped.[56] Compared with genomic microarrays, RNA-Seq has a greater ability to distinguish RNA isoforms, determine allelic expression, and reveal sequence variants.

Chromatin immunoprecipitation with sequencing (ChIP-Seq) can be used to determine the genome-wide location of chromatin-binding transcription factors or specific epigenetic modifications of histones. This has proved to be a very powerful research tool, which to date has not been used for clinical diagnostics. Proteins in contact with genomic DNA are chemically cross-linked (usually with formaldehyde treatment) to their binding sites, the DNA is fragmented, and the proteins cross-linked with DNA are then immunoprecipitated with antibodies specific for the proteins (or specific epigenetic histone modification) of interest. The DNA harvested from the immunoprecipitate is converted into a library for NGS. The obtained reads are mapped to the reference genome of interest to generate a genome-wide protein binding map.[63,64] ChIP-Seq is rapidly replacing chromatin immunoprecipitation and microarray hybridization (ChIP-on-chip) technology[65] because of its higher sensitivity and resolution.[66]

Genomic Microarrays

High-density genomic microarrays are widely used for whole genome assessment of copy number changes, LOH, and genotyping. In array comparative genomic hybridization (aCGH), cloned genomic probes are arrayed onto glass slides and serves as targets for the competitive hybridization of normal and tumor DNA. In the aCGH reaction, tumor DNA and DNA from a normal control sample are labeled with different fluorophores. These samples are denatured and hybridized together to the arrayed single-strand probes. Digital imaging systems are used to quantify the relative fluorescence intensities of the labeled DNA probes that have hybridized to each target probe. The fluorescence ratio of the tumor and control hybridization signals is determined at different positions along the genome, which provides information on the relative copy number of sequences in the tumor genome as compared to the normal genome.[67] This method is able to detect copy number variation, such as deletions, duplications, and gene amplification, but it cannot detect polymorphic allele changes.

An SNP array has the ability to detect LOH profiles in addition to high-resolution detection of copy number aberrations, such as amplifications and deletions. This method employs thousands of unique fluorescent-labeled nucleotide probe sequences arrayed on a chip to which a fragmented single-stranded specimen DNA binds to their complementary partners. Each SNP site is interrogated by complementary sets of probes containing perfect matches and mismatches to each SNP site. Each probe is associated with one of the two alleles of an SNP (also known as A and B). Relative fluorescence intensity depends on both the amount of target DNA in the sample, as well as the affinity between target and probe. An analysis of the raw fluorescence intensity is done by computational

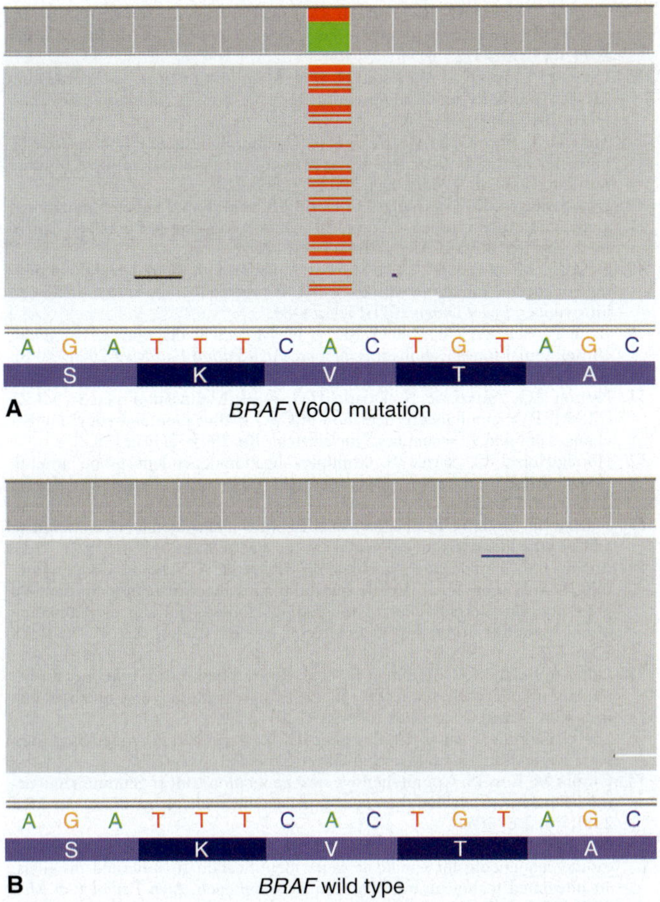

Figure 3.10 Next-generation sequencing (NGS). Hundreds to thousands of sequence reads are mapped and horizontally aligned to specific targeted regions in the reference genome (sequence shown on *bottom* of each panel). A software-assisted analysis assists in the detection of mutations, displayed as colored bars in each read above the mutation site. A wild-type sequence within each read is displayed in *gray*. Mutation frequency correlates to the number of times the mutant sequence is detected compared to the total number of reads at that nucleotide position. Shown are sequencing results from *BRAF* V600E mutation positive **(A)** and negative **(B)** melanomas. The A to T base substitution that leads to the V600E mutation is displayed in red. Patients with metastatic melanoma that harbors the *BRAF*V600E mutation are candidates for targeted therapy.

algorithms that convert the set of probe intensities into genotypes. Deleted genomic regions are identified as having an LOH associated with copy number reduction. A copy-neutral LOH is detected when SNPs expected to be heterozygous in the normal sample are detected as homozygous in the tumor sample without copy number variation. A copy neutral LOH may arise from somatic homologous recombination of a mutated tumor suppressor allele and its surrounding DNA that replaces the other allele (uniparental disomy [UPD]). SNP microarrays are the only genomic microarrays that are able to identify UPD. Array technologies cannot detect true balanced chromosome abnormalities and low-level mosaicism.

Examples of genomic microarrays applications in oncology include the detection of copy number variations and LOH in chronic lymphocytic leukemia[68] and recurrent cytogenetic abnormalities in MDS (e.g., 5q-, -7 or 7q-, +8, 20q-).[69]

Expression Panels

Gene expression signatures of multiple cancer biomarkers are starting to be incorporated into clinical practice as an adjunct to clinical and pathologic information in diverse cancer management settings. An example of a multigene expression–based test in current use includes Oncotype DX, which is a quantitative RT-PCR–based assay that measures the expression of 21 genes in FFPE breast tumors. The test is designed to predict the potential benefit of chemotherapy and the likelihood of distant breast cancer recurrence in women with node negative or node positive, estrogen receptor (ER)-positive, and *HER2*-negative invasive breast cancer. This test has been in-corporated into current American Society of Clinical Oncology (ASCO) and National Comprehensive Cancer Network (NCCN) for breast cancer management.[70] Prospective trials are in progress to evaluate other multigene tests for early stage breast cancer.

With the rapid advances in molecular diagnostic technologies, it is likely that many mutation- and expression-based panels analyzing hundreds if not thousands of genes, or even the complete genome or transcriptome, will enter widespread use. Some of the many challenges to address will be to provide evidence-based, actionable reports that guide the oncologist to more effective therapies, to learn from the results of such testing to improve the algorithms guiding therapy, to handle the incidental findings in such testing in an ethically responsible way, and ultimately, with the drugs available, to provide sufficient improvements in outcomes so that society will be willing to bear the costs.

REFERENCES

1. Lennard L, Cartwright CS, Wade R, et al. Thiopurine methyltransferase genotype-phenotype discordance and thiopurine active metabolite formation in childhood acute lymphoblastic leukaemia. *Br J Clin Pharmacol* 2013;76(1):125–136.
2. Haber DA, Settleman J. Cancer: drivers and passengers. *Nature* 2007; 446(7132):145–146.
3. Hayashi T, Sudo J. Relieving effect of saline on cephaloridine nephrotoxicity in rats. *Chem Pharm Bull (Tokyo)* 1989;37(3):785–790.
4. Brodeur GM, Seeger RC, Schwab M, et al. Amplification of N-myc in untreated human neuroblastomas correlates with advanced disease stage. *Science* 1984;224(4653):1121–1124.
5. Seeger RC, Brodeur GM, Sather H, et al. Association of multiple copies of the N-myc oncogene with rapid progression of neuroblastomas. *N Engl J Med* 1985;313(18):1111–1116.
6. Weinstein JL, Katzenstein HM, Cohn SL. Advances in the diagnosis and treatment of neuroblastoma. *Oncologist* 2003;8(3):278–292.
7. Pui CH, Crist WM, Look AT. Biology and clinical significance of cytogenetic abnormalities in childhood acute lymphoblastic leukemia. *Blood* 1990;76(8):1449–1463.
8. Lee JA, Lupski JR. Genomic rearrangements and gene copy-number alterations as a cause of nervous system disorders. *Neuron* 2006;52(1):103–121.
9. Kuiper RP, Ligtenberg MJ, Hoogerbrugge N, et al. Germline copy number variation and cancer risk. *Curr Opin Genet Dev* 2010;20(3):282–289.
10. Shlien A, Malkin D. Copy number variations and cancer. *Genome Med* 2009;1(6):62.
11. Lynch TJ, Bell DW, Sordella R, et al. Activating mutations in the epidermal growth factor receptor underlying responsiveness of non–small-cell lung cancer to gefitinib. *N Engl J Med* 2004;350(21):2129–2139.
12. Paez JG, Janne PA, Lee JC, et al. EGFR mutations in lung cancer: correlation with clinical response to gefitinib therapy. *Science* 2004;304(5676): 1497–1500.
13. Forbes SA, Bindal N, Bamford S, et al. COSMIC: mining complete cancer genomes in the Catalogue of Somatic Mutations in Cancer. *Nucleic Acids Res* 2011;39(Database issue):D945–950.
14. Van Allen EM, Wagle N, Levy MA. Clinical analysis and interpretation of cancer genome data. *J Clin Oncol* 2013;31(15):1825–1833.
15. Newman B, Mu H, Butler LM, et al. Frequency of breast cancer attributable to BRCA1 in a population-based series of American women. *JAMA* 1998;279(12):915–921.
16. Ford D, Easton DF, Stratton M, et al. Genetic heterogeneity and penetrance analysis of the BRCA1 and BRCA2 genes in breast cancer families. The Breast Cancer Linkage Consortium. *Am J Hum Genet* 1998;62(3): 676–689.
17. Antoniou A, Pharoah PD, Narod S, et al. Average risks of breast and ovarian cancer associated with BRCA1 or BRCA2 mutations detected in case series unselected for family history: a combined analysis of 22 studies. *Am J Hum Genet* 2003;72(5):1117–1130.
18. Chen S, Iversen ES, Friebel T, et al. Characterization of BRCA1 and BRCA2 mutations in a large United States sample. *J Clin Oncol* 2006;24(6):863–871.

19. Bachner P, Hamlin W. Federal regulation of clinical laboratories and the Clinical Laboratory Improvement Amendments of 1988—Part II. *Clin Lab Med* 1993;13(4):987–994.
20. Halling KC, Schrijver I, Persons DL. Test verification and validation for molecular diagnostic assays. *Arch Pathol Lab Med* 2012;136(1):11–13.
21. Jennings L, Van Deerlin VM, Gulley ML, College of American Pathologists Molecular Pathology Resource C. Recommended principles and practices for validating clinical molecular pathology tests. *Arch Pathol Lab Med* 2009;133(5):743–755.
22. Jennings LJ, Smith FA, Halling KC, et al. Design and analytic validation of BCR-ABL1 quantitative reverse transcription polymerase chain reaction assay for monitoring minimal residual disease. *Arch Pathol Lab Med* 2012;136(1):33–40.
23. Pont-Kingdon G, Gedge F, Wooderchak-Donahue W, et al. Design and analytical validation of clinical DNA sequencing assays. *Arch Pathol Lab Med* 2012;136(1):41–46.
24. Saiki RK, Gelfand DH, Stoffel S, et al. Primer-directed enzymatic amplification of DNA with a thermostable DNA polymerase. *Science* 1988;239(4839):487–491.
25. Mullis KB. The unusual origin of the polymerase chain reaction. *Sci Am* 1990;262(4):56–61, 64–65.
26. Bernard PS, Wittwer CT. Real-time PCR technology for cancer diagnostics. *Clin Chem* 2002;48(8):1178–1185.
27. Bench AJ, Baxter EJ, Green AR. Methods for detecting mutations in the human JAK2 gene. *Methods Mol Biol* 2013;967:115–131.
28. Halait H, Demartin K, Shah S, et al. Analytical performance of a real-time PCR-based assay for V600 mutations in the BRAF gene, used as the companion diagnostic test for the novel BRAF inhibitor vemurafenib in metastatic melanoma. *Diagn Mol Pathol* 2012;21(1):1–8.
29. Furtado LV, Weigelin HC, Elenitoba-Johnson KS, et al. Detection of MPL mutations by a novel allele-specific PCR-based strategy. *J Mol Diagn* 2013;15(6):810–818.
30. Lang AH, Drexel H, Geller-Rhomberg S, et al. Optimized allele-specific real-time PCR assays for the detection of common mutations in KRAS and BRAF. *J Mol Diagn* 2011;13(1):23–28.
31. Wang ZY, Chen Z. Acute promyelocytic leukemia: from highly fatal to highly curable. *Blood* 2008;111(5):2505–2515.
32. O'Brien SG, Guilhot F, Larson RA, et al. Imatinib compared with interferon and low-dose cytarabine for newly diagnosed chronic-phase chronic myeloid leukemia. *N Engl J Med* 2003;348(11):994–1004.
33. Hughes TP, Kaeda J, Branford S, et al. Frequency of major molecular responses to imatinib or interferon alfa plus cytarabine in newly diagnosed chronic myeloid leukemia. *N Engl J Med* 2003;349(15):1423–1432.
34. Szankasi P, Jama M, Bahler DW. A new DNA-based test for detection of nucleophosmin exon 12 mutations by capillary electrophoresis. *J Mol Diagn* 2008;10(3):236–241.
35. Furtado LV, Weigelin HC, Elenitoba-Johnson KS, et al. A multiplexed fragment analysis-based assay for detection of JAK2 exon 12 mutations. *J Mol Diagn* 2013;15(5):592–599.
36. Reed GH, Kent JO, Wittwer CT. High-resolution DNA melting analysis for simple and efficient molecular diagnostics. *Pharmacogenomics* 2007;8(6):597–608.
37. Palais RA, Liew MA, Wittwer CT. Quantitative heteroduplex analysis for single nucleotide polymorphism genotyping. *Anal Biochem* 2005;346(1):167–175.
38. Carillo S, Henry L, Lippert E, et al. Nested high-resolution melting curve analysis a highly sensitive, reliable, and simple method for detection of JAK2 exon 12 mutations—clinical relevance in the monitoring of polycythemia. *J Mol Diagn* 2011;13(3):263–270.
39. Ney JT, Froehner S, Roesler A, et al. High-resolution melting analysis as a sensitive prescreening diagnostic tool to detect KRAS, BRAF, PIK3CA, and AKT1 mutations in formalin-fixed, paraffin-embedded tissues. *Arch Pathol Lab Med* 2012;136(9):983–992.
40. Jones AV, Cross NC, White HE, et al. Rapid identification of JAK2 exon 12 mutations using high resolution melting analysis. *Haematologica* Oct 2008;93(10):1560–1564.
41. Sanger F, Nicklen S, Coulson AR. DNA sequencing with chain-terminating inhibitors. *Proc Natl Acad Sci U S A* 1977;74(12):5463–5467.
42. Ronaghi M, Uhlén M, Nyrén P. A sequencing method based on real-time pyrophosphate. *Science* 1998;281(5375):363, 365.
43. Ronaghi M, Shokralla S, Gharizadeh B. Pyrosequencing for discovery and analysis of DNA sequence variations. *Pharmacogenomics* 2007;8(10):1437–1441.
44. Shigaki H, Baba Y, Watanabe M, et al. KRAS and BRAF mutations in 203 esophageal squamous cell carcinomas: pyrosequencing technology and literature review. *Ann Surg Oncol* 2013;20:485–491.
45. Vaughn CP, Zobell SD, Furtado LV, et al. Frequency of KRAS, BRAF, and NRAS mutations in colorectal cancer. *Genes Chromosomes Cancer* 2011;50(5):307–312.
46. Everhard S, Tost J, El Abdalaoui H, et al. Identification of regions correlating MGMT promoter methylation and gene expression in glioblastomas. *Neuro Oncol* 2009;11(4):348–356.
47. Mikeska T, Bock C, El-Maarri O, et al. Optimization of quantitative MGMT promoter methylation analysis using pyrosequencing and combined bisulfite restriction analysis. *J Mol Diagn* 2007;9(3):368–381.
48. Dias-Santagata D, Akhavanfard S, David SS, et al. Rapid targeted mutational analysis of human tumours: a clinical platform to guide personalized cancer medicine. *EMBO Mol Med* 2010;2(5):146–158.
49. Su Z, Dias-Santagata D, Duke M, et al. A platform for rapid detection of multiple oncogenic mutations with relevance to targeted therapy in non–small-cell lung cancer. *J Mol Diagn* 2011;13(1):74–84.
50. Lazar A, Abruzzo LV, Pollock RE, et al. Molecular diagnosis of sarcomas: chromosomal translocations in sarcomas. *Arch Pathol Lab Med* 2006;130(8):1199–1207.
51. Nygren AO, Ameziane N, Duarte HM, et al. Methylation-specific MLPA (MS-MLPA): simultaneous detection of CpG methylation and copy number changes of up to 40 sequences. *Nucleic Acids Res* 2005;33(14):e128.
52. Hömig-Hölzel C, Savola S. Multiplex ligation-dependent probe amplification (MLPA) in tumor diagnostics and prognostics. *Diagn Mol Pathol* 2012;21(4):189–206.
53. Warren JD, Xiong W, Bunker AM, et al. Septin 9 methylated DNA is a sensitive and specific blood test for colorectal cancer. *BMC Med* 2011;9:133.
54. Boland CR, Thibodeau SN, Hamilton SR, et al. A National Cancer Institute Workshop on Microsatellite Instability for cancer detection and familial predisposition: development of international criteria for the determination of microsatellite instability in colorectal cancer. *Cancer Res* 1998;58(22):5248–5257.
55. Umar A, Boland CR, Terdiman JP, et al. Revised Bethesda Guidelines for hereditary nonpolyposis colorectal cancer (Lynch syndrome) and microsatellite instability. *J Natl Cancer Inst* 2004;96(4):261–268.
56. Voelkerding KV, Dames SA, Durtschi JD. Next-generation sequencing: from basic research to diagnostics. *Clin Chem* 2009;55(4):641–658.
57. Cronin M, Ross JS. Comprehensive next-generation cancer genome sequencing in the era of targeted therapy and personalized oncology. *Biomarker Med* 2011;5(3):293–305.
58. Coonrod EM, Durtschi JD, Margraf RL, et al. Developing genome and exome sequencing for candidate gene identification in inherited disorders: an integrated technical and bioinformatics approach. *Arch Pathol Lab Med* 2013;137(3):415–433.
59. Grossmann V, Kohlmann A, Klein HU, et al. Targeted next-generation sequencing detects point mutations, insertions, deletions and balanced chromosomal rearrangements as well as identifies novel leukemia-specific fusion genes in a single procedure. *Leukemia* 2011;25(4):671–680.
60. Marchetti A, Del Grammastro M, Filice G, et al. Complex mutations & subpopulations of deletions at exon 19 of EGFR in NSCLC revealed by next generation sequencing: potential clinical implications. *PloS One* 2012;7(7):e42164.
61. McCourt CM, McArt DG, Mills K, et al. Validation of next generation sequencing technologies in comparison to current diagnostic gold standards for BRAF, EGFR and KRAS mutational analysis. *PloS One* 2013;8(7):e69604.
62. Thol F, Kölking B, Damm F, et al. Next-generation sequencing for minimal residual disease monitoring in acute myeloid leukemia patients with FLT3-ITD or NPM1 mutations. *Genes Chromosomes Cancer* 2012;51(7):689–695.
63. Barski A, Cuddapah S, Cui K, et al. High-resolution profiling of histone methylations in the human genome. *Cell* 2007;129(4):823–837.
64. Schones DE, Zhao K. Genome-wide approaches to studying chromatin modifications. *Nat Rev Genet* 2008;9(3):179–191.
65. Ren B, Robert F, Wyrick JJ, et al. Genome-wide location and function of DNA binding proteins. *Science* 2000;290(5500):2306–2309.
66. Robertson G, Hirst M, Bainbridge M, et al. Genome-wide profiles of STAT1 DNA association using chromatin immunoprecipitation and massively parallel sequencing. *Nat Methods* 2007;4(8):651–657.
67. Shinawi M, Cheung SW. The array CGH and its clinical applications. *Drug Discov Today* 2008;13(17–18):760–770.
68. Iacobucci I, Lonetti A, Papayannidis C, Martinelli G. Use of single nucleotide polymorphism array technology to improve the identification of chromosomal lesions in leukemia. *Curr Cancer Drug Targets* 2013;13(7):791–810.
69. Ahmad A, Iqbal MA. Significance of genome-wide analysis of copy number alterations and UPD in myelodysplastic syndromes using combined CGH - SNP arrays. *Curr Med Chem* 2012;19(22):3739–3747.
70. Goncalves R, Bose R. Using multigene tests to select treatment for early-stage breast cancer. *J Natl Compr Canc Netw* 2013;11(2):174–182.

PART II

Etiology and Epidemiology of Cancer

4 Tobacco

Richard J. O'Connor

INTRODUCTION

Regrettably, tobacco use remains one of the leading causes of death worldwide. It is projected to leave over 1 billion dead in the 21st century, after killing nearly 100 million during the course of the 20th century.[1] Data from the Global Adult Tobacco Survey (GATS), which conducted representative household surveys in 14 low- and middle-income countries (Bangladesh, Brazil, China, Egypt, India, Mexico, Philippines, Poland, Russia, Thailand, Turkey, Ukraine, Uruguay, and Vietnam), suggest 41% of men and 5% of women across these countries currently smoke.[2] Compare this to approximately 24% of men and 16% of women in the United States.[3] A preponderance of the death and disease associated with tobacco use is associated with its combusted forms, particularly the cigarette. However, all forms of tobacco use have negative health consequences, the severity of which can vary among products. From the introduction of the mass-manufactured, mass-marketed cigarette (e.g., Camel in 1913), smoking rates grew, first among men then among women, and peaked in Western countries in the 1960s to 1970s, before beginning a steady decline.[4] The smoking rate among US adults has dropped from its peak in 1965 of 42% to 19% in 2011.[3] Per capita consumption has been dropping almost continuously since the 1960s, although the rate of decline has slowed since the early 2000s.[5] Among youth, smoking rates have been in decline since the 1990s,[6,7] although there is some evidence of growth in use of other forms of tobacco (e.g., cigars, water pipes, electronic cigarettes) in 2011 to 2012 that may be displacing cigarette use.[8]

Tobacco control policy interventions can impact both smoking prevalence and lung cancer incidence.[9] For example, a recent analysis suggests that implementation of graphic health warnings in Canada in 1999 resulted in a significant reduction (up to 4.5 percentage points) in smoking prevalence over a decade.[10] Increases in tobacco taxes have long been shown to reduce youth smoking initiation and to prompt more attempts to quit smoking.[11] Evidence from state comparisons in the United States suggests that comprehensive tobacco control measures effectively implemented (such as in California and Massachusetts) can reduce lung cancer incidence.[12] Indeed, Holford and colleagues[13] have shown that since the seminal 1964 Report of the Surgeon General, an estimated 157 million years of life (approximately 20 years per person) have been saved by tobacco control activities in the United States over 50 years. That is, tobacco control activities are estimated to have averted 8 million premature deaths and extended mean life span by 19 to 20 years.[13] However, the marketing of cigarettes has since shifted focus to the developing world, where smoking rates are on the increase. In an attempt to head off an epidemic of smoking and associated diseases, the World Health Organization initiated a public health treaty, the Framework Convention on Tobacco Control (FCTC), to coordinate international efforts to reduce tobacco use.[14] The FCTC binds parties to enact measures to control the labeling and marketing of tobacco products, create a framework for testing and regulating product contents and emissions, combat smuggling and counterfeiting, and protect nonsmokers from secondhand smoke.[15] To date, the FCTC has been ratified by more than 150 countries. The FCTC provides governments the opportunity to regulate the marketing, labeling, and contents/emissions of tobacco products, as well as control the global trade in tobacco products. In the United States, which is currently not a party to FCTC, the U.S. Food and Drug Administration (FDA) has, since 2009, had authority to regulate tobacco products and their marketing along similar lines.[16]

EPIDEMIOLOGY OF TOBACCO AND CANCER

Linkages between tobacco use and cancers at various sites had been noted for several decades. In the late 1800s, it was believed that excessive cigar use created irritation that led to oral cancers.[17] In the 1930s, German scientists began to establish links between cigarette smoking and lung cancers.[18] However, it was not until the Doll and Hill[19] and Wynder and Graham[20] studies were published that the association was demonstrated in large samples and well-designed studies. Table 4.1 lists the cancers currently recognized by the U.S. Surgeon General as caused by smoking, along with their corresponding estimated mortality statistics.[21–23] Of these, the most well-publicized link is between smoking and lung cancer. In a recent examination of National Health and Nutrition Examination Survey (NHANES) data, Jha[24] showed a hazard ratio for lung cancer in smokers versus nonsmokers of 17.8 in women and 14.6 in men. However, smoking contributes substantially to overall cancer burden across multiple sites, including the oropharynx, cervix, and pancreas. Hazard ratios of 1.7 for women and 2.2 for men are seen for cancers other than in the lung in smokers versus nonsmokers.[24] Emerging evidence also links smoking with breast cancer, although the data are as yet insufficient to make causal conclusions.[23,25] Cancer risks associated with smoking, as well as outcomes and survival, depend on a number of factors. A common index of cancer risk is pack-years, or the number of packs of cigarettes smoked per day multiplied by the number of years smoked in the lifetime. In general, the higher the number of pack-years, the greater the cancer risk. Risks for lung cancer decline with smoking cessation, and the longer a former smoker remains off of cigarettes, the more the risk declines.[26] However, excepting those smokers who quit with relatively few pack years accumulated (typically before age 40), cancer risk rarely approaches that of a never smoker.[24,27]

A recent study using several large cohort studies examined death rates and the relative risks associated with smoking and smoking cessation for 3 epochs (1959 to 1965, 1982 to 1988, and 2000 to 2010).[27] Of most interest here is death from lung cancer. For men, the age-adjusted death rate from lung cancer increased from 1959 through 1965 to 1982 through1988, but then fell for 2000

TABLE 4.1

Level of Evidence for Smoking-Attributable Cancers According to the United States Office of the Surgeon General by Cancer Site and Yearly Smoking-Attributable Mortality at Sites with Available Estimates, United States, 2004

	Cancer Site	Yearly Smoking-Attributable Mortality
Evidence Sufficient to Infer Causal Relationship	Bladder	4,983
	Cervix	447
	Colon and rectum	N/A
	Esophagus	8,592
	Kidney	3,043
	Larynx	3,009
	Leukemia (AML)	1,192
	Liver	N/A
	Lung	125,522
	Oral cavity and pharynx	4,893
	Pancreas	6,683
	Stomach	2,484
Evidence Suggestive but Not Sufficient to Infer Causal Relationship	Breast	
Inadequate to Infer Presence or Absence of Causal Relationship	Ovary	
Evidence Sufficient to Infer No Causal Relationship	Prostate	

N/A, not available; AML, acute myeloid leukemia.

through 2010; for women, the age-adjusted death rate continued to rise over time, with the biggest increase between 1982 through 1988 to 2000 through 2010.[27] In relative risk terms, the likelihood of dying from lung cancer given current smoking has increased from 2.73 to 12.65 to 25.66 among women, and 12.22 to 23.81 to 24.97 for men. Equivalent risks for former smokers increased from 1.3 to 3.85 to 6.7 among women, versus 3.48 to 7.41 to 6.75 for men. These and other analyses suggest that the cancer risks from smoking may have increased with time.[27,28] The histologic subtypes of lung cancer seen in the US population have also shifted with time. Into the early 1980s, squamous cell carcinomas (SCC) were the most common manifestations of lung cancer. However, a rapid rise in adenocarcinomas has been noted, and by the 1990s, had overtaken SCC as the leading type of lung cancer.[23]

Tobacco Use Behaviors

The level of tobacco exposure is ultimately driven by use behaviors, including the number of cigarettes smoked, the patterns of smoking on individual cigarettes, and the number of years smoked. The primary driver of smoking behavior is nicotine—the major addictive substance and primary reinforcer of continued smoking.[29–31] Over time, smokers learn an *acceptable* level of nicotine intake that attains the beneficial effects they seek while avoiding negative withdrawal symptoms. Smokers can affect the amount of nicotine (and accompanying toxicants) they draw from a cigarette by altering the number of puffs taken, puff size, frequency, duration, and velocity (collectively referred to as smoking topography).[32] Smokers tend to consume a relatively stable number of cigarettes per day and to smoke those cigarettes in a relatively consistent manner in order to maintain an acceptable level of nicotine in their system across the day.[33] The number of cigarettes smoked per day and the smoking pattern of an individual may be influenced by the rate of nicotine metabolism.[30] Nicotine is metabolized primarily to cotinine, which is further metabolized to trans-3′-hydroxycotinine (3HC), catalyzed by the liver cytochrome P450 2A6 enzyme.[34] Functional polymorphisms in the genes coding for these enzymes allow for the identification of *fast* metabolizers, who have more rapid nicotine clearance and show greater cigarette intake and more intensive smoking topography profiles relative to *normal* or *slow* metabolizers.[35–37] The ratio of 3HC to cotinine in plasma or saliva can be used as a reliable noninvasive phenotypic marker for CYP2A6 activity.[38,39] CYP2A6 activity is known to vary across racial/ethnic groups, with those of African or Asian descent showing slower metabolism than those of Caucasian descent.[40–42] Clinical trial data clearly show that the metabolite ratio can be used to predict success in quitting, and that the likelihood of quitting decreases as the ratio increases, such that slower metabolizers are more successful at achieving abstinence.[37,41,43] Despite their addiction to nicotine, most smokers in Western countries report that they regret ever starting to smoke and want to quit smoking, and there is evidence for similar regret in developing countries as well.[44–46] However, most smokers are unsuccessful in their attempts to quit smoking; the most effective evidence-based treatments increase the odds of quitting by 3 times, with 12-month cessation rates of approximately 40% relative to placebo.[47]

Evolution of Tobacco Products

Historically, tar was believed to be the main contributor to smoking-caused disease.[48] It is important to note that *tar* is not a specific substance, but simply the collected particulate matter from cigarette smoke, less water and nicotine (in technical reports, it is often referred to as nicotine-free dry particulate matter). Soon after the first studies were done showing that painting mice with cigarette tar caused cancerous tumors, it was theorized that reducing tar yields of cigarettes might also reduce the disease burden of smoking.[48] Concurrently, cigarette manufacturers were seeking to reassure their customers that their products were safe, that if hazardous compounds were identified they would be removed, and that product modifications could help to reduce risks.[4,49–51] Indeed, in the United States and United Kingdom, average tar levels of cigarettes dropped dramatically from the 1960s through the 1990s, and have since leveled off.[52,53] The European Union took the tar reduction mentality to heart in crafting maximum levels of tar in cigarettes that could be sold in member countries, beginning at 15 mg in 1992, then dropping to 12 mg in 1998, and 10 mg in 2005.[54] Unfortunately, these reductions in tar yields have not translated into changes in disease risks among smokers.[55] Despite initial optimism about these products, both laboratory-based and epidemiologic studies indicate neither an individual, nor a public health benefit from *low-tar* cigarettes as compared to *full-flavor* varieties.[56–58] The health consequences of mistakenly accepting the purported benefits of lower tar and nicotine products have been significant. The increases in adenocarcinoma of the lung observed in the United States over recent decades may reflect changes made to the cigarette, such as filters, filter ventilation, and tobacco-specific nitrosamines (TSNA) in smoke produced by the relatively high amount of burley tobacco used in the typical US cigarette blend.[23,59] Tobacco manufacturers engineered cigarettes be *elastic*; that is, cigarettes allow smokers to adjust their puffing patterns to regulate their intake of nicotine, regardless of how the cigarette might perform under the standard testing conditions that drove the labeling and advertising of the products.[55] Researchers have since come to determine that filter vents are the main design feature the industry relied on in creating elastic products.[54,55,60,61] Vents facilitate taking larger puffs and also contribute to sensory perceptions, because they dilute the smoke with air. [62] So, even with a larger puff, the same mass of toxins can seem less harsh and irritating because it is diluted by a proportionate amount of air, which may in turn underscore smokers' beliefs that they are smoking safer cigarettes.[62–64] Other smoke components (e.g., acetaldehyde, ammonia, minor tobacco alkaloids) and aspects of cigarette engineering (e.g., menthol, flavor additives) may further contribute to the addictiveness of cigarettes.[65]

Since the 1980s, manufacturers have introduced products that make more explicit claims about reduced health risks. Examples of modified cigarettelike products include Premier (RJ Reynolds), Eclipse (RJ Reynolds), Accord/Heatbar (Philip Morris), Omni (Vector Tobacco), and Advance (Brown and Williamson).[66] In the 2000s, as evidence of reduced lung cancer incidence and coincident increases in snus use in Sweden appeared,[67,68] manufacturers began to promote smokeless tobacco products as reduced harm alternatives. Most recently, electronic cigarettes, which vaporize a nicotine solution, have gained increasing popularity and generated concern among public health practitioners, particularly with regard to effects on youth.[8,69,70] In the United States, the FDA has authority to authorize marketing claims about reduced risk, which an Institute of Medicine panel concluded should be based on extensive testing of abuse liability, likely health effects, and effects on the whole population.[71]

CARCINOGENS IN TOBACCO PRODUCTS AND PROCESSES OF CANCER DEVELOPMENT

Cigarette smoke has been identified as carcinogenic since the 1950s, and efforts have continued to identify specific carcinogens in smoke and smokeless tobacco products. The International Agency for Research on Cancer (IARC) has classified both cigarette smoke and smokeless tobacco as Group 1 carcinogens.[72,73] IARC has also identified 72 measurable carcinogens in cigarette smoke where evidence is sufficient to classify them as Group 1 (carcinogenic to humans), 2A (probably carcinogenic to humans), or 2B (possibly carcinogenic to humans).[72] The IARC list, in addition to data from the U.S. Environmental Protection Agency (EPA), the National Toxicology Program, and the National Institute for Occupational Safety and Health (NIOSH), informed the FDA's development of a list of Harmful and Potentially Harmful Constituents (HPHC) in tobacco and tobacco smoke, which manufacturers will be required to report.[74] Table 4.2 illustrates the carcinogens listed as HPHC alongside their carcinogenicity classifications by IARC or the EPA.

Compounds of Particular Concern

Research groups have listed components of cigarette smoke theorized to impact health risk, often relying on carcinogenic potency indices and relative concentrations in smoke.[75,76] In these analyses, the N-nitrosamines, benzene, 1,3-butadiene, aromatic amines, and cadmium often rank highly. Polycyclic aromatic hydrocarbons (PAH), many of which are carcinogenic, consist of three or more fused aromatic rings resulting from incomplete combustion of organic (carbonaceous) materials, and are often found in coal tar, soot, broiled foods, and automobile engine exhaust.[77] A compound of particular concern in cigarette smoke historically has been benzo(a)pyrene (BaP), which has substantial carcinogenic activity and is considered carcinogenic to humans by the IARC.[77] In addition to PAH, other hydrocarbons found in significant quantities in cigarette smoke include benzene (a long-established cause of leukemia), 1,3-butadiene (a potent multiorgan carcinogen), naphthalene, and styrene. Carbonyl compounds, such as formaldehyde and acetaldehyde, are found in copious amounts in cigarette smoke, primarily coming from the combustion of sugars and cellulose.[78] However, there are numerous other noncigarette exposures to these compounds, including endogenous formation during metabolism. Smoke contains a number of aromatic amines, such as known bladder carcinogens 2-aminonaphthalene and 4-aminobiphenyl, heterocyclic amines, and furans. Toxic metals, including beryllium, cadmium, lead, and polonium-210, are also present in cigarette smoke in measurable quantities,[79,80] levels of which may depend in part on the region of the world where the tobacco was grown.[81] Much attention has been focused on the N-nitrosamines, primarily because they are well-established carcinogens.[82–85] Nitrosamines form through reactions of nitrite with amino groups. In tobacco, two compounds of concern are 4-(methylnitrosamino)-1-(3-pyridyl)-1-butanone (NNK), which is derived from nitrosation of nicotine, and N′-nitrosonornicotine (NNN), which is derived from nitrosation of nornicotine. Both of these compounds are tobacco specific. NNN and NNK primarily form during the curing process for tobacco, where the leaves are dried through contact with combustion gases from heat (flue) curing or microbial activity in air curing.[78] NNK is known to be a potent lung carcinogen, but also shows tumor induction activity in the nasal cavity, the pancreas, and the liver, whereas NNN has been shown to induce tumors along the respiratory tract and esophagus in various animal models. Because they are produced in the curing process and transfer into smoke, rather than being formed by combustion, it is possible to reduce nitrosamines by changing curing and storage practices.[78,86,87]

Smokeless tobacco products, although they are not burned, nonetheless contain substantial levels of carcinogens, most prominently the N-nitrosamines.[73] Here, product type and composition has an enormous effect on nitrosamine levels. For example, US moist snuff has substantially higher levels than that sold in Sweden (snus), whereas smokeless products available in India are often far higher in nitrosamines.[88] US smokeless products also can contain PAH and carbonyl compounds, likely derived from fire curing the constituent tobacco.[89] Similar to cigarettes, smokeless products would also contain toxic metals.[79,80]

Although tobacco is an exceedingly complex mixture, it is possible to use animal model and epidemiologic evidence to postulate relationships between specific components and known tobacco-induced cancers.[90–92] There is strong evidence from multiple studies to suggest that PAH and N-nitrosamines are involved in lung carcinogenesis. For example, PAH–DNA adducts are observed in lung tissues, and p53 tumor suppressor mutations in lung tumors resemble the damage created by PAH diol epoxide metabolites in vitro.[93–96] NNK appears to preferentially induce lung tumors in the rat, regardless of the route of administration, and DNA–nitrosamine adducts are detectable in lung tissues.[97,98] Most importantly, nitrosamine metabolite levels measured in smokers were prospectively related to the risk of lung cancer in cohort studies, even adjusting for other indices of smoking exposure (e.g., cotinine, pack-years).[98–102] PAH and nitrosamines are also likely to be implicated in cancers along the respiratory tract and the cervix.[103,104] Considerable evidence exist that aromatic amines such as 4-aminobiphenyl and 2-naphthylamine are potent bladder carcinogens, and smokers are known to be at an elevated risk of bladder cancer, so these are presumed to be the primary causative agents.[105–107] Similarly, as benzene is a known cause of leukemia, it is presumed that this is the link to leukemia observed in smokers.

Important to examining the role of various smoke components in cancer is the ability to measure the exposure of smokers to these components. Biomarkers of exposure may also be crucial for examining products for their potential to reduce health risks associated with tobacco use.[71,108,109] Validation of tobacco exposure biomarkers is threefold: method validation, validation with respect to product use, and validation with respect to disease risk.[71]

TABLE 4.2

Carcinogens in Tobacco and Tobacco Smoke Identified as Harmful and Potentially Harmful by the U.S. Food and Drug Administration, with International Agency for Research on Cancer Carcinogenecity (IARC) Classifications as of 2013

Compound	CAS No.	IARC Group	IARC Volume	Year
1,3-Butadiene	106-99-0	1	100F	2012
2-Aminonaphthalene	91-59-8	1	100F	2012
4-(Methylnitrosamino)-1-(3-pyridyl)-1-butanone (NNK)	64091-91-4	1	100E	2012
4-Aminobiphenyl	92-67-1	1	100F	2012
Aflatoxin B1	1162-65-8	1	100F	2012
Arsenic	7440-38-2	1	100C	2012
Benzene	71-43-2	1	100F	2012
Benzo[a]pyrene	50-32-8	1	100F	2012
Beryllium	7440-41-7	1	100C	2012
Cadmium	7440-43-9	1	100C	2012
Chromium (Hexavalent compounds)	18540-29-9	1	100C	2012
Ethylene oxide	75-21-8	1	100F	2012
Formaldehyde	50-00-0	1	100F	2012
N-Nitrosonornicotine (NNN)	16543-55-8	1	100E	2012
Nickel (compounds)		1	100C	2012
o-Toluidine	95-53-4	1	100F	2012
Polonium-210	7440-08-6	1	100D	2012
Uranium (235, 238 Isotopes)	7440-61-1	1	100D	2012
Vinyl chloride	75-01-4	1	100F	2012
Acrylamide	79-06-1	2A	60	1994
Cyclopenta[c,d]pyrene	27208-37-3	2A	92	2010
Dibenz[a,h]anthracene	53-70-3	2A	92	2010
Dibenzo[a,l]pyrene	191-30-0	2A	92	2010
Ethyl carbamate (urethane)	51-79-6	2A	96	2010
IQ (2-Amino-3-methylimidazo[4,5-f]quinoline)	76180-96-6	2A	56	1993
N-Nitrosodiethylamine	55-18-5	2A	SUP 7	1987
N-Nitrosodimethylamine (NDMA)	62-75-9	2A	SUP 7	1987
2-Nitropropane	79-46-9	2B	71	1999
2,6-Dimethylaniline	87-62-7	2B	57	1993
5-Methylchrysene	3697-24-3	2B	92	2010
A-α-C (2-Amino-9H-pyrido[2,3-b]indole)	26148-68-5	2B	SUP 7	1987
Acetaldehyde	75-07-0	2B	71	1999
Acetamide	60-35-5	2B	71	1999
Acrylonitrile	107-13-1	2B	71	1999
Benz[a]anthracene	56-55-3	2B	92	2010
Benz[j]aceanthrylene	202-33-5	2B	92	2012
Benzo[b]fluoranthene	205-99-2	2B	92	2010
Benzo[b]furan	271-89-6	2B	63	1995
Benzo[c]phenanthrene	195-19-7	2B	92	2010
Benzo[k]fluoranthene	207-08-9	2B	92	2010
Caffeic acid	331-39-5	2B	56	1993
Catechol	120-80-9	2B	71	1999
Chrysene	218-01-9	2B	92	2010
Cobalt	7440-48-4	2B	52	1991

(continued)

ETIOLOGY AND EPIDEMIOLOGY OF CANCER

TABLE 4.2

Carcinogens in Tobacco and Tobacco Smoke Identified as Harmful and Potentially Harmful by the U.S. Food and Drug Administration, with International Agency for Research on Cancer Carcinogenecity (IARC) Classifications as of 2013 *(continued)*

Compound	CAS No.	IARC Group	IARC Volume	Year
Dibenzo[a,h]pyrene	189-64-0	2B	92	2010
Dibenzo[a,i]pyrene	189-55-9	2B	92	2010
Ethylbenzene	100-41-4	2B	77	2000
Furan	110-00-9	2B	63	1995
Glu-P-1 (2-Amino-6-methyldipyrido[1,2-a:3′,2′-d]imidazole)	67730-11-4	2B	SUP 7	1987
Glu-P-2 (2-Aminodipyrido[1,2-a:3′,2′-d]imidazole)	67730-10-3	2B	SUP 7	1987
Hydrazine	302-01-2	2B	71	1999
Indeno[1,2,3-cd]pyrene	193-39-5	2B	92	2010
Isoprene	78-79-5	2B	71	1999
Lead	7439-92-1	2B	SUP 7	1987
MeA-α-C (2-Amino-3-methyl)-9H-pyrido[2,3-b]indole)	68006-83-7	2B	SUP 7	1987
N-Nitrosodiethanolamine (NDELA)	1116-54-7	2B	77	2000
N-Nitrosomethylethylamine	10595-95-6	2B	SUP 7	1987
N-Nitrosomorpholine (NMOR)	59-89-2	2B	SUP 7	1987
N-Nitrosopiperidine (NPIP)	100-75-4	2B	SUP 7	1987
N-Nitrosopyrrolidine (NPYR)	930-55-2	2B	SUP 7	1987
N-Nitrososarcosine (NSAR)	13256-22-9	2B	SUP 7	1987
Naphthalene	91-20-3	2B	82	2002
Nickel	7440-02-0	2B	49	1990
Nitrobenzene	98-95-3	2B	65	1996
Nitromethane	75-52-5	2B	77	2000
o-Anisidine	90-04-0	2B	73	1999
PhIP (2-Amino-1-methyl-6-phenylimidazo[4,5-b]pyridine)	105650-23-5	2B	56	1993
Propylene oxide	75-56-9	2B	60	1994
Styrene	100-42-5	2B	82	2002
Trp-P-1 (3-Amino-1,4-dimethyl-5H-pyrido[4,3-b]indole)	62450-06-0	2B	SUP 7	1987
Trp-P-2 (3-Amino-1-Methyl-5H-pyrido[4,3-b]indole)	62450-07-1	2B	SUP 7	1987
Vinyl acetate	108-05-4	2B	63	1995
1-Aminonaphthalene	134-32-7	3	SUP 7	1987
Chromium	7440-47-3	3	49	1990
Crotonaldehyde	4170-30-3	3	63	1995
Dibenzo[a,e]pyrene	192-65-4	3	92	2010
Mercury	7439-97-6	3	58	1993
Quinoline	91-22-5	EPA Group B2		
Cresols (o-, m-, and p-cresol)	1319-77-3	EPA Group C		

Notes: Most recently published IARC monograph for each compound is listed.
Quinoline and cresols have not been evaluated by IARC, but have been evaluated by U.S. Environmental Protection Agency.
IARC Groups: 1, Carcinogenic to humans; 2A, Probably carcinogenic to humans; 2B, Possibly carcinogenic to humans; 3, Not classifiable as to its carcinogenicity to humans; http://monographs.iarc.fr/ENG/Classification/ClassificationsAlphaOrder.pdf
EPA Groups: B2, Likely to be carcinogenic in humans; C, Possible human carcinogen.
CAS No., Chemical Abstracts Service registry number. *CAS Registry Number is a Registered Trademark of the American Chemical Society.* EPA, Environmental Protection Agency.
Quinoline: http://www.epa.gov/iris/subst/1004.htm
Cresols: http://www.epa.gov/iris/subst/0300.htm; http://www.epa.gov/iris/subst/0301.htm; http://www.epa.gov/iris/subst/0302.htm

TABLE 4.3

Commonly Used Biomarkers of Exposure to Carcinogens in Tobacco Smoke

Biomarker	Tobacco Smoke Source	Matrices
Monohydroxy-30butenyl mercapturic acid (MHBMA)	1,3-butadiene	Urine
4-Aminobiphenyl-globin	4-aminobiphenyl	Blood
N-(2-hydroxypropyl)methacrylamide (HPMA)	Acrolein	Urine
Carbamoylethylvaline	Acrylamide	Blood
Cyanoethylvaline	Acrylonitrile	Blood
S-phenylmercapturic acid (SPMA)	Benzene	Urine
Cd	Cadmium	Urine
3-hydroxypropyl mercapturic acid (HBMA)	Crotonaldehyde	Urine
2-hydroxyethyl mercapturic acid (HEMA)	Ethylene oxide	Urine
Nicotine equivalents (nicotine, cotinine, trans 3′-hydroxycotinine, and their respective glucuronides)	Nicotine	Urine
Total 4-(methylnitrosamino)-1-(3-pyridyl)-1-butanol (NNAL) (NNAL + NNAL glucuronide)	NNK	Urine
Total NNN (NNN + NNN glucuronide)	NNN	Urine
1-Hydroxypyrene	Pyrene (representative of other PAH)	Urine

Adapted from Hecht SS, Yuan JM, Hatsukami D. Applying tobacco carcinogen and toxicant biomarkers in product regulation and cancer prevention. *Chem Res Toxicol* 2010;23:1001–1008.

Validation with respect to product use means that levels of a given biomarker differ substantially between users and nonusers, and that biomarker levels decrease substantially when product use is stopped. Validation with respect to disease risk implies that variation in biomarker levels in product users are predictive of variations in disease outcomes. Over the last decade, the development of modern high-throughput, high-resolution mass spectrometry has allowed for the measurement of multiple metabolites of tobacco carcinogens.[110–113] Commonly used biomarkers of tobacco exposure are listed in Table 4.3.

How Tobacco Use Leads to Cancer

A recent U.S. Surgeon General's report provides extensive detail on the current state of knowledge of how smoking causes cancer.[65] Therefore, only a brief overview is provided here. Hecht[101,113–116] has argued for a major pathway by which tobacco use leads to cancer: carcinogen exposure leads to the formation of carcinogen–DNA adducts, which then cause mutations that, if not repaired or removed by apoptosis, will eventually give rise to cancer. It is important to keep perspective that, whereas each cigarette may contain seemingly low levels of a given carcinogen, smoking is, for most people, a long-term addiction. Thus, a mixture of numerous carcinogens is administered multiple times per day over the course of decades. Further, compounds taken in during smokers can be metabolically activated, thus increasing their activity. Cigarette smoke compounds appear to induce the cytochrome P450 system, which facilitates the metabolic activation of carcinogens to electrophilic entities that are able to covalently bind DNA.[117,118] DNA adducts appear to be crucial to the cancer process, and numerous studies show that smoker tissues contain higher levels of DNA adducts than nonsmokers, and that DNA adduct levels are associated with cancer risk.[119,120] At the same time, other systems are involved in the detoxification and deactivation of smoke constituents, typically catalyzed by UDP-glucuronosyltransferases and glutathione-*S*-transferases, resulting in excretion of inactive compounds.[121,122] An individual's balance of activation and deactivation of toxicants may be an important predictor of cancer risk, although evidence for this is mixed in the literature.[123,124] Similarly, DNA repair capacity is an important consideration, because, even if adducts are formed, processes exist to remove such perturbations to normalize DNA structure. Enzymatic processes of DNA repair include alkytransferases, nucleotide excision, and mismatch repair. Polymorphisms in genes coding for these enzymes may relate to individual cancer susceptibility. Table 4.4 outlines the metabolic activation/detoxification, DNA-adduct formation, and repair processes believed to be involved for four tobacco carcinogens (nitrosamines, PAH, benzene, 4-aminobiphenyl).[65,120]

Those DNA adducts that persist can cause miscoding during DNA replication. Smoke carcinogens are known to cause G:A and G:T mutations, and mutations in the *KRAS* oncogene and the *P53* tumor suppressor gene are strongly associated with tobacco-caused cancers.[93,114,125–127] Inactivation of *P53*, together with the activation of *KRAS*, appear to reduce survival in non–small-cell lung cancer.[65] Gene mutations that do not result in apoptosis may go on to influence a number of downstream processes, which may lead to genomic instability, proliferation, and eventually, malignancy.[128–130] Some smoke constituents may also act in ways that indirectly support the development of cancer. Nicotine, although not a carcinogen in itself, is known to reduce apoptosis and increase angiogenesis and transformation processes via nuclear factor kappa B (NF-κB).[65,131] Activation of nicotinic acetylcholine receptors (nAChR) in lung epithelium by nicotine or NNK is associated with survival and proliferation of malignant cells.[65] Nitrosamines also appear to have similar activities via the activation of protein kinases A and B.[132] NNK may bind β-adrenergic receptors to stimulate the release of arachidonic acid, which is converted to prostaglandin E2 by cyclooxygenase (COX)-2. Smoke compounds appear to activate epidermal growth factor receptor (EGFR) and COX-2, both of which are found to be elevated in many cancers.[133] Ciliatoxic, inflammatory, and oxidizing compounds, such as acrolein and ethylene oxide in smoke, may also impact the likelihood of cancer development. Epigenetic changes such as hypermethylation, particularly at P16, may also play a role in lung cancer development.[65]

TABLE 4.4

Key Pathways and Processes Where Selected Smoke Constituents Are Activated and Detoxified

	NNN, NNK	PAH	Benzene	4-ABP
Metabolic Activation	Alpha hydroxylation	Diol epoxide formation	Epoxide/oxepin formation	N-oxidation
Cytochrome P450 Enzymes Involved	2A6, 2A13, 2E1	1A1, 1B1	2E1	1A2
Enzymes Involved in Detoxification/ Activation	UGT	MEH, GST, UGT	MEH, GST	UGT, NAT
DNA Adduct Formation Sites				
Lung	*O6*-POB-deoxyguanosine	BPDE-N2-deoxyguanosine		
Bladder				C-8 deoxyguanosine
DNA Repair Pathways	AGT, BER	NER, MMR	BER, NER, NIR	NER

UGT, uridine-5′-diphosphate-glucuronosyltransferases; MEH, microsomal epoxide hydrolases; NAT, *N*-Acetyltransferases; GST, glutathione-S-transferases; AGT, *O6*-alkylguanine–DNA alkyltransferase; BER, base excision repair; NER, nucleotide excision repair; MMR, mismatch repair; NIR, nucleotide incision repair.

REFERENCES

1. World Health Organization, Research for International Tobacco Control. *WHO Report on the Global Tobacco Epidemic, 2008: the MPOWER Package*. Geneva: World Health Organization; 2008.
2. Giovino GA, Mirza SA, Samet JM, et al. Tobacco use in 3 billion individuals from 16 countries: an analysis of nationally representative cross-sectional household surveys. *Lancet* 2012;380:668–679.
3. Centers for Disease Control and Prevention (CDC). Current cigarette smoking among adults—United States, 2011. *MMWR Morb Mortal Wkly Rep* 2012;61:889–894.
4. Proctor R. *Golden Holocaust: Origins of the Cigarette Catastrophe and the Case for Abolition*. Berkeley: University of California Press; 2011.
5. Centers for Disease Control and Prevention (CDC). Consumption of cigarettes and combustible tobacco—United States, 2000-2011. *MMWR Morb Mortal Wkly Rep* 2012;61:565–569.
6. Centers for Disease Control and Prevention (CDC). Cigarette use among high school students—United States, 1991–2009. *MMWR Morb Mortal Wkly Rep* 2010;59:797–801.
7. Centers for Disease Control and Prevention (CDC). Tobacco use among middle and high school students—United States, 2000–2009. *MMWR Morb Mortal Wkly Rep* 2010;59:1063–1068.
8. Centers for Disease Control and Prevention (CDC). Tobacco product use among middle and high school students—United States, 2011 and 2012. *MMWR Morb Mortal Wkly Rep* 2013;62:893–897.
9. Cummings KM, Fong GT, Borland R. Environmental influences on tobacco use: evidence from societal and community influences on tobacco use and dependence. *Annu Rev Clin Psychol* 2009;5:433–458.
10. Huang J, Chaloupka FJ, Fong GT. Cigarette graphic warning labels and smoking prevalence in Canada: a critical examination and reformulation of the FDA regulatory impact analysis. *Tob Control* 2014;1:i7–i12.
11. Chaloupka FJ, Yurekli A, Fong GT. Tobacco taxes as a tobacco control strategy. *Tob Control* 2012;21:172–180.
12. Centers for Disease Control and Prevention (CDC). State-specific trends in lung cancer incidence and smoking—United States, 1999-2008. *MMWR Morb Mortal Wkly Rep* 2011;60:1243–1247.
13. Holford TR, Meza R, Warner KE, et al. Tobacco control and the reduction in smoking-related premature deaths in the United States, 1964–2012. *JAMA* 2014;311:164–171.
14. Slama K. The FCTC enters into effect in 2005. *Int J Tuberc Lung Dis* 2005;9:119.
15. Liberman J. Four COPs and counting: achievements, underachievements and looming challenges in the early life of the WHO FCTC Conference of the Parties. *Tob Control* 2012;21:215–220.
16. Deyton LR. FDA tobacco product regulations: a powerful tool for tobacco control. *Public Health Rep* 2011;126:167–169.
17. Patterson JT. *The Dread Disease: Cancer and Modern American Culture*. Cambridge, MA: Harvard University Press; 1987.
18. Proctor R. *The Nazi War on Cancer*. Princeton: Princeton University Press; 1999.
19. Doll R, Hill AB. Smoking and carcinoma of the lung: a preliminary report. *BMJ* 1950;2:739–748.
20. Wynder EL, Graham EA. Tobacco smoking as a possible etiologic factor in bronchiogenic carcinoma: a study of six hundred and eighty-four proved cases. *JAMA* 1950;143:329–336.
21. US Department of Health and Human Services. *The Health Consequences of Smoking: A Report of the Surgeon General*. Atlanta: Department of Health and Human Services, Centers for Disease Control and Prevention, National Center for Chronic Disease Prevention and Health Promotion, Office on Smoking and Health; 2004.
22. Centers for Disease Control and Prevention (CDC). Smoking-attributable mortality, years of potential life lost, and productivity losses—United States, 2000-2004. *MMWR Morb Mortal Wkly Rep* 2008;57:1226–1228.
23. US Department of Health and Human Services. *The Health Consequences of Smoking—50 Years of Progress. A Report of the Surgeon General*. Atlanta: U.S. Department of Health and Human Services, Centers for Disease Control and Prevention, National Center for Chronic Disease Prevention and Health Promotion, Office on Smoking and Health; 2014.
24. Jha P, Ramasundarahettige C, Landsman V, et al. 21st-century hazards of smoking and benefits of cessation in the United States. *N Engl J Med* 2013;368:341–350.
25. Gaudet MM, Gapstur SM, Sun J, et al. Active smoking and breast cancer risk: original cohort data and meta-analysis. *J Natl Cancer Inst* 2013;105:515–525.
26. Peto R, Darby S, Deo H, et al. Smoking, smoking cessation, and lung cancer in the UK since 1950: combination of national statistics with two case-control studies. *BMJ* 2000;321:323–329.
27. Thun MJ, Carter BD, Feskanich D, et al. 50-year trends in smoking-related mortality in the United States. *N Engl J Med* 2013;368:351–364.
28. Burns DM, Anderson CM, Gray N. Has the lung cancer risk from smoking increased over the last fifty years? *Cancer Causes Control* 2011;22:389–397.
29. Benowitz NL. Clinical pharmacology of nicotine: implications for understanding, preventing, and treating tobacco addiction. *Clin Pharmacol Ther* 2008;83:531–541.
30. Benowitz NL. Pharmacology of nicotine: addiction, smoking-induced disease, and therapeutics. *Annu Rev Pharmacol Toxicol* 2009;49:57–71.
31. Benowitz NL. Nicotine addiction. *N Engl J Med* 2010;362:2295–2303.
32. Scherer G. Smoking behaviour and compensation: a review of the literature. *Psychopharmacology (Berl)* 1999;145:1–20.
33. Hammond D, Fong GT, Cummings KM, et al. Smoking topography, brand switching, and nicotine delivery: results from an in vivo study. *Cancer Epidemiol Biomarkers Prev* 2005;14:1370–1375.
34. Benowitz NL, Hukkanen J, Jacob P. Nicotine chemistry, metabolism, kinetics and biomarkers. *Handb Exp Pharmacol* 2009:29–60.
35. Benowitz NL, Swan GE, Jacob P, et al. CYP2A6 genotype and the metabolism and disposition kinetics of nicotine. *Clin Pharmacol Ther* 2006;80:457–467.
36. Johnstone E, Benowitz N, Cargill A, et al. Determinants of the rate of nicotine metabolism and effects on smoking behavior. *Clin Pharmacol Ther* 2006;80:319–330.
37. Malaiyandi V, Lerman C, Benowitz NL, et al. Impact of CYP2A6 genotype on pretreatment smoking behaviour and nicotine levels from and usage of nicotine replacement therapy. *Mol Psychiatry* 2006;11:400–409.
38. Lea RA, Dickson S, Benowitz NL. Within-subject variation of the salivary 3HC/COT ratio in regular daily smokers: prospects for estimating CYP2A6 enzyme activity in large-scale surveys of nicotine metabolic rate. *J Anal Toxicol* 2006;30:386–389.
39. St Helen G, Novalen M, Heitjan DF, et al. Reproducibility of the nicotine metabolite ratio in cigarette smokers. *Cancer Epidemiol Biomarkers Prev* 2012;21:1105–1114.

40. Benowitz NL, Dains KM, Dempsey D, et al. Racial differences in the relationship between number of cigarettes smoked and nicotine and carcinogen exposure. *Nicotine Tob Res* 2011;13:772–783.
41. Dempsey DA, St Helen G, Jacob P, et al. Genetic and pharmacokinetic determinants of response to transdermal nicotine in white, black, and asian nonsmokers. *Clin Pharmacol Ther* 2013;94:687–694.
42. Zhu AZ, Renner CC, Hatsukami DK, et al. The ability of plasma cotinine to predict nicotine and carcinogen exposure is altered by differences in CYP2A6: the influence of genetics, race, and sex. *Cancer Epidemiol Biomarkers Prev* 2013;22:708–718.
43. Schnoll RA, Patterson F, Wileyto EP, et al. Nicotine metabolic rate predicts successful smoking cessation with transdermal nicotine: a validation study. *Pharmacol Biochem Behav* 2009;92:6–11.
44. Fong GT, Hammond D, Laux FL, et al. The near-universal experience of regret among smokers in four countries: findings from the International Tobacco Control Policy Evaluation Survey. *Nicotine Tob Res* 2004;6:S341–S351.
45. Lee WB, Fong GT, Zanna MP, et al. Regret and rationalization among smokers in Thailand and Malaysia: findings from the International Tobacco Control Southeast Asia Survey. *Health Psychol* 2009;28:457–464.
46. Sansone N, Fong GT, Lee WB, et al. Comparing the experience of regret and its predictors among smokers in four Asian countries: findings from the ITC surveys in Thailand, South Korea, Malaysia, and China. *Nicotine Tob Res* 2013;15:1663–1672.
47. Tobacco Use and Dependence Guideline Panel. *Treating Tobacco Use and Dependence: 2008 Update.* Rockville, MD: U.S. Department of Health and Human Services; 2008.
48. Wynder EL, Hoffmann D. *Tobacco and Tobacco Smoke.* New York: Academic Press; 1967.
49. Cummings KM, Morley CP, Hyland A. Failed promises of the cigarette industry and its effect on consumer misperceptions about the health risks of smoking. *Tob Control* 2002;11:I110–I117.
50. Pollay RW, Dewhirst T. The dark side of marketing seemingly "Light" cigarettes: successful images and failed fact. *Tob Control* 2002;11:I18–I31.
51. Fairchild A, Colgrove J. Out of the ashes: the life, death, and rebirth of the "safer" cigarette in the United States. *Am J Public Health* 2004;94:192–204.
52. Hoffmann D, Hoffmann I. The changing cigarette, 1950–1995. *J Toxicol Environ Health.* 1997;50:307–364.
53. Jarvis MJ. Trends in sales weighted tar, nicotine, and carbon monoxide yields of UK cigarettes. *Thorax* 2001;56:960–963.
54. O'Connor RJ, Cummings KM, Giovino GA, et al. How did UK cigarette makers reduce tar to 10 mg or less? *BMJ.* 2006;332:302.
55. National Cancer Institute. *Risks Associated with Smoking Cigarettes with Low Machine-Measured Yields of Tar and Nicotine.* Bethesda, MD: The Institute; 2001.
56. Harris JE, Thun MJ, Mondul AM, et al. Cigarette tar yields in relation to mortality from lung cancer in the cancer prevention study II prospective cohort, 1982-8. *BMJ* 2004;328:72.
57. Thun MJ, Burns DM. Health impact of "reduced yield" cigarettes: a critical assessment of the epidemiological evidence. *Tob Control* 2001;10:i4–i11.
58. Benowitz NL, Jacob P, Bernert JT, et al. Carcinogen exposure during short-term switching from regular to "light" cigarettes. *Cancer Epidemiol Biomarkers Prev* 2005;14:1376–1383.
59. Burns DM, Anderson CM, Gray N. Do changes in cigarette design influence the rise in adenocarcinoma of the lung? *Cancer Causes Control* 2011;22:13–22.
60. Kozlowski LT, Mehta NY, Sweeney CT, et al. Filter ventilation and nicotine content of tobacco in cigarettes from Canada, the United Kingdom, and the United States. *Tob Control* 1998;7:369–375.
61. Kozlowski LT, O'Connor RJ, Giovino GA, et al. Maximum yields might improve public health—if filter vents were banned: a lesson from the history of vented filters. *Tob Control* 2006;15:262–266.
62. Kozlowski LT, O'Connor RJ. Cigarette filter ventilation is a defective design because of misleading taste, bigger puffs, and blocked vents. *Tob Control* 2002;11:I40–I50.
63. Kozlowski LT, Goldberg ME, Yost BA, et al. Smokers are unaware of the filter vents now on most cigarettes: results of a national survey. *Tob Control* 1996;5:265–270.
64. O'Connor RJ, Caruso RV, Borland R, et al. Relationship of cigarette-related perceptions to cigarette design features: findings from the 2009 ITC U.S. Survey. *Nicotine Tob Res* 2013;15:1943–1947.
65. Centers for Disease Control and Prevention, National Center for Chronic Disease Prevention and Health Promotion, Office on Smoking and Health. *How Tobacco Smoke Causes Disease: The Biology and Behavioral Basis for Smoking-Attributable Disease: A Report of the Surgeon General.* Rockville, MD: Centers for Disease Control and Prevetion; 2010.
66. Stratton KR. *Clearing the Smoke: Assessing the Science Base for Tobacco Harm Reduction.* Washington, DC: Institute of Medicine, National Academy Press; 2001.
67. Foulds J, Ramstrom L, Burke M, et al. Effect of smokeless tobacco (snus) on smoking and public health in Sweden. *Tob Control* 2003;12:349–359.
68. Henningfield JE, Fagerstrom KO. Swedish Match Company, Swedish snus and public health: a harm reduction experiment in progress? *Tob Control* 2001;10:253–257.
69. Pepper JK, Brewer NT. Electronic nicotine delivery system (electronic cigarette) awareness, use, reactions and beliefs: a systematic review. *Tob Control* 2013 [Epub ahead of print].
70. Schaller K, Ruppert L, Kahnert S, et al. *Electronic Cigarettes—An Overview.* Heidelberg: German Cancer Research Center (DKFZ); 2013. http://www.dkfz.de/en/presse/download/RS-Vol19-E-Cigarettes-EN.pdf
71. Institute of Medicine. *Scientific Standards for Studies on Modified Risk Tobacco Products.* Washington, DC: National Academies Press; 2012.
72. International Agency for Research on Cancer. *Tobacco Smoke and Involuntary Smoking.* Vol 83. Lyon: International Agency for Research on Cancer, World Health Organization; 2004.
73. International Agency for Research on Cancer. *Smokeless Tobacco and Tobacco-Specific Nitrosamines.* Vol 89. Lyon: International Agency for Research on Cancer, World Health Organization; 2007.
74. Center for Tobacco Products. *Reporting Harmful and Potentially Harmful Constituents in Tobacco Products and Tobacco Smoke Under Section 904(a)(3) of the Federal Food, Drug, and Cosmetic Act.* Rockville, MD: Department of Health and Human Services; 2012.
75. Fowles J, Dybing E. Application of toxicological risk assessment principles to the chemical constituents of cigarette smoke. *Tob Control* 2003;12:424–430.
76. Burns DM, Dybing E, Gray N, et al. Mandated lowering of toxicants in cigarette smoke: a description of the World Health Organization tobacco regulation proposal. *Tob Control* 2008;17:132–141.
77. Straif K, Baan R, Gosse Y, et al. Carcinogenicity of polycyclic aromatic hydrocarbons. *Lancet Oncol* 2005;6:931–932.
78. O'Connor RJ, Hurley PJ. Existing technologies to reduce specific toxicant emissions in cigarette smoke. *Tob Control* 2008;17:i39–i48.
79. Pappas RS. Toxic elements in tobacco and in cigarette smoke: inflammation and sensitization. *Metallomics* 2011;3:1181–1198.
80. Marano KM, Naufal ZS, Kathman SJ, et al. Cadmium exposure and tobacco consumption: biomarkers and risk assessment. *Regul Toxicol Pharmacol* 2012;64:243–252.
81. Stephens WE, Calder A, Newton J. Source and health implications of high toxic metal concentrations in illicit tobacco products. *Environ Sci Technol* 2005;39:479–488.
82. Hecht SS, Hoffmann D. Tobacco-specific nitrosamines, an important group of carcinogens in tobacco and tobacco smoke. *Carcinogenesis* 1988;9:875–884.
83. Hecht SS. Biochemistry, biology, and carcinogenicity of tobacco-specific N-nitrosamines. *Chem Res Toxicol* 1998;11:559–603.
84. Hoffmann D, Rivenson A, Hecht SS. The biological significance of tobacco-specific N-nitrosamines: smoking and adenocarcinoma of the lung. *Crit Rev Toxicol* 1996;26:199–211.
85. Nilsson R. The molecular basis for induction of human cancers by tobacco specific nitrosamines. *Regul Toxicol Pharmacol* 2011;60:268–280.
86. Hecht SS, Stepanov I, Hatsukami DK. Major tobacco companies have technology to reduce carcinogen levels but do not apply it to popular smokeless tobacco products. *Tob Control* 2011;20:443.
87. Stepanov I, Knezevich A, Zhang L, et al. Carcinogenic tobacco-specific N-nitrosamines in US cigarettes: three decades of remarkable neglect by the tobacco industry. *Tob Control* 2012;21:44–48.
88. Stanfill SB, Connolly GN, Zhang L, et al. Global surveillance of oral tobacco products: total nicotine, unionised nicotine and tobacco-specific N-nitrosamines. *Tob Control* 2011;20:e2.
89. Stepanov I, Villalta PW, Knezevich A, et al. Analysis of 23 polycyclic aromatic hydrocarbons in smokeless tobacco by gas chromatography-mass spectrometry. *Chem Res Toxicol* 2010;23:66–73.
90. Stanton MF, Miller E, Wrench C, et al. Experimental induction of epidermoid carcinoma in the lungs of rats by cigarette smoke condensate. *J Natl Cancer Inst* 1972;49:867–877.
91. Hoffmann D, Stepanov I, Hecht SS, et al. *Tobacco Carcinogenesis.* New York: Academic Press; 1978.
92. Deutsch-Wenzel R, Brune H, Grimmer G. Experimental studies in rat lungs on the carcinogenicity and dose-response relationships of eight frequently occurring environmental polycyclic aromatic hydrocarbons. *J Natl Cancer Inst* 1983;71:539–544.
93. Pfeiffer GP, Denissenko MF, Olivier M, et al. Tobacco smoke carcinogens, DNA damage and p53 mutations in smoking-associated cancers. *Oncogene* 2002;21:7435–7451.
94. Boysen G, Hecht SS. Analysis of DNA and protein adducts of benzo[a]pyrene in human tissues using structure-specific methods. *Mutat Res* 2003;543:17–30.
95. Phillips DH. Smoking-related DNA and protein adducts in human tissues. *Carcinogenesis* 2002;23:1979–2004.
96. Liu Z, Muehlbauer KR, Schmeiser HH, et al. p53 Mutations in benzo[a]pyrene-exposed human p53 knock-in murine fibroblasts correlate with p53 mutations in human lung tumors. *Cancer Res* 2005;65:2583–2587.
97. Belinsky SA, Foley JF, White CM, et al. Dose-response relationship between O6-methylguanine formation in Clara cells and induction of pulmonary neoplasia in the rat by 4-(methylnitrosamino)-1-(3-pyridyl)-1-butanone. *Cancer Res* 1990;50:3772–3780.
98. Stepanov I, Sebero E, Wang R, et al. Tobacco-specific N-nitrosamine exposures and cancer risk in the Shanghai cohort study: remarkable coherence with rat tumor sites. *Int J Cancer* 2014;134:2278–2283.
99. Yuan JM, Koh WP, Murphy SE, et al. Urinary levels of tobacco-specific nitrosamine metabolites in relation to lung cancer development in two prospective cohorts of cigarette smokers. *Cancer Res* 2009;69:2990–2995.

100. Church TR, Anderson SE, Caporaso NE, et al. A prospectively measured serum biomarker for a tobacco-specific carcinogen and lung cancer in smokers. *Cancer Epidemiol Biomarkers Prev* 2009;18:260–266.
101. Hecht SS, Murphy SE, Stepanov I, et al. Tobacco smoke biomarkers and cancer risk among male smokers in the Shanghai Cohort Study. *Cancer Lett* 2012 [Epub ahead of print].
102. Yuan JM, Butler LM, Gao YT, et al. Urinary metabolites of a polycyclic aromatic hydrocarbon and volatile organic compounds in relation to lung cancer development in lifelong never smokers in the Shanghai Cohort Study. *Carcinogenesis* 2014;35:339–345.
103. Melikian AA, Sun P, Prokopczyk B, et al. Identification of benzo[a]pyrene metabolites in cervical mucus and DNA adducts in cervical tissues in humans by gas chromatography-mass spectrometry. *Cancer Lett* 1999;146: 127–134.
104. Prokopczyk B, Trushin N, Leszczynska J, et al. Human cervical tissue metabolizes the tobacco-specific nitrosamine, 4-(methylnitrosamino)-1-(3-pyridyl)-1-butanone, via alpha-hydroxylation and carbonyl reduction pathways. *Carcinogenesis* 2001;22:107–114.
105. Castelao JE, Yuan JM, Skipper PL, et al. Gender- and smoking-related bladder cancer risk. *J Natl Cancer Inst* 2001;93:538–545.
106. Sugimura T. History, present and future, of heterocyclic amines, cooked food mutagens. *Princess Takamatsu Symp* 1995;23:214–231.
107. Turesky RJ. Heterocyclic aromatic amine metabolism, DNA adduct formation, mutagenesis, and carcinogenesis. *Drug Metab Rev* 2002; 34:625–650.
108. Ashley DL, O'Connor RJ, Bernert JT, et al. Effect of differing levels of tobacco-specific nitrosamines in cigarette smoke on the levels of biomarkers in smokers. *Cancer Epidemiol Biomarkers Prev* 2010;19:1389–1398.
109. Hatsukami DK, Benowitz NL, Rennard SI, et al. Biomarkers to assess the utility of potential reduced exposure tobacco products. *Nicotine Tob Res* 2008;8: 169–191.
110. Carmella SG, Chen M, Han S, et al. Effects of smoking cessation on eight urinary tobacco carcinogen and toxicant biomarkers. *Chem Res Toxicol* 2009;22:734–741.
111. Carmella SG, Ming X, Olvera N, et al. High throughput liquid and gas chromatography-tandem mass spectrometry assays for tobacco-specific nitrosamine and polycyclic aromatic hydrocarbon metabolites associated with lung cancer in smokers. *Chem Res Toxicol* 2013;26:1209–1217.
112. Church TR, Anderson KE, Le C, et al. Temporal stability of urinary and plasma biomarkers of tobacco smoke exposure among cigarette smokers. *Biomarkers* 2010;15:345–352.
113. Hecht SS, Yuan JM, Hatsukami D. Applying tobacco carcinogen and toxicant biomarkers in product regulation and cancer prevention. *Chem Res Toxicol* 2010;23:1001–1008.
114. Hecht SS. Tobacco smoke carcinogens and lung cancer. *J Natl Cancer Inst* 1999;91:1194–1210.
115. Hecht SS. Tobacco carcinogens, their biomarkers, and tobacco-induced cancer. *Nature Rev Cancer* 2003;3:733–744.
116. Hecht SS. Lung carcinogenesis by tobacco smoke. *Int J Cancer* 2012;131: 2724–2732.
117. Guengerich FP. Common and uncommon cytochrome P450 reactions related to metabolism and chemical toxicity. *Chem Res Toxicol* 2001; 14:611–650.
118. Jalas J, Hecht SS, Murphy SE. Cytochrome P450 2A enzymes as catalysts of metabolism of 4-(methylnitrosamino)-1-(3-pyridyl)-1-butanone (NNK), a tobacco-specific carcinogen. *Chem Res Toxicol* 2005;18:95–110.
119. Nebert DW, Dalton TP, Okey AB, et al. Role of aryl hydrocarbon receptor-mediated induction of the CYP1 enzymes in environmental toxicity and cancer. *J Biol Chem* 2004;279:23847–23850.
120. Hang B. Formation and repair of tobacco carcinogen-derived bulky DNA adducts. *J Nucleic Acids* 2010;2010:709521.
121. Burchell B, McGurk K, Brierley CH, et al. *UDP-Glucuronosyltransferases.* Vol 3. New York: Elsevier Science; 1997.
122. Armstrong RN. *Glutathione-S-Transferases.* Vol 3. New York: Elsevier Science; 1997.
123. Vineis P, Veglia F, Benhamou S, et al. CYP1A1 T3801 C polymorphism and lung cancer: a pooled analysis of 2451 cases and 3358 controls. *Int J Cancer* 2003;104:650–657.
124. Carlsten C, Sagoo GS, Frodsham AJ, et al. Glutathione S-transferase M1 (GSTM1) polymorphisms and lung cancer: a literature-based systematic HuGE review and meta-analysis. *Am J Epidemiol* 2008;167:759–774.
125. Ahrendt SA, Decker PA, Alawi EA, et al. Cigarette smoking is strongly associated with mutation of the K-ras gene in patients with primary adenocarcinoma of the lung. *Cancer* 2001;92:1525–1530.
126. Ding L, Getz G, Wheeler DA, et al. Somatic mutations affect key pathways in lung adenocarcinoma. *Nature* 2008;455:1069–1075.
127. Johnson L, Mercer K, Greenbaum D, et al. Somatic activation of the K-ras oncogene causes early onset lung cancer in mice. *Nature* 2001;410:1111–1116.
128. Sekido Y, Fong KW, Minna JD. Progress in understanding the molecular pathogenesis of human lung cancer. *Biochim Biophys Acta* 1998;1378:F21–F59.
129. Bode AM, Dong A. Signal transduction pathways in cancer development and as targets for cancer prevention. *Prog Nucleic Acid Res Mol Biol* 2005;79:237–297.
130. Schuller HM. Mechanisms of smoking-related lung and pancreatic adenocarcinoma development. *Nat Rev Cancer* 2002;2:455–463.
131. Heeschen C, Jang JJ, Weis M, et al. Nicotine stimulates angiogenesis and promotes tumor growth and atherosclerosis. *Nat Med* 2001;7:833–839.
132. West KA, Brognard J, Clark AS, et al. Rapid Akt activation by nicotine and a tobacco carcinogen modulates the phenotype of normal human airway epithelial cells. *J Clin Invest* 2003;111:81–90.
133. Moraitis D, Du B, De Lorenzo MS, et al. Levels of cyclooxygenase-2 are increased in the oral mucosa of smokers: evidence for the role of epidermal growth factor receptor and its ligands. *Cancer Res* 2005;65:664–670.

5 Oncogenic Viruses

Christopher B. Buck and Lee Ratner

PRINCIPLES OF TUMOR VIROLOGY

Viral infections are estimated to play a causal role in at least 11% of all new cancer diagnoses worldwide.[1] A vast majority of cases (>85%) occur in developing countries, where poor sanitation, high rates of cocarcinogenic factors such as HIV/AIDS, and lack of access to vaccines and cancer screening all contribute to increased rates of virally induced cancers. Even in developed countries, where effective countermeasures are widely available, cancers attributable to viral infection account for at least 4% of new cases.[2,3]

Viruses thought to cause various forms of human cancer come from six distinct viral families with a range of physical characteristics (Table 5.1). All known human cancer viruses are capable of establishing durable, long-term infections and cause cancer only in a minority of persistently infected individuals. The low penetrance of cancer induction is consistent with the idea that a virus capable of establishing a durable productive infection would not benefit from inducing a disease that kills the host.[4] The slow course of cancer induction (typically over a course of many years after the initial infection) suggests that viral infection alone is rarely sufficient to cause human malignancy and that virally induced cancers arise only after additional oncogenic "hits" have had time to accumulate stochastically.

In broad terms, viruses can cause cancer through either (or both) of two broad mechanisms: direct or indirect. Direct mechanisms, in which the virus-infected cell ultimately becomes malignant, are typically driven by the effects of viral oncogene expression or through direct genotoxic effects of viral gene products. In most established examples of direct viral oncogenesis, the cancerous cell remains "addicted" to viral oncogene expression for ongoing growth and viability.

A common feature of DNA viruses that depend on host cell DNA polymerases for replication (e.g., papillomaviruses, herpesviruses, and polyomaviruses) is the expression of viral gene products that promote progression into the cell cycle. A typical mechanism of direct oncogenic effects is through the inactivation of tumor suppressor proteins, such as the guardian of the genome, p53, and retinoblastoma protein (pRB). This effectively primes the cell to express the host machinery necessary for replicating the viral DNA. The study of tumor viruses has been instrumental in uncovering the existence and function of key tumor suppressor proteins, as well as key cellular proto-oncogenes, such as Src and Myc.

In theory, viruses could cause cancer via direct hit-and-run effects. In this model, viral gene products may serve to preserve cellular viability and promote cell growth in the face of otherwise proapoptotic genetic damage during the early phases of tumor development. In principle, the precancerous cell might eventually accumulate enough additional genetic hits to allow for cell growth and survival independent of viral oncogene expression. This would allow for stochastic loss of viral nucleic acids from the nascent tumor, perhaps giving a growth advantage due to the loss of "foreign" viral antigens that might otherwise serve as targets for immune-mediated clearance of the nascent tumor. Although hit-and-run effects have been observed in animal models of virally induced cancer,[5] these effects are extremely difficult to address in humans. Currently, there are no clearly established examples of hit-and-run effects in human cancer.

In indirect oncogenic mechanisms, the cells that give rise to the malignant tumor have never been infected by the virus. Instead, the viral infection is thought to lead to cancer by attracting inflammatory immune responses that, in turn, lead to accelerated cycles of tissue damage and regeneration of noninfected cells. In some instances, virally infected cells may secrete paracrine signals that drive the proliferation of uninfected cells. At a theoretical level, it may be difficult to distinguish between indirect carcinogenesis and hit-and-run direct carcinogenesis, because, in both cases, the metastatic tumor may not contain any viral nucleic acids.

A variety of hunting approaches have been used to uncover etiologic roles for viruses in human cancer. The first clues that high-risk human papillomaviruses (HPVs), Epstein-Barr virus (EBV), Kaposi's sarcoma–associated herpesvirus (KSHV), and Merkel cell polyomavirus (MCPyV) might be carcinogenic were based on the detection of virions, viral DNA, or viral RNA in the tumors these viruses cause. A common feature of known virally induced cancers is that they are more prevalent in immunosuppressed individuals, such as individuals suffering from HIV/AIDS or patients on immunosuppressive therapy after organ transplantation. This is thought to reflect the lack of immunologic control over the cancer-causing virus. Studies focused on AIDS-associated cancers provided the first evidence for the carcinogenic potential of KSHV and MCPyV. A theoretical limitation of this approach is that some virally induced cancers may not occur at dramatically elevated rates in all types of immunosuppressed subjects, particularly if the virus causes only a fraction of cases (e.g., HPV-induced head and neck cancers). Fortunately, the unbiased analysis of nucleic acid sequences found in tumors has become substantially more tractable as deep-sequencing methods have continued to fall in price. In the coming years, it should be increasingly possible to search for viral sequences without making the starting assumption that all virally induced tumors are associated with immunosuppression.[6]

One limitation of tumor sequencing approaches is that they might miss undiscovered divergent viral species within viral families known to have extensive sequence diversity[7] and could miss viral families that have not yet been discovered.[8] Tumor-sequencing approaches might also miss viruses that cause cancer by hit-and-run or indirect mechanisms. It is conceivable that this caveat could be addressed by focusing on sequencing early precancerous lesions thought to ultimately give rise to metastatic cancer.

An additional successful approach to hunting cancer viruses involves showing that individuals who are infected with a particular virus have an increased long-term risk of developing particular forms of cancer. This approach was successful for identifying and validating the carcinogenic roles of high-risk HPV types, hepatitis B virus (HBV), hepatitis C virus (HCV), KSHV, and human T-lymphotropic virus 1 (HTLV-1). Although viruses that are extremely prevalent, such as EBV and MCPyV, are not amenable to this approach per se, it may still be possible to draw connections

TABLE 5.1

Oncogenic Viruses

Virus	Taxon	Viral Genome	Virion	Infection Rate	Site of Persistance	Diseases in Normal Hosts	Diseases in Immunocompromised Hosts	Associated Cancers
High-risk human papillomavirus types (e.g., HPV16)	*Alphapapillomavirus*	8 kb circular dsDNA	Nonenveloped	>70%	Anogential mucosa, oral mucosa	Carcinomas of the cervix, penis, anus, vagina, vulva, tonsils, base of tongue	Increased incidence of same diseases	610,000
Hepatitis B virus (HBV)	*Hepadnaviridae*	3 kb ss/dsDNA	Enveloped	2%–8%	Hepatocytes	Cirrhosis, hepatocellular carcinoma	Same diseases, increased incidence with AIDS	380,000
Hepatitis C virus (HCV)	*Flaviviridae*	10 kb +RNA	Enveloped	~3%	Hepatocytes	Cirrhosis, hepatocellular carcinoma, splenic marginal zone lymphoma	Same diseases, increased incidence with AIDS	220,000
Epstein-Barr virus (EBV, HHV-4)	*Gammaherpesvirinae*	170 kb linear DNA	Enveloped	90%	B cells, pharyngeal mucosa	Mononucleosis, Burkitt lymphoma, other non-Hodgkin lymphoma, nasopharyngeal carcinoma	Increased incidence of same diseases, lymphoproliferative disease, other lymphomas, oral hairy leukoplakia, leiomyosarcoma	110,000
Kaposi's sarcoma herpesvirus (KSHV, HHV-8)	*Gammaherpesvirinae*	170 kb linear DNA	Enveloped	2%–60%	Oral mucosa, endothelium, B cells	Kaposi's sarcoma (KS), multicentric Castleman disease (MCD)	Increased KS, MCD incidence, primary effusion lymphoma	43,000
Merkel cell polyomavirus (MCPyV, MCV)	*Orthopolyomavirus*	5 kb circular dsDNA	Nonenveloped	75%	Skin (lymphocytes?)	Merkel cell carcinoma (MCC)	Increased MCC incidence	1,500 (US)
Human T-cell leukemia virus (HTLV-1)	*Deltaretrovirus*	9 kb +RNA (RT)	Enveloped	0.01%–6%	T and B cells	Adult T-cell leukemia/lymphoma, tropical spastic paraparesis, myelopathy, uveitis, dermatitis	Unknown	2,100

Note: Ranges for infection rates imply major variations in prevalence among populations in different world regions. *Associated cancers* indicates the annual number of new cases clearly attributable to viral infection. An estimate for the worldwide incidence of Merkel cell carcinoma is not currently available and an estimate of the annual new cases in the United States alone is given instead.

ds, double-stranded; ss, single-stranded; HHV, human herpesvirus; RT, reverse transcriptase.

Adapted from de Martel C, Ferlay J, Franceschi S, et al. Global burden of cancers attributable to infections in 2008: a review and synthetic analysis. *Lancet Oncol* 2012;13(6):607–615; Schiller JT, Lowy DR. Virus infection and human cancer: an overview. *Recent Results Cancer Res* 2014;193:1–10; Chen CJ, Hsu WL, Yang HI, et al. Epidemiology of virus infection and human cancer. *Recent Results Cancer Res* 2014;193:11–32; and Virgin HW, Wherry EJ, Ahmed R. Redefining chronic viral infection. *Cell* 2009;138(1):30–50.

between cancer risk and either unusually high serum antibody titers against viral antigens or unusually high viral load. Relatively high serologic titers reflect either comparatively poor control of the viral infection in at-risk individuals or expression of viral antigens in tumors or tumor precursor cells.[9,10]

The finding that a virus causes cancer is good news, in the sense that it can suggest possible paths to clinical intervention. These can include the development of vaccines or antiviral agents that prevent, attenuate, or eradicate the viral infection and thereby prevent cancer; the development of methods for early detection or diagnosis of cancer based on assays for viral nucleic acids or gene products; or the development of drugs or immunotherapeutics that treat cancer by targeting viral gene products. Unfortunately, establishing the carcinogenicity of a given viral species is an arduous process that must inevitably integrate multiple lines of evidence.[11] The demonstration that the virus can transform cells in culture and/or cause cancer in animal models provides circumstantial evidence of the oncogenic potential of a virus. All known human cancer viruses meet this criterion. However, it is important to recognize that viruses can theoretically coevolve to be noncarcinogenic in their native host (e.g., humans) and cause cancer only in the dysregulated environment of a nonnative host animal. This caveat may apply to human adenoviruses.

Finding that viral DNA is clonally integrated in a primary tumor and its metastatic lesions helps address the caveat that the virus might merely be a hitchhiker that finds the tumor cell a conducive environment in which to replicate (as opposed to playing a causal carcinogenic role). This caveat is also addressed by the observation that, in most instances, viruses found in tumors have lost the ability to exit viral latency and are functionally unable to produce new progeny virions. An unfortunate consequence of this is that vaccines or antiviral agents that target virion proteins (e.g., vaccines against high-risk HPVs or HBV) or gene products expressed late in the viral life cycle (e.g., herpesvirus thymidine kinase, which is the target of drugs such as ganciclovir) are rarely effective for treating existing virally induced tumors.

Demonstrating that a vaccine or antiviral agent targeting the virus either prevents or treats human cancer is by far the strongest form of evidence that a given virus causes human cancer. This type of proof has fully validated the causal role of HBV in human liver cancer. Compelling clinical trial data also show that antiherpesvirus therapeutics can prevent KSHV- or EBV-associated lymphoproliferative disorders, and that vaccination against HPV can prevent the development of precancerous lesions on the uterine cervix.

PAPILLOMAVIRUSES

History

The idea that cancer of the uterine cervix might be linked to sexual behavior was first proposed in the mid 19th century by Dominico Rigoni-Stern, who observed that nuns rarely contracted cervical cancer, whereas prostitutes suffered from cervical cancer more often than the general populace.[12] Another major milestone in cervical cancer research was Georgios Papanikolaou's development of the so-called Pap smear for early cytologic diagnosis of precancerous cervical lesions.[13] This form of screening, which allows for surgical intervention to remove precancerous lesions, has saved many millions of lives in developed countries, where public health campaigns have made testing widely available.

Although observations in the early 1980s suggested the possibility of a hit-and-run carcinogenic role for herpes simplex viruses in cervical cancer,[14] this hypothesis was abandoned in light of studies led by Harald zur Hausen. Low-stringency hybridization approaches revealed the presence of two previously unknown papillomavirus types, HPV16 and HPV18, in various cervical cancer cell lines, including the famous HeLa cell line.[15,16] There is now overwhelming evidence that a group of more than a dozen sexually transmitted HPV types, including HPV16 and HPV18, play a causal role in essentially all cases of cervical cancer. HPVs associated with a high risk of cancer also cause about half of all penile cancers, 88% of anal cancers, 43% of vulvar cancers, 70% of vaginal cancers,[2] and an increasing fraction of head and neck cancers (see the following). In 2008, zur Hausen was awarded the Nobel Prize for his groundbreaking work establishing the link between HPVs and human cancer.

The viral family *Papillomaviridae* is named for the benign skin warts (papillomas) that some members of the family cause. In the early 1930s, Richard Edwin Shope and colleagues demonstrated viral transmission of papillomas in a rabbit model system.[17] Using this system, Peyton Rous and others showed that cottontail rabbit papillomavirus-induced lesions can progress to malignant skin cancer.[18,19] This was the first demonstration of a cancer-causing virus in mammals, building on Rous' prior work demonstrating a virus capable of causing cancer in chickens (the Rous sarcoma retrovirus).

Tissue Tropism and Gene Functions

Although papillomaviruses can achieve infectious entry into a wide variety of cell types in vitro and in vivo, the late phase of the viral life cycle, during which the viral genome undergoes vegetative replication and the L1 and L2 capsid proteins are expressed, is strictly dependent on host cell factors found only in differentiating keratinocytes near the surface of the skin or mucosa. Interestingly, a majority of HPV-induced cancers appear to arise primarily at zones of transition between stratified squamous epithelia and the single-layer (columnar) epithelia of the endocervix, the inner surface of the anus, and tonsillar crypts. It is thought that the mixed phenotypic milieu in cells at squamocolumnar transition zones may cause dysregulation of the normal coupling of the HPV life cycle to keratinocyte differentiation.

There are nearly 200 known HPV types.[20] In general, each papillomavirus type is a functionally distinct serotype, meaning that serum antibodies that neutralize one HPV type do not robustly neutralize other HPV types. Various HPV types preferentially infect different skin or mucosal surfaces. Different types tend to establish either transient infections that may be cleared over the course of months, or stable infections where virions are chronically shed from the infected skin surface for the lifetime of the host. HPV infections may or may not be associated with the formation of visible warts or other lesions. High-risk HPV types, with clearly established causal links to human cancer, are preferentially tropic for the anogenital mucosa and the oral mucosa, are usually transmitted by sexual contact, rarely cause visible warts, and usually establish only transient infections in a great majority of exposed individuals. The lifetime risk of sexual exposure to a high-risk HPV type has been estimated to be >70%. Individuals who fail to clear their infection with a high-risk HPV type and remain persistently infected are at much greater risk of developing cancer. Polymerase chain reaction (PCR)-based screening for the presence of high-risk HPV types thus serves as a useful adjunct to, or even a replacement for, the traditional Pap test.[21]

A consequence of the strict tissue-differentiation specificity of the papillomavirus life cycle is that HPVs do not replicate in standard monolayer cell cultures. Papillomaviruses also seem to be highly species restricted, and there are no known examples of an HPV type capable of infecting animals.[22] Thus, the investigation of key details of papillomavirus biology has relied almost entirely on modern recombinant DNA and molecular biologic analyses.

Papillomavirus genomes are roughly 8 kb, double-stranded, closed-circular DNA molecules (essentially reminiscent of a plasmid). During the normal viral life cycle, the genome does not adopt a linear form, does not integrate into the host cell chromosome, and remains as an extrachromosomal episome or minichromosome.

All the viral protein-coding sequences are arranged on one strand of the genome. The expression of various proteins is regulated by differential transcription and polyadenylation, as well as effects at the level of RNA splicing, export from the nucleus, and translation. In addition to the late half of the viral genome, which encodes the L1 and L2 capsid proteins, all papillomaviruses encode six key early region genes: E1, E2, E4, E5, E6, and E7.

The master transcriptional regulator E2 serves as a transcriptional repressor, and loss of E2 expression (typically through integration of the viral episome into the host cell DNA) results in the upregulation of early gene expression. The most extensively studied early region proteins are the E6 and E7 oncogenes of HPV16 and HPV18. The E6 protein of high-risk HPV types triggers the destruction of p53 by recruiting a host cell ubiquitin–protein ligase, E6AP.[23–25] Another important oncogenic function of E6 is the activation of cellular telomerase.[26] A wide variety of additional high-risk E6 activities that do not involve p53 have been identified.[27]

Most E7 proteins, including those of many low-risk HPV types, contain a conserved LXCXE motif that mediates interaction with pRB and the related "pocket" proteins p107 and p130.[28] Interestingly, the LXCXE motif is present in a wide variety of other oncogenes, most notably the T antigens of polyomaviruses and the E1A oncogenes of adenoviruses. The interaction of E7 with pRB disrupts the formation of a complex between pRB and E2F transcription factors, thereby blocking the ability of pRB to trigger cell cycle arrest.[29] The E7 proteins of high-risk HPVs can also contribute to chromosomal mis-segregation and aneuploidy, which may in turn contribute to malignant progression.[30] Like E6, E7 interacts with a wide variety of additional cellular targets, the spectrum of which seems to vary with different HPV types.[27]

Some papillomavirus types express an E5 oncogene, which functions as an agonist for cell surface growth factor receptors such as platelet-derived growth factor beta (PDGF-β) and epidermal growth factor (EGF) receptor.[31] Because E5 expression is uncommon in cervical tumors, it is uncertain whether the protein plays a key role in human cancer.

Human Papilloma Virus Vaccines

Two preventive vaccines against cancer-causing HPVs, trade named Gardasil (Merck) and Cervarix (GSK), are currently marketed worldwide for the prevention of cervical cancer. Both vaccines contain recombinant L1 capsid proteins based on HPV16 and HPV18 that are assembled in vitro into virus-like particles (VLPs). Together, HPV16 and HPV18 cause about 70% of all cases of cervical cancer worldwide. Gardasil also includes VLPs based on HPV types 6 and 11, which rarely cause cervical cancer but together cause about 90% of all genital warts. The VLPs contained in the vaccines are highly immunogenic in humans, eliciting high-titer serum antibody responses against L1 that are capable of neutralizing the infectivity of the cognate HPV types represented in the vaccine. It appears that the current HPV vaccines may confer lifelong immunity against new infection with the HPV types represented in the vaccine.[32] The vaccines elicit lower titer cross-neutralizing responses against a subset of cancer-causing HPV types that are closely related to HPV16 and HPV18.[33] Although these cross-neutralizing responses can at least partially protect vaccinees against a new infection with additional high-risk types, such as HPV31 and HPV45, it remains unclear how durable the lower level cross-protection will be.[33]

Because L1 is not expressed in latently infected keratinocyte stem cells residing on the epithelial basement membrane, current HPV vaccines are very unlikely to eradicate existing infections.[34,35] Like keratinocyte stem cells, cervical cancers and precursor lesions rarely or never express L1. Thus, the existing L1-based vaccines seem unlikely to serve as therapeutic agents for treating cervical cancer.

Three types of next-generation HPV vaccines are currently in human clinical trials. Merck has recently announced that a newer version of Gardasil, which contains VLPs based on a total of nine different HPV types, remained highly effective against HPV16 and HPV18 and also prevented 97% of precancerous cervical lesions caused by a wider variety of high-risk HPV types.[36] Another class of second-generation vaccines targets the papillomavirus minor capsid protein L2. An N-terminal portion of L2 appears to represent a highly conserved "Achilles' heel", which contains conserved protein motifs required for key steps of the infectious entry process.[37] Anti-L2 antibodies can neutralize a broad range of different human and animal HPV types, and thus, L2 vaccines are hoped to offer protection against all HPVs that cause cervical cancer, all low-risk HPV types that cause abnormal Pap smear results, as well as the full range of HPV types that cause skin warts. Finally, a wide variety of vaccines that seek to elicit cell-mediated immune responses against the E6 and E7 oncoproteins are aimed at a therapeutic intervention for the treatment of cervical cancer.[38]

Oropharyngeal Cancer

It is well established that tobacco products and alcohol cause head and neck cancer. In the late 1990s, Maura Gillison and colleagues noted a surprising number of new cases of tonsillar cancer in nonsmokers.[39] Many of the tumors found in nonsmokers were found to have wild-type p53 genes, raising the possibility that the tumor might be dependent on a p53-suppressing viral oncogene (as seen in cervical cancer). Gillison and colleagues went on to show that nearly half of all tonsillar cancers contain HPV DNA, most commonly HPV16. Interestingly, HPV-positive oropharyngeal cancers tend to be less lethal than tobacco-associated HPV-negative tumors. This finding has important implications for treatment of HPV-positive head and neck cancers.[40]

Although the incidence of tobacco-associated head and neck cancer has been declining in recent decades due to decreased tobacco use, recent studies suggest an ongoing increase in the incidence of HPV-associated cancers of the tonsils and the base of the tongue. By 2025, the number of new HPV-induced head and neck cancer cases in the United States is expected to roughly equal the number of new cervical cancer cases.[39] Based in part on these observations, the U.S. Centers for Disease Control and Prevention recommends that boys, in addition to girls, should be vaccinated against high-risk HPVs.

Nonmelanoma Skin Cancer

Epidermodysplasia verruciformis (EV) is a rare immunodeficiency that is characterized by the appearance of numerous flat, wartlike lesions across wide areas of skin. The lesions typically contain genus betapapillomaviruses, such as HPV5 or HPV8. EV patients frequently develop squamous cell carcinomas (SCC) in sun-exposed skin areas (suggesting that ultraviolet [UV] light exposure is a cofactor). It is also well established that other immunosuppressed individuals, such as organ transplant recipients and HIV-infected individuals, are at increased risk of developing SCC.[41,42] Although the E6 and E7 proteins of betapapillomaviruses appear to exert a different spectrum of effects than the E6 and E7 proteins of HPV types associated with cervical cancer,[43–45] Betapapillomavirus oncogenes can transform cells in vitro.[46] Although these circumstantial lines of evidence suggest that infectious agents, such as Betapapillomaviruses, might play a causal role in SCC, recent deep sequencing studies have observed few or no viral sequences in SCC tumors.[47] Although the results argue against durable direct oncogenic effects of any known viral species in SCC, an animal model system using bovine papillomavirus type 4 strongly suggests that papillomaviruses can cause cancer by hit and run mechanisms.[5] Thus, the question of whether hit-and-run or indirect oncogenic effects of HPVs may be at play in human SCC remains open.

POLYOMAVIRUSES

History

In the early 1950s, Ludwik Gross showed that a filterable infectious agent could cause salivary gland cancer in laboratory mice.[48] Later work by Bernice Eddy and Sarah Stewart showed that the murine polyoma (Greek for "many tumors") virus caused many different types of cancer in experimentally infected mice.[49] The discovery that murine polyomavirus could be grown in cell culture helped rekindle research interest in tumor virology and interest in the question of whether viruses might cause human cancer.

Like papillomaviruses, polyomaviruses have a nonenveloped capsid assembled from 72 pentamers of a single major capsid protein (VP1). Both viral families also carry circular dsDNA genomes. These physical similarities initially led to the classification of both groups into a single family, *Papovaviridae*. When sequencing studies ultimately revealed that polyomaviruses have a unique genome organization (with early and late genes being arranged on opposing strands of the genome) and almost no sequence homology to papillomaviruses, the two groups of viruses were divided into separate families.

In the early 1960s, Bernice Eddy, Maurice Hilleman, and Benjamin Sweet reported the discovery of simian vacuolating virus 40 (SV40), a previously unknown polyomavirus that was found as a contaminant in vaccines against poliovirus.[50,51] SV40 was derived from the rhesus monkey kidney cells used to amplify poliovirus virions in culture.[52] SV40 rapidly became an important model polyomavirus, and studies of its major and minor tumor antigens (large T [LT]and small t [ST], respectively) have played an important role in understanding various aspects of carcinogenesis. Despite significant alarm about the possible risk SV40 might pose to exposed individuals, a comprehensive, decades long series of studies have failed to uncover compelling evidence that SV40 exposure is causally associated with human cancer.[53]

Two naturally human-tropic polyomaviruses, BK virus (BKV) and John Cunningham virus (JCV), were first reported in back-to-back publications in 1971.[54,55] BKV and JCV are known to cause kidney disease and a lethal brain disease called progressive multifocal leukoencephalopathy, respectively, in immunosuppressed individuals. Although both viruses can cause cancer in experimentally exposed animals, it remains unclear whether either virus plays a causal role in human cancer. Although BKV LT expression can frequently be observed in the inflammatory precursor lesions that are thought to give rise to prostate cancer,[56] there is no evidence for the persistence of BKV DNA in malignant prostate tumors.[57] There have been case studies finding BKV T-antigen expression in bladder cancer,[58] and some reports have indicated the presence of JCV DNA in colorectal tumors. The long history of conflicting evidence concerning possible roles for BKV or JCV in human cancer is reviewed elsewhere.[59,60]

Merkel Cell Polyomavirus

In 2008, Yuan Chang and Patrick Moore reported their lab's discovery of the fifth known human polyomavirus species, which they named Merkel cell polyomavirus (MCV or MCPyV) based on its presence in Merkel cell carcinoma (MCC).[61] The discovery used an RNA deep sequencing approach called digital transcriptome subtraction. Using classic Southern blotting, this report demonstrated the clonal integration of MCPyV in an MCC tumor and its distant metastases. Many other labs worldwide have independently confirmed the presence of MCPyV DNA in about 80% of MCC tumors.[11]

MCC is a rare but highly lethal form of cancer that typically presents as a fast-growing lesion on sun-exposed skin surfaces (Fig. 5.1).[62] The risk of MCC is dramatically higher in HIV/AIDS patients, offering an initial clue that MCC might be a virally induced cancer.[63] Although MCC tumors express neuroendocrine markers associated with sensory Merkel cells of the epidermis, one recent report has shown that some MCC tumors also express B-cell markers, including rearranged antibody loci.[64] Currently, there is no clear evidence for the involvement of MCPyV in other tumors with neuroendocrine features.

In 2012, the International Agency for Research on Cancer (IARC) concluded that MCPyV is a class 2A carcinogen (probably carcinogenic to humans).[10,53] It should be noted that IARC evaluations rely heavily on animal carcinogenicity studies, and the 2A designation was assigned prior to a recent report showing that MCV-positive MCC lines are tumorigenic in a mouse model system.[65]

A great majority of healthy adults have serum antibodies specific for the MCPyV major capsid protein VP1. A majority also shed MCPyV virions from apparently healthy skin surfaces, and there is a strong correlation between individual subjects' serologic titer against VP1 and the amount of MCPyV DNA they shed.[66–68] Interestingly, MCC patients tend to have exceptionally strong serologic titers against VP1.[69] MCC tumors do not express detectable amounts of VP1, so this is unlikely to reflect direct exposure to

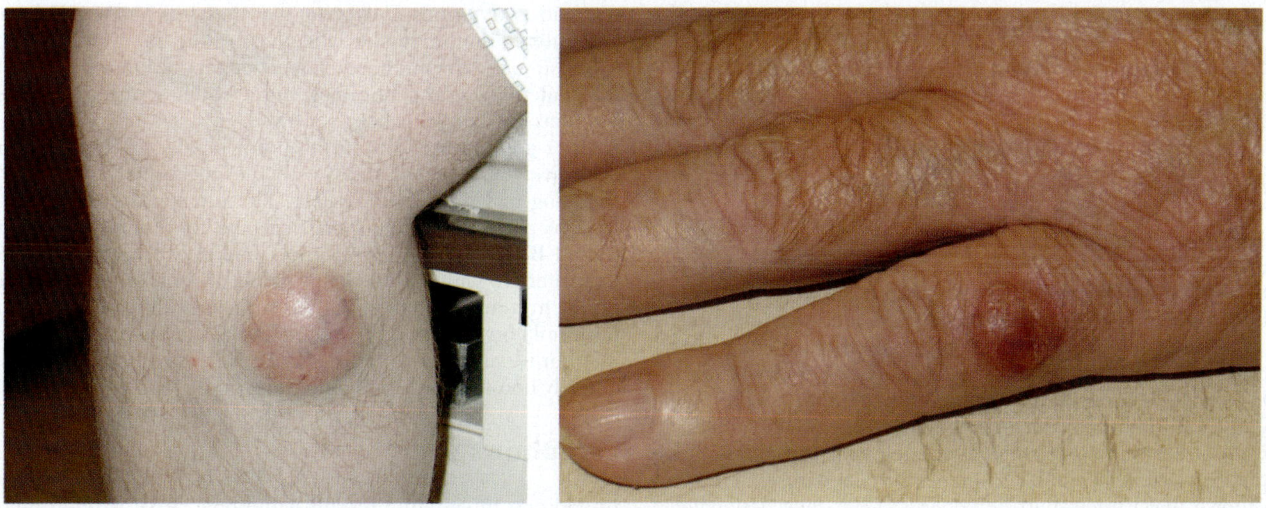

Figure 5.1 Merkel cell carcinoma (MCC). The *left panel* shows an MCC tumor on the calf. The *right panel* shows an MCC tumor on the finger. Photographs provided with permission by Dr. Paul Nghiem (University of Washington, www.merkelcell.org).

the tumor and instead likely represents a history of a high MCPyV load in MCC patients. A recent study of archived serum samples shows that unusually high serologic titers against MCPyV VP1 often precede the development of MCC by many years.[70]

Like the LT protein of SV40 (and the E7 proteins of high-risk HPVs), an N-terminal portion of the MCPyV LT protein contains an LXCXE motif that mediates inactivation of pRB function. In contrast to SV40 LT, which carries a p53-inactivation domain that overlaps the C-terminal helicase domain, MCPyV LT does not appear to inactivate p53 function.[71] Instead, the MCPyV LT helicase domain activates DNA damage responses and induces cell cycle arrest in cultured cell lines.[72] This may explain why the LT genes found in MCC tumors essentially always carry mutations that truncate LT upstream of the helicase domain. siRNA experiments indicate that most (although possibly not all) MCC tumors are "addicted" to the expression of MCPyV T antigens.[73–75] Interestingly, patients with higher levels of MCPyV DNA in their tumors, stronger T-antigen expression, and tumors that have been infiltrated by CD8+ T cells appear to have better prognoses.[76] This is consistent with the idea that cell-mediated immunity can help clear MCC tumors that express MCPyV antigens.

Recent work has shown that the pRB interacting domain of LT mediates increased expression of the cellular gene survivin. The knockdown of survivin using siRNAs results in MCC tumor cell death and YM155, a small molecule inhibitor of survivin expression, protects mice from MCC tumors in a xenograft challenge system.[77,78]

In contrast to SV40, where LT appears to be the dominant oncogene, the MCPyV ST protein appears to play a key role in cell transformation. In addition to modifying the signaling functions of the cellular proto-oncogene PP2A, ST triggers the phosphorylation of eukaryotic translation initiation factor 4E binding protein 1.[79] This results in dysregulation of cap-dependent translation and cellular transformation.

Although there is an intriguing epidemiologic correlation between MCC and chronic lymphocytic leukemia (CLL),[80] there are conflicting reports concerning the presence of MCPyV in CLL and other lymphocytic cancers.[81–83]

Other Human Polyomaviruses

In recent years, the number of known human polyomaviruses has expanded dramatically. Of the 12 currently known HPyV species, only MCPyV has been clearly linked to human cancer. One new HPyV, trichodysplasia spinulosa polyomavirus (TSV or TSPyV) has been found in association with abnormal spiny growths on the facial skin of a small number of immunocompromised individuals.

EPSTEIN-BARR VIRUS

History

In 1958, Denis Burkitt provided the first clear clinical description of an unusual B-cell–derived tumor that frequently affects the jawbones of children in equatorial Africa.[84] After hearing Burkitt give a 1961 lecture entitled "The Commonest Children's Cancer in Tropical Africa – A Hitherto Unrecognized Syndrome," Michael Epstein became interested in the idea that an insect vector-borne infection might account for the high incidence of Burkitt lymphoma in tropical Africa. Epstein, together with then PhD candidate Yvonne Barr, began examining tumor samples sent to them by Burkitt. Electron micrographs of lymphoid cells that grew out of the tumors in culture revealed viral particles with a morphology strikingly similar to herpes simplex viruses.[85] It was soon shown that Epstein-Barr herpesvirus (EBV, later designated human herpesvirus 4 [HHV-4]) can transform cultured B cells and is the agent responsible for infectious mononucleosis.[86–88]

Although the initial conjecture that tropically endemic Burkitt lymphoma depends on a geographically restricted infectious agent ultimately proved correct, it was quickly established that the EBV infection is not restricted to the tropics. It instead appears likely that the malaria parasite *Plasmodium falciparum* is a key geographically restricted cocarcinogen responsible for endemic Burkitt lymphoma.[53] In areas where children suffer repeated malaria infections, it appears that the parasite triggers abnormal B-cell responses, as well as weakened cell-mediated immune function, and these effects of recurring malaria infection in turn promote or allow the development of EBV-induced Burkitt tumors.[11]

Epstein-Barr Virus Life Cycle

EBV chronically infects nearly all humans. In a great majority of individuals, the infection is initially established in early childhood and is never associated with any noticeable symptoms. The infection is typically transmitted when virions, shed in the saliva of a chronically infected individual, come in contact with the oropharyngeal epithelium of a naïve individual. Although infected epithelial cells, such as keratinocytes, might serve to amplify the virus in some circumstances,[89] the establishment of chronic infection is ultimately dependent on mature B cells, as subjects with X-linked agammaglobulinemia (who lack mature B cells) appear to be immune to stable EBV infection.[90] Individuals who escape infection during childhood and instead first become infected during adolescence or adulthood often develop mononucleosis, which is associated with fevers and extreme fatigue lasting for weeks or sometimes months. Interestingly, late-infected individuals who experience mononucleosis and high EBV viral load are at increased risk of developing EBV-positive Hodgkin lymphoma.[91]

EBV-infected B cells can either go on to produce new virions, which are typically associated with cell lysis, or the virus can enter a nonproductive state known as latency. Viral latency is defined as a condition in which the virus expresses few (or possibly no) gene products but can, under some conditions, "reawaken" to express the full range of viral gene products and produce new progeny virions. Latently infected cells are highly resistant to immune clearance.

There are three recognized forms of EBV latency. In latency I, EBV nuclear antigen-1 (EBNA1), which is required for the stable maintenance of the circularized viral DNA minichromosome, is the only viral protein expressed. EBV-derived microRNAs (miRs) may also be expressed. At the other end of the spectrum, latency III is characterized by the expression of EBNA1–6, several latent membrane proteins (LMP1, 2A, and 2B), two noncoding RNAs (EBER1 and 2), the BCL-2 homolog BHRF1, BARF0, and multiple miRs. Although the initial discovery of EBV involved the visualization of virions, indicating that the virus had exited latency and entered the productive lytic phase of the life cycle, viral gene expression in EBV-induced cancers generally follows one of the three latent patterns. The oncogenic activities of various EBV gene products have recently been reviewed.[87,88]

In a great majority of healthy individuals, EBV exists almost exclusively in a latent state, with the occasional asymptomatic shedding of virions in the saliva. The infection is controlled, at least in part, by CD8+ T cells specific for various latency proteins. EBV, like other herpesviruses, expresses a variety of proteins that interfere with cell-mediated immune responses. Intriguingly, results from mouse model systems suggest that the chronic immunostimulatory effects of persistent gammaherpesvirus emergence (or abortive emergence) from latency in healthy hosts can nonspecifically boost immunity to other infections.[92]

Lymphomas

In addition to endemic Burkitt lymphoma, EBV is often present in sporadic cases of Burkitt lymphoma in individuals who have not been exposed to malaria. Although nearly all cases of endemic

Burkitt's lymphoma contain EBV DNA in the tumor (typically in a latency I–like state), only about 20% of sporadic cases arising in immunocompetent individuals contain EBV. Rates of Burkitt lymphoma are elevated in HIV-infected individuals, and HIV-associated Burkitt lymphomas contain EBV in about 30% of cases.

A common hallmark of all types of Burkitt's lymphomas is deregulation of the cellular Myc proto-oncogene. A classic mutation involves chromosomal translocation of the Myc gene to the antibody heavy chain locus. Burkitt's lymphoma tumors that lack detectable EBV DNA tend to carry multiple additional mutations in host cell genes, raising the possibility that an originally EBV-positive precursor cell ultimately accumulated mutations that rendered it independent of viral genes.[88,93]

In addition to Burkitt lymphoma, EBV is associated, to varying extents, with a histologically diverse range of other lymphoid cancers, including Hodgkin lymphoma, natural killer (NK)/T-cell lymphoma, primary central nervous system (CNS) lymphoma, and diffuse large B-cell lymphoma. The incidence of these various forms of lymphoma is significantly increased both in AIDS patients as well as in iatrogenically and congenitally immunosuppressed individuals.[88] In particular, the essentially universal presence of EBV in CNS lymphomas in AIDS patients makes it possible to diagnose the disease with a PCR test for EBV that, together with radiologic findings, can obviate the need for a brain biopsy.

EBV is almost invariably associated with lymphoproliferative disorders, such as plasmacytic hyperplasia and polymorphic B cell hyperplasia, which are often observed in organ transplant recipients. These polyclonal lymphoproliferative responses can, in some instances, progress to oligoclonal or monoclonal lymphomas of various types. The occurrence of EBV-associated lymphoproliferative disease in immunosuppressed patients is generally heralded by the increased detection of EBV DNA in the peripheral blood and the oral cavity. This presumably reflects the failure of cellular immune responses to drive the virus into full latency and perhaps also a failure of cell-mediated immune responses targeting latency-associated EBV gene products present in the nascent tumor.

Carcinomas

In Southern China, NPC affects 25 out of 100,000 people, accounting for 18% of all cancers in China as a whole.[94] Most other world regions have a 25- to 100-fold lower rate of NPC. EBV is present in nearly all cases of NPC, both in endemic and nonendemic regions. Although there is support for the idea that dietary intake of salted fish and other preserved foods is a factor in endemic NPC, it remains possible that genetic traits or as yet unidentified environmental cocarcinogenic factors may play a role as well. Individuals with rising or relatively high IgA antibody responses to EBNA1, DNase, and/or EBV capsid antigens have a dramatically increased risk of developing NPC, offering an early detection method for at-risk individuals.[87]

EBV is also present in a small percentage (5% to 15%) of gastric adenocarcinomas and over 90% of gastric lymphoepithelioma-like carcinomas. In contrast to NPC, the prevalence of EBV-associated gastric cancer is similar in all world regions. As with NPC, elevated antibody responsiveness to EBV antigens may offer a method for identifying individuals at greater risk of gastric cancer.

Prevention and Treatment

The reduction of immunosuppression in response to increasing EBV loads is a standard approach to preventing EBV diseases in T-cell immunosuppressed individuals. Another approach to the prevention of EBV disease relies on ganciclovir (or related antiherpesvirus drugs), which can trigger the death of cells that express the EBV thymidine kinase gene. Pretreating at-risk individuals, such as organ transplant recipients, with ganciclovir has been shown to effectively prevent the development of EBV-induced lymphoproliferative disorders.[95] However, it is important to note that thymidine kinase is only expressed in the lytic phase of the viral life cycle, and drugs of this class are not generally effective for treating existing tumors, presumably due to the fact that EBV gene expression in tumors is typically of a latent type.

Although a recently developed vaccine targeting the EBV gp350 virion surface antigen did not provide sterilizing immunity to EBV infection, vaccinees did experience lower peak EBV viral loads upon infection.[96] Given the strong correlation between high EBV loads and the development of EBV diseases, it is hoped that the vaccine's ability to merely blunt the acute infection may offer significant protection against disease.

Most forms of EBV-associated lymphoid cancers express the B-cell marker CD20, making rituximab (an anti-CD20 mAb) a potentially effective adjunct therapy.[97,98] An emerging treatment approach that has recently entered clinical trials involves stimulating T cells ex vivo against peptides based on EBV antigens or against autologous EBV-transformed B cells.

KAPOSI'S SARCOMA HERPESVIRUS

History and Epidemiology

In the late 19th century, Hungarian dermatologist Moritz Kaposi's described a relatively rare type of indolent pigmented skin sarcoma affecting older men.[99] Kaposi's sarcoma (KS) was later found to be more prevalent in the Mediterranean region and in eastern portions of sub-Saharan Africa.[100] An early clue to the emergence of the HIV/AIDS pandemic in the early 1980s was a dramatic increase in the incidence of highly aggressive forms of KS, particularly in gay men who were much younger than typical KS patients. After the discovery of HIV, it was briefly hypothesized that HIV might be a direct cause of KS. However, this hypothesis failed to explain the existence of KS long prior to the HIV pandemic and the low incidence of KS in individuals who became infected with HIV via blood products. This latter observation was more easily explained by the existence of a sexually transmitted cofactor other than HIV.[101]

Using a subtractive DNA hybridization approach known as representational difference analysis, Yuan Chang, Patrick Moore, and colleagues discovered the presence of a previously unknown herpesvirus in KS tumors.[102] The newly founded field of research rapidly established key lines of evidence supporting the conclusion that KSHV (later designated human herpesvirus-8 [HHV-8]) is a causal factor in KS.[11]

It is now clear that the rate of KSHV infection varies greatly in different world regions.[11,103] In North America and Western Europe, KSHV seroprevalence in the general population ranges from 1% to 7%. Seroprevalence among gay men in these regions is substantially higher (25% to 60%), suggesting a possible link to sexual transmission. KSHV infection is much more prevalent in the general population in central and eastern Africa, where seroprevalence ranges from 23% to 70%. In endemic areas, up to 15% of children are seropositive, suggesting either vertical transmission or transmission via nonsexual casual contact (presumably via saliva). In endemic regions, KS is estimated to be the third most common cancer among adults.[104]

Kaposi's Sarcoma-Associated Herpesvirus in Kaposi's Sarcoma

KS tumors are complex on a number of levels. In contrast to most other forms of cancer, where it is often clear that a single cell type has proliferated out of control, KS tumors are composed of cells from multiple lineages (Fig. 5.2). KSHV-infected cells in the tumor often have a spindle-shaped morphology. Interestingly,

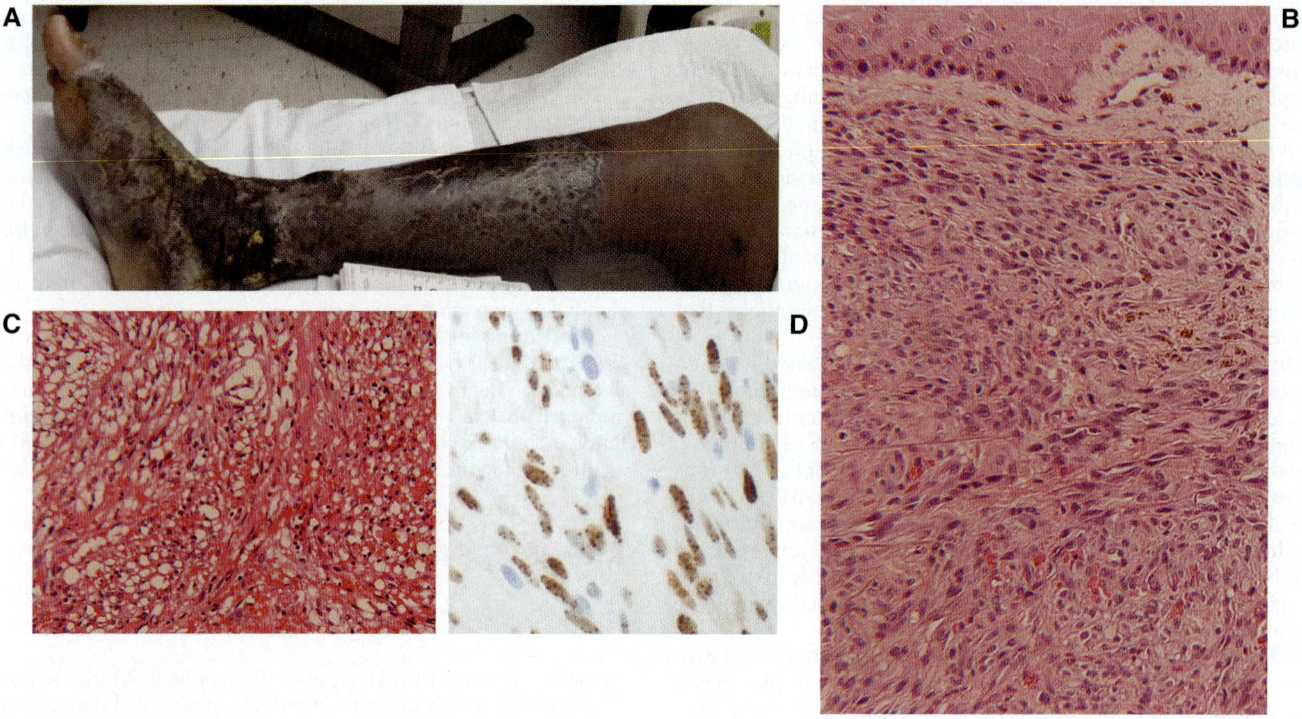

Figure 5.2 Kaposi's sarcoma (KS). **(A)** Photograph of the lower leg of an individual with severe, diffuse KS involving the lower leg. **(B)** Histology of the skin. **(C)** Lung shows a mixture of spindle to epithelioid cells, with slitlike vascular spaces intermixed with red blood cells and red blood cell fragments. **(D)** Immunohistochemical detection of KSHV LANA in the cutaneous tumor. Photographs provided with permission by Drs. Odey Ukpo and Ethel Cesarman.

spindle cells do not exhibit a highly transformed phenotype and tend to show relatively little chromosomal instability. In a culture, the cells are highly dependent on exogenous cytokines and other factors present in the tumor microenvironment in vivo. Although spindle cells express a number of markers of the endothelial lineage, it is uncertain whether they are derived from mature endothelial cells, the early precursor cells that give rise to smooth muscle and vascular endothelial cells, or cells of the lymphatic endothelial lineage. KS tumors also contain infiltrating lymphocytes and monocytes, as well as aberrant neovascular spaces lined with infected and uninfected endothelial cells. The aberrant blood vessels in KS lesion vessels rupture easily and leak red blood cells, giving KS tumors their classic dark red, brown, or purple color.

The latency status of KSHV in KS tumors is also complex, with the expression of gene products typical of latency (e.g., LANA) as well as lytic-phase genes (e.g., RTA/ORF50). Some of these gene products, such as the viral interleukin (IL)-6 homolog (vIL-6), trigger proliferation and secondary cytokine signaling in noninfected cells within the tumor. The tumorigenic effects of individual KSHV gene products have recently been reviewed.[88,103] In contrast to EBV, where tumorigenesis is driven by latency gene expression, it appears that KS pathogenesis is often dependent on lytic phase gene expression. This may explain why ganciclovir, which is not a particularly effective treatment for EBV tumors, was found to prevent the formation of new KS lesions in HIV-positive patients.[105] However, it should be noted that this outcome has more recently proven difficult to reproduce.[106] At present, there are no recommended preventive therapies for individuals at risk of KS, but this is an area of active investigation.

There are a variety of possible explanations for the need for lytic-phase KSHV gene expression during tumor development. For example, infected spindle cells may lose the viral DNA during cell division and require reinfection for ongoing tumorigenicity. Alternatively, factors secreted by a small fraction of tumor cells that enter the lytic phase may be required for tumorigenesis. An important area of current research focus is the role of KSHV gene products in the regulation of angiogenesis in KS lesions[107] and several current trials are investigating inhibitors of angiogenic pathways for the treatment of KS.

Lymphoproliferative Disorders

KSHV causes two forms of B-cell proliferative disorder: multicentric Castleman disease (MCD) and primary effusion lymphoma (PEL). Both diseases are most commonly found in association with HIV infection. In HIV-infected individuals, MCD tumors contain KSHV in nearly all cases, whereas in HIV-negative individuals, the tumor contains KSHV in only about 50% of cases.[108] KSHV in MCD tumors exhibits periodic activation of lytic replication and the expression of lytic phase genes.[109] The expression of vIL-6 during disease flare-ups appears to play a role in MCD pathogenesis, raising the possibility that tocilizumab (a mAb therapeutic that targets the IL-6 receptor) may be of therapeutic benefit.

PEL comprises about 4% of all HIV-associated non-Hodgkin lymphomas.[110] Typically, PEL tumors express markers of both plasma cells (akin to multiple myeloma tumors) and immunoblasts (similar to some EBV-induced tumors). In AIDS patients, essentially all PEL tumors are infected with KSHV and a great majority are also coinfected with EBV.[88] Although PEL is rare in HIV-negative individuals, PEL tumors in such individuals contain KSHV in about 50% of cases.

A common approach to the treatment of all KSHV-associated diseases is the restoration of immune function, either through antiretroviral therapy of HIV/AIDS or through a reduction of immunosuppressive therapy. The general success of immune reconstitution in many KSHV-associated diseases presumably involves an immune-mediated attack of cells expressing KSHV gene products, particularly the many lytic-phase gene products the virus can produce in various disease states.

ANIMAL AND HUMAN RETROVIRUSES

The first oncogenic retroviruses were discovered by Ellerman and Bang in 1908 and by Rous in 1911, but it was many years before the significance of these findings was appreciated.[111] One reason the field was stymied was the failure to identify RNA forms of the viral genome in infected cells. This led to the discovery of the reverse transcriptase independently by Baltimore and Temin in 1970. Another major development was the finding in 1976 of viral oncogenes derived from cellular genes, with the identification by Varmus and Bishop of the first dominant oncogene, *src*. With the discovery of IL-2 by Gallo in 1976, it became possible to culture the first human retrovirus, HTLV-1, from a form of adult T-cell leukemia/lymphoma (ATLL) that was first recognized by Takatsuki and coworkers.[112] These advances opened the door for Montagnier and colleagues' isolation of HIV-1 in 1983, a discovery confirmed independently by Gallo and Levy. This breakthrough led to the first licensed HIV test in 1985.

Retroviruses are positive single-strand RNA viruses that utilize transcription of their RNA genome into a DNA intermediate during virus replication.[111] This accounts for their name, retroviruses, because this is opposite to the normal flow of eukaryotic genetic information. They infect a wide range of vertebrate animal species and are distantly related to repetitive elements in the human genome, known as retrotransposons. Retroviruses are also related to hepadnaviruses, double-stranded DNA viruses, such as hepatitis B virus, which also undergo a reverse transcription step in their replication.

Retroviruses may be classified as *endogenous* or *exogenous* depending on whether they appear in the genome of the host species. There are approximately 100,000 endogenous retroviral elements in the human genome, making up nearly 8% of the genetic information, but their potential roles in disease are unclear.[113] Retroviruses may also be classified as *ecotropic*, *xenotropic*, or *polytropic* depending on whether they infect cells of the same animal species from which they are derived, infect cells of a different species, or both. *Amphotropic* retroviruses infect cells of the species of origin without producing disease, but infect cells of other species and may produce disease.

Retroviruses that produce disease after a long incubation period are termed *lentiviruses* and include human, simian, feline, ovine, caprine, and bovine immunodeficiency viruses. Another group of retroviruses that are not clearly associated with disease are known as *spumaviruses* and include human and simian foamy viruses. HTLV-1, which is classified in the genus Delta, is the only retrovirus known to be oncogenic in humans. A member of the retroviral genus Gamma identified in 2008, designated xenotropic murine leukemia virus-related virus (XMRV), was thought to be associated with human prostate cancer; however, more recent studies showed XMRV to be a lab-derived artifact.[114] A genus betaretrovirus related to the mouse mammary tumor virus has been suggested to be associated with biliary cirrhosis, but this finding requires independent validation.[115]

Retroviruses producing tumors in animals or birds are designated transforming viruses and may be classified as acute or chronic transforming retroviruses. Acute transforming retroviruses have acquired a mutated cellular gene, termed *oncogene*, and induce cancer in an animal within a few weeks. Many dominant acting proto-oncogenes in humans (e.g., *ras*, *myc*, and *erbB*), were first identified as retroviral oncogenes.

Chronic transforming retroviruses integrate almost randomly in the genome, but when integrated in the vicinity of specific genes disrupt their regulation and induce cell proliferation or resistance to apoptosis. Chronic transforming retroviruses induce malignancy only after many weeks to months of infection. The use of a murine leukemia virus vector for gene therapy in children with a form of severe combined immune deficiency syndrome characterized by defective expression of the common gamma chain of the IL-2 receptor resulted in T-cell acute lymphoblastic leukemia. This was found to be the result of persistent expression of the LIM domain only 2 (LMO2) gene triggered by the nearby integration of the retroviral vector.[116]

In addition to acute or chronic transformation mechanisms, retroviruses can transform cells through direct effects on cell physiology mediated by structural or nonstructural viral proteins. Transforming genes of HTLV-1 are nonstructural viral proteins that activate host cell signaling pathways.[117] Because the oncogenic effects of HTLV-1 transforming genes generally take many years to cause cancer, the virus does not fit the precise definition of having either an acute or a chronic oncogenic mechanism.

HIV-1 infection is also associated with a variety of malignancies, but only by indirect effects of suppressing immunity to oncogenic virus infections, such as gammaherpesviruses, high-risk human papillomaviruses, and hepatitis viruses.

Human T-Cell Leukemia Virus Epidemiology

Four species of human T-cell leukemia virus have been identified. HTLV-1 was identified in 1980 as the first human retrovirus associated with cancer, and it is the focus of the remainder of this section.[118] HTLV-2 was discovered in 1982 and shares 70% genomic homology with HTLV-1.[119] HTLV-3 and -4 were sporadically isolated from individuals who had contact with monkeys.[120] HTLV-2, -3, and -4 do not appear to be associated with disease in humans.

HTLV-1 is present in 15 to 20 million individuals worldwide, most commonly in the Caribbean Islands, South America, southern Japan, and parts of Australia, Melanesia, Africa, and Iran.[121] In the United States, Canada, and Europe, 0.01% to 0.03% of blood donors are infected with HTLV-1. It is most commonly found in individuals who emigrated from endemic regions or among African Americans. HTLV-1 is transmitted sexually, by contaminated cell-associated blood products, or by breast-feeding.[122] Only 2% to 5% of HTLV-1–infected individuals develop disease, and ATLL only occurs in individuals who acquired HTLV-1 by breast-feeding.

Human T-Cell Leukemia Virus Molecular Biology

HTLV-1, like other retroviruses, encodes Gag, Protease, Pol, and Envelope proteins.[123] Gag proteins compose the inner nucleocapsid core of the virus. The Pol proteins include the reverse transcriptase and integrase. The reverse transcriptase copies the single-stranded viral RNA into double-stranded DNA, and it is inhibited by several nucleoside analogs, but not by the nonnucleoside reverse transcriptase inhibitors approved for HIV-1.[124] The integrase is responsible for inserting the linear double-stranded DNA product of reverse transcription into the host chromosomal DNA. At least one integrase inhibitor, raltegravir, now approved for HIV-1, is active against HTLV-1.[125] Integration occurs throughout the human genome, but there is preference for integration into transcriptionally active genomic regions.[126] The viral protease proteolytically processes Gag, Protease, and Pol precursor proteins to the mature individual proteins, but it is not affected by inhibitors of HIV-1 protease. The envelope proteins include the transmembrane protein, which anchors the surface envelope protein on the virion, which mediates binding to the viral receptor.[127]

The viral genome also encodes regulatory proteins, including Tax and HTLV-1 bZIP factor (HBZ).[117] Tax is a transcriptional transactivator protein that functions as a coactivator to induce members of the cAMP response element-binding protein/activating transcription factor (CREB/ATF) family, nuclear factor kappa B (NF-κB), and serum response factor (SRF) pathways. Tax activation of the CREB/ATF pathway is responsible for upregulation of the viral promoter. Tax induction of NF-κB promotes cell proliferation and resistance to apoptosis. Tax also binds and activates cyclin-dependent kinases and inhibits cell cycle checkpoint proteins. Tax

ETIOLOGY AND EPIDEMIOLOGY OF CANCER

is important for tumor initiation, whereas HBZ may be important in tumor maintenance.[128]

HTLV-1 preferentially immortalizes CD4+ T lymphocytes and induces tumors in mice.[129] Tax also promotes the leukemia-initiating activity of ATLL cells in mouse models.[130] In immunodeficient mice reconstituted with human hematopoietic cells, HTLV-1 causes CD4+ lymphomas.[131]

Clinical Characteristics and Treatment of HTLV-Associated Malignancies

The diagnosis of HTLV-1 is based on serologic assays.[132] HTLV-1 is associated with various inflammatory disorders, including uveitis, polymyositis, pneumonitis, Sjögren syndrome, and myelopathy. Infected patients are susceptible to certain infectious disorders (e.g. staphylococcal dermatitis) and opportunistic infections such as pneumocystis pneumonia, disseminated cryptococcosis, strongyloidiasis, or toxoplasmosis.[133] Vaccines have not been developed for HTLV infections.

T-lymphocyte proliferative disorders develop in 1% to 5% of infected individuals and are generally CD2+, CD3+, CD4+, CD5+, CD25+, CD29+, CD45RO+, CD52+, HLA-DR+, T-cell receptor αβ+, and variably CD30+, and lack CD7, CD8, and CD26 expression. The virus is clonally integrated in the malignant cells. Complex karyotypes are often found, and cytogenetic analysis is rarely useful. The histologic features of lymph nodes in ATLL may be indistinguishable from those of other peripheral T-cell lymphomas.[134] Circulating tumor "flower cells" are helpful in the diagnosis (Fig. 5.3).

ATLL is categorized in four subtypes.[135] (1) Smoldering ATLL is defined as 5% or more abnormal T lymphocytes and lactate dehydrogenase (LDH) levels up to 1.5× the upper limit of normal, with normal lymphocyte count, calcium, and no lymph node or visceral disease other than skin or pulmonary disease. (2) Chronic ATLL is characterized by lymphocytosis, LDH up to 2× the upper limit of normal, no hypercalcemia, and no CNS, bone, pleural, peritoneal, or gastrointestinal involvement, although the lymph nodes, liver, spleen, skin, or lungs may be involved. The mean survival of these forms of ATLL is 2 to 5 years.[136] No intervention in these subtypes of ATLL has been defined that prevents progression to the more aggressive forms of ATLL. Although chronic or smoldering ATLL may respond to zidovudine and interferon, randomized studies have not been conducted.[137] (3) Lymphoma-type ATLL is characterized by ≤1% abnormal T lymphocytes and features of non-Hodgkin lymphoma. (4) Acute-type ATLL includes the remaining patients. Even with optimal therapy, the median survival of lymphoma and acute-type ATLL is less than 1 year.[138] Lymphoma and acute types of ATLL are the most common presenting subtypes. Other major prognostic factors include performance status, age, the presence of more than three involved lesions, and hypercalcemia.[139]

Combination chemotherapy for lymphoma or acute-type ATLL with the infusional etoposide, prednisone, vincristine, and doxorubicin (EPOCH) regimen or the LSG-15 regimen results in complete remission rates of 15% to 40%.[140,141] However, responses are short lived, with <10% of patients free of disease at 4 years. The addition of anti-CCR4 antibody, mogamulizumab, may improve response rates, but studies are still underway.[142]

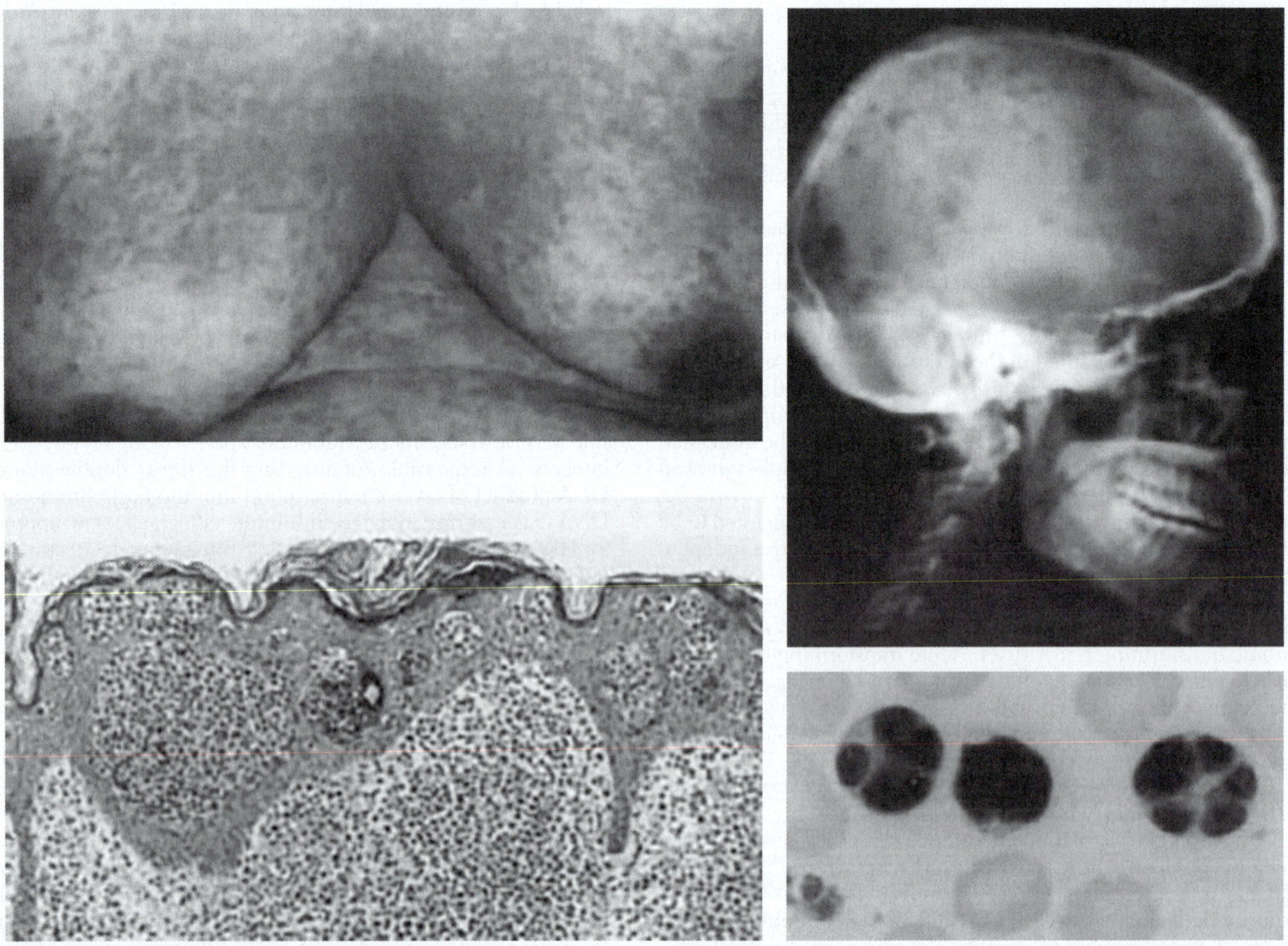

Figure 5.3 Clinical manifestation of adult T-cell leukemia/lymphoma. **(A–B)** Infiltration of malignant T lymphocytes into the skin. **(C)** Lytic bone lesions seen on lateral skull x-ray. **(D)** "Flower cells" in the blood.

The combination of interferon and zidovudine with or without arsenic may result in the remission of acute, but not lymphoma subtypes.[143] Allogenic transplantation may result in long-term, disease-free survival for patients with complete or near complete remission of disease, although infectious complications have been notable in these studies.[144]

HEPATITIS VIRUSES

The earliest record of an epidemic caused by a hepatitis virus was in 1885, occurring in individuals vaccinated for smallpox with lymph from other people.[145] The cause of the epidemic, HBV, was not identified until 1966, when Blumberg discovered the *Australian antigen* now known to be the hepatitis B surface antigen (HBsAg). This was followed by the discovery of the virus particle by Dane in 1970. In the early 1980s, the HBV genome was sequenced and the first vaccines were tested. In the mid 1970s, Alter described cases of hepatitis not due to hepatitis A or B viruses, and the suspected agent was designated non-A, non-B hepatitis virus, now known as HCV.[146] In 1987, Houghton used molecular cloning to identify the HCV genome and develop a diagnostic test, which was licensed in 1990.

Approximately 240 million people are chronically infected with HBV and 150 to 200 million people are infected with HCV worldwide, according to the World Health Organization (WHO). About 1 million deaths per year are attributed to the chronic diseases such as liver cirrhosis and hepatocellular carcinoma (HCC) that result from viral hepatitis infections. HBV and HCV are the leading cause of liver cancer in the world, accounting for almost 80% of the cases. In the United States, Europe, Egypt, and Japan, more than 60% of HCC cases are associated with HCV, and 20% are related to HBV and chronic alcoholism.[147] In Africa and Asia, 60% of HCC is associated with HBV, 20% related to HCV, and the remainder related to other risk factors, such as alcohol and aflatoxin. HCC is the sixth most common cancer worldwide and is the third most common cause of cancer death.[148]

In Asia and Africa, up to 70% of individuals have serologic evidence of current or prior HBV infection, and 8% to 15% of these subjects have a chronic active infection. Rates of HCV infection of >3.5% occur in Central and East Asia, North Africa, and the Middle East. In the United States, 0.8 to 1.4 million individuals are infected with HBV, and 3.2 million with HCV. The incidence of HCC in the United States tripled between 1975 and 2005, particularly in African American and Hispanic males.[149]

HBV is transmitted primarily through exposure to infected blood, semen, and other body fluids, whereas HCV is transmitted primarily by contact with contaminated blood. Acute HCV infection causes mild and vague symptoms in about 15% of individuals and resolves spontaneously in 10% to 50% of cases.[150] Liver enzymes are normal in 5% to 50% of individuals with chronic HCV infection.[151] After 20 years of an HCV infection, the likelihood of cirrhosis is 10% to 15% for men, and 1.5% for women.[152] Cofactors that increase the likelihood of cirrhosis are coinfection with both hepatitis viruses, persistently high levels of HBV or HCV viremia, HBeAg, certain viral genotypes, schistosoma, HIV, alcoholism, male gender, advanced age at the time of infection, diabetes, and obesity.[153,154]

Hepatitis B Virus

HBV is an enveloped DNA virus that is a member of the *Hepadnaviridae* family.[155] HBV has a strong preference for infecting hepatocytes, but small amounts of viral DNA can also be found in kidney, pancreas, and mononuclear cells, although it is not linked to extrahepatic disease. The viral genome is a relaxed circular, partially double-stranded (ds) DNA of 3.2 kb. The genome exists as an episomal covalently closed circular dsDNA (cccDNA) molecule in the nucleus of infected cells, although chromosomal integration of viral genomic sequences can occur during cycles of hepatocyte regeneration and proliferation. In addition to 40 to 42 nm virions, HBV-infected cells also produce noninfectious 20-nm spherical and filamentous particles. The viral genome encodes four open reading frames. The presurface–surface (preS-S) region encodes three proteins from different translational initiation sites; these include the S (HBsAg), M (or pre-S2), and L (or pre-S1) proteins. The L protein is responsible for receptor binding and virion assembly. The precore–core (preC-C) region encodes the HBcAg and HBeAg. The P region encodes the viral polymerase, and the X (HBx) protein modulates host-signal transduction.

After infection, the viral genome is transcribed by host RNA polymerase II, and viral proteins are translated. Nucleocapsids assemble in the cytosol, incorporating a molecule of pregenomic RNA into the viral core, where reverse transcription occurs to produce the dsDNA viral genome. Viral cores are enveloped with intracellular membranes and viral L, M, and S surface antigens, which are exported from the cells.

HBV replication is not cytotoxic. Instead, liver injury is due to the host immune response, primarily T-cell and proinflammatory cytokine responses. Chronic HBV carriers exhibit an attenuated virus-specific T-cells response, although a vigorous humoral response is still evident. About 5% of infections in adults and up to 90% of infections in neonates result in a persistent infection, which may or may not be associated with symptoms and elevated serum aminotransferase levels. About 20% of such individuals develop cirrhosis. Immunosuppressed individuals also have a higher likelihood of a persistent infection.

With acute infection, viral titers of 10^9 to 10^{10} virions per mililiter are present, whereas levels of 10^7 to 10^9 virions per mililiter and HBsAg, and in some cases, HBeAg are present in the blood of individuals with a persistent infection. The resolution of infection, which is associated with declining viral DNA titers, is observed at a rate of 5% to 10% per year in persistently infected individuals. However, even subjects who have resolved the infection continue to have very low levels of viral DNA (10^3 to 10^5 copies per mililiter) for most of their lives.

HBV infection can be managed with alpha interferon or nucleos(t)ide analogs that inhibit the viral polymerase, such as lamivudine, telbivudine, entecavir, adefovir, and tenofovir.[156] Entecavir and tenofovir are both effective at inducing viral suppression, and may be used in combination in patients with high HBV DNA load or multidrug resistance. Because these agents are all associated with some toxicity, current guidelines recommend therapy only when liver disease is clinically apparent, with continued treatment for 6 to 12 months after clearance of HBeAg or HBsAg. Although these drugs effectively control HBV, they typically fail to cure the infection due to the long-term persistence of the cccDNA form of the viral genome. Other nucleos(t)ide analogs are currently in clinical trials, as well as a novel form of interferon (IFN-λ) and an inhibitor of virus release.[157]

Hepatitis D virus (HDV) occurs only in individuals coinfected with HBV. HDV is composed a single-stranded circular viral RNA genome of 1,679 nucleotides, a central core of HDAg, and an outer coat with all three HBV envelope proteins. HDV infection results in more severe complications than infection with HBV alone, with a higher likelihood and more rapid progression to cirrhosis and HCC.

Hepatits C Virus

HCV is an enveloped RNA virus associated with cancer, primarily HCC and, rarely, splenic marginal zone lymphoma.[158] HCV is a positive-sense, single-stranded RNA virus of the *Flaviviridae* family.[159] There are seven genotypes of HCV; in the United States, about 70% of infections are caused by genotype 1.[160] HCV replicates in the cytoplasm and does not integrate into the host cell genome. The viral RNA is 9.6 kb and encodes a single polyprotein of 3,010 amino acids that is proteolytically processed into structural and nonstructural proteins. In addition to the structural roles of the core (C) protein, it has also been reported to affect various host cell functions. The envelope glycoproteins E1 and E2 mediate infectious entry through tetraspanin CD81 and other receptors on hepatocytes and B lymphocytes.

HCV non structural proteins NS2, NS3, NS4A, NS4B, NS5A, NS5B, and p7 are required for virus replication and assembly. NS2 is a membrane-associated cysteine protease. NS3 is a helicase and NTPase that unwinds RNA and DNA substrates. The complex of NS3 with NS4A forms a serine protease. NS4B induces the formation of a membranous web associated with the viral RNA replicase. NS5A is an RNA-binding phosphoprotein, whereas NS5B is the RNA-dependent RNA polymerase. The p7 protein forms a cation channel in infected cells that has a role in particle maturation and release.

Treating an HCV infection typically utilizes 24 to 48 weeks of pegylated IFN-α and ribavirin.[161] Treatment with IFN and ribavirin alone produces sustained virologic responses in 70% to 80% of subjects with genotype 2 or 3 infections. Recently approved inhibitors of the NS3-4A protease (e.g., telaprevir, boceprevir, or simeprevir) may be included in IFN-based regimens, particularly if the patient has failed prior therapy. Protease inhibitors are currently approved for use in IFN/ribavirin combination therapy for HCV genotype 1 or 4 infection. Sofosbuvir, a nucleoside analog inhibitor of the viral NS5B polymerase, has recently been approved for use in combination with ribavirin alone for genotypes 2 or 3, or in triple therapy for genotypes 1 and 4. Recently, IFN-free regimens have also been approved. Additional protease and polymerase inhibitors are currently in development. A recent meta-analysis of eight randomized controlled trials comparing antiviral therapy with placebo suggested that antiviral therapy resulted in a 50% reduced risk of HCC.[162]

Hepatitis Virus Pathogenesis

HBV and HCV depress innate immune responses by inhibiting Toll-like receptor signaling through effects of HBx and NS3-4A.[147] In addition, HCV C inhibits the Janus kinase (JAK)-signal transducer and activator of transcription (STAT) signaling, and NS5A and E2 inhibit IFN signaling. Through an undefined mechanism, HBV can inhibit JAK-STAT signaling as well.

HBV and HCV induce HCC by direct and indirect mechanisms.[147] Both HBV and HCV encode proteins that have pro- and antiapoptotic properties. High levels of HBx block activation of the NF-κB pathway, whereas HCV C and NS5A block apoptosis by the activation of AKT and NF-κB, respectively. The C and NS5A proteins may also induce epithelial–mesenchymal transition (EMT), which is important for liver fibrosis, through effects on transforming growth factor β and Src signaling. Mice transgenic for NS5A develop steatosis and HCC.

HBx and HCV C are associated with mitochondria, where they trigger oxidative stress that induces apoptosis. In addition, HBs and HBx and NS3-4A alter calcium signaling and increase reactive oxygen species, which trigger endoplasmic reticulum (ER) stress, an unfolded protein response, and the production of proinflammatory cytokines that induce collagen synthesis, which drives the development of fibrosis. Autophagy is triggered by both viruses to restore ER integrity, which promotes cell survival and viral persistence.

HBV and HCV also disrupt tumor suppressor proteins. HCV NS5B recruits an ubiquitin ligase protein to modify pRB and induce its degradation, whereas HBx and HCV C proteins both inhibit p16INK4a and p21 cell cycle inhibitors, which leads to the inactivating phosphorylation of pRB. The HBx and HCV C, NS3, and NS5A proteins deregulate p53 tumor suppressor activity, by compromising p53-mediated DNA repair. HBV and HCV also induce alterations in micro-RNAs that are partially responsible for cell cycle effects.

Although not part of the normal virus replication cycle, the tendency of HBV genomic DNA sequences to integrate within the host cell chromosomes also contributes to the pathogenesis of HBV-associated HCC. In most hepatoma cells, HBV replication is extinguished, and integration at certain sites provides a growth or survival advantage, leading to tumors that are clonal with respect to viral integration. Whole-genome sequencing studies have identified a number of cellular loci, including *TERT* and *MLL*, where HBV integration is associated with HCC.[163,164]

Both HBV and HCV promote characteristics of cancer stem cells. HBx promotes the expression of Nanog, Kruppel-like factor 4, octamer-binding transcription factor 4, and Myc. These markers are also induced by HBV and HCV-induced hypoxia and hypoxia-induced factors.

Clinical Characteristics and Treatment of Hepatitis Virus-Associated Malignancies

HBV and HCV infections are diagnosed by serologic assays, and/or antigen assays in the case of HBV.[153] Quantitative HBV DNA and HCV RNA polymerase chain reactions are utilized to measure virus load. No vaccine has been identified that protects against HCV because infections consist of a genetically heterogenous "swarm" of virus particles, some of which escape neutralization. However, a vaccine, which now utilizes a recombinant HBsAg produced in yeast cells, has been available for HBV prevention for more than 30 years. The HBV vaccine reduces the risk of infection by more than 70%.[157] Factors associated with HBV vaccination failure in adults include increased age, obesity, smoking, diabetes, end-stage renal disease, HIV infection, alcoholism, or recipients of liver or kidney transplantation. There have been recent suggestions that emerging HBV strains may be evolving to escape neutralizing antibodies elicited by the current vaccine.[165] Novel vaccine adjuvants are currently in clinical trials, as well as studies of a therapeutic HBV vaccine.

Because an early diagnosis of HCC is key to a successful treatment, there has been extensive research on surveillance techniques in HBV- and HCV-infected individuals.[166] The U.S. Centers for Disease Control and Prevention has recently recommended that all individuals born between 1945 and 1965 be tested for HCV infection. The American Association for the Study of Liver Diseases, as well as the European and Asian Pacific Associations for the Study of the Liver, endorse surveillance in HCV-infected individuals with cirrhosis using ultrasound every 6 months. Viral eradication does not fully eliminate the risk of HCC, and thus, continued surveillance is still recommended in cirrhotic patients.

Therapeutic options for HCC are determined not only by the number and size of HCC nodules as well as the presence or absence of vascular invasion and metastases, but also by liver function and the presence or absence of portal hypertension.[167] HCC amenable to liver transplantation is usually defined as either one tumor measuring ≤50 mm in diameter or two to three tumors measuring ≤30 mm in diameter without vascular extension or metastasis (Milan criteria).[168] Up to 30% of all cases of HCC present with multiple nodules of HCC, suggesting a field carcinogenesis effect of HBV and HCV.[169] HBV- and HCV-infected patients may have a lower survival than noninfected patients after liver transplantation.[170] Hepatitis B immune globulin and nucleos(t)ide analogs are recommended for reinfection prophylaxis in the posttransplant period for HBV-infected individuals.[171] Studies are underway to examine the appropriate use of antiviral therapy for HCV-infected patients undergoing liver transplantation.

Reactivation of HCV can occur with chemotherapy or monoclonal antibody-based immunosuppressive therapies, but is less frequent as compared to HBV infection.[172] Individuals who appear to have cleared an HBV infection and who have an undetectable viral load can experience HBV reactivation on rituximab therapy. Monitoring hepatic function and virus load is indicated during chemoimmunotherapy of HBV- or HCV-positive patients.[173] Although there is controversy regarding the role of virus screening for patients undergoing chemotherapy, antiviral therapy is recommended for high-risk HBV-infected patients undergoing chemoimmunotherapy, such as rituximab-based chemotherapy regimens.[174]

An association between HCV and B-cell non-Hodgkin lymphoma (NHL) has also been demonstrated in highly endemic geographic areas.[175] Lymphoproliferation has been linked to type II mixed cryoglobulinemia in many of these individuals. In addition to diffuse large B-cell lymphoma, marginal zone lymphomas and lymphoplasmacytic lymphomas are the histologic subtypes most frequently associated with HCV infection. Antiviral treatment with IFNα with or without ribavirin has been effective in the treatment of HCV-infected patients with indolent lymphoma, but rarely in individuals with aggressive lymphomas.

CONCLUSION

Oncogenic viruses are important causes of cancer, especially in less industrialized countries and in immunosuppressed individuals. They are common causes of anogenital cancers, lymphomas, oral and hepatocellular carcinomas and are associated with a variety of other malignancies. Vaccines and antiviral agents play an important role in the prevention of virus-induced cancers. Studies of virus pathogenesis will continue to establish paradigms that are critical to our understanding of cancer etiology in general.

REFERENCES

1. de Martel C, Ferlay J, Franceschi S, et al. Global burden of cancers attributable to infections in 2008: a review and synthetic analysis. *Lancet Oncol* 2012;13(6):607–615.
2. Schiller JT, Lowy DR. Virus infection and human cancer: an overview. *Recent Results Cancer Res* 2014;193:1–10.
3. Chen CJ, Hsu WL, Yang HI, et al. Epidemiology of virus infection and human cancer. *Recent Results Cancer Res* 2014;193:11–32.
4. Virgin HW, Wherry EJ, Ahmed R. Redefining chronic viral infection. *Cell* 2009;138(1):30–50.
5. Campo MS, O'Neil BW, Barron RJ, et al. Experimental reproduction of the papilloma-carcinoma complex of the alimentary canal in cattle. *Carcinogenesis* 1994;15(8):1597–1601.
6. Khoury JD, Tannir NM, Williams MD, et al. Landscape of DNA virus associations across human malignant cancers: analysis of 3,775 cases using RNA-Seq. *J Virol* 2013;87(16):8916–8926.
7. zur Hausen H, de Villiers EM. TT viruses: oncogenic or tumor-suppressive properties? *Curr Top Microbiol Immunol* 2009;331:109–116.
8. Mizutani T, Sayama Y, Nakanishi A, et al. Novel DNA virus isolated from samples showing endothelial cell necrosis in the Japanese eel, Anguilla japonica. *Virology* 2011;412(1):179–187.
9. Paulson KG, Carter JJ, Johnson LG, et al. Antibodies to merkel cell polyomavirus T antigen oncoproteins reflect tumor burden in merkel cell carcinoma patients. *Cancer Res* 2010;70:8388–8397.
10. International Agency for Research on Cancer (IARC) Working Group. *IARC Monographs on the Evalation of Carcinogenic Risks to Humans. Malaria and Some Polyomaviruses (SV40, BK, JC, and Merkel Cell Viruses)*, Vol. 104. Lyon, France: IARC; 2013.
11. Moore PS, Chang Y. The conundrum of causality in tumor virology: the cases of KSHV and MCV. *Semin Cancer Biol* 2013;26C:4–12.
12. Rigoni-Stern D. Fatti statistici relativi alle malattie cancrose. *Giornale Service Progr Pathol Terap Ser* 1842;2:507–517.
13. Lowy DR. History of papillomavirus research. In: Garcea RL, DiMaio D, eds. *The Papillomaviruses*. New York, NY: Springer; 2007:13–28.
14. zur Hausen H. Herpes simplex virus in human genital cancer. *Int Rev Exp Pathol* 1983;25:307–326.
15. Durst M, Gissmann L, Ikenberg H, et al. A papillomavirus DNA from a cervical carcinoma and its prevalence in cancer biopsy samples from different geographic regions. *Proc Natl Acad Sci U S A* 1983;80(12):3812–3815.
16. Boshart M, Gissmann L, Ikenberg H, et al. A new type of papillomavirus DNA, its presence in genital cancer biopsies and in cell lines derived from cervical cancer. *Embo J* 1984;3(5):1151–1157.
17. Christensen ND. Cottontail rabbit papillomavirus (CRPV) model system to test antiviral and immunotherapeutic strategies. *Antivir Chem Chemother* 2005;16(6):355–362.
18. Rous P, Beard J. The progression to carcinoma of virus induced rabbit papillomas (Shope). *J Exp Med* 1935;62:523–545.
19. Syverton JT, Berry GP. Carcinoma in the cottontail rabbit following spontaneous virus papilloma (Shope). *Proc Soc Exp Biol Med* 1935;33:399–400.
20. de Villiers EM. Cross-roads in the classification of papillomaviruses. *Virology* 2013;445(1–2):2–10.
21. Bosch FX, Broker TR, Forman D, et al. Comprehensive control of human papillomavirus infections and related diseases. *Vaccine* 2013;31 Suppl 8:I1–I31.
22. Van Doorslaer K. Evolution of the papillomaviridae. *Virology* 2013;445(1–2):11–20.
23. Scheffner M, Werness BA, Huibregtse JM, et al. The E6 oncoprotein encoded by human papillomavirus types 16 and 18 promotes the degradation of p53. *Cell* 1990;63(6):1129–1136.
24. Scheffner M, Huibregtse JM, Vierstra RD, Howley PM. The HPV-16 E6 and E6–AP complex functions as a ubiquitin-protein ligase in the ubiquitination of p53. *Cell* 1993;75(3):495–505.
25. Huibregtse JM, Scheffner M, Howley PM. Cloning and expression of the cDNA for E6–AP, a protein that mediates the interaction of the human papillomavirus E6 oncoprotein with p53. *Mol Cell Biol* 1993;13(2):775–784.
26. Klingelhutz AJ, Foster SA, McDougall JK. Telomerase activation by the E6 gene product of human papillomavirus type 16. *Nature* 1996;380(6569):79–82.
27. White EA, Howley PM. Proteomic approaches to the study of papillomavirus-host interactions. *Virology* 2013;435(1):57–69.
28. Dyson N, Howley PM, Munger K, et al. The human papilloma virus-16 E7 oncoprotein is able to bind to the retinoblastoma gene product. *Science* 1989;243(4893):934–937.
29. Munger K, Howley PM. Human papillomavirus immortalization and transformation functions. *Virus Res* 2002;89(2):213–228.
30. Duensing S, Lee LY, Duensing A, et al. The human papillomavirus type 16 E6 and E7 oncoproteins cooperate to induce mitotic defects and genomic instability by uncoupling centrosome duplication from the cell division cycle. *Proc Natl Acad Sci U S A* 2000;97(18):10002–10007.
31. DiMaio D, Petti LM. The E5 proteins. *Virology* 2013;445(1–2):99–114.
32. Schiller JT, Lowy DR. Understanding and learning from the success of prophylactic human papillomavirus vaccines. *Nat Rev Microbiol* 2012;10(10):681–692.
33. Kemp TJ, Safaeian M, Hildesheim A, et al. Kinetic and HPV infection effects on cross-type neutralizing antibody and avidity responses induced by Cervarix((R)). *Vaccine* 2012;31(1):165–170.
34. Haupt RM, Wheeler CM, Brown DR, et al. Impact of an HPV6/11/16/18 L1 virus-like particle vaccine on progression to cervical intraepithelial neoplasia in seropositive women with HPV16/18 infection. *Int J Cancer* 2011;129(11):2632–2642.
35. Kreuter A, Wieland U. Lack of efficacy in treating condyloma acuminata and preventing recurrences with the recombinant quadrivalent human papillomavirus vaccine in a case series of immunocompetent patients. *J Am Acad Dermatol* 2013;68(1):179–180.
36. Joura E, Team V-S, eds. Abstract SS 8–4: Efficacy and immunogenicity of a novel 9-valent HPV L1 virus-like particle vaccine in 16- to 26-year-old women. Paper presented at: Eurogin 2013 International Multidisciplinary Congress; 2013; Florence, Italy.
37. Wang JW, Roden RB. L2, the minor capsid protein of papillomavirus. *Virology* 2013;445(1–2):175–186.
38. Ma B, Maraj B, Tran NP, et al. Emerging human papillomavirus vaccines. *Expert Opin Emerg Drugs* 2012;17(4):469–492.
39. Scudellari M. HPV: sex, cancer and a virus. *Nature* 2013;503(7476):330–332.
40. Gillison ML, Alemany L, Snijders PJ, et al. Human papillomavirus and diseases of the upper airway: head and neck cancer and respiratory papillomatosis. *Vaccine* 2012;30 Suppl 5:F34–54.
41. Silverberg MJ, Leyden W, Warton EM, et al. HIV infection status, immunodeficiency, and the incidence of non-melanoma skin cancer. *J Natl Cancer Inst* 2013;105(5):350–360.
42. Kempf W, Mertz KD, Hofbauer GF, et al. Skin cancer in organ transplant recipients. *Pathobiology* 2013;80(6):302–309.
43. Wallace NA, Gasior SL, Faber ZJ, et al. HPV 5 and 8 E6 expression reduces ATM protein levels and attenuates LINE-1 retrotransposition. *Virology* 2013;443(1):69–79.
44. White EA, Kramer RE, Tan MJ, et al. Comprehensive analysis of host cellular interactions with human papillomavirus E6 proteins identifies new E6 binding partners and reflects viral diversity. *J Virol* 2012;86(24):13174–13186.
45. White EA, Sowa ME, Tan MJ, et al. Systematic identification of interactions between host cell proteins and E7 oncoproteins from diverse human papillomaviruses. *Proc Natl Acad Sci U S A* 2012;109(5):E260–267.
46. Caldeira S, Zehbe I, Accardi R, et al. The E6 and E7 proteins of the cutaneous human papillomavirus type 38 display transforming properties. *J Virol* 2003;77(3):2195–2206.
47. Arron ST, Ruby JG, Dybbro E, et al. Transcriptome sequencing demonstrates that human papillomavirus is not active in cutaneous squamous cell carcinoma. *J Invest Dermatol* 2011;131(8):1745–1753.
48. Gross L. A filterable agent, recovered from Ak leukemic extracts, causing salivary gland carcinomas in C3H mice. *Proc Soc Exp Biol Med* 1953;83(2):414–421.

49. Eddy BE, Stewart SE. Characteristics of the SE polyoma virus. *Am J Public Health Nations Health* 1959;49:1486–1492.
50. Sweet BH, Hilleman MR. The vacuolating virus, S.V. 40. *Proc Soc Exp Biol Med* 1960;105:420–427.
51. Eddy BE, Borman GS, Grubbs GE, et al. Identification of the oncogenic substance in rhesus monkey kidney cell culture as simian virus 40. *Virology* 1962;17:65–75.
52. Dang-Tan T, Mahmud SM, Puntoni R, et al. Polio vaccines, simian virus 40, and human cancer: the epidemiologic evidence for a causal association. *Oncogene* 2004;23(38):6535–6540.
53. Bouvard V, Baan RA, Grosse Y, et al. Carcinogenicity of malaria and of some polyomaviruses. *Lancet Oncol* 2012;13(4):339–340.
54. Gardner SD, Field AM, Coleman DV, et al. New human papovavirus (B.K.) isolated from urine after renal transplantation. *Lancet*.1971;1(7712): 1253–1257.
55. Padgett BL, Walker DL, ZuRhein GM, et al. Cultivation of papova-like virus from human brain with progressive multifocal leucoencephalopathy. *Lancet* 1971;1(7712):1257–1260.
56. Das D, Wojno K, Imperiale MJ. BK virus as a cofactor in the etiology of prostate cancer in its early stages. *J Virol* 2008;82(6):2705–2714.
57. Akgul B, Pfister D, Knuchel R, et al. No evidence for a role of xenotropic murine leukaemia virus-related virus and BK virus in prostate cancer of German patients. *Med Microbiol Immunol* 2012;201(2):245–248.
58. Alexiev BA, Randhawa P, Vazquez Martul E, et al. BK virus-associated urinary bladder carcinoma in transplant recipients: report of 2 cases, review of the literature, and proposed pathogenetic model. *Human Pathol* 2013;44(5):908–917.
59. Abend JR, Jiang M, Imperiale MJ. BK virus and human cancer: innocent until proven guilty. *Semin Cancer Biol* 2009;19(4):252–260.
60. Maginnis MS, Atwood WJ. JC virus: an oncogenic virus in animals and humans? *Semin Cancer Biol* 2009;19(4):261–269.
61. Feng H, Shuda M, Chang Y, et al. Clonal integration of a polyomavirus in human Merkel cell carcinoma. *Science* 2008;319(5866):1096–1100.
62. Hodgson NC. Merkel cell carcinoma: changing incidence trends. *J Surg Oncol* 2005;89(1):1–4.
63. Engels EA, Frisch M, Goedert JJ, et al. Merkel cell carcinoma and HIV infection. *Lancet* 2002;359(9305):497–498.
64. Zur Hausen A, Rennspiess D, Winnepenninckx V, et al. Early B-cell differentiation in Merkel cell carcinomas: clues to cellular ancestry. *Cancer Res* 2013;73(16):4982–4987.
65. Guastafierro A, Feng H, Thant M, et al. Characterization of an early passage Merkel cell polyomavirus-positive Merkel cell carcinoma cell line, MS-1, and its growth in NOD scid gamma mice. *J Virol Methods* 2013;187(1):6–14.
66. Schowalter RM, Pastrana DV, Pumphrey KA, et al. Merkel cell polyomavirus and two previously unknown polyomaviruses are chronically shed from human skin. *Cell Host Microbe* 2010;7(6):509–515.
67. Faust H, Pastrana DV, Buck CB, et al. Antibodies to Merkel cell polyomavirus correlate to presence of viral DNA in the skin. *J Infect Dis* 2011;203(8):1096–1100.
68. Pastrana DV, Wieland U, Silling S, et al. Positive correlation between Merkel cell polyomavirus viral load and capsid-specific antibody titer. *Med Microbiol Immunol* 2011;201(1):17–23.
69. Pastrana DV, Tolstov YL, Becker JC, et al. Quantitation of human seroresponsiveness to Merkel cell polyomavirus. *PLoS Pathog* 2009;5(9):e1000578.
70. Faust H, Andersson K, Ekstrom J, et al. Prospective study of Merkel cell polyomavirus and risk of Merkel cell carcinoma. *Int J Cancer* 2014;134(4):844–848.
71. Cheng J, Rozenblatt-Rosen O, Paulson KG, et al. Merkel cell polyomavirus large T antigen has growth-promoting and inhibitory activities. *J Virol* 2013;87(11):6118–6126.
72. Li J, Wang X, Diaz J, et al. Merkel cell polyomavirus large T antigen disrupts host genomic integrity and inhibits cellular proliferation. *J Virol* 2013;87(16):9173–9188.
73. Houben R, Shuda M, Weinkam R, et al. Merkel cell polyomavirus-infected Merkel cell carcinoma cells require expression of viral T antigens. *J Virol* 2010;84(14):7064–7072.
74. Houben R, Grimm J, Willmes C, et al. Merkel cell carcinoma and Merkel cell carcinoma polyomavirus: evidence for hit-and-run oncogenesis. *J Invest Dermatol* 2012;132(1):254–256.
75. Shuda M, Chang Y, Moore PS. Merkel cell polyomavirus positive Merkel cell carcinoma requires viral small T antigen for cell proliferation. *J Invest Dermatol* 2013 [Epub ahead of print].
76. Paulson KG, Iyer JG, Tegeder AR, et al. Transcriptome-wide studies of merkel cell carcinoma and validation of intratumoral CD8+ lymphocyte invasion as an independent predictor of survival. *J Clin Oncol* 2011;29(12):1539–1546.
77. Arora R, Shuda M, Guastafierro A, et al. Survivin is a therapeutic target in Merkel cell carcinoma. *Sci Transl Med* 2012;4(133):133ra56.
78. Dresang LR, Guastafierro A, Arora R, et al. Response of merkel cell polyomavirus-positive merkel cell carcinoma xenografts to a survivin inhibitor. *PloS One* 2013;8(11):e80543.
79. Shuda M, Kwun HJ, Feng H, et al. Human Merkel cell polyomavirus small T antigen is an oncoprotein targeting the 4E-BP1 translation regulator. *J Clin Invest* 2011;121(9):3623–3634.
80. Howard RA, Dores GM, Curtis RE, et al. Merkel cell carcinoma and multiple primary cancers. *Cancer Epidemiol Biomarkers Prev* 2006;15(8): 1545–1549.
81. Pantulu ND, Pallasch CP, Kurz AK, et al. Detection of a novel truncating Merkel cell polyomavirus large T antigen deletion in chronic lymphocytic leukemia cells. *Blood* 2010;116(24):5280–5284.
82. Tolstov YL, Arora R, Scudiere SC, et al. Lack of evidence for direct involvement of Merkel cell polyomavirus (MCV) in chronic lymphocytic leukemia (CLL). *Blood* 2010;115(23):4973–4974.
83. Cimino PJ, Jr., Bahler DW, Duncavage EJ. Detection of Merkel cell polyomavirus in chronic lymphocytic leukemia T-cells. *Exp Mol Pathol* 2013;94(1):40–44.
84. Burkitt D. A sarcoma involving the jaws in African children. *Br J Surg* 1958;46(197):218–223.
85. Epstein MA, Achong BG, Barr YM. Virus particles in cultured lymphoblasts from Burkitt's lymphoma. *Lancet* 1964;1(7335):702–703.
86. Henle G, Henle W, Diehl V. Relation of Burkitt's tumor-associated herpesytpe virus to infectious mononucleosis. *Proc Natl Acad Sci U S A* 1968;59(1): 94–101.
87. Longnecker RM, Kieff E, Cohen JI. Epstein-Barr virus. In: Knipe DM, Howley PM, eds. *Fields Virology*. 6th ed. Philadelphia, PA: Lippincott Williams & Wilkins; 2013.
88. Cesarman E. Gammaherpesviruses and lymphoproliferative disorders. *Annu Rev Pathol* 2014;9:349–372.
89. Shannon-Lowe C, Rowe M. Epstein-Barr virus infection of polarized epithelial cells via the basolateral surface by memory B cell-mediated transfer infection. *PLoS Pathog* 2011;7(5):e1001338.
90. Faulkner GC, Burrows SR, Khanna R, et al. X-Linked agammaglobulinemia patients are not infected with Epstein-Barr virus: implications for the biology of the virus. *J Virol* 1999;73(2):1555–1564.
91. Hjalgrim H, Smedby KE, Rostgaard K, et al. Infectious mononucleosis, childhood social environment, and risk of Hodgkin lymphoma. *Cancer Res* 2007;67(5):2382–2388.
92. Barton ES, White DW, Cathelyn JS, et al. Herpesvirus latency confers symbiotic protection from bacterial infection. *Nature* 2007;447(7142):326–329.
93. Giulino-Roth L, Cesarman E. Molecular biology of Burkitt lymphoma. In: Robertson E, ed. *Burkitt's Lymphoma*. New York, NY: Springer; 2013: 211–226.
94. Chang ET, Adami HO. The enigmatic epidemiology of nasopharyngeal carcinoma. *Cancer Epidemiol Biomarkers Prev* 2006;15(10):1765–1777.
95. Murukesan V, Mukherjee S. Managing post-transplant lymphoproliferative disorders in solid-organ transplant recipients: a review of immunosuppressant regimens. *Drugs* 2012;72(12):1631–1643.
96. Cohen JI, Mocarski ES, Raab-Traub N, et al. The need and challenges for development of an Epstein-Barr virus vaccine. *Vaccine* 2013;31(Suppl 2): B194–196.
97. Choquet S, Leblond V, Herbrecht R, et al. Efficacy and safety of rituximab in B-cell post-transplantation lymphoproliferative disorders: results of a prospective multicenter phase 2 study. *Blood* 2006;107(8):3053–3057.
98. Barnes JA, Lacasce AS, Feng Y, et al. Evaluation of the addition of rituximab to CODOX-M/IVAC for Burkitt's lymphoma: a retrospective analysis. *Ann Oncol* 2011;22(8):1859–1864.
99. Kaposi M. Idiopathisches multiples Pigmentsarkom der Haut. *Archiv für Dermatologie und Syphilis* 1872;4(2):265–273.
100. Antman K, Chang Y. Kaposi's sarcoma. *N Engl J Med* 2000;342(14):1027–1038.
101. Beral V, Peterman TA, Berkelman RL, et al. Kaposi's sarcoma among persons with AIDS: a sexually transmitted infection? *Lancet* 1990;335(8682):123–128.
102. Chang Y, Cesarman E, Pessin MS, et al. Identification of herpesvirus-like DNA sequences in AIDS-associated Kaposi's sarcoma. *Science* 1994;266(5192): 1865–1869.
103. Damania BA, Cesarman E. Kaposi's sarcoma-associated herpesvirus. In: Knipe DM, Howley PM, eds. *Fields Virology*. 6th ed. Philadelphia, PA: Lippincott Williams & Wilkins; 2013.
104. Cook-Mozaffari P, Newton R, Beral V, et al. The geographical distribution of Kaposi's sarcoma and of lymphomas in Africa before the AIDS epidemic. *Br J Cancer* 1998;78(11):1521–1528.
105. Martin DF, Kuppermann BD, Wolitz RA, et al. Oral ganciclovir for patients with cytomegalovirus retinitis treated with a ganciclovir implant. Roche Ganciclovir Study Group. *N Engl J Med* 1999;340(14):1063–1070.
106. Krown SE, Dittmer DP, Cesarman E. Pilot study of oral valganciclovir therapy in patients with classic Kaposi sarcoma. *J Infect Dis* 2011;203(8):1082–1086.
107. Sakakibara S, Tosato G. Regulation of angiogenesis in malignancies associated with Epstein-Barr virus and Kaposi's sarcoma-associated herpes virus. *Future Microbiol* 2009;4(7):903–917.
108. Soulier J, Grollet L, Oksenhendler E, et al. Kaposi's sarcoma-associated herpesvirus-like DNA sequences in multicentric Castleman's disease. *Blood* 1995;86(4):1276–1280.
109. Polizzotto MN, Uldrick TS, Wang V, et al. Human and viral interleukin-6 and other cytokines in Kaposi sarcoma herpesvirus-associated multicentric Castleman disease. *Blood* 2013;122(26):4189–4198.
110. Simonelli C, Spina M, Cinelli R, et al. Clinical features and outcome of primary effusion lymphoma in HIV-infected patients: a single-institution study. *J Clin Oncol* 2003;21(21):3948–3954.
111. Coffin JM, Hughes SH, Varmus HE, eds. The interactions of retroviruses and their hosts. *Retroviruses*. Cold Spring Harbor, NY: Cold Spring Harbor Laboratory Press; 1997.
112. Gallo RC. History of the discovery of the first human retroviruses: HTLV-1 and HTLV-2. *Oncogene* 2005;24:5926–5930.
113. Smit AF, Riggs AD. Tiggers and DNA transposon fossils in the human genome. *Proc Natl Acad Sci U S A* 1996;93:1443–1448.
114. Delviks-Frankenberry K, Paprotka T, Cingöz O, et al. Generation of multiple replication-competent retroviruses through recombination between PreXMRV-1 and PreXMRV-2. *J Virol* 2013;87:11525–11537.

115. Mason AL, Zhang G. Linking human beta retrovirus infection with primary biliary cirrhosis. *Gastroenterol Clin Biol* 2010;34:359–366.
116. Hacein-Bey-Abina S, VonKalle C, Schmidt M, et al. LMO2-associated clonal T cell proliferation in two patients after gene therapy for SCID-X1. *Science* 2003;302:415–419.
117. Matsuoka M, Jeang K-T. Human T-cell leukaemia virus type 1 (HTLV-1) infectivity and cellular transformation. *Nat Rev Cancer* 2007;7:270–280.
118. Poiesz BJ, Ruscetti FW, Mier JW, et al. T-cell lines established from human T-lymphocytic neoplasias by direct response to T-cell growth factor. *Proc Natl Acad Sci U S A* 1980;77:6815–6819.
119. Kalyanaraman VS, Sarngadharan MG, Robert-Guroff M, et al. A new subtype of human T-cell leukemia virus (HTLV-II) associated with a T-cell variant of hairy cell leukemia. *Science* 1982;218:571–573.
120. Wolfe ND, Heneine W, Carr JK, et al. Emergence of unique primate T-lymphotropic viruses among central African bushmeat hunters. *Proc Natl Acad Sci U S A* 2005;102:7994–7999.
121. Goncalves DU, Prioietti FA, Ribas JGR, et al. Epidemiology, treatment, and prevention of human T-cell leukemia virus type 1-associated diseases. *Clin Microbiol Rev* 2010;23:577–589.
122. Hino S, Sugiyama H, Doi H, et al. Breaking the cycle of HTLV-1 transmission via carrier mothers' milk. *Lancet Oncol* 1987;2:158–159.
123. Kannian P, Green PL. Human T lymphotropic virus type 1 (HTLV-1): molecular biology and oncogenesis. *Viruses* 2010;2:2037–2077.
124. Hill SA, Lloyd PA, McDonald S, et al. Susceptibility of human T cell leukemia virus type I to nucleoside reverse transcriptase inhibitors. *J Infec Dis* 2003;188:424–427.
125. Seegulam ME, Ratner L. Integrase inhibitors effective against human T-cell leukemia virus type 1. *Antimicrob Agents Chemother* 2011;55:2011–2017.
126. Derse D, Crise B, Li Y, et al. Human T-cell leukemia virus type 1 integration target sites in the human genome: comparison with those of other retroviruses. *J Virol* 2007;81:6731–6741.
127. Jones KS, Lambert S, Bouttieer M, et al. Molecular aspects of HTLV-1 entry: functional domains of the HTLV-1 surface subunit (SU) and their relationships to the entry receptors. *Viruses* 2011;3:794–810.
128. Matsuoka M, Green PL. The HBZ gene, a key player in HTLV-1 pathogenesis. *Retrovirology* 2009;6:71.
129. Grossman WJ, Kimata JT, Wong FH, et al. Development of leukemia in mice transgenic for the tax gene of human T-cell leukemia virus type I. *Proc Natl Acad Sci U S A* 1995;92:1057–1061.
130. El Hajj H, El-Sabban M, Hasegawa H, et al. Therapy-induced selective loss of leukemia-initiating activity in murine adult T cell leukemia. *J Exp Med* 2010;207:2785–2792.
131. Villaudy J, Wencker M, Gadot N, et al. HTLV-1 propels thymic human T cell development in "human immune system" Rag2-/-IL-2Rgammac-/- mice. *PLoS Pathog* 2011;7:e1002231.
132. Costa EAS, Magri MC, Caterino-de-Arujo A. The best algorithm to confirm the diagnosis of HTLV-1 and HTLV-2 in at-risk individuals from Sao Paulo, Brazil. *J Virol Methods* 2011;173:280–286.
133. Barros N, Woll F, Watanabe L, et al. Are increased Foxp3+ regulatory T cells responsible for immunosuppression during HTLV-1 infection? Case reports and review of the literature. *BMJ Case Rep* 2012;bcr2012006574.
134. Cook LB, Rowan AG, Melamed A, et al. HTLV-1-infected T cells contain a single integrated provirus in natural infection. *Blood* 2012;120:3488–3490.
135. Shimoyama M. Diagnostic criteria and classification of clinical subtypes of adult T-cell leukemia-lymphoma: a report from the Lymphoma Study Group. *Br J Hematol* 1991;79:426–437.
136. Takasaki Y, Iwanaga M, Imaizumi Y, et al. Long-term study of indolent adult T cell leukemia lymphoma. *Blood* 2010;115:4337–4343
137. Bazarbachi A, Plumelle Y, Ramos JC, et al. Meta-analysis on the use of zidovudine and interferon-alfa in adult T-cell leukemia/lymphoma showing improved survival in the leukemic subtypes. *J Clin Oncol* 2010;28:4177–4183.
138. Katsuya H, Yamanka T, Ishitsuka K, et al. Prognostic index for acute- and lymphoma-type adult T-cell leukemia/lymphoma. *J Clin Oncol* 2012;30:1635–1640.
139. Tsukasaki K, Hermine O, Bazarbachi A, et al. Definition, prognostic factors, treatment, and reponse criteria of adult T-cell leukemia-lymphoma: a proposal from an international consensus meeting. *J Clin Oncol* 2009;27:453–459.
140. Yamada Y, Tomonaga M, Fukuda H, et al. A new G-CSF supported combination chemotherapy, LSG15, for adult T-cell leukaemia-lymphoma: Japan Clinical Oncology Group Study 9303. *Br J Hematol* 2001;113:375–382.
141. Ratner L, Harrington W, Feng X, et al. Human T cell leukemia virus reactivation with progression of adult T-cell leukemia-lymphoma. AIDS Malignancy Consortium. *PLoS One* 2009;4:e4420.
142. Tatsuro J, Ishida T, Takemoto S, et al., eds. Randomized phase II study of mogamulizumab (KW-0761) plus VCAP-AMP-VECP (mLSG15) versus mLSG15 alone for newly diagnosed aggressive adult T-cell leukemia-lymphoma (ATL). Paper presented at: 2013 ASCO Annual Meeting; 2013; Chicago, IL.
143. Bazarbachi A, Suarez F, Fields P, et al. How I treat adult T-cell leukemia/lymphoma. *Blood* 2011;118:1736–1745.
144. Utsonomiya A, Miyazaki Y, Takasuka Y, et al. Improved outcome of adult T cell leukemia/lymphoma with allogeneic hematopoietic stem cell transplanation. *Bone Marrow Transplant* 2001;27:15–20.
145. Blumberg BS. The discovery of the hepatitis B virus and the intervention of the vaccine: a scientific memoir. *J Gastroenterol Hepatol* 2002;17(Supplement s4):S502–S503.
146. Houghton M. Discovery of the hepatitis C virus. *Liver Int* 2009;29(Supplement 1):82–88.
147. Arzumanyan A, Reis HM, Feitelson MA. Pathogenic mechanisms in HBV- and HCV-associated hepatocellular carcinoma. *Nat Rev Cancer* 2013;13:123–135.
148. Soerjomataram I, Lortet-Tieulent J, Parkin DM, et al. Global burden of cancer in 2008: a systematic analysis of disability-adjusted life-years in 12 world regions. *Lancet* 2012;380:1840–1850.
149. Altekruse SF, McGlynn KA, Reichman ME. Hepatocellular carcinoma incidence, mortality, and survival trends in the United States from 1975 to 2005. *J Clin Oncol* 2009;27:1485–1491.
150. Shiffman ML, ed. *Chronic Hepatitis C Virus: Advances in Treatment, Promise for the Future*. New York: Springer Verlag; 2011.
151. Nicot F, Nassim K, Lionel R, et al. Occult hepatitis C virus infection: Where are we now? *Liver Biopsy in Modern Med* 2004;307–334.
152. Freeman AJ, Dore GJ, Law MG, et al. Estimating progression to cirrhosis in chronic hepatitis C virus infection. *Hepatology* 2001;34:809–816.
153. Wilkins T, Malcom JK, Raina D, et al. Hepatitis C: diagnosis and treatment. *Am Fam Physician* 2010;81:1351–1357.
154. Fallot G, Neuveut C, Buendia M-A. Diverse roles of hepatitis B virus in liver cancer. *Curr Opin Virol* 2012;2:467–473.
155. Ganem D, Prince AM. Hepatitis B virus infection - natural history and clinical consequences. *N Engl J Med* 2004;350:1118–1129.
156. Tujios SR, Lee WM. Update in the management of chronic hepatitis B. *Curr Opin Gastroenterol* 2013;29:250–256.
157. Seto W-K, Fung J, Yuen M-F, et al. Future prevention and treatment of chronic hepatitis B infection. *J Clin Gastroenterol* 2012;46:725–734.
158. Wang WK, Levy S. Hepatitis C virus (HCV) and lymphomagenesis. *Leuk Lymphoma* 2003;44:1113–1120.
159. Fernandez-Garcia M-D, Mazzon M, Jacobs M, et al. Pathogenesis of flavivirus infections: using and abusing the host cell. *Cell Host Microbe* 2009;318: 318–328.
160. Moradpour D, Penin F, Rice CM. Replication of hepatitis c virus. *Nat Rev Microbiol* 2007;5:453–463.
161. Liang TJ, Ghany MG. Current and future therapies for hepatitis C virus infection. *N Engl J Med* 2013;368:1907–1917.
162. Kimer N, Dahl EK, Gluud LL, et al. Antiviral therapy for prevention of hepatocellular carcinoma in chronic hepatitis C: systematic review and meta-analysis of randomised controlled trials. *BMJ Open* 2012;2:e001313.
163. Fujimoto A, Totoki Y, Abe T, et al. Whole-genome sequencing of liver cancers identifies etiological influences on mutation patterns and recurrent mutations in chromatin regulators. *Nat Genet* 2012;44:760–764.
164. Sung WK, Zheng H, Li S, et al. Genome-wide survey of recurrent HBV integration in hepatocellular carcinoma. *Nat Genet* 2012;44:765–769.
165. Devi U, Locarnini S. Hepatitis B antivirals and resistance. *Curr Opin Virol* 2013;3:495–500.
166. Aghemo A, Colombo M. Hepatocellular carcinoma in chronic hepatitis C: from bench to bedside. *Semin Immunopathol* 2013;35:111–120.
167. Bruix J, Sherman M. Management of hepatocellular carcinoma: an update. *Hepatology* 2011;53:1020–1022.
168. Mazzaferro V, Regalia E, Doci R, et al. Liver transplantation for the treatment of small hepatocellular carcinomas in patients with cirrhosis. *N Engl J Med* 1996;334:693–699.
169. Mino M, Lauwers GY. Pathologic spectrum and prognostic significance of underlying liver disease in hepatocellular carcinoma. *Surg Oncol Clin N Am* 2003;12:13–24.
170. Burton JR, Everson GT. Management of the transplant recipient with chronic hepatitis C. *Clin Liver Dis* 2013;17:73–91.
171. Beckebaum S, Kabar I, Cicinnati VR. Hepatitis B and C in liver transplantation: new strategies to combat the enemies. *Rev Med Virol* 2012;23:172–193.
172. Torres HA, Davila M. Reactivation of hepatitis B virus and hepatitis C virus in patients with cancer. *Nat Rev Clin Oncol* 2012;9:156–166.
173. Huang Y-H, Hsaio L-T, Hong Y-C, et al. Randomized controlled trial of entecavir prophylaxis for rituximab-associated hepatitis B virus reactivation in patients with lymhoma and resolved hepatitis. *J Clin Oncol* 2013;31: 2765–2772.
174. Artz AS, Somerfield MR, Feld JJ, et al. American Society of Clinical Oncology provisional clinical opinion: chronic hepatitis B virus infection screening in patients receiving cytotoxic chemotherapy for treatment of malignant diseases. *J Clin Oncol* 2010;28:3199–3202.
175. Forghieri F, Luppi M, Barozzi P, et al. Pathogenetic mechanisms of hepatitis C virus-induced B-cell lymphomagenesis. *Clin Dev Immunol* 2012; 2012:807351.

6 Inflammation

Sahdeo Prasad and Bharat B. Aggarwal

INTRODUCTION

Extensive research over the last half a century indicates that inflammation plays an important role in cancer. Although acute inflammation can play a therapeutic role, low-level chronic inflammation can promote cancer. Different inflammatory cells, the various cell signaling pathways that lead to inflammation, and biomarkers of inflammation have now been well defined. These inflammatory pathways, which are primarily mediated through the transcription factors nuclear factor kappa B (NF-κB) and signal transducer and activator of transcription 3 (STAT3), have been linked to cellular transformation, tumor survival, proliferation, invasion, angiogenesis, and metastasis of cancer. These pathways have also now been linked with chemoresistance and radioresistance. This chapter considers the role of inflammation in cancer and its potential for cancer prevention and treatment.

Inflammation is the complex biologic responses of the body to irritation, injury, or infection. The recognition of inflammation dates back to antiquity. As documented by Aulus Cornelius Celsus, a Roman of the 1st century AD, inflammation is characterized by the tissue response to injury that results in *rubor* (redness, due to hyperemia), *tumor* (swelling, caused by increased permeability of the microvasculature and leakage of protein into the interstitial space), *calor* (heat, associated with increased blood flow and the metabolic activity of the cellular mediators of inflammation), and *dolor* (pain, in part due to changes in the perivasculature and associated nerve endings). Rudolf Virchow subsequently added *functio laesa* (dysfunction of the organs involved) in the 1850s. The process includes increased blood flow with an influx of white blood cells and other chemical substances that facilitate healing. Inflammation is also considered the body's self-protective attempt to remove harmful stimuli, including damaged cells, irritants, or pathogens, and to begin the healing process.

The word inflammation is derived from the Latin *inflammo* (meaning "I set alight, I ignite"). Because inflammation is a stereotyped response, it is considered a mechanism of innate immunity, as compared with adaptive immunity. On the basis of longevity, inflammation is classified as acute or chronic. When inflammation is short term, usually appearing within a few minutes or hours and ceasing upon the removal of the injurious stimulus, it is called acute. However, if it persists longer, it is called chronic inflammation, which leads to simultaneous destruction from the inflammatory process. Inflammation is beneficial when it is acute; however, chronic inflammation leads to several diseases, including cancer. Cancer is primarily a disease of lifestyle, with 30% of all cancers having been linked to smoking, 35% to diet, 14% to 20% to obesity, 18% to infection, and 7% to environmental pollution and radiation (Fig. 6.1).[1] Smoking, obesity, infections, pollution, and radiation are all known to activate proinflammatory pathways.[2] Therefore, understanding how inflammation contributes to cancer etiology is important for both cancer prevention and treatment.[3]

MOLECULAR BASIS OF INFLAMMATION

Although it is clear that inflammation and cancer are closely related, the mechanisms underlying persistent and chronic inflammation in chronic diseases remain unclear. Numerous cytokines have been linked with inflammation, including tumor necrosis factor (TNF), interleukin (IL)-1, IL-6, IL-8, IL-17, and vascular endothelial growth factor (VEGF). Among various cytokines that have been linked with inflammation, TNF is a primary mediator of inflammation linked to cancer.[4] However, it has been shown that proinflammatory transcriptional factors (activator protein [AP]-1, STAT3, NF-κB, hypoxia-inducible factor [HIF]-1, and β-catenin/Wnt) are ubiquitously expressed and control numerous physiologic processes, including development, differentiation, immunity, and metabolism in chronic diseases. Although these transcription factors are regulated by completely different signaling mechanisms, they are activated in response to various stimuli, including stresses and cytokines, and are involved in inflammation-induced tumor development and its metastasis.[5] Interestingly, inflammation plays a role at all stages of tumor development: initiation, progression, and metastasis.[2] In initiation, inflammation induces the release of a variety of cytokines and chemokines that promote the release of inflammatory cells and associated factors. This further causes oxidative damage, DNA mutations, and other changes in the tissue microenvironment, making it more conducive to cell transformation, increased survival, and proliferation. Inflammation also contributes to tissue injury, remodeling of the extracellular matrix, angiogenesis, and fibrosis in diverse target tissues. Among all the inflammatory cell signaling pathways, NF-κB has been shown to play a major role in cancer,[6,7] and TNF is one of the most potent activators of NF-κB.[8,9]

ROLE OF INFLAMMATION IN TRANSFORMATION

Transformation is the process by which the cellular and molecular makeup of a cell is altered as it becomes malignant. Numerous factors are involved in the process of cell transformation, including inflammation. A clinical study has shown that chronic inflammation due to heavy metal deposition in lymph nodes leads to malignant transformation and, finally, to patient death.[10] More recently, chronic exposure to cigarette smoke extract[11] and arsenite[12] has been shown to induce inflammation followed by epithelial–mesenchymal transition and transformation of human bronchial epithelial (HBE) cells. Furthermore, activation of NF-κB and HIF-2α increased the levels of the proinflammatory IL-6, IL-8, and IL-1β, which are essential for the malignant progression of transformed HBE cells. Sox2, another important molecular factor, cooperates with inflammation-mediated STAT3 activation, which precedes the malignant transformation of foregut basal progenitor cells.[13] A clinical study reported that the p53 mutation is a critical event for the malignant transformation of sinonasal inverted papilloma. This p53 mutation resulted in cyclooxygenase (COX)-2–mediated inflammatory signals that contribute to the proliferation

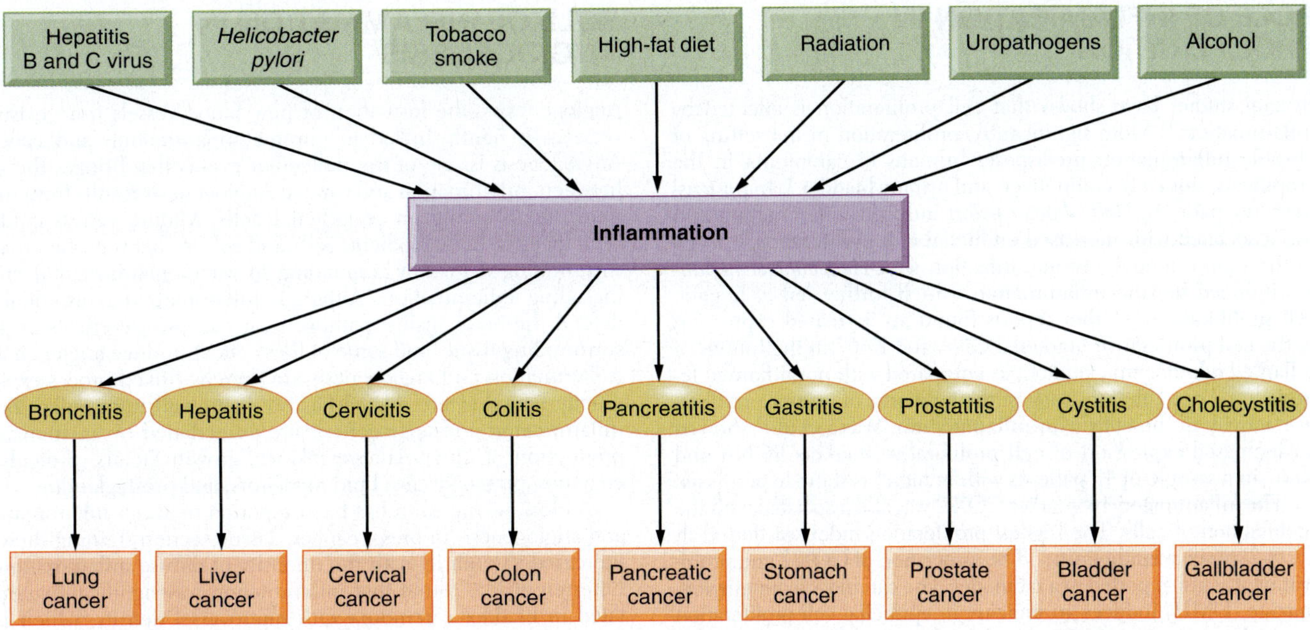

Figure 6.1 Origin of inflammation and its role in various cancers.

of advanced sinonasal inverted papilloma.[14] In another study in patients, the YKL-40 protein was found to be involved in chronic inflammation and oncogenic transformation of human breast tissues.[15] Inflammation-mediated transformation was also found to be regulated by MyD88 in a mouse model through Ras signaling.[16] In addition, inflammation contributed to the activation of the epidermal growth factor receptor (EGFR) and its subsequent interaction with PKCδ, which leads to the transformation of normal esophageal epithelia to squamous cell carcinoma.[17] Activation of Src oncoprotein triggers an inflammatory response mediated by NF-κB that directly activates Lin28 transcription and rapidly reduces let-7 microRNA levels. The inflammatory cytokine IL-6 mediates the activation of STAT3 transcription factor, which results in the transformation of cells.[18]

ROLE OF INFLAMMATION IN SURVIVAL

Numerous findings across different cancer populations have suggested that inflammation has an important role in carcinogenesis and disease progression.[19,20] The important markers of systemic inflammatory response in both in vitro findings and clinical outcomes include plasma C-reactive protein (CRP) concentration,[21,22] hypoalbuminemia,[23] and the Glasgow Prognostic Score (GPS), which combines CRP and albumin.[24,25] In addition to these, hematologic markers of systemic inflammatory response such as absolute white-cell count or its components (neutrophils, neutrophil-to-lymphocyte ratio [NLR]),[26–28] platelets, and a platelet-to-lymphocyte ratio[29,30] are also prognostic indicators for cancer clinical outcomes. Whether these inflammatory biomarkers influence the survival of cancer patients is discussed in this section.

In a study of 416 patients with renal cell carcinoma, with 362 patients included in the analysis, elevated neutrophil count, elevated platelet counts, and a high NLR were found. This inflammatory response was predictive for shorter overall patient survival.[31] Another study in unresectable malignant biliary obstruction (UMBO) found that patients with low GPS (0 and 1) had better postoperative survivals than did patients with a higher GPS. The 6-month and 1-year survival rates were 58.1% to 27.3%, respectively, for patients with low GPS and 25% to 6.2%, respectively, for patients with a higher GPS.[32] It has been also shown that prostate cancer patients with aggressive, clinically significant disease and an elevated GPS[2] had a higher risk of death overall as well as high-grade disease.[33] Other than GPS, age and gastrectomy have also been shown to independently influence the disease-specific and progression-free survival of gastric cancer patients.[34] A biomarker of systemic inflammation, the blood NLR, predicted patient survival with hepatocellular carcinoma (HCC) after transarterial chemoembolization. Patients in whom the NLR remained stable or became normalized after transarterial chemoembolization showed improved overall survival compared with patients showing a persistently abnormal index of NLR.[35]

A further study found that inflammatory transcription factors and cytokines contribute to the overall survival of patients. One study found that 97% of patients with epithelial tumors of malignant pleural mesothelioma and 95% of patients with nonepithelial tumors expressed IL-4Rα protein, and this strong IL-4Rα expression was correlated with a worse survival. In response to IL-4, human malignant pleural mesothelioma cells showed increased STAT6 phosphorylation and increased production of IL-6, IL-8, and VEGF without any effect on proliferation or apoptosis. This finding indicates that high expression of STAT6 as well as STAT3 and cytokines is inversely correlated with survival in patients.[36,37] NF-κB, along with IL-6, contributes to the survival of mammospheres in culture, because NF-κB and IL-6 were hyperactive in breast cancer–derived mammospheres.[38] In addition, elevated CRP and serum amyloid A (SAA) were associated with reduced disease-free survival of breast cancer patients.[39] In gastroesophageal cancer, proinflammatory cytokines IL-1β, IL-6, IL-8, and TNF-α and acute phase protein concentrations (CRP) were found to be elevated, and these levels were associated with reduced survival of patients.[40] Additionally, the Bcl-2 family protein COX-2, which is regulated by inflammatory transcription factors, is also involved in the survival of cancer cells.[41,42] Thus, we conclude that inflammation in general contributes to poor survival of patients.

In contrast to these findings, an in vivo study of dogs with osteosarcoma showed that survival improvement was apparent with inflammation or lymphocyte-infiltration scores >1, as well as in dogs that had apoptosis scores in the top 50th percentile.[43] Also, in patients with epithelioid malignant pleural mesothelioma, a high degree of chronic inflammatory cell infiltration in the stromal component was associated with improved overall survival.[44]

ROLE OF INFLAMMATION IN PROLIFERATION

Several studies have shown that cell proliferation is affected by inflammation.[45] More significantly, proliferation in the setting of chronic inflammation predisposes humans to carcinoma in the esophagus, stomach, colon, liver, and urinary bladder.[46] In postgastrectomy patients, *Helicobacter pylori* induced inflammation and was associated with increased epithelial cell proliferation.[47] Even in the mouse model, chronic infection with *Helicobacter hepaticus* induced hepatic inflammation, which further led to hepatic cell proliferation.[48] Other reports found an increased expression of the cell proliferative markers PCNA and Ki-67 in the linings of inflamed odontogenic keratocysts compared with noninflamed lesions.[49,50] These findings suggest the existence of greater proliferative activity in the cells with inflammation. Wang et al.[51] showed an increased expression of cell proliferative markers PCNA and Ki-67 in a sample of 45 patients with benign prostatic hyperplasia.

The inflammatory biomarker COX-2 was also associated with the proliferation of cells. The highest proliferation index was found in COX-2–positive epithelium.[51] The association of COX-2 and proliferation was also reported in a rat model. The carcinogen dimethylhydrazine (DMH) induces an increase in epithelial cell proliferation and in the expression of COX-2 in the colon of rats.[52] Erbb2, a kinase, regulates inflammation through the induction of NF-κB, Compl, IL-1β, COX-2, and multiple chemokines in the skin by ultraviolet (UV) exposure. This inflammation has been shown to increase the proliferation of skin tissue after UV irradiation.[53]

ROLE OF INFLAMMATION IN INVASION

A characteristic of invasive cancer cells is survival and growth under nonadhesive conditions. This invasion of cancer cells causes the disease to spread, which results in poor patient survival.[54] A strong relationship has been documented between inflammation and cancer cell invasion.[55,56] In a study of 150 patients with HCC, a high GPS score was associated with a high vascular invasion of cancer cells.[57] Another study of colorectal cancer also supports the links between inflammation and the invasion of cancer cells, with a finding that a high GPS increased the invasion of colorectal cancer cells.[58] In patients with esophageal squamous cell carcinoma, a high GPS score also showed a close relationship with lymphatic and venous invasion.[59]

At the molecular level, various proteins are known to be involved in tumor cell invasion. MMP-9, a gelatinase that degrades type IV collagen—the major structural protein component in the extracellular matrix and basement membrane—is thought to play an important role in facilitating tumor invasion, as it is highly expressed in various malignant tumors.[60,61] Additionally, the high expression of HIF-1α has been proposed as being associated with a greater incidence of vascular invasion of HCC. This expression of HIF-1α was further correlated with high expression of the inflammatory molecule COX-2.[62]

Breast cancer invasion has been linked to proteolytic activity at the tumor cell surface. In inflammatory breast cancer (IBC) cells, high expression of cathepsin B, a cell surface proteolytic enzyme, has been shown to be associated with invasiveness of IBC. In addition, a high coexpression of cathepsin B and caveolin-1 was found in IBC patient biopsies. Thus, proteolytic activity of cathepsin B and its coexpression with caveolin-1 contributes to the invasiveness of IBC.[63] In IBC, RhoC GTPase is also responsible for the invasive phenotype.[64] In addition, the PI3K/Akt signaling pathway is crucial in IBC invasion. The molecules involved in cell motility are specifically upregulated in IBC patients compared with stage-matched and cell-type-of-origin–matched non-IBCs patients. Distinctively, RhoC GTPase is a substrate for Akt1, and its phosphorylation is absolutely essential for IBC cell invasion.[65]

ROLE OF INFLAMMATION IN ANGIOGENESIS

Angiogenesis—the formation of new blood vessels from existing vessels—is tightly linked to chronic inflammation and cancer. Angiogenesis is one of the molecular events that bridges the gap between inflammation and cancer. Angiogenesis results from multiple signals acting on endothelial cells. Mature vessels control exchanges of hematopoietic cells and solutes between blood and surrounding tissues by responding to microenvironmental cues, including inflammation. Although inflammation is essential to defend the body against pathogens, it has adverse effects on the surrounding tissue, and some of these effects induce angiogenesis. Inflammation and angiogenesis are thereby linked processes, but exactly how they are related has not been well understood. Both inflammation and angiogenesis are exacerbated by an increased production of chemokines/cytokines, growth factors, proteolytic enzymes, proteoglycans, lipid mediators, and prostaglandins.

A close relationship has been reported between inflammation and angiogenesis in breast cancer. Tissue section staining showed increased vascularity with the intensity of diffuse inflammation.[66] Offersen et al.[67] found that inflammation was significantly correlated in bladder carcinoma with microvessel density, which is a marker of angiogenesis. Leukocytes have been described as mediators of inflammation-associated angiogenesis. In addition, the stable expression of TNF-α in endothelial cells increased angiogenic sprout formation independently of angiogenic growth factors. Furthermore, in work using the Matrigel plug assay in vivo, increased angiogenesis was observed in endothelial TNF-α–expressing mice. Thus, chronic inflammatory changes mediated by TNF-α can induce angiogenesis in vitro and in vivo, suggesting a direct link between inflammation and angiogenesis.[68] TNF-α–induced inhibitor of nuclear factor kappa kinase (IKK)-β activation also activates the angiogenic process. IKK-β activates the mammalian target of rapamycin (mTOR) pathway and enhances angiogenesis through VEGF production.[66] In addition to TNF-α, proinflammatory cytokines IL-1 (mainly IL-1β) and IL-8 were also found to be major proangiogenic stimuli of both physiologic and pathologic angiogenesis.[69,70] Recently, another cytokine macrophage migration inhibitory factor (MIF) was found to play a role in neoangiogenesis/vasculogenesis by endothelial cell activation along with inflammation.[71]

Benest et al.[72] found that a well-known regulator of angiogenesis, angiopoietin-2 (Ang-2), can upregulate inflammatory responses, indicating a common signaling pathway for inflammation and angiogenesis. TGF-β induction was also reported in head and neck epithelia and human head and neck squamous cell carcinomas (HNSCC), with severe inflammation that leads to angiogenesis.[73] The tumor-derived cytokine endothelial monocyte-activating polypeptide II (EMAP-II) has been shown to have profound effects on inflammation as well as on the processes involved in angiogenesis.[74] NF-κB plays an important role in inflammation as well as in angiogenesis, because the suppression of NF-κB and IkB-2A blocks basic fibroblast growth factor–induced angiogenesis in vivo. NF-κB regulates the angiogenic protein VEGF promoted by α5β1 integrin, which coordinately regulates angiogenesis and inflammation.[75] It has been also reported that a coculture of cancer cells with macrophages synergistically increased the production of various angiogenesis-related factors when stimulated by the inflammatory cytokine. This inflammatory angiogenesis was mediated by the activation of NF-κB and activator protein 1 (Jun/Fos), because the administration of either NF-κB–targeting drugs or COX-2 inhibitors or the depletion of macrophages blocked inflammatory angiogenesis.[76]

In a mouse model, cigarette smoke induced the inflammatory protein 5-lipoxygenase (5-LOX), and this induction activated matrix metalloproteinase 2 (MMP-2) and VEGF to induce the angiogenic process.[77] A cellular enzyme, Tank-binding kinase 1

(TBK-1), has been proposed as a putative mediator in tumor angiogenesis. TBK-1 mediates angiogenesis through the upregulation of VEGF and exerts proinflammatory effects via the induction of inflammatory cytokines. Thus, these pathways, including TBK-1, are an important cross-link between angiogenesis and inflammation.[78]

ROLE OF INFLAMMATION IN METASTASIS

Inflammation plays a regulatory role in cancer progression and metastasis. Chronic or tumor-derived inflammation and inflammation-related stimuli within the tumor microenvironment promote blood and lymphatic vessel formation and aid in invasion and metastasis.[79,80] The association of inflammation and metastasis has been observed in several cancer types. In an immunohistochemical analysis of lung cancer tissues, a remarkably high level of metastasis was observed with severe inflammation.[81] A mouse model of breast cancer found that mammary tumors increased the frequency of lung metastases, and this effect was associated with the recruitment of inflammatory cells to the lung as well as elevated levels of IL-6 in the lung airways.[82] In another murine model, implanting human ovarian tumor cells into the ovaries of severe combined immunodeficient mice resulted in peritoneal inflammation and tumor cell dissemination from the ovaries. In addition, enhancement of the inflammatory response with thioglycolate accelerated the development of ascites and metastases, and its suppression with acetylsalicylic acid delayed metastasis.[83] Thus, it can be concluded that inflammation facilitates ovarian tumor metastasis by a mechanism largely mediated by cytokines.

It has been shown that metastatic tumor cells entering a distant organ such as the liver trigger a proinflammatory response involving the Kupffer cell–mediated release of TNF-α and the upregulation of vascular endothelial cell adhesion receptors, such as E-selectin.[84] The physiologic expression of the selectins is tightly controlled to limit the inflammatory response, but dysregulated expression of selectins contributes to inflammatory and thrombotic disorders as well as tumor metastases.[85] Using P-selectin knockout mice, the importance of P-selectin–mediated cell adhesive interactions in the pathogenesis of inflammation and metastasis of cancers has been clearly demonstrated.[86]

Tumor-associated inflammatory monocytes and macrophages are essential promoters of tumor cell migration, invasion, and metastasis.[87] Macrophages and their mediators affect the multistep process of invasion and metastasis, from interaction with the extracellular matrix to the construction of a premetastatic niche. Monocytes are attracted by cytokines and chemokines (e.g., CSF-1, GM-CSF, and MCP 1), which are released by tumor cells or cells of the tumor microenvironment. These monocytes are then induced to express proangiogenic and metastatic factors, including VEGF, fibroblast growth factor (FGF)-2, platelet-derived growth factor (PDGF), intercellular adhesion molecule (ICAM)-1, vascular cell adhesion molecule (VCAM)-1, E-selectin, P- selectin, and MMP-9.[88] Versican, a large extracellular matrix proteoglycan, has been shown to activate tumor-infiltrating myeloid cells through Toll-like receptor (TLR) 2 and its coreceptors TLR6 and CD14 and to elicit the production of proinflammatory cytokines (including TNF-α), which enhance tumor metastasis. TLR2 increases the secretion of IL-8, which potentiates metastatic growth. Ligation of TLR2 by versican induces inflammatory cytokine secretion, providing a link between inflammation and cancer metastasis.[89]

IKK-α has been shown to be important in the inflammation-associated metastasis of cancer cells. Luo et al.[90] demonstrated that activation and nuclear localization of IKK-α by tumor-infiltrating immune cells in prostatic epithelial tumor cells leads to malignant prostatic epithelial cells with a metastatic fate. Src family kinases, when inappropriately activated, promote pathologic inflammatory processes and tumor metastasis, in part through their effects on the regulation of endothelial monolayer permeability.[91] Platelet-activating factor (PAF), an inflammatory biolipid, has also been shown to increase metastasis. In particular, Melnikova et al.[92] demonstrated that PAF receptor antagonists can effectively inhibit the metastatic potential of human melanoma cells in nude mice. Mesenchymal stem cells promote HCC metastasis under the influence of inflammation through TGF-β.[93]

EPIGENETIC CHANGES AND INFLAMMATION

Epigenetics considers the heritable changes in the activity of gene expression without the alteration of DNA sequences, and such changes have been linked to many human diseases, including cancer.[94] DNA methylation and histone modification are well-known epigenetic changes that can lead to gene activation or inactivation.[94–96] DNA methylation occurs primarily at cytosine-phosphate-guanine (CpG) dinucleotides as well as at transcriptional regulatory sites on the gene promoter.[96–98] Epigenetic abnormalities result in dysregulated gene expression and function, which can further lead to cancer. Inflammation and epigenetic abnormalities in cancer are highly associated. Inflammation induces aberrant epigenetic alterations in a tissue early in the process of carcinogenesis, and accumulation of such alterations forms an epigenetic field for cancer. Yara et al.[99] have shown that increased inflammation, as evidenced by the activation of NF-κB, production of IL-6 and COX-2, as well as the decrease of IκB, leads to the promoter's methylation. However, preincubation of cells with a demethylating agent prevented inflammation.

Infectious agents also contribute to inflammation-induced epigenetic changes. Infectious agents such as *H. pylori* and hepatitis C virus as well as intrinsic mediators of inflammatory responses, including proinflammatory cytokines, induce genetic and epigenetic changes, including point mutations, deletions, duplications, recombinations, and methylation of various tumor-related genes. Interestingly, disturbances in cytokine and chemokine signals and the induction of cell proliferation are important ways that inflammation induces aberrant DNA methylation. A study has shown that infection of human gastric mucosae with *H. pylori* induces chronic inflammation and further gastric cancers.[100] This inflammation is associated with high methylation levels or high incidences of methylation.[101–103]

Furthermore, numerous reports have documented the fact that inflammation is linked with epigenetic changes in carcinogenesis. Recently, Achyut[104] reported that inflammation in stromal fibroblasts caused epigenetic silencing of p21 and further tumor progression. Chronic inflammation also led to epigenetic regulation of p16 and activation of DNA damage in a lung carcinogenesis model.[105]

A transient inflammatory signal has been shown to initiate an epigenetic switch from nontransformed cells to cancer cells via a positive feedback loop involving NF-κB, Lin28, let-7, and IL-6. This IL-6 induced STAT3, directly activated miR-21 and miR-181b-1, and further induced the epigenetic switch. Thus, STAT3 underlies the epigenetic switch of mir-21 and mir-181b-1 that links inflammation to cancer.[106] Another report also showed that transient activation of Src oncoprotein mediates an epigenetic switch from immortalized breast cells to a stably transformed line that contained cancer stem cells. Thus, inflammation activates a positive feedback loop that maintains the epigenetic transformed state for many generations in the absence of the inducing signal.[18]

DNA hypermethylation at promoter CpG islands is an important mechanism by which carcinogenesis occurs through the inactivation of tumor-suppressor genes. Aberrant CpG island hypermethylation is also frequently observed in chronic inflammation and precancerous lesions, which again suggests links between inflammation and epigenetic change.[107] In addition, inflammation induced the halogenation of cytosine nucleotide. Damage products of this inflammation-mediated halogenated cytosine interfere with normal epigenetic control by altering DNA-protein interactions that are critical for gene regulation and the heritable transmission of methylation patterns. These inflammation-mediated cytosine damage products also provide a mechanistic link between inflammation and cancer.[108]

ROLE OF INFLAMMATION IN CANCER DIAGNOSIS

Chronic inflammation plays an important role in the etiology and progression of chronic diseases, including cancer. Hence, chronic inflammation may have an important diagnostic role in cancer. Inflammation induced by inflammatory cells such as infiltrating cells and mesothelial cells is mediated via the release of various mediators and proteins, including PDGF, IL-8, monocyte chemotactic peptide (MCP-1), nitric oxide (NO), collagen, antioxidant enzymes, and the plasminogen activation inhibitor (PAI). Furthermore, several inflammatory mediators have been shown to be detected at increased concentrations, thereby aiding in the disease diagnosis.[109]

In one study, numerous inflammatory disorders were detected based on inflammation measured in gastric biopsies of patients by Fourier transform infrared spectroscopy (FT-IR). Using endoscopic samples, gastritis and gastric cancer were diagnosed.[110] Furthermore, the degree of prostate inflammation has been used to determine the level of incidental prostatitis.[111] An assessment of the expression of cytokines and other immune stimulatory molecules that drive B-cell activation provides insight into the etiology of cancers. It has been shown that the dysregulation of cytokine production precedes the diagnosis of non-Hodgkin lymphoma.[112]

Inflammation parameters have been used to diagnose cancer in patients. Inflammation parameters, including CRP, were found to differ in patients with cancer and in those without. In clinical practice, however, such parameters are considered to have modest diagnostic value for cancer.[113] In a study with 1,275 patients, granulomatous inflammation was identified in 154 patients (12.1%), of whom 12 out of 154 (7.8%) had a concurrent diagnosis of cancer.[114] In another study with 173 patients, 52% had lung adenocarcinoma. Patients with high systemic inflammation were more likely to have more than two sites of metastatic disease and to have poor performance status and less likely to receive any chemotherapy. Systemic inflammation at diagnosis is considered to be an independent marker of poor outcome in patients with advanced non-small cell lung cancer (NSCLC).[115]

INFLAMMATION AND GENOMICS

Recently, the genomic landscape of the most common forms of human cancer have been examined.[116] Almost 140 genes and 12 cell signaling pathways have been linked with most cancers. Several of these genes and pathways are directly or indirectly linked with inflammation. A cytokine pattern in patients with cancer has been identified.[117]

INFLAMMATION AND TARGETED THERAPIES

That inflammation can be used as a target for cancer prevention and treatment is indicated by the fact that several drugs approved by the U.S. Food and Drug Administration (FDA) actually modulate proinflammatory pathways. For instance, EGFR, HER2, VEGF, CXCR4, and proteasome have been shown to activate NF-κB–mediated proinflammatory pathways, and their inhibitors have been approved by the FDA for the treatment of various cancers. Similarly, steroids such as dexamethasone, nonsteroidal anti-inflammatory drugs (NSAIDs), and statins that are currently used for prevention or treatment have also been found to suppress the NF-κB pathway. Thus, these observations indicate that inflammatory pathways are excellent targets for cancer.

CONCLUSIONS

According to Colditz et al.,[118] almost 50% of all cancers can be prevented based on what we know today. All the studies summarized previously suggest that inflammation is closely linked to cancer, and the incidence of most cancers can be reduced by controlling inflammation. Proinflammatory conditions such as colitis, bronchitis, hepatitis, and gastritis can all eventually lead to cancer. Thus, one must find ways to treat these conditions before the appearance of cancer. All these studies indicate that an anti-inflammatory lifestyle could play an important role in both the prevention and treatment of cancer.

REFERENCES

1. Anand P, Kunnumakkara AB, Sundaram C, et al. Cancer is a preventable disease that requires major lifestyle changes. *Pharm Res* 2008;25:2097–2116.
2. Aggarwal BB, Gehlot P. Inflammation and cancer: how friendly is the relationship for cancer patients? *Curr Opin Pharmacol* 2009;9:351–369.
3. Coussens LM, Zitvogel L, Palucka AK. Neutralizing tumor-promoting chronic inflammation: a magic bullet? *Science* 2013;339:286–291.
4. Sethi G, Sung B, Aggarwal BB. TNF: a master switch for inflammation to cancer. *Front Biosci* 2008;13:5094–5107.
5. Karin M. Nuclear factor-kappaB in cancer development and progression. *Nature* 2006;441:431–436.
6. Aggarwal BB. Nuclear factor-kappaB: the enemy within. *Cancer Cell* 2004; 6:203–208.
7. Chaturvedi MM, Sung B, Yadav VR, et al. NF-kappaB addiction and its role in cancer: 'one size does not fit all'. *Oncogene* 2011;30:1615–1630.
8. Aggarwal BB. Signalling pathways of the TNF superfamily: a double-edged sword. *Nat Rev Immunol* 2003;3:745–756.
9. Aggarwal BB, Gupta SC, Kim JH. Historical perspectives on tumor necrosis factor and its superfamily: 25 years later, a golden journey. *Blood* 2012; 119:651–665.
10. Iannitti T, Capone S, Gatti A, et al. Intracellular heavy metal nanoparticle storage: progressive accumulation within lymph nodes with transformation from chronic inflammation to malignancy. *Int J Nanomed* 2010;5:955–960.
11. Zhao Y, Xu Y, Li Y, et al. NF-kappaB-mediated inflammation leading to EMT via miR-200c is involved in cell transformation induced by cigarette smoke extract. *Toxicol Sci* 2013;135:265–276.
12. Xu Y, Zhao Y, Xu W, et al. Involvement of HIF-2alpha-mediated inflammation in arsenite-induced transformation of human bronchial epithelial cells. *Toxicol Appl Pharmacol* 2013;272:542–550.
13. Liu K, Jiang M, Lu Y, et al. Sox2 cooperates with inflammation-mediated Stat3 activation in the malignant transformation of foregut basal progenitor cells. *Cell Stem Cell* 2013;12:304–315.
14. Yoon BN, Chon KM, Hong SL, et al. Inflammation and apoptosis in malignant transformation of sinonasal inverted papilloma: the role of the bridge molecules, cyclooxygenase-2, and nuclear factor kappaB. *Am J Otolaryngol* 2013;34:22–30.
15. Roslind A, Johansen JS. YKL-40: a novel marker shared by chronic inflammation and oncogenic transformation. *Methods Mol Biol* 2009;511:159–184.
16. Coste I, Le Corf K, Kfoury A, et al. Dual function of MyD88 in RAS signaling and inflammation, leading to mouse and human cell transformation. *J Clin Invest* 2010;120:3663–3667.
17. Parthasarathy S, Dhayaparan D, Jayanthi V, et al. Aberrant expression of epidermal growth factor receptor and its interaction with protein kinase C delta in inflammation associated neoplastic transformation of human esophageal epithelium in high risk populations. *J Gastroenterol Hepatol* 2011;26:382–390.
18. Iliopoulos D, Hirsch HA, Struhl K. An epigenetic switch involving NF-kappaB, Lin28, Let-7 MicroRNA, and IL6 links inflammation to cell transformation. *Cell* 2009;139:693–706.
19. Colotta F, Allavena P, Sica A, et al. Cancer-related inflammation, the seventh hallmark of cancer: links to genetic instability. *Carcinogenesis* 2009;30: 1073–1081.
20. Hanahan D, Weinberg RA. Hallmarks of cancer: the next generation. *Cell* 2011;144:646–674.
21. Canna K, McMillan DC, McKee RF, et al. Evaluation of a cumulative prognostic score based on the systemic inflammatory response in patients undergoing potentially curative surgery for colorectal cancer. *Br J Cancer* 2004;90: 1707–1709.

22. Hilmy M, Bartlett JM, Underwood MA, et al. The relationship between the systemic inflammatory response and survival in patients with transitional cell carcinoma of the urinary bladder. *Br J Cancer* 2005;92:625–627.
23. Forrest LM, McMillan DC, McArdle CS, et al. Evaluation of cumulative prognostic scores based on the systemic inflammatory response in patients with inoperable non-small-cell lung cancer. *Br J Cancer* 2003;89:1028–1030.
24. Ramsey S, Lamb GW, Aitchison M, et al. Evaluation of an inflammation-based prognostic score in patients with metastatic renal cancer. *Cancer* 2007;109:205–212.
25. Crumley AB, Stuart RC, McKernan M, et al. Comparison of an inflammation-based prognostic score (GPS) with performance status (ECOG-ps) in patients receiving palliative chemotherapy for gastroesophageal cancer. *J Gastroenterol Hepatol* 2008;23:e325–329.
26. Yamanaka T, Matsumoto S, Teramukai S, et al. The baseline ratio of neutrophils to lymphocytes is associated with patient prognosis in advanced gastric cancer. *Oncology* 2007;73:215–220.
27. Halazun KJ, Aldoori A, Malik HZ, et al. Elevated preoperative neutrophil to lymphocyte ratio predicts survival following hepatic resection for colorectal liver metastases. *Eur J Surg Oncol* 2008;34:55–60.
28. Huang ZL, Luo J, Chen MS, et al. Blood neutrophil-to-lymphocyte ratio predicts survival in patients with unresectable hepatocellular carcinoma undergoing transarterial chemoembolization. *J Vasc Interv Radiol* 2011;22:702–709.
29. Heng DY, Xie W, Regan MM, et al. Prognostic factors for overall survival in patients with metastatic renal cell carcinoma treated with vascular endothelial growth factor-targeted agents: results from a large, multicenter study. *J Clin Oncol* 2009;27:5794–5799.
30. Smith RA, Bosonnet L, Raraty M, et al. Preoperative platelet-lymphocyte ratio is an independent significant prognostic marker in resected pancreatic ductal adenocarcinoma. *Am J Surg* 2009;197:466–472.
31. Fox P, Hudson M, Brown C, et al. Markers of systemic inflammation predict survival in patients with advanced renal cell cancer. *Br J Cancer* 2013; 109:147–153.
32. Iwasaki Y, Ishizuka M, Kato M, et al. Usefulness of an inflammation-based prognostic score (mGPS) for predicting survival in patients with unresectable malignant biliary obstruction. *World J Surg* 2013;37:2222–2228.
33. Shafique K, Proctor MJ, McMillan DC, et al. Systemic inflammation and survival of patients with prostate cancer: evidence from the Glasgow Inflammation Outcome Study. *Prostate Cancer Prostatic Dis* 2012;15:195–201.
34. Kunisaki C, Takahashi M, Ono HA, et al. Inflammation-based prognostic score predicts survival in patients with advanced gastric cancer receiving biweekly docetaxel and s-1 combination chemotherapy. *Oncology* 2012;83:183–191.
35. Pinato DJ, Sharma R. An inflammation-based prognostic index predicts survival advantage after transarterial chemoembolization in hepatocellular carcinoma. *Transl Res* 2012;160:146–152.
36. Burt BM, Bader A, Winter D, et al. Expression of interleukin-4 receptor alpha in human pleural mesothelioma is associated with poor survival and promotion of tumor inflammation. *Clin Cancer Res* 2012;18:1568–1577.
37. Sethi G, Shanmugam MK, Ramachandran L, et al. Multifaceted link between cancer and inflammation. *Biosci Rep* 2012;32:1–15.
38. Papi A, Guarnieri T, Storci G, et al. Nuclear receptors agonists exert opposing effects on the inflammation dependent survival of breast cancer stem cells. *Cell Death Differ* 2012;19:1208–1219.
39. Pierce BL, Ballard-Barbash R, Bernstein L, et al. Elevated biomarkers of inflammation are associated with reduced survival among breast cancer patients. *J Clin Oncol* 2009;27:3437–3444.
40. Deans DA, Wigmore SJ, Gilmour H, et al. Elevated tumour interleukin-1beta is associated with systemic inflammation: a marker of reduced survival in gastro-oesophageal cancer. *Br J Cancer* 2006;95:1568–1575.
41. Chen LS, Balakrishnan K, Gandhi V. Inflammation and survival pathways: chronic lymphocytic leukemia as a model system. *Biochem Pharmacol* 2010;80:1936–1945.
42. Sharma-Walia N, Paul AG, Bottero V, et al. Kaposi's sarcoma associated herpes virus (KSHV) induced COX-2: a key factor in latency, inflammation, angiogenesis, cell survival and invasion. *PLoS Pathog* 2010;6:e1000777.
43. Modiano JF, Bellgrau D, Cutter GR, et al. Inflammation, apoptosis, and necrosis induced by neoadjuvant fas ligand gene therapy improves survival of dogs with spontaneous bone cancer. *Mol Ther* 2012;20:2234–2243.
44. Suzuki K, Kadota K, Sima CS, et al. Chronic inflammation in tumor stroma is an independent predictor of prolonged survival in epithelioid malignant pleural mesothelioma patients. *Cancer Immunol Immunother* 2011;60:1721–1728.
45. Hu B, Elinav E, Flavell RA. Inflammasome-mediated suppression of inflammation-induced colorectal cancer progression is mediated by direct regulation of epithelial cell proliferation. *Cell Cycle* 2011;10:1936–1939.
46. Sugar LM. Inflammation and prostate cancer. *Can J Urol* 2006;13(Suppl 1):46–47.
47. Safatle-Ribeiro AV, Ribeiro U, Jr., Clarke MR, et al. Relationship between persistence of *Helicobacter pylori* and dysplasia, intestinal metaplasia, atrophy, inflammation, and cell proliferation following partial gastrectomy. *Dig Dis Sci* 1999;44:243–252.
48. Ihrig M, Schrenzel MD, Fox JG. Differential susceptibility to hepatic inflammation and proliferation in AXB recombinant inbred mice chronically infected with *Helicobacter hepaticus*. *Am J Pathol* 1999;155:571–582.
49. de Paula AM, Carvalhais JN, Domingues MG, et al. Cell proliferation markers in the odontogenic keratocyst: effect of inflammation. *J Oral Pathol Med* 2000;29:477–482.
50. Kaplan I, Hirshberg A. The correlation between epithelial cell proliferation and inflammation in odontogenic keratocyst. *Oral Oncol* 2004;40:985–991.
51. Wang W, Bergh A, Damber JE. Chronic inflammation in benign prostate hyperplasia is associated with focal upregulation of cyclooxygenase-2, Bcl-2, and cell proliferation in the glandular epithelium. *Prostate* 2004;61:60–72.
52. Demarzo MM, Martins LV, Fernandes CR, et al. Exercise reduces inflammation and cell proliferation in rat colon carcinogenesis. *Med Sci Sports Exerc* 2008;40:618–621.
53. Madson JG, Lynch DT, Tinkum KL, et al. Erbb2 regulates inflammation and proliferation in the skin after ultraviolet irradiation. *Am J Pathol* 2006; 169:1402–1414.
54. Bondong S, Kiefel H, Hielscher T, et al. Prognostic significance of L1CAM in ovarian cancer and its role in constitutive NF-kappaB activation. *Ann Oncol* 2012;23:1795–1802.
55. Wu Y, Zhou BP. Inflammation: a driving force speeds cancer metastasis. *Cell Cycle* 2009;8:3267–3273.
56. Aggarwal BB, Vijayalekshmi RV, Sung B. Targeting inflammatory pathways for prevention and therapy of cancer: short-term friend, long-term foe. *Clin Cancer Res* 2009;15:425–430.
57. Kinoshita A, Onoda H, Imai N, et al. The Glasgow Prognostic Score, an inflammation based prognostic score, predicts survival in patients with hepatocellular carcinoma. BMC *Cancer* 2013;13:52.
58. Toiyama Y, Miki C, Inoue Y, et al. Evaluation of an inflammation-based prognostic score for the identification of patients requiring postoperative adjuvant chemotherapy for stage II colorectal cancer. *Exp Ther Med* 2011;2:95–101.
59. Kobayashi T, Teruya M, Kishiki T, et al. Inflammation-based prognostic score, prior to neoadjuvant chemoradiotherapy, predicts postoperative outcome in patients with esophageal squamous cell carcinoma. *Surgery* 2008;144:729–735.
60. Nelson AR, Fingleton B, Rothenberg ML, et al. Matrix metalloproteinases: biologic activity and clinical implications. *J Clin Oncol* 2000;18:1135–1149.
61. Clark ES, Weaver AM. A new role for cortactin in invadopodia: regulation of protease secretion. *Eur J Cell Biol* 2008;87:581–590.
62. Dai CX, Gao Q, Qiu SJ, et al. Hypoxia-inducible factor-1 alpha, in association with inflammation, angiogenesis and MYC, is a critical prognostic factor in patients with HCC after surgery. *BMC Cancer* 2009;9:418.
63. Victor BC, Anbalagan A, Mohamed MM, et al. Inhibition of cathepsin B activity attenuates extracellular matrix degradation and inflammatory breast cancer invasion. *Breast Cancer Res* 2011;13:R115.
64. van Golen KL, Bao LW, Pan Q, et al. Mitogen activated protein kinase pathway is involved in RhoC GTPase induced motility, invasion and angiogenesis in inflammatory breast cancer. *Clin Exp Metastasis* 2002;19:301–311.
65. Lehman HL, Van Laere SJ, van Golen CM, et al. Regulation of inflammatory breast cancer cell invasion through Akt1/PKBalpha phosphorylation of RhoC GTPase. *Mol Cancer Res* 2012;10:1306–1318.
66. Lee DF, Kuo HP, Chen CT, et al. IKK beta suppression of TSC1 links inflammation and tumor angiogenesis via the mTOR pathway. *Cell* 2007;130: 440–455.
67. Offersen BV, Knap MM, Marcussen N, et al. Intense inflammation in bladder carcinoma is associated with angiogenesis and indicates good prognosis. *Br J Cancer* 2002;87:1422–1430.
68. Rajashekhar G, Willuweit A, Patterson CE, et al. Continuous endothelial cell activation increases angiogenesis: evidence for the direct role of endothelium linking angiogenesis and inflammation. *J Vasc Res* 2006;43:193–204.
69. Voronov E, Carmi Y, Apte RN. Role of IL-1-mediated inflammation in tumor angiogenesis. *Adv Exp Med Biol* 2007;601:265–270.
70. Qazi BS, Tang K, Qazi A. Recent advances in underlying pathologies provide insight into interleukin-8 expression-mediated inflammation and angiogenesis. *Int J Inflam* 2011;2011:908468.
71. Asare Y, Schmitt M, Bernhagen J. The vascular biology of macrophage migration inhibitory factor (MIF). Expression and effects in inflammation, atherogenesis and angiogenesis. *Thromb Haemost* 2013;109:391–398.
72. Benest AV, Kruse K, Savant S, et al. Angiopoietin-2 is critical for cytokine-induced vascular leakage. *PLoS One* 2013;8: e70459.
73. Lu SL, Reh D, Li AG, et al. Overexpression of transforming growth factor beta1 in head and neck epithelia results in inflammation, angiogenesis, and epithelial hyperproliferation. *Cancer Res* 2004;64:4405–4410.
74. Berger AC, Tang G, Alexander HR, et al. Endothelial monocyte-activating polypeptide II, a tumor-derived cytokine that plays an important role in inflammation, apoptosis, and angiogenesis. *J Immunother* 2000;23:519–527.
75. Klein S, de Fougerolles AR, Blaikie P, et al. Alpha 5 beta 1 integrin activates an NF-kappa B-dependent program of gene expression important for angiogenesis and inflammation. *Mol Cell Biol* 2002;22:5912–5922.
76. Ono M. Molecular links between tumor angiogenesis and inflammation: inflammatory stimuli of macrophages and cancer cells as targets for therapeutic strategy. *Cancer Sci* 2008;99:1501–1506.
77. Ye YN, Liu ES, Shin VY, et al. Contributory role of 5-lipoxygenase and its association with angiogenesis in the promotion of inflammation-associated colonic tumorigenesis by cigarette smoking. *Toxicology* 2004;203:179–188.
78. Czabanka M, Korherr C, Brinkmann U, et al. Influence of TBK-1 on tumor angiogenesis and microvascular inflammation. *Front Biosci* 2008;13: 7243–7249.
79. Solinas G, Marchesi F, Garlanda C, et al. Inflammation-mediated promotion of invasion and metastasis. *Cancer Metastasis Rev* 2010;29:243–248.
80. Affara NI, Coussens LM. IKKalpha at the crossroads of inflammation and metastasis. *Cell* 2007;129:25–26.
81. Kayser K, Bulzebruck H, Ebert W, et al. Local tumor inflammation, lymph node metastasis, and survival of operated bronchus carcinoma patients. *J Natl Cancer Inst* 1986;77:77–81.

82. Hobson J, Gummadidala P, Silverstrim B, et al. Acute inflammation induced by the biopsy of mouse mammary tumors promotes the development of metastasis. *Breast Cancer Res Treat* 2013;139:391–401.
83. Robinson-Smith TM, Isaacsohn I, Mercer CA, et al. Macrophages mediate inflammation-enhanced metastasis of ovarian tumors in mice. *Cancer Res* 2007;67:5708–5716.
84. Khatib AM, Auguste P, Fallavollita L, et al. Characterization of the host proinflammatory response to tumor cells during the initial stages of liver metastasis. *Am J Pathol* 2005;167:749–759.
85. McEver RP. Selectin-carbohydrate interactions during inflammation and metastasis. *Glycoconj J* 1997;14:585–591.
86. Geng JG, Chen M, Chou KC. P-selectin cell adhesion molecule in inflammation, thrombosis, cancer growth and metastasis. *Curr Med Chem* 2004; 11:2153–2160.
87. Condeelis J, Pollard JW. Macrophages: obligate partners for tumor cell migration, invasion, and metastasis. *Cell* 2006;124:263–266.
88. Siegel G, Malmsten M. The role of the endothelium in inflammation and tumor metastasis. *Int J Microcirc Clin Exp* 1997;17:257–272.
89. Wang W, Xu GL, Jia WD, et al. Ligation of TLR2 by versican: a link between inflammation and metastasis. *Arch Med Res* 2009;40:321–323.
90. Luo JL, Tan W, Ricono JM, et al. Nuclear cytokine-activated IKKalpha controls prostate cancer metastasis by repressing Maspin. *Nature* 2007;446:690–694.
91. Kim MP, Park SI, Kopetz S, et al. Src family kinases as mediators of endothelial permeability: effects on inflammation and metastasis. *Cell Tissue Res* 2009;335:249–259.
92. Melnikova V, Bar-Eli M. Inflammation and melanoma growth and metastasis: the role of platelet-activating factor (PAF) and its receptor. *Cancer Metastasis Rev* 2007;26:359–371.
93. Jing Y, Han Z, Liu Y, et al. Mesenchymal stem cells in inflammation microenvironment accelerates hepatocellular carcinoma metastasis by inducing epithelial-mesenchymal transition. *PLoS One* 2012;7:e43272.
94. Jones PA, Baylin SB. The epigenomics of cancer. *Cell* 2007;128:683–692.
95. Esteller M. Aberrant DNA methylation as a cancer-inducing mechanism. *Annu Rev Pharmacol Toxicol* 2005;45:629–656.
96. Thiagalingam S, Cheng KH, Lee HJ, et al. Histone deacetylases: unique players in shaping the epigenetic histone code. *Ann N Y Acad Sci* 2003; 983:84–100.
97. Li E, Beard C, Jaenisch R. Role for DNA methylation in genomic imprinting. *Nature* 1993;366:362–365.
98. Antequera F, Bird A. Number of CpG islands and genes in human and mouse. *Proc Natl Acad Sci U S A* 1993;90:11995–11999.
99. Yara S, Lavoie JC, Beaulieu JF, et al. Iron-ascorbate-mediated lipid peroxidation causes epigenetic changes in the antioxidant defense in intestinal epithelial cells: impact on inflammation. *PLoS One* 2013;8:e63456.
100. Uemura N, Okamoto S, Yamamoto S, et al. Helicobacter pylori infection and the development of gastric cancer. *N Engl J Med* 2001;345:784–789.
101. Maekita T, Nakazawa K, Mihara M, et al. High levels of aberrant DNA methylation in Helicobacter pylori-infected gastric mucosae and its possible association with gastric cancer risk. *Clin Cancer Res* 2006;12:989–995.
102. Nakajima T, Maekita T, Oda I, et al. Higher methylation levels in gastric mucosae significantly correlate with higher risk of gastric cancers. *Cancer Epidemiol Biomarkers Prev* 2006;15:2317–2321.
103. Perri F, Cotugno R, Piepoli A, et al. Aberrant DNA methylation in non-neoplastic gastric mucosa of H. Pylori infected patients and effect of eradication. *Am J Gastroenterol* 2007;102:1361–1371.
104. Achyut BR, Bader DA, Robles AI, et al. Inflammation-mediated genetic and epigenetic alterations drive cancer development in the neighboring epithelium upon stromal abrogation of TGF-beta signaling. *PLoS Genet* 2013;9:e1003251.
105. Blanco D, Vicent S, Fraga MF, et al. Molecular analysis of a multistep lung cancer model induced by chronic inflammation reveals epigenetic regulation of p16 and activation of the DNA damage response pathway. *Neoplasia* 2007;9:840–852.
106. Iliopoulos D, Jaeger SA, Hirsch HA, et al. STAT3 activation of miR-21 and miR-181b-1 via PTEN and CYLD are part of the epigenetic switch linking inflammation to cancer. *Mol Cell* 2010;39:493–506.
107. Suzuki H, Toyota M, Kondo Y, et al. Inflammation-related aberrant patterns of DNA methylation: detection and role in epigenetic deregulation of cancer cell transcriptome. *Methods Mol Biol* 2009;512:55–69.
108. Valinluck V, Sowers LC. Inflammation-mediated cytosine damage: a mechanistic link between inflammation and the epigenetic alterations in human cancers. *Cancer Res* 2007;67:5583–5586.
109. Kroegel C, Antony VB. Immunobiology of pleural inflammation: potential implications for pathogenesis, diagnosis and therapy. *Eur Respir J* 1997; 10:2411–2418.
110. Li QB, Sun XJ, Xu YZ, et al. Use of Fourier-transform infrared spectroscopy to rapidly diagnose gastric endoscopic biopsies. *World J Gastroenterol* 2005;11:3842–3845.
111. Difuccia B, Keith I, Teunissen B, et al. Diagnosis of prostatic inflammation: efficacy of needle biopsies versus tissue blocks. *Urology* 2005;65:445–448.
112. Vendrame E, Martinez-Maza O. Assessment of pre-diagnosis biomarkers of immune activation and inflammation: insights on the etiology of lymphoma. *J Proteome Res* 2011;10:113–119.
113. Baicus C, Caraiola S, Rimbas M, et al. Utility of routine hematological and inflammation parameters for the diagnosis of cancer in involuntary weight loss. *J Investig Med* 2011;59:951–955.
114. DePew ZS, Gonsalves WI, Roden AC, et al. Granulomatous inflammation detected by endobronchial ultrasound-guided transbronchial needle aspiration in patients with a concurrent diagnosis of cancer: a clinical conundrum. *J Bronchology Interv Pulmonol* 2012;19:176–181.
115. Jafri SH, Shi R, Mills G. Advance lung cancer inflammation index (ALI) at diagnosis is a prognostic marker in patients with metastatic non-small cell lung cancer (NSCLC): a retrospective review. *BMC Cancer* 2013;13:158.
116. Vogelstein B, Papadopoulos N, Velculescu VE, et al. Cancer genome landscapes. *Science* 2013;339:1546–1558.
117. Lippitz BE. Cytokine patterns in patients with cancer: a systematic review. *Lancet Oncol* 2013;14:e218–228.
118. Colditz GA, Wolin KY, Gehlert S. Applying what we know to accelerate cancer prevention. *Sci Transl Med* 2012;4(127):127rv4.

7 Chemical Factors

Stuart H. Yuspa and Peter G. Shields

INTRODUCTION

As early as the 1800s, initial observations of unusual cancer incidences in occupational groups provided the first indications that chemicals were a cause of human cancer, which was then confirmed in experimental animal studies during the early and mid 1900s. However, the extent to which chemical exposures contribute to cancer incidence was not fully appreciated until population-based studies documented differing organ-specific cancer rates in geographically distinct populations and in cohort studies such as those that linked smoking to lung cancer.[1] The most commonly occurring chemical exposures that increase cancer risk are tobacco, alcoholic beverages, diet, and reproductive factors (e.g., hormones). Today, it is recognized that cancer results not solely from chemical exposure (e.g., in the workplace or at home), but that a variety of biologic, social, and physical factors contribute to cancer pathogenesis.[2,3] For some common cancers, it also has been recognized that heritable factors also contribute to cancer risk from chemical exposure (e.g., genes involved in carcinogen metabolism, DNA repair, a variety of cancer pathways).[4] Twin studies show that for common cancers, nongenetic risk factors are dominant, and the best associations for genetic risks of sporadic cancers indicate that the risks for specific genetic traits are typically less than 1.5-fold.[5–7] The role of the tumor microenvironment, the cancer stem cells, and feedback signaling to and from the tumor also have been recently recognized as important contributors to carcinogenesis, although how chemicals affect these have yet been clearly demonstrated.[8–10]

The experimental induction of tumors in animals, the neoplastic transformation of cultured cells by chemicals, and the molecular analysis of human tumors have revealed important concepts regarding the pathogenesis of cancer and how laboratory studies can be used to better understand human cancer pathogenesis.[7,11,12] Chemical carcinogens usually affect specific organs, targeting the epithelial cells (or other susceptible cells within an organ) and causing genetic damage (genotoxic) or epigenetic effects regulating DNA transcription and translation. Chemically related DNA damage and consequent somatic mutations relevant to human cancer can occur either directly from exogenous exposures or indirectly by activation of endogenous mutagenic pathways (e.g., nitric oxide, oxyradicals).[13,14] The risk of developing a chemically induced tumor may be modified by nongenotoxic exogenous and endogenous exposures and factors (e.g., hormones, immunosuppression triggered by the tumor), and by accumulated exposure to the same or different genotoxic carcinogens.[7,15]

Analyses of how chemicals induce cancer in animal models and human populations has had a major impact on human health. Experimental studies have been instrumental in replicating hypotheses generated from human studies and identifying pathobiologic mechanisms. For example, animal experiments confirmed the carcinogenic and cocarcinogenic properties of cigarette smoke and identified bioactive chemical and gaseous components.[1] The transplacental carcinogenicity of diethylstilbestrol and the hazards of specific occupational carcinogens such as vinyl chloride, benzene, aromatic amines, and bis(chloromethyl)ether led to a reduction in allowable exposures of suspected human carcinogens from the workplace and a reduction in cancer rates. Dietary factors that enhance or inhibit cancer development and the contribution of obesity to specific organ sites have been identified in models of chemical carcinogenesis, and alterations in diet and obesity are expected to result in reduced cancer risk. Experimental animal studies are the mainstay of risk assessment as a screening tool to identify potential carcinogens in the workplace and the environment, although these studies do not prove specific chemical etiologies as a cause of human cancer because of interspecies differences and the use of maximally tolerated doses that do not replicate human exposure.

THE NATURE OF CHEMICAL CARCINOGENS: CHEMISTRY AND METABOLISM

The National Toxicology Program, based mostly on experimental animal studies and supported by epidemiology studies when available, lists 45 chemical, physical, and infectious agents as known human carcinogens and about 175 that are reasonably anticipated to be human carcinogens (http://ntp.niehs.nih.gov/?objectid=035E57E7-BDD9-2D9B-AFB9D1CADC8D09C1), whereas the International Agency for Research on Cancer (IARC) lists 113 agents as carcinogenic to humans and 66 that are probably carcinogenic to humans (http://monographs.iarc.fr/ENG/Classification/index.php). Table 7.1 provides a selected list of known human carcinogens, as indicated by the IARC, which are continuously updated.[16] Most chemical carcinogens first undergo metabolic activation by cytochrome P450s or other metabolic pathways so that they react with DNA and/or alter epigenetic mechanisms.[11,17] This process, evolutionarily presumed to have been developed to rid the body of foreign chemicals for excretion, inadvertently generates reactive carcinogenic intermediates that can bind cellular molecules, including DNA, and cause mutations or other alterations.[18] Recent data indicate that metabolizing enzymes also have the ability to cross-talk with transcription factors involved in the regulation of other metabolizing and antioxidant enzymes.[19] DNA is considered the ultimate target for most carcinogens to cause either mutations or gross chromosomal changes, but epigenetic effects, such as altered DNA methylation and gene transcription, also promote carcinogenesis.[20] The formation of DNA adducts, where chemicals bind directly to DNA to promote mutations, is likely necessary but not sufficient to cause cancer.

Genotoxic carcinogens may transfer simple alkyl or complexed (aryl) alkyl groups to specific sites on DNA bases.[18,21] These alkylating and aryl-alkylating agents include, but are not limited to, N-nitroso compounds, aliphatic epoxides, aflatoxins, mustards, polycyclic aromatic hydrocarbons, and other combustion products of fossil fuels and vegetable matter. Others transfer arylamine residues to DNA, as exemplified by aryl aromatic

TABLE 7.1

Known Chemical Carcinogens in Humans[a]

Target Organ	Agents	Industries	Tumor Type
Lung	Tobacco smoke, arsenic, asbestos, crystalline silica, benzo(a)pyrene, beryllium, bis(chloro)methyl ether, 1,3-butadiene, chromium VI compounds, coal tar and pitch, diesel exhaust, nickel compounds, soot, mustard gas, cobalt-tungsten carbide powders	Aluminum production, coal gasification, coke production, painting, hematite mining, painting, grinding in oil and gas	Squamous, large cell, and small cell cancer and adenocarcinoma
Pleura	Asbestos, erionite, painting	Insulation, mining	Mesothelioma
Oral cavity	Tobacco smoke, alcoholic beverages, nickel compounds, betel quid	–	Squamous cell cancer
Esophagus	Tobacco smoke, alcoholic beverages, betel quid	–	Squamous cell cancer
Gastric	Tobacco smoking	Rubber industry	Adenocarcinoma
Colon	Alcohol, tobacco smoking	–	Adenocarcinoma
Liver	Aflatoxin, vinyl chloride, tobacco smoke, alcoholic beverages	–	Hepatocellular carcinoma, hemangiosarcoma
Kidney	Tobacco smoke, trichloroethylene	–	Renal cell cancer
Bladder	Tobacco smoke, 4-aminobiphenyl, benzidine, 2-napthylamine, cyclophosphamide, phenacetin	Magenta manufacturing, auramine manufacturing, painting, rubber production	Transitional cell cancer
Prostate	Cadmium	–	Adenocarcinoma
Skin	Arsenic, benzo(a)pyrene, coal tar and pitch, mineral oils, soot, cyclosporin A, azathioprine, shale oils	–	Squamous cell cancer, basal cell cancer
Bone marrow	Benzene, tobacco smoke, ethylene oxide, antineoplastic agents, cyclosporin A, formaldehyde	Rubber workers	Leukemia, lymphoma

[a] The carcinogen designations are determined by the International Agency for Research on Cancer (http://monographs.iarc.fr/index.php). They do not imply proof of carcinogenicity in individuals. This table is not all inclusive. For additional information, the reader is referred to agency documents and publications.

amines, aminoazo dyes, and heterocyclic aromatic amines. For genotoxic carcinogens, the interaction with DNA is not random, and each class of agents reacts selectively with purine and pyrimidine targets.[7,18,21] Furthermore, targeting carcinogens to particular sites in DNA is determined by nucleotide sequence, by host cell, and by selective DNA repair processes (see later discussion), making some genetic material at risk over others. As expected from this chemistry, genotoxic carcinogens can be potent mutagens and particularly adept at causing nucleotide base mispairing or small deletions, leading to missense or nonsense mutations. Others may cause macrogenetic damage, such as chromosome breaks and large deletions. In some cases, such genotoxic damage may result in changes in transcription and translation that affect protein levels or function, which in turn alter the behavior of the specific host cell type. For example, there may be effects on cell proliferation, programmed cell death, or DNA repair. This is best typified by the signature mutations detected in the p53 gene caused by ingested aflatoxin in human liver cancer[22] and by polycyclic aromatic hydrocarbons human lung cancer caused by the inhalation of cigarette smoke.[15,23,24] Similarly, a distinct pattern of mutations is detected in pancreatic cancers from smokers when compared with pancreatic cancers from nonsmokers.[25]

Some chemicals that cause cancers in laboratory rodents are not demonstrably genotoxic. In general, these agents are carcinogenic in laboratory animals at high doses and require prolonged exposure. Synthetic pesticides and herbicides fall within this group, as do a number of natural products that are ingested. The mechanism of action by nongenotoxic carcinogens is not well understood, and may be related in some cases to toxic cell death and regenerative hyperplasia. They may also induce endogenous mutagenic mechanisms through the production of free radicals, increasing rates of depurination, and the deamination of 5-methylcytosine. In other cases, nongenotoxic carcinogens may have hormonal effects on hormone-dependent tissues. For example, some pesticides, herbicides, and fungicides have endocrine-disrupting properties in experimental models, although the relation to human cancer risk is unknown.

ANIMAL MODEL SYSTEMS AND CHEMICAL CARCINOGENESIS

Most human chemical carcinogens can induce tumors in experimental animals; however, the tumors may not be in the same organ, the exposure pathways may differ from human exposure, and the causative mechanisms may not exist in humans. In many cases, however, the cell of origin, morphogenesis, phenotypic markers, and genetic alterations are qualitatively identical to corresponding human cancers. Furthermore, animal models have revealed the constancy of carcinogen–host interaction among mammalian species by reproducing organ-specific cancers in animals with chemicals identified as human carcinogens, such as coal tar and squamous cell carcinomas, vinyl chloride and hepatic angiosarcomas, aflatoxin and hepatocellular carcinoma, and aromatic amines and bladder cancer. The introduction of genetically modified mice designed to reproduce specific human cancer syndromes and precancer models has accelerated both the understanding of the contributions of chemicals to cancer causation and the identification of potential exogenous carcinogens.[26,27] Furthermore, construction of mouse strains genetically altered to express human drug–metabolizing enzymes has added both to the relevance of mouse studies for understanding human carcinogen metabolism and the prediction of genotoxicity from suspected human carcinogens and other chemical exposures.[28] Together, these studies have indicated that carcinogenic agents can directly activate oncogenes, inactivate tumor suppressor genes, and cause the genomic changes that are associated with autonomous growth, enhanced survival, and modified gene expression profiles that are required for the malignant phenotype.[29]

Genetic Susceptibility to Chemical Carcinogenesis in Experimental Animal Models

The use of inbred strains of rodents and spontaneous or genetically modified mutant strains have led to the identification and characterization of genes that modify risks for cancer development.[30–32] For a variety of tissue sites, including the lungs, the liver, the breast, and the skin, pairs of inbred mice can differ by 100-fold in the risk for tumor development after carcinogen exposure. Genetically determined differences in the affinity for the aryl hydrocarbon hydroxylase (Ah) receptor or other differences in metabolic processing of carcinogens is one modifier that has a major impact on experimental and presumed human cancer risk.[33–35] The development of mice reconstituted with components of the human carcinogen–metabolizing genome should facilitate the extrapolation of metabolic activity by human enzymes and cancer risk.[27,28,36] Such mice also show that other loci regulate the growth of premalignant foci, the response to tumor promoters, the immune response to metastatic cells, and the basal proliferation rate of target cells.[30] In mice susceptible to colon cancer due to a carcinogen-induced constitutive mutation in the APC gene, a locus on mouse chromosome 4 confers resistance to colon cancer.[31] The identification of the phospholipase A2 gene at this locus and subsequent functional testing in transgenic mice revealed an interesting paracrine protective influence on tumor development.[31] This gene, and several other genes mapped for susceptibility to chemically induced mouse tumors (PTPRJ, a receptor type tyrosine phosphatase, and STK6/STK15, an aurora kinase), have now been shown to influence susceptibility to organ-specific cancer induction in humans.[30,31]

MOLECULAR EPIDEMIOLOGY, CHEMICAL CARCINOGENESIS, AND CANCER RISK IN HUMAN POPULATIONS

Molecular epidemiology is the application of biologically based hypotheses using molecular and epidemiologic methods and measures. New technologies continue to allow epidemiologic studies to improve the testing of biologically based hypotheses and to develop large datasets for hypothesis generation, most notably the application of various *–omics* technologies via next-generation sequencing (e.g., genomics, epigenomics, transcriptomics), proteomics, and metabolomics. The greatest challenge now is to develop methods that allow for analysis cutting across various technologies.[37–43] Recent advances now include the role of microRNA and long noncoding RNAs in tumor development and progression because of their impact on the regulation of gene expression.[44,45] Chemical effects on microRNAs and the resultant gene expression is currently being identified.[46] Using such technologies, emerging evidence is noting the importance of the microbiome and associated infections as a risk of human cancer.[47–50] The complexity of environmental exposure and how it interacts with humans to affect numerous biologic pathways has been characterized as the exposome, also expressed as a multidimensional complex dataset.[51] Therefore, the important goal remains: to characterize cancer risk based on gene–environment interactions. However, we remain challenged because cancer is a complex disease of diverse etiologies by multiple exposures causing damage in different genes; for example, $gene^n$–$environment^n$ interactions, for which the variable n is not known.

Two fundamental principles underlie current studies of molecular epidemiology. First, carcinogenesis is a multistage process, and behind each stage are numerous genetic events that occur either due to an exogenous insult such as a chemical exposure or an endogenous insult, such as from free radicals generated via cellular processes or errors in DNA replication. Therefore, identifying a cancer risk factor can be challenging because of the multifactorial nature of carcinogenesis, given that any one risk factor occurs within a background of many risk factors. Second, wide interindividual variation in response to carcinogen exposure and other carcinogenic processes indicate that the human response is not homogeneous, so that experimental models and epidemiology (e.g., the use of a single cell clone to study a gene's effect experimentally or the assumption that the population responds similarly to the mean in epidemiology studies), might not be representative of susceptible and resistant groups within a population.

Genetic Susceptibility

In humans, the determination of genetic susceptibility can be assessed by phenotyping or genotyping methods. Phenotypes generally represent complex genotypes. Examples of phenotypes include the assessment of DNA repair capacity in cultured blood cells, mammographic breast density, or the quantitation of carcinogen-DNA adducts in a target organ. Phenotypes now also include profiles of methylation that affect gene expression, a so-called epigenetic effect, for example, identified though next-generation sequencing or other methods.[52] The contribution of genetics to cancer risk from chemical carcinogens can range from small to large, depending on its penetrance.[4] Highly penetrant cancer-susceptibility genes cause familial cancers, but account for less than 5% of all cancers. Low-penetrant genes cause common sporadic cancers, which have large public health consequences.

A genetic polymorphism (e.g., single nucleotide polymorphisms) is defined as a genetic variant present in at least 1% of the population. Because of the advent of improved genotyping methods that have reduced cost and increased high throughput, haplotyping and whole genomewide association studies are ongoing. Although haplotyping studies, facilitated through the International HapMap Project (www.hapmap.org), have not proven useful for predicting human cancers; high-density, whole genomewide, single nucleotide polymorphism association studies have shown remarkable consistency for many gene loci, although the risk estimates are only 1.0 to 1.4, which are not useful in the clinic for individual risk assessment.[6] For example, the contribution of genetic polymorphisms to cancer risk, at least for breast cancer, appears to improve risk modeling by only a few percent; known breast cancer risk factors account for about 58% of risk, and adding 10 genetic variants increases the risk prediction only to 62%.[53] Genes under study are from pathways that affect behavior, activate and detoxify carcinogens, affect DNA repair, govern cell-cycle control, trigger apoptosis, effect cell signaling, and so forth.

Biomarkers of Cancer Risk

The evaluation of dose and risk estimates in epidemiologic studies can include four components: namely, external exposure measurements, internal exposure measurements, biomarkers estimating the biologically effective dose, and biomarkers of effect or harm. The latter three measurements are biomarkers that improve on the first by quantifying exposure inside the individual and at the cellular level to characterize low-dose exposures in low-risk populations, providing a relative contribution of individual chemical carcinogens from complex mixtures, and/or estimating total burden of a particular exposure where there are many sources.[54]

Chemicals cause genetic damage in different ways, namely in the formation of carcinogen-DNA adducts leading to base mutations or gross chromosomal changes. Adducts are formed when a mutagen, or part of it, irreversibly binds to DNA so that it can cause a base substitution, insertion, or deletion during DNA replication. Gross chromosomal mutations are chromosome breaks, gaps, or translocations. The level of DNA damage is the biologically effective dose in a target organ, and reflects the net result of carcinogen exposure, activation, lack of detoxification, lack of effective DNA repair, and lack of programmed cell death. A variety of assays have been used for determining carcinogen-macromolecular adducts in human tissues; for example, for assessing risk from tobacco smoking for lung cancer and aflatoxin and liver cancer.[55,56] Important considerations for the assessment of biomarkers include sensitivity, specificity, reproducibility, accessibility for human use, and whether it represents a risk measured in a target organ or surrogate tissue. No single biomarker has been considered to be sufficiently validated for use as a cancer risk marker in an individual as it relates to chemical carcinogenesis.[57] However, there is some evidence that DNA adducts are cancer risk factors in both cohort and case-control studies.[58]

People are commonly exposed to N-nitrosamine and other N-nitroso compounds from dietary and tobacco exposures, which are associated with DNA adduct formation and cancer. Exposure can occur through endogenous formation of N-nitrosamines from nitrates in food or directly from dietary sources, cosmetics, drugs, household commodities, and tobacco smoke. Endogenous formation occurs in the stomach from the reaction of nitrosatable amines and nitrate (used as a preservative), which is converted to nitrites by bacteria. The N-nitrosamines undergo metabolic activation by cytochrome P450s (CYP2E1, CYP2A6, and CYP2D6) and form DNA adducts. Biomarkers are available to assess N-nitrosamine exposure from tobacco smoke (e.g., urinary tobacco-specific nitrosamine levels) or DNA, including in target organs such as the lungs. Recent data indicate that increasing levels of tobacco-specific nitrosamine metabolites are associated with increased lung cancer risk.[55]

Heterocyclic amines are formed from the overheating of food with creatine, such as meat, chicken, and fish.[59] Heterocyclic amines, estimated based on consumption of well-done meat, have been associated with breast and colon cancer, presumably through metabolic activation mechanisms and DNA damage.[59] Aflatoxins, another food contaminant, are considered to be a major contributor to liver cancer in China and parts of Africa, especially interacting with hepatitis viruses, and urinary aflatoxin adduct levels are predictors of liver cancer risk.[56]

Aromatic amines are another class of human carcinogens. Aryl aromatic amines have been implicated in bladder carcinogenesis, especially in occupationally exposed cohorts (e.g., dye workers) and tobacco smokers.[60] These compounds are activated by cytochrome P4501A2 and excreted via the N-acetyltransferase 2 gene. They are genotoxic, and the quantitative assessment using biomarkers has been more difficult, but some persons have studied DNA adducts as well.[61]

Polycyclic aromatic hydrocarbons (PAH) are large, aromatic (three or more fused benzene rings) compounds that are a class of more than 200 chemicals. These compounds are ubiquitous in the environment and present in the ambient air. They are formed from overcooking foods, fireplaces, charcoal barbeques, burning of coal and crude oil, tobacco smoke, and can be found in various occupational settings. In order for PAHs to exert their toxic effect, they must undergo metabolic activation via cytochromes P4501A1 and P4503A4 to form DNA adducts, or are excreted via pathways involving the glutathione-S-transferase genes. PAHs are associated with an increased risk of lung and skin cancer in the occupational setting, although risk varies by type of industry and the individual being exposed.[62,63] Benzo(a)pyrene (BaP), the most frequently studied PAH, serves as a model for chemical carcinogens. The bay region diol epoxide binds to DNA, mostly as the N2-deoxyguanosine adduct. The evidence linking BaP-deoxyguanosine adducts with a carcinogenic effect in lung cancer is very strong, including site-specific hotspot mutations in the p53 tumor suppressor gene.[64–68] Various biomarkers of exposure have been developed for assessing PAH exposure. These include measuring DNA adducts, protein adducts, and urinary 1-hydroxypyrene; only the latter is a validated biomarker of exposure and no adducts have been validated as biomarkers of cancer risk. However, recent data indicate that PAH metabolites might be risk factors for lung cancer.[58]

Air pollution has been recently classified by the IARC as a known human lung carcinogen.[69] Studies that support the conclusion include cohort studies that use biomarkers of exposure.[70] Such markers include measurements of 1-hydroxypyrene, DNA adducts, chromosomal aberrations, micronuclei, oxidative damage to nucleobases, and methylation changes.[71]

Epidemiologic and experimental studies have linked benzene to hematologic toxicity, including aplastic anemia, myelodysplastic syndrome, and acute myeloid leukemia.[72–74] Benzene is metabolized by hepatic P4502E1 (CYP2E1), yielding benzene oxide and hydroquinone, among other reactive metabolites. Circulating hydroquinones may be further metabolized to reactive benzoquinones by myeloperoxidase in bone marrow white blood cell precursors and stroma. Benzene metabolites are reported to have a variety of biologic consequences on bone marrow cells, including covalent binding to DNA and protein, alterations in gene expression, cytokine and chemokine abnormalities, and chromosomal aberrations.[75] There are well-established biomarkers of exposure to benzene, but to date, biomarkers of toxicity have not been validated (except for high-level exposure workplaces and effects of peripheral blood counts).

ARISTOLOCHIC ACID AND UROTHELIAL CANCERS AS A MODEL FOR IDENTIFYING HUMAN CARCINOGENS

Aristolochic acids come from the Aristolochia genus of plants, which have been used for herbal remedies (e.g., birthwort, Dutchman's pipe). The case of the carcinogen aristolochic acid, which is identified as a Class 1 human carcinogen by the IARC (http://monographs.iarc.fr/ENG/Monographs/vol100A/mono100A-23.pdf), presents a powerful example of how the forces of epidemiology, classical chemical carcinogenesis, and genomics collaborate to unravel the pathogenesis and prevention of a specific human cancer.[76] In the 1990s, epidemiologists independently reported on three distinct unrelated population groups that developed nephrotoxicity (interstitial fibrosis) and an extraordinary high incidence of urothelial cancer of the upper urinary track after exposure for different reasons and in different parts of the world (Belgium, the Balkans, and China). In Belgian women ingesting an extract from plants of the Aristolochia species for weight reduction, which was provided to them in a weight loss clinic, nearly 50% developed this unusual syndrome. A similar clinical picture (so-called Balkan endemic nephropathy) was reported for residents farming around the Danube River and eating home-baked bread from wheat contaminated with seeds from Aristolochia weeds grown in the same fields. In China, the Aristolochia herbs have been used for centuries in Chinese medicine and are prominently prescribed in Taiwan, a nation with the highest incidence of urothelial cancer in the world, as remedies for ailments of the heart, liver, snake bites, arthritis, gout, childbirth, and others.

Common to all Aristolochia species are one of two major nitrophenanthrene carboxylic acid toxicants, namely, aristolochic acid I and II (http://monographs.iarc.fr/ENG/Monographs/vol100A/

mono100A-23.pdf).[77,78] The oral administration of aristolochic acid to rodents is highly carcinogenic, producing predominantly forestomach cancers and lymphomas, along with cancers of the lung, kidney, and urothelium (http://monographs.iarc.fr/ENG/Monographs/vol100A/mono100A-23.pdf). The major route of excretion of aristolochic acid is through the kidneys. These clinical and experimental observations inspired further analyses of the mechanism of action of these potent human carcinogens. Studies in intact mice and mice reconstituted with humanized P450 revealed that CYP1a and CYP2a were responsible for both the activation and the detoxification of aristolochic acid I and II, and that NAD(P)H:quinone oxidoreductase produced the ultimate reactive aristolactam I nitrenium species.[78] The molecular action of the ultimate carcinogen is remarkably specific, targeting purine nucleotides in DNA to form DNA adducts and binding at the exocyclic amino group of deoxyadenosine and deoxyguanosine with a far greater affinity for dA over dG (Fig. 7.1). DNA adducts from aristolochic acids have been found in both experimental animals and humans. Furthermore, unlike any other human carcinogen, the predominant mutagenic outcome is an A:T transversion with a marked preference for the nontranscribed strand of DNA, notably in the p53 gene.[77,79] The A:T to T:A transversions are extremely uncommon among the mutation spectrum in all eukaryotes. These unique properties of aristolochic acid DNA adducts appear to elude DNA repair mechanisms that commonly focus on transcribing DNA, resulting in persistent carcinogen-DNA adducts in human tissues and surgical tumor specimens, thus confirming the association of exposure with a biologic effect.[80] In experimental models in mice where human p53 is substituted for the mouse gene, multiple sites on p53 are mutated, almost all of which are those unusual A:T transversions.[81] Modern genomic techniques have unraveled other selective properties of this unusual but potent human chemical carcinogen. Whole genome and exome sequencing of multiple aristolochic-associated kidney cancers from patients confirmed the high frequency of the unusual A:T to T:A transversion mutations. Furthermore, an unusual pattern emerges where there is selectivity for mutations at splice sites with a preferable consensus sequence of T/CAG. Among the many mutations detected, certain targets stand out, particularly in p53, MLL2, and other genes the products of which function in regulating gene expression through higher chromosome order.[82,83] This cancer story covers the gamut of all elements of chemical carcinogenesis, and its illumination has opened a door for cancer prevention.

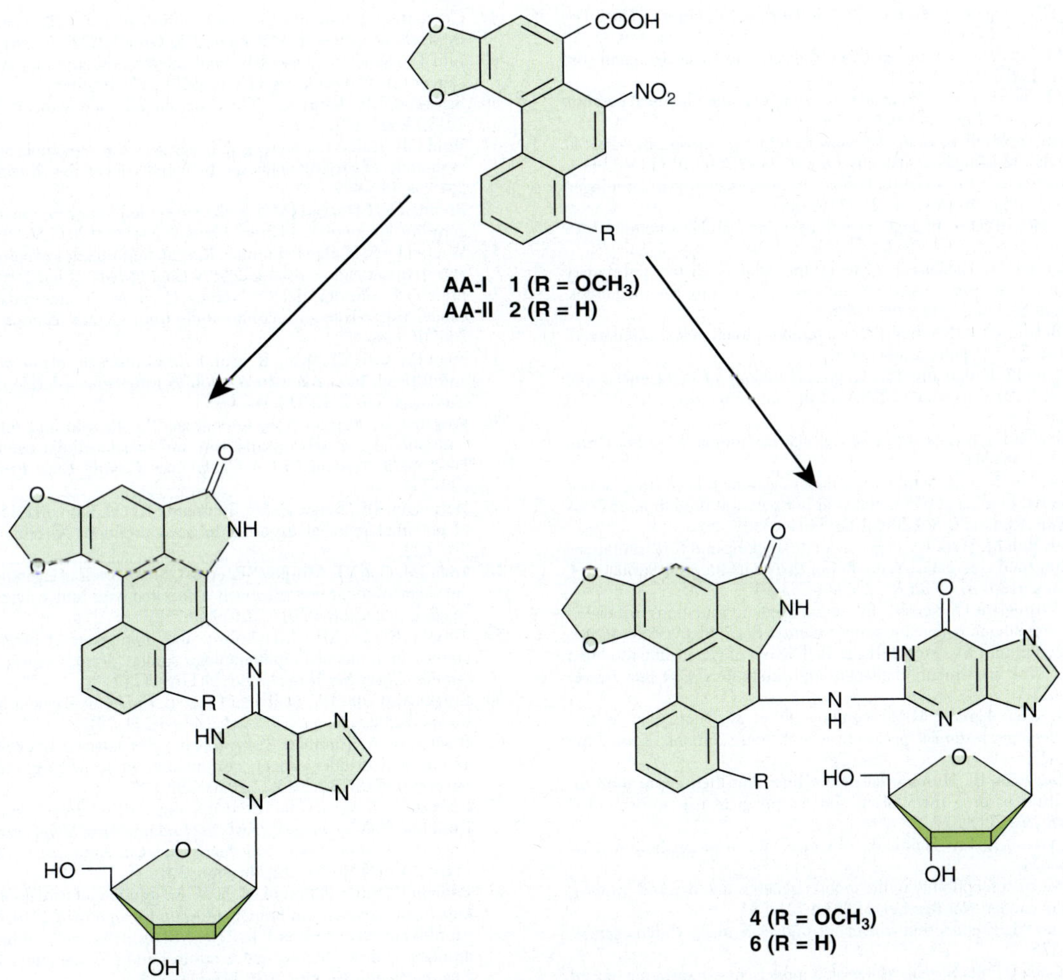

3 ($R = OCH_3$)
5 (R = H)

Figure 7.1 Aristolochic acid I and II form DNA adducts through the exocyclic amino group of deoxyadenosine and deoxyguanosine. The deoxyadenosine adduct is highly favored. For more detailed analysis of the complete metabolic profile, see Attaluri et al.[79]

REFERENCES

1. U.S. Department of Health and Human Services. *The Health Consequences of Smoking: 50 Years of Progress. A Report of the Surgeon General.* Atlanta: Author; 2014.
2. Colditz GA, Wei EK. Preventability of cancer: the relative contributions of biologic and social and physical environmental determinants of cancer mortality. *Annu Rev Public Health* 2012;33:137–156.
3. Lynch SM, Rebbeck TR. Bridging the gap between biologic, individual, and macroenvironmental factors in cancer: a multilevel approach. *Cancer Epidemiol Biomarkers Prev* 2013;22:485–495.
4. Rahman N. Realizing the promise of cancer predisposition genes. *Nature* 2014;505:302–308.
5. Lichtenstein P, Holm NV, Verkasalo PK, et al. Environmental and heritable factors in the causation of cancer—analyses of cohorts of twins from Sweden, Denmark, and Finland. *N Engl J Med* 2000;343:78–85.
6. Hunter DJ, Chanock SJ. Genome-wide association studies and "the art of the soluble." *J Natl Cancer Inst* 2010;102:836–837.
7. Luch A. Nature and nurture - lessons from chemical carcinogenesis. *Nat Rev Cancer* 2005;5:113–125.
8. Taddei ML, Giannoni E, Comito G, et al. Microenvironment and tumor cell plasticity: an easy way out. *Cancer Lett* 2013;341:80–96.
9. Fessler E, Dijkgraaf FE, De Sousa E Melo, et al. Cancer stem cell dynamics in tumor progression and metastasis: is the microenvironment to blame? *Cancer Lett* 2013;341:97–104.
10. Hanahan D, Coussens LM. Accessories to the crime: functions of cells recruited to the tumor microenvironment. *Cancer Cell* 2012;21:309–322.
11. Irigaray P, Belpomme D. Basic properties and molecular mechanisms of exogenous chemical carcinogens. *Carcinogenesis* 2010;31:135–148.
12. Xia HJ, Chen CS. Progress of non-human primate animal models of cancers. *Dongwuxue Yanjiu* 2011;32:70–80.
13. Yi C, He C. DNA repair by reversal of DNA damage. *Cold Spring Harb Perspect Biol* 2013;5:a012575.
14. Dizdaroglu M. Oxidatively induced DNA damage: mechanisms, repair and disease. *Cancer Lett* 2012;327:26–47.
15. Wogan GN, Hecht SS, Felton JS, et al. Environmental and chemical carcinogenesis. *Semin Cancer Biol* 2004;14:473–486.
16. Baan R, Grosse Y, Straif K, et al. A review of human carcinogens—Part F: chemical agents and related occupations. *Lancet Oncol* 2009;10:1143–1144.
17. Rendic S, Guengerich FP. Contributions of human enzymes in carcinogen metabolism. *Chem Res Toxicol* 2012;25:1316–1383.
18. Luch A. The mode of action of organic carcinogens on cellular structures. *EXS* 2006;65–95.
19. Anttila S, Raunio H, Hakkola J. Cytochrome P450-mediated pulmonary metabolism of carcinogens: regulation and cross-talk in lung carcinogenesis. *Am J Respir Cell Mol Biol* 2011;44:583–590.
20. Pogribny IP, Beland FA. DNA methylome alterations in chemical carcinogenesis. *Cancer Lett* 2012 [Epub ahead of print].
21. Shrivastav N, Li D, Essigmann JM. Chemical biology of mutagenesis and DNA repair: cellular responses to DNA alkylation. *Carcinogenesis* 2010;31:59–70.
22. Kew MC. Aflatoxins as a cause of hepatocellular carcinoma. *J Gastrointestin Liver Dis* 2013;22:305–310.
23. Feng Z, Hu W, Hu Y, et al. Acrolein is a major cigarette-related lung cancer agent: preferential binding at p53 mutational hotspots and inhibition of DNA repair. *Proc Natl Acad Sci U S A* 2006;103:15404–15409.
24. Porta M, Crous-Bou M, Wark PA, et al. Cigarette smoking and K-ras mutations in pancreas, lung and colorectal adenocarcinomas: etiopathogenic similarities, differences and paradoxes. *Mutat Res* 2009;682:83–93.
25. Blackford A, Parmigiani G, Kensler TW, et al. Genetic mutations associated with cigarette smoking in pancreatic cancer. *Cancer Res* 2009;69:3681–3688.
26. Eastmond DA, Vulimiri SV, French JE, et al. The use of genetically modified mice in cancer risk assessment: challenges and limitations. *Crit Rev Toxicol* 2013;43:611–631.
27. Boverhof DR, Chamberlain MP, Elcombe CR, et al. Transgenic animal models in toxicology: historical perspectives and future outlook. *Toxicol Sci* 2011;121:207–233.
28. Cheung C, Gonzalez FJ. Humanized mouse lines and their application for prediction of human drug metabolism and toxicological risk assessment. *J Pharmacol Exp Ther* 2008;327:288–299.
29. Hanahan D, Weinberg RA. Hallmarks of cancer: the next generation. *Cell* 2011;144:646–674.
30. Demant P. Cancer susceptibility in the mouse: genetics, biology and implications for human cancer. *Nat Rev Genet* 2003;4:721–734.
31. Klatt P, Serrano M. Engineering cancer resistance in mice. *Carcinogenesis* 2003;24:817–826.
32. Lynch D, Svoboda J, Putta S, et al. Mouse skin models for carcinogenic hazard identification: utilities and challenges. *Toxicol Pathol* 2007;35:853–864.
33. Lash LH, Hines RN, Gonzalez FJ, et al. Genetics and susceptibility to toxic chemicals: do you (or should you) know your genetic profile? *J Pharmacol Exp Ther* 2003;305:403–409.
34. Di PG, Magno LA, Rios-Santos F. Glutathione S-transferases: an overview in cancer research. *Expert Opin Drug Metab Toxicol* 2010;6:153–170.
35. Feng S, Cao Z, Wang X. Role of aryl hydrocarbon receptor in cancer. *Biochim Biophys Acta* 2013;1836:197–210.
36. Jiang XL, Gonzalez FJ, Yu AM. Drug-metabolizing enzyme, transporter, and nuclear receptor genetically modified mouse models. *Drug Metab Rev* 2011;43:27–40.
37. Tuna M, Amos CI. Genomic sequencing in cancer. *Cancer Lett* 2013;340:161–170.
38. MacConaill LE. Existing and emerging technologies for tumor genomic profiling. *J Clin Oncol* 2013;31:1815–1824.
39. Watson IR, Takahashi K, Futreal PA, et al. Emerging patterns of somatic mutations in cancer. *Nat Rev Genet* 2013;14:703–718.
40. Dumas ME. Metabolome 2.0: quantitative genetics and network biology of metabolic phenotypes. *Mol Biosyst* 2012;8:2494–2502.
41. Adamski J, Suhre K. Metabolomics platforms for genome wide association studies—linking the genome to the metabolome. *Curr Opin Biotechnol* 2013;24:39–47.
42. Verma M, Khoury MJ, Ioannidis JP. Opportunities and challenges for selected emerging technologies in cancer epidemiology: mitochondrial, epigenomic, metabolomic, and telomerase profiling. *Cancer Epidemiol Biomarkers Prev* 2013;22:189–200.
43. Edwards SL, Beesley J, French JD, et al. Beyond GWASs: illuminating the dark road from association to function. *Am J Hum Genet* 2013;93:779–797.
44. Di LG, Garofalo M, Croce CM. MicroRNAs in cancer. *Annu Rev Pathol* 2014;9:287–314.
45. Cheetham SW, Gruhl F, Mattick JS, et al. Long noncoding RNAs and the genetics of cancer. *Br J Cancer* 2013;108:2419–2425.
46. Izzotti A, Pulliero A. The effects of environmental chemical carcinogens on the microRNA machinery. *Int J Hyg Environ Health* 2014 [Epub ahead of print].
47. Kostic AD, Gevers D, Pedamallu CS, et al. Genomic analysis identifies association of Fusobacterium with colorectal carcinoma. *Genome Res* 2012;22:292–298.
48. Compare D, Nardone G. Contribution of gut microbiota to colonic and extracolonic cancer development. *Dig Dis* 2011;29:554–561.
49. Ahn J, Chen CY, Hayes RB. Oral microbiome and oral and gastrointestinal cancer risk. *Cancer Causes Control* 2012;23:399–404.
50. Schwabe RF, Jobin C. The microbiome and cancer. *Nat Rev Cancer* 2013;13:800–812.
51. Wild CP, Scalbert A, Herceg Z. Measuring the exposome: a powerful basis for evaluating environmental exposures and cancer risk. *Environ Mol Mutagen* 2013;54:480–499.
52. Brennan K, Flanagan JM. Epigenetic epidemiology for cancer risk: harnessing germline epigenetic variation. *Methods Mol Biol* 2012;863:439–465.
53. Wacholder S, Hartge P, Prentice R, et al. Performance of common genetic variants in breast-cancer risk models. *N Engl J Med* 2010;362:986–993.
54. Boffetta P, van der Hel O, Norppa H, et al. Chromosomal aberrations and cancer risk: results of a cohort study from Central Europe. *Am J Epidemiol* 2007;165:36–43.
55. Yuan JM, Gao YT, Wang R, et al. Urinary levels of volatile organic carcinogen and toxicant biomarkers in relation to lung cancer development in smokers. *Carcinogenesis* 2012;33:804–809.
56. Wogan GN, Kensler TW, Groopman JD. Present and future directions of translational research on aflatoxin and hepatocellular carcinoma. A review. *Food Addit Contam Part A Chem Anal Control Expo Risk Assess* 2012;29:249–257.
57. Hatsukami DK, Benowitz NL, Rennard SI, et al. Biomarkers to assess the utility of potential reduced exposure tobacco products. *Nicotine Tob Res* 2006;8:599–622.
58. Yuan JM, Gao YT, Murphy SE, et al. Urinary levels of cigarette smoke constituent metabolites are prospectively associated with lung cancer development in smokers. *Cancer Res* 2011;71:6749–6757.
59. Turesky RJ, Le ML. Metabolism and biomarkers of heterocyclic aromatic amines in molecular epidemiology studies: lessons learned from aromatic amines. *Chem Res Toxicol* 2011;24:1169–1214.
60. Burger M, Catto JW, Dalbagni G, et al. Epidemiology and risk factors of urothelial bladder cancer. *Eur Urol* 2013;63:234–241.
61. Besaratinia A, Tommasi S. Genotoxicity of tobacco smoke-derived aromatic amines and bladder cancer: current state of knowledge and future research directions. *FASEB J* 2013;27:2090–2100.
62. International Agency for Research on Cancer. *IARC Monographs on the Evaluation of Carcinogenic Risks to Humans: Some Non-Heterocyclic Polycyclic Aromatic Hydrocarbons and Some Related Exposures.* Volume 92. Lyon, France: World Health Organization; 2010.
63. Boffetta P, Autier P, Boniol M, et al. An estimate of cancers attributable to occupational exposures in France. *J Occup Environ Med* 2010;52:399–406.
64. Mordukhovich I, Rossner P Jr, Terry MB, et al. Associations between polycyclic aromatic hydrocarbon-related exposures and p53 mutations in breast tumors. *Environ Health Perspect* 2010;118:511–518.
65. Pfeifer GP, Denissenko MF, Olivier M, et al. Tobacco smoke carcinogens, DNA damage and p53 mutations in smoking-associated cancers. *Oncogene* 2002;21:7435–7451.
66. Pfeifer GP, Hainaut P. On the origin of G →. T transversions in lung cancer. *Mutat Res* 2003;526:39–43.
67. Sjaastad AK, Jorgensen RB, Svendsen K. Exposure to polycyclic aromatic hydrocarbons (PAHs), mutagenic aldehydes and particulate matter during pan frying of beefsteak. *Occup Environ Med* 2010;67:228–232.

68. Hussain SP, Amstad P, Raja K, et al. Mutability of p53 hotspot codons to benzo(a)pyrene diol epoxide (BPDE) and the frequency of p53 mutations in nontumorous human lung. *Cancer Res* 2001;61:6350–6355.
69. Loomis D, Grosse Y, Lauby-Secretan B, et al. The carcinogenicity of outdoor air pollution. *Lancet Oncol* 2013;14:1262–1263.
70. Raaschou-Nielsen O, Andersen ZJ, Beelen R, et al. Air pollution and lung cancer incidence in 17 European cohorts: prospective analyses from the European Study of Cohorts for Air Pollution Effects (ESCAPE). *Lancet Oncol* 2013;14:813–822.
71. Demetriou CA, Raaschou-Nielsen O, Loft S, et al. Biomarkers of ambient air pollution and lung cancer: a systematic review. *Occup Environ Med* 2012;69:619–627.
72. Galbraith D, Gross SA, Paustenbach D. Benzene and human health: A historical review and appraisal of associations with various diseases. *Crit Rev Toxicol* 2010;40:1–46.
73. Vlaanderen J, Portengen L, Rothman N, et al. Flexible meta-regression to assess the shape of the benzene-leukemia exposure-response curve. *Environ Health Perspect* 2010;118:526–532.
74. Vlaanderen J, Lan Q, Kromhout H, et al. Occupational benzene exposure and the risk of chronic myeloid leukemia: a meta-analysis of cohort studies incorporating study quality dimensions. *Am J Ind Med* 2012;55:779–785.
75. Snyder R. Leukemia and benzene. *Int J Environ Res Public Health* 2012;9: 2875–2893.
76. Grollman AP. Aristolochic acid nephropathy: harbinger of a global iatrogenic disease. *Environ Mol Mutagen* 2013;54:1–7.
77. Hollstein M, Moriya M, Grollman AP, et al. Analysis of TP53 mutation spectra reveals the fingerprint of the potent environmental carcinogen, aristolochic acid. *Mutat Res* 2013;753:41–49.
78. Stiborova M, Martinek V, Frei E, et al. Enzymes metabolizing aristolochic acid and their contribution to the development of aristolochic acid nephropathy and urothelial cancer. *Curr Drug Metab* 2013;14:695–705.
79. Attaluri S, Bonala RR, Yang IY, et al. DNA adducts of aristolochic acid II: total synthesis and site-specific mutagenesis studies in mammalian cells. *Nucleic Acids Res* 2010;38:339–352.
80. Sidorenko VS, Yeo JE, Bonala RR, et al. Lack of recognition by global-genome nucleotide excision repair accounts for the high mutagenicity and persistence of aristolactam-DNA adducts. *Nucleic Acids Res* 2012;40:2494–2505.
81. Nedelko T, Arlt VM, Phillips DH, et al. TP53 mutation signature supports involvement of aristolochic acid in the aetiology of endemic nephropathy-associated tumours. *Int J Cancer* 2009;124:987–990.
82. Hoang ML, Chen CH, Sidorenko VS, et al. Mutational signature of aristolochic acid exposure as revealed by whole-exome sequencing. *Sci Transl Med* 2013;5:197ra102.
83. Poon SL, Pang ST, McPherson JR, et al. Genome-wide mutational signatures of aristolochic acid and its application as a screening tool. *Sci Transl Med* 2013;5:197ra101.

8 Physical Factors

Mats Ljungman

INTRODUCTION

Ionizing radiation (IR) and ultraviolet (UV) light have challenged the genetic integrity of all living organisms throughout time. By inducing DNA damage and subsequent mutations, these physical agents have promoted diversity through natural selection, and, as a result, organisms from all kingdoms of life carry genes that encode proteins that repair damaged DNA. In higher, multicellular organisms, many additional mechanisms of genome preservation have evolved, such as cell cycle checkpoints and apoptosis. Despite the many sophisticated mechanisms to safeguard the human genome from the mutagenic actions of DNA-damaging agents, not all exposed cells successfully restore the integrity of their DNA and some cells may subsequently progress into malignant cancer cells. Furthermore, through manmade activities, we are now exposed to many new physical agents, such as radiofrequency and microwave radiation, electromagnetic fields, asbestos, and nanoparticles, for which evolution has not yet had time to deliver genome-preserving response mechanisms. This chapter will highlight the molecular mechanisms by which these physical agents affect cells and how human exposure may lead to cancer.

IONIZING RADIATION

IR is defined as radiation that has sufficient energy to ionize molecules by displacing electrons from atoms. IR can be electromagnetic, such as x-rays and gamma rays, or can consist of particles, such as electrons, protons, neutrons, alpha particles, or carbon ions. Natural sources of IR make up about 80% of human exposure and medical sources make up about 20%.[1] The increased medical use of diagnostic x-rays and computed tomography (CT) scanning procedures likely translates into higher incidences of cancer. Of the natural sources, radon exposure is the most significant exposure risk to humans. Importantly, with better and more comprehensive screening techniques, the human exposure to radon could be dramatically lowered.

Mechanisms of Damage Induction

Linear Energy Transfer

The biologic effects of IR are unique in that the induced damage is clustered due to the local deposition of energy in radiation tracks. The distance between the depositions of energy is biologically very relevant and unique to the energy and the type of radiation. The term *linear energy transfer (LET)* denotes the energy transferred per unit length of a track of radiation. Electromagnetic radiation, such as x-rays or gamma rays, are sparsely ionizing and therefore classified as low LET radiation, whereas particulate radiation, such as neutrons, protons, and alpha particles, are examples of high LET radiation.[1]

Radiation Biochemistry

Radiation-induced damage to cellular target molecules, such as DNA, proteins, and lipids, can be either direct or indirect (Fig. 8.1). The *direct action* of radiation, which is the dominant mode of action of high LET radiation, is due to the deposition of energy directly to the target molecule, resulting in one or more ionization events. The *indirect action* of radiation is due to the radiolysis of water molecules, which, after initial absorption of radiation energy, become excited and generate different types of radiolysis products where the reactive hydroxyl radical (•OH), can damage both DNA and proteins. About two-thirds of the damage induced by low LET radiation is due to the indirect action of radiation. Since the hydroxyl radical is very reactive (half-life is 10^{-9} seconds), it does not diffuse more than a few nanometers after it is formed before it reacts with other molecules, and, thus, only radicals formed in close proximity to the target molecule will contribute to the damage of that target.[2] However, by chemical recombination of the primary radiolysis products, hydrogen peroxide (H_2O_2) is formed, which in turn can produce hydroxyl radicals at a later time through the Fenton reaction, involving free metals. Because H_2O_2 is not very reactive, it can diffuse long distances away from the initial site of energy deposition.

Radical scavengers normally present in cells, such as glutathione, can protect target molecules by reacting with the hydroxyl radical (see Fig. 8.1). Even after the target molecule has been hit and ionized, glutathione can contribute to cell protection by donating a hydrogen atom to the radical, allowing the unpaired electron present in the radical to pair up with the electron from the hydrogen atom. This is considered the simplest of all types of repair and is called *chemical repair.*[3] However, if oxygen molecules are present, they will compete with scavenger molecules for the ionized molecule, and if oxygen reacts with the ionized target molecule before the hydrogen donation occurs, the damage will be solidified as a peroxide, which is not amendable to chemical repair. Instead, this lesion will require enzymatic repair for the restoration of DNA. This augmenting biologic effect of oxygen is called the *oxygen effect* and is considered an important factor for the effectiveness of radiation therapy.[1]

Damage to DNA

The direct and indirect effects of radiation induce more or less identical types of lesions in DNA. However, the density of lesions induced in a stretch of DNA is higher for high LET radiation, and this increased complexity is thought to complicate the repair of these lesions. Radiation-induced lesions consist of more than 100 chemically distinct base lesions, such as the mutagenic lesions thymine glycol and 8-hydroxyguanine.[2,4,5] Furthermore, damage to the sugar moiety in the backbone of DNA and some types of base damage can result in single-strand breaks (SSB). Because the energy deposition of radiation is clustered even for low LET radiation, it is possible that two individual strand breaks are formed in close proximity on opposite strands, resulting in the formation of a double-strand break (DSB). It has been estimated that 1 Gy of ionizing radiation gives rise to about 40 DSBs, 1,000 SSBs, 1,000 base lesions, and 150 DNA-protein cross-links per cell.[2] For a similarly lethal dose of UV light, about 400,000 lesions are required, demonstrating that the lesions induced by IR are much more toxic

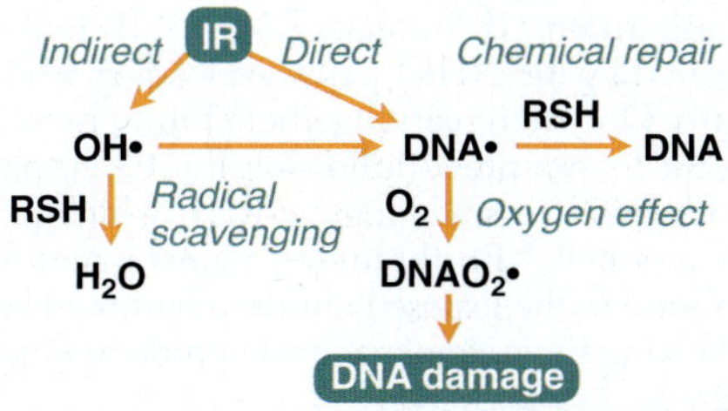

Figure 8.1 Factors affecting the induction of DNA damage by ionizing radiation (IR). Ionizing radiation can ionize DNA either by direct action or by indirect action, in which radiation energy is absorbed by neighboring molecules, such as water, leading to the generation of hydroxyl radicals that attack DNA. Sulfur-containing cellular molecules (RSH), such as glutathione, can scavenge hydroxyl radicals by hydrogen atom donations and thereby protect the DNA from the indirect action of radiation. Glutathione can also donate hydrogen atoms to ionized DNA, thereby restoring the integrity of DNA in a process termed *chemical repair.* Oxygen can compete with chemical repair in a process termed the *oxygen effect,* resulting in the enhancement of the biologic effect of ionizing radiation by the fixation of the initial DNA damage into DNA peroxides ($DNAO_2$•).

than lesions induced by UV light. It is believed that DSBs are the critical lesions that lead to cell lethality following exposure to ionizing radiation.[6]

Damage to Proteins

Although proteins and lipids are subject to damage following exposure to IR, the common belief is that DNA is the critical target for the biologic effects of radiation. Indeed, abrogation of DNA damage surveillance or repair processes in cells results in the enhanced induction of mutations and decreased cell survival following radiation.[5] However, studies of radiation-sensitive and radiation-resistant bacteria imply that mechanisms that suppress protein damage may also play important roles in radiation resistance.[7] *Deinococcus radiodurans* is a bacterium that can survive radiation exposures of up to 17,000 Gy, and its extreme radioresistance has been linked to high intracellular levels of manganese, which protect proteins from oxidation. The thought is that if a cell can limit protein oxidation, then its enzymes will remain active, and cellular functions such as DNA repair will be able to restore the integrity of DNA even after severe DNA damage.[8] It would be interesting to explore whether the concentration of manganese can be manipulated to sensitize tumor cells to radiation therapy. Furthermore, because protein damage due to reactive oxygen species (ROS) accumulate during the aging process, could supplements of manganese turn back the clock on aging?

Cellular Responses

DNA Repair

Ever since organisms started to utilize atmospheric oxygen for metabolic respiration many millions of years ago, they have been forced to deal with the cellular damage induced by ROS. Base excision repair (BER) evolved to remove many of the different types of oxidative base lesions and DNA SSBs induced by ROS. However, ROS seldom induce DSBs unless the generation of hydroxyl radicals is clustered near the DNA molecule. A more important source of intracellular generation of DSBs may instead be the process of DNA replication, and it is possible that homologous recombination (HR) repair primarily evolved to overcome DSBs sporadically induced during the replication process. The other major pathway of DSB repair is the nonhomologous end-joining (NHEJ) pathway, which is utilized by immune cells in the process of antibody generation. Although the HR pathway has high fidelity due to the utilization of homologous sister chromatids to ensure that correct DNA ends are joined, the NHEJ pathway lacks this

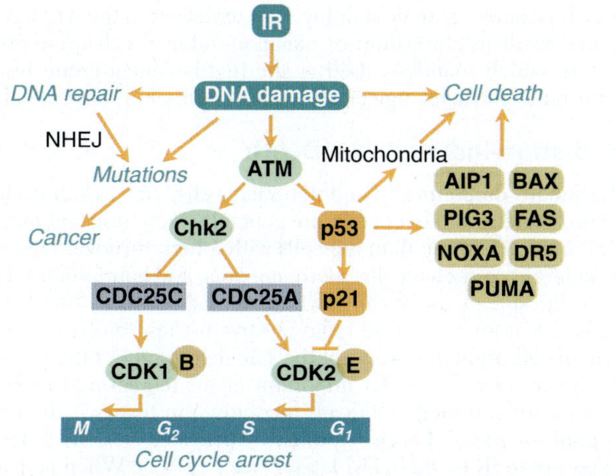

Figure 8.2 Cellular responses to ionizing radiation. Ionizing radiation induces predominantly base lesions and single- and double-strand breaks. Base lesions and single-strand breaks are repaired by base excision repair (BER), whereas double-strand breaks are repaired by nonhomologous end joining (NHEJ) and homologous recombination (HR). If DNA lesions are misrepaired by NHEJ or not repaired at all before cells enter S phase or mitosis, genomic instability is manifested as mutations or chromosome aberrations that promote carcinogenesis. In order for cells to assist DNA repair and safeguard against genetic instability and cancer, cells can induce cell cycle arrest or apoptosis. The ATM kinase is an early responder to DNA damage induced by ionizing radiation that activates the cell cycle checkpoint kinase Chk2 and the tumor suppressor p53. Chk2 inactivates the CDC25A and CDC25C phosphatases that are critical in promoting cell cycle progression by activating the cyclin-dependent kinases CDK2 or CDK1 and thereby arresting the cells at the G_1/S or G_2/M checkpoints. In addition, p53 can arrest cells at the G_1/S checkpoint by inducing the CDK inhibitor p21. p53 also plays a role in promoting apoptosis by inducing a number of proapoptotic proteins as well as translocating to mitochondria where it inhibits the actions of antiapoptotic factors. AIP1, actin interacting protein 1; BAX, bcl-2-like protein; PIG3, p53-inducible gene 3.

control mechanism and therefore occasionally rejoins ends incorrectly. Thus, the NHEJ pathway may contribute to the generation of mutations following radiation (Fig. 8.2). However, NHEJ is the only mechanism available for DSB repair in postmitotic cells and cells in the G_1 phase of the cell cycle because no sister chromatids are available in these cells to support HR repair.

Ataxia-Telangiectasia Mutated and Cell Cycle Checkpoints

Due to the enormous task of replicating the whole genome during the S phase and segregating the chromosomes during mitosis, proliferating cells are generally much more vulnerable to radiation than stationary cells. To prevent cells with damaged DNA from entering into these critical stages of the cell cycle, cells can activate cell cycle checkpoints (see Fig. 8.2). The major sensor of radiation-induced damage in cells is the ataxia-telangiectasia mutated (ATM) kinase, which, following activation, can phosphorylate more than 700 proteins in cells.[9] Two ATM substrates, p53 and Chk2, are critical for the activation of cell cycle arrests at multiple sites in the cell cycle.[10,11] The kinase p53 regulates the gene expression of specific genes such as *p21*, which inhibits cyclin-dependent kinase (CDK)2- and CDK4-mediated phosphorylation of the retinoblastoma protein, resulting in a block in the progression from the G_1 phase to the S phase of the cell cycle.[12,13] The Chk2 kinase promotes checkpoint activation in G_1 by targeting the cell division cycle 25 homolog A (CDC25A) phosphatase[14] and, in G_2/M, by targeting the CDC25C phosphatase.[15] The activation of a cell cycle arrest following DNA damage provides the cell with additional time to repair the DNA before entering critical cell cycle stages, which promotes genetic stability. Loss or defects in the *ATM* or *p53* genes result in abrogation of radiation-induced cell cycle checkpoints, which manifests itself as the highly cancer-prone human syndromes ataxia telangiectasia[16] or Li-Fraumeni,[17] respectively.

Radiation-Induced Cell Death

Terminally differentiated and stationary cells, such as kidney, lung, brain, muscle, and liver cells, are generally more resistant to radiation-induced killing than are cells with a high turnover rate, such as different epithelial cells, spermatogonia, and hair follicles. However, the spleen and thymus, which consist of mostly nondividing cells, are among the most radiosensitive tissues, implying that the rate of cell proliferation is not the sole determiner of the radiation sensitivity of a tissue. An important factor regulating the induction of programmed cell death (apoptosis) in tissues is the tumor suppressor p53.[18] The p53 protein is activated in cells following exposure to IR by the ATM kinase (see Fig. 8.2). When activated, it regulates the expression of multiple genes that have roles in DNA repair, cell cycle arrest, and apoptosis. p53 can also localize to mitochondria following irradiation, where it triggers apoptosis through the inactivation of antiapoptotic regulatory proteins.[19] Not all tissues induce the p53 response to the same degree after similar doses of IR, nor do they activate downstream pathways, such as DNA repair, cell cycle arrest, and apoptosis, in a similar way. For example, thymocytes have an intrinsic setting that favors apoptosis over cell cycle arrest following IR, whereas fibroblasts rarely induce apoptosis, but instead activate a strong and lasting cell cycle arrest.[18]

IR can induce cell death in tissues by many different mechanisms. Apoptosis can occur rapidly in a p53-dependent manner or later in a p53-independent manner. This later wave of radiation-induced apoptosis is often initiated by mitotic catastrophe, which occurs as a result of complications during chromosome segregation. Cell death induced by IR may in some cases be associated with autophagy, also called autophagocytosis, in which cells degrade cellular components via the lysosomal machinery. Whether autophagy is a programmed cell death or occurs in parallel with cell death is not clear. Interestingly, for some cell types, autophagy has been shown to actually protect the cells from radiation-induced death. Finally, tissue can undergo necrotic cell death following exposure to IR. Necrosis is a clinical problem following radiation therapy that can occur in normal tissues many months after treatment and can contribute to the inflammatory response.

Cancer Risks

It is clear from epidemiologic studies of radiation workers and atomic bomb and Chernobyl victims that IR can induce cancer.[20] Twenty years after the atomic bomb explosions in Japan during World War II, significant increases in the incidence of thyroid cancer and leukemia were observed. However, it took almost 50 years before solid tumors appeared in the population as a result of radiation exposure from the atomic bombs.[21] The incidences of solid tumors, such as breast, ovary, bladder, lung, and colon cancers, were estimated to have increased by a factor of 2 in the exposed group during this time period. The epidemiology studies following the nuclear power plant disaster in Chernobyl showed a clear increase in thyroid cancer as early as 4 years after the accident.[22] Young children were the most vulnerable to radiation exposure, with 1-year-old children being 237-fold more susceptible to thyroid cancer than the control group, while 10-year-old children were found to be sixfold more susceptible to thyroid cancer. Many of the thyroid cancers that developed following the Chernobyl disaster could have been prevented if the population had not consumed locally produced milk that was contaminated with radioactive iodine.

The molecular signatures of radiation-induced tumors are complex but involve point mutations that could lead to the activation of the *RAS* oncogene or inactivation of the tumor suppressor gene *p53*. Furthermore, IR induces DNA DSBs that may be unfaithfully repaired by the NHEJ pathway, leading to chromosome rearrangements. One such rearrangement found in 50% to 90% of the thyroid cancers examined following the Chernobyl accident involved the receptor tyrosine kinase c-RET, which promotes cell growth when activated.[22] Furthermore, a great majority of the thyroid cancers found in the exposed children harbored kinase fusion oncogenes affecting the mitogen-activated protein kinase (MAPK) signaling pathway.[23]

The correlation between high exposure to IR and cancer following the atomic bomb explosions and the Chernobyl accident is clear. What about the cancer risk following lower radiation exposures occurring in daily life? There are four theoretical risk models of radiation-induced cancer to consider. First, the *linear, no threshold* (LNT) *model* suggests that the induction of cancer is directly proportional to the dose of radiation, even at low doses of exposure. Second, the *sublinear* or *threshold model* suggests that below a certain threshold dose the risk of radiation-induced cancers is negligible. At these lower doses of radiation exposure, the DNA damage surveillance and repair mechanisms are thought to be fully capable of safeguarding the DNA to avoid the induction of mutations and cancer. Third, the *supralinear* or *stealth model* suggests that doses below a certain threshold or radiation with sufficiently low dose rates may not trigger the activation of DNA damage surveillance and repair mechanisms, resulting in suboptimal activation of cell cycle checkpoints and repair. This would be expected to lead to a higher rate of mutations and cancers than predicted by the LNT model, but may be balanced by a higher incident of cell death. Fourth, the *linear-quadratic model* suggest that radiation effects at low doses are due to a single track of radiation hitting multiple targets, resulting in a linear induction rate, whereas at higher doses, multiple radiation tracks hit multiple cellular targets, resulting in a quadratic induction rate.

The Biological Effects of Ionizing Radiation (BEIR) VII report, released by the Committee on Biological Effects of Ionizing Radiation of the National Academy of Sciences and commissioned by the US Environmental Protection Agency (EPA), is a review of published data regarding human health and cancer risks from exposure to low levels of IR. Although this topic is controversial and not fully settled, the BIER VII report favored the LNT model.[24] Thus, the "official" view is that no level of radiation is safe; therefore, a careful consideration of risks versus benefits is necessary to ensure that the general population only receives radiation doses as low as reasonably achievable. Furthermore, the BIER VII committee concluded that the heritable effects of radiation were not evident in the published data, indicating that an individual is not likely to develop cancer due to radiation exposure of his or her parents.

The largest source of radiation exposure to the population is radon, which is a natural radioactive gas formed as a decay product of radium in the decay chain of uranium. Radon gas can accumulate to high levels in poorly ventilated basements in houses built on rock containing uranium. The major risk with radon is that some of its radioactive decay products can attach to dust particles that accumulate in the lungs, leading to a continuous exposure of the lung tissues to high LET alpha particles. Due to this radiation exposure, the EPA claims that radon is the second leading cause of lung cancer in the United States. Another important source of human exposure to IR is medical x-ray devices, and there is a growing concern about the dramatically increased use of whole body CT scans for diagnostic purposes. For a typical CT scan, a patient will receive about 100-fold more radiation than from a typical mammogram.[24] It is recommended that the use of whole body CT scans for children be very restricted due to the elevated risk of developing radiation-induced cancer for this age group.

Cancer patients who receive radiation therapy are at risk of developing secondary tumors induced by the radiation therapy treatment.[1] This is particularly a concern for young patients since (1) children are more prone to radiation-induced cancer,

(2) children have a relatively good chance of surviving the primary cancer and would have long life expectancies so a secondary tumor would have plenty of time to develop, and (3) many childhood cancers are promoted by genetic defects in DNA damage response pathways, making these patients highly prone to the genotoxic effects of radiation and subsequent secondary cancers. The most sensitive tissues for the development of secondary cancer have been found to be bone marrow (leukemia), the thyroid, breast, and lung.[1]

ULTRAVIOLET LIGHT

Depending on the wavelength, UV light is categorized into UVA (320 to 400 nm), UVB (290 to 320 nm), and UVC (240 to 290 nm) radiation. Most of the UVC light emitted from the sun is absorbed by the ozone layer in the atmosphere, and, thus, living organisms are mostly exposed to UVA and UVB irradiation.

Mechanisms of Damage Induction

UVC light is more damaging to DNA than UVA and UVB because the absorption maximum of DNA is around 260 nm. UVB and UVC induce predominantly pyrimidine dimers and 6-4 photoproducts, which consist of covalent ring structures that link two adjacent pyrimidines on the same DNA strand.[5] The formation of these lesions results in the bending of the DNA helix, resulting in the interference with both DNA and RNA synthesis. UVA light does not induce pyrimidine dimers or 6-4 photoproducts but can induce ROS, which in turn can form SSBs and base lesions in DNA of exposed cells.

Cellular Responses

DNA Repair

The nucleotide excision repair (NER) pathway removes pyrimidine dimers and 6-4 photoproducts from cellular DNA.[5] This pathway involves proteins that recognize the DNA lesions, nucleases that excise the DNA strand that contains the lesion, a DNA polymerase that synthesizes new DNA to fill the gap, and a DNA ligase that joins the backbone in the newly synthesized strand. Genetic defects in the NER pathway result in the human syndrome xeroderma pigmentosum, with individuals more than 1,000-fold more prone to sun-induced skin cancer than normal individuals. In addition, human polymorphisms in certain NER genes are thought to predispose individuals to cancers such as lung cancer, nonmelanoma skin cancer, head and neck cancer, and bladder cancer, indicating that NER is responsible for safeguarding the genome against many types of DNA adducts in addition to UV-induced lesions.[5]

UV-induced lesions formed in the transcribed strand of active genes block the elongation of RNA polymerase II, and if a cell does not restore transcription within a certain time frame, it may undergo apoptosis (Fig. 8.3).[25,26] To rapidly restore RNA synthesis and avoid cell death, NER enzymes are recruited to the sites of blocked RNA polymerase II and the lesions are removed in a process called transcription-coupled repair (TCR).[27] Individuals with Cockayne syndrome (CS), trichothiodystrophy, or the UV-sensitive syndrome, are unable to utilize the TCR pathway following UV irradiation.[5] Cells from these individuals do not recover RNA synthesis following UV irradiation and are therefore very prone to UV-induced apoptosis. Interestingly, despite a clear DNA repair defect, these individuals are not predisposed to UV-induced skin cancer. It is thought that the inability of CS cells to remove the toxic lesions that block transcription following UV irradiation results in the suppression of tumorigenesis by the elimination of damaged cells by apoptosis. However, while protecting against

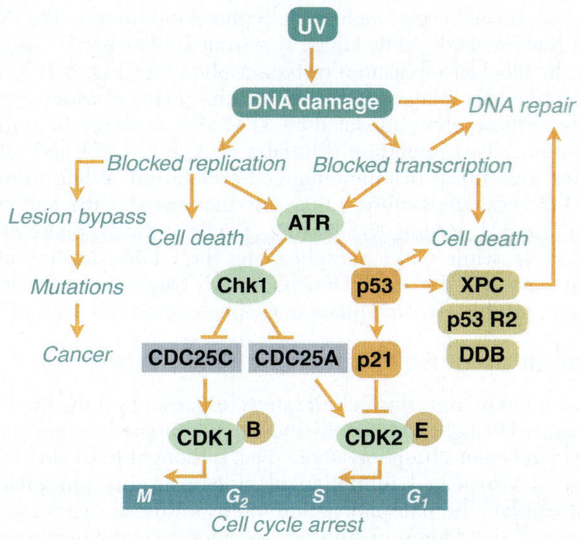

Figure 8.3 Cellular responses to ultraviolet (UV) light–induced DNA damage. UV light predominantly induces bulky DNA lesions that interfere with the processes of DNA replication and transcription. These lesions are removed from the global genome by global genomic nucleotide excision repair (GG-NER) and from transcribed DNA strands by transcription-coupled NER (TC-NER). Lesions blocking replication can be bypassed by exchanging processive DNA polymerases with less processive translesion DNA polymerases. While these polymerases allow cells to continue DNA synthesis and progress through the cell cycle, they have low fidelity, resulting in the potential induction of mutations promoting UV-induced carcinogenesis. To suppress mutations and support DNA repair efforts, the ataxia-telangiectasia and Rad3-related (ATR) kinase is activated in response to blocked replication or transcription. ATR activates the cell cycle checkpoint kinase Chk1, which, similar to Chk2, arrests cells in the G_1/S and G_2/M checkpoints by inhibiting CDC25A and CDC25C. ATR also activates p53, promoting G_1/S checkpoint activation via the induction of the Cdk-inhibitor p21. p53 also stimulates GG-NER by the transactivation of various NER genes and can promote apoptosis by the induction of proapoptotic factors and translocation to mitochondria. Finally, apoptosis is induced if cells do not recover transcription in a certain time frame, potentially due to the loss of survival factors or complications in the S phase when replication encounters stall the transcription complexes.

tumorigenesis, the elevated level of apoptosis in these cells leads to increased cell loss, which in turn may lead to neurologic degeneration.[25,28] Persistent transcription-blocking lesions in the genome have also been linked to aging.[29–31]

Translesion DNA Synthesis

Proliferating skin cells are very vulnerable to UV light because UV lesions block DNA replication (see Fig. 8.3). Cells that have entered the S phase and have initiated DNA synthesis have no choice but to finish replicating the whole genome or they will die. If DNA repair enzymes are not able to remove the blocking lesions from the template, the processive DNA polymerases may be exchanged for other, less processive DNA polymerases that can bypass the lesions. This is part of a "tolerance" mechanism, which allows cells to complete replication and eventually divide.[5] However, the translesion DNA polymerases do not have the same fidelity as the processive DNA polymerases; thus, mutations may occur. This is thought to be a major pathway by which UV light induces mutagenesis and, subsequently, cancer (see Fig. 8.3).

ATM and Rad3-Related Mediated Cell Cycle Checkpoints

In addition to utilizing the NER and BER pathways to repair UV-induced DNA damage, proliferating cells activate cell cycle checkpoints to allow more time for repair before entering critical parts of the cell cycle, such as the S phase and mitosis. The ATM and Rad3-related (ATR) kinase is activated following UV irradiation by blocked replication or transcription (see Fig. 8.3).[32] ATR phosphorylates a large number of proteins, many of which are the same as those phosphorylated by ATM after exposure to ionizing radiation.[9] Two important substrates of ATR are p53 and Chk1, which are critical in promoting cell cycle arrest. When induced by ATR, p53 transactivates the gene that encodes the cell cycle inhibitor p21, leading to the arrest of cells in the G_1 phase of the cell cycle, while Chk1 phosphorylates the CDK-activating phosphatases CDC25A and CDC25C, which targets them for degradation, resulting in an S-phase or G_2-phase arrest (see Fig. 8.3).[33]

Activation of Cell Membrane Receptors

In addition to triggering cellular stress responses by inducing DNA damage, UV light can directly induce membrane receptor signaling by receptor phosphorylation. This is thought to be due to the direct UV-mediated inhibition of protein-tyrosine phosphatases that regulate the phosphorylation levels of various membrane receptors.[34] In addition, membrane receptors may physically aggregate following UV irradiation, leading to the activation of signal transduction pathways that regulate cell growth[35] or apoptosis.[36]

Cell Death

UV light effectively induces apoptosis in skin cells. The mechanism by which UV light induces cell death is not fully understood, but failure to adequately resume RNA synthesis following UV light exposure is strongly linked to apoptosis (see Fig. 8.3).[25] Many potential mechanisms of how blocked transcription results in apoptosis have been suggested, such as a physical clash during the S phase between elongating replication machineries and transcription complexes stalled at UV lesions. Another possible mechanism involves the preferential loss of survival factors coded by highly unstable mRNAs.[37] The induction of p53 may also contribute to UV-induced apoptosis,[38] although p53 appears to protect human fibroblasts[39] and keratinocytes[40] from UV-induced apoptosis. Although complications induced by DNA damage may be the predominant mechanism by which cells die following UV irradiation, UV light may induce apoptosis in certain cell types by directly promoting the physical aggregation of the death receptor Fas/APO1.[36]

Cancer Risks

The incidence of sun-induced skin cancer, especially melanoma, is on the increase due to higher rates of sun exposure in the general population. The link between UV light exposure and skin cancer is very strong, but the role of UV light in the etiology of nonmelanoma and melanoma skin cancer differs. Although the risk of nonmelanoma cancer relates to the cumulative lifetime exposure to UV light, the risk of contracting melanoma appears to be linked to high sunlight exposure during childhood.[41] What makes UV light such a potent carcinogen is that it can initiate carcinogenesis by inducing DNA lesions as well as suppressing the immune system, resulting in a greater probability that initiated cells will survive and grow into tumors.[42,43]

Nonmelanoma Skin Cancer

Basal cell carcinoma (BCC) and squamous cell carcinoma (SCC) are the two most common skin cancer types. BCC and SCC occur predominantly in sun-exposed areas of the skin, but there are examples of these cancers forming in nonexposed areas as well. The tumor suppressor genes *p53* and *p16* are frequently inactivated in BCC and SCC, while the hedgehog-signaling pathway is activated primarily by mutations to the patched gene (percutaneous transhepatic cholangiography [*PTCH*]). This scenario promotes proliferation without the opposition of the cell cycle inhibitors p53 and p16.

Melanoma

Melanoma arises from mutations in epidermal melanocytes and is the most dangerous form of skin cancer because it has the highest propensity to metastasize. It is formed in both sun-exposed and shielded areas of the skin; therefore, the role of UV light as the major carcinogen in melanoma has been controversial.[41] Defects in the NER pathway do not seem to predispose the development of melanoma, suggesting that pyrimidine dimers or 6-4 photoproducts induced by UVB are not the initiators of melanoma carcinogenesis. Instead, ROS induced by UVA may be responsible for the development of melanoma.[41] However, a study using next-generation sequencing techniques to catalog all mutations in a melanoma cell line found a mutational spectrum of the over 33,000 mutations detected that strongly indicated that pyrimidine dimers and 6-4 photoproducts are the major mutagenic lesions in melanoma, whereas a subset of mutations may be induced by ROS.[44] The incidence of mutations in the *p16* and *ARF* genes is high, whereas *p53* and *RAS* mutations are fairly uncommon in melanoma.

Photoimmunosuppression

Studies of transplantation of mouse skin cancers into syngeneic mice revealed that prior UVB irradiation of recipient mice promoted tumor growth, whereas transplantation into naïve nonirradiated mice led to rejection.[43] These studies established that UV light has local immunosuppressing ability, and subsequent studies found that UV light preferentially depletes Langerhans cells from irradiated skin.[42] Langerhans cells play an important role in the immune response by presenting antigens to the immune cells, and, thus, depletion of these cells leads to local immunosuppression. In addition to local immunosuppression, UV light has been shown to promote systemic immunosuppression.[45] This response is complex, but it is known that UV-induced DNA lesions in skin cells contribute to the systemic immunosuppression response.[46] The secretion of the immunosuppressing cytokine interleukin (IL)-10 from irradiated keratinocytes as well as UV-induced structural alteration of the epidermal chromophore urocanic acid may mediate the long-range immunosuppressive effects of UV light.[42,45]

RADIOFREQUENCY AND MICROWAVE RADIATION

Radiofrequency radiation (RFR) is electromagnetic radiation in the frequency range 3 kHz to 300 MHz, whereas microwave radiation (MR) is in the frequency range between 300 MHz to 300 GHz. RFR and MR do not have sufficient energies to cause ionizations in target tissues. Rather, the radiation energy is converted into heat as the radiation energy is absorbed. Sources of radiofrequency and microwave radiation include mobile phones, radio transmitters of wireless communication, radars, medical devices, and kitchen appliances.

Mechanism of Damage Induction

Because human exposure to RFR has increased dramatically in recent years, it is important to know whether this type of radiation gives rise to genotoxic damage. Although there are many studies showing that RFR can induce ROS, leading to genetic damage in cell culture systems, other studies have generated conflicting results.[47] One confounding factor when assessing the genotoxic effect of RFR, and especially MR, is the heating effect that occurs in the tissue when the radiation energy is absorbed. A recent study controlling for the potential heating effect of exposure found that RFR induces ROS and DNA damage in human spermatozoa in vitro, which is an alarming finding considering the potential hereditary implications.[48] It has been suggested that MR may affect the folding of proteins in cells that promote new protein synthesis.[49] Furthermore, exposure of cells to MR has been shown to lead to the phosphorylation of numerous cellular proteins largely through the activation of the p38/MAPK stress response pathway.[50] However, the biologic consequences of these cellular changes are not clear. Epidemiology studies that monitored the genetic effects in individuals exposed to high levels of RF have revealed evidence of increased induction of chromosome aberrations in lymphocytes.[51] However, there is a level of uncertainty in these studies about exposure levels, making it difficult to come to meaningful conclusions.

Cancer Risks

Because the population's exposure to RFR and MR has dramatically increased in recent years, it is of great importance to assess the potential cancer risks of these types of radiation so that appropriate exposure limits can be implemented. A number of studies have focused on the potential cancer risks from mobile phone usage, and some of these studies indicate that long-term mobile phone usage may be associated with increased risks of developing brain tumors (see the following). Other epidemiologic studies of cancer incidences in populations living near radio towers or mobile phone base stations are inconclusive. Some studies have shown a connection between proximity to mobile phone base stations and increased cancer incidence,[52] whereas another study found no association between exposure to RFR from mobile phone base stations and early childhood cancers.[53]

ELECTROMAGNETIC FIELDS

An electromagnetic field (EMF) is a physical field produced by electrically charged objects that can affect other charged objects in the field. Typical sources of EMFs are electric power lines, electrical devices, and magnetic resonance imaging (MRI) machines.

Mechanisms of Damage Induction

A low frequency EMF does not transmit energy high enough to break chemical bonds; therefore, it is not thought to directly damage DNA or proteins in cells. The data obtained from studies to assess the potential genotoxic effects of EMF do not provide a clear conclusion. Some of the results obtained in cell culture studies suggest a harmful effect of EMFs, but the concerns are that these effects may be related to heat production induced by EMFs rather than from the magnetic field itself. A recent in vitro study detected DNA strand breaks in cells exposed to EMFs, but this induction was thought to not be the result of ROS production, but rather due to indirect effects through interference with DNA replication and induction of apoptosis in a subset of cells.[54] A study using an MRI found no evidence of an induced formation of DNA DSBs in cell cultures.[55] EMFs have been shown to induce nongenotoxic effects in cells, such as interference with cellular signaling pathways,[56] which could contribute to neurodegeneration.[57]

Cancer Risks

Studies with rodents have largely failed to detect an association between exposure to EMFs and cancer. This is also true for numerous epidemiology studies, with the only exception being the association between EMF exposure and childhood leukemia where children exposed to doses of 0.4 mcT or above may have about a twofold increased risk of developing leukemia.[58,59] There is no strong link between EMF exposure and increased risks of contracting adult leukemia, brain tumors, or breast cancer.[60,61] Furthermore, a study investigating whether EMF exposure was associated with heritable effects found no correlation between parental exposure and childhood cancer.[62]

Potential Cancer Risks from Mobile Phone Usage

Mobile phones emit RFR and generate EMFs. The biggest health concern with mobile phone usage is its potential role in the development of brain tumors. During mobile phone use, the brain tissue is exposed to doses, giving peak specific absorption rates (SAR) of 4 to 8 W/kg. At these intensities, the induction of DNA damage has been detected in laboratory studies.[63] The current epidemiologic data are largely inconclusive on the association between mobile phone usage and brain tumor incidence. Meta-analysis studies of populations who had used mobile phones for more than 10 years concluded that mobile phone usage was associated with an elevated risk for brain tumors, such as acoustic neuroma and glioma cancer.[64–66] In contrast, other large prospective studies did not observe a correlation between mobile phone usage and incidences of glioma, meningioma, or non–central nervous system (CNS) cancers.[67,68] It is important to point out that, generally, it takes 30 to 40 years for brain tumors to develop, and because mobile phones have only been in general use for about 15 years, there has not been sufficient time to fully evaluate the brain cancer risks of mobile phone usage.

ASBESTOS

Asbestos is a class of naturally occurring silicate minerals that have been widely used in building materials for its heat, sound, and electrical insulating qualities. Asbestos becomes a serious health hazard if the fibers are inhaled over a long period of time, and these health effects are increased dramatically if the exposed individual is a smoker. It was first reported in 1935 that asbestos might be an occupational health hazard that could induce cancer.[69,70] However, it was not until 1986 that the International Labor Organization recommended banning asbestos.[71] The use of asbestos products peaked in the 1970s, yet remains a major health hazard in many places around the world today.

Mechanisms of Damage Induction

Asbestos fibers can enter cells and induce ROS, especially if they contain high levels of iron.[72] In addition, ROS can be generated by "frustrated" phagocytosis, and this in turn can lead to the release of proinflammatory cytokines with subsequent inflammation of the tissue. ROS have been implicated to originate from affected mitochondria leading to induction of SSBs and base damage, such as 8-hydroxyguanine in DNA.[73] Furthermore, if not successfully repaired, asbestos-induced DNA damage has been shown to result in chromosome aberrations, micronuclei formation, and increased rates of sister chromatid exchanges.[74]

Cellular and Tissue Responses

Asbestos-induced ROS cause base lesions and DNA strand breaks, which require base excision repair for the restoration of DNA and for minimizing mutagenesis. In addition to DNA repair, a number of cellular signaling pathways are activated by asbestos. These include the epidermal growth factor receptor (EGFR) and the MAPK pathway, leading to the activation of nuclear factor kappa B

(NF-κB) and transcription factor AP-1.[72,74] Activation of the NF-κB pathway leads to the induction of proinflammatory genes such as tumor necrosis factor (TNF), *IL-6*, *IL-8*, and proliferation-promoting genes such as *c-Myc*, leading to inflammation and increased cell proliferation. Asbestos exposure also stimulates the expression of the transforming growth factor beta (TGF-β), which, in turn, stimulates fibrogenesis in exposed tissues.[74]

Cancer Risks

Lung Cancer

Epidemiologic studies have found a strong link between asbestos exposure and lung cancer.[74] It has been estimated that about 5% to 7% of all lung cancers are attributable to asbestos exposure, and asbestos and tobacco smoking act in synergy to induce lung cancer. Mutational spectra due to 8-hydroxyguanine lesions formed by ROS can be linked to asbestos exposure, and point mutations in the tumor suppressor genes *p53* and *p16/INK4A* and in the *KRAS* oncogene have been found in tumors from asbestos-exposed individuals.

Mesothelioma

After being taken up by lung tissues, asbestos fibers can translocate into the pleura, the body cavity that surrounds the lungs. The pleura are covered with a protective lining, the mesothelium, which consists of squamouslike epithelial cells. Mesothelial cells can internalize asbestos fibers, resulting in the induction of ROS and inflammatory responses, subsequently leading to the initiation and progression of malignant mesothelioma.[75] Asbestos is considered one of the major causes of malignant mesothelioma, and frequent mutations are found in the *p16/INK4A* and *NF2* genes, whereas *p53* mutations are fairly rare.

NANOPARTICLES

Nanoparticles are defined as ultrafine particles of the size range 1 to 100 nm in diameter. Nanoparticle chemistry of a certain compound is different from bulk chemistry of that compound because of the high percentage of atoms at the surface of the particle. The production of nanoparticles has increased dramatically in recent years, and they are found in many industrial and consumer products such as paint, cosmetics, and sunscreens. They also have many potential medical applications, such as delivery vehicles for specific drugs to specific target tissues or tumors.

Mechanisms of DNA Damage Induction

Many of the cellular effects of nanoparticles are similar to the effects exerted by asbestos, such as the generation of ROS and inflammation.[72] Nanoparticles have been shown to induce oxidative DNA damage, such as DNA strand breaks and 8-hydroxyguanine lesions both in cell culture[76, 77] and in vivo.[78] Nanoparticle-induced DNA lesions are manifested as histone γ-H2AX nuclear foci, chromosome deletions, and micronuclei.

Cellular Responses

Nanoparticles induce ROS either directly or indirectly, resulting in DNA lesions, such as 8-hydroxyguanine–base damage and DNA strand breaks. These lesions are repaired by the base excision repair. The phosphorylation of histone H2AX has been shown to occur following exposure of cells to nanoparticles, suggesting that the DNA lesions trigger the activation of ATM or ATR stress kinases.[79] Nanoparticles have also been found to affect the immune system[80] and can induce the release of the proinflammatory cytokine TNF-α from cells.

Cancer Risks

Some nanoparticles, such as titanium dioxide, which is used as pigments in paint, have been classified by the International Agency for Research on Cancer (IARC) as a group 2B carcinogen, "possible carcinogenic to humans." However, rigorous epidemiologic data is lacking to fully evaluate the cancer-inducing potential of nanoparticles.[81]

REFERENCES

1. Hall E, Giaccia A. *Radiobiology for the Radiologist*. Philadelphia: Lippincott Williams & Wilkins; 2012.
2. Ward JF. DNA damage produced by ionizing radiation in mammalian cells: identities, mechanisms of formation, and repairability. *Prog Nucleic Acid Res Mol Biol* 1988;35:95–125.
3. Prutz WA. 'Chemical repair' in irradiated DNA solutions containing thiols and/or disulphides. Further evidence for disulphide radical anions acting as electron donors. *Int J Radiat Biol* 1989;56:21–33.
4. Hutchinson F. Chemical changes induced in DNA by ionizing radiation. *Prog Nucleic Acid Res Mol Biol* 1985;32:115–154.
5. Friedberg E, Walker G, Siede W, et al. *DNA Repair and Mutagenesis*. 2nd ed. Washington, D.C.: ASM Press; 2006.
6. Radford IR. The level of induced DNA double-strand breakage correlates with cell killing after X-irradiation. *Int J Radiat Biol Relat Stud Phys Chem Med* 1985;48:45–54.
7. Daly MJ. A new perspective on radiation resistance based on *Deinococcus radiodurans*. *Nat Rev Microbiol* 2009;7:237–245.
8. Krisko A, Radman M. Biology of extreme radiation resistance: the way of *Deinococcus radiodurans*. *Cold Spring Harb Perspect Biol* 2013;5.
9. Matsuoka S, Ballif BA, Smogorzewska A, et al. ATM and ATR substrate analysis reveals extensive protein networks responsive to DNA damage. *Science* 2007;316:1160–1166.
10. Kastan M, Onyekwere O, Sidransky D, et al. Participation of p53 protein in the cellular response to DNA damage. *Cancer Res* 1991;51:6304–6311.
11. Matsuoka S, Huang M, Elledge SJ. Linkage of ATM to cell cycle regulation by the Chk2 protein kinase. *Science* 1998;282:1893–1897.
12. Harper J, Adami G, Wei N, et al. The p21 cdk-interacting protein Cip1 is a potent inhibitor of G1 cyclin-dependent kinases. *Cell* 1993;75:805–816.
13. El-Deiry W, Tokino T, Velculescu V, et al. WAF1, a potential mediater of p53 tumor suppression. *Cell* 1993;75:817–825.
14. Falck J, Mailand N, Syljuasen RG, et al. The ATM-Chk2-Cdc25A checkpoint pathway guards against radioresistant DNA synthesis. *Nature* 2001;410:842–847.
15. Bartek J, Falck J, Lukas J. Chk2 kinase—a busy messenger [Review]. *Nat Rev Mol Cell Biol* 2001;2:877–886.
16. Savitsky K, Bar-Shira A, Gilad S, et al. A single ataxia telangiectasia gene with a product similar to PI-3 kinase. *Science* 1995;268:1749–1753.
17. Srivastava S, Zou ZQ, Pirollo K, et al. Germ-line transmission of a mutated p53 gene in a cancer-prone family with Li-Fraumeni syndrome. *Nature*.1990;348:747–749.
18. Gudkov AV, Komarova EA. The role of p53 in determining sensitivity to radiotherapy. *Nat Rev Cancer* 2003;3:117–129.
19. Mihara M, Erster S, Zaika A, et al. p53 has a direct apoptogenic role at the mitochondria. *Mol Cell* 2003;11:577–590.
20. Williams D, Baverstock K. Chernobyl and the future: too soon for a final diagnosis. *Nature* 2006;440:993–994.
21. Thompson DE, Mabuchi K, Ron E, et al. Cancer incidence in atomic bomb survivors. Part II: Solid tumors, 1958–1987. *Radiat Res* 1994;137:S17–67.
22. Williams D. Cancer after nuclear fallout: lessons from the Chernobyl accident. *Nat Rev Cancer* 2002;2:543–549.
23. Ricarte-Filho JC, Li S, Garcia-Rendueles ME, et al. Identification of kinase fusion oncogenes in post-Chernobyl radiation-induced thyroid cancers. *J Clin Invest* 2013;123:4935–4944.
24. National Research Council. *Health Risks from Exposure to Low Levels of Ionizing Radiation: BEIR VII Phase 2*. Washington, D.C.: National Academy Press; 2006.
25. Ljungman M, Zhang F. Blockage of RNA polymerase as a possible trigger for u.v. light-induced apoptosis. *Oncogene*.1996;13:823–831.
26. Brash DE, Wikonkal NM, Remenyik E, et al. The DNA damage signal for Mdm2 regulation, Trp53 induction, and sunburn cell formation in vivo originates from actively transcribed genes. *J Invest Derm* 2001;117: 1234–1240.

27. Hanawalt PC, Spivak G. Transcription-coupled DNA repair: two decades of progress and surprises. *Nat Rev Mol Cell Biol* 2008;9:958–970.
28. Lehmann AR. DNA repair-deficient diseases, xeroderma pigmentosum, Cockayne syndrome and trichothiodystrophy. *Biochimie* 2003;85:1101–1111.
29. Andressoo JO, Hoeijmakers JH. Transcription-coupled repair and premature ageing. *Mutat Res* 2005;577:179–194.
30. de Boer J, Andressoo JO, de Wit J, et al. Premature aging in mice deficient in DNA repair and transcription. *Science* 2002;296:1276–1279.
31. Garinis GA, Uittenboogaard LM, Stachelscheid H, et al. Persistent transcription-blocking DNA lesions trigger somatic growth attenuation associated with longevity. *Nat Cell Biol* 2009;11:604–615.
32. Derheimer FA, O'Hagan HM, Krueger HM, et al. RPA and ATR link transcriptional stress to p53. *Proc Natl Acad Sci U S A* 2007;104:12778–12783.
33. Kastan MB, Bartek J. Cell-cycle checkpoints and cancer. *Nature* 2004;432:316–323.
34. Gross S, Knebel A, Tenev T, et al. Inactivation of protein-tyrosine phosphatases as mechanism of UV-induced signal transduction. *J Biol Chem* 1999;274:26378–26386.
35. Sachsenmaier C, Radlerpohl A, Zinck R, et al. Involvement of growth factor receptors in the mammalian UVC response. *Cell* 1994;78:963–972.
36. Rehemtulla A, Hamilton CA, Chinnaiyan AM, et al. Ultraviolet radiation-induced apoptosis is mediated by activation of CD-95 (Fas/APO-1). *J Biol Chem* 1997;272:25783–25786.
37. Ljungman M, Lane DP. Transcription - guarding the genome by sensing DNA damage. *Nat Rev Cancer* 2004;4:727–737.
38. Ziegler A, Jonason AS, Leffell DJ, et al. Sunburn and p53 in the onset of skin cancer. *Nature* 1994;372:773–776.
39. McKay B, Ljungman M. Role for p53 in the recovery of transcription and protection against apoptosis induced by ultraviolet light. *Neoplasia* 1999;1:276–284.
40. Chaturvedi V, Sitailo LA, Qin JZ, et al. Knockdown of p53 levels in human keratinocytes accelerates Mcl-1 and Bcl-x(L) reduction thereby enhancing UV-light induced apoptosis. *Oncogene* 2005;24:5299–5312.
41. Maddodi N, Setaluri V. Role of UV in cutaneous melanoma. *Photochem Photobiol* 2008;84:528–536.
42. Murphy GM. Ultraviolet radiation and immunosuppression. *Br J Dermatol* 2009;161(Suppl 3):90–95.
43. Fisher MS, Kripke ML. Systemic alteration induced in mice by ultraviolet light irradiation and its relationship to ultraviolet carcinogenesis. *Proc Natl Acad Sci U S A* 1977;74:1688–1692.
44. Pleasance ED, Cheetham RK, Stephens PJ, et al. A comprehensive catalogue of somatic mutations from a human cancer genome. *Nature* 2010;463:191–196.
45. Schwarz T. Photoimmunosuppression. *Photodermatol Photoimmunol Photomed* 2002;18:141–145.
46. Kripke ML, Cox PA, Alas LG, et al. Pyrimidine dimers in DNA initiate systemic immunosuppression in UV-irradiated mice. *Proc Natl Acad Sci U S A* 1992;89:7516–7520.
47. Vijayalaxmi, Prihoda TJ. Genetic damage in mammalian somatic cells exposed to radiofrequency radiation: a meta-analysis of data from 63 publications (1990–2005). *Radiat Res* 2008;169:561–574.
48. De Iuliis GN, Newey RJ, King BV, et al. Mobile phone radiation induces reactive oxygen species production and DNA damage in human spermatozoa in vitro. *PLoS One* 2009;4:e6446.
49. Gerner C, Haudek V, Schandl U, et al. Increased protein synthesis by cells exposed to a 1,800-MHz radio-frequency mobile phone electromagnetic field, detected by proteome profiling. *Int Arch Occup Environ Health* 2010;83: 691–702.
50. Leszczynski D, Joenvaara S, Reivinen J, et al. Non-thermal activation of the hsp27/p38MAPK stress pathway by mobile phone radiation in human endothelial cells: molecular mechanism for cancer and blood brain barrier related effects. *Differentiation* 2002;70:120–129.
51. Verschaeve L. Genetic damage in subjects exposed to radiofrequency radiation. *Mutat Res* 2009;681:259–270.
52. Khurana VG, Hardell L, Everaert J, et al. Epidemiological evidence for a health risk from mobile phone base stations. *Int J Occup Environ Health* 2010;16:263–267.
53. Elliott P, Toledano MB, Bennett J, et al. Mobile phone base stations and early childhood cancers: case-control study. *BMJ* 2010;340:c3077.
54. Focke F, Schuermann D, Kuster N, et al. DNA fragmentation in human fibroblasts under extremely low frequency electromagnetic field exposure. *Mutat Res* 2010;683:74–83.
55. Schwenzer NF, Bantleon R, Maurer B, et al. Detection of DNA double-strand breaks using gammaH2AX after MRI exposure at 3 Tesla: an in vitro study. *J Magn Reson Imaging* 2007;26:1308–1314.
56. Girgert R, Hanf V, Emons G, et al. Signal transduction of the melatonin receptor MT1 is disrupted in breast cancer cells by electromagnetic fields. *Bioelectromagnetics* 2010;31:237–245.
57. Consales C, Merla C, Marino C, et al. Electromagnetic fields, oxidative stress, and neurodegeneration. *Int J Cell Biol* 2012;2012:683897.
58. Ahlbom A, Day N, Feychting M, et al. A pooled analysis of magnetic fields and childhood leukaemia. *Br J Cancer* 2000;83:692–698.
59. Malagoli C, Fabbi S, Teggi S, et al. Risk of hematological malignancies associated with magnetic fields exposure from power lines: a case-control study in two municipalities of northern Italy. *Environ Health* 2010;9:16.
60. Kheifets L, Monroe J, Vergara X, et al. Occupational electromagnetic fields and leukemia and brain cancer: an update to two meta-analyses. *J Occup Environ Med* 2008;50:677–688.
61. Chen C, Ma X, Zhong M, et al. Extremely low-frequency electromagnetic fields exposure and female breast cancer risk: a meta-analysis based on 24,338 cases and 60,628 controls. *Breast Cancer Res Treat* 2010;123:569–576.
62. Hug K, Grize L, Seidler A, et al. Parental occupational exposure to extremely low frequency magnetic fields and childhood cancer: a German case-control study. *Am J Epidemiol* 2010;171:27–35.
63. Hardell L, Sage C. Biological effects from electromagnetic field exposure and public exposure standards. *Biomed Pharmacother* 2008;62:104–109.
64. Hardell L, Carlberg M, Hansson Mild K. Mobile phone use and the risk for malignant brain tumors: a case-control study on deceased cases and controls. *Neuroepidemiology* 2010;35:109–114.
65. Hardell L, Carlberg M, Soderqvist F, et al. Meta-analysis of long-term mobile phone use and the association with brain tumours. *Int J Oncol* 2008;32: 1097–1103.
66. Myung SK, Ju W, McDonnell DD, et al. Mobile phone use and risk of tumors: a meta-analysis. *J Clin Oncol* 2009;27:5565–5572.
67. Benson VS, Pirie K, Schuz J, et al. Mobile phone use and risk of brain neoplasms and other cancers: prospective study. *Int J Epidemiol* 2013;42: 792–802.
68. Poulsen AH, Friis S, Johansen C, et al. Mobile phone use and the risk of skin cancer: a nationwide cohort study in Denmark. *Am J Epidemiol* 2013;178: 190–197.
69. Lynch K, Smith W. Pulmonary asbestosis. III. Carcinoma of lung in asbestos-silicosis. *Am J Cancer* 1935;24:56–64.
70. Gloyne S. Two cases of squamous carcinoma of the lung occuring in asbestosis. *Tubercele* 1935;17:5–10.
71. LaDou J. The asbestos cancer epidemic. *Environ Health Perspect* 2004;112: 285–290.
72. Pacurari M, Castranova V, Vallyathan V. Single- and multi-wall carbon nanotubes versus asbestos: are the carbon nanotubes a new health risk to humans? *J Toxicol Environ Health A* 2010;73:378–395.
73. Liu G, Cheresh P, Kamp DW. Molecular basis of asbestos-induced lung disease. *Annu Rev Pathol* 2013;8:161–187.
74. Nymark P, Wikman H, Hienonen-Kempas T, et al. Molecular and genetic changes in asbestos-related lung cancer. *Cancer Lett* 2008;265:1–15.
75. Jaurand MC, Renier A, Daubriac J. Mesothelioma: do asbestos and carbon nanotubes pose the same health risk? *Part Fibre Toxicol* 2009;6:16.
76. Shukla RK, Kumar A, Gurbani D, et al. TiO(2) nanoparticles induce oxidative DNA damage and apoptosis in human liver cells. *Nanotoxicology* 2013;7: 48–60.
77. Horie M, Nishio K, Endoh S, et al. Chromium(III) oxide nanoparticles induced remarkable oxidative stress and apoptosis on culture cells. *Environ Toxicol* 2013;28:61–75.
78. Trouiller B, Reliene R, Westbrook A, et al. Titanium dioxide nanoparticles induce DNA damage and genetic instability in vivo in mice. *Cancer Res* 2009;69:8784–8789.
79. Prasad RY, Chastain PD, Nikolaishvili-Feinberg N, et al. Titanium dioxide nanoparticles activate the ATM-Chk2 DNA damage response in human dermal fibroblasts. *Nanotoxicology* 2013;7:1111–1119.
80. Zolnik BS, Gonzalez-Fernandez A, Sadrieh N, et al. Nanoparticles and the immune system. *Endocrinology* 2010;151:458–465.
81. Shi H, Magaye R, Castranova V, et al. Titanium dioxide nanoparticles: a review of current toxicological data. *Part Fibre Toxicol* 2013;10:15.

9 Dietary Factors

Karin B. Michels and Walter C. Willett

INTRODUCTION

Over two decades ago, Doll and Peto[1] speculated that 35% (range: 10% to 70%) of all cancer deaths in the United States may be preventable by alterations in diet. The magnitude of the estimate for dietary factors exceeded that for tobacco (30%) and infections (10%).

Studies of cancer incidence among populations migrating to countries with different lifestyle factors have indicated that most cancers have a large environmental etiology. Although the contribution of environmental influences differs by cancer type, the incidence of many cancers changes by as much as five- to tenfold among migrants over time, approaching that of the host country. The age at migration affects the degree of adaptation among first-generation migrants for some cancers, suggesting that the susceptibility to environmental carcinogenic influences varies with age by cancer type. Identifying the specific environmental and lifestyle factors most important to cancer etiology, however, has proven difficult.

Environmental factors such as diet may influence the incidence of cancer through many different mechanisms and at different stages in the cancer process. Simple mutagens in foods, such as those produced by the heating of proteins, can cause damage to DNA, but dietary factors can also influence this process by inducing enzymes that activate or inactivate these mutagens, or by blocking the action of the mutagen. Dietary factors can also affect every pathway hypothesized to mediate cancer risk–for example, the rate of cell cycling through hormonal or antihormonal effects, aiding or inhibiting DNA repair, promoting or inhibiting apoptosis, and DNA methylation. Because of the complexity of these mechanisms, knowledge of dietary influences on risk of cancer will require an empirical basis with human cancer as the outcome.

METHODOLOGIC CHALLENGES

Study Types and Biases

The association between diet and the risk of cancer has been the subject of a number of epidemiologic studies. The most prevalent designs are the case-control study, the cohort study, and the randomized clinical trial. When the results from epidemiologic studies are interpreted, the potential for confounding must be considered. Individuals who maintain a healthy diet are likely to exhibit other indicators of a healthy lifestyle, including regular physical activity, lower body weight, use of multivitamin supplements, lower smoking rates, and lower alcohol consumption. Even if the influence of these confounding variables is analytically controlled, residual confounding remains possible.

Ecologic Studies

In ecologic studies or international correlation studies, variation in food disappearance data and the prevalence of a certain disease are correlated, generally across different countries. A linear association may provide preliminary data to inform future research but, due to the high probability of confounding, cannot provide strong evidence for a causal link. Food disappearance data also may not provide a good estimate for human consumption. The gross national product is correlated with many dietary factors such as fat intake.[2] Many other differences besides dietary fat exist between the countries with low fat consumption (less affluent) and high fat consumption (more affluent); reproductive behaviors, physical activity level, and body fatness are particularly notable and are strongly associated with specific cancers.

Migrant Studies

Studies of populations migrating from areas with low incidence of disease to areas with high incidence of disease (or vice versa) can help sort out the role of environmental factors versus genetics in the etiology of a cancer, depending on whether the migrating group adopts the cancer rates of the new environment. Specific dietary components linked to disease are difficult to identify in a migrant study.

Case-Control Studies

Case-control studies of diet may be affected by recall bias, control selection bias, and confounding. In a case-control study, participants affected by the disease under study (cases) and healthy controls are asked to recall their past dietary habits. Cases may overestimate their consumption of foods that are commonly considered "unhealthy" and underestimate their consumption of foods considered "healthy." Giovannucci et al.[3] have documented differential reporting of fat intake before and after disease occurrence. Thus, the possibility of recall bias in a case-control study poses a real threat to the validity of the observed associations. Even more importantly, in contemporary case-control studies using a population sample of controls, the participation rate of controls is usually far from complete, often 50% to 70%. Unfortunately, health-conscious individuals may be more likely to participate as controls and will thus be less overweight, will consume fruits and vegetables more frequently, and will consume less fat and red meat, which can substantially distort associations observed.

Cohort Studies

Prospective cohort studies of the effects of diet are likely to have a much higher validity than retrospective case-control studies because diet is recorded by participants before disease occurrence. Cohort studies are still affected by measurement error because diet consists of a large number of foods eaten in complex combinations. Confounding by other unmeasured or imperfectly measured lifestyle factors can remain a problem in cohort studies.

Now that the results of a substantial number of cohort studies have become available, their findings can be compared with those of case-control studies that have examined the same relations. In many cases, the findings of the case-control studies have not been confirmed; for example, the consistent finding of lower risk of many cancers with higher intake of fruits and vegetables in case-control studies has generally not been seen in cohort studies.[4] These findings suggest that the concerns about biases in case-control studies of diet, and probably many other lifestyle factors, are justified, and findings from such studies must be interpreted cautiously.

Randomized Clinical Trials

The gold standard in medical research is the randomized clinical trial (RCT). In an RCT on nutrition, participants are randomly assigned to one of two or more diets; hence, the association between diet and the cancer of interest should not be confounded by other factors. The problem with RCTs of diet is that maintaining the assigned diet strictly over many years, as would be necessary for diet to have an impact on cancer incidence, is difficult. For example, in the dietary fat reduction trial of the Women's Health Initiative (WHI), participants randomized to the intervention arm reduced their fat intake much less than planned.[5] The remaining limited contrast between the two groups left the lack of difference in disease outcomes difficult to interpret. Furthermore, the relevant time window for intervention and the necessary duration of intervention are unclear, especially with cancer outcomes. Hence, randomized trials are rarely used to examine the effect of diet on cancer but have better promise for the study of diet and outcomes that require a considerably shorter follow-up time (e.g., adenoma recurrence). Also, the randomized design may lend itself better to the study of the effects of dietary supplements such as multivitamin or fiber supplements, although the control group may adopt the intervention behavior because nutritional supplements are widely available. For example, in the WHI trial of calcium and vitamin D supplementation, two-thirds of the study population used vitamin D or calcium supplements that they obtained outside of the trial, again rendering the lack of effect in the trial uninterpretable.

Diet Assessment Instruments

Observational studies depend on a reasonably valid assessment of dietary intake. Although, for some nutrients, biochemical measurements can be used to assess intake, for most dietary constituents, a useful biochemical indicator does not exist. In population-based studies, diet is generally assessed with a self-administered instrument. Since 1980, considerable effort has been directed at the development of standardized questionnaires for measuring diet, and numerous studies have been conducted to assess the validity of these methods. The most widely used diet assessment instruments are the food frequency questionnaire, the 7-day diet record, and the 24-hour recall. Although the 7-day diet record may provide the most accurate documentation of intake during the week the participant keeps a diet diary, the burden of computerizing the information and extracting foods and nutrients has prohibited the use of the 7-day diet record in most large-scale studies. The 24-hour recall provides only a snapshot of diet on one day, which may or may not be representative of the participant's usual diet and is thus affected by both personal variation and seasonal variation. The food frequency questionnaire, the most widely used instrument in large population-based studies, asks participants to report their average intake of a large number of foods during the previous year. Participants tend to substantially overreport their fruit and vegetable consumption on the food frequency questionnaire.[6] This tendency may reflect social desirability bias, which leads to overreporting healthy foods and underreporting less healthy foods. Studies of validity using biomarkers or detailed measurements of diet as comparisons have suggested that carefully designed questionnaires can have sufficient validity to detect moderate to strong associations. Validity can be enhanced by using the average of repeated assessments over time.[7]

THE ROLE OF INDIVIDUAL FOOD AND NUTRIENTS IN CANCER ETIOLOGY

Energy

The most important impact of diet on the risk of cancer is mediated through body weight. Overweight, obesity, and inactivity are major contributors to cancer risk. (A more detailed discussion is provided in Chapter 10.) In the large American Cancer Society Cohort, obese individuals had substantially higher mortality from all cancers and, in particular, from colorectal cancer, postmenopausal breast cancer, uterine cancer, cervical cancer, pancreatic cancer, and gallbladder cancer than their normal-weight counterparts.[8] Adiposity and, in particular, waist circumference are predictors of colon cancer incidence among women and men.[9,10] A weight gain of 10 kg or more is associated with a significant increase in postmenopausal breast cancer incidence among women who never used hormone replacement therapy, whereas a weight loss of comparable magnitude after menopause substantially decreases breast cancer risk.[11] Regular physical activity contributes to a lower prevalence of being overweight and obesity and consequently reduces the burden of cancer through this pathway.

The mechanisms whereby adiposity increases the risk of various cancers are probably multiple. Being overweight is strongly associated with endogenous estrogen levels, which likely contribute to the excess risks of endometrial and postmenopausal breast cancers. The reasons for the association with other cancers are less clear, but excess body fat is also related to higher circulating levels of insulin, insulin-like growth factor (IGF)-1, and C-peptide (a marker of insulin secretion), lower levels of binding proteins for sex hormones and IGF-1, and higher levels of various inflammatory factors, all of which have been hypothesized to be related to risks of various cancers.

Energy restriction is one of the most effective measures to prevent cancer in the animal model. While energy restriction is more difficult to study in humans, voluntary starvation among anorectics and situations of food rationing during famines provide related models. Breast cancer rates were substantially reduced among women with a history of severe anorexia.[12] Although breast cancer incidence was higher among women exposed to the Dutch famine during childhood or adolescence, such short-term involuntary food rationing for 9 months or less was often followed by overnutrition.[13] A more prolonged deficit in food availability during World War II in Norway was associated with a reduction in adult risk of breast cancer if it occurred during early adolescence.[14]

Alcohol

Aside from body weight, alcohol consumption is the best established dietary risk factor for cancer. Alcohol is classified as a carcinogen by the International Agency for Research on Cancer. The consumption of alcohol increases the risk of numerous cancers, including those of the liver, esophagus, pharynx, oral cavity, larynx, breast, and colorectum in a dose-dependent fashion.[15] Evidence is convincing that excessive alcohol consumption increases the risk of primary liver cancer, probably through cirrhosis and alcoholic hepatitis. At least in the developed world, about 75% of cancers of the esophagus, pharynx, oral cavity, and larynx are attributable to alcohol and tobacco, with a marked increase in risk among drinkers who also smoke, suggesting a multiplicative effect. Mechanisms may include direct damage to the cells in the upper gastrointestinal tract; modulation of DNA methylation, which affects susceptibility to DNA mutations; and an increase in acetaldehyde, the main metabolite of alcohol, which enhances the proliferation of epithelial cells, forms DNA adducts, and is a recognized carcinogen. The association between alcohol consumption and breast cancer is notable because a small but significant risk has been found even with one drink per day. Mechanisms may include an interaction with folate, an increase in endogenous estrogen levels, and an elevation of acetaldehyde. Some evidence suggests that the excess risk is mitigated by adequate folate intake possibly through an effect on DNA methylation.[16] Notably, for most cancer sites, no important difference in associations was found with the type of alcoholic beverage, suggesting a critical role of ethanol in carcinogenesis.

Dietary Fat

In recent years, reducing dietary fat has been at the center of cancer prevention efforts. In the landmark 1982 National Academy of Sciences review of diet, nutrition, and cancer, a reduction in fat intake to 30% of calories was the primary recommendation.

Interest in dietary fat as a cause of cancer began in the first half of the 20th century, when studies by Tannenbaum[17] indicated that diets high in fat could promote tumor growth in animal models. Dietary fat has a clear effect on tumor incidence in many models, although not in all; however, a central issue has been whether this is independent of the effect of energy intake. In the 1970s, the possible relation of dietary fat intake to cancer incidence gained greater attention as the large international differences in rates of many cancers were noted to be strongly correlated with apparent per capita fat consumption in ecologic studies.[2] Particularly strong associations were seen with cancers of the breast, colon, prostate, and endometrium, which include the most important cancers not due to smoking in affluent countries. These correlations were observed to be limited to animal, not vegetable, fat.

Dietary Fat and Breast Cancer

Breast cancer is the most common malignancy among women, and incidence has been increasing for decades, although a decline has been noted starting with the new millennium. Rates in most parts of Asia, South America, and Africa have been only approximately one-fifth that of the United States, but in almost all these areas rates of breast cancer are also increasing. Populations that migrate from low- to high-incidence countries develop breast cancer rates that approximate those of the new host country. However, rates do not approach those of the general US population until the second or third generation.[18] This slower rate of change for immigrants may indicate delayed acculturation; although because a similar delay in rate increase is not observed for colon cancer, it may suggest an origin of breast cancer earlier in the life course.

The results from 12 smaller case-control studies that included 4,312 cases and 5,978 controls have been summarized in a meta-analysis.[19] The pooled relative risk (RR) was 1.35 (P <.0001) for a 100-g increase in daily total fat intake, although the risk was somewhat stronger for postmenopausal women (RR, 1.48; P <.001). This magnitude of association, however, could be compatible with biases due to recall of diet or the selection of controls.

Because of the prospective design of cohort studies, most of the methodologic biases of case-control studies are avoided. In an analysis of the Nurses' Health Study that included 121,700 US female registered nurses, no association with total fat intake was observed, and there was no suggestion of any reduction in risk at intakes below 25% of energy.[20] Because repeated assessments of diet were obtained at 2- to 4-year intervals, this analysis provided a particularly detailed evaluation of fat intake over an extended period in relation to breast cancer risk. Similar observations were made in the National Institutes of Health (NIH)–American Association of Retired Persons (AARP) Diet and Health Study including 188,736 postmenopausal women[21] and in the European Prospective Investigation into Cancer and Nutrition (EPIC), which included 7,119 incident cases.[22] In a pooled analysis of seven prospective studies, which included 337,000 women who developed 4,980 incident cases of breast cancer, no overall association was seen for fat intake over the range of less than 20% to more than 45% energy (reflecting the current range observed internationally).[23] A similar lack of association was seen for specific types of fat. This lack of association with total fat intake was confirmed in a subsequent analysis of the pooled prospective studies of diet and breast cancer, which included over 7,000 cases.[24] Therefore, these cohort findings do not support the hypothesis that dietary fat is an important contributor to breast cancer incidence.

Endogenous estrogen levels have now been established as a risk factor for breast cancer. Thus, the effects of fat and other dietary factors on estrogen levels are of potential interest. Vegetarian women, who consume higher amounts of fiber and lower amounts of fat, have lower blood levels and reduced urinary excretion of estrogens, apparently due to increased fecal excretion. A meta-analysis has suggested that a reduction in dietary fat reduces plasma estrogen levels,[25] but the studies included were plagued by the lack of concurrent controls, the short duration, and the negative energy balance. In a large, randomized trial among postmenopausal women with a previous diagnosis of breast cancer, a reduction in dietary fat did not affect estradiol levels when the data were appropriately analyzed.[26]

The WHI Randomized Controlled Dietary Modification Trial similarly suggested no association between fat intake and breast cancer incidence,[5] but these results are difficult to interpret.[27] The data on biomarkers that reflect fat intake suggest little if any difference in fat intake between the intervention and control groups.[28] Even if dietary fat does truly have an effect on cancer incidence and other outcomes, this lack of adherence to the dietary intervention could explain the absence of an observed effect on total cancer incidence and total mortality. In another randomized trial in Canada that tested an intervention target of 15% of calories from fat, a small but significant difference in high-density lipoprotein (HDL) levels was observed after 8 to 9 years of follow-up suggesting a difference in fat intake in the two groups.[29] The incidence of breast cancer in the intervention and the control group did not differ significantly.

Some prospective cohort studies suggest an inverse association between monounsaturated fat and breast cancer. This is an intriguing observation because of the relatively low rates of breast cancer in southern European countries with high intakes of monounsaturated fats due to the use of olive oil as the primary fat. In case-control studies in Spain, Greece, and Italy, women who used more olive oil had reduced risks of breast cancer.

In a report of findings from the Nurses' Health Study II cohort of premenopausal women, a higher intake of animal fat was associated with an approximately 50% greater risk of breast cancer, but no association was seen with intake of vegetable fat.[30] This suggests that factors in foods containing animal fats, rather than fat per se, may account for the findings. In the same cohort, an intake of red meat and total fat during adolescence was also associated with the risk of premenopausal breast cancer.[31,32]

Dietary Fat and Colon Cancer

In comparisons among countries, rates of colon cancer are strongly correlated with a national per capita disappearance of animal fat and meat, with correlation coefficients ranging between 0.8 and 0.9.[2] Rates of colon cancer rose sharply in Japan after World War II, paralleling a 2.5-fold increase in fat intake. Based on these epidemiologic investigations and on animal studies, a hypothesis has developed that higher dietary fat increases the excretion of bile acids, which can be converted to carcinogens or act as promoters. However, evidence from many studies on obesity and low levels of physical activity increasing the risk of colon cancer suggests that at least part of the high rates in affluent countries previously attributed to fat intake is probably due to a sedentary lifestyle.

The Nurses' Health Study suggested an approximately twofold higher risk of colon cancer among women in the highest quintile of animal fat intake than in those in the lowest quintile.[33] In a multivariate analysis of these data, which included red meat intake and animal fat intake in the same model, red meat intake remained significantly predictive of colon cancer risk, whereas the association with animal fat was eliminated. Other cohort studies have supported associations of colon cancer and the consumption of red meat and processed meats but not other sources of fat or total fat.[34–36] Similar associations were also observed for colorectal adenomas. In a meta-analysis of prospective studies, red meat consumption was associated with a risk of colon cancer (RR = 1.24; 95% confidence interval [CI], 1.09 to 1.41 for an increment of 120 g per day).[37] The association with the consumption of processed meats was particularly strong (RR = 1.36; 95% CI, 1.15 to 1.61 for an increment of 30 g per day).

The apparently stronger association with red meat consumption than with fat intake in most large cohort studies needs further confirmation, but such an association could result if the fatty acids or nonfat components of meat (e.g., the heme iron or carcinogens created by cooking) were the primary etiologic factors. This issue has major practical implications because current dietary recommendations support the daily consumption of red meat as long as it is lean.[38]

Dietary Fat and Prostate Cancer

Although further data are desirable, the evidence from international correlations, case-control[39] and cohort studies[40–44] provides some support for an association between the consumption of fat-containing animal products and prostate cancer incidence. This evidence does not generally support a relation with intake of vegetable fat, which suggests that either the type of fat or other components of animal products are responsible. Some evidence also indicates that animal fat consumption may be most strongly associated with the incidence of aggressive prostate cancer, which suggests an influence on the transition from the widespread indolent form to the more lethal form of this malignancy. Data are limited on the relation of fat intake to the probability of survival after the diagnosis of prostate cancer.

Dietary Fat and Other Cancers

Rates of other cancers that are common in affluent countries, including those of the endometrium and ovary, are also correlated with fat intake internationally. In prospective studies between Iowa and Canadian women, no evidence of a relation between fat intake and risk of endometrial cancer was found. Positive associations between dietary fat and lung cancer have been observed in many case-control studies. However, in a pooled analysis of large prospective studies that included over 3,000 incident cases, no association was observed.[45] These findings provide further evidence that the results of case-control studies of diet and cancer are likely to be misleading.

Summary

Largely on the basis of the results of animal studies, international correlations, and a few case-control studies, great enthusiasm developed in the 1980s that modest reductions in total fat intake would have a major impact on breast cancer incidence. As the findings from large prospective studies have become available, however, support for this relation has greatly weakened. Although evidence suggests that a high intake of animal fat early in adult life may increase the risk of premenopausal breast cancer, this is not likely to be due to fat per se because vegetable fat intake was not related to risk. For colon cancer, the associations seen with animal fat intake internationally have been supported in numerous case-control and cohort studies, but this also appears to be explained by factors in red meat other than simply its fat content. Further, the importance of physical activity and leanness as protective factors against colon cancer indicates that international correlations probably overstate the contribution of diet to differences in colon cancer incidence. At present, the available evidence most strongly suggests an association between animal fat consumption and risk of prostate cancer, particularly the aggressive form of this disease. As with colon cancer, the possibility remains that other factors in animal products contribute to risk.

Despite the large body of data on dietary fat and cancer that has accumulated since 1985, any conclusions should be regarded as tentative, because these are disease processes that are poorly understood and are likely to take many decades to develop. Because most of the reported literature from prospective studies is based on fewer than 20 years' follow-up, further evaluations of the effects of diet earlier in life and at longer intervals of observation are needed to fully understand these complex relations. Nevertheless, persons interested in reducing their risk of cancer could be advised, as a prudent measure, to minimize their intake of foods high in animal fat, particularly red meat. Such a dietary pattern is also likely to be beneficial for the risk of cardiovascular disease. On the other hand, unsaturated fats (with the exception of *transfatty* acids) reduce blood low-density lipoprotein cholesterol levels and the risk of cardiovascular disease, and little evidence suggests that they adversely affect cancer risk. Thus, efforts to reduce unsaturated fat intake are not warranted at this time and are likely to have adverse effects on cardiovascular disease risk. Because excess adiposity increases the risk of several cancers and cardiovascular disease, balancing calories from any source with adequate physical activity is extremely important.

Fruits and Vegetables

General Properties

Fruits and vegetables have been hypothesized to be major dietary contributors to cancer prevention because they are rich in potential anticarcinogenic substances. Fruits and vegetables contain antioxidants and minerals and are good sources of fiber, potassium, carotenoids, vitamin C, folate, and other vitamins. Although fruits and vegetables supply less than 5% of total energy intake in most countries worldwide on a population basis, the concentration of micronutrients in these foods is greater than in most others.

The comprehensive report of the World Cancer Research Fund and the American Institute for Cancer Research, published in 2007 and titled *Food, Nutrition, Physical Activity, and the Prevention of Cancer: A Global Perspective,* reached the consensus based on the available evidence: "findings from cohort studies conducted since the mid-1990s have made the overall evidence, that vegetables or fruits protect against cancers, somewhat less impressive. In no case now is the evidence of protection judged to be convincing."[15]

Fruit and Vegetable Consumption and Colorectal Cancer

The association between fruit and vegetable consumption and the incidence of colon or rectal cancer has been examined prospectively in at least six studies. In some of these prospective cohorts, inverse associations were observed for individual foods or particular subgroups of fruits or vegetables, but no consistent pattern emerged and many comparisons revealed no such links. The results from the largest studies, the Nurses' Health Study and the Health Professionals' Follow-Up Study, suggested no important association between the consumption of fruits and vegetables and the incidence of cancers of the colon or rectum during 1,743,645 person-years of follow-up.[46] In these two large cohorts, diet was assessed repeatedly during follow-up with a detailed food frequency questionnaire. Similarly, in the Pooling Project of Prospective Studies of Diet and Cancer, including 14 studies, 756,217 participants, and 5,838 cases of colon cancer, no association with overall colon cancer risk was found.[47]

Fruit and Vegetable Consumption and Stomach Cancer

At least 12 prospective cohort studies have examined the consumption of some fruits and vegetables and the incidence of stomach cancer.[15] Seven of these studies considered total vegetable intake. Three found significant protection from stomach cancer, whereas three did not. All other comparisons were made for subgroups of vegetables and produced inconsistent results. Nine prospective cohort studies investigated the association between fruit consumption and stomach cancer risk. Four studies found an inverse association of borderline statistical significance.

Fruit and Vegetable Consumption and Breast Cancer

The most comprehensive evaluation of fruit and vegetable consumption and the incidence of breast cancer was provided by a pooled analysis of all cohort studies.[48] Data were pooled from eight prospective studies that included 351,825 women, 7,377 of whom developed incident invasive breast cancer during follow-up. The pooled relative risk adjusted for potential confounding variables was 0.93 (95% CI, 0.86 to 1.0; *P* for trend, .08) for the highest versus the lowest quartile of fruit consumption, 0.96 (95% CI, 0.89 to 1.04; *P* for trend, .54) for vegetable intake, and 0.93 (95% CI, 0.86 to 1.0; *P* for trend, .12) for total consumption of fruits and vegetables combined. The EPIC study confirmed this lack of association.[49] In a recent analysis within the Nurses' Health Study, an inverse association was seen between vegetable intake and the risk of estrogen receptor–negative breast cancer.[50] This observation was confirmed in the pooling project of prospective studies: The pooled relative risk for the highest vs. the lowest quintile of total vegetable consumption was 0.82 (95% CI 0.74 to 0.90) for estrogen-receptor negative breast cancer.[51]

Fruit and Vegetable Consumption and Lung Cancer

The relation between fruit and vegetable consumption and the incidence of lung cancer was examined in the pooled analysis of cohort studies.[52] Overall, no association was observed, although a modest increase in lung cancer incidence was evident among participants with the lowest fruit and vegetable consumption.

Fruit and Vegetable Consumption and Total Cancer

An analysis of the Nurses' Health Study and the Health Professionals' Follow-Up Study, including over 9,000 incident cases of cancer, did not reveal a benefit of fruit and vegetable consumption for total cancer incidence.[53] Observations from the EPIC cohort were essentially consistent with these findings.[54] Although there may be no or only a very weak protection conferred for cancer from consuming an abundance of fruits and vegetables, there is a substantial benefit for protection from cardiovascular disease.

Summary

The consumption of fruits and vegetables and some of their main micronutrients appear to be less important in cancer prevention than previously assumed. With an accumulation of data from prospective cohort studies and randomized trials, a lack of association of these foods and nutrients with cancer outcomes has become apparent. A modest association cannot be excluded because of an imperfect measurement of diet, and it remains possible that a high consumption of fruits and vegetables during childhood and adolescence is more effective at reducing cancer risk than consumption in adult life due to the long latency of cancer manifestation.

Conversely, it is possible that, with the fortification of breakfast cereal, flour, and other staple foods, the frequent consumption of fruits and vegetables has become less essential for cancer prevention. Nevertheless, an abundance of fruits and vegetables as part of a healthy diet is recommended, because evidence consistently suggests that it lowers the incidence of hypertension, heart disease, and stroke.

Fiber

General Properties

Dietary fiber was defined in 1976 as "all plant polysaccharides and lignin which are resistant to hydrolysis by the digestive enzymes of men."[55] Fiber, both soluble and insoluble, is fermented by the luminal bacteria of the colon. Among the properties of fiber that make it a candidate for cancer prevention are its "bulking" effect, which reduces colonic transit time, and the binding of potentially carcinogenic luminal chemicals. Fiber may also aid in producing short-chain fatty acids that may be directly anticarcinogenic. Fiber may also induce apoptosis.

Dietary Fiber and Colorectal Cancer

In 1969, Dennis Burkitt hypothesized that dietary fiber is involved in colon carcinogenesis.[56] While working as a physician in Africa, Burkitt noticed the low incidence of colon cancer among African populations whose diets were high in fiber. Burkitt concluded that a link might exist between the fiber-rich diet and the low incidence of colon cancer. Burkitt's observations were followed by numerous case-control studies that seemed to confirm his theories. A combined analysis of 13 case-control studies[57] as well as a meta-analysis of 16 case-control studies[58] suggested an inverse association between fiber intake and the risk of colorectal cancer. The inclusion of studies was selective, however, and effect estimates unadjusted for potential confounders were used for most studies. Moreover, recall bias is a severe threat to the validity of retrospective case-control studies of fiber intake and any disease outcome.

Data from prospective cohort studies have largely failed to support an inverse association between dietary fiber and colorectal cancer incidence. Initial analyses from the Nurses' Health Study and the Health Professionals' Follow-Up Study[36] found no important association between dietary fiber and colorectal cancer. A significant inverse association between fiber intake and incidence of colorectal cancer was reported from the EPIC study. The analysis presented on dietary fiber and colorectal cancer encompassed 434,209 women and men from eight European countries.[59] The analytic model used by the EPIC investigators included adjustments for age, height, weight, total caloric intake, sex, and center assessed at baseline and identified[60] a significant inverse association between fiber intake and colorectal cancer. Applying the same analytic model used in EPIC to data from the Nurses' Health Study and the Health Professionals' Follow-Up Study encompassing 1.8 million person-years of follow-up and 1,572 cases of colorectal cancer revealed associations similar to those found in the EPIC study.[61] After a more complete adjustment for confounding variables, however, the association vanished.[61] Results from the pooled analysis of 13 prospective cohort studies, including 8,081 colorectal cancer cases diagnosed during over 7 million person-years of follow-up, suggested an inverse relation between dietary fiber and colorectal cancer incidence in age-adjusted analyses, but this association disappeared after appropriate adjustment for confounding variables, particularly other dietary factors.[62] The NIH–AARP study, which included 2,974 cases of colorectal cancer, confirmed the lack of association between total dietary fiber and colorectal cancer risk.[63]

The association between dietary fiber and colorectal cancer appears to be confounded by a number of other dietary and nondietary factors. These methodologic considerations must be taken into account when interpreting the evidence. It is possible that other dietary factors such as folate intake are more important for colorectal cancer pathogenesis than dietary fiber.

Dietary Fiber and Colorectal Adenomas

In a few prospective cohort studies, the primary occurrence of colorectal polyps was investigated, but no consistent relation was found.

The study of fiber intake and colorectal adenoma recurrence lends itself to a randomized clinical trial design because of the relatively short follow-up necessary and because fiber can be provided as a supplement. A number of RCTs have explored the effect of fiber supplementation on colorectal adenoma recurrence. Evidence has fairly consistently indicated no effect of fiber intake.[64–68] In one RCT, an increase in adenoma recurrence was observed among participants randomly assigned to use a fiber supplement, which was stronger among those with high dietary calcium.[69]

Dietary Fiber and Breast Cancer

Investigators have speculated that dietary fiber may reduce the risk of breast cancer through a reduction in intestinal absorption of estrogens excreted via the biliary system.

Relatively few epidemiologic studies have examined the association between fiber intake and breast cancer. In a meta-analysis of 10 case-control studies, a significant inverse association was observed. However, these retrospective studies were likely affected by the aforementioned biases—selection and recall bias, in particular. Results from at least six prospective cohort studies consistently suggested no association between fiber intake and breast cancer incidence.[70–75]

Dietary Fiber and Stomach Cancer

The results from retrospective case-control studies of fiber intake and gastric cancer risk are inconsistent. In the Netherlands Cohort Study, dietary fiber was not associated with an incidence of gastric carcinoma.[76] Further investigations through prospective cohort studies must be completed before conclusions about the relation between fiber intake and stomach cancer incidence can be drawn.

Summary

The observational data presently available do not indicate an important role for dietary fiber in the prevention of cancer, although small effects cannot be excluded. The long-held perception that a high intake of fiber conveys protection originated largely from retrospectively conducted studies, which are affected by a number of biases, in particular, the potential for differential recall of diet, and from studies that were not well controlled for potential confounding variables.

OTHER FOODS AND NUTRIENTS

Red Meat

The regular consumption of red meat has been associated with an increased risk of colorectal cancer. In a recent meta-analysis, the increase in risk associated with an increase in intake of 120 g per day was 24% (95% CI, 9% to 41%).[37] The association was strongest for processed meat; the relative risk of colorectal cancer was 1.36 (95% CI, 1.15 to 1.61) for a consumption of 30 g per day.[37] No overall association has been observed between red meat consumption and breast cancer in a pooled analysis of prospective cohorts.[77] However, among premenopausal women in the Nurses' Health Study II, the risk for estrogen-receptor–positive and progesterone-receptor–positive breast cancer doubled with 1.5 servings of red meat per day compared to three or fewer servings per week.[78] No associations have been found in studies on poultry or fish.[15] Mechanisms through which red meat may increase cancer risk include anabolic hormones routinely used in meat production in the United States, heterocyclic amines, and polycyclic aromatic hydrocarbons formed during cooking at high temperatures, the high amounts of heme iron, and nitrates and related compounds in smoked, salted, and some processed meats that can convert to carcinogenic nitrosamines in the colon.

Milk, Dairy Products, and Calcium

Regular milk consumption has been associated with a modest reduction in colorectal cancer in both a pooling project[79] and a meta-analysis of cohort studies,[80] possibly due to its calcium content. In the pooling project of prospective studies of diet and cancer, a modest inverse association was also seen for calcium intake.[79] This finding is consistent with the results of a randomized trial in which calcium supplements reduced the risk of colorectal adenomas.[81] Associations with cheese and other dairy products have been less consistent.[79,80]

Conversely, in multiple studies, a high intake of calcium or dairy products has been associated with an increased risk of prostate cancer,[80,82–86] specifically fatal prostate cancer.[87,88] Similar observations were made in the NIH–AARP study, although the increase in risk there did not reach statistical significance.[89] While the Multiethnic Cohort[90] and the Prostate, Lung, Colorectal, and Ovarian Cancer Screening Trial[91] did not find an important association between dairy consumption and prostate cancer, these cohort studies did not specifically include fatal prostate cancer cases. A meta-analysis of prospective studies generated an overall relative risk of advanced prostate cancer of 1.33 (95% CI, 1.00 to 1.78) for the highest versus the lowest intake categories of dairy products.[92] In another meta-analysis, no significant association was found for cohort studies on dairy or milk consumption, but relative risk estimates suggested a positive association.[93] Thus, although the findings are not entirely consistent and are complicated by the widespread use of prostate-specific antigen (PSA) screening in the United States, the global evidence suggests a positive association between the regular consumption of dairy products and the risk of fatal prostate cancer. Consuming three or more servings of dairy products per day has been associated with endometrial cancer among postmenopausal women not using hormonal therapy.[94] A high intake of lactose from dairy products has also been associated with a modestly higher risk of ovarian cancer.[95]

These observations are particularly important in the context of national dietary recommendations to drink three glasses of milk per day.[38] Possible mechanisms include an increase in endogenous IGF-1 levels[96] and steroid hormones contained in cows' milk.[97]

Vitamin D

In 1980, Garland and Garland[98] hypothesized that sunlight and vitamin D may reduce the risk of colon cancer. Since then, substantial research has been conducted in this area supporting an inverse association between circulating 25-hydroxyvitamin D (25[OH]D) levels and colorectal cancer risk.[99–103] A meta-analysis, including five nested case-control studies with prediagnostic serum, suggested a reduction of colorectal cancer risk by about half among individuals with serum 25(OH)D levels of more than 82 nmol/L compared to individuals with less than 30 nmol/L.[104] A subsequent meta-analysis including eight studies confirmed these associations.[105] These observations are supported by similar findings for colorectal adenomas.[106] Vitamin D levels may particularly affect colorectal cancer prognosis; colorectal cancer mortality was 72% lower among individuals with 25(OH)D concentrations of 80 nmol/L or higher.[107]

The evidence for other cancers has been less consistent. High plasma levels of vitamin D have been associated with a decreased risk of several other cancers, including cancer of the breast[108–111]; prostate, especially fatal prostate cancer[112]; and ovary.[113,114] Whether vitamin D plays a role in pancreatic cancerogenesis remains to be determined with one pooling project, suggesting a positive association,[115] whereas other prospective studies[116] and a pooling project of cohort studies found inverse associations.[117]

The activation of vitamin D receptors by $1,25(OH)^2D$ induces cell differentiation and inhibits proliferation and angiogenesis.[118] Solar ultraviolet B radiation is the major source of plasma vitamin D, and dietary vitamin D without supplementation has a minor effect on plasma vitamin D. To achieve sufficient plasma levels through sun exposure, at least 15 minutes of full-body exposure to bright sunlight is necessary. Physical activity has to be considered as possible confounder of studies on plasma levels of vitamin D and cancer. Sunscreen effectively blocks vitamin D production. Populations who live in geographic areas with limited or seasonal sun exposure may benefit from a vitamin D supplementation of 1,000 IU per day.

Folate

Folate is a micronutrient commonly found in fruits and vegetables, particularly oranges, orange juice, asparagus, beets, and peas. Folate may affect carcinogenesis through various mechanisms: DNA methylation, DNA synthesis, and DNA repair. In the animal model, folate deficiency enhances intestinal carcinogenesis.[119] Folate deficiency is related to the incorporation of uracil into human DNA and to an increased frequency of chromosomal breaks. A number of epidemiologic studies suggest that a diet rich in folate lowers the risk of colorectal adenomas and colorectal cancer.[15] Because the folate content in foods is generally relatively low, is susceptible to oxidative destruction by cooking and food processing, and is not well absorbed, folic acid from supplements and fortification plays an important role. Pooled results from 13 prospective studies suggests that intake of 400 to 500 μg per day is required to minimize risk.[120]

Potential interactions among alcohol consumption, folic acid intake, and methionine intake have been described. Although alcohol consumption has been fairly consistently related to an increase in breast cancer incidence, the potential detrimental effect of alcohol seems to be eliminated in women with high folic acid intake.[16] A similar folic acid or methionine–alcohol interaction has been observed for colorectal cancer risk.[119]

Genetic susceptibility may also modify the relation between folate intake and cancer risk. A polymorphism of the *methylenetetrahydrofolate reductase (MTHFR)* gene (cytosine to thymine transition at position 677) may result in a relative deficiency of methionine. Individuals with the common C677T mutation appear to experience the greatest protection from high folic acid or methionine intake and low alcohol consumption.[121] Although the interaction between this polymorphism and dietary factors needs to be investigated further, the consistently observed association between this polymorphism and the risk of colorectal cancer supports a role of folate in the etiology of colorectal cancer.

Folate levels also affect the availability of methyl groups via S-adenosylmethionine in the one-carbon metabolism.[122] Low red blood cell folate levels are associated with low DNA methylation status among homozygous *MTHFR* 677T/T mutation carriers, whereas at high red blood cell folate levels, the amount of methylated cytosine in DNA is similar to that of the heterozygote *MTHFR* C677T genotype.[123]

Conversely, evidence from animal and human studies suggests that a high folate status may promote the progression of existing neoplasias.[122,124,125] The randomization of folic acid supplements among individuals with a history of colorectal adenoma resulted in either no effect on recurrent adenoma recurrence[126] or an increase in recurrence with over 6 to 8 years of follow-up.[127] The high proliferation rate of neoplastic cells requiring increased DNA synthesis is likely supported by folate, which is necessary for thymidine synthesis.[122,125] The effects of folate on de novo methylation and subsequent gene silencing have been insufficiently studied. An increase in colorectal cancer rates has been observed in the United States and Canada concurrent with the introduction of the folic acid fortification program, but this could be an artifact due to increased use of colonoscopies.[128] The lack of increase in mortality, but an acceleration in a long-term downward trend suggests the latter explanation (http://progressreport.cancer.gov/).

Carotenoids

Carotenoids, antioxidants prevalent in fruits and vegetables, enhance cell-to-cell communication, promote cell differentiation, and modulate immune response. In 1981, Doll and Peto[1] speculated that beta-carotene may be a major player in cancer prevention and encouraged testing its anticarcinogenic properties. Indeed, subsequent observational studies, mostly case-control investigations, suggested a reduced cancer risk—especially of lung cancer—with a high intake of carotenoids. In contrast, clinical trials randomizing the intake of beta-carotene supplements have not revealed the evidence of a protective effect of beta-carotene. In fact, beta-carotene was found to increase the risk of lung cancer and total mortality among smokers in the Finnish Alpha-Tocopherol, Beta-Carotene Cancer Prevention Study.[129] However, these adverse affects disappeared during longer periods of follow-up.[130] In a detailed analysis of prospective studies, no association was seen between the intake of beta-carotene and the risk of lung cancer.[131]

The pooled analysis of 18 cohort studies including more than 33,000 breast cancer cases suggested inverse associations between the intake of several carotenoids (beta-carotene, alpha-carotene, luteine/zeaxanthin) and estrogen-receptor–negative breast cancer incidence, whereas no association was found for estrogen-receptor–positive tumors.[132] Similarly, in a pooled analysis of data from eight prospective studies including about 3,055 breast cancer cases, blood levels of carotenoids were inversely related to estrogen-receptor–negative mammary tumor incidence.[133] Women in the highest quintile of beta-carotene levels had about half the risk of developing estrogen-receptor–negative breast cancer than women in the lowest quintile (hazard ratio [HR] = 0.52; 95% CI, 0.36 to 0.77).

The particularly pronounced antioxidant properties of lycopene, a carotenoid mainly found in tomatoes, may explain the inverse associations with some cancers. The frequent consumption of tomato-based products has been associated with a decreased risk of prostate, lung, and stomach cancers.[134] The bioavailability of lycopene from cooked tomatoes is higher than from fresh tomatoes, making tomato soup and sauce excellent sources of the carotenoid.

Selenium

Selenium has long been of interest in cancer prevention due to its antioxidative properties. Its intake is difficult to estimate because food content depends on the selenium content of the soil it is grown in. Selenium enriches in toenails, which provide an integrative measure of intake during the previous year and therefore are popular biomarkers in epidemiologic studies. Inverse associations with toenail selenium levels have been found in several prospective studies, especially for fatal protate cancer.[135–137] In a recent meta-analysis, plasma/serum selenium was also inversely correlated with prostate cancer.[138] In the Selenium and Vitamin E Cancer Prevention Trial (SELECT), no protective effect of selenium was found for prostate cancer. However, the trial was terminated prematurely after 4 years, which is a short period in which to expect a reduction in cancer.[139]

Soy Products

The role of soy products has been considered for breast carcinogenesis. In Asian countries, which traditionally have a high consumption of soy foods, breast cancer rates have been low until recently. In Western countries, soy consumption is generally low, and between-person variation may be insufficient to allow meaningful comparisons. Soybeans contain isoflavones, which are phytoestrogens that compete with estrogen for the estrogen receptor. Hence, soy consumption may affect estrogen concentrations differently depending on the endogenous baseline level. This mechanism may also contribute to the equivocal results of studies on soy foods and breast cancer risk. In a recent meta-analysis of 18 epidemiologic studies, including over 9,000 breast cancer cases, frequent soy intake was associated with a modest decrease in risk (odds ratio = 0.86; 95% CI, 0.75 to 0.99).[140] Wu et al.[141] observed that childhood intake of soy was more relevant to breast cancer prevention than adult consumption.

Carbohydrates

The Warburg hypothesis postulated in 1924 that tumor cells mainly generate energy by the nonoxidative breakdown of glucose (glucolysis) instead of pyrovate.[142] Carbohydrates with a high glycemic load increase blood glucose levels after consumption, which results in insulin spikes increasing the risk for type 2 diabetes. Several cancers, including colorectal cancer[143] and breast cancer,[144] have been associated with type 2 diabetes. The evidence on the consumption of sucrose and refined, processed flour and cancer incidence is heterogeneous.[145] Whereas in some prospective cohort studies an increase in colon cancer incidence was observed,[146] this was not found in other studies.[147] In large cohort studies, associations have been observed for pancreatic[148] and endometrial[145] cancer risk, but not for postmenopausal breast cancer.[149] Especially in obese, sedentary individuals, abnormal glucose and insulin metabolism may contribute to tumorigenesis.

DIETARY PATTERNS

Foods and nutrients are not consumed in isolation, and, when evaluating the role of diet in disease prevention and causation, it is sensible to consider the entire dietary pattern of individuals. Public health messages may be better framed in the context of a global diet than individual constituents.

The role of vegetarian diets for cancer incidence has been examined in a few studies. In the Adventist Health Study-2, vegetarians had an 8% lower incidence of cancer than nonvegetarians (95% CI, 1 to 15%).[150] The protective association was strongest for cancers of the gastrointestinal tract with 24% (95% CI, 10 to 37%). Vegans had a 16% (95%, 1 to 28%) lower incidence of cancer, with a particular protection conferred to female cancers of 34% (95% CI, 8 to 53%). A combined analysis of data from the Oxford Vegetarian Study and EPIC similarly suggest a 12% (95% CI, 4 to 19%) reduction in cancer incidence among vegetarians compared to meat eaters.[151]

During the past decade, dietary pattern analyses have gained popularity in observational studies. The most commonly employed methods are factor analyses and cluster analyses, which are largely data-driven methods, and investigator-determined methods such as dietary indices and scores. The search for associations between distinct patterns such as the "Western pattern," which is characterized by a high consumption of red and processed meats; high fat dairy products, including butter and eggs; and refined carbohydrates, such as sweets, desserts, and refined grains, and the "prudent pattern," which is defined by the frequent consumption of a variety of fruits and vegetables, whole grains, legumes, fish, and poultry, and the risk of cancer has been largely disappointing. Notable exceptions were the link between a Western dietary pattern and colon cancer incidence and an inverse relation between a prudent diet[152] and estrogen-receptor–negative breast cancer.[153] These findings were subsequently in the California Teachers Study.[154] The general lack of association between global dietary patterns and cancer supports a more modest role of nutrition during adult life in carcinogenesis than previously assumed.

DIET DURING THE EARLY PHASES OF LIFE

Some cancers may originate early in the course of life. A high birth weight is associated with an increase in the risk of childhood leukemia,[155] premenopausal breast cancer,[156] and testicular cancer.[157] Tall height is an indicator of the risk of many cancers and is in part determined by nutrition during childhood.[15] Until recently, most studies focused on the role of diet during adult life. However, the critical exposure period for nutrition to affect cancer risk may be earlier, and because the latent period for cancer may span several decades, diet during childhood and adolescence may be important. However, relating dietary information during early life and cancer outcomes prospectively is difficult because nutrition records from the remote past are not available. Studies in which recalled diet during youth is used have to be interpreted cautiously due to misclassification, although recall has been found reasonably reproducible and consistent with recalls provided by participants' mothers.[158,159] The role of early life diet has been explored in only a few studies in relation to breast cancer risk. In a study nested in the Nurses' Health Study cohorts that used data recalled by mothers, frequent consumption of french fries was associated with an increased risk of breast cancer, whereas whole milk consumption was inversely related to risk.[160] Similarly, an inverse association with milk consumption during childhood was found among younger women (30 to 39 years), but not among older premenopausal women (40 to 49 years) in a Norwegian cohort.[161] Dietary habits during high school recalled by adult participants of the Nurses' Health Study II (but before the diagnosis of breast cancer) suggested a positive association of total fat and red meat consumption.[31,32] More data are needed in this promising area of research.[162]

DIET AFTER A DIAGNOSIS OF CANCER

The role of diet in the secondary prevention of cancer recurrence and survival is generally of great interest to cancer patients because they are highly motivated to make lifestyle changes to optimize their prognosis. The compliance of cancer patients makes the RCTs a more feasible design to evaluate the role of diet than among healthy individuals. However, concurrent cancer treatments may make any effect of diet more difficult to isolate.

Most evidence is available for breast cancer, colorectal, and prostate cancer. Observational data suggest a limited role of diet in the prevention of breast cancer recurrence and survival. The Life After Cancer Epidemiology (LACE) Cohort supported a beneficial role for vitamin C and E supplement use but the effect of other health-seeking behaviors is difficult to exclude.[163] In a pooled analysis, alcohol consumption after a diagnosis did not affect survival.[164] Several randomized trials have addressed the role of diet in breast cancer prognosis. In the Women's Intervention Nutrition Study (WINS), 2,437 women with early stage breast cancer were randomized to a dietary goal of 15% of calories from fat or maintenance of their usual dietary habits.[165] The intervention group received dietary counseling by registered dieticians and, according to self-reports, a difference of 19 g in daily fat intake was maintained between the intervention and the control group after 60 months of follow-up. However, at that time, women in the intervention group were also 6 pounds lighter, making it difficult to separate an effect of dietary fat from a nonspecific effect of intensive dietary intervention, which quite consistently produces weight loss. Breast cancer recurrence was 29% lower in the intervention group (95% CI, 6% to 47%), whereas overall survival was not affected. In the Women's Healthy Eating and Living (WHEL) RCT, 3,088 early stage breast cancer patients were randomly assigned to a target of five vegetable servings, three fruit servings, 30 g fiber per day, and 15% to 20% of calories from fat.[166] After 72 months, the intervention versus control group reports were 5.8 versus 3.6 servings of vegetables, 3.4 versus 2.6 servings of fruit, 24.2 versus 18.9 g fiber per day, and 28.9% versus 32.4% of calories from fat. The total plasma carotenoid concentration, a biomarker of vegetable and fruit intake, was 43% higher in the intervention group than the comparison group after 4 years ($p<0.001$). Neither recurrence rates nor mortality were affected by the intervention after the 7.3-year follow-up. Overall, diet is unlikely a major factor influencing breast cancer prognosis. However, because the prognosis for breast cancer is relatively good, women diagnosed with breast cancer remain at risk for cardiovascular disease and other causes of death that affect those without breast cancer. Thus, among women in the Nurses' Health Study diagnosed with breast cancer, a higher diet quality, which was assessed by the Alternative Healthy Eating Index, was not associated with mortality due to breast cancer but was associated with substantially lower mortality due to other causes.[167] Similarly, among over 4,000 women with breast cancer, intakes of saturated and trans fat, but not of total fat, were associated with significantly greater total mortality but not specifically breast cancer mortality. Thus, there is good reason for women with breast cancer to adopt a healthy diet even if it does not affect the prognosis of breast cancer.

In a systematic review, no consistent association between individual dietary components and colorectal cancer prognosis outcome was found.[168] However, in an observational study including 1,009 patients with stage III colon cancer, a Western dietary pattern was associated with lower rates of disease-free survival, recurrence-free survival, and overall survivals.[169] In the same patient population, higher dietary glycemic load and total carbohydrate intake were significantly associated with an increased risk of recurrence and mortality.[170] These findings support a possible role of glycemic load in colon cancer progression.

In the Physician's Health Study, whole milk consumption among men with incident prostate cancer was associated with double the risk of progression to fatal disease.[171] Among men with nonmetastatic prostate cancer in the Health Professionals' Follow-up Study, replacing 10% of energy intake from carbohydrates with vegetable fat was associated with a lower risk of lethal prostate cancer.[172] A marginally increased risk of progression of localized to lethal prostate cancer among these men was also associated with postdiagnostic poultry and processed red meat consumption,[173] whereas postdiagnostic consumption of fish and tomato sauce were inversely related with a risk of progression.[174] In an intervention study, 93 patients with early stage prostate cancer (PSA = 4 to 10 ng per mililiter and Gleason score <7) were randomized to comprehensive lifestyle changes, including a vegan diet based on 10% of calories from fat and consisting predominantly of vegetables, fruit, whole grains, legumes, and soy protein.[175] Other interventions included moderate exercise, stress management, and relaxation. After 1 year, PSA values decreased 4% in the intervention group, but increased 6% in the control group. Six patients in the control group, but none in the experimental group, underwent conventional prostate cancer treatment. Although the impact of the different intervention components are difficult to separate in this study, further data on diet and the prognosis for patients with localized prostate cancer are needed.

SUMMARY

A considerable proportion of cancers are potentially preventable through lifestyle changes. Besides a curtailment of smoking, the most important strategies are maintaining a healthy body weight and regular physical activity, which contribute to a lower prevalence of being overweight and obesity. The avoidance of a positive energy balance and becoming overweight are the most important nutritional factors in cancer prevention.

Although dietary patterns, including frequent fruit and vegetable consumption, appear to play a modest role in cancer prevention, knowledge gained about some specific foods and nutrients might inform a targeted approach. Vitamin D is a strong candidate to counter carcinogenesis, thus supplementation could be a feasible and safe route to avoid several types of cancer. Although the data on vitamin D and cancer incidence are not conclusive, the prevention of bone fractures is a sufficient reason to maintain good vitamin D status.

Limiting or avoiding red meat, processed meat, and alcohol reduces the risk of breast, colorectal, stomach, esophageal, and other cancers. Although the role of dairy products and milk remains to be more fully elucidated, current evidence suggests a probable increase in the risk of prostate cancer with frequent milk consumption, and possibly endometrial cancer, which raises concern regarding current dietary recommendations of three glasses of milk per day. The relation of calcium and dairy intake to cancer is complex, as the evidence for a reduction in the risk of colorectal cancer is strong, but high intakes appear likely to increase the risk of fatal prostate cancer. The consumption of tomato-based products may contribute to the prevention of prostate cancer. Finally, diet may influence the prognosis of colorectal and prostate cancer, but more data are needed in this area. Because most people with cancer remain at risk of cardiovascular disease and other common conditions related to unhealthy diets, an overall healthy diet can be recommended while further research on diet and cancer survival is ongoing.

LIMITATIONS

Studying the role of diet in health and disease requires overcoming a number of hurdles. Because biomarkers reflecting nutrient intake with sufficient accuracy are largely lacking, assessing nutrition in a population-based study has to rely on self-reports by individuals, which inevitably leads to imprecision or error in the diet assessment. Such misclassification may produce spurious associations in case-control studies or may lead to an underestimation of true associations in prospective cohort studies. Ideally, hypotheses relating dietary factors to cancer risks would be tested in large randomized trials. Besides being extremely expensive, maintaining adherence to assigned diets has been challenging; for example, in the WHI trial that focused on dietary fat reduction, there were no differences between intervention and control groups in blood lipid fractions that are known to change with a reduction in fat intake, indicating a failure to test the hypothesis.[28]

Most observational studies are conducted within populations or countries. Although reasonable variations in nutritional habits exist within populations, allowing for the detection of substantial dietary risk factors for cardiovascular disease and diabetes, these contrasts may be too limited to detect small relative risks as they may exist for cancer. The pooled analysis of large prospective cohort studies across countries and continents attempts to overcome this limitation. Studies taking advantage of the large between-population variation in diets across developed and developing countries would appear to be advantageous, but would be plagued by confounding by other differences in lifestyle factors that might be difficult to assess and control adequately.

Few epidemiologic studies repeatedly capture dietary habits over time and thus account for potential changes in diet over time. Furthermore, the length of follow-up in prospective studies may not be sufficient to capture the impact of diets assessed at baseline. In case-control studies, a recall of dietary habits prior to the disease onset may be influenced by current disease status; moreover, the relevant time for nutrition to act may be decades earlier, which is more difficult to remember.

Most epidemiologic studies of diet and cancer have assessed intake among adults. Due to greater susceptibility to genotoxic influences earlier in life, it is possible that data on diet during childhood or early adolescence are more relevant for carcinogenesis and cancer prevention. Studies that have collected dietary data during childhood and followed the subjects for cancer incidence would be most informative but are virtually nonexistent and will be challenging to conduct.

Finally, data on special diets including organic foods, whole foods, raw foods, and a vegan diet are limited.

FUTURE DIRECTIONS

Some of the most promising research at present is in the areas of vitamin D, milk consumption, and the effect of diet early in life on cancer incidence. Recent nutrition changes in countries previously maintaining a more traditional diet such as Japan and some developing countries have already been followed by increased rates of some cancers (but declines in stomach cancer), providing a setting to study the effect of change over time. Additional insight may come from studies on gene–nutrient interaction and epigenetic changes induced by the diet. To improve observational research methods, refined dietary assessment methods, including the identification of new biomarkers, will be advantageous.

RECOMMENDATIONS

A wealth of data are available from observational studies on diet and cancer, and the current evidence supports suggestions made by Doll and Peto[1] that approximately 30% to 40% of cancers may be avoidable with changes in nutrition; however, much of this risk of cancer is related to being overweight and to inactivity. Excessive energy intake and lack of physical activity, marked by rapid growth in childhood and being overweight, have become growing threats to population health and are important contributors to risks of many cancers. Nevertheless, the cumulative incidence for many cancers has decreased over the past decade, in part due to the decreasing prevalence of smoking and use of hormone therapy.

Dietary recommendations must integrate the goal of overall avoidance of disease and maintenance of health and, thus, should not focus singularly on cancer prevention. The strength of the evidence and magnitude of the expected benefit should also be considered in recommendations. With these considerations in mind, the following recommendations are outlined, which are largely in agreement with the guidelines put forth by the American Cancer Society in 2012:[176]

1. *Engage in regular physical activity.* Physical activity is a primary method of weight control and it also reduces risk of several cancers, especially colon cancer, through independent mechanisms. Moderate to vigorous exercise for at least 30 minutes on most days is a minimum and more will provide additional benefits.
2. *Avoid being overweight and weight gain in adulthood.* A positive energy balance that results in excess body fat is one of the most important contributors to cancer risk. Staying within 10 pounds of body weight at age 20 may be a simple guide, assuming no adolescent obesity.
3. *Limit alcohol consumption.* Alcohol consumption contributes to the risk of many cancers and increases the risk of accidents and addiction, but low to moderate consumption has benefits for coronary heart disease risk. The individual family history of disease as well as personal preferences should be considered.
4. *Consume lots of fruits and vegetables.* Frequent consumption of fruits and vegetables during adult life is not likely to have a major effect on cancer incidence, but will reduce the risk of cardiovascular disease.
5. *Consume whole grains and avoid refined carbohydrates and sugars.* A regular consumption of whole grain products instead of refined flour and a low consumption of refined sugars lower the risk of cardiovascular disease and diabetes. The effect on cancer risk is less clear.
6. *Replace red meat and dairy products with fish, nuts, and legumes.* Red meat consumption increases the risk of colorectal cancer, diabetes, and coronary heart disease and should be largely avoided. Frequent dairy consumption may increase the risk of prostate cancer. Fish, nuts, and legumes are excellent sources of valuable mono- and polyunsaturated fats and vegetable proteins and may contribute to lower rates of cardiovascular disease and diabetes.
7. *Consider taking a vitamin D supplement.* A substantial proportion of the population, especially those living at higher latitudes, are vitamin D deficient. Most adults may benefit from taking 1,000 IU of vitamin D^3 per day during months of low sunlight intensity. Vitamin D supplementation will, at a minimum, reduce bone fracture rates, probably colorectal cancer incidence, and possibly other cancers.

ETIOLOGY AND EPIDEMIOLOGY OF CANCER

REFERENCES

1. Doll R, Peto R. The causes of cancer: quantitative estimates of avoidable risks of cancer in the United States today. *J Natl Cancer Inst* 1981;66:1191–1308.
2. Armstrong B, Doll R. Environmental factors and cancer incidence and mortality in different countries, with special reference to dietary practices. *Int J Cancer* 1975;15:617–631.
3. Giovannucci E, Stampfer MJ, Colditz GA, et al. A comparison of prospective and retrospective assessments of diet in the study of breast cancer. *Am J Epidemiol* 1993;137:502–511.
4. Riboli E, Norat T. Epidemiologic evidence of the protective effect of fruit and vegetables on cancer risk. *Am J Clin Nutr* 2003;78:559S–569S.
5. Prentice RL, Caan B, Chlebowski RT, et al. Low-fat dietary pattern and risk of invasive breast cancer: the Women's Health Initiative Randomized Controlled Dietary Modification Trial. *JAMA* 2006;295:629–642.
6. Michels KB, Bingham SA, Luben R, et al. The effect of correlated measurement error in multivariate models of diet. *Am J Epidemiol* 2004;160:59–67.
7. Willett W. *Nutritional Epidemiology*. 3rd ed. New York: Oxford University Press; 2013.
8. Calle EE, Rodriguez C, Walker-Thurmond K, et al. Overweight, obesity, and mortality from cancer in a prospectively studied cohort of U.S. adults. *N Engl J Med* 2003;348:1625–1638.
9. Giovannucci E, Ascherio A, Rimm EB, et al. Physical activity, obesity, and risk for colon cancer and adenoma in men. *Ann Intern Med* 1995;122:327–334.
10. Martinez ME, Giovannucci E, Spiegelman D, et al. Leisure-time physical activity, body size, and colon cancer in women. Nurses' Health Study Research Group. *J Natl Cancer Inst* 1997;89:948–955.
11. Eliassen AH, Colditz GA, Rosner B, et al. Adult weight change and risk of postmenopausal breast cancer. *JAMA* 2006;296:193–201.
12. Michels KB, Ekbom A. Caloric restriction and incidence of breast cancer. *JAMA* 2004;291:1226–1230.
13. Elias SG, Peeters PH, Grobbee DE, et al. Breast cancer risk after caloric restriction during the 1944–1945 Dutch famine. *J Natl Cancer Inst* 2004;96:539–546.
14. Tretli S, Gaard M. Lifestyle changes during adolescence and risk of breast cancer: an ecologic study of the effect of World War II in Norway. *Cancer Causes Control* 1996;7:507–512.
15. World Cancer Research Fund/American Institute for Cancer Research. *Food, Nutrition, Physical Activity, and the Prevention of Cancer: A Global Perspective*. Washington, D.C.: AICR; 2007.
16. Zhang S, Hunter DJ, Hankinson SE, et al. A prospective study of folate intake and the risk of breast cancer. *JAMA* 1999;281:1632–1637.
17. Tannenbaum A. The genesis and growth of tumors. III. Effects of a high-fat diet. *Cancer Res* 1942;2:468–475.
18. Kolonel L, Hinds M, Hankin J. *Cancer Patterns Among Migrant and Native-Born Japanese in Hawaii in Relation to Smoking, Drinking, and Dietary Habits*. Tokyo: Japan Scientific Societies Press; 1980.
19. Howe GR, Hirohata T, Hislop TG, et al. Dietary factors and risk of breast cancer: combined analysis of 12 case-control studies. *J Natl Cancer Inst* 1990;82:561–569.
20. Kim EH, Willett WC, Colditz GA, et al. Dietary fat and risk of postmenopausal breast cancer in a 20-year follow-up. *Am J Epidemiol* 2006;164:990–997.
21. Thiebaut AC, Kipnis V, Chang SC, et al. Dietary fat and postmenopausal invasive breast cancer in the National Institutes of Health-AARP Diet and Health Study cohort. *J Natl Cancer Inst* 2007;99:451–462.
22. Sieri S, Krogh V, Ferrari P, et al. Dietary fat and breast cancer risk in the European Prospective Investigation into Cancer and Nutrition. *Am J Clin Nutr* 2008;88:1304–1312.
23. Hunter DJ, Spiegelman D, Adami HO, et al. Cohort studies of fat intake and the risk of breast cancer—a pooled analysis. *N Engl J Med* 1996;334:356–361.
24. Smith-Warner SA, Spiegelman D, Adami HO, et al. Types of dietary fat and breast cancer: a pooled analysis of cohort studies. *Int J Cancer* 2001;92:767–774.
25. Wu AH, Pike MC, Stram DO. Meta-analysis: dietary fat intake, serum estrogen levels, and the risk of breast cancer. *J Natl Cancer Inst* 1999;91:529–534.

26. Rose DP, Connolly JM, Chlebowski RT, et al. The effects of a low-fat dietary intervention and tamoxifen adjuvant therapy on the serum estrogen and sex hormone-binding globulin concentrations of postmenopausal breast cancer patients. *Breast Cancer Res Treat* 1993;27:253–262.
27. Michels KB. The women's health initiative—curse or blessing? *Int J Epidemiol* 2006;35:814–816.
28. Michels KB, Willett WC. The Women's Health Initiative Randomized Controlled Dietary Modification Trial: a post-mortem. *Breast Cancer Res Treat* 2009;114:1–6.
29. Martin LJ, Li Q, Melnichouk O, et al. A randomized trial of dietary intervention for breast cancer prevention. *Cancer Res* 2011;71:123–133.
30. Cho E, Spiegelman D, Hunter DJ, et al. Premenopausal fat intake and risk of breast cancer. *J Natl Cancer Inst* 2003;95:1079–1085.
31. Linos E, Willett WC, Cho E, et al. Red meat consumption during adolescence among premenopausal women and risk of breast cancer. *Cancer Epidemiol Biomarkers Prev* 2008;17:2146–2151.
32. Linos E, Willett WC, Cho E, et al. Adolescent diet in relation to breast cancer risk among premenopausal women. *Cancer Epidemiol Biomarkers Prev* 2010;19:689–696.
33. Willett WC, Stampfer MJ, Colditz GA, et al. Relation of meat, fat, and fiber intake to the risk of colon cancer in a prospective study among women. *N Engl J Med* 1990;323:1664–1672.
34. Bostick RM, Potter JD, Kushi LH, et al. Sugar, meat, and fat intake, and non-dietary risk factors for colon cancer incidence in Iowa women (United States). *Cancer Causes Control* 1994;5:38–52.
35. Goldbohm RA, van den Brandt PA, van't Veer P, et al. A prospective cohort study on the relation between meat consumption and the risk of colon cancer. *Cancer Res* 1994;54:718–723.
36. Giovannucci E, Rimm EB, Stampfer MJ, et al. Intake of fat, meat, and fiber in relation to risk of colon cancer in men. *Cancer Res* 1994;54:2390–2397.
37. Norat T, Lukanova A, Ferrari P, et al. Meat consumption and colorectal cancer risk: dose-response meta-analysis of epidemiological studies. *Int J Cancer* 2002;98:241–256.
38. Dietary Guidelines for Americans. DietaryGuidelines.gov Web site. http://www.health.gov/dietaryguidelines/.
39. Whittemore AS, Kolonel LN, Wu AH, et al. Prostate cancer in relation to diet, physical activity, and body size in blacks, whites, and Asians in the United States and Canada. *J Natl Cancer Inst* 1995;87:652–661.
40. Crowe FL, Key TJ, Appleby PN, et al. Dietary fat intake and risk of prostate cancer in the European Prospective Investigation into Cancer and Nutrition. *Am J Clin Nutr* 2008;87:1405–1413.
41. Giovannucci E, Rimm EB, Colditz GA, et al. A prospective study of dietary fat and risk of prostate cancer. *J Natl Cancer Inst* 1993;85:1571–1579.
42. Mills PK, Beeson WL, Phillips RL, et al. Cohort study of diet, lifestyle, and prostate cancer in Adventist men. *Cancer* 1989;64:598–604.
43. Park S-Y, Murphy SP, Wilkens LR, et al. Fat and meat intake and prostate cancer risk: The multiethnic cohort study. *Int J Cancer* 2007;121:1339–1345.
44. Schuurman AG, van den Brandt PA, Dorant E, et al. Association of energy and fat intake with prostate carcinoma risk: results from The Netherlands Cohort Study. *Cancer* 1999;86:1019–1027.
45. Smith-Warner SA, Ritz J, Hunter DJ, et al. Dietary fat and risk of lung cancer in a pooled analysis of prospective studies. *Cancer Epidemiol Biomarkers Prev* 2002;11:987–992.
46. Michels KB, Edward G, Joshipura KJ, et al. Prospective study of fruit and vegetable consumption and incidence of colon and rectal cancers. *J Natl Cancer Inst* 2000;92:1740–1752.
47. Koushik A, Hunter DJ, Spiegelman D, et al. Fruits, vegetables, and colon cancer risk in a pooled analysis of 14 cohort studies. *J Natl Cancer Inst* 2007; 99:1471–1483.
48. Smith-Warner SA, Spiegelman D, Yaun SS, et al. Intake of fruits and vegetables and risk of breast cancer: a pooled analysis of cohort studies. *JAMA* 2001;285:769–776.
49. van Gils CH, Peeters PH, Bueno-de-Mesquita HB, et al. Consumption of vegetables and fruits and risk of breast cancer. *JAMA* 2005;293:183–193.
50. Fung TT, Hu FB, McCullough ML, et al. Diet quality is associated with the risk of estrogen receptor-negative breast cancer in postmenopausal women. *J Nutr* 2006;136:466–472.
51. Jung S, Spiegelman D, Baglietto L, et al. Fruit and vegetable intake and risk of breast cancer by hormone receptor status. *J Natl Cancer Inst* 2013; 105:219–236.
52. Smith-Warner SA, Spiegelman D, Yaun SS, et al. Fruits, vegetables and lung cancer: a pooled analysis of cohort studies. *Int J Cancer* 2003;107:1001–1011.
53. Hung HC, Joshipura KJ, Jiang R, et al. Fruit and vegetable intake and risk of major chronic disease. *J Natl Cancer Inst* 2004;96:1577–1584.
54. Boffetta P, Couto E, Wichmann J, et al. Fruit and vegetable intake and overall cancer risk in the European Prospective Investigation into Cancer and Nutrition (EPIC). *J Natl Cancer Inst* 2010;102:529–537.
55. Trowell H, Southgate DA, Waolever TM, et al. Letter: Dietary fibre redefined. *Lancet* 1976;1:967.
56. Burkitt DP. Related disease—related cause? *Lancet* 1969;2:1229–1231.
57. Howe GR, Benito E, Castelleto R, et al. Dietary intake of fiber and decreased risk of cancers of the colon and rectum: evidence from the combined analysis of 13 case-control studies. *J Natl Cancer Inst* 1992;84:1887–1896.
58. Trock B, Lanza E, Greenwald P. Dietary fiber, vegetables, and colon cancer: critical review and meta-analyses of the epidemiologic evidence. *J Natl Cancer Inst* 1990;82:650–661.
59. Bingham SA, Day NE, Luben R, et al. Dietary fibre in food and protection against colorectal cancer in the European Prospective Investigation into Cancer and Nutrition (EPIC): an observational study. *Lancet* 2003;361: 1496–1501.
60. Fuchs CS, Giovannucci EL, Colditz GA, et al. Dietary fiber and the risk of colorectal cancer and adenoma in women. *N Engl J Med* 1999;340:169–176.
61. Michels KB, Fuchs CS, Giovannucci E, et al. Fiber intake and incidence of colorectal cancer among 76,947 women and 47,279 men. *Cancer Epidemiol Biomarkers Prev* 2005;14:842–849.
62. Park Y, Hunter DJ, Spiegelman D, et al. Dietary fiber intake and risk of colorectal cancer: a pooled analysis of prospective cohort studies. *JAMA* 2005;294:2849–2857.
63. Schatzkin A, Mouw T, Park Y, et al. Dietary fiber and whole-grain consumption in relation to colorectal cancer in the NIH-AARP Diet and Health Study. *Am J Clin Nutr* 2007;85:1353–1360.
64. Alberts DS, Martinez ME, Roe DJ, et al. Lack of effect of a high-fiber cereal supplement on the recurrence of colorectal adenomas. Phoenix Colon Cancer Prevention Physicians' Network. *N Engl J Med* 2000;342: 1156–1162.
65. Jacobs ET, Giuliano AR, Roe DJ, et al. Intake of supplemental and total fiber and risk of colorectal adenoma recurrence in the wheat bran fiber trial. *Cancer Epidemiol Biomarkers Prev* 2002;11:906–914.
66. MacLennan R, Macrae F, Bain C, et al. Randomized trial of intake of fat, fiber, and beta carotene to prevent colorectal adenomas. The Australian Polyp Prevention Project. *J Natl Cancer Inst* 1995;87:1760–1766.
67. McKeown-Eyssen GE, Bright-See E, Bruce WR, et al. A randomized trial of a low fat high fibre diet in the recurrence of colorectal polyps. Toronto Polyp Prevention Group. *J Clin Epidemiol* 1994;47:525–536.
68. Schatzkin A, Lanza E, Corle D, et al. Lack of effect of a low-fat, high-fiber diet on the recurrence of colorectal adenomas. Polyp Prevention Trial Study Group. *N Engl J Med* 2000;342:1149–1155.
69. Bonithon-Kopp C, Kronborg O, Giacosa A, et al. Calcium and fibre supplementation in prevention of colorectal adenoma recurrence: a randomised intervention trial. European Cancer Prevention Organisation Study Group. *Lancet* 2000;356:1300–1306.
70. Graham S, Zielezny M, Marshall J, et al. Diet in the epidemiology of postmenopausal breast cancer in the New York State Cohort. *Am J Epidemiol* 1992;136:1327–1337.
71. Horn-Ross PL, Hoggatt KJ, West DW, et al. Recent diet and breast cancer risk: the California Teachers Study (USA). *Cancer Causes Control* 2002;13: 407–415.
72. Jarvinen R, Knekt P, Seppanen R, et al. Diet and breast cancer risk in a cohort of Finnish women. *Cancer Lett* 1997;114:251–253.
73. Terry P, Jain M, Miller AB, et al. No association among total dietary fiber, fiber fractions, and risk of breast cancer. *Cancer Epidemiol Biomarkers Prev* 2002;11:1507–1508.
74. Verhoeven DT, Assen N, Goldbohm RA, et al. Vitamins C and E, retinol, beta-carotene and dietary fibre in relation to breast cancer risk: a prospective cohort study. *Br J Cancer* 1997;75:149–155.
75. Willett WC, Hunter DJ, Stampfer MJ, et al. Dietary fat and fiber in relation to risk of breast cancer. An 8-year follow-up. *JAMA* 1992;268:2037–2044.
76. Botterweck AA, van den Brandt PA, Goldbohm RA. Vitamins, carotenoids, dietary fiber, and the risk of gastric carcinoma: results from a prospective study after 6.3 years of follow-up. *Cancer* 2000;88:737–748.
77. Missmer SA, Smith-Warner SA, Spiegelman D, et al. Meat and dairy food consumption and breast cancer: a pooled analysis of cohort studies. *Int J Epidemiol* 2002;31:78–85.
78. Cho E, Chen WY, Hunter DJ, et al. Red meat intake and risk of breast cancer among premenopausal women. *Arch Intern Med* 2006;166:2253–2259.
79. Cho E, Smith-Warner SA, Spiegelman D, et al. Dairy foods, calcium, and colorectal cancer: a pooled analysis of 10 cohort studies. *J Natl Cancer Inst* 2004;96:1015–1022.
80. Aune D, Lau R, Chan DS, et al. Dairy products and colorectal cancer risk: a systematic review and meta-analysis of cohort studies. *Ann Oncol* 2012; 23:37–45.
81. Baron JA, Beach M, Mandel JS, et al. Calcium supplements for the prevention of colorectal adenomas. Calcium Polyp Prevention Study Group. *N Engl J Med* 1999;340:101–107.
82. Allen NE, Key TJ, Appleby PN, et al. Animal foods, protein, calcium and prostate cancer risk: the European Prospective Investigation into Cancer and Nutrition. *Br J Cancer* 2008;98:1574–1581.
83. Kurahashi N, Inoue M, Iwasaki M, et al. Dairy product, saturated fatty acid, and calcium intake and prostate cancer in a prospective cohort of Japanese men. *Cancer Epidemiol Biomarkers Prev* 2008;17:930–937.
84. Chan JM, Stampfer MJ, Ma J, et al. Dairy products, calcium, and prostate cancer risk in the Physicians' Health Study. *Am J Clin Nut* 2001;74:549–554.
85. Mitrou PN, Albanes D, Weinstein SJ, et al. A prospective study of dietary calcium, dairy products and prostate cancer risk (Finland). *Int J Cancer* 2007;120:2466–2473.
86. Tseng M, Breslow RA, Graubard BI, et al. Dairy, calcium, and vitamin D intakes and prostate cancer risk in the National Health and Nutrition Examination Epidemiologic Follow-up Study cohort. *Am J Clin Nutr* 2005; 81:1147–1154.
87. Giovannucci E, Liu Y, Stampfer MJ, et al. A prospective study of calcium intake and incident and fatal prostate cancer. *Cancer Epidemiol Biomarkers Prev* 2006;15:203–210.

88. Snowdon DA, Phillips RL, Choi W. Diet, obesity, and risk of fatal prostate cancer. *Am J Epidemiol* 1984;120:244–250.
89. Park Y, Mitrou PN, Kipnis V, et al. Calcium, dairy foods, and risk of incident and fatal prostate cancer: the NIH-AARP Diet and Health Study. *Am J Epidemiol* 2007;166:1270–1279.
90. Park SY, Murphy SP, Wilkens LR, et al. Calcium, vitamin D, and dairy product intake and prostate cancer risk: the Multiethnic Cohort Study. *Am J Epidemiol* 2007;166:1259–1269.
91. Ahn J, Albanes D, Peters U, et al. Dairy products, calcium intake, and risk of prostate cancer in the prostate, lung, colorectal, and ovarian cancer screening trial. *Cancer Epidemiol Biomarkers Prev* 2007;16:2623–2630.
92. Gao X, LaValley MP, Tucker KL. Prospective studies of dairy product and calcium intakes and prostate cancer risk: a meta-analysis. *J Natl Cancer Inst* 2005;97:1768–1777.
93. Huncharek M, Muscat J, Kupelnick B. Dairy products, dietary calcium and vitamin D intake as risk factors for prostate cancer: a meta-analysis of 26,769 cases from 45 observational studies. *Nutr Cancer* 2008;60:421–441.
94. Ganmaa D, Cui X, Feskanich D, et al. Milk, dairy intake and risk of endometrial cancer: a 26-year follow-up. *Int J Cancer* 2012;130:2664–2671.
95. Genkinger JM, Hunter DJ, Spiegelman D, et al. Dairy products and ovarian cancer: a pooled analysis of 12 cohort studies. *Cancer Epidemiol Biomarkers Prev* 2006;15:364–372.
96. Hoppe C, Molgaard C, Juul A, et al. High intakes of skimmed milk, but not meat, increase serum IGF-I and IGFBP-3 in eight-year-old boys. *Eur J Clin Nutr* 2004;58:1211–1216.
97. Ganmaa D, Wang PY, Qin LQ, et al. Is milk responsible for male reproductive disorders? *Med Hypotheses* 2001;57:510–514.
98. Garland CF, Garland FC. Do sunlight and vitamin D reduce the likelihood of colon cancer? *Int J Epidemiol* 1980;9:227–231.
99. Feskanich D, Ma J, Fuchs CS, et al. Plasma vitamin D metabolites and risk of colorectal cancer in women. *Cancer Epidemiol Biomarkers Prev* 2004; 13:1502–1508.
100. Woolcott CG, Wilkens LR, Nomura AM, et al. Plasma 25-hydroxyvitamin D levels and the risk of colorectal cancer: the multiethnic cohort study. *Cancer Epidemiol Biomarkers Prev* 2010;19:130–134.
101. Jenab M, Bueno-de-Mesquita HB, Ferrari P, et al. Association between pre-diagnostic circulating vitamin D concentration and risk of colorectal cancer in European populations: a nested case-control study. *BMJ* 2010; 340:b5500.
102. Wactawski-Wende J, Kotchen JM, Anderson GL, et al. Calcium plus vitamin D supplementation and the risk of colorectal cancer. *N Engl J Med* 2006;354:684–696.
103. Park SY, Murphy SP, Wilkens LR, et al. Calcium and vitamin D intake and risk of colorectal cancer: the Multiethnic Cohort Study. *Am J Epidemiol* 2007;165:784–793.
104. Gorham ED, Garland CF, Garland FC, et al. Optimal vitamin D status for colorectal cancer prevention: a quantitative meta analysis. *Am J Prev Med* 2007;32:210–216.
105. Yin L, Grandi N, Raum E, et al. Meta-analysis: longitudinal studies of serum vitamin D and colorectal cancer risk. *Aliment Pharmacol Ther* 2009;30: 113–125.
106. Wei MY, Garland CF, Gorham ED, et al. Vitamin D and prevention of colorectal adenoma: a meta-analysis. *Cancer Epidemiol Biomarkers Prev* 2008; 17:2958–2969.
107. Freedman DM, Looker AC, Chang SC, et al. Prospective study of serum vitamin D and cancer mortality in the United States. *J Natl Cancer Inst* 2007;99:1594–1602.
108. Bertone-Johnson ER, Chen WY, Holick MF, et al. Plasma 25-hydroxyvitamin D and 1,25-dihydroxyvitamin D and risk of breast cancer. *Cancer Epidemiol Biomarkers Prev* 2005;14:1991–1997.
109. McCullough ML, Rodriguez C, Diver WR, et al. Dairy, calcium, and vitamin D intake and postmenopausal breast cancer risk in the Cancer Prevention Study II Nutrition Cohort. *Cancer Epidemiol Biomarkers Prev* 2005;14: 2898–2904.
110. Chen P, Hu P, Xie D, et al. Meta-analysis of vitamin D, calcium and the prevention of breast cancer. *Breast Cancer Res Treat* 2010;121:469–477.
111. Platz EA, Leitzmann MF, Hollis BW, et al. Plasma 1,25-dihydroxy- and 25-hydroxyvitamin D and subsequent risk of prostate cancer. *Cancer Causes Control* 2004;15:255–265.
112. Shui IM, Mucci LA, Kraft P, et al. Vitamin D-related genetic variation, plasma vitamin D, and risk of lethal prostate cancer: a prospective nested case-control study. *J Natl Cancer Inst* 2012;104:690–699.
113. Tworoger SS, Lee IM, Buring JE, et al. Plasma 25-hydroxyvitamin D and 1,25-dihydroxyvitamin D and risk of incident ovarian cancer. *Cancer Epidemiol Biomarkers Prev* 2007;16:783–788.
114. Toriola AT, Surcel HM, Agborsangaya C, et al. Serum 25-hydroxyvitamin D and the risk of ovarian cancer. *Eur J Cancer* 2010;46:364–369.
115. Stolzenberg-Solomon RZ, Jacobs EJ, Arslan AA, et al. Circulating 25-hydroxyvitamin D and risk of pancreatic cancer: Cohort Consortium Vitamin D Pooling Project of Rarer Cancers. *Am J Epidemiol* 2010; 172:81–93.
116. Skinner HG, Michaud DS, Giovannucci E, et al. Vitamin D intake and the risk for pancreatic cancer in two cohort studies. *Cancer Epidemiol Biomarkers Prev* 2006;15:1688–1695.
117. Wolpin BM, Ng K, Bao Y, et al. Plasma 25-hydroxyvitamin D and risk of pancreatic cancer. *Cancer Epidemiol Biomarkers Prev* 2012;21:82–91.
118. Giovannucci E. Epidemiology of vitamin D and colorectal cancer: casual or causal link? *J Steroid Biochem Mol Biol* 2010;121(1–2):349–354.
119. Giovannucci E. Epidemiologic studies of folate and colorectal neoplasia: a review. *J Nutr* 2002;132:2350S–2355S.
120. Kim D, Smith-Warner S, Spiegelman D, et al. Pooled analysis of 13 prospective cohort studies on folate and colon cancer. *Cancer Causes Control* 2010;21:1919-1930.
121. Chen J, Giovannucci E, Kelsey K, et al. A methylenetetrahydrofolate reductase polymorphism and the risk of colorectal cancer. *Cancer Res* 1996;56:4862–4864.
122. Osterhues A, Holzgreve W, Michels KB. Shall we put the world on folate? *Lancet* 2009;374:959–961.
123. Friso S, Choi SW, Girelli D, et al. A common mutation in the 5,10-methylenetetrahydrofolate reductase gene affects genomic DNA methylation through an interaction with folate status. *Proc Natl Acad Sci U S A* 2002;99:5606–5611.
124. Kim YI. Folate: a magic bullet or a double edged sword for colorectal cancer prevention? *Gut* 2006;55:1387–1389.
125. Mason JB. Folate, cancer risk, and the Greek god, Proteus: a tale of two chameleons. *Nutr Rev* 2009;67:206–212.
126. Wu K, Platz EA, Willett W, et al. A randomized trial on folic acid supplementation and risk of recurrent colorectal adenoma. *Am J Clin Nutr* 2009; 90:1623–1631.
127. Cole BF, Baron JA, Sandler RS, et al. Folic acid for the prevention of colorectal adenomas: a randomized clinical trial. *JAMA* 2007;297:2351–2359.
128. Mason JB, Dickstein A, Jacques PF, et al. A temporal association between folic acid fortification and an increase in colorectal cancer rates may be illuminating important biological principles: a hypothesis. *Cancer Epidemiol Biomarkers Prev* 2007;16:1325–1329.
129. The effect of vitamin E and beta carotene on the incidence of lung cancer and other cancers in male smokers. The Alpha-Tocopherol, Beta Carotene Cancer Prevention Study Group. *N Engl J Med* 1994;330:1029–1035.
130. Virtamo J, Pietinen P, Huttunen JK, et al. Incidence of cancer and mortality following alpha-tocopherol and beta-carotene supplementation: a postintervention follow-up. *JAMA* 2003;290:476–485.
131. Mannisto S, Smith-Warner SA, Spiegelman D, et al. Dietary carotenoids and risk of lung cancer in a pooled analysis of seven cohort studies. *Cancer Epidemiol Biomarkers Prev* 2004;13:40–48.
132. Zhang X, Spiegelman D, Baglietto L, et al. Carotenoid intakes and risk of breast cancer defined by estrogen receptor and progesterone receptor status: a pooled analysis of 18 prospective cohort studies. *Am J Clin Nutr* 2012;95:713–725.
133. Eliassen AH, Hendrickson SJ, Brinton LA, et al. Circulating carotenoids and risk of breast cancer: pooled analysis of eight prospective studies. *J Natl Cancer Inst* 2012;104:1905–1916.
134. Giovannucci E. Tomatoes, tomato-based products, lycopene, and cancer: review of the epidemiologic literature. *J Natl Cancer Inst* 1999;91:317–331.
135. Yoshizawa K, Willett WC, Morris SJ, et al. Study of prediagnostic selenium level in toenails and the risk of advanced prostate cancer. *J Natl Cancer Inst* 1998;90:1219–1224.
136. Amaral AF, Cantor KP, Silverman DT, et al. Selenium and bladder cancer risk: a meta-analysis. *Cancer Epidemiol Biomarkers Prev* 2010;19:2407–2415.
137. Geybels MS, Verhage BA, van Schooten FJ, et al. Advanced prostate cancer risk in relation to toenail selenium levels. *J Natl Cancer Inst* 2013;105:1394–1401.
138. Hurst R, Hooper L, Norat T, et al. Selenium and prostate cancer: systematic review and meta-analysis. *Am J Clinical Nutr* 2012;96:111–122.
139. Lippman SM, Klein EA, Goodman PJ, et al. Effect of selenium and vitamin E on risk of prostate cancer and other cancers: the Selenium and Vitamin E Cancer Prevention Trial (SELECT). *JAMA* 2009;301:39–51.
140. Trock BJ, Hilakivi-Clarke L, Clarke R. Meta-analysis of soy intake and breast cancer risk. *J Natl Cancer Inst* 2006;98:459–471.
141. Wu AH, Wan P, Hankin J, et al. Adolescent and adult soy intake and risk of breast cancer in Asian-Americans. *Carcinogenesis* 2002;23:1491–1496.
142. Warburg O, Posener K, Negelein E. Ueber den Stoffwechsel der Tumoren. *Biochemische Zeitschrift* 1924;152:319.
143. Hu FB, Manson JE, Liu S, et al. Prospective study of adult onset diabetes mellitus (type 2) and risk of colorectal cancer in women. *J Natl Cancer Inst* 1999;91:542–547.
144. Michels KB, Solomon CG, Hu FB, et al. Type 2 diabetes and subsequent incidence of breast cancer in the Nurses' Health Study. *Diabetes Care* 2003;26:1752–1758.
145. Gnagnarella P, Gandini S, La Vecchia C, et al. Glycemic index, glycemic load, and cancer risk: a meta-analysis. *Am J Clinical Nutr* 2008;87:1793–1801.
146. Slattery ML, Benson J, Berry TD, et al. Dietary sugar and colon cancer. *Cancer Epidemiol Biomarkers Prev* 1997;6:677–685.
147. Terry PD, Jain M, Miller AB, et al. Glycemic load, carbohydrate intake, and risk of colorectal cancer in women: a prospective cohort study. *J Natl Cancer Inst* 2003;95:914–916.
148. Michaud DS, Liu S, Giovannucci E, et al. Dietary sugar, glycemic load, and pancreatic cancer risk in a prospective study. *J Natl Cancer Inst* 2002; 94:1293–1300.
149. Jonas CR, McCullough ML, Teras LR, et al. Dietary glycemic index, glycemic load, and risk of incident breast cancer in postmenopausal women. *Cancer Epidemiol Biomarkers Prev* 2003;12:573–577.
150. Tantamango-Bartley Y, Jaceldo-Siegl K, Fan J, et al. Vegetarian diets and the incidence of cancer in a low-risk population. *Cancer Epidemiol Biomarkers Prev* 2013;22:286–294.
151. Key TJ, Appleby PN, Spencer EA, et al. Cancer incidence in British vegetarians. *Br J Cancer* 2009;101:192–197.

152. Fung T, Hu FB, Fuchs C, et al. Major dietary patterns and the risk of colorectal cancer in women. *Arch Intern Med* 2003;163:309–314.
153. Fung TT, Hu FB, Holmes MD, et al. Dietary patterns and the risk of postmenopausal breast cancer. *Int J Cancer* 2005;116:116–121.
154. Link LB, Canchola AJ, Bernstein L, et al. Dietary patterns and breast cancer risk in the California Teachers Study cohort. *Am J Clin Nutr* 2013;98:1524–1532.
155. Caughey RW, Michels KB. Birth weight and childhood leukemia: a meta-analysis and review of the current evidence. *Int J Cancer* 2009;124:2658–2670.
156. Michels KB, Xue F. Role of birthweight in the etiology of breast cancer. *Int J Cancer* 2006;119:2007–2025.
157. Michos A, Xue F, Michels KB. Birth weight and the risk of testicular cancer: a meta-analysis. *Int J Cancer* 2007;121:1123–1131.
158. Chavarro JE, Rosner BA, Sampson L, et al. Validity of adolescent diet recall 48 years later. *Am J Epidemiol* 2009;170:1563–1570.
159. Maruti SS, Feskanich D, Colditz GA, et al. Adult recall of adolescent diet: reproducibility and comparison with maternal reporting. *Am J Epidemiol* 2005;161:89–97.
160. Michels KB, Rosner BA, Chumlea WC, et al. Preschool diet and adult risk of breast cancer. *Int J Cancer* 2006;118:749–754.
161. Hjartaker A, Laake P, Lund E. Childhood and adult milk consumption and risk of premenopausal breast cancer in a cohort of 48,844 women - the Norwegian women and cancer study. *Int J Cancer* 2001;93:888–893.
162. Michels KB, Mohllajee AP, Roset-Bahmanyar E, et al. Diet and breast cancer: a review of the prospective observational studies. *Cancer* 2007;109:2712–2749.
163. Greenlee H, Kwan ML, Kushi LH, et al. Antioxidant supplement use after breast cancer diagnosis and mortality in the Life After Cancer Epidemiology (LACE) cohort. *Cancer* 2012;118:2048–2058.
164. Kwan ML, Chen WY, Flatt SW, et al. Postdiagnosis alcohol consumption and breast cancer prognosis in the after breast cancer pooling project. *Cancer Epidemiol Biomarkers Prev* 2013;22:32–41.
165. Chlebowski RT, Blackburn GL, Thomson CA, et al. Dietary fat reduction and breast cancer outcome: interim efficacy results from the Women's Intervention Nutrition Study. *J Natl Cancer Inst* 2006;98:1767–1776.
166. Pierce JP, Natarajan L, Caan BJ, et al. Influence of a diet very high in vegetables, fruit, and fiber and low in fat on prognosis following treatment for breast cancer: the Women's Healthy Eating and Living (WHEL) randomized trial. *JAMA* 2007;298:289–298.
167. Izano MA, Fung TT, Chiuve SS, et al. Are diet quality scores after breast cancer diagnosis associated with improved breast cancer survival? *Nutr Cancer* 2013;65:820–826.
168. van Meer S, Leufkens AM, Bueno-de-Mesquita HB, et al. Role of dietary factors in survival and mortality in colorectal cancer: a systematic review. *Nutrition Rev* 2013;71:631–641.
169. Meyerhardt JA, Niedzwiecki D, Hollis D, et al. Association of dietary patterns with cancer recurrence and survival in patients with stage III colon cancer. *JAMA* 2007;298:754–764.
170. Meyerhardt JA, Sato K, Niedzwiecki D, et al. Dietary glycemic load and cancer recurrence and survival in patients with stage III colon cancer: findings from CALGB 89803. *J Natl Cancer Inst* 2012;104:1702–1711.
171. Song Y, Chavarro JE, Cao Y, et al. Whole milk intake is associated with prostate cancer-specific mortality among U.S. male physicians. *J Nutr* 2013;143:189–196.
172. Richman EL, Kenfield SA, Chavarro JE, et al. Fat intake after diagnosis and risk of lethal prostate cancer and all-cause mortality. *JAMA Intern Med* 2013;173:1318–1326.
173. Richman EL, Kenfield SA, Stampfer MJ, et al. Egg, red meat, and poultry intake and risk of lethal prostate cancer in the prostate-specific antigen-era: incidence and survival. *Cancer Prev Res (Phila)* 2011;4:2110–2121.
174. Chan JM, Holick CN, Leitzmann MF, et al. Diet after diagnosis and the risk of prostate cancer progression, recurrence, and death (United States). *Cancer Causes Control* 2006;17:199–208.
175. Ornish D, Weidner G, Fair WR, et al. Intensive lifestyle changes may affect the progression of prostate cancer. *J Urol* 2005;174:1065–1070.
176. Kushi LH, Doyle C, McCullough M, et al. American Cancer Society Guidelines on nutrition and physical activity for cancer prevention: reducing the risk of cancer with healthy food choices and physical activity. *CA Cancer J Clin* 2012;62:30–67.

10 Obesity and Physical Activity

Yani Lu, Jessica Clague, and Leslie Bernstein

INTRODUCTION

Evidence showing that physical activity is associated with decreased cancer risk and that obesity is associated with increased cancer risk at certain sites is rapidly accumulating. It is not yet known whether these two factors are interrelated or independent. Physical activity may act to decrease cancer risk primarily by preventing weight gain and obesity. However, physical activity may also have independent effects on cancer risk. In this chapter, we present a summary of the current epidemiologic literature on the possible associations between physical activity and obesity and risk of cancer at several organ sites.

Physical activity is defined as any movement of the body that results in energy expenditure. In this chapter, we focus on recreational physical activity, also called leisure-time physical activity or exercise, and occupational physical activity, including household activity.[1] Occupational physical activity typically occurs over a longer period of time and generally requires less energy expenditure per hour than bouts of strenuous or moderate recreational physical activity. The distinction between recreational and occupational activity is important because increasing mechanization and technologic advances have led to decreased occupational physical activity in developed areas of the world, perhaps contributing to a decrease in overall physical activity.

Obesity is defined as the condition of being extremely overweight. In epidemiologic studies, the usual, but not necessarily the best, measure of body mass in adults is Quetelet's Index, or body mass index (BMI), which is measured as weight in kilograms (kg) divided by the square of height in meters (m^2). In the year spanning 2009 to 2010, the prevalence of obesity, defined by having a BMI of 30 kg/m^2 or greater, in the US population was 35.5% for adult men and 35.8% for adult women.[2] Physical inactivity has likely contributed to the high prevalence of obesity in the United States; data from the 2003 to 2004 National Health and Nutritional Examination Survey, a cross sectional study of a sample of the civilian, noninstitutionalized population of the United States, has indicated that less than 5% of US adults achieve 30 minutes per day of physical activity, and that men are more physically active than women.[3]

Epidemiologic evidence on the associations of physical activity and obesity with cancer come from observational studies, including cohort studies, which follow populations forward in time after collecting exposure information, and case-control studies, which optimally identify a population-based series of newly diagnosed cases and healthy control subjects, collecting information retrospectively on exposures. In both study designs, physical activity information is usually self-reported and measures vary substantially with respect to timing and level of detail. Studies have measured lifetime or long-term physical activity, activity at defined ages or time points in life, and/or current or recent activity. Ideally, a study would capture activity by type (recreational, occupational, or other, such as an activity related to transportation), duration (minutes per session), frequency (sessions per day), and intensity (low, moderate, or strenuous as defined by examples of activity types) across the lifetime. These studies have often measured height and weight by self-report at one time point, such as at the time of study entry. Some studies have collected other or more detailed anthropometric information, such as waist circumference, hip circumference, or weight at an additional time point like at age 18. Anthropometrics are directly measured by trained study personnel in only a few studies.

Epidemiologic evidence for a role of physical activity or obesity in relation to cancer risk exists for cancers of the breast, colon, endometrium, esophagus, kidney, and pancreatic cancer. Evidence is accumulating to link at least one of these "exposures" to the incidence of gallbladder cancer, non-Hodgkin lymphoma (NHL), and advanced prostate cancer. The evidence for an association between either physical activity or obesity and lung and ovarian cancer is inconclusive.

In addition to specific biologic mechanisms pertinent to physical activity or to obesity at each specific organ site, several global mechanisms have been implicated in both relationships across a number of these organ sites. The steroid hormone and insulin/insulinlike growth factor (IGF) pathways are two such global mechanisms hypothesized to be involved in the links between physical activity or obesity and cancer.[4] The role of steroid hormones as a mediator in these relationships is perhaps best understood in the context of breast cancer and endometrial cancer, and will be discussed in those sections. The roles of the insulin and IGF pathways have been discussed in depth with respect to colon cancer and, thus, will be presented in that context. Other global mechanisms have been proposed that have more generalized anticancer impacts and may explain associations between physical activity and several cancer sites; these include heightening immune surveillance, reducing inflammation, increasing insulin sensitivity, controlling growth factor production and activation, decreasing obesity and central adiposity, optimizing DNA repair capacity, and reducing oxidative stress.[5,6] Further, obesity has been shown to produce a proinflammatory state and, thus, inflammation may mediate the relationship between obesity and cancer risk.[7] It is highly plausible that several of these mechanisms act simultaneously and that they interact synergistically to mediate the associations between physical activity, obesity, and cancer.

BREAST CANCER

Low level of physical activity is an established breast cancer risk factor among postmenopausal women and, to a lesser extent, premenopausal women.[4,8,9] The evidence for an association between physical activity and breast cancer has been classified as convincing, with a 20% to 40% reduced risk among physically active women.[10] Obesity appears to have a paradoxical relationship with breast cancer risk in that it is an established breast cancer risk factor among postmenopausal women, but may offer some protection for breast cancer among premenopausal women.[4]

The epidemiologic literature has shown with relative consistency that breast cancer risk is reduced by increasing one's amount of physical activity.[4,8,9,11–13] One of the earliest studies, a case-control study of women age 40 years or younger, showed a dramatic reduction in risk of approximately 50% among women who averaged about 4 hours of activity per week during their reproductive years.[14] Similarly, among postmenopausal women, those with higher levels of recreational physical activity during their lifetimes have been shown to have lower breast cancer risk.[15] A meta-analysis of 29 case-control studies and 19 cohort studies published between 1994 and 2006 provided strong evidence for an inverse association between physical activity and risk of breast cancer, citing that the evidence for an association between physical activity and premenopausal breast cancer was not as strong as that for postmenopausal breast cancer.[8] The conclusion of the meta-analysis was that each additional hour of physical activity per week decreases breast cancer by approximately 6%.

Epidemiologists require that a risk factor demonstrate consistency across populations before considering it as accepted. Recently, studies have been published on the association between physical activity and breast cancer risk among Japanese,[16] Chinese,[17] Mexican,[18] Tunisian,[19] and African American women.[20] All studies showed a decreased risk of breast cancer with increasing physical activity. Interestingly, both Suzuki et al.[17] and Pronk et al.[21] observed the strongest associations among "heavier" women (BMI ≥25 kg/m^2 and 23.73 kg/m^2, respectively). In the California Teachers Study (CTS), a prospective cohort study of over 133,000 female public school professionals, a variable combining strenuous and moderate long-term recreational physical activity was associated with a reduced risk of estrogen receptor (ER)-negative but not ER-positive invasive breast cancer.[11] On the contrary, the Women's Health Initiative (WHI) observed decreases in breast cancer risk associated with recreational physical activity among postmenopausal women with ER-positive breast cancer and triple negative breast cancer, with only results for ER-positive breast cancer demonstrating a 15% statistically significant reduced risk (when comparing the highest versus lowest tertile of moderate-intensity physical activity).[22] Similar but not statistically significant results were observed for strenuous recreational physical activity.[22] A major limitation to this and previous studies stratifying by hormone receptor status is the inability to comprehensively classify triple negative breast cancer due to missing HER2 status (unknown in 40% of cases in the WHI study). The use of hormone therapy did not alter the inverse association between recreational physical activity and invasive breast cancer in the Women's Contraceptive and Reproductive Experiences (CARE) Study.[23] Most recently, in the American Cancer Society Cancer Prevention Study II Nutrition Cohort, it was observed that postmenopausal women who engage in at least 7 hours of walking over the course of a week had a modest decreased risk of breast cancer, even in the absence of more vigorous exercise.[24] Further, this association did not differ by ER status, BMI, adult weight gain, postmenopausal hormone therapy use, or time spent sitting.[24]

Lastly, whether physical activity reduces breast cancer risk by impacting preinvasive disease has been studied by assessing the associations with in situ breast cancer and benign breast disease. In the CTS cohort, increasing levels of long-term strenuous recreational physical activity were associated with a decreasing risk of in situ breast cancer.[11] Furthermore, a report from the Nurses' Health Study II cohort showed that lifetime recreational physical activity was associated with a decreased risk of benign breast disease and columnar cell lesions, which may be precursors to breast cancer.[25]

In summary, epidemiologic studies investigating the association between physical activity and breast cancer risk have produced relatively consistent results showing a reduction in breast cancer risk with increasing level of physical activity. Results to date suggest that moderate-to-strenuous activity may be required for the effect between physical activity and breast cancer risk to be clear; however, clarification of other key details, such as the importance of timing and intensity of activity or variation in effects by tumor characteristics, is pending.

Adult obesity and adult weight gain have both been associated with increased breast cancer risk among postmenopausal women, especially among women who were not current users of menopausal hormone therapy.[4,26,27] Most studies among postmenopausal women show a 1.5- to 2-fold increase in risk of invasive breast cancer when comparing the most obese women or those with the largest weight gain to normal-weight women (BMI: 18.5 to 24.9 kg/m^2) or those with the least weight gain.[4] Paradoxically, overweight or obese premenopausal women have a slightly decreased risk of breast cancer compared with normal-weight or thinner women. Whether larger waist circumference is more important than BMI has been studied in order to separate overall weight gain from abdominal obesity (i.e., visceral fat, which is one element of metabolic syndrome); however, most studies have reported a null association between waist circumference, used as a surrogate for visceral fat, and risk of postmenopausal breast cancer after adjustment for BMI.[26] In contrast to the results for postmenopausal women, waist circumference and a positive association with premenopausal breast cancer was found after adjustment for BMI.[26] A recent analysis of the Nurses' Health Study suggests that self-rated body fatness during youth and BMI at age 18 years are both inversely associated with breast cancer risk, with similar results for premenopausal and postmenopausal breast cancer.[28]

Hormones are central to the discussion of biologic mechanisms linking both physical activity and obesity with breast cancer risk. Physical activity can alter menstrual cycle patterns in premenopausal women, and hormone profiles in both premenopausal and postmenopausal women. Physical activity may lower body fat among children,[29] which in turn may delay age at menarche.[30] Later age at menarche has been associated with reduced breast cancer risk.[31] Physical activity may reduce the frequency of ovulatory cycles.[32] Having less frequent and therefore fewer cumulative ovulatory cycles is likely to reduce the lifetime exposure of the breast to endogenous ovarian hormones,[31] which are proven proliferative agents.[33] Physical activity also can have a direct impact on circulating estrogen levels among postmenopausal women.[34]

In the postmenopausal period, adipose tissue is the primary source of endogenous hormones via aromatization of androstenedione to estrone.[35] Thus, heavier postmenopausal women have higher levels of circulating estrogen than women with less adipose tissue. The involvement of estrogen in the relationship between obesity and breast cancer risk is supported by the observation that obesity does not independently increase breast cancer risk among menopausal hormone therapy users[27]; the obesity-related increase in estrogen over that provided by exogenous estrogens is negligible. The breast tissue of overweight or obese perimenopausal and postmenopausal women with relatively high risk of breast cancer has been shown to have cytologic abnormalities and higher epithelial cell counts than that of normal-weight women.[36] In contrast, obese premenopausal women experience menstrual cycle disturbances, including anovulatory cycles and secondary amenorrhea, thereby lowering their cumulative exposure to estradiol and progesterone.[31] A possible explanation for the inverse association between youth body fatness and breast cancer risk is that youth body size is inversely associated with adult IGF-1 levels.[28]

Other likely mechanisms that may link physical activity[37,38] and obesity[39,40] with breast cancer risk include aspects of immune function, inflammatory mechanisms, oxidative stress and DNA repair capability, metabolic hormones, and growth factors.

COLON AND RECTAL CANCER

An inverse association between physical activity and colon cancer risk has been consistently observed among epidemiologic studies; however, the evidence for rectal cancer remains inconclusive. Historically, comprehensive reviews have estimated that physical activity may reduce colon cancer risk by 20% to 25% when comparing individuals with the highest levels to those with the lowest levels of activity.[41] Risk reductions are greater for case-control studies (24%) than for cohort studies (17%), and risk reductions for occupational activity (22%) and recreational activity (23%) are similar.[41] In cohort studies, colon cancer risk reduction associated with physical activity is greater for men than for women, which may be due to the influence of hormone therapy on colon cancer risk,[42] although case-control studies suggest similar benefits for men and women.[43]

Whether physical activity preferentially protects against proximal or distal colon cancer is of interest. A meta-analysis including 21 cohort and case-control studies that examined associations between physical activity and the risks of proximal colon and distal colon cancers produced results suggesting that physical activity is associated with a reduced risk of both proximal colon and distal colon cancers, and that the magnitude of the association does not differ by subsite.[44]

Although the majority of previous studies have not found an association between physical activity and rectal cancer,[41] the National Institutes of Health (NIH)–AARP Diet and Health Study observed a modest reduction in rectal cancer risk for men but not for women after 6.9 years of follow-up.[45] Further, in a case-control study conducted in Australia, rectal cancer risk was reduced among men but not among women who participated in vigorous recreational physical activity averaging at least 6 metabolic equivalent task (MET)-hours per week during their adult years.[46]

An emphasis has been made on trying to identify risk factors for colon adenomas, which are considered precursor lesions for colon cancer; these are detected and removed during colonoscopy or sigmoidoscopy. Wolin et al. conducted a meta-analysis of 20 studies published through April 2010 that investigated the association between recreational physical activity and colon adenomas.[47] Adenoma risk was reduced by 19% among men and by 13% among women and, when combining men and women, the inverse association with physical activity was strongest for large/advanced polyps.

Obesity is an established risk factor for colon cancer in both men and women, although the relative risks for men have been higher than those for women.[4,26] The adverse impact of being overweight or obese on colon cancer risk is stronger for distal than for proximal colon cancers. In addition, visceral adiposity appears to confer greater risk than general adiposity.[26] In the European Prospective Investigation into Cancer and Nutrition (EPIC) study, abdominal obesity as well as adult weight gain were strongly associated with colon cancer risk in both men and women.[48,49] No association between these adiposity measures and colon cancer risk was evident among postmenopausal women who had used menopausal hormone therapy, and no association was observed between any measure of adiposity and rectal cancer risk.[48] The positive association between obesity and risk of colon cancer was further supported by the findings that both general obesity and abdominal obesity increase the risk of colon adenomas[47] with one study of women indicating that the distal colon is the main target site.[50]

Given that a higher BMI and lack of physical activity are both risk factors for colon cancer, several statistical approaches have been employed to tease apart their joint and independent effects on colon cancer risk. In the Netherlands Cohort Study,[51] colorectal cancer risk was increased at each subsite among larger women in the lowest recreational activity category (<30 minutes per day) than in smaller women in the highest recreational activity category (>90 minutes per day); however, the interaction between physical activity and body size was statistically significant only for proximal tumors. Using different fatness measures for men, the only similar finding was that men with low levels of physical activity whose trouser size was below the median of that for the cohort had an increased risk of distal colon cancer; no differences in risk were noted for other subsites or for men with larger trouser sizes.[51]

The mechanisms explaining the relationship between physical activity and colon cancer are not clearly established, but include the impact on insulin sensitivity and IGF profiles, and inflammation, as well as some colon-specific mechanisms. Physical activity may stimulate stool transit in the colon, thereby decreasing the exposure of colonic mucosa to carcinogens in the stool.[6] Alternatively, physical activity–induced decreases in prostaglandin E_2 may decrease colonic cell proliferation rates and increase colonic motility.[6] In addition to steroid hormones, which have been clearly implicated as biologic modifiers of the effect of physical activity and obesity on colon cancer risk, the insulin and IGF pathways may mediate the associations between these exposures and colon cancer risk. For obesity in particular, the link can be inferred because obesity can lead to insulin resistance,[52] a syndrome characterized by high circulating insulin levels. High insulin levels appear to promote cell proliferation and tumor growth in the colon[7] and may also suppress the expression of IGF-binding proteins 1 and 2, leading to increased bioavailable IGF-1 levels.[53] Another possible mechanism is obesity-enhanced inflammation in which increases in adipose tissue macrophages lead to the secretion of inflammatory cytokines associated with colon cancer risk (e.g., tumor necrosis factor [TNF]-α, monocyte chemoattractant protein [MCP]-1, and interleukin [IL]-6).

ENDOMETRIAL CANCER

The evidence for an association between physical activity and endometrial cancer risk is accumulating[4,54–58] but is not definitive. A meta-analysis of prospective cohort studies results published through 2009 indicates that recreational physical activity lowers endometrial cancer risk by 27%, and occupational activity lowers risk by 21%.[59] Adjustments for BMI minimally change relative risk estimates, suggesting that physical activity is independently associated with endometrial cancer. Although physical activity is associated with a decreased risk of endometrial cancer in both normal-weight and obese women, two recent studies have suggested that this association is more pronounced for obese women.[54,58]

Two meta-analyses of the association between physical activity and endometrial cancer have identified some inconsistencies in dose-response relationships, indicating the importance of differences in activity type and intensity.[55,56] Little evidence exists on how long-term or lifetime physical activity and activity patterns during different life periods might influence endometrial cancer risk; it has been suggested that recent or long-term activity might be more important than activity at early ages.[56] In the CTS, higher levels of recent (at cohort formation) strenuous recreational physical activity was associated with lower levels of endometrial cancer risk; among women exercising >3 hours per week per year, risk was approximately 25% lower than that of women exercising <0.5 hour per week per year.[60] This inverse association was limited to overweight and obese women (BMI ≥25 kg/m^2). Finally, sitting time has been independently associated with increased endometrial cancer risk.[59]

Epidemiologic studies have established a strong association between obesity and endometrial cancer risk.[26] Recent studies have suggested a linear trend between increasing body weight or BMI and increasing endometrial cancer risk among postmenopausal women, whereas among premenopausal women, no trend is observed, but rather, only obese women have an increased risk.[26] Furthermore, the strong association among postmenopausal women is only observed among those who are not using hormone therapy.[26] Finally, BMI appears to exert an effect on the risk of endometrial cancer that is independent of physical activity.[55]

Physical activity and obesity are likely to influence endometrial cancer risk by altering endogenous hormone profiles.[31,53] Heavier postmenopausal women have higher circulating levels of estrogen than do lighter postmenopausal women because of the aromatization of androstenedione to estrone in adipose tissue. This is pertinent to endometrial cancer risk because this aromatization occurs in the absence of progesterone, which opposes the proliferative effects of estrogen on endometrial tissue. Physical activity may counter the proliferative effects of estrogen either directly or by restricting weight gain. Some evidence also links elevated insulin levels and diabetes to endometrial cancer risk.[61] Physical inactivity and obesity play a role in the development of insulin insensitivity and diabetes, providing another mechanism by which they may influence endometrial cancer risk.

ADENOCARCINOMA OF THE ESOPHAGUS

Several case-control studies[62–64] and one cohort study[65] have examined the association between physical activity and risk of adenocarcinoma of the esophagus. Zhang et al.[62] reported a modest association between participation in recreational physical activity more than once per week and a decreased risk of all esophageal cancer (adenocarcinomas and squamous cell tumors), although the result was not statistically significant. Lagergren et al.[63] reported no association between total, usual recreational and occupational physical activity and esophageal adenocarcinoma. Vigen et al.[64] showed that lifetime occupational physical activity was modestly associated with a lower risk of adenocarcinoma of the esophagus: the average annual level of occupational physical activity before age 65 years was associated with an approximately 40% reduction in risk of esophageal adenocarcinoma when the highest was compared with the lowest occupational physical activity category. Results from the NIH–AARP Diet and Health Study also support the hypothesis that physical activity lowers the risk of esophageal adenocarcinoma, but no association between physical activity and the risk of squamous cell esophageal cancer was found.[65]

Obesity is strongly associated with an increased risk of esophageal adenocarcinoma.[66,67] A pooled analysis of existing data showed that individuals with severe obesity (BMI ≥40 kg/m^2) had a 4.8-fold greater risk than individuals who were not overweight (BMI <25 kg/m^2), with similar risk estimates for men and women.[68] Several studies have examined the effect of abdominal adiposity, which have suggested that the risk associated with obesity is driven primarily by abdominal fatness.[26]

It is likely that obesity impacts esophageal adenocarcinoma risk because it is associated with the risk of gastroesophageal reflux disease (GERD). GERD may cause changes in the esophageal epithelium, leading to Barrett esophagus, a well-established precancerous condition for esophageal adenocarcinoma. On the other hand, obesity is associated with a systemic inflammatory state, which includes the exposure to adipocytokines and procoagulant factors released by adipocytes in central fat, which may also contribute to the development of esophageal adenocarcinoma.[67] Physical activity may influence the risk of esophageal adenocarcinoma by increasing digestive track transit time, thus reducing exposure of the esophagus to putative cancer-causing agents.

KIDNEY/RENAL CELL CANCER

Physical activity has been studied in relation to renal cell carcinoma in part because of the known deleterious effects of high BMI and hypertension on the risk of renal cell cancer; however, no association has been firmly established. A review of physical activity and risk of genitourinary cancers noted significant protective effects in 8 of 15 studies of physical activity in relation to renal cell carcinoma, with an average 8% reduction in risk when comparing individuals with the highest level of physical activity to those with the lowest level of activity.[69] Reductions in risk were greater for recreational than for other forms of activity and for activity performed later in life.

Obesity, in addition to high blood pressure and diabetes, is an established risk factor for kidney cancer.[26] It is still uncertain whether a gender difference exists, however. A meta-analysis has suggested a similar impact of BMI on kidney cancer risk among women and men, with an approximate 7% increase in risk per unit increase in BMI.[26] The effect of obesity may differ by histology; a recent study reported an increased risk observed for clear cell and chromophobe cancers, but not papillary renal cell cancer.[70]

PANCREATIC CANCER

Pancreatic cancer is generally diagnosed at an advanced stage and is associated with high mortality rates. A meta-analysis of 28 studies of pancreatic cancer showed that higher total lifetime physical activity and occupational activity were associated with a lower risk.[71] Nonsignificant reductions in risk were observed for recreational physical activity and transportation (walking and cycling as a form of commuting). Significant heterogeneity was present across the studies, making it difficult to find a definitive answer.

Evidence indicating that obesity is a risk factor for pancreatic cancer is convincing. Three large pooled analyses and three of four meta-analyses that encompass a range of well-designed, independent observational epidemiologic studies have demonstrated a positive association between obesity and pancreatic cancer risk.[72,73] Effects were relatively consistent across studies, with an approximate 10% or greater increase in risk for every 5 kg/m^2 increase in BMI. Two of the pooled analyses and one of the meta-analyses assessed measures of adiposity such as waist circumference or waist-to-hip ratio (WHR); each of the results suggested positive associations with pancreatic cancer risk.[72,74,75] The pooled analyses reported at least a 35% greater risk when the fourth quartile of WHR was compared to the first quartile. The meta-analysis study reported an 11% increase in risk associated with each 10-cm increase in waist circumference and a 19% increase in risk for each 0.1-unit increment in WHR.

GALLBLADDER CANCER

Gallbladder cancer occurs more frequently in women than in men, and the major risk factor is a history of gallstones,[10] which has been associated with the use of exogenous estrogens.[76] To date, we have found no epidemiologic literature investigating the possible association of physical activity and gallbladder cancer, although several studies have suggested a positive association between obesity and gallbladder cancer. In a meta-analysis comprised of 3,288 cases derived from eight cohort studies and three case-control studies, obesity was associated with a 66% increased risk of gallbladder cancer, and the increase in risk was larger for women than for men.[77] Further, two studies found that WHR was positively associated with gallbladder cancer risk among men and women with and without a history of gallstones, suggesting that abdominal obesity may be important in the etiology of this disease.[78,79]

NON-HODGKIN LYMPHOMA

Studies addressing physical inactivity and obesity as potential risk factors for NHL have been mixed, in part because they have not had a sufficient number of cases to assess risk by NHL subtype. Generally, studies have shown no overall association between physical activity and NHL risk.[4] The results of four cohort studies, the CTS,[80] WHI,[81] EPIC,[82] and the American Cancer Society Prevention Study-II[83] have been unconvincing, with WHI showing a nonstatistically significant positive association, whereas the other studies showed no association.

In 2008, the International Lymphoma Epidemiology Consortium (InterLymph) published a pooled analysis of 18 case-control studies with more than 10,000 cases reporting no association between BMI around the time of diagnosis and NHL risk overall, but an increased risk of diffuse NHL for severe obesity (BMI ≥40 kg/m^2).[84] The results from meta-analyses of cohort studies suggested a weak positive association overall and for diffuse NHL.[85,86] An analysis of two cohort studies has suggested that body size in early adulthood may be more predictive of NHL risk than that later in life for all NHL and for the diffuse and follicular subtypes.[87]

PROSTATE CANCER

More than 20 studies have assessed the potential association between physical activity and prostate cancer.[4,88,89] Regardless of the different approaches used, the populations studied, or the sample sizes of the studies, the majority of studies have suggested a modest reduction in risk with an increased level of physical activity.[4] In a review of the literature, Friedenreich and Orenstein[88] concluded that prostate cancer risk is reduced 10% to 30% when comparing the most active with the least active men and suggested that it may be high levels of physical activity earlier in life that are most relevant to this disease. An update to this review, based on 22 additional studies, indicates that the majority of recent research studies observed protective effects.[90] Leitzmann and Rohrmann[91] added that the associations with reduced risk may be most apparent for fatal prostate cancer. A current systematic review and meta-analysis, including 19 cohort and 24 case-control studies, agrees.[92] A pooled 19% reduction in risk was observed for occupational physical activity, and a 5% reduction was observed for recreational physical activity comparing the most physically active men to the least active.[92] An issue that somewhat reduces our confidence in these estimates is that considerable heterogeneity between studies was observed. Further, it is not yet clear whether these results reflect a true causal association or whether they are due to confounding by prostate-specific antigen testing, which may be more common among physically active men.

The early epidemiologic literature on the potential association between obesity and prostate cancer provided no consistent evidence of any relationship.[4] Recent studies have suggested that obesity may have a dual effect on prostate cancer risk. One meta-analysis reported that the risk of early-stage prostate cancer decreased by 6%, whereas the risk of advanced prostate cancer increased 9% per 5-kg/m^2 increase in BMI.[93] Another possibility is that obesity may decrease the likelihood of diagnosis of less aggressive prostate cancer. Proposed mechanisms include the paradoxical effects of testosterone on low-grade versus more advanced prostate cancer and alterations in insulin and circulating IGF-1.[94]

LUNG CANCER

Physical activity may reduce lung cancer risk by 30% to 40%,[88] but no definitive conclusion can be drawn because one cannot ignore potential residual confounding or effect modification due to smoking as an explanation for any observed association. Recent studies have attempted to address this issue by estimating risk within subgroups defined by smoking status. A recent review suggests an inverse relationship between heavy lifetime physical activity and lung cancer in former and current smokers that is consistent across all histologies, but is not observed among never smokers.[5] A small case-control study of current and former smokers enrolled in the Cologne Smoking Study came to a similar conclusion, observing a lower risk of lung cancer among participants who were physically active compared to those who were not.[95] In the large NIH–AARP Diet and Health Study, no associations were observed between occupational or recreation physical activity and lung cancer risk among those who never smoked.[96]

Due to sex differences in lung cancer pathology, risk factors, and prognosis, current research has also begun to investigate the association for men and women separately.[97] The recent literature consists of small case-control studies,[98] which lack statistical power to examine risks in subgroups defined by histology, smoking status, or sex, and which may be affected by survival bias in that rapidly fatal cases or those who are too ill to be interviewed are excluded from the study population.

Several studies have suggested the existence of an inverse association between increasing BMI and lung cancer risk.[99–102] Nevertheless, this inverse effect may have been due to residual confounding by smoking because the inverse association was restricted to ever smokers. One meta-analysis showed an inverse association between BMI and lung cancer in nonsmokers[103]; however, caution should be exercised when interpreting the results due to concerns about heterogeneity of risk estimates across studies, the quality of the original studies, and confounding by smoking.[104]

OVARIAN CANCER

The literature on ovarian cancer risk in relation to physical activity and obesity has been inconclusive. More than 18 studies have assessed the impact of physical activity on ovarian cancer risk. A meta-analysis of 12 studies found an approximate 20% decrease in ovarian cancer risk associated with physical activity when the highest category of exercise was compared to the lowest.[105] Four[106–109] of five[110] additional studies found no association; the fifth study found a nonsignificant 10% to 20% reduction in ovarian cancer risk for women who participated in at least 1 hour per week of recreational aerobic activity.

The evidence for an association between obesity and increased ovarian cancer risk is weak, with few studies showing a statistically significant result.[4,111] A meta-analysis of 16 studies indicated that adult obesity increases the risk for ovarian cancer; the overall pooled effect estimate was a 30% increase in ovarian cancer risk associated with adult obesity with a possible dose-response effect, but no variation in risk estimates across histologic subtypes.[111] In contrast, the results from the Ovarian Cancer Association Consortium, based on original data from 15 case-control studies, suggest that obesity only increases the risk of the less common histologic subtypes of ovarian cancer; obesity does not increase risk of high-grade invasive serous cancers, the most common subtype.[112] A pooled analysis of 12 cohort studies reported that BMI was not associated with ovarian cancer risk in postmenopausal women, but was positively associated with risk in premenopausal women.[113] Another meta-analysis, using 47 studies, showed that the positive association between BMI and ovarian cancer was restricted to women who had never used hormone therapy; among these women, risk increased by 10% with every 5 kg/m^2 increase in BMI.[114]

CONCLUSIONS

Table 10.1 illustrates the strength of evidence regarding increased physical activity as a protective factor and obesity as a risk factor

TABLE 10.1

Summary of the Strength of the Observational Epidemiologic Evidence for Physical Activity as a Protective Factor and Obesity as a Risk Factor for Cancer, By Type of Cancer

	Physical Activity	Overweight/ Obesity
Breast, postmenopausal	+++	+++
Breast, premenopausal	++	++ (protection)
Colon	+++	+++
Endometrium	+	+++
Esophagus, adenocarcinoma	?	+++
Kidney/renal cell	?	+++
Gallbladder	?	++
Pancreas	?	+++
Non-Hodgkin lymphoma	?	+
Prostate, aggressive	+	+
Lung	+	?
Ovary	?	?

+++, evidence is convincing; ++, evidence is probable; +, evidence is possible; ?, evidence remains insufficient/inconclusive.

for cancer. The strength of evidence for each exposure is classified as convincing (+++), probable (++), possible (+), or insufficient and inconclusive (?). Overall, for physical activity, convincing evidence exists for an association with postmenopausal breast cancer and colon cancer; for obesity, the evidence is convincing for breast, colon, endometrial, esophageal, and kidney/renal cell cancer. Evidence for associations between these exposures and several other cancer sites is accumulating. Despite some convincing evidence of the effects of physical activity and obesity on the risk of certain cancers, it is difficult to make recommendations as to appropriate changes in lifestyle that will reduce a person's chances of developing cancer. We have no physical activity prescriptions to give at this time. Many questions remain to be answered: What are the ages at which physical activity will provide the most benefit? What types of activity should one do and at what intensity, frequency (times per week), and duration (hours per week)? Similarly, for BMI, is there some threshold below which the individual will not have excess cancer risk? Does purposeful weight loss during the adult years lower the risk associated with being overweight or obese? Finally, necessary research is ongoing to identify the biologic mechanisms that account for these effects and to determine whether all persons are affected equally. For instance, it is possible that genetically defined subgroups of the population respond to physical activity or obesity differently. Understanding mechanisms and population variation in these effects will illuminate appropriate prescriptions for lifestyle change.

REFERENCES

1. Caspersen CJ, Powell KE, Christenson GM. Physical activity, exercise, and physical fitness: definitions and distinctions for health-related research. *Public Health Rep* 1985;100(2):126–131.
2. Flegal KM, Carroll MD, Kit BK, et al. Prevalence of obesity and trends in the distribution of body mass index among US adults, 1999-2010. *JAMA* 2012;307(5):491–497.
3. Troiano RP, Berrigan D, Dodd KW, et al. Physical activity in the United States measured by accelerometer. *Med Sci Sports Exerc* 2008;40(1):181–188.
4. Vainio H, Bianchini F, eds. *IARC Handbooks of Cancer Prevention Volume 6: Weight Control and Physical Activity*. Lyon, France: IARC Press; 2000.
5. Anzuini F, Battistella A, Izzotti A. Physical activity and cancer prevention: a review of current evidence and biological mechanisms. *J Prev Med Hyg* 2011;52(4):174–180.
6. Hardman AE. Physical activity and cancer risk. *Proc Nutr Soc* 2001;60(1):107–113.
7. Gunter MJ, Leitzmann MF. Obesity and colorectal cancer: epidemiology, mechanisms and candidate genes. *J Nutr Biochem* 2006;17(3):145–156.
8. Monninkhof EM, Elias SG, Vlems FA, et al. Physical activity and breast cancer: a systematic review. *Epidemiol* 2007;18(1):137–157.
9. World Cancer Research Fund/American Institute for Cancer Research. *Food, Nutrition, Physical Activity, and the Prevention of Cancer: A Global Perspective*. Washington, D.C.: World Cancer Research Fund/American Institute for Cancer Research; 2007.
10. Ishiguro S, Inoue M, Kurahashi N, et al. Risk factors of biliary tract cancer in a large-scale population-based cohort study in Japan (JPHC study); with special focus on cholelithiasis, body mass index, and their effect modification. *Cancer Causes Control* 2008;19(1):33–41.
11. Dallal CM, Sullivan-Halley J, Ross RK, et al. Long-term recreational physical activity and risk of invasive and in situ breast cancer: The California Teachers Study. *Arch Intern Med* 2007;167(4):408–415.
12. Lahmann P, Friedenreich C, Schuit A, et al. Physical activity and breast cancer risk: The European Prospective Investigation into Cancer and Nutrition. *Cancer Epidemiol Biomarkers Prev* 2007;16(1):36–42.
13. Maruti SS, Willett WC, Feskanich D, et al. A prospective study of age-specific physical activity and premenopausal breast cancer. *J Natl Cancer Inst* 2008;100(10):728–737.
14. Bernstein L, Henderson BE, Hanisch R, et al. Physical exercise and reduced risk of breast cancer in young women. *J Natl Cancer Inst* 1994;86(18):1403–1408.
15. Carpenter CL, Ross RK, Paganini-Hill A, et al. Effect of family history, obesity and exercise on breast cancer risk among postmenopausal women. *Int J Cancer* 2003;106(1):96–102.
16. Iwasaki M, Tsugane S. Risk factors for breast cancer: epidemiological evidence from Japanese studies. *Cancer Sci* 2011;102(9):1607–1614.
17. Pronk A, Ji BT, Shu XO, et al. Physical activity and breast cancer risk in Chinese women. *Br J Cancer* 2011;105(9):1443–1450.
18. Sanchez-Zamorano LM, Flores-Luna L, Angeles-Llerenas A, et al. Healthy lifestyle on the risk of breast cancer. *Cancer Epidemiol Biomarkers Prev* 2011;20(5):912–922.
19. Awatef M, Olfa G, Rim C, et al. Physical activity reduces breast cancer risk: a case-control study in Tunisia. *Cancer Epidemiol* 2011;35(6):540–544.
20. Sheppard VB, Makambi K, Taylor T, et al. Physical activity reduces breast cancer risk in African American women. *Ethn Dis* 2011;21(4):406–411.
21. Suzuki R, Iwasaki M, Yamamoto S, et al. Leisure-time physical activity and breast cancer risk defined by estrogen and progesterone receptor status—the Japan Public Health Center-based Prospective Study. *Prev Med* 2011;52(3-4):227–233.
22. Phipps AI, Chlebowski RT, Prentice R, et al. Body size, physical activity, and risk of triple-negative and estrogen receptor-positive breast cancer. *Cancer Epidemiol Biomarkers Prev* 2011;20(3):454–463.
23. Dieli-Conwright CM, Sullivan-Halley J, Patel A, et al. Does hormone therapy counter the beneficial effects of physical activity on breast cancer risk in postmenopausal women? *Cancer Causes Control* 2011;22(3):515–522.
24. Hildebrand JS, Gapstur SM, Campbell PT, et al. Recreational physical activity and leisure-time sitting in relation to postmenopausal breast cancer risk. *Cancer Epidemiol Biomarkers Prev* 2013;22(10):1906–1912.
25. Jung MM, Colditz GA, Collins LC, et al. Lifetime physical activity and the incidence of proliferative benign breast disease. *Cancer Causes Control* 2011;22(9):1297–1305.
26. Boeing H. Obesity and cancer—the update 2013. *Best Pract Res Clin Endocrinol Metab* 2013;27(2):219–227.
27. Lahmann PH, Schulz M, Hoffmann K, et al. Long-term weight change and breast cancer risk: The European Prospective Investigation into Cancer and Nutrition (EPIC). *Br J Cancer* 2005;93(5):582–589.
28. Harris HR, Tamimi RM, Willett WC, et al. Body size across the life course, mammographic density, and risk of breast cancer. *Am J Epidemiol* 2011;174(8):909–918.
29. Goran MI. Energy metabolism and obesity. *Med Clin North Am* 2000;84(2):347–362.
30. Frisch R, McArthur J. Menstrual cycles: fatness as a determinant of minimum weight for height necessary for their maintenance or onset. *Science* 1974;185:949–951.
31. Bernstein L. Epidemiology of endocrine-related risk factors for breast cancer. *J Mammary Gland Biol Neoplasia* 2002;7(1):3–15.
32. Bernstein L, Ross RK, Lobo RA, et al. The effects of moderate physical activity on menstrual cycle patterns in adolescence: implications for breast cancer prevention. *Br J Cancer* 1987;55(6):681–685.
33. Anderson E, Clarke RB, Howell A. Estrogen responsiveness and control of normal human breast proliferation. *J Mammary Gland Biol Neoplasia* 1998;3(1):23–35.
34. Cauley JA, Gutai JP, Kuller LH, et al. The epidemiology of serum sex hormones in postmenopausal women. *Am J Epidemiol* 1989;129(6):1120–1131.
35. MacDonald PC, Edman CD, Hemsell DL, et al. Effect of obesity on conversion of plasma androstenedione to estrone in postmenopausal women with and without endometrial cancer. *Am J Obstet Gynecol* 1978;130(4):448–455.
36. Seewaldt FL, Goldenberg V, Jones LW, et al. Overweight and obese perimenopausal and postmenopausal women exhibit increased abnormal mammary epithelial cytology. *Cancer Epidemiol Biomarkers Prev* 2007;16:613–616.
37. Bernstein L. Exercise and breast cancer prevention. *Curr Oncol Reports* 2009;11(6):490–496.
38. Neilson HK, Friedenreich CM, Brockton NT, et al. Physical activity and postmenopausal breast cancer: proposed biologic mechanisms and areas for future research. *Cancer Epidemiol Biomarkers Prev* 2009;18(1):11–27.
39. Cleary MP, Grossmann ME. Obesity and breast cancer: the estrogen connection. *Endocrinol* 2009;150(6):2537–2542.
40. Brown KA, Simpson ER. Obesity and breast cancer: progress to understanding the relationship. *Cancer Res* 2010;70(1):4–7.
41. Friedenreich CM, Neilson HK, Lynch BM. State of the epidemiological evidence on physical activity and cancer prevention. *Eur J Cancer* 2010;46(14):2593–2604.
42. Mai PL, Sullivan-Halley J, Ursin G, et al. Physical activity and colon cancer risk among women in the California Teachers Study. *Cancer Epidemiol Biomarkers Prev* 2007;16(3):517–525.
43. Wolin KY, Yan Y, Colditz GA, et al. Physical activity and colon cancer prevention: a meta-analysis. *Br J Cancer* 2009;100(4):611–616.
44. Boyle T, Keegel T, Bull F, et al. Physical activity and risks of proximal and distal colon cancers: a systematic review and meta-analysis. *J Natl Cancer Inst* 2012;104(20):1548–1561.
45. Howard RA, Freedman DM, Park Y, et al. Physical activity, sedentary behavior, and the risk of colon and rectal cancer in the NIH-AARP Diet and Health Study. *Cancer Causes Control* 2008;19(9):939–953.
46. Boyle T, Heyworth J, Bull F, et al. Timing and intensity of recreational physical activity and the risk of subsite-specific colorectal cancer. *Cancer Causes Control* 2011;22(12):1647–1658.
47. Wolin KY, Yan Y, Colditz GA. Physical activity and risk of colon adenoma: a meta-analysis. *Br J Cancer* 2011;104(5):882–885.
48. Pischon T, Lahmann PH, Boeing H, et al. Body size and risk of colon and rectal cancer in the European Prospective Investigation Into Cancer and Nutrition (EPIC). *J Natl Cancer Inst* 2006;98(13):920–931.
49. Aleksandrova K, Pischon T, Buijsse B, et al. Adult weight change and risk of colorectal cancer in the European Prospective Investigation into Cancer and Nutrition. *Eur J Cancer* 2013;49(16):3526–3536.
50. Nimptsch K, Giovannucci E, Willett WC, et al. Body fatness during childhood and adolescence, adult height, and risk of colorectal adenoma in women. *Cancer Prev Res* 2011;4(10):1710–1718.

51. Hughes LA, Simons CC, van den Brandt PA, et al. Body size and colorectal cancer risk after 16.3 years of follow-up: an analysis from the Netherlands Cohort Study. *Am J Epidemiol* 2011;174(10):1127–1139.
52. Abate N. Insulin resistance and obesity. The role of fat distribution pattern. *Diabetes Care* 1996;19(3):292–294.
53. Calle EE, Kaaks R. Overweight, obesity and cancer: epidemiological evidence and proposed mechanisms. *Nat Rev Cancer* 2004;4(8):579–591.
54. Gierach GL, Chang SC, Brinton LA, et al. Physical activity, sedentary behavior, and endometrial cancer risk in the NIH-AARP Diet and Health Study. *Int J Cancer* 2009;124(9):2139–2147.
55. Voskuil DW, Monninkhof EM, Elias SG, et al. Physical activity and endometrial cancer risk, a systematic review of current evidence. *Cancer Epidemiol Biomarkers Prev* 2007;16(4):639–648.
56. Cust AE, Armstrong BK, Friedenreich CM, et al. Physical activity and endometrial cancer risk: a review of the current evidence, biologic mechanisms and the quality of physical activity assessment methods. *Cancer Causes Control* 2007;18(3):243–258.
57. Friedenreich C, Cust A, Lahmann PH, et al. Physical activity and risk of endometrial cancer: The European Prospective Investigation into Cancer and Nutrition. *Int J Cancer* 2007;121(2):347–355.
58. Patel AV, Feigelson HS, Talbot JT, et al. The role of body weight in the relationship between physical activity and endometrial cancer: results from a large cohort of US women. *Int J Cancer* 2008;123(8):1877–1882.
59. Moore SC, Gierach GL, Schatzkin A, et al. Physical activity, sedentary behaviours, and the prevention of endometrial cancer. *Br J Cancer* 2010;103(7):933–938.
60. Dieli-Conwright CM, Ma H, Lacey JV, Jr., et al. Long-term and baseline recreational physical activity and risk of endometrial cancer: The California Teachers Study. *Br J Cancer* 2013;109(3):761–768.
61. Kaaks R, Lukanova A, Kurzer MS. Obesity, endogenous hormones, and endometrial cancer risk: a synthetic review. *Cancer Epidemiol Biomarkers Prev* 2002;11(12):1531–1543.
62. Zhang ZF, Kurtz RC, Sun M, et al. Adenocarcinomas of the esophagus and gastric cardia: medical conditions, tobacco, alcohol, and socioeconomic factors. *Cancer Epidemiol Biomarkers Prev* 1996;5(10):761–768.
63. Lagergren J, Bergstrom R, Nyren O. Association between body mass and adenocarcinoma of the esophagus and gastric cardia. *Ann Intern Med* 1999;130(11):883–890.
64. Vigen C, Bernstein L, Wu AH. Occupational physical activity and risk of adenocarcinomas of the esophagus and stomach. *Int J Cancer* 2006;118(4):1004–1009.
65. Leitzmann MF, Koebnick C, Freedman ND, et al. Physical activity and esophageal and gastric carcinoma in a large prospective study. *Am J Prev Med* 2009;36(2):112–119.
66. Lepage C, Drouillard A, Jouve JL, et al. Epidemiology and risk factors for oesophageal adenocarcinoma. *Dig Liver Dis* 2013;45(8):625–629.
67. Ryan AM, Duong M, Healy L, et al. Obesity, metabolic syndrome and esophageal adenocarcinoma: epidemiology, etiology and new targets. *Cancer Epidemiol* 2011;35(4):309–319.
68. Hoyo C, Cook MB, Kamangar F, et al. Body mass index in relation to oesophageal and oesophagogastric junction adenocarcinomas: a pooled analysis from the International BEACON Consortium. *Int J Epidemiol* 2012;41(6):1706–1718.
69. Leitzmann MF. Physical activity and genitourinary cancer prevention. *Recent Results Cancer Res* 2011;186:43–71.
70. Purdue MP, Moore LE, Merino MJ, et al. An investigation of risk factors for renal cell carcinoma by histologic subtype in two case-control studies. *Int J Cancer* 2013;132(11):2640–2647.
71. O'Rorke MA, Cantwell MM, Cardwell CR, et al. Can physical activity modulate pancreatic cancer risk? A systematic review and meta-analysis. *Int J Cancer* 2010;126(12):2957–2968.
72. Aune D, Greenwood DC, Chan DS, et al. Body mass index, abdominal fatness and pancreatic cancer risk: a systematic review and non-linear dose-response meta-analysis of prospective studies. *Ann Oncol* 2012;23(4):843–852.
73. Bracci PM. Obesity and pancreatic cancer: overview of epidemiologic evidence and biologic mechanisms. *Mol Carcinog* 2012;51(1):53–63.
74. Arslan AA, Helzlsouer KJ, Kooperberg C, et al. Anthropometric measures, body mass index, and pancreatic cancer: a pooled analysis from the Pancreatic Cancer Cohort Consortium (PanScan). *Arch Intern Med* 2010;170(9):791–802.
75. Genkinger JM, Spiegelman D, Anderson KE, et al. A pooled analysis of 14 cohort studies of anthropometric factors and pancreatic cancer risk. *Int J Cancer* 2010;129(7):1708–1717.
76. Uhler ML, Marks JW, Judd HL. Estrogen replacement therapy and gallbladder disease in postmenopausal women. *Menopause* 2000;7(3):162–167.
77. Larsson SC, Wolk A. Obesity and the risk of gallbladder cancer: a meta-analysis. *Br J Cancer* 2007;96(9):1457–1461.
78. Hsing AW, Sakoda LC, Rashid A, et al. Body size and the risk of biliary tract cancer: a population-based study in China. *Br J Cancer* 2008;99(5):811–815.
79. Schlesinger S, Aleksandrova K, Pischon T, et al. Abdominal obesity, weight gain during adulthood and risk of liver and biliary tract cancer in a European cohort. *Int J Cancer* 2013;132(3):645–657.
80. Lu Y, Prescott J, Sullivan-Halley J, et al. Body size, recreational physical activity, and B-cell non-Hodgkin lymphoma risk among women in the California Teachers Study. *Am J Epidemiol* 2009;170(10):1231–1240.
81. Kabat GC, Kim MY, Jean Wactawski W, et al. Anthropometric factors, physical activity, and risk of non-Hodgkin's lymphoma in the Women's Health Initiative. *Cancer Epidemiol* 2012;36(1):52–59.
82. van Veldhoven CM, Khan AE, Teucher B, et al. Physical activity and lymphoid neoplasms in the European Prospective Investigation into Cancer and Nutrition (EPIC). *Eur J Cancer* 2011;47(5):748–760.
83. Teras LR, Gapstur SM, Diver WR, et al. Recreational physical activity, leisure sitting time and risk of non-Hodgkin lymphoid neoplasms in the American Cancer Society Cancer Prevention Study II Cohort. *Int J Cancer* 2012; 131(8):1912–1920.
84. Willett EV, Morton LM, Hartge P, et al. Non-Hodgkin lymphoma and obesity: a pooled analysis from the InterLymph Consortium. *Int J Cancer* 2008;122(9):2062–2070.
85. Larsson SC, Wolk A. Body mass index and risk of non-Hodgkin's and Hodgkin's lymphoma: a meta-analysis of prospective studies. *Eur J Cancer* 2011;47(16):2422–2430.
86. Larsson SC, Wolk A. Obesity and risk of non-Hodgkin's lymphoma: a meta-analysis. *Int J Cancer* 2007;121(7):1564–1570.
87. Bertrand KA, Giovannucci E, Zhang SM, et al. A prospective analysis of body size during childhood, adolescence, and adulthood and risk of non-Hodgkin lymphoma. *Cancer Prev Res* 2013;6(8):864–873.
88. Friedenreich CM, Orenstein MR. Physical activity and cancer prevention: Etiologic evidence and biological mechanisms. *J Nutr* 2002;132(11 Suppl):3456S–3464S.
89. Friedenreich CM, McGregor SE, Courneya KS, et al. Case-control study of lifetime total physical activity and prostate cancer risk. *Am J Epidemiol* 2004;159(8):740–749.
90. Young-McCaughan S. Potential for prostate cancer prevention through physical activity. *World J Urol* 2012;30(2):167–179.
91. Leitzmann MF, Rohrmann S. Risk factors for the onset of prostatic cancer: age, location, and behavioral correlates. *Clin Epidemiol* 2012;4:1–11.
92. Liu Y, Hu F, Li D, et al. Does physical activity reduce the risk of prostate cancer? A systematic review and meta-analysis. *Eur Urol* 2011;60(5):1029–1044.
93. Discacciati A, Orsini N, Wolk A. Body mass index and incidence of localized and advanced prostate cancer—a dose-response meta-analysis of prospective studies. *Ann Oncol* 2012;23(7):1665–1671.
94. Rodriguez C, Freedland SJ, Deka A, et al. Body mass index, weight change, and risk of prostate cancer in the Cancer Prevention Study II Nutrition Cohort. *Cancer Epidemiol Biomarkers Prev* 2007;16(1):63–69.
95. Schmidt A, Jung J, Ernstmann N, et al. The association between active participation in a sports club, physical activity and social network on the development of lung cancer in smokers: A case-control study. *BMC Res Notes* 2012;5:2.
96. Lam TK, Moore SC, Brinton LA, et al. Anthropometric measures and physical activity and the risk of lung cancer in never-smokers: a prospective cohort study. *PLoS One* 2013;8(8):e70672.
97. Tardon A, Lee WJ, Delgado-Rodriguez M, et al. Leisure-time physical activity and lung cancer: a meta-analysis. *Cancer Causes Control* 2005;16(4):389–397.
98. Lin Y, Cai L. Environmental and dietary factors and lung cancer risk among Chinese women: a case-control study in Southeast China. *Nutr Cancer* 2012;64(4):508–514.
99. Bethea TN, Rosenberg L, Charlot M, et al. Obesity in relation to lung cancer incidence in African American women. *Cancer Causes Control* 2013;24(9):1695–1703.
100. Smith L, Brinton LA, Spitz MR, et al. Body mass index and risk of lung cancer among never, former, and current smokers. *J Natl Cancer Inst* 2012;104(10):778–789.
101. Andreotti G, Hou L, Beane Freeman LE, et al. Body mass index, agricultural pesticide use, and cancer incidence in the Agricultural Health Study cohort. *Cancer Causes Control* 2010;21(11):1759–1775.
102. Tarnaud C, Guida F, Papadopoulos A, et al. Body mass index and lung cancer risk: results from the ICARE Study, a large, population-based case-control study. *Cancer Causes Control* 2012;23(7):1113–1126.
103. Yang Y, Dong J, Sun K, et al. Obesity and incidence of lung cancer: a meta-analysis. *Int J Cancer* 2013;132(5):1162–1169.
104. El Zein M, Parent ME, Rousseau MC. Comments on a recent meta-analysis: obesity and lung cancer. *Int J Cancer* 2012;132(8):1962–1963.
105. Olsen CM, Bain CJ, Jordan SJ, et al. Recreational physical activity and epithelial ovarian cancer: A case-control study, systematic review, and meta-analysis. *Cancer Epidemiol Biomarkers Prev* 2007;16(11):2321–2330.
106. Weiderpass E, Margolis KL, Sandin S, et al. Prospective study of physical activity in different periods of life and the risk of ovarian cancer. *Int J Cancer* 2006;118(12):3153–3160.
107. Lahmann PH, Friedenreich C, Schulz M, et al. Physical activity and ovarian cancer risk: The European Prospective Investigation into Cancer and Nutrition. *Cancer Epidemiol Biomarkers Prev* 2009;18(1):351–354.
108. Leitzmann MF, Koebnick C, Moore SC, et al. Prospective study of physical activity and the risk of ovarian cancer. *Cancer Causes Control* 2009;20(5):765–773.
109. Xiao Q, Yang HP, Wentzensen N, et al. Physical activity in different periods of life, sedentary behavior, and the risk of ovarian cancer in the NIH-AARP Diet and Health Study. *Cancer Epidemiol Biomarkers Prev* 2013;22(11):2000–2008.
110. Moorman PG, Jones LW, Akushevich L, et al. Recreational physical activity and ovarian cancer risk and survival. *Ann Epidemiol* 2011;21(3):178–187.
111. Olsen CM, Green AC, Whiteman DC, et al. Obesity and the risk of epithelial ovarian cancer: a systematic review and meta-analysis. *Eur J Cancer* 2007;43(4):690–709.
112. Olsen CM, Nagle CM, Whiteman DC, et al. Obesity and risk of ovarian cancer subtypes: evidence from the Ovarian Cancer Association Consortium. *Endocr Relat Cancer* 2013;20(2):251–262.
113. Schouten LJ, Rivera C, Hunter DJ, et al. Height, body mass index, and ovarian cancer: a pooled analysis of 12 cohort studies. *Cancer Epidemiol Biomarkers Prev* 2008;17(4):902–912.
114. Collaborative Group on Epidemiological Studies of Ovarian Cancer. Ovarian cancer and body size: individual participant meta-analysis including 25,157 women with ovarian cancer from 47 epidemiological studies. *PLoS Med* 2012;9(4):e1001200.

11 Epidemiologic Methods

Xiaomei Ma and Herbert Yu

INTRODUCTION

Epidemiology is the study of the distribution and determinants of health-related states or events in specified populations and the application of this study to control health problems.[1] Epidemiologic principles and methods have long been applied to cancer research, with the assumptions that cancer does not occur at random and the nonrandomness of carcinogenesis can be elucidated through systematic research. An example of such applications is the lung cancer study conducted by Doll and Hill in the early 1950s, which linked tobacco smoking to an increased mortality of lung cancer in over 40,000 medical professionals in the United Kingdom.[2] The observation from this study and many other studies, in conjunction with laboratory findings regarding the underlying biologic mechanisms for the effect of tobacco smoking, helped establish the role of tobacco smoking in the etiology of lung cancer. Epidemiologic methods are also used in clinical settings, where trials are conducted to evaluate the efficacy of new treatment protocols or preventive measures and where observational studies of prognostic factors are done.

Epidemiologic studies can take different forms, but generally they can be classified into two broad categories, observational studies and experimental studies (Fig. 11.1). In experimental studies, an investigator allocates different study regimens to the subjects, usually with randomization (experimental studies without randomization are sometimes referred to as "quasi-experiments").[3] Experimental studies can be individual based or community based. An experimental study most closely resembles laboratory experiments in that the investigator has control over the study condition. Experimental studies can be used to evaluate the efficacy of a treatment protocol (e.g., low-dose compared with standard-dose chemotherapy for non-Hodgkin's lymphoma)[4] or preventive measures (e.g., tamoxifen for women at an increased risk of breast cancer).[5] Although experimental studies are often considered the "gold standard" because of well-controlled study situations, they are only suitable for the evaluation of effects that are beneficial or at least not harmful due to ethical concerns. Experimental studies are discussed in detail in other chapters of this book. This section will focus on observational studies.

Observational studies do not involve the artificial manipulation of study regimens. In an observational study, an investigator stands by to observe what happens or happened to the subjects, in terms of exposure and outcome. Observational studies can be further divided into descriptive and analytical studies (see Fig. 11.1). Descriptive studies focus on the *distribution* of diseases with respect to person, place, and time (i.e., who, where, and when), whereas analytical studies focus on the *determinants* of diseases. Descriptive studies are often used to *generate* hypotheses, whereas analytical studies are often used to *test* hypotheses. However, the two types of studies should not be considered mutually exclusive entities; rather, they are the opposite ends of a continuum. Descriptive studies are discussed in detail in other chapters of this book.

ANALYTICAL STUDIES

Ecologic Studies

As in experimental studies, the unit of analysis can be individuals or groups of people in observational studies. Studies that use groups of people as the unit of analysis are called ecologic studies, which are relatively easy to carry out when group level measures are available. However, a relationship observed between variables on a group level does not necessarily reflect the relationship that exists at an individual level. For example, the fraction of energy supply from animal products was found to be positively correlated with breast cancer mortality in a recent ecologic study, which used preexisting data on both dietary supply and breast cancer mortality rates from 35 countries.[6] Because the data were country based, no reliable inference can be made at an individual level. Within each country, it could be that the people who had a low fraction of energy supply from animal products were actually dying from breast cancer. Results from ecologic studies are useful for inference at an individual level only when the within-group variability of the exposure is low so that a group-level measure can reasonably reflect exposure at an individual level. Alternatively, if the implications for prevention or intervention are at a group level (e.g., taxation of cigarettes to reduce smoking), results from ecologic studies are very useful.

Cross-Sectional Studies

There are three main types of analytical studies in which the unit of analysis is individuals: cross-sectional, cohort, and case-control studies. In a cross-sectional study, the information on various factors is collected from the study population at a given point in time. From a public health perspective, data collected in cross-sectional studies can be of great value in assessing the general health status of a population and allocating resources. For example, the National Health and Nutrition Examination Survey has provided valuable national estimates of health and nutritional status of the US civilian, noninstitutionalized population.[7] Findings from cross-sectional studies can also help generate hypotheses that may be tested later in other types of studies. However, it should be noted that cross-sectional studies have serious methodologic limitations if the research purpose is etiologic inference. Because exposures and disease status are evaluated simultaneously, it is usually not possible to know the temporality of events unless the exposure cannot change over time (e.g., blood type, skin color, race, country of birth). If one observes that more brain cancer patients are depressed than people without brain cancer in a cross-sectional study, the correlation does not necessarily mean that depression causes brain cancer. Depression may simply have resulted from the pathogenesis and diagnosis of brain cancer, or depression may

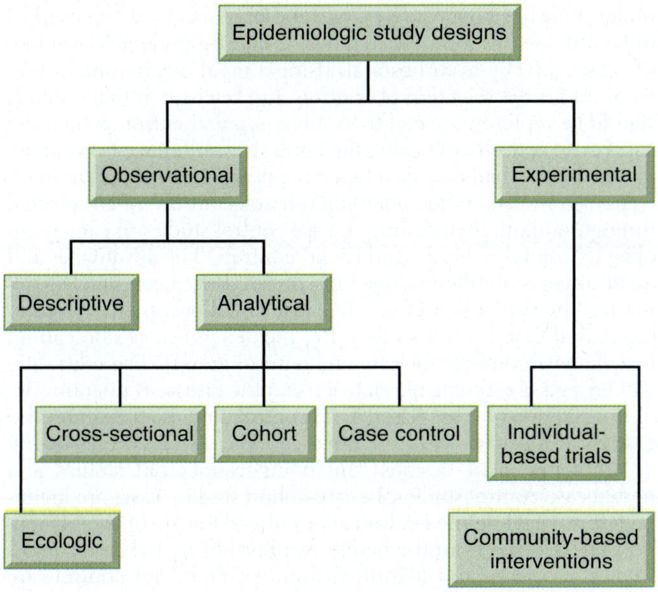

Figure 11.1 Classification of epidemiologic study designs.

have caused brain cancer in some patients and resulted from brain cancer in other patients. Without additional information on the timing of events, no conclusions can be made. Another concern in cross-sectional studies is the enrollment of prevalent cases, who survived different lengths of time after the incidence of disease. Factors that affect survival may also influence incidence. Prevalent cases may not be representative of incident cases, which makes etiologic inferences based on cross-sectional studies suspect at best.

Cohort Studies

In a cohort study, a study population free of a specific disease (or any other health-related condition) is grouped based on their exposure status and followed up for a certain period of time. Then the exposed and unexposed subjects are compared with respect to disease status at the end of the follow-up. The objective of a cohort study is usually to evaluate whether the incidence of a disease is associated with an exposure. The cohort design is fundamental in observational epidemiology and is considered "ideal" in that, if unbiased, cohort data reflect the real-life cause/effect sequence of disease.[8] Subjects in cohort studies may be a sample of the general population in a geographic area, a group of workers who are exposed to certain occupational hazards in a specific industry, or people who are considered at a high risk for a specific disease. A cohort study is considered prospective or concurrent if the investigator starts following up the cohort from the present time into the future, and retrospective or historical if the cohort is established in the past based on existing records (e.g., an occupational cohort based on employment records) and the follow-up ends before or at the time of the study. Alternatively, a cohort study can be ambidirectional in that data collection goes both directions.[9] Whether a cohort study is prospective, retrospective, or ambidirectional, the key feature is that all the subjects were free of the disease at the beginning of the follow-up and the study tracks the subjects from exposure to disease. Follow-up time, ranging from days to decades, is an essential element in cohort studies.

In a cohort study, the incidence of disease in the exposed group and the unexposed group is compared. The incidence measure can be cumulative incidence or incidence density, depending on the availability of data. When comparing the incidence in the two groups, both relative differences and absolute differences can be assessed. In cohort studies, the relative risk of developing the disease is expressed as the ratio of the cumulative incidence in the exposed group to that in the unexposed group, which is also called cumulative incidence ratio or risk ratio. If we have data on the exact person-time of follow-up for every subject, we can also calculate an incidence density ratio (also called rate ratio) in a similar way. The numeric value of the risk or rate ratio reflects the magnitude of the association between an exposure and a disease. For example, a risk ratio of 2 would be interpreted as exposed individuals have a doubled risk of developing a disease than unexposed individuals, whereas a risk ratio of 5 indicates that exposed individuals have 5 times the risk of developing a disease compared with unexposed individuals. To put in another way, a factor with a risk ratio of 5 has a stronger effect than another factor with a risk ratio of 2. In addition to risk ratio and rate ratio, another relative measure called probability odds ratio can be calculated in cohort studies. The probability odds of disease is the number of subjects who developed a disease divided by the number of subjects who did not develop the disease, and the probability odds ratio is the probability odds in the exposed group divided by the probability odds in the unexposed group. Many investigators prefer risk ratio or rate ratio to probability odds ratio in cohort studies, because the ability to directly measure the risk of developing a disease is one of the most significant advantages in cohort studies. In practice, however, a probability odds ratio is often used as an approximation for risk or rate ratio, especially when multivariate logistic regression models are employed to adjust for the effect of other factors that may influence the relationship between an exposure and a disease.

As for absolute differences, a commonly used measure is called attributable risk in the exposed, which is the incidence in the exposed group minus the incidence in the unexposed group. Attributable risk reflects the disease incidence that could be attributed to the exposure in exposed individuals and the reduction in incidence that we would expect if the exposure can be removed from the exposed individuals, provided that there is a causal relationship between the exposure and the disease. Another absolute measure called population attributable risk extends this concept to the general population; it estimates the disease incidence that could be attributed to an exposure in the general population. Because both relative and absolute differences can be assessed in cohort studies, a natural question to ask is what measures to choose. In general, the relative differences are used more often if the main research objective is etiologic inference, and they can be used for the judgment of causality. Once causality is established, or at least assumed, measures of absolute differences are more important from a public health perspective. This point can be illustrated using the following hypothetical example. Assume the following: toxin X in the environment triples the risk of bladder cancer and toxin Y doubles the risk of bladder cancer, the effects of X and Y are entirely independent of each other, the prevalence of exposure to toxin Y in the general population is 20 times higher than the prevalence of exposure to toxin X, and there are only resources available to reduce the exposure to one toxin. It would be more effective to use the resources to reduce the exposure to toxin Y instead of toxin X. This is because the population attributable risk due to Y is higher than that due to X, although the risk ratio associated with toxin Y is smaller than that associated with toxin X.

Cohort studies have many advantages. A cohort design is the best way to study the natural history of a disease.[9] There is usually a clear temporal relationship between an exposure and a disease because all the subjects are free of the disease at the beginning of the follow-up (it can be a problem if a subject has a subclinical disease such as undetected prostate cancer). Furthermore, multiple diseases can be studied with respect to the same exposure. On the other hand, cohort studies, especially prospective cohort studies, are costly in terms of both time and money. A cohort design requires the follow-up of a large number of study participants over a sometimes extremely lengthy period of time and usually extensive data collection through questionnaires, physical measurements, and/or biologic specimens at regular intervals. Participants may be "lost" during the follow-up because they became tired of the study, moved away from the study area, or died from some causes other than the disease under study. If the subjects who were lost during the follow-up are different from those who remained under observation with respect to exposure, disease, or other factors that may influence the relationship between the exposure and the disease, results from the study may be biased. To date, cohort studies have been used to study the etiology of a wide spectrum of diseases, including different types of cancer. If a cohort study is conducted to evaluate the etiology of cancer, usually the study sample size would need to be very large (such as the National Institutes of Health-AARP Diet and Health Study, which included more than half million subjects[10]) and the follow-up time would need to be long, unless the cohort selected is a high-risk population.

For simplicity, we have discussed cohort studies in which the outcome of interest is the incidence of a specific disease and there are only two exposure groups. In practice, any health-related event can be the outcome of interest, and multiple exposure groups can be compared.

Case-Control Studies

Case-control design is an alternative to cohort design for the evaluation of the relationship between an exposure and a disease (or any other health condition). A case-control approach compares the odds of past exposure between cases and noncases (controls) and uses the exposure odds ratio as an estimate for relative risk. A primary goal in a case-control study is to reach the same conclusions as what would have been obtained from a cohort study, if one had been done.[11] If appropriately designed and conducted, a case-control study can optimize speed and efficiency as the need for follow-up is avoided.[8] The starting point of a case-control study is a source population from which the cases arise. Instead of obtaining the denominators for the calculation of risks or rates in a cohort study, a control group is sampled from the entire source population. After selecting control subjects, who ideally would have become cases had they developed the disease, an investigator collects data on past exposures from both the cases and the controls and then calculates an odds ratio, which is the odds of exposure in the cases divided by the odds of exposure in the controls.

There are two main types of case-control studies: case-based case-control studies and case-control studies within defined cohorts.[8] Some variations of the case-control design also exist. For instance, if the effect of an exposure is transient, sometimes a case can be used as his/her own control (case cross-over design). In case-based case-control studies, cases and controls are selected at a given point in time from a hypothetical cohort (e.g., at the end of follow-up). A cross-sectional ascertainment of cases will result in a case group that mostly contains prevalent cases who may have survived for different lengths of time after disease incidence. Cases who died before an investigator began subject ascertainment would not be eligible to be included in the study. As a result, the cases finally included in the study may not be representative of all the cases from the entire hypothetical cohort. Another disadvantage of enrolling prevalent cases is that cases that were diagnosed a long time ago will likely have difficulties recalling exposures that occurred before the disease incidence. In case-control studies, it is preferable to ascertain incident cases as soon as they are diagnosed and to select controls as soon as cases are identified. Case-control studies that enroll only incident cases are sometimes called *prospective* case-control studies because the investigators need to wait for the incident cases to develop and get diagnosed. For cancer studies, the cases can be ascertained from population-based cancer registries or hospitals. A major advantage of using a cancer registry is the completeness of case ascertainment; however, the reporting of cancer cases to registries is usually not instantaneous. There could be a lag time of several months or even over a year, and some cases could have died during the lag time. If the cancer under study has a poor survival rate and/or clinical specimens need to be obtained in a timely manner, it may be preferable to identify cases directly from hospitals using a rapid ascertainment protocol. As for the selection of controls, the key issue is that controls should be representative of the source population from which the cases arise and, theoretically, the controls would have been ascertained as cases had they developed the disease. The most common types of controls include population-based controls (often selected through random digit dialing in case-control studies of cancer etiology), hospital controls, and friend controls. The advantages and disadvantages of different types of controls have been nicely summarized by Wacholder et al.[12] Because no follow-up is involved in case-based case-control studies, the incidence risk or rate cannot be calculated directly for case and control groups. The odds ratio will be a good estimate of relative risk if the disease is uncommon.

In addition to case-based case-control studies, there are also case-control studies within defined cohorts (also known as hybrid or ambidirectional designs), including case-cohort studies and nested case-control studies. In case-cohort studies, cases are identified from a well-defined cohort after some follow-up time, and controls are selected from the baseline cohort. In nested case-control studies, cases are also identified from a cohort, but controls are selected from the individuals at risk at the time each case occurs (i.e., incidence density sampling).[8] In these types of designs, controls are a sample of the cohort and the controls selected can theoretically become cases at some point. The possibility of selection bias in case-control studies within defined cohorts is lower than that in case-based case-control studies because the cases and the controls are selected from the same source population. Because of an increased awareness of the methodological issues inherent in the design of case-based case-control studies and the availability of a growing number of large cohorts, case-control studies within defined cohorts have become more common in recent years. The advantage of case-control studies within cohorts over traditional cohort studies is mainly the efficiency in additional data collection. For instance, a recent nested case-control study evaluated the relationship between endogenous sex hormones and prostate cancer risk.[13] Instead of measuring the serum hormones levels of the entire cohort (over 12,000 subjects), investigators chose to measure 300 cases and 300 controls selected from the cohort. Doing so not only significantly reduced the cost of measurements and the time it took to address the research question, but also helped preserve valuable serum samples for possible analyses in the future. In a case-cohort design, an odds ratio estimates risk ratio; in a nested case-control design, an odds ratio estimates rate ratio. In both designs, the disease under study does not have to be rare for the odds ratio to be a good estimate of the risk ratio or rate ratio.[8,14]

The biggest advantage of a case-control design is the speed and efficiency of obtaining data. It is claimed that investigators implement case-control studies more frequently than any other analytical epidemiologic study.[15] Because most types of cancer are uncommon and take a long time to develop, to date, most epidemiologic studies of cancer have been case-control instead of cohort in design. A case-control study can be conducted to evaluate the relationship between many different exposures and a specific disease, but the study will have limited statistical power if the exposure is rare. In general, a case-control design tends to be more susceptible to biases than a cohort design. Such biases include, but are not limited to, selection bias when choosing and enrolling subjects (especially controls) and recall bias when obtaining data from the subjects. The status of the subjects—that is, case or control—may affect how they recall and report previous exposures, some of which occurred years or even decades ago. It is important for investigators to explicitly define the diagnostic and eligibility criteria for cases, to select controls from the same population as the cases independent of the exposures of interest, to blind data collection staff to the case or control status of subjects and/or the main hypotheses of the study, to ascertain exposure in a similar manner from cases and controls, and to take into account other factors that may influence the relationship between an exposure and a disease.[15]

INTERPRETATION OF EPIDEMIOLOGIC FINDINGS

We have discussed measures of effects in various study designs. However, a risk ratio of 3 from a cohort study or an odds ratio of 2.5 from a case-control study does not necessarily mean that there is an association between an exposure and a disease. Several alternative explanations need to be assessed, including chance (random error), bias (systematic error), and confounding. Potential interaction also needs be evaluated.

Statistical methods are required to evaluate the role of chance. A usual way is to calculate the upper and lower limits of a 95% confidence interval around a point estimate for relative risk (risk ratio, rate ratio, or odds ratio). If the confidence interval does not include one, one would say that the observed association is statistically significant; if the confidence interval includes one, one would say that the observed relationship is not statistically significant. The width of a confidence interval is directly related to the number of participants in a study, which is called sample size. A larger sample size leads to less variability in the data, a tighter confidence interval, and a higher possibility in finding a statistically significant association if one truly exists. A 95% confidence interval means that if the data collection and analysis could be replicated many times, the confidence interval should include the correct value of the measure 95% of the time.[16] It is better to consider a confidence interval to be a general guide to the amount of random error in the data but not necessarily a literal measure of statistical variability.[16]

Bias can be defined as any systematic error in an epidemiologic study that results in an incorrect estimate of the association between exposure and disease, and it can occur in every type of epidemiologic study design. There are two main types of bias: selection bias and information bias. Selection bias is present when individuals included in a study are systematically different from the target population. For example, a selection bias would occur if a study aimed to generate a sample representing all women in the United States, but of the women contacted, more with a family history of breast cancer agreed to participate. This sample would be at a higher risk for breast cancer than the target population. Refusal to participate poses a constant challenge in epidemiologic studies. As individuals have become more concerned about privacy issues and as studies have become more demanding of time, biologic specimens, and other impositions, participation rates have dropped substantially in recent years. If nonparticipants are different from the participants with respect to study-related characteristics, the validity of the study is threatened. Information bias occurs when the data collected from the study subjects are erroneous. Information bias is also known as misclassification if the variable is measured on a categorical scale and the error causes a subject to be placed in a wrong category. Misclassification can happen to both exposure and disease. For example, in a case-control study of previous reproductive history and ovarian cancer, a woman who had an extremely early pregnancy loss might not even realize that she was ever pregnant and would mistakenly report no pregnancy, and another woman who has only subclinical presentations of ovarian cancer might be mistakenly selected as a control. Misclassification can be differential or nondifferential. An exposure misclassification is considered differential if it is related to disease status and nondifferential if not related to disease status. Similarly, a disease misclassification is considered differential if it is related to exposure status and nondifferential if not related to exposure status. If a binary exposure variable and a binary disease variable are analyzed, a nondifferential misclassification will result in an underestimate of the true association. Differential misclassification can either exaggerate or underestimate a true effect. Usually not much can be done to control or correct bias at the data analysis stage; therefore, it is important to establish research protocols that are not prone to bias. The evaluation of potential bias is critical to the interpretation of study results. An invalid estimate is worse than no estimate.

Confounding refers to a situation in which the association between an exposure and a disease (or any health-related condition) is influenced by a third variable. This third variable is considered a confounding variable or confounder. A confounder must fulfill three criteria: (1) be associated with the exposure, (2) be associated with the disease independent of the exposure, and (3) not be an intermediate step between the exposure and the disease (i.e., not on the causal pathway). Unlike bias, which is primarily introduced by the investigator or study participants, confounding is a function of the complex interrelationship between various exposures and disease.[17] In a hypothetical case-control study of the effect of alcohol drinking on lung cancer, we may observe an odds ratio of 2.5 (usually called a "crude" odds ratio in the sense that no other variables were taken into account), which indicates that alcohol drinking increases the risk of lung cancer by 1.5-fold. However, if we classify all study subjects into two strata based on a history of cigarette smoking and then calculate the odds ratio in the two strata (smokers and nonsmokers) separately, we may have two stratum-specific odds ratios both equal to one, indicating that alcohol drinking is not associated with lung cancer risk. In this example, the crude odds ratio calculated to estimate the association between alcohol drinking and lung cancer without considering smoking is simply misleading. Being associated with both the exposure (i.e., alcohol drinking) and the disease (i.e., lung cancer), smoking acted as a confounder in this example. A stratified analysis is needed to evaluate the potential confounding effect of a third variable, whether it is done with pencil and paper or statistical modeling. Usually data are stratified based on the level of a third variable. If the stratum-specific effect measures are similar to each other but different from the crude effect measure, confounding is said to be present. In this section, we have illustrated basic epidemiologic principles using an overly simplified scenario and only considered a single exposure. In practice, most if not all diseases, cancer included, have a multifactorial etiology. Consequently, it is usually necessary to assess the potential confounding effect of a group of variables simultaneously using multivariate statistical models. The effect measure derived from a multivariate model will then be called an "adjusted" one in the sense that the effect of other factors was also adjusted for. Without controlling for the potential effect of other variables, an investigator cannot really judge whether an observed association between a given exposure and a specific disease is spurious.

If the effect of an exposure on the risk of a disease is not homogeneous in strata formed by a third variable, the third variable is considered an effect modifier, and the situation is called interaction or effect modification. Put in other words, interaction exists when the stratum-specific effect measures are different from each other. In the lung cancer example given previously, if the odds ratio for alcohol drinking is 1 in smokers but 3 in nonsmokers, then there is interaction and smoking is an effect modifier. The evaluation of interaction is essentially a stratified analysis, which is similar to the evaluation of confounding. Confounding and interaction can be both present in a given study. However, when interaction occurs, the stratum-specific effect measures should be reported. It is no longer appropriate to report a summary measure in the presence of interaction. Unlike confounding, which is a nuisance that an investigator hopes to remove, interaction is a more detailed description of the true relationship between an exposure and a disease.

CANCER OUTCOMES RESEARCH

The discussion of epidemiologic methods in this section focuses primarily on etiological research, which aims at identifying the risk factors of cancer. However, similar principles and methods are applicable to cancer outcomes research, which aims at studying a variety of factors related to the early identification, treatment, prognosis, health related quality of life, and cost of care. Cancer outcomes research can be experimental or observational in nature. For example, randomized clinical trials have been conducted to assess the impact of screening on prostate cancer mortality[18] and to compare the effect of radical prostatectomy versus observation in patients with localized prostate cancer.[19] Observational studies of cancer outcomes, especially those that build upon preexisting resources,[20,21] can be carried out in a large group of patients with relatively little cost to capture the patterns and cost of care and to address many other research questions that have important clinical implications. Although the findings of such observation studies are subject to bias and confounding inherent in an observational design, these studies are complementary to experimental studies and have their unique value. Given an increasing interest in improving the effectiveness and value of cancer care, more cancer outcomes research is to be expected in the future.

MOLECULAR EPIDEMIOLOGY

Molecular epidemiology involves multidisciplinary and transdisciplinary research that entails not only traditional epidemiology and biostatistics, but also genetics, molecular biology, biochemistry, cellular biology, analytical chemistry, toxicology, pharmacology, and laboratory medicine. Unlike traditional epidemiology research of cancer, which focuses on exposures or risk factors ascertained through questionnaire-based interviews or surveys, molecular epidemiology studies expand the assessment of exposure to a much broader scope that includes an analysis of biomarkers underlying internal exposure of exogenous and endogenous carcinogenic agents or risk factors, molecular alterations in response to exposure, and genetic susceptibility to cancer. The biomarkers often measured in molecular epidemiology research include DNA, RNA, proteins, chromosomes, compound molecules (e.g., DNA and protein adducts), and various metabolites as well as other endogenous and exogenous substances (e.g., steroids, nutrients, chemical or biologic toxins, and phytochemicals). Molecular markers can reflect different aspects of the tumorigenic process, which include biomarkers of internal exposure, biomarkers of molecular or cellular changes in response to exposure, and biomarkers of precursor lesions or early diseases.[22,23] Depending on the source of molecules and location of diseases, surrogates are often used in epidemiologic studies. When using a surrogate marker or tissue, the relevance of a proxy to its underlying target needs to be established or justified.[23] This justification is especially important when conducting population-based epidemiologic studies that focus on organ-specific cancers, because assessing biomarkers in target tissue is difficult for controls; molecular markers from blood samples are often used as substitutes. If a biomarker in the blood does not travel to or act on the tissue or organ of interest, an association between the circulating marker and the cancer may not be relevant. Thus, establishing a close link between a surrogate and its target is crucial in molecular epidemiology research.

Gene-environment interaction plays an essential role in cancer development.[24] Common genetic variations are considered an important determinant of host susceptibility and are a major focus of molecular epidemiology research. Depending on the biologic mechanism involved, genetic variations can influence every aspect of the carcinogenic process, ranging from external and internal exposure to carcinogens or risk factors to molecular and cellular damage, alteration, and response.[22,23] Currently, single nucleotide polymorphisms (SNPs) are the most studied genetic variations. It is believed that even if SNPs confer a small risk, they may still be important at the population level because these variations are common in the general population. It is also important that the impacts of SNPs on cancer are considered under the context of gene–gene and gene–environment interactions. As genotyping technology has advanced substantially with respect to its analytic quality, capacity, and cost, research of genetic polymorphisms has evolved rapidly from investigations of a single SNP to studies of haplotypes and tag SNPs, and from a pathway-based candidate gene approach to genome-wide association studies (GWAS).[25] A GWAS analyzes hundreds of thousands of SNPs simultaneously for hundreds or even thousands of study subjects. When these data are further combined with questionnaire information such as environmental exposures, lifestyle factors, dietary habits, and medical history, enormous information is generated, which requires a huge sample size to allow for a reliable and complete assessment of these variables individually and jointly. A single epidemiologic study can no longer provide sufficient power for this type of investigation. Multicenter investigations or study consortia that pool study information and specimens together are developed to address the sample size issue.[26] False-positive findings resulting from multiple comparisons constitute a major challenge in epidemiologic studies of genetic associations with cancer.[27] A meta-analysis or pooled analysis can be used to address this problem if sufficient studies are already published and available for evaluation. To address this issue at the time of study design, one may adopt a two- or multiphase study design in which study subjects are divided into two or multiple groups for genotyping and data analysis. Selected or genomewide SNPs are first screened in one group of the study subjects (discovery phase), and then the significant findings determined by stringent statistical criteria (usually p values less than 1×10^{-5} or 1×10^{-7}) are reanalyzed in one or several other groups of subjects for verification (validation phase). This study design also lowers the cost of genotyping. False-positive findings can also be addressed with various statistical methods, such as bootstrap, permutation test, estimate of false positive report probability, prediction of false discovery rate, and the use of a much more stringent p value to accommodate multiple comparisons. For epidemiologic studies that are not population based or not conducted strictly following epidemiology principles, population stratification is a potential source of bias that may distort genetic associations.[28]

A large number of GWAS have been completed in search for SNPs that influence host susceptibility to cancer. Considering that more than 5 million SNPs are present in the human genome, the numbers of SNPs that are found to be associated with cancer risk after rigorous validation are much fewer than what one would have anticipated. In addition, the risk associations detected are quite weak, with most of the odds ratios ranging from 1.1 to 1.5, and the functional relevance or biologic implications are unclear for most of the SNPs. Furthermore, not many SNPs associated with cancer risk are located in protein-coding regions, and even fewer are in the loci of candidate genes suspected to be involved in tumorigenesis, such as oncogenes, tumor suppressor genes, DNA repair genes, and xenobiotic metabolizing or detoxification genes. Genes where SNPs are found to be linked to cancer by GWAS include *FGFR2, MAP3K1, MRPS30, LSP1, TNRC9, TOX3, STXBP1*, and *RAD51L1* for breast cancer[29–31]; *JAZF1, HNF1B, MSMB, CTBP2*, and *KLK2/KLK3* for prostate cancer[29,32]; *SMAD7, CRAC1, EIF3H, BMP4, CDH1*, and *RHPN2* for colorectal cancer[29,33]; *CHRNA3* and *CHRNA5* for lung cancer[34,35]; *ABO* for pancreatic cancer[36]; *TACC3* and *PSCA* for bladder cancer[37,38]; and *KRT5* for basal cell carcinoma.[39] Among these genes identified by GWAS, two findings are considered especially interesting. One is the association of lung cancer with *CHRNA3* and *CHRNA5*, which encode neuronal nicotinic acetylcholine receptor subunits. Different genotypes of these receptor subunits appear to influence individual's addiction to tobacco, which further leads to different smoking exposure and lung cancer risk.[40,41] Another is the link of the *ABO* gene to pancreatic cancer. The association between pancreatic cancer risk and ABO blood type was observed 50 years ago. The GWAS finding not only confirms the relationship, but also provides new clues for understanding the underlying biologic mechanism.

Besides intragenic SNPs, GWAS also found many intergenic SNPs in association to cancer risk, which include those in the regions of 8q24, 5p15, 1p11, 1p36, 1q42, 2p15, 2q35, 3p12, 3p24,

3q28, 6p21, 6q25, 7q21, 7q32, 9p21, 9p22, 9p24, 9q22, 10p14, 11q13, 11q23, 14q13, 18q23, and 20p12.[29–31,33,39,42–48] Of these loci, SNPs in 8q24 are associated with several cancer sites, including prostate, breast, colon, and bladder.[29,31–33,47–49] Further analysis of 8q24 indicates that there are nine SNPs in five regions and each region is independently related to different types of cancer, with SNPs in regions 1, 4, and 5 associated exclusively with prostate cancer, a SNP in region 2 related to breast cancer, and SNPs in region 3 linked to prostate, colon, and ovarian cancers.[50] No known genes are located within the region of 8q24, but an oncogene *c-MYC* resides about 330 kb downstream of the region.[51] An initial investigation found no evidence of the SNPs' influence on *c-MYC* expression,[47] but a later study suggests that the SNPs in 8q24 may be distal enhancers of *c-MYC*, interacting with its promoter through a chromatin loop.[52] Another genomic region that is associated with the risk of multiple cancer sites is 5p15, a region involving telomerase reverse transcriptase (TERT) cleft lip and palate transmembrane protein 1–like protein (CLPTM1L). Five types of cancer are found to be linked to this region, including basal cell carcinoma, lung, bladder, prostate, and cervical cancers.[53] TERT extends the length of telomere and is associated with cell proliferation and abnormal telomere maintenance.[54] The risk alleles of TERT are associated with shorter telomere length among the elderly and with higher DNA adduct in the lungs.[53,55]

GWAS has demonstrated its value in identifying disease-related SNPs in unknown regions of the genome, which provides new clues for investigators to interrogate and understand different regions of the human genome, especially in the gene-desert areas. Despite the strength, the low yield of significant findings from the GWAS has raised concerns in several areas, including the SNP coverage in the genome (rare SNPs and SNP representativeness in unknown regions), associations with low statistical significance (p value between 0.01 and 1×10^{-5}, the GWAS cutoff), other forms of genetic variations (copy number variation and other structural variations), cancer subtypes, and genetic interplay with environmental factors (gene–environment interaction).[56,57] To address these issues, investigators propose to perform fine-mapping and resequencing to examine genetic regions more specifically and meticulously. Epidemiologists suggest that detailed environmental exposure and lifestyle factors should be included in the next wave of GWAS. Furthermore, to make the study more reliable and compelling, DNA specimens, instead of convenient samples, should come from well-designed and well-executed epidemiologic studies that pay close attention to the selection of study subjects and the measurement of environmental and lifestyle factors to eliminate or minimize selection bias and measurement errors.

As described earlier, analytical epidemiology has two major study designs: the case-control study and the cohort study. It is important that investigators choose an appropriate study design to investigate molecular markers in epidemiologic studies. Two types of molecular markers, genotypic and phenotypic markers, can be considered. Genotypic markers refer to nucleotide sequences of genomic DNA, and all other molecules are considered phenotypic markers, including most of the chemical modifications on DNA, such as cytosine methylation. The distinction between the two is a marker's status in relation to an outcome variable, usually a disease. Genotypic markers generally do not change over time and are not affected by the development of a disease, whereas phenotypic markers are likely to change over time or be influenced by the presence of a disease, either itself or the treatment associated with it. If measurements of a phenotypic marker are made from the specimens that are collected after or at the time of cancer diagnosis, investigators will have difficulties determining the status of the phenotypic marker before the cancer was diagnosed. A disease condition, however, does not affect genotypic markers such as SNPs; therefore, a temporal relationship can be easily established even if the samples are collected after the disease is diagnosed. Based on this distinction, one can evaluate genotypic markers either in case-control or cohort studies, but a case-control study would be the design of choice because of efficiency and cost-effectiveness. A prospective cohort study design is ideal for phenotypic markers. Investigators, however, may use other study designs if they can demonstrate that the disease status does not influence the phenotypic markers of interest. To reduce study cost, investigators usually use nested case-control or case-cohort designs to avoid analyzing specimens from the entire cohort. The main purpose in choosing a cohort study design for a molecular epidemiology investigation is to ensure that biospecimens are collected before the development of a disease so that a temporal relationship between a marker and disease development can be established.

The differences between molecular epidemiology and genetic epidemiology are the scope of the molecular analysis and the emphasis on heredity. Sometimes molecular and genetic epidemiology both investigate genetic factors in association with cancer risk, but each has its own emphasis. The former assesses genetic involvement, but not necessarily inheritance, whereas the latter focuses mainly on heredity. Because of the difference in focus, study populations are different between the two types of investigation. Molecular epidemiology studies unrelated individuals, whereas genetic epidemiology investigates family members in the format of pedigrees, parent–child trios, or sibling pairs. Given the different research focus between genetic and molecular epidemiology, these investigations evaluate different genetic markers. Genetic epidemiology research is designed to identify genetic markers with high penetrance (strong association with an underlying disease) but low prevalence in the general populations, whereas a molecular epidemiology investigation targets low penetrance markers that are commonly present in the general population. Given the difference in study design, the analysis of genetic marker's link to cancer is also different between the studies. Relative risks or odds ratios are calculated in molecular epidemiology studies because study participants are unrelated individuals, whereas linkage analysis is used in genetic epidemiology because individuals in the study are genetically related family members. Recently, both genetic and molecular epidemiology study designs have been considered in GWAS to improve study validity and to minimize false positive findings. Another difference between genetic and molecular epidemiology research is that molecular epidemiology also studies nongenetic molecules. Thus, the scope of molecular analysis is much broader in molecular epidemiology research than in genetic epidemiology studies.

A laboratory analysis of molecular markers is another integral part of molecular epidemiology research, which has unique features that are different from basic science research. Collecting biologic specimens is difficult and expensive in population-based epidemiologic studies. It not only increases the study cost, but also imposes constraints to multiple areas of epidemiology research. Specimen collection may adversely influence the response rate of study participants, potentially compromising study validity. For organ-specific cancer research, investigating molecular markers in target tissue is difficult. Blood is the most common and versatile specimen used in molecular epidemiology research; other specimens used include urine, stool, nail, hair, sputum, buccal cells, and saliva. Tissue samples, either fresh frozen or chemically fixed, are also used, but the availability of these samples is highly limited to patients or selected subgroups of a general study population. Comparability and generalizability are always problems in epidemiologic studies involving tissue specimens, except for those investigations that focus on cancer prognosis or treatment in which only cancer patients are involved. Attempts have been made to use special body fluids for epidemiologic research, such as nipple aspirate and breast or pulmonary lavage, but the difficulty in specimen collection and preparation makes these samples impractical in large population-based studies.

Given the research value of biologic specimens and the difficulty in collecting them for population-based studies, technical issues related to specimen collection, processing, and storage become especially important in molecular epidemiology research.

These include time and conditions for specimen transportation and processing, a sample aliquot and labeling system, a sample special treatment for storage and analysis, a sample storage and tracking system, as well as backup plans and equipment for unexpected adverse events during long-term storage (e.g., power failure, earthquake, flooding). Laboratory methods used to analyze biomarkers are also important in molecular epidemiology. Because large numbers of specimens are involved, laboratory methods are required to be robust, reproducible, high throughput, low cost, and easy to use. These requirements are often met in the analysis of nucleotide sequences that serve as genotypic markers. However, for phenotypic markers, many methods do not readily meet these requirements. Moreover, many phenotypic markers, such as proteins, require both qualitative and quantitative assessments. An ideal laboratory method should be quantitative (able to measure a wide range of values), sensitive (able to detect a small amount of analyte), specific (able to detect only the molecule of interest, no other molecules), reproducible (high precision and low variation), and versatile (easy to use). In addition, investigators need to implement appropriate quality assurance procedures during sample processing and testing as well as include appropriate quality control samples in specimen analysis.

Host–environment interaction is believed to play a key role in the etiology of most types of cancer. Genetic factors, including mutations and polymorphisms, are initially considered important host factors, but recent developments in cancer research has indicated that epigenetic factors may also play a critical role in cancer as a host factor involved in host–environment interaction. Epigenetic factors, which regulate the function of human genome without altering the physical sequences of nucleotides, include pretranscription regulation through nucleotide modification (e.g., cytosine methylation at CpG sites), chromosome modification (e.g., histone acetylation), and posttranscription regulation by noncoding small RNA (e.g., microRNAs). These epigenetic factors have two unique features that have captured the attention of cancer researchers, especially cancer epidemiologists who are interested in the gene–environment interaction. It is known that epigenetic factors are heritable, but these inherited features are readily modifiable by environmental and lifestyle factors. Monozygotic twins have an identical genome as well as epigenome at birth, but the latter undergoes substantial changes over time, resulting in distinct epigenetic profiles that depend heavily on their environmental exposures.[58] Animal studies also indicated that the maternal intake of dietary nutrients involving one-carbon metabolism could influence offsprings' growth phenotypes, which are regulated by DNA methylation.[59] As evidence mounts on epigenetic involvement in cancer, molecular epidemiologists will start to look for clues in human populations that can link epigenetic factors to both lifestyle factors and cancer risk. Given that epigenetic regulation is tissue specific and time dependent, investigators face challenges in accurately assessing these phenotypic markers in etiologic studies. However, progress in the analysis of circulating methylation markers and microRNAs may provide an alternative to study epigenetic regulation in human cancer. Furthermore, methods for a genome-wide analysis of DNA methylation have been developed and applied in epidemiologic studies, which can substantially accelerate the search for cancer-related DNA methylation. Together with the high-throughput, high-dimensional analysis of DNA methylation, two other evolving fields that will have significant impacts on molecular epidemiology of cancer research are metagenomics and metabolomics. The former focuses on environmental genomics of the microbiome that resides in our body and influences one's biologic functions and health status. The latter refers to the analysis of hundreds or thousands of metabolites in a biologic specimen, including tissue, blood, urine, body fluids, and fecal samples. These new analyses will add tremendous value to epidemiologic studies.

REFERENCES

1. Last J. *A Dictionary of Epidemiology*. 3rd ed. New York: Oxford University Press; 1995.
2. Doll R, Hill AB. Lung cancer and other causes of death in relation to smoking: a second report on the mortality of British doctors. *Br Med J* 1956;12:1071–1081.
3. Kleinbaum D, Kupper L, Morgenstern H. *Epidemiologic Research*. New York: Van Nostrand Reinhold; 1982.
4. Kaplan LD, Straus DJ, Testa MA, et al. Low-dose compared with standard-dose m-BACOD chemotherapy for non-Hodgkin's lymphoma associated with human immunodeficiency virus infection. National Institute of Allergy and Infectious Diseases AIDS Clinical Trials Group. *N Engl J Med* 1997;336:1641–1648.
5. Dunn BK, Kramer BS, Ford LG. Phase III, large-scale chemoprevention trials. Approach to chemoprevention clinical trials and phase III clinical trial of tamoxifen as a chemopreventive for breast cancer—the US National Cancer Institute experience. *Hematol Oncol Clin North Am* 1998;12:1019–1036, vii.
6. Grant WB. An ecologic study of dietary and solar ultraviolet-B links to breast carcinoma mortality rates. *Cancer* 2002;94:272–281.
7. National Center for Health Statistics. Third National Health and Nutrition Examination Survey, 1988-1994, Plan and Operations Procedures Manuals (CD-ROM). Hyattsville, MD: U.S. Department of Health and Human Services (DHHS), Centers for Disease Control and Prevention; 1996.
8. Szklo M, Nieto F. *Epidemiology: Beyond the Basics*. Gaithersburg, MD: Aspen Publishers; 2000.
9. Grimes DA, Schulz KF. Cohort studies: marching towards outcomes. *Lancet* 2002;359:341–345.
10. Schatzkin A, Subar AF, Thompson FE, et al. Design and serendipity in establishing a large cohort with wide dietary intake distributions: the National Institutes of Health-American Association of Retired Persons Diet and Health Study. *Am J Epidemiol* 2001;154:1119–1125.
11. Mantel N, Haenszel W. Statistical aspects of the analysis of data from retrospective studies of disease. *J Natl Cancer Inst* 1959;22:719–748.
12. Wacholder S, Silverman DT, McLaughlin JK, et al. Selection of controls in case-control studies. II. Types of controls. *Am J Epidemiol* 1992;135:1029–1041.
13. Chen C, Weiss NS, Stanczyk FZ, et al. Endogenous sex hormones and prostate cancer risk: a case-control study nested within the Carotene and Retinol Efficacy Trial. *Cancer Epidemiol Biomarkers Prev* 2003;12:1410–1416.
14. Pearce N. What does the odds ratio estimate in a case-control study? *Int J Epidemiol* 1993;22:1189–1192.
15. Schulz KF, Grimes DA. Case-control studies: research in reverse. *Lancet* 2002;359:431–434.
16. Rothman K. *Epidemiology: An Introduction*. New York: Oxford University Press; 2002.
17. Hennekens C, Buring J. *Epidemiology in Medicine*. Boston: Little, Brown and Company; 1987.
18. Andriole GL, Crawford ED, Grubb RL 3rd, et al. Mortality results from a randomized prostate-cancer screening trial. *N Engl J Med* 2009;360:1310–1319.
19. Wilt TJ, Brawer MK, Jones KM, et al. Radical prostatectomy versus observation for localized prostate cancer. *N Engl J Med* 2012;367:203–213.
20. Yu JB, Soulos PR, Herrin J, et al. Proton versus intensity-modulated radiotherapy for prostate cancer: patterns of care and early toxicity. *J Natl Cancer Inst* 2013;105:25–32.
21. Ma X, Wang R, Long JB, et al. The cost implications of prostate cancer screening in the Medicare population. *Cancer* 2014;120(1):96–102.
22. Rundle A, Schwartz S. Issues in the epidemiological analysis and interpretation of intermediate biomarkers. *Cancer Epidemiol Biomarkers Prev* 2003;12:491–496.
23. Shields PG. Tobacco smoking, harm reduction, and biomarkers. *J Natl Cancer Inst* 2002;94:1435–1444.
24. Hunter DJ. Gene-environment interactions in human diseases. *Nat Rev Genet* 2005;6:287–298.
25. Hirschhorn JN, Daly MJ. Genome-wide association studies for common diseases and complex traits. *Nat Rev Genet* 2005;6:95–108.
26. Breast Cancer Association Consortum. Commonly studied single-nucleotide polymorphisms and breast cancer: results from the Breast Cancer Association Consortium. *J Natl Cancer Inst* 2006;98:1382–1396.
27. Wacholder S, Chanock S, Garcia-Closas M, et al. Assessing the probability that a positive report is false: an approach for molecular epidemiology studies. *J Natl Cancer Inst* 2004;96:434–442.
28. Clayton DG, Walker NM, Smyth DJ, et al. Population structure, differential bias and genomic control in a large-scale, case-control association study. *Nat Genet* 2005;37:1243–1246.
29. Easton DF, Eeles RA. Genome-wide association studies in cancer. *Hum Mol Genet* 2008;17:R109–115.
30. Ahmed S, Thomas G, Ghoussaini M, et al. Newly discovered breast cancer susceptibility loci on 3p24 and 17q23.2. *Nat Genet* 2009;41:585–590.
31. Thomas G, Jacobs KB, Kraft P, et al. A multistage genome-wide association study in breast cancer identifies two new risk alleles at 1p11.2 and 14q24.1 (RAD51L1). *Nat Genet* 2009;41:579–584.
32. Thomas G, Jacobs KB, Yeager M, et al. Multiple loci identified in a genome-wide association study of prostate cancer. *Nat Genet* 2008;40:310–315.

33. Le Marchand L. Genome-wide association studies and colorectal cancer. *Surg Oncol Clin N Am* 2009;18:663–668.
34. Hung RJ, McKay JD, Gaborieau V, et al. A susceptibility locus for lung cancer maps to nicotinic acetylcholine receptor subunit genes on 15q25. *Nature* 2008;452:633–637.
35. Amos CI, Wu X, Broderick P, et al. Genome-wide association scan of tag SNPs identifies a susceptibility locus for lung cancer at 15q25.1. *Nat Genet* 2008;40:616–622.
36. Amundadottir L, Kraft P, Stolzenberg-Solomon RZ, et al. Genome-wide association study identifies variants in the ABO locus associated with susceptibility to pancreatic cancer. *Nat Genet* 2009;41:986–990.
37. Kiemeney LA, Sulem P, Besenbacher S, et al. A sequence variant at 4p16.3 confers susceptibility to urinary bladder cancer. *Nat Genet* 2010;42(5):415–419.
38. Wu X, Ye Y, Kiemeney LA, et al. Genetic variation in the prostate stem cell antigen gene PSCA confers susceptibility to urinary bladder cancer. *Nat Genet* 2009;41:991–995.
39. Stacey SN, Sulem P, Masson G, et al. New common variants affecting susceptibility to basal cell carcinoma. *Nat Genet* 2009;41:909–914.
40. Thorgeirsson TE, Geller F, Sulem P, et al. A variant associated with nicotine dependence, lung cancer and peripheral arterial disease. *Nature* 2008;452:638–642.
41. Spitz MR, Amos CI, Dong Q, et al. The CHRNA5-A3 region on chromosome 15q24-25.1 is a risk factor both for nicotine dependence and for lung cancer. *J Natl Cancer Inst* 2008;100:1552–1556.
42. Zheng W, Long J, Gao YT, et al. Genome-wide association study identifies a new breast cancer susceptibility locus at 6q25.1. *Nat Genet* 2009;41:324–328.
43. Gudmundsson J, Sulem P, Gudbjartsson DF, et al. Common variants on 9q22.33 and 14q13.3 predispose to thyroid cancer in European populations. *Nat Genet* 2009;41:460–464.
44. Gudmundsson J, Sulem P, Gudbjartsson DF, et al. Genome-wide association and replication studies identify four variants associated with prostate cancer susceptibility. *Nat Genet* 2009;41:1122–1126.
45. Song H, Ramus SJ, Tyrer J, et al. A genome-wide association study identifies a new ovarian cancer susceptibility locus on 9p22.2. *Nat Genet* 2009;41: 996–1000.
46. Stacey SN, Gudbjartsson DF, Sulem P, et al. Common variants on 1p36 and 1q42 are associated with cutaneous basal cell carcinoma but not with melanoma or pigmentation traits. *Nat Genet* 2008;40:1313–1318.
47. Zanke BW, Greenwood CM, Rangrej J, et al. Genome-wide association scan identifies a colorectal cancer susceptibility locus on chromosome 8q24. *Nat Genet* 2007;39:989–994.
48. Haiman CA, Patterson N, Freedman ML, et al. Multiple regions within 8q24 independently affect risk for prostate cancer. *Nat Genet* 2007;39:638–644.
49. Kiemeney LA, Thorlacius S, Sulem P, et al. Sequence variant on 8q24 confers susceptibility to urinary bladder cancer. *Nat Genet* 2008;40:1307–1312.
50. Ghoussaini M, Song H, Koessler T, et al. Multiple loci with different cancer specificities within the 8q24 gene desert. *J Natl Cancer Inst* 2008;100:962–966.
51. Harismendy O, Frazer KA. Elucidating the role of 8q24 in colorectal cancer. *Nat Genet* 2009;41:868–869.
52. Wright JB, Brown SJ, Cole MD. Upregulation of c-MYC in cis through a large chromatin loop linked to a cancer risk-associated single-nucleotide polymorphism in colorectal cancer cells. *Mol Cell Biol* 2010;30:1411–1420.
53. Rafnar T, Sulem P, Stacey SN, et al. Sequence variants at the TERT-CLPTM1L locus associate with many cancer types. *Nat Genet* 2009;41:221–227.
54. Fernandez-Garcia I, Ortiz-de-Solorzano C, Montuenga LM. Telomeres and telomerase in lung cancer. *J Thorac Oncol* 2008;3:1085–1088.
55. Zienolddiny S, Skaug V, Landvik NE, et al. The TERT-CLPTM1L lung cancer susceptibility variant associates with higher DNA adduct formation in the lung. *Carcinogenesis* 2009;30:1368–1371.
56. Ioannidis JP, Thomas G, Daly MJ. Validating, augmenting and refining genome-wide association signals. *Nat Rev Genet* 2009;10:318–329.
57. Chung CC, Magalhaes WC, Gonzalez-Bosquet J, et al. Genome-wide association studies in cancer—current and future directions. *Carcinogenesis* 2010;31:111–120.
58. Fraga MF, Ballestar E, Paz MF, et al. Epigenetic differences arise during the lifetime of monozygotic twins. *Proc Natl Acad Sci U S A* 2005;102:10604–10609.
59. Dolinoy DC, Weidman JR, Waterland RA, et al. Maternal genistein alters coat color and protects Avy mouse offspring from obesity by modifying the fetal epigenome. *Environ Health Perspect* 2006;114:567–572.

12 Trends in United States Cancer Mortality

Tim E. Byers

INTRODUCTION

Cancer incidence registries now cover nearly all of the US population. State-based vital records systems and aggregate national systems regularly report trends in both cancer incidence and mortality, and national surveys routinely monitor cancer-related risk factors in the population. These surveillance systems have documented substantial changes in both risk factors for cancer and in cancer incidence and mortality rates in the United States over the past 3 decades. In 1996, the American Cancer Society (ACS) set an ambitious challenge for the United States: to reduce cancer mortality rates from their apparent peak in 1990 by 50% in the 25-year period ending in 2015.[1] In 1998, the ACS then challenged the United States to also reduce cancer incidence rates from their peak in 1992 by 25% by the year 2015.[2] In this chapter, we will examine trends in cancer risk factors as well as trends in cancer incidence and mortality rates in the United States over the 25-year period between 1990 and 2015.

CANCER SURVEILLANCE SYSTEMS

Collecting cancer incidence rates is largely a state-based activity in the United States, because cancer is a reportable disease in all states. The Centers for Disease Control and Prevention (CDC) organizes all state-based cancer registries within the National Program of Cancer Registries, which now reports collective data on cancer incidence from over 40 different state-based registries, providing data that meets strict quality standards.[3] The National Cancer Institute has supported high-quality cancer incidence and outcomes registration in selected states and cities since 1973 within the Surveillance, Epidemiology, and End Results (SEER) Program.[4] The most precise measures of long-term trends in cancer incidence come from SEER-9, a set of nine SEER registries that together include about 10% of the US population. The populations included in the SEER-9 registries document the most detailed history of cancer trends beginning in the 1970s based on highly standardized cancer case ascertainment, staging, treatment, and outcomes. Deaths from cancer are well ascertained in all states via state-based vital records, which are aggregated into annual national mortality reports by the CDC's National Center for Health Statistics. [5] Each year, the ACS, the National Cancer Institute, and the CDC publish a *Report to the Nation* on trends in cancer incidence and mortality in the United States.[6] Trends in the prevalence of behavioral factors that affect cancer risk are tracked by the Health Interview Survey, an ongoing, in-person interview of a nationally representative sample of adults, and in annual reports by the Behavioral Risk Factor Surveillance System, a continuously operating telephone-based survey operated by state departments of health and organized by the CDC.[7]

MAKING SENSE OF CANCER TRENDS

Understanding the reasons for cancer trends requires understanding trends in cancer-related risk factors. For factors like tobacco, relating trends in exposure to trends in rates is easy, because those effects are large and single. However, for many other cancer risk factors, because effects are much smaller and multifactorial, simple correlations over time are less apparent. In most situations, all that maybe possible are crude qualitative relationships between temporal trends in cancer risk factors and subsequent trends in cancer rates. Statistical methods such as linear regression joinpoint analysis can tell us when inflections in cancer trends occur, but accounting for the precise reasons for changing rates is often impaired by our incomplete knowledge about the interacting impacts of variations in cancer screening, diagnosis, and treatment, and by uncertainties about latencies between interventions and outcomes.[8]

TRENDS IN CANCER RISK FACTORS AND SCREENING

Trends in major cancer risk factors have been mixed (Table 12.1). Although the downward trends in tobacco smoking among adults that began in the 1960s slowed after 1990, there has been a continuing downward trend in the number of cigarettes smoked per day by continuing smokers.[9] Obesity trends have been adverse among both men and women since the 1970s, with more than a doubling of the prevalence of obesity between 1990 and 2010. Long-term trends in the use of hormone replacement therapy (HRT) are not routinely monitored in the Behavioral Risk Factor Surveillance System (BRFSS), but HRT use increased substantially in the last 2 decades of the 20th century. Then, following the 2002 publication of the Women's Health Initiative trial, which showed clear adverse effects of HRT, there was a rapid and substantial drop in HRT use.[10,11] The use of endoscopic screening for colorectal cancer (sigmoidoscopy or colonoscopy) has increased substantially in recent years, approximately doubling since the mid 1990s, so that, as of 2010, about two-thirds of Americans age 50 and older reported ever having had an endoscopic examination. Mammography use increased progressively through the 1990s, but mammogram rates then leveled off after 2000.[12] Widespread prostate-specific antigen (PSA) testing began in the mid to late 1980s, then increased substantially during the 1990s. By 2002, a majority of US men age 50 and older reported having been tested.

CANCER INCIDENCE AND MORTALITY

In this chapter, we describe and discuss cancer trends for the time period 1990 through 2010 using cancer incidence data from the SEER-9 registry (Table 12.2 and Fig. 12.1) and US cancer mortality data from the National Center for Health Statistics (Table 12.3).[4,5] All rates were age-adjusted to the US 2000 standard population by the direct method, using 10-year age intervals.

Lung Cancer

The lung is the second leading site for cancer incidence and the leading site for cancer death among both men and women in the

TABLE 12.1

Trends in Risk Factors and Cancer Screening Practices in the United States, 1990–2010[a]

	Men		Women		Both Genders	
	Smoking	**PSA Screening**	**Smoking**	**Mammography**	**Obesity**	**CRC Screening**
1990	24.9	—	21.3	58.3	11.6	—
1991	25.1	—	21.3	62.2	12.6	—
1992	24.2	—	21.0	63.1	12.6	—
1993	24.0	—	21.1	66.5	13.7	—
1994	23.9	—	21.6	66.6	14.4	—
1995	24.8	—	20.9	68.6	15.8	29.4
1996	25.5	—	21.9	69.2	16.8	—
1997	25.4	—	21.1	70.3	16.6	32.4
1998	25.3	—	20.9	72.3	18.3	—
1999	24.2	—	20.8	72.8	19.7	43.7
2000	24.4	—	21.2	76.1	20.1	—
2001	25.4	—	21.2	—	21.0	—
2002	25.7	53.9	20.8	75.9	22.1	48.1
2003	24.8	—	20.2	—	—	—
2004	23.0	52.1	19.0	74.7	23.2	53.0
2005	22.1	—	19.2	—	24.4	—
2006	22.2	53.8	18.4	76.5	25.1	57.1
2007	21.2	—	18.4	—	26.3	—
2008	20.3	54.8	16.7	76.0	26.6	61.8
2009	19.5	—	16.7	—	27.1	—
2010	18.5	53.2	15.8	75.2	27.5	65.2

CRC, colorectal cancer; PSA, prostate-specific antigen.

[a] Median percent of the population across all states in the Behavioral Risk Factor Surveillance System. The survey covered such areas as body mass index and was based on self-reported height and weight. Questions included: Are you a regular cigarette smoker? Have you ever had a sigmoidoscopy or proctoscopic examination? For women age 40 and older, the following question was included: Have you had a mammogram in the past 2 years? For men aged 50 and older, the following question was included: Have you had a PSA test in the last 2 years? (From Centers for Disease Control and Prevention. Behavioral Risk Factor Surveillance System Web site. http://cdc.gov/brfss.)

United States.[6] There are now more deaths from lung cancer in the United States than from the sum of colorectal, breast, and prostate cancers. Trends in lung cancer incidence and mortality have been nearly identical because there are few effective treatments for lung cancer, and survival time remains short. Lung cancer trends follow historic declines in tobacco use, lagged by about 20 years.[13] Between 1965 and 1985, tobacco use among US adults dropped substantially, and more in men than in women. Lung cancer mortality rates began to decline among men in 1990, but rates increased among women throughout the 1990s. The stabilization of lung cancer incidence trends among women from 2000 to 2005 and the beginning of a decline in the period 2005 to 2010 foretells a coming persistent decline in lung cancer mortality among women in the United States.

The effectiveness of annual examinations by use of chest radiographs in reducing lung cancer mortality was studied as part of the Prostate, Lung, Colorectal, Ovary (PLCO) trial, and the effectiveness of annual screening by low-dose computed tomography (LDCT) of the lung fields was studied in the National Lung Screening Trial (NLST).[14,15] In brief, screening with standard chest radiography finds more cancers earlier but does not affect mortality, whereas screening with LDCT reduces the risk of death from lung cancer by at least 20%.[14,15] Therefore, both the ACS and the US Preventive Services Task Force have issued recommendations that favor informed decision making for lung cancer screening using LDCT.[16,17]

The major factor that will determine lung cancer incidence in the coming decade is the past history of tobacco use, but future screening will also reduce future mortality rates. Considering all factors, it is likely that over the coming decade the downward trends in mortality from lung cancer will continue at about the same rate among men, and soon will become more apparent among women.

Colorectal Cancer

The colorectum is the third leading site for cancer incidence and the second leading site for cancer death in the United States.[6] Colorectal cancer incidence rates increased until 1985, when they began to decline. The reasons for this decline are not clear, but could be related to downward trends in cigarette smoking and the increasing use of both nonsteroidal anti-inflammatory drugs (NSAIDs) and HRT.[18] The rapid decline in HRT use following the publication of the Women's Health Initiative trial results in 2002 may adversely affect colorectal trends among women in the coming years, because HRT reduces the risk for colorectal cancer among women.[11] Recent trials have demonstrated the potential for NSAIDs to reduce colorectal neoplasia, but adverse effects from these agents will limit their widespread use for that explicit purpose. Nonetheless, even the common sporadic use of NSAIDs for other indications will contribute to continuing declines in colorectal cancer incidence in the coming years.

Screening with either sigmoidoscopy or colonoscopy leads to the identification and removal of adenomas, thus preventing the development of colorectal cancer.[19,20] Medicare included

TABLE 12.2

Trends in Age-Adjusted Cancer Incidence Rates in the United States by Cancer Site, 1990–2010[a]

	Men		Women		Both Genders	
	Lung	**Prostate**	**Lung**	**Breast**	**Colorectal**	**All Sites**
1990	96.9	171.0	47.8	131.8	60.7	482.0
1991	97.2	214.8	49.6	133.9	59.5	503.0
1992	97.2	237.4	49.9	132.1	58.0	510.6
1993	94.0	209.5	49.2	129.2	56.8	493.4
1994	90.9	180.3	50.5	131.0	55.6	483.5
1995	89.8	169.3	50.4	132.6	54.0	476.9
1996	88.0	169.5	50.2	133.7	54.8	479.1
1997	86.3	173.5	52.6	138.0	56.4	486.4
1998	88.0	171.0	53.0	141.4	56.8	488.2
1999	84.6	183.4	52.4	141.5	55.5	490.4
2000	82.1	183.0	51.2	136.4	54.1	486.0
2001	81.4	184.8	51.7	138.7	53.6	489.7
2002	80.4	182.2	52.5	135.6	53.1	487.5
2003	81.0	169.6	53.0	126.8	50.8	475.2
2004	76.2	165.7	52.0	128.0	50.0	476.1
2005	75.8	156.5	53.7	126.4	47.8	471.9
2006	74.2	171.5	53.4	126.0	46.8	475.0
2007	73.5	174.3	53.4	127.9	46.3	480.5
2008	72.0	157.0	51.6	128.0	45.2	473.4
2009	70.2	153.7	51.8	130.3	43.0	470.5
2010	66.8	145.1	49.2	126.0	40.6	457.5
Average annual % change 1990–2010	−1.8	−0.5	+0.2	−0.2	−2.0	−0.2

[a] Data source is the Surveillance, Epidemiology, and End Results-9 populations for cancer incidence. Rates are age-adjusted to the year 2000 population standard. The annual percent change is the mean percent change per year across the 20-year period, 1990 to 2010. (From National Cancer Institute. Surveillance, Epidemiology, and End Results Program Web site. http://seer.cancer.gov.)

coverage for all recommended colorectal screening methods in 2001, and national publicity has substantially increased public interest in screening.[21] Colorectal screening rates have increased over time, now with about two-thirds of adults over age 50 reporting having ever been screened by lower gastrointestinal endoscopy (see Table 12.1).

Decreasing rates of colorectal cancer incidence are occurring in spite of the obesity epidemic, which is an adverse force on colorectal cancer risk, because obesity may account for as much as 20% of colorectal cancer in the United States.[22] Recently, however, obesity trends have stabilized in the United States.[23] As a result of the increased use of lower gastrointestinal endoscopy for colorectal screening and this stabilization of obesity trends, the incidence of colorectal cancer may exceed the ACS goal for 2015 of a 25% reduction, and there is a high likelihood that the rate of decline in deaths from colorectal cancer will be steep enough to reach the 2015 ACS mortality reduction goal of 50%.

Breast Cancer

The breast is the leading site of cancer incidence and the second leading site for cancer death among women in the United States.[6] Over the period 1990 to 2001, no substantial changes in incidence rates were observed, but after 2000, breast cancer incidence began to decline. The decline in breast cancer incidence observed after 2002 seems to have been the result of the sudden decline in the use of HRT following the 2002 publication of the Women's Health Initiative results.[10,11] It is likely that persisting lower rates of HRT use will cause a continued decline in breast cancer incidence in the coming years. Countering this favorable trend, however, are the adverse effects of the obesity epidemic. Obesity, a major risk factor for postmenopausal breast cancer, increased substantially between 1990 and 2005, now with over 25% of US women being obese. However, the slowing of the obesity epidemic since 2005 may have substantial beneficial effects on the future trends in breast cancer incidence.

After persistent increases in the use of mammography over a 20-year period, mammography rates declined modestly between 2000 and 2004, and then leveled off. The downgrading of the evidence recommendations by the US Preventive Services Task Force for mammography for women age 40 to 49 and recommendations for every other year mammographies for women age 50 and older have resulted in lower mammogram utilization, which is likely to continue into the coming decade.[17] This trend will have an adverse effect on breast cancer mortality, but will tend to reduce breast cancer incidence somewhat because of a lack of detection of very early stage cancers.

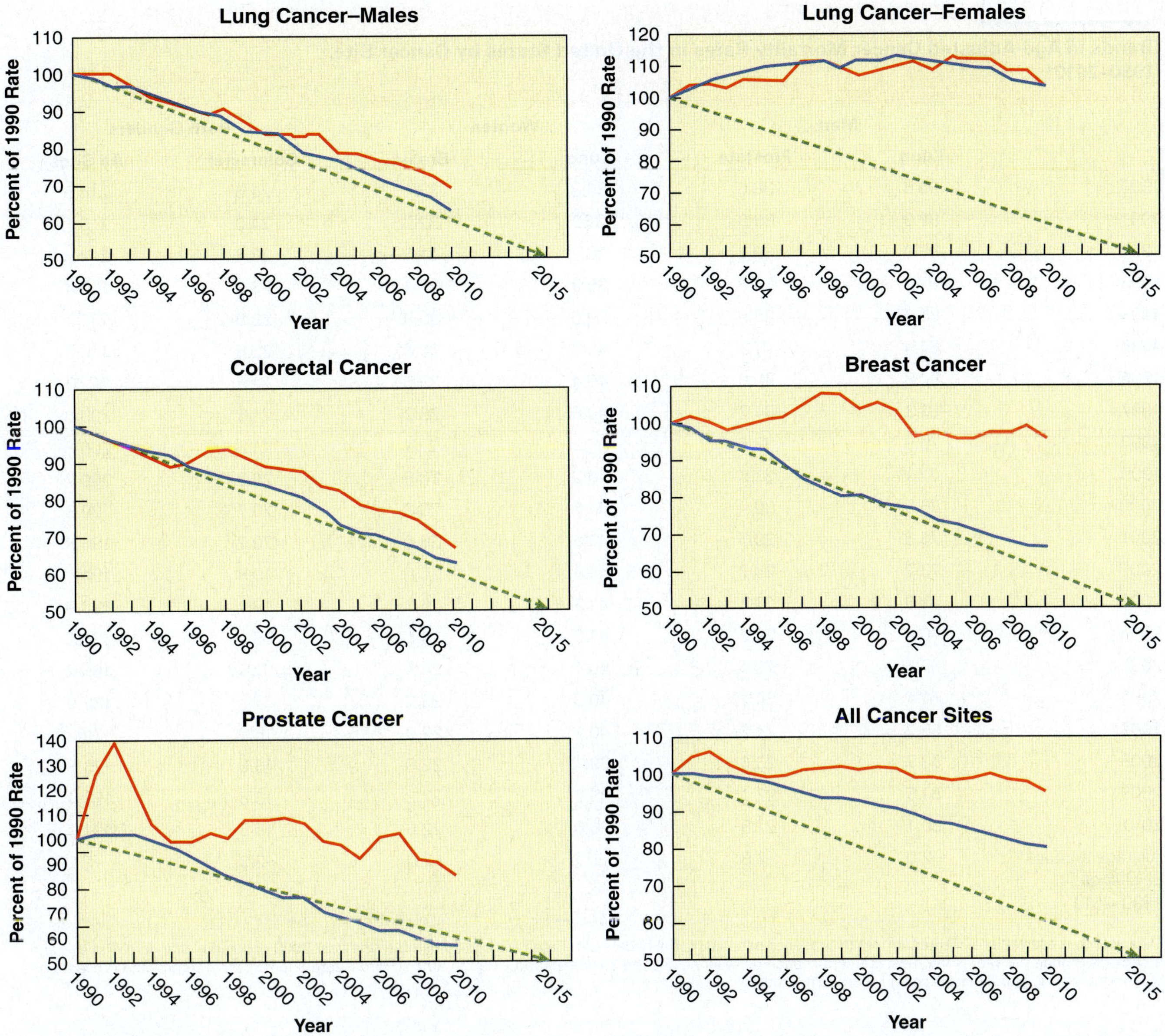

Figure 12.1 **(A–F)** Trends in cancer incidence and mortality between 1990 and 2010. Incidence rates are for the populations in the Surveillance, Epidemiology, and End Results Program; registries and mortality rates are for the entire United States. Rates are age-adjusted to the year 2000 standard. The y-axis rates are expressed as a percentage of the 1990 incidence and mortality rates. The *red lines* represent incidence rates, and the *blue lines* represent mortality rates. The *straight dotted green lines* represent the linear trend that would need to be followed to achieve a 50% mortality reduction between 1990 and 2015. (Data from National Cancer Institute. Surveillance, Epidemiology, and End Results Program Web site. http://seer.cancer.gov, and Centers for Disease Control and Prevention. U.S. mortality data. http://wonder.cdc.gov/ucd-icd10.html)

The antiestrogens tamoxifen and raloxifene have both been shown to reduce the risk of incident breast cancer.[24] The safety profile for tamoxifen discourages its widespread use, but there is a more favorable risk/benefit balance of raloxifene. Nonetheless, neither of these drugs is commonly used for breast cancer prevention among postmenopausal women in the United States.

The average decline in breast cancer death rates of 2% per year since 1990 is the combined result of earlier diagnosis and better treatment.[25] Progress in breast cancer treatment is continuing, especially in the development and application of hormone-targeted therapies. Aromatase inhibitors have largely replaced tamoxifen therapy for breast cancer treatment for postmenopausal women. Because all antiestrogens substantially reduce the incidence of second primary cancers in the contralateral breast, they impact both therapy and prevention. In the coming decade, the longer term effects of decreased HRT use, increased antiestrogen use, reversal of the obesity trends, and continued improvements in therapies will likely lead to continued decreases in both the incidence and mortality rates from breast cancer.

Prostate Cancer

The prostate is the leading site for cancer incidence and the second leading site for cancer death among men in the United States.[6] The incidence of prostate cancer has been extremely variable over the period 1990 to 2010. The incidence spike observed in the early 1990s actually began in the late 1980s, coincident with the advent of PSA testing. The reasons for the 2.8% annual downward trend in prostate cancer mortality since 1990 are uncertain, however, because the ongoing PSA screening trials have not yet demonstrated a mortality benefit from screening anywhere as large as the downward mortality

TABLE 12.3

Trends in Age-Adjusted Cancer Mortality Rates in the United States by Cancer Site, 1990–2010[a]

	Men		Women		Both Genders	
	Lung	**Prostate**	**Lung**	**Breast**	**Colorectal**	**All Sites**
1990	90.6	38.6	36.8	33.1	24.6	214.9
1991	89.9	39.3	37.6	32.7	24.0	215.1
1992	88.0	39.2	38.7	31.6	23.6	213.5
1993	87.6	39.3	39.3	31.4	23.3	213.4
1994	85.7	38.5	39.6	30.9	22.9	211.7
1995	84.4	37.3	40.3	30.6	22.6	210.0
1996	82.8	36.0	40.4	29.5	21.9	207.0
1997	81.3	34.2	40.8	28.2	21.5	203.6
1998	79.9	32.6	41.0	27.5	21.2	200.8
1999	77.0	31.6	40.2	26.6	20.9	200.7
2000	76.5	30.4	41.1	26.6	20.7	198.8
2001	75.3	29.5	41.0	26.0	20.2	196.3
2002	73.7	28.7	41.6	25.6	19.8	194.4
2003	72.0	27.2	41.3	25.3	19.1	190.9
2004	70.4	26.2	41.0	24.5	18.1	186.8
2005	69.5	25.4	40.7	24.1	17.6	185.2
2006	67.4	24.2	40.3	23.6	17.3	182.0
2007	65.2	24.2	40.1	23.0	16.9	179.3
2008	63.7	23.0	39.1	22.6	16.5	176.3
2009	61.5	22.1	38.6	22.2	15.8	173.4
2010	60.1	21.8	38.0	22.0	15.5	171.8
Average annual % change 1990–2010	−2.0	−2.8	+0.2	−2.0	−2.3	−1.1

[a] Data source is the National Center for Health Statistics national mortality data set. Rates are age-adjusted to the year 2000 population standard. The average percentage change per year is the mean percent change per year across the 20-year period, 1990 to 2010. (From Centers for Disease Control and Prevention. U.S. mortality data. http://wonder.cdc.gov/ucd-icd10.html)

decline observed since 1990.[26,27] In fact, the US trial findings suggest that there was virtually no mortality benefit within the first decade following the initiation of screening.[28] Therefore, it is not possible to know how much of this favorable trend was related to early diagnosis, how much was related to improvements in treatment, or how much might have been related to other factors, such as changes in the way cause of death has been listed on death certificates.

The Prostate Cancer Prevention Trial provided an important proof of principle that antiandrogen therapies can reduce prostate cancer risk.[29] Although the net benefits of finasteride for prevention are not clearly demonstrated from this trial, other agents that interfere with androgen effects on prostate cancer growth could prove to be useful for prostate cancer chemoprevention in the future. Prostate cancer incidence trends will likely continue to be largely driven by rates of PSA screening in the coming decade. Longer term results of a clearer benefit to mortality from either the PLCO trial in the United States or the European PSA trial would help to better specify screening recommendations.

Other Cancers

Even though mortality rates have been declining by about 2% per year from the four most common causes of cancer death (lung, colorectal, breast, and prostate), very little progress has been made in reducing death rates from the other half of all adult cancers in the United States. Continuing progress in tobacco control will have beneficial effects on many other types of cancer linked to tobacco, and stopping the obesity epidemic will have favorable effects on many obesity-related cancers that have been increasing in recent years, such as adenocarcinoma of the esophagus and renal cancer.[30] Melanoma incidence rates have been increasing substantially in recent years, likely the result of the combined effects of previous sun exposure and increased awareness and surveillance for pigmented skin lesions, but recent advances in therapy for metastatic melanoma may foretell future declines in melanoma morality. Declining rates of stomach cancer incidence and mortality over several decades may be related to the combined effects of historic improvements in nutrition and the declining prevalence of chronic infection with *Helicobacter pylori*. Liver cancer incidence has been substantially increasing in recent years, likely resulting from historic trends in chronic infection with hepatitis B and C viruses. As a result, liver cancer will likely continue to rise in the United States over the coming decade.

The incidence of thyroid cancer has been increasing in the United States for the past several decades, but thyroid cancer mortality rates have been stable, a pattern most likely due to increased detection from improved diagnostic techniques. Invasive cervical cancer is uncommon in the United States because of widespread screening using Pap smears. Although the vaccination for human papillomavirus (HPV) has been shown to be highly effective in protecting against the serotypes that together account for 70% of cervical cancer cases, so far, HPV vaccine coverage has been low among young women in the United States.[6] For many of the other cancers, such as cancers of the pancreas, brain, ovary, and the hematopoietic malignancies, risk factors are poorly understood, and there are no effective early detection methods. For these cancers, the current hope for improvement resides in the development of better methods for early cancer detection and treatment.

PREDICTING FUTURE CANCER TRENDS

In the United States, cancer is now the leading cause of death under age 85 years. Over the first half of the ACS 25-year challenge period, overall cancer incidence rates have declined by about 0.2% per year, and mortality rates have declined by about 1% per year. The trends in both incidence and mortality from the four leading cancer sites are summarized in Figure 12.1. Using simple linear extrapolation, it therefore seems that the ACS challenge goals of reducing cancer incidence by 25% and mortality by 50% over 25 years may be only half achieved.[31,32] Clearly, though, estimating future trends only by linear extrapolation is a crude way to foretell future events. Projecting cancer trends into the more distant future using complex modeling is possible, however, as knowledge about changes in major cancer risk factors can lead to reasonable predictions about the direction and approximate slope of future trends. One method to incorporate knowledge about trends in risk factors into estimates of future cancer trends is to estimate the impact of changes in the attributable risk (also called the *preventable fraction*) in the population for each risk factor. By making assumptions about latency period, then tying changes in factors to changes in cancer incidence and mortality, cancer trends resulting from risk factor changes can be predicted. For example, if there were a factor that explained 30% of a particular cancer, then cutting that exposure in half would eventually lead to a projected 15% reduction in rates (50% of 30%). This method was used to project cancer mortality trends to 2015 and seems to have projected trends that are quite similar to those observed in recent years.[33]

Progress in cancer prevention, early detection, and treatment since 1990 has been persistent, and there are many reasons to be optimistic about the future. Just how much steeper the future downward slope in cancer death rates can be driven will depend on the extent to which we can discover new factors causing cancer, and effectively deploy ways to better act on our current knowledge about how to prevent and control cancer. Especially important will be progress in reversing the epidemics of tobacco use and obesity, and ensuring that the coming improvements to health care access will lead to access to state-of-the-art cancer screening and therapy for all.

REFERENCES

1. American Cancer Society Board of Directors. ACS Challenge goals for U.S. Cancer Mortality for the Year 2015. *Proceedings of the Board of Directors.* Atlanta, GA: American Cancer Society, 1996.
2. American Cancer Society Board of Directors. ACS Challenge goals for U.S. Cancer Incidence for the Year 2015. *Proceedings of the Board of Directors.* Atlanta, GA: American Cancer Society, 1998.
3. Centers for Disease Control and Prevention. National Program of Cancer Registries (NPCR) Web site. http://cdc.gov/cancer/npcr.
4. National Cancer Institute. Surveillance, Epidemiology, and End Results Program Web site. http://seer.cancer.gov.
5. Centers for Disease Control and Prevention. U.S. mortality data. http://wonder.cdc.gov/ucd-icd10.html
6. Jemal A, Simard E, Dorell C, et al. Annual report to the nation on the status of cancer, 1975–2009, featuring the burden and trends in human papillomavirus (HPV)–associated cancers and HPV vaccination coverage levels. *J Natl Cancer Inst* 2013;105:175–201.
7. Centers for Disease Control and Prevention. Behavioral Risk Factor Surveillance System Web site. http://cdc.gov/brfss.
8. Ward E, Thun M, Hannan L, et al. Interpreting cancer trends. *Ann N Y Acad Sci* 2006;1076:29–53.
9. Centers for Disease Control and Prevention. Smoking & Tobacco Use Web site. http://cdc.gov/tobacco.
10. Rossouw JE, Anderson GL, Prentice RL, et al. Risks and benefits of estrogen plus progestin in healthy postmenopausal women: principal results from the Women's Health Initiative randomized controlled trial. *JAMA* 2002; 288:321–333.
11. Hersh A, Stefanick M, Stafford R. National use of postmenopausal hormone therapy: annual trends and response to recent evidence. *JAMA* 2004;291:47–53.
12. Ryerson AB, Miller J, Eheman CR, et al. Use of mammograms among women aged ≥40 years—United States, 2000–2005. *MMWR* 2007;56:49–51.
13. Giovino GA. Epidemiology of tobacco use in the United States. *Oncogene* 2002;21:7326–7340.
14. Oken M, Hocking W, Kvale P, et al. Screening by chest radiograph and lung cancer mortality. *JAMA* 2011;306:1865–1873.
15. The National Lung Screening Trial Research Team. Reduced lung-cancer mortality with low-dose computed tomographic screening. *N Engl J Med* 2011; 365:395–409.
16. Smith R, Brooks D, Cokkinides V, et al. Cancer screening in the United States, 2013: a review of current American Cancer Society guidelines, current issues in cancer screening, and new guidance on cervical cancer screening and lung cancer screening. *CA Cancer J Clin* 2013;63:88–105.
17. U.S. Preventive Services Task Force. U.S. Preventive Services Task Force Web site. http://uspreventiveservicestaskforce.org.
18. Martinez ME. Primary prevention of colorectal cancer: lifestyle, nutrition, exercise. *Recent Results Cancer Res* 2005;166:177–211.
19. Atkin W, Edwards R, Kralj-Hans I, et al. Once-only flexible sigmoidoscopy screening in prevention of colorectal cancer: a multicentre randomized controlled trial. *Lancet* 2010;375:1624–1633.
20. Schoen RE, Pinsky PF, Weissfeld JL, et al. Colorectal-cancer incidence and mortality with screening flexible sigmoidoscopy. *N Engl J Med* 2012; 366:2345–2357.
21. Cram P, Fendrick A, Inadomi J, et al. The impact of celebrity promotional campaign on the use of colon cancer screening: the Katie Couric effect. *Arch Intern Med* 2003;163(13):1601–1605.
22. World Cancer Research Fund/American Institute for Cancer Prevention. *Policy and Action for Cancer Prevention. Food, Nutrition, and Physical Activity: A Global Perspective.* Washington, DC: AICR; 2009.
23. Ogden CL, Carroll MD, Curtin LR, et al. Prevalence of overweight and obesity in the United States, 1999–2004. *JAMA* 2006;295:1549–1555.
24. Vogel V, Constantino J, Wickerham D, et al. Effects of tamoxifen vs raloxifene on the risks of developing invasive breast cancer and other disease outcomes: the NSABP Study of Tamoxifen and Raloxifene (STAR) P-2 trial. *JAMA* 2006;295:2727–2741.
25. Berry D, Cronin K, Plevritis S, et al. Effect of screening and adjuvant therapy on mortality from breast cancer. *N Engl J Med* 2005;353:1784–1792.
26. Andriole GL, Crawford ED, Grubb RL 3rd, et al. Mortality results from a randomized prostate-cancer screening trial. *N Engl J Med* 2009;360(13):1310–1319.
27. Schröder FH, Hugosson J, Roobol MJ, et al. Screening and prostate-cancer mortality in a randomized European study. *N Engl J Med* 2009;360(13):1320–1328.
28. Andriole G, Crawford D, Grubb R, et al. Prostate cancer screening in the randomized Prostate, Lung, Colorectal, and Ovarian Cancer Screening Trial: mortality results after 13 years of follow-up. *J Natl Cancer Inst* 2012;104: 125–132.
29. Thompson I, Goodman P, Tangen C, et al. Long-term survival of participants in the prostate cancer prevention trial. *N Engl J Med* 2013;369:603–610.
30. International Agency for Cancer Research. *Weight Control and Physical Activity. Handbook 6.* Lyon, France: IARC Press; 2002.
31. Sedjo R, Byers T, Barrera E, et al. A midpoint assessment of the American Cancer Society challenge goal to decrease cancer incidence by 25% between 1992 and 2015. *CA Cancer J Clin* 2007;57:326–340.
32. Byers T, Barrera E, Fontham E, et al. A midpoint assessment of the American Cancer Society challenge goal to halve the U.S. cancer mortality rates between the years 1990 and 2015. *Cancer* 2006;107:396–405.
33. Byers T, Mouchawar J, Marks J, et al. The American Cancer Society challenge goals. How far can cancer rates decline in the U.S. by the year 2015? *Cancer* 1999;86:715–727.

PART III

Cancer Therapeutics

13 Essentials of Radiation Therapy

Meredith A. Morgan, Randall K. Ten Haken, and Theodore S. Lawrence

INTRODUCTION

The beneficial use of radiation was launched by the experiments of Wilhelm Roentgen, who, in 1895, found that x-rays could pass through materials that were impenetrable to light. Emil Grubbe provided one of the early examples of the therapeutic use of radiation by treating an advanced ulcerated breast cancer with x-rays in January 1896. We have made great progress since these early days, which has been strongly influenced by research in radiation chemistry, biology, and physics.

BIOLOGIC ASPECTS OF RADIATION ONCOLOGY

Radiation-Induced DNA Damage

Radiation is administered to cells either in the form of photons (x-rays and gamma rays) or particles (protons, neutrons, and electrons). When photons or particles interact with biologic material, they cause ionizations that can either directly interact with subcellular structures or they can interact with water, the major constituent of cells, and generate free radicals that can then interact with subcellular structures (Fig. 13.1).

The direct effects of radiation are the consequence of the DNA in chromosomes absorbing energy that leads to ionizations. This is the major mechanism of DNA damage induced by charged nuclei (such as a carbon nucleus) and neutrons and is termed *high linear energy transfer* (Fig. 13.2). In contrast, the interaction of photons with other molecules, such as water, results in the production of free radicals, some of which possess a lifetime long enough to be able to diffuse to the nucleus and interact with DNA in the chromosomes. This is the major mechanism of DNA damage induced by x-rays and has been termed *low linear energy transfer*.[1]

A free radical generated through the interaction of photons with other molecules that possess an unpaired electron in their outermost shell (e.g., hydroxyl radicals) can abstract a hydrogen molecule from a macromolecule such as DNA to generate damage. Cells that have increased levels of free radical scavengers, such as glutathione, would have less DNA damage induced by x-rays, but would have similar levels of DNA damage induced by a carbon nucleus that is directly absorbed by chromosomal DNA. Furthermore, a low oxygen environment would also protect cells from x-ray–induced damage because there would be fewer radicals available to induce DNA damage in the absence of oxygen, but this environment would have little impact on DNA damage induced by carbon nuclei.[2]

Cellular Responses to Radiation-Induced DNA Damage

Checkpoint Pathways

The cell cycle must progress in a specific order; checkpoint genes ensure that the initiation of late events is delayed until earlier events are complete. There are three principal places in the cell cycle at which checkpoints induced by DNA damage function: the border between G1 phase and S phase, intra-S phase, and the border between G2 phase and mitosis (Fig. 13.3). Cells with an intact checkpoint function that have sustained DNA damage stop progressing through the cycle and become arrested at the next checkpoint in the cell cycle. For example, cells with damaged DNA in G1 phase avoid replicating that damage by arresting at the G1/S interface. If irradiated cells have already passed the restriction point, a position in G1 phase that is regulated by the phosphorylation of the retinoblastoma tumor suppressor gene (*Rb*) and its dissociation from the E2F family of transcription factors, they will transiently arrest in S phase. The G1/S and intra-S phase checkpoints inhibit the replication of damaged DNA and work in a coordinated manner with the DNA repair machinery to permit the restitution of DNA integrity, thereby increasing cell survival.

The earliest response to radiation is the activation of ataxia-telangiectasia mutated (ATM), which involves a conformational change that results in the activation of its kinase domain and phosphorylation of serine 1981 (see Fig. 13.3).[3] This phosphorylation causes the ATM homodimer to dissociate into active monomers that phosphorylate a wide range of proteins such as 53BP1, the histone variant H2AX, Nbs1 (Nijmegen breakage syndrome; a member of the *MRN complex*, composed of Mre11, Rad50, and Nbs1), BRCA1, and SMC1 (structural maintenance of chromosomes), and these proteins coordinate repair with the cell cycle.[4] In response to DNA damage, H2AX is rapidly phosphorylated by ATM and localizes to sites of DNA double-strand breaks in multiprotein complexes described as foci (Fig. 13.4). Phosphorylation of H2AX by ATM results in the direct recruitment of Mdc1 and forms a complex with H2AX to recruit additional ATM molecules, forming a positive feedback loop.

The G1/S phase checkpoint is the best understood. In response to DNA damage, activated ATM can directly phosphorylate p53 and mdm2, the ubiquitin ligase that targets p53 for degradation. These phosphorylations are important for increasing the stability of the p53 protein. In addition to ATM, checkpoint kinase 2 (Chk2) also phosphorylates p53 and can enhance p53 stability. Activated p53 transcriptionally increases the expression of the $p21^{WAF1/CIP1}$ gene, which results in a sustained inhibition of G1 cyclin/Cdk, and prevents phosphorylation of pRb and progression from G1 into S.[5] Mutations in p53 that are commonly found in solid tumors result in loss of transcriptional activity and compromised checkpoint function.

Control of the S-phase checkpoint is mediated in part by the Cdc25A phosphatase inhibiting Cdk2 activity and the loading of Cdc45 onto chromatin. If Cdc45 fails to bind to chromatin, DNA polymerase α is not recruited to replication origins and replicon initiation fails to occur.[6] A more prominent mechanism for S-phase arrest is signaled through the MRN complex and the cohesin protein SMC1 by ATM.[7] Loss of ATM, MRN components, or SMC1 leads to the loss of the intra-S phase checkpoint function and increased radiosensitivity. Both the CDC45 and ATM pathways represent parallel, but seemingly independent, pathways to protect replication forks from trying to replicate through DNA strand

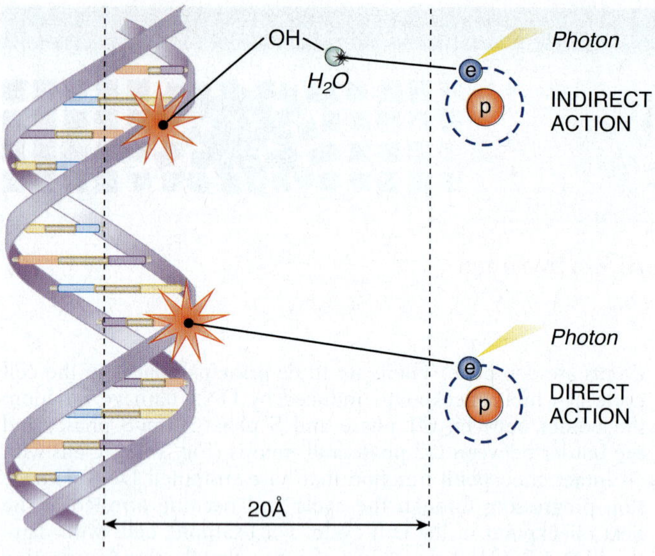

Figure 13.1 The direct and indirect effects of ionizing radiation on DNA. Incident photons transfer part of their energy to free electrons (Compton scattering). These electrons can directly interact with DNA to induce DNA damage, or they can first interact with water to produce hydroxyl radicals that can then induce damage.

breaks. Although ATM has received the lion's share of attention in signaling checkpoint activation in response to ionizing radiation, its family member ATR (ataxia telangiectasia and rad3-related) also plays a role in S-phase checkpoint responses.[8] ATM kinase activity is inducible by radiation, whereas ATR kinase activity is constitutive and does not significantly change with irradiation. (ATR is described in more detail in Chapter 19.) In contrast to Cdc45 and ATM, ATR is probably more important in monitoring

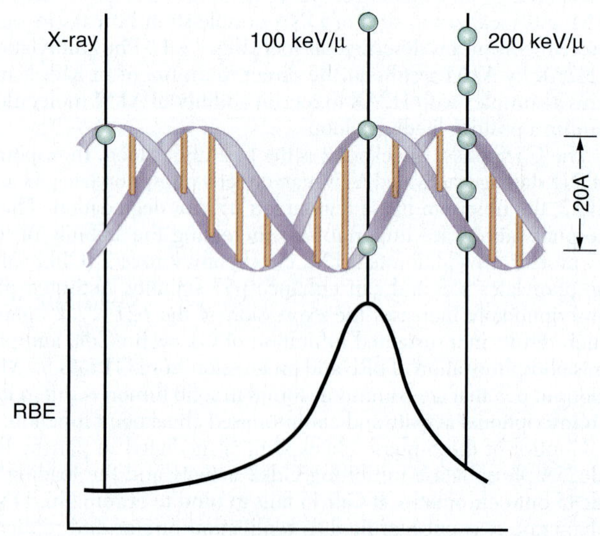

Figure 13.2 Linear energy transfer and DNA damage. Ionizing radiation deposits energy along the track (linear energy transfer [LET]), which causes DNA damage and cell killing. The most biologically potent (highest relative biologic effectiveness [RBE]) LET is 100 keV per μm because the separation between ionizing events is the same as the diameter of the DNA double helix (2 nm). (From Hall EJ, Giaccia AJ. *Radiobiology for the Radiologist*. Philadelphia: Lippincott Williams & Williams; 2012, with permission.)

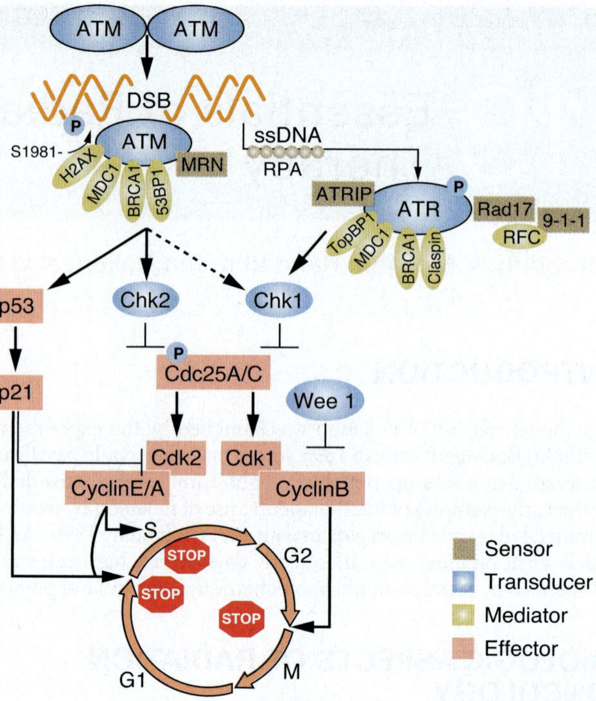

Figure 13.3 In response to DNA damage, the MRN complex—composed of MRE11, Rad50, and NBS1—together with ataxia-telangiectasia mutation (ATM) and H2AX are the earliest proteins recruited to the site of the break. ATM is released from its homodimer complex, activated by transautophosphorylation and, in turn, phosphorylates H2AX. Other members are recruited to the complex such as BRCA1 and 53BP1. As the DNA at the double-strand break (DSB) is resected, single-stranded DNA is formed and bound by replication protein A (RPA), resulting in the activation of the ataxia-telangiectasia and Rad3-related (ATR) pathway. The net result of ATM/ATR activation is the downstream activation of p53, leading to the transcription of the Cdk inhibitor, p21, and the activation of Chk1/Chk2, resulting in the degradation of Cdc25 phosphatases, Cdk-cyclin complex inactivation, and cell cycle arrest at phase G1, intra S, or G2. Note that ATM is also partially activated by changes in chromatin structure induced by DNA double-strand breaks.

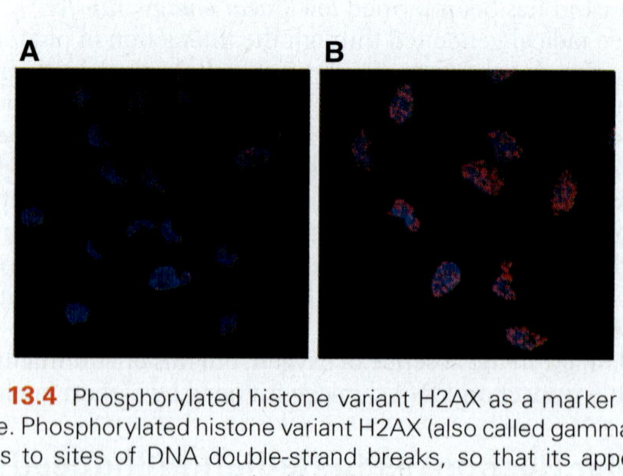

Figure 13.4 Phosphorylated histone variant H2AX as a marker of DNA damage. Phosphorylated histone variant H2AX (also called gamma H2AX) localizes to sites of DNA double-strand breaks, so that its appearance and disappearance correspond with induction and repair of breaks. The cells in panels **A** and **B** have been stained with DAPI (4′,6-diamidino-2-phenylindole) (*blue*) in order to visualize cell nuclei and stained with an antibody, which recognizes *gamma* H2AX (*red*). The cells in **A** are untreated and exhibit little to no gamma H2AX staining, whereas the cells in **B** are treated with 7.5 Gy radiation and exhibit strong gamma H2AX staining at punctate foci in the nuclei, which are thought to correlate with sites of DNA double-strand breaks. (Image provided by Dr. Leslie Parsels, University of Michigan.)

perturbations in replication that are the result of stalled replication forks to prevent the formation of DNA double-strand breaks.

The arrest of cells in the G2 phase following DNA damage is one of the most conserved evolutionary responses to ionizing radiation. It makes sense to have a final checkpoint in the G2 phase to prevent cells from entering into mitosis with damaged DNA that could be transmitted to their progeny. It follows that cells lacking the G2 checkpoint are radiosensitive because they try to divide with damaged chromosomes that cannot be aligned at metaphase to be properly apportioned to daughter cells. At the biochemical level, the regulation of the mitosis-promoting factor cyclin B/Cdk1 is the critical step in the activation of this checkpoint. At the molecular level, ATM and Chk1/2 are activated by DNA damage in the G2 phase and inhibit the activation of Cdc25A and C phosphatases, which are essential for the activation of cyclin B/Cdk1.[9,10] The pololike kinase family (Plk1 and Plk3) also responds to DNA damage and can inhibit Cdc25C activation.[11] A great deal of effort has been focused on the development of small molecules to inhibit checkpoint response proteins, such as Chk1, with the idea that they would inhibit radiation-induced G2 arrest and perhaps repair and thus be used as radiation sensitizers.[12]

DNA Repair

Ionizing radiation causes base damage, single-strand breaks, double-strand breaks, and sugar damage, as well as DNA–DNA, and DNA–protein cross-links. The critical target for ionizing radiation-induced cell inactivation and cell killing is the DNA double-strand break.[13,14] In eukaryotic cells, DNA double-strand breaks can be repaired by two processes: homologous recombination repair (HRR), which requires an undamaged DNA strand as a participant in the repair, and nonhomologous end joining (NHEJ), which mediates end-to-end joining.[15] In lower eukaryotes, such as yeast, HRR is the predominant pathway used for repairing DNA double-strand breaks, whereas mammalian cells use both HHR and non-HHR to repair their DNA. In mammalian cells, the choice of repair is biased by the phase of the cell cycle and by the abundance of repetitive DNA. HRR is used primarily in the late S phase/G2 phases of the cell-cycle, and NHEJ predominates in the G1-phase of the cell cycle (Fig. 13.5). NHEJ and HRR are not mutually exclusive, and both have been found to be active in the late S/G2 phase of the cell cycle, indicating that factors in addition to the cell-cycle phase are important in determining which mechanism will be used to repair DNA strand breaks.

Nonhomologous End Joining. In the G1-phase of the cell cycle, the ligation of DNA double-strand breaks is primarily through NHEJ because a sister chromatid does not exist to provide a template for HRR. The damaged ends of DNA double-strand breaks must first be modified before rejoining. The process of NHEJ can be divided into at least four steps: synapsis, end processing, fill-in synthesis, and ligation (Fig. 13.6).[16] Synapsis is the critical initial step where the Ku heterodimer and the DNA-dependent protein kinase catalytic subunit (DNA-PKcs) bind to the ends of the DNA double-strand break. Ku recruits not only DNA-PKcs to

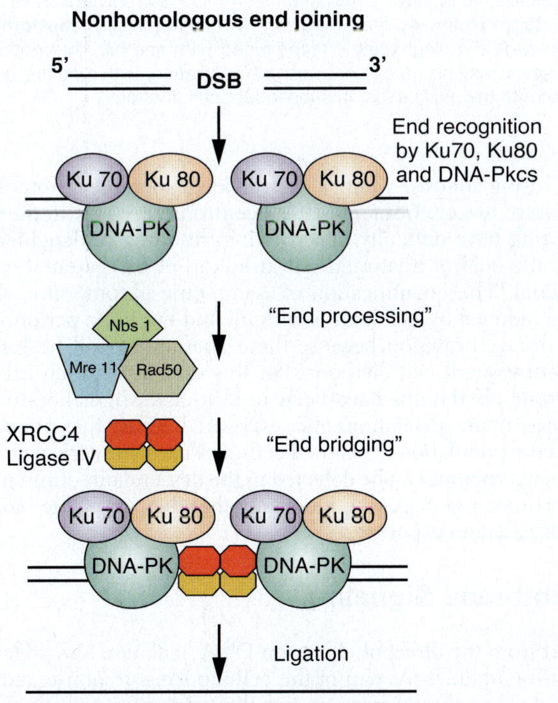

Figure 13.5 Schematic of the critical steps and proteins involved in nonhomologous end joining (NHEJ). The process of NHEJ can be divided into at least four steps: synapsis, end processing, fill-in synthesis, and ligation. DSB, double-strand break.

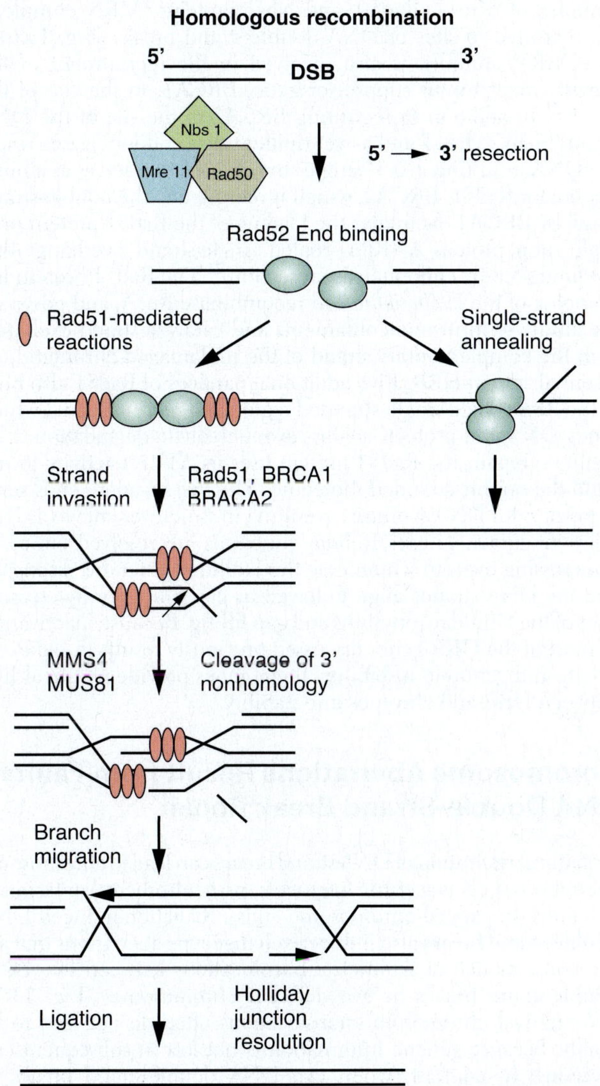

Figure 13.6 Schematic of the critical steps and proteins involved in homologous recombination repair (HRR). The process of HRR can be divided into the following steps: double-strand break (DSB) targeting by H2AX and the MRN complex, recruitment of the ataxia-telangiectasia mutation (ATM) kinase, end processing and protection, strand exchange, single-strand gap filling, and resolution into unique double-stranded molecules.

the DNA ends, but also artemis, a protein that possesses endonuclease activity for 5′ and 3′ overhangs as well as hairpins.[17] DNA-PKcs that is bound to the broken DNA ends phosphorylates artemis and activates its endonuclease activity for end processing. This role of artemis' endonuclease activity in NHEJ may not necessarily be required for the ligation of blunt ends or ends with compatible termini. DNA polymerase μ is associated with the Ku/DNA/XRCC4/DNA ligase IV complex, and is probably the polymerase that is used in the fill-in reaction. The actual rejoining of DNA ends is mediated by a XRCC4/DNA ligase IV complex, which is also probably recruited by the Ku heterodimer.[18,19] Although NHEJ is effective at rejoining DNA double-strand breaks, it is highly error prone. In fact, the main physiologic role of NHEJ is to generate antibodies through V(D)J rejoining, and the error-prone nature of NHEJ is essential for generating antibody diversity.

Homologous Recombination. HRR provides the mammalian genome a high-fidelity pathway of repairing DNA double-strand breaks. In contrast to NHEJ, HRR requires physical contact with an undamaged DNA template, such as a sister chromatid, for repair to occur. In response to a double-strand break, ATM as well as the complex of Mre11, Rad50, and Nbs1 proteins (MRN complex), are recruited to sites of DNA double-strand breaks (Fig. 13.6).[20] The MRN complex is also involved in the recruitment of the breast cancer tumor suppressor gene, *BRCA1*, to the site of the break.[21] In addition to recruiting *BRCA1* to the site of the DNA strand break, Mre11 and as yet unidentified endonucleases resect the DNA, resulting in a 3′ single-strand DNA that serves as a binding site for Rad51. *BRCA2*, which is recruited to the double-strand break by BRCA1, facilitates the loading of the Rad51 protein onto replication protein A (RPA)-coated single-strand overhangs that are produced by endonuclease resection.[22] The Rad51 protein is a homolog of the *Escherichia coli* recombinase RecA, and possesses the ability to form nucleofilaments and catalyze strand exchange with the complementary strand of the undamaged chromatid, an essential step in HRR. Five additional paralogs of Rad51 also bind to the RPA-coated single-stranded region and recruit Rad52, which binds DNA and protects against exonucleolytic degradation.[23] To facilitate repair, the Rad54 protein uses its ATPase activity to unwind the double-stranded molecule. The two invading ends serve as primers for DNA synthesis, resulting in structures known as Holliday junctions. These Holliday junctions are resolved either by noncrossing over, in which case the Holliday junctions disengage and the DNA strands align followed by gap filling, or by crossing over of the Holliday junctions and gap filling. Because inactivation of most of the HRR genes discussed previously results in radiosensitivity and genomic instability, these genes provide a critical link between HRR and chromosome stability.

Chromosome Aberrations Result from Faulty DNA Double-Strand Break Repair

Unfaithful restitution of DNA strand breaks can lead to chromosome aberrations such as acentric fragments (no centromeres) or terminal deletions (uncapped chromosome ends). Radiation-induced DNA double-strand breaks also induce exchange-type aberrations that are the consequence of symmetric translocations between two DNA double-strand breaks in two different chromosomes (Fig. 13.7). Symmetrical chromosome translocations often do not lead to lethality, because genetic information is not lost in subsequent cell divisions. In contrast, when two DNA double-strand breaks in two different chromosomes recombine to form one chromosome with two centromeres and two fragments of chromosomes without centromeres or telomeres, cell death is inevitable. These types of chromosome aberrations are the consequence of asymmetrical chromosome translocations where the genetic material is recombined in what has been termed an *illegitimate* manner (e.g., a chromosome containing an extra centromere).

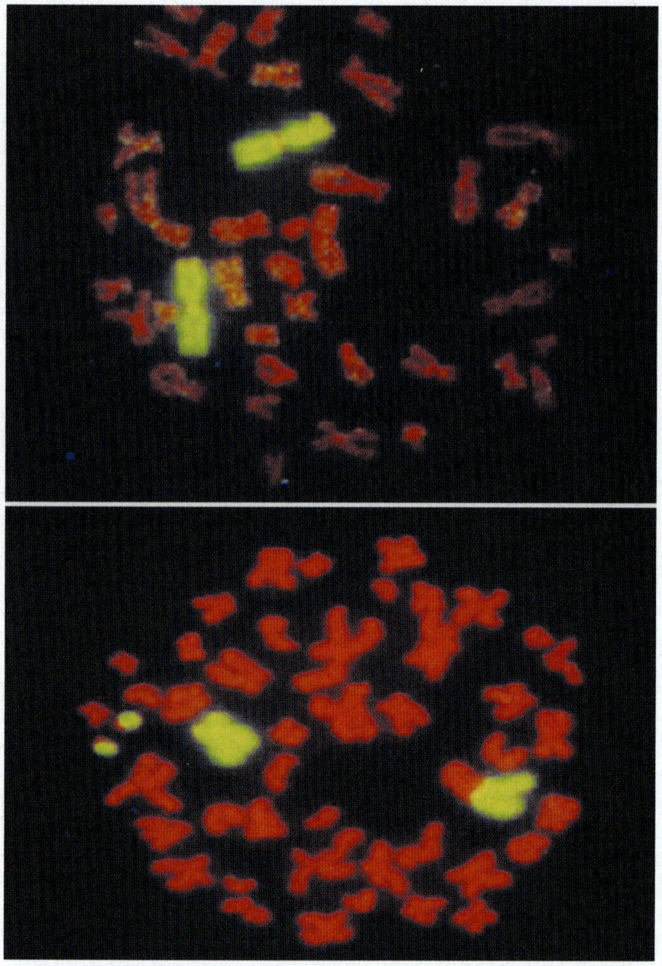

Figure 13.7 Fluorescent in situ hybridization of DNA probes that specifically recognize chromosome 4. In unirradiated cells **(top)**, two chromosome 4s are visualized. In irradiated cells **(bottom)**, one chromosome 4 illegitimately recombined with another chromosome to produce an asymmetrical chromosome aberration, with resulting acentric fragments that will be lost in subsequent cell divisions.

During mitosis, when a cell divides, aberrant chromosomes that have two centromeres, lack a centromere, or are in the shape of a ring have difficulty in separating, resulting in daughter cells with unequal or asymmetric distribution of the parental genetic material. The quantification of asymmetric chromosome aberrations induced by radiation is difficult and has to be performed by the first cell division because these aberrations will be lost during subsequent cell divisions. For this reason, symmetrical chromosome aberrations have been used to assess radiation-induced damage many generations after exposure because they are not lost from the population of exposed cells. In fact, symmetrical chromosome aberrations can be detected in the descendants of survivors of Hiroshima and Nagasaki, indicating that they are stable biomarkers of radiation exposure.[24]

Membrane Signaling

Apart from the direct of effects on DNA, radiation also affects cellular membranes. As part of the cellular stress response, radiation activates membrane receptor signaling pathways such those initiated via epidermal growth factor receptor (EGFR) and transforming growth factor β (TGF-β).[25,26] Activation of these pathways promotes overall survival in response to radiation by promoting DNA damage repair and/or cellular proliferation. In addition,

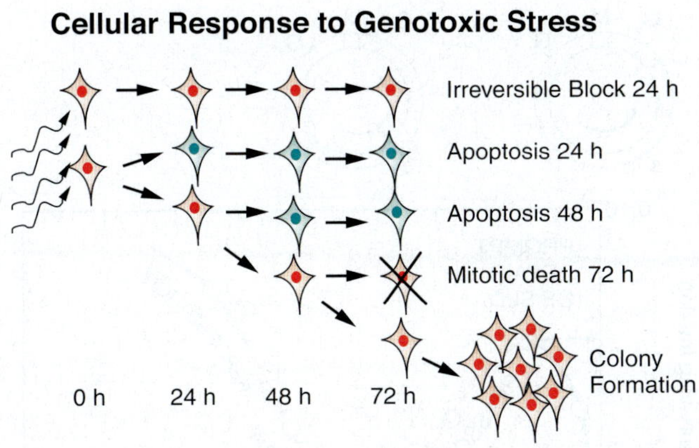

Figure 13.8 Consequences of exposure to ionizing radiation at the cellular level. Cells exposed to ionizing radiation can enter a state of senescence where they are unable to divide, but are still able to secrete growth factors. Alternatively, cells can die through apoptosis, mitotic linked cell death, or they can repair their DNA damage and produce viable progeny.

radiation also induces ceramide production at the membrane via activation of sphingomyelinases, which hydrolyze sphingomyelin to form ceramide. Ceramide production is linked to radiation-induced apoptosis.[27]

The Effect of Radiation on Cell Survival

The major potential consequences of cells exposed to ionizing radiation are normal cell division, DNA damage–induced senescence (reproductively inactive but metabolically active), apoptosis, or mitotic-linked cell death (Fig. 13.8). These manifestations of DNA damage can occur within one or two cell divisions or can manifest at later times after many cell divisions.[28] Effects that occur at later times have been termed *delayed reproductive cell death* and may also be influenced by secreted factors that are induced in response to radiation.[29]

The ability to culture cells derived from both normal and tumor tissues has allowed us to gain insight into how radiosensitivity varies between tissues by analyzing the shape of survival curves. Survival curves of tumor cells often possess a shouldered region at low doses that becomes shallower as the dose increases and eventually becomes exponential. A shoulder on a survival means that these low doses of radiation are less efficient in cell killing, presumably because cells are efficient at repairing DNA strand breaks.[13,14] Killing at low doses of radiation can be described in the form of a linear quadratic equation: $S = e^{-\alpha D-\beta D2}$ (Fig. 13.9).[30] In this equation, S is the fraction of cells that survive a dose (D) of radiation, whereas α and β are constants. Cell killing by the linear and quadratic components are equal when $\alpha D = \beta D^2$ or $D = \alpha/\beta$. Over a larger dose range, the relationship between cell killing and dose is more complex and is described by three different components: an initial slope (D_1), a final slope (D_0), and the width of the shoulder (n, the extrapolation number) or Dq, the quasi-threshold dose (Fig. 13.10). The extrapolation number, n, defines the place where the shoulder intersects the ordinate when the dose is extrapolated to zero, and the quasithreshold dose, Dq, defines the width of the shoulder by cutting the dose axis when there is a survival fraction of unity. In contrast to photons, the shoulder on the survival curve disappears when cells are exposed to densely ionizing radiation from particles, indicating that this form of radiation is highly effective at killing cells at both low and high doses.

In Vivo Survival Determination of Normal Tissue Response to Radiation

Although much of our knowledge on the effects of radiation on cell survival has come from cell culture studies, investigators have also devised experimental approaches to assess the clonogenic survival of normal tissues. The earliest example came from McCulloch and Till,[31] who developed an assay to measure the

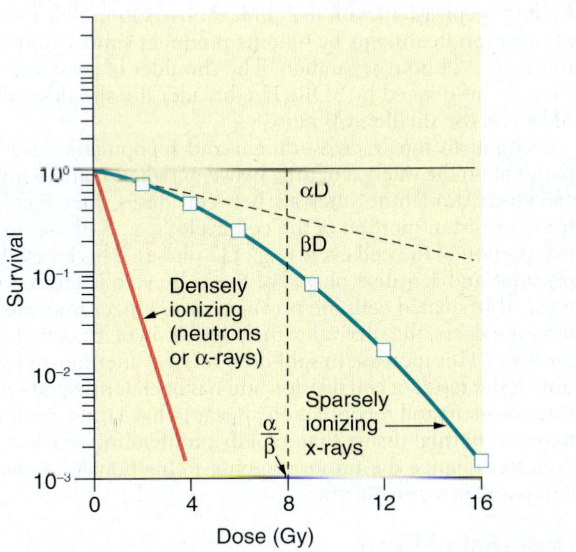

Figure 13.9 An analysis of survival curves for mammalian cells exposed to radiation by the linear quadratic model. The probability of hitting a critical target is proportional to dose (aD): the alpha component. The probability of hitting two critical targets will be the product of those probabilities; therefore, it will be proportional to dose^2 (βD^2): the beta component. The dose at which killing by both the alpha and beta components is equal is defined as $D = \alpha/\beta$. (From Hall EJ, Giaccia AJ. *Radiobiology for the Radiologist*. Philadelphia: Lippincott Williams & Williams; 2012, with permission.)

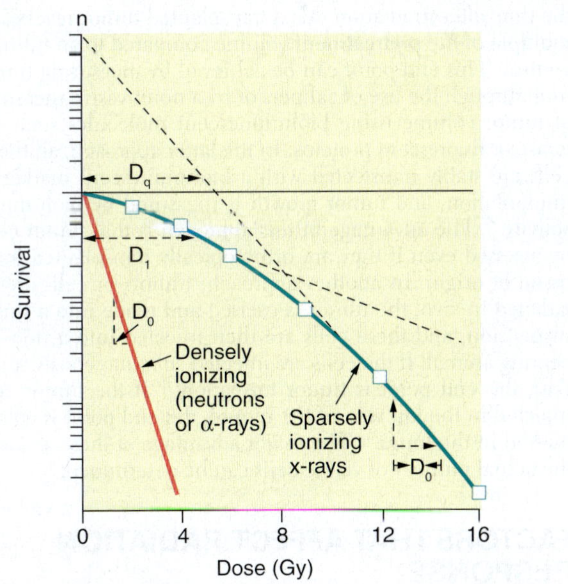

Figure 13.10 An analysis of survival curves for mammalian cells exposed to radiation by the multitarget model. This survival is described by an initial slope (D_1; dose to decreased survival to 37% on initial portion of the curve), a final slope (D_0; dose to decrease survival from starting point to 37% of that point on straight line portion of the curve), an extrapolation number (n; an estimate of the width of the shoulder), and a quasithreshold (D_q; a type of threshold dose below which radiation has no effect). (From Hall EJ, Giaccia AJ. *Radiobiology for the Radiologist*. Philadelphia: Lippincott Williams & Williams; 2012, with permission.)

clonogenic survival of bone marrow–derived cells in response to radiation by injecting them into a recipient mouse and quantifying the number of colonies that developed in the spleen. An analysis of these in vivo spleen assays indicated that bone marrow cells are highly radiosensitive (perhaps the most radiosensitive of all mammalian cells) in that their cell survival curve lacked a shoulder. These experiments represent two important firsts in the radiation sciences: They described the first development of an in vivo assay to assess normal tissue survival to radiation, and they demonstrated the first existence of normal tissue stem cells. Soon after, Withers and colleagues[32] developed an assay to assess the survival of skin stem cells, and Withers and Elkind[33] developed an assay to quantify the viability of small intestinal clonogens.

Because these ingenious approaches cannot be applied to all normal tissues, loss of tissue function instead of clonogenic survival has been used as an end point to assess radiation effects. Effects on tissue function can be grouped into the acute or late variety. Desquamation of skin by radiation is an example of an acute loss of function, whereas loss of spinal cord function is an example of a late functional effect. Acutely sensitive tissues such as skin, bone marrow, and intestinal mucosa possess a significant component of tissue cell division, whereas delayed sensitive tissues, such as spinal cord, breast, and bone, do not possess a significant amount of cell division or turnover and manifest radiation effects at later times.

In Vivo Determination of Tumor Response to Radiation

Assays have also been developed to assess the clonogenic survival of tumor cells in animals. Perhaps the most relevant of these assays is the tumor control dose 50% (TCD_{50}) assay,[34] in which the dose of radiation needed to control the growth of 50% of the tumors is determined in large cohorts of tumor-bearing animals. The TCD_{50} assay in animals most closely approximates the clinical situation because tumors are irradiated in animals and the ability to kill all viable tumor cells is assessed. Unlike assays in which tumor cells are irradiated ex vivo, the TCD_{50} assay takes into account the effects of the tumor microenvironment on tumor response. In contrast to the TCD_{50} assay, the tumor growth delay assay reflects the time after irradiation that a transplanted tumor reaches a fixed multiple of the pretreatment volume compared to an unirradiated control. This end point can be achieved by measuring tumor volume through the use of calipers or by a noninvasive measurement of tumor volume using bioluminescent molecules such as luciferase or fluorescent proteins. In the latter approach, all the tumor cells are stably transfected with a bioluminescent marker before implantation, and tumor growth is measured by bioluminescent activity.[35] The advantage of this approach is that tumor cells can be assessed even if they are orthotopically transplanted into their tissue of origin. In another approach, tumors or cells are first irradiated in vivo, the tumor is excised and made into a single-cell suspension, and these cells are then injected into a non–tumor-bearing animal. If the cells are injected subcutaneously under the skin, the end point is tumor formation.[36] If the tumor cells are injected in the tail vein of the mouse, the end point is colony formation in the lungs.[37] The major advantage of these assays is that the actual number of viable cells can be determined.

FACTORS THAT AFFECT RADIATION RESPONSE

The Fundamental Principles of Radiobiology

Studies on split-dose repair (SDR) by Elkind et al.[38] uncovered three of what we now recognize as the most fundamental principles of fractionated radiotherapy: repair, reassortment, and repopulation (Fig. 13.11). (Reoxygenation, described in the following paragraphs, is the fourth). SDR describes the increased survival

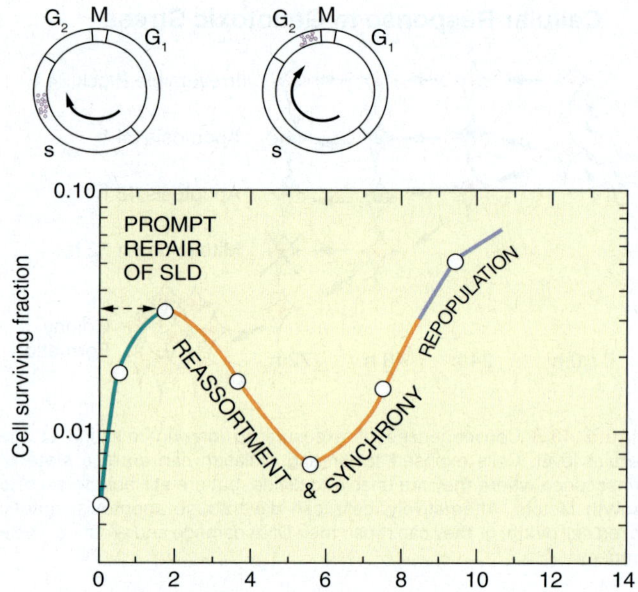

Figure 13.11 Idealized survival curve of rodent cells exposed to two fractions of x-rays. This figure illustrates how the time interval between doses alters the sensitivity of cells when exposed to multiple fractions. In this case, cells move from a resistant phase of the cell cycle (late S phase) to a sensitive phase of the cell cycle (G2 phase). This is known as *reassortment.* If longer periods of time occur between fractions of radiation, cells will undergo division. This latter process is called *repopulation.* SLD, sublethal damage. (From Hall EJ, Giaccia AJ. *Radiobiology for the Radiologist*. Philadelphia: Lippincott Williams & Williams; 2012, with permission.)

or tumor growth delay found if a dose of radiation is split into two fractions compared to the same dose administered in one fraction. This repair is likely due to DNA double-strand break rejoining. Elkind et al. found that the survival of cells increased with an increase in time between doses for up to a maximum of about 6 hours. This finding is consistent with the clinical observation that a separation of radiation treatments by 6 hours produces similar normal tissue injury as a 24-hour separation. The shoulder of a survival curve is strongly influenced by SDR: The broader the shoulder, the more SDR and the smaller α/β ratio.

Similar to repair, reassortment and repopulation are also dependent on the interval of time between radiation fractions. If cells are given short time intervals between doses, they can progress from a resistant portion of the cell cycle (e.g., S phase) to a sensitive portion of the cell cycle (e.g., G2 phase). This transit between resistant and sensitive phases of the cell cycle is termed *reassortment.* If irradiated cells are provided even longer intervals of time between doses, the survival of the population of irradiated cells will increase. This increase in split-dose survival after longer periods of time is the result of cell division and has been termed *repopulation.* Reassortment and repopulation appear to have more protracted kinetics in normal tissues than rapidly proliferating tumor cells, and thereby enhance the tumor response to fractionated radiotherapy compared to normal tissues.

Dose-Rate Effects

For sparsely ionizing radiation, dose rate plays a critical factor in cell killing. Lowering the dose rate, and thereby increasing exposure time, reduces the effectiveness of killing by x-rays because of increased SDR. A further reduction in dose rate results in more SDR and reduces the shoulder of the survival curve. Thus, if one plots the survival for individual doses in a multifraction experiment so that there is sufficient time for SDR to occur, the resulting survival curve would have little shoulder and appear almost linear.[39]

In some cell types, there is a threshold to the lowering of dose rate, and in fact, one paradoxically finds an increase, instead of a decrease, in cell killing. This increase in cell killing under these conditions of protracted dose rate is due to the accumulation of cells in a radiosensitive portion of the cell cycle. In summary, the magnitude of the dose rate effect varies between cell types because of SDR, the redistribution of cells through the cell cycle, and the time for cell division to occur.

Cell Cycle

The phase of the cell cycle at the time of radiation influences the cell's inherent sensitivity to radiation. Cells synchronized in late G1/early S and G2/M phases are most sensitive, whereas cells in G1 and mid to late S phase are more resistant to radiation.[1] These differences in sensitivity during the cell cycle are exploited by the concept of reassortment during fractioned radiotherapy as well by the use of chemotherapeutic agents, which reassort cells into more sensitive phases of the cell cycle in combination with radiation.

Tumor Oxygenation

The major microenvironmental influence on tumor response to radiation is molecular oxygen.[40] Decreased levels of oxygen (hypoxia) in tissue culture result in decreased killing after radiation, which can be expressed as an *oxygen enhancement ratio* (OER). Operationally, OER is defined as the ratio of doses to give the same killing under hypoxic and normoxic conditions. At high doses of radiation, the OER is approximately 3, whereas at low doses, it is closer to 2.[41] Oxygen must be present within 10 μs of irradiation to achieve its radiosensitizing effect. Under hypoxic conditions, damage to DNA can be repaired more readily than under oxic conditions, where damage to DNA is "fixed" because of the interaction of oxygen with free radicals generated by radiation. These changes in radiation sensitivity are detectable at oxygen ranges below 30 mm Hg. Most tumor cells exhibit a survival difference halfway between fully aerobic and fully anoxic cells when exposed to a partial pressure of oxygen between 3 and 10 mm Hg.[1] The presence of hypoxia has greater significance for single-dose fractions used in the treatment of certain primary tumors and metastases and is less important for fractionated radiotherapy, where reoxygenation occurs between fractions. Furthermore, most hypoxic cells are not actively undergoing cell division, thus impeding the efficacy of conventional chemotherapeutic agents that are targeted to actively dividing cells.

Although normal tissue and tumors vary in their oxygen concentrations, only tumors possess levels of oxygen low enough to influence the effectiveness of radiation killing. Although the variations in normal tissue oxygenation are in large part due to physiology governing acute changes in oxygen consumption, the variations in tumor oxygen can be directly attributed to abnormal vasculature that results in a more chronic condition. Thomlinson and Gray[42] observed that variations in tumor oxygen occur because there is insufficient vasculature to provide oxygen to all tumor cells. They hypothesized that oxygen is unable to reach tumor cells beyond 10 to 12 cell diameters from the lumen of a tumor blood vessel because of metabolic consumption by respiring tumor cells. This form of hypoxia caused by metabolic consumption of oxygen has been termed *chronic* or *diffusion-mediated hypoxia*. In contrast, changes in blood flow due either to interstitial pressure changes in tumor blood vessels that lack a smooth muscle component or red blood cell fluxes can cause transient occlusion of blood vessels resulting in *acute* or *transient hypoxia*. Chronically, hypoxic cells will only become reoxygenated when their distance from the lumen of a blood vessel decreases, such as during fractionated radiotherapy when tumor cords shrink. In contrast, tumor cells that are acutely hypoxic because of changes in blood flow or interstitial pressure often cycle in an unpredictable manner between oxic and hypoxic states as blood flow changes.

Based on studies demonstrating that hypoxia can alter radiation sensitivity and decrease tumor control by radiotherapy, strategies have been developed to increase tumor oxygenation. Most importantly, it appears that tumor oxygen levels increase during a course of fractionated radiation. This may be one of the most important benefits of fractionated radiation and is termed *reoxygenation* (the fourth of the four Rs of radiobiology). Tumor reoxygenation during a course of fractionated radiation may also offer an explanation for the general lack of clinical efficacy of hypoxic cell sensitizers despite the clear evidence that hypoxia causes radioresistance.

Aside from using fractionated radiation, the most direct approach to increasing tumor oxygenation is to expose patients receiving radiotherapy to hyperbaric oxygen therapy. The underlying concept is that increasing the amount of oxygen in the bloodstream should result in more oxygen being available for diffusion to the hypoxic regions of tumors. Experimentally, hyperbaric oxygen therapy increases the sensitivity of transplanted tumors to radiation. The results of clinical studies with hyperbaric oxygen therapy, when combined with radiotherapy, showed improvement for two sites—head and neck cancers, and cervix cancers—but failed to show an improvement with other sites, thus calling into question its general usefulness in radiotherapy.[43] In a related approach, erythropoietin (EPO), a hormone released by the kidney that increases red blood cell production, should also increase tumor oxygenation by increasing the delivery of hemoglobin-bound oxygen molecules. EPO has been effective at correcting anemia, but has not been successful in combination with radiation to control head and neck cancer and may, in fact, stimulate tumor growth.[44,45]

Another strategy to increase tumor oxygenation has been the combined use of nicotinamide, which increases tissue perfusion and carbogen (95% O_2 and 5% CO_2) breathing (accelerated radiotherapy with carbogen and nicotinamide [ARCON] therapy). Recently, a randomized phase III clinical trial demonstrated improved regional but not local tumor control in larynx cancer patients treated with nicotinamide, carbogen, and radiation versus radiation alone.[46] Biologics such as antivascular endothelial growth factor (anti-VEGF) therapy have also been demonstrated to increase tumor oxygenation.[47] Anti-VEGF therapy may increase tumor oxygenation by eliminating abnormal vessels that are inadequate in perfusing tumor cells—the so-called *vascular normalization hypothesis*. Although there is solid experimental evidence to support this hypothesis, there appears to be only a short window of time in which it could be effectively combined with radiotherapy.

Because the presence of hypoxia has both prognostic and potential therapeutic implications, a substantial effort has been invested in trying to image hypoxia.[48] The goal of using imaging to "paint" radiation doses to different regions of tumors, although technically possible (as described in the next section, Radiation Physics), faces the problem that changes in oxygenation are dynamic.[49] In the future, hypoxia-directed treatment may evolve from the use of hypoxic cell cytotoxins to targeted drugs that exploit cellular signaling changes induced by hypoxia such as hypoxia-inducible factor 1α (HIF-1α). However, despite the strong rationale supporting their use, at this time, there are no agents used in the clinic that target hypoxia.

Immune Response

The abscopal effects of radiation (i.e., tumor cell killing outside of the radiation field) have been attributed to the activation of antigen and cytokine release by radiation, which subsequently activates a systemic immune response against tumor cells.[50,51] This response begins with the transfer of tumor cell antigens to dendritic cells and, subsequently, the activation of tumor-specific T cells and *immunogenic tumor cell death*. It is likely that radiation dose and fractionation influence the optimal immune response with higher doses and fewer fractions of radiation than those used in conventional fractionation schemes appearing superior in experimental models. Unfortunately, abscopal effects are uncommon because immune system evasion is an inherent characteristic of cancer cells that often dominates, even in the presence of a radiation-induced immune response. Strategies to amplify radiation-induced immune responses, and thus to overcome tumor cell evasion of the immune system, are under investigation. The combination of radiation with immune *checkpoint* modulators such as ipilimumab, an antibody against cytotoxic T-lymphocyte antigen 4 (CTLA-4), have shown promising, albeit anecdotal, clinical effects.

DRUGS THAT AFFECT RADIATION SENSITIVITY

For over 30 years now, chemotherapy and radiotherapy have been administered concurrently. In order to maximize the efficacy of radiochemotherapy, it is necessary to understand the biologic mechanisms underlying radiosensitization by chemotherapeutic agents. The several classes of standard chemotherapeutic agents as well as novel molecularly targeted agents that possess radiosensitizing properties will be discussed in this section.

Antimetabolites

5-fluorouracil is among the most commonly used chemotherapeutic radiation sensitizers. Given in combination with radiation, it has led to clinical improvements in a variety of cancers, including those of the head and neck, the esophagus, the stomach, the pancreas, the rectum, the anus, and the cervix. The combination of 5-fluorouracil with radiation is now a standard therapy for cancers of the stomach (adjuvant), the pancreas (unresectable), and the rectum. For other cancers such as head and neck, esophagus, or anal, 5-fluorouracil and radiation are combined with cisplatin or mitomycin C, respectively. Being an analog of uracil, 5-flourouracil is misincorporated into RNA and DNA. However, the ability of 5-fluorouracil to radiosensitize is related to its ability to inhibit thymidylate synthase, which leads to the depletion of thymidine triphosphate (dTTP) and the inhibition of DNA synthesis. This slowed, inappropriate progression through S phase in response to 5-fluorouracil is thought to be the mechanism underlying radiosensitization.[52] Similar to 5-fluorouracil, the oral thymidylate synthase inhibitor, capecitabine, is also being increasingly used in combination with radiation.

Gemcitabine (2′, 2′-deoxyfluorocytdine [dFdCyd]) is another potent antimetabolite radiosensitizer. Preclinical studies have demonstrated that radiosensitization by gemcitabine involves the depletion of deoxyadenosine triphosphate (dATP) (related to the ability of gemcitabine diphosphate (dFdCDP) to inhibit ribonucleotide reductase) as well as the redistribution of cells into the early S phase of the cell cycle.[53] The combination of gemcitabine with radiation in clinical trials has suggested improved clinical outcomes for patients with cancers of the lung, pancreas, and bladder. Gemcitabine-based chemoradiation has developed into a standard therapy for locally advanced pancreatic cancer. However, in some clinical trials, such as those in lung and head and neck cancers, the combination of gemcitabine with radiation has led to increased mucositis and esophagitis.[54] Thus, it should be emphasized that in the presence of gemcitabine, radiation fields must be defined with great caution. Such is the case with pancreatic cancer, where the combination of full-dose gemcitabine with radiation to the gross tumor can be safely administered if clinically uninvolved lymph nodes are excluded.[55] Conversely, the inclusion of the regional lymphatics in the treatment field in combination with full-dose gemcitabine produces unacceptable toxicities.[56]

Platinums and Temozolomide

Cisplatin is likely the most commonly used chemotherapeutic agent in combination with radiation. Although cisplatin was the prototype for several other platinum analogs, carboplatin is also frequently used in combination with radiation. Cisplatin, in combination with radiation, and sometimes in conjunction with a second chemotherapeutic agent, is indicated for cancers of the head and neck, esophagus (with 5-fluorouracil), the lung, the cervix, and the anus. Radiosensitization by cisplatin is related to its ability to cause inter- and intra-strand DNA cross-links. Removal of these cross-links during the repair process results in DNA strand breaks. Although there are multiple theories to explain the mechanism(s) of radiosensitization by cisplatin, two plausible explanations are that cisplatin inhibits the repair (both homologous and nonhomologous) of radiation-induced DNA double-strand breaks and/or increases the number of lethal radiation-induced double-strand breaks.[57]

Temozolomide in combination with radiation is standard therapy for glioblastoma. Temozolomide is an alkylating agent, which forms methyl adducts at the O^6 position of guanine (as well as at N^7 and N^3-guanine) that are subsequently improperly repaired by the mismatch repair pathway. Radiosensitization by temozolomide involves the inhibition of DNA repair and/or an increase in radiation-induced DNA double-strand breaks due to radiation-induced single-strand breaks in proximity to O^6 methyl adducts. Like cisplatin, temozolomide-mediated radiosensitization does not seem to require cell cycle redistribution.

Taxanes

The taxanes, paclitaxel and docetaxel, act to stabilize microtubules resulting in the accumulation of cells in G2/M, the most radiation-sensitive phase of the cell cycle. The radiosensitizing properties of the taxanes are thought to be attributable to the redistribution of cells into G2/M. Paclitaxel, in combination with radiation (and carboplatin), has demonstrated a clinical benefit in the treatment of resectable lung carcinoma.[58]

Molecularly Targeted Agents

Molecularly targeted agents are especially appealing in the context of radiosensitization because they are generally less toxic than standard chemotherapeutic agents and need to be given in multimodality regimens (given their often inadequate efficacy as single agents). The EGFR has been intensely pursued as a target; both antibody and small molecule EGFR inhibitors, such as cetuximab and erlotinib, respectively, have been developed. The head and neck seem to be the most promising tumor sites for the combination of EGFR inhibitors with radiation therapy. Preclinical data have demonstrated that the schedule of administration of EGFR inhibitors with radiation is important; EGFR inhibition before chemoradiation may produce antagonism.[59] In a randomized phase III trial, cetuximab plus radiation produced a significant survival advantage over radiation alone in patients with locally advanced head and neck cancer.[60] In a subsequent trial, however, cetuximab in combination with concurrent, cisplatin-based chemoradiation failed to produce a survival benefit in head and neck cancer patients.[61] The combination of EGFR inhibitor with cisplatin-radiation requires further preclinical investigation.

Although EGFR inhibition, concurrent with radiation, is by far the best established combination of a molecularly targeted agent with radiation, other exciting molecularly targeted agents are being developed as radiation sensitizers. Targeting DNA damage response pathways is one approach to radiosensitization. Recently, agents that abrogate radiation-induced cell cycle checkpoints, such as Wee1 and Chk1 inhibitors, have been shown to radiosensitize tumor cells and are currently in clinical development in combination with chemotherapy, with clinical trials planned in combination with radiation.[62,63] In addition, poly(ADP-ribose) polymerase (PARP) inhibitors have been demonstrated to preclinically induce radiosensitization, and several clinical trials combining PARP inhibitors with radiation therapy are underway.[64]

Other Agents

Although the most common clinically used agents in combination with radiation have been shown to produce significant clinical benefit, as described previously, other agents with different mechanisms of action have been used as radiation sensitizers as well as radiation protectors. The vinca alkaloids, such as vincristine, possess radiosensitizing properties due to their ability to block mitotic spindle assembly and, thus, arrest cells in M phase. Although vincristine is used in combination with radiation to treat medulloblastoma, rhabdomyosarcoma, and brain stem glioma, its use is principally based on its lack of myelosuppressive side effects, which are dose limiting for radiation in these types of tumors, rather than its potential radiosensitizing properties.

Also worth mention in a discussion of modulators of radiation sensitivity are agents designed to radioprotect normal tissues. One such type of drug, amifostine, is a free radical scavenger with some selectivity toward normal tissues that express more alkaline phosphatase than tumor cells, the enzyme of which converts amifostine to a free thiol metabolite. Clinical trials in head and neck as well as lung cancers have shown a reduction in radiation-related toxicities such as xerostomia, mucositis, esophagitis, and pneumonitis, respectively.[65,66] However, further clinical investigations are necessary to conclusively demonstrate a lack of tumor protection and safety in combination with chemoradiotherapy regimens.

RADIATION PHYSICS

Physics of Photon Interactions

Tumors requiring radiation can be found at depths ranging from zero to 10s of centimeters below the skin. The goal of treatment is to deliver sufficient ionizing radiation to the tumor site, which can result in an absorbed dose. This involves both the availability of treatment beams and delivery techniques, and the methods to plan the treatments and ensure their safe delivery. This section will establish the general physical basis for the use of ionizing radiation in the treatment of tumors, briefly describe some of the treatment equipment, indicate physical qualities of the treatment beams themselves, and summarize the treatment planning process. Those who desire more in-depth details are referred to textbooks and other resources dedicated to medical physics and the technologic aspects of radiation oncology.[67] Most patients who are treated with radiation receive high-energy, external-beam photon therapy. Here, *external* indicates that the treatment beam is generated and delivered from outside of the body. High-energy (6 to 20 MV) photon beams (electromagnetic radiation) penetrate tissue, enabling the treatment of deep-seated tumors. Modern equipment generates these beams with sufficient fluence to ensure delivery of therapeutic fractions of dose in short treatment sessions. Other types of particles and beams also exist for use in treating tumors both externally and internally. They are mentioned briefly later. However, as external photon beams dominate the practice (and as common basic physics principles related to delivered dose exist among the modalities), the focus here will be on photon beam generation and interactions in tissue.

As mentioned earlier, ionizing radiation kills cells via both direct and indirect mechanisms. Radiation therapy aims to instigate those ionizations and events in the tumor cells. Photons are massless, uncharged packets of energy that primarily interact with matter via electromagnetic processes. As a consequence of those interactions, an incident photon can become either entirely absorbed (giving up its energy to the ejection of an atomic electron [photoelectric effect]), or create an energetic electron-positron pair (pair production), or scatter off an electron with a reduction in energy and a change in direction and subsequent transfer of parts of its energy to the free electron (Compton scattering). The secondary electrons generated as a consequence of these interactions have residual energy, mass, and, most importantly, electric charge. They slow down in matter through multiple interactions with (primarily) the electrons of atoms, leading to excitation and ionization of those atoms. These ionizations (hence the term *ionizing radiation*) lead to a local absorption of energy (i.e., dose = energy absorbed per unit mass) and the direct and indirect cell killing effects necessary to treat tumors.

Thus, the use of external photon beams for cancer therapy involves a two-step process: interaction (scattering) of the photons, with subsequent dose deposition via the secondary electrons. The probability of photon interactions is energy dependent. Photoelectric interactions dominate at lower photon energies. Whereas these beams are ideal for diagnostic procedures (for their preferential absorption by tissues of differing atomic number, leading to good subject contrast), they are attenuated too quickly in tissues to supply enough interactions to be useful for therapy for any but the most superficial tumors. Pair production interactions dominate at higher photon energies; however, the probability of interacting in tissues for those high-energy photons is so low as to preclude them from general use as well. In the 10s to 100s of kiloelectron volt (keV) to the few megaelectron volt (MeV) photon energy range, Compton scattering dominates. As will be shown, these beams have sufficient penetration and can be generated with sufficient intensity to be useful for tumor treatments, especially when combined in treatment plans that comprise multiple beams entering the patient from different directions but overlapping at the tumor.

It is useful to point out physical scales of reference for external photon beam therapy. A typical megavoltage photon beam may have an average photon energy near 2 MeV. Those photons primarily undergo Compton scattering with a mean free path in tissue of approximately 20 cm. An average Compton interaction results in a secondary electron with a mean energy near 0.5 MeV (and a Compton scattered photon near 1.5 MeV, which likely escapes or scatters elsewhere in the patient). A typical secondary electron of approximately 0.5 MeV will cause excitations and ionizations of atoms as it dissipates its energy over a path length of approximately 2 mm. This could be expected to lead to approximately 10,000 ionizations, or about 5 ionizations per micron of tissue. As can be seen, therapeutic damage to the DNA of cancer cells (2 nm; see Fig. 13.2) will require very many Compton scatterings with statistical interaction among the ionizations resulting from the slowing down of the secondary electrons.

Photon Beam Generation and Treatment Delivery

As previously mentioned, effective external-beam photon treatments require higher energy beams capable of reaching deep-seated tumors with sufficient fluence to make it likely that the dose deposition will kill the tumor cells. To spare normal tissues and maximize targeting, beams are arranged to enter the patient from several directions and to intersect at the center of the tumor (treatment isocenter). Although machines containing collimated beams from high-intensity radioactive sources (primarily cobalt 60 [^{60}Co]) are still in use, today's modern treatment machine accelerates electrons to high (MeV) energy and impinges them onto an x-ray production target, leading to the generation of intense beams of Bremsstrahlung x-rays. A typical photon beam treatment machine[68,69] (Fig. 13.12) consists of a high-energy (6 to 20 MeV) linear electron accelerator, electromagnetic beam steering and

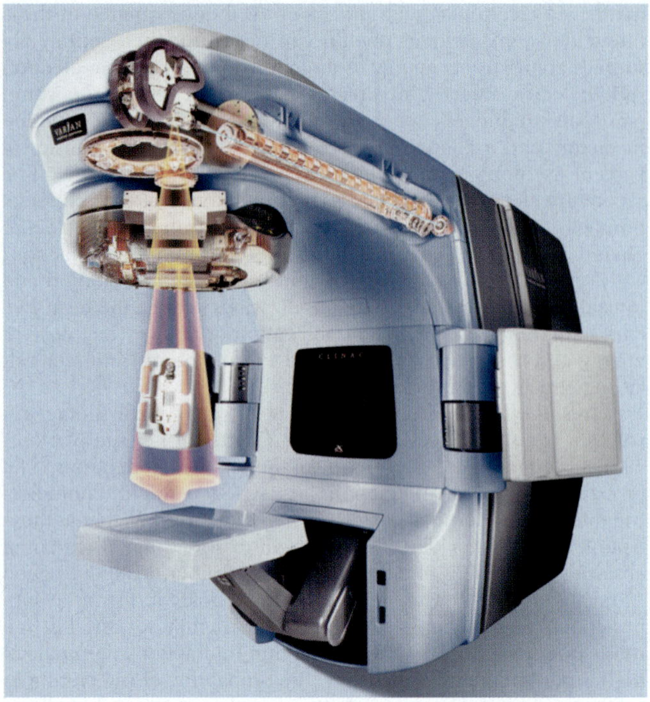

Figure 13.12 A shadow view of a C-arm linear accelerator. The electron beam (originating at upper right) is accelerated through a linear accelerator wave guide, selected for correct energy in a bending magnet, and then impinges on an x-ray production target. The x-ray beam (originating at target upper left) is flattened and collimated before leaving the treatment head. Also illustrated (downstream from the beam) is an electric portal imager that is used to measure (image) the beam exiting a patient. (From Varian Medical Systems, Palo Alto, CA, with permission.)

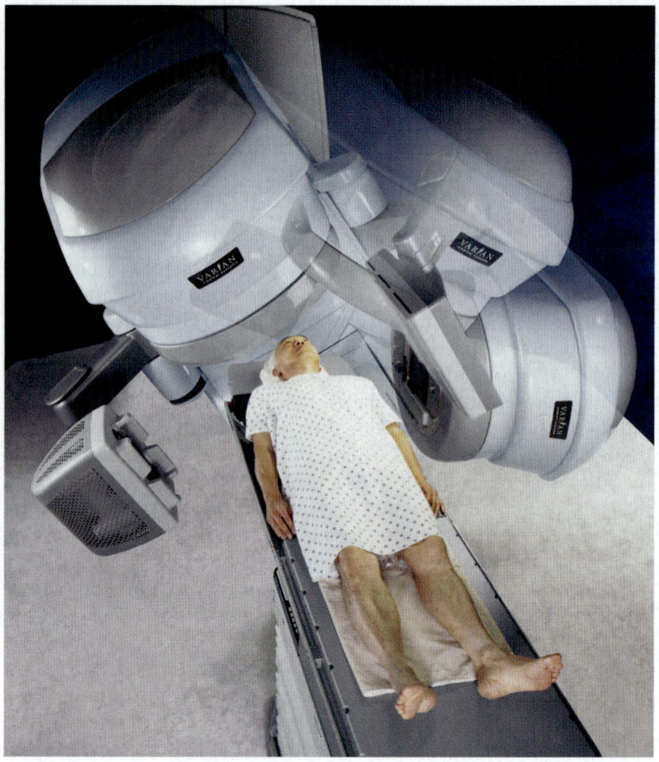

Figure 13.13 Model in treatment position on the patient support table. The treatment delivery head on the gantry's C-arm rotates about the patient, enabling the delivery of beams throughout 360 degrees of rotation. (From Varian Medical Systems, Palo Alto, CA, with permission.)

monitoring systems, x-ray generation targets, high-density treatment field-shaping devices (collimators), and up to a ton of radiation shielding on a mechanical C-arm gantry that can rotate precisely around a treatment couch (Fig. 13.13). These treatment-delivery machines routinely maintain mechanical isocenters for patient treatments to within a sphere of 1 mm radius. The development of *stereotactic radiotherapy*, which will be described in the section titled Clinical Application of Types of Radiation, depends on this level of machine precision.

X-ray production by monoenergetic high-energy electrons results in an x-ray (photon) beam that contains a continuous spectrum of energies with maximum photon energy near that of the incident electron beam. Lower energy photons appear with a much greater probability than do the highest energy ones, but they also become preferentially filtered out of the beam through the absorption in the target and the attenuation in the flattening filter. This generally results in a treatment beam energy spectrum with a mean photon energy of approximately one-third of the initial electron beam energy. In this energy range, the resulting photon beam exits the production target with a narrow angular spread focused primarily in the forward direction. These forward-peaked intensity distributions generally need to be modulated (flattened) to produce a large (up to 40 cm diameter at the patient) photon beam with uniform intensity across the beam. All modern treatment units take advantage of extensive computer control, monitoring, and feedback to produce highly stable and reproducible treatment beams.

The resulting photon beam requires beam shaping for conformal dose delivery. Some combination of primary, high-density field blocks (collimators) together with additional edge blocks generally provide the required shaping and shielding. Modern machines use computer-controlled multileaf collimators (Fig. 13.14)

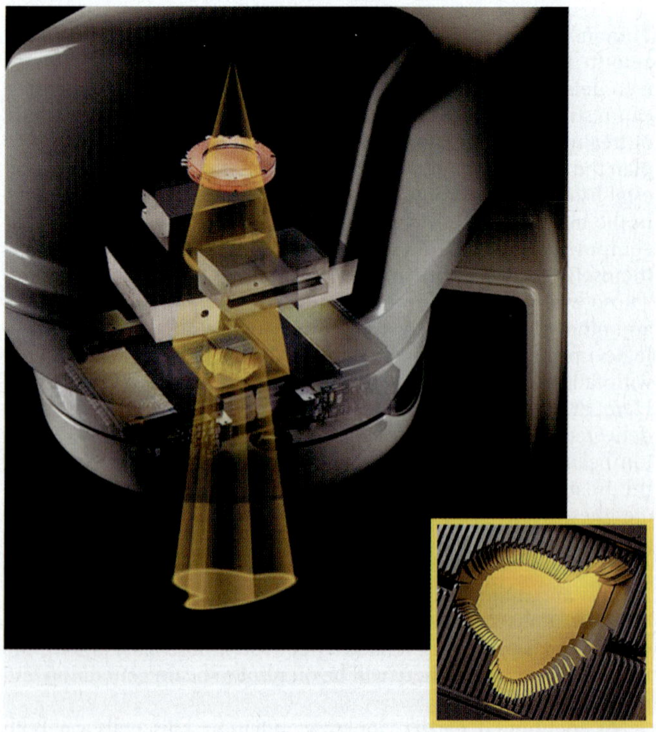

Figure 13.14 Multileaf collimator shaping of an x-ray treatment beam from a linear accelerator. *Inset* shows a view of the multileaf collimator. (From Varian Medical Systems, Palo Alto, CA, with permission.)

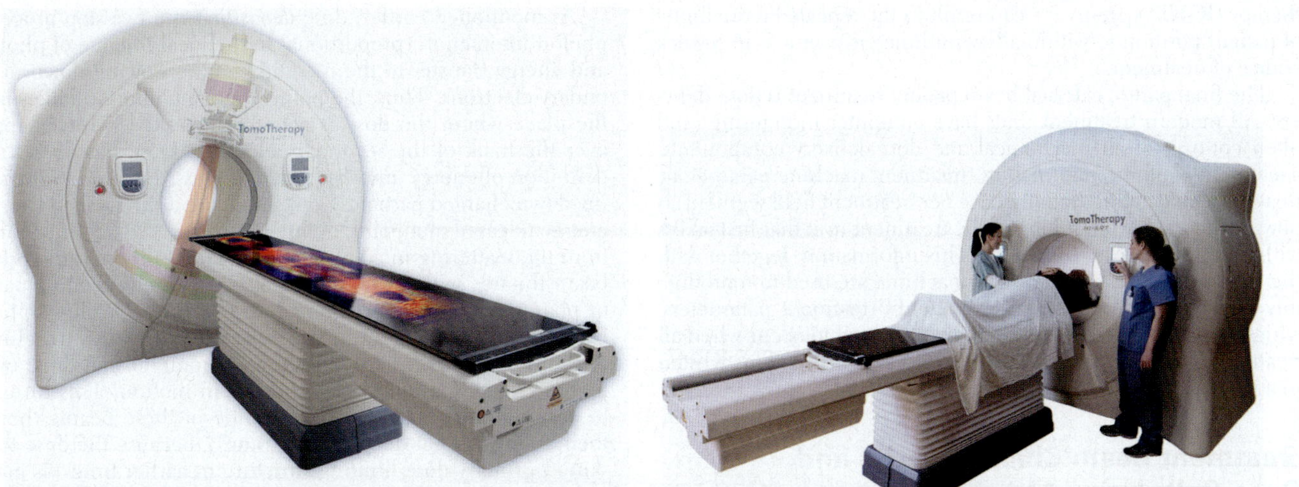

A

B

Figure 13.15 **(A)** A shadow view of linear accelerator, x-ray beam production system, and x-ray fan beam for helical tomotherapy treatment delivery. The beam production system rotates within its enclosed gantry. **(B)** The model patient on treatment table slides into the treatment unit. During treatment, the table moves as the collimated fan beam rotates about the patient, creating a modulated helical dose delivery pattern. (From TomoTherapy, Inc., Madison, WI, with permission.)

for the edge sculpting subsequent to setting the primary collimators for maximal shielding. This computer control provides high precision and reproducibility in the definition of field edges. Additionally, automation allows for a precise reshaping of the treatment beam for each angle of incidence, allowing not only conformation of irradiation to target volumes, but also modulation of the beam intensity patterns across the field (intensity-modulated radiation therapy [IMRT]).

Variations on the standard linear accelerator (linac) plus C-arm scenario that are being used for external-beam radiation treatments throughout the body include helical tomotherapy and nonisocentric miniature linac robotic delivery systems.[70] In helical tomotherapy, the accelerator, photon-production target, and collimation system are mounted on a ring gantry (similar to those found on diagnostic computed tomography [CT] scanners) (Fig. 13.15). It produces a fan beam of photons, and the intensity of each part of the fan being modulated by a binary collimator. As the gantry rotates, the patient simultaneously slides through the bore of the machine (again analogous to modern x-ray/CT imagers), which allows for the continuous delivery of intensity-modulated radiation in a helical pattern from all angles around a patient. Another delivery system uses an industrial robot to hold a miniature accelerator plus photon beam-production system (Fig. 13.16). The bulk of the system is reduced by keeping the field sizes small (spotlike). However, computer control of the robot provides flexibility in irradiating tumors from nearly any position external to the patient. The same control allows for the selection and use of many differing beam angles to build up the dose at the tumor location.

To take advantage of the precision of modern beam delivery, it is crucial to localize the patient's tumor and normal tissue.[71] This process can be divided into patient immobilization (i.e., limiting the motion of the patient) and localization (i.e., knowing the tumor and normal tissue location precisely in space). Although these concepts of immobilization and localization are related, they are not identical. Patients can be held reasonably comfortable in their treatment pose with the aid of foam molds and meshes (i.e., immobilization devices). Traditionally, localization has been achieved by indexing the immobilization device to the computer-controlled treatment couch and by using low-power laser beams aligned to skin marks. These techniques make it possible to reproducibly couple the surface of each patient with the treatment machine isocenter.

However, what is truly needed is to localize the tumor and normal tissues. The development of in-room, online x-ray, ultrasound, and infrared imaging equipment can now be used to ensure that the intended portions of each patient's internal anatomy are correctly positioned at the time of treatment. In particular, the development of rugged, low-profile, active matrix, flat-panel imaging devices, either attached to the treatment gantry or placed in the vicinity of the treatment couch, together with diagnostic x-ray generators or the patient treatment beam (see Fig. 13.13), allows the digital capture of projection x-ray images of patient anatomy with respect to the isocenter and treatment field borders. These digitized electronic images are immediately available for analysis. Software tools allow for a comparison to reference images and the generation of correction coordinates, which are in turn available for downloading to the treatment couch for automated fine adjustment of the patient's treatment position. Other precise localization systems rely on the identification of the positions of small, implanted radiopaque markers or other types of *smart* position-reporting devices. Careful use of these image-guided radiation

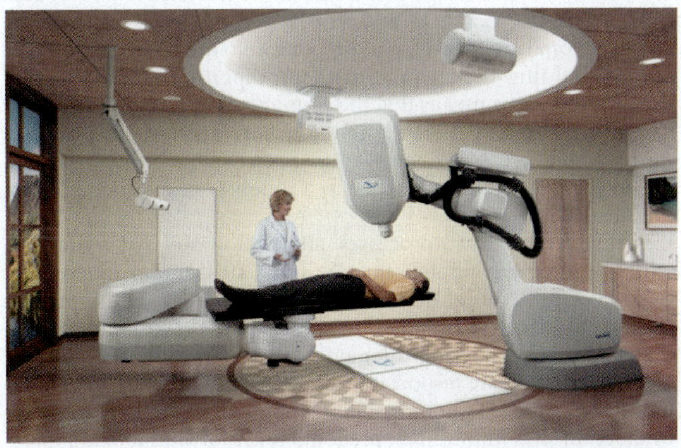

Figure 13.16 A miniature accelerator plus x-ray production system on a robotic delivery arm. Both the treatment table and the treatment head is set by a computer for multiple arbitrary angles of incidence. (From Accuray, Sunnyvale, CA, with permission.)

therapy (IGRT) systems[71, 72] can result in the repeated reducibility of patient position to within a few millimeters over a 5- to 8-week course of treatment.

The final part of external-beam patient treatment is dose delivery. All modern treatment units have computer monitoring (and often control) of all mechanical and dose-delivery components. Treatment-planning information (treatment machine parameters, treatment field configurations, dose per treatment field segment) is downloaded to a work station at the treatment unit that first assists with and then records treatment. This information, together with the readbacks from the treatment machine, are used to reproducibly set up and then verify each patient's treatment parameters, which prevents many of the variations that used to occur when all treatment was performed simply by following instructions written in a treatment chart.

Treatment Beam Characteristics and Dose-Calculation Algorithms

Beyond a basic understanding of the interactions of ionizing radiation with matter lies the requirement of being able to characterize the treatment beams for purposes of planning and verifying treatments. By virtue of a few underlying principles, this generally can be accomplished via a two-step process of absolute calibration of the dose at some reference point in a phantom (i.e., measurement media representative of a patient's tissues), with relative scaling of dose values in other parts of the beam or phantom with respect to that point.

As mentioned earlier, the predominant mode of interaction for therapeutic energy photon beams in tissuelike materials is through Compton scattering. The probability of Compton scattering events is primarily proportional to the relative electron density of the media with which they interact. Because many body tissues are waterlike in composition, it has been possible to make photon beam dosimetric measurements in phantoms consisting mostly of water (water tanks) or tissue-equivalent plastic and to then scale the interactions via relative electron density values (for example, as can be derived from computed x-ray/CT) to other waterlike materials. Thus, the relative fluence of photons in a therapeutic treatment beam is attenuated as it passes through a phantom, primarily via Compton scattering.

It was stated earlier that the photon beam is generated at a small region in the head of the machine. That fluence of photons spreads out through the collimating system before reaching the patient. Thus, without any interactions (e.g., if the beam were in a vacuum), the number of photons crossing any plane perpendicular to the beam direction would remain constant. However, the cross-sectional area of the plane gets larger the farther it is located from the source point. In fact, both the width and length of the cross-sectional area increase in proportion to the distance from the source, and thus the area increases in proportion to the square of the distance. This means that the primary photon fluence per unit area in a plane perpendicular to the beam direction of a pointlike source also decreases as one over the square of the distance, the so-called $1/r^2$ reduction in fluence as a function of distance, r, from the source.

Thus, we have two processes, attenuation and $1/r^2$ reduction, which reduce the photon fluence from an external therapeutic beam as a function of depth in a patient. There is also a process that can increase the photon fluence at a point downstream. Recall that Compton scattering interactions lead not only to secondary electrons (which are responsible for deposition of dose), but also to Compton scattered photons. These photons are scattered from the interaction sites in multiple, predominantly forward-looking directions. Thus, Compton-scattered photons originating from many other places can add to the photon fluence at another point. As the irradiated area (field size) increases, the amount of scattered radiation also increases.

As mentioned earlier, dose *deposition* is a two-step process of photon interaction (proportional to the local fluence of photons) and energy transfer to the medium via the slowing down of secondary electrons. Thus, the point where a photon interacts is not the place where the dose is actually deposited, which happens over the track of the secondary electron. Dose has a very strict definition of energy *absorbed* per unit mass (i.e., due to the slowing down charged particles) and should be distinguished from the energy released at a point, defined as kerma (e.g., energy transfer from the scattering incident photon). Thus, although the photon beam fluence will always be greatest at the entrance to a patient or phantom, the actual *absorbed dose* for a megavoltage photon beam builds up over the first couple of centimeters, reaching a maximum (d-max) at a depth corresponding to the range of the higher energy Compton electrons set in motion. This turns out to be a second desirable characteristic of these beams (beyond their ability to treat deep-seated lesions), because the dose to the skin (a primary dose-limiting structure in earlier times) is greatly reduced.

The relative distributions of dose, normalized to an absolute dose measurement (using a small thimblelike air ionization chamber at a standard depth and for a standard field size according to nationally and internationally accepted protocols), are the major inputs into treatment-planning systems. The major features of these distributions are (1) the initial dose buildup up to a depth of d-max, with a more gradual drop off in dose as a function of depth into the phantom due to the attenuation and $1/r^2$ factors at deeper depths (relative depth dose), and (2) the shape of the dose in the plane perpendicular to the direction of the beams; both as a function of field size. Central axis depth dose curves for typical external photon beams are shown in Figure 13.17 for two beam energies and for both a large and smaller field size. Notice both the expected increase in penetration with increasing beam energy and the increase in dose at a particular depth with increasing field size; the latter effect due to increased numbers of secondary Compton-scattered photons for larger irradiated areas. The change in dose perpendicular to the central axis is less remarkable, because the beams are designed to be uniform across a field as a function of depth.

It is useful to also point out the depth dose characteristics of clinical external treatment beams produced using ionizing

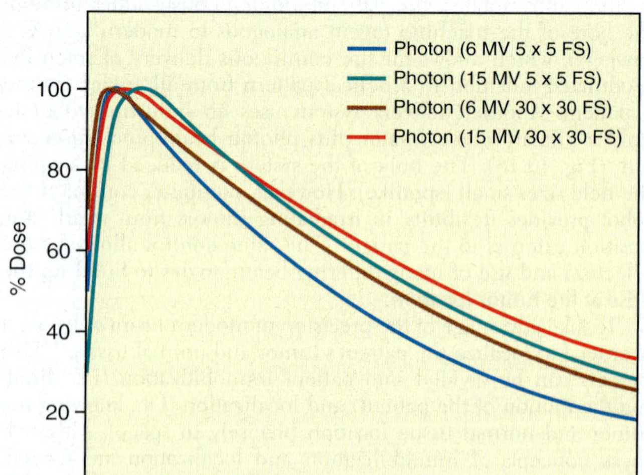

Figure 13.17 Sample depth-dose curves (change in delivered dose as a function of depth) along the central axis of some typical photon treatment beams for low (6 MV) and intermediate (15 MV) energy beams, and large (30 × 30 cm^2) and smaller (5 × 5 cm^2) field sizes (FS).

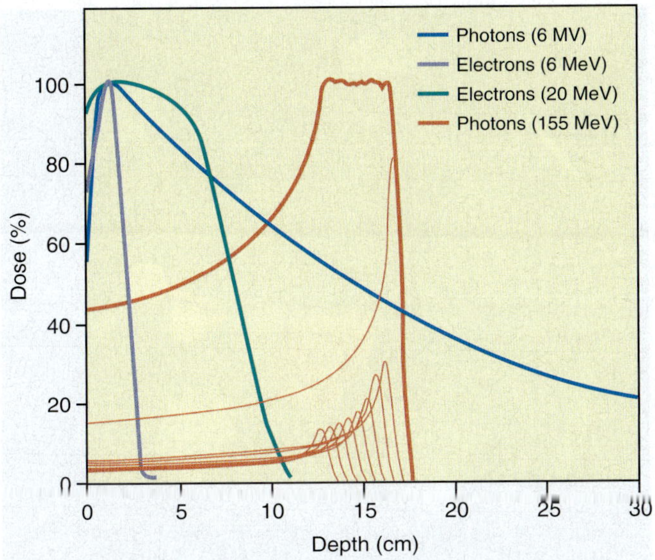

Figure 13.18 Sample depth-dose curves along the central axis of some typical charged particle treatment beams compared with that of a 6-MV proton beam. The spread out Bragg peak at the end of the 155-MeV proton beam (*thick pink curve*) is a composite dose deposition pattern from the addition of the multiple range-shifted proton curves (*thinner pink curves*).

radiations other than photons, primarily through the direct use of charged particles. Those beams (Fig. 13.18) illustrate interesting characteristics, which, when added to the options available for treatment planning (or used by themselves), can produce advantageous results. Relative to the photon beam, the direct use of electron beams leads to deposition of dose over a more localized range, but at the expense of a relative lack of penetration. Thus, electron beams are most widely used for treating, or boosting the treatment of, more superficial tumors and regions (see the section titled Clinical Application of Types of Radiation). The heavier charged particle beams (protons and carbon ions) appear to exhibit even more interesting *depth-dose* characteristics, with the advantage of both (when necessary) being highly penetrating and also lacking a significant dose beyond a certain depth (a depth that can be controlled and purposefully placed, for example, at the distal edge of a target volume).

The results of measurements such as these have been modeled so as to develop dose-calculation algorithms used in treatment-planning systems. These models all use measured beam data to set or adjust parameters used by those algorithms in their dose-distribution computations. Because most of the input data used for beam fitting come from measurements in water phantoms (or waterlike plastic phantoms), patient-specific adjustments are needed for the water phantom data to account for both geometry and tissue properties. It is the task of the dose-calculation algorithms to take those changes into account. The accuracy and precision actually realized for all dose-calculation algorithms generally need to be traded off against the time required to complete the calculation. Although the availability of ever more powerful computers has made calculation time less of a concern for broad, open-beam treatment planning, issues still remain for more specialized planning exercises that use many small beams or parts of beams such as IMRT (discussed later). Typically, relative dose distributions can be computed within patients on the scale of a few millimeters with a precision of better than a few percentage points.

An important area of research is the development of treatment-planning systems that calculate dose based on the principles of how radiation interacts with tissues, rather than simply by fitting data. These approaches use Monte Carlo techniques,[71,73] which build a dose distribution by summing the calculated paths of thousands of photons and scattered electrons. This approach is more accurate than beam-fitting algorithms in regions of differing tissue densities, such as the lung, and therefore, will ultimately replace the current generation of treatment-planning systems, particularly for complex conditions. However, the time to perform these calculations is still prohibitive for a clinic, and it is anticipated that Monte Carlo calculations will be introduced over a period of years by balancing the need for accuracy in a particular clinical situation with the need to initiate patient treatment.

TREATMENT PLANNING

As discussed in the previous section, single-treatment beams usually deposit more of the dose closer to where they enter the patient than they do at depths corresponding to where a deep-seated tumor might be located. The use of multiple beams entering the patient from different directions that overlap at the target produces more dose per unit volume throughout the tumor volume than is received by normal tissues. In fact, as noted earlier, the treatment-delivery machines are designed to make this easy to accomplish. Planning patient treatments under these circumstances should be a somewhat trivial matter of first selecting a sufficient number of beam angles to realize the desired buildup of the dose in the overlap region relative to the doses in the upstream parts of each beam, and then second, designing beam apertures that shape the edges of the beams to match the target. However, dose-limiting normal tissues often also lie in the paths of one or more of the beams. These normal tissues are often more sensitive to radiation damage than the tumor, and regardless, it is best practice to minimize the dose in any case as a general principle. Computerized treatment-planning systems function to develop patient-specific anatomic or geometric models and then use these models together with the beam-specific dose deposition properties (derived from phantom measurements, as previously described) to select beam angles, shapes, and intensities that meet an overall prescribed objective. That is, modern radiation oncology dose prescriptions contain both tumor and normal tissue objectives, and the modern computerized treatment-planning systems make it possible to design treatments that meet these objectives.

The development and use of three-dimensional (3D) models of each patient's anatomy, treatment geometry, and dose distribution led to a paradigm shift in radiation therapy treatment planning. Computerized radiation treatment planning began in the 1980s as a mainly x-ray/CT–based reconstruction of 3D geometries from information manually contoured on multiple two-dimensional (2D) transverse CT images. Today, these models often incorporate imaging data from multiple sources. Geometrically accurate anatomic information from an x-ray/CT scan still anchors these studies (as well as provides tissue density information necessary for dose calculations). However, it is now quite common to also register the CT data set with other studies such as magnetic resonance imaging (MRI), which may add anatomic detail for soft tissues, or functional MRI or positron emission tomography (PET) studies,[74,75] which provide physiologic or molecular information about tumors and normal tissues. Once registered with each other, the unique or complementary information from each data set can be fused for inspection and incorporated into the design of each patient's target and normal tissue volumes (Fig. 13.19). Beyond the ability to more fully define the extent of the primary target volume (for instance, as the encompassing envelope of disease appreciated on all the imaging studies) lies the ability to define subvolumes of the tumor volume that might be appropriate for simultaneous treatment to higher dose. For example, it should soon become possible to define different biologic components of the tumor that could potentially be targeted and then monitored for response using these same imaging techniques.[76]

Current treatment planning makes the tacit assumption that the planning image yields "the truth" about the location and condition

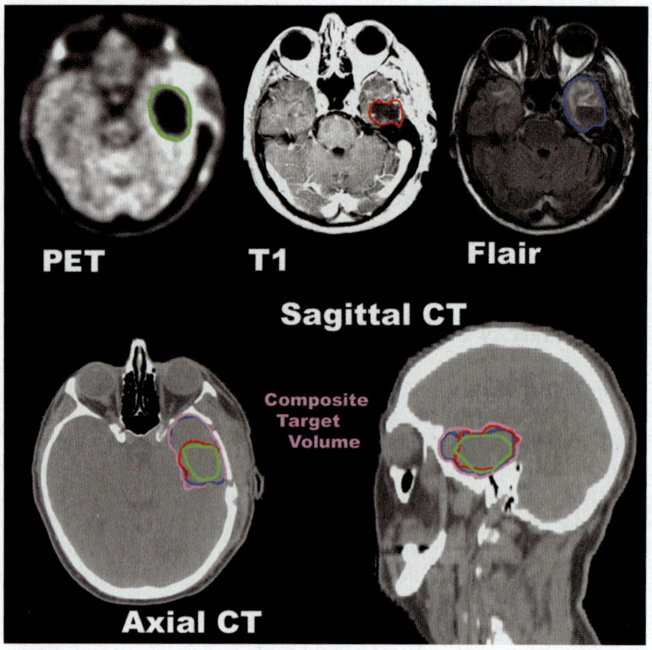

Figure 13.19 An illustration of the brain tumor target volume delineated on coregistered nuclear medicine and magnetic resonance imaging studies fused with computed tomography (CT) data for treatment planning. PET, positron emission tomography.

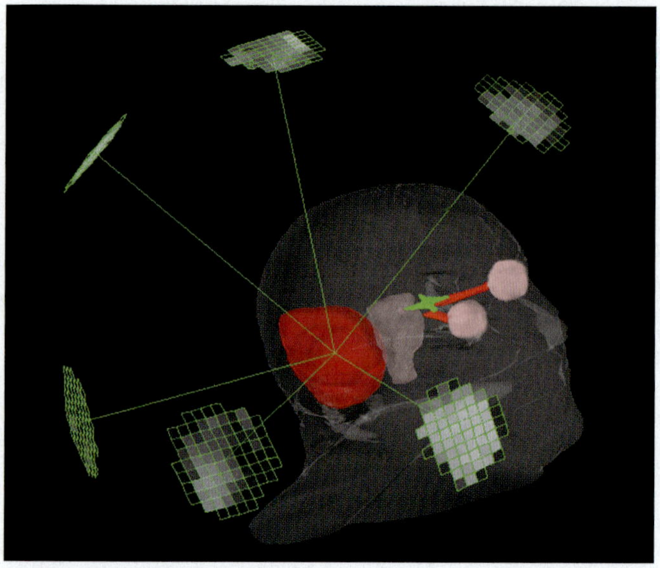

Figure 13.20 Six intensity-modulated treatment ports planned for treatment of a brain tumor (*large object in red*). Differing intensities of the 5 × 5 mm *beamlets* in each port illustrated by gray scale (brighter beamlet = higher intensity). The computer optimization of the beamlet intensities is designed to generate a delivered dose distribution that will conform to the tumor region, yet avoid critical normal tissues such as the brain stem (*dark pink*), optic chiasm (*green*), and optic nerves (*red tubular structures*).

of tumors and normal tissues throughout the course of treatment. However, this ignores the complexity inherent in attempting to build accurate 3D models from multimodality imaging for purposes of planning patient treatments. First, patients breathe and undergo other physiologic processes during a single treatment, changes that require dynamic modeling or other methods of accounting for the changes. Furthermore, the patient's condition may change over time (and hence their model). Thus, a complete design and assessment of a patient undergoing high-precision treatment requires the construction of four-dimensional (4D) patient models. Indeed, the recent ready availability of multidetector CT scanners with subsecond gantry rotations, and even more recently, the availability of cone-beam CT capabilities on the radiation therapy treatment simulators and treatment machines themselves, now makes it possible to construct 4D patient models. A very active area of physics research[72,75] deals with IGRT, including the formation of 4D patient models (including distortions and changes in anatomy) of the motion over time and the determination of the accumulated dose received by a moving tumor as well as the surrounding normal tissues such as uninvolved lung.

Complementary to the availability of these patient and dose models has come a much better understanding of the doses safely tolerated by normal tissues adjacent to a tumor volume (e.g., spinal cord) or surrounding it (e.g., brain, lung, liver).[77] Indeed, not only has knowledge of whole organ tolerances to irradiation been obtained, but it has also become possible to characterize in some detail the complex dependence of the probability of incurring a complication with respect to the highly (intentionally) inhomogeneous dose distributions these normal tissues receive as part of the planning process designed to avoid treating them. Modeling partial organ tolerances to irradiation is of great use in planning patient treatments because it enables[78] integration and manipulation of variable dose and volume distributions with respect to possible clinical outcomes.

Making the vast amount of tumor and normal tissue information useful for planning treatments requires equally sophisticated new ways of planning and delivering dose, potentially preferentially targeting subvolumes of the tumor regions or specifically avoiding selected portions of adjacent organs at risk. As mentioned earlier, modern treatment machines are capable of either varying the intensity of the radiation across each treatment port or projecting many small beams at a targeted region. This modulation of beam intensities (IMRT) from a given beam direction, together with the use of multiple beams (or parts of beams) from different directions, gives many degrees of freedom to create highly sculpted dose distributions, given that a system for designing the intensity modulation is available. Much computer programming and computational analysis has gone into the design of treatment-planning optimization systems to perform these functions.[79,80]

In IMRT, as most often applied, each treatment beam portal is broken down into simple basic components called beamlets, typically 0.5 to 1 cm × 1 cm in size, evenly distributed on a grid over the cross-section of each beam. Optimization begins with precomputation of the relative dose contribution that each of these beamlets gives to every subportion of tumor and normal tissue that the beamlet traverses as it goes through the patient model. Sophisticated optimization engines and search routines then iteratively alter the relative intensities of each beamlet in all the beams to minimize a cost function associated with target and normal tissue treatment goals. These, often hundreds of beamlets (each with its own intensity) (Fig. 13.20), provide the necessary flexibility and degrees of freedom to create dose distributions that can preferentially irradiate subportions of targets and also produce sharp dose gradients to avoid nearby organs at risk (Fig. 13.21). The cost-function approach also facilitates the ability to include factors such as the normal tissue and tumor-response models, mentioned previously in the optimization process, thus integrating the overall effects of the complex dose distributions across whole organ systems or target volumes within the planning process.

OTHER TREATMENT MODALITIES

Other types of external-beam radiation treatments use atomic or nuclear particles rather than photons. Beams of fast neutrons have been used for some cancers,[81] primarily because of the

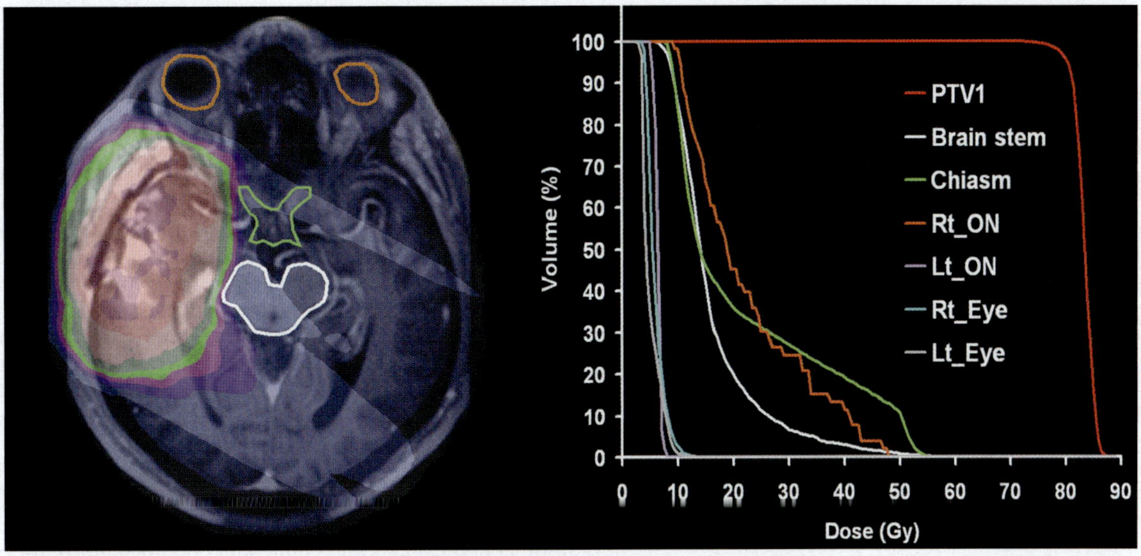

Figure 13.21 Resulting isodose distribution for an optimized intensity-modulated brain treatment. Dose-intensity pattern in the *left panel* is overlaid on the patient's magnetic resonance images used in planning. Also contoured are the optic chiasm (*green*), the brain stem (*white*), and the eyes (*orange*). In the *right panel,* the dose distribution throughout all slices of the patient's anatomy is summarized via cumulative dose-volume histograms for the various tissues and volumes that have been previously segmented. Each location on each curve represents the fraction of the volume of that tissue (%) that receives greater than or the same as the corresponding dose level.

dense ionization patterns they produce as they slow down in tissue (making cell killing less dependent on the indirect effect previously discussed). Being uncharged particles, neutron beams of therapeutic energy penetrate in tissue (have depth-dose characteristics) similar to photon beams, but with denser dose deposition in the cellular scale. Most other external-beam treatments use charged particles, primarily either electrons[82] (produced on the same machines used for photon beam treatments) or protons or heavier particles such as carbon ions.[83,84] The latter beams have desirable dose-deposition properties (see Fig. 13.18), because they can spare tissues downstream from the target volume and generally give less overall dose to normal tissue. There can also be some radiobiologic advantage to the heavier charged particle beams, similar to neutrons. The generation and delivery of proton beams and heavier charged particle beams generally requires an accelerator (in its own vault) plus a beam transport system and some sort of treatment nozzle, often located on an isocentric gantry. The cost of the accelerator is generally leveraged by having it supply beams to multiple treatment rooms, but these units still cost many times that of a standard linear accelerator.

Brachytherapy[85] is a form of treatment that uses direct placement of radioactive sources or materials within tumors (interstitial brachytherapy) or within body or surgical cavities (intracavitary brachytherapy), either permanently (allowing for full decay of short-lived radioactive materials) or temporarily (either in one extended application or over several shorter term applications). The ability to irradiate tumors from close range (even from the inside out) can lead to conformal treatments with low normal tissue doses. The radioactive isotopes most generally used for these treatments are contained within small tubelike or seedlike sealed source enclosures (which prevents direct contamination). They emit photons (gamma and x-rays) during their decay, which penetrate the source cover and interact with tissue via the same physical processes as described for external-beam treatments. The treatments have the advantage of providing a high fluence (and dose) very near each source that drops in intensity as 1 over the square of the distance from the source ($1/r^2$). Radioactive sources decay in an exponential fashion characterized by their individual half-lives. After each half-life ($T_{1/2}$) the strength of each source decreases by half. Brachytherapy treatments are further generally classified into the two broad categories of low–dose-rate and high–dose-rate treatments. Low–dose-rate treatments attempt to deliver tumoricidal doses via continuous irradiation from implanted sources over a period of several days. High–dose-rate treatments use one or more higher activity sources (stored external to the patient) together with a remote applicator or source transfer system to give one or more higher dose treatments on time scales and schedules more like external-beam treatments.

Isotopes for brachytherapy treatments are selected on the basis of a combination of specific activity (i.e., how much activity can be achieved per unit mass [i.e., to keep the source sizes small]), the penetrating ability of the decay photons (together with the $1/r^2$ fall off determines how many sources or source location will be required for treatment), and the half-life of the radioactive material (which must be accounted for in computation of dose, but also determines how often reusable sources will need to be replaced). Table 13.1 lists those isotopes most commonly used, along with some of their primary applications.

The dose-deposition patterns surrounding each type of source can be measured or computed. These data (or the parameterization

TABLE 13.1

Common Isotopes for Brachytherapy Treatment

Isotope	Form	Primary Applications
^{125}I	Implantable sealed seed	LDR: Permanent prostate implants, brain implants, tumor bed implants, eye plaques
^{192}Ir	Implantable sealed seed	LDR: Interstitial solid tumor treatments
^{192}Ir	High activity sealed source on a remote transfer wire	HDR: Intracavitary GYN treatments, intraluminal irradiations
^{137}Cs	Sealed source tubes	LDR: Intracavitary GYN treatments

LDR, low-dose rate; HDR, high-dose rate; GYN, gynecologic; ^{137}Cs, caesium-137.

CANCER THERAPEUTICS

of same) can be stored within a computerized treatment-planning system. Planning a brachytherapy treatment-delivery scheme (desirable source strengths and arrangements) proceeds within the planning system by distributing the sources throughout the treatment area and having the computer add up the contributions of each source to designated tumor and normal tissue locations (e.g., obtained from a CT scan). Source strengths or spacing can be adjusted until an acceptable result is obtained. Indeed, optimization systems are now routinely used to fine tune this process.

Other types of therapeutic treatments with internal sources of ionizing radiation, generally classified as systemic targeted radionuclide therapy (STaRT), use antibodies or other conjugates or carriers such as microspheres to selectively deliver radionuclides to cancer cells.[86] Computing the effective dose to tumors and normal tissues via these techniques requires information on how much of the injected activity reaches the targets (biodistribution) as well as the energy and decay properties of the radionuclide being delivered. Imaging techniques and computer models are aiding in these computations.

CLINICAL APPLICATIONS OF RADIATION THERAPY

In contrast to surgical oncology and medical oncology, which focus on early- or late-stage disease, respectively, the field of radiation oncology encompasses the1p8.49 entire spectrum of oncology. Board certification requires 5 years of postdoctoral training, typically beginning with an internship in internal medicine or surgery, followed by 4 years of radiation oncology residency. Education, as defined by leaders in the field,[87] begins with a thorough knowledge of the biology, physics, and clinical applications of radiation. It also includes training in the theoretical and practical aspects of the administration of radiation protectors and anticancer agents used as radiation sensitizers and the management of toxicities resulting from those treatments. In addition, residents receive education in palliative care, supportive care, and symptom and pain management. This training is in preparation for a practice that, in a given week, might include patients with a 2-mm vocal cord lesion or a 20-cm soft tissue sarcoma, both of whom can be treated with curative intent, as well as a patient with widely metastatic disease who needs palliative radiation, medical care for pain and depression, and discussion of end-of-life issues. More than 50% of (nonskin) cancer patients receive radiation therapy during the course of their illness.[88]

Clinical Application of Types of Radiation

Electrons are now the most widely used form of radiation for superficial treatments. Because the depth of penetration can be well controlled by the energy of the beam, it is possible to treat, for instance, skin cancer, a small part of the breast while sparing the underlying lung, or the cervical lymph nodes but not the spinal cord, which lies several centimeters more deeply. Superficial tumors, such as of skin cancers, can also be treated very effectively with low-energy (kilovoltage) photons, but their use has decreased because a separate machine is required for their production.

The main form of treatment for deep tumors is photons. As described in the Radiation Physics section, photons spare the skin and deposit dose along their entire path until the beam leaves the body. The use of multiple beams that intersect on the tumor permit high doses to be delivered to the tumor with a relative sparing of normal tissue. The pinnacle of this concept is IMRT, which uses hundreds of beams and can treat concave shapes with relative sparing of the central region (see Figs. 13.20 and 13.21). However, as each beam continues on its path beyond the tumor, this use of multiple beams means that a significant volume of normal tissue receives a low dose. There has been considerable debate concerning the magnitude of the risk of second cancers produced by radiating large volumes with low doses of radiation.[89] Charged particle beams (proton and carbon, in this discussion) differ from photons in that they interact only modestly with tissue until they reach the end of their path, where they then deposit the majority of their energy and stop (the Bragg peak; see Fig. 13.18). This ability to stop at a chosen depth decreases the region of low dose. The chief form of charged particle used today is the proton. In the decade from 1980 to 1990, proton therapy could deliver higher doses of radiation to the target than photon therapy because protons could produce a more rapid fall off of dose between the target and the critical normal tissue (e.g., tumor and brain stem). Therefore, initially, their main application was in the treatment uveal melanomas, base-of-skull chondrosarcomas, and chordomas. In contrast, today's IMRT photons are more conformal in the high-dose region than protons due to the range uncertainty of the latter.[90] Thus, it seems unlikely that protons will permit a higher target dose to be delivered than photons. In contrast, protons have the potential to decrease regions of low dose. This would be of particular advantage in the treatment of pediatric malignancies, where low doses of radiation would tend to increase the chance of second cancers and could affect neurocognitive function in the treatment of brain tumors.

A carbon ion beam has an additional potential biologic advantage over protons. As discussed in the section Biologic Aspects of Radiation Oncology, hypoxic cells, which are found in many tumors, are up to 3 times more resistant to photon or proton radiation than well-oxygenated cells. In contrast, hypoxia does not cause resistance to a carbon beam. Whether hypoxia is a cause of clinical resistance to fractionated radiation is still debated.[91] A carbon beam is available at a few sites in Europe and Japan.

Two major issues have affected the widespread acceptance of protons. The most widely recognized is cost. Proton (approximately $120 million) and carbon beam facilities (in excess of $200 million) are substantially more expensive than a similar-sized photon facility (approximately $25 million). The operating costs appear to be significantly higher as well. Although the majority of patients who have received proton therapy have prostate cancer, there is no evidence that protons produce superior results to those obtained with IMRT planned photons.[92,93] The lack of solid evidence that protons are superior to photons for any disease site and the magnitude of these costs are of societal importance.[94] Although less expensive single gantry proton units are under construction, there are no functioning units at the time of this writing. A second, less well-appreciated issue concerns the need to develop full integration of charged particle beams with IGRT, as has already been accomplished with photons, although this feature is being incorporated into second-generation proton units.

Neutron therapy attracted significant interest in the 1980s, based on the principle that it would be more effective than photons against hypoxic cells that some have thought are responsible for radiation resistance of tumors. The effectiveness of neutron therapy has been limited by initial difficulties with collimation and targeting, although there is evidence that they have a role in the treatment of refractory parotid gland tumors.[95]

Brachytherapy refers to the placement of radioactive sources next to or inside the tumor. The chief sites where brachytherapy plays a role are in prostate and cervical cancer, although it has applications in head and neck cancers, soft tissue sarcomas, and other sites. In the case of prostate cancer, most experience is with low–dose-rate permanent implants using iodine-125 (^{125}I) or, more recently, palladium-103 (^{103}Pd). Over the last 5 years, there has been an increasing emphasis on improving the accuracy of seed placement, guided by ultrasound and confirmed by CT or MRI, and in skilled hands, outstanding results can be achieved.[96] In the case of cervical cancer, high–dose-rate treatment, which can be performed in an outpatient setting, has essentially replaced low–dose-rate treatment, which typically requires general anesthesia and a 2-day hospital stay. The results from both techniques appear to be approximately equivalent.

Yttrium microspheres represent a distinct form of brachytherapy. These spheres carry yttrium-90 (^{90}Y), a pure beta emitter with a range of about 1 cm. These have been used to treat both primary hepatocellular cancer and colorectal cancer metastatic to the liver (hepatic arterial or systemic chemotherapy) by administration through the hepatic artery.

TREATMENT INTENT

Radiation doses are chosen so as to maximize the chance of tumor control without producing unacceptable toxicity. The dose of radiation required depends on the tumor type, the volume of disease (number of tumor cells), and the use of radiation-modifying agents (such as chemotherapeutic drugs used as radiation sensitizers). Except for a subset of tumors that are exquisitely sensitive to radiation (e.g., seminoma, lymphoma), doses that are required are often close to the tolerance of the normal tissue. A key fact driving the choice of dose is that a 1-cm^3 tumor contains approximately 1 billion cells. It follows that the reduction of a tumor that is 3 cm in diameter to 3 mm, which would be called a complete response by CT scan, would still leave 1 million tumor cells. Because each radiation fraction appears to kill a fixed fraction of the tumor, the dose to cure occult disease needs to be more similar to the dose for gross disease than one might otherwise expect. Thus, radiation doses (using the standard fractionation) of 45 to 54 Gy are typically used in the adjuvant setting when there is moderate suspicion for occult disease, 60 to 65 Gy for positive margins or when there is a high suspicion for occult disease, and 70 Gy or more for gross disease.

It is common during the course of radiation to give higher doses of radiation to regions that have a higher tumor burden. For example, regions that are suspected of harboring occult disease may be targeted to receive (in once daily 2-Gy fractions) 54 Gy, whereas, to control the gross tumor, the goal may be to administer a total dose of 70 Gy. Because the gross tumor will invariably reside within the region at risk for occult disease, it has become standard practice to deliver 50 Gy to the entire region, and then an additional *boost* dose of 20 Gy to the tumor. This sequence is called the *shrinking field technique*. With the development of IMRT, it has become possible to treat both regions with a different dose each day and achieve both goals simultaneously. For example, on each of the 35 days of treatment, the gross tumor might receive 2 Gy, and the region of occult disease 1.7 Gy, for a total dose of 59.5 Gy, which is of approximately equal biologic effectiveness to 54 Gy in 1.8-Gy fractions because of the lower dose per fraction (see the section Biologic Aspects of Radiation Oncology).

Radiation therapy alone is often used with curative intent for localized tumors. The decision to use surgery or radiation therapy involves factors determined by the tumor (e.g., is it resectable without a serious compromise in function?) and the patient (e.g., is the patient a good operative candidate?). The most common tumor in this group is prostate cancer, but patients with early-stage larynx cancer often receive radiation for voice preservation, and there are many patients with early-stage lung cancer who are not operative candidates. Control rates for these early-stage lesions are in excess of 70% (and as high as 90% for early-stage larynx cancer) and are usually a function of tumor size.

Stereotactic body radiation therapy (SBRT; sometimes called *stereotactic ablative radiation*) uses many (typically more than eight) cross-firing beams and provides an improved method of curing early-stage lung cancer[97] and liver metastases.[98] This approach uses precise localization and image guidance to deliver a small number (less than five) of high doses of radiation, with the concept of ablating the tumor, rather than using fractionation to achieve a therapeutic index (see the section title Fractionation). SBRT can provide long-term, local control rates of >90% for tumors less than 4 to 5 cm with minimal side effects.

Locally advanced or aggressive cancers can be cured with radiation alone or with a combination of radiation and chemotherapy or a molecularly targeted therapy. The most common examples here are locally advanced lung cancer, head and neck, esophageal, and cervix cancers, with cure rates in the 15% to 40% range, and are discussed in detail in their own chapters. A general principle that has emerged during the last decade is that combination chemoradiation has increased the cure rates of locally advanced cancers by 5% to 10% at the cost of increased toxicity.

An important consideration in the use of radiation (with or without chemotherapy) with curative intent is the concept of organ preservation. Perhaps the best example of achieving organ preservation in the face of gross disease involves the use of chemotherapy and radiation to replace laryngectomy in the treatment of advanced larynx cancer. Combined radiation and chemotherapy does not improve overall survival compared with radical surgery; however, the organ-conservation approach permits voice preservation in approximately two-thirds of patients with advanced larynx cancer.[99] The treatment of anal cancer with chemoradiation can also be viewed in this light, with chemoradiotherapy producing organ conservation and cure rates superior to radical surgery used decades ago.[100] Multiple randomized trials have demonstrated that lumpectomy plus radiation for breast cancer produces survival rates equal to that of modified radical mastectomy, while allowing for the preservation of the breast.

In the last decade, it has become clear that some patients with metastatic disease can be cured with radiation (with or without chemotherapy). The concept underlying this approach was established by the surgical practice of resecting a limited number of liver or lung metastases. A significant fraction of patients have a limited number of liver metastases that cannot be resected because of location, but are able to undergo high-dose radiation (often combined with chemotherapy). This radical approach to *oligometastases*[101] can produce 5-year survivals in the range of 20% in selected patients.[102] Patients with a limited number of lung metastases from colorectal cancer or soft tissue sarcomas are now being approached with stereotactic body radiation with a similar concept as has been used to justify surgical resection.[102] In addition to the direct effect of radiation on metastatic tumor, there is now anecdotal but provocative evidence that radiation can stimulate the immune system so that tumors distant from the irradiated tumor can respond. Distant (abscopal) responses have been reported in patients who receive immune checkpoint inhibitors such as ipilimumab.[103]

Radiation therapy can also contribute to the cure of patients when used in an adjuvant setting. If the risk of recurrence after surgery is low or if a recurrence could be easily addressed by a second resection, adjuvant radiation therapy is not usually given. However, when a gross total resection of the tumor is still associated with a high risk of residual occult disease or if local recurrence is morbid, adjuvant treatment is often recommended. A general finding across many disease sites is that adjuvant radiation can reduce local failure rates to below 10%, even in high-risk patients, if a gross total resection is achieved. If gross disease or positive margins remain, higher doses and/or larger volumes may be required, which may be less well tolerated and are less successful in achieving tumor control.

Adjuvant therapy can be delivered before or after definitive surgery. There are some advantages to giving radiation therapy after surgery. The details of the tumor location are known and, with the surgeon's cooperation, clips can be placed in the tumor bed, permitting increased treatment accuracy. In addition, compared with preoperative therapy, postoperative therapy is associated with fewer wound complications. However, in some cases, it is preferable to deliver preoperative radiation. Radiation can shrink the tumor, diminishing the extent of the resection, or making an unresectable tumor resectable. In the case of rectal cancer, the response to treatment may carry more prognostic information than the initial TNM staging.[104] In patients who will undergo significant surgeries (particularly a Whipple procedure or an esophageal resection), preoperative (sometimes called neoadjuvant) therapy can be more reliably administered than postoperative therapy. Most importantly, after resection of abdominal or pelvic tumors (such as rectal cancers or retroperitoneal sarcomas), the small bowel may become fixed by adhesions in the region requiring treatment, thus increasing the morbidity of postoperative treatment. A randomized trial has shown that preoperative therapy produces fewer gastrointestinal side effects and has at least as good efficacy as postoperative adjuvant therapy for locally advanced rectal cancer.[105] Taken together, there appears to be a trend toward preoperative or neoadjuvant therapy in cancers of the gastrointestinal track (esophagus, stomach, pancreas, rectum), postoperative radiation seems to be favored in head and neck, lung, and breast cancer, and soft tissue sarcoma seems equally split.

The effectiveness of adjuvant therapy in decreasing local recurrence has been demonstrated in randomized trials in lung, rectal, and breast cancers. More recently, randomized trials have shown that postmastectomy radiation improved the survival for women with breast cancer and four or more positive lymph nodes, all of whom also received adjuvant chemotherapy. A fascinating analysis has revealed that, across many treatment conditions, each 4% increase in 5-year local control is associated with a 1% increase in 5-year survival.[106] It has been proposed that the long-term survival benefit of radiation in these more recent studies was revealed by the introduction of effective chemotherapy, which prevented such a high fraction of women from dying early with metastatic disease.[107] This concept has been developed into a hypothesis that the effect of adjuvant radiation on survival will depend on the effectiveness of adjuvant chemotherapy. If chemotherapy is either ineffective or very effective, adjuvant radiation may have little influence on the survival in a disease in which systemic relapse dominates survival. Radiation will have its greatest impact on survival when chemotherapy is moderately effective.[108]

In addition to these curative roles, radiation plays an important part in palliative treatment. Perhaps most importantly, emergency irradiation can begin to reverse the devastating effects of spinal cord compression and of superior vena cava syndrome. A single 8-Gy fraction is highly effective for many patients with bone pain from a metastatic lesion. There is increasing evidence of the effectiveness of body stereotactic radiation to treat vertebral body metastases in patients who have a long projected survival or who need retreatment after previous radiation.[109] Stereotactic treatment can relieve symptoms from a small number of brain metastasis, and fractionated whole-brain radiation can mitigate the effects of multiple metastases. Bronchial obstruction can often be relieved by a brief course of treatment as can duodenal obstruction from pancreatic cancer. Palliative treatment is usually delivered in a smaller number of larger radiation fractions (see the section titled Fractionation) because the desire to simplify the treatment for a patient with limited life expectancy outweighs the somewhat increased potential for late side effects.

FRACTIONATION

Two crucial features that influence the effectiveness of a physical dose of radiation are the dose given in each radiation treatment (i.e., the fraction) and the total amount of time required to complete the course of radiation. Standard fractionation for radiation therapy is defined as the delivery of one treatment of 1.8 to 2.25 Gy per day. This approach produces a fairly well-understood chance of tumor control and risk of normal tissue damage (as a function of volume). By altering the fractionation schemes, one may be able to improve the outcome for patients undergoing curative treatment or to simplify the treatment for patients receiving palliative therapy.

Two forms of altered fractionation have been tested for patients undergoing curative treatment: accelerated fractionation and hyperfractionation. Accelerated fractionation emerged from analyses of the control of head and neck cancer as a function of dose administered and total treatment time. It was found that with an increasing dose there was increasing local control, but that protraction of treatment was associated with a loss of local control that was equivalent to about 0.75 Gy per day.[110] The data were best modeled by assuming that, approximately 2 weeks into treatment, tumor cells began to proliferate more rapidly than they were proliferating early in treatment (called *accelerated repopulation*).[111] In accelerated fractionation, the goal is to complete radiation before the accelerated tumor cell proliferation occurs. The most common method of achieving accelerated fractionation is to give a standard fraction to the entire field in the morning and to give a second treatment to the boost field in the afternoon (called *concomitant boost*). As in standard radiation, the boost would be given by extending the length of the treatment course; this concomitant boost approach can shorten treatment from 7 weeks to 5 weeks in head and neck cancer.

The second approach to altering fractionation is called *hyperfractionation*. Hyperfractionation is defined as the use of more than one fraction per day separated by more than 6 hours (see the section titled Biologic Aspects of Radiation Oncology), with a dose per fraction that is less than standard. Hyperfractionation is expected to produce fewer late complications for the same acute effects against both rapidly dividing normal tissues and tumors. Pure hyperfractionation might give 1 Gy twice a day, so that the total dose per day would be 2 Gy, and thus be equal to standard fractionation. In practice, hyperfractionated treatments are usually in the range of 1.2 Gy, which means that, compared with a standard fractionation, a somewhat higher dose is administered during the same period of time (so that most hyperfractionation also includes modest acceleration). The overall effect is to increase the acute toxicity (which resolves) and tumor response, while not increasing the (dose-limiting) late toxicity, which can improve cure rate. Both accelerated fractionation and hyperfractionation have been demonstrated in a meta-analysis to be superior to standard fractionation in the treatment of head and neck cancer with radiation alone.[112] However, a recent randomized trial has shown that there is no increase in control or survival, but there is an increase toxicity using chemotherapy with hyperfractionation compared to standard chemoradiation; therefore, the use of altered fractionation schemes has decreased dramatically during the last few years.[113]

Hypofractionation refers to the administration of a smaller number of larger fractions than is standard. Hypofractionation might be expected to cause more late toxicity for the same antitumor effect than standard or hyperfractionation. In the past, this approach was reserved for palliative cases, with the sense that a modest potential for increased late toxicity was not a major concern in patients with limited life expectancy. However, more recently, it has been proposed that the ability to better exclude normal tissue by using IGRT may permit hypofractionation to be used safely and that, in the specific case of prostate cancer, hypofractionation may have beneficial effects.[114]

ADVERSE EFFECTS

Radiation produces adverse effects in normal tissues. Although these are discussed in detail in later chapters as part of comprehensive discussions of organ toxicity, it is worth making some general comments here from the perspective of how radiation biology relates to the clinical toxicities. The term *radiation toxicity* is used to describe the adverse effects caused by radiation alone and radiation plus chemotherapy. Although this latter toxicity would be better labeled as *combined modality toxicity*, the pattern typically resembles a more severe form of the toxicity produced by radiation alone. Adverse effects from radiation can be divided into acute, subacute, and chronic (or late) effects. Acute effects are common, rarely serious, and usually self-limiting. Acute effects tend to occur in organs that depend on rapid self-renewal, most commonly the skin or mucosal surfaces (oropharynx, esophagus, small intestine, rectum, and bladder). This is due to radiation-induced cell death that occurs during mitosis, so that cells that divide rapidly show the most rapid cell loss. In the treatment of head and neck cancer, mucositis becomes worse during the first 3 to 4 weeks of therapy, but then will often stabilize as the normal mucosa cell proliferation increases in response to mucosal cell loss. It seems likely that normal tissue stem cells are relatively resistant to radiation compared with the more differentiated cells, because these stem cells survive to permit the normal mucosa to reepithelialize. Acute side effects typically resolve within 1 to 2 weeks of treatment completion, although occasionally these effects are so severe that they lead to consequential late effects, as described later.

Because lymphocytes are exquisitely sensitive to radiation, there has been considerable investigation into the effects of radiation on immune function. In contrast to mucosal cell killing, which requires mitosis, radiation kills lymphocytes in all phases of the cell cycle by apoptosis, so that lymphocyte counts decrease within days of initiating treatment. These effects do not tend to put patients at risk for infection, because granulocytes, which are chiefly responsible for combating infections, are relatively unaffected.

Two acute side effects of radiation do not fit neatly into these models relating to cell kill: nausea[115,116] and fatigue.[117,118] The origin of radiation-induced nausea is not related to acute cell loss, because it can occur within hours of the first treatment. Nausea is usually associated with radiation of the stomach, but it can sometimes occur during brain irradiation or from large-volume irradiation that involves neither the brain nor the stomach. Irradiation typically produces fatigue, even if relatively small volumes are irradiated. It seems likely that the origins of both of these *abscopal* effects of radiation (i.e., effects that occur systemically or at a distance for the site of irradiation) are related to the release of cytokines, but little is known.

Radiation can also produce subacute toxicities in the form of radiation pneumonitis and radiation-induced liver disease. These typically occur 2 weeks to 3 months after radiation is completed. The risk of radiation pneumonitis and radiation-induced liver disease is proportional to the mean dose delivered.[119,120] Thus, the 3D tools that permit the calculation of dose-volume histograms (described in the physics section) are currently used to determine the maximum safe treatment that can be delivered in terms of dose and volume. These toxicities appear to be initiated subclinically during the course of radiation as a cascade of cytokines in which TGF-β, tumor necrosis factor α, interleukin 6, and other cytokines play a role.[121] High TGF-β plasma levels during a course of treatment have been found to be associated with a greater risk of radiation pneumonitis.[122] Thus, in the future, we might look toward a combination of physical dose delivery, measured by the dose-volume histogram, the functional imaging of normal tissue damage, and the detection of biomarkers of toxicity, such as TGF-β, to improve the ability to individualize therapy. Attempts to determine the genomic basis of radiation sensitivity, beyond the known rare genetic defects such as ataxia telangiectasia, have not yet been successful.[123]

Late effects, which are typically seen 6 or more months after a course of radiation, include fibrosis, fistula formation, or long-term organ damage. Two theories for the origin of late effects have been put forth: late damage to the microvasculature and direct damage to the parenchyma. Although the vascular damage theory is attractive, it does not account for the differing sensitivities of organs to radiation. Perhaps the microvasculature is unique in each organ.[124] Regardless of the mechanism of toxicity, the tolerance of whole-organ radiation is now fairly well established (Table 13.2). Late complications can also be divided into two categories: consequential and true late effects. The best example of a consequential late effect is fibrosis and dysphagia after high-dose chemoradiation for head and neck cancer. Here, late fibrosis or ulceration appears to be the result of the mucosa becoming denuded for a prolonged time period. Late consequential effects are distinct from true late effects, which can follow a normal treatment course of self-limited toxicity and a 6-month or more symptom-free period. Examples of true late effects are radiation myelitis, radiation brain necrosis, and radiation-induced bowel obstruction. In the past, radiation fibrosis was thought to be an irreversible condition. Therefore, an exciting recent development is that severe radiation-induced breast fibrosis is an active process that can be reversed by drug therapy (pentoxifylline and vitamin E).[125]

TABLE 13.2

Radiation Tolerance Doses for Normal Tissues

	TD 5/5 (Gy)[a]			TD 50/5 (Gy)[b]			
	Portion of Organ Irradiated			Portion of Organ Irradiated			
Site	$^1/_3$	$^2/_3$	$^3/_3$	$^1/_3$	$^2/_3$	$^3/_3$	**Complication End Point(s)**
Kidney	50	30	23	—	40	28	Nephritis
Rain	60	50	45	75	65	60	Necrosis, infarct
Brain stem	60	53	50	—	—	65	Necrosis, infarct
Spinal cord	50 (5–10 cm)	—	47 (20 cm)	70 (5–10 cm)	—	—	Myelitis, necrosis
Lung	45	30	17.5	65	40	24.5	Radiation pneumonitis
Heart	60	45	40	70	55	50	Pericarditis
Esophagus	60	58	55	72	70	68	Stricture, perforation
Stomach	60	55	50	70	67	65	Ulceration, perforation
Small intestine	50	—	40	60	—	55	Obstruction, perforation, fistula
Colon	55	—	45	65	—	55	Obstruction, perforation, fistula, ulceration
Rectum	(100 cm^3 volume)		60	(100 cm^3 volume)		80	Severe proctitis, necrosis, fistula
Liver	50	35	30	55	45	40	Liver failure

[a]TD 5/5, the average dose that results in a 5% complication risk within 5 years.
[b]TD 50/5, the average dose that results in a 50% complication risk within 5 years.
Adapted from Emami B, Lyman J, Brown A, et al. Tolerance of normal tissue to therapeutic irradiation. *Int J Radiat Oncol Biol Phys* 1991;21:109–122.

PRINCIPLES OF COMBINING ANTICANCER AGENTS WITH RADIATION THERAPY

Combining chemotherapy with radiation therapy has produced important improvements in treatment outcome. Randomized clinical trials show improved local control and survival through the use of concurrent chemotherapy and radiation therapy for patients with high-grade gliomas and locally advanced cancers of the head and neck, lung, esophagus, stomach, rectum, prostate, and anus. There are least two proposed reasons why chemoradiotherapy might be successful. The first is radiosensitization. In the laboratory, radiosensitization is defined as a synergistic relationship, using mathematical approaches such as isobologram or median effect analysis.[126,127] The underlying concept is that the observed effect of using chemotherapy and radiation concurrently is greater than simply adding the two together. A second proposed reason to combine radiation and chemotherapy is to realize the benefit of improved local control radiation along with the systemic effect of chemotherapy, a concept called *spatial additivity*.[128]

Clinical results show that both radiosensitization and spatial additivity contribute to varying extents in different clinical settings. In the case of head and neck cancer, radiosensitization predominates. This conclusion is supported by the meta-analysis of head and neck cancer: sequential chemotherapy and radiotherapy produces little if any improvement in survival, whereas concurrent chemoradiation produces a significant increase in survival.[129] Furthermore, in the early positive studies using concurrent chemoradiation, systemic metastases were unaffected even though survival was improved. Radiosensitization may also predominate in the success of chemoradiotherapy for locally advanced lung cancer. For instance, although initial studies indicated that sequential chemotherapy and radiation had some benefit for lung cancer,[130] more recent work indicates that concurrent therapy is superior, and it is now the standard treatment.[131] However, there are also examples of spatial additivity. For example, both radiosensitization and spatial additivity is provided by the use of chemoradiation for locally advanced cervical cancer in that both local and systemic relapses are decreased by combined therapy.[132]

By targeting the aberrant growth factor or proangiogenic pathways that are specific to cancer cells rather than all rapidly proliferating cells, molecularly targeted therapies offer the potential to improve outcome without increasing toxicity. Even a selective cytostatic effect against the tumor would be predicted to act synergistically with radiation (Fig. 13.22). Although preclinical studies (summarized in the previous biology section) have highlighted the potential therapeutic gains that could be achieved by adding EGFR inhibitors to radiation, the best validation of this combination has been from the results of clinical trials in head and neck cancer. A phase III clinical trial demonstrated that, in a cohort of 424 patients with local–regionally advanced squamous cell carcinoma of the head and neck, the addition of cetuximab nearly doubled the median survival of patients (compared to radiotherapy alone), from 28 to 54 months. This study represents the first major success achieved by the addition of an EGFR antagonist to radiotherapy. This improvement was achieved without enhanced toxicity. Notably, the rates of pharyngitis and weight loss were identical in the two arms.[60] Local control was improved rather than the development of metastases, suggesting synergy rather than spatial additivity. Thus, the principle that can be derived from this study is that in tumors expressing high EGFR levels and that are likely to depend on aberrant EGF signaling, combining a true cytotoxic agent such as radiation with a cytostatic agent such as cetuximab has considerable promise.

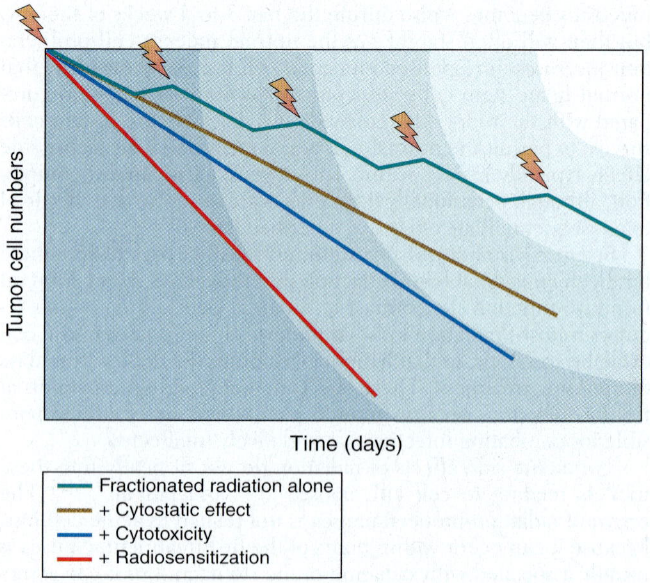

Figure 13.22 Potential mechanisms of synergy between epidermal growth factor receptor (EGFR) inhibitors and radiation. Although each daily radiation treatment kills a fraction of the cells, some cells grow back by the next day, which attenuates the effectiveness of radiation. If an EGFR inhibitor has only a selective cytostatic effect and blocks regrowth between fractions, the result would be a dramatic increase in radiation efficacy. The benefit of the inhibitor would be even greater if it caused tumor cell cytotoxicity or radiosensitization.

Because of the success of chemoradiotherapy, the natural tendency has not been to substitute molecularly targeted agents such as cetuximab for chemotherapy, but to add cetuximab to chemoradiotherapy. Thus, the combination of cisplatin, cetuximab, and radiation was recently found to have the same control rate as cisplatin and radiation for patients with locally advanced head and neck cancer, but the cetuximab arm had greater toxicity. Unfortunately, the triple therapy was never evaluated preclinically, and it has been shown preclinically that when EGFR inhibitors are given prior to chemotherapy, they can produce antagonism.[133] The principles of adding molecularly targeted therapy to chemoradiation are still evolving.[63]

REFERENCES

1. Hall EJ, Giaccia AJ. *Radiobiology for the Radiologist*. Philadelphia: Lippincott Williams & Williams; 2012.
2. Fowler JF. Developing aspects of radiation oncology. *Med Phys* 1981;8:427–434.
3. Lavin MF. Ataxia-telangiectasia: from a rare disorder to a paradigm for cell signalling and cancer. *Nat Rev Mol Cell Biol* 2008;9:759–769.
4. Thompson LH. Recognition, signaling, and repair of DNA double-strand breaks produced by ionizing radiation in mammalian cells: the molecular choreography. *Mutat Res* 2012;751:158–246.
5. Sherr CJ, McCormick F. The RB and p53 pathways in cancer. *Cancer Cell* 2002;2:103–112.
6. Bartek J, Lukas J. Chk1 and Chk2 kinases in checkpoint control and cancer. *Cancer Cell* 2003;3:421–429.
7. Kitagawa R, Bakkenist CJ, McKinnon PJ, et al. Phosphorylation of SMC1 is a critical downstream event in the ATM-NBS1-BRCA1 pathway. *Genes Dev* 2004;18:1423–1438.
8. Abraham RT. Cell cycle checkpoint signaling through the ATM and ATR kinases. *Genes Dev* 2001;15:2177–2196.
9. Mailand N, Podtelejnikov AV, Groth A, et al. Regulation of G(2)/M events by Cdc25A through phosphorylation-dependent modulation of its stability. *EMBO J* 2002;21:5911–5920.
10. Donzelli M, Draetta GF. Regulating mammalian checkpoints through Cdc25 inactivation. *EMBO Rep* 2003;4:671–677.
11. Tsvetkov L. Polo-like kinases and Chk2 at the interface of DNA damage checkpoint pathways and mitotic regulation. *IUBMB Life* 2004;56:449–456.

12. Dai Y, Grant S. New insights into checkpoint kinase 1 in the DNA damage response signaling network. *Clin Cancer Res* 2010;16:376–383.
13. Giaccia A, Weinstein R, Hu J, et al. Cell cycle-dependent repair of double-strand DNA breaks in a gamma-ray-sensitive Chinese hamster cell. *Somat Cell Mol Genet* 1985;11:485–491.
14. Kemp LM, Sedgwick SG, Jeggo PA. X-ray sensitive mutants of Chinese hamster ovary cells defective in double-strand break rejoining. *Mutat Res* 1984;132:189–196.
15. Helleday T, Lo J, van Gent DC, et al. DNA double-strand break repair: from mechanistic understanding to cancer treatment. *DNA Repair (Amst)* 2007;6:923–935.
16. Hefferin ML, Tomkinson AE. Mechanism of DNA double-strand break repair by non-homologous end joining. *DNA Repair (Amst)* 2005;4:639–648.
17. Ma Y, Pannicke U, Schwarz K, et al. Hairpin opening and overhang processing by an Artemis/DNA-dependent protein kinase complex in nonhomologous end joining and V(D)J recombination. *Cell* 2002;108:781–794.
18. Grawunder U, Wilm M, Wu X, et al. Activity of DNA ligase IV stimulated by complex formation with XRCC4 protein in mammalian cells. *Nature* 1997;388:492–495.
19. Chen L, Trujillo K, Sung P, et al. Interactions of the DNA ligase IV-XRCC4 complex with DNA ends and the DNA-dependent protein kinase. *J Biol Chem* 2000;275:26196–26205.
20. Tsukuda T, Fleming AB, Nickoloff JA, et al. Chromatin remodelling at a DNA double-strand break site in Saccharomyces cerevisiae. *Nature* 2005;438:379–383.
21. Yang YG, Saidi A, Frappart PO, et al. Conditional deletion of Nbs1 in murine cells reveals its role in branching repair pathways of DNA double-strand breaks. *EMBO J* 2006;25:5527–5538.
22. Esashi F, Galkin VE, Yu X, et al. Stabilization of RAD51 nucleoprotein filaments by the C-terminal region of BRCA2. *Nat Struct Mol Biol* 2007;14:468–474.
23. Sleeth KM, Sorensen CS, Issaeva N, et al. RPA mediates recombination repair during replication stress and is displaced from DNA by checkpoint signalling in human cells. *J Mol Biol* 2007;373:38–47.
24. Littlefield LG, Kleinerman RA, Sayer AM, et al. Chromosome aberrations in lymphocytes—biomonitors of radiation exposure. *Prog Clin Biol Res* 1991;372:387–397.
25. Toulany M, Rodemann HP. Membrane receptor signaling and control of DNA repair after exposure to ionizing radiation. *Nuklearmedizin* 2010;49:S26–S30.
26. Barcellos-Hoff MH, Akhurst RJ. Transforming growth factor-beta in breast cancer: too much, too late. *Breast Cancer Res* 2009;11:202.
27. Deng X, Yin X, Allan R, et al. Ceramide biogenesis is required for radiation-induced apoptosis in the germ line of *C. elegans*. *Science* 2008;322:110–115.
28. Thompson LH, Suit HD. Proliferation kinetics of x-irradiated mouse L cells studied WITH TIME-lapse photography. II. *Int J Radiat Biol Relat Stud Phys Chem Med* 1969;15:347–362.
29. Sowa Resat MB, Morgan WF. Radiation-induced genomic instability: a role for secreted soluble factors in communicating the radiation response to non-irradiated cells. *J Cell Biochem* 2004;92:1013–1019.
30. Elkind MM. The initial part of the survival curve: does it predict the outcome of fractionated radiotherapy? *Radiat Res* 1988;114:425–436.
31. McCulloch EA, Till JE. The sensitivity of cells from normal mouse bone marrow to gamma radiation in vitro and in vivo. *Radiat Res* 1962;16:822–832.
32. Withers HR. Recovery and repopulation in vivo by mouse skin epithelial cells during fractionated irradiation. *Radiat Res* 1967;32:227–239.
33. Withers HR, Elkind MM. Microcolony survival assay for cells of mouse intestinal mucosa exposed to radiation. *Int J Radiat Biol Relat Stud Phys Chem Med* 1970;17:261–267.
34. Suit H, Wette R. Radiation dose fractionation and tumor control probability. *Radiat Res* 1966;29:267–281.
35. O'Neill K, Lyons SK, Gallagher WM, et al. Bioluminescent imaging: a critical tool in pre-clinical oncology research. *J Pathol* 2010;220:317–327.
36. Hewitt HB, Wilson CW. Survival curves for tumor cells irradiated in vivo. *Ann N Y Acad Sci* 1961;95:818–827.
37. Hill RP, Bush RS. A lung-colony assay to determine the radiosensitivity of cells of a solid tumour. *Int J Radiat Biol Relat Stud Phys Chem Med* 1969;15: 435–444.
38. Elkind MM, Sutton-Gilbert H, Moses WB, et al. Radiation response of mammalian cells grown in culture. V. Temperature dependence of the repair of x-ray damage in surviving cells (aerobic and hypoxic). *Radiat Res* 1965;25: 359–376.
39. Elkind MM, Whitmore GF. *Radiobiology of Cultured Mammalian Cells*. New York: Gordon and Breach; 1967.
40. Mottram JC. Factors of importance in radiosensitivity of tumors. *Br J Radiol* 1936;9:606.
41. Palcic B, Skarsgard LD. Reduced oxygen enhancement ratio at low doses of ionizing radiation. *Radiat Res* 1984;100:328–339.
42. Thomlinson RH, Gray LH. The histological structure of some human lung cancers and the possible implications for radiotherapy. *Br J Cancer* 1955;9:539–549.
43. Overgaard J, Horsman MR. Modification of hypoxia-induced radioresistance in tumors by the use of oxygen and sensitizers. *Semin Radiat Oncol* 1996;6:10–21.
44. Machtay M, Pajak TF, Suntharalingam M, et al. Radiotherapy with or without erythropoietin for anemic patients with head and neck cancer: a randomized trial of the Radiation Therapy Oncology Group (RTOG 99-03). *Int J Radiat Oncol Biol Phys* 2007;69:1008–1017.
45. Henke M, Laszig R, Rube C, et al. Erythropoietin to treat head and neck cancer patients with anaemia undergoing radiotherapy: randomised, double-blind, placebo-controlled trial. *Lancet* 2003;362:1255–1260.
46. Janssens GO, Rademakers SE, Terhaard CH, et al. Accelerated radiotherapy with carbogen and nicotinamide for laryngeal cancer: results of a phase III randomized trial. *J Clin Oncol* 2012;30:1777–1783.
47. Willett CG, Boucher Y, di Tomaso E, et al. Direct evidence that the VEGF-specific antibody bevacizumab has antivascular effects in human rectal cancer. *Nat Med* 2004;10:145–147.
48. Lapi SE, Voller TF, Welch MJ. Positron emission tomography imaging of hypoxia. *PET Clin* 2009;4:39–47.
49. Lee NY, Mechalakos JG, Nehmeh S, et al. Fluorine-18-labeled fluoromisonidazole positron emission and computed tomography-guided intensity-modulated radiotherapy for head and neck cancer: a feasibility study. *Int J Radiat Oncol Biol Phys* 2008;70:2–13.
50. Schaue D, Xie MW, Ratikan JA, et al. Regulatory T cells in radiotherapeutic responses. *Front Oncol* 2012;2:90.
51. Formenti SC, Demaria S. Combining radiotherapy and cancer immunotherapy: a paradigm shift. *J Natl Cancer Inst* 2013;105:256–265.
52. Lawrence TS, Davis MA, Tang HY, et al. Fluorodeoxyuridine-mediated cytotoxicity and radiosensitization require S phase progression. *Int J Radiat Biol* 1996;70:273–280.
53. Lawrence TS, Chang EY, Hahn TM, et al. Radiosensitization of pancreatic cancer cells by 2′,2′-difluoro-2′-deoxycytidine. *Int J Radiat Oncol Biol Phys* 1996;34:867–872.
54. Eisbruch A, Shewach DS, Bradford CR, et al. Radiation concurrent with gemcitabine for locally advanced head and neck cancer: a phase I trial and intracellular drug incorporation study. *J Clin Oncol* 2001;19:792–799.
55. Ben-Josef E, Schipper M, Francis IR, et al. A phase I/II trial of intensity modulated radiation (IMRT) dose escalation with concurrent fixed-dose rate gemcitabine (FDR-G) in patients with unresectable pancreatic cancer. *Int J Radiat Oncol Biol Phys* 2012;84:1166–1171.
56. Wolff RA, Evans DB, Gravel DM, et al. Phase I trial of gemcitabine combined with radiation for the treatment of locally advanced pancreatic adenocarcinoma. *Clin Cancer Res* 2001;7:2246–2253.
57. Wilson GD, Bentzen SM, Harari PM. Biologic basis for combining drugs with radiation. *Semin Radiat Oncol* 2006;16:2–9.
58. Bradley JD, Paulus R, Graham MV, et al. Phase II trial of postoperative adjuvant paclitaxel/carboplatin and thoracic radiotherapy in resected stage II and IIIA non-small-cell lung cancer: promising long-term results of the Radiation Therapy Oncology Group—RTOG 9705. *J Clin Oncol* 2005;23:3480–3487.
59. Nyati MK, Morgan MA, Feng FY, et al. Integration of EGFR inhibitors with radiochemotherapy. *Nat Rev Cancer* 2006;6:876–885.
60. Bonner JA, Harari PM, Giralt J, et al. Radiotherapy plus cetuximab for locoregionally advanced head and neck cancer: 5-year survival data from a phase 3 randomised trial, and relation between cetuximab-induced rash and survival. *Lancet Oncol* 2010;11:21–28.
61. Ang KK, Zhang QE, Rosenthal DI, et al. A randomized phase III trial (RTOG 0522) of concurrent accelerated radiation plus cisplatin with or without cetuximab for stage III-IV head and neck squamous cell carcinomas (HNC). *J Clin Oncol* 2011;29.
62. Engelke CG, Parsels LA, Qian Y, et al. Sensitization of pancreatic cancer to chemoradiation by the Chk1 inhibitor MK8776. *Clin Cancer Res* 2013;19:4412–4421.
63. Morgan MA, Parsels LA, Maybaum J, et al. Improving the efficacy of chemoradiation with targeted agents. *Cancer Discov* 2014;4:280–291.
64. Chalmers AJ, Lakshman M, Chan N, et al. Poly(ADP-ribose) polymerase inhibition as a model for synthetic lethality in developing radiation oncology targets. *Semin Radiat Oncol* 2010;20:274–281.
65. Brizel DM, Wasserman TH, Henke M, et al. Phase III randomized trial of amifostine as a radioprotector in head and neck cancer. *J Clin Oncol* 2000;18:3339–3345.
66. Winczura P, Jassem J. Combined treatment with cytoprotective agents and radiotherapy. *Cancer Treat Rev* 2010;36:268–275.
67. Van Dyk J, ed. Radiation oncology medical physics resources for working, teaching, and learning. In: *The Modern Technology of Radiation Oncology*. Volume 3. Medical Physics Publishing Web site. http://www.medicalphysics.org/vandykch16.pdf. Madison, WI: Medical Physics Publishing; 2013.
68. Karzmark C, Nunan C, Tanabe E. *Medical Electron Accelerators*. New York: McGraw-Hill Ryerson; 1993.
69. Greene D, Williams P. *Linear Accelerators for Radiation Therapy*. 2nd ed. New York: Taylor and Francis Group; 1997.
70. Fenwick JD, Tome WA, Soisson ET, et al. Tomotherapy and other innovative IMRT delivery systems. *Semin Radiat Oncol* 2006;16:199–208.
71. Curran B, Balter J, Chetty I, eds. *Integrating New Technologies into the Clinic: Monte Carlo and Image-Guided Radiation Therapy*. Madison, WI: Medical Physics Publishing; 2006.
72. Bourland J, ed. *Image-Guided Radiation Therapy*. Boca Raton, FL: Taylor & Francis; 2012.
73. Seco J, Verhaegen F, eds. *Monte Carlo Techniques in Radiation Therapy*. Boca Raton, FL: Taylor & Francis; 2013.
74. Kessler ML. Image registration and data fusion in radiation therapy. *Br J Radiol* 2006;79:S99–S108.
75. Brock K, ed. *Image Processing in Radiation Therapy*. Boca Raton, FL: Taylor & Francis Group; 2014.
76. Sovik A, Malinen E, Olsen DR. Strategies for biologic image-guided dose escalation: a review. *Int J Radiat Oncol Biol Phys* 2009;73:650–658.
77. Marks LB, Ten Haken RK, Martel MK. Guest editor's introduction to QUANTEC: a users guide. *Int J Radiat Oncol Biol Phys* 2010;76:S1–S2.

78. Li A, Alber M, Deasy JO, et al. The use and QA of biologically related models for treatment planning: short report of the TG-166 of the therapy physics committee of the AAPM. *Med Phys* 2012;39:1386–1409.
79. Bortfeld T. IMRT: a review and preview. *Phys Med Biol* 2006;51:R363–R379.
80. Webb S. *Contemporary IMRT Developing Physics and Clinical Implementation*. London: IOP Publishing; 2005.
81. Maughan R, Yudelev M. Neutron therapy. In: Van Dyk J, ed. *The Modern Technology of Radiation Oncology*. Madison, WI: Medical Physics Publishing; 1999.
82. Hogstrom KR, Almond PR. Review of electron beam therapy physics. *Phys Med Biol* 2006;51:R455–R489.
83. Schlegel W, Bortfeld T, Grosu A, eds. *New Technologies in Radiation Oncology*. Heidelberg: Springer-Verlag; 2006.
84. Ma C-MC, Lomax T, eds. *Proton and Carbon Ion Therapy*. Boca Raton, FL: Taylor & Francis Group; 2012.
85. Venselaar J, Meigooni A, Baltas D, et al., eds. *Comprehensive Brachytherapy: Physical and Clinical Aspects*. Boca Raton, FL: Taylor & Francis Group; 2012.
86. Meredith RF. Systemic targeted radionuclide therapy symposium introduction. *Int J Radiat Oncol Biol Phys* 2006;66:S7.
87. Tripuraneni P, Watson RL, Ang KK, et al. Intersociety Radiation Oncology Summit-SCOPE II. *Int J Radiat Oncol Biol Phys* 2008;72:323–326.
88. Delaney G, Jacob S, Featherstone C, et al. The role of radiotherapy in cancer treatment: estimating optimal utilization from a review of evidence-based clinical guidelines. *Cancer* 2005;104:1129–1137.
89. Zelefsky MJ, Housman DM, Pei X, et al. Incidence of secondary cancer development after high-dose intensity-modulated radiotherapy and image-guided brachytherapy for the treatment of localized prostate cancer. *Int J Radiat Oncol Biol Phys* 2012;83:953–959.
90. Combs SE, Laperriere N, Brada M. Clinical controversies: proton radiation therapy for brain and skull base tumors. *Semin Radiat Oncol* 2013;23:120–126.
91. Overgaard J. Hypoxic radiosensitization: adored and ignored. *J Clin Oncol* 2007;25:4066–4074.
92. Mouw KW, Trofimov A, Zietman AL, et al. Clinical controversies: proton therapy for prostate cancer. *Semin Radiat Oncol* 2013;23:109–114.
93. Yu JB, Soulos PR, Herrin J, et al. Proton versus intensity-modulated radiotherapy for prostate cancer: patterns of care and early toxicity. *J Natl Cancer Inst* 2013;105:25–32.
94. Brada M, Pijls-Johannesma M, De Ruysscher D. Proton therapy in clinical practice: current clinical evidence. *J Clin Oncol* 2007;25:965–970.
95. Douglas JG, Koh WJ, Austin-Seymour M, et al. Treatment of salivary gland neoplasms with fast neutron radiotherapy. *Arch Otolaryngol Head Neck Surg* 2003;129:944–948.
96. Shilkrut M, Merrick GS, McLaughlin PW, et al. The addition of low-dose-rate brachytherapy and androgen-deprivation therapy decreases biochemical failure and prostate cancer death compared with dose-escalated external-beam radiation therapy for high-risk prostate cancer. *Cancer* 2013;119:681–690.
97. Iyengar P, Timmerman R. Stereotactic ablative radiotherapy for non-small cell lung cancer: rationale and outcomes. *J Natl Compr Canc Netw* 2012;10:1514–1520.
98. Lo SS, Moffatt-Bruce SD, Dawson LA, et al. The role of local therapy in the management of lung and liver oligometastases. *Nat Rev Clin Oncol* 2011;8:405–416.
99. Forastiere AA, Zhang Q, Weber RS, et al. Long-term results of RTOG 91-11: a comparison of three nonsurgical treatment strategies to preserve the larynx in patients with locally advanced larynx cancer. *J Clin Oncol* 2013;31:845–852.
100. Gunderson LL, Winter KA, Ajani JA, et al. Long-term update of US GI intergroup RTOG 98-11 phase III trial for anal carcinoma: survival, relapse, and colostomy failure with concurrent chemoradiation involving fluorouracil/mitomycin versus fluorouracil/cisplatin. *J Clin Oncol* 2012;30:4344–4351.
101. Hellman S, Weichselbaum RR. Oligometastases. *J Clin Oncol* 1995;13:8–10.
102. Hortobagyi GN. Can we cure limited metastatic breast cancer? *J Clin Oncol* 2002;20:620–623.
103. Stamell EF, Wolchok JD, Gnjatic S, et al. The abscopal effect associated with a systemic anti-melanoma immune response. *Int J Radiat Oncol Biol Phys* 2013;85:293–295.
104. Nagtegaal ID, Gosens MJ, Marijnen CA, et al. Combinations of tumor and treatment parameters are more discriminative for prognosis than the present TNM system in rectal cancer. *J Clin Oncol* 2007;25:1647–1650.
105. Sauer R, Becker H, Hohenberger W, et al. Preoperative versus postoperative chemoradiotherapy for rectal cancer. *N Engl J Med* 2004;351:1731–1740.
106. Clarke M, Collins R, Darby S, et al. Effects of radiotherapy and of differences in the extent of surgery for early breast cancer on local recurrence and 15-year survival: an overview of the randomised trials. *Lancet* 2005;366:2087–2106.
107. Hellman S. Stopping metastases at their source. *N Engl J Med* 1997;337:996–997.
108. Marks LB, Prosnitz LR. Postoperative radiotherapy for lung cancer: the breast cancer story all over again? *Int J Radiat Oncol Biol Phys* 2000;48:625–627.
109. Wang XS, Rhines LD, Shiu AS, et al. Stereotactic body radiation therapy for management of spinal metastases in patients without spinal cord compression: a phase 1-2 trial. *Lancet Oncol* 2012;13:395–402.
110. Tarnawski R, Fowler J, Skladowski K, et al. How fast is repopulation of tumor cells during the treatment gap? *Int J Radiat Oncol Biol Phys* 2002;54:229–236.
111. Peters LJ, Withers HR. Applying radiobiological principles to combined modality treatment of head and neck cancer—the time factor. *Int J Radiat Oncol Biol Phys* 1997;39:831–836.
112. Bourhis J, Overgaard J, Audry H, et al. Hyperfractionated or accelerated radiotherapy in head and neck cancer: a meta-analysis. *Lancet* 2006;368:843–854.
113. Bourhis J, Sire C, Graff P, et al. Concomitant chemoradiotherapy versus acceleration of radiotherapy with or without concomitant chemotherapy in locally advanced head and neck carcinoma (GORTEC 99-02): an open-label phase 3 randomised trial. *Lancet Oncol* 2012;13:145–153.
114. Adkison JB, McHaffie DR, Bentzen SM, et al. Phase I trial of pelvic nodal dose escalation with hypofractionated IMRT for high-risk prostate cancer. *Int J Radiat Oncol Biol Phys* 2012;82:184–190.
115. Feyer P, Maranzano E, Molassiotis A, et al. Radiotherapy-induced nausea and vomiting (RINV): antiemetic guidelines. *Support Care Cancer* 2005;13:122–128.
116. Horiot JC. Prophylaxis versus treatment: is there a better way to manage radiotherapy-induced nausea and vomiting? *Int J Radiat Oncol Biol Phys* 2004;60:1018–1025.
117. Hickok JT, Roscoe JA, Morrow GR, et al. Frequency, severity, clinical course, and correlates of fatigue in 372 patients during 5 weeks of radiotherapy for cancer. *Cancer* 2005;104:1772–1778.
118. Schwartz AL, Nail LM, Chen S, et al. Fatigue patterns observed in patients receiving chemotherapy and radiotherapy. *Cancer Invest* 2000;18:11–19.
119. Dawson LA, Ten Haken RK. Partial volume tolerance of the liver to radiation. *Semin Radiat Oncol* 2005;15:279–283.
120. Kong FM, Hayman JA, Griffith KA, et al. Final toxicity results of a radiation-dose escalation study in patients with non-small-cell lung cancer (NSCLC): predictors for radiation pneumonitis and fibrosis. *Int J Radiat Oncol Biol Phys* 2006;65:1075–1086.
121. Fleckenstein K, Gauter-Fleckenstein B, Jackson IL, et al. Using biological markers to predict risk of radiation injury. *Semin Radiat Oncol* 2007;17:89–98.
122. Hart JP, Broadwater G, Rabbani Z, et al. Cytokine profiling for prediction of symptomatic radiation-induced lung injury. *Int J Radiat Oncol Biol Phys* 2005;63:1448–1454.
123. Barnett GC, Coles CE, Elliott RM, et al. Independent validation of genes and polymorphisms reported to be associated with radiation toxicity: a prospective analysis study. *Lancet Oncol* 2012;13:65–77.
124. Fajardo LF. Is the pathology of radiation injury different in small vs large blood vessels? *Cardiovasc Radiat Med* 1999;1:108–110.
125. Delanian S, Porcher R, Rudant J, et al. Kinetics of response to long-term treatment combining pentoxifylline and tocopherol in patients with superficial radiation-induced fibrosis. *J Clin Oncol* 2005;23:8570–8579.
126. Chou TC, Talalay P. Quantitative analysis of dose-effect relationships: the combined effects of multiple drugs or enzyme inhibitors. *Adv Enzyme Regul* 1984;22:27–55.
127. Steel GG, Peckham MJ. Exploitable mechanisms in combined radiotherapy-chemotherapy: the concept of additivity. *Int J Radiat Oncol Biol Phys* 1979;5:85–91.
128. Tannock IF. Treatment of cancer with radiation and drugs. *J Clin Oncol* 1996;14:3156–3174.
129. Blanchard P, Baujat B, Holostenco V, et al. Meta-analysis of chemotherapy in head and neck cancer (MACH-NC): a comprehensive analysis by tumour site. *Radiother Oncol* 2011;100:33–40.
130. Dillman RO, Herndon J, Seagren SL, et al. Improved survival in stage III non-small-cell lung cancer: seven-year follow-up of cancer and leukemia group B (CALGB) 8433 trial. *J Natl Cancer Inst* 1996;88:1210–1215.
131. De Ruysscher D, Belderbos J, Reymen B, et al. State of the art radiation therapy for lung cancer 2012: a glimpse of the future. *Clin Lung Cancer* 2013;14:89–95.
132. Klopp AH, Eifel PJ. Chemoradiotherapy for cervical cancer in 2010. *Curr Oncol Rep* 2011;13:77–85.
133. Chun PY, Feng FY, Scheurer AM, et al. Synergistic effects of gemcitabine and gefitinib in the treatment of head and neck carcinoma. *Cancer Res* 2006;66:981–988.

14 Cancer Immunotherapy

Steven A. Rosenberg, Paul F. Robbins, Giao Q. Phan,
Steven A. Feldman, and James N. Kochenderfer

INTRODUCTION

Progress in understanding basic aspects of cellular immunology and tumor–host immune interactions have led to the development of immune-based therapies capable of mediating the rejection of metastatic cancer in humans. Early studies of allografts and transplanted syngeneic tumors in mice demonstrated that it was the cellular arm of the immune response rather than the action of antibodies (humoral immunity) that was responsible for tissue rejection. Thus, studies of immunotherapy have focused on enhancing antitumor immune responses of T cells that recognize cancer antigens. Antibodies that recognize growth factors on the surface of tumors can contribute to tumor regression, primarily by interfering with growth signals rather than by the direct destruction of tumor cells. The use of monoclonal antibodies in cancer treatment will be considered in Chapter 29.

Evidence for specific tumor recognition by cells of the immune system was obtained in experiments first conducted in the 1940s using murine tumors generated or induced by the mutagen methylcholanthrene (MCA). Mice that received a surgical resection of previously inoculated tumors could be protected against a subsequent tumor challenge with the immunizing tumor but not generally protected against challenge with additional MCA tumors. The observation that CD8+ cytotoxic T cells were primarily responsible for mediating the rejection of MCA-induced tumors in mice led to the identification of genes that encoded tumor rejection antigens expressed on murine tumors as well as the subsequent identification of antigens recognized by human tumor-reactive T cells. The identification of widely shared nonmutated tumor antigens led to the expectation that effective vaccine therapies could be developed for the treatment of cancer patients; however, the response rates in clinical cancer vaccine trials targeting these antigens have, to this point, been disappointingly low. Vaccination with viruslike particles expressing human papilloma virus (HPV) proteins are successful in preventing the establishment of cervical cancer and immunization with peptides derived from the oncogenic HPV E6 and E7 proteins can mediate tumor regression in woman with high vulvar neoplasia.[1] Immune-based therapies have, however, been identified that mediate the regression of large, established tumor metastases. Nonspecific immune stimulation with interleukin-2 (IL-2) administration can lead to objective clinical responses in patients with melanoma and renal cancer,[2] and inhibition of regulatory pathways mediated by CTLA-4[3] or PD-1[4] can lead to tumor regression in patients with metastatic melanoma and lung cancer. The adoptive transfer of melanoma reactive T cells can mediate objective clinical responses in 50% to 70% of patients with melanoma,[5] and the ability to genetically modify antitumor lymphocytes is expanding this cell transfer therapy approach to the treatment of patients with other cancer histologies.[6] Studies aimed at identifying potent tumor rejection antigens, as well as mechanisms that regulate immune responses to cancer, are being actively pursued.

HUMAN TUMOR ANTIGENS

To be recognized by immune lymphocytes, intracellular proteins must be digested and the resulting peptides transported to the cell surface and bound to Class I or II main histocompatibility molecules (Fig. 14.1). A variety of approaches have been used to identify the antigens that are naturally processed and presented on tumor cells. These include evaluating the ability of cells transfected with tumor cDNA library pools along with genes encoding autologous major histocompatibility complex (MHC) molecules, as well as the ability of target cells pulsed with peptides eluted from tumor cell surface MHC molecules for their ability to stimulate tumor reactive T cells. Reverse immunology approaches that involve either repeated in vitro T cell sensitization or in vivo immunization with candidate peptides or proteins have also lead to the identification of tumor antigens. Candidate epitopes identified on the basis of their ability to bind to a particular MHC molecule, however, may not necessarily be naturally processed and presented on the tumor cell surface, and there are conflicting reports on the ability of T cells generated using some candidate epitopes to recognize unmanipulated tumor targets, as discussed further.

Additional tumor antigens have been identified using antisera from cancer patients to screen tumor cell cDNA libraries, a method that has been termed serological analysis of recombinant cDNA expression (SEREX).[7] Although some of the proteins identified using this technique are expressed in a tumor-specific manner, many of these antigens are simply expressed at higher levels in tumor cells than in normal cells. This may occur due to the release of normal self-proteins from necrotic and apoptotic tumor cells leading to the generation of antibodies against intracellular proteins that are normally sequestered from the immune system.

Finally, the use of recently described approaches involving whole exomic sequencing of tumor cells has led to the identification of mutated tumor antigens. These studies will be discussed further in the section devoted to mutated tumor antigens

Cancer/Germ-Line Antigens

The first antigen identified as a target of human tumor reactive T cells was isolated by screening a melanoma genomic DNA library with an autologous cytotoxic T lymphocyte (CTL) clone.[8] The gene that was isolated, termed *MAGE-1*, was found to be a nonmutated gene that was a member of a large, previously unidentified gene family, many of whose members encode antigens recognized by tumor reactive T cells.[9] Members of this family of antigens are expressed in the testes and placenta, both of which lack an expression of MHC molecules, but often not in other normal tissues, which has led to their designation as cancer germ-line (CG) antigens. Members of the MAGE gene family are expressed in a variety of tumor types, including melanoma, breast, prostate, and esophageal cancers. The expression patterns of three

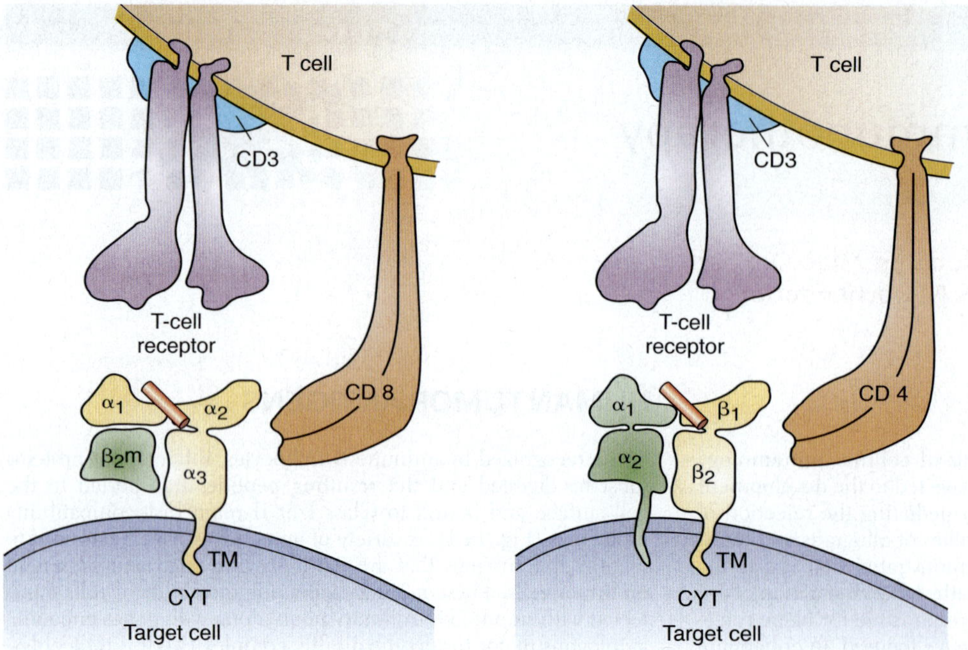

Figure 14.1 CD8 and CD4 cells use different molecules that interact with major histocompatibility complex (MHC) class I and II molecules respectively on the cell surface and serve to potentiate immune reactions.

different cancer/testes antigens in multiple tumor types is shown in Figure 14.2. The NY-ESO-1 antigen—a CG antigen that is unrelated to the MAGE family of genes—is expressed in approximately 30% of breast, prostate, and melanoma tumors, as well as between 70% and 80% of synovial cell sarcomas.[10]

Clinical adoptive immunotherapy trials targeting CG antigens have now been conducted in patients with melanoma as well as other tumor types. In a recent trial, objective clinical responses were seen in approximately 50% of patients with melanoma and 80% of patients with synovial cell sarcoma receiving autologous peripheral blood mononuclear cell (PBMC) transduced with a T-cell receptor directed against an HLA-A*02:01 restricted NY-ESO-1 epitope.[6] A trial targeting a MAGEA3 epitopes was recently carried out using a T-cell receptor (TCR) isolated from an HLA-A*02:01$^+$ transgenic mouse immunized with the MAGEA3:112–120 peptide.[11] Objective clinical responses were observed in five of nine melanoma patients receiving the adoptively transferred PBMC that were transduced with the MAGEA3-reactive TCR.[12] Unexpectedly, neural toxicity was observed in three of the patients treated in this trial, two of whom lapsed into a coma and subsequently died. Autopsy samples of patients' brains revealed that *MAGEA12*, which encodes a cross-reactive epitope recognized by the MAGEA3 TCR, was expressed at low levels in patients' brains, which may have been responsible for the observed neurologic toxicities. In a recent trial carried out using an affinity-enhanced human TCR directed against the

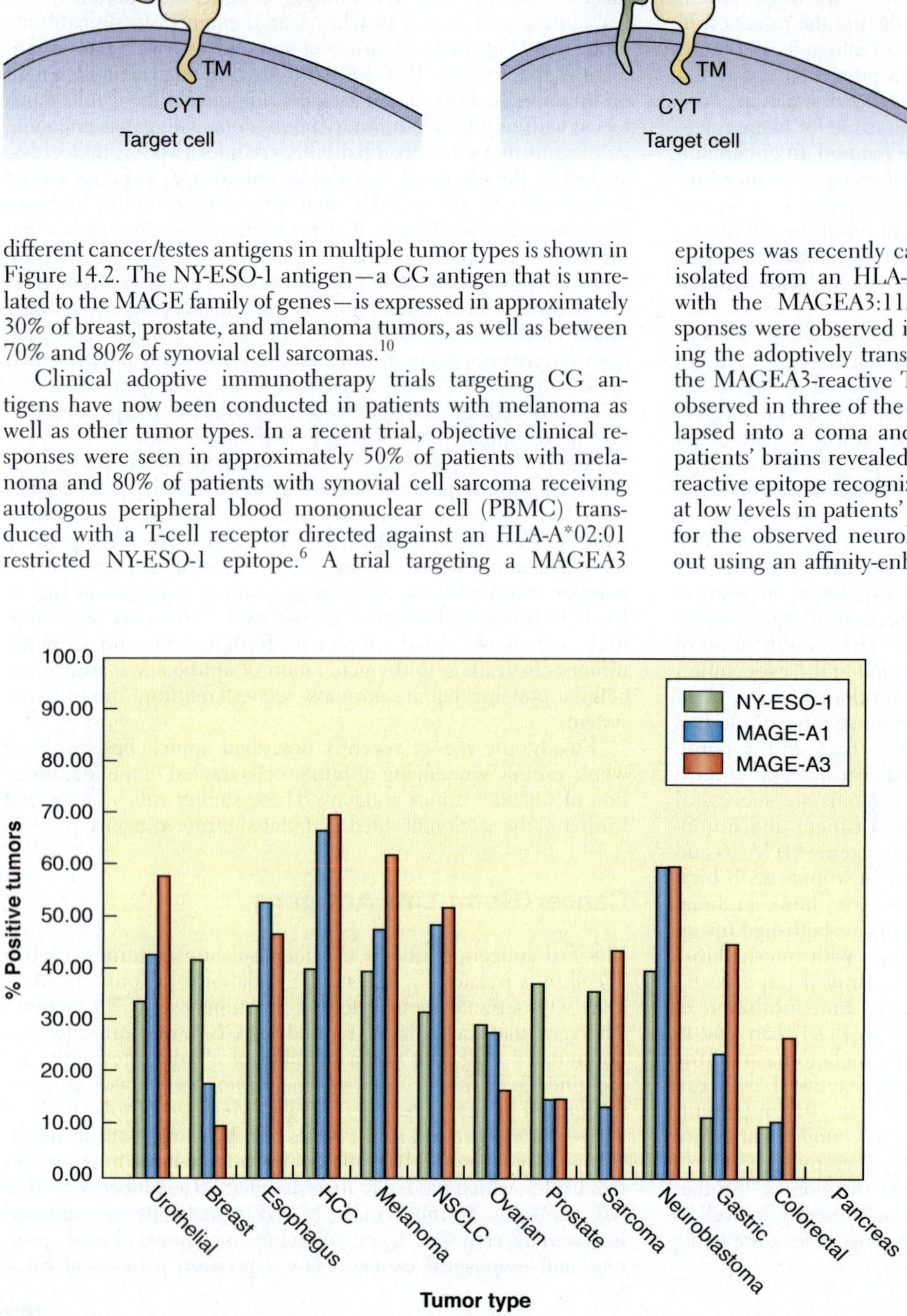

Figure 14.2 Expression of three different cancer/testes antigens in many different tumor types is shown. These data reflect reverse transcription–polymerase chain reaction measurements and is more sensitive than results obtained by immunohistochemistry. NSCLC, non–small-cell lung cancer. (Data compiled by Dr. J. Wargo. Massachusetts General Hospital.)

HLA-A*01:01-restricted, MAGEA3:168-176 epitope, the first two patients receiving TCR-transduced autologous PBMC died of cardiac arrest 4 to 5 days following infusion, which was attributed to cross-reactivity with titin, a protein expressed at high levels in cardimyocytes.[13] Taken together, these findings demonstrate the need for caution in evaluating cross-reactivity of high affinity TCRs recognizing tumor antigens.

Melanocyte Differentiation Antigens

Melanoma-reactive T cells have been frequently found to recognize gene products, termed melanocyte differentiation antigens (MDA), that are expressed in melanomas as well as in normal melanocytes present in the skin, eye, and ear but not in other normal tissues or tumor types. These include epitopes derived from gp100,[14,15] tyrosinase,[16] TRP-1,[17] and TRP-2,[18] proteins that had previously been found to play important roles in melanin synthesis. The screening of melanoma cDNA libraries with an HLA-A2–restricted tumor reactive T cells lead to the isolation of a previously unidentified gene, termed MART-1[19] or Melan-A.[20] The MART-1 antigen, which is expressed in 80% to 90% of fresh melanomas and cultured melanoma cell lines as well as normal melanocytes, represents an MDA of unknown function. The majority of melanoma reactive, HLA-A2–restricted tumor-infiltrating lymphocytes (TIL) recognize a single MART-1 epitope.[21] Studies carried out using a variety of approaches have also resulted in the identification of human leukocyte antigen (HLA) class II restricted epitopes of tyrosinase, TRP-1, TRP-2, and gp100.[9]

Overexpressed Gene Products

Gene products that are expressed at low levels in a variety of normal tissues but are overexpressed in a variety of tumor types have also been shown to be recognized by T cells. Screening of an autologous renal carcinoma cDNA library with a tumor reactive, HLA-A3–restricted T-cell clone resulted in the isolation of FGF5,[22] a protein that was expressed only at low levels in normal tissues but upregulated in multiple renal carcinomas as well as prostate and breast carcinomas. The peptide epitope recognized by FGF5-reactive T cells was generated by protein splicing, a process in which distant protein regions are joined together in the proteasome that had previously only been described in plants[23] and unicellular organisms.[24] Subsequent studies have led to the identification of multiple epitopes that result from protein splicing, suggesting that this represents a general mechanism for generating T-cell epitopes.[25–28] Screening of an autologous cDNA library led to the identification of a previously unknown gene that was termed *PRAME*.[29] This gene product was expressed in relatively high levels in melanomas as well as in additional tumor types but was also expressed at lower levels in a variety of normal tissues that included the testis, endometrium, ovary, and adrenals. The HLA-A24–restricted PRAME reactive T-cell clone, however, expressed the natural killer (NK) inhibitory receptor p58.2, and tumor cell recognition was dependent on the loss of expression of the HLA C*07 allele that represented the ligand for the inhibitory receptor, which may explain the lack of recognition of normal tissues that express relatively high levels of this HLA gene product.

Attempts have also been made to generate T cells directed against overexpressed candidate antigens by repeatedly stimulating PBMC in vitro with peptides that were identified as high binders for particular MHC molecules either using direct binding assays or *in silico* analysis carried out using peptide/MHC binding algorithms.[30,31] Using this approach, candidate epitopes have been identified from a variety of proteins that include prostate-specific antigen (PSA)[32] and prostate-specific membrane antigen (PSMA),[33] as well as Her-2/neu, a protein that is frequently overexpressed in a variety of tumor types, including breast carcinomas. Initial studies indicated that T cells derived by in vitro stimulation with a peptide that was predicted to bind with high affinity to HLA-A*02:01, Her-2/neu:369–377, recognized the appropriate natural tumor targets.[34] In one study, T cells generated following two in vitro stimulations of postvaccination PBMC from three of the four patients who were tested efficiently recognized peptide-pulsed targets but failed to recognize appropriate tumor targets.[35] Similarly, although stimulation with a peptide corresponding to amino acids 540 through 548 of the human telomerase reverse transcriptase (hTERT) catalytic subunit was initially reported to generate tumor-reactive T cells,[36] additional observations indicated that T cells generated using this peptide failed to recognize tumor targets.[37] These factors responsible for these discrepancies remain unresolved, although the in vitro stimulation of T cells with target cells pulsed with relatively high peptide concentrations could have led to the generation of low-avidity T cells that were incapable of recognizing naturally processed antigens.

Alternative screening approaches employed for tumor antigen discovery that may help to address these issues include the use of tandem mass spectrometry to sequence peptides that have been eluted from tumor cell surface MHC molecules. Use of this technique, coupled with microarray gene expression profiling, resulted in the identification of peptides derived from proteins that appeared to be overexpressed in tumor cells.[38] Peptides identified using this approach may, in many cases, not be immunogenic due to the fact that their expression in normal tissues, although lower than in tumor cells, may be high enough to lead to central or peripheral tolerance. Nevertheless, one of the peptides that were identified in this study also appeared to be recognized by human tumor reactive T cells. Recently, a similar approach was used to identify candidate peptides presented on cell surface MHC molecules that appeared to be derived from proteins that were overexpressed on glioblastomas.[39] In a clinical trial involving vaccination of patients with pools of the identified peptides, overall survival was associated with the number of peptides in the vaccine pool that elicited immune response[40]; however, this may simply reflect the fact that T cells from healthier patients can more readily generate peptide-specific responses.

Transgenic mice that express human HLA molecules have also been immunized with candidate antigens in an attempt to identify high avidity tumor-reactive T cells. Immunization of transgenic mice expressing HLA-A*0201 with the native human p53:264–272 peptide that differed from the corresponding murine p53 sequence at a single position lead to the generation of T cells that recognized tumor cells expressing high levels of p53.[41] Human T cells transduced with a murine p53 TCR isolated from an immunized mouse recognized a variety of human tumor cells; however, transduced T cells also recognized normal cells expressing lower p53 levels, indicating the dangers of targeting a normal self-protein whose expression is not strictly limited to tumor cells.[42] Similarly, a TCR that was highly reactive with HLA-A*02:01$^+$ tumor cells expressing the human carcinoembryonic antigen (CEA), a protein that is overexpressed in colon and breast carcinomas, was isolated by immunizing HLA-A*02:01$^+$ transgenic mice with the CEA:691–699 peptide.[43] The adoptive transfer of human PBMC transduced with the CEA-reactive TCR lead to an objective clinical response in one of the three treated patients; however, severe colitis was observed in all three of the treated patients.[44] In general, immunotherapies that target antigens present even in small amounts on normal tissues have led to normal tissue destruction and must be applied with caution.

Mutated Gene Products Recognized by CD8+ and CD4+ T Cells

A variety of mutated antigens have also been identified as targets of tumor reactive T cells. The majority of mutated antigens identified using these approaches appear to be unique or only expressed in a relatively small percentage of cancers, and so do not represent targets that are broadly applicable to the treatment of multiple patients. Nevertheless, these studies have in some cases provided insights into mechanisms involved with tumor development, as the mutations may represent drivers of the transformed phenotype. The CDK4 gene product that was cloned using a CTL clone contained a point mutation that enhanced the binding to the HLA-A2 restriction element.[45] This mutation, which was identified in 1 of an additional 28 melanomas that were analyzed, led to the inhibition of binding to the cell cycle inhibitory protein $p16^{INK4a}$ and may have played a role in the loss of growth control in this tumor cell. A point-mutated product of the β-catenin gene, containing a substitution of phenylalanine for serine at position 37, was isolated by screening a cDNA library with an HLA-24–restricted, melanoma reactive TIL.[46] This mutation was found to stabilize the β-catenin gene product by altering a critical serine phosphorylation site, and 2 of 24 additional melanoma cell lines were found to express transcripts with identical mutations.[47]

The observation that immunization against individual murine tumors did not generally cross-protect against challenge with additional syngeneic murine tumors has provided support for the hypothesis that mutant T-cell epitopes represent the predominant antigens responsible for tumor rejection.[48] Mutated epitopes also represent a foreign antigen, which may render them more immunogenic than the majority of normal self-antigens. Although many of the mutations are specific for individual tumors, T cells have been generated by carrying out in vitro sensitization with peptides encoded at mutational hot spots present in *driver* genes.[49]

Recently, novel approaches have been developed that involve the sequencing of tumor cell DNA to identify potential mutated epitopes. In one study, whole exome sequencing of the murine B16 melanoma led to the identification of mutated epitopes that elicited a T cell that appeared to specifically recognize the mutated but not the corresponding wild-type peptides.[50] In a second study, a mutated antigen was identified by screening candidate epitopes that were expressed by tumors derived from immunodeficient mice that regressed in immune-competent mice.[51] More recently, melanomas from three patients who responded to adoptive immunotherapy were subjected to whole exome sequencing, followed by *in silico* analysis using peptide/MHC binding algorithms to identify candidate epitopes that were predicted to bind to the patients' MHC molecules.[52] Using this approach, a total of seven peptides were identified as targets of the TIL that were administered to these patients. Two mutated epitopes were recently identified by whole exome sequencing of a melanoma from a patient who demonstrated a partial response to treatment with the anti–CTLA-4 antibody ipilimumab, followed by a screening of a panel of mutated candidate peptide/MHC tetramers that were predicted to bind to the patient's HLA-A and B alleles.[53] In addition, a mutated epitope expressed by a bile duct cancer was identified by screening tandem minigenes encoding all mutated epitopes that were identified by whole exome sequencing.[54] The adoptive transfer of T cells directed against this mutation-mediated regression of the patient's cancer. Mutations unique to each cancer represent ideal targets for immunotherapy and can potentially lead to the development of personalized therapies directed against these unique targets.

Antigens Identified in Viral-Associated Cancers

Viruses do not appear to play a role in the development of the majority of human cancers; however, an infection with HPV, a group of double-stranded DNA viruses that infect squamous epithelium, is highly associated with the development of a variety of genital lesions that range from warts to carcinomas, as well as the majority of oropharyngeal carcinomas. Recombinant vaccines have been produced by the generation of viruslike particles (VLP), self-assembling particles that form following the expression of the HPV L1 protein in recombinant viral and yeast systems that were initially found to be protective in animal models. The results of a phase II trial in which 2,392 women between 16 and 23 years of age were immunized with HPV-16 VLPs indicated that 100% of those who were vaccinated were protected against infection with HPV-16.[55,56] Although vaccination with VLP does not lead to the regression of established disease, some success has been seen in therapeutic vaccination trials that target the oncogenic viral proteins E6 and E7. In a trial involving the vaccination of women with HPV-16–positive high-grade vulvar intraepithelial neoplasia with synthetic long peptides that encompass both HLA class I and class II restricted epitopes from the oncogenic HPV proteins E6 and E, clinical responses were observed in 15 of the 19 vaccinated patients, and complete regression of all lesions were seen in 9 of the 19 patients in this trial.[1]

Targeting foreign antigens thus may represent a strategy that can lead to more effective immunotherapies. These include viral epitopes as well as mutated epitopes that are also foreign to the host and therefore may represent more effective targets for these therapies than normal self-antigen.

HUMAN CANCER IMMUNOTHERAPIES

A wide variety of therapies have been evaluated in model systems and are now being developed for the treatment of patients with cancer. These include nonspecific approaches, those that involve direct immunization of patients with a variety of immunogens and approaches that involve the adoptive transfer of activated effector cells (Table 14.1). Much confusion related to the effectiveness of cancer immunotherapy has resulted from the lack of proper evaluation of the results of therapy using standard, accepted oncologic criteria such as the World Health Organization or the Response Evaluation Criteria in Solid Tumors (RECIST). Many clinical trials reported a positive use of *soft* criteria such as lymphoid infiltration or tumor necrosis that can occur in the natural course of cancer growth. Because of the delayed responses seen with some immunotherapy approaches, including tumor regression after initial tumor growth, guidelines have been published suggesting the use of an alternate set of immune-related response criteria for the evaluation of immune-based cancer treatments.[57,58] Other confusion has arisen from the use of inappropriate animal models. Although animal model systems have provided important clues that may lead to improved therapies, model systems that employ artificially introduced foreign antigens or that evaluate protection from tumor challenge do not appear to be relevant to the treatment of patients with bulky metastases. Short-term lung metastasis models involve the treatment of relatively small, nonvascularized tumors and also may not be directly relevant to the majority of tumors that are the targets of current clinical trials.

TABLE 14.1

Three Main Approaches to Cancer Immunotherapy

1. Nonspecific stimulation of immune reactions
   a) Stimulate effector cells
      IL-2 (melanoma and renal cancer)
   b) Inhibit regulatory factors
      Anti-CTLA4 (melanoma)
      Anti–PD-1 (melanoma, lung cancer)
2. Active immunization to enhance antitumor reactions (cancer vaccines)
3. Passively transfer activated immune cells with antitumor activity (adoptive immunotherapy)

Nonspecific Approaches to Cancer Immunotherapy

Progress has surged in the past 10 years in the understanding and utilization of nonspecific immune stimulation for the treatment of metastatic cancers. These agents aim to activate quiescent tumor-reactive immune cells or to remove inhibitory mechanisms to allow immunosuppressed cells to function to their full capacity. Although IL-2 and ipilimumab are currently the only immune stimulants approved by the U.S. Food and Drug Administration (FDA) for the treatment of metastatic renal cell carcinoma (IL-2) and melanoma (IL-2 and ipilimumab), new immune checkpoint inhibitors such as anti–programmed cell death 1 (anti–PD-1) have shown impressive results in recent clinical trials for patients with melanoma, renal cell cancer, and also non–small-cell lung cancer (NSCLC), and will likely be approved in the near future. As expected with nonspecific immunostimulation, systemic and bystander immune-related adverse events such as colitis has been reported with all agents in varying degrees, although most side effects are controllable and reversible if addressed aggressively and promptly by experienced clinicians. Importantly, antitumor responses seen with these immune-based modalities appear to be durable for some patients and may even be potentially curative. As with many therapies for metastatic solid tumors, preliminary trials using combination therapies have suggested better than expected response rates and survival, and confirmatory trials are in process to validate and ensure that toxicities from combining agents would not be prohibitive. Overall, patients with metastatic solid tumors may soon have wider armamentarium of off-the-shelf immunotherapy options.

Interleukin-2

Morgan et al.[59] showed that a *factor* produced in the medium from stimulated normal human blood lymphocytes can allow ex vivo growth and expansion of human T lymphocytes. The identification of this soluble T-cell growth factor (IL-2)[60,61] allowed the ability to culture T cells in vitro. IL-2 is a 15-kd glycoprotein produced in minute amounts by activated peripheral blood lymphocytes, and even with using T-cell hybridomas, minimal quantities could be purified; thus, research using IL-2 was impeded by the limited amounts of purified IL-2 available. The isolation of the cDNA clone in 1983[62] enabled the development in 1984 of recombinant IL-2,[63] which permitted the ability to mass manufacture IL-2. Although murine studies demonstrated the ability of IL-2 to mediate tumor regression,[64] early phase I clinical trials did not show any antitumor response,[65] but was instructive in showing pharmacokinetics and toxicities, which led to more effective regimens. Subsequently, IL-2 was given in higher doses (up to 720,000 IU/kg intravenously every 8 hours) in a landmark trial involving 25 patients, along with nonspecific lymphokine-activated natural killer (LAK) cells, which are non-T and non-B lymphocytes.[66] This report was the first to document the regression of advanced solid cancers (melanoma, renal cell, lung, and colon) using immunotherapy in humans.[66] A follow-up trial randomizing 181 patients to either high-dose IL-2 alone (720,000 IU/kg intravenously every 8 hours) or high-dose IL-2 and LAK cells showed that the tumor response was due to IL-2 alone and not to the nonspecific LAK cells.[67] This study also narrowed the IL-2–sensitive histologies to melanoma and renal cell cancer, which had more consistent responses.

IL-2 Therapy for Metastatic Renal Cell Cancer

Subsequent to the studies discussed previously, high-dose IL-2 was tested by additional centers and in combination with other agents for renal cell cancer. A randomized phase II trial involving 99 kidney cancer patients showed no increase in antitumor responses with the addition of interferon alfa-2b (IFNα-2b). Responses were seen for 12 (17%) of 71 patients who received high-dose IL-2 alone, with 4 complete regressions.[68] A summary report of 227 patients with metastatic renal cell cancer treated with high-dose IL-2 (defined as 600,000 IU/kg or 720,000 IU/kg given intravenously every 8 hours as tolerated up to 15 doses) from 1985 to 1996 at the Surgery Branch of the National Cancer Institute (NCI) documented a total response rate of 19%, with 10% partial and 9% complete; the longest duration of a complete response was over 10 years ongoing (134+ months).[69] Another summary report from seven phase II clinical trials from multiple institutions involving 255 patients with metastatic renal cell cancer receiving high-dose IL-2 showed the overall response rate was 14%, with 9% partial and 5% complete, and responses occurred in all sites of disease, including primary kidney tumors, bone metastases, and bulking visceral tumor burdens.[70] Although the response rates were modest, the durability of the responses was remarkable, with many responses lasting over 5 years ongoing (see Fig. 14.2). Because of the striking durability of the antitumor responses, IL-2 received FDA approval for the treatment of metastatic renal cell cancer in 1992. A follow-up report in 2000 showing the response rates of the 255 renal cell patients in the seven phase II studies to be the same, with complete responses lasting over 10 years ongoing (131+ months for the longest responder), suggesting a potential cure.[71]

To ascertain whether lower doses and/or different administration routes, which would decrease toxicity and obviate the need for inpatient hospitalization for IL-2 therapy, a trial randomizing 400 patients with metastatic renal cell cancer to either standard high-dose intravenous IL-2, low-dose intravenous IL-2 (at 72,000 IU/kg), or low-dose subcutaneous IL-2 (250,000 U/kg per dose daily Monday through Friday in the first week and then 125,000 U/kg per dose daily during the next 5 weeks).[72] Although responses were seen with all three regimens, including complete responses in the low-dose subcutaneous regimen, standard high-dose IL-2 had higher overall response rates (21%) versus low-dose intravenous IL-2 (13%; $p = 0.048$) and low-dose subcutaneous IL-2 (10%; $p = 0.033$), suggesting the superiority of the high-dose intravenous regimen.[72]

The administration of IL-2 represents the only known curative treatment for patients with metastatic renal cell cancer and should be considered as front-line therapy for suitable patients.

IL-2 Therapy for Metastatic Melanoma

Between 1985 and 1993, 270 patients with metastatic melanoma enrolled into eight clinical trials in multiple centers using high-dose IL-2 (defined as 600,000 IU/kg or 720,000 IU/kg given intravenously every 8 hours as tolerated up to 15 doses). Atkins et al.[73] reported overall response rates of 16% (43 patients), with 10% partial and 6% complete; responses occurred at all tumor sites and regardless of initial tumor burden. With median follow-up at that time of 62 months, 20 responders (47%) were still alive, with 15 surviving over 5 years.[73] A follow-up report on those patients in 2000 showed that the response rates were unchanged; with the longest response duration of >12 years ongoing, disease progression was not observed in any patient responding greater than 30 months.[74] As with renal cell cancer, the flat *tail* of the Kaplan-Meier response duration and overall survival curves (Fig. 14.3), showing the potential curative nature of the antitumor responses, was the main compelling reason the FDA approved IL-2 for the treatment of metastatic melanoma in 1998.

Research in subsequent years aimed to increase the response rates of IL-2, led by increasing interests in tumor vaccinations as melanoma-associated antigens were being characterized.[75] Pilot studies suggested that vaccinations using modified melanoma differentiation antigens such as gp100:209–217(210M) could elicit immunologic responses in nearly all patients, and when combined with high-dose IL-2, could elicit potentially higher than expected clinical antitumor responses.[75] A follow-up phase III study[76] randomized 185 patients with HLA*A0201 from 21 centers to either high-dose IL-2 or high-dose IL-2 plus gp100:209–217(210M) concurrent immunization. Although the response rates for the

CANCER THERAPEUTICS

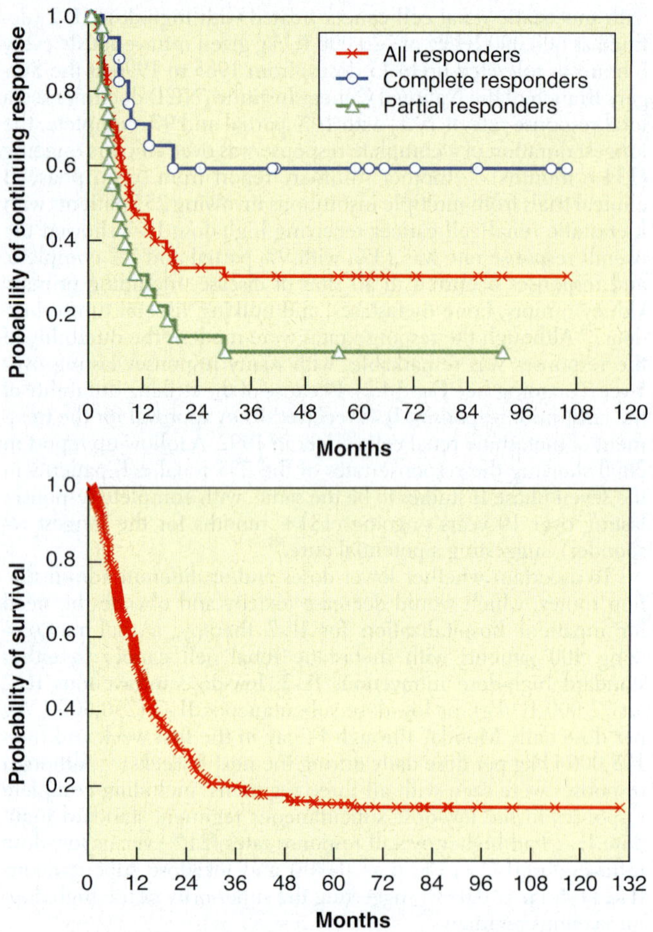

Figure 14.3 Kaplain-Meier plots of response duration (*top*) and overall survival (*bottom*) for 270 patients with metastatic melanoma who were treated with high-dose bolus IL-2 from 1985 to 1993 in eight clinical trials.[73]

IL-2 plus vaccine arm was statistically improved compared to IL-2 alone (16% versus 6%; p = 0.03), the IL-2 alone arm was notable for being much lower than in all prior studies.[76] In addition, a pilot trial of 36 melanoma patients treated high-dose IL-2 concurrently with ipilimumab (an antibody against cytotoxic T lymphocyte–associated antigen 4 discussed in the following section) gave a 25% OR rate, with 17% achieving complete response[77]; however, these data have not been further tested.

Correlative studies suggest that the total doses of IL-2 received during the first treatment course was significantly higher in patients achieving a complete response[69]; however, when limited to patients who were able to complete both cycles of the course, there was no statistical significance, suggesting that patients whose tumors progressed significantly after one cycle (and was not able to complete the second cycle of the course) accounted for some of the difference seen.[78] Responders did have a higher maximal lymphocyte count[69,78] immediately posttherapy and were more likely to develop vitiligo and thyroid dysfunction.[78] There has not been a consistent pretherapy factor that is predictive of response, although one retrospective correlative study involving 374 patients showed that patients with M1a (subcutaneous- and/or cutaneous-only disease) have a response rate of 54% compared with 12% for those with visceral M1b/c ($P_2 < 0.0001$).[78]

Toxicities and Safe Administration of IL-2

High-dose IL-2 has been shown to be associated with adverse events that impact multiple organ systems.[73,79,80] The main component of the toxicities is due to an inflammatory response mediated by the release of cytokines such as IFNγ and tumor necrosis factor alpha (TNF-α)[81] resulting in a capillary-leak syndrome[82] and decreased systemic vascular resistance, which can lead to fever, hypotension, cardiac arrhythmia, lethargy, renal insufficiency, hepatic dysfunction, body edema, pulmonary edema, and confusion; other side effects can also include nausea, diarrhea, rash, anemia, thrombocytopenia, lymphocytosis, and neutrophil chemotactic defect[83] that predispose patients to gram-positive line infections. Since the first clinical trials with IL-2 in 1984, however, much has been learned to permit its safe dosing for appropriately screened patients[82,84,85]; importantly, if patients are appropriately supported, side effects are quickly reversible once IL-2 dosing ceases.[85] Kammula et al.[86] compared the incidences of grade 3/4 toxicities between the 155 patients treated from 1985 to 1986 to 156 patients treated from 1993 through 1997 at the NCI Surgery Branch: grade 3/4 hypotension decreased from 81% to 31%, intubations from 12% to 3%, neuropsychiatric toxicities from 19% to 8%, diarrhea from 92% to 12%, line sepsis from 18% to 4%, cardiac ischemia from 3% to 0%, and mortality from 3% to 0%. In fact, no fatality occurred strictly due to IL-2 therapy since 1989.[86] Overall strategies for the safe administration of high-dose IL-2 include careful screening for appropriately selected patients with adequate cardiopulmonary reserve, having an experienced team of physicians and nurses who are cognizant of the expected toxicities of IL-2, having routine preemptive measures such as prophylactic antibiotics to prevent line infections, and aggressive and prompt management of toxicities.

Checkpoint Modulators

Anti–Cytotoxic T Lymphocyte Antigen 4

CTLA-4 is an immunosuppressive *costimulatory* receptor found on newly activated T cells (and on regulatory T cells) that binds with costimulatory ligands B7-1 and B7-2 on antigen-presenting cells.[87,88] When CTLA-4 is engaged by B7-1 or B7-2, the T cells becomes inhibited,[89,90] suggesting that CTLA-4 likely evolved as a self-protective mechanism to prevent autoimmunity (Fig. 14.4). Thus, overcoming this *checkpoint* molecule was an aim of cancer immunotherapy. After CTLA-4 blockade in murine models led to antitumor immunity,[91,92] anti–CTLA-4 antibodies were tested in clinical trials starting in 2002.

The combination of anti–CTLA-4 blocking antibodies and vaccination worked well in murine models and led to one of the early phase II studies using ipilimumab (a fully human immunoglobulin [IgG_1] monoclonal antibody previously called MDX-010) with two gp100 vaccines, gp100:209–217(210M) and gp100:280–288(288V), in patients with metastatic melanoma.[93] Antitumor regressions were seen (from 11% to 22% overall response rates, with up to 8% complete response rates), along with severe autoimmune toxicities such as colitis, dermatitis, and even hypophysitis,[93–95] as would be expected based on the mechanism of CTLA-4 blockade. In fact, autoimmunity adverse events appeared to correlate with response to ipilimumab.[3] The experience with these early studies led to management strategies to screen aggressively for immune-related adverse events (IRAE), such as routine screening of endocrinopathies, and to treat IRAEs promptly, including high-dose steroids if needed for severe colitis.[96,97] Overall, ipilimumab was in some ways easier to manage for the patients than IL-2 because it was an outpatient infusion given every 3 weeks; IRAEs were unpredictable, however, and can appear suddenly many weeks after receiving a dose.

In 2010, results from a landmark phase III randomized trial comparing three treatment strategies (ipilimumab alone, gp100 peptide vaccine alone, or ipilimumab plus gp100 peptide vaccine) in 676 patients with metastatic melanoma were published showing improvement in median survival in the two arms that received ipilimumab (10 months) compared to the gp100 alone arm (6 months, p <0.001), despite showing a low response rate of 7% (among 540 patients who received ipilimumab).[98] Another

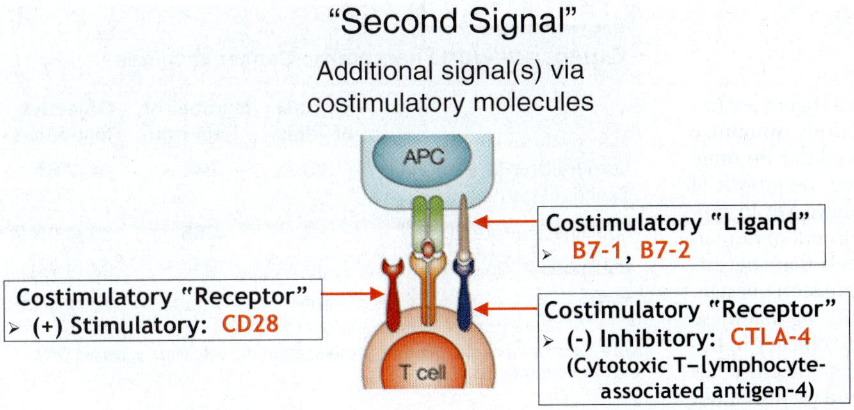

Figure 14.4 Mechanism of action of cytotoxic T-lymphocyte–associated antigen 4 (CTLA-4). When CD28 is engaged on the T cell, reactivity of the T cell is enhanced. When CTLA-4 is engaged on the T cell, reactivity of the T cell is inhibited. Blocking of CTLA-4 with a monoclonal antibody can elicit antitumor immunity but also autoimmunity.

phase III randomized trial comparing dacarbazine plus ipilimumab versus dacarbazine alone again showed improved survival in that arm containing dacarbazine (11.2 months versus 9.1 months; $p < 0.001$).[99] These studies showing survival benefit led to FDA approval of ipilimumab for advanced melanoma in 2011.

The responses seen with ipilimumab appear to be durable.[100] A follow-up study of 177 patients with metastatic melanoma treated on the earliest trials at the NCI Surgery Branch using ipilimumab showed that response duration could last 99+ months ongoing.[77] In fact, 14 out of the 15 complete responders remain disease free 54+ to 99+ months ongoing, suggesting a potential cure for some patients. Interestingly, several patients who were deemed partial responders converted to complete responders several years later, because it look an average of 30 months to have all visible tumor marks on imaging scans to disappear.[77]

Ipilimumab was also tested on other solid tumors, and renal cell cancer again appears to be the only other type beside melanoma that had significant responses. Sixty-one patients with metastatic renal cell cancer were treated, and six developed a response (10%); however, 33% developed grade 3/4 IRAEs.[101] Subsequently, the availability of agents with lower toxicity profiles such as sunitinib and sorafenib prevented further enthusiasm to pursue this drug for renal cell cancer.

Another anti–CTLA-4 antibody, tremelimumab (previously called CP-675,206), has also demonstrated durable responses in melanoma patients.[102,103] A phase III randomized trial randomizing 655 patients with metastatic melanoma to either tremelimumab or physician's choice chemotherapy, however, failed to show a survival difference (despite a significantly different response duration favoring tremelimumab, 35.8 months versus 13.7 months; $p = 0.0011$), possibly due to crossover of chemotherapy patients enrolling into ipilimumab trials and expanded access programs.[103]

Anti–Programmed Death 1 and Anti–Programmed Death Ligand 1

PD-1 is another checkpoint modulator expressed on activated T cells. Although CTLA-4 appears to be involved in the early activation of T cells, PD-1 is involved in the later effector phase of T-cell activation and can function to prevent excessive damage to self by activated T cells in the periphery.[104,105] Interaction with its corresponding ligand, PD-L1 (B7-H1) and PD-L2 (B7-H2) leads to suppressed T-effector function. PD-L1 is expressed on hematopoietic and epithelial cells and is upregulated by cytokines such as IFNγ,[106] whereas PD-L1 is mainly on antigen-presenting cells. Given the clinical results with inhibiting the CTLA-4 checkpoint, recent efforts have focused on inhibiting the PD-1/PD-L1 and PD-1/PD-L2 interactions.

Nivolumab (previously known as BMS-936558, MDX-1106, and ONO-4538) is a fully human anti–PD-1 IgG4 monoclonal antibody that was initially tested in a phase I trial published in 2010 in which 39 patients with advanced solid cancers were treated in escalating doses.[107] Responses were seen in one patient with colon cancer, one with melanoma, and one with renal cell cancer; one patient developed colitis.[108] These hopeful results lead to a larger study in which 236 patients with either NSCLC (74 patients), melanoma (94 patients), or renal cell cancer (33 patients).[4] Objective responses were seen in 18% of patients with NSCLC, 28% with melanoma, and 27% with renal cell cancer.[4] Grade 3/4 adverse events occurred in 14% of patients, including those previously seen with ipilimumab (dermatitis, colitis, hepatitis, thyroiditis, hypophysitis, and pneumonitis). Nine patients developed pneumonitis, six of whom was reversible, and three (1%) with grade 3/4 died despite steroids and infliximab therapy.[4] An update on the status of 107 melanoma patients treated from 2008 to 2012 shows a 31% tumor response rate, with a median response duration of 2 years and a median overall survival of 16.8 months.[109]

Nivolumab was also tested in combination with ipilimumab in melanoma in either concurrent (53 patients) or sequenced (33 patients) regimens. The concurrent group experienced an overall response rate of 40%, whereas the sequenced group had a 20% response rate.[110] The concurrent group also experienced a higher rate of grade 3/4 adverse events (53%), compared to 18% in the sequenced group. Interestingly, 16 of 21 responders in the concurrent group experienced tumor reduction of 80% or greater by 12 weeks,[110] a tempo that is faster than was seen with ipilimumab.

Another anti–PD-1 developed independently, lambrolizumab (previously known as MK-3475, a humanized IgG4κ monoclonal antibody), was tested on 135 patients with metastatic melanoma.[111] The response rate was found to be 38% and was similar between those who had received ipilimumab and those who were ipilimumab naïve,[111] confirming that the antitumor response from lambrolizumab occurs via a different mechanism. Similar to nivolumab, 13% of patients developed grade 3/4 adverse events, with 4% developing pneumonitis, although none developed grade 3/4 pneumonitis.[111]

BMS-936559 is a fully human IgG4 monoclonal antibody that blocks PD-L1 ligation to both PD-1 and CD80. A phase I study was tested in 207 patients (75 with NSCLC, 55 with melanoma, 18 with colon cancer, and 17 with renal cell cancer, 17 with ovarian cancer, 14 with pancreatic cancer, 7 with gastric cancer, and 4 with breast cancer).[112] Among patients who were evaluated for response, objective responses were seen in 16% of melanoma patients, 17% of renal cell cancer patients, 10% of NSCLC patients, and 1 out of 17 ovarian cancer patients. Grade 3/4 toxicities were seen in 9% of patients.[112]

The advent of these checkpoint inhibitors brings additional treatment options to patients with selected advanced cancers, particularly those with histologies deemed previously to be outside the realm of immunotherapy such as NSCLC.[108,113] In addition, a new anti–PD-L1 (MPDL3280A) in clinical trials has also shown some efficacy in melanoma, renal cell cancer, and NSCLC in early reports.

Active Immunization Approaches to Cancer Therapy (Cancer Vaccines)

The molecular characterization of multiple cancer antigens led to a large number of clinical trials that attempted to actively immunize against these antigens with the expectation that cellular immune reactions would be generated capable of inhibiting the growth of established cancers. The results of these efforts have yet to produce significant vaccine efforts of value in the treatment of human cancer. There is a paucity of murine tumor models that suggests that active vaccine approaches can mediate the regression of established vascularized tumors; therefore, it is not surprising that these approaches have, with a few exceptions, shown little efficacy in humans. Enthusiasm about the effectiveness of cancer vaccines has often been grounded in surrogate and subjective end points, rather than reliable objective cancer regressions using standard oncologic criteria. In a review of the world literature, including 107 published cancer vaccine trials involving 2,242 patients, a 3.4% overall objective response rate was observed (Table 14.2).[114,115] In many cases, relatively soft criteria such as stable disease or the regression of individual metastases in the presence of progressive disease at other sites have been reported. A variety of immunizing vectors have been used, including tumor-derived peptides, proteins, whole tumor cells, recombinant viruses, dendritic cells, and heat-shock proteins.[116–122] Although many of these approaches can lead to the development of circulating T cells that can recognize the immunizing tumor antigen, these T cells rarely cause the inhibition of established tumors, a point that has led to much confusion in the field of tumor immunology. The generation of antitumor T cells in vivo is likely a necessary, but certainly not a sufficient criteria for the development of a clinically active immunotherapy. Often, T cells with weak avidity for tumor recognition are generated, and the tolerizing and inhibitory influences that exist in vivo must be overcome for an effective immune response to cause tumor destruction.

A prospective randomized trial of immunization with antigen-presenting cells was carried out by the Dendreon Corporation (Seattle, Washington). This trial used an antigen-presenting cell vaccine loaded with prostatic acid phosphatase linked to GM-CSF compared to placebo in men with hormone-refractory prostate cancer.[123] Of 330 patients who received the vaccine treatment, 1 objective partial response was seen. Only 8 patients experienced a PSA drop of at least 50%. There was no difference in the time to disease progression; however, the vaccine group had a median survival of 25.8 months compared to 21.7 months in the placebo group, and based on this statistically significant survival improvement, this treatment was approved by the FDA (Fig. 14.5).

TABLE 14.2

Experience with Therapeutic Cancer Vaccines

	Number of Trials	Number of Patients	Objective Responses
Surgery Branch, National Cancer Institute	25	541	14 (2.6%)
Published before 2005[114]	33	765	29 (4.0%)
Published 2005–2010[115]	49	936	34 (3.7%)
Total	107	2,242	77 (3.4%)

Note: Vaccines include: peptide, protein, dendritic cell, virus, plasmid DNA, and whole tumor cells.

Adoptive Cell Transfer Immunotherapy

Adoptive cellular immunotherapy refers to the transfer to the tumor-bearing host of immune lymphocytes with anticancer activity. The first successful administration of adoptive cell therapy (ACT) involving TIL, in combination with high-dose IL-2 was carried out at the National Cancer Institute Surgery Branch in 1988.[124] Studies that used cell transfer therapy in patients with metastatic melanoma have provided the clearest evidence of the power of the immune system to mediate the regression of advanced metastatic cancers in humans. Adoptive cell therapy has several theoretical as well as practical advantages.[125] Lymphocytes with antitumor activity can be expanded to very large numbers ex vivo for infusion into cancer patients. These cells can be tested in vitro for antitumor activity, and cells with appropriate properties such as high avidity for tumor recognition and a high proliferative potential

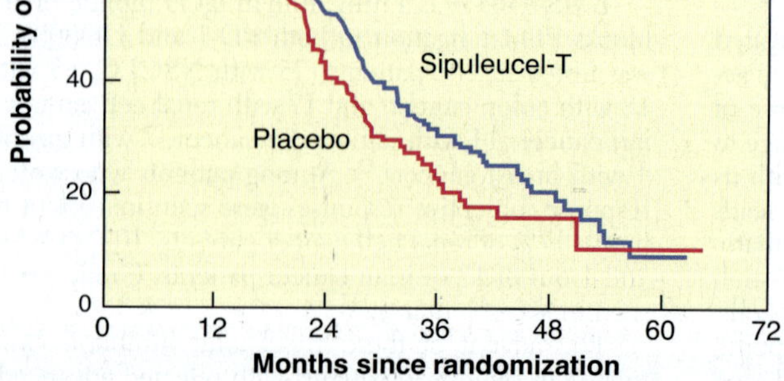

Number at risk

Sipuleucel-T	341	274	129	49	14	1
Placebo	171	123	55	19	4	1

Figure 14.5 Kaplan-Meier estimate of the overall survival in patients with metastatic castration-resistant prostate cancer treated with Sipuleucel-T antigen–presenting cell immunotherapy. A modest but statistically significant improvement in survival was seen ($P = 0.03$).

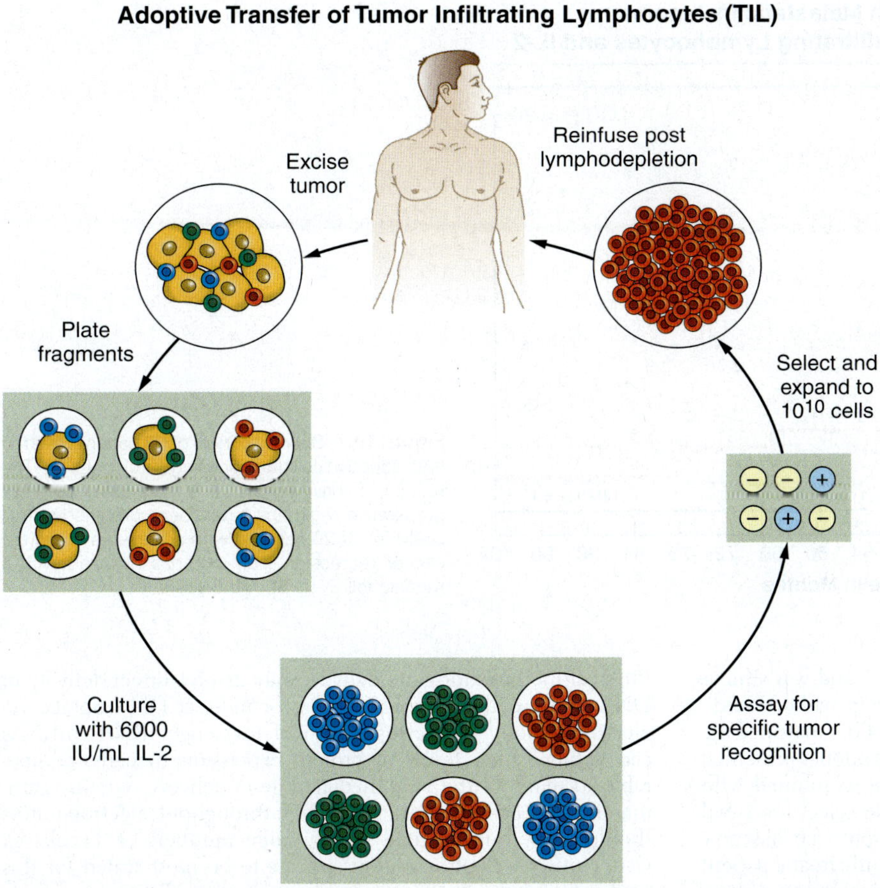

Figure 14.6 Diagram of the adoptive cell therapy of patients with metastatic melanoma. Tumors are resected and individual cultures are grown and tested for antitumor reactivity. Optimal cultures are expanded in vitro and reinfused into the autologous patient who had received a preparative lymphodepleting chemotherapy.

can be identified and selectively expanded for treatment. These cells can be activated in vitro and thus are not subjected to the tolerizing influences that exist in vivo. Perhaps, most important, the host can be manipulated prior to the transfer of the anticancer cells to provide an optimal tumor microenvironment free of in vivo suppressive factors.[125] Studies have shown that the transfer of cultured lymphocytes with antiviral activity can prevent Epstein-Barr virus (EBV) infections as well as the subsequent development of posttransplant lymphoproliferative diseases. Cultured lymphocytes have been used for the treatment of patients with established EBV-induced lymphomas.[126]

The best evidence for the ability of adoptive cell transfer to successfully treat patients with solid tumors comes from the treatment of patients with metastatic melanoma. A diagram that describes the nature of this treatment is shown in Figure 14.6. In patients with metastatic melanoma, TILs can be obtained from resected tumor deposits and individual cultures tested to identify those with optimal anticancer activity.[124,127] These cells are then expanded ex vivo and reinfused along with IL-2, which is the requisite growth factor required for the survival and persistence of these cells. The administration of a preparative lymphodepleting chemotherapy regimen, consisting of cyclophosphamide and fludarabine with or without 2 or 12 Gy total body irradiation, could substantially enhance the survival and persistence of the transferred cells and increase their in vivo antitumor effectiveness.[128,129] In a series of three pilot trials with 93 patients, objective responses were seen in 49% to 72% of patients.[5,130] Of the 93 patients, 20 (22%) experienced a complete regression of all metastatic melanoma. Only 1 of these 20 patients has recurred, and the remaining patients have ongoing complete regressions from 80 to over 104 months (Table 14.3, Fig. 14.7).

TABLE 14.3

Cell Transfer Therapy

Treatment	Total	PR	CR	OR
	Number of Patients (Percentage) (Duration in Months)			
No TBI	43	16 (37%) (84, 36, 29, 28, 14, 12, 11, 7, 7, 7, 7, 4, 4, 2, 2, 2)	5 (12%) (114+, 112+, 111+, 97+, 86+)	21 (49%)
200 TBI	25	8 (32%) (14, 9, 6, 6, 5, 4, 3, 3)	5 (20%) (101+, 98+, 93+, 90+, 70+)	13 (52%)
1,200 TBI	25	8 (32%) (21, 13, 7, 6, 6, 5, 3, 2)	10 (40%) (81+, 78+, 77+, 72+, 72+, 71+, 71+, 70+, 70+, 19)	18 (72%)

Note: 20 complete responses: 19 ongoing at 70 to 114 months.

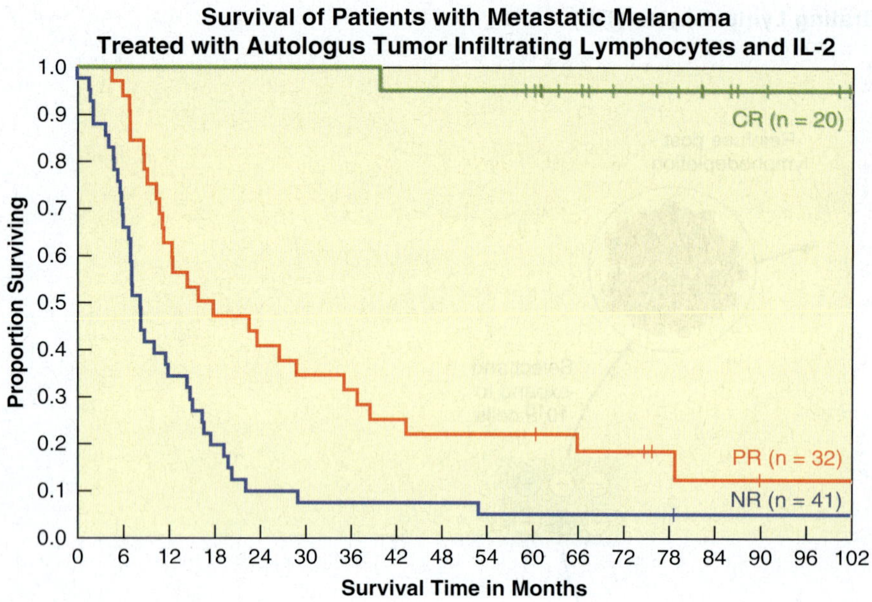

Figure 14.7 Survival curves of 93 patients treated with adoptive cell transfer using autologous TIL. The results of three consecutive trials using different preparative regimens have been combined in this analysis. Of 20 patients who achieved a complete cancer regression, only one has recurred with a median follow-up of over 8 years.[5]

The 5-year survival of these 93 patients was 29% and was similar regardless of the prior treatments that these patients had received.

Extensive genomic studies have shown that TILs that mediate complete cancer regressions recognize mutated epitopes presented by the cancer.[52] The use of exomic sequencing combined with in vitro tests of antitumor activity can be used to select for T-cell populations reactive against the cancer. This approach has now been utilized to identify T cells used to successfully treat a patient with chemotherapy-refractory cholangiocarcinoma and provides a blueprint for the application of cell transfer therapy for a variety of common epithelial cancers.[54]

The difficulty in obtaining TILs with antitumor activity from cancers other than melanoma has also led to the development of approaches using lymphocytes genetically modified using retroviral transduction to insert antitumor T-cell receptors into the normal lymphocytes of patients.[131]

Genetic Modification of Lymphocytes for Use in Adoptive Cell Therapy: Basic Principles and Applications to Solid Tumors

Efforts are in progress to genetically engineer autologous PBMCs through the introduction of exogenous high avidity receptors that specifically recognize tumor antigens (Fig. 14.8). These cells can then be expanded to large numbers in vitro and be readministered back to the patient similar to TILs in order to mediate tumor regression. The use of gene-modified cells for ACT has resulted in objective clinical responses for a variety of cancer histologies including melanoma, synovial sarcoma, and CD19-positive B-cell malignancies.[6,131–133]

There are two key requirements necessary for the use of gene-modified cells for the treatment of solid cancer. The first is the selection of an appropriate gene transfer method in order to achieve high receptor expression levels in the transferred T cells. For this discussion, we will consider both nonviral and viral-based gene delivery platforms. Generally speaking, there are two categories of nonviral gene transfer, chemical and physical. Chemical gene transfer involves the use of positively charged delivery vehicle such as calcium phosphate, cationic lipids, or polymers to form DNA complexes capable of entering a cell through endocytosis.[134] These reagents benefit from their ease of manufacture and ability to form complexes with large DNA sequences; however, low transfection efficiency of human T cells continues to be an issue.

Physical methods for gene delivery may involve direct delivery of DNA into a cell via microinjection or indirect DNA uptake via electroporation.[135] Electroporation of messenger RNA (mRNA) can achieve high levels of protein expression in cells, comparable to many of the viral-mediated gene delivery systems (gammaretroviral or lentiviral).[135,136] High-throughput electroporators should allow one to gene modify large numbers of T cells ex vivo.[137] mRNA electroporation appears to be most suited for this application, because there is significant loss of cell viability following electroporation of large amounts of DNA.[136] The electroporation of mRNA, although gaining traction as a means of redirecting T cell specificity,[137] provides for transient receptor expression because the mRNA will degrade over time. Currently, it is not clear if stable long-term receptor expression is required to mediate tumor regression. However, the main criticism of the non-viral methods described is the lack of stable gene transfer. To overcome this problem, many investigators are now using transposons such as *sleeping beauty* or *piggybac*.[138] Transposons are mobile DNA gene delivery elements encoding a gene of interest (i.e., TCR or chimeric antigen receptors [CAR]) that can randomly integrate into the genome in the presence of the transposase enzyme, thereby allowing for stable gene expression. This technology is currently being used for the ACT of CAR-modified cells targeting B-cell malignancies (see Fig. 14.8B).[139]

Viral-mediated gene delivery is currently the most common method for the genetic modification of immune cells for cancer ACT. Retroviridae is a family of RNA viruses that, upon entry into cells, undergo a process called reverse transcription whereby the viral RNA is converted into DNA as it stably integrates into the host genome. The two most common retroviral vector systems are based on the gammaretrovirus, Moloney murine leukemia virus (MLV), and the lentivirus, HIV type 1 (see Fig. 14.8B). Gammaretroviral vectors have been used in human clinical applications for over 20 years. The only reported toxicity associated with gammaretroviral engineering of human cells involved the retroviral transduction of hematopoietic stem cells for the treatment of children with severe combined immunodeficiency syndrome (X-SCID).[140] There have been no reports of clonal outgrowth following the retroviral transduction of mature T lymphocytes in adults. Highly active vectors have been generated from a variety of murine retroviruses including spleen focus forming virus (SFFV), myeloproliferative sarcoma virus (MPSV), and the murine stem cell virus (MSCV).[141–147] In most cases, these vectors are replication incompetent, but non–self-inactivating in

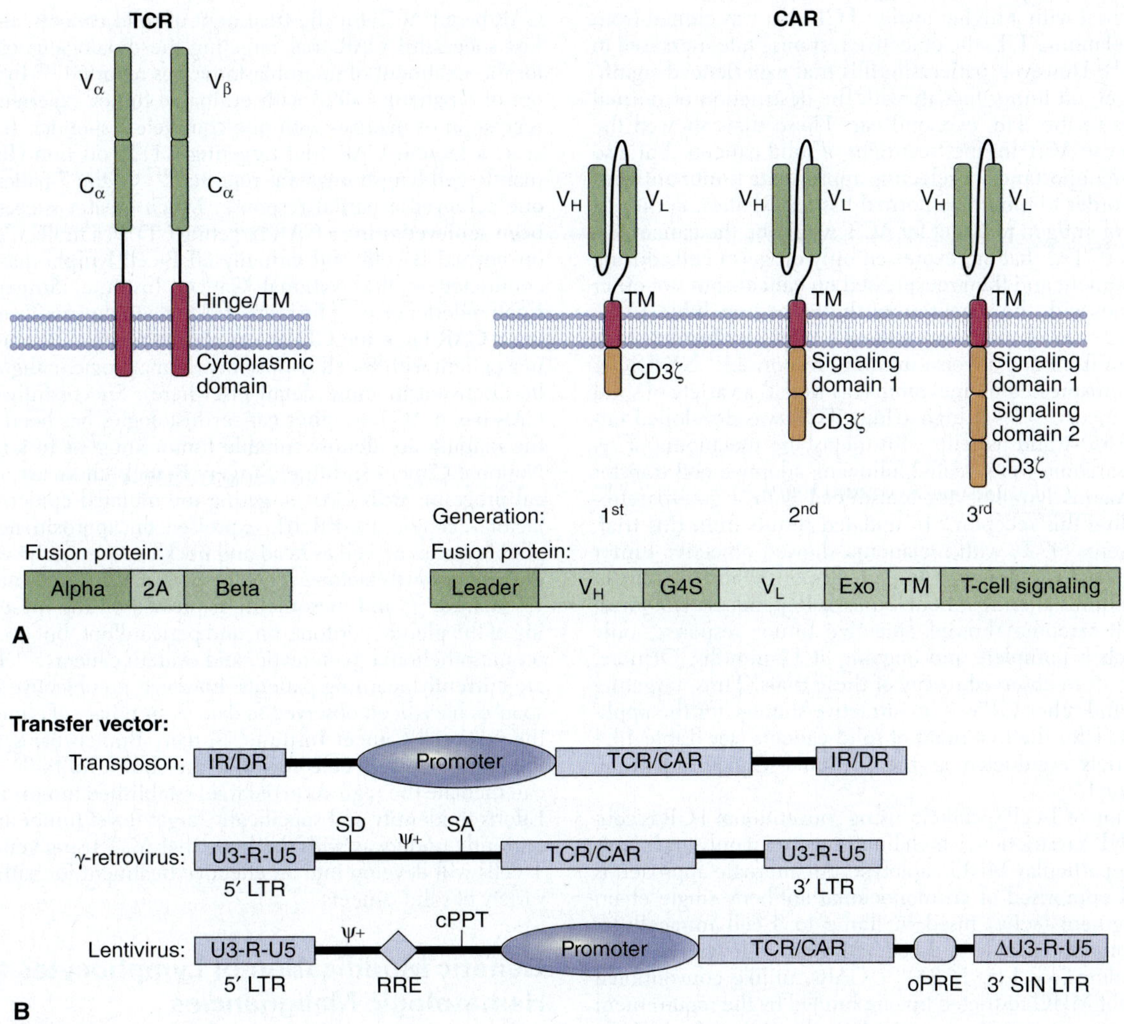

Figure 14.8 Genetic modification of T cells for the treatment of solid cancers. **(A)** In order to gene modify T cells to confer stable tumor-specific reactivity, one can transduce T cells with an exogenous TCR derived from a naturally occurring or murine T-cell clone or a CAR derived from a tumor-specific monoclonal antibody. The TCR or CAR is synthesized as fusion proteins and inserted into the appropriate gene transfer vector. **(B)** Depending on the transfer vector selected, the T cells are then electroporated (transposon) or transduced (viral vector) to confer tumor specificity. V_α, V_β, and C_α, C_β, TCR alpha and beta chain variable and constant regions, respectively; TM, transmembrane domain; V_H and V_L, immunoglobulin variable regions; 2A and G4S, linker sequences; Exo, extracellular spacer domain; SD, splice donor; SA, splice acceptor; Ψ, packaging signal; LTR, long terminal repeat; U3, unique 3′ region; R, repeat region; U5, unique 5′ region; RRE, rev response element; cPPT, central polypurine tract; wPRE, woodchuck hepatitis virus posttranscriptional regulatory element; ΔU3, truncated unique 3′ region; SIN, self-inactivating.

that the promoter for transgene expression is derived from the viral long terminal repeat (LTR). Self-inactivating (SIN) gammaretroviral vectors have been developed that require an internal promoter to drive transgene expression. The advantage of non-SIN vectors is the ability to use a variety of retroviral packaging cell lines (PG13, Phoenix) engineered to constitutively express gag (capsid protein), pol (reverse transcriptase, integrase, and RNase H enzymes) and env (envelope protein). Transduction of these packaging lines with a non-SIN retroviral vector encoding a transgene allows for the generation of a stable packaging cell line that constitutively releases vector into the medium. This platform is easily scaled up to support large-scale vector production efforts. An alternative to the gammaretroviral vector platform is the lentiviral vector platform. There are some advantages to selecting a lentiviral vector for T-cell engineering in that one can transduce large numbers of minimally stimulated T cells,[148] transfer more complex and larger gene expression cassettes, and yield a potentially safer chromosomal integration profile as compared to gammaretroviruses. However, there has been at least one instance of clonal outgrowth following lentiviral vector transduction of CD34+ stem cells.[149] Therefore, more data will be needed to better understand the risk of insertional mutagenesis associated with the use of lentiviral vectors. The major disadvantage with using lentiviral vectors for ACT is the lack of a robust packaging cell line, which requires transient vector production and is difficult to scale up.

The first successful application ACT involved the use of autologous T cells genetically modified with a conventional αβ TCR targeting MART-1 for the treatment of patients with melanoma.[131] The success of this approach relies on the ability to identify naturally occurring TCRs with sufficiently high avidity for the tumor antigen. For this clinical trial, a tumor-specific TCR was cloned directly from melanoma TIL. Exogenous TCR can also be generated from human PBMC following a variety of in vitro sensitization techniques or immunization of transgenic mice expressing HLA molecules. A T-cell clone expressing a low avidity TCR recognizing MART-1 was isolated and the α and β chains cloned into a gammaretroviral vector. The objective response rate from this trial was 13% (2/15).[131] In a follow-up trial with a higher avidity TCR that was cloned from the same melanoma TIL, the objective response rate increased to 30% (6/20).[150] However, patients in this trial experienced significant on-target, off-tumor toxicity with the destruction of normal melanocytes in the skin, eye, and ear. These trials showed the potential to use ACT for the treatment of solid cancers, but also highlight the importance of selecting appropriate tumor antigens to target in order to minimize normal tissue toxicities. Perhaps a better class of antigen to target for ACT would be the cancer testes antigens (CTA) that are expressed only on germ cells during fetal development and then reexpressed on cancers but not other normal tissues with the exception of the testes (see Table 14.1). Because the testes do not express class I MHC molecules, they are protected from any adverse immune response.[151] NY-ESO-1 is a CTA overexpressed on melanoma, as well as a variety of solid epithelial cancers.[152–154] A high-avidity TCR was developed targeting NY-ESO-1 and patients with metastatic melanoma or synovial cell sarcoma were treated following adoptive cell transfer using autologous lymphocytes transduced with a gammaretrovirus encoding this receptor.[6] In updated results from this trial, 8 of 17 patients (47%) with melanoma showed objective tumor responses, two of which were complete responses and ongoing at 51 and 48 months after treatment. Nine of 19 patients (47%) with synovial cell sarcoma showed objective tumor response, only one of which is complete and ongoing at 12 months. Of note, no toxicities were observed in any of these trials. Thus, targeting NY-ESO-1 and other CTAs is an attractive strategy for the application of ACT for the treatment of solid cancers (see Table 14.4 for other trials conducted at the National Cancer Institute, Surgery Branch).

Redirection of T-cell specificity using conventional TCR is constrained by HLA restriction, which limits treatment only to patients expressing a particular MHC haplotype. An alternate approach is to use CAR comprised of an monoclonal antibody single chain variable fragment (scFv) fused in frame to T-cell intracellular signaling domains capable of T-cell activation following antigen-specific binding (see Fig. 14.8A).[155] CARs, unlike conventional TCRs, are not MHC restricted but are limited by the requirement for the tumor antigen to be expressed on the cell surface. CARs can also recognize carbohydrate and lipid moieties further expanding their application. To date, there has been limited success using CAR-based ACT for the treatment of solid cancers. In 2008, the first successful CAR trial targeting the disialoganglioside, GD2, for the treatment of neuroblastoma was reported.[156] In this trial, 4 out of 8 patients (50%) with evaluable tumor experienced tumor regression or necrosis with one complete responder. In that same year, a second CAR trial targeting CD20 on non-Hodgkin and mantle cell lymphomas was reported.[157] Of the 7 patients treated, one achieved a partial response. Much greater success has now been achieved using a CAR targeting CD19, a molecule expressed on normal B cells and virtually all B-cell lymphomas. In a trial conducted at the National Cancer Institute, Surgery Branch, Kochenderfer et al.[132] first reported that autologous T cells expressing a CAR targeting CD19 was able to mediate tumor regression in a patient with B-cell lymphoma (hematologic malignancies will be discussed in more detail elsewhere). Successfully expanding CAR-based ACT to other cancer histologies has been limited by the inability to identify suitable tumor antigens to target. At the National Cancer Institute, Surgery Branch, there are active clinical programs with CAR targeting the mutated epidermal growth factor receptor, EGFRvIII, expressed on approximately 40% of glioblastomas as well as head and neck cancers[158]; the vascular endothelial growth factor-2 receptor, VEGFR-2, expressed on tumor vasculature[159]; and mesothelin, expressed on the mesothelial lining of the pleura, peritoneum, and pericardium, but overexpressed on mesothelioma, pancreatic, and ovarian cancers.[160] These trials are currently accruing patients; however, no objective clinical responses have been observed to date. A summary of clinical trials at the National Cancer Institute, Surgery Branch using gene-modified autologous T cells for ACT are shown in Table 14.4. ACT can mediate the regression of large, established tumors in humans. Efforts to identify and specifically target novel tumor antigens are currently underway with the hope that ACT using gene-modified T cells will develop into an effective treatment for patients with a variety of solid cancers.

Genetic Modification of Lymphocytes to Treat Hematologic Malignancies

Immunologic therapies can be useful treatments for some hematologic malignancies as demonstrated by the effectiveness of mono-

TABLE 14.4

Surgery Branch, National Cancer Institute Program for the Application of Cell Transfer Therapy to a Wide Variety of Human Cancers

Receptor	Type	Cancers	Status
MART-1	TCR	Melanoma	Closed
gp100	TCR	Melanoma	Closed
NY-ESO-1	TCR	Epithelial & sarcomas	Accruing
CEA	TCR	Colorectal	Closed
CD19	CAR	Lymphomas	Accruing
VEGFR2	CAR	All cancers	Accruing
2G-1	TCR	Kidney	Accruing
IL-12	Cytokine	Adjuvant for all receptors	Accruing
MAGE-A3[a]	TCR	Epithelial	In development
EGFRvIII	CAR	Glioblastoma	Accruing
SSX-2	TCR	Epithelial	In development
Mesothelin	CAR	Pancreas & mesothelioma	Accruing
HPV16 (E6&7)	TCR	Cervical, oropharyngeal	In development

[a] MAGE-A3 TCRs; restricted by HLA-A2, A1, Cw7, DP4—covers 80% of patients.
EGFR, epidermal growth factor receptor; VEGFR2, vascular endothelial growth factor 2.

clonal antibodies in treating B-cell malignancies and the fact that allogeneic hematopoietic stem cell transplantation (alloHSCT) can cure a variety of hematologic malignancies.[161–167] The results with monoclonal antibodies and alloHSCT clearly prove that immunologic therapies have significant activity against hematologic malignancies, but monoclonal antibodies are not curative as single agents,[162,166] and alloHSCT has a substantial transplant-related mortality rate due to infections and an immunologic attack against normal tissues known as graft versus host disease (GVHD).[163,165] The proven curative potential of alloHSCT and the effectiveness of autologous T-cell transfer therapies for melanoma have encouraged the development of autologous T-cell therapies for hematologic malignancies.[125,129,163,165] Genetically engineering T cells to specifically recognize antigens expressed by malignant cells has emerged as a very promising strategy for cancer immunotherapy.[125,129,168]

T cells can be genetically engineered to express either of two types of receptors, CARs[168–171] or natural TCRs.[6,131,172] T cells expressing either a CAR or TCR gain the ability to specifically recognize an antigen.[171,172] CARs are artificial fusion proteins that incorporate antigen recognition domains and T-cell activation domains.[168,170,172] The antigen recognition domains are most often derived from monoclonal antibodies.[168,170,172] Antigen recognition by TCRs is major histocompatibility complex restricted.[125,128] In contrast to TCRs, recognition of antigens by CARs is not dependent on MHC molecules. An advantage of TCRs over CARs is that TCRs can recognize intracellular antigens, whereas CARs can only recognize cell-surface antigens.

Chimeric Antigen Receptors

CARs targeting hematopoietic antigens have been extensively studied in preclinical experiments and early-stage clinical trials.[168,170,172,173] For a protein to be a promising target for CAR-expressing T cells, it should be uniformly expressed on the malignant cells being targeted but not expressed on essential normal cells. Many cell-surface proteins with restricted normal tissue expression patterns have been identified on malignant hematologic cells, and CARs targeting many of these proteins are under development (Table 14.5).

Many factors can affect CAR T-cell therapies. The types of gene-therapy vectors encoding the DNA of the CAR could be an important factor. The types of vectors currently being used in clinical trials of CAR T cells are gammaretroviruses, lentiviruses, and transposon-based systems.[132,133,174–181] The design of the CAR fusion protein is another important factor. CAR fusion proteins include an antigen-recognition domain that is most often derived from an antibody, costimulatory domains such as CD28 and 4-1BB, and T-cell activation domains that are usually derived from the CD3z molecule.[168,170,171,182] Other factors that could impact the effectiveness of CAR T-cell therapies include the cell culture method used to prepare the cells and administration of chemotherapy or radiation therapy prior to the CAR T-cell infusions.[170,178,179] In mouse models, a profound enhancement of the antimalignancy activity of infused T cells occurs when the T-cell infusions are preceded by lymphocyte-depleting chemotherapy or radiation therapy.[183–185] Because chemotherapy can have a direct antimalignancy effect against hematologic malignancies, the administration of chemotherapy prior to infusions of T cells is a confounding factor that must always be kept in mind when interpreting the results of clinical trials of T-cell therapies.

Anti-CD19 Chimeric Antigen Receptors

CD19 is an appealing target antigen for CARs because CD19 is expressed on almost all malignant B cells, but CD19 is not expressed on normal cells except B cells.[186] The first preclinical studies of anti-CD19 CARs utilized either gammaretrovirus vectors[174] or plasmid electroporation[176] to insert genes encoding anti-CD19 CARs into human T cells. These studies and subsequent preclinical work by other groups showed that T cells expressing anti-CD19

CANCER THERAPEUTICS

TABLE 14.5

Hematologic Antigens Targeted by Genetically-Modified T-Cells

Antigen	Malignancy Expressing Antigen	Targeted by CAR or TCR	References
CD19	B-cell malignancies	CAR	17, 19, 21, 22, 23, 24, 25, 26, 34, 35, 55, 56
CD20	B-cell malignancies	CAR	36, 37, 38
CD22	B-cell malignancies	CAR	39, 40
CD23	B-cell malignancies	CAR	41
ROR1	B-cell malignancies	CAR	42
Kappa light chain	B-cell malignancies	CAR	43
B-cell maturation antigen (BCMA)	Multiple myeloma	CAR	44
Lewis Y antigen	Multiple myeloma and acute myeloid leukemia (AML)	CAR	45, 46
CD123	AML	CAR	47
CD30	Hodgkin lymphoma	CAR	48, 49
CD70	Hodgkin lymphoma	CAR	50
Wilms tumor-1 (WT1)	AML and acute lymphoid leukemia (ALL)	TCR	51
Aurora kinase-A	AML and chronic myeloid leukemia (CML)	TCR	52
Hyaluronan-mediated motility receptor (HMMR)	AML and ALL	TCR	53

CARs could specifically recognize and kill CD19-expressing malignant B cells in vitro and in vivo.[174–176,187] These preclinical studies compared many different CAR signaling moieties, which led most groups to utilize CARs with T-cell activation domains from the CD3z molecule and costimulatory molecules from either CD28 or 4-1BB (CD137).[165,180,182,187,188] Preclinical studies showed that lymphocyte-depleting radiation therapy administered before anti-CD19 CAR T-cell infusions was critical to the antimalignancy activity of CAR T cells.[183] The addition of lymphocyte-depleting radiation therapy prior to infusions of anti-CD19 CAR T cells increased the percentage of mice cured of lymphoma by the CAR T cells from 0% to 100%.[183] Preclinical experiments with anti-CD19 CARs have led to several early-phase clinical trials.

The first clinical trial to demonstrate in vivo activity of anti-CD19 CAR T cells in humans was conducted in the Surgery Branch of the National Cancer Institute.[132] The gammaretroviral vector used in this trial encoded a CAR with a CD28 costimulatory domain. Patients treated on this clinical trial received cyclophosphamide and fludarabine chemotherapy followed by an infusion of anti-CD19 CAR T cells and a short course of intravenous IL-2.[132,181] Clear antigen-specific activity of the anti-CD19 CAR T cells was demonstrated because blood B cells were selectively eliminated from four of the seven evaluable patients for several months.[181] The duration of B-cell depletion in these patients was much longer than the duration of B-cell depletion caused by the chemotherapy that the patients received.[132,181] This study also generated evidence of an antimalignancy effect by the anti-CD19 CAR T cells because six of seven evaluable patients with advanced B-cell malignancies obtained either complete remissions or partial remissions (Fig. 14.9).[181] One of these remissions is ongoing 45 months after treatment, and another remission is ongoing 31 months after treatment. Significant toxicity, including hypotension and neurologic toxicity, occurred during this clinical trial.[181] The severity of these toxicities correlated with the levels of serum inflammatory cytokines.[181] Except for one patient who died with influenza pneumonia, the toxicities were transient, with all toxicities resolving within 3 weeks of the anti-CD19 CAR T-cell infusions.[181]

Investigators at the Memorial Sloan Kettering Cancer Center treated nine patients with chronic lymphocytic leukemia (CLL) or acute lymphocytic leukemia (ALL) by infusing T cells that expressed a CAR with a CD28 costimulatory domain.[179] The gene therapy vector used in this work was a gammaretrovirus.[179] None of three patients treated with CAR T cells alone experienced a regression of leukemia, and CLL regressed in one of four evaluable patients treated with cyclophosphamide followed by an infusion of CAR T cells. Using the same CAR, the same group went on to treat five patients with ALL.[173] Patients received chemotherapy followed by an infusion of anti-CD19 CAR T cells. Four patients had detectable leukemia prior to their CAR T-cell infusions, and all of these patients became minimal residual disease negative after infusion of CAR T cells. Four of five patients on this trial rapidly underwent allogeneic stem cell transplantation after their CAR T-cell infusions.[173]

Investigators at the Baylor College of Medicine conducted clinical trials of anti-CD19 CAR T cells in which each patient simultaneously received infusions of two types of anti-CD19 CAR T cells.[189] One type of T cell expressed a CAR expressing a CD28 costimulatory domain. The other type of T cell was identical except that the CAR it expressed lacked a CD28 domain. Compared to the T cells lacking a CD28 moiety, the T cells expressing a CAR with a CD28 moiety had higher peak blood levels and longer in vivo persistence.[189] Patients on this trial did not receive chemotherapy, and there were no remissions of malignancy or long-term B-cell depletion.[189]

Investigators at the University of Pennsylvania reported results from three patients with CLL who were treated with chemotherapy followed by infusions of anti-CD19 CAR-expressing T cells.[133,180] The CAR used in this study was encoded by a lentiviral vector and contained a costimulatory domain from the 4-1BB molecule. Two

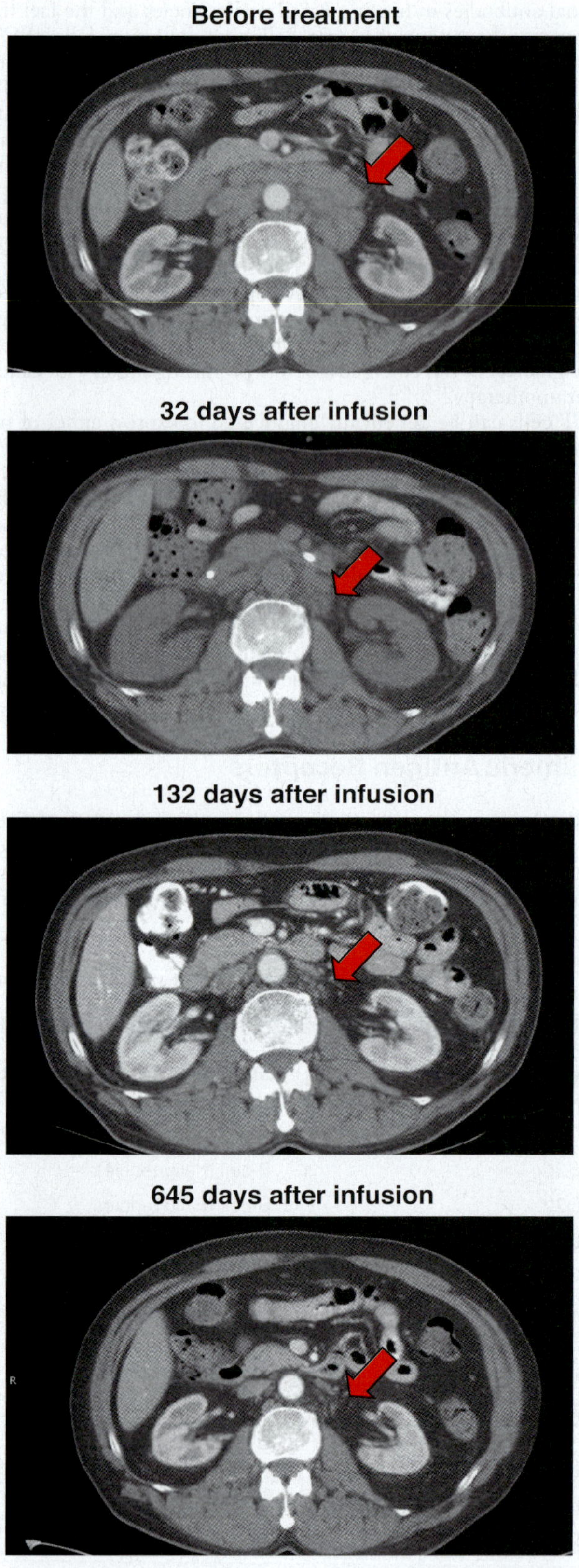

Figure 14.9 Computed tomography (CT) scans show regression of adenopathy in a patient with chronic lymphocytic leukemia (CLL) after treatment with chemotherapy followed by an infusion of autologous anti-CD19 CAR T cells. The time after the cell infusion of each CT scan is indicated. The *arrow* points to a large lymph node mass that resolved completely over time. (Reproduced from Kochenderfer JN, Rosenberg SA. Treating B-Cell cancer with T cells expressing anti-CD19 chimeric antigen receptors. *Nature Rev Clin Oncology* 2013;10:267-276, with permission.)

of the three reported patients obtained prolonged complete remissions.[180] This same CAR design was subsequently evaluated in a clinical trial enrolling patients with ALL.[190] One ALL patient obtained a prolonged complete remission but also experienced significant toxicity that was associated with elevated levels of serum cytokines.[190]

Overall, the early results with anti-CD19 CAR T cells show that this strategy holds great promise to improve the treatment of B-cell malignancies, but anti-CD19 CAR T-cell infusions are also associated with significant toxicity that is usually of short duration. Future progress will require decreasing the toxicity of anti-CD19 CAR T cells while maintaining or enhancing their antimalignancy activity. Parameters that are being studied in an effort to improve anti-CD19 CAR therapy include vector selection, CAR design, cell culture methods, and clinical application.

Chimeric Antigen Receptors and T-Cell Receptors Targeting Hematologic Antigens Other than CD19

CARs and TCRs targeting several hematologic antigens other than CD19 have been evaluated in preclinical or clinical studies. Except for CD19, the B-cell antigen CD20 has been the hematologic antigen most extensively studied as a target of CAR T cells.[191–193] Plasmid electroporation, which is not an optimal method of T-cell genetic modification, was used to transfer the anti-CD20 CAR gene to T cells in these studies. In one trial of anti-CD20 CAR T cells, patients received chemotherapy followed by infusions of T cells expressing a CAR without costimulatory domains.[192] One of seven patients obtained a partial remission that lasted 3 months. In a second trial, patients received chemotherapy followed by anti-CD20 CAR T cells expressing a CAR with both CD28 and 4-1BB costimulatory domains; in this trial, the only evaluable patient obtained a partial remission.[193]

CARs targeting other B-cell antigens including CD22,[157,194] CD23,[195] receptor tyrosine kinase–like orphan receptor-1 (ROR1),[196] and the immunoglobulin kappa light chain[197] have been evaluated in preclinical studies. CARs for treating multiple myeloma are currently being developed. B-cell maturation antigen (BCMA) is expressed on normal and malignant plasma cells, but it is not known to be expressed on other normal cells except for a small subset of mature B cells.[198] CARs targeting BCMA have undergone preclinical testing, and a clinical trial of an anti-BCMA CAR will open soon.[198] Preclinical studies have been performed on CARs targeting the Lewis Y antigen as a treatment for multiple myeloma and acute myeloid leukemia (AML),[199] and activity against AML was recently demonstrated in a phase I clinical trial of a CAR targeting the Lewis Y antigen.[200] CARs targeting the CD123 protein are undergoing preclinical testing for potential use against AML.[201] For Hodgkin lymphoma, CARs have been developed that target the CD30 protein and the CD70 protein, and anti-CD30 CARs are entering early-phase clinical trials.[202–204]

MHC-restricted TCRs targeting some antigens expressed on hematologic malignancies have undergone preclinical testing, but TCRs for treating hematologic malignancies are at a much earlier stage of development than CARs (see Table 14.1). TCRs targeting the Wilms tumor antigen-1 (WT1) are under development to treat ALL and AML.[205] Aurora kinase-A–specific TCRs and hyaluronan-mediated motility receptor (HMMR)-specific TCRs are under preclinical development as leukemia treatments.[206,207]

T-Cell Gene Therapy in the Setting of Allogeneic Hematopoietic Stem Cell Transplantation

A leading cause of death among patients undergoing alloHSCT is relapse of malignancy, and alloHSCT is often complicated by GVHD.[164,165,208] Therefore, a central goal in the field of alloHSCT is to increase the antimalignancy activity of allogeneic T cells without worsening GVHD. One way to accomplish this goal might be to genetically modify T cells to give them the ability to specifically recognize antigens expressed by malignant cells. CARs are well-suited for this task.

Two groups have recently reported promising early results treating B-cell malignancies after alloHSCT with allogeneic donor-derived T cells expressing anti-CD19 CARs.[209,210] Investigators at the National Cancer Institute treated 10 patients with B-cell malignancies that persisted despite alloHSCT and standard donor lymphocyte infusions.[209] Although patients on this trial did not receive chemotherapy before their T-cell infusions, 3 of 10 patients had objective regressions of their malignancies, and 1 patient with CLL remains in CR more than 1 year after treatment.[209] No patient developed GVHD after receiving allogeneic anti-CD19 CAR T cells on this trial.[209] Investigators at the Baylor College of Medicine reported objective antimalignancy responses in two of six patients with relapsed malignancy after infusion of donor-derived allogeneic anti-CD19 CAR T cells that were also specific for viral antigens.[210]

In an effort to improve the safety of infusions of allogeneic lymphocytes by limiting GVHD, investigators have genetically modified T cells to express *suicide genes* that cause death of the T cells containing the suicide gene when certain drugs are administered.[211–214] Suicide gene–expressing T cells are infused to treat malignancy after alloHSCT. This approach has been tested in clinical trials, and rapid abrogation of GVHD has been demonstrated.[211,213,214]

CANCER THERAPEUTICS

REFERENCES

1. Kenter GG, Welters MJ, Valentijn AR, et al. Vaccination against HPV-16 oncoproteins for vulvar intraepithelial neoplasia. *N Engl J Med* 2009;361:1838–1847.
2. Gaffen SL, Liu KD. Overview of interleukin-2 function, production and clinical applications. *Cytokine* 2004;28:109–123.
3. Attia P, Phan GQ, Maker AV, et al. Autoimmunity correlates with tumor regression in patients with metastatic melanoma treated with anti-cytotoxic T-lymphocyte antigen-4. *J Clin Oncol* 2005;23:6043–6053.
4. Topalian SL, Hodi FS, Brahmer JR, et al. Safety, activity, and immune correlates of anti-PD-1 antibody in cancer. *N Engl J Med* 2012;366:2443–2454.
5. Rosenberg SA, Yang JC, Sherry RM, et al. Durable complete responses in heavily pretreated patients with metastatic melanoma using T-cell transfer immunotherapy. *Clin Cancer Res* 2011;17:4550–4557.
6. Robbins PF, Morgan RA, Feldman SA, et al. Tumor regression in patients with metastatic synovial sarcoma and melanoma using genetically engineered lymphocytes reactive with NY-ESO-1. *J Clin Oncol* 2011;29:917–924.
7. Chen YT, Scanlan MJ, Sahin U, et al. A testicular antigen aberrantly expressed in human cancers detected by autologous antibody screening. *Proc Natl Acad Sci U S A* 1997;94:1914–1918.
8. Van der Bruggen P, Traversari C, Chomez P, et al. A gene encoding an antigen recognized by cytolytic T lymphocytes on a human melanoma. *Science* 1991;254:1643–1647.
9. van der Bruggen P, Stroobant V, Vigneron N, et al. Peptide database: T cell-defined tumor antigens. *Cancer Immun* 2013. https://www.cancerimmunity.org/peptide/
10. Gnjatic S, Nishikawa H, Jungbluth AA, et al. NY-ESO-1: review of an immunogenic tumor antigen. *Adv Cancer Res* 2006;95:1–30.
11. Chinnasamy N, Wargo JA, Yu Z, et al. A TCR targeting the HLA-A*0201-restricted epitope of MAGE-A3 recognizes multiple epitopes of the MAGE-A antigen superfamily in several types of cancer. *J Immunol* 2011;186:685–696.
12. Morgan RA, Chinnasamy N, Abate-Daga D, et al. Cancer regression and neurological toxicity following anti-MAGE-A3 TCR gene therapy. *J Immunother* 2013;36:133–151.
13. Linette GP, Stadtmauer EA, Maus MV, et al. Cardiovascular toxicity and titin cross-reactivity of affinity-enhanced T cells in myeloma and melanoma. *Blood* 2013;122:863–871.
14. Cox AL, Skipper J, Chen Y, et al. Identification of a peptide recognized by five melanoma-specific human cytotoxic T cell lines. *Science* 1994;264:716–719.

15. Kawakami Y, Eliyahu S, Jennings C, et al. Recognition of multiple epitopes in the human melanoma antigen gp100 by tumor infiltrating T-lymphocytes associated with in vivo tumor regression. *J Immunol* 1995;154:3961–3968.
16. Brichard V, Van Pel A, Wolfel T, et al. The tyrosinase gene codes for an antigen recognized by autologous cytolytic T lymphocytes on HLA-A2 melanomas. *J Exp Med* 1993;178:489–495.
17. Wang RF, Robbins PF, Kawakami Y, et al. Identification of a gene encoding a melanoma tumor antigen recognized by HLA-A31-restricted tumor-infiltrating lymphocytes. *J Exp Med* 1995;181:799–804.
18. Wang R-F, Appella E, Kawakami Y, et al. Identification of TRP-2 as a human tumor antigen recognized by cytotoxic T lymphocytes. *J Exp Med* 1996;184:2207–2216.
19. Kawakami Y, Eliyahu S, Delgado CH, et al. Cloning of the gene coding for a shared human melanoma antigen recognized by autologous T cells infiltrating into tumor. *Proc Natl Acad Sci U S A* 1994;91:3515–3519.
20. Coulie PG, Brichard V, Van Pel A, et al. A new gene coding for a differentiation antigen recognized by autologous cytolytic T lymphocytes on HLA-A2 melanomas. *J Exp Med* 1992;180:35–42.
21. Kawakami Y, Eliyahu S, Sakaguchi K, et al. Identification of the immunodominant peptides of the MART-1 human melanoma antigen recognized by the majority of HLA-A2-restricted tumor infiltrating lymphocytes. *J Exp Med* 1994;180:347–352.
22. Hanada K, Yewdell JW, Yang JC. Immune recognition of a human renal cancer antigen through post-translational protein splicing. *Nature* 2004;427:252–256.
23. Carrington DM, Auffret A, Hanke DE. Polypeptide ligation occurs during post-translational modification of concanavalin A. *Nature* 1985;313:64–67.
24. Paulus H. Protein splicing and related forms of protein autoprocessing. *Annu Rev Biochem* 2000;69:447–496.
25. Vigneron N, Stroobant V, Chapiro J, et al. An antigenic peptide produced by peptide splicing in the proteasome. *Science* 2004;304:587–590.
26. Warren EH, Vigneron NJ, Gavin MA, et al. An antigen produced by splicing of noncontiguous peptides in the reverse order. *Science* 2006;313:1444–1447.
27. Dalet A, Robbins PF, Stroobant V, et al. An antigenic peptide produced by reverse splicing and double asparagine deamidation. *Proc Natl Acad Sci U S A* 2011;108:E323–E331.
28. Michaux A, Larrieu P, Stroobant V, et al. A spliced antigenic peptide comprising a single spliced amino acid is produced in the proteasome by reverse splicing of a longer peptide fragment followed by trimming. *J Immunol* 2014;192:1962–1971.
29. Ikeda H, Lethe B, Lehmann F. Characterization of an antigen that is recognized on a melanoma showing partial HLA loss by CTL expressing an NK inhibitory receptor. *Immunity* 1999;6:199–208.
30. Lundegaard C, Lamberth K, Harndahl M, et al. NetMHC-3.0: accurate web accessible predictions of human, mouse and monkey MHC class I affinities for peptides of length 8-11. *Nucleic Acids Res* 2008;36:W509–W512.
31. Peters B, Sette A. Generating quantitative models describing the sequence specificity of biological processes with the stabilized matrix method. *BMC Bioinformatics* 2005;6:132.
32. Xue BH, Zhang Y, Sosman JA, et al. Induction of human cytotoxic T lymphocytes specific for prostate-specific antigen. *Prostate* 1997;30:73–78.
33. Horiguchi Y, Nukaya I, Okazawa K, et al. Screening of HLA-A24-restricted epitope peptides from prostate-specific membrane antigen that induce specific antitumor cytotoxic T lymphocytes. *Clin Cancer Res* 2002;8:3885–3892.
34. Peoples GE, Goedegeburre PS, Smith R. Breast and ovarian cancer-specific cytotoxic T lymphocytes recognize the same HER2/neu-derived peptide. *Proc Natl Acad U S A* 1995;92:432–436.
35. Zaks TZ, Rosenberg SA. Immunization with a peptide epitope (p369-377) from HER-2/neu leads to peptide-specific cytotoxic T lymphocytes that fail to recognize HER-2/neu+ tumors. *Cancer Res* 1998;58:4902–4908.
36. Vonderheide RH, Hahn WC, Schultze JL, et al. The telomerase catalytic subunit is a widely expressed tumor-associated antigen recognized by cytotoxic T lymphocytes. *Immunity* 1999;10:673–679.
37. Parkhurst MR, Riley JP, Igarashi T, et al. Immunization of patients with the hTERT:540-548 peptide induces peptide-reactive T lymphocytes that do not recognize tumors endogenously expressing telomerase. *Clin Cancer Res* 2004;10:4688–4698.
38. Weinschenk T, Gouttefangeas C, Schirle M, et al. Integrated functional genomics approach for the design of patient-individual antitumor vaccines. *Cancer Res* 2002;62: 5818–5827.
39. Dutoit V, Herold-Mende C, Hilf N, et al. Exploiting the glioblastoma peptidome to discover novel tumour-associated antigens for immunotherapy. *Brain* 2012;135:1042–1054.
40. Walter S, Weinschenk T, Stenzl A, et al. Multipeptide immune response to cancer vaccine IMA901 after single-dose cyclophosphamide associates with longer patient survival. *Nat Med* 2012;18:1254–1261.
41. Theobald M, Biggs J, Dittmer D, et al. Targeting p53 as a general tumor antigen. *Proc Natl Acad Sci U S A* 1995;92:11993–11997.
42. Theoret MR, Cohen CJ, Nahvi AV, et al. Relationship of p53 overexpression on cancers and recognition by anti-p53 T cell receptor-transduced T cells. *Hum Gene Ther* 2008;19:1219–1231.
43. Parkhurst M, Joo J, Riley JP, et al. Characterization of genetically modified T cell receptors that recognize the CEA:691-699 peptide in the context of HLA-A2.1 on human colorectal cancer cells. *Clin Cancer Res* 2009;15:169–180.
44. Parkhurst MR, Yang JC, Langan RC, et al. T cells targeting carcinoembryonic antigen can mediate regression of metastatic colorectal cancer but induce severe transient colitis. *Mol Ther* 2011;19:620–626.
45. Wolfel T, Hauer M, Schneider J, et al. A p16INK4A-insensitive CDK4 mutant targeted by cytolytic T lymphocytes in a human melanoma. *Science* 1995;269:1281–1284.
46. Robbins PF, El-Gamil M, Li YF, et al. A mutated B-catenin gene encodes a melanoma-specific antigen recognized by tumor infiltrating lymphocytes. *J Exp Med* 1996;183:1185–1192.
47. Rubinfeld B, Robbins P, El-Gamil M. Stabilization of beta-catenin by genetic defects in melanoma cell lines. *Science* 1997;275:1790–1792.
48. Mumberg D, Wick M, Schreiber H. Unique tumor antigens redefined as mutant tumor-specific antigens. *Semin Immunol* 1996;8:289–293.
49. Cheever MA, Chen W, Disis ML, et al. T-cell immunity to oncogenic proteins including mutated ras and chimeric bcr-abl. *Ann N Y Acad Sci* 1993;690: 101–112.
50. Castle JC, Kreiter S, Diekmann J, et al. Exploiting the mutanome for tumor vaccination. *Cancer Res* 2012;72:1081–1091.
51. Matsushita H, Vesely MD, Koboldt DC, et al. Cancer exome analysis reveals a T-cell-dependent mechanism of cancer immunoediting. *Nature* 2012;482: 400–404.
52. Robbins PF, Lu YC, El-Gamil M, et al. Mining exomic sequencing data to identify mutated antigens recognized by adoptively transferred tumor-reactive T cells. *Nat Med* 2013;19:747–752.
53. van Rooij N, van Buuren MM, Philips D, et al. Tumor exome analysis reveals neoantigen-specific T-cell reactivity in an ipilimumab-responsive melanoma. *J Clin Oncol* 2013;31:e439–e442.
54. Tran E, Turcotte S, Gros A, et al. Cancer immunotherapy based on mutation-specific CD4+ T cells in a patient with epithelial cancer. *Science* 2014;344:641–645.
55. Koutsky LA, Ault KA, Wheeler CM, et al. A controlled trial of a human papillomavirus type 16 vaccine. *N Engl J Med* 2002;347:1645–1651.
56. Villa LL, Costa RL, Petta CA, et al. Prophylactic quadrivalent human papillomavirus (types 6, 11, 16, and 18) L1 virus-like particle vaccine in young women: a randomised double-blind placebo-controlled multicentre phase II efficacy trial. *Lancet Oncol* 2005;6:271–278.
57. Wolchok JD, Hoos A, O'Day S, et al. Guidelines for the evaluation of immune therapy activity in solid tumors: immune-related response criteria. *Clin Cancer Res* 2009;15:7412–7420.
58. Hoos A, Eggermont AM, Janetzki S, et al. Improved endpoints for cancer immunotherapy trials. *J Natl Cancer Inst* 2010;102:1388–1397.
59. Morgan DA, Ruscetti FW, Gallo R. Selective in vitro growth of T lymphocytes from normal human bone marrows. *Science* 1976;193:1007–1008.
60. Smith KA, Gilbride KJ, Favata MF. Lymphocyte activating factor promotes T-cell growth factor production by cloned murine lymphoma cells. *Nature* 1980;287:853–855.
61. Smith KA, Lachman LB, Oppenheim JJ, et al. The functional relationship of the interleukins. *J Exp Med* 1980;151:1551–1556.
62. Taniguchi T, Matsui H, Fujita T. Structure and expression of a cloned cDNA for human interleukin-2. *Nature* 1983;302:305–307.
63. Rosenberg SA, Grimm EA, McGrogan M, et al. Biological activity of recombinant human interleukin-2 produced in *Escherichia coli*. *Science* 1984;223:1412–1414.
64. Rosenberg SA, Mule JJ, Spiess PJ, et al. Regression of established pulmonary metastases and subcutaneous tumor mediated by the systemic administration of high dose recombinant IL-2. *J Exp Med* 1985;161:1169–1188.
65. Lotze MT, Matory YL, Ettinghausen SE, et al. In vivo administration of purified human interleukin-2. II. Half life, immunologic effects and expansion of peripheral lymphoid cells in vivo with recombinant IL-2. *J Immunol* 1985;135:2865–2875.
66. Rosenberg SA, Lotze MT, Muul LM, et al. Observations on the systemic administration of autologous lymphokine-activated killer cells and recombinant interleukin-2 to patients with metastatic cancer. *N Engl J Med* 1985;313: 1485–1492.
67. Rosenberg SA, Lotze MT, Yang JC, et al. Prospective randomized trial of high-dose interleukin-2 alone or in conjunction with lymphokine-activated killer cells for the treatment of patients with advanced cancer. *J Natl Cancer Inst* 1993;85:622–632.
68. Atkins MB, Sparano J, Fisher RI, et al. Randomized phase II trial of high-dose interleukin-2 either alone or in combination with interferon alfa-2b in advanced renal cell carcinoma. *J Clin Oncol* 1993;11:661–670.
69. Rosenberg SA, Yang JC, White DE, et al. Durability of complete responses in patients with metastatic cancer treated with high-dose interleukin-2: identification of the antigens mediating response. *Ann Surg* 1998;228:307–319.
70. Fyfe G, Fisher R, Sznol M, et al. Results of treatment of 255 patients with metastatic renal cell carcinoma who received high dose proleukin interleukin-2 therapy. *J Clin Oncol* 1995;13:688–696.
71. Fisher RI, Rosenberg SA, Fyfe G. Long-term survival update for high-dose recombinant interleukin-2 in patients with renal cell carcinoma. *Cancer J Sci Am* 2000;6:S55–S57.
72. Yang JC, Sherry RM, Steinberg SM, et al. Randomized study of high-dose and low-dose interleukin-2 in patients with metastatic renal cancer. *J Clin Oncol* 2003;21:3127–3132.
73. Atkins MB, Lotze MT, Dutcher JP, et al. High-dose recombinant interleukin 2 therapy for patients with metastatic melanoma: analysis of 270 patients treated between 1985 and 1993. *J Clin Oncol* 19991;17:2105–2116.
74. Atkins MB, Kunkel L, Sznol M, et al. High-dose recombinant interleukin-2 therapy in patients with metastatic melanoma: long-term survival update. *Cancer J Sci Am* 2000;6:S11–S14.

75. Rosenberg SA, Yang JC, Schwartzentruber DJ, et al. Immunologic and therapeutic evaluation of a synthetic peptide vaccine for the treatment of patients with metastatic melanoma. *Nat Med* 1998;4:321–327.
76. Schwartzentruber DJ, Lawson DH, Richards JM, et al. gp100 peptide vaccine and interleukin-2 in patients with advanced melanoma. *N Engl J Med* 2011;364:2119–2127.
77. Prieto PA, Yang JC, Sherry RM, et al. CTLA-4 blockade with ipilimumab: long-term follow-up of 177 patients with metastatic melanoma. *Clin Cancer Res* 2012;18:2039–2047.
78. Phan GQ, Attia P, Steinberg SM, et al. Factors associated with response to high-dose interleukin-2 in patients with metastatic melanoma. *J Clin Oncol* 2001;19:3477–3482.
79. Rosenberg SA, Yang JC, Topalian SL, et al. Treatment of 283 consecutive patients with metastatic melanoma or renal cell cancer using high-dose bolus interleukin 2. *JAMA* 1994;271:907–913.
80. Rosenberg SA, Lotze MT, Yang JC, et al. Experience with the use of high-dose interleukin-2 in the treatment of 652 cancer patients. *Ann Surg* 1989;210: 474–484.
81. Gemlo BT, Palladino Jr MA, Jaffe HS, et al. Circulating cytokines in patients with metastatic cancer treated with recombinant interleukin 2 and lymphokine-activated killer cells. *Cancer Res* 1988;48:5864–5867.
82. Pockaj BA, Yang JC, Lotze MT, et al. A prospective randomized trial evaluating colloid versus crystalloid resuscitation in the treatment of the vascular leak syndrome associated with interleukin-2 therapy. *J Immunother Emphasis Tumor Immunol* 1994;15:22–28.
83. Klempner MS, Noring R, Mier JW, et al. An acquired chemotactic defect in neutrophils from patients receiving interleukin-2 immunotherapy. *N Engl J Med* 1990;322:959–965.
84. Lee RE, Lotze MT, Skibber JM, et al. Cardiorespiratory effects of immunotherapy with interleukin-2. *J Clin Oncol* 1989;7:7–20.
85. Schwartzentruber DJ. Guidelines for the safe administration of high-dose interleukin-2. *J Immunother* 2001;24:287–293.
86. Kammula US, White DE, Rosenberg SA. Trends in the safety of high dose bolus interleukin-2 administration in patients with metastatic cancer. *Cancer* 1998;83:797–805.
87. Brunet JF, Denizot F, Luciani MF, et al. A new member of the immunoglobulin superfamily—CTLA-4. *Nature* 1987;328:267–270.
88. Linsley PS, Brady W, Urnes M, et al. CTLA-4 is a second receptor for the B cell activation antigen B7. *J Exp Med* 1991;174:561–569.
89. Walunas TL, Lenschow DJ, Bakker CY, et al. CTLA-4 can function as a negative regulator of T cell activation. *Immunity* 1994;1:405–413.
90. Walunas TL, Bakker CY, Bluestone JA. CTLA-4 ligation blocks CD28-dependent T cell activation. *J Exp Med* 1996;183:2541–2550.
91. van Elsas A, Hurwitz AA, Allison JP. Combination immunotherapy of B16 melanoma using anti-cytotoxic T lymphocyte-associated antigen 4 (CTLA-4) and granulocyte/macrophage colony-stimulating factor (GM-CSF)-producing vaccines induces rejection of subcutaneous and metastatic tumors accompanied by autoimmune depigmentation. *J Exp Med* 1999;190:355–366.
92. Hurwitz AA, Yu TF, Leach DR, et al. CTLA-4 blockade synergizes with tumor-derived granulocyte-macrophage colony-stimulating factor for treatment of an experimental mammary carcinoma. *Proc Natl Acad Sci U S A* 1998;95:10067–10071.
93. Phan GQ, Yang JC, Sherry RM, et al. Cancer regression and autoimmunity induced by cytotoxic T lymphocyte-associated antigen 4 blockade in patients with metastatic melanoma. *Proc Natl Acad Sci U S A* 2003;100:8372–8377.
94. Maker AV, Phan GQ, Attia P, et al. Tumor regression and autoimmunity in patients treated with cytotoxic T lymphocyte-associated antigen 4 blockade and interleukin 2: a phase I/II study. *Ann Surg Oncol* 2005;12:1005–1016.
95. Maker AV, Yang JC, Sherry RM, et al. Intrapatient dose escalation of anti-CTLA-4 antibody in patients with metastatic melanoma. *J Immunother* 2006;29:455–463.
96. Beck KE, Blansfield JA, Tran KQ, et al. Enterocolitis in patients with cancer after antibody blockade of cytotoxic T-lymphocyte-associated antigen 4. *J Clin Oncol* 2006;24:2283–2289.
97. Robinson MR, Chan CC, Yang JC, et al. Cytotoxic T lymphocyte-associated antigen 4 blockade in patients with metastatic melanoma: a new cause of uveitis. *J Immunother* 2004;27:478–479.
98. Hodi FS, O'Day SJ, McDermott DF, et al. Improved survival with ipilimumab in patients with metastatic melanoma. *N Engl J Med* 2010;363:711–723.
99. Robert C, Thomas L, Bondarenko I, et al. Ipilimumab plus dacarbazine for previously untreated metastatic melanoma. *N Engl J Med* 2011;364:2517–2526.
100. Wolchok JD, Weber JS, Maio M, et al. Four-year survival rates for patients with metastatic melanoma who received ipilimumab in phase II clinical trials. *Ann Oncol* 2013;24:2174–2180.
101. Yang JC, Hughes M, Kammula U, et al. Ipilimumab (anti-CTLA4 antibody) causes regression of metastatic renal cell cancer associated with enteritis and hypophysitis. *J Immunother* 2007;30:825–830.
102. Kirkwood JM, Lorigan P, Hersey P, et al. Phase II trial of tremelimumab (CP-675,206) in patients with advanced refractory or relapsed melanoma. *Clin Cancer Res* 2010;16:1042–1048.
103. Ribas A, Kefford R, Marshall MA, et al. Phase III randomized clinical trial comparing tremelimumab with standard-of-care chemotherapy in patients with advanced melanoma. *J Clin Oncol* 2013;31:616–622.
104. Ott PA, Hodi FS, Robert C. CTLA-4 and PD-1/PD-L1 blockade: new immunotherapeutic modalities with durable clinical benefit in melanoma patients. *Clin Cancer Res* 2013;19:5300–5309.
105. Keir ME, Butte MJ, Freeman GJ, et al. PD-1 and its ligands in tolerance and immunity. *Annu Rev Immunol* 2008;26:677–704.
106. Dong H, Strome SE, Salomao DR, et al. Tumor-associated B7-H1 promotes T-cell apoptosis: a potential mechanism of immune evasion. *Nat Med* 2002;8:793–800.
107. Brahmer JR, Drake CG, Wollner I, et al. Phase I study of single-agent anti-programmed death-1 (MDX-1106) in refractory solid tumors: safety, clinical activity, pharmacodynamics, and immunologic correlates. *J Clin Oncol* 2010;28:3167–3175.
108. Brahmer JR. Immune checkpoint blockade: the hope for immunotherapy as a treatment of lung cancer? *Semin Oncol* 2014;41:126–132.
109. Topalian SL, Sznol M, McDermott DF, et al. Survival, durable tumor remission, and long-term safety in patients with advanced melanoma receiving nivolumab. *J Clin Oncol* 2014;32:1020–1030.
110. Wolchok JD, Kluger H, Callahan MK, et al. Nivolumab plus ipilimumab in advanced melanoma. *N Engl J Med* 2013;369:122–133.
111. Hamid O, Robert C, Daud A, et al. Safety and tumor responses with lambrolizumab (anti-PD-1) in melanoma. *N Engl J Med* 2013;369:134–144.
112. Brahmer JR, Tykodi SS, Chow LQ, et al. Safety and activity of anti-PD-L1 antibody in patients with advanced cancer. *N Engl J Med* 2012;366:2455–2465.
113. Drake CG, Lipson EJ, Brahmer JR. Breathing new life into immunotherapy: review of melanoma, lung and kidney cancer. *Nat Rev Clin Oncol* 2014;11:24–37.
114. Rosenberg SA, Yang JC, Restifo NP. Cancer immunotherapy: moving beyond current vaccines. *Nat Med* 2004;10:909–915.
115. Klebanoff CA, Acquavella N, Yu Z, et al. Therapeutic cancer vaccines: are we there yet? *Immunol Rev* 2011;239:27–44.
116. Slingluff CL, Yamshchikov G, Neese P, et al. Phase I trial of a melanoma vaccine with gp100 $_{280-288}$ peptide and tetanus helper peptide in adjuvant: immunologic and clinical outcomes. *Clin Cancer Res* 2001;7:3012–3024.
117. Schaed SG, Klimek VM, Panageas KS, et al. T-cell responses against tyrosinase 368-376(370D) peptide in HLA*A0201$^+$ melanoma patients: randomized trial comparing incomplete Freund's adjuvant, granulocyte macrophage colony-stimulating factor, and QS-21 as immunological adjuvants. *Clin Cancer Res* 2004;8:967–972.
118. Marshall JL, Hoyer RJ, Toomey MA, et al. Phase I study in advanced cancer patients of a diversified prime-and-boost vaccination protocol using recombinant vaccinia virus and recombinant nonreplicating avipox virus to elicit anti-carcinoembryonic antigen immune responses. *J Clin Oncol* 2000;18: 3964–3973.
119. Eder JP, Kantoff PW, Roper K, et al. A phase I trial of a recombinant vaccinia virus expressing prostate-specific antigen in advanced prostate cancer. *Clin Cancer Res* 2003;6:1632–1638.
120. Lurquin C, Lethe B, De Plaen E, et al. Contrasting frequencies of antitumor and anti-vaccine T cells in metastases of a melanoma patient vaccinated with a MAGE tumor antigen. *J Exp Med* 2005;201:249–257.
121. Marincola FM, Rivoltini L, Salgaller ML, et al. Differential anti-MART-1/MelanA CTL activity in peripheral blood of HLA-A2 melanoma patients in comparison to healthy donors: evidence of in vivo priming by tumor cells. *J Immunother Emphasis Tumor Immunol* 1996;19:266–277.
122. Cormier JN, Salgaller ML, Prevette T, et al. Enhancement of cellular immunity in melanoma patients immunized with a peptide from MART-1/Melan A. *Cancer J Sci Am* 1997;3:37–44.
123. Kantoff PW, Higano CS, Shore ND, et al. Sipuleucel-T immunotherapy for castration-resistant prostate cancer. *N Engl J Med* 2010;363:422.
124. Rosenberg SA, Packard BS, Aebersold PM, et al. Use of tumor infiltrating lymphocytes and interleukin-2 in the immunotherapy of patients with metastatic melanoma. Preliminary report. *N Engl J Med* 1988;319:1676–1680.
125. Restifo NP, Dudley ME, Rosenberg SA. Adoptive immunotherapy for cancer: harnessing the T cell response. *Nat Rev Immunol* 2012;12:269–281.
126. Rooney CM, Smith CA, Ng CY, et al. Infusion of cytotoxic T cells for the prevention and treatment of Epstein-Barr virus-induced lymphoma in allogeneic transplant recipients. *Blood* 1998;92:1549–1555.
127. Rosenberg SA, Yannelli JR, Yang JC, et al. Treatment of patients with metastatic melanoma using autologous tumor-infiltrating lymphocytes and interleukin-2. *J Natl Cancer Inst* 1994;86:1159–1166.
128. Dudley ME, Wunderlich JR, Robbins PF, et al. Cancer regression and autoimmunity in patients after clonal repopulation with anti-tumor lymphocytes. *Science* 2002;298:850–854.
129. Dudley ME, Yang JC, Sherry R, et al. Adoptive cell therapy for patients with metastatic melanoma: Evaluation of intensive myeloablative chemoradiation preparative regimens. *J Clin Oncol* 2008;26:5233–5239.
130. Rosenberg SA. Cell transfer immunotherapy for metastatic solid cancer—what clinicians need to know. *Nat Rev Clin Oncol* 2011;8:577–585.
131. Morgan RA, Dudley ME, Wunderlich JR, et al. Cancer regression in patients after transfer of genetically engineered lymphocytes. *Science* 2006;314: 126–129.
132. Kochenderfer JN, Wilson WH, Janik E, et al. Eradication of B-lineage cells and regression of lymphoma in a patient treated with autologous T cells genetically engineered to recognize CD19. *Blood* 2010;116:4099–4102.
133. Porter DL, Levine BL, Kalos M, et al. Chimeric antigen receptor-modified T cells in chronic lymphoid leukemia. *N Engl J Med* 2011;365:725–733.
134. Tiera MJ, Winnik FO, Fernandes JC. Synthetic and natural polycations for gene therapy: state of the art and new perspectives. *Curr Gene Ther* 2006;6:59–71.
135. Birkholz K, Hombach A, Krug C, et al. Transfer of mRNA encoding recombinant immunoreceptors reprograms CD4+ and CD8+ T cells for use in the adoptive immunotherapy of cancer. *Gene Ther* 2009;16:596–604.

136. Zhao Y, Zheng Z, Cohen CJ, et al. High-efficiency transfection of primary human and mouse T lymphocytes using RNA electroporation. *Mol Ther* 2006;13:151–159.
137. Li L, Liu LC, Feller S, et al. Expression of chimeric antigen receptors in natural killer cells with a regulatory-compliant non-viral method. *Cancer Gene Ther* 2010;17:147–154.
138. Zhao Y, Moon E, Carpenito C, et al. Multiple injections of electroporated autologous T cells expressing a chimeric antigen receptor mediate regression of human disseminated tumor. *Cancer Res* 2010;70:9053–9061.
139. Ivics Z, Izsvak Z. Transposons for gene therapy! *Curr Gene Ther* 2006;6:593–607.
140. Singh H, Huls H, Kebriaei P, et al. A new approach to gene therapy using Sleeping Beauty to genetically modify clinical-grade T cells to target CD19. *Immunol Rev* 2014;257:181–190.
141. Hacein-Bey-Abina S, von Kalle C, Schmidt M, et al. A serious adverse event after successful gene therapy for X-linked severe combined immunodeficiency. *N Engl J Med* 2003;348:255–256.
142. Riviere I, Brose K, Mulligan RC. Effects of retroviral vector design on expression of human adenosine deaminase in murine bone marrow transplant recipients engrafted with genetically modified cells. *Proc Natl Acad Sci U S A* 1995;92:6733–6737.
143. Maetzig T, Galla M, Baum C, et al. Gammaretroviral vectors: biology, technology and application. *Viruses* 2011;3:677–713.
144. Schambach A, Swaney WP, van der Loo JC. Design and production of retro- and lentiviral vectors for gene expression in hematopoietic cells. *Methods Mol Biol* 2009;506:191–205.
145. Hughes MS, Yu YYL, Dudley ME, et al. Transfer of a TCR gene derived from a patient with a marked antitumor response conveys highly active T-cell effector functions. *Hum Gene Ther* 2005;16:457–472.
146. Zhang X, Godbey WT. Viral vectors for gene delivery in tissue engineering. *Adv Drug Deliv Rev* 2006;58:515–534.
147. Yu SS, Han E, Hong Y, et al. Construction of a retroviral vector production system with the minimum possibility of a homologous recombination. *Gene Ther* 2003;10:706–711.
148. Cavalieri S, Cazzaniga S, Geuna M, et al. Human T lymphocytes transduced by lentiviral vectors in the absence of TCR activation maintain an intact immune competence. *Blood* 2003;102:497–505.
149. Cavazzana-Calvo M, Payen E, Negre O, et al. Transfusion independence and HMGA2 activation after gene therapy of human beta-thalassaemia. *Nature* 2010;467:318–322.
150. Johnson LA, Morgan RA, Dudley ME, et al. Gene therapy with human and mouse T-cell receptors mediates cancer regression and targets normal tissues expressing cognate antigen. *Blood* 2009;114:535–546.
151. Simpson AJ, Caballero OL, Jungbluth A, et al. Cancer/testis antigens, gametogenesis and cancer. *Nat Rev Cancer* 2005;5:625.
152. Hofmann O, Caballero OL, Stevenson BJ, et al. Genome-wide analysis of cancer/testis gene expression. *Proc Natl Acad Sci U S A* 2008;105: 20422–20427.
153. Zhang Y, Wang Z, Liu H, et al. Pattern of gene expression and immune responses to Semenogelin 1 in chronic hematologic malignancies. *J Immunother* 2003;26:461–467.
154. Jungbluth AA, Antonescu CR, Busam KJ, et al. Monophasic and biphasic synovial sarcomas abundantly express cancer/testis antigen NY-ESO-1 but not MAGE-A1 or CT7. *Int J Cancer* 2001;94:252–256.
155. Gross G, Waks T, Eshhar Z. Expression of immunoglobulin-T-cell receptor chimeric molecules as functional receptors with antibody-type specificity. *Proc Natl Acad Sci U S A* 1989;86:10024–10028.
156. Pule MA, Savoldo B, Myers GD, et al. Virus-specific T cells engineered to coexpress tumor-specific receptors: persistence and antitumor activity in individuals with neuroblastoma. *Nat Med* 2008;14:1264–1270.
157. James SE, Greenberg PD, Jensen MC, et al. Antigen sensitivity of CD22-specific chimeric TCR is modulated by target epitope distance from the cell membrane. *J Immunol* 2008;180:7028–7038.
158. Morgan RA, Johnson LA, Davis JL, et al. Recognition of glioma stem cells by genetically modified T cells targeting EGFRvIII and development of adoptive cell therapy for glioma. *Hum Gene Ther* 2012;23:1043–1053.
159. Chinnasamy D, Yu Z, Theoret MR, et al. Gene therapy using genetically modified lymphocytes targeting VEGFR-2 inhibits the growth of vascularized syngenic tumors in mice. *J Clin Invest* 2010;120:3953–3968.
160. Carpenito C, Milone MC, Hassan R, et al. Control of large, established tumor xenografts with genetically retargeted human T cells containing CD28 and CD137 domains. *Proc Natl Acad Sci U S A* 2009;106:3360–3365.
161. Feugier P, Van HA, Sebban C, et al. Long-term results of the R-CHOP study in the treatment of elderly patients with diffuse large B-cell lymphoma: a study by the Groupe d'Etude des Lymphomes de l'Adulte. *J Clin Oncol* 2005;23:4117–4126.
162. Gribben JG, O'Brien S. Update on therapy of chronic lymphocytic leukemia. *J Clin Oncol* 2011;29:544–550.
163. Sorror ML, Sandmaier BM, Storer BE, et al. Long-term outcomes among older patients following nonmyeloablative conditioning and allogeneic hematopoietic cell transplantation for advanced hematologic malignancies. *JAMA* 2011;306:1874–1883.
164. Van BK. Current status of allogeneic transplantation for aggressive non-Hodgkin lymphoma. *Curr Opin Oncol* 2011;23:681–691.
165. Van BK. Stem cell transplantation for indolent lymphoma: a reappraisal. *Blood Rev* 2011;25:223–228.
166. McLaughlin P, Grillo-Lopez AJ, Link BK, et al. Rituximab chimeric anti-CD20 monoclonal antibody therapy for relapsed indolent lymphoma: half of patients respond to a four-dose treatment program. *J Clin Oncol* 1998;16:2825–2833.
167. Bacher U, Klyuchnikov E, Le-Rademacher J, et al. Conditioning regimens for allotransplants for diffuse large B-cell lymphoma: myeloablative or reduced intensity? *Blood* 2012;120:4256–4262.
168. Dotti G, Gottschalk S, Savoldo B, et al. Design and development of therapies using chimeric antigen receptor-expressing T cells. *Immunol Rev* 2014;257:107–126.
169. Eshhar Z, Waks T, Gross G, et al. Specific activation and targeting of cytotoxic lymphocytes through chimeric single chains consisting of antibody-binding domains and the gamma or zeta subunits of the immunoglobulin and T-cell receptors. *Proc Natl Acad Sci U S A* 1993;90:720–724.
170. Kochenderfer JN, Rosenberg SA. Treating B-cell cancer with T cells expressing anti-CD19 chimeric antigen receptors. *Nat Rev Clin Oncol* 2013;10:267–276.
171. Sadelain M, Brentjens R, Riviere I. The basic principles of chimeric antigen receptor design. *Cancer Discov* 2013;3:388–398.
172. Kershaw MH, Westwood JA, Darcy PK. Gene-engineered T cells for cancer therapy. *Nat Rev Cancer* 2013;13:525–541.
173. Brentjens RJ, Davila ML, Riviere I, et al. CD19-targeted T cells rapidly induce molecular remissions in adults with chemotherapy-refractory acute lymphoblastic leukemia. *Sci Transl Med* 2013;5:177ra38.
174. Brentjens RJ, Latouche JB, Santos E, et al. Eradication of systemic B-cell tumors by genetically targeted human T lymphocytes co-stimulated by CD80 and interleukin-15. *Nat Med* 2003;9:279–286.
175. Milone MC, Fish JD, Carpenito C, et al. Chimeric receptors containing CD137 signal transduction domains mediate enhanced survival of T cells and increased antileukemic efficacy in vivo. *Mol Ther* 2009;17:1453–1464.
176. Cooper LJ, Topp MS, Serrano LM, et al. T-cell clones can be rendered specific for CD19: toward the selective augmentation of the graft-versus-B lineage leukemia effect. *Blood* 2003;101:1637–1644.
177. Kebriaei P, Huls H, Jena B, et al. Infusing CD19-directed T cells to augment disease control in patients undergoing autologous hematopoietic stem-cell transplantation for advanced B-lymphoid malignancies. *Hum Gene Ther* 2012;23:444–450.
178. Wang X, Naranjo A, Brown CE, et al. Phenotypic and functional attributes of lentivirus-modified CD19-specific human CD8+ central memory T cells manufactured at clinical scale. *J Immunother* 2012;35:689–701.
179. Brentjens RJ, Rivière I, Park JH, et al. Safety and persistence of adoptively transferred autologous CD19-targeted T cells in patients with relapsed or chemotherapy refractory B-cell leukemias. *Blood* 2011;118:4817–4828.
180. Kalos M, Levine BL, Porter DL, et al. T cells with chimeric antigen receptors have potent antitumor effects and can establish memory in patients with advanced leukemia. *Sci Transl Med* 2011;3:95ra73.
181. Kochenderfer JN, Dudley ME, Feldman SA, et al. B-cell depletion and remissions of malignancy along with cytokine-associated toxicity in a clinical trial of anti-CD19 chimeric-antigen-receptor-transduced T cells. *Blood* 2011;119:2709–2720.
182. Imai C, Mihara K, Andreansky M, et al. Chimeric receptors with 4-1BB signaling capacity provoke potent cytotoxicity against acute lymphoblastic leukemia. *Leukemia* 2004;18:678–684.
183. Kochenderfer JN, Yu Z, Frasheri D, et al. Adoptive transfer of syngeneic T cells transduced with a chimeric antigen receptor that recognizes murine CD19 can eradicate lymphoma and normal B cells. *Blood* 2010;116:3875–3886.
184. North RJ. Cyclophosphamide-facilitated adoptive immunotherapy of an established tumor depends on elimination of tumor-induced suppressor T cells. *J Exp Med* 1982;155:1063–1074.
185. Gattinoni L, Finkelstein SE, Klebanoff CA, et al. Removal of homeostatic cytokine sinks by lymphodepletion enhances the efficacy of adoptively transferred tumor-specific CD8+ T cells. *J Exp Med* 2005;202:907–912.
186. Uckun FM, Jaszcz W, Ambrus JL, et al. Detailed studies on expression and function of CD19 surface determinant by using B43 monoclonal antibody and the clinical potential of anti-CD19 immunotoxins. *Blood* 1988;71:13–29.
187. Kochenderfer JN, Feldman SA, Zhao Y, et al. Construction and preclinical evaluation of an anti-CD19 chimeric antigen receptor. *J Immunother* 2009;32:689–702.
188. Brentjens RJ, Santos E, Nikhamin Y, et al. Genetically targeted T cells eradicate systemic acute lymphoblastic leukemia xeongrafts. *Clin Cancer Res* 2007;13:5426–5435.
189. Savoldo B, Ramos CA, Liu E, et al. CD28 costimulation improves expansion and persistence of chimeric antigen receptor-modified T cells in lymphoma patients. *J Clin Invest* 2011;121:1822–1826.
190. Grupp SA, Kalos M, Barrett D, et al. Chimeric antigen receptor-modified T cells for acute lymphoid leukemia. *N Engl J Med* 2013;368:1509–1518.
191. Jensen MC, Popplewell L, Cooper LJ, et al. Antitransgene rejection responses contribute to attenuated persistence of adoptively transferred CD20/CD19-specific chimeric antigen receptor redirected T cells in humans. *Biol Blood Marrow Transplant* 2010;16:1245–1356.
192. Till BG, Jensen MC, Wang J, et al. Adoptive immunotherapy for indolent non-Hodgkin lymphoma and mantle cell lymphoma using genetically modified autologous CD20-specific T cells. *Blood* 2008;112:2261–2271.
193. Till BG, Jensen MC, Wang J, et al. CD20-specific adoptive immunotherapy for lymphoma using a chimeric antigen receptor with both CD28 and 4-1BB domains: pilot clinical trial results. *Blood* 2012;119:3940–3950.
194. Haso W, Lee DW, Shah NN, et al. Anti-CD22-chimeric antigen receptors targeting B-cell precursor acute lymphoblastic leukemia. *Blood* 2013;121:1165–1174.
195. Giordano Attianese GM, Marin V, Hoyos V, et al. In vitro and in vivo model of a novel immunotherapy approach for chronic lymphocytic leukemia by anti-CD23 chimeric antigen receptor. *Blood* 2011;117:4736–4745.

196. Hudecek M, Schmitt TM, Baskar S, et al. The B-cell tumor-associated antigen ROR1 can be targeted with T cells modified to express a ROR1-specific chimeric antigen receptor. *Blood* 2010;116: 4532–4541.
197. Vera J, Savoldo B, Vigouroux S, et al. T lymphocytes redirected against the kappa light chain of human immunoglobulin efficiently kill mature B lymphocyte-derived malignant cells. *Blood* 2006;108:3890–3897.
198. Carpenter RO, Evbuomwan MO, Pittaluga S, et al. B-cell maturation antigen is a promising target for adoptive T-cell therapy of multiple myeloma. *Clin Cancer Res* 2013;19:2048–2060.
199. Peinert S, Prince HM, Guru PM, et al. Gene-modified T cells as immunotherapy for multiple myeloma and acute myeloid leukemia expressing the Lewis Y antigen. *Gene Ther* 2010;17:678–686.
200. Ritchie DS, Neeson PJ, Khot A, et al. Persistence and efficacy of second generation CAR T cell against the LeY antigen in acute myeloid leukemia. *Mol Ther* 2013;21:2122–2129.
201. Mardiros A, Dos SC, McDonald T, et al. T cells expressing CD123-specific chimeric antigen receptors exhibit specific cytolytic effector functions and antitumor effects against human acute myeloid leukemia. *Blood* 2013;122:3138–3148.
202. Savoldo B, Rooney CM, Di SA, et al. Epstein Barr virus specific cytotoxic T lymphocytes expressing the anti-CD30zeta artificial chimeric T-cell receptor for immunotherapy of Hodgkin disease. *Blood* 2007;110:2620–2630.
203. Hombach A, Heuser C, Sircar R, et al. An anti-CD30 chimeric receptor that mediates CD3-zeta-independent T-cell activation against Hodgkin's lymphoma cells in the presence of soluble CD30. *Cancer Res* 1998;58:1116–1119.
204. Shaffer DR, Savoldo B, Yi Z, et al. T cells redirected against CD70 for the immunotherapy of CD70-positive malignancies. *Blood* 2011;117:4304–4314.
205. Xue SA, Gao L, Hart D, et al. Elimination of human leukemia cells in NOD/SCID mice by WT1-TCR gene-transduced human T cells. *Blood* 2005;106:3062–3067.
206. Nagai K, Ochi T, Fujiwara H, et al. Aurora kinase A-specific T-cell receptor gene transfer redirects T lymphocytes to display effective antileukemia reactivity. *Blood* 2012;119:368–376.
207. Spranger S, Jeremias I, Wilde S, et al. TCR-transgenic lymphocytes specific for HMMR/Rhamm limit tumor outgrowth in vivo. *Blood* 2012;119: 3440–3449.
208. Hale GA, Shrestha S, Le-Rademacher J, et al. Alternate donor hematopoietic cell transplantation (HCT) in non-Hodgkin lymphoma using lower intensity conditioning: a report from the CIBMTR. *Biol Blood Marrow Transplant* 2012;18:1036–1043.
209. Kochenderfer JN, Dudley ME, Carpenter RO, et al. Donor-derived CD19-targeted T cells cause regression of malignancy persisting after allogeneic hematopoietic stem cell transplantation. *Blood* 2013;122:4129–4139.
210. Cruz CR, Micklethwaite KP, Savoldo B, et al. Infusion of donor-derived CD19-redirected virus-specific T cells for B-cell malignancies relapsed after allogeneic stem cell transplant: a phase 1 study. *Blood* 2013;122:2965–2973.
211. Traversari C, Marktel S, Magnani Z, et al. The potential immunogenicity of the TK suicide gene does not prevent full clinical benefit associated with the use of TK-transduced donor lymphocytes in HSCT for hematologic malignancies. *Blood* 2007;109:4708–4715.
212. Tey S, Dotti G, Rooney CM, et al. Inducible caspase 9 suicide gene to improve the safety of allodepleted T cells after haploidentical stem cell transplantation. *Biol Blood Marrow Transplant* 2007;13:924.
213. Ciceri F, Bonini C, Stanghellini MT, et al. Infusion of suicide-gene-engineered donor lymphocytes after family haploidentical haemopoietic stem-cell transplantation for leukaemia (the TK007 trial): a non-randomised phase I-II study. *Lancet Oncol* 2009;10:489–500.
214. Di Stasi A, Tey SK, Dotti G, et al. Inducible apoptosis as a safety switch for adoptive cell therapy. *N Engl J Med* 2011;365:1673–1683.

15 Pharmacokinetics and Pharmacodynamics of Anticancer Drugs

Alex Sparreboom and Sharyn D. Baker

INTRODUCTION

Drug selection and therapy considerations in oncology were originally solely based on observations of the effects produced.[1] To overcome some of the limitations of this empirical approach and to answer questions related to considerations of dose, frequency, and duration of drug treatment, it is necessary to understand the events that follow drug administration. Preclinical in vitro and in vivo studies have shown that the magnitude of antitumor response is a function of the concentration of drug,[2] and this has led to the suggestion that the therapeutic objective can be achieved by maintaining an adequate concentration at the site of action for the duration of therapy.[3] However, drugs are rarely directly administered at their sites of action. Indeed, most anticancer drugs are given intravenously or orally, and yet are expected to act in the brain, lungs, or elsewhere. Drugs must, therefore, move from the site of administration to the site of action and, moreover, distribute to all other tissues including organs that eliminate them from the body, such as the kidneys and liver. To administer drugs optimally, knowledge is needed not only of the mechanisms of drug absorption, distribution, and elimination, but also of the kinetics of these processes.[4]

The treatment of human malignancies involving drugs can be divided into two pharmacologic phases, a *pharmacokinetic* phase in which the dose, dosage form, frequency, and route of administration are related to drug level–time relationships in the body, and a *pharmacodynamic* phase in which the concentration of drug at the site(s) of action is related to the magnitude of the effect(s) produced. Once both of these phases have been defined, a dosage regimen can be designed to achieve the therapeutic objective, although additional factors need to be taken into consideration (Fig. 15.1). The clinical application of this approach allows distinctions between pharmacokinetic and pharmacodynamic causes of an unusual drug response. A basic tenet of pharmacokinetics is that the magnitude of both the desired response and toxicity are functions of the drug concentration at the site(s) of action. Accordingly, therapeutic failure results when either the concentration is too low, resulting in ineffective therapy, or is too high, producing unacceptable toxicity. Between these limits of concentrations lies a region associated with therapeutic success, the so-called *therapeutic window*.[5] Because the concentration of a drug at the site of action can rarely be measured directly, with the exception of certain hematologic malignancies, plasma or blood is commonly measured instead as a more accessible alternative.

PHARMACOKINETIC CONCEPTS

A drug's pharmacokinetic properties can be defined by two fundamental processes affecting drug behavior over time, *absorption* and *disposition*.

Absorption

Historically, most anticancer drugs have been administered intravenously; however, the use of orally administered agents is growing with the development of small-molecule targeted cancer therapeutics, such as tyrosine kinase inhibitors.[6] Moreover, drugs may also be administered regionally, for example into the pleural or peritoneal cavities,[7] the cerebrospinal fluid, or intra-arterially into a vessel leading to a cancerous tissue.[8] The process by which the unchanged drug moves from the site of administration to the site of measurement within the body is referred to as *absorption*. Loss at any site prior to the site of measurement contributes to a decrease in the apparent absorption of a drug. For an orally administered agent, this complex series of events involves disintegration of the pharmaceutical dosage form, dissolution, diffusion through gastrointestinal fluids, permeation of the gut membrane, portal circulation uptake, passage through the liver, and, finally, entry into the systemic circulation. The loss of drug as it passes for the first time through organs of elimination, such as the gastrointestinal membranes and the liver, during the absorption process is known as the *first-pass effect*.[9]

The pharmacokinetic parameter most closely associated with absorption is availability or bioavailability (F), defined as the fraction (or percent) of the administered dose that is absorbed intact. Bioavailability can be estimated by dividing the area under the plasma concentration–time curve (AUC) achieved following extravascular administration by the AUC observed after intravenous administration, and can range from 0 to 1.0 (or 0% to 100%).

Disposition

Disposition is defined as all the processes that occur subsequent to absorption of a drug; by definition, the components of disposition are *distribution* and *elimination*. Distribution is the process of reversible transfer of a drug to and from the site of measurement. Any drug that leaves the site of measurement and does not return has undergone elimination, which occurs by two processes, *excretion* and *metabolism*. Excretion is the irreversible loss of the chemically unchanged drug, whereas metabolism is the conversion of drug to another chemical species.

The extent of drug distribution can be determined by relating the concentration obtained with a known amount of drug in the body and is, in essence, a dilution space. The apparent volume into which a drug distributes in the body at equilibrium in called the volume of distribution (V_d), and may or may not correspond to an actual physiologic compartment.

The rate and extent to which a drug distributes into various tissues depend on a number of factors, including hydrophobicity, tissue permeability, tissue-binding constants, binding to serum proteins, and local organ blood flow.[10] Large apparent volumes of distribution are common for agents with high tissue binding or high lipid solubility,

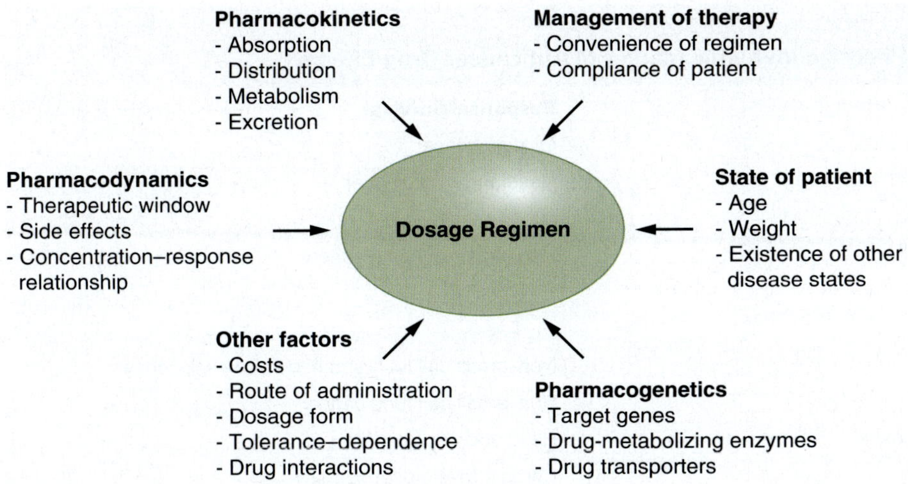

Figure 15.1 Principal determinants of dosage regimen selection for an anticancer drug

although distribution into specific body compartments may be limited by physiologic processes, such as the blood–brain barrier protecting the central nervous system[11,12] or the blood–testes barrier.[13]

Just as V_d is needed as a parameter to relate the concentration to the amount of drug in the body, there is also a need to have a parameter to relate the concentration to the rate of drug elimination, which is known as *clearance* (CL). Of all pharmacokinetic parameters, CL has the most clinical relevance because it defines the key relationship between drug dose and systemic drug exposure (AUC). Derived from V_d and CL is the parameter *elimination rate constant*, which can be regarded as the fractional rate of drug removal. It is, however, more common to refer to the half-life than to the elimination rate constant of a drug. The half-life of a drug is a useful parameter to estimate the time required to reach steady state on a multidose schedule or during a continuous intravenous drug infusion.

Dose Proportionality

When drug concentrations change in strict proportionality to the dose of drug administered, then the condition of dose proportionality (or linear pharmacokinetics) holds. If doubling the dose exactly doubles the plasma concentration or AUC, then pharmacokinetic parameters such V_d, and CL are constant and remain independent of dose and concentration.[14] By strict definition, drugs with linear pharmacokinetics are dose proportional. Dose proportionality is clinically important because it means that dose adjustments will generate predictable changes in systemic drug exposure. For drugs that lack dose proportionality, V_d and CL will demonstrate concentration or time dependence, or both, making it difficult to predict the effect of dose adjustments on drug concentration (Fig. 15.2). Factors that can contribute to a lack of dose proportional pharmacokinetics include saturable oral absorption,[15] capacity-limited distribution or protein binding,[16] and/or saturable metabolism.[17] Dose proportionality of anticancer agents is typically assessed in Phase 1 dose-escalation trials in which small groups of patients are treated at a single dose level using a parallel study design, although the statistical power of such studies to detect deviations from dose proportionality is poor. An alternative, more robust study design is a crossover study in which each patient receives a low dose, an intermediate dose, and a high dose over consecutive cycles of treatment.[18] However, such studies are relatively rare in oncology because of the required use of low, potentially ineffective doses, which may raise ethical concerns for patients.

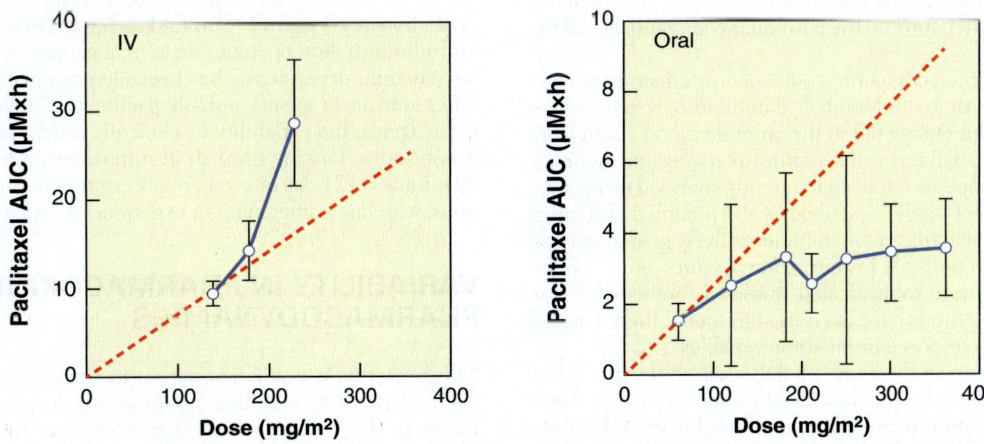

Figure 15.2 Effect of drug dose on systemic exposure to paclitaxel following intravenous (IV) or oral administration in patients with cancer. Data are expressed as mean values (symbols) and standard deviation (error bars). The *dashed line* indicates the hypothetical dose-proportional increase in the area under the plasma concentration time curve (AUC). (Data derived from van Zuylen L, Karlsson MO, Verweij J, et al. Pharmacokinetic modeling of paclitaxel encapsulation in Cremophor EL micelles. *Cancer Chemother Pharmacol* 2001;47:309–318, and Malingre MM, Terwogt JM, Beijnen JH, et al. Phase I and pharmacokinetic study of oral paclitaxel. *J Clin Oncol* 2000;18:2468–2475, respectively.)

TABLE 15.1

Examples of Systemic Exposure as a Pharmacodynamic Marker of Anticancer Drug Effects

Drug	Side Effect	Response/Survival
Carboplatin	Thrombocytopenia	Ovarian cancer
Cisplatin	Nephrotoxicity	Head and neck cancer
Cyclophosphamide	Cardiotoxicity	
Docetaxel	Neutropenia	Non–small-cell lung cancer
Doxorubicin	Neutropenia	
Epirubicin	Neutropenia	
Erlotinib	Skin rash	Non–small-cell lung and head and neck cancer
Etoposide		Non–small-cell lung cancer
5-Fluorouracil	Diarrhea, mucositis	Head and neck cancer
Imatinib		Chronic myeloid leukemia
Irinotecan	Diarrhea, neutropenia	
6-Mercaptopurine		Acute lymphoblastic leukemia
Methotrexate	Mucositis	Acute lymphoblastic leukemia
Nilotinib	Anemia, QT-interval prolongation	
Paclitaxel	Neutropenia	
Sorafenib	Hypertension, hand-foot skin reaction	Renal cell cancer
Sunitinib	Neutropenia	Renal cell cancer
Teniposide		Lymphoma

PHARMACODYNAMIC CONCEPTS

Pharmacodynamic models relate clinical drug effects with drug dose, concentration, or other pharmacokinetic parameters indicative of drug exposures (Table 15.1). In oncology, pharmacodynamic variability may account for substantial differences in clinical outcomes, even when systemic exposures are uniform. Variability in pharmacodynamic response may be heavily influenced by clinical covariates such as age, gender, prior chemotherapy, prior radiotherapy, concomitant medications, or other variables.[19] The pharmacokinetic parameters that are most often correlated with drug effects are markers of drug exposure, such as AUC. In general, the specific parameter used as the independent variable in a pharmacodynamic analysis depends on the particular characteristics of the study drug.

In oncology, pharmacodynamic studies of drug effects have most often focused on toxicity endpoints.[20] Continuous response variables, such as the percentage fall in the absolute blood count from baseline, are easily analyzed using nonlinear regression methods. Dose-limiting neutropenia has been frequently analyzed using a sigmoid maximum effect model described by the modified Hill equation. The pharmacodynamic analysis of subjectively graded clinical endpoints, such as common toxicity criteria scores on a 4-point scale, may require more sophisticated statistical methods.[21,22] Logistical regression methods have been used to model these types of categorical (ordinal) response or outcome variables.

Physiologic pharmacodynamic models describing the severity and time course of drug-related myelosuppression have been derived using population mixed-effect methods for several agents, including paclitaxel[23,24] and pemetrexed.[25] The ability of these models to predict both the severity and duration of drug-induced neutropenia substantially enhances their clinical usefulness.[26] In contrast to small-molecule therapeutics, large-molecule therapeutics such as monoclonal antibodies may not demonstrate toxicities directly related to dose levels. For these agents, a thorough understanding of the pharmacokinetic/pharmacodynamic relationships using modeling approaches may be critical for optimal dose selection.[27]

The antitumor activity of certain chemotherapeutic agents is highly schedule dependent. For such drugs, the dose fractionated over several days can produce a different antitumor response or toxicity profile compared with the same dose given over a shorter period. For example, the efficacy of etoposide in the treatment of small-cell lung cancer is markedly increased when an identical total dose of etoposide is administered by a 5-day divided-dose schedule rather than a 24-hour infusion.[28] Pharmacokinetic analysis in that study showed that both schedules produced very similar overall drug exposure (as measured by AUC), but that the divided-dose schedule produced twice the duration of exposure to an etoposide plasma concentration of >1 μg/mL. This finding has led to the use of prolonged oral administration of etoposide to treat patients with cancer.[29] Similar schedule dependence has been demonstrated for a number of other anticancer agents, notably paclitaxel[30,31] and topotecan.[32] For these agents, the variability in clinically tested treatment schedules is enormous, ranging from short intravenous infusions of less than 30 minutes to 21-day or even 7-week continuous infusion administrations, with large differences in experienced toxicity profiles.

VARIABILITY IN PHARMACOKINETICS/ PHARMACODYNAMICS

There is often a marked variation in drug handling between individual patients, resulting in variability in pharmacokinetic parameters (Fig. 15.3), which will often lead to variability in the pharmacodynamic effects of a given dose of a drug.[33] That is, an identical dose of drug may result in acceptable toxicity in one patient, and unacceptable and possibly life-threatening toxicity in another, or a clinical response in one individual and cancer progression in another. The principal underlying sources of this interindividual pharmacokinetic/pharmacodynamic variability are discussed in the following paragraphs.

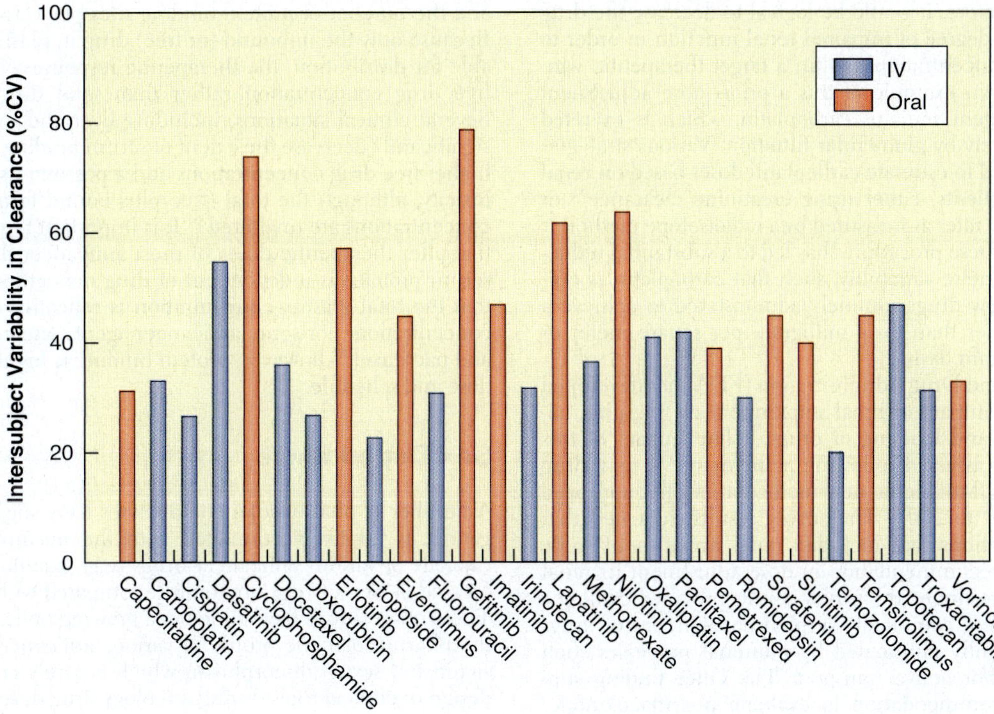

Figure 15.3 Interindividual pharmacokinetic variability of select cytotoxic agents and molecularly targeted agents expressed as a percent coefficient of variation (%CV) in apparent (oral) clearance. IV, intravenous. (Data derived from Mathijssen RH, de Jong FA, Loos WJ, et al. Flat-fixed dosing versus body surface area based dosing of anticancer drugs in adults: does it make a difference? *Oncologist* 2007;12:913–923, and publicly available prescribing information.)

Body Size and Body Composition

The traditional method of individualizing anticancer drug dosage is by using body surface area (BSA).[34] However, the usefulness of normalizing an anticancer drug dose to BSA in adults has been questioned, because, for many drugs, there is no relationship between BSA and CL.[35] Likewise, attempts to replace BSA as a size metric in dose calculation with alternate descriptors such as lean body weight, either in an average population or in individuals at the outer extremes of weight (i.e., frail, severely obese patients) have failed for many anticancer agents.[36,37] It should be pointed out that BSA is a much more important consideration in drug dose calculation for pediatric patients as compared to adults, because of the larger size range in the former population.[38] Based in part on the failure to reduce interindividual pharmacokinetic variability with the use of BSA normalization to obtain a starting dose, many of the more recently developed molecularly targeted agents are currently administered using a flat-fixed dose irrespective of an individual's BSA.[37]

Age

Changes in body composition and organ function at the extremes of age can affect both drug disposition and drug effect.[39] For example, maturational processes in infancy may alter the absorption and distribution of drugs as well as change the capacity for drug metabolism and excretion.[4] The importance of understanding the influence of age on the pharmacokinetics and pharmacodynamics of individual anticancer agents has increased steadily as treatment for the malignancies of infants,[40] adolescents,[41] and the elderly[42] has advanced. Although pediatric cancers remain rare compared with cancers in adults and the elderly population, in particular, optimizing treatment in a patient group with a high cure rate and a long expected survival becomes critical to minimize the incidence of preventable late complications while maintaining efficacy.

Pathophysiologic Changes

Effects of Disease

Pathophysiologic changes associated with particular malignancies may cause dramatic alterations in drug disposition. For example, increases in the clearance of both antipyrine and lorazepam were noted after remission induction compared with the time of diagnosis in children with acute lymphoblastic leukemia (ALL).[43] The clearance of unbound teniposide is lower in children with ALL in relapse than during first remission.[44] Because leukemic infiltration of the liver at the time of diagnosis is common, drugs metabolized by the liver may have a reduced clearance, as has been documented in preclinical models.[45]

Furthermore, in mouse models, certain tumors elicited an acute phase response that coincided with downregulation of human CYP3A4 in the liver as well as the mouse ortholog Cyp3a11.[46] The reduction of murine hepatic Cyp3a gene expression in tumor-bearing mice resulted in decreased Cyp3a protein expression and, consequently, a significant reduction in Cyp3a-mediated metabolism of midazolam. These findings support the possibility that tumor-derived inflammation may alter the pharmacokinetic and pharmacodynamic properties of CYP3A4 substrates, leading to reduced metabolism of drugs in humans.[47] This supports a possible need for disease-specific design of early clinical trials with anticancer drugs,[48] as has been recommended for docetaxel.[49]

Effects of Renal Impairment

The potential impact of pathophysiologic status on interindividual pharmacokinetic variability can be due to either the disease itself or to a dysfunction of specific organs involved in drug elimination. For example, if urinary excretion is an important elimination route for a given drug, any decrement in renal function could lead to decreased drug clearance, which may result in drug accumulation and toxicity.[50] Therefore, it would be logical to decrease the drug dose relative to the degree of impaired renal function in order to maintain plasma concentrations within a target therapeutic window. The best known example of this a priori dose adjustment of an anticancer agent remains carboplatin, which is excreted renally almost entirely by glomerular filtration. Various strategies have been developed to estimate carboplatin doses based on renal function among patients, either using creatinine clearance[51] or glomerular filtration rates as measured by a radioisotope method.[52] The application of these procedures has led to a substantial reduction in pharmacokinetic variability, such that carboplatin is currently one of the few drugs routinely administered to achieve a target exposure rather than on a milligram per square meter or milligram per kilogram basis.

The U.S. Food and Drug Administration (FDA) has developed a guidance on the impact of renal impairment on the pharmacokinetics, dosing, and labeling of drugs.[53] The impact of this guidance has been assessed following a survey of 94 new drug applications for small-molecule new molecular entities approved over the years 2003 to 2007. The survey results indicated that 41% of the applications that included renal impairment study data resulted in a recommendation of dose adjustment in renal impairment.[54] Interestingly, the survey results provided evidence that renal impairment can affect the pharmacokinetics of drugs that are predominantly eliminated by nonrenal processes such as metabolism and/or active transport. The latter finding supports the FDA recommendation to evaluate pharmacokinetic/pharmacodynamic alterations in renal impairment for those drugs that are predominantly eliminated by nonrenal processes, in addition to those that are mainly excreted unchanged by the kidneys. A striking example of a drug in the former category is imatinib, an agent that is predominantly eliminated by hepatic pathways but where predialysis renal impairment is associated with dramatically reduced drug clearance,[55] presumably due to a transporter-mediated process.[56]

Effects of Hepatic Impairment

In contrast to the predictable decline in renal clearance of drugs when glomerular filtration is impaired, it is difficult to make general predictions on the effect of impaired liver function on drug clearance. The major problem is that commonly applied criteria to establish hepatic impairment are typically not good indicators of drug-metabolizing enzyme activity and that several alternative hepatic function tests, such as indocyanine green and antipyrine, have relatively limited value in predicting anticancer drug pharmacokinetics. An alternative dynamic measure of liver function has been proposed, which is based on totaled values (scored to the World Health Organization [WHO] grading system) of serum bilirubin, alkaline phosphatase, and either alanine aminotransferase or aspartate aminotransferase to give a hepatic dysfunction score.[57] Based on pharmacokinetic studies in patients with normal and impaired hepatic function, guidelines have been proposed for dose adjustments of several agents when administered to patients with severe liver dysfunction.[58] It should be emphasized that no uniform criteria have been used in the conduct of these studies and that, ultimately, substantial advances could be made through an a priori determination of the hepatic activity of enzymes of pertinent relevance to the chemotherapeutic drug(s) of interest, as has been done for docetaxel.[59]

Effects of Serum Proteins

The binding of drugs to serum proteins, particularly those that are highly bound, may also have significant clinical implications for a therapeutic outcome.[60] Although protein binding is a major determinant of drug action, it is clearly only one of a myriad of factors that influence the disposition of anticancer drugs.[16] The extent of protein binding is a function of drug and protein concentrations, the affinity constants for the drug–protein interaction, and the number of protein-binding sites per class of binding site. Because only the unbound (or free) drug in plasma water is available for distribution, the therapeutic response will correlate with free drug concentration rather than total drug concentration. Several clinical situations, including liver and renal disease, can significantly decrease the extent of serum binding and may lead to higher free drug concentrations and a possible risk of unexpected toxicity, although the total (free plus bound forms) plasma drug concentrations are unaltered.[61] It is important to realize, however, that after therapeutic doses of most anticancer drugs, binding to serum proteins is independent of drug concentration, suggesting that the total plasma concentration is reflective of the unbound concentration. For some anticancer agents, including etoposide[62] and paclitaxel,[63] however, protein binding is highly dependent on dose and schedule.

Sex Dependence

A number of pharmacokinetic analyses have suggested that male gender is positively correlated with the maximum elimination capacity of various anticancer drugs (e.g., paclitaxel)[8] or with increased clearance (e.g., imatinib)[64] compared with female gender. These observations have added to a growing body of evidence that the pharmacokinetic profile of various anticancer drugs exhibits significant sexual dimorphism, which is rarely considered in the design of clinical trials during oncology drug development.

Drug Interactions

Coadministration of Other Chemotherapeutic Drugs

Favorable and unfavorable interactions between drugs must be considered in developing combination regimens. These interactions may influence the effectiveness of each of the components of the combination, and typically occur when the pharmacokinetic profile of one drug is altered by the other. Such interactions are important in the design of trials evaluating drug combinations because, occasionally, the outcome of concurrent drug administration is diminished therapeutic efficacy or increased toxicity of one or more of the administered agents. Although a recent survey indicated that clinically significant pharmacokinetic interactions are relatively rare in Phase I trials of oncology drug combinations,[65] interactions appear to be more common for combinations of tyrosine kinase inhibitors with cytotoxic chemotherapeutics.[66]

Coadministration of Nonchemotherapeutic Drugs

Many prescription and over-the-counter medications have the potential to cause interactions with anticancer agents by altering their pharmacokinetic characteristics and leading to clinically significant phenotypes. Most clinically relevant drug interactions in this category are due to changes in metabolic routes related to an altered expression or function of cytochrome P450 (CYP) isozymes. This class of enzymes, particularly the CYP3A4 isoform, is responsible for the oxidation of a large proportion of currently approved anticancer drugs. Elevated CYP activity (induction), translated into a more rapid metabolic rate, may result in a decrease in plasma concentrations and to a loss of therapeutic effect. For example, anticonvulsant drugs such as phenytoin, phenobarbital, and carbamazepine can induce drug-metabolizing enzymes and thereby increase the clearance of various anticancer agents.[33]

Conversely, the suppression (inhibition) of CYP activity, for example with ketoconazole,[13,67] may trigger a rise in plasma concentrations and can lead to exaggerated toxicity commensurate with overdose. It should be borne in mind that several pharmacokinetic parameters could be altered simultaneously. Especially in the development of anticancer agents given by the oral route,

TABLE 15.2

Effect of Food on Exposure to Select Oral Anticancer Agents

Drug	Food	Effect on Drug Exposure	Manufacturer's Recommendations
Abiraterone	High-fat meal	↑ AUC 1,000%	Without food
Dasatinib	High-fat meal	↑ AUC 14%	With or without food
Erlotinib	High-fat, high-calorie breakfast	Single dose, ↑ AUC 200% Multiple dose, ↑ AUC 37%–66%	Without food[a]
Gefitinib	High-fat breakfast	↓ AUC 14%, ↓ Cmax 35%	With or without food
	High-fat breakfast	↑ AUC 32%, ↑ Cmax 35%	
Imatinib	High-fat meal	No change	With food and a large glass of water[b]
		Variability (% CV) ↓ 37%	
Lapatinib	Low-fat meal (5% fat, 500 calories)	↑ AUC 167%, ↑ Cmax 142%	Without food[c]
	High-fat meal (50% fat, 1,000 calories)	↑ AUC 325%, ↑ Cmax 203%	
Nilotinib	High-fat meal	↑ AUC 82%	Without food
Sorafenib	Moderate-fat meal (30% fat, 700 calories)	No change in bioavailability	Without food
	High-fat meal (50% fat, 900 calories)	↓ Bioavailability 29%	
Sunitinib	High-fat, high-calorie meal	↑ AUC 18%	With or without food
Everolimus	High-fat meal	↓ AUC 16%, ↓ Cmax 60%	With or without food
Vismodegib	High-fat meal	↑ AUC 74% for single dose; no effect at steady state	With or without food
Vorinostat	High-fat meal	↑ AUC 37%	With food[d]

[a] Recommended without food because the approved dose is the maximum tolerated dose.
[b] Recommended with food to reduce nausea.
[c] Recommended without food to achieve consistent drug exposure; was taken without food in clinical trials.
[d] Was taken with food in clinical trials.
AUC, area under the plasma concentration time curve; Cmax, maximum plasma concentration; CV, coefficient of variation.

oral bioavailability plays a crucial role[9]; this parameter is contingent on adequate absorption and the circumvention of intestinal and, subsequently, hepatic metabolism of the drug. It has been suggested that the prevalence of drug–drug interactions is particularly high in cancer patients receiving oral chemotherapy,[68] especially for agents that are weak bases that exhibit pH-dependent solubility.[69]

An additional consideration is related to a possible influence of food intake on the extent of drug absorption after oral administration, which can increase, decrease, or remain unchanged depending on specific physicochemical properties of the drug in question (Table 15.2). The relatively narrow therapeutic index of most of these agents means that significant inter- and intrapatient variability would predispose some individuals to excessive toxicity or, conversely, inadequate efficacy.[12]

Coadministration of Complementary and Alternative Medicine

Surveys within the past decade estimate the prevalence of complementary and alternative medicine (CAM) use in oncology patients to be as high as 87%, and in many cases the treating physician is not aware of the patients' CAM use.[70] With a larger number of participants to phase I clinical trials[71] using herbal treatments combined with allopathic therapies, the risk for herb–drug interactions is a growing concern, and there is an increasing need to understand possible adverse drug interactions in oncology at the early stages of drug development.

A number of clinically important pharmacokinetic interactions involving CAM and cancer drugs have now been recognized, although causal relationships have not always been established.[72] Most of the observed interactions point to the herbs affecting several isoforms of the CYP family, either through inhibition or induction. In the context of chemotherapeutic drugs, St. John's wort,[73] garlic,[74] milk thistle,[75] and Echinacea[11] have been formally evaluated for their pharmacokinetic drug–interaction potential in cancer patients. However, various other herbs have the potential to significantly modulate the expression and/or activity of drug-metabolizing enzymes and drug transporters (Table 15.3), including ginkgo, ginseng, and kava.[70] Because of the high prevalence of herbal medicine use, physicians should include herb usage in their routine drug histories in order to have an opportunity to outline to individual patients which potential hazards should be taken into consideration prior to participation in a clinical trial.

Inherited Genetic Factors

The discipline of pharmacogenetics describes differences in the pharmacokinetics and pharmacodynamics of drugs as a result of inherited variation in drug metabolizing enzymes, drug transporters, and drug targets between patients.[76] These inherited variations are occasionally responsible for extensive interpatient variability in drug exposure or effects. Severe toxicity might occur in the absence of a typical metabolism of active compounds, while the therapeutic effect of a drug could be diminished in the case of an absence of activation of a prodrug, such as irinotecan.[77] The importance and detectability of polymorphisms for a given enzyme or transporter depends on the contribution of the variant gene product to pharmacologic response, the availability of alternative pathways of elimination, and the frequency of occurrence of the variant allele. Although many substrates have been identified for the known polymorphic drug metabolizing enzymes

TABLE 15.3

Effects of Common Herbal Products on Exposure to Anticancer Agents

Botanical	Concurrent Chemotherapy/Condition (Suspected Effect)
Ephedra	Avoid with all cardiovascular chemotherapy (synergistic increase in blood pressure)
Ginkgo	Caution with camptothecins, cyclophosphamide, TK inhibitors, epipodophyllotoxins, taxanes, and vinca alkaloids (CYP3A4 and CYP2C19 inhibition); discourage with alkylating agents, antitumor antibiotics, and platinum analogs (free-radical scavenging)
Ginseng	Discourage in patients with estrogen-receptor–positive breast cancer and endometrial cancer (stimulation of tumor growth)
Green tea	Discourage with erlotinib and pazopanib (CYP1A2 induction)
Japanese arrowroot	Avoid with methotrexate (ABC and OAT transporter inhibition)
St. John's wort	Avoid with all concurrent chemotherapy (CYP2B6, CYP2C9, CYP2C19, CYP2E1, CYP3A4, and ABCB1 induction)
Valerian	Caution with tamoxifen (CYP2C9 inhibition), cyclophosphamide, and teniposide (CYP2C19 inhibition)
Kava-kava	Avoid in all patients with preexisting liver disease, with evidence of hepatic injury (herb-induced hepatotoxicity), and/or in combination with hepatotoxic chemotherapy; caution with camptothecins, cyclophosphamide, TK inhibitors, epipodophyllotoxins, taxanes, and Vinca alkaloids (CYP3A4 induction)

TK, tyrosine kinase; CYP, cytochrome P450; ABC, ATP-binding cassette; OAT, organic anion transporter.

and transporters, the contribution of a genetically determined source of interindividual pharmacokinetic variability has been established for only a few cancer chemotherapeutic agents. Most of these cases involve agents for which elimination is critically dependent on a rate-limiting breakdown by a polymorphic enzyme (e.g., 6-mercaptopurine by thiopurine-S-methyltransferase; 5-fluorouracil by dihydropyrimidine dehydrogenase) or when a polymorphic enzyme is involved in the formation of a toxic metabolite (e.g., tamoxifen by CYP2D6).[78]

In addition to drug metabolism, pharmacokinetic processes are highly dependent on the interplay with drug transport in organs such as the intestines, kidneys, and liver. Genetically determined variation in drug transporter function or expression is now increasingly recognized to have a significant role as a determinant of intersubject variability in response to various commonly prescribed drugs.[79] The most extensively studied class of drug transporters are those encoded by the family of ATP-binding cassette (ABC) genes, some of which also play a role in the resistance of malignant cells to anticancer agents. Among the 48 known ABC gene products, ABCB1 (P-glycoprotein), ABCC1 (multidrug-resistance associated protein-1 [MRP1]) and its homologue ABCC2 (MRP2; cMOAT), and ABCG2 (breast cancer resistance protein [BCRP]) are known to influence the oral absorption and disposition of a wide variety of drugs.[80] As a result, the expression levels of these proteins in humans have important consequences for an individual's susceptibility to certain anticancer drug–induced side effects, interactions, and treatment efficacy, for example, in the case of genetic variation in ABCG2 in relation to gefitinib-induced diarrhea.[81]

Similar to the discoveries of functional genetic variations in drug efflux transporters of the ABC family, there have been considerable advances in the identification of inherited variants in transporters that facilitate cellular drug uptake in tissues that play an important role in drug elimination, such as the liver (Fig. 15.4). Among these, members of the organic anion-transporting polypeptides (OATP), organic anion transporters (OAT), and organic cation transporters (OCT) can mediate the cellular uptake of a large number of structurally divergent compounds.[82,83] Accordingly, functionally relevant polymorphisms in these influx transporters may contribute to interindividual and interethnic variability in drug disposition and response,[84] for example, in the case of the impact of polymorphic variants in the OCT1 gene *SLC22A1* on the survival of patients with chronic myeloid leukemia receiving treatment with imatinib.[85]

DOSE-ADAPTATION USING PHARMACOKINETIC/PHARMACODYNAMIC PRINCIPLES

Therapeutic Drug Monitoring

Prolonged infusion schedules of anticancer drugs offer a very convenient setting for dose adaptation in individual patients. At the time required to achieve steady-state concentration, it is possible to modify the infusion rate for the remainder of the treatment course if a relationship is known between this steady-state concentration and a desired pharmacodynamic endpoint. This method has been successfully used to adapt the dose during continuous infusions of 5-fluorouracil and etoposide, and for repeated oral administration of etoposide or repeated intravenous administration of cisplatin.[86] Methotrexate plasma concentrations are routinely monitored to identify patients at high risk of toxicity and to adjust leucovorin rescue in patients with delayed drug excretion. This monitoring has significantly reduced the incidence of serious toxicity, including toxic death, and in fact, has improved outcome by eliminating unacceptably low systemic exposure levels.[87] Therapeutic drug monitoring has also been applied to or is currently under investigation for several more recently developed anticancer drugs, including imatinib[88–90] and sorafenib.[91]

Feedback-Controlled Dosing

It remains to be determined how information on interindividual pharmacokinetic variability can eventually be used to devise an optimal dosage regimen of a drug for the treatment of a given disease in an individual patient. Obviously, the desired objective would be most efficiently achieved if the individual's dosage requirements could be calculated prior to administering the drug. While this ideal cannot be met completely in clinical practice, with the notable exception of carboplatin, some success may be achieved by adopting feedback-controlled dosing. In the adaptive dosage with feedback control, population-based predictive models are used initially, but allow the possibility of dosage alteration based on feedback revision. In this approach, patients are first treated with standard dose and, during treatment, pharmacokinetic information is estimated by a limited-sampling strategy and compared with that predicted from the population model with which treatment was initiated. On the basis of the comparison,

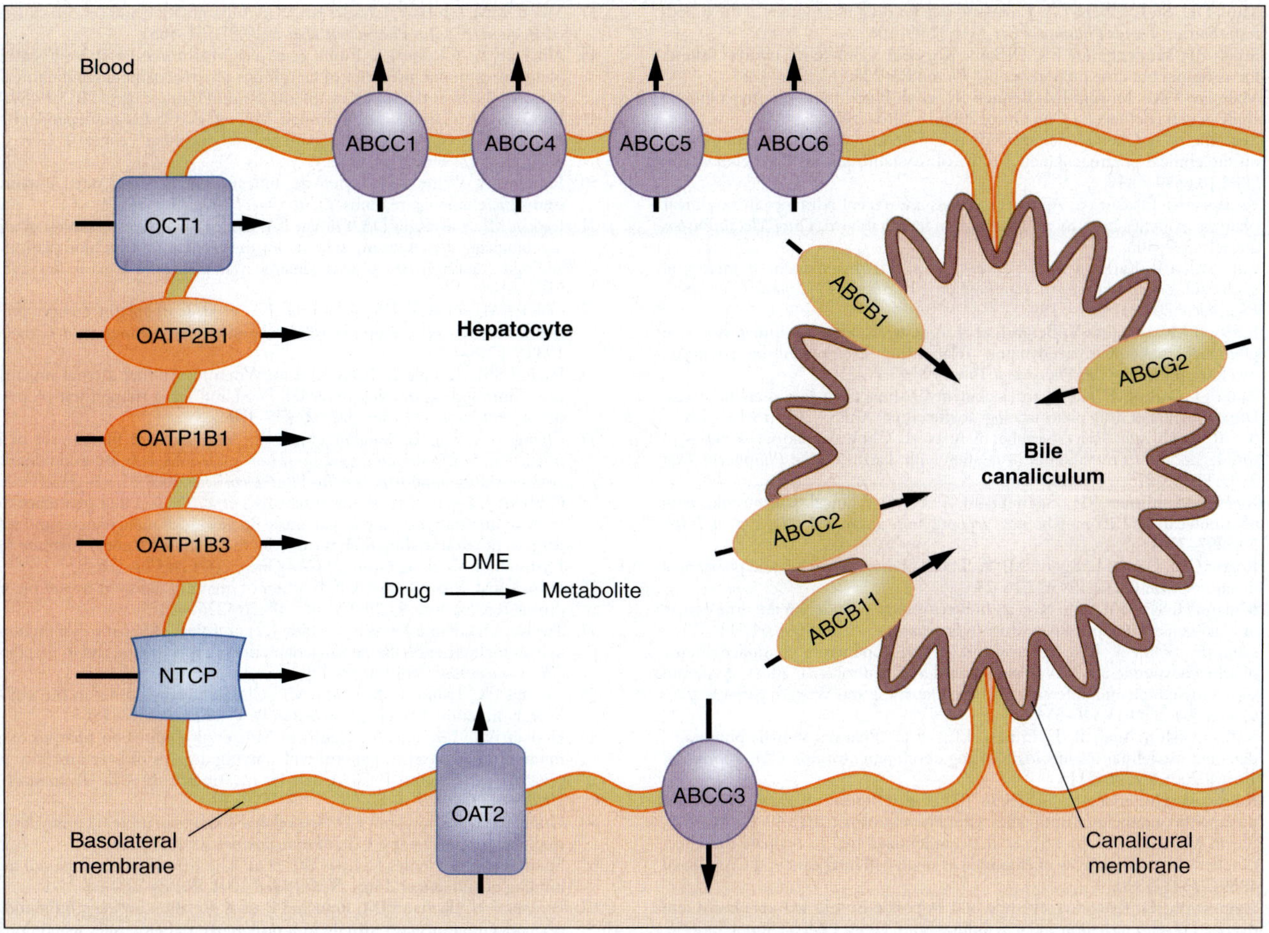

Figure 15.4 Common mechanisms for possible interactions between xenobiotics and anticancer drugs in the liver. DME, drug-metabolizing enzyme(s).

more patient-specific pharmacokinetic parameters are calculated, and dosage is adjusted accordingly to maintain the target exposure measure producing the desired pharmacodynamic effect. Despite its mathematical complexity, this approach may be the only way to deliver the desired and precise exposure of an anticancer agent.

The study of population pharmacokinetics seeks to identify the measurable factors that cause changes in the dose-concentration relationship and the extent of these alterations so that, if these are associated with clinically significant shifts in the therapeutic index, dosage can be appropriately modified in the individual patient. It is obvious that a careful collection of data during the development of drugs and subsequent analyses could be helpful to collect some essential information on the drug. Unfortunately, important information is often lost by failing to analyze this data or due to the fact that the relevant samples or data were never collected. Historically, this has resulted in the notion that tools for the identification of patient population subgroups are inadequate for most of the currently approved anticancer drugs.

However, the use of population pharmacokinetic models is increasingly studied in an attempt to accommodate as much of the pharmacokinetic variability as possible in terms of measurable characteristics. This type of analysis has been conducted for a number of clinically important anticancer drugs, including carboplatin,[92] docetaxel,[93] topotecan,[94] gefitinib,[95] and erlotinib,[96] and provided mathematical equations based on morphometric, demographic, phenotypic enzyme activity, and/or physiologic characteristics of patients, in order to predict drug clearance with an acceptable degree of precision and bias.[97]

REFERENCES

1. DeVita VT, Chu E. A history of cancer chemotherapy. *Cancer Res* 2008;68:8643–8653.
2. Lieu CH, Tan AC, Leong S, et al. From bench to bedside: lessons learned in translating preclinical studies in cancer drug development. *J Natl Cancer Inst* 2013;105:1441–1456.
3. Sparreboom A, Verweij J. Advances in cancer therapeutics. *Clin Pharmacol Ther* 2009;85:113–117.
4. Fujita KI, Sasaki Y. Optimization of cancer chemotherapy on the basis of pharmacokinetics and pharmacodynamics: from patients enrolled in 'clinical trials' to those in the 'real world'. *Drug Metab Pharmacokin* 2014;29(1):20–28.
5. Liliemark J, Peterson C. Pharmacokinetic optimisation of anticancer therapy. *Clin Pharmacokinet* 1991;21:213–231.
6. Stuurman FE, Nuijen B, Beijnen JH, et al. Oral anticancer drugs: mechanisms of low bioavailability and strategies for improvement. *Clin Pharmacokinet* 2013;52:399–414.
7. Hasovits C, Clarke S. Pharmacokinetics and pharmacodynamics of intraperitoneal cancer chemotherapeutics. *Clin Pharmacokinet* 2012;51:203–224.
8. Cai S, Bagby TR, Forrest ML. Development of regional chemotherapies: feasibility, safety and efficacy in clinical use and preclinical studies. *Ther Deliv* 2011;2:1467–1484.
9. DeMario MD, Ratain MJ. Oral chemotherapy: rationale and future directions. *J Clin Oncol* 1998;16:2557–2567.
10. Zou P, Zheng N, Yang Y, et al. Prediction of volume of distribution at steady state in humans: comparison of different approaches. *Exp Opin Drug Metab Toxicol* 2012;8:855–872.
11. Deeken JF, Loscher W. The blood-brain barrier and cancer: transporters, treatment, and Trojan horses. *Clin Cancer Res* 2007;13:1663–1674.
12. Pitz MW, Desai A, Grossman SA, et al. Tissue concentration of systemically administered antineoplastic agents in human brain tumors. *J Neurooncol* 2011;104:629–638.

13. Mruk DD, Su L, Cheng CY. Emerging role for drug transporters at the blood-testis barrier. *Trends Pharmacol Sci* 2011;32:99–106.
14. Smith BP, Vandenhende FR, DeSante KA, et al. Confidence interval criteria for assessment of dose proportionality. *Pharm Res* 2000;17:1278–1283.
15. Malingre MM, Terwogt JM, Beijnen JH, et al. Phase I and pharmacokinetic study of oral paclitaxel. *J Clin Oncol* 2000;18:2468–2475.
16. Sparreboom A, Chen H, Acharya MR, et al. Effects of alpha1-acid glycoprotein on the clinical pharmacokinetics of 7-hydroxystaurosporine. *Clin Cancer Res* 2004;10:6840–6846.
17. Yamaoka K, Takakura Y. Analysis methods and recent advances in nonlinear pharmacokinetics from in vitro through in loci to in vivo. *Drug Metab Dispos* 2004;19:397–406.
18. van Zuylen L, Karlsson MO, Verweij J, et al. Pharmacokinetic modeling of paclitaxel encapsulation in Cremophor EL micelles. *Cancer Chemother Pharmacol* 2001;47:309–318.
19. Karlsson MO, Molnar V, Bergh J, et al. A general model for time-dissociated pharmacokinetic-pharmacodynamic relationship exemplified by paclitaxel myelosuppression. *Clin Pharmacol Ther* 1998;63:11–25.
20. Zhou Q, Gallo JM. The pharmacokinetic/pharmacodynamic pipeline: translating anticancer drug pharmacology to the clinic. *AAPS J* 2011;13:111–120.
21. Xie R, Mathijssen RH, Sparreboom A, et al. Clinical pharmacokinetics of irinotecan and its metabolites in relation with diarrhea. *Clin Pharmacol Ther* 2002;72:265–275.
22. Xie R, Mathijssen RH, Sparreboom A, et al. Clinical pharmacokinetics of irinotecan and its metabolites: a population analysis. *J Clin Oncol* 2002; 20:3293–3301.
23. Kearns CM, Gianni L, Egorin MJ. Paclitaxel pharmacokinetics and pharmacodynamics. *Sem Oncol* 1995;22:16–23.
24. Minami H, Sasaki Y, Saijo N, et al. Indirect-response model for the time course of leukopenia with anticancer drugs. *Clin Pharmacol Ther* 1998;64:511–521.
25. Latz JE, Schneck KL, Nakagawa K, et al. Population pharmacokinetic/pharmacodynamic analyses of pemetrexed and neutropenia: effect of vitamin supplementation and differences between Japanese and Western patients. *Clin Cancer Res* 2009;15:346–354.
26. Karlsson MO, Anehall T, Friberg LE, et al. Pharmacokinetic/pharmacodynamic modelling in oncological drug development. *Basic Clin Pharmacol Toxicol* 2005;96:206–211.
27. Keizer RJ, Huitema AD, Schellens JH, et al. Clinical pharmacokinetics of therapeutic monoclonal antibodies. *Clin Pharmacokinet* 2010;49:493–507.
28. Slevin ML, Clark PI, Joel SP, et al. A randomized trial to evaluate the effect of schedule on the activity of etoposide in small-cell lung cancer. *J Clin Oncol* 1989;7:1333–1340.
29. Hainsworth JD. Extended-schedule oral etoposide in selected neoplasms and overview of administration and scheduling issues. *Drugs* 1999;58 Suppl 3:51–56.
30. Gelderblom H, Mross K, ten Tije AJ, et al. Comparative pharmacokinetics of unbound paclitaxel during 1- and 3-hour infusions. *J Clin Oncol* 2002;20:574–581.
31. Woodward EJ, Twelves C. Scheduling of taxanes: a review. *Curr Clin Pharmacol* 2010;5:226–231.
32. Soepenberg O, Sparreboom A, Verweij J. Clinical studies of camptothecin and derivatives. *Alkaloid Chem Biol* 2003;60:1–50.
33. Undevia SD, Gomez-Abuin G, Ratain MJ. Pharmacokinetic variability of anticancer agents. *Nat Rev Cancer* 2005;5:447–458.
34. Gurney H. Dose calculation of anticancer drugs: a review of the current practice and introduction of an alternative. *J Clin Oncol* 1996;14:2590–2611.
35. Baker SD, Verweij J, Rowinsky EK, et al. Role of body surface area in dosing of investigational anticancer agents in adults, 1991–2001. *J Natl Cancer Inst* 2002;94:1883–1888.
36. Mathijssen RH, Sparreboom A. Influence of lean body weight on anticancer drug clearance. *Clin Pharmacol Ther* 2009;85:23.
37. Sparreboom A, Wolff AC, Mathijssen RH, et al. Evaluation of alternate size descriptors for dose calculation of anticancer drugs in the obese. *J Clin Oncol* 2007;25:4707–4713.
38. Bartelink IH, Rademaker CM, Schobben AF, et al. Guidelines on paediatric dosing on the basis of developmental physiology and pharmacokinetic considerations. *Clin Pharmacokinet* 2006;45:1077–1097.
39. McLeod HL, Relling MV, Crom WR, et al. Disposition of antineoplastic agents in the very young child. *Br J Cancer* 1992;18:S23–S29.
40. Hutson JR, Weitzman S, Schechter T, et al. Pharmacokinetic and pharmacogenetic determinants and considerations in chemotherapy selection and dosing in infants. *Exp Opin Drug Metab Toxicol* 2012;8:709–722.
41. Veal GJ, Hartford CM, Stewart CF. Clinical pharmacology in the adolescent oncology patient. *J Clin Oncol* 2010;28:4790–4799.
42. Lichtman SM. Pharmacology of aging and cancer: how useful are pharmacokinetic tests? *Interdiscip Top Gerontol* 2013;38:104–123.
43. Relling MV, Crom WR, Pieper JA, et al. Hepatic drug clearance in children with leukemia: changes in clearance of model substrates during remission-induction therapy. *Clin Pharmacol Ther* 1987;41:651–660.
44. Evans WE, Rodman JH, Relling MV, et al. Differences in teniposide disposition and pharmacodynamics in patients with newly diagnosed and relapsed acute lymphocytic leukemia. *J Pharmacol Exp Ther* 1992;260:71–77.
45. Powis G, Harris RN, Basseches PJ, et al. Effects of advanced leukemia on hepatic drug-metabolizing activity in the mouse. *Cancer Chemother Pharmacol* 1986;16:43–49.
46. Charles KA, Rivory LP, Brown SL, et al. Transcriptional repression of hepatic cytochrome P450 3A4 gene in the presence of cancer. *Clin Cancer Res* 2006; 12:7492–7497.
47. Moore MM, Chua W, Charles KA, et al. Inflammation and cancer: causes and consequences. *Clin Pharmacol Ther* 2010;87:504–508.
48. Albekairy A, Alkatheri A, Fujita S, et al. Cytochrome P450 3A4FNx011B as pharmacogenomic predictor of tacrolimus pharmacokinetics and clinical outcome in the liver transplant recipients. *Saudi J Gastroenterol* 2013;19:89–95.
49. Franke RM, Carducci MA, Rudek MA, et al. Castration-dependent pharmacokinetics of docetaxel in patients with prostate cancer. *J Clin Oncol* 2010;28:4562–4567.
50. Rahman A, White RM. Cytotoxic anticancer agents and renal impairment study: the challenge remains. *J Clin Oncol* 2006;24:533–536.
51. Egorin MJ, Van Echo DA, Olman EA, et al. Prospective validation of a pharmacologically based dosing scheme for the cis-diamminedichloroplatinum(II) analogue diamminecyclobutanedicarboxylatoplatinum. *Cancer Res* 1985;45: 6502–6506.
52. Calvert AH, Newell DR, Gumbrell LA, et al. Carboplatin dosage: prospective evaluation of a simple formula based on renal function. *J Clin Oncol* 1989;7:1748–1756.
53. Huang SM, Temple R, Xiao S, et al. When to conduct a renal impairment study during drug development: US Food and Drug Administration perspective. *Clin Pharmacol Ther* 2009;86:475–479.
54. Zhang Y, Zhang L, Abraham S, et al. Assessment of the impact of renal impairment on systemic exposure of new molecular entities: evaluation of recent new drug applications. *Clin Pharmacol Ther* 2009;85:305–311.
55. Gibbons J, Egorin MJ, Ramanathan RK, et al. Phase I and pharmacokinetic study of imatinib mesylate in patients with advanced malignancies and varying degrees of renal dysfunction: a study by the National Cancer Institute Organ Dysfunction Working Group. *J Clin Oncol* 2008;26:570–576.
56. Franke RM, Sparreboom A. Inhibition of imatinib transport by uremic toxins during renal failure. *J Clin Oncol* 2008;26:4226–4227.
57. Twelves C, Glynne-Jones R, Cassidy J, et al. Effect of hepatic dysfunction due to liver metastases on the pharmacokinetics of capecitabine and its metabolites. *Clin Cancer Res* 1999;5:1696–1702.
58. Eklund JW, Trifilio S, Mulcahy MF. Chemotherapy dosing in the setting of liver dysfunction. *Oncology (Williston Park)* 2005;19:1057–1063.
59. Hooker AC, Ten Tije AJ, Carducci MA, et al. Population pharmacokinetic model for docetaxel in patients with varying degrees of liver function: incorporating cytochrome P4503A activity measurements. *Clin Pharmacol Ther* 2008;84:111–118.
60. Grandison MK, Boudinot FD. Age-related changes in protein binding of drugs: implications for therapy. *Clin Pharmacokinet* 2000;38:271–290.
61. Sparreboom A, Nooter K, Loos WJ, et al. The (ir)relevance of plasma protein binding of anticancer drugs. *Neth J Med* 2001;59:196–207.
62. Perdaems N, Bachaud JM, Rouzaud P, et al. Relation between unbound plasma concentrations and toxicity in a prolonged oral etoposide schedule. *Eur J Clin Pharmacol* 1998;54:677–683.
63. Sparreboom A, van ZL, Brouwer E, et al. Cremophor EL-mediated alteration of paclitaxel distribution in human blood: clinical pharmacokinetic implications. *Cancer Res* 1999;59:1454–1457.
64. Gardner ER, Burger H, van Schaik RH, et al. Association of enzyme and transporter genotypes with the pharmacokinetics of imatinib. *Clin Pharmacol Ther* 2006;80:192–201.
65. Wu K, House L, Ramirez J, et al. Evaluation of utility of pharmacokinetic studies in phase I trials of two oncology drugs. *Clin Cancer Res* 2013;19:6039–6043.
66. Hu S, Mathijssen RH, de Bruijn P, et al. Inhibition of OATP1B1 by tyrosine kinase inhibitors: in vitro-in vivo correlations. *Br J Cancer* 2014;110(4): 894–898.
67. Kehrer DF, Mathijssen RH, Verweij J, et al. Modulation of irinotecan metabolism by ketoconazole. *J Clin Oncol* 2002;20:3122–3129.
68. van Leeuwen RW, Brundel DH, Neef C, et al. Prevalence of potential drug-drug interactions in cancer patients treated with oral anticancer drugs. *Br J Cancer* 2013;108:1071–1078.
69. Budha NR, Frymoyer A, Smelick GS, et al. Drug absorption interactions between oral targeted anticancer agents and PPIs: is pH-dependent solubility the Achilles heel of targeted therapy? *Clin Pharmacol Ther* 2012;92:203–213.
70. Sparreboom A, Cox MC, Acharya MR, et al. Herbal remedies in the United States: potential adverse interactions with anticancer agents. *J Clin Oncol* 2004;22:2489–2503.
71. Dy GK, Bekele L, Hanson LJ, et al. Complementary and alternative medicine use by patients enrolled onto phase I clinical trials. *J Clin Oncol* 2004;22:4810–4815.
72. Goey AK, Mooiman KD, Beijnen JH, et al. Relevance of in vitro and clinical data for predicting CYP3A4-mediated herb-drug interactions in cancer patients. *Cancer Treat Rev* 2013;39:773–783.
73. Mathijssen RH, Verweij J, De Bruijn P, et al. Effects of St. John's wort on irinotecan metabolism. *J Natl Cancer Inst* 2002;94:1247–1249.
74. Cox MC, Low J, Lee J, et al. Influence of garlic (Allium sativum) on the pharmacokinetics of docetaxel. *Clin Cancer Res* 2006;12:4636–4640.
75. van Erp NP, Baker SD, Zhao M, et al. Effect of milk thistle (*Silybum marianum*) on the pharmacokinetics of irinotecan. *Clin Cancer Res* 2005;11:7800–7806.
76. Wheeler HE, Maitland ML, Dolan ME, et al. Cancer pharmacogenomics: strategies and challenges. *Nat Rev Genet* 2013;14:23–34.
77. Fujita K, Sparreboom A. Pharmacogenetics of irinotecan disposition and toxicity: a review. *Curr Clin Pharmacol* 2010;5:209–217.
78. Huang RS, Ratain MJ. Pharmacogenetics and pharmacogenomics of anticancer agents. *CA Cancer J Clin* 2009;59:42–55.
79. Evans WE, McLeod HL. Pharmacogenomics—drug disposition, drug targets, and side effects. *N Engl J Med* 2003;348:538–549.

80. Sparreboom A, Danesi R, Ando Y, et al. Pharmacogenomics of ABC transporters and its role in cancer chemotherapy. *Drug Resist Updat* 2003;6:71–84.
81. Cusatis G, Gregorc V, Li J, et al. Pharmacogenetics of ABCG2 and adverse reactions to gefitinib. *J Natl Cancer Inst* 2006;98:1739–1742.
82. Kim RB. Organic anion-transporting polypeptide (OATP) transporter family and drug disposition. *Eur J Clin Invest* 2003;33 Suppl 2:1–5.
83. Smith NF, Figg WD, Sparreboom A. Role of the liver-specific transporters OATP1B1 and OATP1B3 in governing drug elimination. *Exp Opin Drug Metab Toxicol* 2005;1:429–445.
84. Sprowl JA, Mikkelsen TS, Giovinazzo H, et al. Contribution of tumoral and host solute carriers to clinical drug response. *Drug Resist Updat* 2012;15:5–20.
85. Kim DH, Sriharsha L, Xu W, et al. Clinical relevance of a pharmacogenetic approach using multiple candidate genes to predict response and resistance to imatinib therapy in chronic myeloid leukemia. *Clin Cancer Res* 2009;15:4750–4758.
86. Canal P, Chatelut E, Guichard S. Practical treatment guide for dose individualisation in cancer chemotherapy. *Drugs* 1998;56:1019–1038.
87. Evans WE, Relling MV, Rodman JH, et al. Conventional compared with individualized chemotherapy for childhood acute lymphoblastic leukemia. *N Engl J Med* 1998;338:499–505.
88. Blasdel C, Egorin MJ, Lagattuta TF, et al. Therapeutic drug monitoring in CML patients on imatinib. *Blood* 2007;110:1699–1701.
89. Larson RA, Druker BJ, Guilhot F, et al. Imatinib pharmacokinetics and its correlation with response and safety in chronic-phase chronic myeloid leukemia: a subanalysis of the IRIS study. *Blood* 2008;111:4022–4028.
90. Picard S, Titier K, Etienne G, et al. Trough imatinib plasma levels are associated with both cytogenetic and molecular responses to standard-dose imatinib in chronic myeloid leukemia. *Blood* 2007;109:3496–3499.
91. Blanchet B, Billemont B, Cramard J, et al. Validation of an HPLC-UV method for sorafenib determination in human plasma and application to cancer patients in routine clinical practice. *J Pharm Biomed Anal* 2009;49:1109–1114.
92. Chatelut E, Canal P, Brunner V, et al. Prediction of carboplatin clearance from standard morphological and biological patient characteristics. *J Natl Cancer Inst* 1995;87:573–580.
93. Bruno R, Hille D, Riva A, et al. Population pharmacokinetics/pharmacodynamics of docetaxel in phase II studies in patients with cancer. *J Clin Oncol* 1998;16:187–196.
94. Gallo JM, Laub PB, Rowinsky EK, et al. Population pharmacokinetic model for topotecan derived from phase I clinical trials. *J Clin Oncol* 2000;18:2459–2467.
95. Li J, Karlsson MO, Brahmer J, et al. CYP3A phenotyping approach to predict systemic exposure to EGFR tyrosine kinase inhibitors. *J Natl Cancer Inst* 2006;98:1714–1723.
96. Lu JF, Eppler SM, Wolf J, et al. Clinical pharmacokinetics of erlotinib in patients with solid tumors and exposure-safety relationship in patients with non-small cell lung cancer. *Clin Pharmacol Ther* 2006;80:136–145.
97. Mathijssen RH, de Jong FA, Loos WJ, et al. Flat-fixed dosing versus body surface area based dosing of anticancer drugs in adults: does it make a difference? *Oncologist* 2007;12:913–923.

16 Pharmacogenomics

Christine M. Walko and Howard L. McLeod

INTRODUCTION

The evolution of understanding cancer biology has yielded many advances that have been translated into cancer treatment. Application of this knowledge has allowed for a shift in chemotherapeutics from traditional cytotoxic agents that worked by killing both healthy and malignant fast growing cells to chemical and biologic therapies aimed at targeting a specific gene or pathway critical to the particular cancer being treated.[1] This age of pathway-directed therapy has been made possible by the increased availability and feasibility of high throughput technology able to provide comprehensive and clinically useful molecular characterization of tumors. Translation of these efforts have resulted in improved degree to disease control for many common cancers including breast, colorectal, lung, and melanoma as well as long-term survival benefits for chronic myelogenous leukemia (CML), gastrointestinal stromal tumors (GIST), and childhood acute lymphoblastic leukemia (ALL).[2]

Pharmacogenomic-guided therapy aims the use information on DNA and RNA integrity to optimize not only the treatment choice for an individual patient, but also the dose and schedule of that treatment. The assessment of both somatic and germ-line mutations contribute to the overall individualization of cancer treatment. Somatic mutations are genetic variations found within the tumor DNA, but not DNA from the normal (germ-line) tissues, which also have functional consequences that influence disease outcomes and/or response to certain therapies. These types of mutations or biomarkers can be classified as either prognostic or predictive. Prognostic biomarkers identify subpopulations of patients with different disease courses or outcomes, independent of treatment. Predictive biomarkers identify subpopulations of patients most likely to have a response to a given therapy.[3] Germline mutations are heritable variations found within the individual and, in practical terms, are focused on DNA markers predictive for toxicity or therapeutic outcomes of a particular therapy as well as inheritable risk of certain cancers.[4] Pharmacogenomic mutations in the germ line provide some explanation for the interindividual and interracial variability in drug response and toxicity. For cancer chemotherapy, where cytotoxic agents are administered at doses close to their maximal tolerable dose, and therapeutic windows are relatively narrow, minor differences in individual drug handling may lead to severe toxicities. Therefore, an understanding of the sources of this variability would lead to the possibility of individualizing dosages or influencing clinical decisions that can improve patient care. Pharmacogenomics has putative utility in therapy selection, clinical study design, and as a tool to improve understanding of the pharmacology of a medication.

The term *pharmacogenetics* was initially used to define inherited differences in drug effects and typically focused on individual candidate genes. The field of pharmacogenomics now includes genomewide association studies and is used to describe genetic variations in all aspects of drug absorption, distribution, metabolism, and excretion in addition to drug targets and their downstream pathways.[5] Table 16.1 illustrates some current clinical examples of genotype-guided cancer chemotherapy. Variations in the DNA sequences encoding these proteins may take the form of deletions, insertions, repeats, frameshift mutations, nonsense mutations, and missense mutations, resulting in an inactive, truncated, unstable, or otherwise dysfunctional protein. The most common change involves single nucleotide substitutions, called single-nucleotide polymorphisms (SNP), which occur at approximately 1 per 1,000 base pairs on the human genome. Variability in toxicity or activity can also be mediated by postgenomic events, at the level of RNA, protein, or functional activity.

PHARMACOGENOMICS OF TUMOR RESPONSE

Tumor response to chemotherapy is regulated by a complex, multigenic network of genes that encompasses inherent characteristics of the tumor, differentially activated pathways of cell signaling, proliferation and DNA repair, factors that control drug delivery to the tumor cells (e.g., metabolism, transport), and cell death. These may in turn be modulated by previously administered treatment or drug exposure, which may upregulate target proteins or activate alternative pathways of drug resistance. The polygenic nature of drug response implies that a better understanding of genotype–phenotype associations would require more than the usual single-gene pharmacogenetic strategies employed to date. However, there are instances where the genomic context of a single gene within a cancer will be of high impact for specific therapeutic agents (see Table 16.1).

Pathway Directed Anticancer Therapy

One of the earliest success stories illustrating pathway-driven therapeutics is with CML. The hallmark chromosomal abnormality of this disease is the translocation of chromosomes 9 and 22 that ultimately produces the fusion gene *BCR-ABL*. This discovery in 1960 eventually led to the development of the targeted tyrosine-kinase inhibitor (TKI) imatinib and its subsequent Food and Drug Administration (FDA) approval for treatment of CML in 2001.[6] The International Randomized Study of Interferon and STI571 (IRIS) trial began enrollment in 2000 and compared imatinib with interferon and low-dose cytarabine, which was the previous standard of care for newly diagnosed patients with chronic-phase CML. All efficacy endpoints favored imatinib, including complete cytogenetic response of 76.2% with imatinib compared with 14.5% with interferon ($p < 0.001$).[7] Overall survival (OS) after 60 months of follow-up was 89% with imatinib.[8] This example is just one of many where a once fatal disease can now be considered more akin to a chronic disease, requiring a daily medication and regular physician follow-up, similar to hypertension or diabetes. Drug development has also kept pace with these advances and now several other agents, including dasatinib, nilotinib, bosutinib, and ponatinib, have joined imatinib as treatment options for CML.

The idea of changing treatment focus from a disease-based model to a pathway-driven model is also evolving. Human epidermal

TABLE 16.1

Clinical Examples of Genotype-Guided Cancer Chemotherapy

Somatic Mutation Examples		
Drug Target	**Drug(s)**	**Malignancy**
EML4-ALK	Crizotinib	Non–small-cell lung cancer
BCR-ABL	Dasatinib, imatinib, nilotinib, bosutinib, ponatinib	Chronic myelogenous leukemia
BRAF	Vemurafenib, dabrafenib	Melanoma
Epidermal growth factor receptor (EGFR)	Erlotinib, afatinib	Non–small-cell lung cancer
HER2	Trastuzumab, lapatinib, pertuzumab, Ado-trastuzumab emtansine	Breast cancer, gastric cancer
Janus kinase 2 (JAK2)	Ruxolitinib	Myelofibrosis
Kirsten rat sarcoma viral oncogene (KRAS)	Cetuximab, panitumumab	Colorectal cancer
Rearranged during transfection (RET)	Vandetanib	Medullary thyroid cancer
Germ-Line Mutation Examples		
Gene Mutation	**Drug**	**Effect**
Cytochrome P450 (CYP) 2C19	Voriconazole	Decreased serum levels of active drug and potential decreased efficacy in patients with high enzyme levels (ultrarapid metabolizers)
CYP2D6	Tamoxifen, codeine, ondansetron	Decreased production of active metabolite and potential decreased efficacy in patients with low enzyme levels
Dihydropyrimidine dehydrogenase (DPYD)	5-Fluorouracil	Decreased elimination and increased risk of myelosuppression, diarrhea, and mucositis in patients with low enzyme levels
Glucose-6-phosphate dehydrogenase (G6PD)	Rasburicase	Risk of severe hemolysis in patients with G6PD deficiency
Thiopurine methyltransferase (TPMT)	Mercaptopurine, thioguanine, azathioprine	Decreased methylation of the active metabolite resulting decreased elimination and increased risk of neutropenia in patients with low enzyme levels
UDP-glucuronosyltransferase (UGT) 1A1	Irinotecan	Decreased glucuronidation of the active metabolite resulting decreased elimination and increased risk of neutropenia and diarrhea in patients with low enzyme levels

growth factor receptor 2 (HER2) is a transmembrane receptor tyrosine kinase that is overexpressed or amplified in up to 25% of breast cancers. Trastuzumab is a humanized monoclonal antibody directed against HER2 and demonstrated improved response rates (RR) and time to disease progression in patients with metastatic HER2 positive breast cancer and improved disease-free survival (DFS) and OS in HER2-positive breast cancer patients treated with adjuvant trastuzumab.[9] Several additional agents are now available to target the HER2 pathway and vary in their pharmacology and mechanism of action. Lapatinib is an oral TKI directed against HER2 and the epidermal growth factor receptor (EGFR), pertuzumab is a humanized monoclonal antibody that binds at a different location than trastuzumab and inhibits the dimerization and subsequent activation of HER2 signaling, and ado-trastuzumab emtansine is an antibody-drug conjugate that targets HER2-positive cells and then releases the cytotoxic antimitotic agent emtansine through liposomal degradation of the linking compound. All of these agents illustrate the progress and pharmacologic diversity of pathway-directed therapy and remain as standard of care options for HER2-positive breast cancer in either the adjuvant and/or metastatic settings.[10] HER2 expression is not limited to breast cancer, however. Though less common, HER2 expression is seen in numerous solid tumors including bladder, gastric, prostate and non–small-cell lung cancer with varying degrees of incidence depending on the method of detection. Based on results from a large, open-label phase III randomized, international trial of 594 patients with gastric or gastroesophageal junction cancer expressing HER2 by either immunohistochemistry or gene amplification by fluorescence in situ hybridization, trastuzumab is also approved for treatment of metastatic gastric or gastroesophageal junction adenocarcinoma that expresses HER2. Patients randomized to chemotherapy in combination with trastuzumab had a median OS of 13.8 months compared with 11.1 months in the patients receiving chemotherapy alone (hazard ratio [HR], 0.74; 0.60 to 0.91, $p = 0.0046$).[11] Numerous examples also support that pathway-directed therapy will cross the boundaries of disease sites and that tumor genetics will become one of the biggest determining factors for treatment.

Simple expression of the drug target does not always translate into desired clinical outcomes though. Cetuximab and panitumumab are monoclonal antibodies directed against EGFR; however, it was found that colorectal cancer (CRC) patients who did not have detectable EGFR still experienced responses to these agents similar in extent to EGFR-positive patients. Kirsten rat sarcoma viral oncogene (KRAS) is a downstream effector of the EGFR pathway. Ligand binding to EGFR on the cell surface activates pathway signaling through the KRAS-RAF-mitogen-activated protein kinase (MAPK) pathway, which is thought to control cell growth, differentiation, and apoptosis.[12] Eventually it was found that CRC patients with a KRAS mutation did not derive benefit from cetuximab or panitumumab. The RR in CRC receiving either cetuximab or panitumumab who were KRAS wild type was 10% to 40% compared with near zero percent in those with KRAS mutations.[13] This finding was the result of a retrospective analysis of small group of patients and was confirmed in large, prospective trials. Additionally, it underscores the importance of tissue collection for biomarker assessment in trials with novel therapeutics. A recent clinical trial genomic analysis suggests that mutations in *NRAS* may also have value in predicting the utility of EGFR antibody therapy in colorectal cancer. Although the predictive value of KRAS mutation status in colorectal cancer has been well established in clinical trials, the role of KRAS in lung cancer and other malignancies is less well elucidated. Lung cancers harboring KRAS mutations have been shown to have less clinical benefit from the EGFR-targeted erlotinib in some trials, although this has not consistently been the case across all trials. Additionally, lung cancer KRAS mutation status does not appear to reproducibly predict clinical benefit from the EGFR-targeted monoclonal antibodies, as is the case in colorectal cancer.[14] Unlike the HER2 example discussed previously, the clinical application of some genetic mutations will differ between tissue of origin.

Deeper investigations and understandings of mutations driving oncogenic pathways can also elucidate mechanisms of resistance and practical therapeutic strategies for treatment and prevention. Approximately half of all cutaneous melanomas carry mutations in *BRAF*, with the most common being the V600E mutation. Vemurafenib is a TKI directed against mutated BRAF that demonstrated improvements in both progression-free survival (PFS) and OS when compared with the cytotoxic agent dacarbazine in previously untreated patients with metastatic melanoma carrying the BRAF V600E mutation. Vemurafenib demonstrated a 63% relative reduction in the risk of death compared with dacarbazine ($p < 0.001$) along with a higher response rate (48% compared with 5% for dacarbazine).[15] Based on these results, vemurafenib was the first BRAF targeted TKI approved by the FDA and was soon joined by dabrafenib. Although dramatic responses to these agents have been observed, relapse almost universally occurs after a median of 6 to 8 months. Activating BRAF mutations, like V600E, result in uncontrolled activity of the MAPK pathway through activation of the downstream kinase MEK, which when phosphorylated, subsequently activates extracellular signal-regulated kinase (ERK), which ultimately translocates to the cell nucleus, resulting in cell proliferation and survival (Fig. 16.1).[16] An assessment of serial biopsies from patients treated with vemurafenib suggested numerous mechanisms for acquired resistance, including the appearance of secondary mutations in MEK.[17] This finding supports the clinical rationale for using combination therapy with a BRAF and a MEK inhibitor. The combination of dabrafenib (BRAF inhibitor) and trametinib (MEK inhibitor) was assessed in 247 metastatic melanoma patients with BRAF V600 mutations compared with dabrafenib alone. Median PFS was 9.4 months in the combination group compared with 5.8 months in the patients who received single agent therapy (HR, 0.39; 0.25 to 0.62, $p < 0.001$). A complete or partial response was also higher in the combination therapy group (76% compared with 54%, $p = 0.03$). The occurrence of cutaneous squamous cell carcinoma, a known side effect of single-agent BRAF inhibitor therapy due to paradoxical activation of RAF in nonmutated cells, was also decreased in the combination therapy group (7% compared with 19%, $p = 0.09$), further supporting the evidence of downstream inhibition.[18] Although combination therapy does prolong the time to disease progression, resistance still occurs in patients through a variety of mechanisms. Utilization of sequential biopsies and a genetic assessment will help to inform rationale combination and sequential pathway-driven therapy trials that will ultimately aid in better understanding and mitigation of common mechanism of resistance.

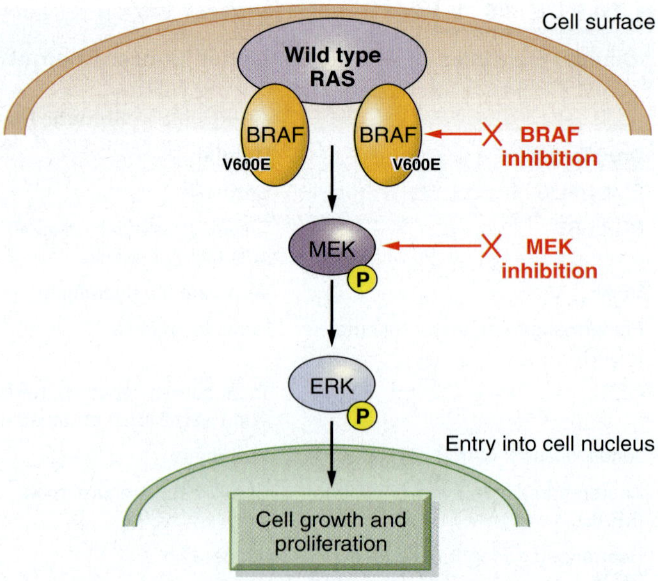

Figure 16.1 MAPK pathway in BRAF mutated melanoma. The BRAF V600E mutation results in activation of the MAPK pathway independent of growth factor binding, initially by phosphorylation (P) of MEK. MEK subsequently phosphorylates ERK. ERK then translocates to the cell nucleus and causes transcription of cellular factors, resulting in cell proliferation and survival. Because one mechanism of resistance to BRAF inhibition is through mutations in MEK, inhibition at both the upstream target of BRAF and the downstream site of MEK can prolong the clinical benefit of the BRAF inhibitor.

Although advances in basic science and drug development have translated many oncogenic driver mutations across tumor types into pathway-directed therapy, this is not the case for the majority. There are numerous examples of functionally relevant recurrent driver mutations that affect protein targets that are not currently druggable. Regardless of malignancy, one of the most commonly mutated tumor suppressors is the protein p53. Mutations can result in p53 acquiring oncogenic functions that enable proliferation, invasion, metastasis, and cell survival as well as coordinating with different proteins, such as EGFR, to enhance or inhibit its effects. However, a clinical application of p53 mutation data or directly targeting p53 has been limited, to date.[19] *PIK3CA* encodes a catalytic subunit of phophoinositol-3 kinase (PI3K), which includes four distinct subfamily kinases involved in regulating cell growth, motility, proliferation, and survival. Direct inhibitors of the kinase, as well as downstream targets, including AKT (protein kinase B [PKB]) and mammalian target of rapamycin (mTOR), are being assessed to target these mutations. Therapeutic challenges include understanding the complex signaling network germane to each cancer and the role of kinases in each subfamily.[20] Both the examples of p53 and PI3K illustrate the challenge of translating the multitude of somatic mutations into applications of available therapeutic agents.

Application of Genomewide Gene Expression Profiling to Guide Therapy

Single gene approaches may not reflect the overall complexity of genetic regulation of chemotherapy responses. Genomic strategies using global gene expression data are able to provide a more complete picture of the tumor through disease classification.[21] These strategies may identify subgroups of patients with early disease that need adjuvant chemotherapy, those who will not benefit from standard therapy, or help with the selection of chemotherapy from a menu of potentially active agents. Oncotype Dx is a 21-gene assay with 16 tumor-associated genes and 5 reference genes used to predict the risk of distant local recurrence in estrogen receptor (ER)-positive, HER2-negative patients with node-negative or select node-positive breast cancer. Additionally, the test also provides predictive information on which patients may benefit from the addition of chemotherapy to hormonal therapy alone. The test ultimately reports a recurrence score (RS) on a continuous scale from zero to 100. Patients with an RS <18 are considered low risk, with a 10-year distant recurrence rate (DRR) of 6.8% (95% confidence interval [CI], 4 to 9.6); RS scores of 18 to 30 are at intermediate risk, with a 10-year DRR of 14.3% (CI, 8.3 to 20.3); and RS scores ≥31 are at high risk, with a 10-year DRR of 30.5% (CI, 23.6 to 37.4).[22] Additionally, high-risk patients have the largest benefit from the addition of chemotherapy to hormonal therapy (HR, 0.26; 0.13 to 0.53), whereas low-risk patients have little benefit from the addition of chemotherapy and could consider hormonal treatment alone (HR, 1.31; 0.46 to 3.78). Intermediate risk patients are harder to classify, and clinical trials are underway to further address treatment recommendations for this group of patients.[23] These type of assays are also in development and in clinical trials for a variety of other solid tumor and hematologic malignancies.

Genetic-Guided Therapy Practical Issues in Somatic Analysis

Currently, targeted DNA capture is the most common type of somatic genetic screening and involves focusing on a few relevant candidate genes followed by deeper sequencing. These types of techniques can reveal common genes associated with a particular malignancy but also may uncover a signaling pathway that would not be obviously associated with a particular histology or tumor site. Application of a next-generation sequencing assay in 40 CRC and 24 non–small-cell lung cancer (NSCLC) tissue samples that assessed 145 cancer-relevant genes demonstrated that somatic mutations were seen in 98% of the CRC tumors and 83% of the NSCLCs (Fig. 16.2).[24] The evolution of sequencing strategies and decreasing costs has made whole genome sequencing more available in the clinical setting, and several companies offer commercially available tumor profiling services. Several limitations exist that currently restrict the broad clinical implementation of these assays, however. Although germ-line genetic assessments can be done on a peripheral blood sample or buccal swab, somatic assessments typically require biopsy tissue, which is often in limited supply and of varying quality or may not be feasible depending on the site of the cancer. Ongoing studies are assessing the value of liquid biopsies of circulating tumor DNA.[25] Optimizing and creating uniformity in quality control of gene panel or whole-genome assessment is also needed to decrease the reporting of uncertain or erroneous identification of mutations. Once sequencing is completed, a predictive analysis is needed for the 25% to 80% of instances where variants of unknown significance are identified in genes of interest. Translation of genomic sequencing into clinical practice will require a diverse team, including pathologists, medical oncologists, surgical oncologists, information technologists, geneticists, and pharmacologists.

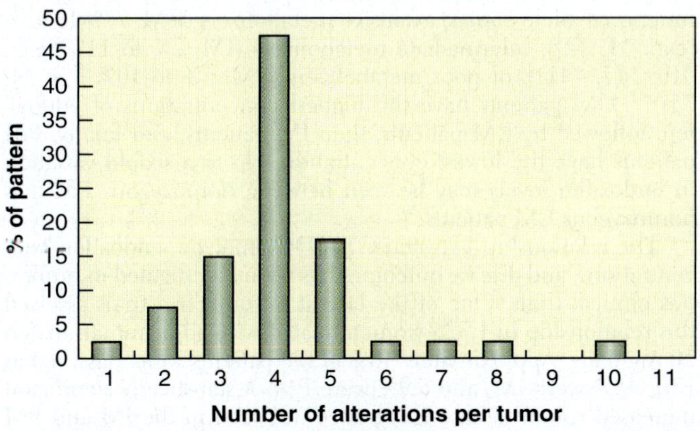

Figure 16.2 Number of alterations per tumor. Deep sequencing of 145 genes in 40 colorectal cancers found a spectrum of incidence of somatic mutations, with more than half occurring in genes that are *druggable* with medication that is either FDA approved or in late stage clinical development.

PHARMACOGENOMICS OF CHEMOTHERAPY DRUG TOXICITY

A drug's disposition and pharmacodynamic effects can be influenced by a number of variables, including patient age, diet, concomitant medications, and underlying disease processes. However, an individual's genetic constitution is an important regulator of variability in drug effect. Differences in drug effects are more pronounced between individuals compared to within an individual. Indeed, studies in monozygotic and dizygotic twins identified that 20% to 80% of the variation in drug disposition is mediated by inheritance.[26] Drug-metabolizing enzymes, cellular transporters, and tissue receptors are governed by genetic variation.

Advances in the treatment of most common malignancies have resulted in the availability of multiple distinct combination chemotherapy regimens with similar or equal anticancer efficacy. Therefore, differences in systemic toxicity have become a major determinant in the selection of therapy. The majority of pharmacogenomic examples affecting adverse events or efficacy from cytotoxic drugs involve hepatic metabolizing enzymes that detoxify or biotransform xenobiotics.[27,28]

Thiopurine Methyltransferase

One of the best-studied pharmacogenetic syndrome involves the metabolism of the thiopurine drugs—6-mercaptopurine (6MP), 6-thioguanine, and azathioprine which have wide applications, including maintenance therapy for childhood ALL and adult leukemias. These prodrugs must be activated to thioguanine nucleotides in order to have antiproliferative effects. However, most of the variability in the formation of active metabolites is mediated by methylation via thiopurine methyltransferase (TPMT).[29] TPMT is a cytosolic enzyme that catalyzes S-methylation of thiopurine agents, resulting in an inactive metabolite. Erythrocyte TPMT activity has a trimodal distribution, with 90% of patients having high activity, 10% intermediate activity, and 0.3% with very low or no detectable activity. TPMT deficiency results in higher intracellular activation of 6MP to form thioguanine nucleotides, resulting in severe or fatal hematologic toxicity from standard doses of therapy.[30] The variable activity results from polymorphism in the TPMT gene, located on chromosome locus 6p22.3. Genetic variants at codon 238 (TPMT*2), codon 719 (TPMT*3C), or both codons 460 and 719 (TPMT*3A) are the most clinically significant, accounting for 95% of the patients with reduced TPMT activity.[31] Heterozygotes (one wild type and one variant allele) are common (10% of patients), and have elevated levels of active metabolites (twofold more than homozygous wild type), and required more cumulative dose reductions of 6MP for maintenance ALL chemotherapy compared to homozygous wild-type patients (Fig. 16.3).[32] Patients with a homozygous variant TPMT genotype are at a fourfold risk of severe toxicity, compared with wild-type patients.[31] TPMT genotype tests are now available commercially in a Clinical Laboratory Improvement Amendments (CLIA)-certified environment. To date, patients homozygous for TPMT variant alleles appear to tolerate 10%, and heterozygotes appear to tolerate 65% of the recommended doses of 6MP, with no apparent

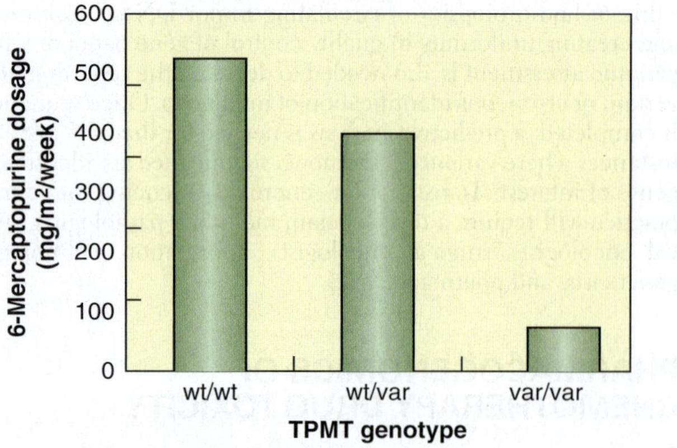

Figure 16.3 Relationship between TPMT genotype and required 6MP dose. Compared with homozygous wild-type patients, those heterozygous for a thiopurine methyltransferase (TPMT) variant allele generally require at least a 30% dose reduction in 6MP, whereas homozygous variant patients require substantial dose reductions of approximately 90% that of wild-type patients.

decrease in clinical efficacy (Fig. 16.3).[32] This has formed the basis for prospective, TPMT genotype-guided dosing of 6MP to avoid severe toxicity. Clinical Pharmacogenomics Implementation Consortium (CPIC) Guidelines recommend that homozygous wild-type patients be started at the full standard dose. Heterozygous patients should start with reduced doses at 30% to 70% of the full dose with adjustments made after 2 to 4 weeks based on myelosuppression and disease-specific guidelines. Homozygous variant patients should start with 10% of the full dose due to the extremely high levels of the active metabolite and potential for fatal toxicity at standard doses. Adjustments should be made after 4 to 6 weeks based on myelosuppression and disease-specific guidelines.[33]

Dihydropyrimidine Dehydrogenase (DPD)

Although 5-fluorouracil (5FU) has been available for over 40 years, it remains the cornerstone of colorectal cancer chemotherapy, both in the adjuvant and metastatic settings. Additionally, the oral prodrug capecitabine ultimately undergoes activation to 5FU and is commonly used in gastrointestinal and breast malignancies. 5FU is a prodrug that is activated intracellularly to 5-fluoro-2′-deoxyuridine monophosphate (5FdUMP), which inhibits thymidylate synthase (TS), among other mechanisms of action. TS inhibition results in impaired de novo pyrimidine synthesis and suppression of DNA synthesis. Approximately 85% of a 5FU dose is catabolized by dihydropyrimidine dehydrogenase (DPD) to inactive metabolites. Therefore, DPD is a primary regulator of 5FU activity. DPD deficiency has been described, resulting in higher 5FU blood levels, greater formation of active metabolites, and severe or fatal clinical toxicity, predominately myelosuppression, mucositis, and cerebellar toxicity.[34] In theory, this toxicity could be reduced or avoided by screening for DPD activity in surrogate tissues, such as peripheral mononuclear cells. However, the technical requirements for preparation of these samples make it impractical for many practice sites. Understanding the molecular basis for DPD deficiency will provide an approach for prospective identification of patients at high risk for severe 5FU toxicity. The gene encoding DPD is composed of 23 exons, and at least 23 SNPs have been found.[35] Studies in DPD-deficient patients have identified several distinct molecular variants associated with low enzyme activity. Many of these are rare, and base substitutions, splicing defects, and frame shift mutations, have been described. The prevalent variation is the splice recognition site in intron 14 (DPYD*2A), where a G to A substitution results in the skipping of exon 14, resulting in an inactive enzyme.[36–38] This polymorphism has been associated with severe DPD deficiency in heterozygous patients, with a homozygous genotype associated with a mental retardation syndrome. Patients with severe 5FU toxicity may harbor one or more variant alleles of DPD, and a recent study showed that 61% of cancer patients experiencing severe 5FU toxicities had decreased DPD activity in peripheral mononuclear cells, and DPYD*2A was commonly found.[39] In the patients with grade 4 neutropenia, 50% harbored at least one DPYD*2A. It is estimated that in the Caucasian population, homozygotes for the variant alleles have an incidence of 0.1% and heterozygotes occur at an incidence of 0.5% to 2%. There are additional DPD mutations that have been associated with impaired enzyme activity, including DPYD *3 and DPYD*13. CPIC guidelines recommend standard dosing for homozygous wild-type patients. Reducing the dose by at least 50% in heterozygous patients (*1/*2A) is recommended, followed by dose adjustment based on toxicity and/or pharmacokinetic testing. The use of an alternative agent is recommended in homozygous-variant patients (*2A/*2A).[34] There are many patients with severe 5FU toxicity that have normal DPD activity. This highlights that many factors, including multiple genes, are potential causes of 5FU toxicity, and there will not be one simple test to avoid this important clinical problem.

Cytochrome P450 2D6

Tamoxifen is a selective estrogen-receptor modulator used in ER-positive breast cancer in both the localized and metastatic settings. It is the drug of choice for premenopausal women and is a treatment option, along with aromatase inhibitors, for postmenopausal women. The low cost of tamoxifen also makes it a preferred therapy regardless of menopausal status in numerous countries. Tamoxifen metabolism is complex, with extensive metabolism through numerous phase I and II enzymes that produce several primary and secondary metabolites and their corresponding isomers, each possessing different antiestrogen effects.[40] The primary active metabolite is believed to be endoxifen, which is produced by the CYP3A4/5 mediated-conversion of tamoxifen to N-desmethyltamoxifen, which is then further converted to endoxifen (4-hydroxy-N-desmethyltamoxifen) via cytochrome P450 2D6 (CYP2D6). A direct relationship between endoxifen concentration and its antiestrogen effects has been demonstrated, potentially suggesting that a threshold concentration may be needed for optimal clinical effect.[41] CYP2D6 is highly polymorphic, with more than 80 allelic CYP2D6 variants described. These alleles vary in enzyme activity and prevalence with respect to race and ethnicity.[42] Based on genotype, patients can be classified by phenotype into ultrarapid metabolizers (UM; approximately 1% to 2% of patients [common alleles include *1xN, *2xN]) who carry more than two functional allele copies, extensive metabolizers (EM; 77% to 92% [e.g., *1, *2]), intermediate metabolizers (IM; 2% to 11% [e.g., *10, *17, *41]), or poor metabolizers (PM; 5% to 10% [*3, *4, *5]).[43] UM patients have the highest concentrations of endoxifen, followed by EM patients, then IM patients, and finally, PM patients have the lowest concentration. Up to a sixfold variation in endoxifen levels may be seen between homozygous PM and homozygous EM patients.[40]

The relationship between CYP2D6 genotype, endoxifen concentrations, and disease outcomes has been investigated in numerous clinical trials. One of the largest retrospective trials assessed this relationship in 1,325 women treated with adjuvant tamoxifen 20 mg daily. Approximately 46% of the patients were classified as EM, 48% were IM, and 5.9% were PM. A statistically significant increased risk of disease recurrence was seen in the IM and PM patients compared with the EM patients (HR, 1.40; 95% CI, 1.04 to 1.90 for IM; and HR 1.90, 95% CI, 1.10 to 3.28 for PM).[44] A large meta-analysis of 4,973 tamoxifen-treated patients across 12 international studies conducted by the International Tamoxifen Pharmacogenomics Consortium also supported this relationship.

CYP2D6 PM phenotypes were associated with decreased DFS (HR 1.25, 95% CI, 1.06 to 1.47, $p = 0.009$) when only considering the data from trials with postmenopausal women with ER-positive breast cancer who received tamoxifen 20 mg daily for 5 years.[45]

Not all trial results have been consistent, however, and dosing guidelines for genotype-guided therapy do not yet exist. Clinical trials do support the potential for genotype-guided therapy. IM patients who received an increased dose of 40 mg daily instead of the standard 20 mg were shown to have endoxifen concentrations similar to that of EM patients ($p = 0.25$).[46] This suggests that genotype-guided therapy with increased dose recommendations may be feasible, but additional prospective trials are needed to determine the clinical efficacy of this intervention.

CONCLUSIONS AND FUTURE DIRECTIONS

Genomic-driven cancer medicine is being translated into clinical practice through increased understanding of somatic mutations in a specific tumor that can be translated to pathway-directed therapeutics as well as germ-line mutations that affect the pharmacokinetics and pharmacodynamics of individual medications. For the practicing oncologist, knowledge of pharmacogenomics is necessary because therapeutic decisions of drug selection and dosage are being based on more molecularly and genetically defined variables than the current phenotypic information of tumor type, immunohistochemistry, and body surface area. Health-care policy changes preferring the bundling of care and reimbursement based on diagnosis coding may further drive individualized therapy where the goal is to optimize both treatment responses while minimizing toxicity. However, with advances always come challenges. Reimbursement for multiplex genomic testing is not universal, so deciding who and when to initiate testing is a consideration. Optimizing turnaround time, especially for referral patients who have had biopsies performed elsewhere, will require requesting this archived tissue prior to or during the initial patient visit to facilitate minimizing treatment delays. Although some variants have strong evidence supporting treatment recommendations, many currently do not yet. Multidisciplinary committees charged with reviewing the level of evidence for each genetic result and providing clinically actionable recommendations will be essential for translating these multigene tumor assay results into routine clinical practice. Decision tools and development of treatment guidelines will further assist with routine integration of this technology, especially for oncologists at smaller practice sites. Oncology fellowship training programs will also need to be expanded to ensure competence of new practitioners in the area of genomic-guided therapies.

Regardless of these challenges, the treatment paradigm of genomic-driven medicine and individualizing therapy has permitted the field of oncology to move beyond the limitations of nonselective cytotoxic therapy and toward the more optimal selection and dosing of oncology agents.

REFERENCES

1. McLeod HL. Cancer pharmacogenomics: early promise, but concerted effort needed. *Science* 2013;339:1563–1566.
2. Garraway LA. Genomics-driven oncology: framework for an emerging paradigm. *J Clin Oncol* 2013;31:1806–1814.
3. Mandrekar SJ, Sargent DJ. Predictive biomarker validation in practice: lessons from real trials. *Clin Trials* 2010;7:567–573.
4. Evans WE, Relling MV. Pharmacogenomics: translating functional genomics into rational therapeutics. *Science* 1999;286:487–491.
5. Wang L, McLeod HL, Weinshilboum RM. Genomics and drug response. *N Engl J Med* 2011;364:1144–1153.
6. Druker BJ. Translation of the Philadelphia chromosome into therapy for CML. *Blood* 2008;112:4808–4817.
7. O'Brien SG, Guilhot F, Larson RA, et al. Imatinib compared with interferon and low-dose cytarabine for newly diagnosed chronic-phase chronic myeloid leukemia. *N Engl J Med* 2003;348:994–1004.
8. Druker BJ, Guilhot F, O'Brien SG, et al. Five-year follow-up of patients receiving imatinib for chronic myeloid leukemia. *N Engl J Med* 2006;355:2408–2417.
9. Hudis CA. Trastuzumab—mechanism of action and use in clinical practice. *N Engl J Med* 2007;357:39–51.
10. Figueroa-Magalhaes MC, Jelovac D, Connolly RM, et al. Treatment of HER2-positive breast cancer. *Breast* 2014;23:128–136.
11. Bang YJ, Van Cutsem E, Feyereislova A, et al. Trastuzumab in combination with chemotherapy versus chemotherapy alone for treatment of HER2-positive advanced gastric or gastro-oesophageal junction cancer (ToGA): a phase 3, open-label, randomised controlled trial. *Lancet* 2010;76:687–697.
12. Bardelli A, Siena S. Molecular mechanisms of resistance to cetuximab and panitumumab in colorectal cancer. *J Clin Oncol* 2010;28:1254–1261.
13. Jimeno A, Messersmith WA, Hirsch FR, et al. KRAS mutations and sensitivity to epidermal growth factor receptor inhibitors in colorectal cancer: practical application of patient selection. *J Clin Oncol* 2009;27:1130–1136.
14. Roberts PJ, Stinchcombe TE, Der CJ, et al. Personalized medicine in non-small-cell lung cancer: is KRAS a useful marker in selecting patients for epidermal growth factor receptor-targeted therapy? *J Clin Oncol* 2010;28:4769–4777.
15. Chapman PB, Hauschild A, Robert C, et al. Improved survival with vemurafenib in melanoma with BRAF V600E mutation. *N Engl J Med* 2011;364:2507–2516.
16. Dhillon AS, Hagan S, Rath O, et al. MAP kinase signalling pathways in cancer. *Oncogene* 2007;26:3279–3290.
17. Trunzer K, Pavlick AC, Schuchter L, et al. Pharmacodynamic effects and mechanisms of resistance to vemurafenib in patients with metastatic melanoma. *J Clin Oncol* 2013;31:1767–1774.
18. Flaherty KT, Infante JR, Daud A, et al. Combined BRAF and MEK inhibition in melanoma with BRAF V600 mutations. *N Engl J Med* 2012;367:1694–1703.
19. Muller PA, Vousden KH. p53 mutations in cancer. *Nat Cell Biol* 2013;15:2–8.
20. Clarke PA, Workman P. Phosphatidylinositide-3-kinase inhibitors: addressing questions of isoform selectivity and pharmacodynamic/predictive biomarkers in early clinical trials. *J Clin Oncol* 2012;30:331–333.
21. Ramaswamy S, Golub T. DNA microarrays in clinical oncology. *J Clin Oncol* 2002;20:1932–1941.
22. Paik S, Shak S, Tang G, et al. A multigene assay to predict recurrence of tamoxifen-treated, node-negative breast cancer. *N Engl J Med* 2004;351:2817–2826.
23. Paik S, Tang G, Shak S, et al. Gene expression and benefit of chemotherapy in women with node-negative, estrogen receptor-positive breast cancer. *J Clin Oncol* 2006;24:3726–3734.
24. Lipson D, Capelletti M, Yelensky R, et al. Identification of new ALK and RET gene fusions from colorectal and lung cancer biopsies. *Nat Med* 2012;18:382–384.
25. Diaz LA Jr, Bardelli A. Liquid biopsies: genotyping circulating tumor DNA. *J Clin Oncol* 2014;32:579–586.
26. Watters J, McLeod H. Cancer pharmacogenomics: current and future applications. *Biochim Biophys Acta* 2003;1603:99–111.
27. Evans W, Relling M. Pharmacogenomics: translating functional genomics into rational therapeutics. *Science* 1999;286:487–491.
28. Deenen MJ, Cats A, Beijnen H, et al. Part 2: pharmacogenetic variability in drug transport and phase I anticancer drug metabolism. *Oncologist* 2011;16:820–834.
29. Krynetski E, Evans W. Drug methylation in cancer therapy: lessons from the TPMT polymorphism. *Oncogene* 2003;22:7403–7413.
30. McLeod H, Krynetski EY, Relling MV, et al. Genetic polymorphism of thiopurine methyltransferase and its clinical relevance for childhood acute lymphoblastic leukemia. *Leukemia* 2000;14:567–572.
31. Evans W, Hon YY, Bomgaars L, et al. Preponderance of thiopurine S-methyltransferase deficiency and heterozygosity among patients intolerant to mercaptopurine or azathioprine. *J Clin Oncol* 2001;19:2293–2301.
32. Relling M, Hancock ML, Rivera GK, et al. Mercaptopurine therapy intolerance and heterozygosity at the thiopurine S-methyltransferase gene locus. *J Natl Cancer Inst* 1999;91:2001–2008.
33. Relling MV, Gardner EE, Sandborn WJ, et al. Clinical pharmacogenetics implementation consortium guidelines for thiopurine methyltransferase genotype and thiopurine dosing: 2013 update. *Clin Pharmacol Ther* 2013;93:324–325.
34. Caudle KE, Thorn CF, Klein TE, et al. Clinical Pharmacogenetics Implementation Consortium guidelines for dihydropyrimidine dehydrogenase genotype and fluoropyrimidine dosing. *Clin Pharmacol Ther* 2013;94:640–645.
35. McLeod H, Collie-Duguid ES, Vreken P, et al. Nomenclature for human DPYD alleles. *Pharmacogenetics* 1998;8:455–459.
36. Wei X, Elizondo G, Sapone A, et al. Characterization of the human dihydropyrimidine dehydrogenase gene. *Genomics* 1998;51:391–400.
37. Ridge S, Sludden J, Wei X, et al. Dihydropyrimidine dehydrogenase pharmacogenetics in patients with colorectal cancer. *Br J Cancer* 1998;77:497–500.
38. Johnson M, Wang K, Diasio R. Profound dihydropyrimidine dehydrogenase deficiency resulting from a novel compound heterozygote genotype. *Clin Cancer Res* 2002;8:768–774.
39. Van Kuilenburg A, Meinsma R, Zoetekouw L, et al. Increased risk of grade IV neutropenia after administration of 5-fluorouracil due to a dihydropyrimidine dehydrogenase deficiency: high prevalence of the IVS14+1g>a mutation. *Int J Cancer* 2002;101:253–258.

40. Mürdter TE, Schroth W, Bacchus-Gerybadze L, et al. Activity levels of tamoxifen metabolites at the estrogen receptor and the impact of genetic polymorphisms of phase I and II enzymes on their concentration levels in plasma. *Clin Pharmacol Ther* 2011;89:708–717.
41. Desta Z, Ward BA, Soukhova NV, et al. Comprehensive evaluation of tamoxifen sequential biotransformation by the human cytochrome P450 system in vitro: prominent roles for CYP3A and CYP2D6. *J Pharmacol Exp Ther* 2004;310:1062–1075.
42. Bradford LD. CYP2D6 allele frequency in European Caucasians, Asians, Africans and their descendants. *Pharmacogenomics* 2002;3:229–243.
43. Crews KR, Gaedigk A, Dunnenberger HM, et al. Clinical Pharmacogenetics Implementation Consortium (CPIC) guidelines for codeine therapy in the context of cytochrome P450 2D6 (CYP2D6) genotype. *Clin Pharmacol Ther* 2012;91:321–326.
44. Schroth W, Goetz MP, Hamann U, et al. Association between CYP2D6 polymorphisms and outcomes among women with early stage breast cancer treated with tamoxifen. *JAMA* 2009;302:1429–1436.
45. Province MA, Goetz MP, Brauch H, et al. CYP2D6 genotype and adjuvant tamoxifen: meta-analysis of heterogeneous study populations. *Clin Pharmacol Ther* 2014;95:216–227.
46. Irvin WJ Jr, Walko CM, Weck KE, et al. Genotype-guided tamoxifen dosing increases active metabolite exposure in women with reduced CYP2D6 metabolism: a multicenter study. *J Clin Oncol* 2011;29:3232–3239.

17 Alkylating Agents

Kenneth D. Tew

PERSPECTIVES

Alkylating agents were the first anticancer molecules developed, and they are still used today. After more than 50 years of use, the basic chemistry and pharmacology of this drug family is well understood and has not changed substantially. The family contains six major classes: nitrogen mustards, aziridines, alkyl sulfonates, epoxides, nitrosoureas, and triazene compounds, although a few nonstandard agents have recently been developed. Most epoxides tend to be quite nonspecific with respect to their reactivity and, as such, few have useful clinical characteristics. This chapter provides perspective on how the limited varieties of alkylating agents continue to be useful in the therapeutic management of cancer patients.

The alkylating agents are a diverse group of anticancer agents with the commonality that they react in a manner such that an electrophilic alkyl group or a substituted alkyl group can covalently bind to cellular nucleophilic sites. Electrophilicity is achieved through the formation of carbonium ion intermediates and can result in transition complexes with target molecules. Ultimately, reactions result in the formation of covalent linkages by alkylation with a broad range of nucleophilic groups, including bases in DNA, and these are believed responsible for ultimate cytotoxicity and therapeutic effect. Although the alkylating agents react with cells in all phases of the cell cycle, their efficacy and toxicity result from interference with rapidly proliferating tissues. From a historical perspective, the vesicant properties of mustard gas used during World War I were shown to be accompanied by the suppression of lymphoid and hematologic functions in experimental animals[1] and led to the development of mechlorethamine as the first alkylating agent used in the management of human cancer.[2] Subsequently, a number of related drugs have been developed, and these have roles in the treatment of a range of leukemias, lymphomas, and solid tumors. Most of the alkylating agents cause dose limiting toxicities to the bone marrow and, to a lesser degree, the intestinal mucosa, with other organ systems also affected contingent on the individual drug, dosage, and duration of therapy. Despite the present trend toward targeted therapies, this class of "nonspecific" drugs maintains an essential role in cancer chemotherapy.

Because of the classic nature of the drug family, there have been relatively few advances in either their use or utility since publication of the previous edition of this book.

CHEMISTRY

Alkylating reactions are generally classified through their kinetic properties as S_N1 (nucleophilic substitution, first order) or S_N2 (nucleophilic substitution, second order) (Fig. 17.1). The first-order kinetics of the S_N1 reactions depend on the concentration of the original alkylating agent. The rate-limiting step is the initial formation of the reactive intermediate, and the rate is essentially independent of the concentration of the substrate. The S_N2 alkylation reaction is a bimolecular nucleophilic displacement with second-order kinetics, where the rate depends on the concentration of both alkylating agent and target nucleophile. Reactivity of electrophiles[3] suggests that the rates of alkylation of cellular nucleophiles (including thiols, phosphates, amino and imidazole groups of amino acids, and various reactive sites in nucleic acid bases) are most dependent on their potential energy states, which can be defined as "hard" or "soft," based on the polarizability of their reactive centers.[4] Although the metabolism and metabolites of nitrogen mustards and nitrosoureas differ, the active alkylating species of each is the alkyl carbonium ion (see Fig. 17.1), a highly polarized hard electrophile as a consequence of its highly positive charge density at the electrophilic center. Alkyl carbonium ions will react most readily with hard nucleophiles (possessing a highly polarized negative charge density), where the high-energy transition state (a potential energy barrier to the reaction) is most favorable. In specific terms, an active alkylating species from a nitrogen mustard will demonstrate selectivity for cellular nucleophiles in the following order: (1) oxygen in phosphate groups of RNA and DNA, (2) oxygens of purines and pyrimidines, (3) amino groups of purine bases, (4) primary and secondary amino groups of proteins, (5) sulfur atoms of methionine, and (6) thiol groups of cysteinyl residues of protein and glutathione.[3] The least favored reactions will still occur, but at much slower rates unless they are catalyzed.

Alkylation through highly reactive intermediates (e.g., mechlorethamine) would be expected to be less selective in their targets than the less reactive S_N2 reagents (e.g., busulfan). However, the therapeutic and toxic effects of alkylating agents do not correlate directly with their chemical reactivity. Clinically useful agents include drugs with S_N1 or S_N2 characteristics, and some with both.[5] These differ in their toxicity profiles and antitumor activity, but more as a consequence of differences in pharmacokinetics, lipid solubility, penetration of the central nervous system (CNS), membrane transport, metabolism and detoxification, and specific enzymatic reactions capable of repairing alkylation sites on DNA.

CLASSIFICATION

The major classes of clinically useful alkylating agents are illustrated in Table 17.1 and summarized in the following sections. Doses and schedules of the various agents are shown in Table 17.2.

Alkyl Sulfonates

Busulfan is used for the treatment of chronic myelogenous leukemia. It exhibits S_N2 alkylation kinetics and shows nucleophilic selectivity for thiol groups, suggesting that it may exert cytotoxicity through protein alkylation rather than through DNA. In contrast to the nitrogen mustards and nitrosoureas, busulfan has a greater effect on myeloid cells than lymphoid cells, thus the reason for its use against chronic myelogenous leukemia.[6]

Aziridines

Aziridines are analogs of ring-closed intermediates of nitrogen mustards and are less chemically reactive, but they have

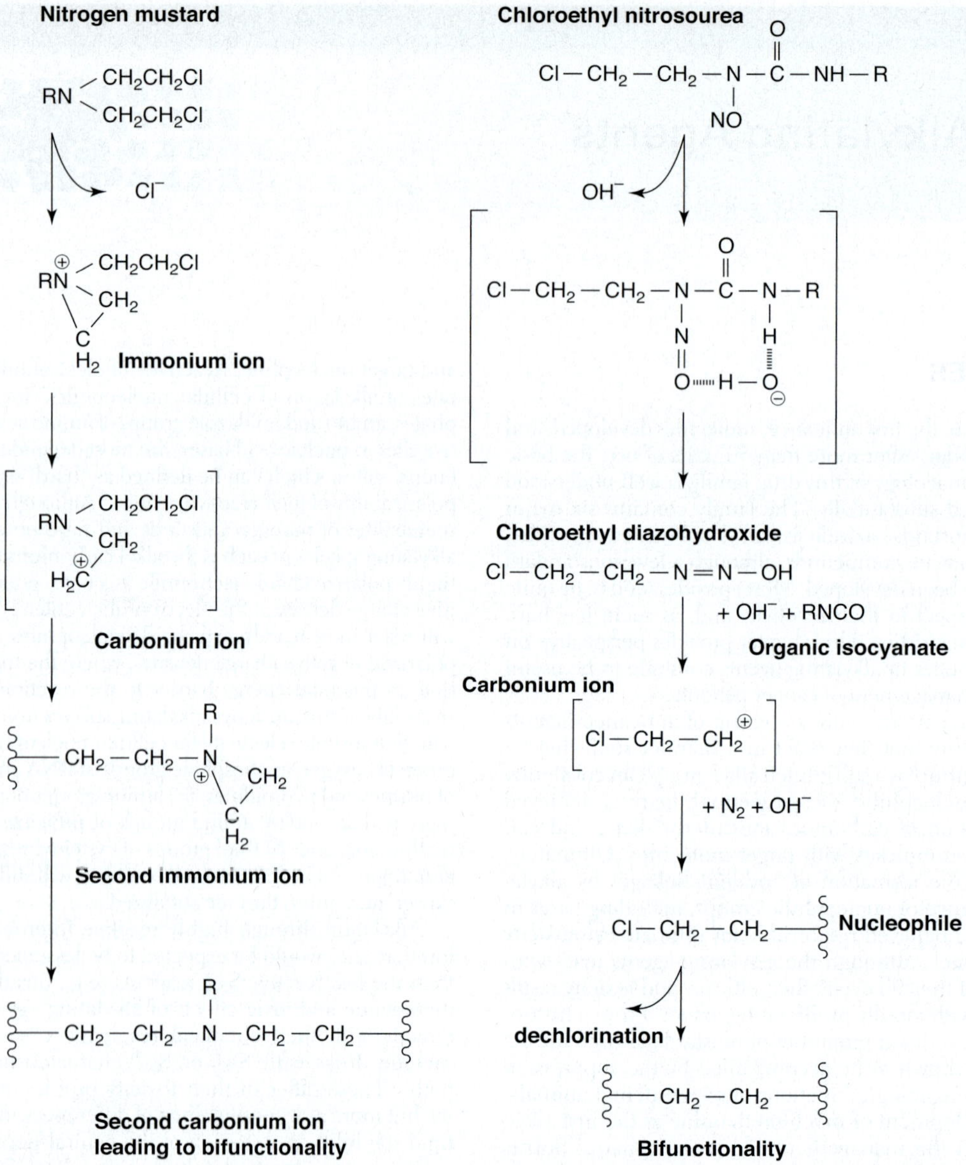

Figure 17.1 Comparative decomposition and metabolism of a typical nitrogen mustard compared to a nitrosourea. Although intermediate metabolites are distinct, the active alkylating species is a carbonium ion in each case. This electrophilic moiety reacts with target cellular nucleophiles.

equivalent therapeutic properties. Thiotepa has been used in the treatment of carcinoma of the breast, ovary, for a variety of CNS diseases, and with increasing frequency as a component of high-dose chemotherapy regimens.[7] Thiotepa and its primary desulfurated metabolite triethylenethiophosphoramide (TEPA) alkylate through aziridine ring openings, a mechanism similar to the nitrogen mustards.

Triazines

Perhaps the newest clinical development in the alkylating agent field is the emergence of temozolomide (TMZ). This agent acts as a prodrug and is an imidazotetrazine analog that undergoes spontaneous activation in solution to produce 5-(3-methyltriazen-1-yl) imidazole-4-carboxamide (MTIC), a triazine derivative. It crosses the blood–brain barrier with concentrations in the CNS approximating 30% of plasma concentrations.[8] Resistance to the methylating agent occurs quite frequently and has adversely affected the rate and durability of the clinical responses of patients. However, because of its favorable toxicity and pharmacokinetics, TMZ is being combined with numerous other classes of anticancer drugs in an effort to improve response rates in diseases such as malignant melanomas, gliomas, brain metastasis from solid tumors, and refractory leukemias. Many of these trials are currently underway.[9]

Nitrogen Mustards

Bischloroethylamines or nitrogen mustards are extensively administered in the clinic. As an initial step in alkylation, chlorine acts as a leaving group and the β-carbon reacts with the nucleophilic nitrogen atom to form the cyclic, positively charged, reactive aziridinium moiety. Reaction of the aziridinium ring with an electron-rich nucleophile creates an initial alkylation product. The remaining chloroethyl group achieves bifunctionality through the formation of a second aziridinium. Melphalan (L-phenylalanine mustard), chlorambucil, cyclophosphamide, and ifosfamide (see Table 17.1) replaced mechlorethamine as primary therapeutic agents. These derivatives have electron-withdrawing groups substituted on the nitrogen atom, reducing the nucleophilicity of the nitrogen and rendering them less reactive, but enhancing their antitumor efficacy.

TABLE 17.1

Major Classes of Clinically Useful Alkylating Agents

Drug	Main Therapeutic Uses	Clinical Pharmacology	Major Toxicities	Notes
ALKYL SULFONATES				
Busulfan	Bone marrow transplantation, especially in chronic myelogenous leukemia	Bioavailability, 80%; protein bound, 33%; $t_{1/2}$, 2.5 h	Pulmonary fibrosis, hyperpigmentation thrombocytopenia, lowered blood platelet count and activity	Oral or parenteral; high dose causes hepatic veno-occlusive disease
ETHYLENEIMINES/METHYLMELAMINES				
Altretamine		Protein bound, 94%; $t_{1/2}$, 5–10 h	Nausea, vomiting, diarrhea, and neurotoxicity	Not widely used
Thio TEPA	Breast, ovarian, and bladder cancer; also bone marrow transplant	$t_{1/2}$, 2.5 h; urinary excretion at 24 h, 25%; substrate for CYP2B6 and CYP2C11	Myelosuppression	Nadirs of leukopenia, occur 2 wk; thrombocytopenia, 3 wk (correlates with AUC of parent drug)
NITROGEN MUSTARDS				
Mechlorethamine	Hodgkin lymphoma		Nausea, vomiting, myelosuppression	Precursor for other clinical mustards
Melphalan (L-phenylalanine mustard)	Multiple myeloma and ovarian cancer, and occasionally malignant melanoma	Bioavailability 25%–90%; $t_{1/2}$, 1.5 h; urinary excretion at 24 h, 13%; clearance, 9 mL/min/kg	Nausea, vomiting, myelosuppression	Causes less mucosal damage than others in class
Chlorambucil	Chronic lymphocytic leukemia	$t_{1/2}$, 1.5 h; urinary excretion at 24 h, 50%	Myelosuppression, gastrointestinal distress, CNS, skin reactions, hepatotoxicity	Oral
Cyclophosphamide	Variety of lymphomas, leukemias, and solid tumors	Bioavailability, >75%; protein bound, >60%; $t_{1/2}$, 3–12 h; urinary excretion at 24 h, <15%	Nausea and vomiting, bone marrow suppression, diarrhea, darkening of the skin/nails, alopecia (hair loss), lethargy, hemorrhagic cystitis	IV; primary excretion route is urine
Ifosfamide	Testicular, breast cancer; lymphoma (non-Hodgkin); soft tissue sarcoma; osteogenic sarcoma; lung, cervical, ovarian, bone cancer	$t_{1/2}$, 15 h; urinary excretion at 24 h, 15%	As for cyclophosphamide	Ifosfamide is often used in conjunction with mesna to avoid cystinuria
NITROSOUREAS				
Carmustine	Glioma, glioblastoma multiforme, medulloblastoma and astrocytoma, multiple myeloma and lymphoma (Hodgkin and non-Hodgkin)	Bioavailability, 25%; protein bound, 80%; $t_{1/2}$, 30 min	Bone marrow and pulmonary toxicities are a function of lifetime cumulative dose	Clinically, nitrosoureas do not share cross-resistance with nitrogen mustards in lymphoma treatment
Streptozotocin	Cancers of the islets of Langerhans	$t_{1/2}$, 35 min; excreted in the urine (15%), feces (<1%), and in the expired air	Nausea and vomiting; nephrotoxicity can range from transient protein urea and azotemia to permanent tubular damage; can also cause aberrations of glucose metabolism	A natural product from *Streptomyces achromogenes*
TRIAZENES				
Dacarbazine	Malignant melanoma and Hodgkin lymphoma	$t_{1/2}$, 5 h; protein bound, 5% hepatic metabolism	Nausea, vomiting, myelosuppression	IV or IM
Temozolomide	Glioblastoma; astrocytoma; metastatic melanoma	Protein bound, 15%; $t_{1/2}$, 1.8 h; clearance, 5.5 l/h/m^2	Nausea, vomiting, myelosuppression	Oral; derivative of imidazotetrazine, prodrug of dacarbazine; rapidly absorbed

$t_{1/2}$, half-life; TEPA, triethylenethiophosphoramide; AUC, area under curve; CNS, central nervous system; IV, intravenous; IM, intramuscular.

TABLE 17.2

Dose and Schedules of Clinically Useful Alkylating Agents

Alkylating Agent	Disease Sites and Dose Ranges Used Clinically	Notes
BCNU (Carmustine)	General antineoplastic 150–200 mg/m^2 (IV, every 6 wks) Cutaneous T-cell lymphoma 200–600 mg (topical solution) Adjunct to surgical resection of brain tumor 61.6 mg (implant)	Infusion 1–2 h; in combination, dose usually reduced by 25%–50% Side effects include irritant dermatitis, telangiectasia, erythema, and bone marrow suppression Up to 8 wafers (7.7 mg of carmustine) implanted
Busulfan	Chronic myelogenous leukemia and myeloproliferative disorders 4–8 mg (daily PO) 1.8 mg/m^2 (daily PO) Bone marrow transplant 640 mg/m^2 (daily PO)	Dispensed over 3–4 d, with cyclophosphamide
Carboplatin	Advanced ovarian cancer—monotherapy 360 mg/m^2 (IV, every 4 wks) Ovarian cancer—combination 300 mg/m^2 (IV, every 4 wks for 6 cycles) Ovarian cancer—IP 200–500 mg/m^2 (IP, 2 L dialysis fluid) Ovarian and other sites phase 1/2 setting—high-dose therapy 800–1,600 mg/m^2 (IV)	With cyclophosphamide Patients usually receive marrow transplantation or peripheral stem cell support
Cisplatin	Metastatic testicular cancer: 20 mg/m^2/d for 5 d of each cycle (IV) Metastatic ovarian cancer: 75–100 mg/m^2 (IV, once every 4 wks) Head and neck cancer: 100 mg/m^2 (IV) Bladder cancer: (combination prior to cystectomy) 50–70; initiate dosing at 50 mg/m^2 (IV, once every 3–4 wks) Metastatic breast cancer: 20 mg/m^2 (IV, days 1–5 every 3 wks) Cervical cancer: 70 mg/m^2 (IV, dosing cycled every 4 wks) Non–small-cell lung cancer: 75 mg/m^2 (IV, every 3 wks) Esophageal cancer: 75 mg/m^2 on day 1 of wks 1, 5, 8, and 11 (IV)	With other antineoplastic agents With cyclophosphamide (600 mg/m^2 once every 4 wks) With vincristine, bleomycin, and fluorouracil With methotrexate and fluorouracil MVAC regimen (methotrexate, vinblastine, doxorubicin, and cisplatin) used for cervical cancer Administration preceded by paclitaxel 135 mg/m^2 every 3 wks With radiation therapy
Cyclophosphamide	General antineoplastic 1–5 mg/kg (daily PO) 40–50 mg/kg (IV, in divided doses over 2–5 d) 40–50 mg/kg (IV, in divided doses over 2–5 d) 10–15 mg/kg (IV, every 7–10 d) 10–15 mg/kg (IV, every 7–10 d) 3–5 mg/kg (IV twice per wk) High-dose regimen in bone marrow transplantation and for other autoimmune disorders 200 mg/kg (IV) 1–2.5 mg/kg (daily PO 7–14 d/mo)	Dose used as monotherapy for patients with no hematologic toxicity
Dacarbazine	General antineoplastic 2–4.5 mg/kg/d (IV) 150 mg/m^2/d (IV)	Administered for 10 d, may be repeated at 4-week intervals With other anticancer agents; treatment lasts 5 d, may be repeated every 4 wks
Etoposide	Testicular cancer 50–100 mg/m^2/day (IV, slow infusion over 30–60+ min for 5 d) Small cell lung cancer 35–50 mg/m^2/day (IV, slow infusion over 30–60+ min for 4–5 d)	Alternatively, 100 mg/m^2/d on days 1, 3, and 5 may be used; doses for combination therapy and are repeated at 3- to 4-wk intervals after recovery from hematologic toxicity Doses are for combination therapy and repeated at 3- to 4-wk intervals after recovery from hematologic toxicity; oral dose is twice the IV, rounded to the nearest 50 mg

(continued)

TABLE 17.2

Dose and Schedules of Clinically Useful Alkylating Agents *(continued)*

Ifosfamide	General antineoplastic 1.2 g/m²/d (IV, for 5 consecutive days)	Repeat every 3 wks
Melphalan	Multiple myeloma: 16 mg/m² (IV, infusion over 15–20 min) 6 mg (daily PO) Epithelial ovarian cancer: 0.2 mg/kg (daily PO)	2-week intervals for 4 doses, 4-wk intervals thereafter After 2–3 wks treatment, should be discontinued for up to 4 wks, then reinstituted at 2–4 mg/d Daily dose for a 5-d course, repeated every 4–5 wks
Streptozotocin	Pancreatic tumors 500 mg/m²/d; 1,000 mg/m²/d (IV; IV)	500 mg for 5 consecutive days every 6 wks, 1,000 mg is for 2 wks, followed by an increase in weekly dose not to exceed 1,500 mg/m²/wk
Temozolomide	Brain tumors 150 mg/m² (daily PO)	Dose adjusted on the basis of blood counts
Thiotepa	General antineoplastic: 0.3–0.4 mg/kg (IV) Papillary carcinoma of the bladder: 60 mg/wk for 4 wks (bladder catheter) Control of serous effusions: 0.6–0.8 mg/kg (intracavitary)	Rapid administration given at 1- to 4-wk intervals 30 or 60 mL should be retained for 2 h, so the patient is usually dehydrated prior to administration of the drug

IV, intravenously; PO, by mouth; IP, intraperitoneal.

One distinguishing feature of melphalan is that an amino acid transporter responsible for uptake influences its efficacy across cell membranes.[10] Although a number of glutathione (GSH) conjugates of alkylating agents are effluxed through adenosine triphosphate–dependent membrane transporters,[11] specific uptake mechanisms are generally rare for cancer drugs. Cyclophosphamide and ifosfamide are prodrugs that require cytochrome P-450 metabolism to release active alkylating species. Cyclophosphamide continues to be the most widely used alkylating agent and has activity against a variety of tumors.[12] A cost saving with equivalent therapeutic activity was recently shown in a modified regimen of high-dose cyclophosphamide plus cyclosporine in patients with severe or very severe aplastic anemia.[13]

Nitrosoureas

The nitrosoureas form a diverse class of alkylating agents that have a distinct metabolism and pharmacology that separates them from others.[14] Under physiologic conditions, proton abstraction by a hydroxyl ion initiates spontaneous decomposition of the molecule to yield a diazonium hydroxide and an isocyanate (see Fig. 17.1). The chloroethyl carbonium ion generated is the active alkylating species. Through a subsequent dehalogenation step, a second electrophilic site imparts bifunctionality.[15] Thus, while cross-linking may occur similar to those lesions caused by nitrogen mustards, the chemistry leading to the endpoint is distinct. The isocyanate species generated are also electrophilic, showing nucleophilic selectivity toward sulfhydryl and amino groups that can inhibit a number of enzymes involved in nucleic acid synthesis and thiol balance.[16] Because carbamoylation is considered of minor importance to the therapeutic efficacy of clinically used nitrosoureas, chlorozotocin and streptozotocin were designed to undergo internal carbamoylation at the 1- or 3-OH group of the glucose ring, with the consequence that no carbamoylating species are produced.[17,18] Streptozotocin is also unusual in that most methylnitrosoureas have only modest therapeutic value. However, its lack of bone marrow toxicity and strong diabetogenic effect in animals led to its use in cancer of the pancreas (see Table 17.1).[19] The dose-limiting toxicities in humans are gastrointestinal and renal, but the drug has considerably less hematopoietic toxicity than the other nitrosoureas. Because of their lipophilicity and capacity to cross the blood–brain barrier, the chloroethylnitrosoureas were found to be effective against intracranially inoculated murine tumors. Indeed, early preclinical studies showed that many mouse tumors were quite responsive to nitrosoureas. The same extent of efficacy was not found in humans. Subsequent analyses demonstrated that an enzyme responsible for repair of O-6-alkyl guanine (O^6-methylguanine-DNA methyltransferase [MGMT], or the Mer/Mex phenotype)[20] was expressed at low levels in mice, but at high levels in humans, a contributory factor in the reduced clinical efficacy of nitrosoureas in humans. In the 1980s, in particular, a number of new nitrosoureas were tested in patients in Europe and Japan, but none established a regular role in standard cancer treatment regimens.

MGMT promoter methylation is crucial in MGMT gene silencing and can predict a favorable outcome in glioblastoma patients receiving alkylating agents.[21] This biomarker is on the verge of entering clinical decision making and is currently used to stratify or even select glioblastoma patients for clinical trials. In other subtypes of glioma, such as anaplastic gliomas, the relevance of MGMT promoter methylation might extend beyond the prediction of chemosensitivity, and could reflect a distinct molecular profile. At this time, the standardization of MGMT assays will be critical in establishing prospective prognostic or predictive effects. In addition, eventual clinical trials will need to determine, for each subtype of glioma, the extent to which methylation patterns are predictive or prognostic and whether such assays could be incorporated into an individualized approach to clinical practice.[21]

CLINICAL PHARMACOKINETICS/ PHARMACODYNAMICS

The pharmacokinetics of the alkylating agents are highly variable depending on the individual agent. Nevertheless, they are generally characterized by high reactivity and short half-lives. Although detailed studies on clinical pharmacology are available,[22] Table 17.1 summarizes some of the primary kinetic characteristics of the major clinically useful drugs. Mechlorethamine is unstable and is administered rapidly in a running intravenous infusion to avoid its rapid breakdown to inactive metabolites. In contrast, chlorambucil and cyclophosphamide are sufficiently stable to be given orally, and are rapidly and completely absorbed from the gastrointestinal tract, whereas others like melphalan have poor and variable

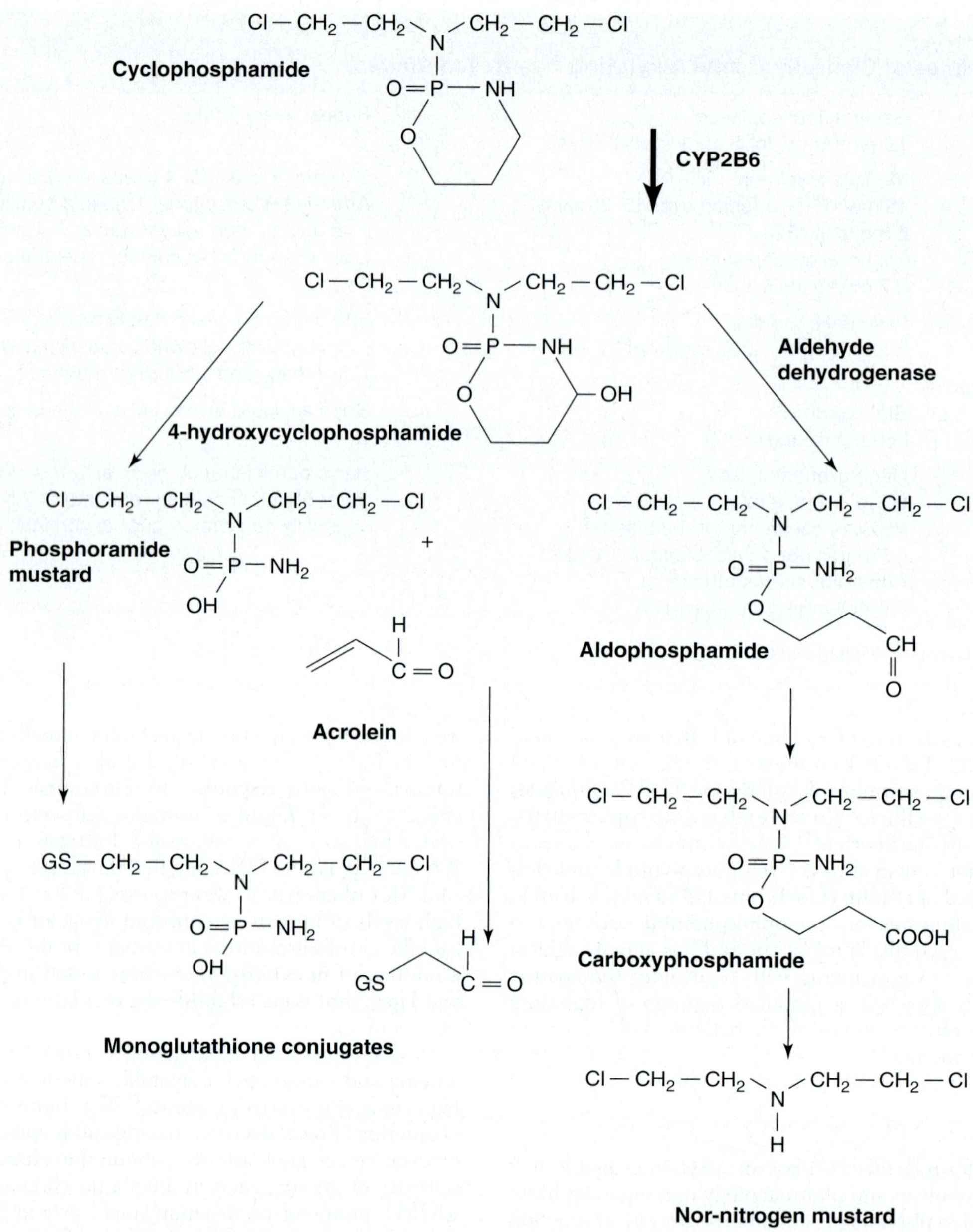

Figure 17.2 Activation and detoxification routes of metabolism for cyclophosphamide.

oral absorption. Cyclophosphamide,[23] ifosfamide, and dacarbazine are unusual in that they require activation by cytochrome P-450 in the liver before they can alkylate cellular constituents. The nitrosoureas also require activation, albeit nonenzymatic. The major route of metabolism of most alkylating agents is spontaneous hydrolysis, although many can also undergo some degree of enzymatic metabolism. This is particularly pertinent for phase II metabolic conversions where reactivity with nucleophilic thiols precedes conversion to mercapturates, with the result that most of the alkylating agents are excreted in the urine. One example of complex multistep metabolism is provided by cyclophosphamide (see Fig. 17.2). Activation by CYP2B6 is followed by the conversion of aldehyde dehydrogenase to reactive alkylating species or possible detoxification through GSH conjugation reactions. The latter is particularly important for acrolein because it is believed to contribute to the bladder toxicities associated with the drug.

The alkylating agents form covalent bonds with a number of nucleophilic groups present in proteins, RNA, and DNA (e.g., amino, carboxyl, sulfhydryl, imidazole, phosphate). Under physiologic conditions, the chloroethyl group of the nitrogen mustards undergoes cyclization, with the chloride acting as a leaving group forming an intermediate carbonium ion that attacks nucleophilic sites (see Fig. 17.1). Bifunctional alkylating agents (with two chloroethyl side chains) can undergo a subsequent cyclization to form a covalent bond with an adjacent nucleophilic group, resulting in DNA–DNA or DNA–protein cross-links. The N7 or O6 positions of guanine are particularly susceptible and may represent primary targets that determine both the cytotoxic and mutagenic consequences of therapy.[24] The nitrosoureas have a similar, but distinct, mechanism of action, spontaneously forming both alkylating and carbamoylating agents in aqueous media (see Fig. 17.1). The carbamoylating moieties are generally believed to be inconsequential to the therapeutic properties of the nitrosoureas.

THERAPEUTIC USES

The alkylating agents are frequently used in combination therapy to treat a variety of types of cancer. Perhaps the most versatile is cyclophosphamide, whereas the other alkylating agents are of more restricted clinical use. Because of early successes, many disease states are managed with drug combinations that contain several alkylating agents. Cyclophosphamide is employed to treat a variety of immune-related diseases and to purge bone marrow in autologous marrow transplant situations.[25] A general summary of the clinical uses of the primary alkylating agents is shown in Table 17.1.

TOXICITIES

The alkylating agents show significant qualitative and quantitative variability in the sites and severities of their toxicities. The primary dose-limiting toxicity is suppression of bone marrow function, with secondary limiting effects on the proliferating cells of the intestinal mucosa.

Contraindications to the use of alkylating agents would identify patients with severely depressed bone marrow function and patients with hypersensitivity to these drugs. Other listed precautions to these drugs include carcinogenic and mutagenic effects and impairment of fertility. Precaution is also advised in patients with (1) leukopenia or thrombocytopenia, (2) previous exposure to chemotherapy or radiotherapy, (3) tumor cell infiltration of the bone marrow, and (4) impaired renal or hepatic function. These drugs can also increase toxicity in adrenalectomized patients and interfere with wound healing. A brief summary of dose-limiting toxicities is shown in Table 17.1, and a narrative of each follows here.

Nausea and Vomiting

Nausea and vomiting are frequent side effects of alkylating agent therapy and are not well controlled by conventional antiemetics.[24] They are a major source of patient discomfort and a significant cause of lack of drug compliance and even discontinuation of therapy. Frequency and extent are highly variable among patients. The overall frequency of nausea and vomiting is directly proportional to the dose of alkylating agent. The onset of nausea may occur within a few minutes of the administration of the drug or may be delayed for several hours.

Bone Marrow Toxicity

Bone marrow toxicity can involve all of the blood elements, leukocytes, platelets, and red cells.[26] The extent and time course of suppression show marked interindividual fluctuation. Relative platelet sparing is a characteristic of cyclophosphamide treatment. Even at the very high doses (<200 mg/kg) of cyclophosphamide (used in preparation for bone marrow transplantation), some recovery of hematopoietic elements occurs within 21 to 28 days. This stem cell–sparing property is further reflected by the fact that cumulative damage to the bone marrow is rarely seen when cyclophosphamide is given as a single agent, and repeated high doses can be given without progressive lowering of leukocyte and platelet counts. The biochemical basis for the stem cell–sparing effect of cyclophosphamide is related to the presence of high levels of aldehyde dehydrogenase in early bone marrow progenitor cells (see Fig. 17.2). Busulfan is particularly toxic to bone marrow stem cells,[26] and treatment can lead to prolonged hypoplasia. The hematopoietic depression produced by the nitrosoureas is characteristically delayed. The onset of leukocyte and platelet depression occurs 3 to 4 weeks after drug administration and may last an additional 2 to 3 weeks.[22,26] Thrombocytopenia appears earlier and usually is more severe than leukopenia. Even if the nitrosourea is given at 6-week intervals, hematopoietic recovery may not occur between courses, and the drug dose often must be decreased when repeated courses are used.

Renal and Bladder Toxicity

Hemorrhagic cystitis is unique to the oxazaphosphorines (cyclophosphamide and ifosfamide) and may range from a mild cystitis to severe bladder damage with massive hemorrhage.[27] This toxicity is caused by the excretion of toxic metabolites (particularly acrolein) (see Fig. 17.2) in the urine, with subsequent direct irritation of the bladder mucosa. The incidence and severity can be lessened by adequate hydration and continuous irrigation of the bladder with a solution containing 2-mercaptoethane sulfonate (MESNA) and frequent bladder emptying.[26] MESNA is given in divided doses every 4 hours in dosages of 60% of those of the alkylating agent.

At high cumulative doses, all commonly used nitrosoureas can produce a dose-related renal toxicity that can result in renal failure and death.[29] In patients developing clinical evidence of toxicity, increases in serum creatinine usually appear after the completion of therapy and may be first detected up to 2 years after treatment.

Interstitial Pneumonitis and Pulmonary Fibrosis

Long-term busulfan therapy can lead to the gradual onset of fever, a nonproductive cough, and dyspnea, followed by tachypnea and cyanosis, and progressing to severe pulmonary insufficiency and death.[30] If busulfan is stopped before the onset of clinical symptoms, pulmonary function may stabilize, but if clinical symptoms are manifest, the condition may be rapidly fatal. Cyclophosphamide, bischloroethylnitrosourea, and methyl-1-(2-chloroethyl)-3-cyclohexyl-1-nitrosourea in cumulative doses exceeding 1,000 mg/m^2 may also lead to similar side effects.[31] Other alkylating agents, including melphalan, chlorambucil, and mitomycin C, can lead to pulmonary fibrosis after therapy.[32] This effect is probably caused by a direct cytotoxicity of the alkylating agent to pulmonary epithelium, resulting in alveolitis and fibrosis.

Gonadal Toxicity, Teratogenesis, and Carcinogenesis

Alkylating agents can have profound toxic effects on reproductive tissue.[33] A depletion of testicular germ (but not Sertoli) cells is accompanied by aspermia. In patients with a total absence of germ cells, an increase in plasma levels of follicle-stimulating hormone occurs. However, patients in remission and off alkylating agents for 2 to 7 years show complete spermatogenesis, indicating that testicular damage is reversible.

In women, a high incidence of amenorrhea and ovarian atrophy is associated with cyclophosphamide or melphalan therapy.[34] This seems to be age related because it developed after lower doses in older compared with younger patients, and was less likely to be reversible in the older cohort. A pathologic analysis reveals the absence of mature or primordial follicles, and endocrinology studies demonstrate decreased estrogen and progesterone levels and elevated serum follicle-stimulating hormone and luteinizing hormone levels typical of menopause.

The DNA-damaging properties of alkylating agents ensure that they are all teratogenic and carcinogenic to some degree. The administration of alkylating agents during the first trimester of pregnancy presents a definitive risk of a malformed fetus, but the administration of such drugs during the second and third trimesters does not increase the risk of fetal malformation above normal.[35]

Development of second cancer as a consequence of alkylating agent therapy has been documented. For example, a fulminant acute myeloid leukemia characterized by a preceding phase of myelodysplasia is found in some patients treated with melphalan, cyclophosphamide (which is much less leukemogenic than melphalan), chlorambucil, and the nitrosoureas.[33] This circumstance probably reflects the fact that these have been the most widely used of the alkylating agents. Also, the preponderance of patients with multiple myeloma, Hodgkin lymphoma, and carcinoma of the ovary in the reports of leukemogenesis is probably because patients with these diseases may have good responses and are often treated with alkylating agents for a number of years. The rate of occurrence of acute leukemia in patients with ovarian cancer who survive for 10 years after treatment with alkylating agents might be as high as 10%. Acute leukemia has been the most frequently described second malignancy, and it usually develops 1 to 4 years after drug exposure.[36] Other malignancies, including solid tumors, also have been reported to develop in patients treated with alkylating agents.[37]

The last four decades have yielded a significant improvement in the survival of children diagnosed with cancer (5-year survival is approximately 80%). As many as two-thirds of the survivors of childhood malignancies can experience delayed drug toxicities that may be severe or even life threatening. Such complications include impairment in growth and development, neurocognitive dysfunction, cardiopulmonary compromise, endocrine dysfunction, renal impairment, gastrointestinal dysfunction, musculoskeletal sequelae, and second cancers.[38]

Alopecia

The degree of alopecia after cyclophosphamide administration may be quite severe, especially when this drug is used in combination with vincristine sulfate or doxorubicin hydrochloride.[39] Regrowth of hair inevitably occurs after the cessation of therapy, but may be associated with a change in the color and greater curl. Use of a tourniquet or ice pack applied to the scalp during and for a short period after cyclophosphamide administration reduces the impact.

Allergic Reactions

Alkylating agents covalently bind to proteins, and these conjugates can act as haptens and produce allergic reactions.[40] An increasing number of reports of skin eruption, angioneurotic edema, urticaria, and anaphylactic reactions after the systemic administration of alkylating agents have appeared.

Immunosuppression

Alkylating agents suppress both humoral and cellular immunity in a variety of experimental systems.[41] The most immunosuppressive is cyclophosphamide, reported to cause (1) selective suppression of B-lymphocyte function, (2) depletion of B-lymphocytes, and (3) suppression of lymphocyte functions that are mediated by T cells, such as the graft-versus-host response and delayed hypersensitivity. Most intermittent antitumor regimens do not uniformly produce profound immunosuppression, and recovery is usually prompt. Sustained drug treatments can lead to severe lymphocyte depletion and profound immunosuppression and may be accompanied by an increase of viral, fungal, and protozoal infections.[41]

COMPLICATIONS WITH HIGH-DOSE ALKYLATING AGENT THERAPY

At standard doses, alkylating agents produce myelosuppression as their dose-limiting toxicity. Less severe effects on the gastrointestinal epithelium, lungs, bladder, and kidneys may become problems with long-term treatment, but rarely limit initial therapy. For this reason, and because of their steep dose response to tumor-killing curves, the alkylating agents have become a logical tool, either alone or in combination, for high-dose chemotherapy regimens in which bone marrow toxicity is expected, and is accommodated by bone marrow transplantation, stem cell reconstitution from peripheral blood monocytes, and growth factor rescue. In this high-dose setting, toxicities that affect the gut, lungs, liver, and CNS become dose limiting and life threatening.[42] The highly lipid-soluble alkylators, especially ifosfamide, busulfan, the nitrosoureas, and thiotepa, cause CNS dysfunction, including seizures, altered mental status, cerebellar dysfunction, cranial nerve palsies, and coma.[43] High-dose ifosfamide is most frequently the cause of neurotoxicity.[44] Clinical manifestations of grade 4 neurotoxicities were reported in approximately one-fourth of those patients receiving ifosfamide. The side-chain N-linked chloroethyl moiety of ifosfamide (see Table 17.1) is more likely than the bischloroethyl group of cyclophosphamide to undergo oxidation and subsequent N-deethylation and lead to the formation of chloroacetaldehyde. High-dose busulfan is also frequently used in a variety of conditioning regimens for hematopoietic cell transplantation. In this setting, busulfan causes neurotoxicity manifesting in seizures that generally are tonic–clonic in character. Phenytoin has been the preferred drug to treat busulfan-induced seizures, although some emerging clinical data support the use of benzodiazepines, most notably clonazepam and lorazepam, to prevent busulfan-induced seizures. Moreover, the second-generation antiepileptic drug levetiracetam possesses the characteristics of optimal prophylaxis for busulfan-induced seizures.[45] At least one recent study has suggested that a polymorphism in the glutathione S-transferase A2 family may be predictive of transplant-related mortality after allogeneic stem cell transplantation,[46] perhaps indicating that a pharmacogenetic approach might be possible in this disease setting. Moreover, in a preclinical setting, a proteomic analysis identified thioredoxin as a potentially important adjuvant therapy in enhancing donor cell graft enhancement in bone marrow transplantation.[47] The possibility that this approach may benefit patients following alkylating agent–based ablation remains to be tested in a clinical setting.

Cyclophosphamide at doses exceeding 100 mg/kg during a 48-hour period (preparatory to bone marrow transplantation) can cause cardiac toxicity.[48] No evidence exists for cumulative damage to the heart after repeated moderate or low doses of the drug. Cardiac toxicity occurs with greatest frequency in patients older than 50 years or in those previously treated with anthracyclines.[48]

ALKYLATING AGENT–STEROID CONJUGATES

Adapting the rationale that steroid receptors may function to localize and concentrate attached drug species intracellularly in hormone-responsive cancers, a number of synthetic conjugates of nitrogen mustards and steroids have been developed. Of these, two made the transition into clinical use.

Prednimustine is an ester-linked conjugate of chlorambucil and prednisolone designed to function as a prodrug for chlorambucil. Release of the alkylating agent occurs after cleavage by serum esterases,[49] which can release the ester link of prednimustine, producing the hormone and active alkylating drug. The elimination phase of chlorambucil in patient plasma is significantly longer after the administration of prednimustine than after chlorambucil. Estramustine is a carbamate ester–linked conjugate of nor-nitrogen mustard and estradiol. Unlike prednimustine, the pharmacology of estramustine is governed by the presence of the carbamate group in the steroid–mustard linkage. The relative resistance of the carbamate bond to enzymatic cleavage eliminates the alkylating activity of the molecule and conveys an entirely new pharmacology.[50] The crystal structural and mechanism of action studies showed that estramustine has antimitotic activity, an activity shared by some other steroids.[51] Estramustine has found a clinical niche used in combination with other antimitotic drugs in the management of hormone refractory prostate cancer.[52]

DRUG RESISTANCE AND MODULATION

As with all drugs, intrinsic or acquired resistance to alkylating agents occurs and limits the therapeutic utility of this class of anticancer drugs.[53] A plethora of preclinical studies have characterized mechanisms by which cells develop resistance and, to a lesser degree, these have been shown to occur clinically. Because alkylating agents have a narrow therapeutic index, the emergence of resistance can have a significant impact on clinical success. Some of the factors that can contribute to the expression of resistance to alkylating agents include (1) alterations in drug uptake or transport, (2) increased repair of drug-induced nucleic acid damage, (3) failure to activate alkylating agent prodrugs, (4) increased scavenging of drug species by nonessential cellular nucleophiles, (5) increased enzymatic detoxification of drug species, and (6) altered expression of genes coding for cellular commitment to apoptosis.

RECENT DEVELOPMENTS

In the era of directed targeted therapies, the lack of specificity of alkylating agents would seem to limit the likelihood that novel drugs will be forthcoming. High toxicities, narrow therapeutic indices, and chemical instabilities are all properties that consign this drug class to the lower echelons of popularity in drug-discovery platforms. Although covalent bonding to specific target sites is one approach to direct targeting, the random electrophilic attraction toward nucleic acids and proteins is not an optimal property by today's standards. Nevertheless, the relative success of the alkylating agents in gaining therapeutic responses to diseases that are difficult to treat continues to serve as an impetus to use alkylating moieties as a means to kill cells. Some novel agents are presently in development. Cyclophosphamide and ifosfamide were prodrugs synthesized in the hope that high levels of phosphoamidase in epithelial tumors would selectively activate the drugs.[27] Other efforts to improve selectivity have centered on the synthesis of antibody–enzyme conjugates that bind to tumor-specific surface antigens. Enzymes frequently associated with the cell surface include peptidases, nitroreductases, and γ-glutamyl transpeptidase; to some degree, each has been targeted to cleave circulating alkylating prodrugs, thereby in a localized fashion releasing active alkylating species. Antibody-directed enzyme prodrug therapy is exemplified by the use of an antibody linked to the peptidase carboxypeptidase G-2, which releases an active alkylator from an inactive γ-glutamyl conjugate.[54] Linkage of the peptidase to any antibody that localizes selectively to a tumor cell membrane is a viable option. Expression of the peptidase on the cell surface then leads to prodrug activation and cell kill. Such approaches have had limited clinical impact to this time; however, their development does continue.

A further rationale for enhancing tumor-specific delivery takes advantage of the observation that glutathione-S-transferase *pi* (GSTP1-1) is preferentially expressed in a number of solid tumors and some lymphomas. In this case, the prodrug consists of an unusual alkylating agent conjugated to a substituted glutathione peptidomimetic. GSTP initiates the cleavage, thereby creating a cytotoxic alkylating species.[55] The initial canfosfamide design strategy relied on the principle that proton-abstracting sites at the active site of GST could initiate a cleavage reaction that would convert an inactive prodrug into a cytotoxic species. The presence of a histidine residue in proximity to the G binding site was integral to the removal of the sulfhydryl proton from the GSH cosubstrate, resulting in the generation of a nucleophilic sulfide anion. This moiety would be more reactive with electrophiles in the absence of GSH. Unlike other standard nitrogen mustard drugs, canfosfamide contains a tetrakis (chloroethyl) phosphorodiamidate moiety. Other compounds bearing this structure have been shown to be more cytotoxic than a similar structure with a single bis-(chloroethyl) amine group.[56]

As in other nitrogen mustards, the chlorines can act as leaving groups, thus creating aziridinium ions with electrophilic characteristics. Although the exact temporal or sequential formation of the four possible chlorine leaving events is not known, the assumption is that these species possess cytotoxic properties through their capacity to alkylate target nucleophiles, such as DNA bases. Tetrafunctionality could result in the formation of cross-links with bonding distances greater than for bifunctional agents. However, a number of caveats apply to this interpretation. For example, alkylating agents, whether mono-, bi-, or putatively tetrafunctional, generally lead to some form of myelosuppression. A number of clinical trials with canfosfamide have now been completed. These include, phase 1,[57] phase 1/2a,[58] phase 2,[59] and phase 3.[60] The phase 3 study was in platinum refractory ovarian cancer patients and proved negative for enhanced survival. Nevertheless, additional trials are still in progress.

Another targeting approach delivers the gene for a cytochrome P-450 isoenzyme to tumors by viral vector, thereby enhancing specific tumor cell activation of cyclophosphamide.[61] Because this therapy has its base in gene delivery technologies, successful development in humans will await further advances in this arena.

Laromustine is in the sulfonylhydrazine class of alkylating agents. It is presently in clinical development for the treatment of malignancies such as acute myelogenous leukemia (AML).[62] Similar to nitrosoureas, laromustine is a prodrug that yields a chloroethylating and a carbamoylating (methyl isocyanate) species. As with nitrosoureas, the cytotoxicity of laromustine is attributed primarily to the chloroethylating-mediated alkylation of DNA and subsequent interstrand cross-links.[63] The carbamoylating species can inhibit DNA repair and other cellular enzyme systems. Phase 1 trials in patients with solid tumors indicated the expected myelosuppression, although few extramedullary toxicities were observed, indicating potential efficacy in the treatment of hematologic malignancies. Phase 2 trials have been completed in patients with untreated AML, high-risk myelodysplastic syndrome, and relapsed AML. The most encouraging results have been found in patients older than 60 years with poor-risk, de novo AML for which no standard treatment exists. Laromustine is currently in phase 2/3 trials for AML and phase 2 trials for myelodysplastic syndrome and solid tumors.[64] Laromustine appears to be a promising agent in elderly patients who do not respond to or are not fit for intensive chemotherapy.

Although not a new drug, bendamustine is a unique cytotoxic agent with structural similarities to alkylating agents and antimetabolites, but it lacks cross-resistance with other established alkylating agents both in vitro and in the clinic.[65] Its mechanism of action is similar to other mustards in causing DNA intra- and interstrand cross-links. In comparison with other more commonly used alkylating agents, such as cyclophosphamide or phenylalanine mustard, more DNA double-strand breaks are formed at equitoxic dosages. Treatment with bendamustine induces a concentration-dependent apoptosis as evidenced by changes in Bcl-2 and Bax expression profiles in chronic B-cell lymphocytic leukemia.[66] DNA damage produced by bendamustine is repaired via base-excision repair mechanisms, implicating an unusual mode of action, which was recently confirmed through gene expression profiling analyses. This also provided an explanation for the lack of cross-resistance with other alkylating agents, as observed in vitro with anthracycline resistant breast cancer and cisplatin-resistant ovarian cancer.[66,67]

Clinical studies conducted in Germany more than 30 years ago suggested activity in indolent non-Hodgkin lymphoma. Subsequent American trials showed responses in more than 70% of patients with drug refractory disease, with the implication that bendamustine may be the most effective drug in this patient population. Combinations of bendamustine and rituximab elicited response rates of 90% to 92%, with complete remission in 55% to 60% in follicular and mantle cell lymphoma. Superiority over chlorambucil in previously untreated patients with chronic lymphocytic leukemia (CLL) led to its recent approval for this disease in the United States. Bendamustine is approved in Germany for the treatment of patients with indolent non-Hodgkin lymphoma, CLL, and multiple myeloma. Activity has also been noted in patients with breast cancer and non–small-cell lung cancer.

Bendamustine has been used both as a single agent and in combination with other agents, including etoposide, fludarabine, mitoxantrone, methotrexate, prednisone, rituximab, and vincristine. A multicenter phase 2 trial in lymphomas had an overall response rate of 89%; (35% complete response and 54% partial response). In previously treated patients. the overall response rate was 76% (38% complete response and 38% partial response). The estimated median progression-free survival was 19 months.[67] In CLL patients, the drug is administered at 100 mg/m^2 intravenously over 30 minutes on days 1 and 2 of a 28-day cycle, for up to six cycles. Efficacy relative to first-line therapies other than chlorambucil has not been established. It is also indicated for the treatment of patients with indolent B-cell non-Hodgkin lymphoma that has progressed during, or within, 6 months of treatment with rituximab or rituximab-containing regimens. As with most alkylating agents, the primary dose-limiting toxicity is myelosuppression; nonhematologic toxicities were mild and included fatigue, nausea, loss of appetite, and vomiting. The optimization of dose and schedule, particularly relative to other drugs, and the management of toxicities has allowed its use in combination with a range of other chemotherapeutic agents, including prednisone, methotrexate, fludarabine, etoposide, mitoxantrone, vinca alkaloids, and rituximab. The availability of bendamustine provides another effective treatment option for patients with lymphoid malignancies, frequently reducing the side effects of the more standard cyclophosphamide, hydroxy doxorubicin, Oncovin, and prednisone (CHOP) regimen.[68] Recent approval by the U.S. Food and Drug Administration has allowed Cephalon, Inc. to market bendamustine under the trade name Treanda and, in combination with mitoxantrone and rituximab, it is now standard of care in indolent lymphomas. Trial results released in 2013 indicated that this combination more than doubled the progression-free survival in this disease[69] and there is early evidence that there may be utility in relapsed or refractory multiple myeloma.[70]

REFERENCES

1. Adair FE, Bagg HJ. Experimental and clinical studies on the treatment of cancer by dichlorethylsulphide (mustard gas). *Ann Surg* 1931;93(1):190–199.
2. Rhoads C. Nitrogen mustards in treatment of neoplastic disease. *JAMA* 1946;131:656–658.
3. Coles B. Effects of modifying structure on electrophilic reactions with biological nucleophiles. *Drug Metab Rev* 1985;15:1307–1334.
4. Pearson R, Songstad J. Application of the principle of hard and soft acids and bases to organic chemistry. *J Am Chem Soc* 1967;89:1827.
5. Ross W. Alkylating agents. In: *Biological Alkylating Agents*. London: Butterworth; 1962.
6. Elson LA. Hematological effects of the alkylating agents. *Ann N Y Acad Sci* 1958;68(3):826–833.
7. Kushner BH, Kramer K, Modak S, et al. Topotecan, thiotepa, and carboplatin for neuroblastoma: failure to prevent relapse in the central nervous system. *Bone Marrow Transplant* 2006;37(3):271–276.
8. Agarwala SS, Kirkwood JM. Temozolomide, a novel alkylating agent with activity in the central nervous system, may improve the treatment of advanced metastatic melanoma. *Oncologist* 2000;5(2):144–151.
9. Tentori L, Graziani G. Recent approaches to improve the antitumor efficacy of temozolomide. *Curr Med Chem* 2009;16(2):245–257.
10. Vistica DT. Cytotoxicity as an indicator for transport mechanism: evidence that murine bone marrow progenitor cells lack a high-affinity leucine carrier that transports melphalan in murine L1210 leukemia cells. *Blood* 1980;56(3):427–429.
11. Dean M, Rzhetsky A, Allikmets R. The human ATP-binding cassette (ABC) transporter superfamily. *Genome Res* 2001;11(7):1156–1166.
12. Sensenbrenner LL, Marini JJ, Colvin M. Comparative effects of cyclophosphamide, isophosphamide, 4-methylcyclophosphamide, and phosphoramide mustard on murine hematopoietic and immunocompetent cells. *J Natl Cancer Inst* 1979;62(4):975–981.
13. Zhang F, Zhang L, Jing L, et al. (2013) High-dose cyclophosphamide compared with antithymocyte globulin for treatment of acquired severe aplastic anemia. *Exp Hematol* 2013;41:328–334.
14. Montgomery JA, James R, McCaleb GS, et al. The modes of decomposition of 1,3-bis(2-chloroethyl)-1-nitrosourea and related compounds. *J Med Chem* 1967;10(4):668–674.
15. Brundrett RB, Cowens JW, Colvin M. Chemistry of nitrosoureas: decomposition of Deuterated 1,3-bis(2-chloroethyl)-1-nitrosourea. *J Med Chem* 1976;19(7):958–961.
16. Tew KD, Kyle G, Johnson A, et al. Carbamoylation of glutathione reductase and changes in cellular and chromosome morphology in a rat cell line resistant to nitrogen mustards but collaterally sensitive to nitrosoureas. *Cancer Res* 1985;45(5):2326–2333.
17. Anderson T, Schein PS, McMenamin MG, et al. Streptozotocin diabetes: correlation with extent of depression of pancreatic islet nicotinamide adenine dinucleotide. *J Clin Invest* 1974;54(3):672–677.
18. Anderson T, McMenamin MG, Schein PS. Chlorozotocin, 2-(3-(2-chloroethyl)-3-nitrosoureido)-D-glucopyranose, an antitumor agent with modified bone marrow toxicity. *Cancer Res* 1975;35(3):761–765.
19. Schein PS, O'Connell MJ, Blom J, et al. Clinical antitumor activity and toxicity of streptozotocin (NSC-85998). *Cancer* 1974;34(4):993–1000.
20. Pieper RO. Understanding and manipulating O6-methylguanine-DNA methyltransferase expression. *Pharmacol Ther* 1997;74(3):285–297.
21. Weller M, Stupp R, Reifenberger G, et al. MGMT promoter methylation in malignant gliomas: ready for personalized medicine? *Nat Rev Neurol* 2010;6(1):39–51.
22. Tew K, Colvin OM, Jones RB. Clinical and high dose alkylating agents. In: Chabner BA, Longo DL, eds. *Cancer: Chemotherapy and Biotherapy: Principles and Practice*. Philadelphia: Lippincott-Raven; 2005: 283.
23. Brookes P, Lawley PD. The reaction of mono- and di-functional alkylating agents with nucleic acids. *Biochem J* 1961;80(3):496–503.
24. Penta JS, Poster DS, Bruno S, et al. Clinical trials with antiemetic agents in cancer patients receiving chemotherapy. *J Clin Pharmacol* 1981;21(8–9 Suppl):11S–22S.
25. Colvin M, Hilton J. Pharmacology of cyclophosphamide and metabolites. *Cancer Treat Rep* 1981;65(Suppl 3):89–95.
26. Elson L. Hematological effects of the alkylating agents. *Ann N Y Acad Sci* 1958;68:826–833.
27. Cox PJ. Cyclophosphamide cystitis—identification of acrolein as the causative agent. *Biochem Pharmacol* 1979;28(13):2045–2049.
28. Andriole GL, Sandlund JT, Miser JS, et al. The efficacy of mesna (2-mercaptoethane sodium sulfonate) as a uroprotectant in patients with hemorrhagic cystitis receiving further oxazaphosphorine chemotherapy. *J Clin Oncol* 1987;5(5):799–803.
29. Schacht RG, Feiner HD, Gallo GR, et al. Nephrotoxicity of nitrosoureas. *Cancer* 1981;48(6):1328–1334.
30. Littler WA, Ogilvie C. Lung function in patients receiving busulphan. *Br Med J* 1970;4(5734):530–532.
31. Mark GJ, Lehimgar-Zadeh A, Ragsdale BD. Cyclophosphamide pneumonitis. *Thorax* 1978;33(1):89–93.
32. Kreisman H, Wolkove N. Pulmonary toxicity of antineoplastic therapy. *Semin Oncol* 1992;19(5):508–520.
33. Kumar R, Biggart JD, McEvoy J, et al. Cyclophosphamide and reproductive function. *Lancet* 1972;1(7762):1212–1214.
34. Miller JJ 3rd, Williams GF, Leissring JC. Multiple late complications of therapy with cyclophosphamide, including ovarian destruction. *Am J Med* 1971;50(4):530–535.
35. Nicholson HO. Cytotoxic drugs in pregnancy: review of reported cases. *J Obstet Gynaecol Br Commonw* 1968;75(3):307–312.
36. Reimer RR, Hoover R, Fraumeni JF Jr, et al. Acute leukemia after alkylating-agent therapy of ovarian cancer. *N Engl J Med* 1977;297(4):177–181.
37. Penn I. Second malignant neoplasms associated with immunosuppressive medications. *Cancer* 1976;37(2 Suppl):1024–1032.
38. Bhatia S, Constine LS. Late morbidity after successful treatment of children with cancer. *Cancer J* 2009;15(3):174–180.
39. Calvert W. Alopecia and cytotoxic drugs. *Br Med J* 1966;2(5517):831.
40. Weiss RB, Bruno S. Hypersensitivity reactions to cancer chemotherapeutic agents. *Ann Intern Med* 1981;94(1):66–72.
41. Santos GW, Sensenbrenner LL, Burke PJ, et al. Marrow transplantation in man following cyclophosphamide. *Transplant Proc* 1971;3(1):400–404.
42. de Jonge ME, Huitema AD, Beijnen JH, et al. High exposures to bioactivated cyclophosphamide are related to the occurrence of veno-occlusive disease of the liver following high-dose chemotherapy. *Br J Cancer* 2006;94(9): 1226–1230.
43. Baruchel S, Diezi M, Hargrave D, et al. Safety and pharmacokinetics of temozolomide using a dose-escalation, metronomic schedule in recurrent paediatric brain tumours. *Eur J Cancer* 2006;42(14):2335–2342.
44. Pratt CB, Goren MP, Meyer WH, et al. Ifosfamide neurotoxicity is related to previous cisplatin treatment for pediatric solid tumors. *J Clin Oncol* 1990;8(8):1399–1401.
45. Eberly AL, Anderson GD, Bubalo JS, et al. Optimal prevention of seizures induced by high-dose busulfan. *Pharmacotherapy* 2008;28(12):1502–1510.
46. Bonifazi F, Storci G, Bandini G, et al. Glutathione transferase-A2 S112T polymorphism predicts survival, transplant-related mortality, busulfan and bilirubin blood levels after allogeneic stem cell transplantation. *Haematologica* 2014;99(1):172–179.

47. An N, Janech MG, Bland AM, et al. Proteomic analysis of murine bone marrow niche microenvironment identifies thioredoxin as a novel agent for radioprotection and for enhancing donor cell reconstitution. *Exp Hematol* 2013;41:944–956.
48. Steinherz LJ, Steinherz PG, Mangiacasale D, et al. Cardiac changes with cyclophosphamide. *Med Pediatr Oncol* 1981;9(5):417–422.
49. Bastholt L, Johansson CJ, Pfeiffer P, et al. A pharmacokinetic study of prednimustine as compared with prednisolone plus chlorambucil in cancer patients. *Cancer Chemother Pharmacol* 1991;28(3):205–210.
50. Tew KD, Glusker JP, Hartley-Asp B, et al. Preclinical and clinical perspectives on the use of estramustine as an antimitotic drug. *Pharmacol Ther* 1992;56(3):323–339.
51. Punzi JS, Duax WL, Strong P, et al. Molecular conformation of estramustine and two analogues. *Mol Pharmacol* 1992;41(3):569–576.
52. Hudes GR, Greenberg R, Krigel RL, et al. Phase II study of estramustine and vinblastine, two microtubule inhibitors, in hormone-refractory prostate cancer. *J Clin Oncol* 1992;10(11):1754–1761.
53. Tew K, Houghton JA, Houghton PJ. *Preclinical and Clinical Modulation of Anticancer Drugs.* Boca Raton, FL: CRC Press; 1993.
54. Friedlos F, Davies L, Scanlon I, et al. Three new prodrugs for suicide gene therapy using carboxypeptidase G2 elicit bystander efficacy in two xenograft models. *Cancer Res* 2002;62(6):1724–1729.
55. Tew KD. TLK-286: a novel glutathione S-transferase-activated prodrug. *Expert Opin Investig Drugs* 2005;14(8):1047–1054.
56. Borch RF, Valente RR. Synthesis, activation, and cytotoxicity of aldophosphamide analogues. *J Med Chem* 1991;34(10):3052–3058.
57. Rosen LS, Laxa B, Boulos L, et al. Phase 1 study of TLK286 (Telcyta) administered weekly in advanced malignancies. *Clin Cancer Res* 2004;10(11):3689–3698.
58. Sequist LV, Fidias PM, Temel JS, et al. Phase 1–2a multicenter dose-ranging study of canfosfamide in combination with carboplatin and paclitaxel as first-line therapy for patients with advanced non-small cell lung cancer. *J Thorac Oncol* 2009;4(11):1389–1396.
59. Kavanagh JJ, Gershenson DM, Choi H, et al. Multi-institutional phase 2 study of TLK286 (TELCYTA, a glutathione S-transferase P1-1 activated glutathione analog prodrug) in patients with platinum and paclitaxel refractory or resistant ovarian cancer. *Int J Gynecol Cancer* 2005;15(4):593–600.
60. Vergote I, Finkler N, del Campo J, et al. Phase 3 randomised study of canfosfamide (Telcyta, TLK286) versus pegylated liposomal doxorubicin or topotecan as third-line therapy in patients with platinum-refractory or -resistant ovarian cancer. *Eur J Cancer* 2009;45(13):2324–2332.
61. Chase M, Chung RY, Chiocca EA. An oncolytic viral mutant that delivers the CYP2B1 transgene and augments cyclophosphamide chemotherapy. *Nat Biotechnol* 1998;16(5):444–448.
62. Vey N, Giles F. Laromustine (cloretazine). *Expert Opin Pharmacother* 2010;11(4):657–667.
63. Pigneux A. Laromustine, a sulfonyl hydrolyzing alkylating prodrug for cancer therapy. *IDrugs* 2009;12(1):39–53.
64. Schiller GJ, O'Brien SM, Pigneux A, et al. Single-agent laromustine, a novel alkylating agent, has significant activity in older patients with previously untreated poor-risk acute myeloid leukemia. *J Clin Oncol* 2010;28(5):815–821.
65. Eichbaum M, Bischofs E, Nehls K, et al. Bendamustine hydrochloride—a renaissance of alkylating strategies in anticancer medicine. *Drugs Today (Barc)* 2009;45(6):431–444.
66. Rasschaert M, Schrijvers D, Van den Brande J, et al. A phase I study of bendamustine hydrochloride administered day 1+2 every 3 weeks in patients with solid tumours. *Br J Cancer* 2007;96(11):1692–1698.
67. Weide R, Hess G, Köppler H, et al. High anti-lymphoma activity of bendamustine/mitoxantrone/rituximab in rituximab pretreated relapsed or refractory indolent lymphomas and mantle cell lymphomas: a multicenter phase II study of the German Low Grade Lymphoma Study Group (GLSG). *Leuk Lymphoma* 2007;48(7):1299–1306.
68. Cheson BD, Rummel MJ. Bendamustine: rebirth of an old drug. *J Clin Oncol* 2009;27(9):1492–1501.
69. van der Jagt R. Bendamustine for indolent non-Hodgkin lymphoma in the front-line or relapsed setting: a review of pharmacokinetics and clinical trial outcomes. *Expert Rev Hematol* 2013;6:525–537.
70. Ponisch W, Heyn S, Beck J, et al. Lenalidomide, bendamustine and prednisolone exhibits a favourable safety and efficacy profile in relapsed or refractory multiple myeloma: final results of a phase 1 clinical trial OSHO - #077. *Br J Haematol* 2013;162:202–209.

18 Platinum Analogs

Peter J. O'Dwyer and A. Hilary Calvert

INTRODUCTION

The platinum drugs represent a unique and important class of antitumor compounds. Alone or in combination with other chemotherapeutic agents, *cis*-diamminedichloroplatinum (II) (cisplatin) and its analogs have made a significant impact on the treatment of a variety of solid tumors for nearly 40 years. The unique activity and toxicity profile observed with cisplatin in early clinical trials fueled the development of platinum analogs that are less toxic and more active against a variety of tumor types, including those that have developed resistance to cisplatin. In addition to cisplatin, two other platinum complexes are currently approved for use in the United States: *cis*-diamminecyclobutanedicarboxylate platinum (II) (carboplatin) and 1,2-diaminocyclohexaneoxalato platinum (II) (oxaliplatin). Several other analogs with unique activities are in various stages of clinical development, and nedaplatin (Japan) and lobaplatin (China) are locally registered. Progress in the development of superior analogs requires a thorough understanding of the chemical, biologic, pharmacokinetic, and pharmacodynamic properties of this important class of drugs.

HISTORY

The realization that platinum complexes exhibited antitumor activity began serendipitously in a series of experiments to investigate the effect of electromagnetic radiation on the growth of bacteria, carried out by Dr. Barnett Rosenberg and colleagues beginning in 1961.[1,2] Exposure of the bacteria to an electric field resulted in a profound change in their morphology; this effect was found not to be from the electric field, but from electrolysis products produced by the platinum electrodes. An analysis of these products resulted in the identification of the cis-isomer of a platinum coordination complex as the active compound. Tests of *cis*-diamminedichloroplatinum (II) in mice bearing several model tumor types indicated that cisplatin exhibited a broad spectrum of antitumor activity. Although early clinical trials demonstrated responses in several tumor types, particularly testicular cancers, the severe renal and gastrointestinal toxicity caused by the drug nearly led to its abandonment. Work at Memorial Sloan-Kettering[3,4] showed that these effects could be ameliorated, in part, by aggressive prehydration, which rekindled interest in its clinical use. Currently, cisplatin is curative in testicular cancer and significantly prolongs survival in combination regimens for ovarian, lung, head and neck, bladder, and upper gastrointestinal (GI) cancers. Its role is being reexamined in other tumors, too, and especially breast cancer.

PLATINUM CHEMISTRY

Platinum exists primarily in either a 2+ or 4+ oxidation state. These oxidation states dictate the stereochemistry of the ligands surrounding the platinum atom. Platinum (II) compounds exhibit a square planar geometry, in which the ammine ligands (also called carrier groups) are relatively stable, whereas the opposite, more polar ligands (leaving groups) are more easily displaced and so confer reactivity toward charged macromolecules, including DNA.[5] The stereochemistry of platinum complexes is critical to their antitumor activity as evidenced by the significantly reduced efficacy observed with *trans*-diamminedichloroplatinum (II).

In an aqueous solution, the chloride leaving groups of cisplatin are subject to mono- and diaqua substitution, particularly at chloride concentrations below 100 mmol, which characterize the intracellular environment. The administration of cisplatin in high chloride solutions (normal saline usually), therefore, contributes to stability. Intracellular formation of partially and fully aquated complexes creates the chloroaqua and hydroxoaqua cisplatin species that bind DNA.[6]

PLATINUM COMPLEXES AFTER CISPLATIN

Early in the clinical development of cisplatin, it became clear that its toxicity was a limitation to its therapeutic effectiveness, and that its activity, although striking in certain diseases, did not extend to all cancers. These observations then motivated a search for structural analogs with less toxicity and a different profile of antitumor activity. In addition, the side effects of cisplatin stimulated the development of antiemetics and other supportive care measures for use with chemotherapy. Progress in understanding the chemistry and pharmacokinetics of cisplatin has guided the development of new analogs. In general, modification of the chloride leaving groups of cisplatin results in compounds with different pharmacokinetics and reactivity towards DNA, whereas modification of the carrier ligands alters the activity of the resulting complex. The features of the more important platinum analogs that have been developed are shown in Figure 18.1.

Carboplatin

The carboplatin molecule has the same ammine carrier ligands as cisplatin. Using a murine screen for nephrotoxicity, Harrap and Calvert discovered that substituting a cyclobutanedicarboxylate moiety for the two chloride ligands of cisplatin resulted in a complex with reduced renal toxicity. This observation was translated to the clinic in the form of carboplatin, a more stable and pharmacokinetically predictable analog.[7,8] The results in humans were accurately predicted by the animal models, and marrow toxicity rather than nephrotoxicity was the principal side effect. At effective doses, carboplatin produced less nausea, vomiting, nephrotoxicity, and neurotoxicity than cisplatin. Furthermore, the myelosuppression was closely associated with the pharmacokinetics. The work of Calvert et al.[9] and Egorin and colleagues[10] showed that toxicity can be made more predictable and dose intensity less variable by dosing strategies based on the exposure. Carboplatin was shown to be indistinguishable from cisplatin in its clinical activity in all but a handful of tumor types and is the most frequently used form of platinum in current use. Cisplatin and carboplatin have almost superimposable profiles of activity in the NCI60 cell line screen, which further emphasizes the dependence of spectrum of activity on the carrier ligand.

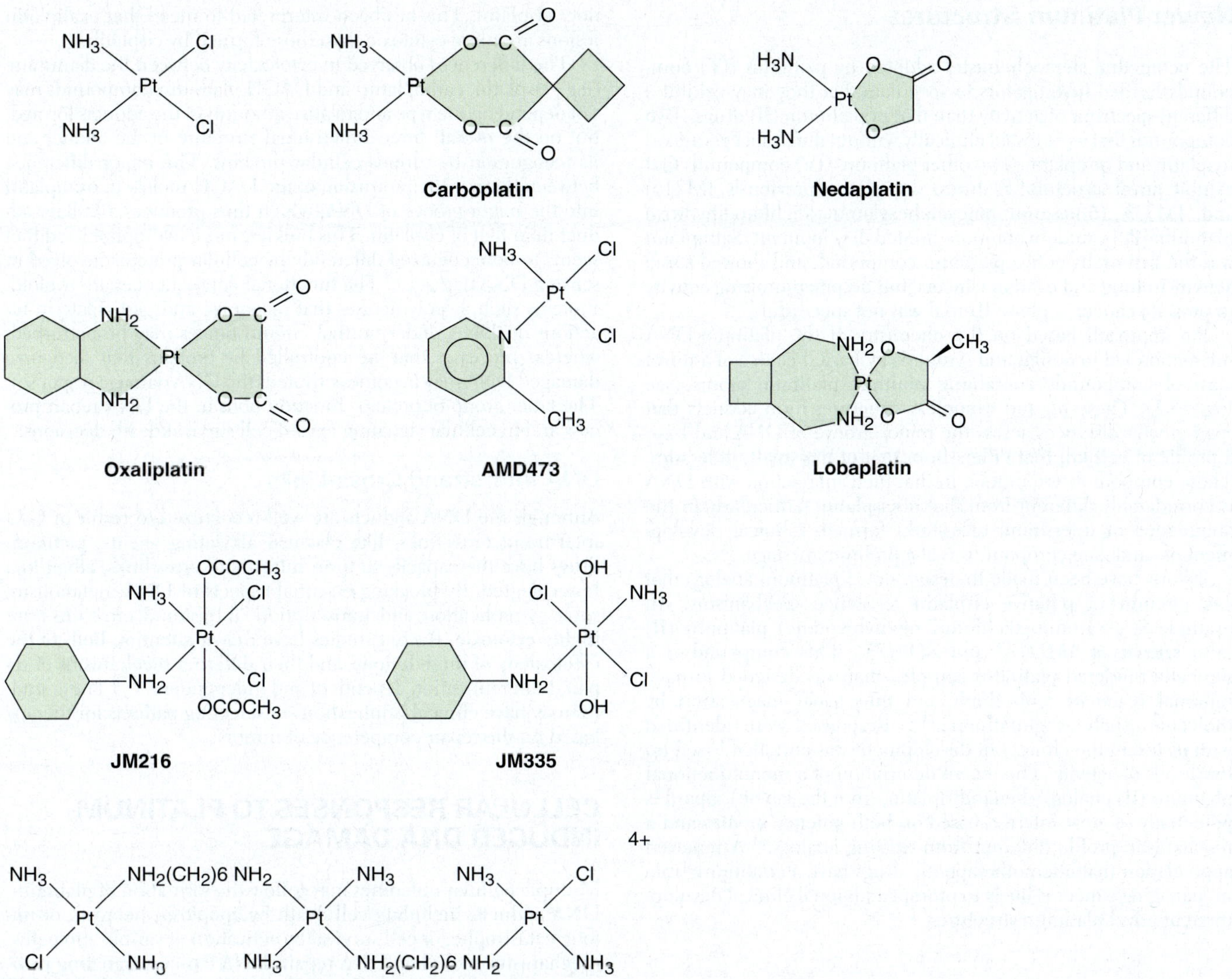

Figure 18.1 Structures of cisplatin, analogs, lobaplatin, and nedaplatin.

Oxaliplatin

Compounds with activity in cisplatin-resistant models emerged from modifications to the carrier group (see left side of the analogs in Fig. 18.1). Connors, in the late 1960s, synthesized platinum coordination compounds with varying physicochemical characteristics and found that the series that possessed a diaminocyclohexane (DACH) carrier group was active in models of cancer in vitro[11] and in vivo.[12] Subsequent studies supported the idea that DACH-based platinum complexes were non–cross-resistant with cisplatin, and DACH derivatives exhibited a unique cytotoxicity profile compared to cisplatin and carboplatin in the National Cancer Institute 60 cell line screen.[13–15] After a number of delays, a DACH analog that had been synthesized by Kidani and colleagues in the early 1970s, was developed in the clinic.[13] Oxaliplatin, a coordination compound of a DACH carrier group and an oxalato leaving group, was active in cisplatin-resistant tumor models. Like cisplatin, oxaliplatin preferentially forms adducts at the N7 position of guanine and, to a lesser extent, adenine. However, there is evidence that the three-dimensional structure of the DNA adducts and biologic response(s) they elicit are different from those of cisplatin. Oxaliplatin demonstrated activity in combination with 5-fluorouracil and leucovorin in colon cancer, a disease that is unresponsive to cisplatin. This finding validated the focus on cisplatin-resistant preclinical models to identify new active molecules. Oxaliplatin is approved for the treatment of advanced colorectal cancer, and enhances cure rates in the adjuvant setting. The therapeutic role of oxaliplatin has been found to extend to pancreatic, gastric, and esophageal cancers, in all of which it is the more active platinum derivative.

Nedaplatin and Lobaplatin

Nedaplatin is cis-diammineglycolatoplatinum, developed as a less nephrotoxic second-generation platinum analog, has been shown to be active in a range of tumors similar to that of cisplatin and carboplatin.[16] As a diammine structure, nedaplatin would fall among the cisplatin analogs analyzed in the NCI60 cell line screen,[17] and this activity is therefore anticipated. Lobaplatin is a platinum (II) complex in which the leaving group is lactic acid and the stable ammine ligand is 1,2-bis(aminomethyl)cyclobutane. In a similar way to oxaliplatin the stable ammine ligand may convey some non–cross-resistance compared to cisplatin or carboplatin. It is licensed in China for the breast cancer, small-cell lung cancer, and chronic myelogenous leukemia. It is unique among the platinum drugs for its approval for breast cancer, but there are few published clinical data and no randomized trials. It has not achieved approval in the United States or Europe.

Newer Platinum Structures

The octahedral stereochemistry adopted by platinum (IV) compounds has led investigators to speculate that they may exhibit a different spectrum of activity than that of platinum (II) drugs. Two compounds that were tested clinically without much success are ormaplatin and iproplatin. Two other platinum (IV) compounds that exhibit novel structural features, satraplatin (previously JM216) and JM335 (*trans*-ammine[cyclohexylamine]dichlorodihydroxo platinum [IV]), underwent more limited development. Satraplatin was the first orally active platinum compound, and showed some activity in lung and ovarian cancers, but despite promising activity in prostate cancer, a phase III trial was not successful.[18,19]

An approach based on the chemistry of the platinum-DNA interaction led to design and synthesis by Farrell et al.[20] of a novel class of compounds containing multiple platinum atoms (see Fig. 18.1). These bi- and trinuclear structures form adducts that span greater distances across the minor groove of DNA and have a profile of cell kill that differs from that of the small molecules. These compounds are unique in that their interaction with DNA is considerably different from that of cisplatin, particularly in the abundance of interstrand cross-links formed. Clinical development of candidate compounds is at a preliminary stage.

Efforts have been made to design novel platinum analogs that can circumvent putative cisplatin resistance mechanisms. An example is *cis*-amminedichloro(2-methylpyridine) platinum (II) (also known as *AMD473* and *ZD0473*). This compound is a sterically hindered platinum complex that was designed to have minimal reactivity with thiols and thus avoid inactivation by molecules such as glutathione.[21,22] Responses were identified with its use in the clinic, but development was curtailed based on low levels of activity. The recent description of a monofunctional platinum (II) analog, phenanthriplatin, from the lab of Lippard is potentially of great interest, based on both potency in vitro and a mechanistic profile different from existing analogs.[23] A renewed appreciation that chemotherapeutic drugs have a continuing role in managing cancer is likely to prompt additional clinical development of novel platinum structures.

MECHANISM OF ACTION

DNA Adduct Formation

DNA has long been thought to be the major therapeutic target for platinum compounds. The cytotoxic effects are determined, in part, by the structure and relative amount of DNA adducts formed. Cisplatin and its analogs react preferentially at the N7 position of guanine and adenine residues to form a variety of monofunctional and bifunctional adducts.[24] The monoadducts may form intrastrand or interstrand cross-links. The predominant lesions that are formed when platinum compounds bind DNA are d(GpG)Pt intrastrand cross-links. Cisplatin also forms interstrand cross-links between guanine residues located on opposite strands, and these account for less than 5% of the total DNA-bound platinum. The formation of adducts and cross-links has been associated with therapeutic efficacy.[25,26] These adducts may contribute to the drug's cytotoxicity because they impede certain cellular processes that require the separation of both DNA strands, such as replication and transcription. The adducts formed in the reaction between carboplatin and DNA in cultured cells are essentially the same as those of cisplatin; however, higher concentrations of carboplatin are required (20- to 40-fold for cells) to obtain equivalent total platinum-DNA adduct levels due to its slower rate of aquation.[27] Oxaliplatin intrastrand adducts form even more slowly due to a slower rate of conversion from monoadducts; however, they are formed at similar DNA sequences and regions as cisplatin adducts. At equitoxic doses, oxaliplatin forms fewer DNA adducts than does cisplatin. This has been interpreted to mean that oxaliplatin lesions are more cytotoxic than those formed by cisplatin.

The differences observed in cytotoxicity between the diammine (e.g., cisplatin, carboplatin) and DACH platinum compounds may not depend on the type and relative amounts of the adducts formed, but on the overall three-dimensional structure of the adduct and its recognition by various cellular proteins. The major difference between them is the protrusion of the DACH moiety of oxaliplatin into the major groove of DNA, which thus produces a bulkier adduct than that of cisplatin. This bulkier, more hydrophobic adduct seems to be recognized differently by cellular proteins involved in sensing DNA damage.[28] The functional consequences are twofold: Proteins such as polymerases that recognize and participate in reactions on DNA under normal circumstances may be perturbed, whereas processes that are controlled by proteins that recognize damaged DNA may become activated (the DNA damage response). The latter group of proteins function both in the DNA repair process and in cellular signaling toward cell survival/death decisions.

DNA Interstrand Cross-Links

Although the DNA adducts are well-recognized to result in G-G interstrand cross-links, like classical alkylating agents, platinum drugs have the capacity to form intrastrand cross-links, albeit to a lesser degree. By blocking essential aspects of DNA metabolism, such as replication and transcription, intrastrand cross-links are highly cytotoxic. Recent studies have drawn attention both to the cytotoxicity of these lesions, and their differing mechanisms of repair, both replication dependent and independent.[29,30] These studies may have clinical implications in selecting patients for therapy based on the repair competence of tumors.

CELLULAR RESPONSES TO PLATINUM-INDUCED DNA DAMAGE

Multiple cellular outcomes may follow the formation of platinum-DNA adducts, including cell death by apoptosis, necrosis, or mitotic catastrophe, or cell survival by activation of various protective mechanisms including DNA repair, DNA damage signaling pathways, cell cycle arrest, and autophagy (the last may have a dual role, possibly context dependent).

Cell Fate

The cellular effects following DNA binding by platinum drugs have been analyzed. The studies of Sorenson and Eastman,[31] using DNA repair-deficient Chinese hamster ovary (CHO) cells, indicated that passage through the S phase is necessary for G2 arrest and cell death, which suggests that DNA replication on a damaged template may result in the accumulation of further damage. An aberrant mitosis was observed before apoptosis in this model.

DNA Damage Recognition

Among the initiation events that ultimately result in platinum drug–induced cell death are the binding of platinum-DNA damage recognition proteins, which then seed the accumulation of a large protein complex capable both of DNA damage signaling (as to cell cycle proteins to halt replication) and repair of the damaged DNA. Among the DNA-binding proteins are the high-mobility group proteins HMG1 and HMG2.[32–34] These proteins are capable of bending DNA as well as recognizing bent DNA structures, such as that produced by cisplatin, and different specificities for cisplatin and for oxaliplatin adducts are observed in structural studies.[35,36] Other candidate platinum-DNA damage recognition proteins include histone H1, RNA polymerase I transcription upstream binding factor (hUBF), the TATA binding protein (TBP), and proteins involved in mismatch repair (MMR). The MMR complex has been implicated in cisplatin sensitivity.[37] Studies have shown that the MSH2 and MLH1 proteins participate in the recognition of DNA adducts formed by cisplatin, but not oxaliplatin, which could contribute to differences in the cytotoxicity profiles observed between these two platinum complexes.

DNA Damage Signaling

A number of signaling events have been shown to occur after treatment of cells with platinum drugs.[38] For example, the ATM- and Rad3-related (ATR) proteins that are involved in cell-cycle checkpoint activation are activated by cisplatin. These kinases phosphorylate and activate several downstream effectors that regulate cell cycle, DNA repair, cell survival, and apoptosis, including p53, CHK2, and members of the mitogen-activated protein kinase (MAPK) pathway (extracellular signal-related kinase [ERK], c-Jun amino-terminal kinase [JNK], and p38 kinase). Recent data especially implicate signaling through the JNK pathway, and inhibition at the level of JNK seems especially relevant to platinum drug cytotoxicity in vitro and in vivo.[39,40] The pleiotropic nature of this stress response only grows, because each of these molecules subsequently controls the activity and expression of many more proteins. As a result of this complexity, acting in the context of variable genomic tumor aberrations, therapeutic strategies directed to these pathways have been slow to emerge. However, clinical trials to investigate specific inhibitors of DNA damage responses are underway and hold promise. It is also relevant to point out that these signaling pathways affect not just the tumor cell, but also may communicate to cells in the microenvironment, the responses of which may also determine the effectiveness of therapy.

IS DNA THE ONLY TARGET?

Early analyses of the action of cytotoxic drugs included a probe of whether effects on DNA were sufficient to explain drug effects. A pioneer in this field was Tritton,[41] who proposed that effects of DNA-intercalating agents on the plasma membrane could underlie the cytotoxicity of the drug. More recently, enucleated cells were shown to be susceptible to cisplatin, and a seminal paper from Voest and colleagues showed that platinum sensitivity was determined not solely by the accumulation of DNA damage in the tumor cell.[42] In analyzing the contribution of cells in the microenvironment of tumors, he showed that tumor infiltration with mesenchymal stem cells could confer drug resistance. A search for secreted factors defined platinum-induced fatty acids, metabolic products in the thromboxane synthetase, and cyclooxygenase-1 pathways as determining the effectiveness of drug therapy. A proteomic study in cisplatin-sensitive and -resistant cells confirmed the substantial effects of drug exposure on lipid metabolites and their relation to susceptibility. A current focus on therapies directed to the microenvironment, including immunologic and anti-inflammatory interventions,[43] has the potential to expand our ability to apply platinum drugs in the clinic.

MECHANISMS OF RESISTANCE

The major limitation to the successful treatment of solid tumors with platinum-based chemotherapy is the emergence of drug-resistant tumor cells.[44] Developments in tumor biology have advanced our thinking with regard to how and when these cells emerge; heterogeneity within a tumor even at its earliest diagnosis reflects the emergence of treatment-resistant clones even in advance of selection pressure and the realization that resistance may not be specific to the DNA-damaging drug. Indeed, this may be reflected clinically in the finding that after progression on initial chemotherapy, the use of second-line therapy is usually associated with a shorter duration of response.

Currently described mechanisms of platinum drug resistance (Fig. 18.2) include reduced cellular accumulation, intracellular detoxification, repair of Pt-DNA lesions, increased damage tolerance, and the activation of cellular defense mechanisms such as autophagy. In addition, we have already alluded to exogenous influences on mechanism, as may be mediated by other cells, metabolites, of physicochemical conditions (such as hypoxia) in the tumor microenvironment. It must be acknowledged, however, that our insights are very limited as to why some tumors respond and others do not to platinum chemotherapy. As genome sequencing yields increasing and often surprising revelations about the genes that drive cancers and the complexity inherent in cancers of a single histologic type, it is likely that when associated with outcomes in large patient populations, patterns will emerge to guide selection of therapies.

Reduced Accumulation

Platinum uptake in cells occurs by simple diffusion and by carrier-mediated mechanisms. Inhibition of transport mechanisms has a marked effect on intracellular platinum accumulation, and Howell's group has shown the importance of the copper transporters CTR-1 and CTR-2 in regulating the influx of various platinum analogs in eukaryotic cells.[45,46] The contribution of these mechanisms to clinical platinum drug resistance is being explored.[47] Accumulation may also be influenced by enhanced efflux, and various transport proteins are upregulated in cell lines selected for acquired resistance, and in platinum-resistant ovarian cancers.

Inactivation

Platinum complexes are highly reactive molecules and bind rapidly to multiple cellular macromolecules. Protection from such chemicals in the environment is afforded by cellular thiols, including

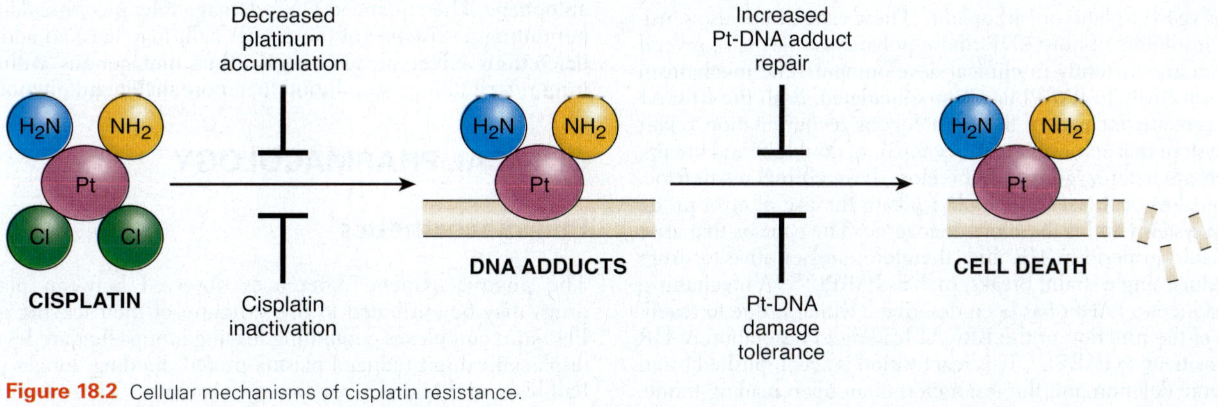

Figure 18.2 Cellular mechanisms of cisplatin resistance.

small peptides such as glutathione (GSH) and larger proteins as exemplified by metallothionein (MT). There are many reports of an association between platinum drug sensitivity and glutathione levels[48–50]; however, reducing intracellular glutathione levels with drugs such as buthionine sulfoximine has resulted in only low to modest potentiation of cisplatin sensitivity.[51] Buthionine sulfoximine was developed for clinical use, and some impact on GSH content of tumors and normal tissues was demonstrated. However, the depletion of GSH was not consistent, and ultimately, the cost of producing the active stereoisomer of the drug was judged prohibitive. Inactivation of the platinum drugs may also occur through binding to the MTs, a family of sulfhydryl-rich, low–molecular-weight proteins that participate in heavy metal binding and detoxification; however, the contribution of MT to clinical platinum drug resistance is unclear, and a therapeutic role has not emerged.

Increased DNA Repair

Once platinum-DNA adducts are formed, cells must either repair or tolerate the damage to survive. In general, the capacity to repair DNA damage seems to play a role in determining a tumor cell's sensitivity to platinum drugs and other DNA-damaging agents. For example, tumors that are unusually sensitive to cisplatin, such as testicular nonseminomatous germ cell tumors, may be deficient in their ability to repair platinum-DNA adducts.[52] The increased repair of platinum-DNA lesions in cisplatin-resistant cell lines as compared to their sensitive counterparts has been shown in several human cancer cell lines, but translation of these observations to the clinic has been difficult. The repair of platinum-DNA adducts appears to occur predominantly by nucleotide excision repair (NER), with a role for MMR under certain circumstances.[53] The molecular basis for the increased repair activity observed in cisplatin-resistant cells is not known precisely, but formation of the ERCC1/XPF protein complex may be a key step. Selvakumaran et al.[54] showed that the downregulation of ERCC-1 using an antisense approach sensitized a platinum-resistant cell line to cisplatin both in vitro and in vivo. There is substantial clinical evidence that implicates *ERCC1* expression in increased NER and cisplatin resistance, and high expression of ERCC1 has been demonstrated to confer a worse outcome after cisplatin treatment in several resistant tumors. The most extensive study of this as a marker has been in non–small-cell lung cancer, results in which were summarized and analyzed by Hubner et al.[55] In gastric cancer also, high levels of ERCC1 are associated with resistance to cisplatin treatment.[56–58] However, a recent reevaluation of discrepant results questioned the reliability of the assays of ERCC1 and their relationship to function.[59] These data suggest that there is a relationship between ERCC1 expression and treatment, but that the lag in marker development precludes implementation of a predictive assay until additional studies have been performed.

Perhaps the most striking evidence that DNA repair is a determinant of platinum drug responses is that breast and ovarian cancers occurring in BRCA1 or BRCA2 mutation carriers are particularly responsive to cisplatin or carboplatin. These cancers are also sensitive to inhibitors of poly(ADP-ribose)polymerase (PARPi), several of which are currently in clinical development. The mechanism of the sensitivity to PARPi has been elucidated. Both the BRCA1 and 2 proteins for part of the homologous recombination repair (HR) system that achieves error-free repair of double strand breaks. Carriers are heterozygous and, therefore, have normal repair function, but loss of the second allele leads to the use of error-prone backup systems and is therefore oncogenic. The cancers that arise are unable to perform HR and, therefore, are sensitive to drugs that induce single strand breaks, such as PARPi.[60,61] A mechanism of resistance to PARPi has been described, which is due to reactivation of the function of the BRCA2 leading to restoration of HR and sensitivity to PARPi.[62] This reactivation is accomplished by an intragenic deletion and the restoration of an open reading frame. It has further been shown that such revertant cells are resistant to cisplatin as well as PARPi. Finally, recurrent cancers in BRCA2 mutation carriers, which have acquired platinum resistance, have been shown to have undergone reversion of the BRCA2 mutation.[63] This clearly shows that the HR system can be one cause of cisplatin resistance. However, not all cisplatin-resistant patients are also resistant to PARPi,[64] showing that there are multiple other causes of cis/carboplatin resistance.

Combinations of platinum drugs with PARPi are being actively pursued in patients with BRCA-related tumors and also in patients whose tumors are likely to have acquired loss of HR function (poorly differentiated serous ovarian cancer and triple negative breast cancer).

Autophagy

After platinum-DNA adduct formation, the cell detects the DNA damage and initiates signaling through multiple pathways, the effects of which include mobilization of repair proteins; arrest of the cell cycle; altered transcriptional programs; redirection of energy production and consumption; activation of cell death pathways and, simultaneously, of pathways that would counter a cell death decision, and so to permit survival. A process recently characterized to perform the last function is autophagy. Initially described as a mechanism of cell death, autophagy represents a regulated dissolution of cellular elements into a characteristic set of subcellular organelles detectable by electron microscopy and linked by a particular profile of gene expression changes.[65] Multiple stimuli precipitate these changes and have in common scarcity of nutrients that are required for survival, from oxygen and glucose withdrawal to less specific calorie deprivation, and inhibition of metabolic pathways. Autophagy is also a consequence of cytotoxic drug treatment and, more recently, has been appreciated as a means by which cells might survive the stress of cellular insults, and so become resistant to treatment.[66] Amaravadi and colleagues[67] demonstrated that autophagy reversal can sensitize tumors to cytotoxic drugs and several trials of platinum compounds along with the autophagy inhibitor hydroxychloroquine are in progress.

Increased DNA Damage Tolerance

The net result of DNA damage signaling in a sensitive tumor cell is engagement of cell death pathways, including apoptosis, and therapeutic benefit. In a resistant tumor cell, the cell survives as a consequence of one or many of these mechanisms, and this can result in platinum-DNA damage tolerance or multidrug resistance phenotype, or both. Contributors to the tolerance might include deficient DNA MMR (which could excise the adduct if NER failed), enhanced replicative bypass (which essentially ignores the adduct, allowing the cell to survive, but could contribute to the increase in mutation frequency observed in chemotherapy-treated cancers), and altered signaling through stress-related kinases such as JNK, which can both alter transcriptional programs and activate autophagy. Indeed JNK, by phosphorylating Bcl-2 or Bcl-XL, and releasing beclin-1 from inhibition, acts as a key switch to turn on autophagy. The enhanced DNA damage tolerance, in addition to permitting persistence of the cancer cell, may have an additional deleterious effect by fostering further mutagenesis within the tumor, facilitating its evolution to a more malignant phenotype.

CLINICAL PHARMACOLOGY

Pharmacokinetics

The pharmacokinetic differences observed between platinum drugs may be attributed to the structure of their leaving groups. Platinum complexes containing leaving groups that are less easily displaced exhibit reduced plasma protein binding, longer plasma half-lives, and higher rates of renal clearance. These features are

TABLE 18.1

Comparative Parmacokinetics of Platinum Analogs After Bolus or Short Intravenous Infusion

	Cisplatin	Carboplatin	Oxaliplatin
$T_{1/2}\alpha$			
Total platinum	14–49 min	12–98 min	26 min
Ultrafiltrate	9–30 min	8–87 min	21 min
$T_{1/2}\beta$			
Total platinum	0.7–4.6 h	1.3–1.7 h	—
Ultrafiltrate	0.7–0.8 h	1.7–5.9 h	—
$T_{1/2}\gamma$			
Total platinum	24–127 h	8.2–40.0 h	38–47 h
Ultrafiltrate	—	—	24–27 h
Protein binding	>90%	24%–50%	85%
Urinary excretion	23%–50%	54%–82%	>50%

$T_{1/2}\alpha$, half-life of first phase; $T_{1/2}\beta$, half-life of second phase; $T_{1/2}\gamma$, half-life of terminal phase.

evident in the pharmacokinetic properties of cisplatin, carboplatin, and oxaliplatin, which are summarized in Table 18.1. Platinum drug pharmacokinetics have been reviewed.[68]

Cisplatin

After intravenous infusion, cisplatin rapidly diffuses into tissues and is covalently bound to plasma protein. More than 90% of platinum is bound to plasma protein at 4 hours after infusion. The disappearance of ultrafilterable platinum is rapid and occurs in a biphasic fashion. Half-lives of 10 to 30 minutes and 0.7 to 0.8 hours have been reported for the initial and terminal phases, respectively. Cisplatin excretion is dependent on renal function, which accounts for the majority of its elimination. The percentage of platinum excreted in the urine has been reported to be between 23% and 40% at 24 hours after infusion. Only a small percentage of the total platinum is excreted in the bile.

Carboplatin

The differences in pharmacokinetics observed between cisplatin and carboplatin depend primarily on the slower rate of conversion of carboplatin to a reactive species. Thus, the stability of carboplatin results in a low incidence of nephrotoxicity. Carboplatin diffuses rapidly into tissues after infusion; however, it is considerably more stable in plasma. Only 24% of a dose was bound to plasma protein at 4 hours after infusion. The disappearance of platinum from plasma after short intravenous infusions of carboplatin has been reported to occur in a biphasic or triphasic manner. The initial half-lives for total platinum, which vary considerably among several studies, are listed in Table 18.1. The half-lives for total platinum range from 12 to 98 minutes during the first phase ($T_{1/2}\alpha$) and from 1.3 to 1.7 hours during the second phase ($T_{1/2}\beta$). Half-lives reported for the terminal phase range from 8.2 to 40 hours. The disappearance of ultrafilterable platinum is biphasic with $T_{1/2}\alpha$ and $T_{1/2}\beta$ values ranging from 7.6 to 87 minutes and 1.7 to 5.9 hours, respectively. Carboplatin is excreted predominantly by the kidneys, and cumulative urinary excretion of platinum is 54% to 82%, most as unmodified carboplatin. The renal clearance of carboplatin is closely correlated with the glomerular filtration rate (GFR).[69] This observation enabled Calvert et al.[9] to design a carboplatin-dosing formula based on the individual patient's GFR.

Oxaliplatin

After oxaliplatin infusion, platinum accumulates into three compartments: plasma-bound platinum, ultrafilterable platinum, and platinum associated with erythrocytes. When specific and sensitive mass spectrometric techniques are used, oxaliplatin itself is undetectable in plasma, even at end infusion.[70] The active forms of the drug have not been extensively characterized. Approximately 85% of the total platinum is bound to plasma protein at 2 to 5 hours after infusion.[71] Plasma elimination of total platinum and ultrafilterates is biphasic. The half-lives for the initial and terminal phases are 26 minutes and 38.7 hours, respectively, for total platinum and 21 minutes and 24.2 hours, respectively, for ultrafilterable platinum (see Table 18.1).[72] Thus, as with carboplatin, substantial differences between total and free platinum kinetics are not observed. As with cisplatin, a prolonged retention of oxaliplatin is observed in red blood cells. However, unlike cisplatin, oxaliplatin does not accumulate to any significant level after multiple courses of treatment.[71] This may explain why neurotoxicity associated with oxaliplatin is reversible. Oxaliplatin is eliminated predominantly by the kidneys, with more than 50% of the platinum being excreted in the urine at 48 hours.

Pharmacodynamics

Pharmacodynamics relates pharmacokinetic indices of drug exposure to biologic measures of drug effect, usually toxicity to normal tissues or tumor cell kill. Two issues to be addressed in such studies are whether the effectiveness of the drug can be enhanced and whether the toxicity can be attenuated by knowledge of the platinum pharmacokinetics in an individual. These questions are appropriate to the use of cytotoxic agents with relatively narrow therapeutic indices. Toxicity to normal tissues can be quantitated as a continuous variable when the drug causes myelosuppression. Thus, the early studies of carboplatin demonstrated a close relationship of changes in platelet counts to the area under the concentration-time curve (AUC) in the individual. The AUC was itself closely related to renal function, which was determined as creatinine clearance. Based on these observations, Egorin et al.,[10] Calvert et al.,[9] and Chatelut and colleagues[73] derived formulas based on creatinine clearance to predict either the percentage change in platelet count or a target AUC. Application of pharmacodynamically guided dosing algorithms for carboplatin has been widely adopted as a means of avoiding overdosage (by producing acceptable nadir platelet counts) and of maximizing dose intensity in the individual. There is good evidence that this approach can decrease the risk of unacceptable toxicity. Accordingly, a dosing strategy based on renal function is recommended for the use of carboplatin.

A key question is whether maximizing carboplatin exposure in an individual can measurably increase the probability of tumor regression or survival. In an analysis by Jodrell et al.,[74] carboplatin AUC was a predictor of response, thrombocytopenia, and leukopenia. The likelihood of a tumor response increased with increasing AUC up to a level of 5 to 7 mg × hour per milliliter, after which a plateau was reached. Similar results were obtained with carboplatin in combination with cyclophosphamide, and neither response rate nor survival was determined by the carboplatin AUC in a cohort of ovarian cancer patients.[75] As a result, most carboplatin recommended doses are based on an AUC in this range (for every 3 to 4 week schedules), and modifications of these are used for more frequent administration (as in combined chemoradiotherapy regimens).

The relationship of pharmacokinetics to response has been sought by investigating the cellular pharmacology of these agents.[76] The formation and repair of the platinum-DNA adducts in human cells are not easily measured. Schellens and colleagues[77,78] analyzed the pharmacokinetic and pharmacodynamic interactions of cisplatin administered as a single agent. In a series of patients with head and neck cancer, they found that cisplatin exposure (measured as the AUC) closely correlated with both the peak DNA adduct content in leukocytes and the area under the DNA-adduct time curve. These measures were important predictors of response, both individually and in logistic regression analysis. However, as an approach to determine who should or should not be treated with platinum drugs, it seems more likely that genomic analyses will provide guidance in the near future.

Pharmacogenomics

Variability in pharmacokinetics and pharmacodynamics of cytotoxic drugs is an important determinant of therapeutic index. This interindividual variation may be attributed in part to genetic differences among patients. Targeted analyses of germ-line DNA and, increasingly, Genome-wide association studies (GWAS) approaches, have yielded genotypic features associated with results of therapy. Detoxification pathways and DNA repair have emerged as having markers attributable to response of lack of it in response to platinum drugs. Single nucleotide polymorphisms (SNP) in genes related to glutathione metabolism and in several DNA repair genes have been identified in lung cancer, breast cancer, and various GI cancers. A concern is that larger trials have not always confirmed early findings. As yet, informative SNPs that could be used to define therapeutic strategies for individual patients have not yet been defined.

FORMULATION AND ADMINISTRATION

Cisplatin (Platinol)

Cisplatin is administered in a chloride-containing solution intravenously over 0.5 to 2.0 hours. To minimize the risk of nephrotoxicity, patients are prehydrated with at least 500 mL of salt-containing fluid. Immediately before cisplatin administration, mannitol (12.5 to 25.0 g) is given parenterally to maximize urine flow. A diuretic such as furosemide may be used also, along with parenteral antiemetics. These currently include dexamethasone together with a 5-hydroxytryptamine (5-HT_3) antagonist. A minimum of 1 L of posthydration fluid is usually given. The intensity of hydration varies somewhat with the dose of cisplatin. High-dose cisplatin (up to 200 mg/m^2 per course) may be administered in a formulation containing 3% sodium chloride, but this method is no longer widely used. Cisplatin may also be administered regionally to increase local drug exposure and diminish side effects. Its intraperitoneal use was defined by Ozols et al.[79] and by Howell and colleagues.[80] Measured drug exposure in the peritoneal cavity is some 50-fold higher compared to levels achieved with intravenous administration. At standard dosages in ovarian cancer patients with low-volume disease, a randomized intergroup trial suggested that intraperitoneal administration is superior to intravenous cisplatin in combination with intravenous cyclophosphamide.[81] The development of combinations of carboplatin and paclitaxel has, however, superseded this technique in the treatment of ovarian cancer, and the intraperitoneal route is now infrequently used. Regional uses also include intra-arterial delivery (as for hepatic tumors, melanoma, and glioblastoma), but none have been adopted as a standard method of treatment. There is growing interest in chemoembolization for the treatment of tumors confined to the liver, and cisplatin is a component of many popular regimens.[82]

Carboplatin (Paraplatin)

Cisplatin treatment over 3 to 6 hours is burdensome for clinical resources and tiring for cancer patients. Previously given as an in-hospital treatment, it is now usually administered in the outpatient setting. The exigencies of the modern health-care environment have contributed to the expanding use of carboplatin as an alternative to cisplatin except in circumstances in which cisplatin is clearly the superior agent. Carboplatin is substantially easier to administer. Extensive hydration is not required because of the lack of nephrotoxicity at standard dosages. Carboplatin is reconstituted in chloride-free solutions (unlike cisplatin, because chloride can displace the leaving groups) and administered over 30 minutes as a rapid intravenous infusion.

Oxaliplatin (Eloxatin)

Oxaliplatin is also uncomplicated in its clinical administration. For bolus infusion, the required dose is administered in 500 mL of chloride-free diluent over a period of 2 hours. Oxaliplatin is most frequently given as a single dose every 2 weeks (85 mg/m^2) or every 3 weeks (130 mg/m^2), alone or with other active agents. It is common to pretreat patients with active antiemetics, such as a 5-HT_3 antagonist, but the nausea is not as severe as with cisplatin. No prehydration is required. Besides a relatively low incidence of myelosuppression, the predominant toxicity of oxaliplatin is cumulative neurotoxicity. The development of an oropharyngeal dysesthesia, often precipitated by exposure to cold, may require prolonging the duration of administration to 6 hours. On occasion, the occurrence of hypersensitivity also requires slowing the infusion.

TOXICITY

A substantial body of literature documents the side effects of platinum compounds. As noted in the section titled History, earlier in this chapter, the toxicity of cisplatin was a driving force both in the search for less toxic analogs and for more effective treatments for its side effects, especially nausea and vomiting. The toxicities associated with cisplatin, carboplatin, and oxaliplatin are described in detail in the following sections and summarized in Table 18.2. Please review the package inserts for these drugs for full prescribing information and delineation of toxic effects.

Cisplatin

The side effects associated with cisplatin (at single doses of more than 50 mg/m^2) include nausea and vomiting, nephrotoxicity, ototoxicity, neuropathy, and myelosuppression. Rare effects include visual impairment, seizures, arrhythmias, acute ischemic vascular events, glucose intolerance, and pancreatitis. The nausea and vomiting stimulated a search for new antiemetics. These effects are currently best managed with 5-HT_3 antagonists, usually given with a glucocorticoid, although other combinations of agents are still widely used. In the weeks after treatment, continuous antiemetic therapy may be required. Nephrotoxicity is ameliorated but not completely prevented by hydration. The renal damage to both glomeruli and tubules is cumulative, and after cisplatin treatment, serum creatinine levels are no longer a reliable guide to GFR. An acute elevation of serum creatinine level may follow a cisplatin dose, but this index returns to normal with time. Tubule damage may be reflected in a salt-losing syndrome that also resolves with time.

Ototoxicity is a cumulative and irreversible side effect of cisplatin treatment that results from damage to the inner ear. The initial audiographic manifestation is loss of high-frequency acuity (4,000 to 8,000 Hz). When acuity is affected in the range of speech, cisplatin

TABLE 18.2

Toxicity Profiles of Platinum Analogs in Clinical Use

Toxicity	Cisplatin	Carboplatin	Oxaliplatin
Myelosuppression		X	
Nephrotoxicity	X		
Neurotoxicity	X		X
Ototoxicity	X		
Nausea and vomiting	X	X	X

should be discontinued under most circumstances and carboplatin substituted where appropriate. Peripheral neuropathy is also cumulative, although less common than with agents such as vinca alkaloids. This neuropathy is usually reversible, although recovery is often slow. A number of agents with the potential for protection from neuropathy have been developed, but none is yet used widely.

Carboplatin

Myelosuppression, which is not usually severe with cisplatin, is the dose-limiting toxicity of carboplatin. The drug is most toxic to the platelet precursors, but neutropenia and anemia are frequently observed. The lowest platelet counts after a single dose of carboplatin are observed 17 to 21 days later, and recovery usually occurs by day 28. The effect is dose dependent, but individuals vary widely in their susceptibility. As shown by Egorin et al.[10] and Calvert et al.,[9] the severity of platelet toxicity is best accounted for by a measure of the drug exposure in an individual, the AUC. Both groups derived pharmacologically based formulas to predict toxicity and guide carboplatin dosing. That of Calvert and colleagues targets a particular exposure to carboplatin:

$$\text{Dose (mg)} = \text{target AUC (mg} \cdot \text{min/mL)} \times (\text{GFR mL/min} + 25)$$

This formula has been widely used to individualize carboplatin dosing and permits targeting an acceptable level of toxicity. Patients who are elderly, have a poor performance status, or have a history of extensive pretreatment have a higher risk of toxicity even when dosage is calculated with these methods, but the safety of drug administration has been enhanced. In the combination of carboplatin and paclitaxel, AUC-based dosing has helped to maximize the dose intensity of carboplatin. Dosages some 30% higher than those using a dosing strategy based solely on body surface area may safely be used. A determination of whether this approach to dosing improves outcomes will require a randomized trial.

The other toxicities of carboplatin are generally milder and better tolerated than those of cisplatin. Nausea and vomiting, although frequent, are less severe, shorter in duration, and more easily controlled with standard antiemetics (i.e., prochlorperazine [Compazine]), dexamethasone, lorazepam) than that after cisplatin treatment. Renal impairment is infrequent, although alopecia is common, especially with the paclitaxel-containing combinations. Neurotoxicity is also less common than with cisplatin, although it is observed more frequently with the increasing use of high-dose regimens. Ototoxicity is also less common.

Oxaliplatin

The dose-limiting toxicity of oxaliplatin is sensory neuropathy, a characteristic of all DACH-containing platinum derivatives. This side effect takes two forms. First, a tingling of the extremities, which may also involve the perioral region, that occurs early and usually resolves within a few days. With repeated dosing, symptoms may last longer between cycles, but do not appear to be cumulative or of long duration. Laryngopharyngeal spasms and cold dysesthesias have also been reported but are not associated with significant respiratory symptoms and can be prevented by prolonging the duration of infusion. A second neuropathy, more typical of that seen with cisplatin, affects the extremities and increases with repeated doses. Definitive physiologic characterization of oxaliplatin-induced neuropathy has proven difficult in large studies. Electromyograms performed in six patients treated by Extra et al.[83] revealed an axonal sensory neuropathy, but nerve conduction velocities were unchanged. Specimens from peripheral nerve biopsies performed in this study showed decreased myelination and replacement with collagen pockets. The neurologic effects of oxaliplatin appear to be cumulative in that they become more pronounced and of greater duration with successive cycles; however, unlike those of cisplatin, they are reversible with drug cessation. In a review of 682 patient experiences, Brienza et al.[84] reported that 82% of patients who experienced grade 2 neurotoxicity or higher had their symptoms regress within 4 to 6 months. In a larger adjuvant trial, de Gramont et al.[85] reported that 12% of patients had grade 3 toxicity at the end of a 6-month treatment period and that the majority of these patients had relief, but not always complete resolution of the symptoms, by 1 year later. The persistence of the neurotoxicity has led to approaches to ameliorate it, including the use of protective agents. The use of calcium and magnesium salts intravenously before and after each infusion has been shown to be ineffective. Ototoxicity is not observed with oxaliplatin. Nausea and vomiting do occur and generally respond to 5-HT_3 antagonists. Myelosuppression is uncommon and is not severe with oxaliplatin as a single agent, but it is a feature of combinations including this drug. Oxaliplatin therapy is not associated with nephrotoxicity.

CANCER THERAPEUTICS

REFERENCES

1. Rosenberg B, VanCamp L, Trosko J, et al. Platinum compounds: a new class of potent antitumor agents. *Nature* 1969;222:385–386.
2. Rosenberg B. Fundamental studies with cisplatin. *Cancer* 1985;55:2303–2316.
3. Cvitkovic E, Spaulding J, Bethune V, et al. Improvement of cis-dichlorodiammineplatinum (NSC 119875): therapeutic index in an animal model. *Cancer* 1977;39:1357–1361.
4. Hayes D, Cvitkovic E, Golbey R, et al. High dose cis-platinum diamine dichloride: amelioration of renal toxicity by mannitol diuresis. *Cancer* 1977;39:1372–1381.
5. Roberts J, Thomson A. The mechanism of action of antitumor platinum compounds. *Nucleic Acids Res* 1979;22:71–133.
6. Martin R. Platinum complexes: hydrolysis and binding to N(7) and N(1) of purines. In: Lippert B, ed. *Cisplatin: Chemistry and Biochemistry of a Leading Anticancer Drug*. Zurich: Verlag Helvetica Chimica Acta; 1999:183.
7. Harrap K. Preclinical studies identifying carboplatin as a viable cisplatin alternative. *Cancer Treat Rev* 1985;12:A21–A33.
8. Harrap K. Initiatives with platinum- and quinazoline-based antitumor molecules—Fourteenth Bruce F. Cain Memorial Award Lecture. *Cancer Res* 1995;55:2761–2768.
9. Calvert A, Newell D, Gumbrell L, et al. Carboplatin dosage: prospective evaluation of a simple formula based on renal function. *J Clin Oncol* 1989;7:1748–1756.
10. Egorin M, Echo DV, Olman E, et al. Prospective validation of a pharmacologically based dosing scheme for the cis-diamminedichloroplatinum(II) analogue diamminecyclobutanedicarboxylatoplatinum. *Cancer Res* 1985;45:6502–6506.
11. Connors T, Jones M, Ross W, et al. New platinum complexes with anti-tumour activity. *Chem Biol Interact* 1972;5:415–424.
12. Burchenal J, Kalaker K, Dew K, et al. Rationale for development of platinum analogs. *Cancer Treat Rep* 1979;63:1493–1498.
13. Kidani Y, Inagaki K, Tsukagoshi S. Examination of antitumor activities of platinum complexes of 1,2-diaminocyclohexane isomers and their related complexes. *Gann* 1976;67:921–922.
14. Burchenal J, Irani G, Kern K, et al. 1,2-Diaminocyclohexane platinum derivatives of potential clinical value. *Rec Res Cancer Res* 1980;74:146–155.
15. Rixe O, Ortuzar W, Alvarez M, et al. Oxaliplatin, tetraplatin, cisplatin, and carboplatin: spectrum of activity in drug-resistant cell lines and in the cell lines of the National Cancer Institute's anticancer drug screen panel. *Biochem Pharmacol* 1996;52:1855–1865.
16. Shimada M, Itamochi H, Kigawa J. Nedaplatin: a cisplatin derivative in cancer therapy. *Cancer Manag Res* 2013;5:67–76.
17. Fojo T, Farrell N, Ortuzar W, et al. Identification of non-cross-resistant platinum compounds with novel cytotoxicity profiles using the NCI anticancer drug screen and clustered image map visualizations. *Crit Rev Oncol Hematol* 2005;53:25–34.
18. Bates SE, Amiri-Kordestani L, Giaccone G. Drug development: portals of discovery. *Clin Cancer Res* 2012;18:23–32.
19. Kelland L. The development of orally active platinum drugs. In: Lippert B, ed. *Cisplatin: Chemistry and Biochemistry of a Leading Anticancer Drug*. Zurich: Verlag Helvetica Chimica Acta; 1999:497.
20. Farrell N, Qu Y, Bierbach U, et al. Structure-activity relationships within di- and trinuclear platinum phase-I clinical anticancer agents. In: Lippert B, ed. *Cisplatin: Chemistry and Biochemistry of a Leading Anticancer Drug*. Zurich: Verlag Helvetica Chimica Acta; 1999;477–496.
21. Holford J, Sharp S, Murrer B, et al. In vitro circumvention of cisplatin resistance by the novel sterically hindered platinum complex AMD473. *Br J Cancer* 1998;77:366–373.
22. Flaherty KT, Stevenson JP, Redlinger M, et al. A phase I, dose escalation trial of ZD0473, a novel platinum analogue, in combination with gemcitabine. *Cancer Chemother Pharmacol* 2004;53:404–408.
23. Park GY, Wilson JJ, Song Y, et al. Phenanthriplatin, a monofunctional DNA-binding platinum anticancer drug candidate with unusual potency and cellular activity profile. *Proc Natl Acad Sci U S A* 2012;109:11987–11992.

24. Eastman A. The formation, isolation and characterization of DNA adducts produced by anticancer platinum complexes. *Pharmacol Ther* 1987;34:155–166.
25. Zhu G, Song L, Lippard SJ. Visualizing inhibition of nucleosome mobility and transcription by cisplatin-DNA interstrand crosslinks in live mammalian cells. *Cancer Res* 2013;73:4451–4460.
26. Martens-de Kemp SR, Dalm SU, Wijnolts FM, et al. DNA-bound platinum is the major determinant of cisplatin sensitivity in head and neck squamous carcinoma cells. *PLoS One* 2013;8:e61555.
27. Blommaert F, van Kijk-Knijnenburg H, Dijt F, et al. Formation of DNA adducts by the anticancer drug carboplatin: different nucleotide sequence preferences in vitro and in cells. *Biochemistry* 1995;34:8474–8480.
28. Scheef E, Briggs J, Howell S. Molecular modeling of the intrastrand guanine-guanine DNA adducts produced by cisplatin and oxaliplatin. *Mol Pharmacol* 1999;56:633–643.
29. Enoiu M, Jiricny J, Schärer OD. Repair of cisplatin-induced DNA interstrand crosslinks by a replication-independent pathway involving transcription-coupled repair and translesion synthesis. *Nucleic Acids Res* 2012;40:8953–8964.
30. Zhu G, Song L, Lippard SJ. Visualizing inhibition of nucleosome mobility and transcription by cisplatin-DNA interstrand crosslinks in live mammalian cells. *Cancer Res* 2013;73:4451–4460.
31. Sorenson C, Eastman A. Mechanism of cis-diamminedichloroplatinum (II)-induced cytotoxicity: role of G2 arrest and DNA double-strand breaks. *Cancer Res* 1988;48:4484–4488.
32. Toney J, Donahue B, Kellett P, et al. Isolation of cDNAs encoding a human protein that binds selectively to DNA modified by the anticancer drug cis-diamminedichloroplatinum. *Proc Natl Acad Sci U S A* 1989;86:8328–8332.
33. Bruhn S, Pil P, Essigmann J, et al. Isolation and characterization of human cDNA clones encoding a high mobility group box protein that recognizes structural distortions to DNA caused by binding of the anticancer agent cisplatin. *Proc Natl Acad Sci U S A* 1989;89:2307–2311.
34. Hughes EN, Engelsberg BN, Billings PC. Purification of nuclear proteins that bind to cisplatin-damaged DNA. Identity with high mobility group proteins 1 and 2. *J Biol Chem* 1992;267:13520–13527.
35. Ramachandran S, Temple BR, Chaney SG, et al. Structural basis for the sequence-dependent effects of platinum-DNA adducts. *Nucleic Acids Res* 2009;37:2434–2448.
36. Ramachandran S, Temple B, Alexandrova AN, et al. Recognition of platinum-DNA adducts by HMGB1a. *Biochemistry* 2012;51:7608–7617.
37. Fink D, Zheng H, Nebel S, et al. In vitro and in vivo resistance to cisplatin in cells that have lost DNA mismatch repair. *Cancer Res* 1997;57:1841–1845.
38. Kelland L. The resurgence of platinum-based cancer chemotherapy. *Nat Rev Cancer* 2007;7:573–584.
39. Vasilevskaya IA, Rakitina TV, O'Dwyer PJ. Quantitative effects on c-Jun N-terminal protein kinase signaling determine synergistic interaction of cisplatin and 17-allylamino-17-demethoxygeldanamycin in colon cancer cell lines. *Mol Pharmacol* 2004;65:235–243.
40. Vasilevskaya IA, Selvakumaran M, O'Dwyer PJ. Disruption of signaling through SEK1 and MKK7 yields differential responses in hypoxic colon cancer cells treated with oxaliplatin. *Mol Pharmacol* 2008;74:246–254.
41. Maestre N, Tritton TR, Laurent G, et al. Cell surface-directed interaction of anthracyclines leads to cytotoxicity and nuclear factor kappaB activation but not apoptosis signaling. *Cancer Res* 2001;61:2558–2561.
42. Roodhart JM, Daenen LG, Stigter EC, et al. Mesenchymal stem cells induce resistance to chemotherapy through the release of platinum-induced fatty acids. *Cancer Cell* 2011;20:370–383.
43. Beatty GL, Chiorean EG, Fishman MP, et al. CD40 regulates cancer inflammation and induces regression of pancreatic carcinoma in mice and humans. *Science* 2011;331:1612–1616.
44. Galluzzi L, Senovilla L, Vitale I, et al. Molecular mechanisms of cisplatin resistance. *Oncogene* 2012;31:1869–1883.
45. Lin X, Okuda T, Holzer A, et al. The copper transporter CTR1 regulates cisplatin uptake in Saccharomyces cerevisiae. *Mol Pharmacol* 2002;62:1154–1159.
46. Blair BG, Larson CA, Safaei R, et al. Copper transporter 2 regulates the cellular accumulation and cytotoxicity of cisplatin and carboplatin. *Clin Cancer Res* 2009;15:4312–4321.
47. Samimi G, Varki NM, Wilczynski S, et al. Increase in the expression of the copper transporter ATP7A during platinum drug-based treatment is associated with poor survival in ovarian cancer patients. *Clin Cancer Res* 2003;9:5853–5859.
48. Britten RA, Green JA, Broughton C, et al. The relationship between nuclear glutathione levels and resistance to melphalan in human ovarian tumour cells. *Biochem Pharmacol* 1991;41:647–649.
49. Mistry P, Kelland L, Abel G, et al. The relationships between glutathione, glutathione-S-transferase and cytotoxicity of platinum drugs and melphalan in eight human ovarian carcinoma cell lines. *Br J Cancer* 1991;64:215–220.
50. Godwin A, Meister A, O'Dwyer P, et al. High resistance to cisplatin in human ovarian cancer cell lines is associated with marked increase in glutathione synthesis. *Proc Natl Acad Sci U S A* 1992;89:3070–3074.
51. Hamilton T, Winker M, Louie K, et al. Augmentation of adriamycin, melphalan and cisplatin cytotoxicity in drug-resistant and -sensitive human ovarian cancer cell lines by buthionine sulfoximine mediated glutathione depletion. *Biochem Pharmacol* 1985;34:2583–2586.
52. Koberle B, Grimaldi K, Sunters A, et al. DNA repair capacity and cisplatin sensitivity of human testis tumour cells. *Int J Cancer* 1997;70:551–555.
53. Martin LP, Hamilton TC, Schilder RJ. Platinum resistance: the role of DNA repair pathways. *Clin Cancer Res* 2008;14:1291–1295.
54. Selvakumaran M, Piscarcik DA, Bao R, et al. Enhanced cisplatin cytotoxicity by disturbing the nucleotide excision repair pathway in ovarian cancer cell lines. *Cancer Res* 2003;63:1311–1316.
55. Hubner RA, Riley RD, Billingham LJ, et al. Excision repair cross-complementation group 1 (ERCC1) status and lung cancer outcomes: a meta-analysis of published studies and recommendations. *PLoS One* 2011;6:e25164.
56. De Dosso S, Zanellato E, Nucifora M, et al. ERCC1 predicts outcome in patients with gastric cancer treated with adjuvant cisplatin-based chemotherapy. *Cancer Chemother Pharmacol* 2013;72:159–165.
57. Squires MH 3rd, Fisher SB, Fisher KE, et al. Differential expression and prognostic value of ERCC1 and thymidylate synthase in resected gastric adenocarcinoma. *Cancer* 2013;119:3242–3250.
58. Yamada Y, Boku N, Nishina T, et al. Impact of excision repair cross-complementing gene 1 (ERCC1) on the outcomes of patients with advanced gastric cancer: correlative study in Japan Clinical Oncology Group Trial JCOG9912. *Ann Oncol* 2013;24:2560–2565.
59. Friboulet L, Olaussen KA, Pignon JP, et al. ERCC1 isoform expression and DNA repair in non–small-cell lung cancer. *N Engl J Med* 2013;368:1101–1110.
60. Bryant HE, Schultz N, Thomas HD, et al. Specific killing of BRCA2-deficient tumours with inhibitors of poly(ADP-ribose) polymerase. *Nature* 2005;434:913–917.
61. Farmer H, McCabel N, Lord C, et al. Targeting the DNA repair defect in BRCA mutant cells as a therapeutic strategy. *Nature* 2005;434:917–921.
62. Edwards SL, Brough R, Lord CJ, et al. Resistance to therapy caused by intragenic deletion in BRCA2. *Nature* 2008;451:1111–1116.
63. Sakai W, Swisher EM, Karlan BM, et al. Secondary mutations as a mechanism of cisplatin resistance in BRCA2-mutated cancers. *Nature* 2008;451:1116–1121.
64. Gelmon KA, Tischkowitz M, Mackay H, et al. Olaparib in patients with recurrent high-grade serous or poorly differentiated ovarian carcinoma or triple-negative breast cancer: a phase 2, multicentre, open-label, non-randomised study. *Lancet Oncology* 2011;12:852–861.
65. Levine B, Kroemer G. Autophagy in the pathogenesis of disease. *Cell* 2008;132:27–42.
66. Matthew R, Karantza-Wadsworth V, White E. Role of autophagy in cancer. *Nat Rev Cancer* 2007;7:961–967.
67. Amaravadi RK, Yu D, Lum JJ, et al. Autophagy inhibition enhances therapy-induced apoptosis in a Myc-induced model of lymphoma. *J Clin Invest* 2007;117:326–336.
68. Duffull S, Robinson B. Clinical pharmacokinetics and dose optimization of carboplatin. *Clin Pharmacokinet* 1997;33:161–183.
69. Harland S, Newell D, Siddik Z, et al. Pharmacokinetics of cis-diammine-1,1-cyclobutane dicarboxylate platinum(II) in patients with normal and impaired renal function. *Cancer Res* 1984;44:1693–1697.
70. Graham MA, Lockwood GF, Greenslade D, et al. Clinical pharmacokinetics of oxaliplatin: a critical review. *Clin Cancer Res* 2000;6:1205–1218.
71. Gamelin E, Bouil A, Boisdron-Celle M, et al. Cumulative pharmacokinetic study of oxaliplatin, administered every three weeks, combined with 5-fluorouracil in colorectal cancer patients. *Clin Cancer Res* 1997;3:891–899.
72. Extra JM, Marty M, Brienza S, et al. Pharmacokinetics and safety profile of oxaliplatin. *Semin Oncol* 1998;25:13–22.
73. Chatelut E, Canal P, Brunner V, et al. Prediction of carboplatin clearance from standard morphological and biological patient characteristics. *J Natl Cancer Inst* 1995;87:573–580.
74. Jodrell D, Egorin M, Canetta R, et al. Relationships between carboplatin exposure and tumor response and toxicity in patients with ovarian cancer. *J Clin Oncol* 1992;10:520–528.
75. Reyno L, Egorin M, Canetta R, et al. Impact of cyclophosphamide on relationships between carboplatin exposure and response or toxicity when used in the treatment of advanced ovarian cancer. *J Clin Oncol* 1993;11:1156–1164.
76. Shen DW, Pouliot LM, Hall MD, et al. Cisplatin resistance: a cellular self-defense mechanism resulting from multiple epigenetic and genetic changes. *Pharmacol Rev* 2012;64:706–721.
77. Ma J, Verweij J, Planting A, et al. Current sample handling methods for measurement of platinum-DNA adducts in leucocytes in man lead to discrepant results in DNA adduct levels and DNA repair. *Br J Cancer* 1995;71:512–517.
78. Schellens J, Ma J, Planting A, et al. Relationship between the exposure to cisplatin, DNA-adduct formation in leucocytes and tumour response in patients with solid tumours. *Br J Cancer* 1996;73:1569–1575.
79. Ozols R, Corden B, Jacob J, et al. High-dose cisplatin in hypertonic saline. *Ann Intern Med* 1984;100:19–24.
80. Howell S, Pfeifle C, Wung W, et al. Intraperitoneal cis-diamminedichloroplatinum with systemic thiosulfate protection. *Cancer Res* 1983;43:1426–1431.
81. Alberts D, Liu P, Hannigan E, et al. Intraperitoneal cisplatin plus intravenous cyclophosphamide versus intravenous cisplatin plus intravenous cyclophosphamide for stage III ovarian cancer. *N Engl J Med* 1996;335:1950–1955.
82. Solomon B, Soulen M, Baum R, et al. Chemoembolization of hepatocellular carcinoma with cisplatin, doxorubicin, mitomycin-C, Ethiodol, and polyvinyl alcohol: prospective evaluation of response and survival in a US population. *J Vasc Interv Radiol* 1999;10:793–798.
83. Extra J, Marty M, Brienza S, et al. Pharmacokinetics and safety profile of oxaliplatin. *Semin Oncol* 1998;25:13–22.
84. Brienza S, Vignoud J, Itzhaki M, et al. Oxaliplatin (L-OHP): global safety in 682 patients. *Proc Am Soc Clin Oncol* 1995;14:209.
85. André T, Boni C, Mounedji-Boudiaf L, et al. Oxaliplatin, fluorouracil, and leucovorin as adjuvant treatment for colon cancer. *N Engl J Med* 2004;350:2343–2351.

19 Antimetabolites

M. Wasif Saif and Edward Chu

ANTIFOLATES

Reduced folates play a key role in one-carbon metabolism, and they are essential for the biosynthesis of purines, thymidylate, and protein biosynthesis. Aminopterin was the first antimetabolite with documented clinical activity in the treatment of children with acute leukemia in the 1940s. This antifolate analog was subsequently replaced by methotrexate (MTX), the 4-amino, 10-methyl analog of folic acid, which remains the most widely used antifolate analog, with activity against a wide range of cancers (Table 19.1), including hematologic malignancies (acute lymphoblastic leukemia and non-Hodgkin's lymphoma) and many solid tumors (breast cancer, head and neck cancer, osteogenic sarcoma, bladder cancer, and gestational trophoblastic cancer).

Pemetrexed is a pyrrolopyrimidine, multitargeted antifolate analog that targets multiple enzymes involved in folate metabolism, including thymidylate synthase (TS), dihydrofolate reductase (DHFR), glycinamide ribonucleotide (GAR) formyltransferase, and aminoimidazole carboxamide (AICAR) formyltransferase.[1,2] This agent has broad-spectrum activity against solid tumors, including malignant mesothelioma and breast, pancreatic, head and neck, non–small-cell lung, colon, gastric, cervical, and bladder cancers.[3–5]

The third antifolate compound to have entered clinical practice is pralatrexate (10-propargyl-10-deazaaminopterin), a 10-deazaaminopterin antifolate that was rationally designed to bind with higher affinity to the reduced folate carrier (RFC)-1 transport protein, when compared with MTX, leading to enhanced membrane transport into tumor cells. It is also an improved substrate for the enzyme folylpolyglutamyl synthetase (FPGS), resulting in enhanced formation of cytotoxic polyglutamate metabolites.[6,7] When compared with MTX, this analog is a more potent inhibitor of multiple enzymes involved in folate metabolism, including TS, DHFR, and GAR and AICAR formyltransferases. This agent is presently approved for the treatment of relapsed or refractory peripheral T-cell lymphomas.[8]

Mechanism of Action

The antifolate compounds are tight-binding inhibitors of DHFR, a key enzyme in folate metabolism.[1] DHFR plays a pivotal role in maintaining the intracellular folate pools in their fully reduced form as tetrahydrofolates, and these compounds serve as one-carbon carriers required for the synthesis of thymidylate, purine nucleotides, and certain amino acids.

The cytotoxic effects of MTX, pemetrexed, and pralatrexate are mediated by their respective polyglutamate metabolites, with up to 5 to 7 glutamyl groups in a γ-peptide linkage. These polyglutamate metabolites exhibit prolonged intracellular half-lives, thereby allowing for prolonged drug action in tumor cells. Moreover, these polyglutamate metabolites are potent, direct inhibitors of several folate-dependent enzymes, including DHFR, TS, AICAR formyltransferase, and GAR formyltransferase.[1]

Mechanisms of Resistance

The development of cellular resistance to antifolates remains a major obstacle to its clinical efficacy.[9,10] In experimental systems, resistance to antifolates arises from several mechanisms, including an alteration in antifolate transport because of either a defect in the reduced folate carrier or folate receptor systems, decreased capacity to polyglutamate the antifolate parent compound through either decreased expression of FPGS or increased expression of the catabolic enzyme γ-glutamyl hydrolase, and alterations in the target enzymes DHFR and/or TS through increased expression of wild-type protein or overexpression of a mutant protein with reduced binding affinity for the antifolate. Gene amplification is a common resistance mechanism observed in various experimental systems, including tumor samples from patients. In in vitro and in vivo experimental model systems, the levels of DHFR and/or TS protein acutely increase after exposure to MTX and other antifolate compounds. This acute induction of target protein in response to drug exposure is mediated, in part, by a translational regulatory mechanism, which may represent a clinically relevant mechanism for the acute development of cellular drug resistance.

Clinical Pharmacology

The oral bioavailability of MTX is saturable and erratic at doses greater than 25 mg/m^2. MTX is completely absorbed from parenteral routes of administration, and peak serum levels are achieved within 30 to 60 minutes of administration.

The distribution of MTX into third-space fluid collections, such as pleural effusions and ascitic fluid, can substantially alter MTX pharmacokinetics. The slow release of accumulated MTX from these third spaces over time prolongs the terminal half-life of the drug, leading to potentially increased clinical toxicity. It is advisable to evacuate these fluid collections before treatment and monitor plasma drug concentrations closely.

Renal excretion is the main route of drug elimination, and this process is mediated by glomerular filtration and tubular secretion. About 80% to 90% of an administered dose is eliminated unchanged in the urine. Doses of MTX, therefore, should be reduced in proportion to reductions in creatinine clearance. Renal excretion of MTX is inhibited by probenecid, penicillins, cephalosporins, aspirin, and nonsteroidal anti-inflammatory drugs.

Pemetrexed enters the cell via the RFC system and, to a lesser extent, by the folate receptor protein. As with MTX, it undergoes polyglutamation within the cell to the pentaglutamate form, which is at least 60-fold more potent than the parent compound. This agent is mainly cleared by renal excretion, and in the setting of renal dysfunction, the terminal drug half-life is significantly prolonged to up to 20 hours. Pemetrexed, therefore, should be used with caution in patients with renal dysfunction. In addition, renal excretion is inhibited in the presence of other agents including probenecid, penicillins, cephalosporins, aspirin, and nonsteroidal anti-inflammatory drugs.

TABLE 19.1

Antimetabolites: Indications, Doses and Schedules, and Toxicities

Drug	Main Therapeutic Uses	Main Doses and Schedule	Major Toxicities
Methotrexate	Non-Hodgkin's lymphoma Primary CNS lymphoma Acute lymphoblastic leukemia Breast cancer Bladder cancer Osteogenic sarcoma Gestational trophoblastic cancer	Low dose: 10–50 mg/m^2 IV every 3–4 weeks Low dose weekly: 25 mg/m^2 IV weekly Moderate dose: 100–500 m/m^2 IV every 2–3 weeks High dose: 1–12 gm/m^2 IV over a 3- to 24-hour period every 1–3 weeks Intrathecal (IT): 10–15 mg IT 2 times weekly until CSF is clear, then weekly dose for 2–6 weeks, followed by monthly dose	Mucositis, diarrhea, myelosuppression, acute renal failure, transient elevations in serum transaminases and bilirubin, pneumonitis, neurologic toxicity
Pemetrexed	Mesothelioma Non–small-cell lung cancer	500 mg/m^2 IV, every 3 weeks	Myelosuppression, skin rash, mucositis, diarrhea, fatigue
Pralatrexate	Peripheral T-cell lymphoma	30 mg/m^2 IV, weekly for 6 weeks; cycles repeated every 7 weeks	Myelosuppression, skin rash, mucositis, diarrhea, elevation of serum transaminases and bilirubin, mild nausea/vomiting
5-Fluorouracil	Breast cancer Colorectal cancer Anal cancer Gastroesophageal cancer Hepatocellular cancer Pancreatic cancer Head and neck cancer	Bolus monthly schedule: 425–450 mg/m^2 IV on days 1–5 every 28 days Bolus weekly schedule: 500–600 mg/m^2 IV every week for 6 weeks every 8 weeks Infusion schedule: 2,400–3,000 mg/m^2 IV over 46 hours every 2 weeks 120-hour infusion: 1,000 mg/m^2/d IV on days 1–5 every 21–28 d Protracted continuous infusion: 200–400 mg/m^2/d IV	Nausea/vomiting, diarrhea, mucositis, myelosuppression, neurotoxicity, coronary artery vasospasm, conjunctivitis
Capecitabine	Breast cancer Colorectal cancer Gastroesophageal cancer Hepatocellular cancer Pancreatic cancer	Recommended dose for monotherapy is 1,250 mg/m^2 PO bid for 2 weeks with 1 wk rest May decrease dose of capecitabine to 850–1,000 mg/m^2 bid on days 1–14 to reduce risk of toxicity without compromising efficacy An alternative dosing schedule for monotherapy is 1,250–1,500 mg/m^2 PO bid for 1 week on and 1 week off; this schedule appears to be well tolerated, with no compromise in clinical efficacy Capecitabine should be used at lower doses (850–1,000 mg/m^2 bid on days 1–14) when used in combination with other cytotoxic agents, such as oxaliplatin and lapatinib	Diarrhea, hand-foot syndrome, myelosuppression, mucositis, nausea/vomiting, neurologic toxicity, coronary artery vasospasm
Cytarabine	Hodgkin's lymphoma Non-Hodgkin's lymphoma Acute myelogenous leukemia Acute lymphoblastic leukemia	Standard dose: 100 mg/m^2/day IV on days 1–7 as a continuous IV infusion, in combination with an anthracycline as induction chemotherapy for acute myelogenous leukemia High-dose: 1.5–3.0 gm/m^2 IV q 12 hours for 3 days as a high dose, intensification regimen for acute myelogenous leukemia SC: 20 mg/m^2 SC for 10 days per month for 6 months, associated with IFN-α for treatment of chronic myelogenous leukemia IT: 10–30 mg IT up to 3 times weekly in the treatment of leptomeningeal carcinomatosis secondary to leukemia or lymphoma.	Nausea/vomiting, myelosuppression, cerebellar ataxia, lethargy, confusion, acute pancreatitis, drug infusion reaction, hand-foot syndrome High-dose therapy: noncardiogenic pulmonary edema, acute respiratory distress and *Streptococcus viridans* pneumonia, conjunctivitis, and keratitis
Gemcitabine	Pancreatic cancer Non–small-cell lung cancer Breast cancer Bladder cancer Hodgkin's lymphoma Ovarian cancer Soft tissue sarcoma	Pancreatic cancer: 1,000 mg/m^2 IV every week for 7 weeks with 1 week rest Treatment then continues weekly for 3 weeks followed by 1 week off Bladder cancer: 1,000 mg/m^2 IV on days 1, 8, and 15 every 28 days Non–small-cell lung cancer: 1,000-1,200 mg/m^2 IV on days 1 and 8 every 21 days	Nausea/vomiting, myelosuppression, flulike syndrome, elevation of serum transaminases and bilirubin, pneumonitis, infusion reaction, mild proteinuria, and rarely, hemolytic-uremic syndrome and thrombotic thrombocytopenic purpura

(continued)

TABLE 19.1

Antimetabolites: Indications, Doses and Schedules, and Toxicities *(continued)*

Drug	Main Therapeutic Uses	Main Doses and Schedule	Major Toxicities
6-Mercaptopurine	Acute lymphoblastic leukemia	Induction therapy: 2.5 mg/kg PO daily Maintenance therapy: 1.5–2.5 mg/kg PO daily	Myelosuppression, nausea/vomiting, mucositis and diarrhea, hepatotoxicity, immunosuppression
6-Thioguanine	Acute myelogenous leukemia Acute lymphoblastic leukemia	Induction: 100 mg/m^2 PO every 12 hours on days 1–5, usually in combination with cytarabine Maintenance: 100 mg/m^2 PO every 12 hours on days 1–5, every 4 weeks, usually in combination with other agents Single agent: 1–3 mg/kg PO daily	Myelosuppression, nausea/vomiting, mucositis and diarrhea, hepatotoxicity, immunosuppression
Fludarabine	Chronic lymphocytic leukemia Non-Hodgkin's lymphoma	25 mg/m^2 IV on days 1–5 every 28 days For oral usage, the recommended dose is 40 mg/m^2 PO on days 1–5 every 28 days	Myelosuppression, immunosuppression with increased risk of opportunistic infections, mild nausea/vomiting, hypersensitivity reaction
Cladribine	Hairy cell leukemia Chronic lymphocytic leukemia Non-Hodgkin's lymphoma	Usual dose is 0.09 mg/kg/d IV via continuous infusion for 7 days; one course is usually administered	Myelosuppression, immunosuppression, mild nausea/vomiting, fever
Clofarabine	Acute lymphoblastic leukemia	52 mg/m^2 IV daily for 5 days every 2–6 weeks	Myelosuppression nausea/vomiting, diarrhea, systemic inflammatory response syndrome, increased risk of opportunistic infections, renal toxicity

CNS, central nervous system; IV, intravenously; CSF, cerebrospinal fluid; PO, by mouth; bid, twice daily; SC, subcutaneously; IFN-α, interferon alpha.

As with other antifolate analogs, pralatrexate is transported into the cell by the RFC carrier protein and then metabolized by FPGS to form longer chain polyglutamates, with up to four additional glutamate residues attached to the parent molecule. About 34% of the parent drug is cleared in the urine during the first 24 hours after drug administration. As such, caution is advised when using pralatrexate in patients with renal dysfunction. As with MTX and pemetrexed, the concomitant administration of other agents such as probenecid, penicillins, cephalosporins, aspirin, and nonsteroidal anti-inflammatory drugs, may inhibit renal clearance.

Toxicity

The main side effects of MTX are myelosuppression and gastrointestinal (GI) toxicity, which are usually completely reversed within 14 days, unless drug-elimination mechanisms are impaired. In patients with compromised renal function, even small doses of MTX may result in serious toxicity. MTX-induced nephrotoxicity is thought to result from the intratubular precipitation of MTX and its metabolites in acidic urine. Antifolates may also exert a direct toxic effect on the renal tubules. Vigorous hydration and urinary alkalinization have greatly reduced the incidence of renal failure in patients on high-dose regimens. Acute elevations in hepatic enzyme levels and hyperbilirubinemia are often observed during high-dose therapy, but these levels usually return to normal within 10 days. Methotrexate given concomitantly with radiotherapy may increase the risk of soft tissue necrosis and osteonecrosis.

The original rationale for high-dose MTX therapy was based on the concept of selective rescue of normal tissues by the reduced folate leucovorin (LV). However, recent data suggest that high-dose MTX may also overcome resistance mechanisms caused by impaired active transport, decreased affinity of DHFR for MTX, increased levels of DHFR resulting from gene amplification, and/or decreased polyglutamation of MTX.

The main toxicities of pemetrexed and pralatrexate include dose limiting myelosuppression, mucositis, and skin rash, usually in the form of the hand-foot syndrome (HFS). Other toxicities include reversible transaminasemia, anorexia and fatigue syndrome, and GI toxicity. These side effects are reduced by supplementation with folic acid (350 μg orally daily) and vitamin B_{12} (1,000 mg subcutaneously given at least 1 week before starting therapy, and then repeated every three cycles). To date, there is no evidence to suggest that vitamin supplementation adversely affects the clinical efficacy of pemetrexed or pralatrexate.

5-FLUOROPYRIMIDINES

The fluoropyrimidine, 5-fluorouracil (5-FU) was synthesized by Charles Heidelberger in the mid 1950s. Uracil is a normal component of RNA; as such, the rationale leading to the development of the drug was that cancer cells might be more sensitive to *decoy* molecules that mimic the natural compound than normal cells. 5-FU and its derivatives are an integral part of treatment for a broad range of solid tumors (see Table 19.1), including GI malignancies (esophageal, gastric, pancreatic, colorectal, anal, and hepatocellular cancers), breast, head and neck, and skin cancers.[11] It continues to serve as the main backbone for combination regimens used to treat metastatic colorectal cancer (mCRC) and as adjuvant therapy of early-stage colon cancer.

Mechanism of Action

5-FU enters cells via the facilitated uracil base transport mechanism and is then anabolized to various cytotoxic nucleotide forms

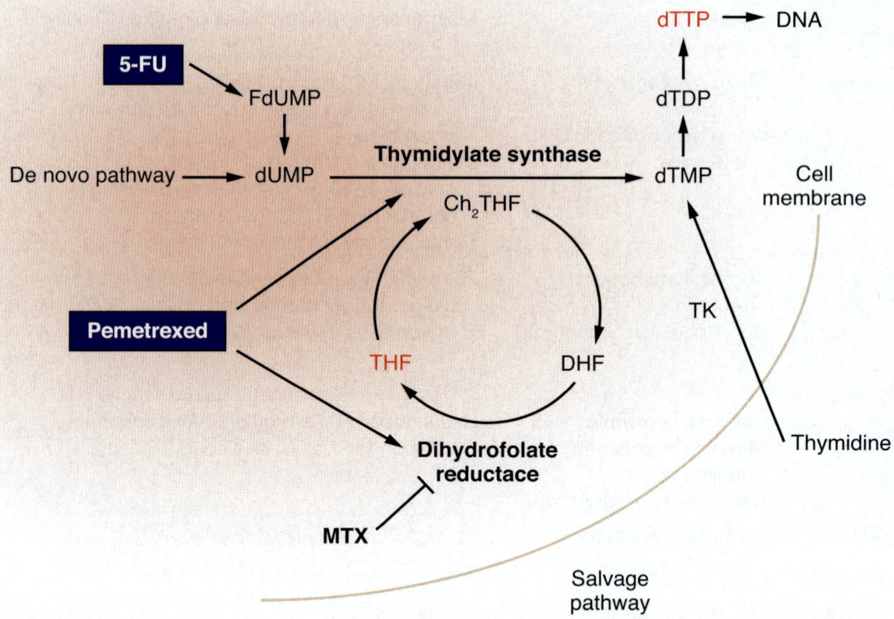

Figure 19.1 Antifolates and 5-fluorouracil (5-FU) sites of action. FdUMP, fluorodeoxyuridine monophosphate; dUMP, deoxyuridine monophosphate; dTTP, deoxythymidine triphosphate; dTDP, deoxyuridine diphosphate; dTMP, deoxythymidine monophosphate; TK, thymidine kinase; CH_2THF, 5,10-methylenetetrahydrofolate; THF, tetrahydrofolate; DHF, dihydrofolate.

by several biochemical pathways. It is thought that 5-FU exerts its cytotoxic effects through various mechanisms, including (1) the inhibition of TS, (2) incorporation into RNA, and (3) incorporation into DNA (Fig. 19.1). In addition to these mechanisms, the genotoxic stress resulting from TS inhibition may also activate programmed cell-death pathways in susceptible cells, which leads to the induction of parental DNA fragmentation.

Mechanisms of Resistance

Several resistance mechanisms to 5-FU have been identified in experimental and clinical settings. Alterations in the target enzyme TS represent the most commonly described mechanism of resistance. In vitro, in vivo, and clinical studies have documented a strong correlation between the levels of TS enzyme activity/TS protein and chemosensitivity to 5-FU. In this regard, cell lines and tumors with higher levels of TS are relatively more resistant to 5-FU. Mutations in the TS protein have been identified that lead to reduced binding affinity of the 5-FU metabolite fluorodeoxyuridine monophosphate (FdUMP) to the TS protein. Reduced expression and/or diminished activity of key activating enzymes may interfere with the formation of cytotoxic 5-FU metabolites. Decreased expression of mismatch repair enzymes, such as human mutL homolog 1 (hMLH1) and human mutS homolog 2 (hMSH2), and increased expression of the catabolic enzyme dihydropyrimidine dehydrogenase (DPD) are associated with fluoropyrimidine resistance. At this time, the relative contribution of each of these mechanisms in the development of cellular resistance to 5-FU in the actual clinical setting remains unclear.

Clinical Pharmacology

5-FU is not orally administered, given its erratic bioavailability resulting from high levels of the catabolic enzyme DPD present in the gut mucosa. After intravenous bolus doses, metabolic elimination is rapid, with a half-life of 8 to 14 minutes. More than 85% of an administered dose of 5-FU is enzymatically inactivated by DPD, the rate-limiting enzyme in the catabolism of 5-FU.

A pharmacogenetic syndrome has been identified in which partial or compete deficiency in the DPD enzyme is present in 3% to 5% and 0.1% of the general population, respectively. As DPD catalyzes the rate-limiting step in the catabolic pathway of 5-FU, a deficiency of DPD can result in a clinically dangerous increase in the anabolic products of 5-FU. Unfortunately, patients with DPD deficiency do not manifest a phenotype only until they are treated with 5-FU, and in that setting, they can develop severe GI toxicity in the form of mucositis and/or diarrhea, myelosuppression, neurologic toxicity, and in rare cases, death. In patients being treated with 5-FU or any other fluoropyrimidine, it is important to consider DPD deficiency in patients who present with excessive, severe toxicity.[12] It is now increasingly appreciated that DPD mutations are unable to account for all of the observed cases of excessive 5-FU toxicity, because up to 50% of patients who experience 5-FU toxicity will have no documented alterations in the *DPD* gene. Moreover, individuals with normal DPD enzyme activity may be diagnosed with high plasma levels of 5-FU, resulting in increased toxicity. Although DPD enzyme activity can be assayed from peripheral blood mononuclear cells in a specialized laboratory, routine phenotypic and genotypic screenings for DPD deficiency prior to 5-FU therapy are not yet available.

Biomodulation of 5-FU

Significant efforts have focused on enhancing the antitumor activity of 5-FU through biochemical modulation in which 5-FU is combined with various agents, including leucovorin, MTX, N-phosphonacetyl-L-aspartic acid, interferon-α, interferon-γ, and

TABLE 19.2

Toxicities of Different Forms of 5-FU

Route	Schedule	Dose	DLT
IV	Daily × 5, bolus	400–500 (mg/m²/d)	⇓ BM D M
IV	Weekly bolus	450–500 (mg/m²/d)	⇓ BM
IV	Daily × 5, CI	750–1,000 (mg/m²/d)	M D
IV	PCI	200–400 (mg/m²/d)	M HFS
HAI	Daily × 14–21, CI	750–1,000 (mg/m²/d)	M D
IP	32–120 hr	5 nM	M D
Oral (Xeloda)	14–21 d	2,000–2,500 (mg/m²/d)	HFS

DLT, dose limiting toxicity; IV, intravenous; BM, bone marrow; D, diarrhea; M, mucositis; CI, continuous infusion; PCI, protracted continuous infusion; HFS, hand-foot syndrome; HAI, hepatic artery infusion; IP, intraperitoneal.

a whole host of other agents.[13] For the past 20 to 25 years, the reduced folate LV has been the main biochemical modulator of 5-FU. An alternative approach has been to alter the schedule of 5-FU administration. Given the S-phase specificity of this agent, prolonged exposure of tumor cells to 5-FU would increase the fraction of cells being exposed to the drug. Overall response rates are significantly higher in patients treated with infusional schedules of 5-FU than in those treated with bolus 5-FU, and this improvement in response rate has translated into an improved progression-free survival. Moreover, the overall safety profile is improved with infusional regimens. A hybrid schedule of bolus and infusional 5-FU was originally developed in France, and this regimen has shown superior clinical activity compared with bolus 5-FU schedules. This hybrid schedule has now been simplified by using only the 46-hour infusion of 5-FU and completely eliminating the 5-FU bolus doses.

Toxicity

The spectrum of 5-FU toxicity is dose- and schedule-dependent (Table 19.2). The main side effects are diarrhea, mucositis, and myelosuppression. The dermatologic HFS is more commonly observed with infusional 5-FU therapy. Acute neurologic symptoms have also been reported, and they include somnolence, cerebellar ataxia, and upper motor signs. Treatment with 5-FU can, on rare occasions, cause coronary vasospasm, resulting in a syndrome of chest pain, cardiac enzyme elevations, and electrocardiographic changes. Cardiac toxicity seems to be related more to infusional 5-FU than bolus administration.[14]

CAPECITABINE

Capecitabine is an oral fluoropyrimidine carbamate that was rationally designed to allow for selective 5-FU activation in tumor tissue.[15] This oral agent was initially approved in anthracycline- and taxane-resistant breast cancer and subsequently approved for use in combination with docetaxel as second-line therapy in metastatic breast cancer and in combination with lapatinib, a tyrosine-kinase inhibitor of human epidermal growth factor receptor type 2 (HER2) and epidermal growth factor receptor (EGFR) in women with HER2-positive metastatic breast cancer following progression on trastuzumab-based therapy.[16] This agent is also approved by the U.S. Food and Drug Administration (FDA) for the first-line treatment of mCRC and as adjuvant therapy for stage III colon cancer when fluoropyrimidine therapy alone is preferred.[17] In Europe and throughout much of the world, the combination of capecitabine plus oxaliplatin (XELOX) is approved for the treatment of mCRC as well as for the adjuvant therapy of stage III colon cancer.[18] In addition, recent studies have documented the noninferiority of capecitabine to 5-FU when combined with cisplatin in the treatment of metastatic gastric cancer.

Clinical Pharmacology

Capecitabine is rapidly and extensively absorbed by the gut mucosa, with nearly 80% oral bioavailability. It is inactive in its parent form and undergoes enzymatic conversion via three successive steps. Of note, the third and final step occurs in tumor tissue and involves the conversion of 5′-deoxy-5-fluorouridine to 5-FU by the enzyme thymidine phosphorylase (TP), which is expressed at much higher levels in tumors when compared with corresponding normal tissue. Capecitabine and capecitabine metabolites are primarily excreted by the kidneys, and in contrast to 5-FU, caution must be taken in the presence of renal dysfunction, with appropriate dose modification. The use of capecitabine is absolutely contraindicated in patients whose creatinine clearance is less than 30 mL per minute. The FDA and Roche have added a black box warning and strengthened the precautions section on the capecitabine label about the drug–drug interaction between warfarin and capecitabine-based chemotherapy. It is generally recommended to do weekly monitoring of the coagulation parameters (prothrombin time/international normalized ratio [PT/INR]) for all patients receiving concomitant warfarin and capecitabine, with an appropriate adjustment of warfarin dose.

Toxicity

Similar to what is observed with infusional 5-FU, the main side effects of capecitabine include diarrhea and HFS. Of note, the incidence of myelosuppression, neutropenic fever, mucositis, alopecia, and nausea/vomiting is lower with capecitabine when compared with 5-FU. Elevations in indirect serum bilirubin can be observed, but are usually transient and clinically asymptomatic. Patients in the United States appear to be unable to tolerate as high doses of capecitabine as European patients, either as monotherapy or in combination with other cytotoxic chemotherapy.[19] Although the underlying reasons for this discrepancy are not known, it may in part be related to the increased fortification of the US diet with folate and the increased focus on vitamin and folic acid supplementation.

S-1

S-1 is an oral fluoropyrimidine that consists of tegafur (FT), a prodrug of 5-FU, combined with two 5-FU biochemical modulators: 5-chloro-2,4-dihydroxypyridine (gimeracil or CDHP), a competitive inhibitor of DPD, and oteracil potassium, which inhibits phosphorylation of 5-flurouracil in the GI tract, thereby decreasing serious GI toxicities such as nausea/vomiting, mucositis, and diarrhea.[20] As with other oral agents, S-1 offers several advantages over 5-FU, including ease of administration, no risks associated with use of central venous access such as infection, thrombosis, etc., and reduced toxicities, especially neurotoxicity. Although S-1 has yet to be approved by the FDA, it has been approved for the treatment of gastric cancer, head and neck, colorectal cancer (CRC), non–small-cell lung, breast, pancreatic, and biliary tract cancers in several countries in Asia and for the treatment of advanced gastric cancer in combination with cisplatin in a large number of European countries.

Clinical Pharmacology

S-1 was designed to provide continuous 5-FU plasma exposure comparable to the intravenous (IV) infusion. FT, the 5-FU prodrug, is absorbed in the small intestine and converted to 5-FU through the liver microsomal P-450 metabolizing enzyme system (CYP2A6). Most of the 5-FU is degraded (85%) by DPD, leading to the formation of fluoro-beta-alanine (FBAL).[21] CDHP inhibits DPD, thus allowing higher concentrations of 5-FU to enter the anabolic pathway and enhance its therapeutic effect. Additionally, the inhibition of DPD leads to a decreased amount of FBAL formation, which presumably leads to reduced neurotoxicity. Oteracil is the final component of the S-1 formulation, and it inhibits orotate phosphoribosyltransferase in the GI mucosa, which prevents the formation of fluorouridine monophosphate (FUMP), thereby decreasing GI toxicity.

The maximum tolerated dose was established at 80 mg/m^2 in two divided doses for a Japanese population and 25 mg/m^2 twice a day for a Caucasian population. This interethnic variability of S-1 pharmacokinetics and pharmacodynamics has been attributed to differences in the CYP2A6 genotypes.[22] Studies have demonstrated a high frequency of allelic variants CYP2A6*4, *7, and *9 in East Asians than in Caucasians, which might be associated with reduced enzymatic activity and decreased activation of FT. On the other hand, higher FT metabolism is seen in Caucasian patients due to higher CYP2A6 activity. However, investigators have established similar 5-FU exposure between these two ethnic groups. These findings were explained by higher CDHP exposure in Asians, resulting in increased DPD inhibition and slower catabolism of 5-FU, despite having low CYP2A6 activity, whereas Caucasians had higher CYP2A6 activity but faster 5-FU clearance.

Clinical Toxicity

Clinical studies have shown that the GI toxicities associated with S-1, such as diarrhea, nausea, vomiting, and hyperbilirubinemia, are more prominent in Western patients, whereas hematologic toxicities are more prevalent in Japanese patients. The difference in safety profile cannot be explained by differences in 5-FU exposure, because pharmacokinetic studies have shown that overall drug exposures are similar. A potential explanation might involve interethnic variations in TS promoter enhancer region polymorphisms, which are more frequently seen in Asians or in Caucasians on a higher folate diet.

CYTARABINE

Cytarabine (ara-C) is a deoxycytidine nucleoside analog isolated from the sponge *Cryptotethya crypta*, and it differs from its physiologic counterpart by virtue of a stereotypic inversion of the 2′-hydroxyl group of the sugar moiety.[23] A regimen of ara-C, combined with an anthracycline and given as a 5- or 7-day continuous infusion, is considered the standard induction treatment for acute myeloid leukemia (AML). Ara-C is active against other hematologic malignancies, such as non-Hodgkin's lymphoma, chronic myelogenous leukemia, and acute lymphocytic leukemia (see Table 19.1). However, this agent has absolutely no activity against solid tumors.

Mechanism of Action

Ara-C enters cells via nucleoside transport proteins, the most important one being the equilibrative inhibitor-sensitive (ES) receptor. Once inside the cell, ara-C requires activation for its cytotoxic effects.[23,24] The first metabolic step is the conversion of ara-C to the monophosphate form ara-cytidine monophosphate (ara-CMP) by the enzyme deoxycytidine kinase (dCK) with subsequent phosphorylation to the di- and triphosphate metabolites, respectively. Ara-cytidine triphosphate (ara-CTP) is a potent inhibitor of DNA polymerases α, β, and γ, which in turn interferes with DNA chain elongation, DNA synthesis, and DNA repair. Ara-CTP is also incorporated directly into DNA and functions as a DNA chain terminator, interfering with chain elongation. Catabolism of ara-C involves two key enzymes, cytidine deaminase and deoxycytidylate deaminase. These breakdown enzymes convert ara-C and ara-CMP into the inactive metabolites, ara-uridine (ara-U) and ara-uridine monophosphate (ara-UMP), respectively. The balance between intracellular activation and degradation is critical in determining the amount of drug that is ultimately converted to ara-CTP and, thus, its subsequent cytotoxic and antitumor activity.

Mechanisms of Resistance

Several resistance mechanisms to ara-C have been described. An impaired transmembrane transport, a decreased rate of anabolism, and an increased rate of catabolism may result in the development of ara-C resistance.[23,25,26] The level of cytidine deaminase enzyme activity has been shown to correlate with clinical response in patients with AML undergoing induction chemotherapy with ara-C–containing regimens.

Clinical Pharmacology

Ara-C has poor oral bioavailability given its extensive deamination within the GI tract. Thus, ara-C is administered intravenously via continuous infusion. After administration, ara-C undergoes extensive metabolism in the liver, plasma, and peripheral tissues. Within 24 hours, up to 80% of drug is recovered in the urine as the ara-U metabolite. Ara-C crosses the blood–brain barrier when used at high doses, with cerebrospinal fluid levels between 7% and 14% of plasma levels and reaching peak levels of up to 10 μM.

Toxicity

The toxicity profile of ara-C is highly dependent on the dose and schedule of administration. Myelosuppression is dose-limiting with a standard 7-day regimen. Leukopenia and thrombocytopenia are observed most frequently, with nadirs occurring between days 7 and 14 after drug administration. GI toxicity commonly manifests as a mild-to-moderate degree of anorexia, nausea, and vomiting along with mucositis, diarrhea, and abdominal pain. In rare cases, acute pancreatitis has been observed. The ara-C syndrome has been described in pediatric patients with hematologic malignancies, usually begins within 12 hours after the start of drug infusion, and is characterized by fever, myalgia, bone pain, maculopapular rash, conjunctivitis, malaise, and occasional chest pain.

The administration of ara-C at high doses (2 to 3 g/m^2 with each dose) is associated with profound myelosuppression.[27] Severe GI toxicity in the form of mucositis and/or diarrhea is also observed. Neurologic toxicity is significantly more common with high-dose ara-C than with standard doses, and presents with seizures, cerebral and cerebellar dysfunction, and peripheral neuropathy. Clinical signs of cerebellar dysfunction occur in up to 15% of patients and include dysarthria, dysmetria, and ataxia. Change in alertness and cognitive ability, memory loss, and frontal lobe release signs reflect cerebral toxicity. Despite discontinuation of therapy, clinical recovery is incomplete in up to 30% of affected patients. Pulmonary complications may include noncardiogenic pulmonary edema, acute respiratory distress, and pneumonia, resulting from *Streptococcus viridans* infection. Other side effects associated with high-dose ara-C include conjunctivitis (often responsive to topical corticosteroids), a painful HFS, and rarely, anaphylactic reactions.

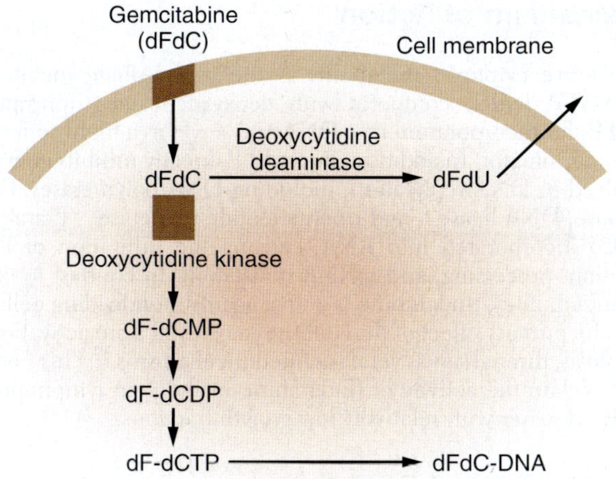

Figure 19.2 Transport and metabolism of gemcitabine. dFdC, gemcitabine; dFdU, 2′,2′-difluorodeoxyuridine; dF-dCMP, gemcitabine monophosphate; dF-dCDP, gemcitabine diphosphate; dF-dCTP, gemcitabine triphosphate.

GEMCITABINE

Gemcitabine (2′,2′-difluorodeoxycytidine) is a difluorinated deoxycytidine analog. Despite its similarity in structure, metabolism, and mechanism of action to ara-C, the spectrum of antitumor activity of gemcitabine is much broader.[23,28] This compound has significant clinical activity against several human solid tumors, including pancreatic, bile duct, gall bladder, small cell and non–small-cell lung, bladder, ovary, and breast cancers as well as hematologic malignancies, namely Hodgkin's and non-Hodgkin's lymphoma (see Table 19.1).

Mechanism of Action

The transport of gemcitabine into cells requires the nucleoside transporter system. Gemcitabine is inactive in its parent form and requires intracellular activation for its cytotoxic effects. The steps involved in the metabolic activation of gemcitabine are similar to those observed with ara-C, with both drugs being activated by the same enzymatic machinery to the active triphosphate metabolite (see Fig. 19.2). Gemcitabine triphosphate is then incorporated into DNA, resulting in chain termination and the inhibition of DNA synthesis and function, or the triphosphate form can directly inhibit DNA polymerases α, β, and γ, which in turn, interferes with DNA chain elongation, DNA synthesis, and DNA repair. The triphosphate metabolite is also a potent inhibitor of ribonucleotide reductase, which further mediates inhibition of DNA biosynthesis by reducing the levels of key deoxynucleotide pools.[29]

Mechanisms of Resistance

Several mechanisms of resistance to gemcitabine have been described in various preclinical experimental models.[30] Gemcitabine is a polar nucleoside analog that requires the activity of human equilibrative nucleoside transporter 1 (hENT1) to enter cells and exert its cytotoxic effects. Preclinical data in human pancreatic cancer cell lines showed that gemcitabine resistance is negatively correlated with hENT1 expression and can be induced by specific inhibitors of hENT1.[31] Clinical data also support the concept that a lack of hENT1 may be predictive of resistance to gemcitabine. CO-101, a lipid-drug conjugate of gemcitabine, was rationally designed to enter cells independently of hENT1. Unfortunately, two studies in pancreatic cancer failed to show any benefit of CO-101.

Additionally, several enzymes involved in the intracellular metabolism of gemcitabine have been implicated in the development of cellular drug resistance, including reduced expression and/or deficiency in dCK enzyme activity as well as increased expression and/or activity of the catabolic enzymes cytidine deaminase and dCMP deaminase. Recent studies have also identified a subset of CD44-positive cancer stem cells within pancreatic tumors that sustain tumor formation and growth, and are resistant to gemcitabine therapy.[33]

Clinical Pharmacology

Gemcitabine is administered via the intravenous route, typically over a 30-minute intravenous infusion, and it undergoes extensive metabolism by deamination to the catabolic metabolite, difluorodeoxyuridine (dFdU), with more than 90% of the metabolized drug being recovered in urine. Plasma clearance is about 30% lower in women and in elderly patients, and this pharmacokinetic difference may result in an increased risk of toxicity in these respective patient populations. The initial findings from pilot pharmacokinetic studies suggested that gemcitabine, when given at a fixed dose rate (FDR) intravenous infusion of 10 mg/m^2 per minute, produced the highest accumulation of active dFdCTP metabolites in peripheral blood mononuclear cells, which led to a randomized phase II trial that compared gemcitabine 1,500 mg/m^2 by FDR or 2,200 mg/m^2 of gemcitabine over 30 minutes. Although this phase II study suggested an improved overall survival with FDR, a subsequent phase III trial failed to confirm the survival advantage of gemcitabine by FDR over its conventional administration schedule.[34]

Toxicity

Gemcitabine is a relatively well-tolerated drug when used as a single agent. The main dose-limiting toxicity is myelosuppression, with neutropenia more commonly experienced than thrombocytopenia. Toxicity is schedule dependent, with longer infusions producing greater hematologic toxicity. Transient flulike symptoms, including fever, headache, arthralgias, and myalgias, occur in 45% of patients. Asthenia and transient transaminasemia may occur. Renal microangiopathy syndromes, including hemolytic-uremic syndrome and thrombotic thrombocytopenic purpura, have been reported rarely.

6-THIOPURINES

The development of the purine analogs in cancer chemotherapy began in the early 1950s with the synthesis of the thiopurines, 6-mercaptopurine (6-MP) and 6-thioguanine (6-TG). 6-MP has an important role in maintenance therapy for acute lymphoblastic leukemia, whereas 6-TG is active in remission induction and in maintenance therapy for AML (see Table 19.1).

Mechanism of Action

The thiopurines, 6-MP and 6-TG, act similarly with respect to their cellular biochemistry.[34] In their respective monophosphate nucleotide forms, they inhibit enzymes involved in de novo purine synthesis and purine interconversion reactions. The triphosphate nucleotide forms can get directly incorporated into either cellular RNA or DNA, leading to the inhibition of RNA and DNA synthesis and function, respectively.

Mechanisms of Resistance

The development of cellular resistance to 6-thiopurines results from a decreased level of key cytotoxic nucleotide metabolites, either through decreased formation or increased breakdown. Resistant cells have been identified that express either complete or partial deficiency of the activating enzyme hypoxanthine-guanine phosphoribosyltransferase (HGPRT). In clinical samples derived from patients with AML, drug resistance has been associated with increased concentrations of a membrane-bound alkaline phosphatase or a conjugating enzyme, 6-thiopurine methyltransferase (TPMT), the end-result being reduced formation of cytotoxic thiopurine nucleotides. Finally, the decreased expression of mismatch repair enzymes, including hMLH1 and hMSH2, has been associated with cellular drug resistance.

Clinical Pharmacology

Oral absorption of 6-MP is highly erratic, and the relatively poor oral bioavailability is mainly related to rapid first-pass metabolism in the liver. The major route of drug elimination is via metabolism by several enzymatic pathways. 6-MP is oxidized to the inactive metabolite 6-thiouric acid by xanthine oxidase. Enhanced 6-MP toxicity may result from the concomitant administration of 6-MP and the xanthine oxidase inhibitor allopurinol. In patients receiving both 6-MP and allopurinol, the 6-MP dose must be reduced by at least 50% to 75%. 6-MP also undergoes S-methylation by the enzyme TPMT to yield 6-methylmercaptopurine.[35]

6-TG is administered orally in the treatment of AML. Its oral bioavailability is erratic, with peak plasma levels occurring 2 to 4 hours after ingestion. The catabolism of 6-TG differs from 6-MP in that it is not a direct substrate for xanthine oxidase.

TPMT enzyme activity may vary considerably among patients as a result of point mutations or loss of alleles of TPMT.[36] Approximately 0.3% of the Caucasian population expresses either a homozygous deletion or a mutation of both alleles of the *TPMT* gene. In these patients, grossly elevated thiopurine nucleotides concentrations, profound myelosuppression with pancytopenia, and extensive GI symptoms are observed after only a brief course of thiopurine treatment. An estimated 10% of patients may be at increased risk for toxicity because of heterozygous loss of the gene or a mutant allele coding for a less enzymatically active TPMT.

Toxicity

The major dose-related toxicities of the thiopurines are myelosuppression and GI toxicity in the form of nausea/vomiting, anorexia, diarrhea, and stomatitis.[37] In TPMT-deficient patients, dosage reduction to 5% to 25% of the standard dosage is necessary to prevent severe excessive toxicity. Thiopurine hepatotoxicity occurs in up to 30% of adult patients and presents mainly as cholestatic jaundice, although elevations of hepatic transaminases may also be seen. Combinations of thiopurines with other known hepatotoxic agents should be avoided, and liver function should be closely monitored. The thiopurines are also potent suppressors of cell-mediated immunity, and prolonged therapy results in an increased predisposition to bacterial and parasitic infections.

FLUDARABINE

Fludarabine (9-β-D-arabinosyl-2-fluoroadenine monophosphate, F-ara-AMP) is an active agent in the treatment of chronic lymphocytic leukemia (CLL) (see Table 19.1).[38,39] It is also active against indolent non-Hodgkin's lymphoma, prolymphocytic leukemia, cutaneous T-cell lymphoma, and Waldenström macroglobulinemia. This agent has also shown promising activity in mantle cell lymphoma. In contrast to its activity in hematologic malignancies, this compound has virtually no activity against solid tumors.

Mechanism of Action

The active cytotoxic metabolite is the triphosphate metabolite F-ara-ATP, which competes with deoxyadenosine triphosphate (dATP) for incorporation into DNA and serves as a highly effective chain terminator. In addition, F-ara-ATP directly inhibits enzymes involved in DNA replication, including DNA polymerases, DNA primase, DNA ligase I, and ribonucleotide reductase.[37] F-ara-ATP is also incorporated into RNA, causing the inhibition of RNA function, processing, and mRNA translation. In contrast to other antimetabolites, fludarabine is active against nondividing cells. In fact, the primary effect of fludarabine may result from activation of apoptosis, through an as yet ill-defined mechanisms.[39] This finding may explain the activity of fludarabine in indolent lymphoproliferative diseases with relatively low growth fractions.

Mechanisms of Resistance

The decreased expression of the activating enzyme dCK resulting in diminished intracellular formation of F-ara-AMP is one of the main resistance mechanisms identified in preclinical models.[38] A high degree of cross-resistance develops to multiple nucleoside analogs, requiring activation by dCK, including cytarabine, gemcitabine, cladribine, and clofarabine. Reduced cellular transport of drug has also been identified as a resistance mechanism.

Clinical Pharmacology

Peak concentrations of F-ara-A are reached 3 to 4 hours after intravenous administration.[40] The main route of elimination is via the kidneys, with about 25% of a given dose of drug being excreted unchanged in the urine.

Toxicity

Myelosuppression and immunosuppression are the major side effects of fludarabine as highlighted by dose-limiting and possibly cumulative lymphopenia and thrombocytopenia. Suppression of the immune system affects T-cell function more than B-cell function. Fevers, often in the setting of neutropenia, occur in 20% to 30% of patients. Lymphocyte counts, specifically CD4-positive cells, decrease rapidly after the initiation of therapy, and recovery of CD4-positive cells to normal levels may take longer than 1 year. Common opportunistic pathogens include the varicella-zoster virus, *Candida*, and *Pneumocystis carinii*. In general, patients are empirically placed on sulfamethoxazole trimethoprim prophylaxis to prevent the development of *P. carinii* infection.

CLADRIBINE

Cladribine (2-CdA) is a purine deoxyadenosine analog, and it is the drug of choice for hairy cell leukemia with activity in low-grade lymphoproliferative disorders (see Table 19.1).[41,42] Salvage treatment of patients previously treated with interferon-α or splenectomy is as effective as first-line treatment. Retreatment with cladribine results in a complete response in up to 60% of relapsing patients. In addition, this agent has promising activity in patients with CLL and non-Hodgkin's lymphoma.

Mechanism of Action

Upon entry into the cell, 2-CdA undergoes an initial conversion to cladribine-monophosphate (Cd-AMP) via the reaction catalyzed by dCK, and Cd-AMP is subsequently metabolized to the active metabolite, cladribine-triphosphate. The triphosphate metabolite competitively inhibits incorporation of the normal dATP nucleotide into DNA, a process that results in the termination of chain elongation.[43] Progressive accumulation of the triphosphate metabolite leads to an imbalance in deoxyribonucleotide pools, thereby inhibiting further DNA synthesis and repair. Finally, the triphosphate metabolite is a potent inhibitor of ribonucleotide reductase, which further facilitates the inhibition of DNA biosynthesis.

Mechanisms of Resistance

Resistance to 2-CdA has been attributed to altered intracellular drug metabolism. A reduction in the activity of dCK, the enzyme responsible for generating cytotoxic nucleotide metabolites, is a major determinant of acquired resistance. The monophosphate and triphosphate metabolites are dephosphorylated by the cytoplasmic enzyme 5′-nucleotidase. Interestingly, resistant cells derived from a patient with CLL exhibited both low levels of dCK expression and high levels of 5′-nucleotidase.

Clinical Pharmacology

2-CdA is orally bioavailable, with 50% of an administered dose orally absorbed. Approximately 50% of an administered dose of drug is cleared by the kidneys, and 20% to 35% of the drug is excreted unchanged in the urine. Of note, this nucleoside can cross the blood–brain barrier with penetration into the cerebrospinal fluid.

Toxicity

At conventional doses, myelosuppression is dose limiting. After a single course of drug, recovery from thrombocytopenia usually occurs within 2 to 4 weeks, whereas recovery from neutropenia takes place in 3 to 5 weeks. GI toxicities are generally mild, with nausea/vomiting and diarrhea. Mild-to-moderate neurotoxicity occurs in 15% of patients and is at least partly reversible with discontinuation of the drug. Immunosuppression accounts for the late morbidity observed in 2-CdA–treated patients. Lymphocyte counts, particularly CD4-positive cells, decrease within 1 to 4 weeks of drug administration and may remain depressed for several years.[44] After discontinuation of 2-CdA, a median time of up to 40 months may be required for complete recovery of normal CD4-positive counts. Although opportunistic infections occur, they do so less frequently than with fludarabine therapy. Infectious complications correlate with decreases in the CD4-positive count, and they include herpes zoster, *Candida*, *Pneumocystis*, *Pseudomonas aeruginosa*, *Listeria monocytogenes*, *Cryptococcus neoformans*, *Aspergillus*, *P. carinii*, and cytomegalovirus.

CLOFARABINE

Clofarabine is a purine deoxyadenosine nucleoside analog, and it is approved for the treatment of pediatric patients with relapsed or refractory acute lymphoblastic leukemia (see Table 19.1).[45] Ongoing studies are exploring the benefit of clofarabine alone and in combination with other agents in less heavily pretreated patients and in the use of different dose schedules for other hematologic malignancies.[46]

Mechanism of Action

Clofarabine is inactive in its parent form and, like other purine analogs, it requires intracellular activation by dCK to form the monophosphate nucleotide, which undergoes further metabolism to the cytotoxic triphosphate metabolite. Clofarabine triphosphate is then incorporated into DNA, resulting in chain termination, and inhibition of DNA synthesis and function or the triphosphate form can directly inhibit DNA polymerases α, β, and γ, which in turn, interferes with DNA chain elongation, DNA synthesis, and DNA repair. The triphosphate metabolite is also a potent inhibitor of ribonucleotide reductase, further mediating the inhibition of DNA biosynthesis by reducing the levels of key deoxyribonucleotide pools.

Mechanisms of Resistance

Several resistance mechanisms have been identified in various preclinical systems, and they include decreased activation of the drug through the reduced expression of the anabolic enzyme deoxycytidine kinase, the decreased transport of drug into cells via the nucleoside transporter protein, and the increased expression of CTP synthetase activity resulting in increased concentrations of competing physiologic nucleotide substrate dCTP. To date, the precise resistance mechanism(s) that are relevant in the clinical setting remain to be determined.

Clinical Pharmacology

Approximately 50% to 60% of an administered dose of drug is excreted unchanged in the urine, and the terminal half-life is on the order of 5 hours. To date, the pathways for nonrenal elimination have not been well defined. Caution should be exercised in patients with abnormal renal function, and concomitant use of medications known to cause renal toxicity should be avoided during drug treatment.

Toxicity

Myelosuppression is dose limiting with neutropenia, anemia, and thrombocytopenia. The capillary leak syndrome (systemic inflammatory response syndrome) presents with tachypnea, tachycardia, pulmonary edema, and hypotension.[47] In essence, this adverse event is part of the tumor lysis syndrome and results from rapid cytoreduction of peripheral leukemic cells following treatment.[47] Other side effects may include nausea/vomiting, reversible liver dysfunction (hyperbilirubinemia and elevated serum transaminases), renal dysfunction (approximately 10%), and cardiac toxicity in the form of tachycardia and acute pump dysfunction.

REFERENCES

1. Wright DL, Anderson AC. Antifolate agents: a patent review (2006–2010). *Expert Opin Ther Pat* 2011;21:1293–1308.
2. Chattopadhyay S, Moran RG, Goldman ID. Pemetrexed: biochemical and cellular pharmacology, mechanisms, and clinical applications. *Mol Cancer Ther* 2007;6:404–417.
3. Vogelzang NJ, Rusthoven JJ, Symanowski J, et al. Phase III study of pemetrexed in combination with cisplatin versus cisplatin alone in patients with malignant pleural mesothelioma. *J Clin Oncol* 2003;21:2636–2644.
4. Kindler HL. Systemic treatments for mesothelioma: standard and novel. *Curr Treat Options Oncol* 2008;9:171–179.
5. Joerger M, Omlin A, Cerny T, et al. The role of pemetrexed in advanced non small-cell lung cancer: special focus on pharmacology and mechanism of action. *Curr Drug Targets* 2010;11:37–47.
6. Zain J, O'Connor O. Pralatrexate: basic understanding and clinical development. *Expert Opin Pharmacother* 2010;11:1705–1714.
7. Sirotnak FM, DeGraw JI, Moccio DM, et al. New folate analogs of the 10-deaza-aminopterin series. Basis for structural design and biochemical and pharmacologic properties. *Cancer Chemother Pharmacol* 1984;12:18–25.
8. O'Connor OA. Pralatrexate: an emerging new agent with activity in T-cell lymphomas. *Curr Opin Oncol* 2006;18:591–597.

9. Bertino JR, Göker E, Gorlick R, et al. Resistance mechanisms to methotrexate in tumors. *Oncologist* 1996;1:223–226.
10. Zhao R, Goldman ID. Resistance to antifolates. *Oncogene* 2003;22:7431–7457.
11. Grem JL. 5-Fluorouracil: forty-plus and still ticking. A review of its preclinical and clinical development. *Invest New Drugs* 2000;18:299–313.
12. Saif MW, Ezzeldin H, Vance K, et al. DPYD*2A mutation: the most common mutation associated with DPD deficiency. *Cancer Chemother Pharmacol* 2007;60:503–507.
13. Grem JL. Biochemical modulation of 5-FU in systemic treatment of advanced colorectal cancer. *Oncology (Williston Park)* 2001;15:13–19.
14. Saif MW, Shah MM, Shah AR. Fluoropyrimidine-associated cardiotoxicity: revisited. *Expert Opin Drug Saf* 2009;8:191–202.
15. Saif MW, Eloubeidi MA, Russo S, et al. Phase I study of capecitabine with concomitant radiotherapy for patients with locally advanced pancreatic cancer: expression analysis of genes related to outcome. *J Clin Oncol* 2005;23:8679–8687.
16. Geyer CE, Forster J, Lindquist D, et al. Lapatinib plus capecitabine for *HER2*-positive advanced breast cancer. *N Engl J Med* 2006;355:2733–2743.
17. Saif MW, Katirtzoglou NA, Syrigos KN. Capecitabine: an overview of the side effects and their management. *Anticancer Drugs* 2008;19:447–464.
18. Van Custem E, Verslype C, Tejpar S. Oral capecitabine: bridging the Atlantic divide in colon cancer treatment. *Semin Oncol* 2005;32:43–51.
19. Haller DG, Cassidy J, Clarke SJ, et al. Potential regional differences for the tolerability profiles of fluoropyrimidines. *J Clin Oncol* 2008;26:2118–2123.
20. Saif MW, Syrigos KN, Katirtzoglou NA. S-1: a promising new oral fluoropyrimidine derivative. *Expert Opin Investig Drugs* 2009;18:335–348.
21. Saif MW, Rosen LS, Saito K, et al. A phase I study evaluating the effect of CDHP as a component of S-1 on the pharmacokinetics of 5-fluorouracil. *Anticancer Res* 2011;31:625–632.
22. Daigo S, Takahashi Y, Fujieda M, et al. A novel mutant allele of the CYP2A6 gene (CYP2A6*11) found in a cancer patient who showed poor metabolic phenotype towards tegafur. *Pharmacogenetics* 2002;12:299–306.
23. Reiter A, Hochhaus A, Berger U, et al. AraC-based pharmacotherapy of chronic myeloid leukaemia. *Expert Opin Pharmacother* 2001;2:1129–1135.
24. Braess J, Wegendt C, Feuring-Buske M, et al. Leukemic blasts differ from normal bone marrow mononuclear cells and CD34+ hematopoietic stem cells in their metabolism of cytosine arabinoside. *Br J Haematol* 1999;105:388–393.
25. Momparler RL, Laliberte J, Eliopoulos N, et al. Transfection of murine fibroblast cells with human cytidine deaminase cDNA confers resistance to cytosine arabinoside. *Anticancer Drugs* 1996;7:266–274.
26. Cai J, Damaraju VL, Groulx N, et al. Two distinct molecular mechanisms underlying cytarabine resistance in human leukemic cells. *Cancer Res* 2008;68:2349–2357.
27. Kern W, Estey EH. High-dose cytosine arabinoside in the treatment of acute myeloid leukemia: review of three randomized trials. *Cancer* 2006;107:116–124.
28. Mini E, Nobili S, Caciagli B, et al. Cellular pharmacology of gemcitabine. *Ann Oncol* 2006;17:v7–v12.
29. Saif MW, Sellers S, Li M, et al. A phase I study of bi-weekly administration of 24-h gemcitabine followed by 24-h irinotecan in patients with solid tumors. *Cancer Chemother Pharmacol* 2007;60:871–882.
30. Bergman AM, Pinedo HM, Peters GJ. Determinants of resistance to 2′, 2′-difluorodeoxycytidine (gemcitabine). *Drug Resist Update* 2002;5:19–33.
31. Saif MW, Lee Y, Kim R. Harnessing gemcitabine metabolism: a step towards personalized medicine for pancreatic cancer. *Ther Adv Med Oncol* 2012;4: 341–346.
32. Hong SP, Wen J, Bang S, et al. CD44-positive cells are responsible for gemcitabine resistance in pancreatic cancer cells. *Int J Cancer* 2009;125: 2323–2331.
33. Poplin E, Feng Y, Berlin J, et al. Phase III, randomized study of gemcitabine and oxaliplatin versus gemcitabine (fixed-dose rate infusion) compared with gemcitabine (30-minute infusion) in patients with pancreatic carcinoma E6201: a trial of the Eastern Cooperative Oncology Group. *J Clin Oncol* 2009;27:3778–3785.
34. Hande KR. Purine antimetabolites. In: Chabner BA, Longo DL, eds. *Cancer Chemotherapy and Biotherapy: Principles and Practice*, 4th ed. Philadelphia: Lippincott–Raven; 2006: 212.
35. Evans WE. Pharmacogenetics of thiopurine S-methyltransferase and thiopurine therapy. *Ther Drug Monitor* 2004;26:186–191.
36. Wang L, Weinshilboum R. Thiopurine S-methyltransferase pharmacogenetics: insights, challenges, and future directions. *Oncogene* 2006;25:1629–1638.
37. Vora A, Mitchell CD, Lennard L, et al. Toxicity and efficacy of 6-thioguanine versus 6-mercaptopurine in childhood lymphoblastic leukaemia: a randomised trial. *Lancet* 2006;368:1339–1348.
38. Montillo M, Ricci F, Tedeschi A. Role of fludarabine in hematological malignancies. *Expert Rev Anticancer Ther* 2006;6:1141–1161.
39. Gandhi V, Plunkett W. Cellular and clinical pharmacology of fludarabine. *Clin Pharmacokinet* 2002;41:93–103.
40. van den Neste E, Cardoen S, Offner F, et al. Old and new insights into the mechanism of action of two nucleoside analogs active in lymphoid malignancies: fludarabine and cladribine. *Int J Oncol* 2005;27:1113–1124.
41. Gidron A, Tallman MS. 2-CdA in the treatment of hairy cell leukemia: a review of long-term follow-up. *Leuk Lymphoma* 2006;47:2301–2307.
42. Huang P, Robertson LE, Wright S, et al. High molecular weight DNA fragmentation: a critical event in nucleoside analog-induced apoptosis in leukemia cells. *Clin Cancer Res* 1995;1:1005–1013.
43. Grevz N, Saven A. Cladribine: from the bench to the bedside: focus on hairy cell leukemia. *Expert Rev Anticancer Ther* 2004;4:745–757.
44. Seto S, Carrera CJ, Kubota M, et al. Mechanism of deoxyadenosine and 2-chlorodeoxyadenosine toxicity to nondividing human lymphocytes. *J Clin Invest* 1985;75:377–383.
45. Bonate PL, Arthaud L, Cantrell WR Jr, et al. Discovery and development of clofarabine: a nucleoside analogue for treating cancer. *Nat Rev Drug Discov* 2006;5:855–863.
46. Faderi S, Gandhi V, Keating MJ, et al. The role of clofarabine in hematologic and solid malignancies: development of a next generation nucleoside analog. *Cancer* 2005;102:1985–1995.
47. Baytan B, Ozdemir O, Gunes AM, et al. Clofarabine-induced capillary leak syndrome in a child with refractory acute lymphoblastic leukemia. *J Pediatr Hematol Oncol* 2010;32:144–146.

20 Topoisomerase Interactive Agents

Khanh T. Do, Shivaani Kummar, James H. Doroshow, and Yves Pommier

CLASSIFICATION, BIOCHEMICAL, AND BIOLOGIC FUNCTIONS OF TOPOISOMERASES

Nucleic acids (DNA and RNA) being long polymers, topoisomerases fulfill the need for cellular DNA to be densely packaged in the cell nucleus, transcribed, replicated, and evenly distributed between daughter cells following replication without tangles. Topoisomerases are ubiquitous and essential for all organisms as they prevent and resolve DNA and RNA entanglements and resolve DNA supercoiling during transcription and replication. This chapter first summarizes the basic elements necessary to understand the mechanism of action of topoisomerases and their inhibitors. More detailed information can be found in recent reviews[1–7] and two recent books.[8,9] The second part of the chapter summarizes the use of topoisomerase inhibitors as anticancer drugs.

Classification of Topoisomerases

Human cells contain six topoisomerase genes (Table 20.1), which have been numbered historically. The commonly used abbreviations are Top1 for topoisomerases I (Top1mt being the mitochondrial topoisomerase whose gene is encoded in the cell nucleus),[10] Top2 for topoisomerases II, and Top3 for topoisomerases III. Top1 was the first eukaryotic topoisomerase discovered by Champoux and Dulbecco.[11] Topoisomerases solve DNA topologic problems by cutting the DNA backbone and religating without the assistance of any additional ligase. Top1 and Top3 act by cleaving/religating a single strand of the DNA duplex, whereas Top2 enzymes cleave and religate both strands, making a four–base pair reversible staggered cut (Fig. 20.1). It is convenient to remember that odd-numbered topoisomerases (Top1 and Top3) cleave and religate one strand, whereas the even numbered topoisomerases (Top2s) cleave and religate both strands.

Biochemical Characteristics and Cleavage Complexes of the Different Topoisomerases

The DNA cutting/relegation mechanism is common to all topoisomerases and utilizes an enzyme catalytic tyrosine residue acting as a nucleophile and becoming covalently attached to the end of the broken DNA. These catalytic intermediates are referred to as cleavage complexes (see Fig. 20.1B, E). The reverse religation reaction is carried out by the attack of the ribose hydroxyl ends toward the tyrosyl-DNA bond.

Top1 (and Top1mt) attaches to the 3′-end of the break, whereas the other topoisomerases (Top2 and Top3) have opposite polarity and covalently attach to the 5′-end of the breaks (see Table 20.1 [second column] and Fig. 20.1B, E). Topoisomerases have distinct biochemical requirements. Top1 and Top1mt are the simplest, nicking/closing, and relaxing DNA as monomers in the absence of cofactor, and even at ice temperature. Top2 enzymes, on the other hand, are the most complex topoisomerases working as dimers, requiring ATP binding and hydrolysis, and a divalent metal (Mg^{2+}) for catalysis. Top3 enzymes also require Mg^{2+} for catalysis but function as monomers without ATP requirement. Notably, the DNA substrates differ for Top3 enzymes. Whereas both Top1 and Top2 process double-stranded DNA, the Top3 substrates need to be single-stranded nucleic acids (DNA for Top3α and DNA or RNA for Top3β).[10,12,13]

Differential Topoisomerization Mechanisms: Swiveling Versus Strand Passage, DNA Versus RNA Topoisomerases

Topoisomerases use two main mechanisms to change nucleic topology. The first is by "untwisting" the DNA duplex. This mechanism is unique to Top1, which, by an enzyme-associated single-strand break, allows the broken strand to rotate around the intact strand (see Fig. 20.1B) until DNA supercoiling is dissipated. At this point, the stacking energy of adjacent DNA bases realigns the broken ends, and the 5′-hydroxyl end attacks the 3′-phosphotyrosyl end, thereby relegating the DNA. A remarkable feature of this Top1 untwisting mechanism is its extreme efficiency with a rotation speed around 6,000 rpm and relative independence from torque, thereby allowing full relaxation of DNA supercoiling.[14]

The second topologic mechanism is by "strand passage." This mechanism allows the passage of a double- or a single-stranded DNA (or RNA) through the cleavage complexes. Top2α and Top2β both act by allowing the passage of an intact DNA duplex through the DNA double-strand break generated by the enzymes. After which, Top2 religates the broken duplex. Such reactions permit DNA decatenation, unknotting, and relaxation of supercoils.[3] Top3 enzymes also act by strand passage but only pass one nucleic acid strand through the single-strand break generated by the enzymes. In the case of Top3α, the substrate is a single-stranded DNA segment (such as a double-Holliday junction), whereas in the case of Top3β, the substrate can be a single-stranded RNA segment, with Top3β acting as a RNA topoisomerase.[13,15]

TOPOISOMERASE INHIBITORS AS INTERFACIAL POISONS

Topoisomerase Inhibitors Act as Interfacial Inhibitors by Binding at the Topoisomerase–DNA Interface and Trapping Topoisomerase Cleavage Complexes

Relegation of the cleavage complexes is dependent on the structure of the ends of the broken DNA (i.e., the realignment of the broken ends). Binding the drugs at the enzyme–DNA interface misaligns the ends of the DNA and precludes relegation, resulting in the stabilization of the topoisomerase cleavage complexes (Top1cc and Top2cc). Crystal structures of drug-bound cleavage complexes have firmly established this mechanism for both Top1- and Top2-targeted drugs.[16]

TABLE 20.1

Classification of Human Topoisomerases and Topoisomerase Inhibitors

Type	Polarity	Mechanism	Genes	Proteins	Main Functions	Drugs
IB	3′-PY	Rotation/ swiveling	*TOP1*	Top1	DNA supercoiling relaxation, replication, and transcription	Camptothecins, noncamptothecins
			TOP1MT	Top1mt		
IIA	5′-PY	Strand passage ATPase	*TOP2A*	Top2α	Decatenation/replication	Anthracyclines, anthracenediones, epipodophyllotoxins
			TOP2B	Top2β	Transcription	
IA	5′-PY	Strand passage	*TOP3A*	Top3α	DNA replication with BLM	None
			TOP3B	Top3β	RNA topoisomerase	

Top1mt, mitochondrial DNA topoisomerase; BLM, Bloom's syndrome helicare.

It is critical to understand that the cytotoxic mechanism of topoisomerase inhibitors requires the drugs to trap the topoisomerase cleavage complexes rather than block catalytic activity. This sets apart topoisomerase inhibitors from classical enzyme inhibitors such as antifolates. Indeed, knocking out Top1 renders yeast cells totally immune to camptothecin,[17,18] and reducing enzyme levels in cancer cells confers drug resistance. Conversely, in breast cancers, amplification of TOP2A, which is on the same locus as HER2, contributes to the efficacy of doxorubicin.[19] Also, cellular mutations of Top1 and Top2 that renders cells insensitive to the trapping of topoisomerase cleavage complexes produce high resistance to Top1 or Top2 inhibitors. Based on this trapping of cleavage complexes mechanism, we refer to topoisomerase inhibitors as topoisomerase cleavage complex-targeted drugs.

Top1cc-Targeted Drugs (Camptothecin and Noncamptothecin Derivatives) Kill Cancer Cells by Replication Collisions

Top1cc are cytotoxic by their conversion into DNA damage by replication and transcription fork collisions. This explains why cytotoxicity is directly related to drug exposure and why arresting DNA replication protects cells from camptothecin.[20,21] The collisions arise from the fact that the drugs, by slowing down the nicking/closing activity of Top1, uncouple the kinetics of Top1 with the polymerases and helicases, which lead polymerases to collide into Top1cc (Fig. 20.2A). Such collisions have two consequences. They generate double-strand breaks (replication and transcription runoff) and irreversible Top1–DNA adducts (see Fig. 20.2B). The replication double-strand breaks are repaired by homologous recombination, which explains the hypersensitivity of BRCA-deficient cancer cells to Top1cc-targeted drugs.[22] The Top1-covalent complexes can be removed by two pathways, the excision pathway centered around tyrosyl-DNA-phosphodiesterase 1 (TDP1)[23] and the endonuclease pathway involving 3′-flap endonucleases such as XPF-ERCC1.[24] It is also possible that drug-trapped Top1cc directly generate DNA double-strand breaks when they are within 10 base pairs on opposite strands of the DNA duplex or when they occur next to a preexisting single-strand break on the opposite strand. Finally, it is not excluded that topologic defects contribute to the cytotoxicity of Top1cc-targeted drugs (the accumulation of supercoils[25] and the formation of alternative structures such as R-loops) (see Fig. 20.2D).[26]

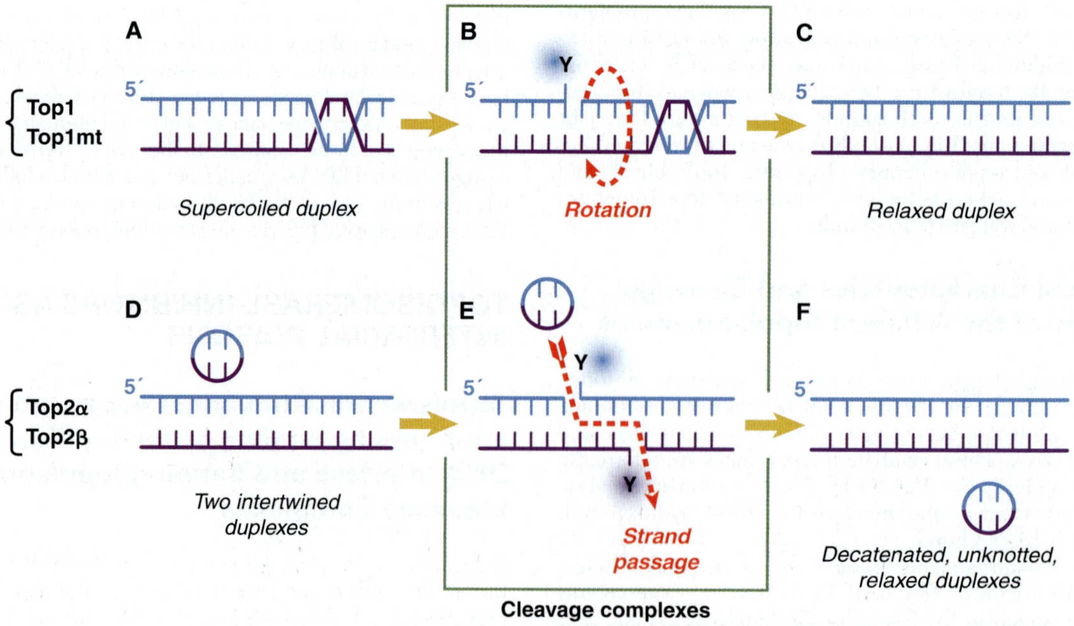

Figure 20.1 Mechanisms of action of topoisomerases. **(A–C)** Topoisomerases I (Top1 for nuclear DNA and Top1mt for mitochondrial DNA) relax supercoiled DNA **(A)** by reversibly cleaving one DNA strand, forming a covalent bond between the enzyme catalytic tyrosine and the 3′ end of the nicked DNA (the Top1 cleavage complex [Top1cc]) **(B).** This reaction allows the swiveling of the broken strand around the intact strand. Rapid religation allows the dissociation of Top1. **(D–F)** Topoisomerases II (Top2α and Top2β) act on two DNA duplexes **(A).** They act as homodimers, cleaving both strands and forming a covalent bond between their catalytic tyrosine and the 5′ end of the DNA break (Top2cc) **(E).** This reaction allows the passage of the intact duplex through the Top2 homodimer *(red dotted arrow)* **(E).** Top2 inhibitors trap the Top2cc and prevent the normal religation **(F).**

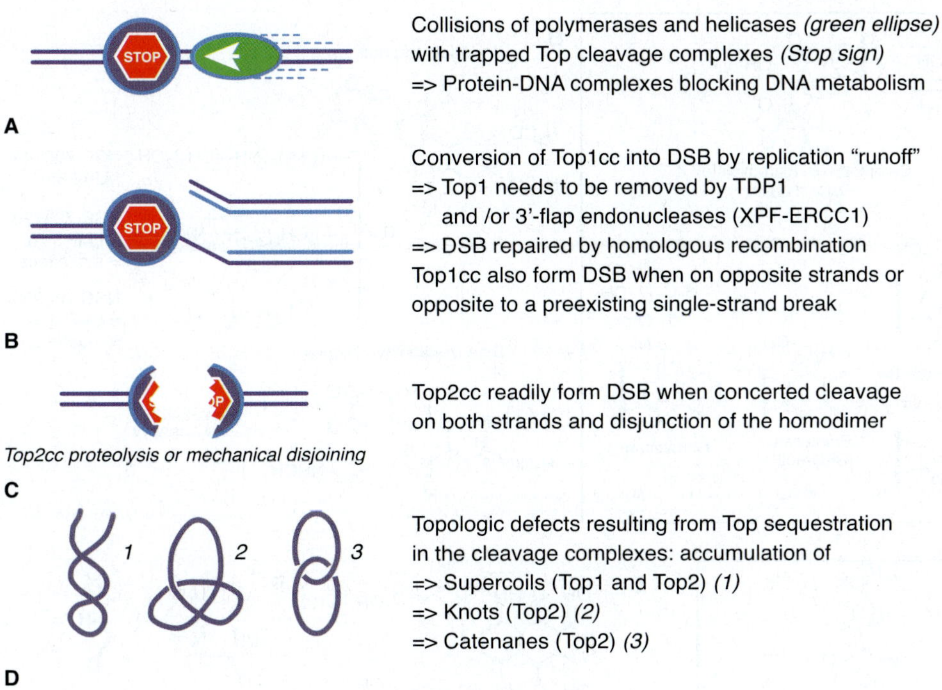

Figure 20.2 Mechanisms of action of topoisomerase inhibitors beyond the trapping of topoisomerase cleavage complexes. **(A)** Stalled or slow cleavage complexes lead to collisions with replication and transcription complexes. **(B)** Collisions of replication complexes with Top1cc on the leading strand for DNA synthesis generate DNA double-strand breaks by replication runoff. Top1cc can also form DNA double-strand breaks (DSBs) when they occur opposite to another Top1cc or preexisting nick. **(C)** Top2cc, which are normally held together by Top2 homodimers, can be converted to free DSBs upon Top2cc proteolysis or dimer disjunction. **(D)** Topologic defects resulting from functional topoisomerase deficiencies play a minor role in the anticancer activity of topoisomerase cleavage complex targeted drugs.

Cytotoxic Mechanisms of Top2cc-Targeted Drugs (Intercalators and Demethyl Epipodophyllotoxins)

Contrary to camptothecins, Top2 inhibitors kill cancer cells without requiring DNA replication fork collisions. Indeed, even after a 30-minute exposure, doxorubicin and other Top2cc-targeted drugs can kill over 99% of the cells, which is in vast excess of the fraction of S-phase cells in tissue culture (generally less than 50%).[27,28] The collision mechanism in the case of Top2cc-targeted drugs (see Fig. 20.2A) appears to involve transcription and proteolysis of both Top2 and RNA polymerase II.[29] Such situation would then lead to DNA double-strand breaks by disruption of the Top2 dimer interface (see Fig. 20.2C). Alternatively, the Top2 homodimer interface could be disjoined by mechanical tension (see Fig. 20.2C). Yet, it is important to bear in mind that 90% of Top2cc trapped by etoposide are not concerted and, therefore, consist in single-strand breaks,[3,30,31] which is different from doxorubicin, which traps both Top2 monomers and produces a majority of DNA double-strand breaks.[32] Finally, it is not excluded that topologic defects resulting from Top2 sequestration by the drug-induced cleavage complexes could contribute to the cytotoxicity of Top2cc-targeted drugs (see Fig. 20.2D). Such topologic defects would include persistent DNA knots and catenanes, potentially leading to chromosome breaks during mitosis.

TOPOISOMERASE I INHIBITORS: CAMPTOTHECINS AND BEYOND

Camptothecin is an alkaloid identified in the 1960s by Wall and Wani[33] in a screen of plant extracts for antineoplastic drugs. The two water-soluble derivatives of camptothecin containing the active lactone form are topotecan and irinotecan, which are approved by the U.S. Food and Drug Administration (FDA) for the treatment of several cancers. In addition, several Top1cc-targeting drugs are in clinical development, including camptothecin derivatives and formulations (including high–molecular-weight conjugates or liposomal formulations), as well as noncamptothecin compounds that exhibit greater potency or noncross resistance to irinotecan and topotecan in preclinical cancer models.[31,34–36]

Irinotecan

Irinotecan, a prodrug containing a bulky dipiperidine side chain at C-10 (Fig. 20.3), is cleaved by a carboxylesterase-converting enzyme in the liver and other tissues to generate the active metabolite, SN-38. Irinotecan is FDA approved for the treatment of colorectal cancer in the metastatic setting as first-line treatment in combination with 5-fluorouracil/leucovorin (5-FU/LV) and as a single agent in the second-line treatment of progressive colorectal cancer after 5-FU–based therapy (see Table 20.1).[37,38] Newer therapeutic uses of irinotecan include a combination with oxaliplatin and 5-FU as first-line treatment in pancreatic cancer.[39] Irinotecan is additionally used in combination with cisplatin or carboplatin in extensive-stage small-cell lung cancer[40,41] as well as refractory esophageal and gastroesophageal junction (GEJ) cancers, gastric cancer, cervical cancer, anaplastic gliomas and glioblastomas, and non–small-cell lung cancer (Table 20.2). Irinotecan is usually administered intravenously at a dose of 125 mg/m^2 for 4 weeks with a 2-week rest period in combination with bolus 5-FU/LV, 180 mg/m^2 every 2 weeks in combination with an infusion of 5-FU/LV, or 350 mg/m^2 every 3 weeks as a single agent.

Diarrhea and myelosuppression are the most common toxicities associated with irinotecan administration. Two mechanisms explain irinotecan-induced diarrhea. Acute cholinergic effects resulting in abdominal cramping and diarrhea occur within 24 hours of drug administration are the result of acetylcholinesterase inhibition by the prodrug, and can be treated with the administration of atropine. Direct mucosal cytotoxicity with diarrhea is typically observed after 24 hours and can result in significant morbidity. Symptoms are managed with loperamide. Hepatic metabolism and biliary excretion accounts for >70% of the elimination of the administered dose, with renal excretion accounting for the remainder of the dose. SN-38 is glucuronidated in the liver by UGT1A1, and deficiencies in this pathway increase the risk of diarrhea and myelosuppression. Dose reductions are recommended for patients who are homozygous for the UGT1A1*28 allele, for which an FDA-approved test for detection of the UGT1A1*28 allele in patients is available.[42,43] Additionally, dose reductions of irinotecan are recommended for patients with hepatic dysfunction, with bilirubin greater than 1.5 mg/mL.[44]

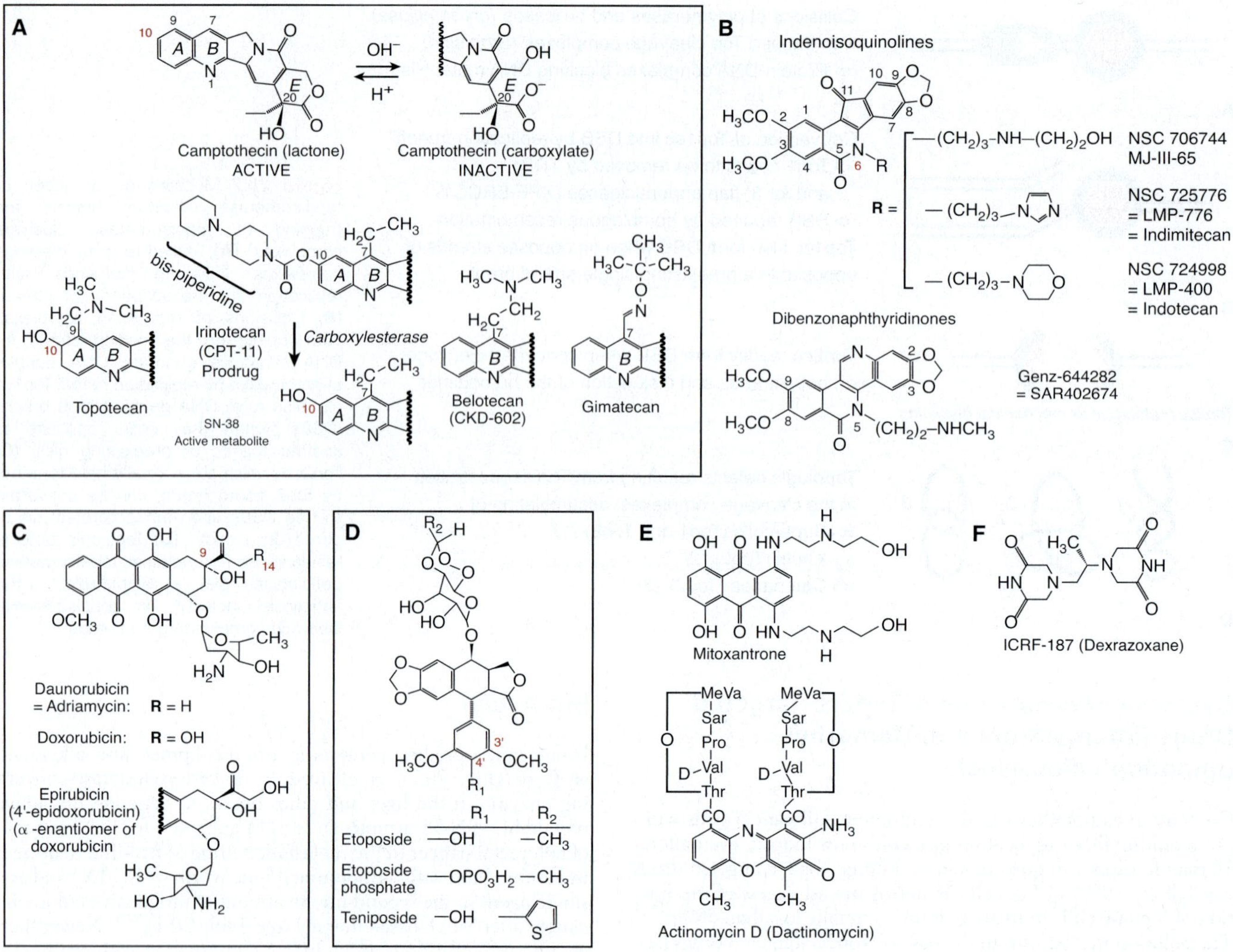

Figure 20.3 Structure of topoisomerase inhibitors. **(A)** Camptothecin derivatives are instable at physiologic pH with the formation of a carboxylate derivative within minutes. Irinotecan is a prodrug and needs to be converted to SN-38 to trap Top1cc. **(B)** Non-camptothecin derivatives in clinical trials. **(C)** Anthracycline derivatives. **(D)** Demethyl epipodophyllotoxin derivatives. **(E)** Other intercalating Top2 inhibitors acting by trapping Top2cc. **(F)** Structure of dexrazoxane, which acts as a catalytic inhibitor of Top2.

Topotecan

Topotecan contains a basic side chain at position C-9 that enhances its water solubility (see Fig. 20.3). Topotecan is approved for the treatment of ovarian cancer,[45] small-cell lung cancer,[46] and as a single agent and in combination with cisplatin for cervical cancer.[47] Additionally, it is active in acute myeloid leukemia (AML) and myelodysplastic syndrome (see Table 20.2). Topotecan is administered intravenously as a single agent at a dose of 1.5 mg/m^2 as a 30-minute infusion daily for 5 days, followed by a 2-week period of rest for the treatment of solid tumors or at a dose of 0.75 mg/m^2 as a 30-minute infusion daily for 3 days in combination with cisplatin on day 1, every 3 weeks, for the treatment of cervical cancer.

Myelosuppression is the most common dose-limiting toxicity. Extensive prior radiation or previous bone marrow–suppressive chemotherapy increases the risk of topotecan-induced myelosuppression. Other toxicities include nausea, vomiting, diarrhea, fatigue, alopecia, and transient hepatic transaminitis.

Topotecan and its metabolites are primarily cleared by the kidneys, requiring dose reduction in patients with renal dysfunction. A 50% dose reduction is recommended for patients with moderate renal impairment (creatinine clearance 20 to 39 mL per minute). There are no formal guidelines for dose reductions in patients with hepatic dysfunction (defined as serum bilirubin >1.5 mg/dL to <10 mg/dL). Topotecan additionally penetrates the blood-brain barrier, achieving concentrations in cerebrospinal fluid that are approximately 30% that of plasma levels.[48]

Camptothecin Conjugates and Analogs

New formulations of camptothecin conjugates and analogs are currently in clinical development in an effort to improve the therapeutic index (Table 20.3). The development of camptothecin conjugates is based on the notion that the addition of a bulky conjugate would allow for a more consistent delivery system and extend the half-life of the molecule.

CRLX101, formerly IT-101, a covalent cyclodextrin-polyethylene glycol copolymer camptothecin conjugate, has plasma concentrations and area under the curve (AUC) that are approximately 100-fold higher than camptothecin, with a half-life in the range of 17 to 20 hours compared to 1.3 hours for camptothecin.[49] It has demonstrated antitumor activity in preclinical studies in irinotecan-resistant tumors with complete tumor regression in human non–small-cell lung cancer, Ewing sarcoma, and

TABLE 20.2

U.S. Food and Drug Administration–Approved Camptothecin Analogs

Irinotecan (Camptosar)	FDA approved for: Metastatic colorectal cancer	First-line therapy in combination with 5-FU/LV Second-line therapy as a single agent	Diarrhea (dose reductions are recommended for patients who are homozygous for the UGT1A1*28 allele) Myelosuppression
	Category 2A[a] recommendations: Pancreatic cancer	First-line therapy in combination with oxaliplatin, 5-FU/LV	
	Extensive-stage small-cell lung cancer	First-line therapy in combination with cisplatin or carboplatin	
	Category 2B[b] recommendations: Esophageal and GEJ cancers, gastric cancer, cervical cancer, anaplastic gliomas and glioblastomas, non–small-cell lung cancer, ovarian cancer		
Topotecan (Hycamtin)	FDA approved for: Cervical cancer	Stage IVB, recurrent, or persistent carcinoma of the cervix not amenable to curative treatment with surgery and/or radiation therapy	Myelosuppression
	Ovarian cancer	After failure of initial therapy	
	Small-cell lung cancer	After failure of initial therapy	
	Class 2B recommendations: AML, MDS		

[a] Category 2A: Recommendations are based upon lower-level evidence, there is uniform National Comprehensive Cancer Network consensus that the intervention is appropriate.
[b] Category 2B: Recommendations are based upon lower-level evidence, there is National Comprehensive Cancer Network consensus that the intervention is appropriate.
MDS, myelodysplastic syndrome.

lymphoma xenograft models.[50] Preliminary data from Phase 1 studies indicate that CRLX101 is well tolerated at a dose of 15 mg/m^2 administered in a biweekly administration schedule.[51] It is currently being studied in Phase 2 studies as a single agent and in combination with chemotherapeutic agents in lung, renal cell cancer, and gynecologic malignancies.[52–54]

Etirinotecan pegol (NKTR-102), an irinotecan polymer conjugate, has a longer plasma circulation time with a lower maximum concentration of SN-38 compared with irinotecan. It was evaluated in a Phase 2 study in platinum-resistant refractory epithelial ovarian cancer at a dose of 145 mg/m^2 administered on a schedule of every 21 days; a median progression-free survival of 5.3 months and median overall survival of 11.7 months was observed.[55] Two schedules of administration, 145 mg/m^2 administered every 14 days versus every 21 days, have been tested in a Phase 2 study of NKTR-102 in patients with previously treated metastatic breast cancer.[56] Of the 70 patients evaluated in this study, 20 patients achieved an objective response (29%; 95% confidence interval [CI] 18.4 to 40.6). For both these studies, the most common adverse events on the 21-day administration schedule were dehydration and diarrhea. Etirinotecan pegol is currently being evaluated in several phase 2 studies in lung cancer, colorectal cancer, and high-grade gliomas,[57–60] with evidence of clinical activity in refractory solid tumors. A Phase 3 trial (The BEACON Study) is underway evaluating NKTR-102 against the physicians' choice in refractory breast cancer.[61]

TABLE 20.3

Topoisomerase I Inhibitors in Development

Camptothecin Conjugates	Camptothecin Analogs	Noncamptothecin Agents
CRLX101	Belotecan	Indenoisoquinoline
NKTR-102	Gimatecan	Indotecan (LMP-400)
MM-398	Homocamptothecin	Indimitecan (LMP-776)
	Elomotecan	Dibenzo naphthyridine
	Diflomotecan	Genz-644282

As an alternative to macromolecular conjugates, attempts have also been made to alter the camptothecin pentacyclic ring structure with modifications of the A and B ring (see Fig. 20.3A) in an effort to improve solubility and enhance antitumor activity. Structure–activity relationship studies have shown that substitutions at the 7, 9, and 10 positions serve to enhance the antitumor activity of camptothecin.[62] Belotecan, a novel camptothecin analog, has a water-solubilizing group at the 7 position of the B ring of camptothecin (see Fig. 20.3A). Several Phase 2 studies have evaluated belotecan in combination with carboplatin in recurrent ovarian cancer[63] and in combination with cisplatin in extensive-stage small-cell lung cancer,[64] demonstrating activity in these cancers; however, these combinations were associated with prominent hematologic toxicities. Phase 2 studies evaluating belotecan as a single agent in patients with recurrent or progressive carcinoma of the uterine cervix failed to show activity.[65] Gimatecan is a lipophilic oral camptothecin analog (see Fig. 20.3A). Pharmacokinetic studies demonstrate that gimatecan is primarily present in plasma as the lactone form (>85%), and has a long half-life of 77.1 +/− 29.6 hours, with an increase in maximum concentration (Cmax) and AUC of three- to six-fold after multiple dosing.[66] Phase 2 studies show that gimatecan has demonstrated activity in previously treated ovarian cancer, with myelosuppression as the main toxicity.[67]

Newer development of analogs have attempted to modify the E-ring through introduction of an electron-withdrawing group at the α position in an effort to overcome the instability of the E-ring while maintaining the binding capability of the camptothecin analog to the Top1-DNA cleavage complex. Collectively called homocamptothecin analogs, two have been tested in clinical trials and include diflomotecan[68] and elomotecan.[69] The dose-limiting toxicity in the Phase I study of elomotecan was neutropenia. A five-member E-ring derivative has also been developed and has reached a Phase 1 clinical trial.[70,71]

Noncamptothecin Topoisomerase I Inhibitors

Noncamptothecin Top1 inhibitors are in clinical development, and include indenoisoquinolines and dibenzonaphthyridines (see Fig. 20.3B). Two indenoisoquinoline derivatives are currently in clinical development, indotecan (LMP400) and indimitecan (LMP776).[72,73] Early in vitro studies show enhanced potency compared with camptothecins, and persistence of Top1 cleavage complexes.[74] Genz-644282, a dibenzonaphthyridine derivative, demonstrated enhanced antitumor activity in preclinical studies[75] and is currently being evaluated in Phase 1 clinical trials.[76]

TOPOISOMERASE II INHIBITORS: INTERCALATORS AND NONINTERCALATORS

Topoisomerase II inhibitors can be classified in two main classes: DNA intercalators, which encompass different chemical classes (Fig. 20.3C, E), and nonintercalators represented by the epipodophyllotoxin derivatives (see Fig. 20.3D). Although both act by trapping Top2 cleavage complexes (Top2cc), DNA intercalators exhibit a second effect as drug concentrations increase above low micromolar values: they block the formation of Top2cc by intercalating into DNA and destabilizing the binding of Top2 to DNA. This explains why Top2α and Top2β are trapped over a relatively narrow concentration range by anthracyclines, and why intercalators have additional effects besides trapping Top2cc, namely inhibition of a broad range of DNA processing enzymes including helicases, polymerase, and even nucleosome destabilization.

Doxorubicin

Doxorubicin and daunorubicin were the first anthracyclines discovered in the 1960s and remain among the most widely used anticancer agents over a broad spectrum of malignancies. Although doxorubicin only differs by one hydroxyl substitution on position 14 (see Fig. 20.3C), doxorubicin has a much broader anticancer activity than daunorubicin. Anthracyclines are natural products derived from *Streptomyces peucetius* variation *caesius*. They were found to target Top2 well after their clinical approval.[77] Subsequent searches for less toxic drugs and formulations led to the approval of liposomal doxorubicin, idarubicin, and epirubicin.

Anthracyclines are flat, planar molecules that are relatively hydrophobic. The quinone structure of anthracyclines (see Fig. 20.3C) enhances the catalysis of oxidation-reduction reactions, thereby promoting the generation of oxygen free radicals, which may be involved in antitumor effects as well as the cardiotoxicity associated with these drugs.[78,79] Anthracyclines are also substrates for P-glycoprotein and Mrp-1, and drug efflux is thought to be a major drug resistance determinant.[80,81]

Doxorubicin is available in a standard salt form and as a liposomal formulation. FDA-labeled indications for standard doxorubicin include acute lymphocytic leukemia (ALL), AML, chronic lymphoid leukemia, Hodgkin lymphoma, non-Hodgkin lymphoma, mantle cell lymphoma, multiple myeloma, mycosis fungoides, Kaposi sarcoma, breast cancer (adjuvant therapy and advanced), advanced prostate cancer, advanced gastric cancer, Ewing sarcoma, thyroid cancer, advanced nephroblastoma, advanced neuroblastoma, advanced non–small-cell lung cancer, advanced ovarian cancer, advanced transitional cell bladder cancer, cervical cancer, and Langerhans cell tumors. Doxorubicin has activity in other malignancies as well, including soft tissue sarcoma, osteosarcoma, carcinoid, and liver cancer (Table 20.4). Doxorubicin is typically administered at a recommended dose of 30 to 75 mg/m^2 every 3 weeks intravenously.

Major acute toxicities of doxorubicin include myelosuppression, mucositis, alopecia, nausea, and vomiting. Myelosuppression is the acute dose-limiting toxicity. Other toxicities, including diarrhea, nausea, vomiting, mucositis, and alopecia, are dose and schedule related. Prophylactic antiemetics are routinely given with bolus doses of doxorubicin, and longer infusions are associated with less nausea and less cardiotoxicity. Patients should also be warned to expect their urine to redden after drug administration. Doxorubicin is a potent vesicant, and extravasation can lead to severe necrosis of skin and local tissues, requiring surgical debridement and skin grafts. Infusions via a central venous catheter are recommended. Other toxicities of doxorubicin include *radiation recall* and the risk of developing secondary leukemia. *Radiation recall* is an inflammatory reaction at sites of previous radiation and can lead to pericarditis, pleural effusion, and skin rash. Secondary leukemias are thought to be a result of balanced translocations that result from Top2 poisoning by the anthracyclines, albeit to lesser degree than other Top2 poisons, such as the epipodophyllotoxins (see the following).[82]

Anthracyclines are cleared mainly by metabolism to less active forms and by biliary excretion. Less than 10% of the administered dose is cleared by the kidneys. Dose reductions should be made in patients with elevated plasma bilirubin. Doxorubicin should be dose reduced by 50% for plasma bilirubin concentrations ranging from 1.2 to 3.0 mg/dL, by 75% for values of 3.1 to 5.0 mg/dL, and withheld for values greater than 5 mg/dL.

Liposomal Doxorubicin

Doxorubicin is also available in a polyethylene glycol (PEG)ylated liposomal form, which allows for enhancement of drug delivery. Use of liposomal doxorubicin has been associated with less cardiotoxicity even at doses exceeding 500 mg/m^2.[83] Additionally, liposomal doxorubicin produces less nausea and vomiting and relatively mild myelosuppression compared to doxorubicin. Unique to the liposomal formulation is the risk of hand–foot syndrome and an acute infusion reaction manifested by flushing, dyspnea, edema, fever, chills, rash, bronchospasm, and hypertension. These infusion reactions are related to the rate of infusion; therefore, the recommended administration schedule is set at an initial rate of 1 mg per minute for the first 10 to 15 minutes. The rate may be slowly increased to complete infusion over 60 minutes if no reaction occurs. Typical dosing schedules include 50 mg/m^2 intravenous infusion every 4 weeks for four courses in ovarian cancer, 20 mg/m^2 intravenous infusion every 3 weeks in AIDS-related Kaposi sarcoma, and 30 mg/m^2 intravenous infusion in combination with bortezomib to be given on days 1, 4, 8, and 11 every 3 weeks in multiple myeloma.

Daunorubicin

Despite its chemical similarity (see Fig. 20.3C), daunorubicin is considerably less active in solid tumors compared to doxorubicin. It is FDA approved for the treatment of ALL and AML. Daunorubicin is typically administered via intravenous push over 3 to 5 minutes at a dose of 30 to 45 mg/m^2 per day on 3 consecutive days in combination chemotherapy. For induction therapy for pediatric acute lymphoblastic leukemia, daunorubicin is dosed at 25 mg/m^2 intravenously in combination with vincristine and prednisone. In children less than 2 years of age or in those who have a body surface area less than 0.5 m^2, current recommendations are based on

TABLE 20.4

U.S. Food And Drug Administration–Approved Topoisomerase II Inhibitors in Clinical Use

Compound	Tumor Type	Clinical Indication	Major Toxicities
I. Anthracyclines			
Doxorubicin (Adriamycin)	Breast carcinoma	Adjuvant setting with axillary LN involvement following resection of primary breast cancer	Dose-dependent cardiotoxicity Myelosuppression
	ALL AML Wilms' tumor Neuroblastoma Sarcomas Ovarian cancer Transitional cell bladder cancer Thyroid cancer Gastric cancer Hodgkin lymphoma Non-Hodgkin lymphoma	In combination with other cytotoxic agents	
Pegylated liposomal doxorubicin (Doxil)	Ovarian cancer	After failure of platinum-based chemotherapy	Myelosuppression Stomatitis Hand-foot syndrome Dosage reduction recommended with hepatic dysfunction
	AIDS-related Kaposi sarcoma	After failure of prior systemic chemotherapy	
	Multiple myeloma	In combination with bortezomib	
Daunorubicin (Cerubidine)	ALL AML	Induction therapy	Dose-dependent cardiotoxicity Myelosuppression
Epirubicin (Ellence)	Breast cancer	Adjuvant therapy in patients with evidence of axillary node tumor involvement following primary resection	Dose-dependent cardiotoxicity Myelosuppression
Idarubicin (Idamycin)	AML	Induction therapy	Dose-dependent cardiotoxicity Myelosuppression
II. Anthracenediones			
Mitoxantrone (Novantrone)	Prostate cancer AML	Hormone-refractory prostate cancer	Myelosuppression
Dactinomycin (Cosmegen)	Wilms' tumor Rhabdomyosarcoma Ewing sarcoma Nonseminomatous testicular cancer Gestational trophoblastic neoplasia		Myelosuppression
III. Epipodophyllotoxins			
Etoposide (VePesid)	Small-cell lung cancer Testicular cancer	First-line in combination First-line in combination	Myelosuppression
Teniposide (Vumon)	Pediatric lymphoblastic leukemia	Refractory setting	Myelosuppression

LN, lymph node.

body mass index (1 mg/kg) rather than body surface area. A higher dose of daunorubicin at 60 mg/m^2 per day to 90 mg/m^2 per day intravenously for 3 consecutive days is currently recommended as part of the induction combination regimen for the treatment of acute myeloblastic leukemia. Daunorubicin has similar toxicities to doxorubicin, including myelosuppression, cardiac toxicity, nausea, vomiting, alopecia, and is also a vesicant. Daunorubicin is metabolized by the liver and undergoes substantial elimination by the kidneys, requiring dose reductions for both renal and hepatic dysfunction. A 50% dose reduction is recommended for either serum creatinine or bilirubin greater than 3 mg/dL, and a 25% reduction in dose for bilirubin concentrations ranging from 1.2 to 3.0 mg/dL.

Epirubicin

Epirubicin is an epimer of doxorubicin (see Fig. 20.3C) with increased lipophilicity. It is FDA approved for adjuvant therapy of breast cancer but is also used in combination for the treatment of a variety of malignancies. Epirubicin is administered intravenously at doses ranging from 60 to 120 mg/m^2 every 3 to 4 weeks. Epirubicin has a similar toxicity profile to doxorubicin but is overall better tolerated.

In addition to being converted to an enol by an aldose reductase, epirubicin has a unique steric orientation of the C-4 hydroxyl group that allows it to serve as a substrate for conjugation reactions mediated by liver glucuronosyltransferases and sulfatases. As such, dose adjustments are recommended in the setting of hepatic dysfunction. For patients with serum bilirubin of 1.2 to 3 mg/dL or aspartate aminotransferase of 2 to 4 times the upper limit of normal, a 50% dose reduction is recommended. For patients with bilirubin greater than 3 mg/dL or aspartate aminotransferase greater than 4 times the upper limit of normal, a dose reduction of 75% is recommended. Due to limited data, no specific dose recommendations are currently available for patients with renal impairment, although current recommendations are for consideration of dose adjustments in patients with serum creatinine greater than 5 mg/dL.

Idarubicin

Idarubicin is a synthetic derivative of daunorubicin, but lacks the 4-methoxy group (see Fig. 20.3C). It is FDA approved as part of combination chemotherapy regimen for AML and is also active in ALL. It is given intravenously at a dose of 12 mg/m^2 for 3 consecutive days, typically in combination with cytarabine. Idarubicin has similar toxicities as daunorubicin. Its primary active metabolite is idarubicinol, and elimination is mainly through the biliary system and, to a lesser extent, through renal excretion. A 50% dose reduction is recommended for serum bilirubin of 2.6 to 5 mg/dL and idarubicin should not be given if the bilirubin is greater than 5 mg/dL. Additionally, dose reductions in renal impairment are advised, but specific guidelines are not available.

Cardiac Toxicity of Anthracyclines

Anthracyclines are responsible for cardiac toxicities, and special considerations are necessary to minimize this severe side effect. Acute doxorubicin cardiotoxicity is reversible, and clinical signs include tachycardia, hypotension, electrocardiogram changes, and arrhythmias. It develops during or within days of anthracycline infusion, and its incidence can be significantly reduced by slowing doxorubicin infusion rates.

Chronic and delayed cardiotoxicity is more common and more severe because it is irreversible. Chronic cardiotoxicity with congestive heart failure peaks at 1 to 3 months but can occur even years after therapy. Myocardial damage has been shown to occur by several mechanisms. The classical mechanism is by the direct generation of reactive oxygen species (ROS) during the electron transfer from the semiquinone to quinone moieties of the anthracycline,[84] which leads to myocardial damage. ROS can also be generated by mitochondrial damage resulting from drug-mediated inactivation of the oxidative phosphorylation chain because doxorubicin accumulates not only in chromatin, but also in mitochondria.[78,79] A recent study has also related doxorubicin cardiotoxicity to the poisoning of Top2β cleavage complexes in myocardiocytes.[85] Endomyocardial biopsy is characterized by a predominant finding of multifocal areas of patchy and interstitial fibrosis (stellate scars) and occasional vacuolated myocardial cells (Adria cells). Myocyte hypertrophy and degeneration, loss of cross-striations, and the absence of myocarditis are also characteristic of this diagnosis.[86] The incidence of cardiomyopathy is related to both the cumulative dose and the schedule of administration, and predisposition to cardiac damage includes a previous history of heart disease, hypertension, radiation to the mediastinum, age greater than 65 years or younger than 4 years, prior use of anthracyclines or other cardiac toxins, and coadministration of other chemotherapy agents (e.g., paclitaxel, cyclophosphamide, or trastuzumab).[87,88] Sequential administration of paclitaxel followed by doxorubicin in breast cancer patients is associated with cardiomyopathy at total doxorubicin doses above 340 to 380 mg/m^2, whereas the reverse sequence of drug administration did not yield the same systemic toxicities at these doses.[89] When doxorubicin is given in a low-dose weekly regimen (10 to 20 mg/m^2 per week) or by slow continuous infusion over 96 hours, cumulative doses of more than 500 mg/m^2 can be given. Doses of epirubicin less than 1,000 mg/m^2 and daunorubicin less than 550 mg/m^2 are considered safe. Additionally, liposomal doxorubicin is associated with less cardiac toxicity.

Cardiac function can be monitored during treatment with anthracyclines by electrocardiography, echocardiography, or radionuclide scans. Numerous studies have established the danger of embarking on anthracycline therapy in patients with underlying cardiac disease (e.g., a baseline left ventricular ejection fraction of less than 50%) and of continuing therapy after a documented decrease in the ejection fraction by more than 10% (if this decrease falls below the lower limit of normal). Because anthracycline-induced cardiotoxicity has been related to the generation of free radicals, efforts have been aimed at attenuating this effect through the targeting of redox response and reduction in oxidative stress. Dexrazoxane is a metal chelator that decreases the myocardial toxicity of doxorubicin in breast cancer patients. In two multicenter, double-blind studies, advanced breast cancer patients were randomized to chemotherapy with dexrazoxane or a placebo; dexrazoxane was shown to have a cardioprotective effect based on serial, noninvasive cardiac testing during the course of the trial and is approved for that use by the FDA.[90] Dexrazoxane chelates iron and copper, thereby interfering with the redox reactions that generate free radicals and damage myocardial lipids. Notably, dexrazoxane is also a Top2 catalytic inhibitor (see Fig. 20.3F), which potentially might minimize the therapeutic activity of anthracyclines by interfering with the trapping of Top2 cleavage complexes by anthracyclines.[2,3,91] Other agents currently in use include β-blockers and statins. A recent meta-analysis of 12 randomized controlled trials and 2 observational studies involving the use of agents to prevent the cardiotoxicity associated with anthracyclines demonstrated relatively similar efficacy regardless of which prophylactic treatment was used.[92]

Anthracenediones

Mitoxantrone (see Fig. 20.3E) is currently the only clinically approved anthracenedione. Compared to anthracyclines, mitoxantrone is less cardiotoxic owing to a decreased ability to undergo oxidation-reduction reactions and form free radicals.

Mitoxantrone is FDA approved for the treatment of advanced hormone-refractory prostate cancer[93] and AML.[94] It is typically administered intravenously at a dose of 12 to 14 mg/m^2 every 3 weeks in the treatment of prostate cancer, and at a dose of 12 mg/m^2 in combination with cytosine arabinoside for 3 days in the treatment of AML.

Toxicities are generally less severe compared to doxorubicin and include myelosuppression, nausea, vomiting, alopecia, and mucositis. Cardiac toxicity can be seen at cumulative doses greater than 160 mg/m^2.[95] Mitoxantrone is rapidly cleared from the plasma and is highly concentrated in tissues. The majority of the drug is eliminated in the feces, with a small amount undergoing renal excretion. Dose adjustments for hepatic dysfunction are recommended, but formal guidelines are currently not available.

Dactinomycin

Dactinomycin was the first antibiotic shown to have antitumor activity[96] and consists of a planar phenoxazone ring attached to two peptide side chains. This unique structure allows for tight intercalation into DNA between adjacent guanine–cytosine bases, leading to Top2 and Top1 poisoning and transcription inhibition.[97] Dactinomycin was one of the first drugs shown to be transported by P-glycoprotein, and represents the major mechanism of resistance.[98]

Dactinomycin is FDA approved for Ewing sarcoma,[99] gestational trophoblastic neoplasm,[100] metastatic nonseminomatous testicular cancer,[101] nephroblastoma,[102] and rhabdomyosarcoma.[103] Typically, it is administered intravenously at doses of 15 μg/kg for 5 days in combination with other chemotherapeutic agents for the treatment of nephroblastoma, rhabdomyosarcoma, and Ewing sarcoma; at does of 12 μg/kg intravenously as a single agent in the treatment of gestational trophoblastic neoplasias; and at doses of 1,000 μg/m^2 intravenously on day 1 as part of a combination regimen with cyclophosphamide, bleomycin, vinblastine, and cisplatin in the treatment of metastatic nonseminomatous testicular cancer. Toxicities include myelosuppression, veno-occlusive disease of the liver, nausea, vomiting, alopecia, erythema, and acne. Additionally, similar to doxorubicin, dactinomycin can cause radiation recall and severe tissue necrosis in cases of extravasation. Dactinomycin is largely excreted unchanged in the feces and urine. Guidelines for dosing in patients with impaired renal or liver function are currently not available.

Epipodophyllotoxins

Epipodophyllotoxins are glycoside derivatives of podophyllotoxin, an antimicrotubule agent extracted from the mandrake plant. Two derivatives, demethylated on the pendant ring (see R1 in Fig. 20.3D), etoposide and teniposide were shown to primarily function as Top2 poisons rather than through antimicrotubule mechanisms.[104,105] Epipodophyllotoxins poison Top2 through a mechanism distinct from that of anthracyclines and other DNA intercalators.[106] without intercalating into normal DNA in the absence of Top2. Therefore, they are "cleaner" Top2 inhibitors than the anthracyclines, anthracenediones, and dactinomycin. However, etoposide and teniposide trap Top2 cleavage complexes by base stacking in a ternary complex at the interface of the DNA and the Top2 homodimer. Mechanisms that have been implicated in resistance to etoposide include drug efflux, because epipodophyllotoxins are substrates for P-glycoprotein[107]; altered localization of Top2α; decreased cellular expression of Top2α[108]; and impaired phosphorylation of Top2.[109]

Etoposide

Etoposide (see Fig. 20.3D) is available in intravenous and oral forms. It is FDA approved for the treatment of small-cell lung cancer[110] and refractory testicular cancer.[111] It also has activity in hematologic malignancies and various solid tumors. The intravenous form is generally administered at doses of 35 to 50 mg/m^2 for 4 to 5 days every 3 to 4 weeks in combination therapy for small-cell lung cancer, and 50 to 100 mg/m^2 for 5 days every 3 to 4 weeks in combination therapy for refractory testicular cancer. The dose of oral etoposide is usually twice the intravenous dose. Oral bioavailability is highly variable due to dependence on intestinal P-glycoprotein.[112]

The dose-limiting toxicity for etoposide is myelosuppression, with white blood cell count nadirs typically occurring on days 10 to 14. Thrombocytopenia is less common than leukopenia. Additionally, mild to moderate nausea, vomiting, diarrhea, mucositis, and alopecia are associated with etoposide. Among topoisomerase inhibitors, epipodophyllotoxins have the greatest association with secondary malignancies, with etoposide having the highest risk, with an estimated 4% 6-year cumulative risk.[113] The majority of etoposide is cleared unchanged by the kidneys, and a 25% dose reduction is recommended in patients with a creatinine clearance of 15 to 50 mL per minute. A 50% dose reduction is recommended in patients with a creatinine clearance less than 15 mL per minute. Because the unbound fraction of etoposide is dependent on albumin and bilirubin concentrations, dose adjustments for hepatic dysfunction are advised, but consensus guidelines are currently not available.

Teniposide

Teniposide contains a thiophene group in place of the methyl group on the glucose moiety of etoposide (Fig. 20.3D). Teniposide is FDA approved for refractory pediatric ALL.[114,115] In pediatric ALL studies, doses ranged from 165 mg/m^2 intravenously in combination with cytarabine to 250 mg/m^2 intravenously weekly in combination with vincristine and prednisone. Similar to etoposide, the dose-limiting toxicity of teniposide is myelosuppression. Additional toxicities include mild-to-moderate nausea, vomiting, diarrhea, alopecia, and secondary leukemia. Teniposide is associated with greater frequency of hypersensitivity reactions compared to etoposide.

Teniposide is 99% bound to albumin and, as compared to etoposide, undergoes hepatic metabolism more extensively and renal clearance less extensively. No specific guidelines are currently available on dose adjustments for renal or hepatic dysfunction.

THERAPY-RELATED SECONDARY ACUTE LEUKEMIA

One of the major complications of Top2 inhibitor therapies, especially for etoposide and mitoxantrone, is acute secondary leukemia, which occurs in approximately 5% of patients. Therapy-related AMLs (t-AML) are characterized by their relatively rapid onset (they can occur only a few months after therapy) and the presence of recurrent balanced translocations involving the mixed lineage leukemia (MLL) locus on 11q23 and over 50 partner genes.[116] The molecular mechanism is likely from the disjoining of two drug-trapped Top2 cleavage complexes on different chromosomes (see Fig. 20.2C) in relationship with transcription collisions and illegitimate relegation.[117] Top2β, rather than Top2α, has been implicated in the generation of these disjoined cleavage complexes.[117,118]

FUTURE DIRECTIONS

Current challenges in the development of topoisomerase inhibitors lie in the inherent chemical instability of current and established agents. In addition to recent developments designed to enhance the stability with semisynthetic analogs and the development of novel delivery systems in an effort to achieve higher intratumoral concentrations, attention is also being focused on targeting other topoisomerase isoenzymes. Driving this trend has been the recent elucidation of the role of Top2β inhibition in the development of treatment-related cardiotoxicity and secondary AML.[86,117,118] In addition to combination chemotherapy regimens already in use, attempts have also been made for the sequential inhibition of Top1 and Top2. Based on early preclinical models suggesting synergy with sequential inhibition of Top1 and Top2,[120] phase I studies have evaluated the sequential administration of topotecan and etoposide in extensive-stage small-cell lung cancer and ovarian cancer, with significant myelosuppression as the dose-limiting toxicity.[121,122] Future rational drug combinations include targeting DNA repair pathways in combination with Top1 inhibition, although further characterization is needed of the specific DNA repair and stress response pathways invoked in response to DNA damage as a result of Top1 inhibition. However, one such attempt of combining topotecan with veliparib, a small molecule inhibitor of poly (ADP-ribose) polymerase, was poorly tolerated due to significant myelosuppression, thus limiting the doses of topotecan that could be safely administered.[123]

Molecular characterization of tumors to better define patient selection and the development of pharmacodynamic biomarkers to monitor the response to treatment and to optimize the combination dose and schedules is needed for the further clinical development of topoisomerase inhibitors. Validated assays have been developed to evaluate topoisomerase 1 levels and levels of phosphorylated histone H2AX (gamma-H2AX) as a marker of DNA damage response to topoisomerase inhibition,[124,125] and are being incorporated in current phase I studies of indenoisoquinolines.[72,73]

REFERENCES

1. Nitiss JL. DNA topoisomerase II and its growing repertoire of biological functions. *Nat Rev Cancer* 2009;9(5):327–337.
2. Nitiss JL. Targeting DNA topoisomerase II in cancer chemotherapy. *Nat Rev Cancer* 2009;9(5):338–350.
3. Pommier Y, Leo E, Zhang H, et al. DNA topoisomerases and their poisoning by anticancer and antibacterial drugs. *Chem Biol* 2010;17(5):421–433.
4. Fortune JM, Osheroff N. Topoisomerase II as a target for anticancer drugs: when enzymes stop being nice. *Prog Nucleic Acid Res Mol Biol* 2000;64:221–253.
5. Wang JC. A journey in the world of DNA rings and beyond. *Annu Rev Biochem* 2009;78:31–54.
6. Wang JC. Cellular roles of DNA topoisomerases: a molecular perspective. *Nat Rev Mol Cell Biol* 2002;3(6):430–440.
7. Champoux JJ. DNA topoisomerases: structure, function, and mechanism. *Annu Rev Biochem* 2001;70:369–413.
8. Wang JC. *Untangling the Double Helix: DNA Entanglements and the Action of DNA Topoisomerases.* Cold Spring Harbor, NY: Cold Spring Harbor Laboratory Press; 2009.
9. Pommier Y. DNA Topoisomerases and cancer. In: Teicher BA, ed. *Cancer Discovery and Development.* New York: Springer & Humana Press; 2012.
10. Zhang H, Barceló JM, Lee B, et al. Human mitochondrial topoisomerase I. *Proc Natl Acad Sci U S A* 2001;98(10):10608–10613.
11. Champoux JJ, Dulbecco R. An activity from mammalian cells that untwists superhelical DNA—a possible swivel for DNA replication (polyoma-ethidium bromide-mouse-embryo cells-dye binding assay). *Proc Natl Acad Sci U S A* 1972;69(1):143–146.
12. Chen SH, Wu CH, Plank JL, et al. Essential functions of C terminus of Drosophila Topoisomerase IIIα in double Holliday junction dissolution. *J Biol Chem* 2012;287(23):19346–19353.
13. Xu D, Shen W, Guo R, et al. Top3β is an RNA topoisomerase that works with fragile X syndrome protein to promote synapse formation. *Nat Neurosci* 2013;16(9):1238–1247.
14. Seol Y, Gentry AC, Osheroff N, et al. Chiral discrimination and writhe-dependent relaxation mechanism of human topoisomerase IIα. *J Biol Chem* 2013;288(19):13695–13703.
15. Stoll G, Pietiläinen OP, Linder B, et al. Deletion of TOP3b, a component of FMRP-containing mRNPs, contributes to neurodevelopmental disorders. *Nat Neurosci* 2013;16(9):1228–1237.
16. Pommier Y, Marchand C. Interfacial inhibitors: targeting macromolecular complexes. *Nat Rev Drug Discov* 2011;11(1):25–36.
17. Nitiss J, Wang JC. DNA topoisomerase-targeting antitumor drugs can be studied in yeast. *Proc Natl Acad Sci U S A* 1988;85(20):7501–7505.
18. Bjornsti MA, Benedetti P, Vigilanti GA, et al. Expression of human DNA topoisomerase I in yeast cells lacking yeast DNA topoisomerase I: restoration of sensitivity of the cells to the antitumor drug camptothecin. *Cancer Res* 1989;49(22):6318–6323.
19. Dressler LG, Berry DA, Broadwater G, et al. Comparison of HER2 status by fluorescence in situ hybridization and immunohistochemistry to predict benefit from dose escalation of adjuvant doxorubicin-based therapy in node-positive breast cancer patients. *J Clin Oncol* 2005;23(19):4287–4297.
20. Holm C, Covey JM, Kerrigan D, et al. Differential requirement of DNA replication for the cytotoxicity of DNA topoisomerase I and II inhibitors in Chinese hamster DC3F cell. *Cancer Res* 1989;49(22):6365–6368.
21. Hsiang YH, Lihou MG, Liu LF. Arrest of DNA replication by drug-stabilized topoisomerase I-DNA cleavable complexes as a mechanism of cell killing by camptothecin. *Cancer Res* 1989;49(18):5077–5082.
22. Maede Y, Shimizu H, Fukushima T, et al. Differential and common DNA repair pathways for topoisomerase I- and II-targeted drug in a genetic DT40 repair screen panel. *Mol Cancer Ther* 2014;13(1):214–220.
23. Huang SN, Pommier Y, Marchand C. Tyrosyl-DNA Phosphodiesterase 1(Tdp1) inhibitors. *Expert Opinion Ther Pat* 2011;21(9):1285–1292.
24. Zhang YW, Regairaz M, Seiler JA, et al. Poly(ADP-ribose) polymerase and XPF-ERCC1 participate in distinct pathways for the repair of topoisomerase I-induced DNA damage in mammalian cells. *Nucleic Acids Res* 2011;39(9):3607–3620.
25. Koster DA, Palle K, Bot ES, et al. Antitumor drugs impede DNA uncoiling by topoisomerase I. *Nature* 2007;448(7150):213–217.
26. Sordet O, Redon CE, Guirouilh-Barbat J, et al. Ataxia telangiectasia mutated activation by transcription- and topoisomerase I-induced DNA double-strand breaks. *EMBO Rep* 2009;10(8):887–893.
27. Pommier Y, Zwelling LA, Mattern MR, et al. Effects of dimethyl sulfoxide and thiourea upon intercalator-induced DNA single-strand breaks in mouse leukemia (L1210) cells. *Cancer Res* 1983;43(12 Pt 1):5718–5724.
28. Long BH, Musial ST, Brattain MG. Comparison of cytotoxicity and DNA breakage activity of congeners of podophyllotoxin including VP16-213 and VM26: a quantitative structure-activity relationship. *Biochemistry* 1984;23(6):1183–1188.
29. Ban Y, Ho CW, Lin RK, et al. Activation of a novel ubiquitin-independent proteasome pathway when RNA polymerase II encounters a protein roadblock. *Mol Cell Biol* 2013;33(20):4008–4016.
30. Long BH, Musial ST, Brattain MG. Single- and double-strand DNA breakage and repair in human lung adenocarcinoma cells exposed to etoposide and teniposide. *Cancer Res* 1985;45(7):3106–3112.
31. Pommier Y. Drugging topoisomerases: lessons and challenges. *ACS Chem Biol* 2013;8(1):82–95.
32. Zwelling LA, Michaels S, Erickson LC, et al. Protein-associated deoxyribonucleic acid strand breaks in L1210 cells treated with the deoxyribonucleic acid intercalating agents 4'-(9-acridinylamino) methanesulfon-m-anisidide and adriamycin. *Biochemistry* 1981;20(23):6553–6563.
33. Wall ME, Wani MC. Camptothecin and taxol: discovery to clinic—thirteenth Bruce F. Cain Memorial Award Lecture. *Cancer Res* 1995;55:753–760.
34. Pommier Y. Topoisomerase I inhibitors: camptothecins and beyond. *Nat Rev Cancer* 2006;6(10):789–802.
35. Teicher BA. Next generation topoisomerase I inhibitors: rationale and biomarker strategies. *Biochem Pharmacol* 2008;75(6):1262–1271.
36. Pommier Y, Cushman M. The indenoisoquinoline noncamptothecin topoisomerase I inhibitors: update and perspectives. *Mol Cancer Ther* 2009;8(5):1008–1014.
37. Douillard JY, Cunningham D, Roth AD, et al. Irinotecan combined with fluorouracil compared with fluorouracil alone as first-line treatment for metastatic colorectal cancer: a multicentre randomised trial. *Lancet* 2000;355:1041–1047.
38. Saltz LB, Cox JV, Blanke C, et al. Irinotecan plus fluorouracil and leucovorin for metastatic colorectal cancer. Irinotecan Study Group. *N Engl J Med* 2000;343:905–914.
39. Conroy T, Desseigne F, Tchou M, et al. FOLFIRINOX versus gemcitabine for metastatic pancreatic cancer. *N Engl J Med* 2011;364:1817–1825.
40. Hanna N, Bunn PA Jr, Langer C, et al. Randomized phase III trial comparing irinotecan/cisplatin with etoposide/cisplatin in patients with previously untreated extensive-stage disease small-cell lung cancer. *J Clin Oncol* 2006;24:2038–2043.
41. Schmittel A, Fischer von Weikersthal L, Sebastian M, et al. A randomized phase II trial of irinotecan plus carboplatin versus carboplatin treatment in patients with extended disease small-cell lung cancer. *Ann Oncol* 2006;17:663–667.
42. Iyer L, King CD, Whitington PF, et al. Genetic predisposition to the metabolism of irinotecan (CPT-11). Role of uridine diphosphate glucuronosyltransferase isoform 1A1 in the glucuronidation of its active metabolite (SN-38) in human liver microsomes. *J Clin Invest* 1998;101:847–854.
43. Innocenti F, Undevia SD, Iyer L, et al. Genetic variants in the UDP-glucuronosyltransferase 1A1 gene predict the risk of severe neutropenia of irinotecan. *J Clin Oncol* 2004;22:1382–1388.
44. Schaaf LJ, Hammond LA, Tipping SJ, et al. Phase 1 and pharmacokinetic study of intravenous irinotecan in refractory solid tumor patients with hepatic dysfunction. *Clin Cancer Res* 2006;12:3782–3791.
45. ten Bokkel Huinink W, Gore M, Carmichael J, et al. Topotecan versus paclitaxel for the treatment of recurrent epithelial ovarian cancer. *J Clin Oncol* 1997;15:2183–2193.
46. Ardizzoni A, Hansen H, Dombernowsky P, et al. Topotecan, a new active drug in the second-line treatment of small-cell lung cancer: a phase II study in patients with refractory and sensitive disease. The European Organization for Research and Treatment of Cancer Early Clinical Studies Group and New Drug Development Office, and the Lung Cancer Cooperative Group. *J Clin Oncol* 1997;15:2090–2096.
47. Long HJ 3rd, Bundy BN, Grendys EC Jr, et al. Randomized phase III trial of cisplatin with or without topotecan in carcinoma of the uterine cervix: a Gynecologic Oncology Group Study. *J Clin Oncol* 2005;23:4626–4633.
48. Baker SD, Heideman RL, Crom WR, et al. Cerebrospinal fluid pharmacokinetics and penetration of continuous infusion topotecan in children with central nervous system tumors. *Cancer Chemother Pharmacol* 1996;37:195–202.
49. Schluep T, Cheng J, Khin KT, et al. Pharmacokinetics and biodistribution of the camptothecin-polymer conjugate IT-101 in rats and tumor-bearing mice. Cancer *Chemother Pharmacol* 2006;57:654–662.
50. Young C, Schluep T, Hwang J, et al. CRLX101 (formerly IT-101)-A novel nanopharmaceutical of camptothecin in clinical development. *Curr Bioact Compd* 2011;7:8–14.
51. Weiss GJ, Chao J, Neidhart JD, et al. First-in-human phase 1/2a trial of CRLX101, a cyclodextrin-containing polymer-camptothecin nanopharmaceutical in patients with advanced solid tumor malignancies. *Invest New Drugs* 2013;31:986–1000.
52. University of Chicago. A randomized phase II study of IV Topotecan versus CRLX101 in the second line treatment of recurrent small cell lung cancer. ClinicalTrials.gov Identifier: NCT01803269.
53. Cerulean Pharma Inc. A randomized, phase 2, study to assess the safety and activity of CRLX101, a nanoparticle formulation of camptothecin, in patients with advanced non-small cell lung cancer who have failed one or two previous regimens of chemotherapy. ClinicalTrials Identifier: NCT01380769.
54. Massachusetts General Hospital. A Phase II, 2-stage Trial of CRLX101-202 in recurrent ovarian, tubal and peritoneal cancer. ClinicalTrials.gov Identifier: NCT01652079.
55. Vergote IB, Garcia A, Micha J et al. Randomized multicentre phase II trial comparing two schedules of etirinotecan pegol (NKTR-102) in women with recurrent platinum-resistant/refractory epithelial ovarian cancer. *J Clin Oncol* 2013;31(32):4060–4066.
56. Awada A, Garcia AA, Chan S et al. Two schedules of etirinotecan pegol (NKTR-102) in patients with previously treated metastatic breast cancer: a randomized phase 2 study. *Lancet Oncol* 2013;14(12):1216–1225.
57. Roswell Park Cancer Institute. A phase II study of single agent topoisomerase-I inhibitor polymer conjugate, Etirinotecan Pegol (NKTR-102), in patients with relapsed small cell lung cancer. ClinicalTrials Identifier: NCT01876446.
58. Abramson Cancer Center of the University of Pennsylvania. Phase 2 study of Etirinotecan Pegol (NKTR-102) in the treatment of patients with metastatic and recurrent non-small cell lung cancer (NSCLC) after failure of 2nd line treatment. ClinicalTrials Identifier: NCT01773109.

59. Nektar Therapeutics. A multicentre, open-label, randomized, phase 2 study to evaluate the efficacy and safety of NKTR-102 versus irinotecan in patients with second-line, irinotecan-naive, KRAS-mutant, metastatic colorectal cancer (mCRC). ClinicalTrials Identifier: NCT00856375.
60. Lawrence Recht. A phase II, single arm, open label study of NKTR-102 in bevacizumab-resistant high-grade glioma. ClinicalTrials Identifier: NCT01663012.
61. Nektar Therapeutics. The BEACON study (breast cancer outcomes with NKTR-102): a phase 3 open-label, randomized, multicenter study of NKTR-102 versus treatment of physician's choice (TPC) in patients with locally recurrent or metastatic breast cancer previously treated with an anthracycline, a taxane and capecitabine. ClinicalTrials Identifier: NCT01492101.
62. Basili S, Moro S. Novel camptothecin derivatives as topoisomerase I inhibitors. *Expert Opin Ther Pat* 2009;19:555–574.
63. Choi CH, Lee YY, Song TJ, et al. Phase II study of belotecan, a camptothecin analogue, in combination with carboplatin for the treatment of recurrent ovarian cancer. *Cancer* 2011;117:2104–2111.
64. Rhee CK, Lee SH, Kim JS, et al. A multicentre phase II study of belotecan, a new camptothecin analogue, as a second-line therapy in patients with small cell lung cancer. *Lung Cancer* 2011;72(1):64–67.
65. Hwang JH, Lim MC, Seo SS, et al. Phase II study of belotecan (CKD 602) as a single agent in patients with recurrent or progressive carcinoma of the uterine cervix. *Jpn J Clin Oncol* 2011;41:624–629.
66. Frapolli R, Zucchetti M, Sessa C, et al. Clinical pharmacokinetics of the new oral camptothecin gimatecan: the inter-patient variability is related to alpha1-acid glycoprotein plasma levels. *Eur J Cancer* 2010;46:505–516.
67. Pecorelli S, Ray-Coquard I, Tredan O, et al. Phase II of oral gimatecan in patients with recurrent epithelial ovarian, fallopian tube or peritoneal cancer, previously treated with platinum and taxanes. *Ann Oncol* 2010;21:759–765.
68. Graham JS, Falk S, Samuel LM et al. A multi-centre dose escalation and pharmacokinetic study of diflomotecan in patients with advanced malignancy. *Cancer Chemother Pharmacol* 2009;63:945–952.
69. Trocóniz IF, Cendrós JM, Soto E, et al. Population pharmacokinetic/pharmacodynamics modeling of drug-induced adverse effects of a novel homocamptothecin analog, elomotecan (BN80927), in a Phase I dose finding study in patients with advanced solid tumors. *Cancer Chemother Pharmacol* 2012;70:239–250.
70. Takagi K, Dexheimer TS, Redon C, et al. Novel E-ring camptothecin keto analogues (S38809 and S39625) are stable, potent, and selective topoisomerase I inhibitors without being substrates of drug efflux transporters. *Mol Cancer Ther* 2007;6(12 Pt 1):3229–3238.
71. Lansiaux A, Léonce S, Kraus-Berthier L, et al. Novel stable camptothecin derivatives replacing the E-ring lactone by a ketone function are potent inhibitors of topoisomerase I and promising antitumor drugs. *Mol Pharmacol* 2007;72(2):311–319.
72. National Cancer Institute. A Phase I Study of Indenoisoquinolines LMP400 and LMP776 in Adults With Relapsed Solid Tumors and Lymphomas. ClinicalTrials Identifier: NCT01051635.
73. National Cancer Institute. A phase I trial of weekly Indenoisoquinolines LMP400 in adults with relapsed solid tumors and lymphomas. ClinicalTrials Identifier: NCT01794104.
74. Antony S, Agama KK, Miao ZH, et al. Novel indenoisoquinolines NSC 725776 and NSC 724998 produce persistent topoisomerase I cleavage complexes and overcome multidrug resistance. *Cancer Res* 2007;67:10397–10405.
75. Kurtzberg LS, Roth S, Krumbholz R, et al. Genz-644282, a novel non-camptothecin topoisomerase I inhibitor for cancer treatment. *Clin Cancer Res* 2011;17:2777–2787.
76. Genzyme, a Sanofi Company. Dose Escalation Study to Assess the Safety and Tolerability of Genz-644282 in Patients With Solid Tumors. ClinicalTrials Identifier: NCT00942799.
77. Capranico G, Zunino F, Kohn KW, et al. Sequence-selective topoisomerase II inhibition by anthracycline derivatives in SV40 DNA: relationship with DNA binding affinity and cytotoxicity. *Biochemistry* 1990;29(2):562–569.
78. Davies KJ, Doroshow JH. Redox cycling of anthracyclines by cardiac mitochondria. I. Anthracycline radical formation by NADH dehydrogenase. *J Biol Chem* 1986;261(7):3060–3067.
79. Doroshow JH, Davies KJ. Redox cycling of anthracyclines by cardiac mitochondria. II. Formation of superoxide anion, hydrogen peroxide, and hydroxyl radical. *J Biol Chem* 1986;261:3068–3074.
80. Schneider E, Cowan KH. Multiple drug resistance in cancer therapy. *Med J Aust* 1994;160(6):371–373.
81. Alvarez M, Paull K, Monks A, et al. Generation of a drug resistance profile by quantitation of mdr-1/P-glycoprotein in the cell lines of the National Cancer Institute Anticancer Drug Screen. *J Clin Invest* 1995;95(5):2205–2214.
82. Felix CA, Kolaris CP, Osheroff N. Topoisomerase II and the etiology of chromosomal translocations. *DNA Repair* 2006;5:1093–1108.
83. O'Brien ME, Wigler N, Inbar M, et al. Reduced cardiotoxicity and comparable efficacy in a phase III trial of pegylated liposomal doxorubicin HCl (CAELYX/Doxil) versus conventional doxorubicin for first-line treatment of metastatic breast cancer. *Ann Oncol* 2004;15(3):440–449.
84. Doroshow JH. Effect of anthracycline antibiotics on oxygen radical formation in rat heart. *Cancer Res* 1983;43(2):460–472.
85. Zhang S, Liu X, Bawa-Khalfe T, et al. Identification of the molecular basis of doxorubicin-induced cardiotoxicity. *Nat Med* 2012;18:1639–1642.
86. Speyer J, Wasserheit C. Strategies for reduction of anthracycline cardiac toxicity. *Sem Oncol* 1998;25:525–537.
87. Chanan-Khan A, Srinivasan S, Czuczman MS. Prevention and management of cardiotoxicity from antineoplastic therapy. *J Support Oncol* 2004;2:251–256.
88. Von Hoff DD, Layard MW, Basa P, et al. Risk factors for doxorubicin-induced congestive heart failure. *Ann Intern Med* 1979;91:710–717.
89. Shan K, Lincoff AM, Young JB. Anthracycline-induced cardiotoxicity. *Ann Intern Med* 1996;125:47–58.
90. Swain SM, Whaley FS, Gerber MC, et al. Cardioprotection with dexrazoxane for doxorubicin-containing therapy in advanced breast cancer. *J Clin Oncol* 15(4):1318–1332.
91. Andoh T, Ishida R. Catalytic inhibitors of DNA topoisomerase II. *Biochim Biophys Acta* 1998;1400(1–3):155–171.
92. Kalam K, Marwick TH. Role of cardioprotective therapy for prevention of cardiotoxicity with chemotherapy: a systematic review and meta-analysis. *Eur J Cancer* 2013;49:2900–2909.
93. Tannock IF, Osoba D, Stockler MR, et al. Chemotherapy with mitoxantrone plus prednisone or prednisone alone for symptomatic hormone-resistant prostate cancer: a Canadian randomized trial with palliative end points. *J Clin Oncol* 1996;14:1756–1764.
94. Reece DE, Elmongy MB, Barnett MJ, et al. Chemotherapy with high-dose cytosine arabinoside and mitoxantrone for poor-prognosis myeloid leukemias. *Cancer Invest* 1993;11:509–516.
95. Shenkenberg TD, Von Hoff DD. Mitoxantrone: a new anticancer drug with significant clinical activity. *Ann Intern Med* 1986;105:67–81.
96. Hollstein U. Actinomycin. Chemistry and mechanism of action. *Chem Rev* 1974;74(6):625–652.
97. Wassermann K, Markovits J, Jaxel C, et al. Effects of morpholinyl doxorubicins, doxorubicin, and actinomycin D on mammalian DNA topoisomerases I and II. *Mol Pharmacol* 1990;38(1):38–45.
98. Biedler JL, Riehm H. Cellular resistance to actinomycin D in Chinese hamster cells in vitro: cross-resistance, radioautographic, and cytogenetic studies. *Cancer Res* 1970;30:1174–1184.
99. Jaffe N, Paed D, Traggis D, et al. Improved outlook for Ewing's sarcoma with combination chemotherapy (vincristine, actinomycin D and cyclophosphamide) and radiation therapy. *Cancer* 1976;38(5):1925–1930.
100. Turan T, Karacay O, Tulunay G, et al. Results of EMA/CO (etoposide, methotrexate, actinomycin D, cyclophosphamide, vincristine) chemotherapy in gestational trophoblastic neoplasia. *Int J Gynecol Cancer* 2006;16(3): 1432–1438.
101. Early KS, Albert DJ. Single agent chemotherapy (actinomycin D) in the treatment of metastatic testicular carcinoma. *South Med J* 1976;69(8):1017–1021.
102. Fernbach DJ, Martyn DT. Role of dactinomycin in the improved survival of children with Wilm's tumor. *JAMA* 1966;195(1222):1005–1009.
103. Maurer HM, Moon T, Donaldson M, et al. The intergroup rhabdomyosarcoma study: a preliminary report. *Cancer* 1977;40(5):2015–2026.
104. Chen GL, Yang L, Rowe TC, et al. Nonintercalative antitumor drugs interfere with the breakage-reunion reaction of mammalian DNA topoisomerase. *J Biol Chem* 1984;259(21):13560–13566.
105. Long BH, Musial ST, Brattain MG. Comparison of cytotoxicity and DNA breakage activity of cogeners of podophyllotoxin including VP16-213 and VM26: a quantitative structure-activity relationship. *Biochemistry* 1984;23(6): 1183–1188.
106. Ross W, Rowe T, Glisson B, et al. Role of topoisomerase II in mediating epipodophyllotoxin-induced DNA cleavage. *Cancer Res* 1984;44:5857–5860.
107. Meresse P, Dechaux E, Monneret C, et al. Etoposide: discovery and medicinal chemistry. *Curr Med Chem* 2004;11:2443–2466.
108. Valkov NI, Gump JL, Engel R, et al. Cell density-dependent VP-16 sensitivity of leukaemic cells is accompanied by the translocation of topoisomerase IIalpha from the nucleus to the cytoplasm. *Br J Haematol* 2000;108:331–345.
109. Takano H, Kohno K, Ono M, et al. Increased phosphorylation of DNA topoisomerase II in etoposide-resistant mutants of human cancer KB cells. *Cancer Res* 1991;51:3951–3957.
110. Sundstrøm S, Bremnes RM, Kaasa S, et al. Cisplatin and etoposide regimen is superior to cyclophosphamide, epirubicin, and vincristine regimen in small-cell lung cancer: results from a randomized phase III trial with 5 years' follow-up. *J Clin Oncol* 2002;20:4665–4672.
111. Nichols CR, Catalano PJ, Crawford ED, et al. Randomized comparison of cisplatin and etoposide and either bleomycin or ifosfamide in treatment of advanced disseminated germ cell tumors: an Eastern Cooperative Oncology Group, Southwest Oncology Group, and Cancer and Leukemia Group B Study. *J Clin Oncol* 1998;16:1287–1293.
112. Leu BL, Huang JD. Inhibition of intestinal P-glycoprotein and effects on etoposide absorption. *Cancer Chemother Pharmacol* 1995;35:432–436.
113. Smith MA, Rubinstein L, Anderson JR, et al. Secondary leukemia or myelodysplastic syndrome after treatment with epipodophyllotoxins. *J Clin Oncol* 1999;17:569–577.
114. Maluf PT, Odone Filho V, Cristofani LM, et al. Teniposide plus cytarabine as intensification therapy and in continuation therapy for advanced nonlymphoblastic lymphomas of childhood. *J Clin Oncol* 1994;12:1963–1968.
115. Rivera G, Bowman WP, Murphy SB, et al. VM-26 with prednisone and vincristine for treatment of refractory acute lymphocytic leukemia. *Med Pediatr Oncol* 1982;10:439–446.
116. Lovett BD, Lo Nigro L, Rappaport EF, et al. Near-precise interchromosomal recombination and functional DNA topoisomerase II cleavage sites at MLL and AF-4 genomic breakpoints in treatment-related acute lymphoblastic leukemia with t(4;11) translocation. *Proc Natl Acad Sci U S A* 2001;98(17):9802–9807.
117. Cowell IG, Sondka Z, Smith K, et al. Model for MLL translocations in therapy-related leukemia involving topoisomerase IIb-mediated DNA strand breaks and gene proximity. *Proc Natl Acad Sci U S A* 2012;109(23):8989–8994.

118. Azarova AM, Lyu YL, Lin CP, et al. Roles of DNA topoisomerases II isozymes in chemotherapy and secondary malignancies. *Proc Natl Acad Sci U S A* 2007;104:11014–11019.
119. Changela A, DiGate RJ, Mondragón A. Structural studies of E. Coli topoisomerase III-DNA complexes reveal a novel type IA topoisomerase-DNA conformational intermediate. *J Mol Biol* 2007;368:105–118.
120. Bertrand R, O'Connor PM, Kerrigan D, et al. Sequential administration of camptothecin and etoposide circumvents the antagonistic cytotoxicity of simultaneous drug administration in slowly growing human colon carcinoma HT-29 cells. *Eur J Cancer* 1992;28A(4–5):743–748.
121. Miller AA, Al Omari A, Murry DJ, et al. Phase I and pharmacologic study of sequential topotecan-carboplatin-etoposide in patients with extensive stage small cell lung cancer. *Lung Cancer* 2006;54:379–385.
122. Rose PG, Markham M, Bell JG, et al. Sequential prolonged oral topotecan and prolonged oral etoposide as second-line therapy in ovarian or peritoneal carcinoma: a phase I Gynecologic Oncology Study Group study. *Gynecol Oncol* 2006;102:236–239.
123. Kummar S, Chen A, Ji J, et al. Phase I study of PARP inhibitor ABT-888 in combination with topotecan in adults with refractory solid tumors and lymphomas. *Cancer Res* 2011;71(17):5626–5634.
124. Pfister TD, Hollingshead M, Kinders RJ, et al. Development and validation of an immunoassay for quantification of topoisomerase I in solid tumor tissues. *PLoS One* 2012;7:e50494.
125. Kinders RJ, Hollingshead M, Lawrence S, et al. Development of a validated immunofluorescence assay for gH2AX as a pharmacodynamics marker of topoisomerase I inhibitor activity. *Clin Cancer Res* 2010;16:5447–5457.

21 Antimicrotubule Agents

Christopher J. Hoimes and Lyndsay N. Harris

MICROTUBULES

Microtubules are vital and dynamic cytoskeletal polymers that play a critical role in cell division, signaling, vesicle transport, shape, and polarity, which make them attractive targets in anticancer regimens and drug design.[1] Microtubules are composed of 13 linear protofilaments of polymerized α/β-tubulin heterodimers arranged in parallel around a cylindrical axis and associated with regulatory proteins such as microtubule-associated proteins, tau, and motor proteins kinesin and dynein.[2] The specific biologic functions of microtubules are due to their unique polymerization dynamics. Tubulin polymerization is mediated by a nucleation-elongation mechanism. One end of the microtubules, termed the *plus end*, is kinetically more dynamic than the other end, termed the *minus end* (Fig. 21.1). Microtubule dynamics are governed by two principal processes driven by guanosine 5′-triphosphate (GTP) hydrolysis: *treadmilling* or *poleward flux* is the net growth at one end of the microtubule and the net shortening at the opposite end, and *dynamic instability*, which is a process in which the microtubule ends switch spontaneously between states of slow sustained growth and rapid depolymerization.[2] Antimicrotubule agents are tubulin-binding drugs that directly bind tubules, inhibitors of tubulin-associated scaffold kinases, or inhibitors of their associated mitotic motor proteins to, ultimately, disrupt microtubule dynamics. They are broadly classified as microtubule stabilizing or microtubule destabilizing agents according to their effects on tubulin polymerization.

TAXANES

Taxanes were the first-in-class microtubule stabilizing drugs. Ancient medicinal attempts at cardiac pharmacotherapy using material from the toxic coniferous yew tree, *Taxus* spp., were likely related to the plant's alkaloid *taxine* effect on sodium and calcium channels. Taxane compounds are the result of a drug screening of 35,000 plant extracts in 1963 that led to the identification of activity from the bark extract of the Pacific yew tree, *Taxus brevifolia*. Paclitaxel was identified as the active constituent with a report of its activity in carcinoma cell lines in 1971.[3] Motivation to identify taxanes derived from the more abundant and available needles of *Taxus baccata* led to the development of docetaxel, which is synthesized by the addition of a side chain to 10-deacetylbaccatin III, an inactive taxane precursor.[4] The taxane rings of paclitaxel and docetaxel are linked to an ester side chain attached to the C13 position of the ring, which is essential for antimicrotubule and antitumor activity. Nanoparticle albumin-bound paclitaxel (nab-paclitaxel) is a formulation that avoids the solvent related side effects of non–water-soluble paclitaxel and docetaxel. Overcoming docetaxel and paclitaxel's susceptibility to the P-glycoprotein efflux pump led to the development of cabazitaxel.[5] Cabazitaxel is synthesized by adding two methoxy groups to the 10-deacetylbaccatin III, which results in the inhibition of the 5′-triphosphate–dependent efflux pump of P-glycoprotein.

Paclitaxel initially received regulatory approval in the United States in 1992 for the treatment of patients with ovarian cancer after failure of first-line or subsequent chemotherapy (Table 21.1).[1,4] Subsequently, it has been approved for several other indications, including advanced breast cancer after anthracycline-based regimens[6]; combination chemotherapy of lymph node–positive breast cancer in the adjuvant setting[7]; advanced ovarian cancer in combination with a platinum compound; second-line treatment of AIDS-related Kaposi sarcoma; and first-line treatment of non–small-cell lung cancer (NSCLC) in combination with cisplatin[8] (see Table 21.1). In addition to the U.S. Food and Drug Administration (FDA) on-label indications, paclitaxel is widely used for several other tumor types, such as cancers of unknown origin, bladder, esophagus, gastric, head and neck, and cervical cancers. The U.S. patent for paclitaxel expired in 2002, and a generic form of paclitaxel is now available.

Docetaxel was first approved for use in the United States in 1996 for patients with metastatic breast cancer that progressed or relapsed after anthracycline-based chemotherapy, which was later broadened to a general second-line indication (see Table 21.1).[4,6] Subsequently, it received regulatory approval in adjuvant chemotherapy of stage II breast cancer in combination with Adriamycin and cyclophosphamide (TAC)[9], and first-line treatment for locally advanced or metastatic breast cancer.[10] In addition, docetaxel has indications in nonresectable, locally advanced, or metastatic NSCLC after failure of or in combination with cisplatin therapy; metastatic castration-resistant prostate cancer in combination with prednisone[11]; first-line treatment of gastric adenocarcinoma, including gastroesophageal junction adenocarcinoma in combination with cisplatin and 5-fluorouracil (5-FU)[12]; and inoperable locally advanced squamous cell cancer of the head and neck in combination with cisplatin and 5-FU (see Table 21.1). Docetaxel came off patent in 2010 and a generic form is available.

Mechanism of Action

The unique mechanism of action for paclitaxel was initially defined by Schiff et al.[13] in 1979, who showed that it bound to the interior surface of the microtubule lumen at binding sites completely distinct from those of exchangeable GTP, colchicine, podophyllotoxin, and the vinca alkaloids.[14] The taxanes profoundly alter the tubulin dissociation rate constants at both ends of the microtubule, suppressing treadmilling and dynamic instability. Dose-dependent taxane β-tubular binding induces mitotic arrest at the G2/M transition and induces cell death. By stabilizing microtubules, they also can stall ligand-dependent intracellular trafficking, as shown in sequestration of the androgen receptor to the cytosol in metastatic prostate cancer patients treated with docetaxel, and is associated with decreased androgen-regulated gene expression, such as prostate-specific antigen (PSA).[15,16] Peripheral neuropathy is a common dose-limiting toxicity across the antimicrotubule agents and likely is a result of their direct effect on microtubules. Studies

CANCER THERAPEUTICS

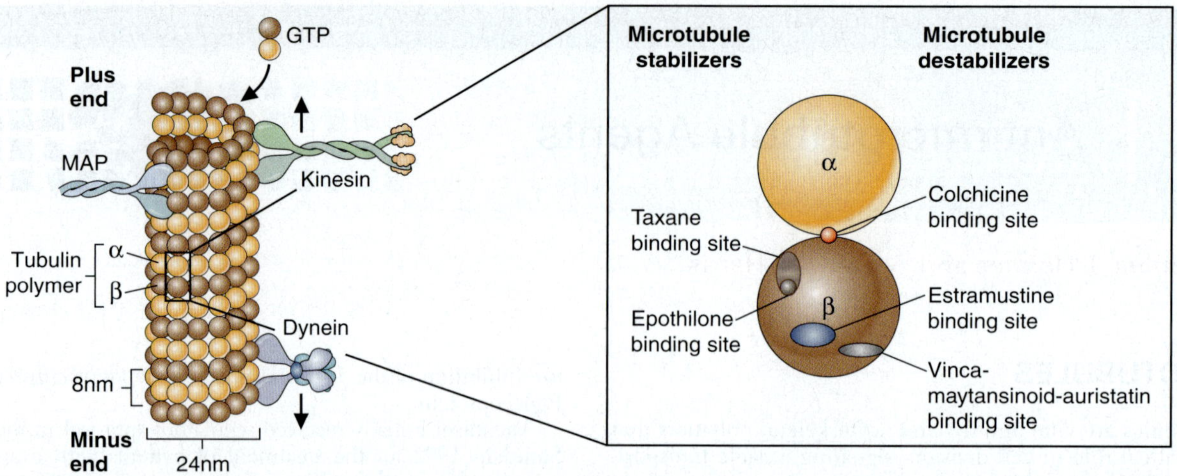

Figure 21.1 Antimicrotubule agents bind tubulin directly or inhibit its associated proteins. Taxanes and epothilones have distinct binding pockets within the same site on the interior surface of the tubule. Estramustine has a distinct site on β-tubulin, although it also directly binds microtubule-associated proteins (MAP). (Adapted from Lieberman M, Marks A. *Mark's Basic Medical Biochemistry: A Clinical Approach.* 3rd ed. Philadelphia: Lippincott Williams & Wilkins; 2009.)

have shown that they inhibit anterograde and/or retrograde fast axonal transport and can explain the demyelinating "dying back" pattern seen and the vulnerability of sensory neurons with the longest axonal projections.[17]

Recent evidence suggests that microtubule inhibitors have collateral effects during interphase that lead to cell death. For instance, paclitaxel-stabilized microtubules serve as a scaffold for the binding of the death-effector domain of pro-caspase-8, and thereby enabling a caspase-8 downstream proteolytic cascade.[18,19] This caspase-8–dependent mechanism also serves as an important basis for the understanding of the loss of function and/or low expression of the breast cancer 1, early onset gene (*BRCA1*) association with resistance to taxane therapy.[20]

Another mechanism of the anticancer effect of taxanes is currently being elaborated and is tied to the B-cell lymphoma-2 (Bcl-2) antiapoptosis family of proteins. Paclitaxel has been shown to cause the phosphorylation of Bcl-2 and the sequestration of Bak and Bim; however, this seemingly cancer-protective phosphorylation needs to be reconciled and likely correlates with Bcl-2–expression levels.[21–23] Interestingly, neutralizing Bcl-2 homology 3 (BH3) domains with compounds such as ABT-737 is synergistic with docetaxel.[24]

Clinical Pharmacology

Paclitaxel

With prolonged infusion schedules (6 and 24 hours), drug disposition is a biphasic process with values for alpha and beta half-lives averaging approximately 20 minutes and 6 hours, respectively.[4] When administered as a 3-hour infusion, the pharmacokinetics are nonlinear and may lead to unexpected toxicity with a small dose escalation, or a disproportionate decrease in drug exposure and loss of tumor response with a dose reduction. Approximately 71% of an administered dose of paclitaxel is excreted in the stool via the enterohepatic circulation over 5 days as either the parent compound or metabolites in humans. Renal clearance of paclitaxel and metabolites is minimal, accounting for 14% of the administered dose. In humans, the bulk of drug disposition is metabolized by cytochrome P-450 mixed-function oxidases—specifically, the isoenzymes CYP2C8 and CYP3A4, which metabolize paclitaxel to hydroxylated 3′p-hydroxypaclitaxel (minor) and 6α-hydroxypaclitaxel (major), as well as dihydroxylated metabolites.

Nanoparticle Albumin-Bound Paclitaxel

Nab-paclitaxel is a solvent-free colloidal suspension made by homogenizing paclitaxel with 3% to 4% albumin under high pressure to form nanoparticles of ~130 nm that disperse in plasma to ~10 nm (see Table 21.1).[25] It received regulatory approval in the United States in 2005 based on results in patients with metastatic breast cancer, and is now also approved in combination with carboplatin for first-line treatment of locally advanced or metastatic NSCLC, and in combination with gemcitabine for first-line treatment of metastatic pancreatic adenocarcinoma.[26–28] The improved responses seen with nab-paclitaxel, when compared to solvent-based paclitaxel, are not fully understood. Nab-paclitaxel likely capitalizes on several mechanisms, which include an improved pharmacokinetic profile with a larger volume of distribution and a higher maximal concentration of circulating, unbound, free drug; improved tumor accumulation by the enhanced permeability and retention (EPR) effect; and receptor-mediated transcytosis via an albumin-specific receptor (gp60) for endothelial transcytosis and binding of secreted protein acidic and rich in cysteine (SPARC) in the tumor interstitium.[29,30] In contrast to cremophor/ethanol (CrEL) solvent-based paclitaxel, nab-paclitaxel exhibits an extensive extravascular volume of distribution exceeding that of water, indicating extensive tissue and extravascular protein distribution. Some studies show that nab-paclitaxel achieves 33% higher drug concentration over CrEL-paclitaxel.[31] Additionally, the maximum concentration (Cmax), the mean plasma half-life of 15 to 18 hours, the area under curve (AUC), and the dose-independent plasma clearance correspond to linear pharmacokinetics over 80 to 300 mg/m^2.[29,32] The improved deposition of a nanoparticle, such as nab-paclitaxel in a tumor tissue, can occur passively through an EPR effect in areas of leaky vasculature, sufficient vascular pore size, and decreased lymphatic flow.[25,33] Once in the tissue, the nab-paclitaxel nanovehicle can deliver the drug locally or benefit from further receptor-mediated targeting to SPARC, which has been shown to be overexpressed, and correlates with disease progression in many tumor types.[34–38] Although preclinical models, as well as one clinical trial, have shown how nanoparticle therapy can benefit from this targeted approach,[39,40] correlative data for nab-paclitaxel is limited. The high stromal SPARC level was associated with longer survival in patients treated with nab-paclitaxel in the phase I/II study of patients with pancreatic cancer; however, this correlative analysis was not included in the phase III trial report and requires validation.[28,41]

TABLE 21.1

Antimicrotubule Agents: Dosages and Toxicities

Chemotherapeutic Agent	Dosage	Indications	Common Toxicities
Paclitaxel	135–200 mg/m^2 IV over 3 h or 135 mg/m^2 IV over 24 h every 3 wk; or 80 mg/m^2 IV over 1 h weekly	Adjuvant therapy of node-positive breast cancer; metastatic breast, ovarian, non–small-cell lung, bladder, esophagus, cervical, gastric, and head and neck cancer; AIDS-related Kaposi sarcoma; cancer of unknown origin	Myelosuppression, hypersensitivity, nausea and vomiting, alopecia, arthralgia, myalgia, peripheral neuropathy
Docetaxel	60–100 mg/m^2 IV over 1 h every 3 wk	Adjuvant therapy of node-positive breast cancer; metastatic breast, gastric, head and neck, prostate, non–small-cell lung, and ovarian cancer	Myelosuppression, hypersensitivity, edema, alopecia, nail damage, rash, diarrhea, nausea, vomiting, asthenia, neuropathy
Cabazitaxel	25 mg/m^2 IV every 3 wk over 1 h	Docetaxel-refractory metastatic castration resistant prostate cancer	Neutropenia, infections, myelosuppression, diarrhea, nausea, vomiting, constipation, abdominal pain, asthenia
Nab-paclitaxel	260 mg/m^2 IV over 30 min every 3 wk; or 125 mg/m^2 IV weekly on days 1, 8, and 15 every 28 d	Metastatic breast cancer, non–small-cell lung cancer, pancreatic cancer	Myelosuppression, nausea, vomiting, alopecia, myalgia, peripheral neuropathy
Ixabepilone	40 mg/m^2 IV over 3 h every 3 wk	Metastatic and locally advanced breast cancer	Myelosuppression, fatigue/asthenia, myalgia/arthralgia, alopecia, nausea, vomiting, stomatitis/mucositis, diarrhea, musculoskeletal pain
Vincristine	0.5–1.4 mg/m^2/wk IV (maximum 2 mg per dose); or 0.4 mg/d continuous infusion for 4 d	Lymphoma, acute leukemia, neuroblastoma, rhabdomyosarcoma, AIDS-related Kaposi sarcoma, multiple myeloma, testicular cancer	Constipation, nausea, vomiting, alopecia, diplopia, myelosuppression
Vinblastine	6 mg/m^2 IV on days 1 and 15 as part of the ABVD regimen; 0.15 mg/kg IV on days 1 and 2 as part of the PVB regimen; 3 mg/m^2 IV as part of days 2, 15, 22 MVAC regimen	Hodgkin and non-Hodgkin lymphoma; Kaposi sarcoma; breast, testicular, bladder, prostate, and renal cell cancer	Myelosuppression, constipation, alopecia, malaise, bone pain
Vinorelbine	25–30 mg/m^2 IV weekly	Non–small-cell lung, breast, cervical, and ovarian cancer	Alopecia, diarrhea, nausea, vomiting, asthenia, neuromyopathy
Estramustine	14 mg/kg PO daily in 3 or 4 divided doses	Metastatic prostate cancer	Nausea, vomiting, gynecomastia, fluid retention
Ado-trastuzumab emtansine	3.6 mg/kg IV every 3 wk	Metastatic breast cancer	Thrombocytopenia, nausea, constipation or diarrhea, peripheral neuropathy, fatigue, increased AST/ALT
Brentuximab vedotin	1.8 mg/kg every 3 wk, maximum dose 180 mg	Refractory Hodgkin lymphoma, refractory systemic anaplastic large cell lymphoma	Neutropenia, anemia, thrombocytopenia, fatigue, fever, peripheral neuropathy

ABVD, doxorubicin (Adriamycin), bleomycin, vinblastine, dacarbazine; PVB, cisplatin, vinblastine, bleomycin; MVAC, methotrexate, vinblastine, doxorubicin (Adriamycin), cisplatin; IV, intravenous; PO, by mouth; AST/ALT, aspartate amniotransferase–alanine amniotransferase.

Docetaxel

The pharmacokinetics of docetaxel on a 1-hour schedule is triexponential and linear at doses of 115 mg/m^2 or less.[4] Terminal half-lives ranging from 11.1 to 18.5 hours has been reported. The most important determinants of docetaxel clearance were the body surface area (BSA), hepatic function, and plasma α_1-acid glycoprotein concentration. Plasma protein binding is high (greater than 80%), and binding is primarily to α_1-acid glycoprotein, albumin, and lipoproteins. The hepatic cytochrome P-450 mixed-function oxidases, particularly isoforms CYP3A4 and CYP3A5, are principally involved in biotransformation. The principal pharmacokinetic determinants of toxicity, particularly neutropenia, are drug exposure and the time that plasma concentrations exceed biologically relevant concentrations. The baseline level of α_1-acid glycoprotein may be elevated as an acute phase reactant in advanced disease and is an independent predictor of response and a major objective prognostic factor of survival in patients with non–small-cell lung cancer treated with docetaxel chemotherapy.

Cabazitaxel

Cabazitaxel is a semisynthetic derivative of the natural taxoid 10-deacetylbaccatin III. It binds to and stabilizes the β-tubulin subunit, resulting in the inhibition of microtubule depolymerization and cell division, cell cycle arrest in the G_2/M phase, and the inhibition of tumor cell proliferation.[5] It is active against diverse cancer cell lines and tumor models that are sensitive and resistant to docetaxel, including prostate, mammary, melanoma, kidney, colon, pancreas, lung, gastric, and head and neck.[5] Cabazitaxel is a poor substrate for the membrane-associated, multidrug resistance P-glycoprotein efflux pump; therefore, is useful for treating docetaxel-refractory prostate cancer for which it gained FDA approval in 2010.[5] In addition, it penetrates the blood–brain barrier.[42] Pharmacokinetics of cabazitaxel is similar to docetaxel; however, cabazitaxel has a larger volume of distribution and a longer terminal half-life (mean 77.3 hours versus 11.2 hours for docetaxel).[43,44]

Tesetaxel

Tesetaxel (DJ-927, XRP6258) is a semisynthetic, orally bioavailable taxane currently in clinical trials in breast, gastric, and prostate cancer. Administration in phase I and II trials has been once per week or every 3 weeks and not associated with hypersensitivity and possibly less neurotoxicity compared to other taxanes. Dose-limiting toxicity has been neutropenia. Overall responses in phase II studies have been 50% and 38% in patients treated for first- and second-line breast cancer, respectively. A phase I/II study in advanced NSCLC showed an overall response rate of 5.6%. Tesetaxel activity is independent of P-glycoprotein expression.[45] Pharmacokinetics on a schedule of every 3 weeks have an AUC of ~1,750 ng/mL per hour, a half life of ~170 hours, and no drug interactions that have been noted.[46]

Drug Interactions

Sequence-dependent pharmacokinetic and toxicologic interactions between paclitaxel and several other chemotherapy agents have been noted. The sequence of cisplatin followed by paclitaxel (on a 24-hour schedule) induces more profound neutropenia than the reverse sequence, which is explained by a 33% reduction in the clearance of paclitaxel after cisplatin.[47] Treatment with paclitaxel on either a 3- or 24-hour schedule followed by carboplatin has been demonstrated to produce equivalent neutropenia and less thrombocytopenia as compared to carboplatin as a single agent, which is not explained by pharmacokinetic interactions. Neutropenia and mucositis are more severe when paclitaxel is administered on a 24-hour schedule before doxorubicin, compared to the reverse sequence, which is most likely due to an approximately 32% reduction in the clearance rates of doxorubicin and doxorubicinol when doxorubicin is administered after paclitaxel. Several agents that inhibit cytochrome P-450 mixed-function oxidases interfere with the metabolism of paclitaxel and docetaxel in human microsomes in vitro; however, the clinical relevance of these findings is not known.[47]

Toxicity

Paclitaxel

The micelle-forming CrEL vehicle, which is required for suspension and intravenous delivery of paclitaxel, causes its nonlinear pharmacokinetics and thereby impacts its therapeutic index. CrEL causes hypersensitivity reactions, with major reactions usually occurring within the first 10 minutes after the first treatment and resolving completely after stopping the treatment. All patients should be premedicated with steroids, diphenhydramine, and an H2 antagonist, although up to 3% will still have reactions. Those who have major reactions have been rechallenged successfully after receiving high doses of corticosteroids.

Neuropathy is the principal toxicity of paclitaxel. Paclitaxel induces a peripheral neuropathy that presents in a symmetric stocking glove distribution, at first transient and then persistent.[48] A neurologic examination reveals sensory loss, and neurophysiologic studies reveal axonal degeneration and demyelination.[48] Compared with cisplatin, a loss of deep tendon reflexes occurs less commonly; however, autonomic and motor changes can occur. Severe neurotoxicity is uncommon when paclitaxel is given alone at doses below 200 mg/m^2 on a 3- or 24-hour schedule every 3 weeks, or below 100 mg/m^2 on a continuous weekly schedule. There is no convincing evidence that any specific measure is effective at ameliorating existing manifestations or preventing the development or worsening of neurotoxicity.[48]

Neutropenia is also frequent with paclitaxel. The onset is usually on days 8 to 11, and recovery is generally complete by days 15 to 21 with an every 3 weeks dosing regimen. Neutropenia is noncumulative, and the duration of severe neutropenia—even in heavily pretreated patients—is usually brief. Severity of neutropenia is related to the duration of exposure above the biologically relevant levels of 0.05 to 0.10 μM/L, and paclitaxel's nonlinear pharmacokinetics should be considered whenever adjusting dose.[49]

The most common cardiac rhythm disturbance, a transient sinus bradycardia, can be observed in up to 30% of patients. Routine cardiac monitoring during paclitaxel therapy is not necessary but is advisable for patients who may not be able to tolerate bradyarrhythmias. Drug-related gastrointestinal effects, such as vomiting and diarrhea, are uncommon. Severe hepatotoxicity and pancreatitis have also been noted rarely. Pulmonary toxicities, including acute bilateral pneumonitis, have been reported. Extravasation of large volumes can cause moderate soft tissue injury. Paclitaxel also induces reversible alopecia of the scalp in a dose-related fashion. Nail disorders have also been reported with paclitaxel use and include ridging, nail bed pigmentation, onychorrhexis, and onycholysis. These side effects have been reported more commonly with dose-intensified paclitaxel regimens.

Recent studies have suggested a role for the adenosine triphosphatase (ATP)-binding cassette (ABC) transporter polymorphisms in the development of neuropathy and neutropenia. Sissung et al.[50] reported that patients carrying two reference alleles for the *ABCB1* (P-glycoprotein, MDR1) 3435C greater than T polymorphism had a reduced risk to develop neuropathy as compared to patients carrying at least one variant allele ($P = .09$). Data from a large controlled trial to evaluate these and other candidate polymorphisms failed to detect a significant association between genotype and outcome or toxicity for any of the genes analyzed, although the correlative studies were retrospective and the sample size was inadequate to rule out smaller differences.[51] A large randomized trial of the CALGB 40101 using an integrated genomewide associate study found two polymorphisms associated with paclitaxel-induced polyneuropathy.[52] Both are involved in nerve development and maintenance, including the hereditary peripheral neuropathy Charcot-Marie-Tooth disease gene, *FGD4*. Further studies are required to adequately assess the role of these variants in predicting toxicity from taxane therapy.

Nab-paclitaxel

Hypersensitivity reactions have not been observed during the infusion period and, therefore, steroid premedications are not necessary. The main dose-limiting toxicities are neutropenia and sensory neuropathy. In a trial comparing weekly paclitaxel 90 mg/m^2 to nab-paclitaxel 150 mg/m^2 to ixabepilone in patients with metastatic breast cancer, there was more hematologic toxicity and peripheral neuropathy in the nab-paclitaxel arm compared to the paclitaxel arm, although median progression-free survival was not significantly different at the 12-month follow-up.[53] This led to dose reductions in 45% of patients in the nab-paclitaxel arm compared with 15% for the paclitaxel arm.[53] Other toxicities include alopecia, diarrhea, nausea and vomiting, elevations in liver enzymes, arthralgia, myalgia, and asthenia.

Docetaxel

Neutropenia is the main toxicity of docetaxel.[4] When docetaxel is administered on an every 3 weeks schedule, the onset of neutropenia is usually noted on day 8, with complete resolution by days 15 to 21. Neutropenia is significantly less when low doses are administered weekly. FDA black box warnings include increased toxicity in patients with abnormal liver function and, in select NSCLC patients that received prior platinum, severe hypersensitivity reactions and severe fluid retention despite dexamethasone at-home premedication.

Hypersensitivity reactions were noted in approximately 31% of patients who received the drug without premedications in early studies.[4] Symptoms include flushing, rash, chest tightness, back pain, dyspnea, and fever or chills. Severe hypotension, bronchospasm, generalized rash, and erythema may also occur.[54] Major reactions usually occur during the first two courses and within minutes after the start of treatment. Signs and symptoms generally resolve within 15 minutes after cessation of treatment, and docetaxel can usually be reinstituted without sequelae after treatment with diphenhydramine and an H2-receptor antagonist. Docetaxel induces a unique fluid retention syndrome characterized by edema, weight gain, and third-space fluid collection. Fluid retention is cumulative and is due to increased capillary permeability. Prophylactic treatment with corticosteroids has been demonstrated to reduce the incidence of fluid retention. Aggressive and early treatment with diuretics has been successfully used to manage fluid retention. Skin toxicity may occur in as many as 50% to 75% of patients; however, premedication may reduce the overall incidence of this effect.[4] Other cutaneous effects include palmar–plantar erythrodysesthesia and onychodystrophy. Docetaxel produces neurotoxicity, which is qualitatively similar to that of paclitaxel; however, neurosensory and neuromuscular effects are generally less frequent and less severe than with paclitaxel. Mild-to-moderate peripheral neurotoxicity occurs in approximately 40% of untreated patients.[55] Asthenia has been a prominent complaint in patients who have been treated with large cumulative doses. Stomatitis appears to occur more frequently with docetaxel than with paclitaxel. Other reported toxicities of note include necrotizing enterocolitis, interstitial pneumonitis, and organizing pneumonia.[56,57]

Cabazitaxel

A phase III multi-institutional study of men with metastatic castration-resistant prostate cancer who had failed docetaxel improved overall median survival on cabazitaxel compared to mitoxantrone.[58] Cabazitaxel was approved by the FDA in June 2010 to treat metastatic castration-resistant prostate cancer in those who had received prior chemotherapy. This was despite a higher rate of adverse deaths (4.9%), a third of which were due to neutropenic sepsis. Cabazitaxel was associated with more grade 3 or 4 neutropenia (82%) than mitoxantrone (58%). Side effects reported in more than 20% of patients treated with cabazitaxel included myelosuppression, diarrhea, nausea, vomiting, constipation, abdominal pain, or asthenia. FDA black box warnings are similar to those for docetaxel.

VINCA ALKALOIDS

The vinca alkaloids have been some of the most active agents in cancer chemotherapy since their introduction 40 years ago. The naturally occurring members of the family, vinblastine (VBL) and vincristine (VCR), were isolated from the leaves of the periwinkle plant *Catharanthus roseus G. Don*. In the late 1950s, their antimitotic and, therefore, cancer chemotherapeutic potential was discovered by groups both at Eli Lilly Research Laboratories and at the University of Western Ontario, and they came into widespread use for the single-agent treatment of childhood hematologic and solid malignancies and, shortly after, for adult hematologic malignancies (see Table 21.1).[1] Their clinical efficacy in several combination therapies has led to the development of various novel semisynthetic analogs, including vinorelbine (VRL), vindesine (VDS), and vinflunine (VFL).

Mechanism of Action

In contrast to the taxanes, the vinca alkaloids depolymerize microtubules and destroy mitotic spindles.[1] At low but clinically relevant concentrations, VBL does not depolymerize spindle microtubules, yet it powerfully blocks mitosis. This has been suggested to occur as a result of the suppression of microtubule dynamics rather than microtubule depolymerization. This group of compounds binds to the β subunit of tubulin dimers at a distinct region called the vinca-binding domain. Importantly, VBL binding induces a conformational change in tubulin in connection with tubulin self-association. In mitotic spindles, the slowing of the growth and shortening or treadmilling dynamics of the microtubules block mitotic progression. Disruption of the normal mitotic spindle assembly leads to delayed cell cycle progress with chromosomes stuck at the spindle poles and unable to pass from metaphase into anaphase, which eventually induces to apoptosis. The naturally occurring vinca alkaloids VCR and VBL, the semisynthetic analog VRL, and a novel bifluorinated analog VFL have similar mechanisms of action.

Tissue and tumor sensitivities to the vinca alkaloids, which, in part, relate to differences in drug transport and accumulation, also vary. Intracellular or extracellular concentration ratios range from five- to 500-fold depending on the individual cell type, lipophilicity, tissue-specific factors such as tubulin isotype composition, and tissue-specific microtubule-associated proteins (MAP).[59–61] Although the vinca alkaloids are retained in cells for long periods of time and thus may have prolonged cellular effects, intracellular retention is markedly different among the various vinca alkaloids. For instance, VBL appears to be retained in lipophilic tissue much more than either VCR or VDS.[59] Newer theories of antimicrotubule agents' mechanism of action have emerged, suggesting that the more important target of these drugs may be the tumor vasculature, as reviewed in the next section.

Clinical Pharmacology

The vinca alkaloids are usually administered intravenously as a brief infusion, and their pharmacokinetic behavior in plasma has generally been explained by a three-compartment model. The vinca alkaloids share many pharmacokinetic properties, including large volumes of distribution, high clearance rates, and long terminal half-lives that reflect the high magnitude and avidity of drug binding in peripheral tissues. VCR has the longest terminal half-life and the lowest clearance rate; VBL has the shortest terminal half-life and the highest clearance rate; and VDS has intermediate characteristics. Although prolonged infusion schedules may avoid excessively toxic peak concentrations and increase the duration of drug exposure in plasma above biologically relevant threshold concentrations, there is little evidence to support the notion that prolonged infusions are more effective than bolus schedules. The longest half-life and lowest clearance rate of VCR may account for its greater propensity to induce neurotoxicity, but there are many other nonpharmacokinetic determinants of tissue sensitivity, as discussed in the previous section.

Vincristine

After conventional doses of VCR (1.4 mg/m^2) given as brief infusions, peak plasma levels approach 0.4 μmol. Plasma clearance is slow, and terminal half-lives that range from 23 to 85 hours have been reported. VCR is metabolized and excreted primarily by the

CANCER THERAPEUTICS

hepatobiliary system. The nature of the VCR metabolites identified to date, as well as the results of metabolic studies in vitro, indicate that VCR metabolism is mediated principally by hepatic cytochrome P-450 CYP3A5.

Vinblastine

The clinical pharmacology of VBL is similar to that of VCR. VBL binding to plasma proteins and formed elements of blood is extensive.[62,63] Peak plasma drug concentrations are approximately 0.4 μm after rapid intravenous injections of VBL at standard doses. Distribution is rapid, and terminal half-lives range from 20 to 24 hours. Like VCR, VBL disposition is principally through the hepatobiliary system with excretion in feces (approximately 95%); however, fecal excretion of the parent compound is low, indicating that hepatic metabolism is extensive.[59]

Vinorelbine

The pharmacologic behavior of VRL is similar to that of the other vinca alkaloids, and plasma concentrations after rapid intravenous administration have been reported to decline in either a biexponential or triexponential manner.[64] After intravenous administration, there is a rapid decay of VRL concentrations followed by a much slower elimination phase (terminal half-life, 18 to 49 hours). Plasma protein binding, principally to α_1-acid glycoprotein, albumin, and lipoproteins, has been reported to range from 80% to 91%, and drug binding to platelets is extensive.[64] VRL is widely distributed, and high concentrations are found in virtually all tissues, except the central nervous system.[64] The wide distribution of VRL reflects its lipophilicity, which is among the highest of the vinca alkaloids. As with other vinca alkaloids, the liver is the principal excretory organ, and up to 80% of VRL is excreted in the feces, whereas urinary excretion represents only 16% to 30% of total drug disposition, the bulk of which is unmetabolized VRL. Studies in humans indicate that 4-O-deacetyl-VRL and 3,6-epoxy-VRL are the principal metabolites, and several minor hydroxy-VRL isomer metabolites have been identified. Although most metabolites are inactive, the deacetyl-VRL metabolite may be as active as VRL. The cytochrome P-450 CYP3A isoenzyme appears to be principally involved in biotransformation.

Vinflunine

VFL is a novel semisynthetic microtubule inhibitor with a fluorinated catharanthine moiety, which translates into lower affinity for the vinca binding site on tubulin and, therefore, different quantitative effects on microtubule dynamics.[65] The low affinity for tubulin may be responsible for its reduced clinical neurotoxicity. Despite this lower affinity, it is more active in vivo than other vinca alkaloids, and resistance develops more slowly. VFL is a new vinca and still under clinical development. Its volume of distribution is large, and has a terminal half-life of nearly 40 hours.[65] The only active metabolite is 4-O-deacetylvinflunine, which has a terminal half-life approximately 5 days longer than that of the parent compound.[65]

Drug Interactions

Methotrexate accumulation in tumor cells is enhanced in vitro by the presence of VCR or VBL, an effect mediated by a vinca alkaloid–induced blockade of drug efflux; however, the minimal concentrations of VCR required to achieve this effect occur only transiently in vivo.[66] The vinca alkaloids also inhibit the cellular influx of the epipodophyllotoxins in vitro, resulting in less cytotoxicity. However, the clinical implications of this potential interaction are unknown. L-asparaginase may reduce the hepatic clearance of the vinca alkaloids, which may result in increased vinca-related toxicity. To minimize the possibility of this interaction, the vinca alkaloids should be given 12 to 24 hours before L-asparaginase. The combined use of mitomycin C and the vinca alkaloids has been associated with acute dyspnea and bronchospasm. The onset of these pulmonary toxicities has ranged from within minutes to hours after treatment with the vinca alkaloids, or up to 2 weeks after mitomycin C.

Treatment with the vinca alkaloids has precipitated seizures associated with subtherapeutic plasma phenytoin concentrations.[66] Reduced plasma phenytoin levels have been noted from 24 hours to 10 days after treatment with VCR and VBL. Because of the importance of the cytochrome P-450 CYP3A isoenzyme in vinca alkaloid metabolism, administration of the vinca alkaloids with erythromycin and other inhibitors of CYP3A may lead to severe toxicity.[67] Concomitantly administered drugs, such as pentobarbital and H_2-receptor antagonists, may also influence VCR clearance by modulating hepatic cytochrome P-450 metabolic processes.[66]

Toxicity

Despite close similarities in structure, the vinca alkaloids differ in their safety profiles. Neutropenia is the principal dose-limiting toxicity of VBL and VRL. Thrombocytopenia and anemia occur less commonly. The onset of neutropenia is usually day 7 to 11, with recovery by day 14 to 21, and can be potentiated by hepatic dysfunction. Gastrointestinal autonomic dysfunction, as manifested by bloating, constipation, ileus, and abdominal pain, occur most commonly with VCR or high doses of the other vinca alkaloids. Mucositis occurs more frequently with VBL than with VRL and is least common with VCR. Nausea, vomiting, diarrhea,[31,43,45] and pancreatitis[53,54] also occur to a lesser extent.

VCR principally induces neurotoxicity characterized by a peripheral, symmetric mixed sensory motor and autonomic polyneuropathy.[68,69] Toxic manifestations include constipation, abdominal cramps, paralytic ileus, urinary retention, orthostatic hypotension, and hypertension. Its primary neuropathologic effects are due to interference with axonal microtubule function. Early symmetric sensory impairment and paresthesias can progress to neuritic pain and loss of deep tendon reflexes with continued treatment, which may be followed by foot drop, wrist drop, motor dysfunction, ataxia, and paralysis. Cranial nerves are rarely affected because the uptake of VCR into the central nervous system is low. Severe neurotoxicity occurs infrequently with VBL and VDS. VRL has been shown to have a lower affinity for axonal microtubules than either VCR or VBL, which seems to be confirmed by clinical observations.[70] Mild-to-moderate peripheral neuropathy, principally characterized by sensory effects, occurs in 7% to 31% of patients, and constipation and other autonomic effects are noted in 30% of patients, whereas severe toxicity occurs in 2% to 3%.

In adults, neurotoxicity may occur after treatment with cumulative doses as little as 5 to 6 mg, and manifestations may be profound after cumulative doses of 15 to 20 mg. Patients with delayed biliary excretion or hepatic dysfunction, and those with antecedent neurologic disorders, such as Charcot-Marie-Tooth disease, hereditary and sensory neuropathy type 1, and Guillain-Barré syndrome, are predisposed to neurotoxicity.

The vinca alkaloids are potent vesicants. To decrease the risk of phlebitis, the vein should be adequately flushed after treatment. If extravasation is suspected, treatment should be discontinued, aspiration of any residual drug remaining in the tissues should be attempted, and prompt application of heat (*not* ice) for 1 hour four times daily for 3 to 5 days can limit tissue damage.[71] Hyaluronidase, 150 to 1,500 U (15 U/mL in 6 mL 0.9% sodium chloride solution) subcutaneously, through six clockwise injections in a circumferential manner using a 25-gauge needle (changing the needle with each new injection) into the surrounding tissues may minimize discomfort and latent cellulitis. A surgical consultation to consider early debridement is also recommended. Mild and reversible alopecia occurs in approximately 10% and 20% of patients treated with VLR and VCR, respectively. Acute cardiac ischemia, chest pains without evidence of ischemia, fever, Raynaud syndrome, hand–foot syndrome, and pulmonary and liver toxicity (transaminitis and hyperbilirubinemia) have also been reported with use of the vinca alkaloids. All of the vinca alkaloids can cause a syndrome of inappropriate secretion of antidiuretic hormone (SIADH), and patients who are receiving intensive hydration are particularly prone to severe hyponatremia secondary to SIADH.

MICROTUBULE ANTAGONISTS

Estramustine Phosphate

Estramustine is a conjugate of nor-nitrogen mustard linked to 17β-estradiol by a carbamate ester bridge. Estramustine phosphate received regulatory approval in the United States in 1981 for treating patients with castration-resistant prostate cancer (CRPC). Although the recommended daily dose of estramustine phosphate is 14 mg/kg per day, patients are usually treated in the daily dosing range of 10 to 16 mg/kg in three to four divided daily doses (see Table 21.1). Estramustine has significant activity in CRPC and had been used in combination with VBL or docetaxel. However, phase III trials in patients with CRPC showed that when combined with docetaxel, there is no added benefit to overall survival compared to docetaxel alone.[72,73]

Estramustine binds to β-tubulin at a site distinct from the colchicine and vinca alkaloid binding sites. This agent depolymerizes microtubules and microfilaments, binds to and disrupts MAPs, and inhibits cell growth at high concentrations, resulting in mitotic arrest and apoptosis in tumor cells. The selective accumulation and actions of estramustine phosphate and its metabolite, *estromustine*, in specific tissues appear to be dependent on the expression of the estramustine-binding protein (EMBP). The disposition of estramustine is principally by rapid oxidative metabolism of the parent compound to estromustine. Estromustine concentrations in plasma are maximal within 2 to 4 hours after oral administration, and the mean elimination half-life of estromustine is 14 hours. Estromustine and estramustine are principally excreted in the feces, with only small amounts of conjugated estrone and estradiol detected in the urine (less than 1%).

In general, this agent has a manageable safety profile. Nausea and vomiting are the principal toxicities encountered. In contrast to the taxanes and the vinca alkaloids, myelosuppression is rarely clinically relevant. Common estrogenic side effects include gynecomastia, nipple tenderness, and fluid retention. Thromboembolic complications may occur in up to 10% of patients.

Epothilones

The epothilones are macrolide compounds that were initially isolated from the mycobacterium *Sorangium cellulosum*. They exert their cytotoxic effects by promoting tubulin polymerization and inducing mitotic arrest.[74] In general, the epothilones are more potent than the taxanes. In contrast to the taxanes and vinca alkaloids, overexpression of the efflux protein P-glycoprotein minimally affects the cytotoxicity of epothilones. Epothilones include the natural epothilone B (patupilone; EPO906) and several semisynthetic epothilone compounds such as aza-epothilone B (ixabepilone; BMS-247550), epothilone D (deoxyepothilone B, KOS-862), and a fully synthetic analog, sagopilone (ZK-EPO).[75]

Ixabepilone has been evaluated in several schedules using a cremophor-based formulation and is FDA approved for the treatment of patients with breast cancer.[75] It is active in breast cancer previously treated with paclitaxel or docetaxel. The principal toxicities observed include neutropenia and peripheral neuropathy, in addition to fatigue, nausea, emesis, and diarrhea.[55,74] It also has been evaluated in other solid tumors such as ovarian, prostate, and renal cell carcinomas.[75] Epothilones are still undergoing evaluations in several clinical trials. Pharmacokinetic studies based on patupilone have shown large volume of distribution (41-fold the total body water) and low body clearance (13% of hepatic blood flow).[76] There do not appear to be active metabolites once the parent drug is hydrolyzed, which is the main elimination pathway.[76]

Maytansinoids and Auristatins: DM1, MMAE

Antibody drug conjugates (ADC) were first attempted with delivery of doxorubicin. Although tissue localization seemed promising, it became clear that the delivery of more potent chemotherapeutics was necessary.[77,78] One of the major advances for the promise of ADC came with the discovery and development of highly potent anticancer compounds such as calicheamicins, maytansinoids, and auristatins.[78] The next necessary advance was a linker that released the drug only when intended, and avoiding, or in some cases capitalizing on, in vivo proteases, oxidizing, or reducing environments. Gemtuzumab ozogamicin was the first ADC using calicheamicin, a potent DNA minor groove binder (and not a microtubule agent), approved in 2000 although withdrawn from the market in 2013 due to failed confirmatory studies. Maytansinoids and auristatins are unrelated, although are both tubulin-binding agents of the vinca binding site and inhibit tubulin polymerization.[78] They are 100- to 1,000-fold more cytotoxic that most cancer chemotherapeutics.[79]

Drug maytansinoid-1 (DM1) is the chemotherapeutic delivered using a thioether linker in the ADC ado-trastuzumab emtansine (T-DM1) that was FDA approved for patients with HER2- positive metastatic breast cancer previously treated with trastuzumab and taxane chemotherapy.[80,81] In the international phase III study, there was a 3.2-month improved progression-free survival among patients that received T-DM1 compared to those receiving standard treatment with capecitabine and lapatinib.[81] Despite a potent chemotherapeutic, the tolerability was much better in the experimental arm, which was dosed at 3.6 mg/kg intravenously every 21 days. The most common side effects in the trial were thrombocytopenia (12.8%), transient transaminitis (4.3%), as well as nausea, fatigue, myalgias, and arthralgias.[81]

Monomethyl auristatin E (MMAE) is linked to a monoclonal antibody against CD30 as an ADC (brentuximab vedotin, SGN35) and approved for refractory Hodgkin lymphoma or anaplastic large cell lymphoma. The linker is a peptide-based substrate for cathepsin-B and thereby designed to detect the lysosome/endosome compartment for drug release.[82,83] Dose-limiting toxicities include thrombocytopenia, hyperglycemia, diarrhea, and vomiting, and the most common side effects in this heavily pretreated population (including autologous stem cell transplant) includes peripheral neuropathy (42%), nausea (35%), and fatigue (34%).[84] The FDA black box warning includes contraindicated use with bleomycin due to increased pulmonary toxicity and the risk of John Cunningham (JC) virus–induced progressive multifocal leukoencephalopathy. Reports of severe pancreatitis are also emerging.[85]

MITOTIC MOTOR PROTEIN INHIBITORS

Aurora Kinase and Pololike Kinase Inhibitors

Aurora kinases are serine/threonine kinases crucial for mitosis in their recruitment of mitotic motor proteins for spindle formation. They are particularly overexpressed in high growth rate tumors. Aurora A and B kinases are expressed globally throughout all tissues, and Aurora C kinase is expressed in testes and participates in meiosis. Aurora A kinase is expressed and frequently amplified in many epithelial tumors and implicated in the microtubule-targeted agent-resistant phenotype.[86] Aurora A kinase interacts with p53, and there is evidence that p53 wild-type tumors are more sensitive to aurora A kinase inhibitors than p53 mutant tumors.[87] MLN-8237 has an IC_{50} of 1 nm for aurora A kinase and >200 nm for aurora B kinase and is in clinical development for treatment-related neuroendocrine prostate cancer.[86,88] The main dose-limiting toxicity of these agents is neutropenia. Pololike kinases (PLKs) are serine or threonine kinases crucial for cell cycle process. Overexpression of PLKs has been shown to be related to histologic grading and poor prognosis in several types of cancer. BI-2536 and ON01910 are PLK inhibitors in early clinical development.[89]

Kinesin Spindle Protein Inhibitor

Ispinesib

Kinesin spindle protein (KSP; also known as EG5) is a kinesin motor protein required to establish mitotic-spindle bipolarity.[90] Several KSP inhibitors have been evaluated in early phase clinical trials. SB-715992 (ispinesib) is a small-molecule inhibitor of KSP ATPase and has been evaluated in two different schedules.[89] The dose-limiting toxicity is neutropenia. Ispinesib was found to be inactive in phase 2 studies evaluating efficacy in patients with castration-resistant and largely docetaxel-resistant prostate cancer, advanced renal cancer, and head and neck cancer.[90–92]

MECHANISMS OF RESISTANCE TO MICROTUBULE INHIBITORS

Drug resistance is often complex and multifaceted and can involve diverse mechanisms such as (1) factors that reduce the ability of drugs to reach their cellular target (e.g., activation of detoxification pathways and decreased drug accumulation); (2) modifications in the drug target; and (3) events downstream of the target (e.g., decreased sensitivity to, or defective, apoptotic signals). Many tubulin binding agents are substrates for multidrug transporters such as P-glycoprotein and the multidrug resistance gene (*MDR1*).[93,94]

The *MDR1*-encoded gene product MDR1 (ABC subfamily B1; ABCB1) and MDR2 (ABC subfamily ABCB4) are the best-characterized ABC transporters thought to confer drug resistance to taxanes.[94,95] MDR-related taxane resistance can be reversed by many classes of drugs, including the calcium channel blockers, cyclosporin A, and antiarrhythmic agents.[94,95] However, the clinical utility of this approach has never been proven, despite several clinical trials. The role of ABC transporters in resistance to microtubule inhibitors remains to be determined.[96]

An increasing number of studies suggest that the expression of individual tubulin isotypes are altered in cells resistant to antimicrotubule drugs and may confer drug resistance.[93,97] Inherent differences in microtubule dynamics and drug interactions have been observed with some isotypes in vitro and in vivo.[98] Several taxane-resistant mutant cell lines that have structurally altered α- and β-tubulin proteins and an impaired ability to polymerize into microtubules have also been identified.[99] Mutations of tubulin isotype genes, gene amplifications, and isotype switching have also been reported in taxane-resistant cell lines.[99] In patients, levels of class III β-tubulin have been shown to correlate with response—those with high RNA levels have poor response—and immunohistochemical stains can correlate and may be predictive.[96,100,101] As opposed to taxanes, resistance to vinca alkaloids has been associated with decreased class II β-tubulin expression.[97,98]

MAPs are important structural and regulatory components of microtubules that act in concert to remodel the microtubule network by stabilizing or destabilizing microtubules during mitosis or cytokinesis. Alterations in the activity and/or balance of stabilizing or destabilizing MAPs can profoundly affect microtubule function.[99,102] The overexpression of stathmin, a destabilizing protein, has been reported to decrease sensitivity to paclitaxel and vinblastine.[1] An analysis of predictive or prognostic factors in a large phase 3 study (National Surgical Adjuvant Breast and Bowel Project NSABP-B 28) in patients with node-positive breast cancer showed that MAP-tau, a stabilizing protein, was a prognostic factor; however, it was not predictive for benefit from paclitaxel-based chemotherapy.[1,93] In a separate randomized controlled trial in breast cancer (TAX 307), where the only variable was docetaxel, MAP-tau was also shown to be prognostic, but not predictive of taxane benefit.[103]

Additional studies have shown a correlation with *BRCA1* loss measured by gene or protein expression, or gene signatures, with resistance to taxane and sensitivity to DNA-damaging agents (such as cisplatin and anthracyclines).[104–107] *BRCA1* is a tumor-suppressor gene with DNA damage response and repair, as well as cell cycle checkpoint activation, which explains why its loss leads to enhanced cisplatin sensitivity.[20] *BRCA1* also indirectly regulates microtubule dynamics and stability and can favorably control how microtubules respond to paclitaxel treatment via their association with pro-caspase-8. The loss of *BRCA1* can lead to impaired taxane-induced activation of apoptosis due to microtubules that are more dynamic and less susceptible to taxane-induced stabilization and proximity-induced activation of caspase-8 signaling.[20]

In addition to resistance, certain tumor subtypes may be sensitive to the taxane dosing schedule. In two randomized trials of low-dose, weekly paclitaxel, the luminal breast cancer subtype was found to have a better outcome compared with the control arm. This suggests that not only the drug, but also the schedule may influence the response to therapy and that genomic approaches may reveal these insights.[108]

REFERENCES

1. Kavallaris M. Microtubules and resistance to tubulin-binding agents. *Nat Rev Cancer* 2010;10:194–204.
2. Nogales E. Structural insights into microtubule function. *Ann Rev Biophys Biomol Struct* 2001;30:397–420.
3. Wani MC, Taylor HL, Wall ME, et al. Plant antitumor agents. VI. Isolation and structure of taxol, a novel antileukemic and antitumor agent from Taxus brevifolia. *J Am Chem Soc* 1971;93:2325–2327.
4. Rowinsky E, Donehower R. Antimicrotubule agents. In: DeVita VT, Hellmann S, Rosenberg SA, eds. *Cancer: Principles and Practice of Oncology*. 5th ed. Philadelphia: Lippincott-Raven;1997.
5. Vrignaud P, Sémiond D, Lejeune P, et al. Preclinical antitumor activity of cabazitaxel, a semisynthetic taxane active in taxane-resistant tumors. *Clin Cancer Res* 2013;19:2973–2983.
6. Sparano JA. Taxanes for breast cancer: an evidence-based review of randomized phase II and phase III trials. *Clin Breast Cancer* 2000;1:32–40.
7. Mamounas E, Leinbersky B, Bryant J, et al. Paclitaxel after doxorubicin plus cyclophosphamide as adjuvant chemotherapy for node-positive breast cancer: results from NSABP B-28. *J Clin Oncol* 2005;23:3686–3696.
8. Bonomi P, Kim KM, Fairclough D, et al. Comparison of survival and quality of life in advanced non-small-cell lung cancer patients treated with two dose levels of paclitaxel combined with cisplatin versus etoposide with cisplatin: results of an Eastern Cooperative Oncology Group trial. *J Clin Oncol* 2000;18:623–631.
9. Martin M, Pienkowski T, Mackey J, et al. Adjuvant docetaxel for node-positive breast cancer. *N Engl J Med* 2005;352:2302–2313.
10. Jones SE, Erban J, Overmoyer B, et al. Randomized phase III study of docetaxel compared with paclitaxel in metastatic breast cancer. *J Clin Oncol* 2005;23:5542–5551.
11. Tannock IF, de Wit R, Berry WR, et al. Docetaxel plus prednisone or mitoxantrone plus prednisone for advanced prostate cancer. *N Engl J Med* 2004;351:1502–1512.
12. Van Cutsem E, Moiseyenko V, Tjulandin S, et al. Phase III study of docetaxel and cisplatin plus fluorouracil compared with cisplatin and fluorouracil as first-line therapy for advanced gastric cancer: a report of the V325 Study Group. *J Clin Oncol* 2006;24:4991–4997.
13. Schiff PB, Fant J, Horwitz SB. Promotion of microtubule assembly in vitro by taxol. *Nature* 1979;277:665–667.

14. Nogales E. Structural insight into microtubule function. *Annu Rev Biophys Biomol Struct* 2001;30:397–420.
15. Darshan MS, Loftus MS, Thadani-Mulero M, et al. Taxane-induced blockade to nuclear accumulation of the androgen receptor predicts clinical responses in metastatic prostate cancer. *Cancer Res* 2011;71:6019–6029.
16. Hoimes CJ, Kelly WK. Redefining hormone resistance in prostate cancer. *Ther Adv Med Oncol* 2010;2:107–123.
17. LaPointe NE, Morfini G, Brady ST, et al. Effects of eribulin, vincristine, paclitaxel and ixabepilone on fast axonal transport and kinesin-1 driven microtubule gliding: Implications for chemotherapy-induced peripheral neuropathy. *Neurotoxicology* 2013;37:231–239.
18. Mielgo A, Torres VA, Clair K, et al. Paclitaxel promotes a caspase 8-mediated apoptosis through death effector domain association with microtubules. *Oncogene* 2009;28:3551–3562.
19. Komlodi-Pasztor E, Sackett D, Wilkerson J, et al. Mitosis is not a key target of microtubule agents in patient tumors. *Nat Rev Clin Oncol* 2011;8:244–250.
20. Sung M, Giannakakou P. BRCA1 regulates microtubule dynamics and taxane-induced apoptotic cell signaling. *Oncogene* 2014;33(11):1418–1428.
21. Strobel T, Kraeft SK, Chen LB, et al. BAX expression is associated with enhanced intracellular accumulation of paclitaxel: a novel role for BAX during chemotherapy-induced cell death. *Cancer Res* 1998;58:4776–4781.
22. Srivastava RK, Mi QS, Hardwick JM, et al. Deletion of the loop region of Bcl-2 completely blocks paclitaxel-induced apoptosis. *Proc Natl Acad Sci U S A* 1999;96:3775–3780.
23. Dai H, Ding H, Meng XW, et al. Contribution of Bcl-2 phosphorylation to Bak binding and drug resistance. *Cancer Res* 2013;73(23)6998–7008.
24. Oakes SR, Vaillant F, Lim E, et al. Sensitization of BCL-2–expressing breast tumors to chemotherapy by the BH3 mimetic ABT-737. *Proc Natl Acad Sci* 2012;109:2766–2771.
25. Chauhan VP, Stylianopoulos T, Martin JD, et al. Normalization of tumour blood vessels improves the delivery of nanomedicines in a size-dependent manner. *Nat Nanotechnol* 2012;7:383–388.
26. Gradishar W, Tjulandin S, Davidson N, et al. Phase III trial of nanoparticle albumin-bound paclitaxel compared with polyethylated castor oil-based paclitaxel in women with breast cancer. *J Clin Oncol* 2005;23:7794–7803.
27. Socinski MA, Bondarenko I, Karaseva NA, et al. Weekly nab-paclitaxel in combination with carboplatin versus solvent-based paclitaxel plus carboplatin as first-line therapy in patients with advanced non–small-cell lung cancer: final results of a Phase III trial. *J Clin Oncol* 2012;30:2055–2062.
28. Von Hoff DD, Ervin T, Arena FP, et al. Increased survival in pancreatic cancer with nab-paclitaxel plus gemcitabine. *N Engl J Med* 2013;369:1691–1703.
29. Sparreboom A, Scripture CD, Trieu V, et al. Comparative preclinical and clinical pharmacokinetics of a cremophor-free, nanoparticle albumin-bound paclitaxel (ABI-007) and paclitaxel formulated in cremophor (Taxol). *Clin Cancer Res* 2005;11:4136–4143.
30. Yardley DA. nab-Paclitaxel mechanisms of action and delivery. *J Control Release* 2013;170:365–372.
31. Desai N, Trieu V, Yao Z, et al. Increased antitumor activity, intratumor paclitaxel concentrations, and endothelial cell transport of cremophor-free, albumin-bound paclitaxel, ABI-007, compared with cremophor-based paclitaxel. *Clin Cancer Res* 2006;12:1317–1324.
32. Nyman DW, Campbell KJ, Hersh E, et al. Phase I and pharmacokinetics trial of ABI-007, a novel nanoparticle formulation of paclitaxel in patients with advanced nonhematologic malignancies. *J Clin Oncol* 2005;23:7785–7793.
33. Cheng CJ, Saltzman WM. Nanomedicine: downsizing tumour therapeutics. *Nat Nanotechnol* 2012;7:346–347.
34. Infante JR, Matsubayashi H, Sato N, et al. Peritumoral fibroblast SPARC expression and patient outcome with resectable pancreatic adenocarcinoma. *J Clin Oncol* 2007;25:319–325.
35. Kato Y, Nagashima Y, Baba Y, et al. Expression of SPARC in tongue carcinoma of stage II is associated with poor prognosis: an immunohistochemical study of 86 cases. *Int J Mol Med* 2005;16:263–268.
36. Lau CPY, Poon RTP, Cheung ST, et al. SPARC and Hevin expression correlate with tumour angiogenesis in hepatocellular carcinoma. *J Pathol* 2006;210:459–468.
37. Thomas R, True LD, Bassuk JA, et al. Differential expression of osteonectin/SPARC during human prostate cancer progression. *Clin Cancer Res* 2000;6:1140–1149.
38. Watkins G, Douglas-Jones A, Bryce R, et al. Increased levels of SPARC (osteonectin) in human breast cancer tissues and its association with clinical outcomes. *Prostaglandins Leukot Essent Fatty Acids* 2005;72:267–272.
39. Cheng CJ, Saltzman WM. Enhanced siRNA delivery into cells by exploiting the synergy between targeting ligands and cell-penetrating peptides. *Biomaterials* 2011;32:6194–6203.
40. Davis ME, Zuckerman JE, Choi CH, et al. Evidence of RNAi in humans from systemically administered siRNA via targeted nanoparticles. *Nature* 2010;464:1067–1070.
41. Von Hoff DD, Ramanathan RK, Borad MJ, et al. Gemcitabine Plus nab-paclitaxel is an active regimen in patients with advanced pancreatic cancer: a Phase I/II trial. *J Clin Oncol* 2011;29:4548–4554.
42. Mita A, Denis L, Rowinsky E, et al. Phase I and pharmacokinetic study of XRP6258 (RPR 116258A), a novel taxane, administered as a 1-hour infusion every 3 weeks in patients with advanced solid tumors. *Clin Cancer Res* 2009;15:723–730.
43. Diéras V, Lortholary A, Laurence V, et al. Cabazitaxel in patients with advanced solid tumours: results of a Phase I and pharmacokinetic study. *Eur J Cancer* 2013;49:25–34.
44. Mita AC, Denis LJ, Rowinsky EK, et al. Phase I and pharmacokinetic study of XRP6258 (RPR 116258A), a novel taxane, administered as a 1-hour infusion every 3 weeks in patients with advanced solid tumors. *Clin Cancer Res* 2009;15:723–730.
45. Yared JA, Tkaczuk KH. Update on taxane development: new analogs and new formulations. *Drug Des Devel Ther* 2012;6:371–384.
46. Baas P, Szczesna A, Albert I, et al. Phase I/II study of a 3 weekly oral taxane (DJ-927) in patients with recurrent, advanced non-small cell lung cancer. *J Thorac Oncol* 2008;3:745–750.
47. Vigano L, Locatelli A, Grasselli G, et al. Drug interactions of paclitaxel and docetaxel and their relevance for the design of combination therapy. *Invest New Drugs* 2001;19:179–196.
48. Kudlowitz D, Muggia F. Defining risks of taxane neuropathy: insights from randomized clinical trials. *Clin Cancer Res* 2013;19:4570–4577.
49. Henningsson A, Karlsson MO, Viganò L, et al. Mechanism-based pharmacokinetic model for paclitaxel. *J Clin Oncol* 2001;19:4065–4073.
50. Sissung T, Mross K, Steinberg S, et al. Association of ABCB1 genotypes with paclitaxel-mediated peripheral neuropathy and neutropenia. *Eur J Cancer* 2006;42:2893–2896.
51. Marsh S, Paul J, King C, et al. Pharmacogenetic assessment of toxicity and outcome after platinum plus taxane chemotherapy in ovarian cancer: the Scottish Randomised Trial in Ovarian Cancer. *J Clin Oncol* 2007;25:4528–4535.
52. Baldwin RM, Owzar K, Zembutsu H, et al. A genome-wide association study identifies novel loci for paclitaxel-induced sensory peripheral neuropathy in CALGB 40101. *Clin Cancer Res* 2012;18:5099–5109.
53. Rugo H, Barry W, Moreno Aspitia A, et al. CALGB 40502/NCCTG N063H: Randomized phase III trial of weekly paclitaxel (P) compared to weekly nanoparticle albumin bound nab-paclitaxel (NP) or ixabepilone (Ix) with or without bevacizumab (B) as first-line therapy for locally recurrent or metastatic breast cancer (MBC). *J Clin Oncol* 2012;30.
54. Baker J, Ajani J, Scotté F, et al. Docetaxel-related side effects and their management. *Eur J Oncol Nurs* 2009;13:49–59.
55. Lee J, Swain S. Peripheral neuropathy induced by microtubule-stabilizing agents. *J Clin Oncol* 2006;24:1633–1642.
56. Alsamarai S, Charpidou AG, Matthay RA, et al. Pneumonitis related to docetaxel: case report and review of the literature. *In Vivo* 2009;23:635–637.
57. Dumitra S, Sideris L, Leclerc Y, et al. Neutropenic enterocolitis and docetaxel neoadjuvant chemotherapy. *Ann Oncol* 2009;20:795–796.
58. de Bono JS, Oudard S, Ozguroglu M, et al. Prednisone plus cabazitaxel or mitoxantrone for metastatic castration-resistant prostate cancer progressing after docetaxel treatment: a randomised open-label trial. *Lancet* 2010;376:1147–1154.
59. Zhou XJ, Placidi M, Rahmani R. Uptake and metabolism of vinca alkaloids by freshly isolated human hepatocytes in suspension. *Anticancer Res* 1994;14:1017–1022.
60. Zhou J, Giannakakou P. Targeting microtubules for cancer chemotherapy. *Curr Med Chem Anticancer Agents* 2005;5:65–71.
61. Jordan MA, Wilson L. Microtubules as a target for anticancer drugs. *Nat Rev Cancer* 2004;4:253–265.
62. Bender RA, Castle MC, Margileth DA, et al. The pharmacokinetics of [3H]-vincristine in man. *Clin Pharmacol Ther* 1977;22:430–435.
63. Zhou XJ, Martin M, Placidi M, et al. In-vivo and in-vitro pharmacokinetics and metabolism of vinca alkaloids in rat. II. Vinblastine and vincristine. *Eur J Drug Metab Pharmacokinet* 1990;15:323–332.
64. Rowinsky EK, Noe DA, Trump DL, et al. Pharmacokinetic, bioavailability, and feasibility study of oral vinorelbine in patients with solid tumors. *J Clin Oncol* 1994;12:1754–1763.
65. Fumoleau P, Guiu S. New vinca alkaloids in clinical development. *Curr Breast Cancer Rep* 2013;5:69–72.
66. Chan JD. Pharmacokinetic drug interactions of vinca alkaloids: summary of case reports. *Pharmacotherapy* 1998;18:1304–1307.
67. Tobe SW, Siu LL, Jamal SA, et al. Vinblastine and erythromycin: an unrecognized serious drug interaction. *Cancer Chemother Pharmacol* 1995;35:188–190.
68. Peltier A, Russell J. Recent advances in drug-induced neuropathies. *Curr Opin Neurol* 2002;15:633–638.
69. Quasthoff S, Hartung H. Chemotherapy-induced peripheral neuropathy. *J Neurol* 2002;249:9–17.
70. Lobert S, Vulevic B, Correia JJ. Interaction of vinca alkaloids with tubulin: a comparison of vinblastine, vincristine, and vinorelbine. *Biochemistry* 1996;35:6806–6814.
71. Schrijvers DL. Extravasation: a dreaded complication of chemotherapy. *Ann Oncol* 2003;14:iii26–iii30.
72. Petrylak D, Hussain MHA, Tangen C, et al. Docetaxel and estramustine compared with mitoxantrone and prednisone for advanced refractory prostate cancer. *N Engl J Med* 2004;351:1513–1520.
73. Tannock IF, de Wit R, Berry WR, et al. Docetaxel plus prednisone or mitoxantrone plus prednisone for advanced prostate cancer. *N Engl J Med* 2004;351:1502–1512.
74. Lee JJ, Kelly WK. Epothilones: tubulin polymerization as a novel target for prostate cancer therapy. *Nat Clin Pract Oncol* 2009;6:85–92.
75. Kelly WK. Epothilones in prostate cancer. *Urol Oncol* 2011;29:358–365.
76. Kelly K, Zollinger M, Lozac'h F, et al. Metabolism of patupilone in patients with advanced solid tumor malignancies. *Invest New Drugs* 2013;31:605–615.
77. Trail PA, Willner D, Lasch SJ, et al. Cure of xenografted human carcinomas by BR96-doxorubicin immunoconjugates. *Science* 1993;261:212–215.

78. Carter PJ, Senter PD. Antibody-drug conjugates for cancer therapy. *Cancer J* 2008;14:154–169.
79. Doronina SO, Toki BE, Torgov MY, et al. Development of potent monoclonal antibody auristatin conjugates for cancer therapy. *Nat Biotechnol* 2003;21: 778–784.
80. Lewis Phillips GD, Li G, Dugger DL, et al. Targeting HER2-positive breast cancer with trastuzumab-DM1, an antibody–cytotoxic drug conjugate. *Cancer Res* 2008;68:9280–9290.
81. Verma S, Miles D, Gianni L, et al. Trastuzumab emtansine for HER2-positive advanced breast cancer. *N Engl J Med* 2012;367:1783–1791.
82. Okeley NM, Miyamoto JB, Zhang X, et al. Intracellular activation of SGN-35, a potent anti-CD30 antibody-drug conjugate. *Clin Cancer Res* 2010;16:888–897.
83. Younes A, Bartlett NL, Leonard JP, et al. Brentuximab vedotin (SGN-35) for relapsed CD30-positive lymphomas. *N Engl J Med* 2010;363:1812–1821.
84. Younes A. Brentuximab vedotin for the treatment of patients with Hodgkin lymphoma. *Hematol Oncol Clin North Am* 2014;28:27–32.
85. Gandhi M, Evens AM, Fenske TS, et al. Pancreatitis in patients treated with brentuximab vedotin: a previously unrecognized serious adverse event. *Blood* 2013;122:4380.
86. Mosquera JM, Beltran H, Park K, et al. Concurrent AURKA and MYCN gene amplifications are harbingers of lethal treatment-related neuroendocrine prostate cancer. *Neoplasia* 2013;15:1–10.
87. Ujhazy P, Stewart D. DNA Repair. *J Thorac Oncol* 2009;4:S1068–S1070.
88. Green MR, Woolery JE, Mahadevan D. Update on aurora kinase targeted therapeutics in oncology. *Expert Opin Drug Discov* 2011;6:291–307.
89. Jackson JR, Patrick DR, Dar MM, et al. Targeted anti-mitotic therapies: can we improve on tubulin agents? *Nat Rev Cancer* 2007;7:107–117.
90. Tang PA, Siu LL, Chen EX, et al. Phase II study of ispinesib in recurrent or metastatic squamous cell carcinoma of the head and neck. *Invest New Drugs* 2008;26:257–264.
91. Beer TM, Goldman B, Synold TW, et al. Southwest oncology group phase II study of ispinesib in androgen-independent prostate cancer previously treated with taxanes. *Clin Genitourin Cancer* 2008;6:103–109.
92. Lee RT, Beekman KE, Hussain M, et al. A university of chicago consortium phase II trial of SB-715992 in advanced renal cell cancer. *Clin Genitourin Cancer* 2008;6:21–24.
93. Perez EA. Microtubule inhibitors: differentiating tubulin-inhibiting agents based on mechanisms of action, clinical activity, and resistance. *Mol Cancer Ther* 2009;8:2086–2095.
94. Gottesman MM, Fojo T, Bates SE. Multidrug resistance in cancer: role of ATP-dependent transporters. *Nat Rev Cancer* 2002;2:48–58.
95. Fojo AT, Menefee M. Microtubule targeting agents: basic mechanisms of multidrug resistance (MDR). *Semin Oncol* 2005;32:S3–S8.
96. Mozzetti S, Ferlini C, Concolino P, et al. Class III beta-tubulin overexpression is a prominent mechanism of paclitaxel resistance in ovarian cancer patients. *Clin Cancer Res* 2005;11:298–305.
97. Drukman S, Kavallaris M. Microtubule alterations and resistance to tubulin-binding agents (review). *Int J Oncol* 2002;21:621–628.
98. Verrills NM, Kavallaris M. Improving the targeting of tubulin-binding agents: lessons from drug resistance studies. *Curr Pharm Des* 2005;11:1719–1733.
99. Orr GA, Verdier-Pinard P, McDaid H, et al. Mechanisms of Taxol resistance related to microtubules. *Oncogene* 2003;22:7280–7295.
100. Monzó M, Rosell R, Sánchez JJ, et al. Paclitaxel resistance in non-small-cell lung cancer associated with beta-tubulin gene mutations. *J Clin Oncol* 1999;17:1786–1793.
101. Seve P, Mackey J, Isaac S, et al. Class III beta-tubulin expression in tumor cells predicts response and outcome in patients with non-small cell lung cancer receiving paclitaxel. *Mol Cancer Ther* 2005;4:2001–2007.
102. Baquero MT, Hanna JA, Neumeister V, et al. Stathmin expression and its relationship to microtubule-associated protein tau and outcome in breast cancer. *Cancer* 2012;118:4660–4669.
103. Baquero MT, Lostritto K, Gustavson MD, et al. Evaluation of prognostic and predictive value of microtubule associated protein tau in two independent cohorts. *Breast Cancer Res* 2011;13(5):R85.
104. Quinn JE, James CR, Stewart GE, et al. BRCA1 mRNA expression levels predict for overall survival in ovarian cancer after chemotherapy. *Clin Cancer Res* 2007;13:7413–7420.
105. Byrski T, Gronwald J, Huzarski T, et al. Response to neo-adjuvant chemotherapy in women with BRCA1-positive breast cancers. *Breast Cancer Res Treat* 2008; 108:289–296.
106. Font A, Taron M, Gago JL, et al. BRCA1 mRNA expression and outcome to neoadjuvant cisplatin-based chemotherapy in bladder cancer. *Ann Oncol* 2011;22:139–144.
107. Reguart N, Cardona AF, Carrasco E, et al. BRCA1: a new genomic marker for non-small-cell lung cancer. *Clin Lung Cancer* 2008;9:331–339.
108. Martin M, Prat A, Rodriguez-Lescure A, et al. PAM50 proliferation score as a predictor of weekly paclitaxel benefit in breast cancer. *Breast Cancer Res Treat* 2013;138:457–466.

22 Kinase Inhibitors as Anticancer Drugs

Charles L. Sawyers

INTRODUCTION

In 2001, the first tyrosine-kinase inhibitor imatinib was approved for clinical use in chronic myeloid leukemia. The spectacular success of this first-in-class agent ushered in a transformation in cancer drug discovery from efforts that were largely based on novel cytotoxic chemotherapy agents to an almost exclusive focus on molecularly targeted agents across the pharmaceutical and biotechnology industry and academia. This chapter summarizes this remarkable progress in this field over ~15 years, with the focus on the concepts underlying this paradigm shift as well as the considerable challenges that remain (Table 22.1). Readers in search of more specific details on individual drugs and their indications should consult the relevant disease-specific chapters elsewhere in this volume as well as references cited within this chapter. Readers should also note that the epidermal growth factor receptor (EGFR) and human epidermal growth factor receptor 2 (HER2) receptor tyrosine kinases covered here have also been successfully targeted by monoclonal antibodies that engage these proteins at the cell surface. These drugs, referred to as biologics rather than small molecule inhibitors, are covered in other chapters. The chapter is organized around kinase targets rather than diseases and, intentionally, has a historical flow to make certain thematic points and to illustrate the broad lessons that have been and continue to be learned through the clinical development of these exciting agents.

Perhaps the most stunning discovery from the clinical trials of the Abelson murine leukemia (ABL) kinase inhibitor imatinib was the recognition that tumor cells acquire exquisite dependence on the breakpoint cluster region protein BCR-ABL fusion oncogene, created by the Philadelphia chromosome translocation.[1] Although this may seem intuitive at first glance, consider the fact that the translocation arises in an otherwise normal hematopoietic stem cell, the survival of which is regulated by a complex array of growth factors and interactions with the bone marrow microenvironment. Although BCR-ABL clearly gives this cell a growth advantage that, over years, results in the clinical phenotype of chronic myeloid leukemia, there was no reason to expect that these cells would depend on BCR-ABL for their survival when confronted with an inhibitor. In the absence of BCR-ABL, these tumor cells could presumably rely on the marrow microenvironment, just like their normal, nontransformed neighbors. Thus, it seemed more likely that, by shutting down the driver oncogene, BCR-ABL inhibitors might halt the progression of chronic myeloid leukemia but not eliminate the preexisting tumor cells. In fact, chronic myeloid leukemia (CML) progenitors are eliminated after just a few months of anti–BCR-ABL therapy, indicating they are dependent on the driver oncogene for their survival and have "forgotten" how to return to normal. This phenomenon, subsequently documented in a variety of human malignancies, is colloquially termed *oncogene addiction*.[2] Although the molecular basis for this addiction still remains to be defined, the notion of finding an Achilles' heel for each cancer continues to captivate the cancer research community and has spawned a broad array of efforts to elucidate the molecular identity of these targets and discover relevant inhibitors.

EARLY SUCCESSES: TARGETING CANCERS WITH WELL-KNOWN KINASE MUTATIONS (BCR-ABL, KIT, HER2)

From the beginning, clinical trials of imatinib were restricted to patients with Philadelphia chromosome–positive chronic myeloid leukemia. For what seem like obvious reasons, there was never any serious discussion about treating patients with Philadelphia chromosome–negative leukemia because the assumption was that only patients with the BCR-ABL fusion gene would have a chance of responding. This was clearly a wise decision because hematologic response rates approached 90% and cytogenetic remissions were seen in nearly half of the patients in the early phase studies.[3] It was obvious that the drug worked, and imatinib was approved in record time. Unwittingly, the power of genome-based patient selection was demonstrated in the clinical development of the very first kinase inhibitor. As we will see, it took nearly a decade for this lesson to be fully learned. Today, the much larger clinical experience, with an array of different kinase inhibitors across many tumor types, has led to a much better understanding of the principles that dictate oncogene addiction that, in retrospect, were staring us in the face. Foremost among them is the notion that tumors with a somatic mutation or amplification of a kinase drug target are much more likely to be dependent on that target for survival. Hence, a patient whose tumor has such a mutation is much more likely to respond to treatment with the appropriate inhibitor. This has also led to a new paradigm at the regulatory level of drug approval requiring codevelopment of a *companion diagnostic* (a molecularly based diagnostic test that reliably identifies patients with the mutation) with the new drug.

After chronic myeloid leukemia, the next example to illustrate this principle was gastrointestinal stromal tumor (GIST), which is associated with mutations in the KIT tyrosine-kinase receptor or, more rarely, in the platelet-derived growth factor (PDGF) receptor.[4,5] Serendipitously, imatinib inhibits both KIT and the PDGF receptor; therefore, the clinical test of KIT inhibition in GIST followed quickly on the heels of the success in CML.[6] In retrospect, the rapid progress made in these two diseases was based, in part, on the fact that the driver molecular lesion (BCR-ABL or KIT mutation, respectively) is present in nearly all patients who are diagnosed with these two diseases. The molecular analysis merely confirmed the diagnosis that was made using standard clinical and histologic criteria. Consequently, clinicians could identify the patients most likely to respond based on clinical criteria rather than rely on an elaborate molecular profiling infrastructure to prescreen patients. Consequently, clinical trials evaluating kinase inhibitors in CML and GIST accrued quickly, and the therapeutic benefit became clear almost immediately.

The notion that molecular alteration of a driver kinase determines sensitivity to a cognate kinase inhibitor was further validated during the development of the dual EGFR/HER2 kinase inhibitor lapatinib. Clinical trials of this kinase inhibitor were conducted in women with advanced HER2-positive breast cancer based on earlier success in these same patients with the monoclonal antibody trastuzumab, which targets the extracellular domain of the HER2

TABLE 22.1

Kinase Inhibitors: Approved or Anticipated Approval In 2014

Target	Drug	Approved Indications	Anticipated Future Indications
ALK	Crizotinib Ceritinib	ALK mutant lung cancer	ALK mutant neuroblastoma, anaplastic lymphoma
BCR-ABL	Imatinib Dasatinib Nilotinib Bosutinib Ponatinib	Chronic myeloid leukemia Philadelphia chromosome–positive acute lymphoid leukemia T315 mutation only (ponatinib)	
BRAF	Vemurafenib Dabrafenib	BRAF mutant melanoma	Other BRAF mutant tumors
BTK	Ibrutinib	Chronic lymphocytic leukemia Mantle cell lymphoma	
EGFR	Gefitinib Erlotinib Afatinib	Lung adenocarcinoma with EGFR mutation	
HER2	Lapatinib	$Her2^+$ breast cancer	
JAK2	Ruxolitinib	JAK2 mutant myelofibrosis	
KIT	Imatinib Sunitinib	Gastrointestinal stromal tumor	
MEK	Trametinib	BRAF mutant melanoma	
PI3K delta[a]	Idelalisib	Chronic lymphocytic leukemia Indolent non-Hodgkin lymphoma	
PDGFR- α/β	Imatinib	Chronic myelomonocytic leukemia (with TEL-PDGFR-β fusion) hypereosinophilic syndrome (with PDGFR-β fusion) Dermatofibrosarcoma protuberans	
RET	Vandetanib Sorafenib Cabozantinib	Medullary thyroid cancer	
TORC1	Sirolimus (rapamycin)	Kidney cancer	
(mTOR)	Everolimus Temsirolimus	Breast cancer Tuberous sclerosis	
VEGF Receptor	Sorafenib Sunitinib Axitinib Pazopanib	Kidney cancer Hepatocellular carcinoma (sorafenib only) Pancreatic neuroendocrine tumors (sunitinib)	

[a] Approval is anticipated based on positive phase 3 data and announcement of accepted Food and Drug Administration submission by the sponsor.

kinase. Lapatinib was initially approved in combination with the cytotoxic agent capecitabine for women with resistance to trastuzumab,[7] and then was subsequently approved for frontline use in metastatic breast cancer in combination with chemotherapy or hormonal therapy, depending on estrogen receptor status. A key ingredient that enabled the clinical development of lapatinib was the routine use of HER2 gene amplification testing in the diagnosis of breast cancer, pioneered during the development of trastuzumab several years earlier. This widespread clinical practice allowed for the rapid identification of those patients most likely to benefit. If lapatinib trials had been conducted in unselected patients, the clinical signal in breast cancer would likely have been missed.

The Serendipity of Unexpected Clinical Responses: EGFR in Lung Cancer

In contrast to the logical development of imatinib and lapatinib in molecularly defined patient populations, the EGFR kinase inhibitors gefitinib and erlotinib entered the clinic without the benefit of such a focused clinical development plan. Although considerable preclinical data implicated EGFR as a cancer drug target, there was little insight into which patients were most likely to benefit. The first clue that EGFR inhibitors would have a role in lung cancer came from the recognition by several astute clinicians of remarkable responses in a small fraction of patients with lung adenocarcinoma.[8] Further studies revealed the curious clinical circumstance that those patients most likely to benefit tended to be those who never smoked, women, and those of Asian ethnicity.[9] Clearly, there was a strong clinical signal in a subgroup of patients, who could perhaps be enriched based on these clinical features, but it seemed that a unifying molecular lesion must be present. Three academic groups simultaneously converged on the answer. Mutations in the EGFR gene were detected in the 10% to 15% of patients with lung adenocarcinoma who had radiographic responses.[10–12] It may seem surprising that mutations in a gene as highly visible as EGFR and in such a prevalent cancer had not been detected earlier. But the motivation to search aggressively for EGFR mutations was not there until the clinical responses were seen. Perhaps even more surprising was the failure of the pharmaceutical company sponsors of the two most advanced compounds, gefitinib and erlotinib, to embrace this important discovery and refocus future clinical development plans on patients with EGFR mutant lung adenocarcinoma.

But that was 2004, when the prevailing approach to cancer drug development was an empiric one originally developed (with great success) for cytotoxic agents. Typically, small numbers of patients with different cancers were treated in *all comer* phase I studies (no enrichment for subgroups) with the goal of eliciting a clinical signal in at least one tumor type. A single-agent response rate of 20% to 30% in a disease-specific phase II trial would justify a randomized phase III registration trial, where the typical endpoint for drug approval is time to progression or survival. Cytotoxics were also typically evaluated in combination with existing standard of care treatment (typically approved chemotherapy agents) with the goal of increasing the response rate or enhancing the duration of response. (Note: The use of the past tense here is intentional. As we will see later in this chapter, nearly all cancer drug development today is based on selecting patients with a certain molecular profile.)

The clinical development of gefitinib and erlotinib followed the cytotoxic model. Both drugs had similarly low but convincing single-agent response rates (10% to 15%) in chemotherapy-refractory, advanced lung cancer. Indeed, gefitinib was originally granted accelerated approval by the U.S. Food and Drug Administration (FDA) in 2003 based on the impressive nature of these responses, contingent on the completion of formal phase III studies with survival endpoints.[13] The sponsors of both drugs, therefore, conducted phase III registration studies in patients with chemotherapy-refractory, advanced stage lung cancer but without prescreening patients for EGFR mutation status. (In fairness, these trials were initiated prior to the discovery of EGFR mutations in lung cancer but study amendments could have been considered.) Erlotinib was approved in 2004 on the basis of a modest survival advantage over placebo (the BR.21 trial); however, gefitinib failed to demonstrate a survival advantage in essentially the same patient population.[14,15] This difference in outcome was surprising because the two drugs have highly similar chemical structures and biologic properties. Perhaps the most important difference was drug dose. Erlotinib was given at the maximum tolerated dose, which produces a high frequency of rash and diarrhea. Both side effects are presumed *on target* consequences of EGFR inhibition because EGFR is highly expressed in skin and gastrointestinal epithelial cells. In contrast, gefitinib was dosed slightly lower to mitigate these toxicities, with the rationale that responses were clearly documented at lower doses.

In parallel with the single-agent phase III trials in chemotherapy-refractory patients, both gefitinib and erlotinib were studied as an upfront therapy for advanced lung cancer to determine if either would improve the efficacy of standard *doublet* (carboplatin/paclitaxel or gemcitabine/cisplatin) chemotherapy when all three drugs were given in combination. These trials, termed INTACT-1 and INTACT-2 (gefitinib with either gemcitabine/cisplatin or with carboplatin/paclitaxel) and TRIBUTE (erlotinib with carboplatin/paclitaxel), collectively enrolled over 3,000 patients.[16–18] Excitement in the oncology community was high based on the clear single-agent activity of both EGFR inhibitors. But, both trials were spectacular failures; neither drug showed any benefit over chemotherapy alone. The fact that EGFR mutations are present in only 10% to 15% of patients (i.e., those likely to benefit) provided a logical explanation. The clinical signal from those whose tumors had EGFR mutations was likely diluted out by all the patients whose tumors had no EGFR alterations, many of whom benefited from chemotherapy.

The convergence of the EGFR mutation discovery with these clinical trial results will be remembered as a remarkable time in the history of targeted cancer therapies, not just for the important role of these agents as lung cancer therapies, but also for missteps in deciding that the EGFR genotype should drive treatment selection. Perhaps the most egregious error came from a retrospective analysis of tumors from patients treated on the BR.21 trial, which concluded that EGFR mutations did *not* predict for a survival advantage.[19] (EGFR gene amplification *was* associated with survival, but only in a univariate analysis.) This conclusion was concerning because less than 30% of patients on the trial had tissue available for EGFR mutation analysis, raising questions about the adequacy of the sample size. Furthermore, the EGFR mutation assay used by the authors was subsequently criticized because a significant number of the EGFR mutations reported in these patients were in residues not previously found by others, who had sequenced thousands of tumors. Many of these mutations were suspected to be an artifact of working from formalin-fixed biopsies. Fortunately, recent advances in DNA mutation detection, using massively parallel next-generation sequencing technology, have largely eliminated this concern. These new platforms are now being used in the clinical setting.

Clinical investigators in Asia, where a greater fraction of lung cancers (roughly 30%) are positive for EGFR mutations, addressed the question of whether mutations predict for clinical benefit in a prospective trial. In this study known as IPASS, gefitinib was clearly superior to standard doublet chemotherapy as frontline therapy for patients with advanced EGFR mutation–positive lung adenocarcinoma.[20] Conversely, EGFR mutation–negative patients fared much worse with gefitinib and benefited from chemotherapy. In addition, EGFR mutation–positive patients had a more favorable overall prognosis regardless of treatment, indicating that EGFR mutation is also a prognostic biomarker. The IPASS trial serves as a compelling example of a properly designed (and executed) biomarker-driven clinical trial. Although the rationale for this clinical development strategy had been demonstrated years earlier with BCR-ABL in leukemia, KIT in GIST, and HER2 in breast cancer, it was difficult to derail the empiric approach that had been used for decades in developing cytotoxic agents.

A Mix of Science and Serendipity: PDGF Receptor–Driven Leukemias and Sarcoma

The discovery of EGFR mutations in lung cancer (motivated by dramatic clinical responses in a subset of patients treated with EGFR kinase inhibitors) is the most visible example of the power of bedside-to-bench science, but it is not the only (or the first) such example from the kinase inhibitor era. Shortly after the approval of imatinib for CML in 2001, two case reports documented dramatic remissions in patients with hypereosinophilic syndrome (HES), a blood disorder characterized by prolonged elevation of eosinophil counts and subsequent organ dysfunction from eosinophil infiltration, when treated with imatinib.[21,22] Although HES resembles myeloproliferative diseases such as CML, the molecular pathogenesis of HES was completely unknown at the time. Reasoning that these clinical responses must be explained by inhibition of a driver kinase, a team of laboratory-based physician/scientists quickly searched for mutations in the three kinases known to be inhibited by imatinib (ABL, KIT, and PDGF receptor). ABL and KIT were quickly excluded, but the PDGF receptor α (PDGFR-α) gene was targeted by an interstitial deletion that fused the upstream FIP1L1 gene to PDGFR-α[23] FIP1L1-PDGFR-α is a constitutively active tyrosine kinase, analogous to BCR-ABL, and is also inhibited by imatinib. As with EGFR-mutant lung cancer, the molecular pathophysiology of HES was discovered by dissecting the mechanism of response to the drug used to treat it.

The HES/FIP1L1-PDGFR-α story serves as a nice bookend to an earlier discovery that the t(5,12) chromosome translocation, found rarely in patients with chronic myelomonocytic leukemia, creates the TEL-PDGFR-β fusion tyrosine kinase.[24] Similar to HES, treatment of patients with t(5,12) translocation-positive leukemias with imatinib has also proven successful.[25] A third example comes from dermatofibrosarcoma protuberans, a sarcoma characterized by a t(17,22) translocation that fuses the COL1A gene to the PDGFB *ligand* (not the receptor). COL1A-PDGFB is oncogenic through autocrine stimulation of the normal PDGF receptor in these tumor cells. Patients with dermatofibrosarcoma protuberans respond to imatinib therapy because it targets the PDGF receptor, just one step downstream from the oncogenic lesion.[26]

Exploiting the New Paradigm: Searching for Other Kinase-Driven Cancers

The benefits of serendipity notwithstanding, the growing number of examples of successful kinase inhibitor therapy in tumors with a mutation or amplification of the drug target begged for a more rational approach to drug discovery and development. In 2002, the list of human tumors known to have mutations in kinases was quite small. Due to advances in automated gene sequencing, it became possible to ask whether a much larger fraction of human cancers might also have such mutations through a brute force approach. To address this question comprehensively, one would have to sequence all of the kinases in the genome in hundreds of samples of each tumor type. Several early pilot studies demonstrated the potential of this approach by revealing important new targets for drug development. Perhaps the most spectacular was the discovery of mutations in the BRAF kinase in over half of patients with melanoma, as well as in a smaller fraction of colon and thyroid cancers.[27] Another was the discovery of mutations in the JAK2 kinase in nearly all patients with polycythemia vera, as well as a significant fraction of patients with myelofibrosis and essential thrombocytosis.[28–30] A third example was the identification of PIK3CA mutations in a variety of tumors, with the greatest frequencies in breast, endometrial, and colorectal cancers.[31] PIK3CA encodes a lipid kinase that generates the second messenger phosphatidyl inositol 3-phosphate (PIP3). PIP3 activates growth and survival signaling through the AKT family of kinases as well as other downstream effectors. Coupled with the well-established role of the phosphatase and tensin homolog (PTEN) lipid phosphatase in dephosphorylating PIP3, the discovery of PIK3CA mutations focused tremendous attention on developing inhibitors at multiple levels of this pathway, as discussed further in the follow paragraphs.

Each of these important discoveries—BRAF, JAK2, and PIK3CA—came from relatively small efforts (less than 100 tumors) and generally focused on resequencing only those exons that coded for regions of kinases where mutations had been found in other kinases (typically, the juxtamembrane and kinase domains). These restricted searches were largely driven by the high cost of DNA sequencing using the Sanger method. In 2006, a comprehensive effort to sequence all of the exons in all kinases in 100 tumors could easily exceed several million dollars. Financial support for such projects could not be obtained easily through traditional funding agencies because the risk/reward was considered too high. Furthermore, substantial infrastructure for sample acquisition, microdissection of the tumors from normal tissue, nucleic acid preparation, high throughput automated sequencing, and computational analysis of the resulting data was essential. Few institutions were equipped to address these challenges. In response, the National Cancer Institute in the United States (in partnership with the National Human Genome Research Institute) and an international group known as the International Cancer Genome Consortium (ICGC) launched large-scale efforts to sequence the complete genomes of thousands of cancers. In parallel, next-generation sequencing technologies resulted in massive reductions in cost, allowing a more comprehensive analysis of much larger numbers of tumors. At the time of this writing, the US effort (called The Cancer Genome Atlas [TCGA]) had reported data on 29 different tumor types (https://tcga-data.nci.nih.gov/tcga/). The international consortium has committed to sequencing 25,000 tumors representing 50 different cancer subtypes.[32] Both groups have enforced immediate release of all sequence information to the research community free of charge so that the entire scientific community can learn from the data. This policy enabled *pan cancer* mutational analyses that give an overall view of the genomic landscape of cancer, serving as a blueprint for the community of cancer researchers and drug developers.[33,34]

Rounding Out the Treatment of Myeloproliferative Disorders: JAK2 and Myelofibrosis

Taken together with the BCR-ABL translocation in CML and FIP1L1-PDGFR-α in HES, the discovery of JAK2 mutations in polycythemia, essential thrombocytosis, and myelofibrosis provided a unifying understanding of myeloproliferative disorders as diseases of abnormal kinase activation. The JAK family kinases are the primary effectors of signaling through inflammatory cytokine receptors and, therefore, had been considered compelling targets for anti-inflammatory drugs. But the JAK2 mutation discovery immediately shifted these efforts toward developing JAK2 inhibitors for myeloproliferative disorders. Because most patients have a common JAK2 V617F mutation, these efforts could rapidly focus on screening for activity against a single genotype. Progress has been rapid. Myelofibrosis was selected as the initial indication (instead of essential thrombocytosis or polycythemia vera) because the time to registration is expected to be the shortest. Currently, ruxolitinib is approved for myelofibrosis based on shrinkage in spleen size as the primary endpoint. Clinical trials in essential thrombocytosis and polycythemia vera (versus hydroxyurea) are ongoing. Other JAK2 inhibitors are also in clinical development.

BRAF Mutant Melanoma: Several Missteps Before Finding the Right Inhibitor

As with JAK2 mutations in myeloproliferative disorders, the discovery of BRAF mutations in patients with melanoma launched widespread efforts to find potent BRAF inhibitors. One early candidate was the drug sorafenib, which had been optimized during drug discovery to inhibit RAF kinases. (Sorafenib also inhibits vascular endothelial growth factor (VEGF) receptors, which led to its approval in kidney cancer, as discussed later in this chapter.) Despite the compelling molecular rationale for targeting BRAF, clinical results of sorafenib in melanoma were extremely disappointing and reduced enthusiasm for pursuing BRAF as a drug target.[35] In hindsight, this concern was completely misguided. Sorafenib dosing is limited by toxicities that preclude achieving serum levels in patients that potently inhibit RAF, but are sufficient to inhibit VEGF receptors. In addition, patients were enrolled without screening for BRAF mutations in their tumors. Although the frequency of BRAF mutations in melanoma is high, the inclusion of patients without the BRAF mutation diluted the chance of seeing any clinical signal. In short, the clinical evaluation of sorafenib in melanoma was poorly designed to test the hypothesis that BRAF is a therapeutic target. The danger is that negative data from such clinical experiments can slow subsequent progress. It is critical to know the pharmacodynamic properties of the drug and the molecular phenotype of the patients being studied when interpreting the results of a negative study.

The fact that RAF kinases are intermediate components of the well-characterized RAS/ mitogen-activated protein (MAP) kinase pathway (transducing signals from RAS to RAF to MEK to ERK) raised the possibility that tumors with BRAF mutations might respond to inhibitors of one of these downstream kinases (Fig. 22.1). Preclinical studies revealed that tumor cell lines with BRAF mutation were exquisitely sensitive to inhibitors of the downstream kinase MEK.[36] (Sorafenib, in contrast, does not show this profile of activity.[37] Thus, proper preclinical screening would have revealed the shortcomings of sorafenib as a BRAF inhibitor.) Curiously, cell lines with a mutation or amplification of EGFR or HER2, which

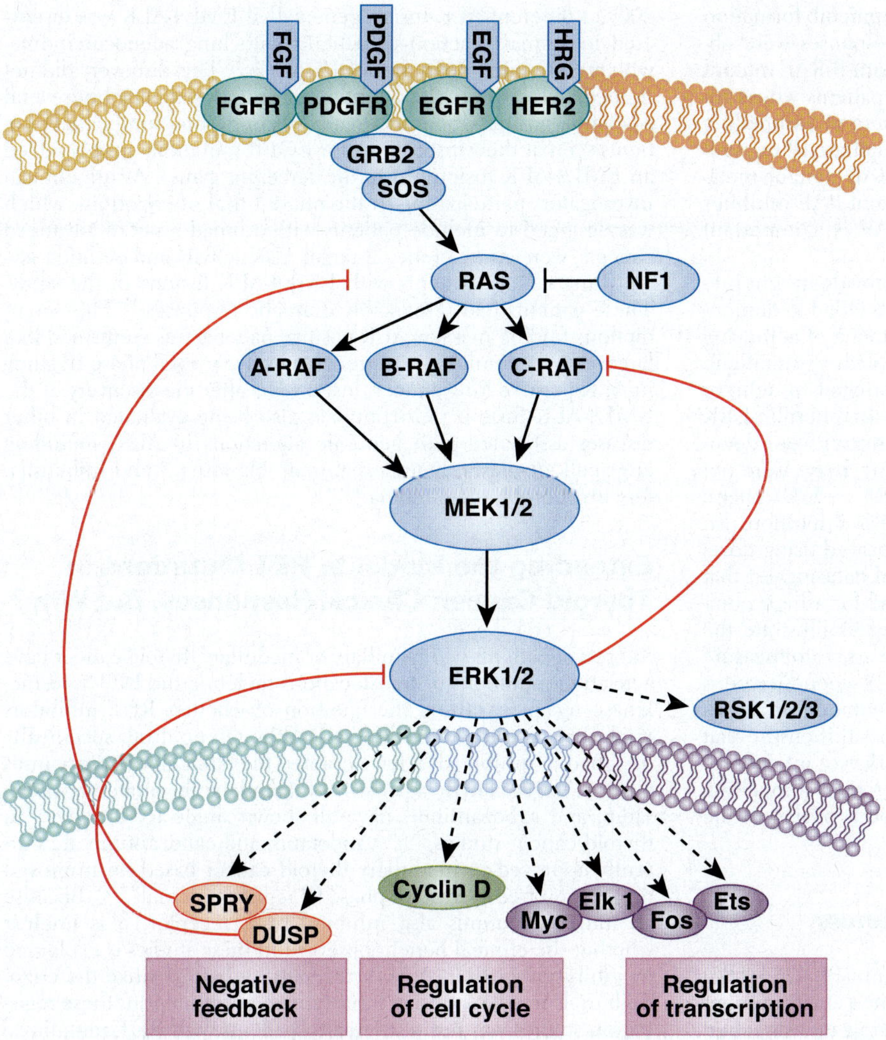

Figure 22.1 The RAS–RAF–MEK–ERK signaling pathway. The classical mitogen-activated protein kinase (MAPK) pathway is activated in human tumors by several mechanisms, including the binding of ligand to receptor tyrosine kinases (RTK), the mutational activation of an RTK, by loss of the tumor suppressor NF1, or by mutations in RAS, BRAF, and MEK1. Phosphorylation and, thus, activation of ERK regulates the transcription of target genes that promote cell cycle progression and tumor survival. The ERK pathway contains a classical feedback loop in which the expression of feedback elements such as SPRY and DUSP family proteins are regulated by the level of ERK activity. Loss of expression of SPRY and DUSP family members due to promoter methylation or deletion is thus permissive for persistently elevated pathway output. In the case of tumors with mutant BRAF, pathway output is enhanced by impaired upstream feedback regulation. FGF, fibroblast growth factor; HRG, heregulin; NF1, neurofibromatosis 1. (From Bernt KM, Zhu N, Sinha AU, et al. MLL-rearranged leukemia is dependent on aberrant H3K79 methylation by DOT1L. *Cancer Cell* 2011;20(1):66–78, with permission.)

function upstream in the pathway, were insensitive to MEK inhibition. Even tumor lines with RAS mutations were variably sensitive. In short, the preclinical data made a strong case that MEK inhibitors should be effective in BRAF mutant melanoma, but not in other subtypes. The reason that HER2, EGFR, and RAS mutant tumors were not sensitive to MEK inhibitors is explained, at least in part, by the existence of negative feedback loops that modulate the flux of signal transduction through MEK.[38]

In parallel with the generation of these preclinical findings, clinical trials of several MEK inhibitors were initiated. Patients with various cancers were enrolled in the early studies, but there was a strong bias to include melanoma patients. Significant efforts were made to demonstrate MEK inhibition in tumor cells by measuring the phosphorylation status of the direct downstream substrate ERK using an immunohistochemical analysis of biopsies from patients with metastatic disease. Phase I studies of the two earliest compounds in clinical development (PD325901 and AZD6244) documented reduced phospho-ERK staining at multiple dose levels in several patients for whom baseline and treatment biopsies were obtained.[39,40] (In the following, we will learn that these pharmacodynamic studies, while well intentioned, were not quantitative enough to document the magnitude of MEK inhibition in these patients.) Furthermore, clinical responses were observed in a few patients with BRAF mutant melanoma. Armed with this confidence, a randomized phase II clinical trial of AZD6244 was conducted in advanced melanoma, with the chemotherapeutic agent temozolomide (which is approved for glioblastoma) as the comparator arm. (The clinical development of PD325901 was discontinued because of safety concerns about ocular and neurologic toxicity.) Disappointingly, patients receiving AZD6244 had no benefit in progression-free survival when compared to temozolomide-treated patients, raising further concerns about the viability of BRAF as a drug target.[41] A closer examination of the data revealed that clinical responses were, indeed, seen in patients receiving AZD6244. The fact that BRAF mutation status was not required for study entry likely diminished the clinical signal in the AZD6244 arm, a lesson learned from the EGFR inhibitor trials in lung cancer. Indeed, a different MEK inhibitor, trametinib, received FDA approval in 2013 based on activity in melanoma patients with the BRAF mutation.[42]

All doubts about BRAF as a target vanished in 2009 to 2010 when dramatic clinical responses were observed with a novel BRAF inhibitor vemurafenib (PLX4032). Like sorafenib, this compound was optimized to inhibit RAF, but with an additional focus on mutant BRAF. Vemurafenib differs dramatically from sorafenib because it potently inhibits BRAF without the additional broad range of activities that sorafenib has against other kinases like the VEGF receptor.[43] The greater selectivity of vemurafenib relative to sorafenib resulted in a much greater tolerability, such that it could be given at high doses while avoiding significant toxicity. The early days of vemurafenib clinical development were plagued by challenges in maximizing the oral bioavailability of the drug.[44] Consequently, the initial phase I clinical trial was temporarily halted to develop a novel formulation (i.e., the coingredients in the drug capsule or tablet that improve solubility and absorption through the gastrointestinal tract). Much higher serum levels were obtained in patients who received the new vemurafenib formation and, shortly thereafter, complete and partial responses were observed in about 80% of the melanoma patients with B-RAF mutant tumors. Strikingly, no activity was observed in patients whose tumors were wild type for BRAF.[45,46] The data were so compelling that vemurafenib was immediately advanced to a phase III registration trial. Similarly impressive responses in BRAF mutant melanoma patients were observed with a second potent RAF inhibitor dabrafenib,[47] providing further proof that BRAF is a important cancer target.

The vemurafenib and dabrafenib data also provide insight into why sorafenib and the early MEK inhibitor trials failed to demonstrate activity. One lesson is the critical importance of achieving adequate target inhibition. Clinical responses with vemurafenib were observed only after the drug was reformulated to achieve substantially higher serum levels. Reductions in phospho-ERK staining (as documented by immunohistochemistry) were documented in the earlier trials but, in retrospect, the assays were not sensitive enough to distinguish between modest (~50%) kinase inhibition versus more complete BRAF or MEK inhibition. Efficacy in preclinical models is significantly improved using doses that give >80% inhibition, and the human trial data suggest that this degree of pathway blockade is also required for a high clinical response rate.[46] Collectively, these experiences illustrate the critical need for quantitative pharmacodynamic assays to measure target inhibition early in clinical development. A second lesson is the importance of genotyping all patients for mutation or amplification of the relevant drug target. Not only does this ensure that a sufficient number of patients with the biomarker of interest are included in the study, but also that the results provide compelling evidence early in clinical development in support (or not) of the preclinical hypothesis.

Getting It Right: ALK and Lung Cancer

The development of the ALK inhibitor crizotinib (PF-02341066) illustrates how an unexpected signal obtained in a small number of patients can quickly shift a program in an entirely new direction with a high probability of success. The key ingredient is this story is a familiar one—a strong molecular hypothesis backed up by clinical response data in a small number of carefully selected patients. Crizotinib emerged from a drug discovery program at Pfizer that was focused on finding inhibitors of the MET receptor tyrosine kinase and entered the clinic with this target as its lead indication.[48] As we previously learned with imatinib, essentially all kinase inhibitors have activity against other targets (so called *off-target* activities), which can sometimes prove to be advantageous. Off-target activities are typically discovered by screening compounds against a large panel of kinases to establish profiles of relative selectivity against the intended target. Off-target activity, potency, and pharmaceutical properties (bioavailability, half-life) are all factors that influence the decision of which compound to advance to clinical development. The primary off-target activity of crizotinib is against the ALK tyrosine kinase.

ALK was first identified as a candidate driver oncogene in 1994 through the cloning of the t(2,5) chromosomal translocation associated with anaplastic large cell lymphoma, which creates the nucleophosmin/anaplastic lymphoma kinase (NPM-ALK) fusion gene.[49] This discovery, together with the demonstration that NPM-ALK causes lymphoma in mice, made a compelling case for ALK as a drug target in this disease. But there was limited interest in developing ALK inhibitors because this particular lymphoma subtype is rare and most commonly found in children. (Companies are generally reluctant to develop drugs solely for pediatric indications because of complexities related to dose selection and additional regulatory guidelines. Efforts to streamline this development process are underway, such as the Creating Hope Act, which provides new incentives for companies to pursue pediatric indications.) In 2007, a different ALK fusion gene called EML4-ALK was discovered in a small fraction of patients with lung adenocarcinoma, with an estimated frequency of 1% to 5%.[50] This discovery did not immediately capture the attention of drug developers, but several academic groups who had already begun testing lung cancer patients seen at their institutions for EGFR mutations simply added an EML4-ALK fusion test to the screening panel. Astute clinical investigators participating in the phase I trial of crizotinib, which was designed to include patients with a broad array of advanced cancers, were aware of the off-target ALK activity and enrolled several lung cancer patients with EML4-ALK fusions in the study. These patients had remarkably dramatic responses.[51] This serendipitous finding in a few ALK-positive patients was confirmed in a larger cohort, resulting in a strongly positive pivotal phase III study in ALK-positive lung cancer, just 2 years after the discovery of the EML4-ALK fusion.[52] Crizotinib is also being evaluated in other diseases associated with genomic alterations in ALK, including large-cell anaplastic lymphoma, neuroblastoma,[53] and inflammatory myofibroblastic sarcoma.[54]

Extending the Model to RET Mutations in Thyroid Cancer: Clinical Responses, But Why?

Subsets of patients with papillary or medullary thyroid cancer have activating mutations or translocations targeting the RET tyrosine-kinase receptor, raising the question of whether RET inhibitors might have a role in this disease.[55] Although no drugs specifically designed to inhibit RET have entered the clinic, four compounds with off-target activity against RET (vandetanib, sorafenib, motesanib, and cabozantinib) have all shown single-agent activity in thyroid cancer studies.[56–60] Vandetanib and cabozantinib are currently approved in medullary thyroid cancer based on improved progression-free survival in phase III registration trials.[61,62] Because all four compounds also inhibit VEGF receptor, it is unclear whether the clinical benefit observed in these studies is explained by inhibition of RET, VEGF receptor, or both. Unlike the crizotinib trials in ALK-positive lung cancer, enrollment in these registration studies was not restricted to patients with RET mutations. In addition to the fact that thyroid cancer patients are not routinely screened for these mutations, the primary reason for including all comers in these studies is that clinical responses are observed in a larger fraction of patients than can be accounted for based on the suspected frequency of an RET mutation. Responses in patients without RET mutation (if they occur) might be explained by mutations in other genes in the RAS-MAP kinase pathway such as BRAF or HRAS, which are found in a substantial fraction of patients and typically do not overlap with RET alterations.[55] Clearly, detailed genotype/response correlations, as demonstrated in lung cancer and melanoma, will clarify the role of these mutations in predicting the response to these drugs. Thyroid cancer is also a compelling indication for the BRAF and MEK inhibitors discussed previously in melanoma.

FLT3 Inhibitors in Acute Myeloid Leukemia: Did the Genomics Mislead Us?

Shortly after the success of imatinib, the receptor tyrosine–kinase FLT3 emerged as a compelling drug candidate based on the presence of activating mutations in about one-third of patients with acute myeloid leukemia.[63] Laboratory studies documented that FLT3 alleles bearing these mutations, which occur as internal tandem duplications (ITD) of the juxtamembrane domain or a point mutation in the kinase domain, function as driver oncogenes in mouse models, giving phenotypes analogous to BCR-ABL.[64] As with RET in thyroid cancer, no compounds had been specifically optimized to target FLT3, but several drugs with off-target FLT3 activity were redirected to acute myeloid leukemia (AML).

Disappointingly, the first three of the compounds tested (midostaurin, lestaurtinib, and sunitinib) showed only marginal single-agent activity in relapsed AML patients, even in those with FLT3 mutations.[65–67] Despite the strong molecular rationale for FLT3 as a driver lesion, questions were raised about the viability of FLT3 as a drug target. Pharmacodynamic studies showed evidence of FLT3 kinase inhibition in tumor cells, but the magnitude and duration of these effects were difficult to quantify, raising the possibility of inadequate target inhibition.[65] Indeed, the dose of all three compounds was limited by toxicities believed to be independent of FLT3. A more pessimistic interpretation was that FLT3, although presumably important for the initiation of AML, was no longer required for tumor maintenance due to the accumulation of additional driver genomic alterations. If true, even a complete FLT3 blockade with a highly selective inhibitor would be expected to fail. But this view was not supported by the fact that clinical responses were observed in the somewhat analogous situation of single-agent ABL kinase inhibitor treatment of CML in blast crisis, where BCR-ABL is just one of many additional genomic alterations that contribute to disease progression, yet complete remissions are observed in many patients.

Despite this pessimism about FLT3 as a viable drug target, several drugs are now advancing toward drug registration trials. Midostaurin, one of the early compounds that showed disappointing single-agent activity in relapsed AML, is being evaluated in a randomized phase III trial in newly diagnosed AML combined with standard induction chemotherapy. A single-arm phase II study showed higher and more durable remission rates in FLT3 mutant patients when compared to historical controls.[68] The second compound, quizartinib (AC220), is a next-generation FLT3 inhibitor with greater potency and specificity and with single-agent activity in FLT3 mutant relapsed AML—precisely the population where midostaurin and others failed.[69,70] The fact that some responder patients have relapsed with drug-resistant gatekeeper mutations in the FLT3 kinase domain provides formal proof that FLT3 is the relevant target.[71] Assuming these compounds prove successful in AML, it will be important to examine their activity in the rare cases of pediatric acute lymphoid leukemia associated with FLT3 mutation. Although the jury is still out on FLT3 inhibitors, the failure of early compounds in AML is reminiscent of the failures of early RAF and MEK inhibitors in melanoma. Collectively, these examples emphasize the importance of using optimized compounds to test a molecularly based hypothesis in patients and to focus enrollment on those patients with the relevant molecular lesion.

Kidney Cancer: Targeting the Tumor and the Host With Mammalian Target of Rapamycin and VEGF Receptor Inhibitors

A recurring theme in this chapter is the critical role of driver kinase mutations in guiding the development of kinase inhibitors. Ironically, several kinase inhibitors have been approved for kidney cancer over the past 5 years in a tumor type with no known kinase mutations. The most common molecular alteration in kidney cancer is a loss of function in the Von Hippel-Lindau (VHL) tumor suppressor gene, resulting in the activation of the hypoxia inducible factor[68] pathway.[72] As a consequence of VHL loss, which normally targets hypoxia-inducible factor (HIF) proteins for proteasomal degradation, HIF-1α and HIF-2α are constitutively active transcription factors that function as oncogenes through activation of an array of downstream target genes. Among these is the angiogenesis factor VEGF, which is secreted by HIF-expressing cells and promotes the development and maintenance of tumor neovasculature. HIF-mediated secretion of VEGF by tumor cells likely explains the highly vascular histopathology of clear cell renal carcinoma. All three currently approved angiogenesis inhibitors (the monoclonal antibody bevacizumab targeting VEGF and the kinase inhibitors sorafenib and sunitinib targeting or its receptor VEGF receptor) have single-agent clinical activity in clear cell carcinoma.[73–75] The high specificity of bevacizumab for VEGF leaves little doubt that the activity of this drug is explained by antiangiogenic effects. In contrast, the off-target activities of sorafenib and sunitinib include several kinases expressed in kidney tumor cells, stroma, and inflammatory cells (PDGFR, RAF, RET, FLT3, and others). Interestingly, the primary effect of bevacizumab in kidney cancer is disease stabilization, whereas sorafenib and sunitinib have substantial partial response rates. This raises the question of whether the superior antitumor activity of the VEGF receptor kinase inhibitors is due to the concurrent inhibition of other kinases. However, partial responses rates with next-generation VEGF receptor inhibitors (axitinib, pazopanib, and tivozanib), all of which have greater potency and selectivity for the VEGF receptor, are similarly high, and reinforce the importance of the VEGF receptor as the critical target in kidney cancer.[76–78] Pazopanib is approved for advanced kidney cancer, whereas axitinib is approved as second-line therapy.

Two inhibitors of the mammalian target of rapamycin (mTOR) kinase (temsirolimus and everolimus) are also approved for advanced renal cell carcinoma.[79,80] Both temsirolimus and everolimus are known as rapalogs because both are chemical derivatives of the natural product sirolimus (rapamycin). Sirolimus was approved more than 10 years ago to prevent graft rejection in transplant recipients based on its immunosuppressive properties against T cells. Sirolimus also has potent antiproliferative effects against vascular endothelial cells and, on that basis, is incorporated into drug-eluting cardiac stents to prevent coronary artery restenosis following angioplasty.[81] Rapalogs differ from all the other kinase inhibitors discussed in this chapter in that they inhibit the kinase through an allosteric mechanism rather than by targeting the mTOR kinase domain. Because rapalogs also inhibit the growth of cancer cell lines from different tissues of origin, clinical trials were initiated to study their potential role as anticancer agents in a broad range of tumor types. Based on responses in a few phase I patients with different tumor types (including kidney cancer), exploratory phase II studies were conducted in several diseases. Single-agent activity of temsirolimus was observed in a phase II kidney cancer study,[82] then confirmed in a phase III registration trial.[79] The phase III everolimus trial, which was initiated after temsirolimus, was noteworthy because clinical benefit was demonstrated in patients who had progressed on the VEGF receptor inhibitors sorafenib or sunitinib.[80]

In parallel with the empirical clinical development of rapalogs, various laboratories explored the molecular basis for mTOR dependence in cancer cells. mTOR functions at the center of a complex network that integrates signals from growth factor receptors and nutrient sensors to regulate cell growth and size (Fig. 22.2). It does so, in part, by controlling the translation of various mRNAs with complex 5′ untranslated regions into protein. mTOR exists in two distinct complexes known as TOR complex 1 (TORC1) and TORC2. Rapalogs only inhibit the TORC1 complex, which is largely responsible for downstream phosphorylation of targets such as S6K1/2 and 4EBP1/2 that regulate protein translation.[83] The TORC2 complex contributes to the activation of AKT by phosphorylating the important regulatory serine residue S473 and is unaffected by rapalogs.

Two hypotheses have emerged to explain the clinical activity of rapalogs in kidney cancer. The antiproliferative activity of these compounds against endothelial cells suggests an antiangiogenic mechanism, which is consistent with the clinical activity of the VEGF receptor inhibitors. But rapalogs also inhibit the growth of kidney cancer cell lines in laboratory models where the effects on tumor angiogenesis have been eliminated. Interestingly, mRNAs for HIF1/2 are among those whose translation is impaired by rapalogs, and this effect has been implicated as the primary mechanism of rapalog activity in kidney cancer xenograft models.[84] As with the VEGF receptor inhibitors, a detailed molecular annotation of tumors from responders and nonresponders will shed light on these issues.

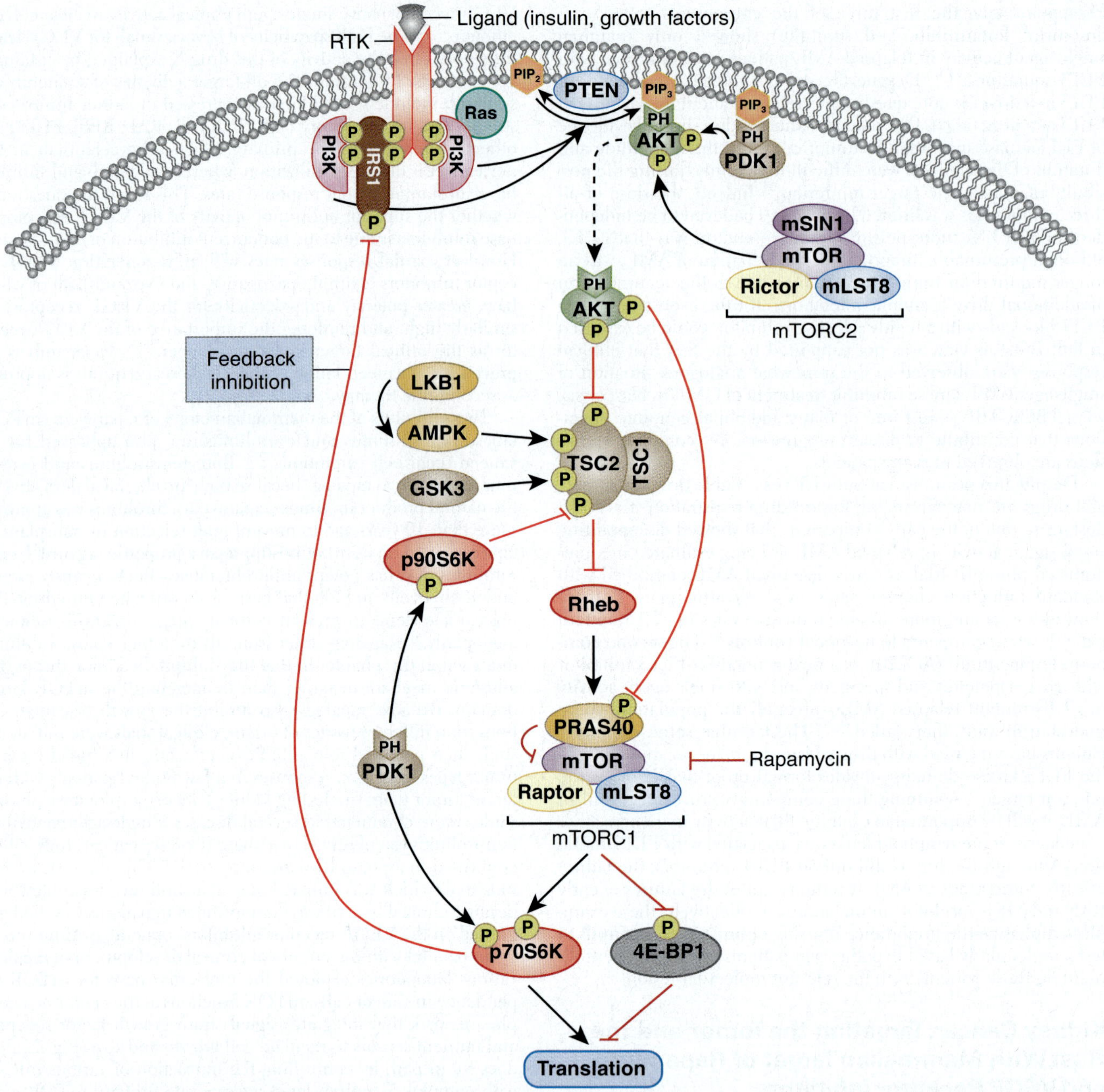

Figure 22.2 Feedback inhibition of the phosphatidylinositol 3-kinase (PI3K) pathway. Activated AKT regulates cellular growth through mammalian target of rapamycin (mTOR), a key player in protein synthesis and translation. mTOR forms part of two distinct complexes known as mTORC1, which contains mTOR, Raptor, mLST8, and PRAS40, and mTORC2, which contains mTOR, Rictor, mLST8, and mSIN1. mTORC1 is sensitive to rapamycin and controls protein synthesis and translation, at least in part, through p70S6K and eukaryotic translation initiation factor 4E–binding protein 1 (4E-BP1). AKT phosphorylates and inhibits tuberous sclerosis complex 2 (TSC2), resulting in increased mTORC1 activity. AKT also phosphorylates PRAS40, thus relieving the PRAS40 inhibitory effect on mTOR and the mTORC1 complex. mTORC2 and 3-phosphoinositide–dependent kinase (PDK1) phosphorylate AKT on Ser473 and Thr308, respectively, rendering it fully active. mTORC1-activated p70S6K can phosphorylate insulin receptor substrate 1 (IRS1), resulting in inhibition of PI3K activity. In addition, PDK1 phosphorylates and activates p70S6K and p90S6K. The latter has been shown to inhibit TSC2 activity through direct phosphorylation. Conversely, LKB1-activated AMP-activated protein kinase (AMPK) and glycogen synthase kinase 3 (GSK3) activate the TSC1/TSC2 complex through direct phosphorylation of TSC2. Thus, signals through PI3K as well as through LKB1 and AMPK converge on mTORC1. Inhibition of mTORC1 can lead to increased insulin receptor–mediated signaling, and inhibition of PDK1 may lead to activation of mTORC1 and may, paradoxically, promote tumor growth. (From Daigle SR, Olhava EJ, Therkelsen CA, et al. Selective killing of mixed lineage leukemia cells by a potent small-molecule DOT1L inhibitor. *Cancer Cell* 2011;20(1):53–65, with permission.)

Other Indications for mTOR Inhibitors: Breast Cancer and Tuberous Sclerosis Complex Mutant Cancers

Two other indications for mTOR have emerged, both based on fundamental insights from laboratory studies but from quite different angles. Preclinical studies of estrogen receptor (ER) therapy in breast cancer suggested that phosphatidylinositol 3-kinase (PI3K) pathway activation may be a mechanism of resistance and that this resistance could be prevented or overcome by combined treatment with ER-based drugs and rapalogs such as everolimus. Based on evidence that some women with progressive disease while receiving the aromatase inhibitor letrozole have clinical benefit from the addition of everolimus, randomized trials were initiated comparing everolimus + exemestane to exemestane alone (called BOLERO-2), or everolimus + tamoxifen to tamoxifen alone (called TAMRAD). Both studies demonstrated substantial improvements in time to progression in women with metastatic breast cancer who had already failed one aromatase inhibitor,[85,86] resulting in FDA approval of the everolimus/exemestane combination. Evidence of cross-talk between the PI3K pathway and hormone receptor signaling (ER in breast cancer, androgen receptor in prostate cancer) provides a molecular rationale for the clinical benefit of combination therapy and is currently under investigation in metastatic prostate cancer.[87]

Yet another indication for rapalog therapy emerged from the genetics of children with tuberous sclerosis caused by a loss of function mutations in tuberous sclerosis complex 1 (TSC1) or TSC2, which encode the proteins hamartin and tuberin that function in the PI3K signaling pathway just upstream of mTOR. Based on laboratory studies showing that TSC1- or TSC2-deficient cells are exquisitely sensitive to rapalogs, a clinical trial was conducted in tuberous sclerosis patients with benign subependymal giant-cell astrocytomas (SEGA) that showed tumor shrinkage in 21 of 28 patients.[88] This genetic dependence on mTOR in tumors with tuberous sclerosis complex (TSC) loss has also been observed in bladder cancer. In a remarkable example of the power of comprehensive DNA sequencing to provide insight into rare clinical phenotypes, investigators examined the tumor genome of the single complete responder patient on a phase II trial of everolimus in bladder cancer and discovered somatic mutations in TSC2 as well as a second gene, NF2, that also controls mTOR activity.[89] This plus other examples of how a retrospective genomic analysis of *extraordinary responders* has led to a national effort to capture these cases, as well as prospective clinical trials of patients with the relevant tumor genotype regardless of histology (called *basket* trials).

It is unclear why rapalogs have failed in other tumor types. One explanation is the concurrence of PI3K pathway mutations with alterations in other pathways that mitigate sensitivity to rapalogs. Another possibility is the disruption of negative feedback loops regulated by mTOR that inhibit signaling from upstream receptor tyrosine kinases. Rapalogs paradoxically *increase* signaling through PI3K due to loss of this negative feedback. A primary consequence is *increased* AKT activation, which signals to an array of downstream substrates that can enhance cell proliferation and survival (other than TORC1, which remains inhibited by rapalog) (see Fig. 22.2). This problem might be overcome by combining rapalogs with an inhibitor of an upstream kinase in the feedback loop, such as HER kinases or the insulinlike growth factor receptor (IGFR), to block this undesired effect of rapalogs on PI3K activation.[90]

DIRECTLY TARGETING THE PI3K PATHWAY

Mutations or copy number alterations (e.g., amplification or deletion of oncogenes or tumor suppressor genes) in PI3K pathway genes (PIK3CA, PIK3R1, PTEN, AKT1, and others) are among the most common abnormalities in cancer. Consequently, intensive efforts at many pharmaceutical companies have been devoted to the discovery of small-molecule inhibitors targeting kinases in the PI3K pathway. Inhibitors of PI3K, AKT, and ATP-competitive (rather than allosteric) inhibitors of mTOR that target both the TORC1 and TORC2 complex are all in clinical development. Phase I clinical trials have, in general, established that the pathway can be efficiently targeted without serious toxicity other than easily manageable effects on glucose metabolism (which is anticipated based on the importance of PI3K signaling in insulin signaling). Unfortunately, there has been no evidence to date of dramatic single-agent clinical activity with any of these agents, although early results with PI3K alpha selective inhibitor BYL719 in PIK3CA mutant breast cancer appear promising.[91]

However, the first approval of a direct PI3K inhibitor in cancer is likely to come in chronic lymphocytic leukemia and in lymphoma, but not on the basis of tumor genomics. Normal and malignant B cells are dependent on PI3K delta as well as Bruton tyrosine kinase (BTK) for proliferation and survival, raising the possibility that inhibitors of these kinases might be broadly active in B-cell malignancies. Concerns about toxicity on normal B cells were alleviated, in part, by the earlier clinical success of the CD20 antibody rituximab in lymphoma, which also eliminates normal circulating B cells, but without significant clinical sequelae. The first such PI3K delta inhibitor, idelalisib, has shown impressive activity in indolent non-Hodgkin lymphoma as a single agent and in relapsed chronic lymphocytic leukemia when given in combination with rituximab. The BTK inhibitor ibrutinib, following a similar clinical development path, was recently approved as second-line therapy for chronic lymphocytic leukemia and for mantle cell lymphoma.[92,93]

COMBINATIONS OF KINASE INHIBITORS TO INDUCT RESPONSE AND PREVENT RESISTANCE

Preclinical studies indicate that combinations of kinase inhibitors are required to realize their full potential as anticancer agents. The most common rationale is to address the problem of concurrent mutations in different pathways that alleviate dependence on a single-driver oncogene. The best examples are cancers with mutations in both the RAS/MAP kinase pathway (RAS or BRAF) and the PI3K pathway (PIK3CA or PTEN). In mouse models, such doubly mutant tumors fail to respond to single-agent treatment with either an AKT inhibitor or a MEK inhibitor. However, combination treatment can give dramatic regressions.[94] Similarly, genetically engineered mice that develop KRAS-driven lung cancer respond only to combination therapy with a PI3K inhibitor and a MEK inhibitor.[95] To date, clinical trials combining different PI3K pathway and RAS/MAP kinase pathway inhibitors have been challenging due to toxicities associated with continuous, concurrent PI3K and RAS/MAP kinase pathway inhibition.

Many of the tumor types discussed in this chapter *do* respond to treatment with a single-agent kinase, but relapse despite continued inhibitor therapy. Research into the causes of "acquired" kinase inhibitor resistance has revealed two primary mechanisms: (1) novel mutations in the kinase domain of the drug target that preclude inhibition, or (2) *bypass* of the driver kinase signal by activation of a parallel kinase pathway. In both cases, the solution is combination therapy to prevent the emergence of resistance. An elegant demonstration of this approach comes from CML where resistance to imatinib is primarily caused by mutations in the BCR-ABL kinase domain.[96,97] The second-generation ABL inhibitors dasatinib and nilotinib are effective against most imatinib-resistant BCR-ABL mutants and were initially approved as single-agent therapy for imatinib-resistant CML.[98,99] Very recently, both drugs have proven superior to imatinib in the upfront treatment of CML due to increased potency and fewer mechanisms of acquired resistance.[100–102] However, one BCR-ABL mutation called T315I is resistant to all three drugs. The third-generation ABL kinase inhibitor ponatinib blocks T315I and showed activity in a phase II clinical trial that included CML patients with the T315I mutation,[103] resulting in FDA approval. However, subsequent reports of severe vascular occlusive events, such as stroke and heart failure, led to withdrawal from the market, followed by approval for restricted use in T315I-mutant patients. Analogous approaches are ongoing in other diseases such as EGFR-mutant lung cancer, where acquired resistance to the frontline kinase inhibitor is also associated with mutations in the target kinase.[104,105] Promising clinical results have been reported with irreversible EGFR inhibitors such as CO-1686 and AZD9291.

The clinical development of kinase inhibitor combinations to prevent acquired resistance is relatively straightforward. Because the frontline drug is already approved, success would be determined by an improvement in response duration using the combination. The situation is more complex when two experimental compounds (e.g., a PI3K pathway inhibitor and a MEK inhibitor) are combined, neither of which shows significant single-agent activity. Older regulatory guidelines required a four-arm study that compared each single agent to the combination and to a control group in order to obtain approval of the combination. Recognizing that this design could discourage drug developers as well as patients from moving forward because it requires a large sample size, the FDA has issued new guidelines for the development of novel combinations that require a two-arm registration study comparing the combination to standard of care http://www.fda.gov/downloads/Drugs/GuidanceComplianceRegulatoryInformation/Guidances/UCM236669.pdf. A more challenging issue may be dose optimization and dose schedule that is needed to safely combine two investigational drugs. Much like the development of combination chemotherapy several decades ago, it may be important to select compounds with nonoverlapping toxicities to allow for sufficient doses of each drug to be achieved.

SPECULATIONS ON THE FUTURE ROLE OF KINASE INHIBITORS IN CANCER MEDICINE

The role of genomics in predicting a response to kinase inhibitor therapy is now irrefutable. As the number of kinase driver mutations continues to grow, the field is likely to move away from the current strategy of a *companion diagnostic* for each drug. Rather, comprehensive mutational profiling platforms that query each tumor for hundreds of potential cancer mutations are more likely to emerge as the diagnostic platform. The number of directly *actionable* mutations (meaning the presence of a mutation defines a treatment decision supported by clinical trial data) remains low, but this number will undoubtedly grow. In addition, it is becoming apparent that many patients have rare mutations (defined as rare in that histologic tumor type) but are, in theory, actionable. Because these examples are unlikely to be formally evaluated in clinical trials, many centers have opened *basket* studies (with eligibility based solely on mutation profile) to capture these cases with some reports of remarkable success.

More effort must be devoted to manipulating the dose and schedule of kinase inhibitor therapy to maximize efficacy and minimize toxicity. To date, all kinase inhibitors have been developed based on the assumption that a 24/7 coverage of the target is required for efficacy. Consequently, most compounds are optimized to have a long serum half-life (12 to 24 hours). Phase II doses are then selected based on the maximum tolerated dose determined with daily administration. But a recent clinical of the ABL inhibitor dasatinib in CML indicates that equivalent antitumor activity can be achieved with intermittent therapy.[106] By giving larger doses intermittently, higher peak drug concentrations were achieved that resulted in equivalent and possibly superior efficacy.[107] Similar results were observed in laboratory studies of EGFR inhibitors in EGFR-mutant lung cancer. Clinically robust, quantitative assays of target inhibition are needed to hasten progress in this area.

Although the focus of this chapter is kinase inhibitors, the themes developed here should apply broadly to inhibitors of other cancer targets. Inhibitors of the G-protein coupled receptor smoothened (SMO) in patients with metastatic basal cell carcinoma or medulloblastoma establish that the driver mutation hypothesis extends beyond kinase inhibitors. SMO is a component in the Hedgehog pathway, which is constitutively activated in subsets of patients with basal cell carcinoma and medulloblastoma due to mutations in the Hedgehog ligand-binding receptor Patched-1. Treatment with the SMO inhibitor vismodegib led to impressive responses in basal cell carcinoma and medulloblastoma patients whose tumors had Patched-1 mutations,[108,109] resulting in FDA approval. Other novel cancer targets are emerging from cancer genome sequencing projects. Somatic mutations in the Krebs cycle enzyme isocitrate dehydrogenase (IDH1/2) were found in subsets of patients with glioblastoma, AML, chondrosarcoma, and cholangiocarcinoma,[110–112] and the first IDH2 inhibitor has entered clinical trials in leukemia. Mutations in enzymes involved in chromatin remodeling, such as the histone methyltransferase EZH2, have been reported in lymphoma and have spurred the ongoing development of EZH2 inhibitors.[113,114] Inhibitors of another histone methyltransferase DOT1L, which is required for the maintenance of mixed lineage leukemia (MLL) fusion leukemias, are also in clinical development.[115,116] Kinase inhibitors are just the first wave of molecularly targeted drugs ushered in by our understanding of the molecular underpinnings of cancer cells. There is much more to follow.

REFERENCES

1. Sawyers CL. Shifting paradigms: the seeds of oncogene addiction. *Nat Med* 2009;15(10):1158–1161.
2. Weinstein IB. Cancer. Addiction to oncogenes—the Achilles heal of cancer. *Science* 2002;297(5578):63–64.
3. Druker BJ, Talpaz M, Resta DJ, et al., Efficacy and safety of a specific inhibitor of the BCR-ABL tyrosine kinase in chronic myeloid leukemia. *N Engl J Med* 2001;344(14):1031–1037.
4. Hirota S, Isozaki K, Moriyama Y, et al. Gain-of-function mutations of c-kit in human gastrointestinal stromal tumors. *Science* 1998;279(5350):577–580.
5. Heinrich MC, Corless CL, Duensing A, et al. PDGFRA activating mutations in gastrointestinal stromal tumors. *Science* 2003;299(5607):708–710.
6. Demetri GD, von Mehren M, Blanke CD, et al. Efficacy and safety of imatinib mesylate in advanced gastrointestinal stromal tumors. *N Engl J Med* 2002;347(7):472–480.
7. Geyer CE, Forster J, Lindquist D, et al. Lapatinib plus capecitabine for HER2-positive advanced breast cancer. *N Engl J Med* 2006;355(26):2733–2743.
8. Kris MG, Natale RB, Herbst RS, et al. Efficacy of gefitinib, an inhibitor of the epidermal growth factor receptor tyrosine kinase, in symptomatic patients with non-small cell lung cancer: a randomized trial. *JAMA* 2003;290(16):2149–2158.
9. Miller VA, Kris MG, Shah N, et al. Bronchioloalveolar pathologic subtype and smoking history predict sensitivity to gefitinib in advanced non-small-cell lung cancer. *J Clin Oncol* 2004;22(6):1103–1109.
10. Paez JG, Jänne PA, Lee JC, et al. EGFR mutations in lung cancer: correlation with clinical response to gefitinib therapy. *Science* 2004;304(5676):1497–1500.
11. Lynch TJ, Bell DW, Sordella R, et al. Activating mutations in the epidermal growth factor receptor underlying responsiveness of non-small-cell lung cancer to gefitinib. *N Engl J Med* 2004;350(21):2129–2139.
12. Pao W, Miller V, Zakowski M, et al. EGF receptor gene mutations are common in lung cancers from "never smokers" and are associated with sensitivity of tumors to gefitinib and erlotinib. *Proc Natl Acad Sci U S A* 2004;101(36):13306–13311.
13. Cohen MH, Willliams GA, Sridhara R, et al. FDA drug approval summary: gefitinib (ZD1839) (Iressa) tablets. *Oncologist* 2003;8(4):303–306.
14. Shepherd FA, Rodrigues Pereira J, Ciuleanu T, et al. Erlotinib in previously treated non-small-cell lung cancer. *N Engl J Med* 2005;353(2):123–132.

15. Thatcher N, Chang A, Parikh P, et al. Gefitinib plus best supportive care in previously treated patients with refractory advanced non-small-cell lung cancer: results from a randomised, placebo-controlled, multicentre study (Iressa Survival Evaluation in Lung Cancer). *Lancet* 2005;366(9496):1527–1537.
16. Herbst RS, Giaccone G, Schiller JH, et al. Gefitinib in combination with paclitaxel and carboplatin in advanced non-small-cell lung cancer: a phase III trial—INTACT 2. *J Clin Oncol* 2004;22(5):785–794.
17. Giaccone G, Herbst RS, Manegold C, et al. Gefitinib in combination with gemcitabine and cisplatin in advanced non-small-cell lung cancer: a phase III trial—INTACT 1. *J Clin Oncol* 2004;22(5):777–784.
18. Herbst RS, Prager D, Hermann R, et al. TRIBUTE: a phase III trial of erlotinib hydrochloride (OSI-774) combined with carboplatin and paclitaxel chemotherapy in advanced non-small-cell lung cancer. *J Clin Oncol* 2005;23(25):5892–5899.
19. Tsao MS, Sakurada A, Cutz JC, et al. Erlotinib in lung cancer - molecular and clinical predictors of outcome. *N Engl J Med* 2005;353(2):133–144.
20. Mok TS, Wu YL, Thongprasert S, et al. Gefitinib or carboplatin-paclitaxel in pulmonary adenocarcinoma. *N Engl J Med* 2009;361(10):947–957.
21. Schaller JL, Burkland GA. Case report: rapid and complete control of idiopathic hypereosinophilia with imatinib mesylate. *MedGenMed* 2001;3(5):9.
22. Ault P, Cortes J, Koller C, et al. Response of idiopathic hypereosinophilic syndrome to treatment with imatinib mesylate. *Leuk Res* 2002;26(9):881–884.
23. Cools J, DeAngelo DJ, Gotlib J, et al. A tyrosine kinase created by fusion of the PDGFRA and FIP1L1 genes as a therapeutic target of imatinib in idiopathic hypereosinophilic syndrome. *N Engl J Med* 2003;348(13):1201–1214.
24. Golub TR, Barker GF, Lovett M, et al. Fusion of PDGF receptor beta to a novel ets-like gene, tel, in chronic myelomonocytic leukemia with t(5;12) chromosomal translocation. *Cell* 1994;77(2):307–316.
25. Apperley JF, Gardembas M, Melo JV, et al. Response to imatinib mesylate in patients with chronic myeloproliferative diseases with rearrangements of the platelet-derived growth factor receptor beta. *N Engl J Med* 2002;347(7):481–487.
26. Rutkowski P, Van Glabbeke M, Rankin CJ, et al. Imatinib mesylate in advanced dermatofibrosarcoma protuberans: pooled analysis of two phase II clinical trials. *J Clin Oncol* 2010;28(10):1772–1779.
27. Davies H, Bignell GR, Cox C, et al. Mutations of the BRAF gene in human cancer. *Nature* 2002;417(6892):949–954.
28. Baxter EJ, Scott LM, Campbell PJ, et al., Acquired mutation of the tyrosine kinase JAK2 in human myeloproliferative disorders. *Lancet* 2005;365(9464):1054–1061.
29. James C, Ugo V, Le Couédic JP, et al. A unique clonal JAK2 mutation leading to constitutive signalling causes polycythaemia vera. *Nature* 2005;434(7037):1144–1148.
30. Levine RL, Wadleigh M, Cools J, et al. Activating mutation in the tyrosine kinase JAK2 in polycythemia vera, essential thrombocythemia, and myeloid metaplasia with myelofibrosis. *Cancer Cell* 2005;7(4):387–397.
31. Samuels Y, Wang Z, Bardellli A, et al. High frequency of mutations of the PIK3CA gene in human cancers. *Science* 2004;304(5670):554.
32. International Cancer Genome Consortium, Hudson TJ, Anderson W, et al. International network of cancer genome projects. *Nature* 2010;464(7291):993–998.
33. Vogelstein B, Papadopoulos N, Velculescu VE, et al. Cancer genome landscapes. *Science* 2013;339(6127):1546–1558.
34. Lawrence MS, Stojanov P, Mermel CH, et al. Discovery and saturation analysis of cancer genes across 21 tumour types. *Nature* 2014;505(7484):495–501.
35. Eisen T, Ahmad T, Flaherty KT, et al. Sorafenib in advanced melanoma: a Phase II randomised discontinuation trial analysis. *Br J Cancer* 2006;95(5):581–586.
36. Solit DB, Garraway LA, Pratilas CA, et al. BRAF mutation predicts sensitivity to MEK inhibition. *Nature* 2006;439(7074):358–362.
37. McDermott U, Sharma SV, Dowell L, et al. Identification of genotype-correlated sensitivity to selective kinase inhibitors by using high-throughput tumor cell line profiling. *Proc Natl Acad Sci U S A* 2007;104(50):19936–19941.
38. Pratilas CA, Taylor BS, Ye Q, et al. (V600E)BRAF is associated with disabled feedback inhibition of RAF-MEK signaling and elevated transcriptional output of the pathway. *Proc Natl Acad Sci U S A* 2009;106(11):4519–4524.
39. LoRusso PM, Krishnamurthi SS, Rinehart JJ, et al. Phase I pharmacokinetic and pharmacodynamic study of the oral MAPK/ERK kinase inhibitor PD-0325901 in patients with advanced cancers. *Clin Cancer Res* 2010;16(6):1924–1937.
40. Adjei AA, Cohen RB, Franklin W, et al. Phase I pharmacokinetic and pharmacodynamic study of the oral, small-molecule mitogen-activated protein kinase kinase 1/2 inhibitor AZD6244 (ARRY-142886) in patients with advanced cancers. *J Clin Oncol* 2008;26(13):2139–2146.
41. Dummer R, Chapman PB, Sosman JA, et al. AZD6244 (ARRY-142886) vs temozolomide (TMZ) in patients (pts) with advanced melanoma: An open-label, randomized, multicenter, phase II study. *J Clin Oncol* 2008;26(May 20 suppl):9033.
42. Flaherty KT, Robert C, Hersey P, et al. Improved survival with MEK inhibition in BRAF-mutated melanoma. *N Engl J Med* 2012;367(2):107–114.
43. Joseph EW, Pratillas CA, Poulikakos PI, et al. The RAF inhibitor PLX4032 inhibits ERK signaling and tumor cell proliferation in a V600E BRAF-selective manner. *Proc Natl Acad Sci U S A* 2010;107(33):14903–14908.
44. Flaherty K, Puzanov I, Sosman J, et al. Phase I study of PLX4032: proof of concept for V600E BRAF mutation as a therapeutic target in human cancer. *J Clin Oncol* 2009;27(15s):abstract 9000.
45. Flaherty KT, Puzanov I, Kim KB, et al. Inhibition of mutated, activated BRAF in metastatic melanoma. *N Engl J Med* 2010;363(9):809–819.
46. Bollag G, Hirth P, Tsai J, et al. Clinical efficacy of a RAF inhibitor needs broad target blockade in BRAF-mutant melanoma. *Nature* 2010;467(7315):596–599.
47. Hauschild A, Grob JJ, Demidov LV, et al. Dabrafenib in BRAF-mutated metastatic melanoma: a multicentre, open-label, phase 3 randomised controlled trial. *Lancet* 2012;380(9839):358–365.
48. Kwak EL, Camidge DR, Clark J, et al. Clinical activity observed in a phase I dose escalation trial of an oral c-MET and ALK inhibitor, PF-02341066. *J Clin Oncol* 2009;27(Suppl):148s.
49. Morris SW, Kirstein MN, Valentine MB, et al. Fusion of a kinase gene, ALK, to a nucleolar protein gene, NPM, in non-Hodgkin's lymphoma. *Science* 1994;263(5151):1281–1284.
50. Soda M, Choi YL, Enomoto M, et al. Identification of the transforming EML4-ALK fusion gene in non-small-cell lung cancer. *Nature* 2007;448(7153):561–566.
51. Bang Y, Kwak EL, Shaw AT, et al. Clinical activity of the oral ALK inhibitor PF-02341066 in ALK-positive patients with non-small cell lung cancer (NSCLC). *J Clin Oncol* 2010;28:18s.
52. Shaw AT, Kim DW, Nakagawa K, et al. Crizotinib versus chemotherapy in advanced ALK-positive lung cancer. *N Engl J Med* 2013;368(25):2385–2394.
53. Chen Y, Takita J, Choi YL, et al. Oncogenic mutations of ALK kinase in neuroblastoma. *Nature* 2008;455(7215):971–974.
54. Sirvent N,Hawkins AL, Moeglin D, et al. ALK probe rearrangement in a t(2;11;2)(p23;p15;q31) translocation found in a prenatal myofibroblastic fibrous lesion: toward a molecular definition of an inflammatory myofibroblastic tumor family? *Genes Chromosomes Cancer* 2001;31(1):85–90.
55. Fagin JA, Mitsiades N. Molecular pathology of thyroid cancer: diagnostic and clinical implications. *Best Pract Res Clin Endocrinol Metab* 2008;22(6):955–969.
56. Wells SA Jr, Gosnell JE, Gagel RF, et al. Vandetanib for the treatment of patients with locally advanced or metastatic hereditary medullary thyroid cancer. *J Clin Oncol* 28(5):767–772.
57. Lam ET, Ringel MD, Kloos RT, et al. Phase II clinical trial of sorafenib in metastatic medullary thyroid cancer. J *Clin Oncol* 28(14):2323–2330.
58. Kloos RT, Ringel MD, Knopp MV, et al. Phase II trial of sorafenib in metastatic thyroid cancer. *J Clin Oncol* 2009;27(10):1675–1684.
59. Schlumberger MJ, Elisei R, Bastholt L, et al. Phase II study of safety and efficacy of motesanib in patients with progressive or symptomatic, advanced or metastatic medullary thyroid cancer. *J Clin Oncol* 2009;27(23):3794–3801.
60. Kurzrock R, Cohen EE, Sherman SI, et al. Long-term results in a cohort of medullary thyroid cancer (MTC) patients (pts) in a phase I study of XL184 (BMS 907351), an oral inhibitor of MET, VEGFR2, and RET. *J Clin Oncol* 2010;28(Suppl):15s.
61. Wells SA Jr, Robinson BG, Gagel RF, et al. Vandetanib in patients with locally advanced or metastatic medullary thyroid cancer: a randomized, double-blind phase III trial. *J Clin Oncol* 2012;30(2):134–141.
62. Elisei R, Schlumberger MJ, Müller SP, et al. Cabozantinib in progressive medullary thyroid cancer. *J Clin Oncol* 2013;31(29):3639–3646.
63. Sawyers CL. Finding the next Gleevec. FLT3 targeted kinase inhibitor therapy for acute myeloid leukemia. *Cancer Cell* 2002;1(5):413–415.
64. Kelly LM, Qing L, Jeffery L, et al. FLT3 internal tandem duplication mutations associated with human acute myeloid leukemias induce myeloproliferative disease in a murine bone marrow transplant model. *Blood* 2002;99(1):310–318.
65. Stone RM, DeAngelo DJ, Klimek V, et al. Patients with acute myeloid leukemia and an activating mutation in FLT3 respond to a small-molecule FLT3 tyrosine kinase inhibitor, PKC412. *Blood* 2005;105(1):54–60.
66. Knapper S, Burnett AK, Littlewood T, et al. A phase 2 trial of the FLT3 inhibitor lestaurtinib (CEP701) as first-line treatment for older patients with acute myeloid leukemia not considered fit for intensive chemotherapy. *Blood* 2006;108(10):3262–3270.
67. Fiedler W, Serve H, Döhner H, et al. A phase 1 study of SU11248 in the treatment of patients with refractory or resistant acute myeloid leukemia (AML) or not amenable to conventional therapy for the disease. *Blood* 2005;105(3):986–993.
68. Stone RM, Fischer T, Paquette R, et al. A Phase 1b study of midostaurin (PKC412) in combination with daunorubicin and cytarabine induction and high-dose cytarabine consolidation in patients under age 61 with newly diagnosed de novo acute myeloid leukemia: overall survival of patients whose blasts have FLT3 mutations is similar to those with wild-type FLT3. Paper presented at: 2009 American Society of Hematology Annual Meeting; 2009; New Orleans, LA.
69. Zarrinkar PP, Gunawardane RN, Cramer MD, et al. AC220 is a uniquely potent and selective inhibitor of FLT3 for the treatment of acute myeloid leukemia (AML). *Blood* 2009;114(14):2984–2992.
70. Cortes J, et al. AC220, a potent, selective, second generation FLT3 receptor tyrosine kinase (RTK) inhibitor, in a first-in-human (FIH) phase 1 AML study. Paper presented at: 2009 American Society of Hematology Annual Meeting; 2009; New Orleans, LA.
71. Smith CC, Wang Q, Chin CS, et al. Validation of ITD mutations in FLT3 as a therapeutic target in human acute myeloid leukaemia. *Nature* 2012;485(7397):260–263.
72. Kaelin WG Jr. The von Hippel-Lindau tumour suppressor protein: O2 sensing and cancer. *Nat Rev Cancer* 2008;8(11):865–873.
73. Yang JC, Haworth L, Sherry RM, et al. A randomized trial of bevacizumab, an anti-vascular endothelial growth factor antibody, for metastatic renal cancer. *N Engl J Med* 2003;349(5):427–434.

74. Escudier B, Eisen T, Stadler WM, et al. Sorafenib in advanced clear-cell renal-cell carcinoma. *N Engl J Med* 2007;356(2):125–134.
75. Motzer RJ, Hutson TE, Tomczak P, et al. Sunitinib versus interferon alfa in metastatic renal-cell carcinoma. *N Engl J Med* 2007;356(2):115–124.
76. Rini BI, Wilding G, Hudes G, et al. Phase II study of axitinib in sorafenib-refractory metastatic renal cell carcinoma. *J Clin Oncol* 2009;27(27):4462–4468.
77. Sonpavde G, Hutson TE, Sternberg CN. Pazopanib, a potent orally administered small-molecule multitargeted tyrosine kinase inhibitor for renal cell carcinoma. *Expert Opin Investig Drugs* 2008;17(2):253–261.
78. Bhargava P, Esteves B, Al-Adhami M, et al. Activity of tivozanib (AV-951) in patients with renal cell carcinoma (RCC): Subgroup analysis from a phase II randomized discontinuation trial (RDT). *J Clin Oncol* 2010;28(suppl):15s.
79. Hudes G, Carducci M, Tomczak P, et al. Temsirolimus, interferon alfa, or both for advanced renal-cell carcinoma. *N Engl J Med* 2007;356(22):2271–2281.
80. Motzer RJ, Escudier B, Oudard S, et al. Efficacy of everolimus in advanced renal cell carcinoma: a double-blind, randomised, placebo-controlled phase III trial. *Lancet* 2008;372(9637):449–456.
81. McKeage K, Murdoch D, Goa FL. The sirolimus-eluting stent: a review of its use in the treatment of coronary artery disease. *Am J Cardiovasc Drugs* 2003;3(3):211–230.
82. Atkins MB, Hidalgo M, Stadler WM, et al. Randomized phase II study of multiple dose levels of CCI-779, a novel mammalian target of rapamycin kinase inhibitor, in patients with advanced refractory renal cell carcinoma. *J Clin Oncol* 2004;22(5):909–918.
83. Guertin DA, Sabatini DM. Defining the role of mTOR in cancer. *Cancer Cell* 2007;12(1):9–22.
84. Thomas GV, Tran C, Mellinghoff IK, et al. Hypoxia-inducible factor determines sensitivity to inhibitors of mTOR in kidney cancer. *Nat Med* 2006;12(1):122–127.
85. Bachelot T, Bourgier C, Cropet C, et al. Randomized phase II trial of everolimus in combination with tamoxifen in patients with hormone receptor-positive, human epidermal growth factor receptor 2-negative metastatic breast cancer with prior exposure to aromatase inhibitors: a GINECO study. *J Clin Oncol* 2012;30(22):2718–2724.
86. Baselga J, Campone M, Piccart M, et al. Everolimus in postmenopausal hormone-receptor-positive advanced breast cancer. *N Engl J Med* 2012;366(6):520–529.
87. Carver BS, Chapinski C, Wongvipat J, et al. Reciprocal feedback regulation of PI3K and androgen receptor signaling in PTEN-deficient prostate cancer. *Cancer Cell* 2011;19(5):575–586.
88. Krueger DA, Care MM, Holland K, et al. Everolimus for subependymal giant-cell astrocytomas in tuberous sclerosis. *N Engl J Med* 2010;363(19):1801–1811.
89. Iyer G, Hanrahan AL, Milowsky MI, et al. Genome sequencing identifies a basis for everolimus sensitivity. *Science* 2012;338(6104):221.
90. O'Reilly KE, Rojo F, She QB, et al. mTOR inhibition induces upstream receptor tyrosine kinase signaling and activates Akt. *Cancer Res* 2006;66(3):1500–1508.
91. Gonzalez-Angulo AM, Juric D, Argilis G, et al. Safety, pharmacokinetics, and preliminary activity of the alpha-specific P13K inhibitor BYL719: results from the first-in-human study. *J Clin Oncol* 2013;31(15 Suppl):2531.
92. Byrd JC, Furman RR, Coutre SE, et al. Targeting BTK with ibrutinib in relapsed chronic lymphocytic leukemia. *N Engl J Med* 2013;369(1):32–42.
93. Wang ML, Rule S, Martin P, et al. Targeting BTK with ibrutinib in relapsed or refractory mantle-cell lymphoma. *N Engl J Med* 2013;369(6):507–516.
94. She QB, Halilovic E, Ye Q, et al. 4E-BP1 is a key effector of the oncogenic activation of the AKT and ERK signaling pathways that integrates their function in tumors. *Cancer Cell* 18(1):39–51.
95. Engelman JA, Chen L, Tan X, et al. Effective use of PI3K and MEK inhibitors to treat mutant Kras G12D and PIK3CA H1047R murine lung cancers. *Nat Med* 2008;14(12):1351–1356.
96. Gorre ME, Mohammed M, Ellwood K, et al. Clinical resistance to STI-571 cancer therapy caused by BCR-ABL gene mutation or amplification. *Science* 2001;293(5531):876–880.
97. Shah NP, Nicoll JM, Nagar B, et al. Multiple BCR-ABL kinase domain mutations confer polyclonal resistance to the tyrosine kinase inhibitor imatinib (STI571) in chronic phase and blast crisis chronic myeloid leukemia. *Cancer Cell* 2002;2(2):117–125.
98. Shah NP, Tran C, Lee FY, et al. Overriding imatinib resistance with a novel ABL kinase inhibitor. *Science* 2004;305(5682):399–401.
99. Talpaz M, Shah NP, Kantarjian H, et al. Dasatinib in imatinib-resistant Philadelphia chromosome-positive leukemias. *N Engl J Med* 2006;354(24):2531–2541.
100. Kantarjian H, Shah NP, Hochhaus A, et al. Dasatinib versus imatinib in newly diagnosed chronic-phase chronic myeloid leukemia. *N Engl J Med* 2010;362(24):2260–2270.
101. Sawyers CL. Even better kinase inhibitors for chronic myeloid leukemia. *N Engl J Med* 2010;362(24):2314–2315.
102. Saglio G, Kim DW, Issaragrisil S, et al. Nilotinib versus imatinib for newly diagnosed chronic myeloid leukemia. *N Engl J Med* 362(24):2251–2259.
103. Cortes JE, Kim DW, Pinilla-Ibarz J, et al. A phase 2 trial of ponatinib in Philadelphia chromosome-positive leukemias. *N Engl J Med* 2013;369(19): 1783–1796.
104. Pao W, Miller VA, Politi KA, et al. Acquired resistance of lung adenocarcinomas to gefitinib or erlotinib is associated with a second mutation in the EGFR kinase domain. *PLoS Med* 2005;2(3):e73.
105. Antonescu CR, Besmer P, Guo T, et al. Acquired resistance to imatinib in gastrointestinal stromal tumor occurs through secondary gene mutation. *Clin Cancer Res* 2005;11(11):4182–4190.
106. Shah NP, Kantarjian HM, Kim DW, et al. Intermittent target inhibition with dasatinib 100 mg once daily preserves efficacy and improves tolerability in imatinib-resistant and -intolerant chronic-phase chronic myeloid leukemia. *J Clin Oncol* 2008;26(19):3204–3212.
107. Shah NP, Kasap C, Weier C, et al. Transient potent BCR-ABL inhibition is sufficient to commit chronic myeloid leukemia cells irreversibly to apoptosis. *Cancer Cell* 2008;14(6):485–493.
108. Von Hoff DD, LoRusso PM, Rudin CM, et al. Inhibition of the hedgehog pathway in advanced basal-cell carcinoma. *N Engl J Med* 2009;361(12): 1164–1172.
109. Rudin CM, Hann CL, Laterra J, et al. Treatment of medulloblastoma with hedgehog pathway inhibitor GDC-0449. *N Engl J Med* 2009;361(12): 1173–1178.
110. Parsons DW, Jones S, Zhang X, et al. An integrated genomic analysis of human glioblastoma multiforme. *Science* 2008;321(5897):1807–1812.
111. Mardis ER, Ding L, Dooling DJ, et al. Recurring mutations found by sequencing an acute myeloid leukemia genome. *N Engl J Med* 2009;361(11): 1058–1066.
112. Ward PS, Patel J, Wise DR, et al. The common feature of leukemia-associated IDH1 and IDH2 mutations is a neomorphic enzyme activity converting alpha-ketoglutarate to 2-hydroxyglutarate. *Cancer Cell* 2010;17(3):225–234.
113. McCabe MT, Ott HM, Ganji G, et al. EZH2 inhibition as a therapeutic strategy for lymphoma with EZH2-activating mutations. *Nature* 2012;492(7427): 108–112.
114. Morin RD, Johnson NA, Severson TM, et al. Somatic mutations altering EZH2 (Tyr641) in follicular and diffuse large B-cell lymphomas of germinal-center origin. *Nat Genet* 2010;42(2):181–185.
115. Bernt KM, Zhu N, Sinha AU, et al. MLL-rearranged leukemia is dependent on aberrant H3K79 methylation by DOT1L. *Cancer Cell* 2011;20(1):66–78.
116. Daigle SR, Olhava EJ, Therkelsen CA, et al. Selective killing of mixed lineage leukemia cells by a potent small-molecule DOT1L inhibitor. *Cancer Cell* 2011;20(1):53–65.

23 Histone Deacetylase Inhibitors and Demethylating Agents

Steven D. Gore, Stephen B. Baylin, and James G. Herman

INTRODUCTION

The past decade has seen an explosive growth, especially at a genome-wide level, in our understanding of the role of chromatin in the normal regulation of gene expression and in the concept of the *epigenome*.[1–3] Concomitant with these advances has been the increasing appreciation of the role of epigenetic abnormalities in the progression of cancer[4–7] and the concept of the *cancer epigenome*. The translational consequences of this research include the possibilities for developing therapies in cancer that target epigenetic abnormalities. These are being explored in clinical trials and several have entered clinical practice.[4,5,7,8] Of these epigenetic abnormalities, the most thoroughly examined is the occurrence of abnormal cytosine guanine (CpG) promoter region DNA methylation and associated altered chromatin involving histone modifications, in the transcriptional silencing of genes, including a group of well-defined tumor suppressor genes.[4,5,7,8] However, targeting epigenetic processes to downregulate the action of overexpressed genes is also an emerging area of research.[9,10] This chapter describes the basis of epigenetic changes in cancer and discusses some of the latest approaches that target epigenetic abnormalities in cancer,[11] including those designed to induce the reexpression of silenced genes, for cancer therapy. The two approaches most mature in development are the inhibition of DNA methyltransferases, which mediate the abnormal promoter DNA methylation, and the inhibition of histone deacetylases, which remove histone modifications associated with active chromatin that alone, or in association with DNA methylation, are associated with transcriptional repression.[4,5,7,8] However, several exciting newer approaches are now in clinical trials and these will be mentioned.

Aberrant gene function and altered patterns of gene expression are key features of cancer.[4] Although genetic alterations remain the best characterized in the development and progression of cancer, increasingly it is appreciated that epigenetic abnormalities cooperate with genetic alterations in multiple ways to cause dysfunction of key regulatory pathways. Through genomic approaches to mutation discovery, there is growing recognition of the frequency of mutations in genes encoding for proteins that regulate the epigenome.[12] This chapter will outline the understanding of how each of these epigenetic alterations contribute to cancer and how derivation of therapeutic approaches may depend on understanding the biology of these changes.

EPIGENETIC ABNORMALITIES AND GENE EXPRESSION CHANGES IN CANCER

Epigenetic changes are defined as heritable alterations of gene expression patterns and cell phenotypes, which are not accompanied by changes in DNA sequence.[13] This definition clearly delineates the two key features of epigenetic regulation important for an understanding of therapies described in this chapter. Specifically, in contrast to genetic alterations (point mutations, deletions, or translocations), epigenetic changes do not alter the coding sequence of targeted genes. Thus, reversal of epigenetic changes can potentially restore the normal function of affected genes and their encoded proteins. Second, the heritable nature of epigenetic changes—that is, the ability of a cell to pass on regulation of gene expression through DNA replication—suggests that such changes, while relatively stable, can be reversed. Thus, therapeutic reprogramming of patterns of gene expression could theoretically result in a long-term change in the cancer cell phenotype, even after the inducing drugs are removed, although to date, this has not been accomplished.

The fundamental unit that determines epigenetic states is the nucleosome that contains an octamer of histone proteins around which approximately 160 base pairs of DNA are wrapped.[13] It is the positioning of these structures, and the three-dimensional aspects of their spacing, and the regulation of this process by posttranslational modifications of the constituent histones that underpins the functions of the epigenome.[13,14]

Abnormal Gene Silencing

One key alteration in cancer, which can be associated with altered epigenetic control, is abnormal gene silencing. Normally, such silencing is fundamental and required at the level of chromatin and DNA methylation regulation for the life of multicellular eukaryotic organisms. The silencing is critical for regulating important biologic processes, including all aspects of development, differentiation, imprinting, and silencing of large chromosomal domains, including the X chromosome of female mammals.[13] For example, the diversity of structure and function of cells derived from epithelial or mesenchymal origin, ultimately differentiating into cells lining the intestine or lung or forming mature granulocytes and myocytes, result from heritable changes in gene expression that are not the result of a change in DNA sequence. Although in many species, silencing can be initiated and maintained solely by processes involving the covalent modifications of histones and other chromatin components, vertebrates utilize an additional layer of gene regulation. This process involves the only natural covalent modification of DNA in humans and is characterized by DNA cytosine methylation that occurs nearly exclusively at the fifth position of the cytosine ring in cytosines preceding guanine, the so-called CpG dinucleotide (Fig. 23.1).[13,15]

Like most biologic processes, the normal patterns of silencing can be altered, resulting in the development of disease states. Thus, activation of genes normally not expressed, or silencing of a gene that should be expressed, can contribute to the dysregulation of gene function that characterizes cancer and, when stably present, represent epigenetic alterations.[4–7] Most studies have focused on the silencing of normally expressed genes. For the purposes of understanding the rationale behind epigenetic therapy, it is important to understand the mechanisms through which such silencing occurs. Alterations in gene expression associated with epigenetic changes that give rise to a growth advantage would be expected to be selected for in the host tissue, leading to progressive dysregulated

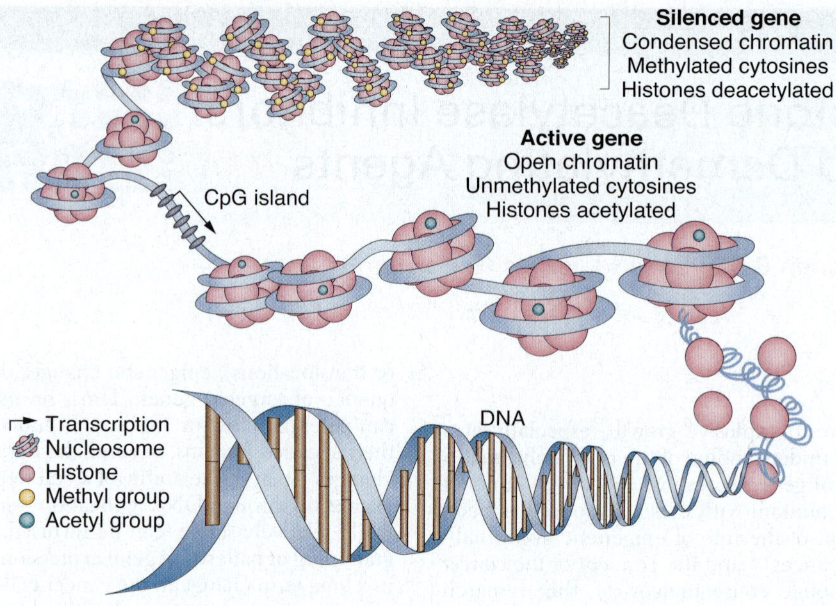

Figure 23.1 Epigenetic regulation of gene expression. In the promoter region, gene expression is controlled by a combination of DNA methylation and chromatin configuration. In normal cells, gene expression is silenced by condensing chromatin, methylating DNA, and deacetylating histones. By contrast, active genes are those with open nucleosome spacing around the transcription start site, are unmethylated, and are associated with acetylated histones. In cancer cells, CpG islands that are rich in cytosine and guanine—and are typically unmethylated to promote gene expression—can be epigenetically silenced by hypermethylation. (Redrawn with permission from Azad N, Zahnow CA, Rudin CM, et al. The future of epigenetic therapy in solid tumours—lessons from the past. *Nat Rev Clin Oncol* 2013;10:256–266.)

growth of the tumor. Such dysregulation is commonly associated with increases in promoter region DNA methylation and is associated with repressive chromatin changes.

Changes in DNA Methylation

The importance of abnormal cytosine methylation and gene silencing has been clearly established in the past 2 decades and been shown convincingly to be involved in cancer development.[4–7] The CpG dinucleotide, usually underrepresented in the genome, is clustered in the promoter regions of approximately 50% of human genes in regions termed *CpG islands*. These regions are largely protected from DNA methylation in normal cells, with the exception of genes on the inactive X chromosome and imprinted genes.[16] This protection is critical, because the methylation of promoter region CpG islands is associated with a loss of gene expression.[4–7] Abnormal de novo DNA methylation of gene promoter CpG islands is a very frequent abnormality in virtually all cancer types and is associated with a process that can serve as an alternative mechanism for loss of tumor suppressor gene function.[4–7] Although a limited number of classic tumor suppressor genes can be affected by this process, a patient's individual cancer may harbor hundreds of such genes.[4–7] Which of these latter genes are drivers of cancer, individually or in groups, versus those which are passengers reflecting only the widespread effects of a global epigenetic abnormality is a leading question in the field and the target of much research.[5,6] A clue to the importance of at least groups of the previous DNA hypermethylated genes may come from the fact that an inordinate number of them are involved in holding normal embryonic and adult stem cells in the self-renewal state and/or rendering such cells refractory to differentiation cues.[17,18] Normally, these genes are then in a poised expression state and can be induced to be activated or repressed as needed for changes in cell state.[18] Abnormal promoter DNA methylation of such genes renders them more repressed and could be a factor in the fact that cancers inevitably exhibit cell populations with enhanced self-renewal or refractoriness to full differentiation.[18]

Recent studies have also suggested that DNA regions other than promoter CpG islands may undergo changes of DNA methylation in cancer. For example, non–CpG-rich sequences surrounding promoter CpG islands, termed CpG island shores, are abnormally methylated in cancers[19] and may be altered in stem cell populations.[20] Thus, the relative cancer specificity of changes of DNA methylation in multiple CpG regions makes reversal of these changes by targeting DNA methyltransferases, the enzymes that catalyze DNA methylation, logical for cancer therapeutics.

As a key example of the previous points, perhaps the most studied tumor suppressor gene for promoter hypermethylation is the *p16* gene, currently designated *CDKN2A*, a cyclin-dependent kinase inhibitor that functions in the regulation of the phosphorylation of the Rb protein. Hypermethylation associated with loss of expression of the *CDKN2A* gene has been found to be one of the most frequent alterations in neoplasia being common in the lung, head and neck, gliomas, colorectal, and breast carcinomas[21,22] and other cancer types. A member of the same gene family, *p15* or *CDKN2B*, also regulates Rb and is silenced in association with promoter methylation in many forms of leukemia and in the chronic myeloid neoplasm myelodysplastic syndrome (MDS).[23] These two previous changes are of much relevance for the clinical uses of epigenetic therapies discussed later.

As mentioned, many hundreds of genes may be inactivated in a single cancer by promoter methylation,[5,6,18,24] providing potential targets for gene reactivation using epigenetic therapies.[25–27] The latter represents one of the potential ways in which epigenetic therapy may be effective: Multiple genes and gene pathways, all

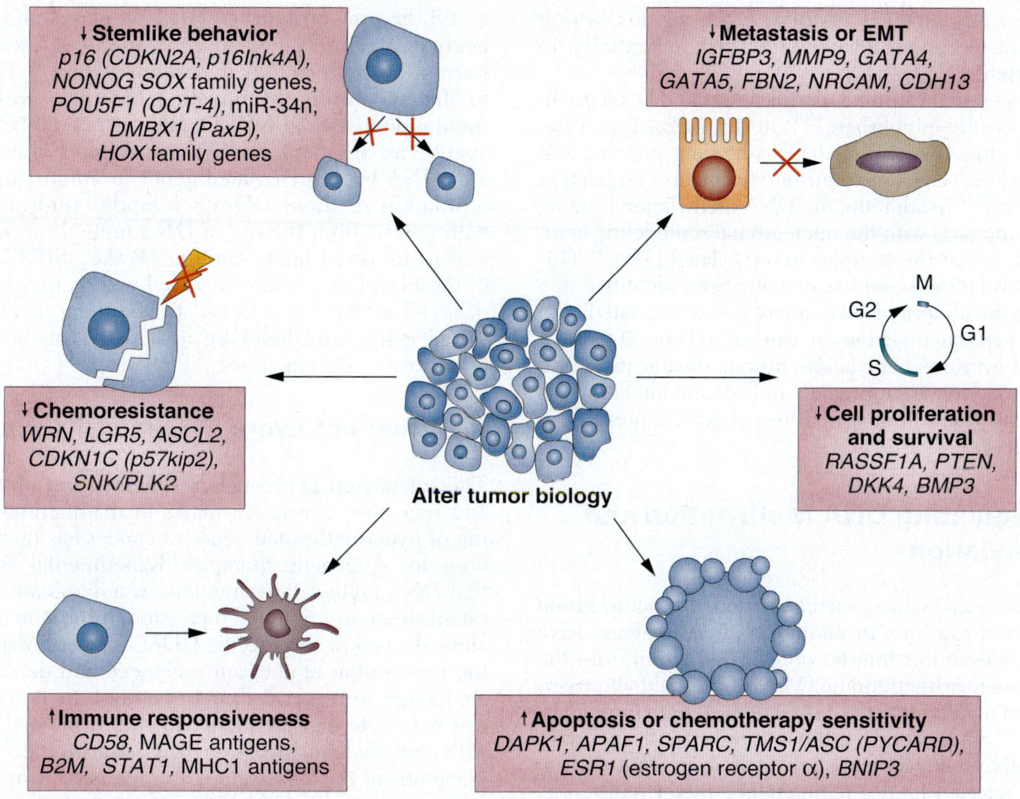

Figure 23.2 Concurrent widespread changes in gene expression with epigenetic therapy. Anticancer efficacy of treatment with epigenetic-modulating agents is associated with extensive changes in gene expression that influence several biologic processes. Gene expression is increased through the direct reversal of epigenetic modifications of genomic DNA, whereas for cancer-promoting genes, gene expression is reduced by the regression of their regulatory genes. EMT, epithelial-membrane transition. (Redrawn with permission from Azad N, Zahnow CA, Rudin CM, et al. The future of epigenetic therapy in solid tumours—lessons from the past. *Nat Rev Clin Oncol* 2013;10:256–266.)

repressed by changes in DNA methylation and chromatin modification, can be reactivated by DNA methyltransferase inhibitors and histone deacetylase (HDAC) inhibitors (HDACi), thereby restoring normal cell cycle control, differentiation, and apoptotic signaling (Fig. 23.2).[8,26,28] In general, methylated CpG islands are not capable of the initiation of transcription unless the methylation signal can be overridden by alterations in factors that modulate chromatin, such as the removal of methylated cytosine-binding proteins. However, reversal of DNA methylation with secondary changes in histone modification or directed reversal of repressive histone modifications represent a target for epigenetic therapies.[8,26,28]

Most studies of DNA methylation, particularly in the study of cancer, have focused on CpG island promoter methylation. However, about 40% of human genes do not contain bona fide CpG islands in their promoters.[29] The primary focus on CpG islands has resulted from the clear demonstration that CpG-island promoter methylation permanently silences genes both physiologically and pathologically in mammalian cells. However, recent work has shown correlations between tissue-specific expression and methylation of non-CpG islands, including, for example, the maspin gene,[30] and as mentioned previously, regions near CpG islands,[19,20] suggesting that many additional genes could be regulated, either normally or abnormally, by changes in DNA methylation.

An exciting new area of DNA methylation research involves the role of this change in regulating gene enhancers: small DNA regions that regulate the expression of multiple target genes.[31–33] The presence of DNA methylation in these areas, which can reside considerable distances from the genes that are being regulated, generally works together with histone modifications to mediate a repressive state for that enhancer.[31–33] The status of enhancers is also emerging as important for cancer risk states.[34]

Chromatin in Gene Regulation

Heritable gene silencing involves the interplay between DNA methylation and histone covalent modifications. Complexes of proteins that can regulate how nucleosomes are positioned perform nucleosomal remodeling.[35–37] What was initially termed the *histone code*, with reference to how histones are modified, has emerged to be much more complex than originally envisioned. An explosion of research findings during the last several years now allows for an appreciation of how the epigenome is controlled by a complex interplay between a myriad of posttranslational histone modifications that occur on key amino acid residues of these proteins.[37] Acetylation, deacetylation, methylation, phosphorylation, and other modifications all modify chromatin structure and thereby alter gene expression.[38] Some of the enzymes that catalyze these modifications include HDACs, histone methyltransferases (HMT), and most recently, histone demethylases.[13,14,39,40] These modifications help establish heritable states at the start site of genes, but also at enhancers and other transcribed DNA regions not encoding for canonical genes. The latter areas contain noncoding RNAs (ncRNAs) and micro-RNAs (miRNAs), which play key modulatory roles for overall gene expression and protein patterns that can be altered in cancer.[41–43] Again, much research is being focused on epigenetic changes in these DNA regions, which may be important to cancer development and, potentially, to cancer management.

A link between covalent histone modifications and DNA methylation has been clearly established.[44–46] In this interaction, cytosine methylation attracts methylated DNA-binding proteins and HDACs to methylated CpG sites during chromatin compaction and gene silencing.[46,47] In addition, the DNA methylation binding protein (MBD2) interacts with the nucleosomal remodeling complex (NuRD) and directs the complex to methylated DNA.[48] This complex also binds HDACs and has recently been identified as a central player for the abnormal silencing of genes associated with promoter DNA hypermethylation in cancer.[47] Thus, the three processes of DNA cytosine methylation, histone modification, and nucleosomal remodeling are intimately linked, and alterations in these processes can result in abnormalities of gene expression in cancer-relevant genes.

Enzymes Regulating DNA Methylation and Histone Acetylation

DNA methylation involves the covalent addition of a methyl group to the 5′ position of cytosine. In mammals, three enzymes have been shown to catalyze this transfer of a methyl group from the methyl donor S-adenosylmethionine. Most of the methyltransferase activity present in differentiated cells is derived from the expression of DNMT1.[49] This enzyme is thought to be most important in maintaining DNA methylation patterns following DNA replication and thus is referred to as a maintenance methyltransferase. However, the enzyme does possess the ability to methylate previously unmethylated DNA sequences (de novo activity).[50] In contrast, the other enzymes, DNMT3a and DNMT3b, are efficient at methylating previously unmethylated DNA and thus are considered de novo methyltransferases. Each of these enzymes possesses a similar catalytic site,[51] a fact important for the inhibition of DNMT enzymes by nucleoside analogs, discussed later in this chapter.

DNA methylation is closely associated with changes in the histone modifications. As previously discussed, histone proteins are the central components of the nucleosome, and modifications of the histone tails of core histones are associated with active or repressed chromatin.[52] Although it is beyond the scope of this chapter to fully discuss the complex series of modifications to the histone tails of histone H3 and H4, a few well-characterized modifications should be mentioned that are relevant to therapies designed to target epigenetic abnormalities in cancer. In reference to currently investigated epigenetic therapies, changes in histone acetylation are of importance. Acetylation of histones H3 and H4 at key amino acids is associated with the active chromatin present at the promoters of transcribed genes, whereas the absence of histone acetylation is associated with repressed, silenced genes.[13,14,53] Histone acetyltransferases (HAT) HDACs have opposing functions to maintain the proper level of histone acetylation for gene expression.[13,14,53] HDACs specifically deacetylate the lysine residues of the histone tails, and this deacetylation is associated with condensation of nucleosome positions in what is termed a closed chromatin formation. This scenario is key to transcriptional repression. There are four classes of HDACs.[53] Class I HDACs are characterized by their similarity to the yeast Rpd3 HDAC. In humans, this class of enzymes includes HDAC1, -2, -3, and -8. These HDACs are thought to be ubiquitously expressed in tissue throughout the body. In contrast, class II HDACs are similar to yeast Hda1 and include HDAC4, -5, -6, -7, -9, and -10, and they have a greater degree of tissue specificity. Class III HDACs are similar to yeast Sir2 and are set apart from the other classes by their dependence on nicotinamide adenine dinucleotide (NAD+) as a cofactor. Finally, class IV includes HDAC11.[53]

Of the previously listed HDACs, class I and 2 HDACs have been most closely tied to gene silencing associated with abnormal promoter DNA hypermethylation.[48] These are bound to the nucleosome remodeling complex, NuRD.[48,49] Experimental decreases in NURD, after use of a DNA demethylating agent, can augment reactivation of many abnormally silenced and DNA hypermethylated genes in colon cancer cells.[48] Manipulation of these HDACs is under study in clinical trials, with and without the use of DNA methyltransferase inhibitors, and is discussed later. Another HDAC, SIRT1 in the class III of these proteins, is also involved with gene silencing.[54,55] This deacetylase has been linked to silencing of DNA hypermethylated genes, and blocking its activity can be associated with reactivation of such genes.[55]

Reversal of Layers of Gene Silencing

The interaction between DNA methylation and HDAC activity and repressive chromatin marks in maintaining aberrant silencing of hypermethylated genes in cancer has therapeutic implications for epigenetic therapies. Experimental evidence suggests that DNA methylation functions as a dominant event that stably establishes transcriptional repression. Inhibition of HDAC activity alone, by potent and specific HDACis, does not generally result in the reactivation of aberrantly silenced and densely hypermethylated genes in tumor cells.[56] In contrast, treatment with HDACis can reactivate densely silenced genes if the cells are first treated with demethylating drugs, such as 5-azacitidine.[56] The clinical implications of this observation are discussed in more detail in the following section (Table 23.1).

DNA Methyltransferase Inhibitors

Originally synthesized as cytotoxic antimetabolite drugs in the 1960s,[57] azacytosine nucleosides were recognized as inhibitors of DNA methylation in the early 1980s. The inhibitors 5-azacitidine (5AC) and 2′-deoxy-5-azacytidine induced muscle, fat, and chondrocyte differentiation in mouse embryo cells, in association with a reversal of DNA methylation.[58,59] The incorporation of azacytosine nucleosides into DNA in lieu of cytosine residues was shown to be associated with inhibition of DNMT activity.[59,60] DNMT inhibition requires the incorporation of decitabine triphosphate into DNA. The incorporated azacytosine nucleoside forms an irreversible inactive adduct with DNMT. The sequential reversal of DNA methylation then results when DNA replication proceeds in the absence of active DNMT.[61] The inhibitor 5AC must be phosphorylated and converted to decitabine diphosphate by ribonucleotide reductase before it can be activated through triphosphorylation, whereas decitabine does not require ribonucleotide reductase. The inhibitor 5AC can also be incorporated into RNA. DNMT2, a misnamed protein that is actually an RNA-specific methyltransferase,[62] becomes inhibited, leading to the depletion of methylated tRNA.[60] This may contribute to the inhibition of protein synthesis and is a potential difference between azacitidine and decitabine.[63] The previous DNA methyltransferase inhibitors not only block the catalytic activities of DNMTs, but also trigger degradation of these proteins, especially DNMTs 1 and 3B.[64–68] This latter activity is potentially important for their activities for gene reexpression because each of these two proteins, experimentally, possess transcriptional repression properties independent of their DNA methylation catalytic sites.[69,70]

The azacytosine nucleosides exhibit complex dose–response characteristics. At low concentrations (0.2 to 1 μM), the *epigenetic* activities of these drugs predominate, with dose-dependent reversal of DNA methylation[71,72] and induction of terminal differentiation in some systems.[28,71] As concentrations are increased, DNA damage and apoptosis become more prominent.[28,72] Cell lines with 30-fold resistance to the cytotoxic effects of doxifluridine,

TABLE 23.1

Small Molecules Targeting Epigenetic Abnormalities in Clinical Development

Drug	Class	Target	Dose Range	Schedule	Route of Administration
5-Azacitidine	Nucleoside	DNA methyl-transferase	30–75 mg/m²/d	Daily × 7–14 d/28 d	Subcutaneous or intravenous
2′-Deoxy-5-azacytidine	Nucleoside	DNA methyl-transferase	10–45 mg/m²/d	Daily × 3–5 d/4–6 wk	Intravenous
SG110	Nucleoside	DNA methyl-transferase	Being determined	Being determined	Subcutaneous
Valproic acid	Small chain fatty acid	Histone deacetylase (class I and II)	25–50 mg/kg/d	Daily	Oral or intravenous
Vorinostat	Hydroxamic acid	Histone deacetylase (class I and II)	400–600 mg/d	Divided doses	Oral
Entinostat	Benzamide	Histone deacetylase (class I)	2–8 mg/m²	Weekly	Oral
Belinostat	Hydroxamic acid	Histone deacetylase (class I and II)	600–1,000 mg/m²	Daily × 5/28 d	Intravenous
Romidepsin	Cyclic tetrapeptide	Histone deacetylase (class I and II)	13–18 mg/m²	Weekly	Intravenous
LBH-589	Hydroxamic acid	Histone deacetylase (class I and II)	5–11 mg/m²	Daily × 3	Intravenous
MGCD-0103	Benzamide	Histone deacetylase (class I)	40–125 mg/m²	Twice weekly	Oral
CI-994	Benzamide	Histone deacetylase (class I)	5–8 mg/m²	Daily	Oral

adriamycin, cyclophosphamide (DAC) continue to reverse methylation in response to this nucleoside, suggesting that the methylation reversing and cytotoxic activities of this compound can be separated.[73] The ability of these drugs to inhibit the cell cycle, at least in part through induction of $p21^{WAF1/CIP1}$ expression, complicates the goal of reversing DNA methylation, because the latter requires DNA replication with the azacytosine nucleoside incorporated into the DNA.

The importance of low doses of the two azacytosine nucleosides to achieve a targeted therapeutic effect has been recently explored in a series of laboratory observations. Transient exposure of both leukemia and solid tumor cells to submicromolar doses induce such cells to undergo cellular reprogramming, accompanied by decreases in ability to clone in long-term self-renewal assays and to grow as explants in immune-incompetent mice.[28] These effects occur with partial genome-wide DNA demethylation and changes in gene expression in multiple pathways potentially key for driving tumorigenesis.

The pharmacokinetic properties of the two azacytosine nucleosides are also very important to consider for their clinical use. In this regard, a major potential challenge for their usage is the fact that these drugs are highly unstable in an aqueous solution, resulting in their rapid hydrolysis and resultant inactivation.[74] In clinical practice, the drugs must be administered shortly after reconstitution. The drugs are also metabolized by cytidine deaminase,[74] leading to a short half-life in plasma. When injected subcutaneously, 5AC reaches a maximal plasma concentration at 30 minutes, with a terminal half-life of 1.5 to 2.3 hours.[75,76] At the U.S. Food and Drug Administration (FDA) approved dose of 5AC (75 mg/m² administered subcutaneously daily for 7 days), peak plasma concentrations were 3 to 5 μM, which is well within the range of DNMT inhibitory concentrations.[75,76] Intravenous (IV) administration of the same dose has led to higher peak plasma concentrations (11 μM) with a shorter half-life (approximately 22 minutes).[75] DAC given over 1 hour IV at 15 to 20 mg/m² produced plasma concentrations of 1.1 to 1.6 μM during the infusion,[77] whereas in a phase 1 study in patients with thoracic malignancies, patients were treated with escalating doses of decitabine for 72-hour IV infusions for two 35-day cycles. The maximum tolerated total dose was 60 to 75 mg/m² with neutropenia as the dose-limiting toxicity. Steady-state plasma concentrations ranged from 25 to 40 nM, which is less than those usually used to induce expression of methylated genes in tissue culture models.[78] An oral formulation of 5AC has also been studied. The oral bioavailability of oral azacitidine ranged from 6% to 20%. Nonetheless, MDS and acute myelogenous leukemia (AML) patients receiving oral azacitidine developed clinical responses similar to patients receiving parenteral azacitidine. Oral azacitidine has also been safely administered on 14-daily and 21-daily schedules repeated monthly. The extended administration of lower daily doses may provide favorable pharmacodynamics of DNA methylation reversal given the need for ongoing cell cycling to effect methylation reversal.[79]

SGI-110 is a dinucleoside that acts as a prodrug for decitabine. This drug is being studied in myelodysplasia and AML.[80]

HISTONE DEACETYLASE INHIBITORS

The increasing recognition of the critical importance of histone modifications in regulating the transcriptional permissively of chromatin has led to intense interest in compounds that can inhibit the activity of HDAC proteins, facilitating the acetylation of lysines associated with transcriptional activation of genes. As with the DNMT inhibitors discussed previously, there are multiple, sometimes dose-dependent, effects of HDACis in preclinical studies. Some of these may truly be epigenetic, others strictly cytotoxic, and others a combination of both.[9,81–84] Some actions of HDACis may relate to altering how chromatin is central to the repair of DNA. Thus, at especially high doses, these compounds can blunt efficient repair and even induce DNA breaks.[84,85] These effects may underlie cell cycle arrest and induction of cell death as is often observed in preclinical studies of HDACis.[81–84]

Perhaps novel uses of these drugs may be inferred by results from recent studies suggesting they could be extremely powerful epigenetic therapy agents when used in proper doses, for targeted purposes, and at key time intervals. Recent studies by Settleman and colleagues[86] suggest that histone acetylation changes, and thus epigenetic mechanisms, could be a key factor for cancer therapy resistance to both targeted therapy agents and conventional chemotherapy. The mechanisms involved may involve the emergence of drug-tolerant stem-like cells.[86] In such cells, gene expression studies suggest that a protein upregulated in resistance is a histone demethylase, which diminishes a key histone modification for active transcription, H3K4methyl.[86] A very similar enzyme has been shown in other studies to be central to self-renewal of stem-like melanoma cells.[87] Key to the therapies under discussion is that, in the previous drug-resistance studies, low doses of HDACis, could reversibly reduce drug-resistant cells induced by the various anticancer drugs.[86] It is essential going forward to sort out which of these effects are dose-related off-target effects and which are desired on-target effects that can be optimized for efficacious therapy strategies.

Types of Histone Deacetylase Inhibitors

Small Chain Fatty Acids

The earliest report of the use of an HDACi to treat leukemia described the treatment of a child with refractory AML with intravenous sodium butyrate, with a concomitant clearance of peripheral blood blast cells and a decrement in bone marrow blasts.[88] No responses developed in a subsequent study of nine AML patients who were treated with intravenous butyrate.[89] Phase 1 studies of sodium phenylbutyrate (NaPB) in MDS and AML explored 7-day continuous infusions administered monthly or biweekly, and 21-day continuous infusions administered monthly.[90,91] At the maximum tolerated dose (375 mg per kilogram per day), the mean steady-state plasma concentration was 0.3 mM, within the range of HDAC inhibition.[90–92] Isolated patients developed hematologic improvement in response to NaPB.

Similar to NaPB, valproic acid (VPA) requires near millimolar concentrations to effectively inhibit HDACs. Of 18 patients with MDS or AML with trilineage dysplasia treated with VPA to target plasma concentrations of 0.3 to 0.7 mM, 6 patients developed hematologic improvement.[93] Of 20 elderly patients with AML treated with VPA, only 11 could remain in control long enough to be considered evaluable for response. Five had improvement in platelet counts.[94] VPA induced hematologic improvement in combination with all-transretinoic acid in two of eight patients treated with AML; a fluorescence in situ hybridization analysis showed definitive evidence of terminal differentiation of the malignant cells.[95] A larger study of this combination induced hematologic response in only 2 of 26 elderly patients with AML.[96] It appears unlikely that the small chain fatty acids will develop an important role in the treatment of malignancy given the availability of HDACis with vastly greater potency.

Hydroxamic Acids

The FDA approved vorinostat as the first commercially available HDACi. The approval was based on activity of this agent in cutaneous T-cell lymphoma (CTCL). Thirty-three patients with a median number of five prior systemic therapy regimens received one of three dose schedules of vorinostat in a single institution study.[97] Eight patients achieved a partial response, with a median time to response of 12 weeks and a median duration of response of 15 weeks. Overall, 45% of patients had relief of pruritus. Fatigue, diarrhea, nausea, and thrombocytopenia were common toxicities. In a multicenter phase 2 trial, 74 patients with relapsed or refractory CTCL were treated with 400 mg daily.[98] Similar to the prior study, 29% of patients responded, consisting almost entirely of partial responses. Median time to response was 56 days, and median duration of response was greater than 6 months. In phase 1 trials, responses to vorinostat have developed in other non-Hodgkin's and Hodgkin's lymphoma cases.[99] More recently, in a trial combining vorinostat with carboplatin and paclitaxel in patients with untreated, advanced, non–small-cell lung cancer (NSCLC), response rates increased significantly from 12.5% to 34%, and a trend to improved progression-free survival and overall survival was observed.[100]

Panobinostat (LBH589), a cinnamic hydroxamic acid HDACi, reduced peripheral blood blast percentage but did not induce remissions in a phase 1 trial of daily times 7 oral dosing in patients with a variety of relapsed hematologic malignancies.[101] Asymptomatic changes in electrocardiographic T waves developed in 80% of treated patients. Gastrointestinal symptoms and thrombocytopenia were common. Panobinostat has recently been approved by the FDA for the treatment of multiple myeloma.[102]

Cyclic Tetrapeptides

Romidepsin is FDA approved for the treatment of CTCL[103] and peripheral T-cell lymphoma.[104,105] Antitumor activity, including tumor lysis syndrome, was demonstrated in a phase 1 study that enrolled patients with chronic lymphocytic leukemia and AML, but no complete or partial remissions were seen.[75] The administration of romidepsin induces electrocardiographic changes, including T-wave flattening and ST-T wave depression in greater than half of the posttreatment tracings; however, no changes in serum cardiac troponin levels or left ventricular ejection fraction have been reported.[106]

Benzamides

Entinostat, formerly known as MS-275, was administered weekly times four to patients with relapsed and refractory AML in a phase 1 study. Infections, unsteady gate, and somnolence were dose-limiting toxicities. No clinical responses developed, although improvements in neutrophil counts were observed.[107] Entinostat did not increase the response rate in patients with higher risk MDS and AML with MDS-related changes when combined with azacitidine compared to azacitidine alone.[108] Most recently, however, studies NSCLC suggest that entinostat could be a valuable therapeutic agent in solid tumors when used with established therapies. When combined with the epidermal growth factor inhibitor erlotinib, in a randomized phase 2 trial for patients with recurrent advanced NSCLC, entinostat was not efficacious alone but appeared to combine with erlotinib to benefit a group of patients whose tumors contained baseline high E-cadherin levels. Overall survival in these latter patients yielded an increased survival benefit of 9.4 versus 5.4 months.[109] Finally, entinostat significantly increased survival when combined with an aromatase inhibitor in a phase 2 trial for patients with breast cancer.[110]

Pharmacodynamic Properties

The administration of oral vorinostat was associated with a transient increase in acetylation of histone H3 in peripheral blood lymphocytes, which peaked at 2 hours post dosing and reverted to baseline by 8 hours; similar changes were observed in the lymph node of a treated patient with lymphoma.[99] Treatment with vorinostat was associated with translocation of phosphorylated signal transducer and activator of transcription 3 (STAT-3) from nucleus to cytoplasm in responding patients and with reduced microvessel density.[97]

Similar changes in the acetylation of histones 2B and 3 were observed in peripheral blood cells from patients treated with LBH589.[101] Romidepsin induced acetylation of H3 and H4 in peripheral blood tumor cells within 4 hours of dosing[111]; of interest, p21$^{WAF1/CIP1}$ protein levels also increased, associated with an increase in acetylation of H4 at the p21 promoter (using chromatin immunoprecipitation). Treatment with entinostat led to increased acetylation of H3 and H4 in both peripheral blood and bone marrow. This increase was detectable within 8 hours and remained above baseline throughout the treatment cycle. Thus, this compound may provide the most prolonged inhibition of protein deacetylation of HDACis and is under current investigation.[107] Increases in p21$^{WAF1/CIP1}$ and activation of caspase 3 were also demonstrated in these samples.

EPIGENETIC THERAPY FOR HEMATOLOGIC MALIGNANCIES

DNA Methyltransferase Inhibitors

Epigenetic therapy has seen the most widespread use to date and achieved the greatest efficacy in hematologic malignancies. The therapeutic efficacy of 5AC and DAC for patients with the chronic myeloid neoplasm myelodysplasia (MDS) and AML has been well reviewed.[26,27] Their FDA approval for MDS/AML emerged only after doses were reduced, with resultant diminishing toxicities for patients. The successful development of 5AC for the treatment of MDS can be credited largely to Silverman et al.[25,112,114] in the Cancer and Leukemia Group B (CALGB). The inhibitor 5AC had successfully induced the expression of hemoglobin F in patients with sickle cell anemia.[25,112] Viewing this compound as a potential inducer of terminal differentiation, Silverman et al. conducted a series of phase 2 trials of 5AC administered as a continuous intravenous infusion or as subcutaneous injections for the treatment of MDS.[113,114] Based on significant hematologic responses, the group performed a phase 2 trial (CALGB 9221) in which patients with low- and high-risk MDS with significant hematopoietic compromise were randomly assigned to receive subcutaneous 5AC (75 mg/m^2 per day daily for 7 days, repeated on a 28-day cycle) or observation. Patients on the observation arm with progressive disease could cross over to receive 5AC. This study firmly established the ability of 5AC to induce hematologic improvement, and, less frequently, complete and partial responses.[113,115] The median time to development of AML (defined by 30% bone marrow blast cells) or death was greater in the 5AC arm by 9 months (21 versus 12 months); of note, the observation arm included patients who subsequently crossed over to 5AC treatment.

In a subsequent phase 3 trial (AZA001),[116] patients with higher risk myelodysplastic syndromes were randomly assigned one-to-one to receive 5AC (75 mg/m^2 per day for 7 days every 28 days) or conventional care (best supportive care, low-dose cytarabine, or intensive chemotherapy as selected by investigators before randomization). Three hundred fifty-eight patients were randomly assigned to receive 5AC (n = 179) or conventional care regimens (n = 179). After a median follow-up of 21.1 months (interquartile range [IQR] 15.1 to 26.9), median overall survival was 24.5 months (9.9 not reached) for the azacitidine group versus 15.0 months (5.6 to 24.1) for the conventional care group (hazard ratio [HR] 0.58; 95% confidence interval [CI], 0.43 to 0.77; $p = 0.0001$). At 2 years, on the basis of Kaplan-Meier estimates, 50.8% (95% CI, 42.1 to 58.8) of patients in the 5AC group were alive compared with 26.2% (95% CI, 18.7 to 34.3) in the conventional care group ($p < 0.0001$). Median time to AML transformation was 17.8 months (IQR 8.6 to 36.8; 95% CI, 13.6 to 23.6) in the 5AC group compared with 11.5 months (4.9 not reached; 8.3 to 14.5) in the conventional care group (HR 0.50; 95% CI, 0.35 to 0.70; $p < 0.0001$). Subsequent unplanned analyses of AZA001 included an examination of elderly patients with what would now be classified as AML (blast count 20% to 30%). In these 113 patients, there remains a statistically significant improvement in survival of 24.5 months versus 16.0 months (HR 0.47; 95% CI; $p = 0.0001$).[117]

The early development of decitabine in MDS took place primarily in Europe under the leadership of Wijermans et al.[118,119] These investigators pursued intravenous scheduling of decitabine administered three times daily for 3 days (45 mg/m^2 per day total dose). This cycle was repeated every 6 weeks. Phase 2 studies suggested a response rate of approximately 50% in MDS patients. In a randomized trial of DAC versus observation, patients with International Prognostic Score risk categories intermediate 1 to high received the previously listed schedule of decitabine or observation. No crossover was allowed in this trial. Response rates reported were: complete response: 9%, partial response: 8%, and hematologic improvement: 13%.[120] A 10% induction death rate occurred, suggesting that this schedule of DAC may be more toxic than the CALGB schedule of 5AC (1% induction mortality). DAC has also been investigated in low-dose daily intravenous dosing[121] and in daily-times-five schedules. The latter appears convenient and well tolerated. A daily-times-five schedule (20 mg/m^2 per day) has been FDA approved[121]; 99 patients with MDS (de novo or secondary) of any French-American-British (FAB) subtype and an International Prognostic Scoring System (IPSS) score equal to or greater than 0.5 were treated, with an overall response rate of 32% (17 complete responses [CR] plus 15 marrow CRs [mCR]).[122] Among patients who improved, 82% demonstrated responses by the end of cycle two. This well-tolerated regimen allows outpatient administration and, as noted previously, provides plasma levels of decitabine that inhibit DNMTs.

The 3-day intravenous schedule of DAC has been studied in two randomized trials compared to supportive care in patients with higher risk MDS. The first trial confirmed the hematologic activity of decitabine in this patient population but failed to show an improvement in survival in the DAC-treated patients.[123] Survival was also not increased in the subsequent trial, performed by the European Organization for Research and Treatment of Cancer (EORTC).[124] The failure of the randomized decitabine trials to show a survival benefit may be partially due to study design. Both randomized trials of 5AC continued treatment until disease progression for patients who did not achieve complete remission; in fact, this meant that most patients received maintenance therapy. In contrast, both randomized trials of decitabine allowed a maximum of eight cycles of treatment. The need for maintenance therapy in patients treated with DNMT inhibitors has not been tested in prospective randomized trials. An additional difference in the conduct of the two sets of DNMT inhibitor trials involves the duration of therapy administered. The median number of cycles of treatment administered in the two randomized trials of decitabine was three, compared to nine in the azacytidine trials. This may reflect greater toxicity of the originally 3-day schedule of decitabine compared to that of the approved schedule of 5AC. Although the differences in survival may reflect differences in trial design and trial conduct, emerging data suggests that despite similarities in methylation reversal, the two drugs differ in other potentially important biologic parameters, which may contribute to clinical outcomes.[62,63,125]

Two randomized phase 3 trials have been published treating elderly AML patients (greater than 20% blasts) with decitabine, both demonstrating improvement in survival that was not statistically significant. In the European study, 233 patients received either

DAC at 15 mg/m^2 × 9 doses over 3 days on 42-day cycles or best supportive care. The patients received a median of 4 cycles (0 to 9), and the overall survival was improved in the decitabine-treated patients, but did not reach statistical significance (median overall survival [OS], 10.1 versus 8.5 months, respectively; HR, 0.88; 95% CI, 0.66 to 1.17; two-sided, log-rank p = 0.38).[126] In the M.D. Anderson Cancer Center–led multicenter trial,[127] 485 patients 65 years or older were randomly assigned to receive decitabine 20 mg/m^2 per day as a 1-hour intravenous infusion for 5 consecutive days every 4 weeks or best supportive care or low-dose cytarabine (20 mg/m^2 per day for 10 days every 4 weeks). There was a similar improvement in OS with decitabine (7.7 months; 95% CI, 6.2 to 9.2) versus the control group (5.0 months; 95% CI, 4.3 to 6.3; p = 0.108; HR, 0.85; 95% CI, 0.69 to 1.04).[127]

The azacytosine nucleosides require prolonged administration to demonstrate hematologic improvement in MDS. Median time to development of first clinical response in the CALGB studies of 5AC was three cycles; 90% of responses developed by cycle six.[114] In the phase 3 trial of decitabine, the median time to response was two cycles,[123] as also seen in the alternative regimen of decitabine.[122] It is, therefore, extremely important when treating patients with azacytosine nucleosides to commit to administering between four and six cycles of therapy before determining whether a patient is responding to treatment. Furthermore, survival benefit is seen even in patients not showing bone marrow improvement for 5AC, perhaps related to decreased transfusion requirements or delayed progression to AML.[116]

Because AML in the context of MDS is arbitrarily defined based on marrow blast count, activity of the azanucleoside analogs in AML should not be surprising. In CALGB 9221, 20 patients were reclassified upon central pathology review as meeting criteria for AML (greater than 30% blasts). Their outcomes were comparable to the overall population in the study.[115] In all three CALGB studies among patients meeting current World Health Organization (WHO) criteria for AML (greater than 20% blasts), a complete response was achieved in 9% and hematologic improvement in 26%.[114] A retrospective review of 20 patients with AML, including 8 patients with bone marrow blasts greater than 29% treated with 5AC, reported a complete remission in 4 patients, a partial response in 5, and a hematologic improvement in 3. The median duration of response was 8 months (range: 3 to 33 months).[128] DAC induced a complete hematologic response in 2 of 20 patients treated who had the blastic phase of chronic myeloid leukemia.[129] These studies suggest activity of the azacytosine nucleosides in the treatment of a subset of AML patients. Current studies do not allow for the determination of whether this subset is limited to MDS-associated AML (AML with MDS-related changes), which tends to have low white blood cell counts and have a low proliferative rate, or whether these compounds are also active for those with AML without a history of antecedent hematologic disorder. Several reports describe the sensitivity MDS and AML, characterized by abnormalities of chromosome 7 and associated with poor outcomes in response to cytarabine-based therapy to azanucleosides. In one nonrandomized retrospective study, survival of such patients following the administration of DNMT inhibitors surpassed survival in response to conventional cytotoxic chemotherapy, similar to the outcomes of AZA001.[130–132]

Although the mechanisms underlying the clinical activity of azacytosine analogs may involve reversal of gene methylation, other actions need to be considered. The administration of DAC has been shown to induce transient decrements of methylation in noncoding regions, including long interspersed nuclear element (LINE) and ALU elements.[133] Early studies that examined methylation reversal of the target gene p15^{INK4B} in response to DAC showed no correlation between methylation reversal and clinical response.[134,135] Clinical responders to DAC developed significantly higher expression of this gene following treatment, and certainly key biologic roles for this gene and its low basal expression are probable. Moreover, in one study, the clinical response was closely associated with the reversal of methylation of p15 or CDH-1 during the first cycle of treatment with 5AC followed by the HDACi NaPB.[25] In that study, it was noteworthy that the administration of 5AC prior to the addition of an HDACi was associated with the induction of histone acetylation. Although the mechanism underlying this activity is unknown, histone acetylation has been observed following DNA damage due to gamma irradiation.[136] Subsequent studies have found demethylation following treatment with either DAC or 5AC[137–140] but not consistently associated with response.[137,138,140] More work will be required to answer the important mechanistic question underpinning the clinical activity of azacytosine analogs.

Combining Inhibitors in the Treatment of Hematologic Malignancies

It is almost certain that the biggest promise of epigenetic therapy lies in strategies to combine existing and newer drugs with each other and with current chemotherapies and targeted therapies. To date, the example for existing agents is the combination of DNMT inhibitors and HDAC inhibitors based on the hypothesis from the laboratory that this paradigm leads to optimal reexpression of transcriptionally silenced genes with promoter methylation.[56,141] This in vitro treatment paradigm has led to a variety of clinical studies that have attempted to apply this concept to the treatment of hematologic malignancies. Much remains to be determined with regard to its efficacy and precisely what determines this. The first study of sequential DNMT/HDAC inhibitors administered a variety of doses of 5AC for 5 to 14 days followed by 7 days of NaPB by continuous infusion at its maximum tolerated dose to patients with MDS and AML.[25] The combination was well tolerated, and clinical responses were frequent in patients receiving 5AC at 50 mg/m^2 per day daily for 10 days and 25 mg/m^2 per day daily for 14 days, with 5 of 14 patients at those dose schedules achieving complete or partial response.

In a pilot study, 10 patients with MDS or AML were treated with 5AC at 75 mg/m^2 per day daily times seven followed by 5 days of NaPB given at 200 mg per kilogram per day as a 1- to 2-hour infusion. Three patients developed a partial response.[142]

In a similar study, investigators at the M.D. Anderson Cancer Center treated leukemic patients with decitabine (15 mg/m^2 per day IV daily times 10) and concomitant VPA at a variety of doses. Of 54 patients, 12 achieved complete remission or complete remission with incomplete platelet recovery.[143] The inhibitors 5AC, VPA, and all-transretinoic acid have been administered to patients with AML and MDS. Of 33 previously untreated patients, 14 over the age of 60 years developed a complete remission or a complete remission with inadequate platelet recovery.[144] A subsequent study of 5AC and VPA suggests increased efficacy of this combination in high-risk MDS.[145]

Entinostat has been successfully combined with azacytidine in patients with myeloid malignancies.[140] The US Leukemia Intergroup recently completed a randomized phase 2 trial of this combination compared with 5AC alone. In this study, of 149 patients, the primary endpoint of hematologic normalization was statistically similar, with 32% (95% CI, 22% to 44%) of the 5AC group reaching hematologic normalization (HN) versus 27% (95% CI, 17% to 39%) in the AZA + entinostat group. Median overall survivals were 18 months for the AZA group and 13 months for the AZA + entinostat group, but were also not statistically significant.[108] In the latter study, the administration of the combination was associated with less DNA methylation reversal compared to azacitidine monotherapy, likely due to cell cycle inhibitory effects of the HDACi. This highlights the complexity of effectively targeting epigenetic gene regulation.

It remains to be established whether combination therapies are more effective than single-agent demethylating therapies.

Epigenetically Targeted Therapy in Nonhematologic Malignancies

The efficacies that have emerged in the application of epigenetically targeted drugs to hematologic malignancies has spurred interest in using epigenetic therapy for other types of cancer. As outlined as follows, laboratory studies and clinical trials support this approach. Studies in the lab have been directed by lessons learned from therapy in hematologic malignancies, suggesting that low doses of drugs like DAC and 5AC, in the nanomolar range, may avoid excess toxicities due to off-target effects of the drugs and may maximize epigenetic effects of the agents.[28] The desired effects may require minimizing initial cellular cytotoxicity, giving tumor cells time to accrue maximal cellular reprogramming responses to the inhibition of DNMTs.[28] DAC and 5AC are effective only when they have been incorporated into DNA, after which they irreversibly inhibit DNMT catalytic activity and target these proteins for degradation.[64–68] In cell culture and mouse explants, low nanomolar doses appear to induce both human leukemic and solid tumor cells to exhibit blunting of self-renewal and tumorigenic activity of tumor stem-like cells.[28] These preclinical results suggest a key possibility that use of epigenetic therapies might inhibit these latter cell populations, which often are difficult to eradicate and are a factor in resistance to many standard cancer therapies.[146] Exhaustion of such cells over time during therapy with DAC or 5AC might explain the observation that most patients with MDS/AML take several months to reach best response.[147] Leukemic stem cells were not eliminated in one study in MDS and AML patients treated with 5AC in combination with VPA, although their frequency decreased in clinical responders.[148]

Clinical trials for common solid tumors, informed through the previous laboratory studies, have been initiated including phase 2 designs using low-dose strategies with 5AC often combined with use of histone deacetylase inhibitors. Sixty-five patients with advanced, multiply treated NSCLCs were treated with 5AC plus entinostat.[149] Only 3% of patients developed Response Evaluation Criteria (RECIST)-measureable responses; however, these two patients had durable responses, with survival of 3 to 4 years.[149] Upregulation of immunogenic pathways in NSCLC and other solid tumor cells, observed in laboratory studies, suggest a potential for sequencing DNMT inhibitors with immune checkpoint inhibitors.[150] This drug is also reported to induce antitumor responses and immune recognition in a model of pancreatic cancer.[151] Other laboratory results and emerging clinical trials also suggest the promise of combining epigenetic therapy approaches to sensitize cancers other than NSCLC to subsequent therapies. Low-dose DAC appears able to upregulate a key mediator of 5-fluorouracil (5FU) action, uridine monophosphate (UMP) kinase, in colorectal cancer cell lines.[152] These increases correlated with a reversal of 5FU resistance. Similar to studies discussed previously, DAC plus the HDACi, trichostatin A, decreased marker identified self-renewal populations in ovarian cancer while simultaneously inducing increased sensitivity to cisplatin.[153] In advanced ovarian cancer, 5AC or DAC plus carboplatin have yielded durable responses and induced stable disease in ovarian cancer patients.[154,155] These early results are being extrapolated for verification in larger, ongoing clinical trials.

NEW APROACHES TO EPIGENETIC THERAPY

As we have outlined previously, the emerging promise for epigenetic therapy and the future of the approaches may lie in combinatorial drug strategies. Although this is already being explored with older agents, new drugs for new targets are now entering the picture.[9,11,156–158] In these efforts, several themes we have introduced in this chapter will likely dominate.

Most epigenetic therapies will not induce, when used at truly targeting doses, immediate cytotoxic effects. Therapeutic efficacy based on cellular reprogramming may require significant time to manifest. Clinical trial designs may need adaptation so that effective therapies are not discarded due to premature response evaluations. Finally, the ultimate promise for epigenetic therapy may lie with newer drugs now entering clinical trials. Outcomes with DNMT inhibitors may be improved with alternative scheduling of oral azacitidine or through prolonged pharmacokinetics of the decitabine prodrug SGI110.[79] Also, drugs targeting other proteins including BET family bromodomain proteins are generating much excitement.[9,82,156–159] BET inhibitors may interfere with localization of the oncogene *C-MYC* to acetylated lysines in regulatory regions of target genes.[9,82,156–159] These inhibitors are now entering clinical trials. Other promising approaches include the use of inhibitors of EZH2, the enzyme in the PcG system, which catalyzes the repressive histone mark H3K27me3.[9,82,156–159] Another clinical trial underway employs targeting of the translocation in which the protein mixed lineage leukemia (MLL) is fused with several targets, such as in infant leukemias. These translocations result in abnormal recruitment of the histone methyltransferase, DOT1L, to target genes like *HOXA9*.[158] This fusion induces hypermethylation of H3K79 and abnormal activation of MLL target genes.[158,160] Very selective inhibitors of DOT1L are now in clinical trials.

Epigenetically targeted therapies continue to hold great promise that reprogramming of malignant cells could alter approaches to cancer management. Strategies to merge older drugs, which we have focused on in this chapter, with the newer agents briefly discussed in this section, will underpin future trials to test this approach.

CANCER THERAPEUTICS

REFERENCES

1. Bernstein BE, Meissner A, Lander ES. The mammalian epigenome. *Cell* 2007;128:669–681.
2. Young RA. Control of the embryonic stem cell state. *Cell* 2011;144:940–954.
3. Suva ML, Riggi N, Bernstein BE. Epigenetic reprogramming in cancer. *Science* 2013;339:1567–1570.
4. Herman JG, Baylin SB. Gene silencing in cancer in association with promoter hypermethylation. *N Engl J Med* 2003;349:2042–2054.
5. Jones PA, Baylin SB. The epigenomics of cancer. *Cell* 2007;128:683–692.
6. Baylin SB, Jones PA. A decade of exploring the cancer epigenome — biological and translational implications. *Nat Rev Cancer* 2011;11:726–734.
7. Esteller M. Cancer epigenomics: DNA methylomes and histone-modification maps. *Nat Rev Genet* 2007;8:286–298.
8. Yoo CB, Jones PA. Epigenetic therapy of cancer: past, present and future. *Nat Rev Drug Discov* 2006;5:37–50.
9. Dawson MA, Kouzarides T. Cancer epigenetics: from mechanism to therapy. *Cell* 2012;150:12–27.
10. Dawson MA, Kouzarides T, Huntly BJ. Targeting epigenetic readers in cancer. *N Engl J Med* 2012;367:647–657.
11. Bradner J. New targets for hematologic malignancies. *Clin Adv Hematol Oncol* 2013;11:375–376.
12. You JS, Jones PA. Cancer genetics and epigenetics: two sides of the same coin? *Cancer Cell* 2012;22:9–20.
13. Allis C, Jenuwein T, Reinberg D. *Epigenetics*, Vol. 1. Cold Spring Harbor, NY: Cold Spring Harbor Laboratory Press; 2007.

14. Kouzarides T. Chromatin modifications and their function. *Cell* 2007;128: 693–705.
15. Baylin SB, Jones PA. Epigenetic determinants of cancer. In: Allis CD, Jenuwein T, Reinberg D, eds. *Epigenetics*. Cold Spring Harbor, NY: Cold Spring Harbor Laboratory Press; 2006: 457–476.
16. Bird AP. CpG-rich islands and the function of DNA methylation. *Nature* 1986;321:209–213.
17. Morey L, Pascual G, Cozzuto L, et al. Nonoverlapping functions of the Polycomb group Cbx family of proteins in embryonic stem cells. *Cell Stem Cell* 2012;10:47–62.
18. Easwaran H, Johnstone SE, Van Neste L, et al. A DNA hypermethylation module for the stem/progenitor cell signature of cancer. *Genome Res* 2012;22: 837–849.
19. Irizarry RA, Ladd-Acosta C, Wen B, et al. The human colon cancer methylome shows similar hypo- and hypermethylation at conserved tissue-specific CpG island shores. *Nat Genet* 2009;41:178–186.
20. Doi A, Park IH, Wen B, et al. Differential methylation of tissue- and cancer-specific CpG island shores distinguishes human induced pluripotent stem cells, embryonic stem cells and fibroblasts. *Nat Genet* 2009;41:1350–1353.
21. Herman JG, Merlo A, Mao L, et al. Inactivation of the CDKN2/p16/MTS1 gene is frequently associated with aberrant DNA methylation in all common human cancers. *Cancer Res* 1995;55:4525–4530.
22. Merlo A, Herman JG, Mao L, et al. 5′ CpG island methylation is associated with transcriptional silencing of the tumour suppressor p16/CDKN2/MTS1 in human cancers. *Nat Med* 1995;1:686–692.
23. Herman JG, Civin CI, Issa JP, et al. Distinct patterns of inactivation of p15INK4B and p16INK4A characterize the major types of hematological malignancies. *Cancer Res* 1997;57:837–841.
24. Costello JF, Fruhwald MC, Smiraglia DJ, et al. Aberrant CpG-island methylation has non-random and tumour-type-specific patterns. *Nat Genet* 2000;24:132–138.
25. Gore SD, Baylin S, Sugar E, et al. Combined DNA methyltransferase and histone deacetylase inhibition in the treatment of myeloid neoplasms. *Cancer Res* 2006;66:6361–6369.
26. Azad N, Zahnow CA, Rudin CM, et al. The future of epigenetic therapy in solid tumours—lessons from the past. *Nat Rev Clin Oncol* 2013;10:256–266.
27. Issa JP, Kantarjian HM. Targeting DNA methylation. *Clin Cancer Res* 2009;15:3938–3946.
28. Tsai HC, Li H, Van Neste L, et al. Transient low doses of DNA-demethylating agents exert durable antitumor effects on hematological and epithelial tumor cells. *Cancer Cell* 2012;21:430–446.
29. Takai D, Jones PA. Comprehensive analysis of CpG islands in human chromosomes 21 and 22. *Proc Natl Acad Sci U S A* 2002;99:3740–3745.
30. Futscher BW, Oshiro MM, Wozniak RJ, et al. Role for DNA methylation in the control of cell type specific maspin expression. *Nat Genet* 2002;31:175–179.
31. Feldmann A, Ivanek R, Murr R, et al. Transcription factor occupancy can mediate active turnover of DNA methylation at regulatory regions. *PLoS Genet* 2013;9:e1003994.
32. Aran D, Hellman A. Unmasking risk loci: DNA methylation illuminates the biology of cancer predisposition: analyzing DNA methylation of transcriptional enhancers reveals missed regulatory links between cancer risk loci and genes. *Bioessays* 2014;36:184–190.
33. Ziller MJ, Gu H, Muller F, et al. Charting a dynamic DNA methylation landscape of the human genome. *Nature* 2013;500:477–481.
34. Akhtar-Zaidi B, Cowper-Sal-lari R, Corradin O, et al. Epigenomic enhancer profiling defines a signature of colon cancer. *Science* 2012;336:736–739.
35. Kingston R, Tamkun JW. Transcriptional regulation by trithorax group. In: Allis CD, Jenuwein T, Reinberd D, eds. *Epigenetics*. Cold Spring Harbor, NY: Cold Spring Harbor Laboratory Press; 2006: 231–248.
36. Becker PB, Workman JL. Nucleosome remodeling and epigenetics. *Cold Spring Harb Perspect Biol* 2013;5.
37. Petty E, Pillus L. Balancing chromatin remodeling and histone modifications in transcription. *Trends Genet* 2013;29:621–629.
38. Jones PA. Functions of DNA methylation: islands, start sites, gene bodies and beyond. *Nat Rev Genet* 2012;13:484–492.
39. Bannister AJ, Kouzarides T. Reversing histone methylation. *Nature* 2005; 436:1103–1106.
40. Bannister AJ, Kouzarides T. Regulation of chromatin by histone modifications. *Cell Res* 2011;21:381–395.
41. Di Leva G, Garofalo M, Croce CM. MicroRNAs in cancer. *Annu Rev Pathol* 2014;9:287–314.
42. Han BW, Chen YQ. Potential pathological and functional links between long noncoding RNAs and hematopoiesis. *Sci Signal* 2013;6:re5.
43. Xi JJ. MicroRNAs in Cancer. *Cancer Treat Res* 2013;158:119–137.
44. Nan X, Ng HH, Johnson CA, et al. Transcriptional repression by the methyl-CpG-binding protein MeCP2 involves a histone deacetylase complex. *Nature* 1998;393:386–389.
45. Jones PL, Veenstra GJ, Wade PA, et al. Methylated DNA and MeCP2 recruit histone deacetylase to repress transcription. *Nat Genet* 1998;19:187–191.
46. Parry L, Clarke AR. The Roles of the Methyl-CpG Binding Proteins in Cancer. *Genes Cancer* 2011;2:618–630.
47. Lopez-Serra L, Esteller M. Proteins that bind methylated DNA and human cancer: reading the wrong words. *Br J Cancer* 2008;98:1881–1885.
48. Cai Y, Geutjes EJ, de Lint K, et al. The NuRD complex cooperates with DNMTs to maintain silencing of key colorectal tumor suppressor genes. *Oncogene* 2014;33:2157–2168.
49. Bestor TH. Cloning of a mammalian DNA methyltransferase. *Gene* 1998; 74:9–12.
50. Jair KW, Bachman KE, Suzuki H, et al. De novo CpG island methylation in human cancer cells. *Cancer Res* 2006;66:682–692.
51. Rius M, Lyko F. Epigenetic cancer therapy: rationales, targets and drugs. *Oncogene* 2012;31:4257–4265.
52. Jenuwein T, Allis CD. Translating the histone code. *Science* 2001;293: 1074–1080.
53. Bolden JE, Peart MJ, Johnstone RW. Anticancer activities of histone deacetylase inhibitors. *Nat Rev Drug Discov* 2006;5:769–784.
54. Vaquero A, Scher M, Erdjument-Bromage H, et al. SIRT1 regulates the histone methyl-transferase SUV39H1 during heterochromatin formation. *Nature* 2007;450:440–444.
55. Pruitt K, Zinn RL, Ohm JE, et al. Inhibition of SIRT1 reactivates silenced cancer genes without loss of promoter DNA hypermethylation. *PLoS Genet* 2006;2:344–352.
56. Cameron EE, Bachman KE, Myohanen S, et al. Synergy of demethylation and histone deacetylase inhibition in the re-expression of genes silenced in cancer. *Nat Genet* 1999;21:103–107.
57. Sorm F, Piskala A, Cihak A, et al. 5-Azacytidine, a new, highly effective cancerostatic. *Experientia* 1964;20:202–203.
58. Taylor SM, Jones PA. Multiple new phenotypes induced in 10T1/2 and 3T3 cells treated with 5-azacytidine. *Cell* 1979;17:771–779.
59. Jones PA, Taylor SM. Hemimethylated duplex DNAs prepared from 5-azacytidine-treated cells. *Nucleic Acids Res* 1981;9:2933–2947.
60. Lu SH, Ohshima H, Bartsch H. Recent studies on N-nitroso compounds as possible etiological factors in oesophageal cancer. *IARC Sci Publ* 1984;947–953.
61. Taylor SM, Jones PA. Mechanism of action of eukaryotic DNA methyltransferase. Use of 5-azacytosine-containing DNA. *J Mol Biol* 1982;162:679–692.
62. Schaefer M, Hagemann S, Hanna K, et al. Azacytidine inhibits RNA methylation at DNMT2 target sites in human cancer cell lines. *Cancer Res* 2009; 69:8127–8132.
63. Hollenbach PW, Nguyen AN, Brady H, et al. A comparison of azacitidine and decitabine activities in acute myeloid leukemia cell lines. *PLoS One* 2010; 5:e9001.
64. Kelly TK, De Carvalho DD, Jones PA. Epigenetic modifications as therapeutic targets. *Nat Biotechnol* 2010;28:1069–1078.
65. Ferguson AT, Vertino PM, Spitzner JR, et al. Role of estrogen receptor gene demethylation and DNA methyltransferase. DNA adduct formation in 5-aza-2′deoxycytidine-induced cytotoxicity in human breast cancer cells. *J Biol Chem* 1997;272:32260–32266.
66. Gabbara S, Bhagwat AS. The mechanism of inhibition of DNA (cytosine-5-)-methyltransferases by 5-azacytosine is likely to involve methyl transfer to the inhibitor. *Biochem J* 1995;307:87–92.
67. Santi DV, Norment A, Garrett CE. Covalent bond formation between a DNA-cytosine methyltransferase and DNA containing 5-azacytosine. *Proc Natl Acad Sci U S A* 1984;81:6993–6997.
68. Ghoshal K, Datta J, Majumder S, et al. 5-Aza-deoxycytidine induces selective degradation of DNA methyltransferase 1 by a proteasomal pathway that requires the KEN box, bromo-adjacent homology domain, and nuclear localization signal. *Mol Cell Biol* 2005;25:4727–4741.
69. Rountree MR, Bachman KE, Baylin SB. DNMT1 binds HDAC2 and a new co-repressor, DMAP1, to form a complex at replication foci. *Nat Genet* 2000;25:269–277.
70. Bachman KE, Rountree MR, Baylin SB. Dnmt3a and Dnmt3b are transcriptional repressors that exhibit unique localization properties to heterochromatin. *J Biol Chem* 2001;276:32282–32287.
71. Jones PA, Taylor SM. Cellular differentiation, cytidine analogs and DNA methylation. *Cell* 1980;20:85–93.
72. Berg T, Guo Y, Abdelkarim M, et al. Reversal of p15/INK4b hypermethylation in AML1/ETO-positive and -negative myeloid leukemia cell lines. *Leuk Res* 2007;31:497–506.
73. Flatau E, Gonzales FA, Michalowsky LA, et al. DNA methylation in 5-aza-2′-deoxycytidine-resistant variants of C3H 10T1/2 C18 cells. *Mol Cell Biol* 1984;4:2098–2102.
74. Chan KK, Giannini DD, Staroscik JA, et al. 5-Azacytidine hydrolysis kinetics measured by high-pressure liquid chromatography and 13C-NMR spectroscopy. *J Pharm Sci* 1979;68:807–812.
75. Gore SD, Weng LJ, Figg WD, et al. Impact of prolonged infusions of the putative differentiating agent sodium phenylbutyrate on myelodysplastic syndromes and acute myeloid leukemia. *Clin Cancer Res* 2002;8:963–970.
76. Yu L, Liu C, Vandeusen J, et al. Global assessment of promoter methylation in a mouse model of cancer identifies ID4 as a putative tumor-suppressor gene in human leukemia. *Nat Genet* 2005;37:265–274.
77. Blum W, Klisovic RB, Hackanson B, et al. Phase I study of decitabine alone or in combination with valproic acid in acute myeloid leukemia. *J Clin Oncol* 2007;25:3884–3891.
78. Schrump DS, Fischette MR, Nguyen DM, et al. Phase I study of decitabine-mediated gene expression in patients with cancers involving the lungs, esophagus, or pleura. *Clin Cancer Res* 2006;12:5777–5785.
79. Garcia-Manero G, Gore SD, Cogle C, et al. Phase I study of oral azacitidine in myelodysplastic syndromes, chronic myelomonocytic leukemia, and acute myeloid leukemia. *J Clin Oncol* 2011;29:2521–2527.
80. Issa JP, Roboz G, Rizzieri D, et al. Abstract LB-214: Interim results from a randomized Phase 1-2 first-in-human (FIH) study of PK/PD guided escalating doses of SGI-110, a novel subcutaneous (SQ) second generation hypomethylating

agent (HMA) in relapsed/refractory MDS and AML. *Cancer Res* 2012;72: LB–214.
81. Mund C, Lyko F. Epigenetic cancer therapy: Proof of concept and remaining challenges. *Bioessays* 2010;32:949–957.
82. Popovic R, Licht JD. Emerging epigenetic targets and therapies in cancer medicine. *Cancer Discov* 2012;2:405–413.
83. Verbrugge I, Johnstone RW, Bots M. Promises and challenges of anticancer drugs that target the epigenome. *Epigenomics* 2011;3:547–565.
84. Robert C, Rassool FV. HDAC inhibitors: roles of DNA damage and repair. *Adv Cancer Res* 2012;116:87–129.
85. Kachhap SK, Rosmus N, Collis SJ, et al. Downregulation of homologous recombination DNA repair genes by HDAC inhibition in prostate cancer is mediated through the E2F1 transcription factor. *PLoS One* 2010;5:e11208.
86. Sharma SV, Lee DY, Li B, et al. A chromatin-mediated reversible drug-tolerant state in cancer cell subpopulations. *Cell* 2010;141:69–80.
87. Villanueva J, Vultur A, Lee JT, et al. Acquired resistance to BRAF inhibitors mediated by a RAF kinase switch in melanoma can be overcome by cotargeting MEK and IGF-1R/PI3K. *Cancer Cell* 2010;18:683–695.
88. Novogrodsky A, Dvir A, Ravid A, et al. Effect of polar organic compounds on leukemic cells. Butyrate-induced partial remission of acute myelogenous leukemia in a child. *Cancer* 1983;51:9–14.
89. Miller AA, Kurschel E, Osieka R, et al. Clinical pharmacology of sodium butyrate in patients with acute leukemia. *Eur J Cancer Clin Oncol* 1987; 23:1283–1287.
90. Gore SD, Weng LJ, Zhai S, et al. Impact of the putative differentiating agent sodium phenylbutyrate on myelodysplastic syndromes and acute myeloid leukemia. *Clin Cancer Res* 2001;7:2330–2339.
91. Gore SD, Weng LJ, Figg WD, et al. Impact of prolonged infusions of the putative differentiating agent sodium phenylbutyrate on myelodysplastic syndromes and acute myeloid leukemia. *Clin Cancer Res* 2002;8:963–970.
92. DiGiuseppe JA, Weng LJ, Yu KH, et al. Phenylbutyrate-induced G1 arrest and apoptosis in myeloid leukemia cells: structure-function analysis. *Leukemia* 1999;13:1243–1253.
93. Kuendgen A, Strupp C, Aivado M, et al. Treatment of myelodysplastic syndromes with valproic acid alone or in combination with all-trans retinoic acid. *Blood* 2004;104:1266–1269.
94. Pilatrino C, Cilloni D, Messa E, et al. Increase in platelet count in older, poor-risk patients with acute myeloid leukemia or myelodysplastic syndrome treated with valproic acid and all-trans retinoic acid. *Cancer* 2005;104:101–109.
95. Fizzotti M, Cimino G, Pisegna S, et al. Detection of homozygous deletions of the cyclin-dependent kinase 4 inhibitor (p16) gene in acute lymphoblastic leukemia and association with adverse prognostic features. *Blood* 1995; 85:2685–2690.
96. Xu GL, Bestor TH, Bourc'his D, et al. Chromosome instability and immunodeficiency syndrome caused by mutations in a DNA methyltransferase gene. *Nature* 1999;402:187–191.
97. Duvic M, Talpur R, Ni X, et al. Phase 2 trial of oral vorinostat (suberoylanilide hydroxamic acid, SAHA) for refractory cutaneous T-cell lymphoma (CTCL). *Blood* 2007;109:31–39.
98. Olsen EA, Kim YH, Kuzel TM, et al. Phase IIb multicenter trial of vorinostat in patients with persistent, progressive, or treatment refractory cutaneous T-cell lymphoma. *J Clin Oncol* 2007;25:3109–3115.
99. O'Connor OA, Heaney ML, Schwartz L, et al. Clinical experience with intravenous and oral formulations of the novel histone deacetylase inhibitor suberoylanilide hydroxamic acid in patients with advanced hematologic malignancies. *J Clin Oncol* 2006;24:166–173.
100. Ramalingam SS, Maitland ML, Frankel P, et al. Carboplatin and Paclitaxel in combination with either vorinostat or placebo for first line therapy of advanced non-small-cell lung cancer. *J Clin Oncol* 2010;28:56–62.
101. Giles F, Fischer T, Cortes J, et al. A phase I study of intravenous LBH589, a novel cinnamic hydroxamic acid analogue histone deacetylase inhibitor, in patients with refractory hematologic malignancies. *Clin Cancer Res* 2006; 12:4628–4635.
102. Richardson PG, Hungria VTM, Yoon S-S, et al. Panorama 1: A randomized, double-blind, phase 3 study of panobinostat or placebo plus bortezomib and dexamethasone in relapsed or relapsed and refractory multiple myeloma. *ASCO Meeting Abstracts* 2014;32:8510.
103. Piekarz RL, Robey R, Sandor V, et al. Inhibitor of histone deacetylation, depsipeptide (FR901228), in the treatment of peripheral and cutaneous T-cell lymphoma: a case report. *Blood* 2001;98:2865–2868.
104. Coiffier B, Pro B, Prince HM, et al. Romidepsin for the treatment of relapsed/refractory peripheral T-cell lymphoma: pivotal study update demonstrates durable responses. *J Hematol Oncol* 2014;7:11.
105. Coiffier B, Pro B, Prince HM, et al. Results from a pivotal, open-label, phase II study of romidepsin in relapsed or refractory peripheral T-cell lymphoma after prior systemic therapy. *J Clin Oncol* 2012;30:631–636.
106. Piekarz RL, Frye AR, Wright JJ, et al. Cardiac studies in patients treated with depsipeptide, FK228, in a phase II trial for T-cell lymphoma. *Clin Cancer Res* 2006;12:3762–3773.
107. Gojo I, Jiemjit A, Trepel JB, et al. Phase 1 and pharmacologic study of MS-275, a histone deacetylase inhibitor, in adults with refractory and relapsed acute leukemias. *Blood* 2007;109:2781–2790.
108. Prebet T, Sun Z, Figueroa ME, et al. Prolonged administration of azacitidine with or without entinostat for myelodysplastic syndrome and acute myeloid leukemia with myelodysplasia-related changes: results of the US Leukemia Intergroup Trial E1905. *J Clin Oncol* 2014;32:1242–1248.
109. Witta SE, Jotte RM, Konduri K, et al. Randomized phase II trial of erlotinib with and without entinostat in patients with advanced non-small-cell lung cancer who progressed on prior chemotherapy. *J Clin Oncol* 2012;30:2248–2255.
110. Yardley DA, Ismail-Khan RR, Melichar B, et al. Randomized phase II, double-blind, placebo-controlled study of exemestane with or without entinostat in postmenopausal women with locally recurrent or metastatic estrogen receptor-positive breast cancer progressing on treatment with a nonsteroidal aromatase inhibitor. *J Clin Oncol* 2013;31:2128–2135.
111. Byrd JC, Marcucci G, Parthun MR, et al. A phase 1 and pharmacodynamic study of depsipeptide (FK228) in chronic lymphocytic leukemia and acute myeloid leukemia. *Blood* 2005;105:959–967.
112. Charache S, Dover G, Smith K, et al. Treatment of sickle cell anemia with 5-azacytidine results in increased fetal hemoglobin production and is associated with nonrandom hypomethylation of DNA around the gamma-delta-beta-globin gene complex. *Proc Natl Acad Sci U S A* 1983;80:4842–4846.
113. Silverman LR, Holland JF, Weinberg RS, et al. Effects of treatment with 5-azacytidine on the in vivo and in vitro hematopoiesis in patients with myelodysplastic syndromes. *Leukemia* 1993;7:21–29.
114. Silverman LR, McKenzie DR, Peterson BL, et al. Further analysis of trials with azacitidine in patients with myelodysplastic syndrome: studies 8421, 8921, and 9221 by the Cancer and Leukemia Group B. *J Clin Oncol* 2006;24:3895–3903.
115. Silverman LR, Demakos EP, Peterson BL, et al. Randomized controlled trial of azacitidine in patients with the myelodysplastic syndrome: a study of the Cancer and Leukemia Group B. *J Clin Oncol* 2002;20:2429–2440.
116. Fenaux P, Mufti GJ, Hellstrom-Lindberg E, et al. Efficacy of azacitidine compared with that of conventional care regimens in the treatment of higher-risk myelodysplastic syndromes: a randomised, open-label, phase III study. *Lancet Oncol* 2009;10:223–232.
117. Fenaux P, Mufti GJ, Hellstrom-Lindberg E, et al. Azacitidine prolongs overall survival compared with conventional care regimens in elderly patients with low bone marrow blast count acute myeloid leukemia. *J Clin Oncol* 2010;28: 562–569.
118. Wijermans P, Lubbert M, Verhoef G, et al. Low-dose 5-aza-2′-deoxycytidine, a DNA hypomethylating agent, for the treatment of high-risk myelodysplastic syndrome: a multicenter phase II study in elderly patients. *J Clin Oncol* 2000;18:956–962.
119. Wijermans PW, Krulder JW, Huijgens PC, et al. Continuous infusion of low-dose 5-Aza-2′-deoxycytidine in elderly patients with high-risk myelodysplastic syndrome. *Leukemia* 1997;11:1–5.
120. Kantarjian HM, O'Brien S, Cortes J, et al. Results of decitabine (5-aza-2′deoxycytidine) therapy in 130 patients with chronic myelogenous leukemia. *Cancer* 2003;98:522–528.
121. Kantarjian H, Oki Y, Garcia-Manero G, et al. Results of a randomized study of 3 schedules of low-dose decitabine in higher-risk myelodysplastic syndrome and chronic myelomonocytic leukemia. *Blood* 2007;109:52–57.
122. Steensma DP, Baer MR, Slack JL, et al. Multicenter study of decitabine administered daily for 5 days every 4 weeks to adults with myelodysplastic syndromes: the alternative dosing for outpatient treatment (ADOPT) trial. *J Clin Oncol* 2009;27:3842–3848.
123. Kantarjian H, Issa JP, Rosenfeld CS, et al. Decitabine improves patient outcomes in myelodysplastic syndromes: results of a phase III randomized study. *Cancer* 2006;106:1794–1803.
124. WijerMans P, Suciu S, Baila L, et al. Low-dose decitabine versus best supportive care in elderly patients with intermediate or high risk MDS not eligible for intensive chemotherapy: final results of the randomized phase III study (06011) of the EORTC Leukemia and German MDS Study Groups. *ASH Annual Meeting Abstracts* 2008;112:226.
125. Flotho C, Claus R, Batz C, et al. The DNA methyltransferase inhibitors azacitidine, decitabine and zebularine exert differential effects on cancer gene expression in acute myeloid leukemia cells. *Leukemia* 2009;23:1019–1028.
126. Lübbert M, Suciu S, Baila L, et al. Low-dose decitabine versus best supportive care in elderly patients with intermediate- or high-risk myelodysplastic syndrome (MDS) ineligible for intensive chemotherapy: final results of the randomized phase III study (06011) of the European Organisation for Research and Treatment of Cancer Leukemia Group and the German MDS Study Group. *J Clin Oncol* 2011;29:1987–1996.
127. Kantarjian HM, Thomas XG, Dmoszynska A, et al. Multicenter, randomized, open-label, phase III trial of decitabine versus patient choice, with physician advice, of either supportive care or low-dose cytarabine for the treatment of older patients with newly diagnosed acute myeloid leukemia. *J Clin Oncol* 2012;30:2670–2677.
128. Sudan N, Rossetti JM, Shadduck RK, et al. Treatment of acute myelogenous leukemia with outpatient azacitidine. *Cancer* 2006;107:1839–1843.
129. Kantarjian HM, O'Brien SM, Keating M, et al. Results of decitabine therapy in the accelerated and blastic phases of chronic myelogenous leukemia. *Leukemia* 1997;11:1617–1620.
130. Ruter B, Wijermans P, Claus R, et al. Preferential cytogenetic response to continuous intravenous low-dose decitabine (DAC) administration in myelodysplastic syndrome with monosomy 7. *Blood* 2007;110:1080–1082.
131. Raj K, John A, Ho A, et al. CDKN2B methylation status and isolated chromosome 7 abnormalities predict responses to treatment with 5-azacytidine. *Leukemia* 2007;21:1937–1944.
132. Ravandi F, Issa JP, Garcia-Manero G, et al. Superior outcome with hypomethylating therapy in patients with acute myeloid leukemia and high-risk myelodysplastic syndrome and chromosome 5 and 7 abnormalities. *Cancer* 2009;115:5746–5751.

133. Yang AS, Doshi KD, Choi SW, et al. DNA methylation changes after 5-aza-2′-deoxycytidine therapy in patients with leukemia. *Cancer Res* 2006;66:5495–5503.
134. Yang AS, Estecio MR, Doshi K, et al. A simple method for estimating global DNA methylation using bisulfite PCR of repetitive DNA elements. *Nucleic Acids Res* 2004;32:e38.
135. Daskalakis M, Nguyen TT, Nguyen C, et al. Demethylation of a hypermethylated P15/INK4B gene in patients with myelodysplastic syndrome by 5-Aza-2′-deoxycytidine (decitabine) treatment. *Blood* 2002;100:2957–2964.
136. Bakkenist CJ, Kastan MB. DNA damage activates ATM through intermolecular autophosphorylation and dimer dissociation. *Nature* 2003;421:499–506.
137. Borthakur G, Ahdab SE, Ravandi F, et al. Activity of decitabine in patients with myelodysplastic syndrome previously treated with azacitidine. *Leuk Lymphoma* 2008;49:690–695.
138. Shen L, Kantarjian H, Guo Y, et al. DNA methylation predicts survival and response to therapy in patients with myelodysplastic syndromes. *J Clin Oncol* 2010;28:605–613.
139. Figueroa ME, Skrabanek L, Li Y, et al. MDS and secondary AML display unique patterns and abundance of aberrant DNA methylation. *Blood* 2009;114:3448–3458.
140. Fandy TE, Herman JG, Kerns P, et al. Early epigenetic changes and DNA damage do not predict clinical response in an overlapping schedule of 5-azacytidine and entinostat in patients with myeloid malignancies. *Blood* 2009;114:2764–2773.
141. Schuebel KE, Chen W, Cope L, et al. Comparing the DNA hypermethylome with gene mutations in human colorectal cancer. *PLoS Genet* 2007;3:1709–1723.
142. Maslak P, Chanel S, Camacho LH, et al. Pilot study of combination transcriptional modulation therapy with sodium phenylbutyrate and 5-azacytidine in patients with acute myeloid leukemia or myelodysplastic syndrome. *Leukemia* 2006;20:212–217.
143. Garcia-Manero G, Kantarjian HM, Sanchez-Gonzalez B, et al. Phase I/II study of the combination of 5-aza-2′-deoxycytidine with valproic acid in patients with leukemia. *Blood* 2006;108:3271–3279.
144. Soriano AO, Yang H, Faderl S, et al. Safety and clinical activity of the combination of 5-azacytidine, valproic acid, and all-trans retinoic acid in acute myeloid leukemia and myelodysplastic syndrome. *Blood* 2007;110:2302–2308.
145. Voso MT, Santini V, Finelli C, et al. Valproic acid at therapeutic plasma levels may increase 5-azacytidine efficacy in higher risk myelodysplastic syndromes. *Clin Cancer Res* 2009;15:5002–5007.
146. Sharma S, Kelly TK, Jones PA. Epigenetics in cancer. *Carcinogenesis* 2010;31:27–36.
147. Silverman LR, Fenaux P, Mufti GJ, et al. Continued azacitidine therapy beyond time of first response improves quality of response in patients with higher-risk myelodysplastic syndromes. *Cancer* 2011;117:2697–2702.
148. Craddock C, Quek L, Goardon N, et al. Azacitidine fails to eradicate leukemic stem/progenitor cell populations in patients with acute myeloid leukemia and myelodysplasia. *Leukemia* 2013;27:1028–1036.
149. Juergens RA, Wrangle J, Vendetti FP, et al. Combination epigenetic therapy has efficacy in patients with refractory advanced non-small cell lung cancer. *Cancer Discov* 2011;1: 598–607.
150. Wrangle J, Wang W, Koch A, et al. Alterations of immune response of Non-Small Cell Lung Cancer with Azacytidine. *Oncotarget* 2013;4:2067–2079.
151. Shakya R, Gonda TA, Quante M, et al. Hypomethylating therapy in an aggressive stroma-rich model of pancreatic carcinoma. *Cancer Res* 2013;73: 885–896.
152. Humeniuk R, Menon LG, Mishra PJ, et al. Decreased levels of UMP kinase as a mechanism of fluoropyrimidine resistance. *Mol Cancer Ther* 2009;8: 1037–1044.
153. Meng F, Sun G, Zhong M, et al. Anticancer efficacy of the combination of low-dose cisplatin and trichostatin A or 5-aza-2′-deoxycytidine in ovarian cancer cells. Paper presented at: 2012 ASCO Annual Meeting; 2012; Chicago, IL.
154. Matei D, Fang F, Shen C, et al. Epigenetic resensitization to platinum in ovarian cancer. *Cancer Res* 2012;72:2197–2205.
155. Fu S, Hu W, Iyer R, et al. Phase 1b-2a study to reverse platinum resistance through use of a hypomethylating agent, azacitidine, in patients with platinum-resistant or platinum-refractory epithelial ovarian cancer. *Cancer* 2011;117:1661–1669.
156. Chung CW, Coste H, White JH, et al. Discovery and characterization of small molecule inhibitors of the BET family bromodomains. *J Med Chem* 2011;54:3827–3838.
157. Bernt KM, Zhu N, Sinha AU, et al. MLL-rearranged leukemia is dependent on aberrant H3K79 methylation by DOT1L. *Cancer Cell* 2011;20:66–78.
158. Daigle SR, Olhava EJ, Therkelsen CA, et al. Selective killing of mixed lineage leukemia cells by a potent small-molecule DOT1L inhibitor. *Cancer Cell* 2011;20:53–65.
159. Spannhoff A, Hauser AT, Heinke R, et al. The emerging therapeutic potential of histone methyltransferase and demethylase inhibitors. *ChemMedChem* 2009;4:1568–1582.
160. Okada Y, Feng Q, Lin Y, et al. hDOT1L links histone methylation to leukemogenesis. *Cell* 2005;121:167–178.

24 Proteasome Inhibitors

Christopher J. Kirk, Brian B. Tuch, Shirin Arastu-Kapur, and Lawrence H. Boise

BIOCHEMISTRY OF THE UBIQUITIN-PROTEASOME PATHWAY

The ubiquitin proteasome system is involved in the degradation of more than 80% of cellular proteins, including those that control cell-cycle progression, apoptosis, DNA repair, and the stress response.[1] A key step in this process is the *tagging* of proteins targeted for degradation with multiple copies of ubiquitin, a 76–amino acid protein whose primary sequence and structure is highly conserved in organisms ranging from yeasts to mammals.[2,3] Once polyubiquitinated, proteins targeted for degradation bind to the 26S proteasome, a holoenzyme composed of two 19S regulatory complexes capping a central 20S proteolytic core. The 20S core is a hollow "barrel" consisting of four stacked heptameric rings. The subunits of the rings are classified as either β subunits (outer two rings) or β subunits (inner two rings). The 19S regulatory complex consists of a lid that recognizes ubiquitinated protein substrates with high fidelity, and a base that contains six adenosine triphosphatases, unfolds protein substrates, removes the polyubiquitin tag, and threads them into the catalytic chamber of the 20S particle in an adenosine triphosphate–dependent manner.[4,5] Unlike typical proteases, the 20S proteasome in eukaryotic cells contains multiple proteolytic activities resulting in the cleavage of protein targets after many different amino acids. In most cells, the 20S core particle contains the catalytic subunits β5 (PSMB5), β1 (PSMB1), and β2 (PSMB2), accounting for chymotrypsin-like (CT-L), caspaselike (C-L), and trypsinlike (T-L) activities, respectively, each differing in their substrate preference.[6] However, in cells of hematopoietic origin, such as lymphocytes and monocytes, the proteasome catalytic subunits are encoded by homologous gene products: LMP7 (PSMB8), LMP2 (PSMB9), and MECL-1 (PSMB10).[7] These immunoproteasome subunits are also induced in nonhematopoietic cells following exposure to inflammatory cytokines such as interferon-γ (IFN-γ) and tumor necrosis factor alpha (TNF-α).[8] In the immunoproteasome, the 19S regulatory complex can be replaced with proteasome activators such as PA28, whose expression is also induced in cells following exposure to IFN-γ. Hybrid proteasomes, both for the catalytic subunits and regulatory particles, have been described.[9]

Given its key role in maintaining cellular homeostasis, the ubiquitin proteasome system appeared to be an unlikely target for pharmaceutical intervention. However, a variety of groundbreaking studies in the 1990s suggested that inhibitors of proteasome function might prove to be viable therapeutic agents.[10] Initial studies used substrate-related peptide aldehydes to investigate the proteolytic functions and specificity of the proteasome.[11] In vitro and in vivo studies with these inhibitors demonstrated their ability to induce apoptosis as well as inhibit tumor growth.[12–15] It was subsequently discovered that several natural products with antitumor activity exert their action via proteasome inhibition, providing additional rationale for the development of selective proteasome inhibitors (PIs).[16,17]

PROTEASOME INHIBITORS

Chemical Classes of Proteasome Inhibitors in Clinical Development

As of the writing of this overview, six different proteasome inhibitors comprising three distinct chemical classes have been tested in clinical trials (Table 24.1) and include: (1) dipeptide boronic acids, (2) peptide epoxy ketones, and (3) β-lactones.[18,19] Bortezomib (PS-341, Velcade), a dipeptide boronic acid, was developed by Millennium Pharmaceuticals (Cambridge, MA) and was the first PI approved for clinical use.[20] Two additional dipeptide boronic acids have entered clinical development, ixazomib/MLN 9708 (Millennium), currently in phase III studies, and delanzomib/CEP-18770 (Teva Pharmaceuticals; Frazer, PA), the clinical development of which has been halted. Carfilzomib (Onyx Pharmaceuticals; San Francisco, CA), a tetrapeptide epoxy ketone, received U.S. Food and Drug Administration (FDA) approval in 2012.[21] A second peptide epoxy ketone proteasome inhibitor, oprozomib (Onyx), entered clinical study in 2010. The third class of proteasome inhibitors, β-lactones, is represented by NPI-0052 (salinosporamide A [Marizomib]) and is currently being developed by Nereus Pharmaceuticals, Inc. (San Diego, CA). The initial approvals for both bortezomib and carfilzomib were in multiple myeloma (MM), a plasma cell neoplasm and the second most common hematologic cancer. However, the activity of PIs in other B-cell neoplasms has resulted in an expansion of the clinical utilization of this drug class.

Preclinical Activity of Proteasome Inhibitors

Each of the three classes of inhibitors has a distinct chemical mechanism of proteasome inhibition.[22] Peptide boronates form stable but reversible tetrahedral intermediates with the γ-hydroxyl (γ-OH) group of the catalytic N-terminal threonine of the proteasome active sites.[23,24] β-lactones also interact with this γ-OH, but form a completely irreversible interaction.[25] Similarly, peptide epoxy ketones form irreversible covalent adducts with the active site threonine but do so via a dual covalent adduction of γ-OH group and the free amine.[26] This interaction is highly specific for N-terminal threonine-containing hydrolases and renders peptide epoxy ketones the most selective proteasome inhibitors yet described.[27,28]

The primary targets of these PIs within the constitutive and immunoproteasomes are the CT-L subunits, β5 and LMP7, respectively. Despite accounting for less than 50% of total protein turnover by the proteasome, these subunits are essential for cell survival.[29] In MM cell lines, inhibiting both subunits (β5 and LMP7) is necessary and sufficient for tumor cell death.[30] Cytotoxicity of other tumor cell types requires the inhibition of multiple active sites beyond the CT-L activity. The combination of inhibitors specific for either the T-L or C-L activities, which have no cytotoxic activity on their own, augments the cytotoxic potential of the CT-L–specific inhibitors.[31,32]

TABLE 24.1

Proteasome Inhibitors in Clinical Development

Agent	Other Names	Drug Class	Stage of Development	Tumor Types	Route of Administration	Dose Levels	Schedule of Administration
Bortezomib	Velcade PS-341	Peptide boronate	FDA/EMEA approved	Multiple myeloma, mantle cell lymphoma	Intravenous, subcutaneous	1.3 mg/m^2	Days 1, 4, 8, & 11 (21-day cycle)
Ixazomib	MLN 9708 MLN 2238	Peptide boronate	Phase III	Multiple myeloma, AL, amyloidosis	Oral	4 mg	Once weekly (21-day cycle)
Delanzomib	CEP-18770	Peptide boronate	Phase I (discontinued)	Multiple myeloma	Intravenous	0.1–1.8 mg/m^2	Days 1, 4, 8, & 11 (21-day cycle)
Carfilzomib	Kyprolis PR-171	Peptide epoxy ketone	FDA approved, phase III	Multiple myeloma	Intravenous	20/27 mg/m^2	Days 1, 2, 8, 9, 15, & 16 (28-day cycle)
Oprozomib	ONX 0912 PR-047	Peptide epoxy ketone	Phase I/II	Multiple myeloma	Oral	150–240 mg (dose escalation ongoing)	Days 1, 2, 8, & 9 (14-day cycle) Days 1–5 (14-day cycle)
Marizomib	NPI-0052 Salinosporamide A	β-lactone	Phase II	Multiple myeloma	Intravenous	0.075–0.6 mg/m^2	Days 1, 4, 8, & 11 (21-day cycle)

EMEA, European Medicines Agency; AL, amyloid light chain.

Given its status as the first proteasome inhibitor approved for marketed use, the antitumor potential and preclinical activity of other proteasome inhibitors have generally been compared to bortezomib.[19] Carfilzomib showed equivalent antitumor activity to bortezomib in vitro against a panel of tumor cell lines under standard culture conditions but was >10-fold more potent at inducing tumor cell death when cells were exposed to drug for a 1-hour pulse, which mimics the pharmacokinetics of both compounds.[33] MLN2238 (the active agent of ixazomib) was active in the same mouse models of human tumors as bortezomib, but demonstrated greater levels of proteasome inhibition in the tumors.[34] In biochemical assays of proteasome activity, delanzomib had an identical potency and subunit activity profile to bortezomib, but in tumor cytotoxicity assays, potency relative to bortezomib was 2- to 10-fold less.[35] In addition, delanzomib appeared to be less cytotoxic than bortezomib to normal cells and had a differential effect on cytokine release in bone marrow stromal cells, suggesting a different pharmacologic activity. Oprozomib is 10-fold less potent than carfilzomib in proteasome activity assays, but showed similar antitumor activity in mouse tumor models.[36,37] Marizomib displayed greater potency against the non–CT-L active sites of the proteasome than bortezomib.[38] Interestingly, this agent synergized with bortezomib in killing tumor cells in vitro.[39] All of the second-generation inhibitors have shown activity in tumor cells made resistant to bortezomib and/or MM cells isolated from patients relapsed from bortezomib-based therapies[35,36,40–42]

The inhibition of tumor cells with proteasome inhibitors induces cell death via the induction of apoptosis through death effector caspase activation.[10] Although the mechanism underlying the induction of cell death remains to be fully elucidated, extensive research suggests a complex interplay of multiple pathways. PIs have been shown to affect the half-life of the *BH3-only* members of the Bcl-2 family, specifically BH3–interacting-domain death agonist (Bid) and Bcl-2 interacting killer (Bik).[43] Moreover the BH3-only protein NOXA is upregulated at the transcription level by PIs.[44–48] Proteasome inhibition also upregulates the expression of several key cell-cycle checkpoint proteins that include p53 (an inducer of G0/G1 cell-cycle arrest through accumulation of the cyclin-dependent kinase [CDK] inhibitor p27); the CDK inhibitor p21; mammalian cyclins A, B, D, and E; and transcription factors E2F and Rb.[49,50] The transcription factor nuclear factor kappa B (NF-κB), an important regulator of cell survival and cytokine/growth factor production,[51] is also affected by proteasome inhibition in multiple ways. The net effect on NF-κB signaling is not consistent across various assays and cell lines, and its relative importance in the antitumor effects of PIs remains unclear. Although it is interesting to note that patients whose myeloma harbor NF-κB–activating mutations (~20%) respond better to bortezomib than those without NF-κB–activating mutations.[52–54] In MM cell lines, there is growing evidence that the major determinant of sensitivity to proteasome inhibition is the relative load of protein flux to the proteasome.[55–57] These data suggest that induction of the terminal unfolded protein response may drive cell death. Whether proteotoxic stress induced cell death reflects sensitivity to proteasome inhibitors in other tumor types remains to be determined.

Pharmacokinetics and Pharmacodynamics of Proteasome Inhibitors in Animals

Following intravenous (IV) administration to animals and humans, proteasome activity is inhibited in a dose-dependent fashion within minutes; however, PIs such as bortezomib and carfilzomib are also rapidly cleared from circulation.[55,56,58–61] Recovery of proteasome activity in animals occurs in tissues with a half-life of approximately 24 hours, mirroring the recovery time of cells exposed to sublethal concentrations of PIs in vitro and likely reflecting new protein synthesis.[33,62]

PROTEASOME INHIBITORS IN CANCER

Clinical Activity of Bortezomib

Bortezomib is typically administered on days 1, 4, 8, and 11 of a 3-week cycle either as an IV bolus or subcutaneous administration. Increasing doses of bortezomib inhibit proteasome activity in blood in a dose-dependent fashion, reaching a maximum of 74% inhibition at a dose of 1.38 mg/m^2. Daily dosing schedules in animal studies have been associated with severe toxicity and have not been attempted in humans. In clinical trials, thrombocytopenia and peripheral neuropathy (PN) were common adverse events.[20,63,64] Bortezomib has shown remarkable single-agent antitumor activity in a wide range of B-cell neoplasms, including MM, non Hodgkin lymphoma (NHL), and Waldenström macroglobulinemia (WM). In 2003, bortezomib was approved by the FDA for use as a single agent for the treatment of patients with MM following two prior therapies and who demonstrated disease progression with their most recent therapy. The primary efficacy data for this approval was derived from the SUMMIT trial in which 202 patients with heavily pretreated disease were treated with bortezomib at 1.3 mg/m^2.[65] In this trial, the overall response rate (ORR), defined as patients achieving at least a 50% reduction in serum or urine levels of the myeloma M protein, was 35%. This clinical trial was supported by the CREST trial, in which the activity of 1.3 mg/m^2 dose was determined to be superior to a dose of 1.0 mg/m^2.[66] Bortezomib is also active as a single agent in earlier stage MM patient populations. A single-agent ORR of 38%, with a 6% complete response (CR) rate, was seen in the phase III APEX study in early relapsed MM, with a time to progression (TTP) of 6.2 months and a median duration of response of 8 months.[67] In this study, the major grade 3 and 4 toxicities were PN, 12%; dysesthesia and related symptoms, 8% to 10%; anemia, 8%; diarrhea, 8%; neutropenia, 14%; and fatigue, 12%. In the frontline setting, bortezomib demonstrated a single-agent response rate of 41% (5% CR rate).[68]

Bortezomib is also approved for newly diagnosed MM in combination with velcade, melphalan and prednisone (VMP). The phase III VISTA trial evaluated VMP in patients with untreated MM who were ineligible for high-dose therapy.[69] The addition of bortezomib to the melphalan prednisone (MP) backbone significantly improved response rates in this setting with an ORR of 71% for VMP (including 30% CR) versus 35% (with only 4% CR) for MP.[52] VMP was associated with a TTP of ~24 months, compared with ~16.6 months with MP. After a 5-year follow-up, there was a 31% reduced risk of death for the VMP group versus MP-treated patients.[70]

Bortezomib has also shown promise when combined with other agents in relapsed and refractory MM patients. The combination of bortezomib with pegylated doxorubicin (Doxil, Centocor Ortho Biotech Products, L.P.; Horsham, PA) resulted in an ORR of 79% in relapsed patients, and toxicities were similar to those observed with each agent administered separately.[71] A phase III study in 646 patients with relapsed and refractory MM compared this treatment with bortezomib alone; the combination produced a 44% ORR and extended the TTP from 6 to 9.3 months.[72,73] The combination of bortezomib with revlimid, lenalidomide and dexamethasone (Rd), a standard of care in the treatment of MM, resulted in an ORR of 64% and a median duration of response of 8.7 months.[74] This activity is striking given that 53% of patients had received prior bortezomib and 75% of patients had received prior thalidomide, a closely related analog of lenalidomide. Other agents tested in combination with bortezomib include vorinostat, the anti-CS1 mAb, elotuzumab, the Hsp90 inhibitor tanespimycin, and the Akt inhibitor perifosine.[75]

Frontline combinations with bortezomib in MM patients have shown high ORRs with a notable improvement in CR rates. In longer term studies, CR rates with bortezomib-based combinations have been shown to be associated with improved clinical outcomes.[63,64] A community-based phase IIIb study evaluating bortezomib + dexamethasone (VD) versus bortezomib + thalidomide + dexamethasone (VTD) versus VMP found similar ORR (60%, 70%, and 52%, respectively) and CR rates (13%, 18%, and 15%, respectively).[63] Bortezomib + melphalan + prednisone + thalidomide (VMPT) followed by bortezomib + thalidomide (VT) maintenance resulted in a superior CR rate compared with VMP with no maintenance (34% versus 21%) and improved 2-year progression-free survival (70% versus 58.2%).[64] A protocol modification in this trial involved changing from twice weekly to weekly bortezomib administration, which yielded similar TTP but reduced the incidence (21% versus 43%) and severity of PN (2% grade 3/4 versus 14%).[64] The bortezomib, lenalidomide, and dexamethasone combination in newly diagnosed MM resulted in a ORR of 100% in 66 patients, 29% of whom achieved a CR.[76]

Bortezomib has also shown activity in other hematologic cancers, most notably mantle cell lymphoma (MCL).[77,78] As a single agent in 155 relapsed and refractory MCL patients, bortezomib yielded an ORR of 33% (8% CR), a median duration of response of 9.2 months, and a TTP of 6.2 months.[78] Toxicities observed were similar to those seen in patients with MM and included thrombocytopenia, PN, and fatigue. When bortezomib was used to treat both newly diagnosed and refractory MCL, a response rate of 46% was observed in both populations,[77] leading to FDA approval late in 2006.

Bortezomib has been tested in a variety of solid tumors in phase I and II studies.[79] Partial responses (PR) were reported in 8% of patients with refractory non–small-cell lung cancer (NSCLC), although the TTP was 1.5 months.[80] Exacerbation of PN was common. Bortezomib was subsequently tested in combination with paclitaxel, irinotecan, and gemcitabine/carboplatin; however, results have not been encouraging. Bortezomib continues to be tested in combination with other agents in a variety of tumor types.[81,82]

Recent clinical activity and preclinical data suggest that proteasome inhibition may extend to nononcology applications. Single-agent bortezomib therapy in kidney transplant patients undergoing antibody-mediated rejection resulted in a reduction of donor-specific antibodies and improved renal function.[83] In mouse models of lupus nephritis, bortezomib resulted in a reduction of pathogenic plasma cells and the prevention of disease progression.[84] These data suggest that PIs may be useful in a wide range of B-cell–mediated diseases. However, toxicities with bortezomib, particularly PN, may prevent wider application of this particular agent.

Carfilzomib

Parallel phase I studies of carfilzomib have been conducted in patients with multiple tumor types, and two phase I dose-finding studies targeting B-cell malignancies have been completed. The first study used daily IV bolus dosing with doses up to 20 mg/m^2 for 5 consecutive days followed by 9 days of rest and resulted in substantial inhibition of proteasome activity.[85] In the second study, carfilzomib was administered daily for 2 days for 3 consecutive weeks (days 1, 2, 8, 9, 15, and 16), followed by 12 days of recovery.[86] Hematologic toxicities were the most frequent adverse events, observed along with transient, noncumulative elevations in serum creatinine, usually with increases in serum urea nitrogen and consistent with a *prerenal* etiology. New onset PN was infrequent. Among 20 evaluable patients (including bortezomib-refractory patients), 4 PRs and 1 minor response were seen. Responses were also durable, lasting more than 1 year in some cases. Although the maximum tolerated dose of carfilzomib was not established in this study, a dose of 20 mg/m^2 was initially selected for the phase II studies.

Based on the phase I studies, an open-label, single-arm, phase II study of single-agent carfilzomib in relapsed and refractory MM was initiated in 2007.[87,88] Carfilzomib was administered as an IV bolus on the twice-weekly dose schedule. Patients enrolled in the initial phase of the study (003-A0) had received a median of five prior therapies, and 78% of patients had grade 1/2 PN at entry.[87] Among 39 evaluable patients in 003-A0, 10 (26%) achieved a minor response or better, including 5 PRs, and 16 additional patients with stable disease. Based on new safety information from phase I studies, the protocol was amended and the carfilzomib dose was escalated to 27 mg/m^2 after the first cycle (003-A1).[89] In this trial, 266 patients were enrolled and all patients had previously been treated with an immunomodulatory agent (IMiD) and bortezomib and were refractory to their last therapy. An ORR of 24% with a median duration of response of 8 months was reported. Adverse events were predominantly hematopoietic (thrombocytopenia, lymphopenia, and anemia) and there was a <1% rate of grade 3 PN, despite 77% having a history of PN. Based on these findings, carfilzomib was granted conditional approval by the FDA in 2012 for the treatment of patients with relapsed and refractory myeloma who had received prior bortezomib and IMiD therapy.

The parallel PX-171-004 trial enrolled patients with relapsed MM following one to three prior treatments and who may have been refractory to one or more of these therapies.[90,91] Of the 155 patients enrolled in this trial, 120 had not received prior bortezomib-based therapy. In patients with relapsed disease, nonhematologic and hematologic toxicity profiles were similar. Despite high rates of baseline PN, reports of worsening neuropathic symptoms were infrequent (2% incidence of grade 3 and no grade 4 events). Carfilzomib demonstrated considerable activity in bortezomib-naïve patients, inducing PR or better in 46% of 54 evaluable patients at 20 mg/m^2 and 53% of patients at 27 mg/m^2.[91] The response rate in patients previously exposed to bortezomib was lower (18%).[90] Responses across groups are durable, typically 8 to 9 months.[90,91]

Based on findings in animal studies in which a 30-minute infusion of carfilzomib resulted in reduced toxicities,[61] the effect of infusional administration was tested in patients with relapsed and refractory myeloma. In a dose escalation study, PX-171-007, the MTD dose of carfilzomib was determined to be 56 mg/m^2, more than twice the dose used in the studies described previously. In a cohort of 24 patients receiving this dose and who had received a median of five prior lines of therapy (including two prior bortezomib-containing regimens), the ORR was 60%.[92] This enhanced efficacy also correlated with a greater level of inhibition of all three subunits of the immunoproteasome measured in isolated peripheral blood mononuclear cells (Lee S, et al., unpublished).[93] This same dose and infusion time is currently being explored in a phase III trial of nearly 900 patients comparing carfilzomib plus low-dose dexamethasone (Cd) to bortezomib plus low-dose dexamethasone (Vd) in MM patients with relapsed disease.

Trials of carfilzomib in combination with other agents in MM have been initiated, including a phase Ib/II safety and efficacy study of carfilzomib in combination with lenalidomide and low-dose dexamethasone (CRd) in relapsed and/or refractory MM. At the maximum planned dose, the ORR was 77% with a median duration of response of 22 months.[94] The CRd combination is now being tested in an international, multicenter, randomized, open-label phase III study in comparison with lenalidomide and low-dose dexamethasone (Rd) in approximately 780 patients with relapsed MM following one to three prior therapies. The CRd regimen has also been explored in newly diagnosed MM patients.[95] When carfilzomib is combined with Rd at a dose of 36 mg/m^2, 62% of the 53 patients treated achieved a CR. In addition, 20 of 21 patients analyzed for signs of minimal residual disease (MRD), utilizing multiparameter flow cytometry were determined to be free of MRD.

Ixazomib

Initial clinical studies of ixazomib involved dose escalation studies in patients with hematologic malignancies and explored both weekly and twice weekly dosing schedules.[96,97] Oral administration resulted in potent proteasome inhibition of ~65%. Clinical activity in patients with relapsed MM was 16%.[98] In patients with newly diagnosed MM, ixazomib plus lenalidomide and low-dose dexamethasone resulted in an ORR of 93% with 24% achieving a CR.[99] This combination is also being investigated in a phase III trial comparing this to Rd in patients with relapsed MM.

Oprozomib

Initial clinical testing of oprozomib in patients with solid tumors investigated a dosing schedule consisting of a 14-day cycle with once daily administration for 5 consecutive days.[100] In patients with relapsed and/or refractory B-cell neoplasms, two dosing schedules are being utilized: the schedule described previously and one involving 2 consecutive days of dosing repeated weekly.[101] Proteasome inhibition following the administration of oprozomib reached >80% and clinical activity was noted in patients with MM and WM. In patients receiving the 5 consecutive day schedule, 5 of 19 MM patients (26%) and 8 of 10 WM patients (80%) achieved a partial response or better. Exploration of the dose and schedule continues as a single agent and in combination with other anti-MM therapies.

Biomarkers for Proteasome Inhibitors

As described previously, PI-based therapies have proven highly effective in the treatment of MM and other B-cell neoplasms. Given that response rates in single-agent trials are generally <50%, there would be a distinct clinical benefit to identify those patients most likely to respond to proteasome inhibition prior to treatment initiation. Gene expression analysis from bone marrow–derived MM tumor cells from 169 bortezomib-treated patients and 70 dexamethasone-treated patients revealed a 100-gene signature that provided a stratification for patients likely to respond that performed better than standard staging systems.[102] However, this signature provided only a modest increase in predictive power for treatment with bortezomib versus dexamethasone. More recently, Keats et al.[54] reanalyzed this dataset based on a pathway analysis of NF-κB and the realization that TRAF3, a key regulatory of the noncanonical NF-κB pathway, is a tumor suppressor in MM cell lines. They found a dramatic enrichment for response to bortezomib in patients with low levels of TRAF3 expression. However, these data remain to be validated in a separate sample set. A transcriptomic analysis of samples derived from single-agent carfilzomib trials suggest that patients with the highest level of immunoglobulin heavy chain expression were the most sensitive to carfilzomib therapy.[103] Similar findings were noted in the expression data from bortezomib-treated patients described previously.[103] These data are supported by phenotypic data from patients progressing on bortezomib-based therapy, in which resistance to bortezomib was associated with a dedifferentiated (and lower immunoglobulin expressing) B-cell phenotype.[104] Taken together, these findings suggest that biomarkers, potentially those involving an analysis of protein load of immunoglobulin expression, may be developed to predict those patients most likely to respond to PIs.

REFERENCES

1. Ciechanover A. Intracellular protein degradation: from a vague idea thru the lysosome and the ubiquitin-proteasome system and onto human diseases and drug targeting. *Biochim Biophys Acta* 2012;1824:3–13.
2. Kopp F, Hendil KB, Dahlmann B, et al. Subunit arrangement in the human 20S proteasome. *Proc Natl Acad Sci U S A* 1997;94:2939–2944.
3. Wilkinson KD. Ubiquitination and deubiquitination: targeting of proteins for degradation by the proteasome. *Semin Cell Dev Biol* 2000;11:141–148.
4. Braun BC, Glickman M, Kraft R, et al. The base of the proteasome regulatory particle exhibits chaperone-like activity. *Nat Cell Biol* 1999;1:221–226.
5. Groll M, Ditzel L, Lowe J, et al. Structure of 20S proteasome from yeast at 2.4 A resolution. *Nature* 1997;386:463–471.
6. Borissenko L, Groll M. 20S proteasome and its inhibitors: crystallographic knowledge for drug development. *Chem Rev* 2007;107:687–717.
7. Kloetzel PM, Ossendorp F. Proteasome and peptidase function in MHC-class-I-mediated antigen presentation. *Curr Opin Immunol* 2004;16:76–81.
8. Griffin TA, Nandi D, Cruz M, et al. Immunoproteasome assembly: cooperative incorporation of interferon gamma (IFN-gamma)-inducible subunits. *J Exp Med* 1998;187:97–104.

9. Tanahashi N, Murakami Y, Minami Y, et al. Hybrid proteasomes. Induction by interferon-gamma and contribution to ATP-dependent proteolysis. *J Biol Chem* 2000;275:14336–14345.
10. Adams J. The proteasome: a suitable antineoplastic target. *Nat Rev Cancer* 2004;4:349–360.
11. Vinitsky A, Michaud C, Powers JC, et al. Inhibition of the chymotrypsin-like activity of the pituitary multicatalytic proteinase complex. *Biochemistry* 1992;31:9421–9428.
12. Orlowski RZ, Eswara JR, Lafond-Walker A, et al. Tumor growth inhibition induced in a murine model of human Burkitt's lymphoma by a proteasome inhibitor. *Cancer Res* 1998;58:4342–4348.
13. Imajoh-Ohmi S, Kawaguchi T, Sugiyama S, et al. Lactacystin, a specific inhibitor of the proteasome, induces apoptosis in human monoblast U937 cells. *Biochem Biophys Res Commun* 1995;217:1070–1077.
14. Shinohara K, Tomioka M, Nakano H, et al. Apoptosis induction resulting from proteasome inhibition. *Biochem J* 1996;317:385–388.
15. Delic J, Masdehors P, Omura S, et al. The proteasome inhibitor lactacystin induces apoptosis and sensitizes chemo- and radioresistant human chronic lymphocytic leukaemia lymphocytes to TNF-alpha-initiated apoptosis. *Br J Cancer* 1998;77:1103–1107.
16. Meng L, Mohan R, Kwok BH, et al. Epoxomicin, a potent and selective proteasome inhibitor, exhibits in vivo antiinflammatory activity. *Proc Natl Acad Sci U S A* 1999;96:10403–10408.
17. Meng L, Kwok BH, Sin N, et al. Eponemycin exerts its antitumor effect through the inhibition of proteasome function. *Cancer Res* 1999;59:2798–2801.
18. Dick LR, Fleming PE. Building on bortezomib: second-generation proteasome inhibitors as anti-cancer therapy. *Drug Discov Today* 2010;15:243–249.
19. Kirk CJ. Discovery and development of second-generation proteasome inhibitors. *Semin Hematol* 2012;49:207–214.
20. Bross PF, Kane R, Farrell AT, et al. Approval summary for bortezomib for injection in the treatment of multiple myeloma. *Clin Cancer Res* 2004;10:3954–3964.
21. Herndon TM, Deisseroth A, Kaminskas E, et al. U.S. Food and Drug Administration approval: carfilzomib for the treatment of multiple myeloma. *Clin Cancer Res* 2013;19:4559–4563.
22. Bennett MK, Kirk CJ. Development of proteasome inhibitors in oncology and autoimmune diseases. *Curr Opin Drug Discov Devel* 2008;11:616–625.
23. Adams J, Behnke M, Chen S, et al. Potent and selective inhibitors of the proteasome: dipeptidyl boronic acids. *Bioorg Med Chem Lett* 1998;8:333–338.
24. Groll M, Berkers CR, Ploegh HL, et al. Crystal structure of the boronic acid-based proteasome inhibitor bortezomib in complex with the yeast 20S proteasome. *Structure* 2006;14:451–456.
25. Groll M, Huber R, Potts BC. Crystal structures of Salinosporamide A (NPI-0052) and B (NPI-0047) in complex with the 20S proteasome reveal important consequences of beta-lactone ring opening and a mechanism for irreversible binding. *J Am Chem Soc* 2006;19:5136–5141.
26. Groll M, Kim KB, Kairies N, et al. Crystal structure of epoxomicin: 20S proteasome reveals a molecular basis for selectivity of a' b'-epoxyketone proteasome inhibitors. *J Am Chem Soc* 2000;122:1237–1238.
27. Kisselev AF, van der Linden WA, Overkleeft HS. Proteasome inhibitors: an expanding army attacking a unique target. *Chem Biol* 2012;19:99–115.
28. Arastu-Kapur S, Anderl JL, Kraus M, et al. Nonproteasomal targets of the proteasome inhibitors bortezomib and carfilzomib: a link to clinical adverse events. *Clin Cancer Res* 2011;17:2734–2743.
29. Kisselev AF, Callard A, Goldberg AL. Importance of the different proteolytic sites of the proteasome and the efficacy of inhibitors varies with the protein substrate. *J Biol Chem* 2006;281:8582–8590.
30. Parlati F, Lee SJ, Aujay M, et al. Carfilzomib can induce tumor cell death through selective inhibition of the chymotrypsin-like activity of the proteasome. *Blood* 2009;114:3439–3447.
31. Britton M, Lucas MM, Downey SL, et al. Selective inhibitor of proteasome's caspase-like sites sensitizes cells to specific inhibition of chymotrypsin-like sites. *Chem Biol* 2009;16:1278–1289.
32. Mirabella AC, Pletnev AA, Downey SL, et al. Specific cell-permeable inhibitor of proteasome trypsin-like sites selectively sensitizes myeloma cells to bortezomib and carfilzomib. *Chem Biol* 2011;18:608–618.
33. Demo SD, Kirk CJ, Aujay MA, et al. Antitumor activity of PR-171, a novel irreversible inhibitor of the proteasome. *Cancer Res* 2007;67:6383–6391.
34. Kupperman E, Lee EC, Cao Y, et al. Evaluation of the proteasome inhibitor MLN9708 in preclinical models of human cancer. *Cancer Res* 2010;70:1970–1980.
35. Piva R, Ruggeri B, Williams M, et al. CEP-18770: A novel, orally active proteasome inhibitor with a tumor-selective pharmacologic profile competitive with bortezomib. *Blood* 2008;111:2765–2775.
36. Chauhan D, Singh AV, Aujay M, et al. A novel orally active proteasome inhibitor ONX 0912 triggers in vitro and in vivo cytotoxicity in multiple myeloma. *Blood* 2010;116:4906–4915.
37. Zhou HJ, Aujay MA, Bennett MK, et al. Design and synthesis of an orally bioavailable and selective peptide epoxyketone proteasome inhibitor (PR-047). *J Med Chem* 2009;52:3028–3038.
38. Chauhan D, Catley L, Li G, et al. A novel orally active proteasome inhibitor induces apoptosis in multiple myeloma cells with mechanisms distinct from Bortezomib. *Cancer Cell* 2005;8:407–419.
39. Chauhan D, Singh A, Brahmandam M, et al. Combination of proteasome inhibitors bortezomib and NPI-0052 trigger in vivo synergistic cytotoxicity in multiple myeloma. *Blood* 2008;111:1654–1664.
40. Chauhan D, Tian Z, Zhou B, et al. In vitro and in vivo selective antitumor activity of a novel orally bioavailable proteasome inhibitor MLN9708 against multiple myeloma cells. *Clin Cancer Res* 2011;17:5311–5321.
41. Kuhn DJ, Chen Q, Voorhees PM, et al. Potent activity of carfilzomib, a novel, irreversible inhibitor of the ubiquitin-proteasome pathway, against preclinical models of multiple myeloma. *Blood* 2007;110:3281–3290.
42. Suzuki E, Demo S, Deu E, et al. Molecular mechanisms of bortezomib resistant adenocarcinoma cells. *PLoS One* 2011;6:e27996.
43. Zhang HG, Wang J, Yang X, et al. Regulation of apoptosis proteins in cancer cells by ubiquitin. *Oncogene* 2004;23:2009–2015.
44. Fernandez Y, Verhaegen M, Miller TP, et al. Differential regulation of noxa in normal melanocytes and melanoma cells by proteasome inhibition: therapeutic implications. *Cancer Res* 2005;65:6294–6304.
45. Nikiforov MA, Riblett M, Tang WH, et al. Tumor cell-selective regulation of NOXA by c-MYC in response to proteasome inhibition. *Proc Natl Acad Sci U S A* 2007;104:19488–19493.
46. Qin JZ, Ziffra J, Stennett L, et al. Proteasome inhibitors trigger NOXA-mediated apoptosis in melanoma and myeloma cells. *Cancer Res* 2005;65:6282–6293.
47. Wang Q, Mora-Jensen H, Weniger MA, et al. ERAD inhibitors integrate ER stress with an epigenetic mechanism to activate BH3-only protein NOXA in cancer cells. *Proc Natl Acad Sci U S A* 2009;106:2200–2205.
48. Mannava S, Zhuang D, Nair JR, et al. KLF9 is a novel transcriptional regulator of bortezomib- and LBH589-induced apoptosis in multiple myeloma cells. *Blood* 2012;119:1450–1458.
49. Koepp DM, Harper JW, Elledge SJ. How the cyclin became a cyclin: regulated proteolysis in the cell cycle. *Cell* 1999;97:431–434.
50. Pagano M, Tam SW, Theodoras AM, et al. Role of the ubiquitin-proteasome pathway in regulating abundance of the cyclin-dependent kinase inhibitor p27. *Science* 1995;269:682–685.
51. Wan F, Lenardo MJ. The nuclear signaling of NF-kappaB: current knowledge, new insights, and future perspectives. *Cell Res* 2010;20:24–33.
52. Annunziata CM, Davis RE, Demchenko Y, et al. Frequent engagement of the classical and alternative NF-kappaB pathways by diverse genetic abnormalities in multiple myeloma. *Cancer Cell* 2007;12:115–130.
53. Chapman MA, Lawrence MS, Keats JJ, et al. Initial genome sequencing and analysis of multiple myeloma. *Nature* 2011;471:467–472.
54. Keats JJ, Fonseca R, Chesi M, et al. Promiscuous mutations activate the noncanonical NF-kappaB pathway in multiple myeloma. *Cancer Cell* 2007;12:131–144.
55. Meister S, Schubert U, Neubert K, et al. Extensive immunoglobulin production sensitizes myeloma cells for proteasome inhibition. *Cancer Res* 2007;67:1783–1792.
56. Obeng EA, Carlson LM, Gutman DM, et al. Proteasome inhibitors induce a terminal unfolded protein response in multiple myeloma cells. *Blood* 2006;107:4907–4916.
57. Shabaneh TB, Downey SL, Goddard AL, et al. Molecular basis of differential sensitivity of myeloma cells to clinically relevant bolus treatment with bortezomib. *PLoS One* 2013;8:e56132.
58. Papadopoulos KP, Burris HA III, Gordon M, et al. A phase I/II study of carfilzomib 2-10-min infusion in patients with advanced solid tumors. *Cancer Chemother Pharmacol* 2013;72:861–868.
59. Papandreou CN, Daliani DD, Nix D, et al. Phase I trial of the proteasome inhibitor bortezomib in patients with advanced solid tumors with observations in androgen-independent prostate cancer. *J Clin Oncol* 2004;22:2108–2121.
60. Wang Z, Yang J, Kirk C, et al. Clinical pharmacokinetics, metabolism, and drug-drug interaction of carfilzomib. *Drug Metab Dispos* 2013;41:230–237.
61. Yang J, Wang Z, Fang Y, et al. Pharmacokinetics, pharmacodynamics, metabolism, distribution, and excretion of carfilzomib in rats. *Drug Metab Dispos* 2011;39:1873–1882.
62. Meiners S, Heyken D, Weller A, et al. Inhibition of proteasome activity induces concerted expression of proteasome genes and de novo formation of mammalian proteasomes. *J Biol Chem* 2003;278:21517–21525.
63. Lonial S, Waller EK, Richardson PG, et al. Risk factors and kinetics of thrombocytopenia associated with bortezomib for relapsed, refractory multiple myeloma. *Blood* 2005;106:3777–3784.
64. Richardson PG, Briemberg H, Jagannath S, et al. Frequency, characteristics, and reversibility of peripheral neuropathy during treatment of advanced multiple myeloma with bortezomib. *J Clin Oncol* 2006;24:3113–3120.
65. Richardson PG, Barlogie B, Berenson J, et al. A phase 2 study of bortezomib in relapsed, refractory myeloma. *N Engl J Med* 2003;348:2609–2617.
66. Jagannath S, Barlogie B, Berenson J, et al. A phase 2 study of two doses of bortezomib in relapsed or refractory myeloma. *Br J Haematol* 2004;127:165–172.
67. Richardson PG, Sonneveld P, Schuster MW, et al. Bortezomib or high-dose dexamethasone for relapsed multiple myeloma. *N Engl J Med* 2005;352:2487–2498.
68. Jagannath S, Brian D, Wolf JL, et al. A phase 2 study of bortezomib as first-line therapy in patients with multiple myeloma. *Blood* 2004;104:333.
69. San Miguel JF, Schlag R, Khuageva NK, et al. Bortezomib plus melphalan and prednisone for initial treatment of multiple myeloma. *N Engl J Med* 2008;359:906–917.
70. San Miguel JF, Schlag R, Khuageva NK, et al. Persistent overall survival benefit and no increased risk of second malignancies with bortezomib-melphalan-prednisone versus melphalan-prednisone in patients with previously untreated multiple myeloma. *J Clin Oncol* 2013;31:448–455.
71. Orlowski RZ, Voorhees PM, Garcia RA, et al. Phase 1 trial of the proteasome inhibitor bortezomib and pegylated liposomal doxorubicin in patients with advanced hematologic malignancies. *Blood* 2005;105:3058–3065.

72. Orlowski RZ, Nagler A, Sonneveld P, et al. Randomized phase III study of pegylated liposomal doxorubicin plus bortezomib compared with bortezomib alone in relapsed or refractory multiple myeloma: combination therapy improves time to progression. *J Clin Oncol* 2007;25:3892–3901.
73. Sonneveld P, Hajek R, Nagler A, et al. Combined pegylated liposomal doxorubicin and bortezomib is highly effective in patients with recurrent or refractory multiple myeloma who received prior thalidomide/lenalidomide therapy. *Cancer* 2008;112:1529–1537.
74. Richardson PG, Xie W, Jagannath S, et al. A phase II trial of lenalidomide, bortezomib and dexamethasone in patients with relapsed and relapsed/refractory myeloma. *Blood* 2014;123:1461–1469.
75. Kapoor P, Ramakrishnan V, Rajkumar SV. Bortezomib combination therapy in multiple myeloma. *Semin Hematol* 2012;49:228–242.
76. Richardson PG, Weller E, Lonial S, et al. Lenalidomide, bortezomib, and dexamethasone combination therapy in patients with newly diagnosed multiple myeloma. *Blood* 2010;116:679–686.
77. Belch A, Kouroukis CT, Crump M, et al. A phase II study of bortezomib in mantle cell lymphoma: the National Cancer Institute of Canada Clinical Trials Group trial IND.150. *Ann Oncol* 2007;18:116–121.
78. Fisher RI, Bernstein SH, Kahl BS, et al. Multicenter phase II study of bortezomib in patients with relapsed or refractory mantle cell lymphoma. *J Clin Oncol* 2006;24:4867–4874.
79. Milano A, Iaffaioli RV, Caponigro F. The proteasome: a worthwhile target for the treatment of solid tumours? *Eur J Cancer* 2007;43:1125–1133.
80. Fanucchi MP, Fossella FV, Belt R, et al. Randomized phase II study of bortezomib alone and bortezomib in combination with docetaxel in previously treated advanced non-small-cell lung cancer. *J Clin Oncol* 2006;24:5025–5033.
81. Ramaswamy B, Phelps MA, Baiocchi R, et al. A dose-finding, pharmacokinetic and pharmacodynamic study of a novel schedule of flavopiridol in patients with advanced solid tumors. *Invest New Drugs* 2012;30:629–638.
82. Luu T, Chow W, Lim D, et al. Phase I trial of fixed-dose rate gemcitabine in combination with bortezomib in advanced solid tumors. *Anticancer Res* 2010;30:167–174.
83. Everly MJ, Everly JJ, Susskind B, et al. Bortezomib provides effective therapy for antibody- and cell-mediated acute rejection. *Transplantation* 2008; 86:1754–1761.
84. Neubert K, Meister S, Moser K, et al. The proteasome inhibitor bortezomib depletes plasma cells and protects mice with lupus-like disease from nephritis. *Nat Med* 2008;14:748–755.
85. O'Connor OA, Stewart AK, Vallone M, et al. A phase 1 dose escalation study of the safety and pharmacokinetics of the novel proteasome inhibitor carfilzomib (PR-171) in patients with hematologic malignancies. *Clin Cancer Res* 2009;15: 7085–7091.
86. Alsina M, Trudel S, Furman RR, et al. A phase I single-agent study of twice-weekly consecutive-day dosing of the proteasome inhibitor carfilzomib in patients with relapsed or refractory multiple myeloma or lymphoma. *Clin Cancer Res* 2012;18:4830–4840.
87. Jagannath S, Vij R, Stewart AK, et al. An open-label single-arm pilot phase II study (PX-171-003-A0) of low-dose, single-agent carfilzomib in patients with relapsed and refractory multiple myeloma. *Clin Lymphoma Myeloma Leuk* 2012;12:310–318.
88. Siegel DS, Martin T, Wang M, et al. A phase 2 study of single-agent carfilzomib (PX-171-003-A1) in patients with relapsed and refractory multiple myeloma. *Blood* 2012;120:2817–2825.
89. Siegel DS, Martin T, Wang M, et al. Results of PX-171-003-A1, an open-label, single-arm, phase 2 (Ph 2) study of carfilzomib (CFZ) in patients (pts) with relapsed and refractory multiple myeloma (MM). *Blood* 2012;120:2817–2825.
90. Vij R, Siegel DS, Jagannath S, et al. An open-label, single-arm, phase 2 study of single-agent carfilzomib in patients with relapsed and/or refractory multiple myeloma who have been previously treated with bortezomib. *Br J Haematol* 2012;158:739–748.
91. Vij R, Wang M, Kaufman JL, et al. An open-label, single-arm, phase 2 (PX-171-004) study of single-agent carfilzomib in bortezomib-naive patients with relapsed and/or refractory multiple myeloma. Blood 2012;119:5661–5670.
92. Papadopoulos K, Capua Siegel DS, Singhal SB, et al. Phase 1b evaluation of the safety and efficacy of a 30-minute IV infusion of carfilzomib in patients with relapsed and/or refractory multiple myeloma. *Blood* 2010;116:3024.
93. Lee SJ, Levitsky K, Parlati F, et al. Clinical activity of carfilzomib correlates with inhibition of multiple proteasome subunits: application of a novel pharmacodynamics assay. (In press).
94. Wang M, Martin T, Bensinger W, et al. Phase 2 dose-expansion study (PX-171-006) of carfilzomib, lenalidomide, and low-dose dexamethasone in relapsed or progressive multiple myeloma. *Blood* 2013;122:3122–3128.
95. Jakubowiak AJ, Dytfeld D, Griffith KA, et al. A phase 1/2 study of carfilzomib in combination with lenalidomide and low-dose dexamethasone as a frontline treatment for multiple myeloma. *Blood* 2012;120:1801–1809.
96. Richardson PG, Baz R, Wang L, et al. Investigational agent MLN9708, an oral proteasome inhibitor, in patients (Pts) with relapsed and/or refractory multiple myeloma (MM): results from the expansion cohorts of a phase 1 dose-escalation study. *Blood* 2011;118:301.
97. Richardson PG, Spencer A, Cannell P, et al. Phase 1 clinical evaluation of twice-weekly marizomib (NPI-0052), a novel proteasome inhibitor, in patients with relapsed/refractory multiple myeloma (MM). *Blood* 2011;118:302.
98. Roy V, Reeder C, LaPlant BR, et al. Phase 2 trial Of single agent MLN9708 in patients with relapsed multiple myeloma not refractory to bortezomib. *Blood* 2013;122:1944.
99. Hofmeister CC, Rosenbaum CA, Htut M, et al. Twice-weekly oral MLN9708 (ixazomib citrate), an investigational proteasome inhibitor, in combination with lenalidomide (len) and dexamethasone (dex) in patients (pts) with newly diagnosed multiple myeloma (MM): final phase 1 results and phase 2 data. *Blood* 2013;122:535.
100. Papadopoulos KP, Mendelson DS, Tolcher AW, et al. A phase I, open-label, dose-escalation study of the novel oral proteasome inhibitor (PI) ONX 0912 in patients with advanced refractory or recurrent solid tumors. *Blood* 2011;29:3075.
101. Kaufman JL, Siegel DS, Vij R, et al. Clinical profile of single-agent modified-release oprozomib tablets in patients (pts) with hematologic malignancies: updated results from a multicenter, open-label, dose escalation phase 1b/2 study. *Blood* 2013;122:3184.
102. Mulligan G, Mitsiades C, Bryant B, et al. Gene expression profiling and correlation with outcome in clinical trials of the proteasome inhibitor bortezomib. *Blood* 2007;109:3177–3188.
103. Loehr A, Degenhardt JD, Kwei KA, et al. Immunoglobulin expression is a major determinant of patient sensitivity to proteasome inhibitors. *Blood* 2013;122:1903.
104. Leung-Hagesteijn C, Erdmann N, Cheung G, et al. Xbp1s-negative tumor B cells and pre-plasmablasts mediate therapeutic proteasome inhibitor resistance in multiple myeloma. *Cancer Cell* 2013;24:289–304.

25 Poly (ADP-ribose) Polymerase Inhibitors

Alan Ashworth

INTRODUCTION

Cancer cells may harbor defects in DNA repair pathways leading to genomic instability. This can foster tumorigenesis but also provides a weakness that can be exploited therapeutically. Tumors with compromised ability to repair double-strand DNA breaks by homologous recombination, including those with defects in the *BRCA1* and *BRCA2* genes, are highly sensitive to blockade of the repair of DNA single-strand breaks, via the inhibition of the enzyme poly(ADP-ribose) (PARP). This provides the basis for a *synthetic lethal* approach to cancer therapy, which is showing considerable promise in the clinic.

CELLULAR DNA REPAIR PATHWAYS

DNA is continually damaged by environmental exposures and endogenous activities, such as DNA replication and cellular free-radical generation, which cause diverse lesions including base modifications, double-strand breaks (DSB), single-strand breaks (SSB), and intrastrand and interstrand cross-links.[1] These aberrations are repaired by distinct repair pathways, which are coordinated to maintain the stability and integrity of the genome. This faithful repair of DNA damage is an essential prerequisite for the maintenance of genomic integrity and cellular and organismal viability. Where one DNA strand is affected and the intact complementary strand is available as a template, the base-excision repair (BER), nucleotide-excision repair, or mismatch repair pathways are used and these pathways are highly efficient at repairing damage. DSBs, more problematic than SSBs because the complementary strand is not available as a template, are repaired by the homologous recombination (HR) or nonhomologous end-joining (NHEJ) pathways.[1]

Endogenous base damage, including SSBs, is the most common DNA aberration and it has been estimated that the average cell may repair 10,000 such lesions every day. BER is an important pathway for the repair of SSBs and involves the sensing of the lesion followed by the recruitment of a number of other proteins. PARP-1 (poly[ADP]ribose polymerase) is a critical component of the major "short-patch" BER pathway. PARP is an enzyme, discovered over 40 years ago,[2] that produces large branched chains of poly(ADP) ribose (PAR) from NAD^+. In humans, there are 17 members of the PARP gene family but most of these are poorly characterized.[3,4] The abundant nuclear protein PARP-1 senses and binds to DNA nicks and breaks, resulting in activation of catalytic activity causing poly(ADP)ribosylation of PARP-1 itself as well as other acceptor proteins including histones. This modification may signal the recruitment of other components of DNA repair pathways as well as modify their activity. The highly negatively charged PAR that is produced around the site of damage may also serve as an antirecombinogenic factor. In addition to the BER pathway PARP enzymes have been implicated in numerous cellular pathways.[3,4]

Two main DSB repair pathways are available within eukaryotic cells: NHEJ and HR.[5,6] HR can be further subdivided into the gene conversion (GC) and single-strand annealing (SSA) subpathways.[1] Both GC and SSA rely on sequence homology for repair whereas NHEJ uses no, or little, homology.[2,3] NHEJ is the most important pathway for the repair of DSBs during G_0, G_1, and early S phases of the cell cycle, although it is likely active throughout the cell cycle.[7,8] This form of DSB repair usually results in changes in DNA sequence at the break site and, occasionally, in the joining of previously unlinked DNA molecules, potentially resulting in gross chromosomal rearrangements such as translocations.[9] GC uses a homologous sequence, preferably the sister chromatid, as a template to resynthesize the DNA surrounding the DSB, and therefore generally results in accurate repair of the break. Repair by GC is critically dependent on the recombinase function of RAD51 and is facilitated by a number of other proteins. SSA also involves the use of homologous sequences for the repair of DSBs, but unlike GC, SSA is RAD51-independent and involves the annealing of DNA strands formed after resection at the DSB. The detailed mechanism of SSA is still obscure but it frequently results in the loss of one of the homologous sequences and deletion of the intervening sequence.[9] SSA is a potentially important pathway of mutagenesis because a significant fraction of mammalian genomes consist of repetitive elements. GC and SSA are cell-cycle regulated and are most active in S-G_2 phases of the cell cycle.[10]

THE DEVELOPMENT OF PARP INHIBITORS

PARP inhibitors were originally developed as chemopotentiators, which are agents that enhance the effects of DNA damage—a common mechanism of action of drugs used to treat cancer. The rationale was that inhibition of the repair of chemotherapy-induced DNA damage might give greater efficacy. Early studies using relatively nonspecific PARP inhibitors such as 3-aminobenzamide, demonstrated potential synergy with alkylating agents.[11] Subsequent studies with more potent PARP inhibitors demonstrated synergy with temozolomide, an observation that was taken into a clinical trial with AG014699,[12] a PARP inhibitor developed by Pfizer. This agent is now being developed by Clovis. Although the major focus of this chapter is the use of PARP inhibitors in synthetic lethal therapeutic strategies, their use in chemopotentiation in combination with chemotherapy remains under active investigation, as described later.

BRCA1 AND *BRCA2* MUTATIONS AND DNA REPAIR

Heterozygous germline mutations in the *BRCA1* and *BRCA2* genes confer a high risk of breast (up to 85% lifetime risk) and ovarian (10% to 40%) cancer in addition to a significantly increased risk of pancreatic, prostate, and male breast cancer.[13] The genes have been classified as tumor suppressors, because the wild-type *BRCA* allele is frequently lost in tumors, a phenomenon that occurs by a variety of mechanisms. The *BRCA1* and *BRCA2* genes encode large proteins that likely function in multiple cellular pathways, including transcription, cell-cycle regulation, and the maintenance of genome integrity. However, the roles of BRCA1 and BRCA2 in DNA repair have been best documented.[14]

BRCA1- and BRCA2-deficient cells are highly sensitive to ionizing radiation and display chromosomal instability, which is likely to be a direct consequence of unrepaired DNA damage.[14] The similar genomic instability in BRCA1- and BRCA2-deficient cells and the interaction of both BRCA1 and BRCA2 with RAD51 suggested a functional link between the three proteins in the RAD51-mediated DNA damage repair process. However, although BRCA2 is directly involved in RAD51-mediated repair, affecting the choice between GC and SSA, BRCA1 acts upstream of these pathways[15]; both GC and SSA are reduced in BRCA1-deficient cells, placing BRCA1 before the branch point of GC and SSA.[15]

BRCA1 has a role in signaling DNA damage and cell-cycle checkpoint regulation,[14,15] whereas BRCA2 has a more direct role in DNA repair itself. BRCA2 is thought to promote genomic stability through a role in the error-free repair of DSBs by GC via association with RAD51. Aberrations in *BRCA2*-deficient cells arise at least in part by the use of the SSA pathway. NHEJ, however, is apparently unaffected in BRCA2-deficient cells.[14,15] Loss of BRCA2, therefore, results in the repair of DSBs by preferential utilization of an error-prone mechanism, which potentially explains the apparent chromosome instability associated with *BRCA2* deficiency.[15]

The physical interaction between BRCA2 and RAD51 is essential for error-free DSB repair. BRCA2 is required for the localization of RAD51 to sites of DNA damage, where RAD51 forms the nucleoprotein filament required for recombination. The foci of the RAD51 protein are apparent in the nucleus after certain forms of DNA damage and these likely represent sites of repair by HR; BRCA2-deficient cells do not form RAD51 foci in response to DNA damage.[15] Two different domains within BRCA2 interact with RAD51, the eight BRC repeats in the central part of the protein and a distinct domain, TR2, at the C-terminus.[16]

PARP-1 INHIBITION AS A SYNTHETIC LETHAL THERAPEUTIC STRATEGY FOR THE TREATMENT OF BRCA-DEFICIENT CANCERS

Synthetic lethality is defined as the situation when a mutation in either of two genes individually has no effect, but combining the mutations leads to death.[17] This effect was first described and studied in genetically tractable organisms such as *Drosophila* and yeast.[17,18] This effect can arise because of a number of different gene–gene interactions. Examples include two genes in separate semiredundant or cooperating pathways, and two genes acting in the same pathway where loss of both critically affects flux through the pathway. The implication is that targeting one of these genes in a cancer where the other is defective should be selectively lethal to the tumor cells but not toxic to the normal cells. In principle, this should lead to a large therapeutic window.[19] The original suggestion that the concept of synthetic lethality could be used in the selection or development of cancer therapeutics came from Hartwell et al.,[18] and from experiments performed in yeast. Synthetic lethal screens have now been performed in a number of model organisms[20] and in human cells,[21] and these have revealed multiple potential gene–gene interactions, some of which could be exploited clinically. However, synthetic lethal therapies have not been clinically used until recently, when evidence has been provided for PARP-1 inhibition as a potential synthetic lethal approach for the treatment of *BRCA*-mutation–associated cancers.

PARP-1 inhibition causes failure of the repair of SSB lesions but does not affect DSB repair.[22] However, a persistent DNA SSB encountered by a DNA replication fork will cause stalling of the fork and may result in either fork collapse or the formation of a DSB.[23] Therefore, the loss of PARP-1 increases the formation of DNA lesions that might be repaired by GC. As a loss of function of either BRCA1 or BRCA2 impairs GC,[14,15] a loss of PARP-1 function in a BRCA1- or BRCA2-defective background could result in the generation of replication-associated DNA lesions normally repaired by sister chromatid exchange. If so, this might lead to cell-cycle arrest and/or cell death. Therefore, PARP inhibitors could be selectively lethal to cells lacking functional BRCA1 or BRCA2 but might be minimally toxic to normal cells. This would indicate a synthetic lethal interaction between PARP and BRCA1 or BRCA2. Exemplifying this principle, potent inhibitors of PARP were applied to cells deficient in either BRCA1 or BRCA2. Cell survival assays showed that cell lines lacking wild-type BRCA1 or BRCA2 were extremely sensitive to these agents compared with heterozygous mutant or wild-type cells.[24,25]

To explain these observations, a model was proposed whereby persistent single-strand gaps in DNA caused by PARP inhibition when encountered by a replication fork might trigger fork arrest, collapse, and/or a DSB.[26] Alternatively, PARP-1 trapped on DNA by the inhibition of enzyme activity might also cause a fork collapse. Normally, these DSBs would be repaired by RAD51-dependent GC.[14,15] However, in the absence of BRCA1 or BRCA2, the replication fork cannot be restarted and collapses, causing persistent chromatid breaks. When repaired by the alternative error-prone DSB repair mechanisms of SSA or NHEJ, large numbers of chromatid aberrations would be induced, leading to cell lethality.[26] The idea that the defect in GC is being targeted in BRCA-deficient cells is supported by the demonstration that deficiency in other genes implicated in HR also confers sensitivity to PARP inhibitors.[27] This further suggests that this approach may be more widely applicable in the treatment of sporadic cancers with impairments of the HR pathway or *BRCAness*[28] (see the following).

INITIAL CLINICAL RESULTS TESTING SYNTHETIC LETHALITY OF PARP INHIBITORS AND BRCA MUTATION

Phase I studies[29] established that olaparib (AstraZeneca, London, UK; formerly KU-0059436, KuDOS Pharmaceuticals, Cambridge, UK) could be administered safely as a single agent at a dose of 400 mg twice per day. Side effects were classified as mild and were unlike those typically experienced with cytotoxic chemotherapy. Significant and durable responses were observed in patients with germ-line *BRCA1* or *BRCA2* mutations and breast ovary or prostate cancer. Of the 19 mutation carriers enrolled, 9 had an objective response defined by Response Evaluation Criteria in Sold Tumors (RECIST) criteria and 12 had stable disease for more than 4 months in duration. A similar magnitude of clinical responses was observed in an expanded cohort.[30] These observations are impressive because the cohort had been heavily pretreated and most were resistant to a wide range of chemotherapies.[29,30]

Phase II studies were subsequently performed in advanced breast and ovarian cancers arising in *BRCA1* and *BRCA2* mutation carriers.[31,32] The reported response rate was 41% in the breast study and 52% in the ovarian group; both groups had been heavily pretreated. Again, the drug was well tolerated. Another study of *BRCA1/2* carriers with ovarian cancer compared olaparib with pegylated liposomal doxorubicin (PLD).[33] There was no significant difference in the response rates, but there were some differences in the patient characteristics and an unexpectedly high rate of response to PLD.

There are also reports of responses to PARP inhibitors in *BRCA2* mutation carriers with prostate[34] and pancreatic[35] cancer. A number of other PARP inhibitors are in clinical development (Table 25.1), and some of these have shown efficacy in the treatment of cancers arising in *BRCA1* or *BRCA2* mutation carriers.[36,37]

TABLE 25.1

PARP Inhibitors in Late Stage Clinical Development

Agent	Company	Phase III Trials
Olaparib	AstraZeneca (formerly KuDOS)	*BRCA*-mutant ovarian cancer
Niraparib	Tesaro (formerly Merck)	Platinum sensitive ovarian cancer *BRCA*-mutant breast cancer
Rucaparib	Clovis (formerly Pfizer)	Platinum sensitive ovarian cancer
Veliparib	AbbVie (formerly Abbot)	Undisclosed
BMN673	BioMarin (formerly Lead)	*BRCA*-mutant breast cancer

Adapted from Garber, K. PARP inhibitors bounce back. *Nat Rev Drug Discov* 2013;12:725–727.

THE USE OF PARP INHIBITORS IN SPORADIC CANCERS

Germline mutations in *BRCA1* or *BRCA2* are relatively common in hereditary breast and ovarian cancer. However, inactivation of *BRCA* genes by mutation in sporadic cancers is rare, at least in breast cancer, which may seem to limit the application of PARP inhibitors to a wider range of patients. However, many tumors display features in common with BRCA-deficient tumors, including similar defects in DNA repair due to either epigenetic mutation of *BRCA1*, such as promoter methylation, or mutation of other components of BRCA-associated pathways.[28] This *BRCAness* may make these tumors also susceptible to PARP inhibition.[28] For example, phosphatase and tensin homolog (*PTEN*) mutations, which occur with a frequency estimated at 50% to 80% in sporadic tumors,[38] may cause PARP inhibitor sensitivity in preclinical models, possibly because PTEN-null cells display BRCAness phenotypes, such as the inability to efficiently repair certain forms of DNA damage.[39]

Traditional histopathologic methods and, more recently, gene expression profiling approaches have shown the phenotypic overlap between triple-negative breast cancers, basal-like breast cancers, and *BRCA1* familial breast cancers.[40,41] In gene expression profiling studies, it has been observed that *BRCA1* familial cancers strongly segregate with basal-like tumors and share features such as high-grade and pushing margins.[28,40,41] Although the overlap is not absolute, it leads to the hypothesis that there may be a subset of sporadic breast cancers that exhibits features of BRCAness, including deficiencies in HR and that may be susceptible to treatment with drugs such as PARP inhibitors.[26]

There have been several studies of PARP inhibitors in sporadic ovarian cancer. A study by Lederman[42] showed in a maintenance study following the response to platinum therapy a significant benefit in terms of progression-free survival (PFS) of olaparib compared to placebo. This was even more pronounced when the subgroup of BRCA mutation carriers were examined.[43] In both cases, the overall survival (OS) advantage was less than the PFS, but in the case of the BRCA mutation group, this reached statistical significance. Gelmon[44] also showed activity in sporadic ovarian cancer. In contrast, a study in sporadic triple-negative breast cancer failed to observe any benefit, although the study was small and the patients were heavily pretreated.[44]

Iniparib (initially reported as a PARP inhibitor) showed an overall survival benefit in a Phase II trial of triple-negative breast cancer in combination with gemcitabine and carboplatin compared with chemotherapy alone.[45] However, a subsequent Phase III study showed no improvement in PFS.[45] The reasons for this are uncertain, but significant questions have been raised about whether iniparib is indeed a bona fide PARP inhibitor. Therefore, it is now generally conceded that studies of iniparib have no implications for PARP inhibitors as a drug class.[46]

Which population of patients lacking a *BRCA1* or *BRCA2* mutation might benefit from PARP inhibitors remains unclear. This is likely to require the development of a clinical test to identify prospectively tumors with intrinsic sensitivity. Presently, most efforts are directed at developing assays of DNA repair deficiency.[47]

MECHANISMS OF RESISTANCE TO PARP INHIBITORS

Resistance to targeted therapy frequently occurs, but it was unclear how resistance might arise to a synthetic lethal therapy.[48] Potential mechanisms of resistance to PARP inhibitors have, however, been elucidated both directly in vitro, in mouse models, and in the clinic.[48] An in vitro model for resistance was developed by producing cells from the highly PARP inhibitor–sensitive BRCA2-deficient cell line CAPAN1, which carries a c.6174delT *BRCA2* frameshift mutation. CAPAN1 cells cannot form damage-induced RAD51 foci, are defective for HR, and are extremely sensitive to treatment with PARP inhibitors.[49] PARP inhibitor–resistant clones were highly resistant (over 1,000-fold) to the drug and were also cross-resistant to the DNA cross-linking agent cisplatin, but not to the microtubule-stabilizing drug docetaxel. PARP inhibitors and cisplatin both exert their effects on BRCA-deficient cells by increasing the frequency of misrepaired DSBs in the absence of effective HR. Therefore, this observation indicates that the resistance of PARP inhibitor–resistant clones to PARP inhibitors might be because of restored HR. This contention was supported by the acquisition in PARP inhibitor–resistant clone cells of the ability to form RAD51 foci after PARP inhibitor treatment or exposure to irradiation.

DNA sequencing of PARP inhibitor–resistant clones revealed the unexpected presence of novel *BRCA2* alleles that resulted in the elimination of the c.6174delT mutation and restoration of an open reading frame.[49] Therefore, in this case, resistance arises because of gain of function mutations in the synthetic lethal partner (BRCA2) rather than the direct drug target (PARP). Alternative mechanisms of PARP inhibitor resistance have also been described.[48] A mouse model of *BRCA1*-associated mammary gland cancer demonstrated the efficacy of olaparib in vivo and was used to study mechanisms of resistance.[50] Resistance seemed to be caused by the upregulation of *ABCB1a/b*, which encode P-glycoprotein pumps; this effect could be reversed with the P-glycoprotein inhibitor tariquidar. In addition, other alterations in DNA repair pathways have been proposed to compensate for BRCA1 deficiency resulting in PARP inhibitor deficiency.[48]

Studies of the mechanisms of resistance to PARP inhibitors in patient material are still at an early stage. Initial studies addressed the mechanism of resistance to platinum salts in *BRCA* mutation carriers. Cisplatin and carboplatin are part of the standard of care for the treatment of ovarian cancer, including individuals with *BRCA1* or *BRCA2* mutations. Platinum salts are thought to exert their BRCA-selective effects by a similar mechanism to PARP inhibitors.[15] Clinical observations suggest that *BRCA* mutation carriers with ovarian cancer usually respond better to these agents than patients without *BRCA* mutations[51,52]; however, resistance does eventually occur. To investigate this effect, *BRCA1* and *BRCA2* have been sequenced in tumor material from mutation carriers.[49,53] These studies revealed mutations in *BRCA1* or *BRCA2* that restored the open reading frame and likely contributed to platinum resistance. These observations suggest that specific mutations in *BRCA1* or *BRCA2* and sensitivity to therapeutics in cell lines and patients can be suppressed by intragenic deletion. Pre-

CANCER THERAPEUTICS

sumably, these mutations occur randomly and are then selected for by differential drug sensitivity. Therefore, the best use of these agents is likely to be earlier in the disease process when the disease burden is smaller, which will reduce the probability of resistance based on stochastic genetic reversion. Recently, similar observations of revertant *BRCA* alleles were made in two patients who became resistant after an initial response to olaparib.[54] Although preliminary, these results suggest that this mechanism is responsible for at least some of the clinical resistance observed. Doubtless, as with other targeted therapies, multiple resistance mechanisms will be implicated as further patients are studied.[48]

PROSPECTS

Currently, the treatments for cancers arising in carriers of *BRCA1* or *BRCA2* mutations are the same as those that occur sporadically matched for tumor pathology and age of onset. However, tumors in *BRCA1* or *BRCA2* mutation carriers lack wild-type *BRCA1* or *BRCA2*, but normal tissues retain a single wild-type copy of the relevant gene. This is a potentially targetable alteration that provides the basis for new mechanism-based approaches to the treatment of cancer. The biochemical difference in capacity to carry out HR between the tumor and normal tissues, in a *BRCA1* or *BRCA2* carrier, provides the rationale for this approach. Inhibiting the DNA repair protein PARP results in the generation of specific DNA lesions that require BRCA1 and BRCA2 specialized repair function(s) for their removal. Preclinical data indicate that tumors defective in wild-type BRCA1 or BRCA2 could be much more sensitive to PARP inhibition than unaffected heterozygous tissues, providing a potentially large therapeutic window. The safety and efficacy of this approach is currently being tested in clinical trials, which, if successful, may lead to registration for routine clinical use of one or more PARP inhibitors.[37]

Synthetic lethality by combinatorial targeting of DNA repair pathways may have usefulness as a therapeutic approach beyond familial cancers. The majority of solid tumors also exhibit genomic instability and aneuploidy. This suggests that pathways involved in the maintenance of genomic stability are dysfunctional in a significant proportion of neoplastic disorders.[47] Understanding which specialized DNA damage response and repair pathways are abrogated in sporadic tumor subtypes may allow for the development of therapies that target the residual repair pathways on which the cancer, but not normal tissue, is now completely dependent. These potential therapies may significantly improve response rates while causing fewer treatment-related toxicities. However, these approaches may be associated with mechanism-associated resistance, and careful consideration of their optimal use will be required.

REFERENCES

1. Hoeijmakers JH. Genome maintenance mechanisms for preventing cancer. *Nature* 2001;411:366–374.
2. Chambon P, Weill JD, Mandel P. Nicotinamide mononucleotide activation of new DNA-dependent polyadenylic acid synthesizing nuclear enzyme. *Biochem Biophys Res Commun* 1963;11:39–43.
3. Amé JC, Spenlehauer C, de Murcia G. The PARP superfamily. *Bioessays* 2004;26:882–893.
4. Otto H, Reche PA, Bazan F, et al. In silico characterization of the family of PARP-like poly(ADP-ribosyl)transferases (pARTs). *BMC Genomics* 2005;6:139.
5. van Gent DC, Hoeijmakers JH, Kanaar R. Chromosomal stability and the DNA double-stranded break connection. *Nat Rev Genet* 2001;2:196–206.
6. Shin DS, Chahwan C, Huffman JL, et al. Structure and function of the double-strand break repair machinery. *DNA Repair (Amst)* 2004;3: 863–873.
7. Takata M, Sasaki MS, Sonoda E, et al. Homologous recombination and non-homologous end-joining pathways of DNA double-strand break repair have overlapping roles in the maintenance of chromosomal integrity in vertebrate cells. *EMBO J* 1998;17:5497–5508.
8. Rothkamm K, Krüger I, Thompson LH, et al. Pathways of DNA double-strand break repair during the mammalian cell cycle. *Mol Cell Biol* 2003;23: 5706–5715.
9. Stark JM, Pierce AJ, Oh J, et al. Genetic steps of mammalian homologous repair with distinct mutagenic consequences. *Mol Cell Biol* 2004;24: 9305–9316.
10. Elliott B, Richardson C, Jasin M. Chromosomal translocation mechanisms at intronic alu elements in mammalian cells. *Mol Cell* 2005;17:885–894.
11. Durkacz BW, Omidiji O, Gray DA, et al. (ADP-ribose)n participates in DNA excision repair. *Nature* 1980;283(5747):593–596.
12. Tertoli L, Graziani G. Chemosensitisation by PARP inhibitors in cancer therapy. *Pharmacol Res* 2005;52:25–33.
13. Wooster R, Weber BL. Breast and ovarian cancer. *N Engl J Med* 2003;348: 2339–2347.
14. Gudmundsdottir K, Ashworth A. The roles of BRCA1 and BRCA2 and associated proteins in the maintenance of genomic stability. *Oncogene* 2006;25: 5864–5874.
15. Tutt AN, Lord CJ, McCabe N, et al. Exploiting the DNA repair defect in BRCA mutant cells in the design of new therapeutic strategies for cancer. *Cold Spring Harb Symp Quant Biol* 2005;70:139–148.
16. Lord CJ, Ashworth A. RAD51, BRCA2 and DNA repair: a partial resolution. *Nat Struct Mol Biol* 2007;14:461–462.
17. Dobzhansky T. Genetics of natural populations: Xiii. Recombination and variability in populations of *Drosophila pseudoobscura*. *Genetics* 1946;31:269–290.
18. Hartwell LH, Szankasi P, Roberts CJ, et al. Integrating genetic approaches into the discovery of anticancer drugs. *Science* 1997;278:1064–1068.
19. Kaelin WG Jr. The concept of synthetic lethality in the context of anticancer therapy. *Nat Rev Cancer* 2005;5:689–698.
20. Ooi SL, Pan X, Peyser BD, et al. Global synthetic-lethality analysis and yeast functional profiling. *Trends Genet* 2006;22:56–63.
21. Iorns E, Lord CJ, Turner N, et al. Utilizing RNA interference to enhance cancer drug discovery. *Nat Rev Drug Discov* 2007;6:556–568.
22. Noël G, Giocanti N, Fernet M, et al. Poly(ADP-ribose) polymerase (PARP-1) is not involved in DNA double-strand break recovery. *BMC Cell Biol* 2003;4:7.
23. Haber JE. DNA recombination: the replication connection. *Trends Biochem Sci* 1999;24:271–275.
24. Farmer H, McCabe N, Lord CJ, et al. Targeting the DNA repair defect in BRCA mutant cells as a therapeutic strategy. *Nature* 2005;434:917–921.
25. Bryant HE, Schultz N, Thomas HD, et al. Specific killing of *BRCA2*-deficient tumours with inhibitors of poly(ADP-ribose) polymerase. *Nature* 2005;434: 913–917.
26. Ashworth A. A synthetic lethal therapeutic approach: PARP inhibitors for the treatment of cancers deficient in double-strand break repair. *J Clin Oncol* 2008;26:3785–3790.
27. McCabe N, Turner NC, Lord CJ, et al. Deficiency in the repair of DNA damage by homologous recombination and sensitivity to poly(ADP-ribose) polymerase inhibition. *Cancer Res* 2006;66:8109–8115.
28. Turner N, Tutt A, Ashworth A. Hallmarks of 'BRCAness' in sporadic cancers. *Nat Rev Cancer* 2004;4:814–819.
29. Fong PC, Boss DS, Yap TA, et al. Inhibition of poly(ADP-ribose) polymerase in tumors from BRCA mutation carriers. *N Engl J Med* 2009;361:123–134.
30. Fong PC, Yap TA, Boss DS, et al. Poly(ADP)-ribose polymerase (PARP) inhibition: frequent durable responses in BRCA carrier ovarian cancer correlating with platinum-free interval. *J Clin Oncol* 2010;28:2512–2519.
31. Audeh MW, Carmichael J, Penson RT, et al. Oral poly(ADP-ribose) polymerase inhibitor olaparib in patients with *BRCA1* or *BRCA2* mutations and recurrent ovarian cancer: a proof-of-concept trial. *Lancet* 2010;376:245–251.
32. Tutt A, Robson M, Garber JE, et al. Oral poly(ADP-ribose) polymerase inhibitor olaparib in patients with *BRCA1* or *BRCA2* mutations and advanced breast cancer: a proof-of-concept trial. *Lancet* 2010;376:235–244.
33. Kaye SB, Lubinski J, Matulonis U, et al. Phase II, open-label, randomized, multicenter study comparing the efficacy and safety of olaparib, a poly (ADP-ribose) polymerase inhibitor, and pegylated liposomal doxorubicin in patients with BRCA1 or BRCA2 mutations and recurrent ovarian cancer. *J Clin Oncol* 2012;30:372–379.
34. Sandhu SK, Omlin A, Hylands L et al. Poly (ADP-ribose) polymerase (PARP) inhibitors for the treatment of advanced germline BRCA2 mutant prostate cancer. *Ann Oncol* 2013;24:1416–1418.
35. Fogelman DR, Wolff RA, Kopetz S, et al. Evidence for the efficacy of Iniparib, a PARP-1 inhibitor, in BRCA2-associated pancreatic cancer. *Anticancer Res* 2011;31:1417–1420.
36. Maxwell KN, Domchek SM. Cancer treatment according to BRCA1 and BRCA2 mutations *Nat Rev Clin Oncol* 2012;9:520–528.
37. Garber K. PARP inhibitors bounce back. *Nat Rev Drug Discov* 2013;12: 725–727.
38. Salmena L, Carracedo A, Pandolfi PP. Tenets of PTEN tumor suppression. *Cell* 2008;133:403–414.
39. Mendes-Pereira AM, Martin SA, Brough R, et al. Synthetic lethal targeting of PTEN mutant cells with PARP inhibitors. *EMBO Mol Med* 2009;1:315–322.
40. Foulkes WD, Stefansson IM, Chappuis PO, et al. Germline BRCA1 mutations and a basal epithelial phenotype in breast cancer. *J Natl Cancer Inst* 2003;95:1482–1485.

41. Turner NC, Reis-Filho JS. Basal-like breast cancer and the BRCA1 phenotype. *Oncogene* 2006;25:5846–5853.
42. Ledermann J, Harter P, Gourley C, et al. Olaparib maintenance therapy in platinum-sensitive relapsed ovarian cancer. *N Engl J Med* 2012;366:1382–1392.
43. Ledermann JA, Harter P, Gourley C. Olaparib maintenance therapy in patients with platinum-sensitive relapsed serous ovarian cancer (SOC) and a BRCA mutation (BRCAm). *J Clin Oncol* 2013;31 (suppl; abstr 5505).
44. Gelmon KA, Tischkowitz M, Mackay H, et al. Olaparib in patients with recurrent high-grade serous or poorly differentiated ovarian carcinoma or triple-negative breast cancer: a phase 2, multicentre, open-label, non-randomised study. *Lancet Oncol* 2011;12:852–861.
45. O'Shaughnessy J, Osborne C, Pippen J, et al. Iniparib plus chemotherapy in metastatic triple-negative breast cancer. *N Engl J Med* 2011;3:205–214.
46. Mateo J, Ong M, Tan DS, et al. Appraising iniparib, the PARP inhibitor that never was—what must we learn? *Nat Rev Clin Oncol* 2013;10:688–696.
47. Lord CJ, Ashworth A. The DNA damage response and cancer therapy. *Nature* 2012;481:287–294.
48. Lord CJ, Ashworth A. Mechanisms of resistance to therapies targeting BRCA-mutant cancers. *Nat Med* 2013;19:1381–1388.
49. Edwards S, Brough R, Lord CJ, et al. Resistance to therapy caused by intragenic deletion in *BRCA2*. *Nature* 2008;451(7182):1111–1115.
50. Rottenberg S, Jaspers JE, Kersbergen A, et al. High sensitivity of *BRCA1*-deficient mammary tumors to the PARP inhibitor AZD2281 alone and in combination with platinum drugs. *Proc Natl Acad Sci U S A* 2008;105: 17079–17084.
51. Cass I, Baldwin RL, Varkey T, et al. Improved survival in women with BRCA-associated ovarian carcinoma. *Cancer* 2003;97:2187–2195.
52. Pal T, Permuth-Wey J, Kapoor R, et al. Improved survival in BRCA2 carriers with ovarian cancer. *Fam Cancer* 2007;6:113–119.
53. Sakai W, Swisher EM, Karlan BY, et al. Secondary mutations as a mechanism of cisplatin resistance in *BRCA2*-mutated cancers. *Nature* 2008;451: 1116–1120.
54. Barber LJ, Sandhu S, Chen L, et al. Secondary mutations in BRCA2 associated with clinical resistance to a PARP inhibitor. *J Pathol* 2013;229:422–429.

26 Miscellaneous Chemotherapeutic Agents

M. Sitki Copur, Scott Nicholas Gettinger, Sarah B. Goldberg, and Hari A. Deshpande

HOMOHARRINGTONINE AND OMACETAXINE

Homoharringtonine and its congener, harringtonine, are cephalotaxine esters isolated from the evergreen tree *Cephalotaxus hainanensis*, which are distributed throughout southern and northeastern China. The two differ only by a single methylene group, but both have a similar activity against murine leukemia.[1] The primary action of homoharringtonine appears to be the inhibition of protein synthesis and chain elongation through binding to 80S ribosome in eukaryotic cells.[2] DNA effects may also be important, involving a block in progression of cells from G1 phase into S phase and from G2 phase into M phase.[3] Homoharringtonine exhibits a triphasic plasma decay with a terminal half-life of 65.3 hours and apparent volume of distribution of 2.4 L/kg.[4] In early phase I studies, homoharringtonine was administered as a 10 to 360 minute infusion daily for 10 days.[5] Dose-limiting cardiovascular toxicity with hypotension began 4 or more hours after drug administration, which was alleviated by interrupting the infusion or by fluid administration and prolonging the duration of administration. Initial clinical studies with homoharringtonine in China showed activity against acute myeloid leukemia (AML) and chronic phase chronic myeloid leukemia (CML).[6] Variable activity was observed in the initial series of phase II trials in pediatric and adult patients with acute leukemia. In early studies of homoharringtonine, a continuous intravenous (IV) infusion at 2.5 mg/m^2 per day for 10 to 14 days per month induced complete hematologic and cytogenetic responses in 72% and 31% of patients, respectively, with chronic phase CML.[7]

The greater availability of homoharringtonine led to its further testing and the development of a semisynthetic cephalotaxine ester, omacetaxine mepesuccinate.[2] The mechanism of action of omacetaxine includes inhibition of protein synthesis and is independent of direct Bcr-Abl binding. In vitro, it reduces protein levels of the Bcr-Abl oncoprotein and Mcl-1, an antiapoptotic B-cell lymphoma 2 (Bcl-2) family member. The antileukemic effect of omacetaxine is not affected by the presence of mutations in Bcr-Abl.[8] Omacetaxine is absorbed following subcutaneous administration of 1.25 mg/m^2 twice daily for 11 days with a mean half-life of 6 hours, and a volume of distribution of 141 +/−93.4 L. A phase 2 trial assessed the efficacy of omacetaxine in CML patients with T315I and tyrosine–kinase inhibitor failure. Patients received subcutaneous omacetaxine 1.25 mg/m^2 twice daily on days 1 through 14, every 28 days until hematologic response or a maximum of 6 cycles, and then days 1 through 7 every 28 days as maintenance. Complete hematologic response was achieved in 77%, with a median response duration of 9.1 months. Of patients, 23% achieved a major cytogenetic response, including a complete cytogenetic response in 16%. Hematologic toxicity included thrombocytopenia (76%), neutropenia (44%), and anemia (39%) and was typically manageable by dose reduction. Nonhematologic adverse events were mostly grade 1/2 and included infection, diarrhea, and nausea.[9]

L-ASPARAGINASE

L-Asparaginase (L-asparagine aminohydrolase, EC 3.5.1.1), which catalyzes the hydrolysis of the essential amino acid L-asparagine to L-aspartic acid and ammonia, is a naturally occurring enzyme in some microorganisms.[10,11] Although cancer cells depend on an exogenous source of L-asparagine for survival, normal cells can synthesize asparagine. In addition to the depletion of L-asparagine, it may exert its antitumor activity through a glutaminase effect, depleting essential glutamine stores and leading to the inhibition of DNA biosynthesis. It comes in three preparations, two of which are native forms purified from bacterial sources, *Escherichia coli* and *Erwinia carotovora*. A third preparation, pegylated (PEG)-L-asparaginase, is a chemically modified form of the enzyme in which native *E. coli* L-asparaginase has been covalently conjugated to polyethylene glycol.[12]

After an intramuscular (IM) injection, peak plasma levels, approximately one-half of those achieved with IV administration, are reached within 14 to 24 hours. Plasma protein binding is 30%. The pharmacokinetics vary depending on the source of the enzyme.[13] Pharmacokinetic studies in newly diagnosed children with acute lymphocytic leukemia (ALL) have shown peak serum concentrations in the range of 1 to 10 IU/mL in 24 to 48 hours of a single dose of 2,500 to 25,000 IU/m^2 of the enzyme derived from *E. coli*. After a single dose of 25,000 IU/m^2, peak serum levels are reached within 24 hours. PEG-L-asparaginase, when administered at a dose of 2,500 IU/m^2, achieves peak drug levels at 72 to 96 hours and has a significantly longer half-life (5.7 days) than the *E. coli* L-asparaginase preparation.[13] Clinical trials have demonstrated the efficacy, safety, and tolerability of PEG-L-asparaginase administered intramuscularly, subcutaneously, or intravenously as part of multiagent chemotherapy regimens in the management of newly diagnosed and relapsed pediatric and adult ALL. L-Asparaginase can antagonize antineoplastic effects of methotrexate if given concurrently or immediately before. These two drugs should be administered sequentially at least 24 hours apart. L-Asparaginase has also been shown to inhibit the metabolic clearance of vincristine and can result in increased neurotoxicity. Toxicity is less pronounced if L-asparaginase is administered after vincristine. Hypersensitivity reactions occur in up to 25% of patients as a skin rash and urticaria or serious anaphylactic reactions. The risk increases with repeat exposure, and as a single-agent use without steroids. PEG-L-asparaginase is less immunogenic than the native nonpegylated forms of the enzyme. A number of other side effects are observed that are secondary to the inhibitory effects of L-asparaginase on cellular protein synthesis. Decreased serum levels of insulin, key lipoproteins, and albumin have been reported. L-Asparaginase can cause alterations in thyroid function tests as early as 2 days after an administered dose, possibly secondary to a reduction in the serum levels of thyroxine-binding globulin. Alterations in coagulation parameters with prolonged thrombin time, prothrombin time, and partial thromboplastin time have been observed. Patients treated with L-asparaginase are at an increased risk for bleeding or thromboembolic events.[14] L-Asparaginase is contraindicated in patients with a prior history of pancreatitis, because there is a 10% incidence of acute pancreatitis. Neurologic toxicity includes lethargy, confusion, agitation, hallucinations, and/or coma. In contrast to the other anticancer agents used to treat ALL, myelosuppression is rare.

BLEOMYCIN

Bleomycin is a glycopeptide antibiotic produced by the bacterium *Streptomyces verticillus*. The most active chemotherapeutical forms are bleomycin A_2 and B_2.[15] The effect of bleomycin is cell cycle specific, because its main effects are mediated in the G_2 and M phases of the cell cycle.[16] The exact mechanism for DNA strand scission has been suggested to be due to bleomycin's chelating of metal ions (primarily iron) and producing a pseudoenzyme that reacts with oxygen to produce superoxide- and hydroxide-free radicals, thus cleaving DNA. Alternatively, bleomycin may bind at specific sites in the DNA strand and induce scission by abstracting the hydrogen atom from the base, resulting in strand cleavage as the base undergoes a Criegee-type rearrangement, or bleomycin may form an alkali-labile lesion.[17] Bleomycin is used in the treatment of Hodgkin lymphoma (as a component of the ABVD and BEACOPP regimen), squamous cell carcinomas, and testicular cancer; in the treatment of plantar warts,[18] as a means of effecting pleurodesis,[19] as well as an intralesional agent with electrochemotherapy in the management of cutaneous malignancies.[20]

The oral bioavailability is poor. It must be administered via IV or IM routes. The initial distribution half-life is 10 to 20 minutes with a terminal half-life of 3 hours. Bleomycin can be administered via the intracavitary route to control malignant pleural effusions or ascites, or both. Approximately 45% to 55% of an administered intracavitary dose of bleomycin is absorbed into the systemic circulation. Elimination is primarily via the kidneys, and approximately 60% to 70% of an administered dose is excreted unchanged in the urine. Dose reductions are required if creatinine clearance is less than 25 mL per minute.

Bleomycin-induced pneumonitis, the dose-limiting toxicity of the drug, occurs in 10% of patients, and is dependent on the cumulative dose.[21] The risk increases in patients older than 70 years and in those who receive a total cumulative dose greater than 400 U. In addition, patients with an underlying lung disease, prior irradiation to the chest or mediastinum, and exposure to high concentrations of inspired oxygen are at increased risk. Increased use of granulocyte colony-stimulating factor (G-CSF) has been paralleled by an increased incidence of bleomycin-induced pulmonary toxicity. The exacerbating effects of G-CSFs seem to be associated with a marked infiltration of activated neutrophils along with the lung injury caused by the direct effects of bleomycin.[22,23] In a retrospective review, 18% of a total of 141 patients with Hodgkin lymphoma treated with a bleomycin-containing regimen developed pulmonary toxicity. G-CSF use was one of the key factors associated with the development of this complication, and omission of bleomycin had no impact on clinical outcomes.[24] Similarly the combination of brentuximab vedotin and ABVD was associated with excessive pulmonary toxicity, indicating that brentuximab vedotin and bleomycin should not be used together.[25]

Patients with bleomycin-induced pulmonary toxicity may present with cough, dyspnea, dry inspiratory crackles, and infiltrates on chest radiograph. Pulmonary function testing is the most sensitive approach to monitor patients, and pulmonary function tests should be obtained at baseline and before each cycle of therapy, with a specific focus on the carbon monoxide diffusion capacity and vital capacity. A decrease greater than 15% in either diffusion capacity of carbon monoxide or vital capacity should mandate immediate discontinuation of bleomycin. Early clinical trials and isolated case reports suggest that bleomycin-induced acute hypersensitivity reactions occur in 1% of patients with lymphoma and less than 0.5% of those with solid tumors. The reactions are mainly characterized by high-grade fever, chills, hypotension, and, in a few cases, cardiovascular collapse, which can lead to death. The exact mechanism of these reactions is unclear, but is thought to be related to the release of endogenous pyrogens from the host cells. Supportive care, including hydration, steroids, antipyretics, and antihistamines, may resolve the symptoms.

Clinicians should monitor their patients for any signs and symptoms of acute hyperpyrexic reactions during bleomycin administration. Because the onset of the reactions can occur with any dose of bleomycin and at any time, routine test dosing does not seem to predict when drug reactions may occur.[26] Mucocutaneous toxicity presents as mucositis, erythema, hyperpigmentation, induration, hyperkeratosis, and skin peeling, which may progress to ulceration, and usually develops in the 2nd and 3rd week of treatment and after a cumulative dose of 150 to 200 U of the drug. Levels of bleomycin hydrolase are relatively low in lung and skin tissue, perhaps offering an explanation as to why these normal tissues are more adversely affected by bleomycin. Myelosuppression and immunosuppression are relatively mild. In rare cases, vascular events, including myocardial infarction, stroke, and Raynaud phenomenon, have been reported.

PROCARBAZINE

Originally prepared as a monoamine oxidase inhibitor, procarbazine is a prodrug, which after oxidation of the hydrazine in the liver, undergoes a complex enzymatic and chemical breakdown to its alkylating and methylating species.[27,28] The precise mechanism of action is uncertain, but may involve damaging the DNA, RNA or transfer RNA, and the inhibition of protein synthesis. Procarbazine is a cell-cycle phase-nonspecific antineoplastic agent. This agent was initially approved by the U.S. Food and Drug Administration (FDA) in 1969 as part of the MOPP (mechlorethamine, vincristine, procarbazine, and prednisone) regimen for the treatment of Hodgkin lymphoma. Since then, it has also demonstrated clinical activity in non-Hodgkin lymphoma, cutaneous T-cell lymphoma, and brain tumors.

Procarbazine is rapidly and completely absorbed from the gastrointestinal tract. Following oral administration, peak drug levels are reached within 10 to 15 minutes. Procarbazine crosses the blood–brain barrier and rapidly equilibrates between plasma and cerebrospinal fluid after oral administration. Peak cerebrospinal fluid drug concentrations are reached within 30 to 90 minutes after drug administration. The biologic half-life of procarbazine hydrochloride in both plasma and cerebrospinal fluid is approximately 1 hour. Procarbazine is metabolized to active and inactive metabolites by chemical breakdown in an aqueous solution and the liver microsomal P-450 system. Approximately 70% of procarbazine is excreted in urine within 24 hours, and less than 5% to 10% of the drug is eliminated in an unchanged form.[29,30]

A careful food and drug history is required before starting a patient on procarbazine therapy, because there are several potential drug–drug and drug–food interactions. Patients should avoid tyramine-containing foods, such as dark beer, wine, cheese, yogurt, bananas, and smoked foods. Procarbazine produces a disulfiramlike reaction with concurrent use of alcohol. Acute hypertensive reactions may occur with coadministration of tricyclic antidepressants and sympathomimetic drugs. Concurrent use of procarbazine with antihistamines and other central nervous system (CNS) depressants can result in CNS and/or respiratory depression.

Dose-limiting toxicity is myelosuppression, more commonly thrombocytopenia, and the nadir in platelet count is generally observed at 4 weeks. Patients with glucose-6-phosphate dehydrogenase deficiency can develop hemolytic anemia while receiving procarbazine therapy. Stepwise dose increments over the first few days of drug administration may minimize gastrointestinal intolerance. On rare occasions, procarbazine may induce interstitial pneumonitis, which mandates the discontinuation of therapy. Azoospermia and infertility after treatment with MOPP can be attributed, in part, to procarbazine. Procarbazine is associated with an increased risk of secondary malignancies, especially acute leukemia.

VISMODEGIB

Vismodegib (Erivedge, GDC-0449, Genentech) is a first-in-class, small-molecule inhibitor of the Hedgehog pathway. It binds to and inhibits smoothened, a transmembrane protein that is involved in Hedgehog signaling.[31] Pharmacodynamic downmodulation in the Hedgehog pathway was shown by a 90% decrease in transcription factor Gli1 mRNA in basal-cell carcinoma biopsy specimens of patients treated for a month. One-month vismodegib treatment also significantly reduced tumor proliferation, as assessed by Ki-67 expression, but did not change apoptosis, as assessed by cleaved caspase 3. The extent of Gli1 downmodulation does not seem to correlate with pharmacokinetic levels of vismodegib in individual patients. Vismodegib is absorbed from the gastrointestinal tract, with an oral bioavailability of 32%. Food does not affect drug exposure. Elimination is mainly hepatic, with excretion in feces. The median steady-state concentration is not changed by increasing the dose from 150 mg to 270 mg, and the median time to steady state is 14 days. The half-life is estimated at 8 days after a single dose. Intermittent doses (e.g., three times per week or once per week) were associated with a decrease of 50% and 80% in effective plasma levels of unbound drug, respectively, thus reinforcing the recommended dose and schedule of 150 mg orally daily.[32] Vismodegib is approved for the treatment of adults with metastatic basal-cell carcinoma that has recurred following surgery or in those who are not candidates for surgery and who are not candidates for radiation.[33]

No dose-limiting toxic effects or grade 5 events have been observed. However, 54% of patients receiving vismodegib discontinued the medication owing to side effects, and only one out of give eligible patients was able to continue vismodegib for 18 months. Abdominal pain, fatigue, weight loss, dysgeusia, and anorexia were reasons for discontinuation of the drug. When vismodegib was withdrawn, dysgeusia and muscle cramps ceased within 1 month, and scalp and body hair started to regrow within 3 months. Other side effects reported include hyponatremia, dyspnea, muscle spasm, atrial fibrillation, aspiration, back pain, corneal abrasion, dehydration, keratitis, lymphopenia, pneumonia, urinary tract infection, and a prolonged QT interval.[34]

ADO-TRASTUZUMAB EMTANSINE

Ado-trastuzumab emtansine (T-DM1), is a HER2-targeted antibody-drug conjugate (ADC). It is a novel compound composed of trastuzumab, a stable thioether linker, and DM1. DM1, a derivative of maytansine, is a microtubule polymerization inhibitor with activity similar to that of vinca alkaloids. T-DM1 is taken up into cells after binding to HER2, allowing for cytotoxic drug delivery specifically to cells overexpressing HER2. It has a drug-to-antibody ratio of approximately 3.5:1. T-DM1 is administered intravenously every 3 weeks and has been tested in a phase I trial at doses ranging from 0.3 to 4.8 mg/kg. The maximally tolerated dose is 3.6 mg/kg, which was the dose used in further phase II–III trials. T-DM1 is metabolized by the liver, via CYP3A4/5, and has a half-life of 3.5 days.[35]

T-DM1 is approved for use in patients with metastatic HER2-positive breast cancer who have received prior trastuzumab and a taxane. This approval was based on the results of the EMILIA trial, which randomized 991 patients with HER2-positive unresectable, locally advanced or metastatic breast cancer to T-DM1 3.6 mg/kg IV every 21 days or lapatinib 1,250 mg daily plus capecitabine 1,000 mg/m^2 on days 1 through 14 every 21 days. All patients were previously treated with trastuzumab and a taxane. T-DM1 resulted in a progression-free survival of 9.6 months compared to 6.4 months for lapatinib plus capecitabine (hazard ratio [HR] 0.65; 95% confidence interval [CI] 0.55 to 0.77; p <0.001). The response rate and overall survival was also higher with T-DM1 compared to lapatinib plus capecitabine.[36]

Although maytansine itself is associated with significant toxicity, T-DM1 is very well tolerated overall, which is likely due to the targeted nature of the compound. Side effects from T-DM1 include thrombocytopenia, hepatotoxicity, hypersensitivity/infusion reactions, and cardiotoxicity. Nausea, fatigue, headaches, and anemia are also common. The left ventricular ejection fraction should be monitored prior to and at least every 3 months during therapy because of the potential for cardiac dysfunction.

SIROLIMUS AND TEMSIROLIMUS

Sirolimus (rapamycin) was isolated from the soil bacteria *Streptomyces hygroscopicus*, in the mid 1970s.[37] This bacterial macrolide later became the preferred immunosuppressant for kidney transplantation, because it was mildly immunosuppressive; however, in contrast to cyclosporine A, it did not enhance tumor incidence.[38] Sirolimus is the prototypic inhibitor of the mammalian target of rapamycin (mTOR), a serine/threonine protein kinase that is a highly conserved regulatory protein involved in cell-cycle progression, proliferation, and angiogenesis.[39] Signaling pathways both upstream and downstream of mTOR have been shown to be commonly dysregulated in cancer. mTOR functions through two main mechanisms, depending on the presence and activity of the mTOR-associated protein complexes, mTORC1 and mTORC2. Sirolimus and its analog compounds, temsirolimus and everolimus, form a complex with the FK-binding protein (FKBP) and inhibit activation of a subset of mTOR proteins residing within mTORC1. In contrast, mTORC2 holds mTOR in a form that is not as readily inhibited by these rapamycin analogs, and upregulation of mTORC2 may represent a mechanism by which resistance can develop to this class of compounds.

Temsirolimus (CCI-779), a novel functional ester of sirolimus, is a water-soluble dihydroxymethyl propionic acid compound that rapidly undergoes hydrolysis to sirolimus after IV administration, reaching peak concentrations within 0.5 to 2.0 hours.[40] This drug is widely distributed in tissues, and steady-state drug levels are reached in 7 to 8 days. Temsirolimus is metabolized primarily in the liver by CYP3A4 microsomal enzymes to yield sirolimus as the main metabolite. The terminal half-life of temsirolimus is 17 hours, whereas that of sirolimus is approximately 55 hours. When bound to temsirolimus, mTOR is unable to phosphorylate the key protein translation factors, such as 4E-BP1 and S6K1, leading to translational inhibition of several critical regulatory proteins involved in cell-cycle control. Several other cellular proteins involved in the regulation of angiogenesis, such as hypoxia-inducible factor-1α (HIF-1α) and vascular endothelial growth factor (VEGF), are suppressed through mTOR inhibition by temsirolimus.

Phase I studies of temsirolimus have investigated various schedules and doses, ranging from 7.5 mg to 220 mg given as weekly 30-minute infusions.[40] A phase II study in patients with cytokine-refractory renal cell cancer (RCC) investigated the efficacy and safety of three different dose levels (25 mg, 75 mg, and 250 mg, respectively) administered on a weekly schedule. This study showed promising antitumor activity for all three dose levels with no significant difference in efficacy or toxicity.[41] As a result, the 25-mg dose was eventually selected as the monotherapy dose for further study. A phase III randomized trial compared interferon, temsirolimus, and the combination of the two agents in previously untreated patients with advanced RCC who had at least three of six poor prognostic features.[42] Once-weekly IV temsirolimus, 25 mg, prolonged the median overall survival of patients with poor prognostic features by 49% from 7.3 months (95% CI, 6.1 to 8.8 months) in the interferon arm to 10.9 months (95% CI, 8.6 to 12.7 months) in the temsirolimus arm (P = .008). The temsirolimus arm also had a prolonged median progression-free survival of 5.5 months compared to 3.1 months in the interferon arm (P <.001). Moreover, temsirolimus was effective for both clear cell and non–clear cell histologies.[43,44]

Mantle cell lymphoma was the first hematologic malignancy in which mTOR inhibition was explored as a treatment strategy. The rationale for this approach was that mantle cell lymphoma is characterized by overexpression of cyclin D1, which is a cyclin whose expression appears to be tightly regulated by mTOR signaling. The early-phase clinical trials of temsirolimus showed promising activity against non-Hodgkin lymphomas, multiple myeloma, and myeloid leukemias, with some evidence of success thus far.[45]

In terms of the safety profile, the most common adverse events associated with temsirolimus were asthenia and fatigue, dry skin with acneiform skin rash, nausea/vomiting, mucositis, and anorexia. Hyperlipidemia with increased serum triglycerides and/or cholesterol as well as hyperglycemia occur in up to 90% of patients. Allergic, hypersensitivity reactions have been observed in about 10% of patients, and pulmonary toxicity, presenting as increased cough, dyspnea, fever, and pulmonary infiltrates, is a relatively rare event, occurring in less than 1% of patients. However, the risk of pulmonary toxicity increases in patients with an underlying pulmonary disease.[46]

EVEROLIMUS

Everolimus (RAD001) is an orally active hydroxyethyl ether analog of rapamycin that contains a 2-hydroxyethyl chain substitution. This molecule is significantly more water soluble than sirolimus. As with sirolimus and temsirolimus, everolimus targets mTOR by forming a complex with mTOR and FKBP, resulting in inhibition of mTOR activity. Few data are available regarding the actual differences in the ability of temsirolimus and everolimus to inhibit mTOR. One preclinical in vitro study showed that the binding of everolimus to FKBP was approximately threefold weaker than that of sirolimus.[47] In vivo studies, however, have documented similar efficacy of the two agents in terms of immunosuppressive activity as well as antitumor activity. In preclinical models, the administration of everolimus results in the inhibition of mTOR, similar to what has been observed with the other rapamycin analogs.[48] In terms of clinical pharmacology, peak drug levels are achieved within 1 to 2 hours after oral administration, and food with a high fat content reduces oral bioavailability by up to 20%. This compound is metabolized in the liver, mainly by the CYP3A4 system, and six main metabolites have been identified. In general, these metabolites are less active than the parent compound. Elimination is mainly hepatic with excretion in feces, and caution should be used in patients with moderate liver impairment (Child-Pugh class B).[49] In this setting, the daily dose of drug should be reduced to 5 mg. In patients with severe liver dysfunction (Child-Pugh class C), the use of this drug is contraindicated.

Encouraging clinical activity was initially observed in phase 1/2 trials in patients with non–small-cell lung, gastric, and esophageal cancers, sarcomas, pancreatic neuroendocrine tumors, as well as hematologic malignancies.[50–53] Presently, everolimus is indicated and approved for the treatment of adults with advanced RCC after failure with sunitinib or sorafenib; advanced hormone receptor-positive, HER2-negative breast cancer in combination with exemestane; and progressive unresectable, locally advanced, or metastatic neuroendocrine tumors of pancreatic origin (PNET).[54,55] The recommended dose of everolimus for these indications is 10 mg taken orally once daily.

The safety profile of everolimus is similar to what has been observed with temsirolimus. The most common adverse events include asthenia and fatigue, dry skin with acneiform skin rash, nausea/vomiting, mucositis, and anorexia. Hyperlipidemia with increased serum triglycerides and/or cholesterol as well as hyperglycemia occur in up to 90% of patients. Allergic, hypersensitivity reactions have been observed in about 10% of patients, and pulmonary toxicity, presenting as increased cough, dyspnea, fever, and pulmonary infiltrates, are a relatively rare event, occurring in less than 1% of patients. However, the risk of pulmonary toxicity increases in patients with an underlying pulmonary disease.

THALIDOMIDE, LENALIDOMIDE, AND POMALIDOMIDE

Thalidomide and its amino-substituted analogs, lenalidomide and pomalidomide, are small-molecule glutamic acid derivatives that possess a wide range of biologic properties, including immunomodulating, antiangiogenic, and epigenetic effects. They are classified as class I (non–phosphophodiesterase-4 inhibitory) immunomodulatory drugs (IMiDs). Although their primary mechanism of activity against malignancy is uncertain, it is believed that IMiDs exert their anticancer effects both directly on cancer cells and indirectly via effects on the tumor microenvironment and host antitumor immunity. Specific mechanisms include the inhibition of nuclear factor kappa B (NF-κB) transcriptional activity in malignant cells with a resultant decrease in the production of antiapoptotic molecules; the inhibition of surface adhesion molecule expression on both multiple myeloma cells and bone marrow stromal cells; the inhibition of the production and release of various growth factors (including vascular endothelial growth factor, basic fibroblast growth factor, tumor necrosis factor alpha, and interleukin [IL] 6) that regulate angiogenesis and tumor cell proliferation; and costimulation of IL-2 and interferon gamma (IFN-γ) release with T-helper 1 subset skewing and augmentation of cytotoxic T-cell and natural killer cell effector function.[56,57] Unlike thalidomide, both lenalidomide and pomalidomide result in cell cycle arrest and apoptosis of myeloma cells in vitro, believed in part to be related to epigenetic effects.[58] They are also more potent stimulators of IL-2 and INF-γ production and T-cell proliferation than thalidomide, and appear to additionally inhibit T-regulatory cells.[57] Clinically, lenalidomide has activity in patients with thalidomide-resistant multiple myeloma, and pomalidomide has additional activity in patients with lenalidomide-resistant disease.[59,60] Recently, the protein cereblon (cerebral protein with lon protease), a highly conserved E3 ligase, was recognized as a primary target of IMiDs teratogenic effect, and appears to be an important target of IMiD anticancer activity.[61–63] Efforts are currently under way to evaluate the expression of Cereblon as a predictive biomarker of response to IMiDs.[63] Due to the potential risk of significant teratogenicity, thalidomide, lenalidomide, and pomalidomide can only be prescribed by licensed prescribers who are registered in restricted distribution programs.

Thalidomide

Thalidomide (2-[2,6-dioxopiperidin-3-yl]-2,3-dihydro-1H-isoindole-1,3-dione; Thalomid) is a synthetic glutamic acid derivative that was initially synthesized in 1953. It was used widely in Europe between 1956 and 1962 as a sleeping aid and antiemetic for pregnant women before it was discovered to cause severe congenital malformations. Initial reports of its efficacy in multiple myeloma were published in 1999, and the 200-mg daily dose combined with pulse dexamethasone (40-mg daily dose on days 1 through 4, 9 through 12, and 17 through 20 on a 28-day schedule) was approved by the FDA in 2006 for newly diagnosed multiple myeloma. The use of thalidomide has dropped precipitously in the United States with the FDA approval of more efficacious and less toxic therapies for myeloma. Thalidomide is poorly soluble, and it is absorbed slowly from the gastrointestinal tract, reaching peak plasma concentration in 3 to 6 hours, with 55% to 66% bound to plasma proteins. The exact metabolic route and fate of thalidomide is not known. Thalidomide does not appear to be hepatically metabolized, but rather undergoes spontaneous nonenzymatic hydrolysis in plasma to multiple metabolites, with a half-life of elimination ranging from 5 to 7 hours. These metabolites are believed to be responsible for the antitumor effects of thalidomide. Less than 1% is excreted into the urine as unchanged drug.[64]

Thalidomide frequently causes drowsiness, constipation, and fatigue. Peripheral neuropathy is a common and potentially severe and irreversible side effect occurring in up to 30% of patients. Increased incidences of venous thromboembolic events, such as deep venous thrombosis and pulmonary embolus, have also been observed with thalidomide, particularly when used in combination with dexamethasone or anthracycline-based chemotherapy. Patients who are appropriate candidates may benefit from concurrent prophylactic anticoagulation or aspirin treatment.[65] Other side effects of thalidomide include rash, nausea, dizziness, orthostatic hypotension, bradycardia, and mood changes. In 2013, additional alerts were released linking thalidomide to an increased risk of developing second primary malignancies (both acute myelogenous leukemia and myelodysplastic syndrome) and arterial thromboembolic events.

Lenalidomide

Lenalidomide (3-[4-amino-1-oxo-2,3-dihydro-1H-isoindol-2-yl]piperidine-2,6-dione; Revlimid) is a thalidomide derivative that shares the immunomodulatory and antineoplastic properties of its parent compound. However, lenalidomide appears to be more potent in vitro with less nonhematologic toxicities in clinical studies. It initially received FDA approval (10-mg daily dose) in 2005 for the treatment of patients with transfusion-dependent anemia secondary to low or intermediate risk myelodysplastic syndromes associated with a deletion 5q cytogenetic abnormality, with or without additional cytogenetic abnormalities. In 2006, lenalidomide (25-mg daily dose on days 1 through 21 of a 28-day cycle) in combination with dexamethasone (40-mg daily dose on days 1 through 4, 9 through 12, and 17 through 20 on each 28-day cycle for the first four cycles, then 40 mg daily on days 1 through 4 every 28 days) was approved by the FDA for the treatment of patients with multiple myeloma who had received at least one prior therapy for multiple myeloma. In 2013, lenalidomide 25 mg daily (days 1 through 21 on repeated 28-day cycles) was additionally approved for use in refractory mantle cell lymphoma (after relapse/ progression on two lines of therapy, one of which contained bortezomid). Lenalidomide is administered orally and is rapidly absorbed from the gastrointestinal tract. Maximum plasma concentration is reached 0.625 to 1.5 hours after dosing, with approximately 30% bound to plasma proteins. The half-life of elimination is approximately 3 hours, with little information currently available concerning metabolism. Approximately 70% of an administered dose is excreted unchanged by the kidneys.[66]

Compared with thalidomide, lenalidomide is associated with less sedation, constipation, and peripheral neuropathy. However, myelosuppression in the form of neutropenia and thrombocytopenia can be dose limiting. As with thalidomide, the incidence of thromboembolic events is significant with the combination of dexamethasone and lenalidomide. A pooled analysis of 691 patients enrolled in two randomized studies reported a 12% incidence of thrombotic or thromboembolic events with the combination, compared with 4% with dexamethasone alone.[67]

Pomalidomide

Pomalidomide (4-amino-2-[2,6-dioxopiperidin-3-yl]-2,3-dihydro-1H-isoindole-1,3-dione; Pomalyst) is another thalidomide derivative designed to be more portent and less toxic than both thalidomide and lenalidomide. It is currently FDA approved (4-mg once daily dose orally on days 1 through 21 of a 28-day cycle, with or without dexamethasone) for use in patients with progressive multiple myeloma who have received at least two prior therapies, including lenalidomide and bortezomid. Pomalidomide is administered orally and is rapidly absorbed. Maximum plasma concentration is reached 2 to 3 hours after ingestion, with approximately 12% to 44% protein binding.[68] The half-life of elimination is between 7.5 and 9.5 hours. Pomalidomide is metabolized in the liver,via CYP1A2/CYP3A4 (major) and CYP2C19/CYP2D6 (minor), and excretion occurs primarily through the kidneys (73%; 2% as unchanged drug).

Like lenalidomide, pomalidomide is better tolerated than thalidomide at approved doses with less constipation, fatigue, and neuropathy.[69] The primary toxicity appreciated in myeloma trials has been myelosuppression, particularly neutropenia, which can be dose limiting. The risk of thromboembolic events is similar to that seen with thalidomide and lenalidomide. Unlike thalidomide or lenalidomide, dermatologic toxicity is rare with pomalidomide. A summary of the characteristics of the miscellaneous drugs mentioned in this chapter is provided in Table 26.1. A summary of all hematology oncology drug approvals since the last edition of the textbook can be viewed in Table 26.2.

TABLE 26.1

Miscellaneous Chemotherapeutic Agents

	Main Therapeutic Uses	Clinical Pharmacology	Major Toxicities	Notes
Omacetaxine	CML	Mean half-life of 6 h after subcutaneous injection	Thrombocytopenia, anemia, nausea, diarrhea	Efficacy shown in Bcr-Abl–mutated CML
L-Asparaginase	Pediatric and adult ALL	Peak concentration 7–12 h after IV administration; 30% plasma protein binding; PEG form has longer half-life of 5.7 days; antagonize effects of methotrexate if given before or concurrently	Hypersensitivity reactions, alterations in thyroid function, prolonged PT/PTT, decreased levels of vitamin K–dependent factors, acute pancreatitis	Myelosuppression is rare; hypersensitivity reaction risk increases with repeated exposure and when used as single agent; PEG form is less immunogenic
Bleomycin	Hodgkin disease, neoplastic pleural effusion, non-Hodgkin lymphoma, squamous cell carcinoma of cervix, squamous cell carcinoma of nasopharynx, squamous cell carcinoma of penis, squamous cell carcinoma of the head and neck, squamous cell carcinoma of vulva, testicular cancer	Terminal half-life of 3h; can be given intracavitary; 45%–55% of intracavitary dose absorbed systemically; elimination via kidneys if CrCl <25–35 mL/min dose reduction required	Pulmonary toxicity dose-limiting; more if age >70 y; cumulative dose >400 U; acute hypersensitivity reactions rare (1%); mucositis, erythema, hyperpigmentation	Not myelosuppressive; immunosuppressive; metabolizing enzyme; bleomycin hydrolase enzyme low in lung and skin tissue; G-CSF use seems to exacerbate pulmonary toxicity

(continued)

TABLE 26.1

Miscellaneous Chemotherapeutic Agents *(continued)*

	Main Therapeutic Uses	Clinical Pharmacology	Major Toxicities	Notes
Procarbazine	Hodgkin lymphoma	Rapid complete oral absorption; peak concentration, 10–15 min; crosses blood–brain barrier; half-life 1 h; several drug–drug and food–drug interactions; metabolized by hepatic microsomal P-450 system; 70% excreted in urine	Dose-limiting toxicity is myelosuppression, more commonly thrombocytopenia nadir at 4 wk; G-6PD–deficient patients can develop hemolytic anemia, nausea, vomiting, diarrhea, flulike symptoms, peripheral neuropathy, hypersensitivity reactions	Avoid tyramine-containing foods; disulfiramlike reaction with concurrent alcohol use; hypertensive reaction with concurrent tricyclic antidepressant use; increased risk for azoospermia/infertility and secondary malignancy
Vismodegib	Basal cell carcinoma of the skin	Oral bioavailability 32%; not affected by food	No dose limiting toxicity; abdominal pain, fatigue, weight loss, dysgeusia	Hedgehog-signaling pathway inhibitor
Ado-trastuzumabemtansine	Advanced HER2-positive breast cancer	Peak concentration near the end of infusion metabolized by CYP3A4/5; half-life, 3.5 days	Thrombocytopenia, hepatotoxicity, cardiac toxicity fatigue, nausea	Monitor cardiac function
Temsirolimus	Advanced renal cancer	Peak concentration, 0.5–2 h; widely distributed in tissues; steady-state levels reached in 7–8 d; half-life, 17 h	Asthenia, fatigue, dry skin, acneiform skin rash, mucositis, anorexia, hyperlipidemia, hyperglycemia	Efficacy shown for both clear cell and non–clear-cell histologies; efficacy in hematologic malignancies (mantle cell lymphoma, non-Hodgkin lymphoma, multiple myeloma)
Everolimus	Advanced renal cell carcinoma, breast cancer, pancreatic neuroendocrine tumor	Peak concentration, 1–2 hr; reduced bioavailability with high fat content food; metabolized by CYP3A4 system; mainly hepatic excretion	Asthenia, dry skin, nausea, vomiting, mucositis, hyperlipidemia, hyperglycemia, allergic hypersensitivity reaction, pulmonary toxicity	Contraindicated in Child-Pugh class C patients; encouraging activity in gastric, non–small-cell, lung, esophageal cancers, sarcomas; approved for organ rejection prophylaxis
Thalidomide	Multiple myeloma, erythema nodosum leprosum	Oral absorption slow; peak concentration, 3–6 h; 55%–66% bound to plasma proteins; half-life, 5–7 h, spontaneous nonenzymatic hydrolysis in plasma	Drowsiness, constipation, fatigue, skin rash, increased risk for thromboembolic complications	Pregnancy category X; may be present in semen; serious skin reactions including Stevens-Johnson syndrome
Lenalidomide	Low-to-intermediate risk myelodysplastic syndrome associated with 5q deletion, multiple myeloma	Rapid oral absorption; peak concentration, 0.6–1.5 h; half-life, 3 h; 70% excreted unchanged by kidneys	Less sedation, drowsiness, constipation than thalidomide; myelosuppression; thromboembolic events; peripheral neuropathy	Pregnancy category X; caution in patients with renal function impairment; neutropenia; thrombocytopenia may be dose limiting
Pomalidomide	Multiple myeloma who have received at least two prior therapies	Rapid oral absorption; peak concentration, 2–3 h; half-life, 7.5 h	Myelosuppression; thromboembolic events; skin toxicity rare	Better tolerated than thalidomide; effective in prior bortezomib- and lenalidomide-receiving patients

PT, prothrombin time; PTT, partial thromboplastin time; CrCl, creatinine clearance.

TABLE 26.2

U.S. Food And Drug Administration Hematology Oncology Drug Approvals 2010–2013

Drug/Manufacturer	Indication	Approval Date
Sorafenib (NEXAVAR tablets, Bayer Healthcare Pharmaceuticals Inc.)	For the treatment of locally recurrent or metastatic, progressive, differentiated thyroid carcinoma (DTC) refractory to radioactive iodine treatment.	November 22, 2013
Crizotinib (Xalkori, Pfizer, Inc.) capsules	For the treatment of patients with metastatic non–small-cell lung cancer (NSCLC) whose tumors are anaplastic lymphoma kinase (ALK) positive as detected by an FDA-approved test.	November 20, 2013
Ibrutinib (IMBRUVICA, Pharmacyclics, Inc.)	For the treatment of patients with mantle cell lymphoma (MCL) who have received at least one prior therapy.	November 13, 2013
Obinutuzumab (GAZYVA injection, for intravenous use, Genentech, Inc.; previously known as GA101)	For use in combination with chlorambucil for the treatment of patients with previously untreated chronic lymphocytic leukemia (CLL).	November 1, 2013
Pertuzumab injection (PERJETA, Genentech, Inc.)	For use in combination with trastuzumab and docetaxel for the neoadjuvant treatment of patients with HER2-positive, locally advanced, inflammatory, or early stage breast cancer (either greater than 2 cm in diameter or node positive) as part of a complete treatment regimen for early breast cancer.	September 30, 2013
Paclitaxel protein-bound particles (albumin-bound) (Abraxane for injectable suspension, Abraxis BioScience, LLC, a wholly owned subsidiary of Celgene Corporation)	In combination with gemcitabine for the first-line treatment of patients with metastatic adenocarcinoma of the pancreas.	September 6, 2013
Afatinib (Gilotrif tablets, Boehringer Ingelheim Pharmaceuticals, Inc.)	For the first-line treatment of patients with metastatic NSCLC whose tumors have epidermal growth factor receptor (EGFR) exon 19 deletions or exon 21 (L858R) substitution mutations as detected by an FDA-approved test. The safety and efficacy of afatinib have not been established in patients whose tumors have other EGFR mutations.	July 12, 2013
Denosumab (Xgeva injection, for subcutaneous use, Amgen Inc.)	For the treatment of adults and skeletally mature adolescents with a giant cell tumor of bone that is unresectable or where surgical resection is likely to result in severe morbidity.	June 13, 2013
Lenalidomide capsules (REVLIMID, Celgene Corporation)	For the treatment of patients with MCL whose disease has relapsed or progressed after two prior therapies, one of which included bortezomib.	June 5, 2013
Trametinib (MEKINIST tablet, GlaxoSmithKline, LLC)	For the treatment of patients with unresectable or metastatic melanoma with BRAF V600E or V600K mutation as detected by an FDA-approved test.	May 29, 2013
Dabrafenib (TAFINLAR capsule, GlaxoSmithKline, LLC)	For the treatment of patients with unresectable or metastatic melanoma with BRAF V600E mutation as detected by an FDA-approved test.	May 29, 2013
Radium Ra 223 dichloride (Xofigo Injection, Bayer HealthCare Pharmaceuticals Inc.)	For the treatment of patients with castration-resistant prostate cancer, symptomatic bone metastases, and no known visceral metastatic disease.	May 15, 2013
Erlotinib (Tarceva, Astellas Pharma Inc.)	For the first-line treatment of metastatic NSCLC patients whose tumors have EGFR exon 19 deletions or exon 21 (L858R) substitution mutations.	May 14, 2013
Ado-trastuzumab emtansine (KADCYLA for injection, Genentech, Inc.)	For use as a single agent for the treatment of patients with HER2-positive, metastatic breast cancer who previously received trastuzumab and a taxane, separately or in combination.	February 22, 2013
Pomalidomide (POMALYST capsules, Celgene Corporation)	For the treatment of patients with multiple myeloma who have received at least two prior therapies, including lenalidomide and bortezomib, and have demonstrated disease progression on or within 60 days of completion of the last therapy.	February 8, 2013

(continued)

TABLE 26.2

U.S. Food And Drug Administration Hematology Oncology Drug Approvals 2010–2013 *(continued)*

Drug/Manufacturer	Indication	Approval Date
Doxorubicin hydrochloride liposome injection (Sun Pharma Global FZE), a generic version of DOXIL Injection (doxorubicin hydrochloride liposome; Janssen Products, L.P.)	For the treatment of ovarian cancer in patients whose disease has progressed or recurred after platinum-based chemotherapy and for AIDS-related Kaposi sarcoma after failure of prior systemic chemotherapy or intolerance to such therapy.	February 4, 2013
Bevacizumab (Avastin, Genentech U.S., Inc.)	For use in combination with fluoropyrimidine–irinotecan- or fluoropyrimidine–oxaliplatin-based chemotherapy for the treatment of patients with metastatic colorectal cancer (mCRC) whose disease has progressed on a first-line bevacizumab-containing regimen.	January 23, 2013
Ponatinib (Iclusig tablets, ARIAD Pharmaceuticals, Inc.)	For the treatment of adult patients with chronic phase, accelerated phase, or blast phase chronic myeloid leukemia (CML) that is resistant or intolerant to prior tyrosine–kinase inhibitor (TKI) therapy or Philadelphia chromosome–positive acute lymphoblastic leukemia (Ph+ ALL) that is resistant or intolerant to prior TKI therapy.	December 17, 2012
Abiraterone acetate (Zytiga Tablets, Janssen Biotech, Inc.)	In combination with prednisone for the treatment of patients with metastatic castration-resistant prostate cancer.	December 10, 2012
Cabozantinib (COMETRIQ capsules, Exelixis, Inc.)	For the treatment of patients with progressive metastatic medullary thyroid cancer (MTC).Cabozantinib is a small molecule that inhibits the activity of multiple tyrosine kinases, including RET, MET, and VEGF receptor 2.	November 29, 2012
Omacetaxine mepesuccinate (SYNRIBO for injection, for subcutaneous use, Teva Pharmaceutical Industries Ltd.)	For the treatment of adult patients with chronic or accelerated phase CML with resistance and/or intolerance to two or more TKIs.	October 26, 2012
Paclitaxel protein-bound particles for injectable suspension, albumin-bound (ABRAXANE for injectable suspension; Abraxis Bioscience a wholly owned subsidiary of Celgene Corporation)	For use in combination with carboplatin for the initial treatment of patients with locally advanced or metastatic NSCLC who are not candidates for curative surgery or radiation therapy.	October 11, 2012
Regorafenib (Stivarga tablets, Bayer HealthCare Pharmaceuticals, Inc.)	For the treatment of patients with mCRC who have been previously treated with fluoropyrimidine-, oxaliplatin-, and irinotecan-based chemotherapy, an anti-VEGF therapy, and, if KRAS wild-type, an anti-EGFR therapy.	September 27, 2012
Bosutinib tablets (Bosulif, Pfizer, Inc.)	for the treatment of chronic, accelerated, or blast phase Ph+ CML in adult patients with resistance or intolerance to prior therapy.	September 4, 2012
Enzalutamide (XTANDI Capsules, Medivation, Inc., and Astellas Pharma US, Inc.)	For the treatment of patients with metastatic castration-resistant prostate cancer who have previously received docetaxel.	August 31, 2012
Everolimus tablets for oral suspension (Afinitor Disperz, Novartis Pharmaceuticals Corp.)	For the treatment of pediatric and adult patients with tuberous sclerosis complex (TSC) who have subependymal giant cell astrocytoma (SEGA) that requires therapeutic intervention, but that cannot be curatively resected.	August 30, 2012
Vincristine sulfate LIPOSOME injection (Marqibo, Talon Therapeutics, Inc.)	For the treatment of adult patients with Ph- ALL in second or greater relapse or whose disease has progressed following two or more antileukemia therapies.	August 9, 2012
Ziv-aflibercept injection (ZALTRAP, Sanofi U.S., Inc.)	For use in combination with 5-fluorouracil, leucovorin, irinotecan (FOLFIRI) for the treatment of patients with mCRC that is resistant to or has progressed following an oxaliplatin-containing regimen.	August 3, 2012
Everolimus tablets (Afinitor, Novartis Pharmaceuticals Corporation)	For the treatment of postmenopausal women with advanced hormone receptor–positive, HER2-negative breast cancer in combination with exemestane, after failure of treatment with letrozole or anastrozole.	July 20, 2012

(continued)

TABLE 26.2

U.S. Food And Drug Administration Hematology Oncology Drug Approvals 2010–2013 *(continued)*

Drug/Manufacturer	Indication	Approval Date
Carfilzomib injection (Kyprolis, Onyx Pharmaceuticals)	For the treatment of patients with multiple myeloma who have received at least two prior therapies, including bortezomib and an immunomodulatory agent, and have demonstrated disease progression on or within 60 days of the completion of the last therapy.	July 20, 2012
Cetuximab (Erbitux, ImClone LLC, a wholly owned subsidiary of Eli Lilly and Co.)	For use in combination with FOLFIRI for first-line treatment of patients with K-ras mutation-negative (wild-type), EGFR-expressing mCRC as determined by FDA-approved tests for this use.	July 9, 2012
Pertuzumab injection (PERJETA, Genentech, Inc.)	For use in combination with trastuzumab and docetaxel for the treatment of patients with HER2-positive metastatic breast cancer who have not received prior anti-HER2 therapy or chemotherapy for metastatic disease.	June 8, 2012
Pazopanib tablets (VOTRIENT, a registered Trademark of GlaxoSmithKline)	For the treatment of patients with advanced soft tissue sarcoma (STS) who have received prior chemotherapy.	April 26, 2012
Everolimus (Afinitor tablets, Novartis)	For the treatment of adults with renal angiomyolipoma, associated with TSC who do not require immediate surgery.	April 26, 2012
Imatinib mesylate tablets (Gleevec, Novartis Pharmaceuticals)	For the adjuvant treatment of adult patients following complete gross resection of Kit (CD117)-positive gastrointestinal stromal tumors (GIST).	January 31, 2012
Vismodegib (ERIVEDGE Capsule, Genentech, Inc.)	For the treatment of adults with metastatic basal cell carcinoma or with locally advanced basal cell carcinoma that has recurred following surgery or who are not candidates for surgery and who are not candidates for radiation.	January 30, 2012
Axitinib tablets (Inlyta, Pfizer, Inc.)	For the treatment of advanced renal cell carcinoma after failure of one prior systemic therapy.	January 27, 2012
Glucarpidase injection (Voraxaze, BTG International Inc.)	For the treatment of toxic plasma methotrexate concentrations (>1 μmol/L) in patients with delayed methotrexate clearance due to impaired renal function.	January 17, 2012
Asparaginase *Erwinia chrysanthemi* (Erwinaze, injection, EUSA Pharma [USA], Inc.)	As a component of a multiagent chemotherapeutic regimen for the treatment of patients with ALL who have developed hypersensitivity to *E. coli*–derived asparaginase.	November 18, 2011
Ruxolitinib (Jakafi oral tablets, Incyte Corporation)	For the treatment of intermediate and high risk myelofibrosis, including primary myelofibrosis, postpolycythemia vera myelofibrosis, and postessential thrombocythemia myelofibrosis.	November 16, 2011
Cetuximab (Erbitux, ImClone LLC, a wholly-owned subsidiary of Eli Lilly and Company)	In combination with platinum-based therapy plus 5-fluorouracil (5-FU) for the first-line treatment of patients with recurrent locoregional disease and/or metastatic squamous cell carcinoma of the head and neck (SCCHN).	November 7, 2011
Eculizumab (Soliris, Alexion, Inc.)	For the treatment of pediatric and adult patients with atypical hemolytic uremic syndrome (aHUS).	September 23, 2011
Denosumab (Prolia, Amgen Inc.)	As a treatment to increase bone mass in patients at high risk for fracture receiving androgen-deprivation therapy (ADT) for nonmetastatic prostate cancer or adjuvant aromatase inhibitor (AI) therapy for breast cancer.	September 16, 2011
Crizotinib (XALKORI Capsules, Pfizer Inc.)	For the treatment of patients with locally advanced or metastatic NSCLC that is ALK-positive as detected by an FDA-approved test.	August 26, 2011

(continued)

TABLE 26.2

U.S. Food And Drug Administration Hematology Oncology Drug Approvals 2010–2013 *(continued)*

Drug/Manufacturer	Indication	Approval Date
Brentuximab vedotin (Adcetris for injection, Seattle Genetics, Inc.)	For treatment of patients with Hodgkin lymphoma after failure of autologous stem cell transplant (ASCT) or after failure of at least two prior multiagent chemotherapy regimens in patients who are not ASCT candidates and treatment of patients with systemic anaplastic large cell lymphoma (ALCL) after failure of at least one prior multiagent chemotherapy regimen.	August 19, 2011
Vemurafenib tablets (ZELBORAF, Hoffmann-La Roche Inc.)	For the treatment of patients with unresectable or metastatic melanoma with the BRAFV600E mutation as detected by an FDA-approved test.	August 17, 2011
Sunitinib (Sutent capsules, Pfizer, Inc.)	For the treatment of progressive, well-differentiated pancreatic neuroendocrine tumors (pNET) in patients with unresectable, locally advanced, or metastatic disease.	May 20, 2011
Everolimus (Afinitor tablets, Novartis Pharmaceuticals Corporation)	For the treatment of progressive PNET in patients with unresectable, locally advanced, or metastatic disease.	May 5, 2011
Abiraterone acetate (Zytiga tablets, Centocor Ortho Biotech, Inc.)	For use in combination with prednisone for the treatment of patients with metastatic castration-resistant prostate cancer (mCRPC) who have received prior chemotherapy containing docetaxel.	April 28, 2011
Vandetanib tablets (Vandetanib tablets, AstraZeneca Pharmaceuticals LP)	For the treatment of symptomatic or progressive medullary thyroid cancer in patients with unresectable, locally advanced, or metastatic disease.	April 6, 2011
Peginterferon alfa-2b (Sylatron, Schering Corporation, Kenilworth, NJ 07033)	For the treatment of patients with melanoma with microscopic or gross nodal involvement within 84 days of definitive surgical resection including complete lymphadenectomy.	March 29, 2011
Ipilimumab injection (YERVOY, Bristol-Myers Squibb Company)	For the treatment of unresectable or metastatic melanoma.	March 25, 2011
Rituximab (Rituxan, Genentech, Inc.)	For maintenance therapy in patients with previously untreated follicular, CD-20 positive, B-cell non-Hodgkin lymphoma who achieve a response to rituximab in combination with chemotherapy.	January 28, 2011
Eribulin mesylate (Halaven injection, Eisai Inc.)	For the treatment of patients with metastatic breast cancer who have previously received an anthracycline and a taxane in either the adjuvant or metastatic setting, and at least two chemotherapeutic regimens for the treatment of metastatic disease.	November 15, 2010
Everolimus (Afinitor, Novartis), an mTOR inhibitor	For patients with SEGA associated with tuberous sclerosis (TS) who require therapy but who are not candidates for surgical resection.	October 29, 2010
Dasatinib (Sprycel, Bristol-Myers Squibb)	For the treatment of newly diagnosed adult patients with Ph+ CML in chronic phase (CP-CML).	October 28, 2010
Trastuzumab (Herceptin, Genentech, Inc.)	In combination with cisplatin and a fluoropyrimidine (capecitabine or 5-FU), for the treatment of patients with HER2-overexpressing metastatic gastric or gastroesophageal (GE) junction adenocarcinoma, who have not received prior treatment for metastatic disease.	October 20, 2010
Nilotinib (Tasigna capsules, Novartis Pharmaceuticals Corporation)	For the treatment of adult patients with newly diagnosed Ph+ CP-CML.	June 17, 2010
Cabazitaxel (Jevtana injection, Sanofi-Aventis)	For use in combination with prednisone for treatment of patients with metastatic hormone-refractory prostate cancer (mHRPC) previously treated with a docetaxel-containing regimen.	June 17, 2010

REFERENCES

1. Powell RG, Weisleder D, Smith CR, et al. Antitumor alkaloids from *Cephalotaxus harringtonia* structure and activity. *J Pharm Sci* 1972;61:1227–1230.
2. Huang MT. Harringtonine, an inhibitor of initiation of protein biosynthesis. *Mol Pharmacol* 1975;11:511–519.
3. Baaske DM, Heinstein P. Cytotoxicity and cell cycle specificity of homoharrintonine. *Antimicrob Agents Chemother* 1977;12:298–300.
4. Savaraj N, Lu K, Dimery I, et al. Clinical pharmacology of homoharringtonine. *Cancer Treat Rep* 1986;70:1403–1407.
5. Neidhart JA, Young DC, Derocher D, et al. Phase I trial of homoharringtonine. *Cancer Treat Rep* 1983;67:801–804.
6. Grem JL, Cheson BD, King SA, et al. Cephalotoxine esters: antileukemic advance of therapeutic failure. *J Natl Cancer Inst* 1988;80:1095–1103.
7. O'Brien S, Kantarjian H, Keating M, et al. Homoharringtonine therapy indices responses in patients with chronic myelogenous leukemia in late chronic phase. *Blood* 1995;86:3322–3326.
8. Legros L, Hayette S, Nicolini FE, et al. BCR-ABL(T315I) transcript disappearance in an imatinib-resistant CML patient treated with homoharringtonine: a new therapeutic challenge? *Leukemia* 2007;21(10):2204–2206.
9. Jorge Cortes J, Lipton JF, Rea D, et al. Phase 2 study of subcutaneous omacetaxine mepesuccinate after TKI failure in patients with chronic-phase CML with T315I mutation. *Blood* 2012;120:2573–2580.
10. Labrou NE, Papageorgiou AC, Avramis VI. Structure-function relationships and clinical applications of L-Asparaginases. *Curr Med Chem* 2010;17: 2183–2195.
11. Verma N, Kumar K, Kaur G, et al. L-Asparaginase: a promising chemotherapeutic agent. *Crit Rev Biotechnol* 2007;27:45–62.
12. Zeidan A, Wang ES, Wetzler M. Pegasparaginase: where do we stand? *Expert Opin Biol Ther* 2009;9:111–119.
13. Avramis VI, Panosyan EH. Pharmacokinetic/pharmacodynamic relationships of asparaginase formulations: the past, the present and recommendations for the future. *Clin Pharmacokinet* 2005;44:367–393.
14. Appel IM, Hop WC, Pieters R. Changes in hypercoagulability by asparaginase: a randomized study between two asparaginases. *Blood Coagul Fibrinolysis* 2006;17:139–146.
15. Evans WE, Yee GC, Crom WR, et al. Clinical pharmacology of bleomycin and cisplatin. *Head Neck Surg* 1981;4:98–110.
16. Chen J, Stubbe J. Bleomycins: towards better therapeutics. *Nat Rev Cancer* 2005;2:102–112.
17. Hecht SM. Bleomycin: new perspectives on the mechanism of action. *J Nat Prod* 2000;63:158–168.
18. Lewis TG, Nydorf ED. Intralesional bleomycin for warts: a review. *J Drugs Dermatol* 2006;5:499–504.
19. Shaw P, Agarwal R. Pleurodesis for malignant pleural effusions. *Cochrane Database Syst Rev* 2004;(1):CD002916.
20. Good LM, Miller MD, High WA. Intralesional agents in the management of cutaneous malignancy: a review. *J Am Acad Dermatol* 2011;64:413–422
21. Kawai K, Akaza H. Bleomycin-induced pulmonary toxicity in chemotherapy for testicular cancer. *Expert Opin Drug Saf* 2003;2:587–596.
22. Azulay E, Herigault S, Levame M, et al. Effect of granulocyte colony-stimulating factor on bleomycin-induced acute lung injury and pulmonary fibrosis. *Crit Care Med* 2003;31:1442–1448.
23. Adachi K, Suzuki M, Sugimoto T, et al. Effects of granulocyte colony-stimulating factor on the kinetics of inflammatory cells in the peripheral blood and pulmonary lesions during the development of bleomycin-induced lung injury in rats. *Exp Toxicol Pathol* 2003;55:21–32.
24. Martin WG, Ristow KM, Habermann TM, et al. Bleomycin pulmonary toxicity has a negative impact on the outcome of patients with Hodgkin's lymphoma. *J Clin Oncol* 2005;23:7614–7620.
25. Younes A, Connors JM, Park SI et al. Brentuximab vedotin combined with ABVD or AVD for patients with newly diagnosed Hodgkin's lymphoma: a phase 1, open-label, dose-escalation study. *Lancet Oncol* 2013;14:1348–1356.
26. Lam MS. The need for routine bleomycin test dosing in the 21st century. *Ann Pharmacother* 2005;39:1897–1902.
27. Swaffar DS, Horstman MG, Jaw JY, et al. Methylazoxyprocarbazine, the active metabolite responsible for the anticancer activity of procarbazine against L1210 leukemia. *Cancer Res* 1989;49:2442–2447.
28. Patterson LH, Murray GI. Tumour cytochrome P450 and drug activation. *Curr Pharm Des* 2002;8:1335–1347.
29. Swaffar DS, Pomerantz SC, Harker WG, et al. Non-enzymatic activation of procarbazine to active cytotoxic species. *Oncol Res* 1992;4:49–58.
30. Preiss R, Baumann F, Regenthal R, et al. Plasma kinetics of procarbazine and azo-procarbazine in humans. *Anticancer Drugs* 2006;17:75–80.
31. Von Hoff DD, LoRusso PM, Rudin CM, et al. Inhibition of the hedgehog pathway in advanced basal-cell carcinoma. *N Engl J Med* 2009;361: 1164–1172.
32. Rudin CM. Vismodegib. *Clin Cancer Res* 2012;18:1–5.
33. U.S. Food and Drug Administation. News & Events: FDA News Release: FDA approves new treatment for most common types of skin cancer. http://www.fda.gov/NewsEvents/Newsroom/PressAnnouncements/ucm289545.htm. Published January 30, 2012. Updated January 31, 2012.
34. Tang JY, Mackay-Wiggan JM, Aszterbaum M, et al. Inhibiting the Hedgehog pathway in patients with the basal-cell nevus syndrome. *N Engl J Med* 2012;366:2180–2188.
35. Krop IE, Beeram M, Modi S, et al. Phase I study of trastuzumab-DM1, an HER2 antibody-drug conjugate, given every 3 weeks to patients with HER2-positive metastatic breast cancer. *J Clin Oncol* 2010;28:2698–2704.
36. Verma S, Miles D, Gianni L, et al. Trastuzumab emtansine for HER2-positive advanced breast cancer. *N Engl J Med* 2012;367:1783–1791.
37. Sehgal SN, Baker H, Vézina C. Rapamycin (AY-22,989), a new antifungal antibiotic. II. Fermentation, isolation and characterization. *J Antibiot (Tokyo)* 1975;28:727–732.
38. Sehgal SN, Molnar-Kimber K, Ocain TD, et al. Rapamycin: a novel immunosuppressive macrolide. *Med Res Rev* 1994;14:1–22.
39. Wullschleger S, Loewith R, Hall MN. TOR signaling in growth and metabolism. *Cell* 2006;124:471–484.
40. Raymond E, Alexandre J, Faivre S, et al. Safety and pharmacokinetics of escalated doses of weekly intravenous infusion of CCI-779, a novel mTOR inhibitor in patients with cancer. *J Clin Oncol* 2004;22:2336–2347.
41. Zeng Z, Sarbassov dos D, Samudio IJ, et al. Rapamycin derivatives reduce mTORC2 signaling and inhibit AKT activation in AML. *Blood* 2007;109: 3509–3512.
42. Kapoor A, Figlin RA. Targeted inhibition of mammalian target of rapamycin for the treatment of advanced renal cell carcinoma. *Cancer* 2009;115: 3618–3630.
43. Atkins MB, Hidalgo M, Stadler WM, et al. Randomized phase II study of multiple dose levels of CCI-779, a novel mammalian target of rapamycin kinase inhibitor, in patients with advanced refractory renal cell carcinoma. *J Clin Oncol* 2004;22:909–918.
44. Hudes G, Carducci M, Tomczak P, et al. Temsirolimus, interferon alfa, or both for advanced renal-cell carcinoma. *N Engl J Med* 2007;356: 2271–2281.
45. Smith SM, van Besien K, Karrison T, et al. Temsirolimus has activity in non-mantle cell non-Hodgkin's lymphoma subtypes: The University of Chicago phase II consortium. *J Clin Oncol* 2010;28:4740–4746.
46. Duran I, Siu LL, Oza AM, et al. Characterization of the lung toxicity of the cell cycle inhibitor temsirolimus. *Eur J Cancer* 2006;42:1875–1880.
47. Schuler W, Sedrani R, Cottens S, et al. SDZ RAD, a new rapamycine derivative: pharmacological properties in vitro and in vivo. *Transplantation* 1997;64: 36–42.
48. Dudkin L, Dilling MB, Cheshire PJ, et al. Biochemical correlates of mTOR inhibition by the rapamycin ester CCI-779 and tumor growth inhibition. *Clin Cancer Res* 2001;7:1758–1764.
49. Kirchner GI, Meier-Wiedenbach I, Manns MP. Clinical pharmacokinetics of everolimus. *Clin Pharmacokinet* 2004;43:83–95.
50. Doi T, Muro K, Boku N, et al. Multicenter phase II study of everolimus in patients with previously treated metastatic gastric cancer. *J Clin Oncol* 2010;28: 1904–1910.
51. Yao JC, Lombard-Bohas C, Baudin E, et al. Daily oral everolimus activity in patients with metastatic pancreatic neuroendocrine tumors after failure of cytotoxic chemotherapy: a phase II trial. *J Clin Oncol* 2010;28:69–76.
52. Yee KW, Zeng Z, Konopleva M, et al. Phase I/II study of the mammalian target of rapamycin inhibitor everolimus(RAD001) in patients with relapsed or refractory hematological malignancies. *Clin Cancer Res* 2008;12: 5165–5173.
53. Okuno S. Mammalian target of rapamycin inhibitors in sarcomas. *Curr Opin Oncol* 2006;18:360–362.
54. Yao JC, Shah MH, Ito T, et al. Everolimus for advanced pancreatic neuroendocrine tumors. *N Engl J Med* 2011;364:514–523.
55. Baselga J, Campone M, Piccart M, et al. Everolimus in postmenopausal hormone-receptor-positive advanced breast cancer. *N Engl J Med* 2012;366: 520–529.
56. Shortt J, Hsu AK, Johnstone RW. Thalidomide-analogue biology: immunological, molecular and epigenetic targets in cancer therapy. *Oncogene* 2013;32: 4191–4202.
57. Zhu YX, Kortuem KM, Stewart AK. Molecular mechanism of action of immune-modulatory drugs thalidomide, lenalidomide and pomalidomide in multiple myeloma. *Leuk Lymphoma* 2013;54:683–687.
58. Escoubet-Lozach L, Lin IL, Jensen-Pergakes K, et al. Pomalidomide and lenalidomide induce p21 WAF-1 expression in both lymphoma and multiple myeloma through a LSD1-mediated epigenetic mechanism. *Cancer Res* 2009; 69:7347–7356.
59. Madan S, Lacy MQ, Dispenzieri A, et al. Efficacy of retreatment with immunomodulatory drugs (IMiDs) in patients receiving IMiDs for initial therapy of newly diagnosed multiple myeloma. *Blood* 2011;118:1763–1765.
60. Lacy MQ, Tefferi A. Pomalidomide therapy for multiple myeloma and myelofibrosis: an update. *Leuk Lymphoma* 2011;52:560–566.
61. Ito T, Ando H, Suzuki T, et al. Identification of a primary target of thalidomide teratogenicity. *Science* 2010;327:1345–1350.
62. Zhu YX, Braggio E, Shi CX, et al. Cereblon expression is required for the antimyeloma activity of lenalidomide and pomalidomide. *Blood* 2011;118: 4771–4779.
63. Lopez-Girona A, Mendy D, Ito T, et al. Cereblon is a direct protein target for immunomodulatory and antiproliferative activities of lenalidomide and pomalidomide. *Leukemia* 2012;26:2326–2335.
64. Schuster SR, Kortuem KM, Zhu YX, et al. Cereblon expression predicts response, progression free and overall survival after pomalidomide and

dexamethasone therapy in multiple myeloma. *ASH Ann Meeting Abstracts* 2012;120:194.

65. Bennett CL, Angelotta C, Yarnold PR, et al. Thalidomide- and lenalidomide-associated thromboembolism among patients with cancer. *JAMA #2006;296:* 2558–2560.
66. Rao KV. Lenalidomide in the treatment of multiple myeloma. *Am J Health Syst Pharm* 2007;64:1799–1807.
67. Lenalidomide. Drugs@FDA. Food and Drug Administration Web site. http://www.accessdata.fda.gov/drugsatfda_docs/label/2009/021880s006s016s017lbl.pdf. Published December 2008.
68. Pomalidomide. Drugs@FDA. Food and Drug Administration Web site. http://www.accessdata.fda.gov/drugsatfda_docs/label/2013/204026lbl.pdf. Revised February 2013.
69. Lacy MQ, McCurdy AR. Pomalidomide. *Blood* 2013;122:2305–2309.

CANCER THERAPEUTICS

27 Hormonal Agents

Matthew P. Goetz, Charles Erlichman, Charles L. Loprinzi, and Manish Kohli

INTRODUCTION

Hormonal agents are commonly used as a treatment of hormonally responsive cancers, such as breast, prostate, or endometrial carcinomas. Other uses for some hormonal therapies include the treatment of paraneoplastic syndromes, such as carcinoid syndrome, and symptoms caused by cancer, including anorexia. This chapter discusses the major hormonal agents for such therapy, first with an overview of their use in practice, then with more detailed pharmacologic information regarding them (Table 27.1).

SELECTIVE ESTROGEN RECEPTOR MODULATORS

Tamoxifen

Tamoxifen continues to be an important hormonal therapy for the prevention and treatment of breast cancer worldwide. The continued importance of tamoxifen is reflected in the fact that it is the only hormonal agent approved by the U.S. Food and Drug Administration (FDA) for the prevention of premenopausal breast cancer,[1] the treatment of ductal carcinoma in situ (DCIS),[2] and the treatment of surgically resected premenopausal estrogen receptor (ER)–positive breast cancer.[3]

The standard daily dose of tamoxifen is 20 mg, and the optimal duration depends on the underlying clinical setting. Although the recommended duration in the prevention and DCIS settings is 5 years, recently published prospective studies have demonstrated that for the adjuvant treatment of invasive breast cancer, a duration of 10 years (compared to 5 years) further reduced the risk of breast cancer mortality and improved overall survival.[4]

The most common toxicity from tamoxifen is hot flashes, affecting approximately 50% of treated women. These hot flashes are of varying intensity and duration. Tamoxifen-induced hot flashes appear to increase over the first 3 months of therapy and then plateau. They appear to be more prominent in women with a history of hot flashes or estrogen replacement use. Tamoxifen-induced hot flashes can be ameliorated by a number of different pharmacotherapies, including low doses of megestrol[5]; antidepressants such as venlafaxine,[6] desvenlafaxine,[7] citalopram,[8] escitalopram,[9] and paroxetine[10]; and the anticonvulsant drugs gabapentin[11] and pregabalin.[12] There is evidence that drugs that inhibit CYP2D6 (e.g., paroxetine) alter the metabolic activation of tamoxifen to endoxifen, a critical metabolite associated with in vivo tamoxifen efficacy.[13]

The estrogenic properties of tamoxifen are responsible for both beneficial and deleterious side effects. Tamoxifen increases the incidence of endometrial cancer in postmenopausal (but not premenopausal) women, with the increase in the annual incidence of endometrial cancer being approximately 2.58 (ratio of incidence rates).[14] The absolute risk depends on the duration of tamoxifen administration. For women who receive 10 years of adjuvant tamoxifen, the cumulative risk is 3.1% (mortality, 0.4%) versus 1.6% (mortality, 0.2%) for 5 years of tamoxifen.[4] The incidence of a rarer form of uterine cancer, uterine sarcoma, is also increased after tamoxifen use.[15] This form of endometrial cancer comprises approximately 15% of all uterine malignancies that develop after tamoxifen use.[15] Beneficial estrogenic effects from tamoxifen include a decrease in total cholesterol[16] and the preservation of bone density in postmenopausal women.[17] In premenopausal women, however, tamoxifen has a negative effect on bone density.[18] Although most patients do not complain of vaginal symptoms, a few complain of vaginal dryness, whereas others have increased vaginal secretions and discharge, the latter of which is an indication of the estrogenic activity of tamoxifen on the vagina. In the Arimidex, Tamoxifen, Alone or in Combination (ATAC) trial, a commonly observed tamoxifen side effect was vaginal bleeding, leading to a higher hysterectomy rate for patients randomized to tamoxifen (5%) compared to anastrozole (1%).[19] An uncommon effect from tamoxifen is retinal toxicity. This drug can also increase the risk of cataracts. However, no difference in the rate of vision-threatening ocular toxicity has been seen among prospectively treated tamoxifen patients.[20] Tamoxifen predisposes patients to thromboembolic phenomena, especially if used with concomitant chemotherapy. Depression has also been described, but the association with tamoxifen is not clear. Although liver cancers have been noted in laboratory animals, there is no established association between tamoxifen and liver cancers in humans.

Pharmacology

Tamoxifen acts by blocking estrogen stimulation of breast cancer cells, inhibiting both translocation and nuclear binding of the ER. This alters transcriptional and posttranscriptional events mediated by this receptor.[21] Tamoxifen has agonistic, partial agonistic, or antagonistic effects depending on the species, tissue, or endpoints that have been assessed. Additionally, there are marked differences between the antiproliferative properties of tamoxifen and its metabolites.[22]

Resistance to tamoxifen can be intrinsic or acquired, and the potential mechanisms for this resistance are reviewed in the following paragraphs. At each step of the signal transduction pathway with which tamoxifen or its metabolites interferes, there is the potential for an alteration in response. The most important factor appears to be the level of ER, which is highly predictive for a response to tamoxifen. Tamoxifen is ineffective in ER-negative breast cancer. Although decreased or absent expression of the progesterone receptor (PR) is associated with a worse prognosis, the relative risk reduction in tamoxifen-treated patients is the same regardless of the presence or absence of the PR.

Following binding to the ER, subsequent translocation of the tamoxifen/ER complex to the nucleus and binding to an estrogen-response element may occur. This binding prevents transcriptional activation of estrogen-responsive genes. Laboratory and clinical data have demonstrated that ER-positive breast cancers that overexpress HER2 may be less responsive to tamoxifen and

TABLE 27.1

Overview of Major Hormonal Agents Used in Cancer

Class of Drug	Individual Drug	Dose	Route of Delivery	Frequency of Delivery
Selective estrogen receptor modulator	Tamoxifen Toremifene Raloxifene	20 mg 60 mg 60 mg	Oral Oral Oral	Once daily Once daily Once daily
Aromatase inhibitor	Anastrozole Letrozole Exemestane	1 mg 2.5 mg 25 mg	Oral Oral Oral	Once daily Once daily Once daily
Estrogen receptor downregulator	Fulvestrant	500 mg	IM	Once monthly
Luteinizing hormone releasing hormone agonist	Goserelin Leuprolide	7.5 3.6	IM IM	Once monthly[a] Once monthly[a]
GnRH antagonist	Degarelix	240 mg loading dose	SC	80 mg SC monthly maintenance dose
Antiandrogen	Flutamide Bicalutamide Nilutamide	250 mg 50 mg 300 mg for 30 d then 150 mg	Oral Oral Oral	Three times daily Once daily Once daily
Cytochrome P45017 alpha inhibitors	Abiraterone Acetate	1,000 mg (four 250 mg capsules)	Oral	Once Daily
AR "super antagonists"	Enzalutamide	160–240 mg	Oral	Daily
Androgen	Fluoxymesterone	10 mg	Oral	Twice daily
Estrogen	Estradiol	10 mg	Oral	Up to three times daily
Somatostatin analog	Octreotide	Varies	SC or IV	Up to three times daily[b]
Progestational agents	Megestrol Medroxyprogesterone acetate	Varies Varies	Oral Oral or IM	Once daily Varies

[a] Longer acting depot preparations (every 3 months) are available.
[b] Depot formulations are available.
IM, intramuscular; SC, subcutaneous; GnRH, gonadotropin-releasing hormone; CYP, cytochrome P-450; AR, androgen receptor.

to hormonal therapy in general.[23–26] In these tumors, ligand-independent activation of the ER by mitogen-activated protein kinase (MAPK) pathways may contribute to resistance.[27–29] In addition, the expression of AIB1, an estrogen-receptor coactivator, has been associated with tamoxifen resistance in patients whose breast cancers overexpress HER2.[30] In some cases, resistance may result from a decrease or loss of ER expression.[31,32] Although mutations in the ER ligand binding domain (LBD) are rare in newly diagnosed breast cancer, ER mutations are present in up to 20% of recurrent breast cancers.[33–36] These mutations lead to a conformational change in the LBD, which mimics the conformation of activated ligand-bound receptor and constitutive, ligand-independent transcriptional activity, resulting in resistance to hormonal therapy. Preclinical studies suggest that some of these mutations, although insensitive to aromatase inhibitors, retain sensitivity to higher dose selective estrogen-receptor modulators (SERM), such as endoxifen, as well as fulvestrant.[35]

The carcinogenic potential of tamoxifen has been recognized in rat studies[37–39] and in humans (endometrial cancer).[40] It has been proposed that the generation of reactive intermediates that bind covalently to macromolecules underlies the process. Such reactive intermediates have been demonstrated in vitro.[40–43] In addition, the induction of covalent DNA adducts in rat livers treated with tamoxifen has been reported.[44] Both constitutive and inducible cytochrome P-450 (CYP) enzymes have been implicated in the formation of metabolites with tamoxifen,[45,46] and the flavone-containing monooxygenase has been implicated in the formation of the N-oxide of tamoxifen. Reactive intermediates from such metabolic steps are being evaluated for their carcinogenic potential in vitro and in vivo.

Multiple studies to evaluate tumor gene expression profiling have identified gene expression patterns or specific genes associated with resistance to tamoxifen therapy. A commonly utilized gene expression assay, Oncotype DX 21 gene assay (Genomic Health, Redwood City, California), measures the expression of genes known to be involved in estrogen signaling (e.g., ER, PR), HER2, proliferation (e.g., Ki-67), and others. In multiple different data sets, the recurrence score has been associated with a higher risk of breast cancer recurrence in patients treated with hormonal therapy (e.g., tamoxifen or aromatase inhibitors) without concomitant chemotherapy.[47–49]

The pharmacokinetics of tamoxifen is complex. The chemical structure and metabolic pathway of tamoxifen are shown in Figure 27.1. Metabolic activation of tamoxifen is associated with greater pharmacologic activity. The two most active tamoxifen metabolites are 4-hydroxytamoxifen (4-OH tamoxifen) and 4-OH-N-desmethyltamoxifen (endoxifen). A series of studies carried out to characterize endoxifen pharmacology have demonstrated that it has equivalent potency in vitro to 4-hydroxytamoxifen in ER-α and -beta (ER-β) binding,[50] for the suppression of ER-dependent human breast cancer cell line proliferation,[22,50] and in global ER-responsive gene expression.[51] A recent study suggests that endoxifen's effect on the ER may differ from 4-hydroxytamoxifen based on the observation of ER-α degradation.[52]

In women who receive tamoxifen at a dose of 20 mg per day, plasma endoxifen steady-state concentrations are generally 6 to

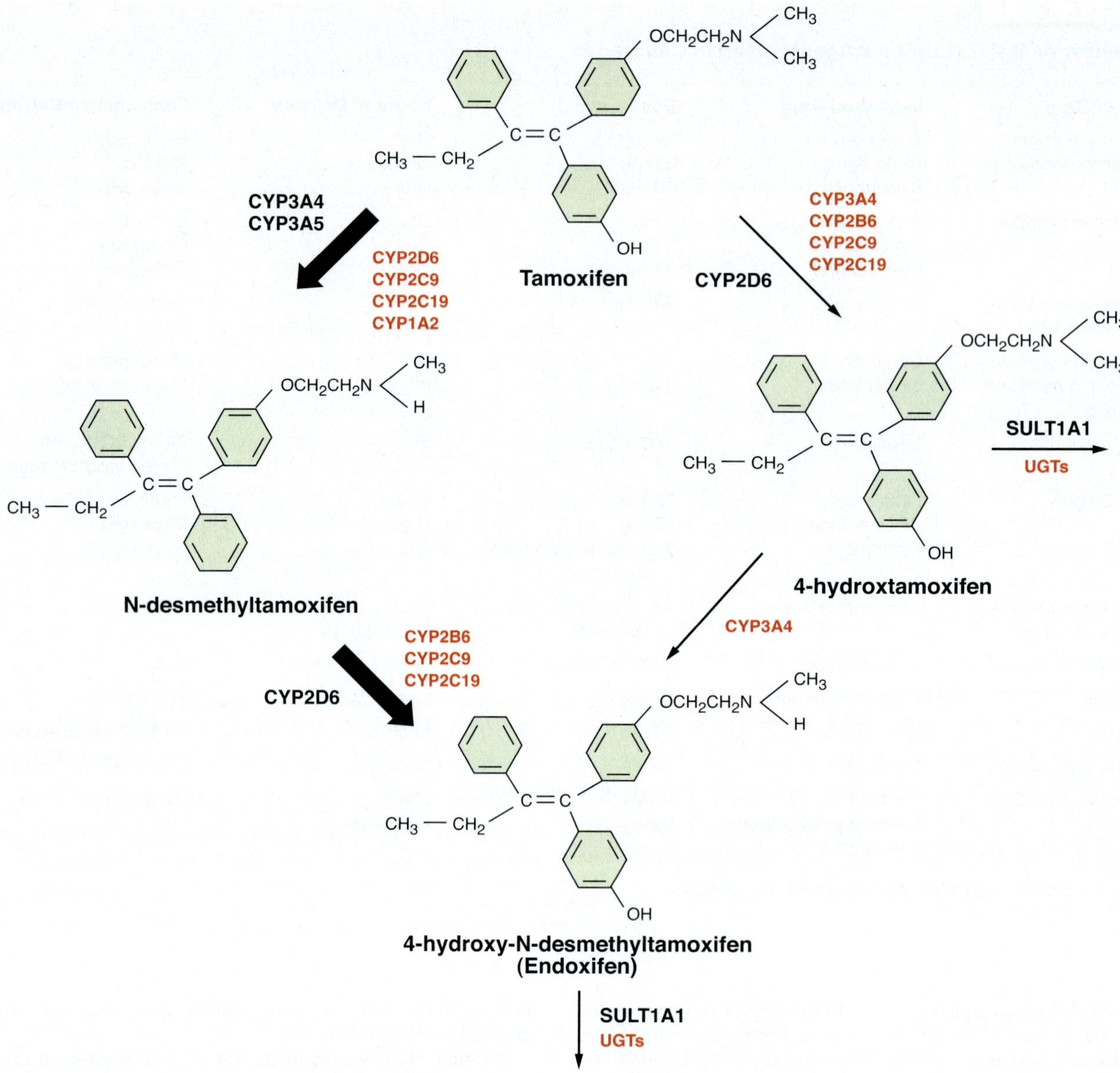

Figure 27.1 Metabolic pathway of tamoxifen biotransformation. (From Sideras K, Ingle JN, Ames MM, et al. Coprescription of tamoxifen and medications that inhibit CYP2D6. *J Clin Oncol* 2010;28:2768–2776.)

10 times higher than 4-hydroxytamoxifen.[53] Although the metabolism of tamoxifen to 4-OH-tamoxifen is catalyzed by multiple enzymes, endoxifen is formed predominantly by the CYP2D6-mediated oxidation of N-desmethyltamoxifen, the most abundant tamoxifen metabolite (see Fig. 27.1).[54] Multiple clinical studies have demonstrated that common *CYP2D6* genetic variation (leading to low or absent CYP2D6 activity) or the drug-induced inhibition of CYP2D6 significantly lowers endoxifen concentrations.[53,55] The *CYP2D6* gene is highly polymorphic, with more than 70 major alleles with four well-defined phenotypes: poor metabolizers (PM), intermediate metabolizers (IM), extensive metabolizers (EM), and ultrarapid metabolizers (UM).

The clinical studies to evaluate the association between *CYP2D6* polymorphisms and tamoxifen outcomes have yielded conflicting results. Initial[56] and follow-up data[57,58] demonstrated that CYP2D6 PM had an approximately two- to threefold higher risk of breast cancer recurrence (compared to CYP2D6 EM) and these data led an FDA special emphasis panel to recommend a tamoxifen label change to incorporate data that the *CYP2D6* genotype was an important biomarker associated with tamoxifen efficacy.[5] However, this label change has been delayed, in part because of conflicting data from secondary analyses of 5-year tamoxifen prospective trials (ATAC,[59] BIG 1-98,[60] and ABCSG8[61]) as well as meta-analyses,[62] which demonstrate that the *CYP2D6* genotype is associated with tamoxifen efficacy when tamoxifen is administered as monotherapy for the adjuvant treatment of postmenopausal, ER-positive breast cancer. Additional support for the importance of endoxifen concentrations came from a secondary analysis of a prospective study, which demonstrated a higher risk of recurrence for women with low endoxifen concentrations.[13]

Many drugs are known to inhibit CYP2D6 activity. In tamoxifen-treated women, the coadministration of potent CYP2D6 inhibitors, such as paroxetine, converts a patient with normal CYP2D6 metabolism to a phenotypic PM.[63] Many other clinically important drugs have been reported to inhibit the CYP2D6 enzyme system, but their effects on tamoxifen metabolism have not been prospectively studied. As with the data regarding *CYP2D6* genotype, the data regarding CYP2D6 inhibitors has additionally been controversial, including two studies that reported opposite findings with regard to CYP2D6 inhibitor use and breast cancer recurrence or death.[64,65] Although the *CYP2D6* data remain controversial, we conclude that until results from prospective adjuvant studies are available, women should be counseled regarding the potential impact of the *CYP2D6* genotype on the effectiveness of adjuvant tamoxifen, and potent CYP2D6 inhibitors should be avoided. Additional caution should be used with drugs that induce CYP3A, such as rifampicin, as a these drugs have been demonstrated to substantially reduce (up to 86%) the concentrations of tamoxifen and its metabolites.[66]

Strategies to overcome low endoxifen concentrations include dose escalation of tamoxifen to 40 mg per day, which has been demonstrated to significantly increase endoxifen concentrations,[67,68] as well as the direct administration of endoxifen itself. The latter strategy is ongoing in multiple different clinical trials, and early reports suggest clinical activity in aromatase inhibitors (AI)-resistant breast cancer.[69]

Following the metabolic activation of tamoxifen, the hydroxylated metabolites undergo both glucuronidation and sulfation. Peak plasma levels of tamoxifen (maximum concentration [Cmax]) are seen 3 to 7 hours after oral administration. Assuming an oral bioavailability of 30%, the volume of distribution has been calculated to be 20 L/kg, and plasma clearance ranges from 1.2 to 5.1 L per hour.[70] The terminal half-life of tamoxifen has been reported to range between 4 and 11 days.[71,72] The elimination half-life of tamoxifen increases with successive doses, which is consistent with saturable kinetics.[71,73] The drug's distribution in tissues is extensive. Levels of the parent drug and metabolites have been reported to be higher in tissue than in plasma in animal studies.[74,75] Reports of tamoxifen concentrations 10- to 60-fold higher than plasma concentrations in the liver, lungs, brain, pancreas, skin, and bones are reported.[76,77] Elevated levels of tamoxifen with biliary obstruction have been reported.[78]

Tamoxifen has been reported to interact with warfarin,[73,79–81] digitoxin, phenytoin,[82] and medroxyprogesterone.[73] Tamoxifen-induced activation of human transcription factor pregnane X receptor (hPXR), resulting in the induction of CYP3A4, may increase the elimination of concomitantly administered CYP3A substrates,[83] such as anastrozole.[84]

Toremifene

Toremifene is an agent similar to tamoxifen. It is available in the United States for the treatment of patients with metastatic breast cancer, and is approved in other countries for the adjuvant treatment of ER-positive breast cancer. Clinical trials have demonstrated no difference in either disease free or overall survival when toremifene was compared with tamoxifen for the treatment of ER-positive breast cancer,[85,86]and evidence exists for major cross-resistance between tamoxifen and toremifene.[87,88]

Pharmacology

Toremifene is an antiestrogen with a chemical structure that differs from that of tamoxifen by the substitution of a chlorine for a hydrogen atom that is retained when toremifene undergoes metabolism.[89] Like tamoxifen, toremifene is metabolized by CYP3A,[90] with a secondary metabolism to form hydroxylated metabolites that appear to have similar binding affinities to 4-OH tamoxifen.[89,91] The importance of these metabolites or the role of metabolism to the hydroxylated metabolites is unknown, but may play a role given the structural similarity of toremifene to tamoxifen. Although the oral bioavailability has not been defined, toremifene's oral absorption appears to be good. The time to peak plasma concentrations after oral administration ranges from 1.5 to 6.0 hours,[92] with the terminal half-lives for toremifene and one metabolite, 4-hydroxytoremifene, being 5 to 6 days.[93,94] The apparent clearance is 5.1 L per hour. The terminal half-life for the major metabolite, N-desmethyltoremifene, is 21 days.[95] The time to reach plasma steady-state concentrations is 1 to 5 weeks. Plasma protein binding is more than 99%. As with tamoxifen, toremifene is present at higher concentrations in tissues compared to plasma with a high apparent volume of distribution (958 L). Seventy percent of the drug is excreted in feces as metabolites. Studies in patients with impaired liver function or those on anticonvulsants known to induce CYP3A have demonstrated that hepatic dysfunction decreases the clearance of toremifene and N-desmethyltoremifene,[95] whereas those patients on anticonvulsants had an increased clearance. Although toremifene appeared to be less carcinogenic than tamoxifen in preclinical models,[43,96,97] of the rates of endometrial cancer in the adjuvant studies have been similar to tamoxifen.[85]

Raloxifene

Raloxifene is an estrogen agonist and antagonist originally developed to treat osteoporosis. Large placebo-controlled randomized trials demonstrated reduced rates of osteoporosis and a reduction in new breast cancers in treated women, leading to the development of a second-generation breast cancer chemoprevention trial (National Surgical Adjuvant Breast and Bowel Project, NSAPB P2) in which raloxifene was compared with tamoxifen in high-risk postmenopausal women. In this study, tamoxifen was superior to raloxifene in terms of both invasive and noninvasive cancer events, but was associated with a higher risk of thromboembolic events and endometrial cancer.[98]

Pharmacology

Raloxifene is partially estrogenic in bone[99] and lowers cholesterol.[100] It is antiestrogenic in mammary tissue[101,102] and uterine tissue.[103]

The pharmacokinetics of raloxifene have been studied principally in postmenopausal women.[104–106] Pharmacokinetic parameters of raloxifene show considerable interindividual variation. Limited information is available on the pharmacokinetics of raloxifene in individuals with hepatic impairment, renal impairment, or both.

Raloxifene is rapidly absorbed from the gastrointestinal tract. Because raloxifene undergoes extensive first-pass glucuronidation, oral bioavailability of unchanged drug is low. Although approximately 60% of an oral dose is absorbed, the absolute bioavailability as unchanged raloxifene is only 2%. However, systemic availability of raloxifene may be greater than that indicated in bioavailability studies, because circulating glucuronide conjugates are converted back to the parent drug in various tissues.

After the oral administration of a single 120- or 150-mg dose of raloxifene hydrochloride, peak plasma concentrations of raloxifene and its glucuronide conjugates are achieved at 6 hours and 1 hour, respectively. After the oral administration of radiolabeled raloxifene, less than 1% of total circulating radiolabeled material in plasma represents the parent drug.

Results of a single-dose study in patients with liver dysfunction indicate that plasma raloxifene concentrations correlate with serum bilirubin concentrations and are 2.5 times higher than individuals with normal hepatic function. In postmenopausal women who received raloxifene in clinical trials, plasma concentrations of raloxifene and the glucuronide conjugates in those with renal impairment (i.e., estimated creatinine clearance values as low as 23 mL per minute) were similar to values in women with normal renal function.

Raloxifene and its monoglucuronide conjugates are more than 95% bound to plasma proteins. Raloxifene binds to albumin and α_1-acid glycoprotein. Raloxifene undergoes extensive first-pass metabolism to the glucuronide conjugates raloxifene 4′-glucuronide, 6-glucuronide, and 6,4′-diglucuronide. UGT1A1 and -1A8 have been found to catalyze the formation of both the 6-β-and 4′-β-glucuronides, whereas UGT1A10 formed only the 4′-β-glucuronide.[107] The metabolism of raloxifene does not ap-

CANCER THERAPEUTICS

pear to be mediated by CYP enzymes (such as CYP2D6), because metabolites other than glucuronide conjugates have not been identified.

The plasma elimination half-life of raloxifene at steady state averages 32.5 hours (range, 15.8 to 86.6 hours). Raloxifene is excreted principally in feces as an unabsorbed drug and via biliary elimination as glucuronide conjugates, which, subsequently, are metabolized by bacteria in the gastrointestinal tract to the parent drug. After oral administration, less than 0.2% of a raloxifene dose is excreted as the parent compound and less than 6% as glucuronide conjugates in urine.

Fulvestrant

Fulvestrant is an ER antagonist that has no known agonist activity and results in ER downregulation.[108–111] Like tamoxifen, fulvestrant competitively binds to the ER but with a higher affinity—approximately 100 times greater than that of tamoxifen,[108,112–114]—thus preventing endogenous estrogen from exerting its effect in target cells.

Results from two phase III clinical trials using the 250 mg per month dose demonstrated fulvestrant to be as effective as anastrozole in the treatment of postmenopausal women with advanced hormone receptor–positive breast cancer previously treated with antiestrogen therapy (mainly tamoxifen).[112–116] In the setting of first-line hormone-responsive metastatic breast cancer, a randomized phase III clinical trial to compare tamoxifen to fulvestrant (250 mg per month) demonstrated no differences in response or time to progression.[117] Because of pharmacology data (discussed in the following paragraphs), the 500 mg per day dose was developed. A randomized trial comparing the 250 mg per month with 500 mg per month dose demonstrated a 4-month improvement in median overall survival advantage for the higher dose.[118] For this reason, the higher dose is now the standard recommended dose.

Fulvestrant is well tolerated. The most common drug-related events (greater than 10% incidence) from the randomized phase III studies were injection-site reactions and hot flashes. Common events (1% to 10% incidence) included asthenia, headache, and gastrointestinal disturbances such as nausea, vomiting, and diarrhea, with minor gastrointestinal disturbances being the most commonly described adverse event.

Pharmacology

Fulvestrant is a steroidal molecule derived from E_2 with an alkylsulphonyl side chain in the 7-α position (Fig. 27.2). Because fulvestrant is poorly soluble and has low and unpredictable oral bioavailability, a parenteral formulation of fulvestrant was developed in an attempt to maximize delivery of the drug.[111] The intramuscular formulation provides prolonged release of the drug over several weeks. The pharmacokinetics of three different single doses of fulvestrant (50, 125, and 250 mg) have been published.[111] In this phase I/II multicenter study, postmenopausal women with primary breast cancer who were awaiting curative surgery received either fulvestrant, tamoxifen, or placebo. After single intramuscular injections of fulvestrant, the time of maximal concentration (t_{max}) ranged from 2 to 19 days, with the median being 7 days for each dose group. At the interval of 28 days, Cmin values were two- to fivefold lower than the Cmax values. For most patients in the 125- and 250-mg dose groups, significant levels of fulvestrant were still measurable 84 days after administration. Pharmacokinetic modeling of the pooled data from the 250-mg cohort was best described by a two-compartment model in which a longer terminal phase began approximately 3 weeks after administration. Because of the long time needed to reach a steady state, the 500-mg loading dose regimen was prospectively studied and determined to be superior to the 250 mg per month dose, both in terms of steady state concentrations achieved within 1 month[119]as well as progression-free and overall survival.[118]

AROMATASE INHIBITORS

At menopause, the synthesis of ovarian hormones ceases. However, estrogen continues to be converted from androgens (produced by the adrenal glands) by aromatase, an enzyme of the CYP superfamily. Aromatase is the enzyme complex responsible for the final step in estrogen synthesis via the conversion of androgens, androstenedione and testosterone, to estrogens, estrone (E_1) and E_2. This biologic pathway served as the basis for the development of the antiaromatase class of compounds. Alterations in aromatase expression have been implicated in the pathogenesis of estrogen-dependent disease, including breast cancer, endometrial cancer, and endometriosis. The importance of this enzyme is also highlighted by the fact that selective aromatase inhibitors are commonly used as first-line therapy for the treatment of postmenopausal women with estrogen-responsive breast cancer. Aminoglutethimide was the first clinically used aromatase inhibitor. When it became available, it was used to cause a *medical adrenalectomy*. Because of the lack of selectivity for aromatase and the resultant suppression of aldosterone and cortisol, aminoglutethimide is no longer recommended for treating metastatic breast cancer. Aminoglutethimide is also occasionally used to try to reverse excess hormone production by adrenocortical cancers.[120]

Aromatase (cytochrome P-450 19 [CYP19]) is encoded by the *CYP19* gene, which is highly polymorphic. Some of these variants are functionally important[121] and may have clinical significance.[122,123]

Aromatase inhibitors have been classified in a number of different ways, including first, second, and third generation; steroidal and nonsteroidal; and reversible (ionic binding) and irreversible (suicide inhibitor, covalent binding).[124] The nonsteroidal aromatase inhibitors include aminoglutethimide (first generation), rogletimide and fadrozole (second generation), and anastrozole, letrozole, and vorozole (third generation). The steroidal aromatase inhibitors include formestane (second generation) and exemestane (third generation).

Steroidal and nonsteroidal aromatase inhibitors differ in their modes of interaction with, and their inactivation of, the aromatase enzyme. Steroidal inhibitors compete with the endogenous

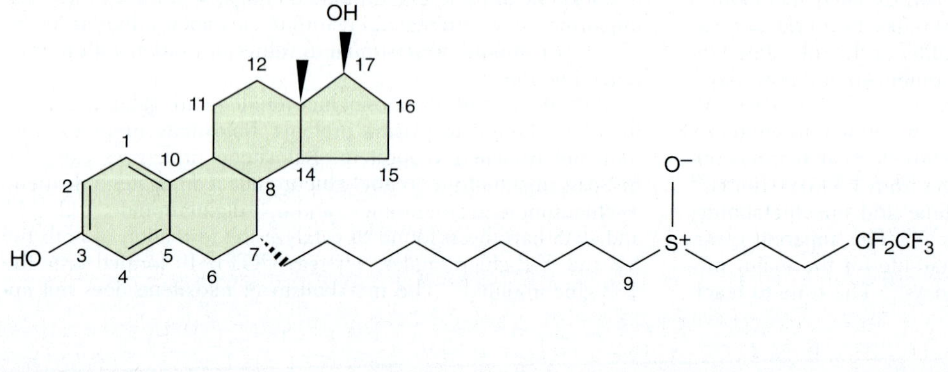

Figure 27.2 Structure of fulvestrant.

substrates, androstenedione and testosterone, for the active site of the enzyme and are processed into intermediates that bind irreversibly to the active site, causing irreversible enzyme inhibition.[19] Nonsteroidal inhibitors also compete with the endogenous substrates for access to the active site, where they then form a reversible bond to the heme iron atom so that enzyme activity can recover if the inhibitor is removed; however, inhibition is sustained whenever the inhibitor is present.[19]

Letrozole and Anastrozole

Both letrozole and anastrozole have been extensively studied in the metastatic and adjuvant settings. When compared to tamoxifen, both letrozole and anastrozole have demonstrated superior response rates and progression-free survival in the metastatic setting.[124,125] In the adjuvant setting, two trials have been performed and demonstrated superiority in terms of relapse-free survivals of both anastrozole (ATAC)[126] and letrozole (BIG 1-98).[127] Additionally, anastrozole has been studied in a sequential approach, and the sequence of tamoxifen followed by anastrozole is superior to 5 years of tamoxifen alone.[128] Anastrozole has recently been compared to placebo in women at an increased risk of developing breast cancer and was demonstrated to significantly reduce the incidence of invasive breast cancer.[129]

The side effects of both anastrozole and letrozole are similar and include arthralgias and myalgias in up to 50% of patients. Both letrozole and anastrozole are associated with a higher rate of bone fracture, compared with the tamoxifen.[130] At the present time, minimal long-term (longer than 5 years) clinical data regarding the effect of aromatase inhibitors on bones are available. When offering anastrozole for extended periods of time to patients with early breast cancer, attention to bone health is paramount, and bone density should be monitored in all patients. Prospective studies have demonstrated that bisphosphonates prevent aromatase-inhibitor–induced bone loss and a meta-analysis presented at the 2013 San Antonio Breast Cancer Symposium demonstrated that bisphosphonates reduce bone recurrences and prolong overall survival. Therefore, bisphosphonates should be considered in AI-treated patients, both in those with and without an increased risk of bone fractures.

A meta-analysis of toxicities comparing aromatase inhibitors with tamoxifen has demonstrated a 30% increase in grade 3 and 4 cardiac events with aromatase inhibitors.[131] However, prospective data demonstrate no differences in myocardial events comparing anastrozole with placebo, although an increase in hypertension was observed.[129]

No impact has been seen with anastrozole on adrenal steroidogenesis at up to 10 times the clinically recommended dose.[132] Although letrozole may decrease basal and adrenocorticotropic hormone–stimulated cortisol synthesis,[133,134] the clinical effect appears to be minimal. Aromatase inhibitors appear to have differential effects on lipids. In a study of over 900 patients with metastatic disease, anastrozole showed no marked effect on lipid profiles compared with baseline.[135] Conversely, the administration of letrozole in women with advanced breast cancer resulted in significant increases in total cholesterol and low-density lipoprotein, from baseline, after 8 and 16 weeks of therapy.[136] In the Breast International Group 1-98 trial, more women who received letrozole experienced grade 1 hypercholesterolemia compared to women who received tamoxifen.[127]

Letrozole is a nonsteroidal aromatase inhibitor with a high specificity for the inhibition of estrogen production (Fig. 27.3). Letrozole is 180 times more potent than aminoglutethimide as an inhibitor of aromatase in vitro. Aldosterone production in vitro is inhibited by concentrations 10,000 times higher than those required for inhibition of estrogen synthesis.[137,138] In a normal male volunteer study, letrozole was shown to decrease E_2 and serum E_1 levels to 10% of baseline with a single 3-mg dose. In phase I studies, letrozole caused a significant decline in plasma E_1 and E_2 within 24 hours of a single oral dose of 0.1 mg.[139,140] After 2 weeks of treatment, the blood levels of E_2, E_1, and estrone sulfate were suppressed 95% or more from baseline. This continued over the 12 weeks of therapy. There was no apparent alteration in plasma levels of cortisol and aldosterone with letrozole or after corticotropin stimulation.[139] In postmenopausal women with advanced breast cancer, the drug did not have any effect on follicle-stimulating hormone (FSH), luteinizing hormone (LH), thyrotropin (previously thyroid-stimulating hormone), cortisol, 17-α-hydroxyprogesterone, androstenedione, or aldosterone blood concentrations.[141,142]

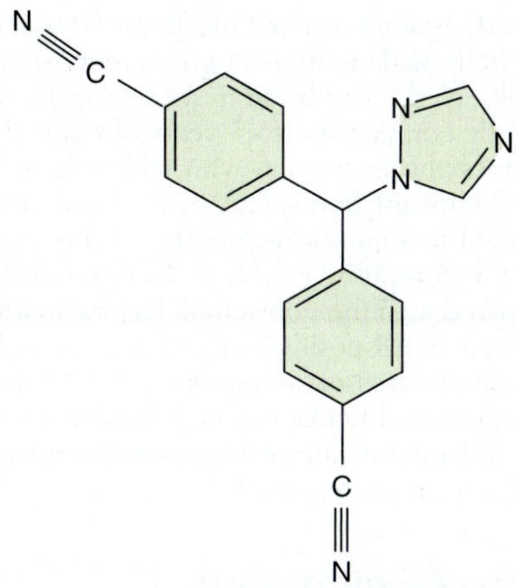

Figure 27.3 Structure of letrozole.

Anastrozole is a nonsteroidal aromatase inhibitor that is 200-fold more potent than aminoglutethimide.[143] No effect on the adrenal glands has been detected. In human studies, the t_{max} is 2 to 3 hours after oral ingestion.[144] Elimination is primarily via hepatic metabolism, with 85% excreted by that route and only 10% excreted unchanged in urine. The main circulating metabolite is triazole after cleavage of the two rings in anastrozole by N-dealkylation. Linear pharmacokinetics have been observed in the dose range of 1 to 20 mg and do not change with repeat dosing. The terminal half-life is approximately 50 hours, and steady-state concentrations are achieved in approximately 10 days with once-a-day dosing and are three to four times higher than peak concentrations after a single dose. Plasma protein binding is approximately 40%.[145] In one study, anastrozole 1 mg and 10 mg daily, inhibited in vivo aromatization by 96.7% and 98.1%, respectively, and plasma E_1 and E_2 levels were suppressed 86.5% and 83.5%, respectively, regardless of dose.[146] Thus, 1 mg of anastrozole achieves near maximal aromatase inhibition and plasma estrogen suppression in breast cancer patients.

A recent prospective study to evaluate the pharmacokinetics of anastrozole (1 mg per day) demonstrated large interindividual variations in plasma anastrozole and anastrozole metabolite concentrations, as well as pretreatment and postdrug plasma E_1, E_2, and E_1 conjugate and estrogen precursor (androstenedione and testosterone) concentrations.[147] Further research is needed to determine the basis for the wide variability in the pharmacokinetics of anastrozole and whether these findings are clinically relevant.

Exemestane

Exemestane has a steroidal structure and is classified as a type 1 aromatase inhibitor, also known as an *aromatase inactivator*, because it irreversibly binds with and permanently inactivates the enzyme.[134] Exemestane has been compared to tamoxifen in both the metastatic and adjuvant settings. In the setting of tamoxifen-refractory metastatic breast cancer, exemestane is superior to

CANCER THERAPEUTICS

megestrol acetate, as demonstrated in a phase III trial in which improvements in both median time to tumor progression and median survival were observed.[148] In the adjuvant setting, the international exemestane study compared 2 to 3 years of tamoxifen with 2 to 3 years of exemestane in women who had previously competed 2 to 3 years of adjuvant tamoxifen. In this trial, a switch to exemestane resulted in superior disease-free and overall survival in the hormone receptor–positive subtype. Furthermore, exemestane has been compared with the nonsteroidal agent anastrozole in the adjuvant treatment of ER-positive breast cancer, and there were no differences in disease-free or overall survival.[149] Finally, exemestane has been compared to placebo in patients at increased risk of breast cancer, and a significant reduction in the risk of developing invasive breast cancer was observed.[150]

Side Effects of Exemestane

Although preclinical studies have suggested that exemestane prevented bone loss in ovariectomized rats,[151] the Intergroup Exemestane adjuvant trial still demonstrated a higher rate of bone fracture for patients randomized to the exemestane arm and there were no differences in fracture rates comparing anastrozole with exemestane.[149] Side effects, including arthralgias and myalgias, appear to be similar to the other AIs. With regard to steroidogenesis, no impact on either cortisol or aldosterone levels was seen in a small study after the administration of exemestane for 7 days.[152] Finally, exemestane has weak androgenic properties, and its use at higher doses has been associated with steroidal-like side effects, such as weight gain and acne.[153,154] However, these side effects have not been observed with the FDA-approved dose (25 mg per day).[155]

Pharmacology

Exemestane is administered once daily by mouth, with the recommended daily dose being 25 mg. The time needed to reach maximal E_2 suppression is 7 days,[156] and its half-life is 27 hours.[157] At daily doses of 10 to 25 mg, exemestane suppresses estrogen concentrations to 6% to 15% of pretreatment levels. This activity is more pronounced than that produced by formestane and comparable to that produced by the nonsteroidal AIs, anastrozole and letrozole.[158–160] Exemestane does not appear to affect cortisol or aldosterone levels when evaluated after 7 days of treatment based on dose-ranging studies, including doses from 0.5 to 800 mg.[152] Exemestane is metabolized by CYP3A4.[134] Although drug–drug interactions have not been formally reported for exemestane, there is the potential for interactions with drugs that affect CYP3A4.[134]

GONADOTROPIN-RELEASING HORMONE ANALOGS

Gonadotropin-releasing hormone (GnRH) analogs result in a *medical orchiectomy* in men and are used as a means of providing androgen ablation for hormone-sensitive and castration refractory metastatic prostate cancer.[161] Because the initial agonist activity of GnRH analogs can cause a *tumor flare* from temporarily increased androgen levels, concomitant use of the antiandrogen flutamide or bicalutamide has been used to prevent this effect. GnRH analogs can also cause tumor regressions in hormonally responsive breast cancers[162] and have received FDA approval for the treatment of metastatic breast cancer in premenopausal women. Data suggest that these drugs may be useful as adjuvant therapy of premenopausal women with resected breast cancer.[163] The use of these drugs in combination with tamoxifen or exemestane in premenopausal women with primary breast cancer is the subject of large, ongoing, international clinical trials. The primary toxicities of GnRH analogs are secondary to the ablation of sex steroid concentrations and include hot flashes, sweating, and nausea.[164] These symptoms can be reversed with low doses of progesterone analogs.[5] In males treated with GnRH analogs for prostate cancer, an alternate strategy of intermittent schedule of GnRH administration may result in improved tolerability and quality of life, with comparable efficacy compared with continuous GnRH analog administration in well-selected advanced prostate cancer patient cohorts.[165] However, in a recent trial comparing intermittent with continuous androgen ablation in newly diagnosed metastatic hormone sensitive prostate cancer patients, a greater risk for death from an intermittent strategy could not be conclusively ruled out although intermittent therapy resulted in small improvements in quality of life.[166]

GnRH analogs available for clinical use include goserelin[167,168] and leuprolide.[169] Both are available in depot intramuscular preparations to be given at monthly intervals. The recommended monthly dose of leuprolide is 7.5 mg and of goserelin is 3.6 mg. There are also longer acting depot preparations to be administered every 3, 4, 6, and 12 months.

Pharmacology

Analogs of the decapeptide GnRH[167,169,170] have been synthesized by modifications of position 6 in which the l-glycine has been exchanged for a d-amino acid and the C-terminal amino acid has been either replaced by an ethylamide or substituted for a modified amino acid. These changes increase the affinity of the analog for the GnRH receptor and decrease the susceptibility to enzymatic degradation. There is an amino acid structure of GnRH with the substitutions for leuprolide and goserelin. Initial administration of these compounds results in stimulation of gonadotropin release. However, prolonged administration has led to profound inhibition of the pituitary–gonadal axis.[170] Plasma E_2 and progesterone are consistently suppressed to postmenopausal or castrate levels after 2 to 4 weeks of treatment with goserelin or leuprolide.[164,171] These drugs are administered intramuscularly or subcutaneously in a parenteral sustained-release microcapsule preparation, because parenteral administration of the parent drug is otherwise associated with rapid clearance. The GnRH analogs are metabolized in the liver, kidney, hypothalamus, and pituitary gland by neutral peptidase cleavage of the peptide bond between the tyrosine in the 5 position and the amino acid in position 6 and by a postproline-cleaving enzyme that cleaves the peptide bond between proline in the 9 position and the glycine-NH_2 in the 10 position. Substitutions at the glycine 6 position and modification of the C-terminal make these analogs more resistant to this enzymatic cleavage.

Leuprolide is approximately 80 to 100 times more potent than endogenous GnRH. It induces castrate levels of testosterone in men with prostate cancer within 3 to 4 weeks of drug administration after an initial sharp increase in LH and FSH. The mechanisms of action include pituitary desensitization after a reduction in pituitary GnRH receptor binding sites and possibly a direct antitumor effect in ER-positive human breast cancer cells.[169] The depot form results in a dose rate of 210 μg per day of leuprolide. Peak concentrations of the depot form, achieved approximately 3 hours after drug administration, have been reported to range between 13.1 and 54.5 μg/L. There appears to be a linear increase in the area under the curve (AUC) for doses of 3.75, 7.5, and 15.0 mg in the depot form. The parenteral bioavailability of subcutaneously injected leuprolide is 94%. The volume of distribution ranges from 27.4 to 37.1 L. In human studies, leuprolide urinary excretion as a metabolite was the primary route of clearance.

Goserelin is approximately 100 times more potent than the naturally occurring GnRH. Like leuprolide, it causes the stimulation of LH and FSH acutely, and with subsequent administration, GnRH receptor numbers decrease, and the pituitary becomes desensitized with decreasing LH and FSH levels. Castrate levels of testosterone are achieved within 1 month. In women, goserelin inhibits ovarian androgen production, but serum levels of dehydroepiandrosterone sulfate and, to a lesser extent, androstenedione, are preserved. In vitro, goserelin has demonstrated antitumor activity in estrogen-dependent MCF7 human breast cancer cells and LNCaP2 prostate cancer cells. The drug is released at a continuous mean rate of 120 μg per day in the depot form, with peak concentrations in the range of 2 to 3 μg/L achieved. The mean volume of distribution in six patients has been reported to be 13.7 L,[172] which is consistent with extracellular fluid volume. Goserelin is principally excreted in the urine, with a mean total body clearance of 8 L per hour in patients with normal renal function. The total body clearance is reduced by approximately 75%, with renal dysfunction and the elimination half-life increased two- or threefold. However, dose adjustment for renal insufficiency does not appear to be necessary. The 5 to 10 hexapeptide and the 4 to 10 hexapeptide were detected in urine in animal studies.[173] The terminal half-life of goserelin is approximately 5 hours after subcutaneous injection. Protein binding is low, and no known drug interactions have been documented.

GONADOTROPIN-RELEASING HORMONE ANTAGONISTS

Modification to the structure of GnRH has resulted in the development of GnRH antagonist compounds that are currently being used in the treatment of prostate cancer. Abarelix was initially approved by the FDA in 2003 as the first depot-injectable GnRH antagonist, but was subsequently withdrawn in 2005. Degarelix is a synthetically modified compound with GnRH antagonist activity that was approved for use by the FDA in 2008 for the management of prostate cancer.[174] Its effect in prostate cancer treatment is to block the GnRH receptor, and thereby prevent the trigger for the production of LH, which mediates androgen synthesis. In contrast to GnRH analogs, degarelix does not cause *tumor flare* symptoms secondary to temporary increased androgen production. A large randomized clinical trial demonstrated that degarelix was associated with a rapid and sustained reduction in serum testosterone, prostate-specific antigen (PSA), FSH, and LH levels, with a loading dose of 240 mg subcutaneously, followed by a monthly maintenance dose of 80 mg[175] with comparable efficacy to leuprolide.[176] The most common side effects (greater than 10%) were hot flashes and pain at the injection site[176] when patients were provided degarelix for a 12-month period. It is unknown if degarelix will have a similar chronic side effect profile known to be associated with long-term GnRH analog use.

Pharmacology

The recommended loading dose of degarelix is 240 mg, administered as two injections of 120 mg each subcutaneously. Monthly maintenance doses of 80 mg as a 20 mg/mL solution is started 28 days after the loading dose. In an analysis of pharmacokinetic/pharmacodynamic (PK/PD) properties of degarelix in 60 healthy males, after a single subcutaneous dose, a terminal half life of 47 days was observed.[177] PK properties of degarelix have been evaluated when administered as a subcutaneous depot of drug as a gel in six different doses to 48 healthy males and when administered intravenously. Using data from several clinical trials, the rate of drug diffusion from subcutaneous administration results in detectable drug up to 60 days after a single dose compared to less than 4 days when the drug is injected intravenously.

ANTIANDROGENS

Flutamide

The antiandrogen flutamide is used in men with metastatic prostate cancer either as initial therapy, combined with GnRH analog administration, or when the metastatic prostate cancer is unresponsive, despite androgen ablation therapy. The recommended dose is 250 mg by mouth three times a day. In patients whose prostate cancer is growing despite flutamide use, stopping flutamide can sometimes cause a flutamide-withdrawal response.

The most common toxicity seen with flutamide is diarrhea, with or without abdominal discomfort. Gynecomastia, which can be tender, frequently occurs in men who are not receiving concomitant androgen ablation therapy.[178] Flutamide can rarely cause hepatotoxicity, a condition that is reversible if detected early, but this toxicity can also be fatal.[179] There is no accepted, clinically recommended testing schedule to screen for flutamide-induced hepatotoxicity other than being aware of this phenomenon and testing for liver function if hepatic symptoms develop.

Pharmacology

Flutamide is a pure antiandrogen with no intrinsic steroidal activity.[180] Flutamide's mechanism of action is as an androgen-receptor antagonist. This binding prevents dihydrotestosterone binding and subsequent translocation of the androgen-receptor complex into the nuclei of cells. Because it is a pure antiandrogen, it acts only at the cellular level. The administration of flutamide alone leads to increased LH and FSH production and a concomitant increase in plasma testosterone and E_2 levels. Plasma protein binding ranges between 94% and 96% for flutamide and between 92% and 94% for 2-hydroxyflutamide, its major metabolite. When the drug is administered three times a day, steady state levels are achieved by day 6. The elimination half-life at steady state is 7.8 hours, and 2-hydroxyflutamide achieves concentrations 50 times higher than the parent drug at steady state and has equal or greater potency than that of flutamide.[180] The elimination half-life for the metabolite is 9.6 hours. The high plasma concentrations of 2-hydroxyflutamide, as compared with flutamide, suggest that the therapeutic benefits of flutamide are mediated primarily through its active metabolite.[181]

Bicalutamide

Bicalutamide is another nonsteroidal antiandrogen that has been approved by the FDA for use in the United States. The recommended dose is one 50-mg tablet per day. One randomized trial reported that bicalutamide compared favorably with flutamide in patients with advanced prostate cancer.[182] Bicalutamide appears to be relatively well tolerated and is associated with a lower incidence of diarrhea than is flutamide.

Pharmacology

Bicalutamide has a binding affinity to the androgen receptor in the rat prostate that is four times greater than that of 2-hydroxyflutamide.[183,184] In vivo, bicalutamide caused a marked inhibition of growth of accessory sex organs in rats, with a potency 5 to 10 times greater than that of flutamide. Unlike flutamide, bicalutamide did not cause a significant increase in LH or testosterone in rats. In humans, the drug has a long plasma half-life of 5 to 7 days, so it may be administered on a weekly schedule. Pharmacokinetics of the drug showed a dose-dependent increase in mean peak plasma concentrations, and the AUC increased linearly with the dose. The half-life of bicalutamide in humans was approximately 6 days, and the drug clearance was not saturable at plasma concentrations up to 1,000 ng/mL. Daily dosing of the drug led to an approximately tenfold accumulation after 12 weeks of administration. In contrast to results in rats, serum concentrations of testosterone and LH increased significantly from baseline at all dose levels tested in humans. Whereas serum FSH concentrations remained essentially unchanged, the median serum E_2 concentrations increased significantly.[185]

Nilutamide

Nilutamide represents the third variation of an antiandrogen available for use in patients with prostate cancer. The observation of unique toxicities, night blindness, and pulmonary toxicity has limited its use.

NOVEL ANTIANDROGENS

Although testosterone depletion remains an unchallenged standard for advanced stage hormone-sensitive disease, evidence has emerged that *castration-recurrent* prostate cancer remains androgen receptor (AR) dependent and is neither *hormone refractory* nor *androgen independent*, which were commonly used terms to define the progression of advanced stage disease following androgen deprivation therapy. Recognition of AR functioning despite the paucity of circulating androgens is evidenced by the elevation of AR messenger RNA in castration-recurrent tumor tissue relative to androgen-dependent tumors and reexpression of some androgen-regulated genes during clinical castration resistance. Recently, the AR axis has been the focus of therapeutic targeting.

Abiraterone Acetate

After the failure of initial androgen manipulation with GnRH analogs and peripheral antiandrogens, prostate cancer continues to respond to a variety of second- and third-line hormonal interventions. Based on this observation, CYP17, a key enzyme in androgen and estrogen synthesis, was targeted using ketoconazole, which is a weak, reversible, and nonspecific inhibitor of CYP17 resulting in modest antitumor activity of short durability. More recently, abiraterone, a more potent (i.e., 20 times more than ketoconazole), selective, and irreversible inhibitor of CYP17, has been investigated in castration-recurrent prostate cancer, and significant objective responses have been observed.[186] Chemically, it is a 3-pyridyl steroid pregnenolone–derived compound available in an oral prodrug form of abiraterone acetate. Its main toxicity is from symptoms of mineralocorticoid excess (including hypokalemia, hypertension, and fluid overload), because continuous CYP17 blockade results in raising adrenocorticotrophic hormone (ACTH) levels that increase steroid levels upstream of CYP17, including corticosterone and deoxycorticosterone. These adverse effects are best avoided by the coadministration of steroids.

The established dose of abiraterone is 1,000 mg a day (four 250 mg tablets). Following oral administration of abiraterone acetate, the median time to maximum plasma abiraterone concentrations is 2 hours. At the dose of 1,000 mg daily, steady state values (mean ± standard deviation [SD]) of Cmax were 226 ± 178 ng/mL and of AUC were 1173 ± 690 ng.hr/mL. Abiraterone is highly bound (>99%) to the human plasma proteins, albumin and alpha-1 acid glycoprotein. The apparent steady state volume of distribution (mean ± SD) is 19,669 ± 13,358 L. No major deviation from dose proportionality was observed in the dose range of 250 mg to 1,000 mg. However, the exposure was not significantly increased when the dose was doubled from 1,000 to 2,000 mg (8% increase in mean AUC). The two main circulating metabolites of abiraterone in human plasma are abiraterone sulfate (inactive) and N-oxide abiraterone sulfate (inactive), which each account for about 43% of exposure. CYP3A4 and SULT2A1 are enzymes involved in the formation and conjugation of N-oxide abiraterone.

Enzalutamide

Enzalutamide is a new diarylthiohydantoin compound that binds AR with an affinity that is several-fold greater than the antiandrogens bicalutamide and flutamide. This class of novel AR inhibitor also disrupts the nuclear translocation of AR and impairs DNA binding to androgen response elements and the recruitment of coactivators.[187] In early clinical trials, promising results have been observed in castrate refractory and chemotherapy-resistant settings. The major metabolite of enzalutamide is N-desmethyl enzalutamide, and CYP2C8 is responsible for the formation of the active metabolite, N-desmethyl enzalutamide. Enzalutamide pharmacokinetics, in the studied dose range between 30 mg to 480 mg, exhibited a linear, two-compartmental model with first-order kinetics. In patients with mCRPC, the mean (% coefficient of variation [CV]) predose Cmin values for enzalutamide and N-desmethyl enzalutamide were 11.4 (25.9%) μg/mL and 13.0 (29.9%) μg/mL, respectively. Enzalutamide is mainly metabolized by CYP2C8 and CYP3A4. Doses ranging from 30 to 600 mg daily have been evaluated, with dose-limiting toxicities including fatigue, seizure, asthenia, anemia, and arthralgia occurring at higher dose levels. At present, enzalutamide has been approved for treating advanced castrate-recurrent prostate cancer[188] after a failure of docetaxel chemotherapy at a dose of 160 mg (four, 40 mg oral capsules). Clinical trials are ongoing to evaluate the efficacy of enzalutamide in castrate-recurrent patients who are chemotherapy naïve.

Galeterone and Orteronel

Novel CYP17 inhibitors that are more selective for 17,20-lyase over 17 α-hydroxylase are currently being developed. Orteronel (TAK-700) is an example of a highly selective 17,20 lyase, which is currently undergoing phase III clinical trials in a pre- and post-chemotherapy castrate-recurrent setting after the failure of androgen-deprivation therapy.[189] Other novel agents being developed include galeterone, which is an inhibitor of CYP 17 α-hydroxylase and C17,20 lyase. Survival mechanisms of prostate cancer cells targeted by galeterone include its binding to AR, competitive inhibition of testosterone binding, and a reduction in the quantity of AR protein within the prostate cancer cells. It can also enhance the degradation of constitutively active splice variants. Therefore, taken together, it diminishes the ability of the cells to respond to the low levels of androgenic growth signals. This agent is currently in early clinical safety and efficacy testing for advanced stage prostate cancer.

OTHER SEX STEROID THERAPIES

Fluoxymesterone

Fluoxymesterone is an androgen that has been used in women with metastatic breast cancer who have hormonally responsive cancers and who have progressed on other hormonal therapies such as tamoxifen, an aromatase inhibitor, or megestrol acetate. The usual dose is 10 mg given twice daily. Although the overall response rate is low for fluoxymesterone used in this clinical situation,[190] there are some patients who have substantial antitumor responses lasting for months or even years.

Toxicities associated with fluoxymesterone are those that would be expected with an androgen: hirsutism, male-pattern baldness, voice lowering (hoarseness), acne, enhanced libido, and erythrocytosis. Fluoxymesterone can also cause elevated liver function test results in some patients and, rarely, has been associated with hepatic neoplasms.

Pharmacology

Fluoxymesterone is a chlorinated synthetic analog of testosterone with potent androgenic and anabolic activity in humans. Limited pharmacologic information is available on this agent. Colburn,[191] using a radioimmunoassay, studied two patients after a single oral administration of a 50-mg dose. Peak serum concentrations were achieved between 1 and 3 hours after administration, with the average peak concentrations being 335 ng/mL. By 5 hours after drug administration, serum levels had declined to approximately 50% of the peak concentration. Urinary excretion of a 10-mg dose can be detected for 24 hours, and at least 6-hydroxy, 4-ene, 3-β, and 11-hydroxy metabolites of fluoxymesterone have been detected.[192]

Estrogens: Diethylstilbestrol and Estradiol

Diethylstilbestrol (DES) had been the primary hormonal therapy for postmenopausal metastatic breast cancer. Randomized comparative trials demonstrated it had a similar response rate to that of tamoxifen.[193,194] However, based on these trials, DES use was supplanted by tamoxifen, primarily because DES has more toxicity. DES is occasionally used in metastatic breast cancer patients who have hormonally sensitive cancers that have failed to respond to multiple other hormonal therapies. The usual dose in this situation is 15 mg per day, either as a single dose or as divided doses. DES was also used as androgen ablation therapy in men with metastatic prostate cancer.[195] Doses of approximately 3 mg per day result in testosterone levels that are seen in an anorchid state.

DES toxicities include nausea and vomiting, breast tenderness, and a darkening of the nipple–areolar complex. DES increases the risk of thromboembolic phenomenon, which may result in life-threatening complications. Although DES is not clinically available in the United States, similar antitumor effects and toxicities are seen with estradiol, with a target dose of 10 mg by mouth three times a day. The pharmacology of E_2 has been extensively described elsewhere.[196]

Medroxyprogesterone and Megestrol

Medroxyprogesterone and megestrol are 17-OH-progesterone derivatives differing in a double bond between C6 and C7 positions in megestrol. Historically, megestrol was used as a hormonal agent for patients with advanced breast cancer, usually at a total daily dose of 160 mg. Additionally, it is still used for the treatment of hormonally responsive metastatic endometrial cancer, at a dose of 320 mg per day. In addition, doses of 160 mg per day are occasionally used as a hormonal therapy for prostate cancer.[197] Megestrol has also been extensively evaluated for the treatment of anorexia/cachexia related to cancer or AIDS.[198–201] Various dosages ranging from 160 to 1,600 mg per day have been used. A prospective study has demonstrated a dose–response relationship with doses up to 800 mg per day.[202] Low dosages of megestrol (20 to 40 mg per day) have been shown to be an effective means of reducing hot flashes in women with breast cancer and in men who have undergone androgen ablation therapy.[5] Although megestrol had historically been commonly administered four times per day, the long terminal half-life supports once-per-day dosing.

Megestrol is a relatively well-tolerated medication, with its most prominent side effects being appetite stimulation and resultant weight gain. Although these may be beneficial effects in patients with anorexia/cachexia, they can be important problems in patients with breast or endometrial cancers. Another side effect of megestrol acetate is the marked suppression of adrenal steroid production by suppression of the pituitary–adrenal axis.[203] Although this appears to be asymptomatic in the majority of patients, reports suggest that this adrenal suppression can cause clinical problems in some patients.[204] This drug has been abruptly stopped for decades without the recognition of untoward sequelae in patients, and it seems reasonable to continue this practice. Nonetheless, if Addisonian signs or symptoms develop after drug discontinuation, corticosteroids should be administered. Furthermore, if patients who receive megestrol have a significant infection, experience trauma, or undergo surgery, then corticosteroid coverage should be administered. There appears to be a slightly increased incidence of thromboembolic phenomena in patients receiving megestrol alone.[202] This risk appears to be higher if megestrol is administered with concomitant cytotoxic therapy.[205] There are conflicting reports regarding megestrol-causing edema.[206] If it does, the edema is generally minimal and easily handled with a mild diuretic. Megestrol may cause impotence in some men.[207] The incidence of this is controversial, although it is generally agreed that this is a reversible situation. Megestrol can cause menstrual irregularities, the most prominent of which is withdrawal menstrual bleeding within a few weeks of drug discontinuation.[5] Although nausea and vomiting have sometimes been attributed as a toxicity of this drug, there are data to demonstrate that this drug has antiemetic properties.[200,201,205] In terms of magnitude, megestrol appears to decrease both nausea and vomiting in advanced-stage cancer patients by approximately two thirds.

Medroxyprogesterone has many of the same properties, clinical uses, and toxicities as megestrol acetate. It has never been commonly used in the United States for the treatment of breast cancer but has been used more in Europe. Medroxyprogesterone is available in 2.5- and 10-mg tablets and in injectable formulations of 100 and 400 mg/L. Dosing for the treatment of metastatic breast or prostate cancer has commonly been 400 mg per week or more and 1,000 mg per week or more for metastatic endometrial cancer. Injectable or daily oral doses have been used for controlling hot flashes.

Pharmacology

The exact mechanism of antitumor effect of medroxyprogesterone and megestrol is unclear. These drugs have been reported to suppress adrenal steroid synthesis,[208] suppress ER levels,[209] alter tumor hormone metabolism,[210] enhance steroid metabolism,[211] and directly kill tumor cells.[212] In addition, progestins may influence some growth factors,[213] suppress plasma estrone sulfate formation, and, at high concentrations, inhibit P-glycoprotein.

The oral bioavailability of these progestational agents is unknown, although absorption appears to be poor for medroxyprogesterone relative to megestrol.

The terminal half-life for megestrol is approximately 14 hours,[214,215] with a t_{max} of 2 to 5 hours after oral ingestion.[216] The AUC for a single megestrol dose of 160 mg is between 2.5- and 8-fold higher than that for single-dose medroxyprogesterone at 1,000 mg with a radioactive dose of megestrol; 50% to 78% is found in the urine after oral administration, and 8% to 30% is found in the feces.

Metabolism and excretion of medroxyprogesterone have been incompletely characterized. In humans, 20% to 50% of a [^{3}H]medroxyprogesterone dose is excreted in the urine and 5% to 10% in the stool after intravenous administration.[217–219] Metabolism of medroxyprogesterone occurs via hydroxylation, reduction, demethylation, and combinations of these reactions.[220] The major urinary metabolite is a glucuronide. Less than 3% of the dose is excreted as unconjugated medroxyprogesterone in humans. Clearance of medroxyprogesterone has been reported to range between 27 and 70 L per hour.[219] The initial volume of distribution is between 4 and 8 L in humans. The mean terminal half-life is 60 hours. The t_{max} for medroxyprogesterone occurs 2 to 5 hours after oral administration. Medroxyprogesterone appears to be concentrated in the small intestine, the colon, and in adipose tissue in human autopsy studies.[221] Drug interactions of medroxyprogesterone have been reported with aminoglutethimide, which decreases plasma medroxyprogesterone levels.[222] Medroxyprogesterone may reduce the concentration of the N-desmethyltamoxifen metabolite concentration. Progestational agents also may increase plasma warfarin levels.[223] These reports are consistent with CYP3A being the site of interaction.

OTHER HORMONAL THERAPIES

Octreotide

Octreotide is a somatostatin analog that is administered for the treatment of carcinoid syndrome and other hormonal excess syndromes associated with some pancreatic islet cell cancers and acromegaly. Response rates (measured in terms of a reduction in diarrhea and flushing) are high and can last for several months to years. Occasionally, antitumor responses temporarily related to octreotide are seen with these tumors. Octreotide may be useful to alleviate 5-fluorouracil–associated diarrhea.[224–226]

Octreotide can be administered intravenously or subcutaneously. Initial doses of 50 μg are given two to three times on the first day. The dose is titrated upward, with a usual daily dose of 300 to 450 μg per day for most patients. A depot preparation is available, allowing doses to be administered at monthly intervals. Octreotide is generally well tolerated overall. It appears to cause more toxicity in acromegalic patients, with such problems as bradycardia, diarrhea, hypoglycemia, hyperglycemia, hypothyroidism, and cholelithiasis.

Pharmacology

Octreotide is an 8-amino acid synthetic analog of the 14-amino acid peptide somatostatin.[227] Octreotide has a similar high affinity for somatostatin receptors, as does its parent compound, with a concentration that inhibits the receptor by 50% in the subnanomolar range. Octreotide inhibits insulin, glucagon, pancreatic polypeptide, gastric inhibitory polypeptide, and gastrin secretion. It has a much longer duration of action than the parent compound because of its greater resistance to enzymatic degradation. Its absorption after subcutaneous administration is rapid, and bioavailability is 100% after subcutaneous injection. Peak concentrations of 4 μg/L after a 100-μg dose occur within 20 to 30 minutes of subcutaneous injection and are 20% to 40% of the corresponding intravenous injection. Both peak concentration and AUC for octreotide increase linearly with dose. The total body clearance in healthy volunteers is 9.6 L per hour. Hepatic metabolism of octreotide accounts for 30% to 40% of the drug's disposition, and 11% to 20% is excreted unchanged in the urine. The volume of distribution ranges between 18 and 30 L, and the terminal half-life is reported to be between 72 and 98 minutes. Sixty-five percent of the drug is protein bound primarily to the lipoprotein fraction.[227,228] Because of the short half-life, classic octreotide is administered subcutaneously two or three times per day.[229] A slow-release form of octreotide, designed for once-per-month administration, controls the symptoms of carcinoid syndrome at least as well as three-times-per-day octreotide.[230]

REFERENCES

1. Fisher B, Costantino JP, Wickerham DL, et al. Tamoxifen for the prevention of breast cancer: current status of the National Surgical Adjuvant Breast and Bowel Project P-1 study. *J Natl Cancer Inst* 2005;97:1652–1662.
2. Fisher B, Dignam J, Wolmark N, et al. Tamoxifen in treatment of intraductal breast cancer: National Surgical Adjuvant Breast and Bowel Project B-24 randomised controlled trial. *Lancet* 1999;353:1993–2000.
3. Colleoni M, Gelber S, Goldhirsch A, et al. Tamoxifen after adjuvant chemotherapy for premenopausal women with lymph node-positive breast cancer: International Breast Cancer Study Group Trial 13-93. *J Clin Oncol* 2006;24:1332–1341.
4. Davies C, Pan H, Godwin J, et al. Long-term effects of continuing adjuvant tamoxifen to 10 years versus stopping at 5 years after diagnosis of oestrogen receptor-positive breast cancer: ATLAS, a randomised trial. *Lancet* 2013;381:805–816.
5. Loprinzi CL, Michalak JC, Quella SK, et al. Megestrol acetate for the prevention of hot flashes. *N Engl J Med* 1994;331:347–352.
6. Loprinzi CL, Kugler JW, Sloan JA, et al. Venlafaxine in management of hot flashes in survivors of breast cancer: a randomised controlled trial. *Lancet* 2000;356:2059–2063.
7. Archer DF, Dupont CM, Constantine GD, et al. Desvenlafaxine for the treatment of vasomotor symptoms associated with menopause: a double-blind, randomized, placebo-controlled trial of efficacy and safety. *Am J Obstet Gynecol* 2009;200:238.e1–238e10.
8. Barton DL, LaVasseur BI, Sloan JA, et al. Phase III, placebo-controlled trial of three doses of citalopram for the treatment of hot flashes: NCCTG trial N05C9. *J Clin Oncol* 2010;28:3278–3283.
9. Freeman EW, Guthrie KA, Caan B, et al. Efficacy of escitalopram for hot flashes in healthy menopausal women: a randomized controlled trial. *JAMA* 2011;305:267–274.
10. Stearns V, Beebe KL, Iyengar M, et al. Paroxetine controlled release in the treatment of menopausal hot flashes: a randomized controlled trial. *JAMA* 2003;289:2827–2834.
11. Pandya KJ, Morrow GR, Roscoe JA, et al. Gabapentin for hot flashes in 420 women with breast cancer: a randomised double-blind placebo-controlled trial. *Lancet* 2005;366:818–824.
12. Loprinzi CL, Qin R, Balcueva EP, et al. Phase III, randomized, double-blind, placebo-controlled evaluation of pregabalin for alleviating hot flashes, N07C1. *J Clin Oncol* 2010;28:641–647.
13. Madlensky L, Natarajan L, Tchu S, et al. Tamoxifen metabolite concentrations, CYP2D6 genotype, and breast cancer outcomes. *Clin Pharmacol Ther* 2011;89:718–725.
14. Tamoxifen for early breast cancer: an overview of the randomised trials. Early Breast Cancer Trialists' Collaborative Group. *Lancet* 1998;351:1451–1467.
15. Wickerham DL, Fisher B, Wolmark N, et al. Association of tamoxifen and uterine sarcoma. *J Clin Oncol* 2002;20:2758–2760.
16. Dewar JA, Horobin JM, Preece PE, et al. Long term effects of tamoxifen on blood lipid values in breast cancer. *BMJ* 1992;305:225–226.
17. Love RR, Mazess RB, Barden HS, et al. Effects of tamoxifen on bone mineral density in postmenopausal women with breast cancer. *N Engl J Med* 1992;326:852–856.
18. Powles TJ, Hickish T, Kanis JA, et al. Effect of tamoxifen on bone mineral density measured by dual-energy x-ray absorptiometry in healthy premenopausal and postmenopausal women. *J Clin Oncol* 1996;14:78–84.
19. Buzdar A, Howell A, Cuzick J, et al. Comprehensive side-effect profile of anastrozole and tamoxifen as adjuvant treatment for early-stage breast cancer: long-term safety analysis of the ATAC trial. *Lancet Oncol* 2006;7:633–643.
20. Gorin MB, Day R, Costantino JP, et al. Long-term tamoxifen citrate use and potential ocular toxicity. *Am J Ophthalmol* 1998;125:493–501.
21. Tonetti DA, Jordan VC. Possible mechanisms in the emergence of tamoxifen-resistant breast cancer. *Anticancer Drugs* 1995;6:498–507.
22. Lim YC, Desta Z, Flockhart DA, et al. Endoxifen (4-hydroxy-N-desmethyl-tamoxifen) has anti-estrogenic effects in breast cancer cells with potency similar to 4-hydroxy-tamoxifen. *Cancer Chemother Pharmacol* 2005;55:471–478.
23. Benz CC, Scott GK, Sarup JC, et al. Estrogen-dependent, tamoxifen-resistant tumorigenic growth of MCF-7 cells transfected with HER2/neu. *Breast Cancer Res Treat* 1993;24:85–95.
24. Borg A, Baldetorp B, Ferno M, et al. ERBB2 amplification is associated with tamoxifen resistance in steroid-receptor positive breast cancer. *Cancer Lett* 1994;81:137–144.
25. Houston SJ, Plunkett TA, Barnes DM, et al. Overexpression of c-erbB2 is an independent marker of resistance to endocrine therapy in advanced breast cancer. *Br J Cancer* 1999;79:1220–1226.
26. Lipton A, Ali SM, Leitzel K, et al. Serum HER-2/neu and response to the aromatase inhibitor letrozole versus tamoxifen. *J Clin Oncol* 2003;21:1967–1972.
27. Bunone G, Briand PA, Miksicek RJ, et al. Activation of the unliganded estrogen receptor by EGF involves the MAP kinase pathway and direct phosphorylation. *Embo J* 1996;15:2174–2183.
28. Kato S, Endoh H, Masuhiro Y, et al. Activation of the estrogen receptor through phosphorylation by mitogen-activated protein kinase. *Science* 1995;270:1491–1494.
29. Pietras RJ, Arboleda J, Reese DM, et al. HER-2 tyrosine kinase pathway targets estrogen receptor and promotes hormone-independent growth in human breast cancer cells. *Oncogene* 1995;10:2435–2446.
30. Osborne CK, Bardou V, Hopp TA, et al. Role of the estrogen receptor coactivator AIB1 (SRC-3) and HER-2/neu in tamoxifen resistance in breast cancer. *J Natl Cancer Inst* 2003;95:353–361.
31. Encarnacion CA, Ciocca DR, McGuire WL, et al. Measurement of steroid hormone receptors in breast cancer patients on tamoxifen. *Breast Cancer Res Treat* 1993;26:237–246.
32. Watts CK, Handel ML, King RJ, et al. Oestrogen receptor gene structure and function in breast cancer. *J Steroid Biochem Mol Biol* 1992;41:529–536.
33. Zhang QX, Borg A, Wolf DM, et al. An estrogen receptor mutant with strong hormone-independent activity from a metastatic breast cancer. *Cancer Res* 1997;57:1244–1249.
34. Toy W, Shen Y, Won H, et al. ESR1 ligand-binding domain mutations in hormone-resistant breast cancer. *Nat Genet* 2013;45:1439–1445.
35. Robinson DR, Wu YM, Vats P, et al. Activating ESR1 mutations in hormone-resistant metastatic breast cancer. *Nat Genet* 2013;45:1446–1451.

36. Merenbakh-Lamin K, Ben-Baruch N, Yeheskel A, et al. D538G mutation in estrogen receptor-alpha: a novel mechanism for acquired endocrine resistance in breast cancer. *Cancer Res* 2013;73:6856–6864.
37. Fendl KC, Zimniski SJ. Role of tamoxifen in the induction of hormone-independent rat mammary tumors. *Cancer Res* 1992;52:235–237.
38. Williams GM. Tamoxifen experimental carcinogenicity studies: implications for human effects. *Proc Soc Exp Biol Med* 1995;208:141–143.
39. Williams GM, Iatropoulos MJ, Djordjevic MV, et al. The triphenylethylene drug tamoxifen is a strong liver carcinogen in the rat. *Carcinogenesis* 1993;14:315–317.
40. Rutqvist LE, Johansson H, Signomklao T, et al. Adjuvant tamoxifen therapy for early stage breast cancer and second primary malignancies. Stockholm Breast Cancer Study Group. *J Natl Cancer Inst* 1995;87:645–651.
41. Mani C, Kupfer D. Cytochrome P-450-mediated activation and irreversible binding of the antiestrogen tamoxifen to proteins in rat and human liver: possible involvement of flavin-containing monooxygenases in tamoxifen activation. *Cancer Res* 1991;51:6052–6058.
42. Mani C, Pearce R, Parkinson A, et al. Involvement of cytochrome P4503A in catalysis of tamoxifen activation and covalent binding to rat and human liver microsomes. *Carcinogenesis* 1994;15:2715–2720.
43. Styles JA, Davies A, Lim CK, et al. Genotoxicity of tamoxifen, tamoxifen epoxide and toremifene in human lymphoblastoid cells containing human cytochrome P450s. *Carcinogenesis* 1994;15:5–9.
44. Han XL, Liehr JG. Induction of covalent DNA adducts in rodents by tamoxifen. *Cancer Res* 1992;52:1360–1363.
45. Mani C, Hodgson E, Kupfer D. Metabolism of the antimammary cancer antiestrogenic agent tamoxifen. II. Flavin-containing monooxygenase-mediated N-oxidation. *Drug Metab Dispos* 1993;21:657–661.
46. Mani C, Gelboin HV, Park SS, et al. Metabolism of the antimammary cancer antiestrogenic agent tamoxifen. I. Cytochrome P-450-catalyzed N-demethylation and 4-hydroxylation. *Drug Metab Dispos* 1993;21:645–656.
47. Albain KS, Barlow WE, Shak S, et al. Prognostic and predictive value of the 21-gene recurrence score assay in postmenopausal women with node-positive, oestrogen-receptor-positive breast cancer on chemotherapy: a retrospective analysis of a randomised trial. *Lancet Oncol* 2010;11:55–65.
48. Dowsett M, Cuzick J, Wale C, et al. Prediction of risk of distant recurrence using the 21-gene recurrence score in node-negative and node-positive postmenopausal patients with breast cancer treated with anastrozole or tamoxifen: a TransATAC study. *J Clin Oncol* 2010;28:1829–1834.
49. Paik S, Shak S, Tang G, et al. A multigene assay to predict recurrence of tamoxifen-treated, node-negative breast cancer. *N Engl J Med* 2004;351:2817–2826.
50. Johnson MD, Zuo H, Lee KH, et al. Pharmacological characterization of 4-hydroxy-N-desmethyl tamoxifen, a novel active metabolite of tamoxifen. *Breast Cancer Res Treat* 2004;85:151–159.
51. Lim YC, Li L, Desta Z, et al. Endoxifen, a secondary metabolite of tamoxifen, and 4-OH-tamoxifen induce similar changes in global gene expression patterns in MCF-7 breast cancer cells. *J Pharmacol Exp Ther* 2006;318:503–512.
52. Wu X, Hawse JR, Subramaniam M, et al. The tamoxifen metabolite, endoxifen, is a potent antiestrogen that targets estrogen receptor alpha for degradation in breast cancer cells. *Cancer Res* 2009;69:1722–1727.
53. Jin Y, Desta Z, Stearns V, et al. CYP2D6 genotype, antidepressant use, and tamoxifen metabolism during adjuvant breast cancer treatment. *J Natl Cancer Inst* 2005;97:30–39.
54. Desta Z, Ward BA, Soukhova NV, et al. Comprehensive evaluation of tamoxifen sequential biotransformation by the human cytochrome P450 system in vitro: prominent roles for CYP3A and CYP2D6. *J Pharmacol Exp Ther* 2004;310:1062–1075.
55. Stearns V, Johnson MD, Rae JM, et al. Active tamoxifen metabolite plasma concentrations after coadministration of tamoxifen and the selective serotonin reuptake inhibitor paroxetine. *J Natl Cancer Inst* 2003;95:1758–1764.
56. Goetz MP, Rae JM, Suman VJ, et al. Pharmacogenetics of tamoxifen biotransformation is associated with clinical outcomes of efficacy and hot flashes. *J Clin Oncol* 2005;23:9312–9318.
57. Schroth W, Antoniadou L, Fritz P, et al. Breast cancer treatment outcome with adjuvant tamoxifen relative to patient CYP2D6 and CYP2C19 genotypes. *J Clin Oncol* 2007;25:5187–5193.
58. Schroth W, Goetz MP, Hamann U, et al. Association between CYP2D6 polymorphisms and outcomes among women with early stage breast cancer treated with tamoxifen. *JAMA* 2009;302:1429–1436.
59. Rae JM, Drury S, Hayes DF, et al. CYP2D6 and UGT2B7 genotype and risk of recurrence in tamoxifen-treated breast cancer patients. *J Natl Cancer Inst* 2012;104:452–460.
60. Regan MM, Leyland-Jones B, Bouzyk M, et al. CYP2D6 genotype and tamoxifen response in postmenopausal women with endocrine-responsive breast cancer: the breast international group 1-98 trial. *J Natl Cancer Inst* 2012;104:441–451.
61. Goetz MP, Suman VJ, Hoskin TL, et al. CYP2D6 metabolism and patient outcome in the Austrian Breast and Colorectal Cancer Study Group trial (ABCSG) 8. *Clin Cancer Res* 2013;19:500–507.
62. Province MA, Goetz MP, Brauch H, et al. CYP2D6 Genotype and adjuvant tamoxifen: meta-analysis of heterogeneous study populations. *Clin Pharmacol Ther* 2014;95:216–227.
63. Borges S, Desta Z, Li L, et al. Quantitative effect of CYP2D6 genotype and inhibitors on tamoxifen metabolism: implication for optimization of breast cancer treatment. *Clin Pharmacol Ther* 2006;80:61–74.
64. Dezentje VO, van Blijderveen NJ, Gelderblom H, et al. Effect of concomitant CYP2D6 inhibitor use and tamoxifen adherence on breast cancer recurrence in early-stage breast cancer. *J Clin Oncol* 2010;28:2423–2429.
65. Kelly CM, Juurlink DN, Gomes T, et al. Selective serotonin reuptake inhibitors and breast cancer mortality in women receiving tamoxifen: a population based cohort study. *BMJ* 2010;340:c693.
66. Binkhorst L, van Gelder T, Loos WJ, et al. Effects of CYP induction by rifampicin on tamoxifen exposure. *Clin Pharmacol Ther* 2012;92:62–67.
67. Irvin WJ Jr., Walko CM, Weck KE, et al. Genotype-guided tamoxifen dosing increases active metabolite exposure in women with reduced CYP2D6 metabolism: a multicenter study. *J Clin Oncol* 2011;29:3232–3239.
68. Kiyotani K, Mushiroda T, Imamura CK, et al. Dose-adjustment study of tamoxifen based on CYP2D6 genotypes in Japanese breast cancer patients. *Breast Cancer Res Treat* 2012;131:137–145.
69. Goetz MP, Suman VA, Reid JR, et al. A first-in-human phase I study of the tamoxifen (TAM) metabolite, Z-endoxifen hydrochloride (Z-Endx) in women with aromatase inhibitor (AI) refractory metastatic breast cancer (MBC) (NCT01327781). *Cancer Res* 2013;73(24 Suppl): Abstract nr PD3-4.
70. Lien EA, Anker G, Lonning PE, et al. Decreased serum concentrations of tamoxifen and its metabolites induced by aminoglutethimide. *Cancer Res* 1990;50:5851–5857.
71. Adam HK, Patterson JS, Kemp JV. Studies on the metabolism and pharmacokinetics of tamoxifen in normal volunteers. *Cancer Treat Rep* 1980;64:761–764.
72. Patterson JS, Settatree RS, Adam HK, et al. Serum concentrations of tamoxifen and major metabolite during long-term nolvadex therapy, correlated with clinical response. *Eur J Cancer Suppl* 1980;1:89–92.
73. Camaggi CM, Strocchi E, Canova N, et al. Medroxyprogesterone acetate (MAP) and tamoxifen (TMX) plasma levels after simultaneous treatment with 'low' TMX and 'high' MAP doses. *Cancer Chemother Pharmacol* 1985;14:229–231.
74. Lien EA, Solheim E, Lea OA, et al. Distribution of 4-hydroxy-N-desmethyltamoxifen and other tamoxifen metabolites in human biological fluids during tamoxifen treatment. *Cancer Res* 1989;49:2175–2183.
75. Lien EA, Solheim E, Ueland PM. Distribution of tamoxifen and its metabolites in rat and human tissues during steady-state treatment. *Cancer Res* 1991;51:4837–4844.
76. Daniel P, Gaskell SJ, Bishop H, et al. Determination of tamoxifen and biologically active metabolites in human breast tumours and plasma. *Eur J Cancer Clin Oncol* 1981;17:1183–1189.
77. Robinson SP, Langan-Fahey SM, Johnson DA, et al. Metabolites, pharmacodynamics, and pharmacokinetics of tamoxifen in rats and mice compared to the breast cancer patient. *Drug Metab Dispos* 1991;19:36–43.
78. DeGregorio MW, Wiebe VJ, Venook AP, et al. Elevated plasma tamoxifen levels in a patient with liver obstruction. *Cancer Chemother Pharmacol* 1989;23:194–195.
79. Lodwick R, McConkey B, Brown AM. Life threatening interaction between tamoxifen and warfarin. *Br Med J (Clin Res Ed)* 1987;295:1141.
80. Ritchie LD, Grant SM. Tamoxifen-warfarin interaction: the Aberdeen hospitals drug file. *BMJ* 1989;298:1253.
81. Tenni P, Lalich DL, Byrne MJ. Life threatening interaction between tamoxifen and warfarin. BMJ 1989;298:93.
82. Rabinowicz AL, Hinton DR, Dyck P, et al. High-dose tamoxifen in treatment of brain tumors: interaction with antiepileptic drugs. *Epilepsia* 1995;36:513–515.
83. Desai PB, Nallani SC, Sane RS, et al. Induction of cytochrome P450 3A4 in primary human hepatocytes and activation of the human pregnane X receptor by tamoxifen and 4-hydroxytamoxifen. *Drug Metab Dispos* 2002;30:608–612.
84. Dowsett M, Cuzick J, Howell A, et al. Pharmacokinetics of anastrozole and tamoxifen alone, and in combination, during adjuvant endocrine therapy for early breast cancer in postmenopausal women: a sub-protocol of the 'Arimidex and tamoxifen alone or in combination' (ATAC) trial. *Br J Cancer* 2001;85:317–324.
85. Pagani O, Gelber S, Price K, et al. Toremifene and tamoxifen are equally effective for early-stage breast cancer: first results of International Breast Cancer Study Group Trials 12-93 and 14-93. *Ann Oncol* 2004;15:1749–1759.
86. Hayes DF, Van Zyl JA, Hacking A, et al. Randomized comparison of tamoxifen and two separate doses of toremifene in postmenopausal patients with metastatic breast cancer. *J Clin Oncol* 1995;13:2556–2566.
87. Stenbygaard LE, Herrstedt J, Thomsen JF, et al. Toremifene and tamoxifen in advanced breast cancer—a double-blind cross-over trial. *Breast Cancer Res Treat* 1993;25:57–63.
88. Vogel CL, Shemano I, Schoenfelder J, et al. Multicenter phase II efficacy trial of toremifene in tamoxifen-refractory patients with advanced breast cancer. *J Clin Oncol* 1993;11:345–350.
89. Kangas L. Review of the pharmacological properties of toremifene. *J Steroid Biochem* 1990;36:191–195.
90. Berthou F, Dreano Y, Belloc C, et al. Involvement of cytochrome P450 3A enzyme family in the major metabolic pathways of toremifene in human liver microsomes. *Biochem Pharmacol* 1994;47:1883–1895.
91. Simberg NH, Murai JT, Siiteri PK. In vitro and in vivo binding of toremifene and its metabolites in rat uterus. *J Steroid Biochem* 1990;36:197–202.
92. Kohler PC, Hamm JT, Wiebe VJ, et al. Phase I study of the tolerance and pharmacokinetics of toremifene in patients with cancer. *Breast Cancer Res Treat* 1990;16 Suppl:S19–S26.
93. Tominaga T, Abe O, Izuo M. A phase I study of toremifene. *Breast Cancer Res Treat* 1990;16 (Suppl):27.
94. Wiebe VJ, Benz CC, Shemano I, et al. Pharmacokinetics of toremifene and its metabolites in patients with advanced breast cancer. *Cancer Chemother Pharmacol* 1990;25:247–251.

95. Anttila M, Laakso S, Nylanden P, et al. Pharmacokinetics of the novel antiestrogenic agent toremifene in subjects with altered liver and kidney function. *Clin Pharmacol Ther* 1995;57:628–635.
96. Hard GC, Iatropoulos MJ, Jordan K, et al. Major difference in the hepatocarcinogenicity and DNA adduct forming ability between toremifene and tamoxifen in female Crl:CD(BR) rats. *Cancer Res* 1993;53:4534–4541.
97. Montandon F, Williams GM. Comparison of DNA reactivity of the polyphenylethylene hormonal agents diethylstilbestrol, tamoxifen and toremifene in rat and hamster liver. *Arch Toxicol* 1994;68:272–275.
98. Vogel VG, Costantino JP, Wickerham DL, et al. Update of the National Surgical Adjuvant Breast and Bowel Project Study of Tamoxifen and Raloxifene (STAR) P-2 Trial: Preventing Breast Cancer. *Cancer Prev Res (Phila)* 2010;3:696–706.
99. Delmas PD, Balena R, Confravreux E, et al. Bisphosphonate risedronate prevents bone loss in women with artificial menopause due to chemotherapy of breast cancer: a double-blind, placebo-controlled study. *J Clin Oncol* 1997;15:955–962.
100. Draper MW, Flowers DE, Huster WJ, et al. A controlled trial of raloxifene (LY139481) HCl: impact on bone turnover and serum lipid profile in healthy postmenopausal women. *J Bone Miner Res* 1996;11:835–842.
101. Anzano MA, Peer CW, Smith JM, et al. Chemoprevention of mammary carcinogenesis in the rat: combined use of raloxifene and 9-cis-retinoic acid. *J Natl Cancer Inst* 1996;88:123–125.
102. Gottardis MM, Jordan VC. Antitumor actions of keoxifene and tamoxifen in the N-nitrosomethylurea-induced rat mammary carcinoma model. *Cancer Res* 1987;47:4020–4024.
103. Black LJ, Jones CD, Falcone JF. Antagonism of estrogen action with a new benzothiophene derived antiestrogen. *Life Sci* 1983;32:1031–1036.
104. Allerheiligen S, Geiser J, Knadler M. Raloxifen (RAL) pharmacokinetics and the associated endocrine effects in premenopausal women treated during the follicular, ovulatory, and luteal phases of the menstrual cycle. *Pharmaceut Res* 1996;13:S430.
105. Forgue ST, Rudy AC, Knadler MP. Raloxifene pharmacokinetics in healthy postmenopausal women. *Pharmaceut Res* 1996;13:S430.
106. Ni L, Allerheiligen S, Basson R. Pharacokinetics of raloxifene in men and postmenopausal women volunteers. *Pharmaceut Res* 1996;13:S430.
107. Kemp DC, Fan PW, Stevens JC. Characterization of raloxifene glucuronidation in vitro: contribution of intestinal metabolism to presystemic clearance. *Drug Metab Dispos* 2002;30:694–700.
108. Coopman P, Garcia M, Brunner N, et al. Anti-proliferative and anti-estrogenic effects of ICI 164,384 and ICI 182,780 in 4-OH-tamoxifen-resistant human breast-cancer cells. *Int J Cancer* 1994;56:295–300.
109. Howell A, DeFriend DJ, Robertson JF, et al. Pharmacokinetics, pharmacological and anti-tumour effects of the specific anti-oestrogen ICI 182780 in women with advanced breast cancer. *Br J Cancer* 1996;74:300–308.
110. Howell A, Osborne CK, Morris C, et al. ICI 182,780 (Faslodex): development of a novel, "pure" antiestrogen. *Cancer* 2000;89:817–825.
111. Robertson JF, Odling-Smee W, Holcombe C, et al. Pharmacokinetics of a single dose of fulvestrant prolonged-release intramuscular injection in postmenopausal women awaiting surgery for primary breast cancer. *Clin Ther* 2003;25:1440–1452.
112. Piccart M, Parker LM, Pritchard KI. Oestrogen receptor downregulation: an opportunity for extending the window of endocrine therapy in advanced breast cancer. *Ann Oncol* 2003;14:1017–1025.
113. Wakeling AE, Bowler J. Steroidal pure antioestrogens. *J Endocrinol* 1987;112:R7–R10.
114. Wakeling AE, Dukes M, Bowler J. A potent specific pure antiestrogen with clinical potential. *Cancer Res* 1991;51:3867–3873.
115. Howell A, Robertson JF, Quaresma Albano J, et al. Fulvestrant, formerly ICI 182,780, is as effective as anastrozole in postmenopausal women with advanced breast cancer progressing after prior endocrine treatment. *J Clin Oncol* 2002;20:3396–3403.
116. Osborne CK, Pippen J, Jones SE, et al. Double-blind, randomized trial comparing the efficacy and tolerability of fulvestrant versus anastrozole in postmenopausal women with advanced breast cancer progressing on prior endocrine therapy: results of a North American trial. *J Clin Oncol* 2002;20:3386–3395.
117. Howell A, Robertson JF, Abram P, et al. Comparison of fulvestrant versus tamoxifen for the treatment of advanced breast cancer in postmenopausal women previously untreated with endocrine therapy: a multinational, double-blind, randomized trial. *J Clin Oncol* 2004;22:1605–1613.
118. Leo AD, Jerusalem G, Petruzelka L, et al. Final overall survival: fulvestrant 500 mg vs 250 mg in the randomized CONFIRM trial. *J Natl Cancer Inst* 2014;106:djt337.
119. McCormack P, Sapunar F. Pharmacokinetic profile of the fulvestrant loading dose regimen in postmenopausal women with hormone receptor-positive advanced breast cancer. *Clin Breast Cancer* 2008;8:347–351.
120. Schteingart DE, Cash R, Conn JW. Amino-glutethimide and metastatic adrenal cancer. Maintained reversal (six months) of Cushing's syndrome. *JAMA* 1996;198:1007–1010.
121. Ma CX, Adjei AA, Salavaggione OE, et al. Human aromatase: gene resequencing and functional genomics. *Cancer Res* 2005;65:11071–11082.
122. Colomer R, Monzo M, Tusquets I, et al. A single-nucleotide polymorphism in the aromatase gene is associated with the efficacy of the aromatase inhibitor letrozole in advanced breast carcinoma. *Clin Cancer Res* 2008;14:811–816.
123. Wang L, Ellsworth KA, Moon I, et al. Functional genetic polymorphisms in the aromatase gene CYP19 vary the response of breast cancer patients to neoadjuvant therapy with aromatase inhibitors. *Cancer Res* 2010;70:319–328.
124. Goss PE, Ingle JN, Martino S, et al. A randomized trial of letrozole in postmenopausal women after five years of tamoxifen therapy for early-stage breast cancer. *N Engl J Med* 2003;349:1793–1802.
125. Mouridsen H, Gershanovich M, Sun Y, et al. Phase III study of letrozole versus tamoxifen as first-line therapy of advanced breast cancer in postmenopausal women: analysis of survival and update of efficacy from the International Letrozole Breast Cancer Group. *J Clin Oncol* 2003;21:2101–2109.
126. Howell A, Cuzick J, Baum M, et al. Results of the ATAC (Arimidex, Tamoxifen, Alone or in Combination) trial after completion of 5 years' adjuvant treatment for breast cancer. *Lancet* 2005;365:60–62.
127. Thurlimann B, Keshaviah A, Coates AS, et al. A comparison of letrozole and tamoxifen in postmenopausal women with early breast cancer. *N Engl J Med* 2005;353:2747–2757.
128. Jakesz R, Jonat W, Gnant M, et al. Switching of postmenopausal women with endocrine-responsive early breast cancer to anastrozole after 2 years' adjuvant tamoxifen: combined results of ABCSG trial 8 and ARNO 95 trial. *Lancet* 2005;366:455–462.
129. Cuzick J, Sestak I, Forbes JF, et al. Anastrozole for prevention of breast cancer in high-risk postmenopausal women (IBIS-II): an international, double-blind, randomised placebo-controlled trial. *Lancet* 2014;383:1041–1048.
130. Baum M, Budzar AU, Cuzick J, et al. Anastrozole alone or in combination with tamoxifen versus tamoxifen alone for adjuvant treatment of postmenopausal women with early breast cancer: first results of the ATAC randomised trial. *Lancet* 2002;359:2131–2139.
131. Amir E, Seruga B, Nira S, et al. Toxicity of adjuvant endocrine therapy in postmenopausal breast cancer patients: a systematic review and meta-analysis. *J Natl Cancer Inst* 2011;103:1299–1309.
132. Plourde PV, Dyroff M, Dukes M. Arimidex: a potent and selective fourth-generation aromatase inhibitor. *Breast Cancer Res Treat* 1994;30:103–111.
133. Bisagni G, Cocconi G, Scaglione F, et al. Letrozole, a new oral non-steroidal aromastase inhibitor in treating postmenopausal patients with advanced breast cancer. A pilot study. *Ann Oncol* 1996;7:99–102.
134. Buzdar AU. Pharmacology and pharmacokinetics of the newer generation aromatase inhibitors. *Clin Cancer Res* 2003;9:468S–472S.
135. Dewar JA, Nabholtz JM, Bonneterre J, et al. The effect of anastrozole (Arimidex) on serum lipids: data from a randomized comparison of anastrozole (AN) versus tamoxifen (TAM) in postmenopausal (PM) women with advanced breast cancer (ABC). *Breast Cancer Res Treat* 2000;64:51.
136. Elisaf MS, Bairaktari ET, Nicolaides C, et al. Effect of letrozole on the lipid profile in postmenopausal women with breast cancer. *Eur J Cancer* 2001;37:1510–1513.
137. Bhatnagar AS, Hausler A, Schieweck K. Inhibition of aromatase in vitro and in vivo by aromatase inhibitors. *J Enzyme Inhib* 1990;4:179–186.
138. Bhatnagar AS, Hausler A, Schieweck K, et al. Highly selective inhibition of estrogen biosynthesis by CGS 20267, a new non-steroidal aromatase inhibitor. *J Steroid Biochem Mol Biol* 1990;37:1021–1027.
139. Demers LM. Effects of Fadrozole (CGS 16949A) and Letrozole (CGS 20267) on the inhibition of aromatase activity in breast cancer patients. *Breast Cancer Res Treat* 1994;30:95–102.
140. Lipton A, Demers LM, Harvey HA, et al. Letrozole (CGS 20267). A phase I study of a new potent oral aromatase inhibitor of breast cancer. *Cancer* 1995;75:2132–2138.
141. Iveson TJ, Smith IE, Ahern J, et al. Phase I study of the oral nonsteroidal aromatase inhibitor CGS 20267 in postmenopausal patients with advanced breast cancer. *Cancer Res* 1993;53:266–270.
142. Trunet PF, Muller PH, Bhatnagar A. Phase I study in healthy male volunteers with the non-steroidal aromatase inhibitor GCS 20267. *Eur J Cancer* 1990;26:173.
143. Dukes M, Edwards PN, Large M, et al. The preclinical pharmacology of "Arimidex" (anastrozole; ZD1033)—a potent, selective aromatase inhibitor. *J Steroid Biochem Mol Biol* 1996;58:439–445.
144. Yates RA, Dowsett M, Fisher GV, et al. Arimidex (ZD1033): a selective, potent inhibitor of aromatase in postmenopausal female volunteers. *Br J Cancer* 1996;73:543–548.
145. Lonning PE, Geisler J, Dowsett M. Pharmacological and clinical profile of anastrozole. *Breast Cancer Res Treat* 1998;49:S53–S57.
146. Geisler J, King N, Dowsett M, et al. Influence of anastrozole (Arimidex), a selective, non-steroidal aromatase inhibitor, on in vivo aromatisation and plasma oestrogen levels in postmenopausal women with breast cancer. *Br J Cancer* 1996;74:1286–1291.
147. Ingle JN, Buzdar AU, Schaid DJ, et al. Variation in anastrozole metabolism and pharmacodynamics in women with early breast cancer. *Cancer Res* 2010;70:3278–3286.
148. Kaufmann M, Bajetta E, Dirix LY, et al. Exemestane is superior to megestrol acetate after tamoxifen failure in postmenopausal women with advanced breast cancer: results of a phase III randomized double-blind trial. The Exemestane Study Group. *J Clin Oncol* 2000;18:1399–1411.
149. Goss PE, Ingle JN, Pritchard KI, et al. Exemestane versus anastrozole in postmenopausal women with early breast cancer: NCIC CTG MA.27—a randomized controlled phase III trial. *J Clin Oncol* 2013;31:1398–1404.
150. Goss PE, Ingle JN, Ales-Martinez JE, et al. Exemestane for breast-cancer prevention in postmenopausal women. *N Engl J Med* 2011;364:2381–2391.
151. Goss PE, Grynpas M, Qi S, et al. The effects of exemestane on bone and lipids in the ovariectomized rat. *Breast Cancer Res Treat* 2001;69:224.
152. Evans TR, Di Salle E, Ornati G, et al. Phase I and endocrine study of exemestane (FCE 24304), a new aromatase inhibitor, in postmenopausal women. *Cancer Res* 1992;52:5933–5939.

153. Bajetta E, Zilembo N, Noberasco C, et al. The minimal effective exemestane dose for endocrine activity in advanced breast cancer. *Eur J Cancer* 1997;33:587–591.
154. Michaud LB, Buzdar AU. Risks and benefits of aromatase inhibitors in postmenopausal breast cancer. *Drug Saf* 1999;21:297–309.
155. Coombes RC, Hall E, Gibson LJ, et al. A randomized trial of exemestane after two to three years of tamoxifen therapy in postmenopausal women with primary breast cancer. *N Engl J Med* 2004;350:1081–1092.
156. Demers LM, Lipton A, Harvey HA, et al. The efficacy of CGS 20267 in suppressing estrogen biosynthesis in patients with advanced stage breast cancer. *J Steroid Biochem Mol Biol* 1993;44:687–691.
157. Spinelli R, Jannuzzo MG, Poggesi I, et al. Pharmacokinetics (PK) of Aromasin (Exemestane, EXE) after single and repeated doses in healthy postmenopausal volunteers (HPV). *Eur J Cancer* 1999;35:S295.
158. Buzdar A, Howell A. Advances in aromatase inhibition: clinical efficacy and tolerability in the treatment of breast cancer. *Clin Cancer Res* 2001;7:2620–2635.
159. Johannessen DC, Engan T, Di Salle E, et al. Endocrine and clinical effects of exemestane (PNU 155971), a novel steroidal aromatase inhibitor, in postmenopausal breast cancer patients: a phase I study. *Clin Cancer Res* 1997;3:1101–1108.
160. Jones S, Vogel C, Arkhipov A, et al. Multicenter, phase II trial of exemestane as third-line hormonal therapy of postmenopausal women with metastatic breast cancer. Aromasin Study Group. *J Clin Oncol* 1999;17:3418–3425.
161. Ahmann FR, Citrin DL, deHaan HA, et al. Zoladex: a sustained-release, monthly luteinizing hormone-releasing hormone analogue for the treatment of advanced prostate cancer. *J Clin Oncol* 1987;5:912–917.
162. Corbin A. From contraception to cancer: a review of the therapeutic applications of LHRH analogues as antitumor agents. *Yale J Biol Med* 1982;55:27–47.
163. Kaufmann M, Jonat W, Blamey R, et al. Survival analyses from the ZEBRA study. Goserelin (Zoladex) versus CMF in premenopausal women with node-positive breast cancer. *Eur J Cancer* 2003;39:1711–1717.
164. Harvey HA, Lipton A, Max DT, et al. Medical castration produced by the GnRH analogue leuprolide to treat metastatic breast cancer. *J Clin Oncol* 1985;3:1068–1072.
165. Abrahamsson PA. Potential benefits of intermittent androgen suppression therapy in the treatment of prostate cancer: a systematic review of the literature. *Eur Urol* 2010;57:49–59.
166. Hussain M, Tangen CM, Berry DL, et al. Intermittent versus continuous androgen deprivation in prostate cancer. *N Engl J Med* 2013;368:1314–1325.
167. Brogden RN, Faulds D. Goserelin. A review of its pharmacodynamic and pharmacokinetic properties and therapeutic efficacy in prostate cancer. *Drugs Aging* 1995;6:324–343.
168. Vogelzang NJ, Chodak GW, Soloway MS, et al. Goserelin versus orchiectomy in the treatment of advanced prostate cancer: final results of a randomized trial. Zoladex Prostate Study Group. *Urology* 1995;46:220–226.
169. Plosker GL, Brogden RN. Leuprorelin. A review of its pharmacology and therapeutic use in prostatic cancer, endometriosis and other sex hormone-related disorders. *Drugs* 1994;48:930–967.
170. Nillius SJ. *The Therapeutic Uses of Gonadotropin-Releasing Hormone and Its Analogues*. London: Butterworth; 1981.
171. Klijn JG, DeJong FH, Blankenstein MA. Anti-tumor and endocrine effects of chronic LHRH agonist treatment (buserelin) with or without tamoxifen in premenopausal metastatic breast cancer. *Breast Cancer Res Treat* 1984;4:209.
172. Clayton RN, Bailey LC, Cottam J, et al. A radioimmunoassay for GnRH agonist analogue in serum of patients with prostate cancer treated with D-Ser (tBu)6 AZA Gly10 GnRH. *Clin Endocrinol (Oxf)* 1985;22:453–462.
173. Chrisp P, Goa KL. Goserelin. A review of its pharmacodynamic and pharmacokinetic properties, and clinical use in sex hormone-related conditions. *Drugs* 1991;41:254–288.
174. Samant MP, Hong DJ, Croston G, et al. Novel gonadotropin-releasing hormone antagonists with substitutions at position 5. *Biopolymers* 2005;80:386–391.
175. Van Poppel H, Tombal B, de la Rosette JJ, et al. Degarelix: a novel gonadotropin-releasing hormone (GnRH) receptor blocker—results from a 1-yr, multicentre, randomised, phase 2 dosage-finding study in the treatment of prostate cancer. *Eur Urol* 2008;54:805–813.
176. Klotz L, Boccon-Gibod L, Shore ND, et al. The efficacy and safety of degarelix: a 12-month, comparative, randomized, open-label, parallel-group phase III study in patients with prostate cancer. *BJU Int* 2008;102:1531–1538.
177. Steinberg M. Degarelix: a gonadotropin-releasing hormone antagonist for the management of prostate cancer. *Clin Ther* 2009;31:2312–2331.
178. Brogden RN, Clissold SP. Flutamide. A preliminary review of its pharmacodynamic and pharmacokinetic properties, and therapeutic efficacy in advanced prostatic cancer. *Drugs* 1989;38:185–203.
179. Wysowski DK, Freiman JP, Tourtelot JB, et al. Fatal and nonfatal hepatotoxicity associated with flutamide. *Ann Intern Med* 1993;118:860–864.
180. Brogden RN, Chrisp P. Flutamide. A review of its pharmacodynamic and pharmacokinetic properties, and therapeutic use in advanced prostatic cancer. *Drugs Aging* 1991;1:104–115.
181. Radwanski E, Perentesis G, Symchowicz S, et al. Single and multiple dose pharmacokinetic evaluation of flutamide in normal geriatric volunteers. *J Clin Pharmacol* 1989;29:554–558.
182. Schellhammer PF, Sharifi R, Block NL, et al. A controlled trial of bicalutamide versus flutamide, each in combination with luteinizing hormone-releasing hormone analogue therapy, in patients with advanced prostate carcinoma. Analysis of time to progression. CASODEX Combination Study Group. *Cancer* 1996;78:2164–2169.
183. Furr BJ. Casodex (ICI 176,334)—a new, pure, peripherally-selective anti-androgen: preclinical studies. *Horm Res* 1989;32:69.
184. Furr BJ. Casodex: preclinical studies. *Eur Urol* 1990;18:2.
185. Kennealey GT, Furr BJ. Use of the nonsteroidal anti-androgen Casodex in advanced prostatic carcinoma. *Urol Clin North Am* 1991;18:99–110.
186. Attard G, Reid AH, A'Hern R, et al. Selective inhibition of CYP17 with abiraterone acetate is highly active in the treatment of castration-resistant prostate cancer. *J Clin Oncol* 2009;27:3742–3748.
187. Tran C, Ouk S, Clegg NJ, et al. Development of a second-generation antiandrogen for treatment of advanced prostate cancer. *Science* 2009;324:787–790.
188. Scher HI, Fizazi K, Saad F, et al. Increased survival with enzalutamide in prostate cancer after chemotherapy. *N Engl J Med* 2012;367:1187–1197.
189. Zhu H, Garcia JA. Targeting the adrenal gland in castration-resistant prostate cancer: a case for orteronel, a selective CYP-17 17,20-lyase inhibitor. *Curr Oncol Rep* 2013;15:105–112.
190. Kennedy BJ. Hormonal therapies in breast cancer. *Semin Oncol* 1974;1:119–130.
191. Colburn WA. Radioimmunoassay for fluoxymesterone (Halotestin). *Steroids* 1975;25:43–52.
192. Kammerer RC, Merdink JL, Jagels M, et al. Testing for fluoxymesterone (Halotestin) administration to man: identification of urinary metabolites by gas chromatography-mass spectrometry. *J Steroid Biochem* 1990;36:659–666.
193. Ingle JN, Ahmann DL, Green SJ, et al. Randomized clinical trial of diethylstilbestrol versus tamoxifen in postmenopausal women with advanced breast cancer. *N Engl J Med* 1981;304:16–21.
194. Stewart HJ, Forrest AP, Gunn JM, et al. The tamoxifen trial - a double-blind comparison with stilboestrol in postmenopausal women with advanced breast cancer. *Eur J Cancer* 1980;Suppl 1:83–88.
195. Byar DP. Proceedings: The Veterans Administration Cooperative Urological Research Group's studies of cancer of the prostate. *Cancer* 1973;32:1126–1130.
196. Loose-Mitchell DS, Stancel GM. *Estrogens and Progestins*. 10 ed. New York: McGraw-Hill; 2001.
197. Bonomi P, Pessis D, Bunting N, et al. Megestrol acetate used as primary hormonal therapy in stage D prostatic cancer. *Semin Oncol* 1985;12:36–39.
198. Bruera E, Macmillan K, Kuehn N, et al. A controlled trial of megestrol acetate on appetite, caloric intake, nutritional status, and other symptoms in patients with advanced cancer. *Cancer* 1990;66:1279–1282.
199. Feliu J, Gonzalez-Baron M, Berrocal A, et al. Usefulness of megestrol acetate in cancer cachexia and anorexia. A placebo-controlled study. *Am J Clin Oncol* 1992;15:436–440.
200. Loprinzi CL, Ellison NM, Schaid DJ, et al. Controlled trial of megestrol acetate for the treatment of cancer anorexia and cachexia. *J Natl Cancer Inst* 1990;82:1127–1132.
201. Tchekmedyian NS, Hickman M, Siau J, et al. Megestrol acetate in cancer anorexia and weight loss. *Cancer* 1992;69:1268–1274.
202. Loprinzi CL, Michalak JC, Schaid DJ, et al. Phase III evaluation of four doses of megestrol acetate as therapy for patients with cancer anorexia and/or cachexia. *J Clin Oncol* 1993;11:762–767.
203. Loprinzi CL, Jensen MD, Jiang NS, et al. Effect of megestrol acetate on the human pituitary-adrenal axis. *Mayo Clin Proc* 1992;67:1160–1162.
204. Leinung MC, Liporace R, Miller CH. Induction of adrenal suppression by megestrol acetate in patients with AIDS. *Ann Intern Med* 1995;122:843–845.
205. Rowland KM Jr., Loprinzi CL, Shaw EG, et al. Randomized double-blind placebo-controlled trial of cisplatin and etoposide plus megestrol acetate/placebo in extensive-stage small-cell lung cancer: a North Central Cancer Treatment Group study. *J Clin Oncol* 1996;14:135–141.
206. Loprinzi CL, Johnson PA, Jensen M. Megestrol acetate for anorexia and cachexia. *Oncology* 1992;49:46–49.
207. Von Roenn JH, Armstrong D, Kotler DP, et al. Megestrol acetate in patients with AIDS-related cachexia. *Ann Intern Med* 1994;121:393–399.
208. Alexieva-Figusch J, Blankenstein MA, Hop WC, et al. Treatment of metastatic breast cancer patients with different dosages of megestrol acetate; dose relations, metabolic and endocrine effects. *Eur J Cancer Clin Oncol* 1984;20:33–40.
209. Tseng L, Gurpide E. Effects of progestins on estradiol receptor levels in human endometrium. *J Clin Endocrinol Metab* 1975;41:402–404.
210. Gurpide E, Tseng L, Gusberg SB. Estrogen metabolism in normal and neoplastic endometrium. *Am J Obstet Gynecol* 1977;129:809–816.
211. Gordon GG, Altman K, Southren AL, et al. Human hepatic testosterone A-ring reductase activity: effect of medroxyprogesterone acetate. *J Clin Endocrinol Metab* 1971;32:457–461.
212. Allegra JC, Kiefer SM. Mechanisms of action of progestational agents. *Semin Oncol* 1985;12:3–5.
213. Ewing TM, Murphy LJ, Ng ML, et al. Regulation of epidermal growth factor receptor by progestins and glucocorticoids in human breast cancer cell lines. *Int J Cancer* 1989;44:744–752.
214. Adlercreutz H, Eriksen PB, Christensen MS. Plasma concentration of megestrol acetate and medroxyprogesterone acetate after single oral administration to healthy subjects. *J Pharm Biomed Anal* 1983;1:153.
215. Martin F, Adlercreutz H, eds. *Aspects of Megestrol Acetate and Medroxyprogesterone Acetate Metabolism*. New York: Raven Press; 1977.
216. Gaver RC, Pittman KA, Reilly CM, et al. Bioequivalence evaluation of new megestrol acetate formulations in humans. *Semin Oncol* 1985;12:17–19.
217. Fotherby K, Kamyab S, Littleton P. Metabolism of synthetic progestational compounds in humans. *J Reprod Fertil* 1968;5:51–61.

218. Fukushima DK, Ievin J, Liang JS, et al. Isolation and partial synthesis of a new metabolite of medroxyrogesterone acetate. *Steroids* 1979;34:57–72.
219. Utaaker E, Lundgren S, Kvinnsland S, et al. Pharmacokinetics and metabolism of medroxyprogesterone acetate in patients with advanced breast cancer. *J Steroid Biochem* 1988;31:437–441.
220. Sturm G, Haberlein H, Bauer T, et al. Mass spectrometric and high-performance liquid chromatographic studies of medroxyprogesterone acetate metabolites in human plasma. *J Chromatogr* 1991;562:351–362.
221. Pannuti F, Camaggi CM, Strocchi E, eds. *Medroxyprogesterone Acetate Pharmacokinetics.* New York: Raven Press; 1984.
222. Lundgren S, Lonning PE, Aakvaag A, et al. Influence of aminoglutethimide on the metabolism of medroxyprogesterone acetate and megestrol acetate in postmenopausal patients with advanced breast cancer. *Cancer Chemother Pharmacol* 1990;27:101–105.
223. Lundgren S, Kvinnsland S, Utaaker E, et al. Effect of oral high-dose progestins on the disposition of antipyrine, digitoxin, and warfarin in patients with advanced breast cancer. *Cancer Chemother Pharmacol* 1986;18:270–275.
224. Cascinu S, Fedeli A, Fedeli SL, et al. Control of chemotherapy-induced diarrhoea with octreotide in patients receiving 5-fluorouracil. *Eur J Cancer* 1992;28:482–483.
225. Cascinu S, Fedeli A, Fedeli SL, et al. Octreotide versus loperamide in the treatment of fluorouracil-induced diarrhea: a randomized trial. *J Clin Oncol* 1993;11:148–151.
226. Gebbia V, Carreca I, Testa A, et al. Subcutaneous octreotide versus oral loperamide in the treatment of diarrhea following chemotherapy. *Anticancer Drugs* 1993;4:443–445.
227. Harris AG. Somatostatin and somatostatin analogues: pharmacokinetics and pharmacodynamic effects. *Gut* 1994;35:S1–S4.
228. Chanson P, Timsit J, Harris AG. Clinical pharmacokinetics of octreotide. Therapeutic applications in patients with pituitary tumours. *Clin Pharmacokinet* 1993;25:375–391.
229. Marbach P, Briner U, Lemaire M. From somatostatin to Sandostatin: pharmacodynamics and pharmacokinetics. *Digestion* 1993;54:9–13.
230. Rubin J, Ajani J, Schirmer W, et al. Octreotide acetate long-acting formulation versus open-label subcutaneous octreotide acetate in malignant carcinoid syndrome. *J Clin Oncol* 1999;17:600–606.

28 Antiangiogenesis Agents

Cindy H. Chau and William Douglas Figg, Sr.

INTRODUCTION

Blood vessels are indispensable for tumor growth and metastasis, and the formation of a new network of blood vessels from the existing vasculature, termed *angiogenesis*, is one of the essential hallmarks of cancer development.[1] Indeed, it was over 70 years ago that the existence of tumor-derived factors responsible for promoting new vessel growth was postulated,[2] and that tumor growth is essentially dependent on vascular induction and the development of a neovascular supply.[3] By the late 1960s, Dr. Judah Folkman and colleagues[4] had begun the search for a tumor angiogenesis factor. In the 1971 landmark report, Folkman[5] proposed that inhibition of angiogenesis by means of holding tumors in a nonvascularized dormant state would be an effective strategy to treat human cancer, and hence laid the groundwork for the concept behind the development of *antiangiogenesis* agents. This fostered the search for angiogenic factors, regulators of angiogenesis, and antiangiogenic molecules over the next few decades and shed light on angiogenesis as an important therapeutic target for the treatment of cancer and other diseases.

A decade has passed since the regulatory approval of the first antiangiogenic drug bevacizumab, and while initial results were regarded as highly promising, clinical evidence indicated that antiangiogenic therapy also had limitations. Successful development and clinical translation of this novel class of agents depends on the complete understanding of the biology of angiogenesis and the regulatory proteins that govern this angiogenic process, topics that have been covered in greater detail in another section of this textbook. This chapter will briefly review the mechanisms underlying tumor angiogenesis followed by an in-depth discussion of antiangiogenic therapy, the modes of action of angiogenesis inhibitors, and the successes and challenges of this treatment modality.

UNDERSTANDING THE ANGIOGENIC PROCESS

Angiogenic Switch and Regulatory Proteins

Tumor development and progression depend on angiogenesis. Recruitment of new blood vessels to the tumor site is required for the delivery of nutrients and oxygen to the cancerous growths and for the removal of waste products.[6] Cancer cells promote angiogenesis at an early stage of tumorigenesis, beginning with the release of molecules that send signals to the surrounding normal host tissue and stimulate the migration of microvascular endothelial cells (EC) in the direction of the angiogenic stimulus. These angiogenic factors not only mediate EC migration, but also EC proliferation and microvessel formation in tumors undergoing the switch to the angiogenic phenotype.[7] Experimental evidence for this *angiogenic switch* was observed when hyperplastic islets in transgenic mice (RIP-Tag model) switch from small (<1 mm), white microscopic dormant tumors to red, rapidly growing tumors.[7] Dormant tumors have been discovered during autopsies of individuals who died of causes other than cancer.[8] These autopsy studies suggest that the vast majority of microscopic in situ cancers never switch to the angiogenic phenotype during a normal lifetime. Such incipient tumors are usually not neovascularized and can remain harmless to the host for long periods of time as microscopic lesions that are in a state of dormancy.[9,10] These nonangiogenic tumors cannot expand beyond the initial microscopic size and cannot become clinically detectable, lethal tumors until they have switched to the angiogenic phenotype[11–13] through neovascularization and/or blood vessel cooption.[14] Depending on the tumor type and the environment, this switch can occur at different stages of the tumor progression pathway and ultimately depends on a net balance of positive and negative regulators. Thus, the angiogenic phenotype may result from the production of growth factors by tumor cells and/or the downregulation of negative modulators.

Changes in this angiogenic balance affecting the levels of activator and inhibitor molecules dictate whether an EC will be in a quiescent or an angiogenic state. Normally, the inhibitors predominate, thereby blocking growth. Once the balance shifts in favor of the angiogenic state, proangiogenic factors prompts the activation, growth, and division of vascular ECs, resulting in the formation of new blood vessels. Activated ECs produce and release matrix metalloproteinases (MMP) into the surrounding tissue to break down the extracellular matrix to allow the ECs to migrate and organize themselves into hollow tubes that eventually evolve into a mature network of blood vessels. Proangiogenic factors or positive regulators of angiogenesis include vascular endothelial growth factor (VEGF), basic fibroblast growth factor (PlGF), platelet-derived growth factor (PDGF), placental growth factor, transforming growth factor-β, pleiotrophins, and others.[15] Activation of the hypoxia-inducible factor 1 (HIF-1) via tumor-associated hypoxic conditions is also involved in the upregulation of several angiogenic factors.[16] The angiogenic switch also involves the downregulation of angiogenesis suppressor proteins, which include endostatin, angiostatin, thrombospondin, and others.[17,18] Most notably, however, is the link between many oncogenes and angiogenesis and the significant role oncogenes play in driving the angiogenic switch.[19,20] These proangiogenic oncogenes not only induce the expression of stimulators, but may also downregulate inhibitors of angiogenesis.[21]

Endogenous Inhibitors of Angiogenesis

The infrequency of microscopic in situ tumors that actually undergo the angiogenic switch (<1%) suggests that naturally occurring endogenous inhibitors exist in the body to defend against the angiogenic switch in pathologic conditions and to limit physiologic angiogenesis.[9] These circulating endogenous inhibitors could also prevent microscopic metastases from growing into visible tumors. Early studies by Langer et al.[22,23] demonstrated the possible existence of such inhibitors through the extraction of a functional inhibitor from cartilage, a tissue that is poorly vascularized. Since then, dozens of endogenous angiogenesis inhibitors have been identified, some of which are listed in Table 28.1.[17,18,24] Many of the endogenous inhibitors of angiogenesis that have been discovered to date are proteolytically cleaved fragments of larger proteins that are members of either the clotting/coagulation system

CANCER THERAPEUTICS

TABLE 28.1

Examples of Endogenous Inhibitors of Angiogenesis

Alphastatin
Angiostatin
Antithrombin III (cleaved)
Arrestin
Canstatin
Endostatin
Interferon alpha/beta (IFN-α/β)
2-Methoxyestradiol (2-ME)
Pigment epithelial-derived factor (PEDF)
Platelet factor 4 (PF-4)
Tetrahydrocortisol-S
Thrombospondin 1
Tissue inhibitor of metalloproteinase 2 (TIMP-2)
Tumstatin
Vasohibin

or members of the extracellular matrix family of glycoproteins. Endostatin is the most well-studied endogenous angiogenesis inhibitor.[25,26] Other potent endogenous angiogenesis inhibitors include thrombospondin-1[27] and tumstatin.[28] The discovery of vasohibin, an endogenous inhibitor that is selectively induced in ECs by proangiogenic stimulatory growth factors such as VEGF, demonstrated the existence of an intrinsic and EC-specific feedback inhibitor control mechanism,[29,30] whereas most endogenous inhibitors of angiogenesis are extrinsic to ECs. More recently, a second endothelium-produced negative regulator of angiogenesis has been discovered, the Dll4-Notch signaling system.[31,32] Both intrinsic factors have since been shown to control tumor angiogenesis by an autoregulatory or negative-feedback mechanism. The Dll4-Notch axis has emerged as a critical regulator of tumor angiogenesis, and inhibitors of this pathway (e.g., demcizumab, the anti-Dll4 monoclonal antibody) are currently being investigated in early phase trials of solid tumors.[33]

Perhaps the most compelling genetic evidence that endogenous inhibitors suppress pathologic angiogenesis was observed in studies using mice deficient in tumstatin, endostatin, or thrombospondin 1 (TSP-1).[34] These experiments demonstrate that normal physiologic levels of the inhibitors can retard the tumor growth and that their absence leads to enhanced angiogenesis and increased tumor growth by two- to threefold, strongly suggesting that endogenous inhibitors of angiogenesis can act as endothelium-specific tumor suppressors. The connection between a tumor suppressor protein and angiogenesis is best illustrated by the classic tumor suppressor p53. p53 inhibits angiogenesis by increasing the expression of TSP-1[35] by repressing VEGF[36] and basic fibroblast growth factor–binding protein,[37] and by degrading HIF-1,[38] which blocks the downstream induction of VEGF expression. New evidence suggests that p53 also indirectly downregulates VEGF expression via the retinoblastoma pathway in a p21-dependent manner during sustained hypoxia.[39] Furthermore, p53-mediated inhibition of angiogenesis may also occur in part via the antiangiogenic activity of endostatin and tumstatin.[40] This landmark finding clearly demonstrates that p53 not only controls cell proliferation, but can also repress tumor angiogenesis through enzymatic mobilization of these endogenous angiogenesis inhibitor proteins to prevent ECs from being recruited into the dormant, microscopic tumors, thereby preventing the switch to the angiogenic phenotype.[41] The discovery that these endogenous angiogenesis inhibitors can suppress the growth of primary tumors raises the possibility that such inhibitors might also be able to slow tumor metastasis. Indeed, the inhibition of angiogenesis by angiostatin significantly reduced the rate of metastatic spread.

DRUG DEVELOPMENT OF ANGIOGENESIS INHIBITORS

The first angiogenesis inhibitor was reported in 1980 and involved the low-dose administration of interferon α (IFN-α).[42–44] Over the next decade, several compounds were discovered to have potent antiangiogenic activity, including protamine and platelet factor 4,[45] trahydrocortisol,[46] and the fumagillin analog TNP-470.[47] The proof of concept that targeting angiogenesis is an effective strategy for treating cancer came with the approval of the first angiogenesis inhibitor, bevacizumab, by the U.S. Food and Drug Administration (FDA). Since then, several antiangiogenic agents have received FDA approval for cancer treatment (Table 28.2), and three additional agents (pegaptanib, ranibizumab, and aflibercept) are approved for the treatment of wet age-related macular degeneration.

Rationale for Antiangiogenic Therapy

Antiangiogenic therapy stems from the fundamental concept that tumor growth, invasion, and metastasis are angiogenesis dependent; thus, blocking blood vessel recruitment to starve primary and metastatic tumors is a rational approach. The microvascular EC recruited by a tumor has become an important second target in cancer therapy. Unlike the cancer cell (the primary target of cytotoxic chemotherapy), which is genetically unstable with unpredictable mutations, the genetic stability of ECs may make them less susceptible to acquired drug resistance.[48] Moreover, ECs in the microvascular bed of a tumor may support 50 to 100 tumor cells. Coupling this amplification potential together with the lower toxicity of most angiogenesis inhibitors results in the use of antiangiogenic therapy, which should be significantly less toxic than conventional chemotherapy. However, the variable responses of antiangiogenic therapy observed in different tumor types and the fact that angiogenesis inhibitors have not delivered the benefits initially envisaged suggest that the precise mechanism of action of angiogenesis inhibitors is complex and remains incompletely understood.

Modes of Action of Antiangiogenic Agents

Various strategies for the development of antiangiogenic drugs have been investigated over the years, with these agents being classified into several different categories depending on their modes of action. Some inhibit ECs directly, whereas others inhibit the angiogenesis signaling cascade or block the ability of ECs to break down the extracellular matrix. Inhibitors may block one main angiogenic protein, two or three angiogenic proteins, or have a broad-spectrum effect by blocking a range of angiogenic regulators that can be located in both the tumor and ECs.[49] In some cases, the antiangiogenic activity is discovered as a secondary function after the drug has received regulatory approval for a different primary function. For example, bortezomib is a proteasome inhibitor that is approved for multiple myeloma and was later found to possess antiangiogenic activity via inhibiting VEGF. Some small-molecule drugs may display their antiangiogenic activity through inducing the expression of endogenous angiogenesis inhibitors such as celecoxib, a cyclooxygenase-2 (COX-2) inhibitor, which inhibits angiogenesis by increasing levels of endostatin.[25]

Some drugs possess antiangiogenic properties but with mechanisms that are not completely understood, such as thalidomide and its analogs, lenalidomide and pomalidomide, referred to as immunomodulatory drugs. Thalidomide was originally shown to inhibit angiogenesis by D'Amato et al.[50] in 1994 and this was subsequently confirmed in several different in vitro and ex vivo

TABLE 28.2

Antiangiogenic Agents that Have Received U.S. Food and Drug Administration Approval for Cancer Treatment

Drug	Class	Mechanism (Cellular Targets)	Year of Approval	Indications	Dosages
Bevacizumab (Avastin)	Anti-VEGF mAB	VEGF	2004	First- and second-line metastatic CRC	5 mg/kg IV q2wk + bolus IFL; 10 mg/kg IV q2wk + FOLFOX4
			2006	First-line NSCLC	15 mg/kg IV q3wk + carboplatin/ paclitaxel
			2009	Second-line GBM	10 mg/kg IV q2wk
			2009	Metastatic RCC	10 mg/kg IV q2wk + IFN
			2013	Second-line metastatic CRC (after prior bevacizumab-containing regimen)	5 mg/kg IV q2wk or 7.5 mg/kg IV q3wk + fluoropyrimidine–irinotecan or fluoropyrimidine-oxaliplatin–based regimen
Ziv-aflibercept (Zaltrap, VEGF Trap)	Anti-VEGF mAB	VEGFA, VEGFB, PIGF1, PIGF2	2012	Metastatic CRC (after prior oxaliplatin-containing regimen)	4 mg/kg IV q2wk (1-hr infusion)
Sorafenib (Nexavar, BAY439006)	Small-molecule TKI	VEGFR2, VEGFR3, PDGFR, FLT3, c-Kit	2005	Advanced RCC	400 mg PO bid (w/o food)
			2007	Unresectable HCC	400 mg PO bid (w/o food)
			2013	RAI-refractory DTC	400 mg PO bid (w/o food)
Sunitinib (Sutent, SU11248)	Small-molecule TKI	VEGFR1, VEGFR2, VEGFR3, PDGFR, FLT3, c-Kit, RET	2006	Imatinib-resistant or -intolerant GIST	50 mg PO qd, 4 wk on/2 wk off
			2006	Advanced RCC	50 mg PO qd, 4 wk on/2 wk off
			2011	Advanced pNET	37.5 mg PO qd
Pazopanib (Votrient)	Small-molecule TKI	VEGFR1, VEGFR2, VEGFR3, PDGFR, Itk, Lck, c-Fms	2009	Advanced RCC	800 mg PO qd (w/o food)
			2012	Advanced soft tissue sarcoma	800 mg PO qd (w/o food)
Vandetanib (Caprelsa)	Small molecule TKI	RET, VEGFR, EGFR, BRK, TIE2	2011	Advanced MTC	300 mg PO qd
Axitinib (Inlyta)	Small molecule TKI	VEGFR1, VEGFR2, VEGFR3	2012	Advanced RCC (after failure of prior therapy)	5 mg PO bid
Cabozantinib (XL184, Cometriq)	Small molecule TKI	MET, VEGFR2, RET, KIT, AXL, FLT3	2012	Progressive, metastatic MTC	140 mg PO qd (w/o food)
Regorafenib (Stivarga)	Small molecule TKI	RET, VEGFR1, VEGFR2, VEGFR3, TIE2, KIT, PDGFR	2012	Previously treated metastatic CRC	160 mg PO qd × 21days (q28-day cycle)
			2013	GIST	160 mg PO qd × days 1–21 (q28-day cycle)
Temsirolimus (Torisel)	mTOR inhibitor	mTOR	2007	Advanced RCC	25 mg IV qwk (infused over 30–60 min)
Everolimus (Afinitor, RAD-001)[a]	mTOR inhibitor	mTOR	2009	Second-line advanced RCC (after VEGFR TKI failure)	10 mg PO qd
			2010	SEGA associated w/TSC	4.5 mg/m^2 PO qd
			2011	pNET	10 mg PO qd
			2012	Advanced HR+, HER2- breast cancer	10 mg PO qd
			2012	AML associated w/TSC	10 mg PO qd

[a] Afinitor Disperz (everolimus tablets for oral suspension) was approved in 2012 for children aged 1 and older who have SEGA + TSC.
mAB, monoclonal antibody; CRC, colorectal cancer; IV, intravenous; IFL, irinotecan, 5-fluorouracil, and leucovorin; FOLFOX4, 5-flourouracil, leucovorin, and oxaliplatin; NSCLC, non–small-cell lung cancer; GBM, glioblastoma multiforme; RCC, renal cell carcinoma; VEGFA, vascular endothelial growth factor A; PIGF, placental growth factor; TKI, tyrosine–kinase inhibitor; VEGFR, VEGF receptor; PDGFR, platelet-derived growth factor receptor; FLT, Fms-like tyrosine kinase; c-Kit, stem cell factor receptor; HCC, hepatocellular carcinoma; RAI, radioactive iodine; DTC, differentiated thyroid carcinoma; PO, orally; RET, glial cell line-derived neurotrophic factor receptor; pNET, pancreatic neuroendocrine tumor; GIST, gastrointestinal stromal tumor; qd, every day; Itk, interleukin-2 receptor inducible T-cell kinase; Lck, leukocyte-specific protein tyrosine kinase; c-Fms, transmembrane glycoprotein receptor tyrosine kinase; bid, twice daily; EGFR, epidermal growth factor receptor; BRK, protein tyrosine kinase 6; MTC, medullary thyroid cancer; mTOR, mammalian target of rapamycin; SEGA, subependymal giant cell astrocytoma; TSC, tuberous sclerosis complex; HR, hormone receptor; HER2, human epidermal growth factor receptor 2; AML, angiomyolipoma.

assays.[51–54] Interestingly, unlike other mechanisms of action, the antiangiogenic activity of thalidomide is believed to require enzymatic activation. The extent to which the antiangiogenic properties of thalidomide and its analogs play a role in its antimyeloma activity is not clearly understood. Several mechanisms have been proposed that involve the downregulation of cytokines in EC, the inhibition of EC proliferation, the decrease in the level of circulating ECs, or the modulation of adhesion molecules between the multiple myeloma cells and the endogenous bone marrow stromal cells, thereby decreasing the production of VEGF and interleukin 6 (IL-6).[55–59] The immunomodulatory agents are discussed in greater detail in another section of this textbook. Examples of the various types of angiogenesis inhibitors are highlighted in Table 28.3.

Drugs with antiangiogenic activity may be classified as either direct or indirect angiogenesis inhibitors. A direct angiogenesis inhibitor blocks vascular ECs from proliferating, migrating, or increasing their survival in response to proangiogenic proteins. They target the activated endothelium directly and inhibit multiple angiogenic proteins. Examples of direct angiogenesis inhibitors include many of the endogenous inhibitors of angiogenesis, such as endostatin, angiostatin, and TSP-1. Indirect angiogenesis inhibitors decrease or block expression of a tumor cell product, neutralize the tumor product itself, or block its receptor on ECs. The limitation to indirect inhibitors is that, over time, tumor cells may acquire mutations that lead to increased expression of other proangiogenic proteins that are not blocked by the indirect inhibitor. This may give the appearance of drug resistance and warrants the addition of a second antiangiogenic agent, one that would target the expression of these upregulated proangiogenic proteins. Examples of drugs that interfere with the angiogenesis-signaling pathway include the anti-VEGF monoclonal antibodies and small-molecule tyrosine–kinase inhibitors. These drugs target the major signaling pathways in tumor angiogenesis: VEGF, PDGF, and their respective receptors, as well as other growth factors and/or signaling pathways.

VEGF (also known as vascular permeability factor) is a potent proangiogenic growth factor and its expression is upregulated by most cancer cell types. It stimulates EC proliferation, migration, and survival as well as induces increased vascular permeability. The different forms of VEGF bind to transmembrane receptor tyrosine kinases (RTK) on ECs: VEGFR1 (Flt-1), VEGFR2 (KDR/Flk-1 or kinase insert domain receptor/fetal liver kinase 1), or VEGFR3 (Flt-4).[60] This results in receptor dimerization, activation, and autophosphorylation of the tyrosine–kinase domain, thereby triggering downstream signaling pathways. Other signaling molecules that may represent attractive therapeutic targets include PDGF and the angiopoietins (Ang1, Ang2). PDGF-B/PDGF receptor (R)-β plays an important role in the recruitment of pericytes and maturation of the microvasculature.[61] Ang2, which binds the Tie-2 receptor, is mostly expressed in tumor-induced neovasculature, whereby its selective inhibition results in reduced EC proliferation.[62] The angiopoietins are also involved in lymphangiogenesis, the formation of new lymphatic vessels, which plays a key role in tumor metastasis. An increased Ang2/Ang1 ratio correlates with tumor angiogenesis and poor prognosis in many cancers, thus making the angiopoietins an attractive therapeutic target. Angiopoietin inhibitors are currently under investigation in the preclinical and clinical setting.

Other strategies for targeting angiogenesis involve the tumor microenvironment. Breakdown of the extracellular matrix is required to allow ECs to migrate into surrounding tissues and proliferate into new blood vessels; thus, drugs that target MMPs, enzymes that catalyze the breakdown of the matrix, can also inhibit angiogenesis. However, clinical development of MMP inhibitors (MMPI) has yielded disappointing results.[63–66]

Integrins are cell surface adhesion molecules that play an essential role in cell–cell and cell–matrix adhesion as well as in transmitting signals important for cell migration, invasion, proliferation, and survival. The involvement of integrin in tumor angiogenesis was demonstrated in studies that show the β-4 subunit of integrin promoting endothelial migration and invasion.[67] Agents that target integrins (inhibitors of $\alpha_v\beta_3$ and $\alpha_v\beta_5$) have been evaluated as potential therapeutic options and include etaracizumab, cilengitide, and intetumumab. However, all three integrin inhibitors have proven to be largely ineffective in various early and late stage cancer trials.[68–73] In summary, the downstream effects of antiangiogenic agents, in addition to blocking angiogenesis, may involve inducing vessel regression, promoting sensitization to radiotherapy and chemotherapy by depriving ECs of VEGF's prosurvival signals, and inhibiting the recruitment of proangiogenic bone marrow–derived cells as well as reducing the self-renewal capability of cancer stem cells.[74]

TABLE 28.3

Examples of Drugs that Possess Antiangiogenic Activity or Inhibit Angiogenesis as a Secondary Function

Drug	Class
Cetuximab Panitumumab Trastuzumab	EGFR/HER monoclonal antibodies
Gefitinib Erlotinib	EGFR small-molecule tyrosine–kinase receptor inhibitors
Everolimus Temsirolimus	mTOR inhibitors
Thalidomide Lenalidomide Pomalidomide	Immunomodulatory agents
Belinostat (PXD101) LBH589 Vorinostat (SAHA)	HDAC inhibitors
Celecoxib	COX-2 inhibitors
Bortezomib	Proteasome inhibitors
Zoledronic acid	Bisphosphonates
Rosiglitazone	PPAR-γ agonists
Doxycycline	Antibiotic

EGFR, epidermal growth factor receptor; mTOR, mammalian target of rapamycin HDAC, histone deacetylase; COX-2, cyclooxygenase-2; PPAR, peroxisome proliferator–activated receptor.

CLINICAL UTILITY OF APPROVED ANTIANGIOGENIC AGENTS IN CANCER THERAPY

The following section reviews the current FDA-approved angiogenesis inhibitors (Table 28.2). These agents include: (1) the monoclonal anti-VEGF antibodies (bevacizumab and ziv-aflibercept); (2) small-molecule tyrosine–kinase inhibitors (TKI) (sorafenib, sunitinib, pazopanib, vandetanib, axitinib, cabozantinib, and regorafenib); and (3) the mammalian target of rapamycin (mTOR) inhibitors (temsirolimus and everolimus), as examples of drugs that possess antiangiogenic activity. Other approved drugs that also inhibit angiogenesis as a secondary function, such as thalidomide, are discussed in greater detail in another section of this textbook and are presented in Table 28.3.

Anti-VEGF Therapy

Bevacizumab

Bevacizumab is a recombinant humanized anti–VEGF-A monoclonal antibody that received FDA approval in February 2004 for use in combination therapy with fluorouracil-based regimens for metastatic colorectal cancer. Bevacizumab binds VEGF and prevents the interaction of VEGF to its receptors (Flt-1 and KDR) on the surface of ECs. It is the first antiangiogenic agent clinically proven to extend survival following a large, randomized, double-blind, phase III study in which bevacizumab was administered in combination with bolus irinotecan, 5-fluorouracil, and leucovorin (IFL) as first-line therapy for metastatic colorectal cancer (CRC).[75] In 2006, its approval extended to first- or second-line treatment of patients with metastatic carcinoma of the colon or rectum. This recommendation is based on the demonstration of a statistically significant improvement in overall survival (OS) in patients receiving bevacizumab plus FOLFOX4 (5-flourouracil, leucovorin, and oxaliplatin) when compared to those receiving FOLFOX4 alone. In January 2013, it was further approved to treat mCRC for second-line treatment when used with fluoropyrimidine-based (combined with irinotecan or oxaliplatin) chemotherapy after disease progression following a first-line treatment with a bevacizumab-containing regimen based on clinical benefits observed in the randomized phase III study (ML18147).[76] Despite the benefit in the metastatic setting, the addition of bevacizumab did not improve clinical outcomes in the adjuvant setting in CRC.[77,78] In 2006, bevacizumab received an additional approval for use in combination with carboplatin and paclitaxel, and is indicated for first-line treatment of patients with unresectable, locally advanced, recurrent, or metastatic nonsquamous, non–small-cell lung cancer (NSCLC) based on the demonstration of a statistically significant improvement in OS in patients in the bevacizumab arm compared to those receiving chemotherapy alone.[79] In February 2008, the FDA granted a conditional, accelerated approval for bevacizumab to be used in combination with paclitaxel for the treatment of patients who have not received chemotherapy for metastatic human epidermal growth factor receptor 2 (*HER2*)-negative breast cancer. However, additional clinical trials were conducted and the new data showed only a small effect on progression free survival (PFS) without evidence of an improvement in OS or a clinical benefit to patients sufficient to outweigh the risks; thus, the FDA rescinded its approval and removed the breast cancer indication from the drug's label in November 2011.[80–82] This controversial decision continues to be debated with ongoing subgroup analyses to identify patients who would likely benefit from bevacizumab.

Bevacizumab received another accelerated approval as a single agent for patients with glioblastoma multiforme (GBM) with progressive disease following therapy in May 2009. The approval was based on the demonstration of durable objective response rates observed in two single-arm trials, AVF3708g and NCI 06-C-0064E.[83] Currently, no data have shown whether bevacizumab improves disease-related symptoms or survival in people previously treated for GBM. Moreover, phase III trials of bevacizumab in newly diagnosed GBM (RTOG 8025 and AVAglio) have shown a 3- to 4-month improvement of PFS, but no OS advantage over the standard of care.[84] The AVAglio trial improved patients' quality of life, whereas the RTOG 0825 did not and instead increased the burden of symptoms with a negative impact on cognition. Although these two studies showed that bevacizumab had a modest benefit as the initial therapy for GBM, it remained effective to treat recurrences where treatment options are limited. In July 2009, bevacizumab was approved for use in combination with IFN-α for the treatment of patients with metastatic renal cell carcinoma (RCC). Results from the AVOREN trial demonstrated a 5-month improvement in median PFS in patients treated with bevacizumab plus IFN-α-2a versus IFN-α-2a plus placebo.[85] Another phase III trial (CALGB 90206) of bevacizumab plus IFN-α versus IFN-α monotherapy was conducted in patients with previously untreated, metastatic clear cell RCC. Median PFS was 8.4 months versus 4.9 months in favor of the bevacizumab arm.[86] Both studies did not demonstrate a statistically significant advantage in OS.[87,88]

Clinical studies of bevacizumab in combination with oxaliplatin-containing and 5-fluorouracil–based regimens have shown that combination therapy is well tolerated with toxicity not being substantially greater than that of the chemotherapy alone.[89] Side effects included grade 3 hypertension, grade 1 or 2 proteinuria, a slight increase (less than two percentage points) in grade 3 or 4 bleeding, and impaired surgical wound healing in patients who underwent surgery during treatment with bevacizumab. However, potentially life-threatening events (e.g., arterial and venous thromboembolic events, gastrointestinal perforation, hemoptysis, risk of ovarian failure) have occurred in some patients, thus requiring close patient monitoring in individuals who are at greater risk of adverse events.[90] In a recent meta-analysis of RCTs, bevacizumab in combination with chemotherapy or biologic therapy, compared with chemotherapy alone, was associated with increased treatment-related mortality.[91]

Although four phase III randomized studies have demonstrated improvements in PFS for ovarian cancer (OC)—two first-line trials (GOG 218 and ICON7) and two in recurrent OC [*platinum-resistant* (AURELIA Trial) or *platinum-sensitive* (OCEANS Trial)]—the role of bevacizumab in OC remains controversial. Bevacizumab is approved for use in combination with chemotherapy in the first- and second-line treatment of advanced OC in Europe, but it is not currently licensed in the United States for this indication. Mature OS data and predictive biomarkers are key to defining the subsets of patients who will most like benefit from this therapy. More recently, a randomized, phase III trial (GOG240) has demonstrated for the first time that bevacizumab can prolong OS and PFS for women with advanced, recurrent, or persistent cervical cancer that was not curable with standard chemotherapy. At the time of writing, there are currently over 400 actively recruiting, ongoing trials investigating the clinical benefits of bevacizumab in combination with chemotherapeutic regimens or as adjuvant therapy in various stages and types of cancer (http://clinicaltrial.gov).

Ziv-aflibercept

Ziv-aflibercept (previously known as aflibercept or VEGFTrap) is a recombinant humanized fusion protein of the extracellular domains of VEGF receptor 1 (VEGFR1) and VEGFR2 with the constant region (Fc) of human immunoglobulin (Ig)G1 that binds to VEGF-A, VEGF-B, PlGF1, and PlGF2, thereby preventing these ligands from binding to and activating their cognate receptors.[97] Ziv-aflibercept has a higher VEGF-A binding affinity and more potent blockade of VEGFR1 or VEGFR2 activation than bevacizumab.[93] In tumor models, ziv-aflibercept exerts its antiangiogenic effects through regressing tumor vasculature and size, remodeling or normalizing surviving vasculature, and inhibiting ascites formation.[94] In August 2012, ziv-aflibercept received regulatory approval for use in combination with 5-fluorouracil, leucovorin, and irinotecan (FOLFIRI) for the treatment of patients with metastatic CRC that is resistant to or that has progressed following treatment with an oxaliplatin-containing regimen. Results from the pivotal phase III VELOUR trial showed that ziv-aflibercept plus FOLFIRI statistically and significantly improved PFS (median PFS, 6.90 versus 4.67 months, respectively), OS (median OS, 13.50 versus 12.06 months, respectively), and overall response rates (19% versus 11.1%, respectively) relative to placebo plus FOLFIRI.[95] Toxicities related to ziv-aflibercept were consistent with those expected from the anti-VEGF drug class. The frequency of vascular-related adverse events appeared to be higher with ziv-aflibercept than bevacizumab treatment when compared across trials. Current clinical data are insufficient to directly compare ziv-aflibercept and bevacizumab in the first- or second-line setting for metastatic CRC.

Tyrosine–Kinase Inhibitor Therapy

Sorafenib

Sorafenib is a small-molecule Raf kinase and VEGF receptor kinase (VEGFR2 and VEGFR3) inhibitor. It has been shown to exhibit broad-spectrum effects on multiple targets (PDGF receptor (PDGFR), stem cell factor (c-KIT) receptor, p38) that affect the maintenance of the tumor vasculature and angiogenesis.[96] In December 2005, the FDA granted approval for sorafenib, which is considered the first multikinase inhibitor, for the treatment of patients with advanced RCC. Safety and efficacy of sorafenib was proven in the largest randomized phase III study conducted in advanced RCC that showed prolong PFS in favor of sorafenib.[97,98] In November 2007, sorafenib was approved for the treatment of patients with unresectable hepatocellular carcinoma (HCC) based on the study results in patients with advanced HCC who had not received previous systemic treatment. Median survival and the time to radiologic progression were nearly 3 months longer for patients treated with sorafenib than for those given placebo.[99] In November 2013, sorafenib received a new indication under the FDA's priority review program for the treatment of locally recurrent or metastatic, progressive differentiated thyroid carcinoma (DTC) refractory to radioactive iodine (RAI) treatment based on positive results from the phase III DECISION trial. Treatment with sorafenib improved PFS (the primary endpoint of the trial) by 41% compared with placebo (10.8 versus 5.8 months, respectively; hazard ratio [HR], 0.587, 95% confidence interval [CI] [0.454 to 0.758]; p <0.0001).[100] The overall response rates were 12% for patients who received sorafenib versus 1% for the placebo arm. Although only about 5% to 15% of thyroid cancer patients become refractory to RAI, no standard treatments are available and, thus, sorafenib is the first agent specifically approved for RAI-resistant DTC. Sorafenib was generally well tolerated with a predictable safety profile. Common adverse events include diarrhea, rash/desquamation, fatigue, hand–foot skin reaction, alopecia, and nausea/vomiting. Grade 3/4 adverse events were 38% for sorafenib versus 28% for placebo. Sorafenib-induced hypertension occurred in patients with metastatic RCC. The treatment-related hypertension was noted to be a class effect observed not only with VEGFR inhibitors, but also with the VEGF monoclonal antibody as well.[90] No significant relationship between previously described mediators of blood pressure and the magnitude of increase was found in a study evaluating the mechanism of sorafenib-induced hypertension in patients.[101]

Sunitinib

Sunitinib (SU11248) is a small-molecule, multitargeted TKI that exhibits potent antitumor and antiangiogenic activity and inhibits VEGFR-1, -2, -3, c-KIT, PDGFR; FLT-3; colony-stimulating factor receptor type 1 receptor; and the glial cell line–derived neurotrophic factor receptor. It was rationally designed and chosen for its high bioavailability and its nanomolar-range potency against the antiangiogenic RTKs. Sunitinib received its first U.S. regulatory approval in 2006 for the treatment of gastrointestinal stromal tumor (GIST) after disease progression on, or intolerance to, imatinib and accelerated approval for the treatment of advanced RCC.[102] Sunitinib demonstrated significant efficacy (prolonged median time to progression) in imatinib-resistant or -intolerant GIST in a randomized phase III trial.[103] The accelerated approval for RCC was based on durable partial responses, with a response rate of 26% to 37%, and a median duration of response of 54 weeks from two phase II, single-arm trials of patients with cytokine-refractory RCC.[104] The accelerated approval was converted to regular approval in 2007 following confirmation of an improvement in PFS and OS in a phase III trial of sunitinib for first-line treatment of patients with treatment-naïve, metastatic RCC.[105,106] In May 2011, the drug received a new indication for the treatment of progressive, well-differentiated pancreatic neuroendocrine tumors (pNET) in patients with unresectable, locally advanced, or metastatic disease. The randomized phase III trial was discontinued early after the independent data monitoring committee observed more serious adverse events and deaths in the placebo group as well as a difference in PFS favoring sunitinib. The median PFS for patients treated with sunitinib was 10.2 months, compared with 5.4 months for patients treated with placebo (HR, 0.427, 95% CI, 0.271 to 0.673], p <0.001).[107] Common adverse effects, including diarrhea, mucositis, asthenia, skin abnormalities, and altered taste, were more common in patients receiving sunitinib. In addition, a decrease in left ventricular ejection fraction and severe hypertension were also more commonly reported in the sunitinib arm. Grade 3 or 4 treatment-emergent adverse events were reported in 56% versus 51% of patients on sunitinib versus placebo, respectively.

Pazopanib

Pazopanib is a second-generation, multitargeted TKI that binds to VEGFR-1, -2, -3, PDGFR-α and -β, c-KIT, and several other key proteins responsible for angiogenesis, tumor growth, and cell survival. Pazopanib exhibited in vivo and in vitro activity against tumor growth, and early clinical trials demonstrated potent antitumor and antiangiogenic activity.[108] A phase III clinical trial in treatment-naïve and cytokine-pretreated patients with advanced and/or metastatic RCC showed a significant improvement in PFS and tumor response compared with placebo,[109] leading to the approval of pazopanib in the United States in October 2009. A recent, randomized phase III trial (COMPARZ) compared the efficacy and safety of pazopanib and sunitinib as first-line therapy involving patients with metastatic RCC and demonstrated that both pazopanib and sunitinib have similar efficacy, but the safety and quality-of-life profiles favor pazopanib.[110] In April 2012, pazopanib was approved for the treatment of patients with metastatic nonadipocytic soft tissue sarcoma who have received prior chemotherapy following a phase III trial that demonstrated a statistically significant improvement in PFS. The median PFS was 4.6 months for patients receiving pazopanib versus 1.6 months for the placebo arm.[111] The drug is generally well tolerated, with the most common adverse events being diarrhea, fatigue, anorexia, hypertension, and hair depigmentation, as well as laboratory abnormalities in elevated aspartate aminotransferase and alanine aminotransferase. Pazopanib has shown clinical activity in a variety of tumors, including breast cancer, thyroid cancer, HCC, and cervical cancer.[112] Ongoing phase II and III trials are further evaluating pazopanib in these malignancies.

Vandetanib

Vandetanib is an oral, small-molecule TKI that inhibits the activity of RET kinase, VEGFR, epidermal growth factor receptor (EGFR), protein tyrosine kinase 6 (BRK), TIE2, members of the ephrin (EPH) receptors kinase family, and members of the Src family of tyrosine kinases.[113] Vandetanib reduced endothelial cell migration, proliferation, survival, and angiogenesis in vitro, and it decreased tumor vessel permeability and inhibited tumor growth and metastasis in vivo. In April 2011, vandetanib received U.S. regulatory approval for the treatment of symptomatic or progressive medullary thyroid cancer (MTC) in patients with unresectable, locally advanced, or metastatic disease. Until the approval of vandetanib, no systemic therapy was approved for the treatment of unresectable MTC, making it the first molecularly targeted agent approved for this disease. Results of a randomized phase III trial of patients with unresectable, locally advanced, or metastatic MTC demonstrated statistically significant and clinically meaningful improvements in PFS for vandetanib compared with placebo (HR, 0.46; 95% CI, 0.31 to 0.69; p <0.001).[114] Common grade 3 and 4 toxicities (>5%) were diarrhea and/or colitis, hypertension and hypertensive crisis, fatigue, hypocalcemia, rash, and corrected QT interval (QTc) prolongation. Given the toxicity profile, which includes QTc prolongation and sudden death, vandetanib is only available through a restricted distribution program. Vandetanib is also the first targeted drug to show evidence of efficacy in a randomized phase II trial in patients with locally advanced or metastatic differentiated thyroid carcinoma,[115] and a phase III trial is currently underway. Early phase studies are also being conducted in solid tumors, including GIST and kidney and pancreatic cancers.

Axitinib

Axitinib is a potent and selective second-generation inhibitor of VEGFR-1, -2, and -3. The in vitro half-maximal inhibitory concentration (IC50) of axitinib is 10-fold lower for the VEGF family of receptors than for other TKIs such as pazopanib, sunitinib, or sorafenib.[116] In January 2012, axitinib received approval for the treatment of advanced RCC after the failure of one prior systemic therapy based on a phase III trial (AXIS) comparing the efficacy and safety of axitinib versus sorafenib as a second-line treatment for metastatic RCC.[117,118] The median PFS was 6.7 months with axitinib compared to 4.7 months with sorafenib (HR, 0.67; 95% CI, 0.54, 0.81; one-sided p <0.0001). This improvement in PFS was greater in the cytokine-pretreated subgroup in comparison with the sunitinib-pretreated subgroup. The most frequent adverse events with axitinib were diarrhea (all grade), hypertension (all grade), fatigue, decreased appetite, nausea, and dysphonia. Moreover, hypertension, nausea, dysphonia, and hypothyroidism were more common with axitinib, whereas palmar–plantar erythrodysesthesia, alopecia, and rash were more frequent with sorafenib. A phase III trial (AGILE) comparing axitinib with sorafenib as first-line therapy in patients with treatment-naïve metastatic RCC demonstrated no significant difference in median PFS between patients treated with axitinib or sorafenib.[119] Additionally, axitinib is being studied as a single agent as well as in combination with chemotherapy across several tumor types including HCC, NSCLC, and pancreatic and thyroid cancers.

Cabozantinib

Cabozantinib (XL184) is a small-molecule TKI with potent activity toward the MET receptor and VEGFR2, as well as a number of other receptor tyrosine kinases, including RET, KIT, AXL, and FLT-3. MET is the only known receptor for hepatocyte growth factor (HGF), and its signaling activity plays a key role in tumorigenic growth, metastasis, and therapeutic resistance. The dysregulated expression and/or activation of MET and HGF have been implicated in the development of numerous human cancers including glioma; melanoma; and hepatocellular, renal, gastric, pancreatic, prostate, ovarian, breast, and lung cancers, and is often correlated with poor prognosis.[120] Recent studies have determined that the MET pathway plays an important role in the development of resistance to VEGF pathway inhibition and that the use of VEGFR inhibitors, such as sunitinib, sorafenib, or a VEGFR2-targeting antibody, can result in the development of an aggressive tumor phenotype characterized by increased invasiveness and metastasis.[121–123] Thus, there is an advantage to targeting both the MET and VEGF pathways to disrupt angiogenesis, tumorigenesis, and cancer progression. In November 2012, cabozantinib received U.S. regulatory approval for progressive metastatic MTC based on the phase III trial that demonstrated a statistically significant PFS prolongation for the cabozantinib-treatment arm.[124] The estimated median PFS was 11.2 months for cabozantinib versus 4.0 months for placebo (HR, 0.28; 95% CI, 0.19 to 0.40; p <0.001). Manageable toxicities included diarrhea, palmar–plantar erythrodysesthesia, decreased weight and appetite, nausea, and fatigue. Cabozantinib has been effective against several solid cancers, including MTC, breast, NSCLC, melanoma, and liver cancer, and is currently being studied in clinical trials in a number of tumor types, with the most significant results observed in the reduction of bone metastatic lesions in castration-resistant prostate cancer.[125]

Regorafenib

Regorafenib is a small-molecule TKI of multiple membrane-bound and intracellular kinases including RET, VEGFR1, VEGFR2, VEGFR3, KIT, PDGFR-α, PDGFR-β, FGFR1, FGFR2, TIE2, DDR2, TrkA, Eph2A, RAF-1, BRAF, BRAFV600E, SAPK2, PTK5, and Abl pathways.[126] Regorafenib is structurally related to sorafenib and differs from the latter by the presence of a fluorine atom in the center phenyl ring, resulting in higher inhibitory potency against various proangiogenic receptors than sorafenib, including VEGFR2 and FGFR1. In September 2012, regorafenib was approved for the treatment of patients with mCRC who have been previously treated with fluoropyrimidine-, oxaliplatin-, and irinotecan-based chemotherapy, with an anti-VEGF therapy, and if KRAS wild type, with an anti-EGFR therapy. The phase III CORRECT trial that resulted in approval of the drug demonstrated a median OS of 6.4 months in the regorafenib group versus 5.0 months in the placebo group (HR, 0.77; 95% CI, 0.64 to 0.94; one-sided p = 0.0052).[127] Regorafenib is the first TKI with survival benefits in mCRC that has progressed after all standard therapies. In February 2013, it received another indication for the treatment of patients with locally advanced, unresectable, or metastatic GIST who have been previously treated with imatinib and sunitinib. This was based on positive findings of the phase III GRID trial that demonstrated a median PFS of 4.8 months for regorafenib and 0.9 months for placebo (HR, 0.27, 95% CI, 0.19 to 0.39; p <0.0001).[128] In both studies, regorafenib provided significant improvements in PFS to highly refractory patient populations who have progressed on standard treatments. The most common adverse events that were grade 3 or higher and related to regorafenib were hand–foot skin reaction, fatigue, diarrhea, hypertension, and rash or desquamation. Its clinical development as a single agent or in combination with standard chemotherapeutic agents in various malignant tumors is ongoing and includes a phase III trial in patients with HCC whose disease has progressed after treatment with sorafenib.

mTOR Inhibitors

The mTOR pathway is a central component of the PI3K/Akt signaling pathway and a regulator of many biologic processes that are essential for angiogenesis, cell proliferation, and metabolism.[129] Inhibition of the mTOR kinase prevents downstream signaling via the Akt pathway, resulting in inhibition of protein translation and cell growth. mTOR plays a key role in angiogenesis and specifically regulates the expression of HIF-1, which is upregulated by the loss of the von Hippel–Lindau gene in RCC. In May 2007, temsirolimus was approved for the treatment of advanced RCC. Efficacy and safety were demonstrated in a phase III study in previously untreated patients (n = 626) with poor risk features of metastatic RCC assigned to one of three treatment arms: IFN-α alone, temsirolimus 25 mg alone, or the combination of temsirolimus (15 mg) and IFN-α.[130] Single-agent temsirolimus was associated with a statistically significant improvement in OS when compared with IFN; the addition of temsirolimus to IFN did not improve OS. The results of the phase III INTORSECT trial compared the efficacy of temsirolimus and sorafenib in the second-line treatment of metastatic RCC after disease progression on sunitinib demonstrated that temsirolimus did not improve survival over sorafenib in the second-line setting.[131] The significant OS difference in favor of sorafenib (stratified HR, 1.31; 95% CI, 1.05 to 1.63; two-sided p = 0.01) suggested that VEGFR inhibition may be a better option than mTOR inhibitors for patients progressing on sunitinib. The most common adverse reactions that occurred were rash, asthenia, mucositis, nausea, edema, and anorexia. Rare, but serious adverse reactions associated with temsirolimus included interstitial lung disease, bowel perforation, and acute renal failure.

Everolimus (RAD001) was approved in March 2009 for patients with advanced RCC whose disease had progressed on VEGFR-targeted therapy (sunitinib or sorafenib). Efficacy was demonstrated in a phase 3 trial that study met its primary endpoint with a median PFS of 4.9 and 1.9 months in the everolimus and placebo arms, respectively (HR, 0.33; p <0.0001).[132] Everolimus is also indicated for subependymal giant cell astrocytoma (SEGA) associated with tuberous sclerosis complex (TSC), renal angiomyolipoma with TSC, progressive neuroendocrine tumors of pancreatic origin, and advanced hormone receptor-positive, HER2-negative breast cancer in combination with exemestane.[133] The most common adverse reactions were stomatitis, infections, asthenia, fatigue, cough, and diarrhea. The most common grade 3/4 adverse reactions were infections, dyspnea, fatigue, stomatitis, dehydration, pneumonitis, abdominal pain, and asthenia. Both temsirolimus and everolimus are currently being evaluated in phase I through III studies of various cancer types. By downregulating HIF-1 in the tumor cell, mTOR inhibitors may complement the effects of TKIs at the level of the EC; thus, the combination of mTOR inhibitors with other targeted agents such as bevacizumab or sorafenib/sunitinib are also being investigated.

On the Horizon: Anti-VEGFR2 Monoclonal Antibody

Ramucirumab (IMC-1121B) is a fully human IgG1 monoclonal antibody that binds with high affinity to the extracellular VEGF-binding domain of VEGFR-2. In a phase III trial (REGARD), ramucirumab monotherapy conferred a statistically significant benefit in OS and PFS compared to placebo in patients with advanced gastric or gastroesophageal junction adenocarcinoma in the second-line setting with an acceptable safety profile.[134] The survival advantage is the first to be elicited by a single-agent biologic treatment in this setting and, based on these findings, the FDA has assigned a priority review designation for ramucirumab. An ongoing phase III trial (RAINBOW) of ramucirumab in combination with chemotherapy as second-line treatment for patients with advanced gastric cancer is currently underway, and preliminary results demonstrated the trial met both its primary (OS) and secondary (PFS) endpoints. In April 2014, the U.S. FDA approved ramucirumab for use as a single agent for the treatment of patients with advanced or metastatic, gastric or gastroesophageal junction adenocarcinoma with disease progression on or after prior treatment with fluoropyrimidine- or platinum-containing chemotherapy. The recommended ramucirumab dose and schedule is 8 mg/kg administered as a 60-minute intravenous infusion every 2 weeks. The drug also marginally improved survival in the second-line treatment of NSCLC in an ongoing phase III (REVEL) trial.

COMBINATION THERAPIES

Tumor angiogenesis is a highly complex process involving multiple growth factors and their receptor signaling pathways. Based on current evidence, with a few exceptions, effective therapy will probably rely on a combinatorial approach that involves targeting multiple pathways simultaneously. However, a recent study has demonstrated that simultaneous inhibition of the VEGF and EGF pathways in combination with chemotherapy shortens rather than prolongs PFS as compared to inhibition of the VEGF pathway alone in combination with chemotherapy.[135] Whether other targeted agents exhibit beneficial effects when combined with VEGF inhibitors remains to be investigated. Moreover, a number of studies have shown that antiangiogenic agents in combination with chemotherapy or radiotherapy result in additive or synergistic effects. Several models have been proposed to explain the mechanism responsible for this potentiation, keying in on the chemosensitizing effects of antiangiogenic therapy.[136] One hypothesis is that antiangiogenic therapy may normalize the tumor vasculature, thus resulting in improved oxygenation, better blood perfusion, and consequently, improved delivery of chemotherapeutic drugs.[137] A second model suggests that chemotherapy delivered at low doses and at close, regular intervals with no extended drug-free break periods preferentially damages ECs in the tumor neovasculature.[138,139] and suppresses circulating endothelial progenitor cells.[140,141] This regimen, also called metronomic chemotherapy, sustains antiangiogenic activity and reduces acute toxicity.[142] Thus, the efficacy of metronomic chemotherapy may increase when administered in combination with specific antiangiogenic drugs. Another model addresses the use of antiangiogenic drugs to slow down tumor cell repopulation between successive cycles of cytotoxic chemotherapy.[143] This model underscores the importance of timing and sequence in achieving the maximal therapeutic benefit from combination therapies. In fact, a preclinical study in murine tumor models demonstrated that the administration of sunitinib markedly reduced chemotherapy-induced bone marrow toxicity, suggesting that the sequential treatment regimen (delivery of antiangiogenics followed by chemotherapy) showed superior survival benefits compared with the simultaneous administration of two drugs.[144] Finally, other mechanisms that might also contribute to the synergism include angiogenesis inhibitor–induced tumor blood vessel regression, the prevention of tumor coopting of vessels from surrounding healthy tissues, and the formation of abnormal vessels in the tumor microenvironment.[145] Nevertheless, it remains a challenge to determine why bevacizumab has proved largely ineffective as a single agent, whereas VEGF RTK inhibitors have repeatedly failed in randomized phase III trials when used in combination with chemotherapy. Furthermore, an additional challenge is to determine the optimal dose and duration of antiangiogenic drugs as well as the impact of drug sequencing in combination regimens. Studies are warranted to delineate the discrepancy of bevacizumab's efficacy in the macrometastatic versus micrometastatic disease settings.[146,147]

BIOMARKERS OF ANTIANGIOGENIC THERAPY

Antiangiogenic therapy has created a need to develop effective biomarkers to assess the activity of these inhibitors. Biomarkers of tumor angiogenesis activity are important to guide clinical development of these agents and to select patients most likely to benefit from this approach. Although there are currently no validated biomarkers for clinically assessing the efficacy of or selecting patients who will respond to antiangiogenic therapies, a number of candidate markers, including tissue, imaging, and circulating biomarkers, are emerging that need to be prospectively validated.[148,149] Several avenues are currently being investigated and include tumor biopsy analysis, microvessel density, noninvasive vascular imaging modalities (positron-emission tomography, dynamic contrast-enhanced magnetic resonance imaging), and measuring circulating biomarkers (levels of angiogenic factors in serum, plasma, urine, or circulating ECs and their precursors).[150–152] Recent research efforts have focused on identifying genetic and toxicity biomarkers to predict which patients will benefit from anti-VEGF/VEGFR therapy and identify patients at risk of adverse events. The existence of VEGF single-nucleotide polymorphisms (SNP) and their association with clinical outcomes may be predictive of patient response to bevacizumab. A recent study identified a locus in VEGFR1 that correlated with increased VEGFR1 expression and poor bevacizumab treatment outcomes.[153] Moreover, a breast cancer study (E2100) reported the VEGF-2578 AA and VEGF-1154 AA genotypes predicted an improved median OS, whereas the VEGF-634 CC and VEGF-1498 TT genotypes predicted protection from grade 3/4 hypertension in the combination-treatment arm.[154] The degree of hypertension can serve as a predictive biomarker of survival in patients after bevacizumab or TKI treatment. Although an association between hypertension and anti-VEGF therapy has been described, the clinical implications of this association and the predictive value of hypertension remains to be validated prospectively. A retrospective analysis of hypertension and efficacy outcomes was conducted in seven large phase III trials ($n = 6{,}486$ patients) and, in six of seven studies, early treatment-related blood pressure increase was neither predictive of clinical benefit from bevacizumab nor prognostic for the course of the disease.[155] However, one study (AVF2107g) showed early increased blood pressure was associated with longer PFS and OS. Because genetics play a significant role in modifying the risk of hypertension,[156] it remains to be determined whether polymorphisms in the VEGF/VEGFR pathway may function as potential biomarkers to predict the association between treatment-related hypertension and response to anti-VEGF therapy, as previously implicated in the E2100 trial.[154] Other biomarkers of response include elevated VEGF and placental growth factor levels,[148,152] whereas biomarkers of resistance, including circulating basic fibroblast growth factor, stromal cell-derived factor 1α, and viable circulating endothelial cells, increased when tumors escaped treatment.[157] A first prospective biomarker study (MERiDiAN) in metastatic breast cancer is currently underway to evaluate the impact of bevacizumab in patients stratified for plasma short VEGF-A isoforms. If validated, these findings could help identify which subgroup of patients should receive antiangiogenic therapy and could lead the way to possible future tailoring of individualized antiangiogenic therapy.

RESISTANCE TO ANTIANGIOGENIC THERAPY

Despite a decade of trials with angiogenesis inhibitors, clinical experience reveals that VEGF-targeted therapy often prolongs the survival of cancer patients by only months because tumors elicit evasive resistance.[145,158] Resistance to VEGF inhibitors may be observed in late-stage tumors when tumors regrow during treatment after an initial period of growth suppression from these antiangiogenic agents. This resistance involves the reactivation of tumor angiogenesis and increased expression of other proangiogenic factors. As the disease progresses, it is possible that redundant pathways might be implicated, with VEGF being replaced by other angiogenic pathways, warranting the addition of a second angiogenesis inhibitor that would target these secondary growth factors and/or their activated receptor pathways, or the use of a multitargeted TKI antiangiogenic drug (e.g., sunitinib, sorafenib). However, resistance to these drugs eventually occurs, implicating the existence of additional pathways mediating resistance to antiangiogenic therapies. Moreover, tumor cells bearing genetic alterations of the *p53* gene may display a lower apoptosis rate under hypoxic conditions, which might reduce their reliance on vascular supply and, therefore, their responsiveness to antiangiogenic therapy.[159] The selection and overgrowth of tumor-variant cells that are hypoxia resistant and, thus, less dependent[159] on angiogenesis and vasculature remodeling, resulting in vessel stabilization,[160] could also explain the resistance to antiangiogenic drugs. Other possible mechanisms for acquired resistance include tumor vessels becoming less sensitive to antiangiogenic agents, tumor regrowth via rebound revascularization, and vessel cooption.[161–166] Perhaps one of the most intriguing findings is that, although ECs are assumed to be genetically stable, they may under some circumstances harbor genetic abnormalities and thus acquire resistance as well.[167,168]

Recent studies report that VEGF-targeted therapies not only induce primary tumor shrinkage and inhibit tumor progression, but can also initiate mechanisms that increase malignancy to promote tumor invasiveness and metastasis.[122,123,169] These mechanisms of resistance to antiangiogenic therapy involve tumor- and host-mediated pathways and may allow for differential efficacy in different stages of disease progression.[163] Specifically, antiangiogenic drug–resistance mechanisms involve pathways mediated by the tumor, whether intrinsic or acquired in response to therapy or by the host, which is either responding directly to therapy or indirectly to tumoral cues. Taken together, antiangiogenic therapy can enhance tumor invasiveness and metastasis to facilitate and/or accelerate disease in microscopic tumors and, hence, reduce OS benefit. Understanding the mechanisms of resistance, whether intrinsic or acquired, after exposure to antiangiogenic drug treatment is essential for developing strategies that will allow for optimal exploitation of VEGF inhibitors. It is equally important to identify biomarkers of drug resistance and factors mediating this resistance because the development of reliable biomarkers can be invaluable to monitor the development of evasive resistance to angiogenesis inhibitors.

REFERENCES

1. Hanahan D, Weinberg RA. Hallmarks of cancer: the next generation. *Cell* 2011;144:646–674.
2. Ide AG, Baker NH, Warren SL. Vascularization of the Brown Pearce rabbit epithelioma transplant as seen in the transparent ear chamger. *Am J Roentgenol* 1939;42:891–899.
3. Algire GH, Chalkley HW, Legallais FY, et al. Vascular reactions of normal and malignant tissues in vivo. I. Vascular reactions of mice to wounds and to normal and neoplastic transplants. *J Natl Cancer Inst* 1945;6:73–85.
4. Folkman J, Merler E, Abernathy C, et al. Isolation of a tumor factor responsible for angiogenesis. *J Exp Med* 1971;133:275–288.
5. Folkman J. Tumor angiogenesis: therapeutic implications. *N Engl J Med* 1971;285:1182–1186.
6. Papetti M, Herman IM. Mechanisms of normal and tumor-derived angiogenesis. *Am J Physiol Cell Physiol* 2002;282:C947–C970.
7. Hanahan D, Folkman J. Patterns and emerging mechanisms of the angiogenic switch during tumorigenesis. *Cell* 1996;86:353–364.
8. Black WC, Welch HG. Advances in diagnostic imaging and overestimations of disease prevalence and the benefits of therapy. *N Engl J Med* 1993;328:1237–1243.
9. Folkman J, Kalluri R. Cancer without disease. *Nature* 2004;427:787.
10. Weidner N, Semple JP, Welch WR, et al. Tumor angiogenesis and metastasis—correlation in invasive breast carcinoma. *N Engl J Med* 1991;324:1–8.
11. Holmgren L, O'Reilly MS, Folkman J. Dormancy of micrometastases: balanced proliferation and apoptosis in the presence of angiogenesis suppression. *Nat Med* 1995;1:149–153.
12. Naumov GN, Bender E, Zurakowski D, et al. A model of human tumor dormancy: an angiogenic switch from the nonangiogenic phenotype. *J Natl Cancer Inst* 2006;98:316–325.
13. Udagawa T, Fernandez A, Achilles EG, et al. Persistence of microscopic human cancers in mice: alterations in the angiogenic balance accompanies loss of tumor dormancy. *Faseb J* 2002;16:1361–1370.
14. Holash J, Maisonpierre PC, Compton D, et al. Vessel cooption, regression, and growth in tumors mediated by angiopoietins and VEGF. *Science* 1999; 284:1994–1998.
15. Relf M, LeJeune S, Scott PA, et al. Expression of the angiogenic factors vascular endothelial cell growth factor, acidic and basic fibroblast growth factor, tumor growth factor beta-1, platelet-derived endothelial cell growth factor, placenta growth factor, and pleiotrophin in human primary breast cancer and its relation to angiogenesis. *Cancer Res* 1997;57:963–969.
16. Carmeliet P, Dor Y, Herbert JM, et al. Role of HIF-1alpha in hypoxia-mediated apoptosis, cell proliferation and tumour angiogenesis. *Nature* 1998; 394:485–490.
17. Folkman J. Endogenous angiogenesis inhibitors. *Apmis* 2004;112:496–507.
18. Nyberg P, Xie L, Kalluri R. Endogenous inhibitors of angiogenesis. *Cancer Res* 2005;65:3967–3979.
19. Rak J, Yu JL. Oncogenes and tumor angiogenesis: the question of vascular "supply" and vascular "demand". *Semin Cancer Biol* 2004;14:93–104.
20. Bottos A, Bardelli A. Oncogenes and angiogenesis: a way to personalize antiangiogenic therapy? *Cell Mol Life Sci* 2013;70:4131–4140.
21. Rak J, Yu JL, Klement G, et al. Oncogenes and angiogenesis: signaling three-dimensional tumor growth. *J Investig Dermatol Symp Proc* 2000;5:24–33.
22. Langer R, Brem H, Falterman K, et al. Isolations of a cartilage factor that inhibits tumor neovascularization. *Science* 1976;193:70–72.
23. Langer R, Conn H, Vacanti J, et al. Control of tumor growth in animals by infusion of an angiogenesis inhibitor. *Proc Natl Acad Sci U S A* 1980;77: 4331–4335.
24. Ribatti D. Endogenous inhibitors of angiogenesis: a historical review. *Leuk Res* 2009;33:638–644.
25. Folkman J. Antiangiogenesis in cancer therapy—endostatin and its mechanisms of action. *Exp Cell Res* 2006;312:594–607.
26. Karamouzis MV, Moschos SJ. The use of endostatin in the treatment of solid tumors. *Expert Opin Biol Ther* 2009;9:641–648.
27. Lawler J. Thrombospondin-1 as an endogenous inhibitor of angiogenesis and tumor growth. *J Cell Mol Med* 2002;6:1–12.
28. Maeshima Y, Manfredi M, Reimer C, et al. Identification of the anti-angiogenic site within vascular basement membrane-derived tumstatin. *J Biol Chem* 2001; 276:15240–15248.
29. Kerbel RS. Vasohibin: the feedback on a new inhibitor of angiogenesis. *J Clin Invest* 2004;114:884–886.
30. Sato Y. The vasohibin family: a novel family for angiogenesis regulation. *J Biochem* 2013;153:5–11.

31. Noguera-Troise I, Daly C, Papadopoulos NJ, et al. Blockade of Dll4 inhibits tumour growth by promoting non-productive angiogenesis. *Nature* 2006;444:1032–1037.
32. Ridgway J, Zhang G, Wu Y, et al. Inhibition of Dll4 signalling inhibits tumour growth by deregulating angiogenesis. *Nature* 2006;444:1083–1087.
33. Kuhnert F, Kirshner JR, Thurston G. Dll4-Notch signaling as a therapeutic target in tumor angiogenesis. *Vasc Cell* 2011;3:20.
34. Sund M, Hamano Y, Sugimoto H, et al. Function of endogenous inhibitors of angiogenesis as endothelium-specific tumor suppressors. *Proc Natl Acad Sci U S A* 2005;102:2934–2939.
35. Dameron KM, Volpert OV, Tainsky MA, et al. Control of angiogenesis in fibroblasts by p53 regulation of thrombospondin-1. *Science* 1994;265:1582–1584.
36. Zhang L, Yu D, Hu M, et al. Wild-type p53 suppresses angiogenesis in human leiomyosarcoma and synovial sarcoma by transcriptional suppression of vascular endothelial growth factor expression. *Cancer Res* 2000;60:3655–3661.
37. Sherif ZA, Nakai S, Pirollo KF, et al. Downmodulation of bFGF-binding protein expression following restoration of p53 function. *Cancer Gene Ther* 2001;8:771–782.
38. Ravi R, Mookerjee B, Bhujwalla ZM, et al. Regulation of tumor angiogenesis by p53-induced degradation of hypoxia-inducible factor 1alpha. *Genes Dev* 2000;14:34–44.
39. Farhang Ghahremani M, Goossens S, Nittner D, et al. p53 promotes VEGF expression and angiogenesis in the absence of an intact p21-Rb pathway. *Cell Death Differ* 2013;20:888–897.
40. Teodoro JG, Parker AE, Zhu X, et al. p53-mediated inhibition of angiogenesis through up-regulation of a collagen prolyl hydroxylase. *Science* 2006;313:968–971.
41. Folkman J. Tumor suppression by p53 is mediated in part by the antiangiogenic activity of endostatin and tumstatin. *Sci STKE* 2006;2006:pe35.
42. Brouty-Boye D, Zetter BR. Inhibition of cell motility by interferon. *Science* 1980;208:516–518.
43. Dvorak HF, Gresser I. Microvascular injury in pathogenesis of interferon-induced necrosis of subcutaneous tumors in mice. *J Natl Cancer Inst* 1989;81:497–502.
44. Sidky YA, Borden EC. Inhibition of angiogenesis by interferons: effects on tumor- and lymphocyte-induced vascular responses. *Cancer Res* 1987;47:5155–5161.
45. Taylor S, Folkman J. Protamine is an inhibitor of angiogenesis. *Nature* 1982; 297:307–312.
46. Crum R, Szabo S, Folkman J. A new class of steroids inhibits angiogenesis in the presence of heparin or a heparin fragment. *Science* 1985;230:1375–1378.
47. Ingber D, Fujita T, Kishimoto S, et al. Synthetic analogues of fumagillin that inhibit angiogenesis and suppress tumour growth. *Nature* 1990;348:555–557.
48. Kerbel RS. Inhibition of tumor angiogenesis as a strategy to circumvent acquired resistance to anti-cancer therapeutic agents. *Bioessays* 1991;13:31–36.
49. Folkman J. Angiogenesis: an organizing principle for drug discovery? *Nat Rev Drug Discov* 2007;6:273–286.
50. D'Amato RJ, Loughnan MS, Flynn E, et al. Thalidomide is an inhibitor of angiogenesis. *Proc Natl Acad Sci U S A* 1994;91:4082–4085.
51. Bauer KS, Dixon SC, Figg WD. Inhibition of angiogenesis by thalidomide requires metabolic activation, which is species-dependent. *Biochem Pharmacol* 1998;55:1827–1834.
52. Figg WD. The 2005 Leon I. Goldberg Young Investigator Award Lecture: development of thalidomide as an angiogenesis inhibitor for the treatment of androgen-independent prostate cancer. *Clin Pharmacol Ther* 2006;79:1–8.
53. Kenyon BM, Browne F, D'Amato RJ. Effects of thalidomide and related metabolites in a mouse corneal model of neovascularization. *Exp Eye Res* 1997;64:971–978.
54. Price DK, Ando Y, Kruger EA, et al. 5'-OH-thalidomide, a metabolite of thalidomide, inhibits angiogenesis. *Ther Drug Monit* 2002;24:104–110.
55. Dredge K, Marriott JB, Macdonald CD, et al. Novel thalidomide analogues display anti-angiogenic activity independently of immunomodulatory effects. *Br J Cancer* 2002;87:1166–1172.
56. Gupta D, Treon SP, Shima Y, et al. Adherence of multiple myeloma cells to bone marrow stromal cells upregulates vascular endothelial growth factor secretion: therapeutic applications. *Leukemia* 2001;15:1950–1961.
57. Ng SS, Gutschow M, Weiss M, et al. Antiangiogenic activity of N-substituted and tetrafluorinated thalidomide analogues. *Cancer Res* 2003;63:3189–3194.
58. Zhang H, Vakil V, Braunstein M, et al. Circulating endothelial progenitor cells in multiple myeloma: implications and significance. *Blood* 2005;105: 3286–3294.
59. De Sanctis JB, Mijares M, Suarez A, et al. Pharmacological properties of thalidomide and its analogues. *Recent Pat Inflamm Allergy Drug Discov* 2010;4:144–148.
60. Ferrara N, Gerber HP, LeCouter J. The biology of VEGF and its receptors. *Nat Med* 2003;9:669–676.
61. Lindahl P, Johansson BR, Leveen P, et al. Pericyte loss and microaneurysm formation in PDGF-B-deficient mice. *Science* 1997;277:242–245.
62. Oliner J, Min H, Leal J, et al. Suppression of angiogenesis and tumor growth by selective inhibition of angiopoietin-2. *Cancer Cell* 2004;6:507–516.
63. Fingleton B. MMPs as therapeutic targets—still a viable option? *Semin Cell Dev Biol* 2008;19:61–68.
64. Roy R, Yang J, Moses MA. Matrix metalloproteinases as novel biomarkers and potential therapeutic targets in human cancer. *J Clin Oncol* 2009;27:5287–5297.
65. Shi ZG, Li JP, Shi LL, et al. An updated patent therapeutic agents targeting MMPs. *Recent Pat Anticancer Drug Discov* 2012;7:74–101.
66. Gialeli C, Theocharis AD, Karamanos NK. Roles of matrix metalloproteinases in cancer progression and their pharmacological targeting. *FEBS J* 2011;278:16–27.
67. Nikolopoulos SN, Blaikie P, Yoshioka T, et al. Integrin beta4 signaling promotes tumor angiogenesis. *Cancer Cell* 2004;6:471–483.
68. Bradley DA, Daignault S, Ryan CJ, et al. Cilengitide (EMD 121974, NSC 707544) in asymptomatic metastatic castration resistant prostate cancer patients: a randomized phase II trial by the prostate cancer clinical trials consortium. *Invest New Drugs* 2011;29:1432–1440.
69. Desgrosellier JS, Cheresh DA. Integrins in cancer: biological implications and therapeutic opportunities. *Nat Rev Cancer* 2010;10:9–22.
70. Hersey P, Sosman J, O'Day S, et al. A randomized phase 2 study of etaracizumab, a monoclonal antibody against integrin alpha(v)beta(3), + or − dacarbazine in patients with stage IV metastatic melanoma. *Cancer* 2010;116: 1526–1534.
71. Heidenreich A, Rawal SK, Szkarlat K, et al. A randomized, double-blind, multicenter, phase 2 study of a human monoclonal antibody to human alphanu integrins (intetumumab) in combination with docetaxel and prednisone for the first-line treatment of patients with metastatic castration-resistant prostate cancer. *Ann Oncol* 2013;24:329–336.
72. O'Day S, Pavlick A, Loquai C, et al. A randomised, phase II study of intetumumab, an anti-alphav-integrin mAb, alone and with dacarbazine in stage IV melanoma. *Br J Cancer* 2011;105:346–352.
73. Stupp R, Hegi M, Gorlia T, et al. Standard chemoradiotherapy ± cilengitide in newly diagnosed glioblastoma (GBM): updated results and subgroup analyses of the international randomized phase III CENTRIC trial (EORTC trial #26071-22072/Canadian Brain Tumor Consortium). Program and abstracts presented at: 2013 European Cancer Congress; 2013; Amsterdam.
74. Ellis LM, Hicklin DJ. VEGF-targeted therapy: mechanisms of anti-tumour activity. *Nat Rev Cancer* 2008;8:579–591.
75. Hurwitz H, Fehrenbacher L, Novotny W, et al. Bevacizumab plus irinotecan, fluorouracil, and leucovorin for metastatic colorectal cancer. *N Engl J Med* 2004;350:2335–2342.
76. Bennouna J, Sastre J, Arnold D, et al. Continuation of bevacizumab after first progression in metastatic colorectal cancer (ML18147): a randomised phase 3 trial. *Lancet Oncol* 2013;14:29–37.
77. Allegra CJ, Yothers G, O'Connell MJ, et al. Phase III trial assessing bevacizumab in stages II and III carcinoma of the colon: results of NSABP protocol C-08. *J Clin Oncol* 2011;29:11–16.
78. de Gramont A, Van Cutsem E, Schmoll HJ, et al. Bevacizumab plus oxaliplatin-based chemotherapy as adjuvant treatment for colon cancer (AVANT): a phase 3 randomised controlled trial. *Lancet Oncol* 2012;13:1225–1233.
79. Sandler A, Gray R, Perry MC, et al. Paclitaxel-carboplatin alone or with bevacizumab for non-small-cell lung cancer. *N Engl J Med* 2006;355:2542–2550.
80. Miles DW, Chan A, Dirix LY, et al. Phase III study of bevacizumab plus docetaxel compared with placebo plus docetaxel for the first-line treatment of human epidermal growth factor receptor 2-negative metastatic breast cancer. *J Clin Oncol* 2010;28:3239–3247.
81. Robert NJ, Dieras V, Glaspy J, et al. RIBBON-1: randomized, double-blind, placebo-controlled, phase III trial of chemotherapy with or without bevacizumab for first-line treatment of human epidermal growth factor receptor 2-negative, locally recurrent or metastatic breast cancer. *J Clin Oncol* 2011;29:1252–1260.
82. Brufsky AM, Hurvitz S, Perez E, et al. RIBBON-2: a randomized, double-blind, placebo-controlled, phase III trial evaluating the efficacy and safety of bevacizumab in combination with chemotherapy for second-line treatment of human epidermal growth factor receptor 2-negative metastatic breast cancer. *J Clin Oncol* 2011;29:4286–4293.
83. Cohen MH, Shen YL, Keegan P, et al. FDA drug approval summary: bevacizumab (Avastin) as treatment of recurrent glioblastoma multiforme. *Oncologist* 2009;14:1131–1138.
84. Soffietti R, Trevisan E, Ruda R. What have we learned from trials on antiangiogenic agents in glioblastoma? *Expert Rev Neurother* 2014;14:1–3.
85. Escudier B, Pluzanska A, Koralewski P, et al. Bevacizumab plus interferon alfa-2a for treatment of metastatic renal cell carcinoma: a randomised, double-blind phase III trial. *Lancet* 2007;370:2103–2111.
86. Rini BI, Halabi S, Rosenberg JE, et al. Bevacizumab plus interferon alfa compared with interferon alfa monotherapy in patients with metastatic renal cell carcinoma: CALGB 90206. *J Clin Oncol* 2008;26:5422–5428.
87. Escudier B, Bellmunt J, Negrier S, et al. Phase III trial of bevacizumab plus interferon alfa-2a in patients with metastatic renal cell carcinoma (AVOREN): final analysis of overall survival. *J Clin Oncol* 2010;28:2144–2150.
88. Rini BI, Halabi S, Rosenberg JE, et al. Phase III trial of bevacizumab plus interferon alfa versus interferon alfa monotherapy in patients with metastatic renal cell carcinoma: final results of CALGB 90206. *J Clin Oncol* 2010;28: 2137–2143.
89. Hurwitz H, Saini S. Bevacizumab in the treatment of metastatic colorectal cancer: safety profile and management of adverse events. *Semin Oncol* 2006;33:S26–S34.
90. Chen HX, Cleck JN. Adverse effects of anticancer agents that target the VEGF pathway. *Nat Rev Clin Oncol* 2009;6:465–477.
91. Ranpura V, Hapani S, Wu S. Treatment-related mortality with bevacizumab in cancer patients: a meta-analysis. *JAMA* 2011;305:487–494.
92. Holash J, Davis S, Papadopoulos N, et al. VEGF-Trap: a VEGF blocker with potent antitumor effects. *Proc Natl Acad Sci U S A* 2002;99:11393–11398.
93. Papadopoulos N, Martin J, Ruan Q, et al. Binding and neutralization of vascular endothelial growth factor (VEGF) and related ligands by VEGF Trap, ranibizumab and bevacizumab. *Angiogenesis* 2012;15:171–185.
94. Gaya A, Tse V. A preclinical and clinical review of aflibercept for the management of cancer. *Cancer Treat Rev* 2012;38:484–493.

95. Van Cutsem E, Tabernero J, Lakomy R, et al. Addition of aflibercept to fluorouracil, leucovorin, and irinotecan improves survival in a phase III randomized trial in patients with metastatic colorectal cancer previously treated with an oxaliplatin-based regimen. *J Clin Oncol* 2012;30:3499–3506.
96. Wilhelm SM, Carter C, Tang L, et al. BAY 43-9006 exhibits broad spectrum oral antitumor activity and targets the RAF/MEK/ERK pathway and receptor tyrosine kinases involved in tumor progression and angiogenesis. *Cancer Res* 2004;64:7099–7109.
97. Escudier B, Eisen T, Stadler WM, et al. Sorafenib in advanced clear-cell renal-cell carcinoma. *N Engl J Med* 2007;356:125–134.
98. Escudier B, Eisen T, Stadler WM, et al. Sorafenib for treatment of renal cell carcinoma: Final efficacy and safety results of the phase III treatment approaches in renal cancer global evaluation trial. *J Clin Oncol* 2009;27:3312–3318.
99. Llovet JM, Ricci S, Mazzaferro V, et al. Sorafenib in advanced hepatocellular carcinoma. *N Engl J Med* 2008;359:378–390.
100. Brose MS, Nutting C, Jarzab B, et al. Sorafenib in locally advanced or metastatic patients with radioactive iodine refractory differentiated thyroid cancer: the phase III DECISION trial. *J Clin Oncol* 2013;31.
101. Veronese ML, Mosenkis A, Flaherty KT, et al. Mechanisms of hypertension associated with BAY 43-9006. *J Clin Oncol* 2006;24:1363–1369.
102. Goodman VL, Rock EP, Dagher R, et al. Approval summary: sunitinib for the treatment of imatinib refractory or intolerant gastrointestinal stromal tumors and advanced renal cell carcinoma. *Clin Cancer Res* 2007;13:1367–1373.
103. Demetri GD, van Oosterom AT, Garrett CR, et al. Efficacy and safety of sunitinib in patients with advanced gastrointestinal stromal tumour after failure of imatinib: a randomised controlled trial. *Lancet* 2006;368:1329–1338.
104. Motzer RJ, Michaelson MD, Redman BG, et al. Activity of SU11248, a multitargeted inhibitor of vascular endothelial growth factor receptor and platelet-derived growth factor receptor, in patients with metastatic renal cell carcinoma. *J Clin Oncol* 2006;24:16–24.
105. Motzer RJ, Hutson TE, Tomczak P, et al. Sunitinib versus interferon alfa in metastatic renal-cell carcinoma. *N Engl J Med* 2007;356:115–124.
106. Motzer RJ, Hutson TE, Tomczak P, et al. Overall survival and updated results for sunitinib compared with interferon alfa in patients with metastatic renal cell carcinoma. *J Clin Oncol* 2009;27:3584–3590.
107. Raymond E, Dahan L, Raoul JL, et al. Sunitinib malate for the treatment of pancreatic neuroendocrine tumors. *N Engl J Med* 2011;364:501–513.
108. Kumar R, Knick VB, Rudolph SK, et al. Pharmacokinetic-pharmacodynamic correlation from mouse to human with pazopanib, a multikinase angiogenesis inhibitor with potent antitumor and antiangiogenic activity. *Mol Cancer Ther* 2007;6:2012–2021.
109. Sternberg CN, Davis ID, Mardiak J, et al. Pazopanib in locally advanced or metastatic renal cell carcinoma: results of a randomized phase III trial. *J Clin Oncol* 2010;28:1061–1068.
110. Motzer RJ, Hutson TE, Cella D, et al. Pazopanib versus sunitinib in metastatic renal-cell carcinoma. *N Engl J Med* 2013;369:722–731.
111. van der Graaf WT, Blay JY, Chawla SP, et al. Pazopanib for metastatic soft-tissue sarcoma (PALETTE): a randomised, double-blind, placebo-controlled phase 3 trial. *Lancet* 2012;379:1879–1886.
112. Schutz FA, Choueiri TK, Sternberg CN. Pazopanib: Clinical development of a potent anti-angiogenic drug. *Crit Rev Oncol Hematol* 2011;77:163–171.
113. Thornton K, Kim G, Maher VE, et al. Vandetanib for the treatment of symptomatic or progressive medullary thyroid cancer in patients with unresectable locally advanced or metastatic disease: U.S. Food and Drug Administration drug approval summary. *Clin Cancer Res* 2012;18:3722–3730.
114. Wells SA, Jr., Robinson BG, Gagel RF, et al. Vandetanib in patients with locally advanced or metastatic medullary thyroid cancer: a randomized, double-blind phase III trial. *J Clin Oncol* 2012;30:134–141.
115. Leboulleux S, Bastholt L, Krause T, et al. Vandetanib in locally advanced or metastatic differentiated thyroid cancer: a randomised, double-blind, phase 2 trial. *Lancet Oncol* 2012;13:897–905.
116. Gross-Goupil M, Francois L, Quivy A, et al. Axitinib: a review of its safety and efficacy in the treatment of adults with advanced renal cell carcinoma. *Clin Med Insights Oncol* 2013;7:269–277.
117. Rini BI, Escudier B, Tomczak P, et al. Comparative effectiveness of axitinib versus sorafenib in advanced renal cell carcinoma (AXIS): a randomised phase 3 trial. *Lancet* 2011;378:1931–1939.
118. Motzer RJ, Escudier B, Tomczak P, et al. Axitinib versus sorafenib as second-line treatment for advanced renal cell carcinoma: overall survival analysis and updated results from a randomised phase 3 trial. *Lancet Oncol* 2013;14:552–562.
119. Hutson TE, Lesovoy V, Al-Shukri S, et al. Axitinib versus sorafenib as first-line therapy in patients with metastatic renal-cell carcinoma: a randomised open-label phase 3 trial. *Lancet Oncol* 2013;14:1287–1294.
120. Graveel CR, Tolbert D, Vande Woude GF. MET: a critical player in tumorigenesis and therapeutic target. *Cold Spring Harb Perspect Biol* 2013;5.
121. Shojaei F, Lee JH, Simmons BH, et al. HGF/c-Met acts as an alternative angiogenic pathway in sunitinib-resistant tumors. *Cancer Res* 2010;70:10090–10100.
122. Ebos JM, Lee CR, Cruz-Munoz W, et al. Accelerated metastasis after short-term treatment with a potent inhibitor of tumor angiogenesis. *Cancer Cell* 2009;15:232–239.
123. Paez-Ribes M, Allen E, Hudock J, et al. Antiangiogenic therapy elicits malignant progression of tumors to increased local invasion and distant metastasis. *Cancer Cell* 2009;15:220–231.
124. Elisei R, Schlumberger MJ, Muller SP, et al. Cabozantinib in progressive medullary thyroid cancer. *J Clin Oncol* 2013;31:3639–3646.
125. Smith DC, Smith MR, Sweeney C, et al. Cabozantinib in patients with advanced prostate cancer: results of a phase II randomized discontinuation trial. *J Clin Oncol* 2013;31:412–429.
126. Strumberg D, Schultheis B. Regorafenib for cancer. *Expert Opin Investig Drugs* 2012;21:879–889.
127. Grothey A, Van Cutsem E, Sobrero A, et al. Regorafenib monotherapy for previously treated metastatic colorectal cancer (CORRECT): an international, multicentre, randomised, placebo-controlled, phase 3 trial. *Lancet* 2013;381:303–312.
128. Demetri GD, Reichardt P, Kang YK, et al. Efficacy and safety of regorafenib for advanced gastrointestinal stromal tumours after failure of imatinib and sunitinib (GRID): an international, multicentre, randomised, placebo-controlled, phase 3 trial. *Lancet* 2013;381:295–302.
129. Gibbons JJ, Abraham RT, Yu K. Mammalian target of rapamycin: discovery of rapamycin reveals a signaling pathway important for normal and cancer cell growth. *Semin Oncol* 2009;36 Suppl 3:S3–S17.
130. Hudes G, Carducci M, Tomczak P, et al. Temsirolimus, interferon alfa, or both for advanced renal-cell carcinoma. *N Engl J Med* 2007;356:2271–2281.
131. Hutson TE, Escudier B, Esteban E, et al. Randomized phase III trial of temsirolimus versus sorafenib as second-line therapy after sunitinib in patients with metastatic renal cell carcinoma. *J Clin Oncol* 2014;32:760–767.
132. Motzer RJ, Escudier B, Oudard S, et al. Efficacy of everolimus in advanced renal cell carcinoma: a double-blind, randomised, placebo-controlled phase III trial. *Lancet* 2008;372:449–456.
133. Lebwohl D, Anak O, Sahmoud T, et al. Development of everolimus, a novel oral mTOR inhibitor, across a spectrum of diseases. *Ann N Y Acad Sci* 2013;1291:14–32.
134. Fuchs CS, Tomasek J, Yong CJ, et al. Ramucirumab monotherapy for previously treated advanced gastric or gastro-oesophageal junction adenocarcinoma (REGARD): an international, randomised, multicentre, placebo-controlled, phase 3 trial. *Lancet* 2014;383:31–39.
135. Tol J, Koopman M, Cats A, et al. Chemotherapy, bevacizumab, and cetuximab in metastatic colorectal cancer. *N Engl J Med* 2009;360:563–572.
136. Kerbel RS. Antiangiogenic therapy: a universal chemosensitization strategy for cancer? *Science* 2006;312:1171–1175.
137. Jain RK. Normalization of tumor vasculature: an emerging concept in antiangiogenic therapy. *Science* 2005;307:58–62.
138. Browder T, Butterfield CE, Kraling BM, et al. Antiangiogenic scheduling of chemotherapy improves efficacy against experimental drug-resistant cancer. *Cancer Res* 2000;60:1878–1886.
139. Klement G, Baruchel S, Rak J, et al. Continuous low-dose therapy with vinblastine and VEGF receptor-2 antibody induces sustained tumor regression without overt toxicity. *J Clin Invest* 2000;105:R15–R24.
140. Bertolini F, Paul S, Mancuso P, et al. Maximum tolerable dose and low-dose metronomic chemotherapy have opposite effects on the mobilization and viability of circulating endothelial progenitor cells. *Cancer Res* 2003;63:4342–4346.
141. Mancuso P, Colleoni M, Calleri A, et al. Circulating endothelial-cell kinetics and viability predict survival in breast cancer patients receiving metronomic chemotherapy. *Blood* 2006;108:452–459.
142. Kerbel RS, Kamen BA. The anti-angiogenic basis of metronomic chemotherapy. *Nat Rev Cancer* 2004;4:423–436.
143. Hudis CA. Clinical implications of antiangiogenic therapies. *Oncology (Williston Park)* 2005;19:26–31.
144. Zhang D, Hedlund EM, Lim S, et al. Antiangiogenic agents significantly improve survival in tumor-bearing mice by increasing tolerance to chemotherapy-induced toxicity. *Proc Natl Acad Sci U S A* 2011;108:4117–4122.
145. Kerbel RS. Tumor angiogenesis. *N Engl J Med* 2008;358:2039–2049.
146. Mountzios G, Pentheroudakis G, Carmeliet P. Bevacizumab and micrometastases: Revisiting the preclinical and clinical rollercoaster. *Pharmacol Ther* 2014;141:117–124.
147. Ebos JM, Kerbel RS. Antiangiogenic therapy: impact on invasion, disease progression, and metastasis. *Nat Rev Clin Oncol* 2011;8:210–221.
148. Jain RK, Duda DG, Willett CG, et al. Biomarkers of response and resistance to antiangiogenic therapy. *Nat Rev Clin Oncol* 2009;6:327–338.
149. Murukesh N, Dive C, Jayson GC. Biomarkers of angiogenesis and their role in the development of VEGF inhibitors. *Br J Cancer* 2010;102:8–18.
150. Davis DW, McConkey DJ, Abbruzzese JL, et al. Surrogate markers in antiangiogenesis clinical trials. *Br J Cancer* 2003;89:8–14.
151. Wehland M, Bauer J, Magnusson NE, et al. Biomarkers for anti-angiogenic therapy in cancer. *Int J Mol Sci* 2013;14:9338–9364.
152. Lambrechts D, Lenz HJ, de Haas S, et al. Markers of response for the antiangiogenic agent bevacizumab. *J Clin Oncol* 2013;31:1219–1230.
153. Lambrechts D, Claes B, Delmar P, et al. VEGF pathway genetic variants as biomarkers of treatment outcome with bevacizumab: an analysis of data from the AViTA and AVOREN randomised trials. *Lancet Oncol* 2012;13:724–733.
154. Schneider BP, Wang M, Radovich M, et al. Association of vascular endothelial growth factor and vascular endothelial growth factor receptor-2 genetic polymorphisms with outcome in a trial of paclitaxel compared with paclitaxel plus bevacizumab in advanced breast cancer: ECOG 2100. *J Clin Oncol* 2008;26:4672–4678.
155. Hurwitz HI, Douglas PS, Middleton JP, et al. Analysis of early hypertension and clinical outcome with bevacizumab: results from seven phase III studies. *Oncologist* 2013;18:273–280.
156. Levy D, Ehret GB, Rice K, et al. Genome-wide association study of blood pressure and hypertension. *Nat Genet* 2009;41:677–687.

157. Batchelor TT, Sorensen AG, di Tomaso E, et al. AZD2171, a pan-VEGF receptor tyrosine kinase inhibitor, normalizes tumor vasculature and alleviates edema in glioblastoma patients. *Cancer Cell* 2007;11:83–95.
158. Sennino B, McDonald DM. Controlling escape from angiogenesis inhibitors. *Nat Rev Cancer* 2012;12:699–709.
159. Yu JL, Rak JW, Coomber BL, et al. Effect of p53 status on tumor response to antiangiogenic therapy. *Science* 2002;295:1526–1528.
160. Glade Bender J, Cooney EM, Kandel JJ, et al. Vascular remodeling and clinical resistance to antiangiogenic cancer therapy. *Drug Resist Updat* 2004;7:289–300.
161. Bergers G, Hanahan D. Modes of resistance to anti-angiogenic therapy. *Nat Rev Cancer* 2008;8:592–603.
162. Crawford Y, Ferrara N. Tumor and stromal pathways mediating refractoriness/resistance to anti-angiogenic therapies. *Trends Pharmacol Sci* 2009;30:624–630.
163. Ebos JM, Lee CR, Kerbel RS. Tumor and host-mediated pathways of resistance and disease progression in response to antiangiogenic therapy. *Clin Cancer Res* 2009;15:5020–5025.
164. Kerbel RS, Yu J, Tran J, et al. Possible mechanisms of acquired resistance to anti-angiogenic drugs: implications for the use of combination therapy approaches. *Cancer Metastasis Rev* 2001;20:79–86.
165. Shojaei F, Ferrara N. Role of the microenvironment in tumor growth and in refractoriness/resistance to anti-angiogenic therapies. *Drug Resist Updat* 2008;11:219–230.
166. Sweeney CJ, Miller KD, Sledge GW Jr. Resistance in the anti-angiogenic era: nay-saying or a word of caution? *Trends Mol Med* 2003;9:24–29.
167. Hida K, Hida Y, Amin DN, et al. Tumor-associated endothelial cells with cytogenetic abnormalities. *Cancer Res* 2004;64:8249–8255.
168. Streubel B, Chott A, Huber D, et al. Lymphoma-specific genetic aberrations in microvascular endothelial cells in B-cell lymphomas. *N Engl J Med* 2004;351:250–259.
169. Loges S, Mazzone M, Hohensinner P, et al. Silencing or fueling metastasis with VEGF inhibitors: antiangiogenesis revisited. *Cancer Cell* 2009;15:167–170.

29 Monoclonal Antibodies

Hossein Borghaei, Matthew K. Robinson, Gregory P. Adams, and Louis M. Weiner

INTRODUCTION

Antibody-based therapeutics are important components of the cancer therapeutic armamentarium. Early antibody therapy studies attempted to explicitly target cancers based on the structural and biologic properties that distinguish neoplastic cells from their normal counterparts. The immunogenicity and inefficient effector functions of the first-generation murine monoclonal antibodies (MAb) that were evaluated in clinical trials limited their effectiveness.[1–3] Patients developed human antimouse antibody (HAMA) responses against the therapeutic agents that rapidly cleared it from the body and limited the number of times the therapy could be administered. The development of engineered chimeric, humanized, and fully human MAbs has identified a number of important and useful applications for antibody-based cancer therapy. Currently, the U.S. Food and Drug Administration (FDA) has approved 14 MAbs and MAb-conjugates for the treatment of cancer (Table 29.1) and many more are under evaluation in late-stage clinical trials.[4] Antibodies provide an important means by which to exploit the immune system by specifically recognizing and directing antitumor responses.

Antibodies are produced by B cells and arise in response to exposures to a variety of structures, termed antigens, as a result of a series of recombinations of V, D, and J germline genes. Immunoglobulin-G (IgG) molecules are most commonly employed as the working backbones of current therapeutic monoclonal antibodies, although various other isotypes of antibodies have specialized functions (e.g., IgA molecules play important roles in mucosal immunity, IgE molecules are involved in anaphylaxis). The advent of hybridoma technology by Kohler and Milstein[5] made it possible to produce large quantities of antibodies with high purity and monospecificity for a single binding region (epitope) on an antigen.

The mechanisms that antibody based therapeutics employ to elicit antitumor effects include focusing components of the patient's immune system to attack tumor cells[6,7] and methods to alter signal transduction pathways that drive tumor progression.[8,9] Antibody-based conjugates employ the targeting specificity of antibodies to deliver toxic compounds, such as chemotherapeutics, specifically to the tumor sites.

IMMUNOGLOBULIN STRUCTURE

Structural and Functional Domains

An IgG molecule is typically divided into three domains consisting of two identical antigen-binding (Fab) domains connected to an effector or Fc domain by a flexible hinge sequence. Figure 29.1 shows the structure of an IgG molecule. IgG antibodies are comprised of two identical light chains and two identical heavy chains, with the chains joined by disulfide bonds, resulting in a bilaterally symmetrical complex. The Fab domains mediate the binding of IgG molecules to their cognate antigens and are composed of an intact light chain and half of a heavy chain. Each chain in the Fab domain is further divided into variable and constant regions, with the variable region containing hypervariable, or complementarity determining regions (CDR) in which the antigen-contact residues reside. The light and heavy chain variable regions each contain three CDRs (CDR1, CDR2, and CDR3). All six CDRs form the antigen-binding pocket and are collectively defined in immunologic terms as the idiotype of the antibody. In the majority of cases, the variable heavy chain CDR3 plays a dominant role in binding.[10]

The different isotypes of immunoglobulins are defined by the structure and function of their Fc domains. The Fc domain, composed of the CH2 and CH3 regions of the antibody's heavy chains, is the critical determinant of how an antibody mediates effector functions, transports across cellular barriers, and persists in circulation.[7,11]

MODIFIED ANTIBODY-BASED MOLECULES

Advances in antibody engineering and molecular biology have facilitated the development of many novel antibody-based structures with unique physical and pharmacokinetic properties (see Fig. 29.1). These include chimeric human-murine antibodies with human-constant regions and murine-variable regions,[12] humanized antibodies in which murine CDR sequences have been grafted into human IgG molecules, and entirely human antibodies derived from human hybridomas and, more recently, from transgenic mice expressing human immunoglobulin genes.[13] An accepted naming scheme based on "stems" was developed by the World Health Organization's International Nonproprietary Names (INN) for pharmaceuticals and is employed in the United States (Table 29.2). Engineering has also facilitated the development of antibody-based fragments. In addition to the classic, enzymatically derived Fab and $F(ab')_2$ molecules, a plethora of promising IgG-derivatives have been developed that retain antigen-binding properties of intact antibodies (see Fig. 29.1; for review see Robinson et al.[14]). The basic building block for these molecules is the 25 kDa, monovalent single-chain Fv (scFv) that is comprised of the variable domains (V_H and V_L) of an antibody fused together with a short peptide linker. Novel, bispecific antibody-based structures can facilitate binding to two tumor antigens or bridge tumor cells with immune effector cells to focus antibody-dependent cell-mediated cytotoxicity (ADCC) or killing by T cells. An example of the former is MM-111, a bispecific gene-fused molecule composed of an anti-HER2 scFv connected to an anti-HER3 scFv via a modified form of human serum albumin.[15] Examples of the latter mechanism include small scFv-based bispecific T-cell engagers (BiTE) such as the anti-CD3/anti-CD19 molecule blinatumomab[16] and larger MAb-based antibodies such as catumaxomab, a rat/mouse anti-CD3/EpCAM bispecific MAb produced via quadroma technology.[17] Both classes of bispecifics endow selectivity and targeting properties that are not obtainable with natural antibody formats.

TABLE 29.1

FDA Approved Antibodies for the Treatment of Cancer

Generic Name (Trade Name)	Origin	Isotype (Conjugate)	Indication	Target	Initial Approval
Unconjugated MAbs					
Rituximab (Rituxan)	Chimeric	IgG1	NHL	CD20	1997
Trastuzumab (Herceptin)	Humanized	IgG1	BrCa	HER2	1998
Alemtuzumab (Campath-1H)	Humanized	IgG1	CLL	CD52	2001
Cetuximab (Erbitux)	Chimeric	IgG1	CRC, SCCHN	EGFR	2004
Bevacizumab (Avastin)	Humanized	IgG1	CRC, NSCLC, RCC, GBM	VEGF	2004
Panitumumab (Vectibix)	Human (XenoMouse)	IgG2	CRC	EGFR	2006
Ofatumumab (Arzerra)	Human (XenoMouse)	IgG1	CLL	CD20	2009
Denosumab (Prolia/Xgeva)	Human	IgG2	Metastasis-related SREs, ADT/AI-associated osteoporosis, GCT	RANKL	2010
Pertuzumab (Perjeta)	Humanized	IgG1	BrCa	HER2	2012
Immunoconjugates					
Gemtuzumab ozogamicin (Mylotarg)	Humanized	IgG4 (calicheamicin)	AML	CD33	2000[a]
Ibritumomab tiuxetan (Zevalin)	Murine	IgG1 (^{90}Y)	NHL	CD20	2002
Tositumomab (Bexxar)	Murine	IgG2A (^{131}I)	NHL	CD20	2003
Brentuximab vedotin (Adcetris)	Chimeric	IgG1 (MMAE)	HL, sALCL	CD30	2011
Ado-trastuzumab emtansine (Kadcyla)	Humanized	IgG1 (DM1)	BrCa	HER2	2013

[a] Withdrawn from the US market in June 2010.
NHL, non-Hodgkin lymphoma; BrCa, breast cancer; CLL, chronic lymphocytic leukemia; CRC, colorectal cancer; SCCHN, squamous cell carcinoma of head and neck; EGFR, epidermal growth factor receptor; NSCLC, non–small-cell lung cancer; RCC, renal cell carcinoma; GBM, glioblastoma multiforme; VEGF, vascular endothelial growth factor; SREs, skeletal-related events; ADT, androgen deprivation therapy; AI, aromatase inhibitor; GCT, giant cell tumor; RANKL, RANK ligand; AML, acute myelogenous leukemia; ^{90}Y, yttrium-90; ^{131}I, iodine-131; MMAE, Monomethyl auristatin E; HL, Hodgkin lymphoma; sALCL, systemic anaplastic large-cell lymphoma.

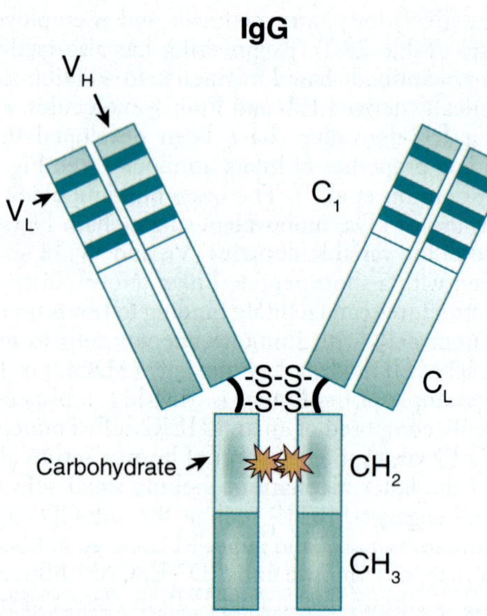

Figure 29.1 Structure of an IgG. C, constant; V, variable; H, heavy chain; L, light chain.

TABLE 29.2

Rules for Naming MAb for the Treatment of Cancer

The International Nonproprietary Names (INN) for monoclonal antibodies (MAbs) are composed of "stems" that indicate their origin, specificity, and modifications. The names include a random prefix to provide distinction from other names, a substem indicating the target specificity *(-t[u]-* for tumor), a substem indicating the species of origin (see the following) and a suffix (*-mab*), which indicates the presence of an immunoglobulin variable domain.

Substem Indication of the Species on Which the Immunoglobulin Sequence Is Based	
-o-	mouse
-xi-	chimeric
-zu-	humanized
-xizu-	chimeric/humanized
-u-	human

FACTORS REGULATING ANTIBODY-BASED TUMOR TARGETING

Antibody Size

Nonuniform distribution of systemically administered antibody is generally observed in biopsied specimens of solid tumors. Heterogeneous tumor blood supply limits uniform antibody delivery to tumors, and elevated interstitial pressures in the center of tumors oppose inward diffusion.[18] This high interstitial pressure slows the diffusion of molecules from their vascular extravasation site in a size-dependent manner.[19,20] The relatively large transport distances in the tumor interstitium also substantially increase the time required for large IgG macromolecules to reach target cells.[21]

Tumor Antigens

Access to the target antigen is undoubtedly a critical determinant of therapeutic effect of antibody-based applications. Such access is regulated by the heterogeneity of antigen expression by tumor cells. Shed antigen in the serum, tumor microenvironment, or both may saturate the antibody's binding sites and prevent binding to the cell surface. Alternatively, a rapid internalization of an antibody/antigen complex, although critical for antibody–drug conjugates (ADC), may deplete the quantity of cell surface MAb capable of initiating ADCC or cytotoxic signal transduction events. Finally, target antigens are normally *tumor associated* rather than *tumor specific*. Tumor-specific antigens are both highly desirable and rare. Typically, such antigens arise as a result of unique tumor-based genetic recombinations, such as clonal immunoglobulin idiotypes expressed on the surface of B-cell lymphomas.[22]

Antibody affinity for its target antigen has complex effects on tumor targeting. The *binding-site barrier* hypothesis postulates that antibodies with extremely high affinity for target antigen would bind irreversibly to the first antigen encountered upon entering the tumor, which would limit the diffusion of the antibody into the tumor and accumulate instead in regions surrounding the tumor vasculature.[23,24] Similarly, in tumor spheroids, the in vitro penetration of engineered antibodies is primarily limited by internalization and degradation.[25] The valence of an antibody molecule can increase the functional affinity of the antibody through an avidity effect.[26–28]

Half-Life/Clearance Rate

The concentration of intact IgG in mammalian serum is maintained at constant levels with half-lives of IgGs measured in days. This homeostasis is regulated in part by the major histocompatibility complex (MHC)-class I–related Fc receptor, FcRn (n = neonatal), a saturable, pH-dependent salvage mechanism that regulates quality and quantity of IgG in serum. This mechanism can be exploited via mutations in the Fc portion of an IgG to modulate IgGs pharmacokinetics.[29,30] Indeed, multiple strategies have been developed to increase the serum persistence of antibody-based fragments and other classes of protein therapeutics.[14,31]

Glycosylation

IgGs undergo N-linked glycosylation at the conserved Asn residue at position 297 within the C_H2 domain of the constant region. Glycosylation status of the residue has long been known to impact the ability of IgGs to bind effector ligands such as FcγR and C1q, which, in turn, affects their ability to participate in Fc-mediated functions such as ADCC and complement-dependent cytotoxicity (CDC).[32–34] The glycosylation of MAbs can be altered to increase ADCC by producing them in a cell line engineered to express β(1,4)-N-acetylglucosaminyltransferase III (GnTIII), the enzyme required to add the bisecting GlcNAc residues.[33] Defucosylation of antibody Fc domains is also associated with enhanced ADCC, and in a recently completed multicenter phase II trial of a defucosylated anti-CC chemokine receptor 4 (CCR4), MAb was associated with meaningful antitumor activity, including complete responses and enhanced progression-free survival (PFS).[35]

UNCONJUGATED ANTIBODIES

The majority of monoclonal antibodies approved for clinical use display intrinsic antitumor effects that are mediated by one or more of the following mechanisms.

Cell-Mediated Cytotoxicity

As components of the immune system, effector cells such as natural killer (NK) cells and monocytes/macrophages represent natural lines of defense against oncologically transformed cells. These effector cells express Fcγ receptors (FcγR) on their cell surfaces, which interact with the Fc domain of IgG molecules. This family is comprised of three classes (type I, II, and III) that are further divided into subclasses (IIa/IIb and IIIa/IIIb).[36] Recognition of transformed cells by immune effector cells leads to cell-mediated killing through processes such as ADCC and phagocytosis, as shown in Figure 29.2, and can be mediated by FcγRI (CD64), a high affinity receptor capable of binding to monomeric IgG, or FcγRII (CD32) and FcγRIII (CD16), which are low affinity receptors that preferentially bind multimeric complexes of IgG. Signaling through type I, IIa, and IIIa receptors results in the activation of effector cells due to associated immunoreceptor tyrosine-based activation motifs (ITAM), whereas the engagement of type IIb receptors inhibits cell activation through associated immunoreceptor tyrosine-based inhibitory motifs (ITIM).[36] Clinical results support the idea that ADCC can play a role in the efficacy of antibody-based therapies. Naturally occurring polymorphisms in FcγRs alter their affinity for human IgG1 and have been linked to clinical response.[37,38] A polymorphism in the FCGR3A gene results in either a valine or phenylalanine at position 158 of FcγRIIIa. Human IgG1 binds more strongly to FcγRIIIa 158V than FcγRIIIa-158F, and likewise to NK cells from individuals that are either homozygous for 158F or heterozygous for this polymorphism.[39] The FcγRIIIa-158v was a predictor of early response and was associated with improved PFS.

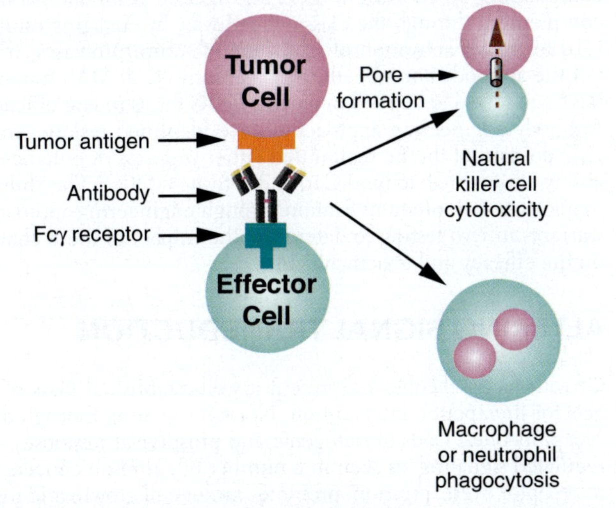

Figure 29.2 Antibody-dependent cellular cytotoxicity. The antibody engages the tumor antigen and the Fc domain binds to cellular Fc receptors to bridge effector and target cells. This bridging induces effector cell activation, resulting in natural killer cell cytotoxicity or phagocytosis by neutrophils, monocytes, or macrophages.

CANCER THERAPEUTICS

A second polymorphism, FcγRIIa-131H/R, did not predict early response but was an independent predictor of time to progression (TTP).[38] Taken together, these data suggest that modulating the affinity of MAbs for FcγRIIIa, FcγRIIa, or both may increase the efficacy of therapeutic MAbs.

Each class of FcγR exhibits a characteristic specificity for IgG subclasses.[40] Many groups have focused on modifying the Fc domain of IgGs to optimize the engagement of subclasses of FcγR and the induction of ADCC, based on the findings of Shields et al.,[29] who performed a series of mutagenesis experiments to map the residues required for IgG1-FcγR interaction. Antibodies such as ocrelizumab, a humanized version of rituximab, have increased binding to low affinity FcγRIIIa variants and are now in clinical trials.

An alternative to modifying the Fc region of MAbs is to create bispecific antibodies (bsAbs) that recognize both a tumor-associated antigen and a *trigger antigen* present on the surface of an immune effector cell.[43] Simultaneous engagement of both antigens can redirect the cytotoxic potential of the effector cell against the tumor.[41–43] Such antibodies are capable of eliciting effector function against tumor cell lines in vitro and in animal models. Two HER-2 directed bispecific antibodies, 2B1 and MDX-H210, have been tested in phase I clinical trials.[44,45]

Bispecific antibodies have a number of distinctive properties, including flexible choices of cytotoxic trigger molecules,[46] recruitment of effector function in the presence of excess IgG,[42] and custom tailoring of the affinity of the bsAb to match effector cell characteristics. These advantages have been facilitated by improved methods of bsAb production.[47] BiTE antibodies represent a novel class of bispecific, single-chain Fv antibodies.[48] Promising results have been seen in early phase clinical trials with at least two BiTE antibodies, one of which, blinatumomab, targets CD19/CD3.[49] Promising phase I results have also been reported in an interim analysis of an anti-EpCAM/anti-CD3 MT110 BiTE in the setting of advanced lung and gastrointestinal tumors.[50]

Complement-Dependent Cytotoxicity

In addition to cell-mediated killing (see previous), MAbs can recruit the complement cascade to kill cells via CDC. Although IgM is the most effective isotype for complement activation, it is not widely used in clinical oncology. Similar to ADCC, the human IgG subclass used to construct a therapeutic MAb dictates its ability to elicit CDC; IgG1 is extremely efficient at fixing complement, in contrast to IgG2 and IgG4.[51] Antibodies activate complement through the classical pathway, by engaging multiple C1q to trigger activation of a cascade of serum proteases, which kill the antibody-bound cells.[52,53] The anti-CD20 MAb rituximab has been found to depend in part on CDC for its *in vivo* efficacy.[54] Antibody engineering approaches have identified residues in the C_H2 domain of the Fc region that either suppress or enhance the ability of rituximab to bind C1q and activate CDC.[55] The ability to manipulate complement fixation through engineering approaches warrants *in vivo* testing to determine the impact of these changes on the efficacy and toxicity of MAbs.

ALTERING SIGNAL TRANSDUCTION

Growth factor receptors represent a well-established class of targets for therapeutic intervention. Normal signaling through these receptors often leads to mitogenic and prosurvival responses. Unregulated signaling, as seen in a number of common cancers due to receptor overexpression, promotes tumor cell growth and insensitivity to chemotherapeutic agents. Clinically relevant MAbs can modulate signaling through their target receptors to normalize cell growth rates and sensitize tumor cells to cytotoxic agents. The binding of cetuximab or panitumumab to the epidermal growth factor receptor (EGFR) physically blocks ligand binding[56] and prevents the receptor from assuming the extended conformation required for dimerization.[57] Pertuzumab binds to the dimerization domain of HER-2, thereby sterically inhibiting subsequent receptor heterodimerization with other ligand-bound family members.[58] Alternatively, signaling through growth factor receptors can be indirectly modified by MAbs that bind to activating ligands, as is seen with the anti–vascular endothelial growth factor (VEGF) MAb, bevacizumab.[59]

IMMUNOCONJUGATES

MAbs that are not capable of directly eliciting antitumor effects, either by altering signal transduction or directing immune system cells, can still be effective against tumors by delivering cytotoxic payloads. MAbs have been employed to deliver a wide variety of agents, including chemotherapy, toxins, radioisotopes, and cytokines (for review see Adams and Weiner[60]). In theory, the appropriate combination of toxic agents and MAbs could lead to a synergistic effect. For example, delivery of a therapeutic radioisotope by a MAb would be significantly enhanced if, by binding to its target antigen, the MAb also activated a signaling event that increased the target cell's sensitivity to ionizing radiation.

Catalytic toxins derived from plants catalytic toxins derived from plants (e.g., ricin) and microorganisms (e.g., Pseudomonas) represent two classes of cytotoxic agent that have been investigated for their utility in immunoconjugate strategies.[61] Although there are promising preclinical studies,[62] few successful clinical trials have been reported using this approach. In a phase I clinical trial in hairy cell leukemia patients who were resistant to cladribine, 11 of 16 patients exhibited complete remissions with minimal side effects with an anti-CD22 immunotoxin with a truncated form of *Pseudomonas exotoxin*.[63] Clinical trials with other immunotoxins have been associated with unacceptable neurotoxicity[64] and life-threatening vascular leak syndrome.[65]

Immunocytokine fusions have also been investigated as an approach to direct the patient's immune response to his or her own tumor.[66] A number of cytokines have been incorporated into antibody-based constructs, including interleukin-2 (IL-2),[67,68] interferon γ (IFN-γ),[69] tumor necrosis factor α (TFN-α),[69] VEGF,[70] and IL-12.[71]

Antibody–Drug Conjugates

The first ADC, gemtuzumab ozogamicin (Mylotarg), was approved by the FDA in 2000 for the treatment of patients with relapsed CD33-positive acute myeloid leukemia, but was voluntarily withdrawn from the US market by its manufacturer in 2010 after a confirmatory phase III trial (SWOG S0106) recommended, based on results of a planned interim analysis, that Mylotarg randomizations be terminated due to a lack of efficacy in the presence of enhanced toxicity.[72] Although two additional randomized trials[73,74] suggested that some patient populations may benefit from Mylotarg therapy, the drug remains off the market in the United States.

The majority of ADCs under development employ potent cytotoxic agents that block the polymerization of tubulin (e.g., auristatins or maytansines) or damage DNA (e.g., calicheamicins or pyrrolobenzodiazepines) by employing a variety of linkers and conjugation strategies.[75]

A variety of ADCs specific for a wide range of oncology targets are currently in clinical evaluation, with the majority of the more advanced agents being tested in the setting of diffuse malignancies.[76] The majority of these employ auristatins or maytansines as their payloads. Early observations suggest that cumulative, dose-related peripheral sensory neuropathy can result when auristatins are conjugated to an antibody via a cleavable linker, and dose-limiting thrombocytopenia can result when auristatins and maytansinoids are conjugated to the antibody via an uncleavable linker.[76,77]

Two ADCs are now approved for use in clinical practice. Ado-trastuzumab emtansine (T-DM1, Kadcyla), an ADC composed of the anti-HER2 MAb trastuzumab linked to DM1,[78] is now approved for the treatment of patients with refractory HER2/neu expressing breast cancers. The other, brentuximab vedotin (SGN-35, Adcetris), is an ADC consisting of the anti-CD30 chimeric MAb cAC10 that is linked to three to five molecules of the microtubule-disrupting agent Monomethyl auristatin E. At this point, this drug is approved for use in patients with recurrent systemic anaplastic large cell lymphoma. The clinical data associated with both of these ADCs will be discussed in subsequent sections of this chapter.

Antibodies also can be used to target liposome-encapsulated drugs[79] and other cytotoxic agents, such as antisense RNA[80] or radionuclides to tumors.

Radioimmunoconjugates

Two anti-CD20 radioimmunoconjugates have been FDA approved for radioimmunotherapy (RIT) of non-Hodgkin lymphoma (NHL). Ibritumomab (Zevalin) and tositumomab (Bexxar) are murine MAbs labeled with yttrium-90 (^{90}Y) and iodine-131 (^{131}I), respectively. Both are associated with impressive clinical efficacy.[81,82] Although these radioimmunoconjugates are effective therapeutics, cumbersome logistics surrounding their administration have significantly limited their use. Despite significant preclinical evidence supporting the use of RIT for solid malignancies, clinical results have not demonstrated consistent antitumor activity.[60]

ANTIBODIES APPROVED FOR USE IN SOLID TUMORS

Trastuzumab

Trastuzumab (Herceptin) is a humanized IgG1[83] that targets domain IV of the HER2/ErbB2 member of the EGFR/ErbB family of receptor tyrosine kinases. Gene amplification as judged by fluorescence in situ hybridization (FISH) with concomitant overexpression of HER2 protein measured by immunohistochemistry (IHC) is seen in approximately 25% of breast cancers.[84,85] HER2 amplification and overexpression is now recognized to also be a critical driver in a subset (7% to 34%) of gastric cancers.[86] Trastuzumab inhibits tumor cell growth by binding to HER2 and blocking the unregulated HER2 signaling that is associated with its high level overexpression.

Trastuzumab became the first FDA-approved monoclonal antibody for the treatment of solid tumors based on a series of studies carried out in the setting of HER2-positive metastatic breast cancer.[87,88] A subsequent phase III trial investigating trastuzumab in combination with cytotoxic chemotherapy demonstrated an improved response rate compared to chemotherapy alone, from 25.0% to 57.3% with a taxane regimen.[89]

Trastuzumab is also approved for use in the adjuvant setting based on an approximately 50% reduction in recurrence after 1 year in multiple phase III trials.[90–92] Myocardial dysfunction, seen with anthracycline therapy, was observed with increased frequency in patients receiving antibody alone[93] or with doxorubicin or epirubicin.

Recognition of HER2 as a driver in a subset of gastric cancers led to an open-label, randomized, phase III trial (ToGA) that investigated the addition of trastuzumab to standard of care chemotherapy[94] and showed increased median overall survival with higher levels of HER2 expression. A study by Gomez-Martin et al.[95] in 99 patients with metastatic gastric cancer being treated with first-line trastuzumab plus chemotherapy identified a mean HER2/CEP17 ratio of 4.7 to be an optimal cut-off to discriminate between trastuzumab-sensitive and refractory patients.

Pertuzumab

Pertuzumab (Perjeta) is a humanized IgG1 MAb that binds to domain II of HER2 and blocks ligand-dependent dimerization of HER2 with other members of the EGFR family.[96] Pertuzumab, in combination with trastuzumab and docetaxel, is approved for use as first-line therapy in HER2-positive metastatic breast cancer patients. Use of the combination is also approved for the treatment of HER2-positive, locally advanced, inflammatory, or high-risk early breast cancer (>2 cm node negative or node positive) in the neoadjuvant setting.

FDA-approval of pertuzumab was based on results of a phase III trial (CLEOPATRA) of 808 patients with locally recurrent, unresectable, or metastatic breast cancer randomized to receive trastuzumab plus docetaxel with or without the addition of pertuzumab. Inclusion of pertuzumab increased the independently assessed PFS by 6.1 months from 12.4 to 18.5 (hazard ratio [HR], 0.62 (95% confidence interval [CI], 0.51, 0.75), $p < 0.0001$], with a trend toward improved overall survival[97] that reached statistical significance ($p = 0.0008$) after an additional year of follow-up.[98] The addition of pertuzumab did increase rates of grade 3 adverse events (AE), but it did not adversely affect cardiac function. Accelerated approval was granted for use of pertuzumab in combination with trastuzumab and docetaxel for the neoadjuvant treatment of high-risk early-stage breast cancer. This approval was based on results from a four-arm, open-label phase II study of 417 patients randomized to receive trastuzumab plus docetaxel, pertuzumab plus docetaxel, pertuzumab plus trastuzumab, or the triple combination. The triple combination improved the pathologic complete response (pCR) rate by 17.8% over the trastuzumab plus docetaxel arm (39.3% versus 21.5%) in the pertuzumab arm.[99] Follow-up studies to confirm a correlation between pCR and long-term clinical benefit are ongoing.

Cetuximab

Cetuximab (Erbitux) targets the EGFR. This chimeric IgG1 binds to domain III of the EGFR, with roughly a tenfold higher affinity than either EGF or transforming growth factor α (TGF-α) ligands and thereby inhibits ligand-induced activation of this tyrosine kinase receptor. Cetuximab may also function to downregulate EGFR-dependent signaling by stimulating EGFR internalization.[100] Cetuximab is approved for the treatment of colorectal cancer (CRC) and, more recently, for the treatment of squamous cell cancer of the head and neck (SCCHN).

The efficacy and safety of cetuximab against CRC was demonstrated alone and in combination with irinotecan in a phase II, multicenter, randomized, and controlled trial of 329 patients.[101] The combination of irinotecan plus cetuximab increased both the overall response and the median duration of response as compared to cetuximab alone. Additionally, patients with irinotecan refractory disease responded to treatment with the combination regimen. Recent studies in patients with colorectal cancers have indicated that patients with KRAS mutations in codon 12 or 13 should not receive anti-EGFR therapy.[101,102]

An international, multicenter, phase III trial comparing definitive radiotherapy to radiotherapy plus cetuximab in SCCHN demonstrated that EGFR blockade with radiotherapy significantly reduced the risk of locoregional failure by 32% and the risk of death by 26%. In advanced stage non–small-cell lung cancer (NSCLC) expressing EGFR, the combination of cetuximab and standard doublet chemotherapy (cisplatin plus vinorelbine) was studied in a prospective randomized phase III trial.[103] The addition of cetuximab was associated with a slight, but statistically significant, benefit in overall survival over chemotherapy alone (median overall survival 10.1 versus 11.3 months). A similar study using the carboplatin plus paclitaxel backbone in combination with cetuximab did not meet its primary endpoint of improved PFS, although cetuximab-treated patients exhibited higher objective response rates.[104] Therefore, the benefit of adding cetuximab to standard chemotherapy for patients with advanced NSCLC is unclear.

Panitumumab

Panitumumab (Vectibix) is a fully human IgG2 monoclonal antibody that binds to EGFR. Similar to cetuximab, panitumumab inhibits EGFR activation by blocking the binding of EGF and TGF-α. However, it does so by binding to EGFR with a higher affinity than cetuximab (5×10^{-11} M versus 1×10^{-10} M). As previously mentioned, the IgG2 class of antibodies does not induce activation of the immune system cell via the Fc-receptor mechanism, so panitumumab's primary action appears to be interference with EGFR–ligand interactions.

A phase III trial of 463 patients with metastatic colorectal cancer compared panitumumab plus best supportive care (BSC) to BSC alone.[105] A partial-response rate of 8% and a stable-disease rate of 28% were reported for the panitumumab arm compared with a 10% stable-disease rate in the best supportive care arm of the study. As with cetuximab, patients with metastatic colorectal cancers who have KRAS mutations in codons 12 or 13 are not routinely offered therapy with panitumumab.[106]

Bevacizumab

Bevacizumab (Avastin or rhuMAb VEGF) is a humanized monoclonal antibody targeting VEGF. VEGF is a critical determinant of tumor angiogenesis, a process that is a necessary component of tumor invasion, growth, and metastasis. VEGF expression by invasive tumors has been shown to correlate with vascularity and cellular proliferation and is prognostic for several human cancers.[107–109] Interestingly, the inhibition of VEGF signaling via bevacizumab treatment may normalize tumor vasculature, promoting a more effective delivery of chemotherapy agents.[110] Bevacizumab is approved for use as a first-line therapy for metastatic colorectal cancer and NSCLC when given in combination with appropriate cytotoxic chemotherapy regimens. Phase III clinical trials leading to the approval of bevacizumab for the treatment of colorectal cancer demonstrated improved response rates from 35% to 45% compared to fluorouracil (5-FU)–based chemotherapy alone. Enhanced response durations and improved patient survival were seen in patients treated with chemotherapy plus bevacizumab as compared to patients receiving chemotherapy alone.[111] A survival benefit was also seen in the setting of NSCLC. A randomized phase III trial (ECOG 4599) of paclitaxel and carboplatin with or without bevacizumab in patients with advanced nonsquamous NSCLC led to a significant improvement in median survival (12.5 months versus 10.2 months; $p = 0.0075$) for patients in the bevacizumab arm,[112] with significantly higher response rates. A higher incidence of bleeding was associated with bevacizumab (4.5% versus 0.7%). Five of 10 treatment-related deaths occurred as a result of hemoptysis, all in the bevacizumab arm.

A phase III trial randomized 722 patients with metastatic breast cancer with no prior chemotherapy for advanced disease to either paclitaxel or paclitaxel and bevacizumab.[113] PFS was significantly better in the paclitaxel plus bevacizumab arm (median, 11.8 versus 5.9 months; HR for progression, 0.60; $p < 0.001$) with an increased response rate (36.9% versus 21.2%, $p < 0.001$). Overall survival, however, was similar.

In contrast,[114] in a randomized phase III trial, capecitabine/bevacizumab increased response rates compared with capecitabine alone in 462 anthracycline and taxane pretreated metastatic breast cancer patients but did not meet its primary endpoint of improved PFS. Overall survival and time to deterioration in quality of life were comparable in both treatment groups.

Bevacizumab has not demonstrated activity in the adjuvant colorectal and breast cancer settings.[115,116] There was no improvement in overall survival between the two groups and the rate of invasive disease-free survival was also not significantly different between the treatment groups.

Bevacizumab is also approved for the management of recurrent glioblastomas based on results of phase II studies.[117]

Ado-Trastuzumab Emtansine

Ado-trastuzumab emtansine (T-DM1, Kadcyla) is an ADC composed of the anti-HER2 MAb trastuzumab linked to DM1, a highly potent derivative of maytansine, through a stable thioether linker.[78]

Based on two single-agent phase II trials of T-DM1[118,119] that demonstrated single-agent activity in the setting of metastatic breast cancer, two separate phase III studies were conducted. The 991 patient EMILIA trial demonstrated that T-DM1 significantly prolongs both PFS and overall survival as compared to a regimen of lapatinib plus capecitabine when used in the setting of metastatic breast cancer that had progressed after treatment with trastuzumab plus a taxane.[120] Grade 3 and worse AEs were lower in the T-DM1 arm (200, 40.8%) as compared to the lapatinib plus capecitabine arm (278, 57%). Results are still awaited from the ongoing MARIANNE trial that is assessing first-line efficacy and safety of T-DM1 alone and T-DM1 plus pertuzumab versus trastuzumab plus taxane (NCT01120184).

Denosumab

Denosumab (Xgeva) is a fully human IgG2 RANK ligand (RANKL) neutralizing antibody. Denosumab is FDA-approved for use in adults and skeletally mature adolescents who have either surgically unsalvageable giant cell tumors of the bone (GCTB) or where resection is anticipated to result in severe morbidity. Approval was based in part on two open-label, phase II trials examining subcutaneous administration of 120 mg q4 week with additional loading doses on days 8 and 15 of the first cycle.[121,122] Serious adverse events were seen in 9% of patients ($n = 25$). Of 187 patients, 47 (25%) exhibited partial objective responses based on modified Response Evaluation Criteria in Solid Tumors (RECIST) criteria.

Denosumab is also approved in for use in two supportive care settings based on three randomized, double-blind, placebo-controlled phase III trials evaluating its efficacy versus zoledronic acid[123–125] to reduce bone metastasis-related skeletal-related events (SRE). Based on data from two phase III trials, a second formulation and dosing schedule of denosumab is approved to increase bone mass in prostate cancer[126] and breast cancer[127] patients at high risk for bone fracture due to hormone-ablation therapies.

ANTIBODIES USED IN HEMATOLOGIC MALIGNANCIES

Rituximab

Rituximab (Rituxan) is a chimeric anti-CD20 monoclonal antibody that was the first MAb to be approved by the FDA for use in human malignancy.[128,129] Studies have shown that multiple doses can be safely administered, and *in vitro* studies have demonstrated multiple mechanisms by which anti-CD20 antibodies can lead to cell death.[130] Efficacy of rituximab monotherapy is well established.[131]

Rituximab has been tested in conjunction with chemotherapy based on supportive preclinical data.[132,133] The combination of rituximab with cyclophosphamide, doxorubicin, vincristine, and prednisolone (CHOP) resulted in a 95% overall response rate (55% complete response, 40% partial response) among 40 patients with low-grade or follicular B-cell non–Hodgkin lymphoma, with molecular complete remissions observed.[134] A long-term study of elderly patients with previously untreated diffuse large-cell lymphoma randomized to either CHOP chemotherapy plus rituximab (R-CHOP) or CHOP alone demonstrated a significant improvement in event-free survival, PFS, disease-free survival, and overall survival for the combination arm.[135] No significant differences in long-term toxicity were noted.

Low-grade B-cell lymphoma patients possessing the 158V/V polymorphism in FcγRIII experience superior response rates and outcomes when treated with rituximab.[37,38] These findings signify that antibody Fc domain::Fc receptor interactions underlie at least some of the clinical benefit of rituximab, and indicate a possible role for ADCC that depends on such interactions.

A combination of active agents (such as lenalidomide and thalidomide) that are also immune modulating may be additive with rituximab,[136] and perhaps synergize by increasing ADCC.[137] Cytokines such as interleukin-2 (IL-2), IL-12, or IL-15 and myeloid growth factors may also enhance therapeutic antibody activity as suggested by preclinical data demonstrating that IL-2 can promote NK cell proliferation and activation and can enhance rituximab activity[138] and clinical efficacy.[139,140] Myeloid growth factors, in combination with rituximab, may also activate ADCC.[141] Alternative approaches to induce effector cell activity by combining Toll-like receptors (TLR) agonists, such as CpG oligonucleotides, have been investigated.[142] Altering the balance of proapoptotic and antiapoptotic signals could generate more rituximab-induced cytotoxicity. BCL-2 downregulation by antisense oligonucleotides was found to enhance rituximab efficacy in preclinical testing.[143,144] However, small molecules that bind to the BH-3 domain common to many members of the BCL-2 family of proteins may be better therapeutic agents.[145–147]

Ofatumumab

The anti-CD20 ofatumumab[148] is a fully human antibody that binds an epitope on CD20 distinct from that bound by rituximab and is engineered for better complement activation, although it induces less ADCC. Ofatumumab has received regulatory approval for the treatment of patients with fludarabine-refractory chronic lymphocytic leukemia (CLL). In a recently reported, planned interim analysis that included 138 CLL patients with treatment-refractory disease or bulky (>5 cm) lymphadenopathy, treatment with ofatumumab led to an overall response rate (primary endpoint) of 47% in patients with bulky disease and 5% in patients refractory to both alemtuzumab and fludarabine.[149]

Additional humanized anti-CD20 antibodies (veltuzumab[150] and ocrelizumab) are under development.

Alemtuzumab

Alemtuzumab (Campath-1H) targets the CD52 glycopeptide, which is highly expressed on T and B lymphocytes. It has been tested as a therapeutic agent for CLL and promyelocytic leukemias, as well as other non–Hodgkin lymphomas.

Brentuximab Vedotin

Brentuximab vedotin (SGN-35, Adcetris) is an ADC consisting of the anti-CD30 chimeric MAb cAC10 that is linked to three to five molecules of the microtubule-disrupting agent Monomethyl auristatin E (MMAE). MMAE is a highly potent derivative of dolastatin. Linkage of MMAE to cAC10 occurs through a protease-cleavable linter.[151] Brentuximab vedotin is approved for treating systemic, chemotherapy-refractory anaplastic large-cell lymphomas (sALCL). It is also approved to treat patients with Hodgkin lymphoma who have progressed after an autologous stem cell transplant (ASCT). Patients ineligible for ASCT must have failed two prior multidrug chemotherapy regimens.

Brentuximab vedotin received accelerated approval in 2011 based in part on the results of two phase II trials. In a multicenter trial conducted by Pro et al.,[152] 58 patients with relapsed or refractory sALCL received brentuximab vedotin (1.8 mg per kilogram per week), and 86% of patients achieved objective response. Complete responses occurred in 57% of patients, with a median duration of 13.2 months. An additional 17 patients (29%) had partial responses. Median overall response was 12.6 months. Most common grade 3 and 4 adverse events (AE) were neutropenia (21%), thrombocytopenia (14%), and peripheral sensory neuropathy (12%). A similar trial, in Hodgkin lymphoma, was reported by Younes et al.[153] Patients (n = 102) that had failed ASCT received brentuximab vedotin on the same schedule as listed previously and were assessed for the objective response rate. In this setting, 75% of patients had objective responses, with 34% being complete remissions. The median duration of complete responses was 20.5 months, and 31 patients were progression free after a median follow-up of 1.5 years. Phase III trials to assess the known risk of neuropathy (AETHERA) and to confirm overall clinical benefit seen in the phase II trials (ECHELON-2, or ClinicalTrials.gov Identifier NCT01712490) are ongoing.

CONCLUSION

In the 35 years since Kohler and Milstein first developed the hybridoma technology that enabled antibody-based therapeutics, the field has made remarkable progress. Numerous antibody-based molecules are currently in clinical trials and many more are in development. Multiple therapeutic antibodies have a proven clinical benefit and have been licensed by the FDA. The thoughtful application of advances in cancer biology and antibody engineering suggest that this progress will continue.

REFERENCES

1. Badger CC, Anasetti C, Davis J, et al. Treatment of malignancy with unmodified antibody. *Pathol Immunopathol Res* 1987;6:419–434.
2. Khazaeli MB, Conry RM, Lobuglio AF. Human immune-response to monoclonal-antibodies. *J Immunother Emphasis Tumor Immunol* 1994;15:42–52.
3. Lee J, Fenton BM, Koch CJ, et al. Interleukin 2 expression by tumor cells alters both the immune response and the tumor microenvironment. *Cancer Res* 1998;58:1478–1485.
4. Reichert JM, Dhimolea E. The future of antibodies as cancer drugs. *Drug Discov Today* 2012;17:954–963.
5. Kohler G, Milstein C. Continuous cultures of fused cells secreting antibody of predefined specificity. *Nature* 1975;256:495–497.
6. Houghton AN, Mintzer D, Cordon-Cardo C, et al. Mouse monoclonal IgG3 antibody detecting GD3 ganglioside: a phase I trial in patients with malignant melanoma. *Proc Natl Acad Sci U S A* 1985;82:1242–1246.
7. Steplewski Z, Lubeck MD, Koprowski H. Human macrophages armed with murine immunoglobulin G2a antibodies to tumors destroy human cancer cells. *Science* 1983;221:865–867.
8. Trauth BC, Klas C, Peters AM, et al. Monoclonal antibody-mediated tumor regression by induction of apoptosis. *Science* 1989;245:301–305.
9. Yang XD, Jia XC, Corvalan JR, et al. Eradication of established tumors by a fully human monoclonal antibody to the epidermal growth factor receptor without concomitant chemotherapy. *Cancer Res* 1999;59:1236–1243.
10. Komissarov AA, Calcutt MJ, Marchbank MT, et al. Equilibrium binding studies of recombinant anti-single-stranded DNA Fab. Role of heavy chain complementarity-determining regions. *J Biol Chem* 1996;271:12241–12246.
11. Ghetie V, Popov S, Borvak J, et al. Increasing the serum persistence of an IgG fragment by random mutagenesis. *Nat Biotechnol* 1997;15:637–640.
12. LoBuglio AF, Wheeler RH, Trang J, et al. Mouse/human chimeric monoclonal antibody in man: kinetics and immune response. *Proc Natl Acad Sci U S A* 1989;86:4220–4224.
13. Kudo T, Saeki H, Tachibana T. A simple and improved method to generate human hybridomas. *J Immunol Methods* 1991;145:119–125.
14. Robinson MK, Weiner LM, Adams GP. Improving monoclonal antibodies for cancer therapy. *Drug Dev Res* 2004;61:172–187.
15. Denlinger CS, Beeram M, Tolcher AW, et al. A phase I/II and pharmacologic study of MM-111 in patients with advanced, refractory HER2-positive (HER2+) cancers. *J Clin Oncol* 2010;28:15s.
16. Nagorsen D, Bargou R, Ruttinger D, et al. Immunotherapy of lymphoma and leukemia with T-cell engaging BiTE antibody blinatumomab. *Leuk Lymphoma* 2009;50:886–891.
17. Goere D, Flament C, Rusakiewicz S, et al. Potent immunomodulatory effects of the trifunctional antibody catumaxomab. *Cancer Res* 2013;73:4663–4673.
18. Jain RK. Transport of molecules in the tumor interstitium: a review. *Cancer Res* 1987;47:3039–3051.

19. Jain RK. Physiological barriers to delivery of monoclonal antibodies and other macromolecules in tumors. *Cancer Res* 1990;50:814s–819s.
20. Jain RK, Baxter LT. Mechanisms of heterogeneous distribution of monoclonal antibodies and other macromolecules in tumors: significance of elevated interstitial pressure. *Cancer Res* 1988;48:7022–7032.
21. Jain RK. Transport of molecules across tumor vasculature. *Cancer Metastasis Rev* 1987;6:559–593.
22. Miller RA, Maloney DG, Warnke R, et al. Treatment of B-cell lymphoma with monoclonal anti-idiotype antibody. *N Engl J Med* 1982;306:517–522.
23. Fujimori K, Covell DG, Fletcher JE, et al. A modeling analysis of monoclonal antibody percolation through tumors: a binding site barrier. *J Nucl Med* 1990;31:1191–1198.
24. Rudnick SI, Lou J, Shaller CC, et al. Influence of affinity and antigen internalization on the uptake and penetration of Anti-HER2 antibodies in solid tumors. *Cancer Res* 2011;71:2250–2259.
25. Thurber GM, Wittrup KD. Quantitative spatiotemporal analysis of antibody fragment diffusion and endocytic consumption in tumor spheroids. *Cancer Res* 2008;68:3334–3341.
26. Adams GP, Tai MS, McCartney JE, et al. Avidity-mediated enhancement of in vivo tumor targeting by single-chain Fv dimers. *Clin Cancer Res* 2006;12:1599–1605.
27. Wolff EA, Schreiber GJ, Cosand WL, et al. Monoclonal antibody homodimers: enhanced antitumor activity in nude mice. *Cancer Res* 1993;53:2560–2565.
28. Werlen RC, Lankinen M, Offord RE, et al. Preparation of a trivalent antigen-binding construct using polyoxime chemistry: improved biodistribution and potential for therapeutic application. *Cancer Res* 1996;56:809–815.
29. Shields RL, Namenuk AK, Hong K, et al. High resolution mapping of the binding site on human IgG1 for Fc gamma RI, Fc gamma RII, Fc gamma RIII, and FcRn and design of IgG1 variants with improved binding to the Fc gamma R. *J Biol Chem* 2001;276:6591–6604.
30. Kenanova V, Olafsen T, Crow DM, et al. Tailoring the pharmacokinetics and positron emission tomography imaging properties of anti-carcinoembryonic antigen single-chain Fv-Fc antibody fragments. *Cancer Res* 2005;65:622–631.
31. McDonagh CF, Huhalov A, Harms BD, et al. Antitumor activity of a novel bispecific antibody that targets the ErbB2/ErbB3 oncogenic unit and inhibits heregulin-induced activation of ErbB3. *Mol Cancer Ther* 2012;11:582–593.
32. Lund J, Takahashi N, Pound JD, et al. Multiple interactions of IgG with its core oligosaccharide can modulate recognition by complement and human Fc gamma receptor I and influence the synthesis of its oligosaccharide chains. *J Immunol* 1996;157:4963–4969.
33. Umana P, Jean-Mairet J, Moudry R, et al. Engineered glycoforms of an antineuroblastoma IgG1 with optimized antibody-dependent cellular cytotoxic activity. *Nat Biotechnol* 1999;17:176–180.
34. Wright A, Morrison SL. Effect of glycosylation on antibody function: implications for genetic engineering. *Trends Biotechnol* 1997;15:26–32.
35. Ishida T, Joh T, Uike N, et al. Defucosylated anti-CCR4 monoclonal antibody (KW-0761) for relapsed adult T-cell leukemia-lymphoma: a multicenter phase II study. *J Clin Oncol* 2012;30:837–842.
36. Raghavan M, Bjorkman PJ. Fc receptors and their interactions with immunoglobulins. *Annu Rev Cell Dev Biol* 1996;12:181–220.
37. Cartron G, Dacheux L, Salles G, et al. Therapeutic activity of humanized anti-CD20 monoclonal antibody and polymorphism in IgG Fc receptor FcgammaRIIIa gene. *Blood* 2002;99:754–758.
38. Weng WK, Levy R. Two immunoglobulin G fragment C receptor polymorphisms independently predict response to rituximab in patients with follicular lymphoma. *J Clin Oncol* 2003;21:3940–3947.
39. Koene HR, Kleijer M, Algra J, et al. Fc gammaRIIIa-158V/F polymorphism influences the binding of IgG by natural killer cell Fc gammaRIIIa, independently of the Fc gammaRIIIa-48L/R/H phenotype. *Blood* 1997;90:1109–1114.
40. Gessner JE, Heiken H, Tamm A, et al. The IgG Fc receptor family. *Ann Hematol* 1998;76:231–248.
41. Keler T, Graziano RF, Mandal A, et al. Bispecific antibody-dependent cellular cytotoxicity of HER2/neu-overexpressing tumor cells by Fcgamma receptor type I-expressing effector cells. *Cancer Res* 1997;57:4008–4014.
42. Weiner LM, Holmes M, Richeson A, et al. Binding and cytotoxicity characteristics of the bispecific murine monoclonal antibody 2B1. *J Immunol* 1993;151:2877–2886.
43. Shalaby MR, Shepard HM, Presta L, et al. Development of humanized bispecific antibodies reactive with cytotoxic lymphocytes and tumor cells overexpressing the HER2 protooncogene. *J Exp Med* 1992;175:217–225.
44. Valone FH, Kaufman PA, Guyre PM, et al. Phase Ia/Ib trial of bispecific antibody MDX-210 in patients with advanced breast or ovarian cancer that overexpresses the proto-oncogene HER-2/neu. *J Clin Oncol* 1995;13:2281–2292.
45. Weiner LM, Clark JI, Davey M, et al. Phase I trial of 2B1, a bispecific monoclonal antibody targeting c-erbB-2 and FcgammaRIII. *Cancer Res* 1995;55:4586–4593.
46. Liu MA, Kranz DM, Kurnick JT, et al. Heteroantibody duplexes target cells for lysis by cytotoxic T lymphocytes. *Proc Natl Acad Sci U S A* 1985;82:8648–8652.
47. Carter P. Bispecific human IgG by design. *J Immunol Methods* 2001;248:7–15.
48. Mack M, Riethmuller G, Kufer P. A small bispecific antibody construct expressed as a functional single-chain molecule with high tumor cell cytotoxicity. *Proc Natl Acad Sci U S A* 1995;92:7021–7025.
49. Bargou R, Leo E, Zugmaier G, et al. Tumor regression in cancer patients by very low doses of a T cell-engaging antibody. *Science* 2008;321:974–977.
50. Fiedler W, Hönemann D, Ritter B, et al. Safety and pharmacology of the EpCAM/CD3-bispecific BiTE antibody MT110 in patients with metastatic colorectal, gastric, and lung cancer. *Eur J Cancer* 2009;7:136–137.
51. Presta LG. Engineering antibodies for therapy. *Curr Pharm Biotechnol* 2002;3:237–256.
52. Makrides SC. Therapeutic inhibition of the complement system. *Pharmacol Rev* 1998;50:59–87.
53. Walport MJ. Complement, First of two parts. *N Engl J Med* 2001;344:1058–1066.
54. Di Gaetano N, Cittera E, Nota R, et al. Complement activation determines the therapeutic activity of rituximab in vivo. *J Immunol* 2003;171:1581–1587.
55. Idusogie EE, Presta LG, Gazzano-Santoro H, et al. Mapping of the C1q binding site on Rituxan, a chimeric antibody with a human IgG1 Fc. *J Immunol* 2000;164:4178–4184.
56. Sunada H, Magun BE, Mendelsohn J, et al. Monoclonal antibody against epidermal growth factor receptor is internalized without stimulating receptor phosphorylation. *Proc Natl Acad Sci U S A* 1986;83:3825–3829.
57. Li S, Schmitz KR, Jeffrey PD, et al. Structural basis for inhibition of the epidermal growth factor receptor by cetuximab. *Cancer Cell* 2005;7:301–311.
58. Franklin MC, Carey KD, Vajdos FF, et al. Insights into ErbB signaling from the structure of the ErbB2-pertuzumab complex. *Cancer Cell* 2004;5:317–328.
59. Presta LG, Chen H, O'Connor SJ, et al. Humanization of an anti-vascular endothelial growth factor monoclonal antibody for the therapy of solid tumors and other disorders. *Cancer Res* 1997;57:4593–4599.
60. Adams GP, Weiner LM. Monoclonal antibody therapy of cancer. *Nat Biotechnol* 2005;23:1147–1157.
61. Reiter Y, Pastan I. Recombinant Fv immunotoxins and Fv fragments as novel agents for cancer therapy and diagnosis. *Trends Biotechnol* 1998;16:513–520.
62. Kreitman RJ, Wang QC, FitzGerald DJ, et al. Complete regression of human B-cell lymphoma xenografts in mice treated with recombinant anti-CD22 immunotoxin RFB4(dsFv)-PE38 at doses tolerated by cynomolgus monkeys. *Int J Cancer* 1999;81:148–155.
63. Kreitman RJ, Wilson WH, Bergeron K, et al. Efficacy of the anti-CD22 recombinant immunotoxin BL22 in chemotherapy-resistant hairy-cell leukemia. *N Engl J Med* 2001;345:241–247.
64. Pai LH, Bookman MA, Ozols RF, et al. Clinical evaluation of intraperitoneal Pseudomonas exotoxin immunoconjugate OVB3-PE in patients with ovarian cancer. *J Clin Oncol* 1991;9:2095–2103.
65. Baluna R, Vitetta ES. Vascular leak syndrome: a side effect of immunotherapy. *Immunopharmacology* 1997;37:117–132.
66. Lode HN, Xiang R, Becker JC, et al. Immunocytokines: a promising approach to cancer immunotherapy. *Pharmacol Ther* 1998;80:277–292.
67. Hornick JL, Khawli LA, Hu P, et al. Pretreatment with a monoclonal antibody/interleukin-2 fusion protein directed against DNA enhances the delivery of therapeutic molecules to solid tumors. *Clin Cancer Res* 1999;5:51–60.
68. Lode HN, Xiang R, Duncan SR, et al. Tumor-targeted IL-2 amplifies T cell-mediated immune response induced by gene therapy with single-chain IL-12. *Proc Natl Acad Sci U S A* 1999;96:8591–8596.
69. Sharifi J, Khawli LA, Hu P, et al. Generation of human interferon gamma and tumor necrosis factor alpha chimeric TNT-3 fusion proteins. *Hybrid Hybridomics* 2002;21:421–432.
70. Halin C, Niesner U, Villani ME, et al. Tumor-targeting properties of antibody-vascular endothelial growth factor fusion proteins. *Int J Cancer* 2002;102:109–116.
71. Halin C, Rondini S, Nilsson F, et al. Enhancement of the antitumor activity of interleukin-12 by targeted delivery to neovasculature. *Nature Biotechnol* 2002;20:264–269.
72. Petersdorf SH, Kopecky KJ, Slovak M, et al. A phase 3 study of gemtuzumab ozogamicin during induction and postconsolidation therapy in younger patients with acute myeloid leukemia. *Blood* 2013;121:4854–4860.
73. Burnett AK, Hills RK, Milligan D, et al. Identification of patients with acute myeloblastic leukemia who benefit from the addition of gemtuzumab ozogamicin: results of the MRC AML15 trial. *J Clin Oncol* 2011;29:369–377.
74. Castaigne S, Pautas C, Terre C, et al. Effect of gemtuzumab ozogamicin on survival of adult patients with de-novo acute myeloid leukaemia (ALFA-0701): a randomised, open-label, phase 3 study. *Lancet* 2012;379:1508–1516.
75. Ducry L, Stump B. Antibody-drug conjugates: linking cytotoxic payloads to monoclonal antibodies. *Bioconjug Chem* 2010;21:5–13.
76. Lambert JM. Drug-conjugated antibodies for the treatment of cancer. *Br J Clin Pharmacol* 2013;76:248–262.
77. van de Donk NW, Dhimolea E. Brentuximab vedotin. *MAbs* 2012;4:458–465.
78. LoRusso PM, Weiss D, Guardino E, et al. Trastuzumab emtansine: a unique antibody-drug conjugate in development for human epidermal growth factor receptor 2-positive cancer. *Clin Cancer Res* 2011;17:6437–6447.
79. Park JW, Hong K, Kirpotin DB, et al. Anti-HER2 immunoliposomes: enhanced efficacy attributable to targeted delivery. *Clin Cancer Res* 2002;8:1172–1181.
80. Rodriguez M, Coma S, Noe V, et al. Development and effects of immunoliposomes carrying an antisense oligonucleotide against DHFR RNA and directed toward human breast cancer cells overexpressing HER2. *Antisense Nucleic Acid Drug Dev* 2002;12:311–325.
81. Juweid ME. Radioimmunotherapy of B-cell non-Hodgkin's lymphoma: from clinical trials to clinical practice. *J Nucl Med* 2002;43:1507–1529.
82. Witzig TE, White CA, Wiseman GA, et al. Phase I/II trial of IDEC-Y2B8 radioimmunotherapy for treatment of relapsed or refractory CD20(+) B-cell non-Hodgkin's lymphoma. *J Clin Oncol* 1999;17:3793–3803.

83. Carter P, Presta L, Gorman CM, et al. Humanization of an anti-p185HER2 antibody for human cancer therapy. *Proc Natl Acad Sci U S A* 1992;89: 4285–4289.
84. Slamon DJ, Clark GM, Wong SG, et al. Human breast cancer: correlation of relapse and survival with amplification of the HER-2/neu oncogene. *Science* 1987;235:177–182.
85. Dawood S, Broglio K, Buzdar AU, et al. Prognosis of women with metastatic breast cancer by HER2 status and trastuzumab treatment: an institutional-based review. *J Clin Oncol* 2010;28:92–98.
86. Tanner M, Hollmen M, Junttila TT, et al. Amplification of HER-2 in gastric carcinoma: association with Topoisomerase IIalpha gene amplification, intestinal type, poor prognosis and sensitivity to trastuzumab. *Ann Oncol* 2005;16:273–278.
87. Baselga J, Tripathy D, Mendelsohn J, et al. Phase II study of weekly intravenous recombinant humanized anti-p185HER2 monoclonal antibody in patients with HER2/neu-overexpressing metastatic breast cancer. *J Clin Oncol* 1996;14:737–744.
88. Cobleigh MA, Vogel CL, Tripathy D, et al. Multinational study of the efficacy and safety of humanized anti-HER2 monoclonal antibody in women who have HER2-overexpressing metastatic breast cancer that has progressed after chemotherapy for metastatic disease. *J Clin Oncol* 1999;17:2639–2648.
89. Slamon D, Leyland-Jones B, Shak S, et al. Addition of Herceptin™ (humanized anti-HER2 antibody) to first line chemotherapy for HER2 overexpressing metastatic breast cancer (HER21/MBC) markedly increases anticancer activity: a randomized multinational controlled phase III trial. *Proc Am Soc Clin Oncol* 1998;17:A377.
90. Piccart-Gebhart MJ, Procter M, Leyland-Jones B, et al. Trastuzumab after adjuvant chemotherapy in HER2-positive breast cancer. *N Engl J Med* 2005;353:1659–1672.
91. Romond EH, Perez EA, Bryant J, et al. Trastuzumab plus adjuvant chemotherapy for operable HER2-positive breast cancer. *N Engl J Med* 2005;353:1673–1684.
92. Smith I, Procter M, Gelber RD, et al. 2-year follow-up of trastuzumab after adjuvant chemotherapy in HER2-positive breast cancer: a randomised controlled trial. *Lancet* 2007;369:29–36.
93. Ewer MS, Gibbs HR, Swafford J, et al. Cardiotoxicity in patients receiving transtuzumab (Herceptin): primary toxicity, synergistic or sequential stress, or surveillance artifact? *Semin Oncol* 1999;26:96–101.
94. Bang YJ, Van Cutsem E, Feyereislova A, et al. Trastuzumab in combination with chemotherapy versus chemotherapy alone for treatment of HER2-positive advanced gastric or gastro-oesophageal junction cancer (ToGA): a phase 3, open-label, randomised controlled trial. *Lancet* 2010;376:687–697.
95. Gomez-Martin C, Plaza JC, Pazo-Cid R, et al. Level of HER2 gene amplification predicts response and overall survival in HER2-positive advanced gastric cancer treated with trastuzumab. *J Clin Oncol* 2013;10:4445–4452.
96. Agus DB, Akita RW, Fox WD, et al. Targeting ligand-activated ErbB2 signaling inhibits breast and prostate tumor growth. *Cancer Cell* 2002;2:127–137.
97. Baselga J, Cortes J, Kim SB, et al. Pertuzumab plus trastuzumab plus docetaxel for metastatic breast cancer. *N Engl J Med* 2012;366:109–119.
98. Swain SM, Kim SB, Cortes J, et al. Pertuzumab, trastuzumab, and docetaxel for HER2-positive metastatic breast cancer (CLEOPATRA study): overall survival results from a randomised, double-blind, placebo controlled, phase 3 study. *Lancet Oncol* 2013;14:461–471.
99. Gianni L, Pienkowski T, Im YH, et al. Efficacy and safety of neoadjuvant pertuzumab and trastuzumab in women with locally advanced, inflammatory, or early HER2-positive breast cancer (NeoSphere): a randomised multicentre, open-label, phase 2 trial. *Lancet Oncol* 2012;13:25–32.
100. Waksal HW. Role of an anti-epidermal growth factor receptor in treating cancer. *Cancer Metastasis Rev* 1999;18:427–436.
101. Van Cutsem ELI, D'haens G. KRAS status and efficacy in the first line treatment of patients with metastatic colorectal cancer (metastatic CRC) treated with FOLFIRI with or without cetuximab: The CRYSTAL experience. Abstract 2. *J Clin Oncol* 2008;26:5s.
102. Bokemeyer CBI, Hartmann JT. KRAS status and efficacy of first-line treatment of patients with metastatic colorectal cancer (metastatic CRC) with FOLFOX with or without cetuximab: The OPUS experience. Abstract 4000. *J Clin Oncol* 2008;26:178s.
103. Pirker R, Pereira JR, Szczesna A, et al. Cetuximab plus chemotherapy in patients with advanced non-small-cell lung cancer (FLEX): an open-label randomised phase III trial. *Lancet* 2009;373:1525–1531.
104. Lynch TJ, Patel T, Dreisbach L, et al. Cetuximab and first-line taxane/carboplatin chemotherapy in advanced non-small-cell lung cancer: results of the randomized multicenter phase III trial BMS099. *J Clin Oncol* 2010;28: 911–917.
105. Gibson TB, Ranganathan A, Grothey A. Randomized phase III trial of panitumumab, a fully human anti-epidermal growth factor receptor monoclonal antibody, in metastatic colorectal cancer. *Clin Colorectal Cancer* 2006;6: 29–31.
106. Amado RG, Wolf M, Peeters M, et al. Wild-type KRAS is required for panitumumab efficacy in patients with metastatic colorectal cancer. *J Clin Oncol* 2008;26:1626–1634.
107. Brown LF, Berse B, Jackman RW, et al. Expression of vascular permeability factor (vascular endothelial growth factor) and its receptors in breast cancer. *Hum Pathol* 1995;26:86–91.
108. Obermair A, Kohlberger P, Bancher-Todesca D, et al. Influence of microvessel density and vascular permeability factor/vascular endothelial growth factor expression on prognosis in vulvar cancer. *Gynecol Oncol* 1996;63:204–209.
109. Takahashi Y, Tucker SL, Kitadai Y, et al. Vessel counts and expression of vascular endothelial growth factor as prognostic factors in node-negative colon cancer. *Arch Surg* 1997;132:541–546.
110. Jain RK. Normalization of tumor vasculature: an emerging concept in antiangiogenic therapy. *Science* 2005;307:58–62.
111. Hurwitz H, Fehrenbacher L, Novotny W, et al. Bevacizumab plus irinotecan, fluorouracil, and leucovorin for metastatic colorectal cancer. *N Engl J Med* 2004;350:2335–2342.
112. Sandler A, Gray R, Perry MC, et al. Paclitaxel-carboplatin alone or with bevacizumab for non-small-cell lung cancer. *N Engl J Med* 2006;355:2542–2550.
113. Miller K, Wang M, Gralow J, et al. Paclitaxel plus bevacizumab versus paclitaxel alone for metastatic breast cancer. *N Engl J Med* 2007;357:2666.
114. Miller KD, Chap LI, Holmes FA, et al. Randomized phase III trial of capecitabine compared with bevacizumab plus capecitabine in patients with previously treated metastatic breast cancer. *J Clin Oncol* 2005;23: 792–799.
115. Allegra CJ, Yothers G, O'Connell MJ, et al. Initial safety report of NSABP C-08: A randomized phase III study of modified FOLFOX6 with or without bevacizumab for the adjuvant treatment of patients with stage II or III colon cancer. *J Clin Oncol* 2009;27:3385–3390.
116. Cameron D, Brown J, Dent R, et al. Adjuvant bevacizumab-containing therapy in triple-negative breast cancer (BEATRICE): primary results of a randomised, phase 3 trial. *Lancet Oncol* 2013;14:933–942.
117. Kreisl TN, Kim L, Moore K, et al. Phase II trial of single-agent bevacizumab followed by bevacizumab plus irinotecan at tumor progression in recurrent glioblastoma. *J Clin Oncol* 2009;27:740–745.
118. Burris HA 3rd, Rugo HS, Vukelja SJ, et al. Phase II study of the antibody drug conjugate trastuzumab-DM1 for the treatment of human epidermal growth factor receptor 2 (HER2)-positive breast cancer after prior HER2-directed therapy. *J Clin Oncol* 2011;29:398–405.
119. Krop IE, LoRusso P, Miller KD, et al. A phase II study of trastuzumab emtansine in patients with human epidermal growth factor receptor 2-positive metastatic breast cancer who were previously treated with trastuzumab, lapatinib, an anthracycline, a taxane, and capecitabine. *J Clin Oncol* 2012;30: 3234–3241.
120. Verma S, Miles D, Gianni L, et al. Trastuzumab emtansine for HER2-positive advanced breast cancer. *N Engl J Med* 2012;367:1783–1791.
121. Thomas D, Carriere P, Jacobs I. Safety of denosumab in giant-cell tumour of bone. *Lancet Oncol* 2012;11:815.
122. Chawla S, Henshaw R, Seeger L, et al. Safety and efficacy of denosumab for adults and skeletally mature adolescents with giant cell tumour of bone: interim analysis of an open-label, parallel-group, phase 2 study. *Lancet Oncol* 2013;14:901–908.
123. Fizazi K, Carducci M, Smith M, et al. Denosumab versus zoledronic acid for treatment of bone metastases in men with castration-resistant prostate cancer: a randomised, double-blind study. *Lancet* 2011;377:813–822.
124. Henry DH, Costa L, Goldwasser F, et al. Randomized, double-blind study of denosumab versus zoledronic acid in the treatment of bone metastases in patients with advanced cancer (excluding breast and prostate cancer) or multiple myeloma. *J Clin Oncol* 2011;29:1125–1132.
125. Stopeck AT, Lipton A, Body JJ, et al. Denosumab compared with zoledronic acid for the treatment of bone metastases in patients with advanced breast cancer: a randomized, double-blind study. *J Clin Oncol* 2010;28:5132–5139.
126. Smith MR, Egerdie B, Hernandez Toriz N, et al. Denosumab in men receiving androgen-deprivation therapy for prostate cancer. *N Engl J Med* 2009;361: 745–755.
127. Ellis GK, Bone HG, Chlebowski R, et al. Randomized trial of denosumab in patients receiving adjuvant aromatase inhibitors for nonmetastatic breast cancer. *J Clin Oncol* 2008;26:4875–4882.
128. Maloney D, Grillo-López A, Bodkin D, et al. IDEC-C2B8: results of a phase I multiple-dose trial in patients with relapsed non-Hodgkin's lymphoma. *J Clin Oncol* 1997;15:3266–3274.
129. Maloney D, Grillo-López A, White C, et al. IDEC-C2B8 (Rituximab) anti-CD20 monoclonal antibody therapy in patients with relapsed low-grade non-Hodgkin's lymphoma. *Blood* 1997;90:2188–2195.
130. Shan D, Ledbetter J, Press O. Signaling events involved in anti-CD20-induced apoptosis of malignant human B cells. *Cancer Immunol Immunother* 2000;48:673–683.
131. Coiffier B, Haioun C, Ketterer N, et al. Rituximab (anti-CD20 monoclonal antibody) for the treatment of patients with relapsing or refractory aggressive lymphoma: a multicenter phase II study. *Blood* 1998;92:1927–1932.
132. Czuczman MS, Grillo-López AJ, White CA, et al. Treatment of patients with low-grade B-cell lymphoma with the combination of chimeric anti-CD20 monoclonal antibody and CHOP chemotherapy. *J Clin Oncol* 1999;17: 268–276.
133. Demidem A, Lam T, Alas S, et al. Chimeric anti-CD20 (IDEC-C2B8) monoclonal antibody sensitizes a B cell lymphoma cell line to cell killing by cytotoxic drugs. *Cancer Biother Radiopharm* 1997;12:177–186.
134. Gribben JG, Freedman A, Woo SD, et al. All advanced stage non-Hodgkin's lymphomas with a polymerase chain reaction amplifiable breakpoint of bcl-2 have residual cells containing the rearrangement at evaluation and after treatment. *Blood* 1991;78:3275–3280.
135. Feugier P, Van Hoof A, Sebban C, et al. Long-term results of the R-CHOP study in the treatment of elderly patients with diffuse large B-cell lymphoma: a study by the Groupe d'Etude des Lymphomes de l'Adulte. *J Clin Oncol* 2005;23:4117–4126.

136. Kaufmann H, Raderer M, Wohrer S, et al. Antitumor activity of rituximab plus thalidomide in patients with relapsed/refractory mantle cell lymphoma. *Blood* 2004;104:2269–2271.
137. Reddy N, Hernandez-Ilizaliturri FJ, Deeb G, et al. Immunomodulatory drugs stimulate natural killer-cell function, alter cytokine production by dendritic cells, and inhibit angiogenesis enhancing the anti-tumour activity of rituximab in vivo. *Br J Haematol* 2008;140:36–45.
138. Hooijberg E, Sein JJ, van den Berk PC, et al. Eradication of large human B cell tumors in nude mice with unconjugated CD20 monoclonal antibodies and interleukin 2. *Cancer Res* 1995;55:2627–2634.
139. Friedberg JW, Neuberg D, Gribben JG, et al. Combination immunotherapy with rituximab and interleukin 2 in patients with relapsed or refractory follicular non-Hodgkin's lymphoma. *Br J Haematol* 2002;117:828–834.
140. Khan KD, Emmanouilides C, Benson DM Jr., et al. A phase 2 study of rituximab in combination with recombinant interleukin-2 for rituximab-refractory indolent non-Hodgkin's lymphoma. *Clin Cancer Res* 2006;12:7046–7053.
141. van der Kolk LE, Grillo-López AJ, Baars JW, et al. Treatment of relapsed B-cell non-Hodgkin's lymphoma with a combination of chimeric anti-CD20 monoclonal antibodies (rituximab) and G-CSF: final report on safety and efficacy. *Leukemia* 2003;17:1658–1664.
142. Warren TL, Dahle CE, Weiner GJ. CpG oligodeoxynucleotides enhance monoclonal antibody therapy of a murine lymphoma. *Clin Lymphoma* 2000;1:57–61.
143. Smith MR, Jin F, Joshi I. Enhanced efficacy of therapy with antisense BCL-2 oligonucleotides plus anti-CD20 monoclonal antibody in scid mouse/human lymphoma xenografts. *Mol Cancer Ther* 2004;3:1693–1699.
144. Ramanarayanan J, Hernandez-Ilizaliturri FJ, Chanan-Khan A, et al. Pro-apoptotic therapy with the oligonucleotide Genasense (oblimersen sodium) targeting Bcl-2 protein expression enhances the biological anti-tumour activity of rituximab. *Br J Haematol* 2004;127:519–530.
145. van Delft MF, Wei AH, Mason KD, et al. The BH3 mimetic ABT-737 targets selective Bcl-2 proteins and efficiently induces apoptosis via Bak/Bax if Mcl-1 is neutralized. *Cancer Cell* 2006;10:389–399.
146. Paoluzzi L, Gonen M, Gardner JR, et al. Targeting Bcl-2 family members with the BH3 mimetic AT-101 markedly enhances the therapeutic effects of chemotherapeutic agents in in vitro and in vivo models of B-cell lymphoma. *Blood* 2008;111:5350–5358.
147. Nguyen M, Marcellus RC, Roulston A, et al. Small molecule obatoclax (GX15-070) antagonizes MCL-1 and overcomes MCL-1-mediated resistance to apoptosis. *Proc Natl Acad Sci U S A* 2007;104:19512–19517.
148. Coiffier B, Lepretre S, Pedersen LM, et al. Safety and efficacy of ofatumumab, a fully human monoclonal anti-CD20 antibody, in patients with relapsed or refractory B-cell chronic lymphocytic leukemia: a phase 1-2 study. *Blood* 2008;111:1094–1100.
149. Wierda WG, Kipps TJ, Mayer J, et al. Ofatumumab as single-agent CD20 immunotherapy in fludarabine-refractory chronic lymphocytic leukemia. *J Clin Oncol* 2010;28:1749–1755.
150. Stein R, Qu Z, Chen S, et al. Characterization of a new humanized anti-CD20 monoclonal antibody, IMMU-106, and its use in combination with the humanized anti-CD22 antibody, epratuzumab, for the therapy of non-Hodgkin's lymphoma. *Clin Cancer Res* 2004;10:2868–2878.
151. Senter PD, Sievers EL. The discovery and development of brentuximab vedotin for use in relapsed Hodgkin lymphoma and systemic anaplastic large cell lymphoma. *Nat Biotechnol* 2012;30:631–637.
152. Pro B, Advani R, Brice P, et al. Brentuximab vedotin (SGN-35) in patients with relapsed or refractory systemic anaplastic large-cell lymphoma: results of a phase II study. *J Clin Oncol* 2012;30:2190–2196.
153. Younes A, Gopal AK, Smith SE, et al. Results of a pivotal phase II study of brentuximab vedotin for patients with relapsed or refractory Hodgkin's lymphoma. *J Clin Oncol* 2012;30:2183–2189.

30 Assessment of Clinical Response

Antonio Tito Fojo and Susan E. Bates

INTRODUCTION

Approaches to response assessments have become increasingly important over the past decade as the drug development pipeline has steadily increased in volume. In 2012, an estimated 981 medicines were in development for cancer, and the number is certainly higher today.[1] The challenge is, first, how to measure the activity of an agent in the research setting, and, second, how to measure activity in the standard of care setting.

The "modern era" of drug development began in 1976 when 16 experienced oncologists treating lymphoma gathered to decide what would be considered a reliable measure of response to a therapy.[2] Each oncologist measured 12 *simulated tumor masses* employing *usual clinical methods* (i.e., calipers or rulers). A principal goal was to identify the amount of shrinkage that *could not* be ascribed to operator error and that *would not* be found if a *placebo* was administered. Moertel and Hanley recommended that *to avoid error, a 50% reduction in the product of perpendicular diameters be employed as the criterion for efficacy*.[2] It was from this beginning that our current methodologies of response assessment evolved. The important point to note is that the decision to use a 50% reduction in the product of perpendicular diameters as a measure of efficacy was made so as to reduce error and *not because it represented a value that conferred clinical benefit.*

From Calipers and Rulers in Lymphoma to the Bidimensional World Health Organization Criteria

In 1981, five years after the Moertel and Hanley report,[2] a World Health Organization (WHO) initiative developed standardized approaches for the "reporting of response, recurrence and disease-free interval."[3] The WHO criteria, like Moertel and Hanley, recommended that malignant disease be measured in two dimensions. Complete response (CR) was defined as the disappearance of all known disease, and a partial response (PR) was scored if there occurred a *"50% decrease in the sum of the products of the perpendicular diameters of the multiple lesions."* Thus, the 50% reduction initially chosen as an operationally optimal value became institutionalized as the threshold for declaring efficacy in the majority of cancers. This measure of efficacy was perpetuated in 2000 with the now widely used Response Evaluation Criteria in Solid Tumors (RECIST), but shifting to one dimension.[4] The authors noted "the definition of a partial response, in particular, is an arbitrary convention—there is no inherent meaning for an individual patient of a 50% decrease in overall tumor load." Nevertheless, the threshold chosen—a 30% reduction in one dimension—was comparable in volume to the 50% decrease in the sum of the products of the perpendicular diameters and thus perpetuated the 1976 standard. In spite of its arbitrary origins, the 50% reduction has held up over time. But the major impact of the WHO criteria was that it marked the beginning of a common language of response. These criteria have been revisited and refined over time, as technology and medicine advanced. Table 30.1 compares the WHO criteria with those of RECIST 1.0 and RECIST 1.1 and three modifications of RECIST, whereas Figure 30.1 provides a visual presentation of the RECIST threshold required to qualify as response or progression.[3–9]

ASSESSING RESPONSE

RECIST 1.1

The RECIST 1.0 guidelines were updated as RECIST 1.1 in 2009, with a number of differences between the two response criteria highlighted. RECIST 1.1 preserves the same categories of response found in RECIST 1.0:

- Complete response: Complete disappearance of all disease
- Partial response: ≥30% reduction in the sum of the longest diameter of target lesions
- Stable disease: Change not meeting criteria for response or progression
- Progression: ≥20% increase in the sum of the longest diameter of target lesions

However, a decade of experience with RECIST identified several problems with the criteria, some of which could be corrected. In RECIST 1.0, minimum size varied between 1 and 2 cm depending on technique; in RECIST 1.1, a 1-cm lesion is the minimum measurable. In RECIST 1.0, 10 lesions were to be measured, 5 per organ; RECIST 1.1 reduced that to 5 lesions, 2 per organ. Response criteria in RECIST 1.0 did not address lymph nodes; in RECIST 1.1, lymph nodes decreasing to <1 cm in their short axis could constitute a complete response. Disease progression in nontarget disease was further defined to indicate that in addition to a 20% increase in target lesions over the smallest sum on study, there must be an absolute increase of 5 mm, and that an increase of a single nontarget lesion should not trump an overall disease status assessment based on target lesions.

Variations of the RECIST Criteria

The RECIST criteria have been widely used for standardizing the reporting of clinical trial results and have improved reproducibility. However, the increasing precision and codification of RECIST has led to recognition of its limitations. For example, there are unique challenges in central nervous system (CNS) disease, relating response to tumor size measurements based on contrast enhancement. Pseudoprogression refers to an increase in contrast enhancement due to a transient increase in vascular permeability after irradiation, whereas pseudoresponse is a decrease in contrast enhancement that may occur due to a reduction in vascular permeability following corticosteroids or an antiangiogenic agent such as bevacizumab.[10–12] The McDonald criteria, traditionally used in determining glioma response based

TABLE 30.1

Key Features of Response Criteria

	WHO[3]	RECIST 1.0[4]	RECIST 1.1[5]	CNS RANO Criteria[7]	RECIST Mesothelioma[8]	RECIST Immunotherapy[9]
Dimension	Uni- and bidimensional	Unidimensional	Unidimensional	Bidimensional	Unidimensional	Bidimensional
Measurable Lesion	Not defined	Longest diameter, ≥20 mm with most modalities; ≥10 mm with spiral CT	Longest diameter ≥10 mm on CT or on skin if using calipers; ≥20 mm if using CXR	Two perpendicular diameters of contrast enhancing lesions ≥10 mm	Tumor thickness perpendicular to chest wall or mediastinum, measured in two positions at three levels on transverse cuts of CT scan	Longest perpendicular diameters
Measurable Lymph Nodes	Not defined	Not defined	≥15 mm short axis	—	—	—
Disease Burden to be Assessed at Baseline	All (not specified)	Measurable target lesions up to 10 total (5 per organ); other lesions nontarget	Measurable target lesions up to 5 total (2 per organ); other lesions nontarget	Two to five lesions in patients with several lesions	Pleural disease in perpendicular diameter; nodal, subcutaneous, and other bidimensional lesions measured unidimensionally as per the RECIST criteria	5 lesions per organ, up to 10 visceral lesions and five cutaneous lesions
Sum	*Sum of the products* of bidimensional diameters or sum of linear unidimensional diameters	Sum of longest diameters of all measurable lesions	Sum of the longest diameters of target lesions with only exception use of short axis for lymph nodes	Sum of the products of perpendicular diameters of all measurable enhancing target lesions	Sum of the six measurements defines a pleural unidimensional measure	SPD with new lesions incorporated into baseline; tumor burden = $SPD_{index\ lesions}$ + $SPD_{new\ lesions}$
Complete Response	Disappearance all known disease	Disappearance all known disease	Disappearance all known disease; lymph nodes <10 mm	—	Disappearance all target lesions with no evidence of tumor elsewhere	Disappearance all lesions in two consecutive observations
Partial Response	≥50% decrease	≥30% decrease; all other no evidence of progression	≥30% decrease; all other disease, no evidence of progression	≥50% reduction; stable or decreased steroid use compared to baseline	≥30% reduction in total tumor measurement	≥50% decrease compared with baseline in two observations
Response Confirmation?	≥4 weeks apart	≥4 weeks apart	≥4 weeks apart (if response primary end point); no, if secondary endpoint	≥4 weeks apart	Repeat on two occasions ≥4 weeks apart	≥4 weeks apart

(continued)

TABLE 30.1

Key Features of Response Criteria *(continued)*

	WHO[3]	RECIST 1.0[4]	RECIST 1.1[5]	CNS RANO Criteria[7]	RECIST Mesothelioma[8]	RECIST Immunotherapy[9]
Progressive Disease	≥25% increase in size of one or more measurable lesions or appearance of new lesions	≥20% increase, taking as reference smallest sum in study; or appearance of new lesions	≥20% increase, with absolute increase ≥5 mm, taking as reference smallest sum in study; or appearance of new lesions	≥25%, or any new lesions	≥20% increase in the total tumor measurement over the nadir measurement, or the appearance of one or more new lesions	≥25% increase compared with nadir confirmed ≥4 weeks apart; up to five new lesions (≥5 × 5 mm) per organ incorporated into tumor burden
	Nonmeasurable disease: Estimated increase of ≥25%	Nonmeasurable disease: unequivocal progression	Nonmeasurable disease: unequivocal progression	Nonmeasurable disease: >5 mm increase in maximal diameter; ≥25% increase in SPD; or significant increase in nonenhancing lesions on same or lower dose of corticosteroids	—	New, nonmeasurable lesions (i.e., <5 × 5 mm) do not define progression
Stable Disease	Stable disease or non-PR and non-PD ≥4 weeks	Non-PR, non-PD; minimum time defined by protocol	Non-PR, non-PD; minimum time defined by protocol	—	Non-PR, non-PD	Non-irPR, non-irPD

CXR, Chest X-ray; SPD, sum of products of two largest perpendicular diameters; PD, progressive disease; irPR, immune-related partial response; irPD, immune-related progressive disease.

on two-dimensional measurements, have been recently updated as part of the Response Assessment in Neuro-Oncology (RANO) response criteria and extended to include a response assessment for metastatic CNS disease.[7,13]

Other examples where RECIST is limited include mesothelioma, gastrointestinal stromal tumors (GIST), hepatocellular cancers, among others. The pleural disease of mesothelioma increases in depth while following the pleural surface. GIST tumors may remain unchanged in size after treatment, whereas the center of the tumor mass undergoes necrosis, and progression may occur in the remaining rim.[14] Hepatocellular cancers are often treated with local–regional therapy in which the goal is tumor necrosis and treatment failure occurs in surviving viable tumor.[15] Different strategies have emerged to quantify these diseases, including modifications of RECIST, quantifying positron-emission tomography (PET) imaging, and biomarker criteria, as will be discussed. The RECIST adaptation for mesothelioma, growing along the pleural surface, is to measure the diameter perpendicular to the chest wall or mediastinum, and to measure at three levels.[8] The adaptation for hepatocellular cancer following local therapy is measurement of the longest diameter of the tumor that shows enhancement on the arterial phase of the scan, bypassing the dense, homogeneous Lipiodol-containing necrotic area.[15]

Investigators have also observed that following immunotherapy, tumor lesions may increase in size due to the increased infiltration of T cells, even meeting criteria for RECIST-defined progressive

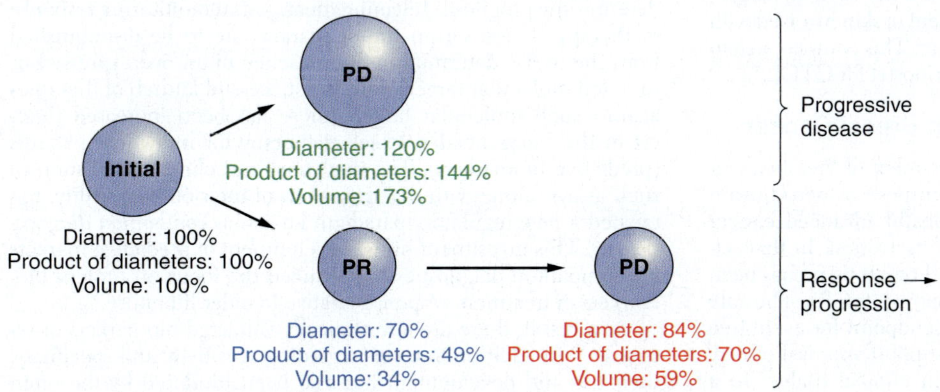

Figure 30.1 RECIST thresholds in three parameters: diameter, product of diameters, and volume. In the figure, spheres meeting RECIST criteria for progressive disease (PD) and for PR are shown with the percentage relative to the baseline calculated for each parameter. To meet the threshold for PD, the longest diameter must increase to 120%, which is equivalent to a 144% increase in the product of the perpendicular diameters and a 173% increase in the volume of a sphere. Although PR definitions are almost identical to those employed with WHO, RECIST has a higher threshold to meet PD.[6]

disease (PD). Previously radiographically undetectable lesions may appear. Departing from conventional RECIST, which defines any new lesion as PD, the immune response criteria allow the appearance of new lesions, adding them to the total tumor burden.[9] An increase in total tumor burden of >25% relative to baseline or nadir is required to define PD.

International Working Group Criteria for Lymphoma

Revised guidelines for lymphoma assessment were promulgated by the International Working Group (IWG) in 2007.[16] These guidelines incorporated 18F-fluorodeoxyglucose (FDG)-PET assessments in metabolically active lymphomas.[16] Although a CR requires the complete disappearance of detectable disease, a post-treatment residual mass is permitted if it is negative on FDG-PET and was positive at baseline. For lymphomas that are not consistently FDG avid, or if FDG avidity is unknown, a CR requires that nodes >1.5 cm before therapy regress to <1.5 cm, and nodes that were 1.1 to 1.5 cm in long axis and >1.0 cm in the short axis shrink to ≤1.0 cm in short axis. The definition of PR resembles the WHO criteria, in that a ≥50% decrease in the sum of the product of the diameters in up to six nodal masses or in hepatic or splenic nodules must be documented. Although RECIST 1.1 now includes lymph node assessment, the IWG criteria remain the assessment method typically used in lymphoma clinical trials.

ALTERNATE RESPONSE CRITERIA

The previous examples represent attempts to more accurately measure tumor burden. Evolving imaging technology enabling volumetric measurements of tumor masses may eventually resolve some of these problems, but effective therapeutic agents are required to enable validation and utilization of response assessment tools. The lack of an agent that can mediate substantial tumor shrinkage underlies the concept of *clinical benefit response* (CBR) as an endpoint in pancreatic cancer. Clinical benefit was defined as a combination of improvement in pain, performance status, and weight; the assessment of CBR supported the U.S. Food and Drug Administration (FDA) approval of gemcitabine in pancreatic cancer.[17,18] Better therapies for pancreatic cancer that result in tumor shrinkage or eradication should include and then eclipse clinical benefit.

Response criteria may be specific to a particular disease or clinical setting. Some diseases by their nature require specific strategies for response assessment.

Severity-Weighted Assessment Tool Score in Cutaneous T-Cell Lymphoma

Cutaneous T-cell lymphoma (CTCL) is a disease that can involve the entire epidermis, or comprise individual skin lesions varying widely in severity rather than size. The severity-weighted assessment tool (SWAT) assigns a factor for skin lesion severity—patch, plaque, or tumor—multiplies this factor by the percent of skin involved with each lesion type and then adds these together. This complex system formed the basis of the FDA approval of vorinostat for CTCL.[19]

Pathologic Complete Response in Breast Cancer

One unique response endpoint is the assessment of breast cancer treated in the neoadjuvant setting. The purpose of neoadjuvant therapy is to improve survival, render locally advanced cancer amenable to surgery, or to aid in breast conservation. In that setting, the absence of cancer cells in resected breast tissue has been used to define a pathologic complete response (pCR). The rate of pCR has been proposed as a surrogate endpoint for event-free survival (EFS) or overall survival (OS) to support approval of new agents or combinations of agents tested in clinical trials.[20] In a pooled analysis of 11,955 patients enrolled on 12 neoadjuvant trials, individual patients with pCR had improved EFS and OS.[21] However, at the trial level, pCR rates did not correlate with EFS or OS, a problem likely due to heterogeneity of breast cancer subtypes among the trials. Despite this, pCR rates were recently used to support the approval of pertuzumab and trastuzumab in the neoadjuvant setting.[21,22]

Computed Tomography-Based Tumor Density

One approach, often called the Choi criteria, advocates assessing tumor response in GIST, renal cell cancer, or hepatocellular cancer based on density on computed tomography (CT) scans (Table 30.2). This variation was prompted by the evident response to treatment with imatinib but with minimal tumor shrinkage.[23] The Choi criteria are still considered exploratory in GIST,[24,25] and it is too soon to know of benefits in other histologies.[26,27] Further study should determine its utility, although it will likely be confined to specific tumor types with specific drugs.

FDG-PET

Although widely used in clinical practice, FDG-PET has become part of standardized response criteria for clinical trials only in lymphoma (see Table 30.2). In solid tumors, FDG-PET can aid in the detection of new or recurrent sites of disease, and can be used as an adjunct during assessments for disease progression when using RECIST criteria.[3] Although FDG uptake is a powerful diagnostic tool and its uptake reflects a tumor's metabolic activity, it has some limitations: Some tumors have variable FDG avidity; differences can occur due to variations in patient activity, carbohydrate intake, blood glucose, and timing; and there are several benign sources of uptake, including inflammatory and postsurgical sites. Multiple methods of quantitating FDG-PET and assessing response have been proposed, but to date there is no consensus, particularly regarding the definition of a metabolic response.[28–33]

The two most widely used response criteria—the European Organisation for the Research and Treatment of Cancer (EORTC) criteria and PET Response Criteria in Solid Tumors (PERCIST) (see Table 30.2)—have been evaluated in specific disease types, but unifying FDG-PET response criteria remains a challenge in anticancer drug development.[28,30] We would note that, as shown in Figure 30.1, a 30% reduction in the diameter of a sphere—the magnitude of change required to score a response according to RECIST—represents a 65% decrease in volume. If an standardized uptake value (SUV) decrease is directly equated to a volume decrease, a reduction of 25% translates to a 10% reduction in diameter, a value that likely constitutes an insufficient response.

Serum Biomarkers of Response

The ideal response assessment method is an assay that could measure tumor quantity by a simple blood test (see Table 30.2). Circulating protein biomarkers have been identified and studied for several decades for screening, early detection of recurrent disease, determining prognosis, selecting therapy, and monitoring response to therapy. These serum tumor markers are to be distinguished from the assays determining the presence of an overexpressed or mutated molecular target. With the successful launch of therapies against such molecular targets, there has been increased interest in the assays needed to select therapy for individual patients (predictive biomarkers). The analytical and clinical validation of such assays, along with determination of their clinical utility, has created a new regulatory paradigm known as *companion diagnostics*.[34,35] This investment in the development of predictive markers for companion diagnostics has reduced the focus on protein biomarkers of treatment response relative to older literature.

As a result, there are few clinically validated biomarkers of response.[36] In addition to issues regarding sensitivity and specificity, their use and development has also been hindered by the often

TABLE 30.2

Alternate Response Criteria: Biomarkers

Criterion	Baseline	Response	Progression
CA-125 in ovarian cancer (GCIG criteria)[43]	CA 125 >2× ULN	CA 125 decline ≥50% confirmed at 28 days	2× nadir OR 2× ULN if normalized on therapy on two occasions 1 wk apart
PSA in prostate cancer (PSA WG1)[45,a]	PSA ≥5 ng/mL and documentation of two consecutive increases in PSA 1 wk apart	PSA decline of 50% from baseline (measured twice 3–4 wks apart)	After decrease from baseline, a 50% increase AND an increase ≥5 ng/mL, or back to baseline, whichever is lower
PSA in prostate cancer (PCWG2)[46,a]	PSA ≥2.0 ng/mL; estimate pretreatment PSA-DT: Need ≥3 values ≥4 wks apart	Report percent change from baseline (rise or fall) at 12 weeks, and separately, the maximal change (rise or fall) at any time using a waterfall plot	PSA increase ≥25% and absolute increase by ≥2 ng/mL above the nadir, confirmed by a second value ≥3 wks later (i.e., confirmed rising trend) OR PSA increase ≥25% and ≥2 ng/mL above baseline >12 wks
hCG and AFP in testicular cancer[50–51]		Decrease consistent with marker half-life: 2–3 d for hCG, 5–7 d for AFP	Rising levels usually indicate need to change therapy
		Choi Criteria for CT Imaging	
Choi criteria[24–27]		≥10% decrease in tumor size OR ≥15% reduction in tumor density	An increase in tumor size ≥10% and does not meet criteria of PR by tumor attenuation on CT
		FDG-PET Criteria	
EORTC criteria[29–31]	ROI should be drawn, SUV calculated	**CMR:** Complete resolution of uptake **PMR:** SUV reduction ≥25% **SMD:** SUV increase <25% and decrease <15%	**PMD:** SUV increase >25% in regions defined on baseline, or appearance of new FDG-avid lesions
PERCIST criteria[29]	SUL peak >1.5× normal liver	**CMR:** Complete resolution of uptake **PMR:** SUL reduction ≥30%	**PMD:** SUL increase >30% in regions defined on baseline, or appearance of new FDG avid lesions

[a] Guidelines for PSA assessment have evolved from those of the PSAWG1, where responses were dichotomized based on the percent decline, to those in the PCWG2 where PSA response is considered a continuous variable. Recently, emphasis has shifted to assessing PSA doubling time.
CA-125, cancer antigen 125; GCIG, Gynecologic Cancer InterGroup; ULN, upper limit of normal; PSA, prostate-specific antigen; PSAWG1, PSA Working Group 1; PCWG2, Prostate Cancer Working Group 2; PSA-DT, PSA-doubling time; hCG, human chorionic gonatropin; AFP, alpha-fetoprotein; EORTC, European Organisation for the Research and Treatment of Cancer; ROI, regions of interest; SUV, standardized uptake value; CMR, complete metabolic response; PMR, partial metabolic response, SMD, stable metabolic disease; PMD, progressive metabolic disease; PERCIST, PET response criteria in solid tumors; SUL, SUV normalized to lean body mass.

limited efficacy of therapies; response biomarkers are of little value without highly effective primary and salvage therapies. For example, a recent clinical trial indicates that in *asymptomatic patients* with ovarian cancer whose only evidence of disease progression is an isolated rising CA-125, nothing is gained by instituting treatment before there is other evidence of progression.[37,38]

- **Cancer Antigen 125 (CA-125):** Despite recognized limitations, CA-125 is widely used. For example, the Gynecologic Cancer InterGroup (GCIG) criteria have evolved to help determine whether a patient's tumor has responded to therapy.[39–41] Response is defined as a 50% decline from an elevated baseline value, whereas progression is defined as a doubling over the nadir or the upper limit of normal.[42] In clinical practice, CA-125 levels are followed as part of standard management, but making clinical decisions on marker changes alone is not recommended.[43]
- **Prostate-Specific Antigen (PSA):** Similar issues have confronted investigators caring for patients with prostate cancer. The PSA Working Group 1 (PCWG1) guidelines, first published in 1999, established PSA criteria, particularly for use in patients with disease that was difficult to quantify.[44] There followed a second working group (PCWG2) that recommended plotting the percent PSA change for each patient in a waterfall plot so as to avoid creating a dichotomous variable from the changes in PSA.[45] PCWG2 also recommended keeping patients on trial until evidence of a change in clinical status—either symptomatic or radiographic progression. The latter addressed concerns with patients in whom PSA changes did not reflect clinical status, particularly those with transient increases in the first 12 weeks of a new therapy.
- **Human Chorionic Gonadotropin (hCG) and alpha fetoprotein (AFP):** Because testicular cancer is a highly curable disease with validated biomarkers, outcome assessment has focused on the rapid detection of patients whose tumors have a poor response to therapy. Because both markers have relatively short half-lives—2 to 3 days for hCG and 5 to 7 days for serum AFP—the rate of decline can be determined. Various methods have demonstrated that a rapid decline or early normalization of marker levels is indicative of a good

outcome, without any one method achieving widespread acceptance.[46–48] Nonetheless, the 2010 American Society of Clinical Oncology (ASCO) guidelines on serum tumor markers concluded there was still insufficient evidence to recommend changing therapy solely on the basis of a slow marker decline.[49] Rising levels after two cycles of therapy (outside the first week of treatment when rises can be due to tumor lysis) can be considered an indication to change the treatment plan.[49,50]

Circulating Tumor Cells and Circulating Tumor DNA

Two response endpoints under recent investigation show a potential to detect the impact of therapy. One is the measurement of circulating tumor cells (CTC) in the bloodstream, enriched by one or more capture strategies, including one that has received FDA approval.[51] The number of CTCs in the blood has been shown to be prognostic, with higher levels conferring a poor prognosis, and to correlate with a response to therapy. A second approach is the determination of levels of circulating tumor DNA (ctDNA) in the blood. This is detected by quantitating the number of DNA molecules carrying a given mutation or gene rearrangement in the blood, typically detected through targeted sequencing of common mutations, or of a previously identified *mutation signature* or gene rearrangement. The amount of ctDNA appears to correlate with tumor burden, increases with stage, and in one study, was deemed more sensitive than CTC detection.[52–54] Whether these tests will ultimately prove to be more sensitive and accurate than the serum biomarkers discussed previously remains to be determined. Because targeted sequencing can be very sensitive, one concern is that false-positive ctDNA detection may occur after treatment, or intermittently in the setting of enlarging tumor masses. At the least, detection of CTCs and ctDNA is advancing our understanding of cancer biology, as studies reveal evidence of metastatic heterogeneity, clonal heterogeneity, and emergence of resistance mutations in clinical samples.

DETERMINING OUTCOME

The response measures described previously represent different approaches to quantitate tumor burden. What happens after those data are obtained varies depending on the clinical setting. In the community, less emphasis is placed on strict criteria. In the setting of a clinical trial, tumor size is measured and the response categorized. For FDA submission, these are but factors in the risk-benefit equation needed for drug approvals. The FDA conveys full approval to new agents based on true *clinical benefit* (i.e., an improvement in a *survival* endpoint or symptom relief).[55] Surrogates for clinical benefit, such as response rate, may support either regular approval or accelerated approval, depending on the setting.

Overall Response Rate, Duration of Response, and Stable Disease

Overall response rate (ORR) is the proportion of patients with a tumor size reduction of a predefined amount for a minimum time period. The FDA has generally defined ORR as the sum of PRs and CRs. Although OS remains the gold standard, ORR is often used both in drug development and in clinical practice to indicate antitumor efficacy of a given therapy. Table 30.3 summarizes the attributes and drawbacks of using ORR as a method of assessment. Using standardized definitions of response, it has been shown that ORR often correlates with OS, although ORR usually explains only a fraction of the variability of the survival benefits.[56–58] Equally important, however, is the duration of response, a value that is measured from the time of initial response until documented tumor progression, and which assumes added importance when ORR is the endpoint for regulatory approval.

Unlike PR and CR, the FDA has generally not been willing to include *stable disease (SD)*, defined as shrinkage that qualifies as neither response nor progression, as part of the ORR, feeling it is often indicative of the underlying disease biology rather than a drug's therapeutic effect.[55,59] Nevertheless, in reporting data, investigators are increasingly using the term *CBR*, which includes CR + PR + SD and which is a misuse of the term *clinical benefit* because neither CR, PR, or SD are *objective tumor findings* that address the true *clinical benefit* of a therapy.[58,60] In the absence of standardized definitions for SD that are shown to effect meaningful changes in a clinical outcome, SD should not be used as a response endpoint. A better approach is to use nondichotomized response assessments, such as the waterfall plot or one of the kinetic analyses, discussed later.

Progression-Free Survival, Time to Progression, and Time to Treatment Failure

In cancer drug development, one usually finds ORR assessed as an indicator of activity in phase II trials, whereas randomized phase III trials rely on other endpoints such as progression-free survival (PFS) and time to progression (TTP) (see Table 30.3). Although PFS and TTP attempt to assess efficacy in close proximity to a therapy, they score outcomes differently and are not interchangeable. TTP is defined as the time from randomization to *the time of disease progression.*[55] *In TTP analyses, deaths are censored either at the time of death or at an earlier visit.* In contrast, PFS is defined from the time of randomization to the time of *disease progression or death*. Although patients who discontinue trial participation for adverse events might be censored in both analyses, patients who die while on study are censored only in the TTP analysis. Those who favor TTP argue that if a patient dies without their tumor meeting criteria for progression, one cannot accurately estimate when progression might have occurred, so the data should be censored. However, those who favor PFS argue that, in some cases, death might be an adverse effect of the therapy. High-dose therapies represent an example of why PFS might be a preferable (regulatory) endpoint. If in a given tumor there is evidence of a dose-response relationship for an active drug, then high doses may have a greater response. However, such high doses may also be responsible for a greater number of deaths. Assessing only those who survive the high dose therapy and ignoring those who die (i.e., TTP) may lead to the conclusion that the high-dose therapy is more effective. The balance sheet that includes death (i.e., PFS) would clearly demonstrate this efficacy came at too great a price.

Although many have argued that PFS and TTP should be acceptable endpoints for cancer clinical trials, in the majority of tumors there is no convincing evidence PFS is a surrogate for OS, and in those where there is some evidence, its value is arguable.[61] Table 30.3 presents the attributes and drawbacks of PFS and TTP. Note that the definition of progression is often difficult, particularly in some tumor types, and that investigator bias can influence PFS and TTP. Problems with ascertainment bias and censoring, depicted in Figure 30.2, can also impact outcomes.

Alternate endpoints include time to treatment failure (TTF), defined as a composite endpoint measuring time from randomization to discontinuation of treatment for any reason, including disease progression, treatment toxicity, and death. The FDA has not recommended TTF as a regulatory endpoint for drug approval. However, the high rates of censoring due to toxicity seen in phase III clinical trails may lead to a reassessment of this position given that most can agree that not only is efficacy important, but so too is tolerability, and TTF can capture both of these attributes.

TABLE 30.3

A Comparison of Important Cancer Approval Endpoints

Regulatory Evidence	Endpoints	Advantages	Disadvantages
Clinical benefit used for regular approvals	Overall survival (OS)	▪ Universally accepted direct measure of clinical benefit ▪ Easily measured ▪ Includes treatment-related mortality that can obscure benefit in a subset ▪ Precisely measured; unambiguous ▪ Not dependent on assessment intervals	▪ May involve larger studies ▪ May require long follow-up ▪ May be affected by crossover and/or sequential therapies ▪ Includes noncancer deaths
	Symptom endpoints (patient-reported outcomes)	▪ Patient perspective of direct clinical benefit	▪ Blinding is often difficult ▪ Data are frequently missing or incomplete ▪ Clinical significance of small changes is unknown ▪ Multiple analyses ▪ Lack of validated instruments
Surrogates used for accelerated approvals or regular approvals	Disease-free survival (DFS)	▪ Smaller sample size and shorter follow-up necessary compared with survival studies	▪ Not statistically validated as surrogate for survival in all settings ▪ Not precisely measured; subject to assessment bias, particularly in open-label studies ▪ Definitions vary among studies
	Objective response rate (ORR)	▪ Can be assessed in single-arm studies ▪ Assessed earlier and in smaller studies compared with survival studies ▪ Effect attributable to drug, not natural history	▪ Not a direct measure of benefit ▪ Not a comprehensive measure of drug activity ▪ Only a subset of patients who benefit
	Complete response (CR)	▪ Can be assessed in single-arm studies ▪ Durable complete responses can represent clinical benefit ▪ Assessed earlier and in smaller studies compared with survival studies ▪ Definition of progressive disease (PD) identifies uniform time to end treatment and data capture	▪ Not a direct measure of benefit in all cases ▪ Not a comprehensive measure of drug activity ▪ Small subset of patients with benefit ▪ Requires prospective, consistent definition. Meaningful response durations not standardized ▪ Definition of PD is arbitrary without evidence it actually represents end of benefit period
	Progression-free survival (PFS) or time to progression (TTP)[a]	▪ Smaller sample size and shorter follow-up necessary compared with survival studies ▪ Measurement of stable disease included ▪ Not confounded by crossover or subsequent therapies ▪ Generally based on objective and quantitative assessment	▪ Statistically validated as surrogate for survival only in some settings ▪ Not precisely measured; subject to assessment bias particularly in open-label studies ▪ Definitions vary among studies; little agreement on magnitude of difference that constitutes clinical benefit ▪ Requires frequent and consistent radiological or other assessments ▪ Involves balanced timing of assessments among treatment arms

[a] Progression-free survival includes all deaths; time to progression censors deaths that occur before progression.
Adapted from U.S. Department of Health and Human Services, Food and Drug Administration, Center for Drug Evaluation and Research (CDER), Center for Biologics Evaluation and Research (CBER). *Guidance from Industry. Clinical Trial Endpoints for the Approval of Cancer Drugs and Biologics.* 2007. http://www.fda.gov/downloads/Drugs/.../Guidances/ucm071590.pdf.

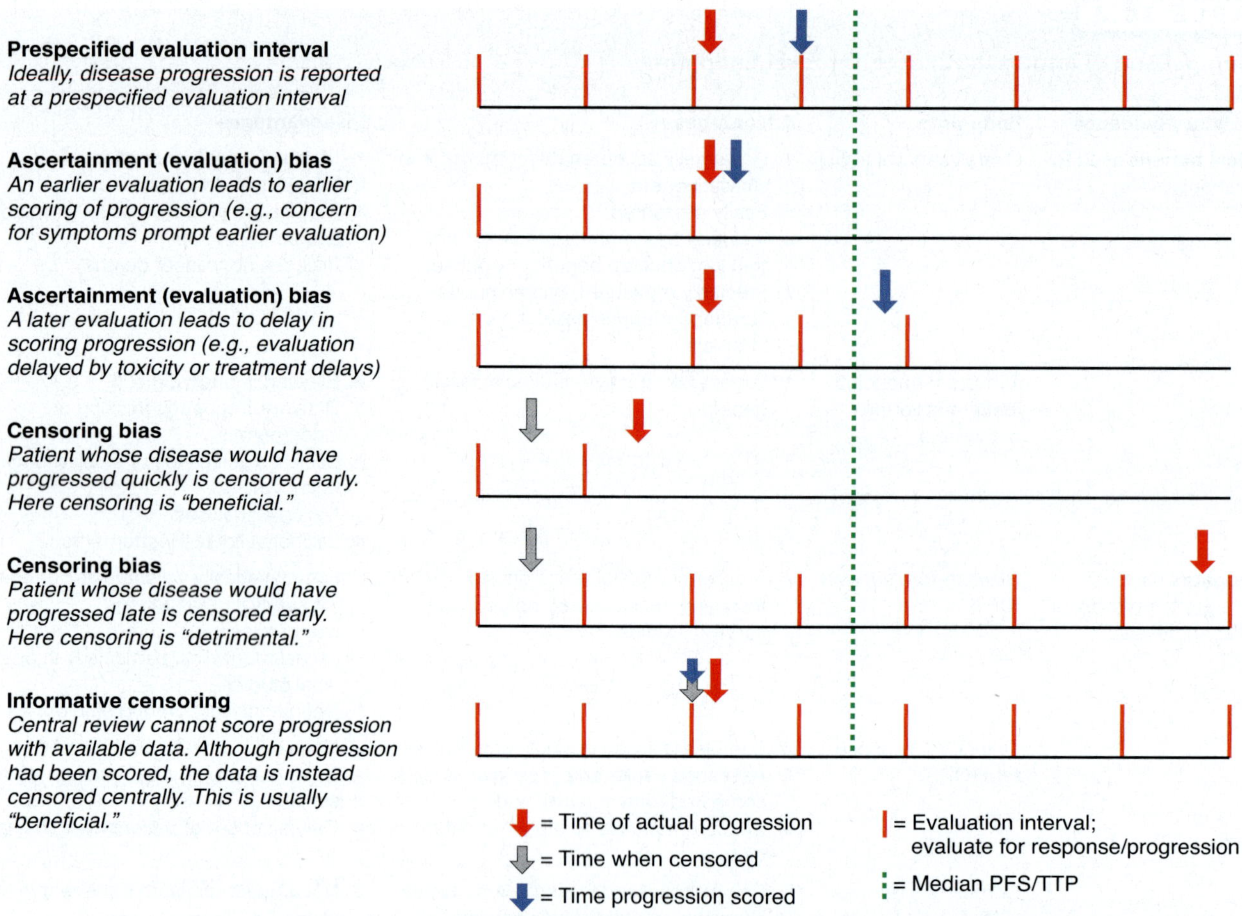

Figure 30.2 The potential problems encountered when PFS is used as an endpoint. Ideally, as depicted at the *top*, response assessment will be conducted at a prespecified time. However, the date at which progression is scored may suffer from either ascertainment or censoring bias. Ascertainment bias can occur if either an evaluation occurs before the prespecified date or if it is delayed. For example, a clinician concerned about a patient who is not experiencing side effects and has likely been randomized to placebo may be more inclined to investigate symptoms early and document progression before the prespecified time, while delaying the evaluation of a patient randomized to the experimental arm who experiences some toxicity. Similarly, censoring—an increasing problem in randomized trials—may impact the outcome of a given study arm by either censoring patients who would experience early progression (beneficial impact) or censoring those who would have remained progression free for a long time (detrimental impact). Finally, informative censoring can occur when independent radiologic review cannot concur with an investigator's assessment of progression and censors the patient. This outcome is usually beneficial, because a patient who is very close to experiencing progression is censored. (Adapted from Villaruz LC, Socinski MA. The clinical viewpoint: definitions, limitations of RECIST, practical considerations of measurement. *Clin Cancer Res* 2013;19:2629–2636.)

Overall Survival

Defined as the time from randomization to death, OS has been considered the gold standard of clinical trial endpoints (see Table 30.3). In part, this is so because it is unambiguous and does not suffer from interpretation bias. An additional advantage of the survival endpoint is that it can balance the effect of therapies with high treatment-related mortality even if tumor control is substantially better with the new treatment. However, some worry that because patients may receive multiple lines of therapy following the clinical trial, the results may be confounded by those subsequent therapies. The latter concern is often cited as the reason why an advantage in PFS/TTP *disappears* when one looks to OS. But as a review of clinical trials confirms,[62] the magnitude of the difference does not disappear, only the statistical validity (Fig. 30.3).[63,64]

When evaluating a randomized controlled trial, it is important that the OS as well as the PFS analyses are always by intention to treat (ITT). In an ITT analysis, often described as *once randomized, always analyzed,* all patients assigned to a group at the time of randomization are analyzed regardless of what occurred subsequently.[65] An ITT analysis avoids the bias introduced by omitting dropouts and noncompliant patients that can negate randomization and overestimate clinical effectiveness.

Kaplan–Meier Plots

In a typical clinical trial, data are often presented as a Kaplan–Meier plots. In discrete time intervals, the number of patients in each group who are progression free and alive (PFS analysis) or alive (OS analysis) at the end of the interval are counted and divided by the total number of patients in that group at the beginning of the time interval. One excludes from this calculation patients censored for a reason other than progressive disease or death during the same interval. This has the advantage that it allows one to include censored patients in estimates of the probability of PFS or OS up to the point when they were censored (i.e., they are excluded only beyond the point of censoring). In most clinical trials, a fraction of patients are typically censored.

In constructing the Kaplan–Meier plot, probabilities are calculated for each interval of time. The probability of surviving

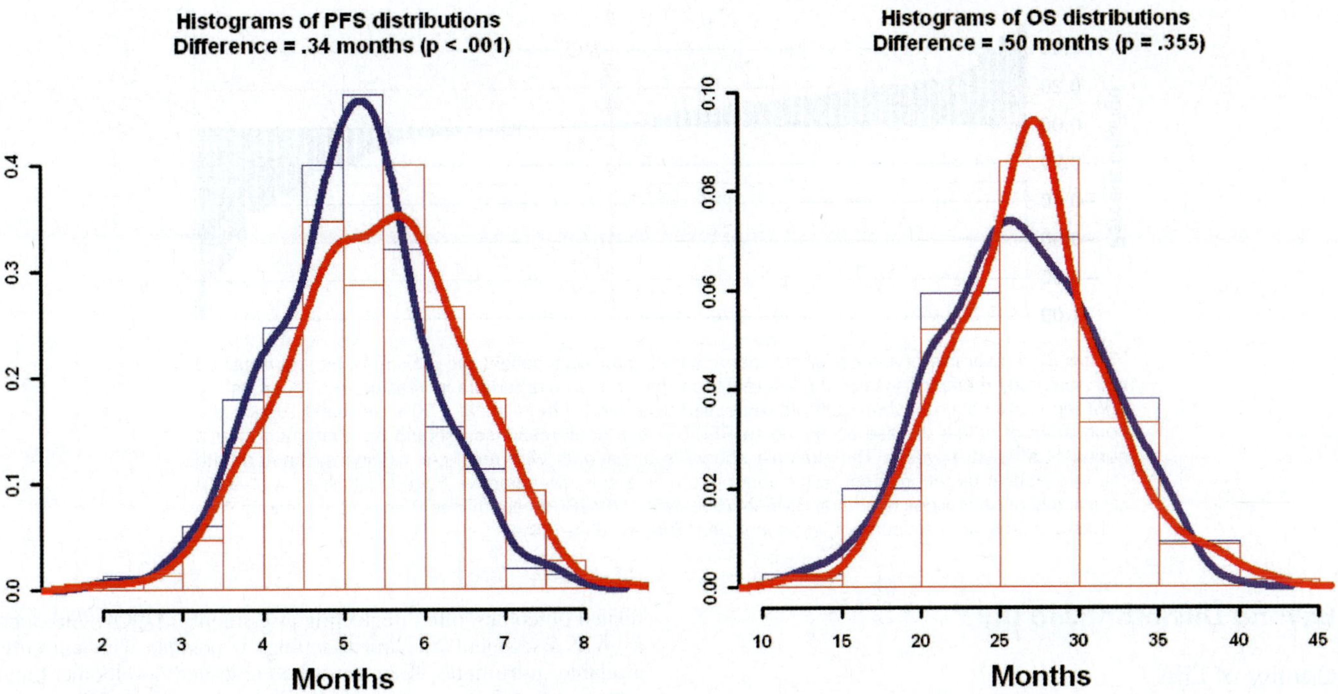

Figure 30.3 Hypothetical distribution of PFS and OS data demonstrating the *disappearance of PFS benefit*. Because chemotherapy does not exert a lasting effect on the underlying tumor biology and because PFS is a shorter interval (measured in increments, not daily as is OS) PFS differences often disappear. The *hypothetical example* shown illustrates this phenomenon. The *left panel* shows a histogram of PFS distributions with a difference of 0.34 months that nevertheless achieves statistical significance over the short interval when PFS is measured. The *right panel* depicts similar histograms for OS captured over a longer time period. Despite a larger absolute difference of 0.5 months, the OS difference does not reach statistical significance. For these hypothetical curves, random number generated data sets (with normal distribution), histograms, and density plots were generated using R version 2.11.1 (2010-05-31).[75] The differences were deliberately chosen to be small, but a similar disappearance can also occur with larger differences. As can be seen, what disappears is not the absolute benefit, but the statistical validity.

progression free or being counted as a survivor to the end of any interval of assessment is the product of the probabilities of surviving in all the preceding assessment intervals multiplied by the probability for the interval of interest. One might ask to what extent the two curves in each study differ. One measure that is of value is the median PFS or OS—a value calculated in most studies from a Kaplan–Meier plot.

Hazard Ratios

Increasingly, however, hazard ratios are cited in preference to the more traditional measures of efficacy such as the median PFS and median OS. *However, because a hazard ratio is a value that has no dimensions, it has very limited value, informing the reader only with regard to the reliability and uniformity of the data.* It does not quantify the magnitude of the benefit. A physician and, especially, a patient want to know the magnitude of the benefit (i.e., the extent to which a life will be prolonged), not what a dimensionless hazard ratio is. By definition, the *hazard ratio* is a ratio of the *hazard rates*. The hazard rate quantifies the likelihood that a patient will experience a *hazardous event* or a hazard during a defined interval of observation, and this is expressed as a rate or percent. For example, if during a given period of observation 20 of 100 patients receiving a reference or control therapy experience progression or death, their hazard rate during this interval is 0.2 (20/100). If during this same interval, only 10 of the 100 patients receiving the experimental therapy experience progression or death, their hazard rate is 0.1 (10/100). In this simple example, the hazard ratio for the interval, calculated as *the ratio of the hazard rates* is 0.5 (0.1/0.2) and indicates the likelihood of experiencing a hazardous event is reduced by 50% in the experimental arm. As commonly presented, and as this simple example illustrates, the lower the hazard ratio, the better the experimental therapy. To determine whether the hazard ratio has statistical significance, one can (1) use a log-rank test to show that the null hypothesis that the two treatments lead to the same survival probabilities is wrong, or (2) use a parametric approach writing a regression model and fitting the data to the model so that one can establish the hazard ratio for the whole trial and its statistical significance. In many cases, the Cox proportional hazard model is used. Although the ideal hazard ratio would capture the differential benefit throughout the period of study, in practice, the extremes depicted in a Kaplan–Meier plot may not be analyzed.

Forest Plots

Interest in determining whether there is heterogeneity in a treatment effect, such that better outcomes occur in some subgroups, has led to the use of Forest plots to display treatment effects across subgroups. Although simple in concept, these plots are subject to error because subgroups are composed of smaller numbers and the confidence intervals are therefore wider than those for the entire group. The most common presentation includes a vertical line at the *no effect point* (e.g., a hazard ratio of 1.0), with symbols of varying size representing the subgroups, each with its confidence interval depicted by a line that stretches from the symbol to both sides (the symbol size is usually proportional to the size of the subgroup). If the confidence interval for a subgroup crosses the no effect point, this is commonly interpreted (not necessarily correctly) as a lack of effect in the subgroup. *The information one seeks from a Forest plot is whether the effect size for different subgroups varies significantly from the main effect, which is determined by a test for heterogeneity.*[66]

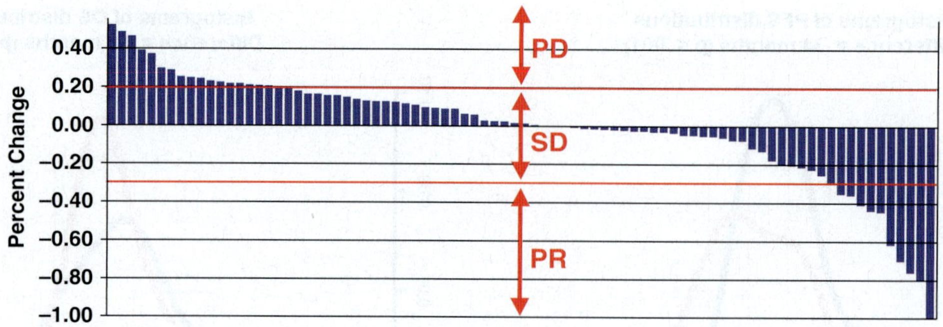

Figure 30.4 Example of a waterfall plot demonstrating for each patient the maximum benefit obtained with the study therapy. Those to the *left* represent patients whose tumors increased, and those on the *right* represent patients whose tumors regressed. The *vertical red lines* at +20% and -30% define the boundaries of stable disease according to RECIST. Ideally, all responses should be confirmed after a period of at least 4 weeks. The example shown is of patients with renal cell carcinoma treated with the microtubule targeting agent ixabepilone. (From Huang H, Menefee M, Edgerly M, et al. A phase II clinical trial of ixabepilone [Ixempra; BMS-247550; NSC 710428], an epothilone B analog, in patients with metastatic renal cell carcinoma. *Clin Cancer Res* 2010;16:1634–1641.)

Beyond Dichotomized Data

Quality of Life

The assessment of cancer patients enrolled on a clinical trial can be said to consist of two sets of endpoints: cancer outcomes and patient outcomes. Cancer outcomes measure the response of the tumor to treatment, the duration of the response, the symptom-free period, and the early recognition of relapse. In contrast, patient outcomes assess the benefit achieved with a given therapy by measuring the increase in survival and the quality of life (QOL) before and after therapy. Unfortunately, physicians tend to concentrate on cancer-related outcomes, often neglecting assessments of QOL. Although a QOL assessment in clinical settings is possible with currently available instruments, there must be continued development and refinement of these instruments. Such development must focus not only on extracting valuable information in an unbiased manner, but also and equally important, developing an instrument that is user friendly and will be completed in a high percentage of encounters.

Waterfall Plots

The arbitrary nature of the 50% cutoff set by Moertel and Hanley and its evolution to the current RECIST threshold of 30%

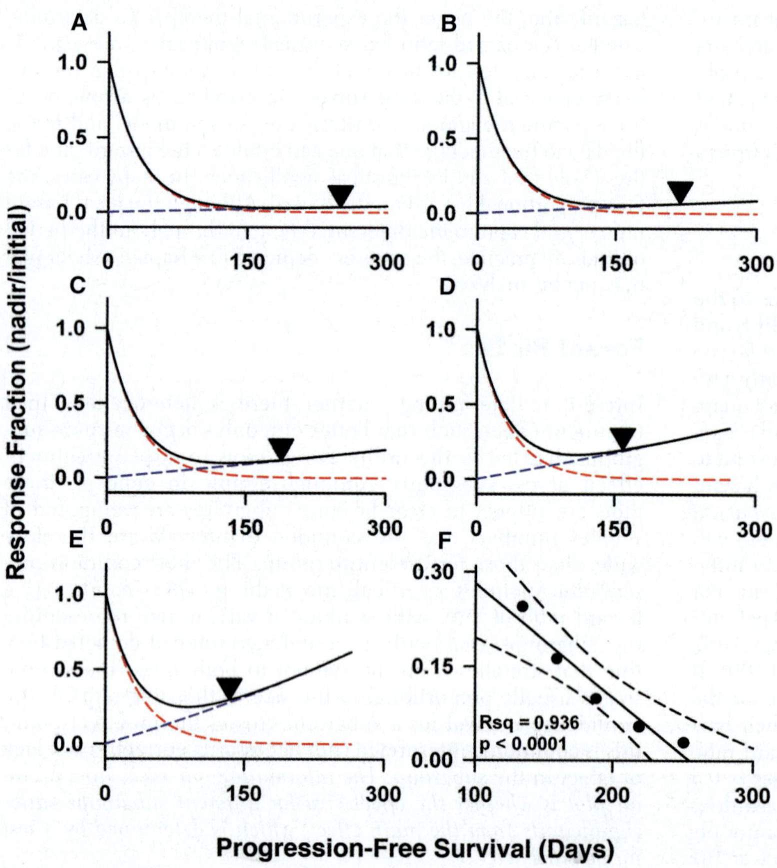

Figure 30.5 The effect of the growth rate constant, *g*, on two commonly reported clinical values: maximum tumor shrinkage and PFS. Tumor measurements obtained in patients can be analyzed mathematically. **(A–E)** The *black line* depicts idealized clinical data using tumor quantities measured as patients received chemotherapy. Actually, clinical measurements comprise concurrent tumor regression *(dashed red line)* and growth *(dashed blue line)* that can be described by a rate constant and a first order kinetic equation, $f(t) = \exp^{(-d \cdot t)} + \exp^{(g \cdot t)} - 1$, where *exp* is the base of the natural logarithm, e = 2.7182. . . , and *f* is the percent change in tumor measurement at time *t*, normalized to the value when treatment began. The rate constant ***d*** accounts for exponential decrease, whereas the rate constant ***g*** accounts for exponential growth occurring during treatment.[68,69] To demonstrate the correlation between the growth rate, tumor shrinkage and PFS, the *same* regression rate **(*d*)** has been modeled in panels *A* through *E*, whereas the growth rate constant, ***g***, *increases* in each successive panel. The *black triangles* depict the point at which tumor size is 20% above the nadir (RECIST definition of PD). As the growth rate increases (i.e., faster tumor growth) from **A** to **E**, the nadir is reached sooner, and the depth of the nadir is less. **(F)** The correlation between PFS and maximum tumor shrinkage (nadir) is shown, plotting the correlation between PFS and response fraction, which is defined as the ratio of nadir to initial value.[68,69] Although idealized plots are given, the curves are based firmly on data obtained from patients enrolled on clinical trials.

reduction in the size of the maximum diameter raises valid queries as to why 30% is valuable and not 29% or 25%. On this background, waterfall plots such as the one shown in Figure 30.4 have become increasingly popular because they depict the benefit or lack thereof in all patients as a continuum of response, rather than a dichotomized response rate.[67] Waterfall plots can be generated from any quantitative assessment. If ctDNA or tumor cells prove to be as quantitative as hoped, the maximum decline could be plotted as a waterfall plot.

Growth Kinetics

Efforts to quantify tumor kinetic parameters from clinical data have been investigated in recent years. Different equations have been applied to describe the two-phase curve based on tumor size as observed in most solid tumor trials, where there is first shrinkage followed by regrowth (Fig. 30.5). These models show exponential tumor shrinkage after treatment, followed by tumor regrowth that is either exponential or linear and have been shown to correlate with OS and to discriminate effective therapies as well as individual patients within trials.[68–73] A major advantage is that more of the data are used, relative to dichotomized response assessment, and regression or growth rates can be determined even in patients who are censored in a Kaplan–Meier analysis. Equations that model both regression and growth rates confirm the clinical intuition that resistant disease is emerging even as overall tumor volume is reduced. Further, "the strategy of studying tumor growth kinetics circumvents one weakness of 'progression criteria,' which is that they inherently dichotomize a complex biological process that may be better characterized using a continuous function."[74] As shown in Figure 30.5, the response of a tumor to a therapy is exemplified by the nadir, the time to the nadir, and the time to progression or PFS, and these are all are all dependent on the growth rate.

REFERENCES

1. America's Biopharmaceutical Research Companies. *Medicines in Development for Cancer*. PhRMA Web site. http://www.phrma.org/sites/default/files/pdf/phrmamedicinesindevelopmentcancer2012.pdf.
2. Moertel CG, Hanley JA. The effect of measuring error on the results of therapeutic trials in advanced cancer. *Cancer* 1976;38:388–394.
3. Miller AB, Hoogstraten B, Staquet M, et al. Reporting results of cancer treatment. *Cancer* 1981;47:207–214.
4. Therasse P, Arbuck SG, Eisenhauer EA, et al. New guidelines to evaluate the response to treatment in solid tumors. European Organization for Research and Treatment of Cancer, National Cancer Institute of the United States, National Cancer Institute of Canada. *J Natl Cancer Inst* 2000;92:205–216.
5. Eisenhauer EA, Therasse P, Bogaerts J, et al. New response evaluation criteria in solid tumours: revised RECIST guideline (version 1.1). *Eur J Cancer* 2009;45:228–247.
6. Mazumdar M, Smith A, Schwartz LH. A statistical simulation study finds discordance between WHO criteria and RECIST guideline. *J Clin Epidemiol* 2004;57:358–365.
7. Wen PY, Macdonald DR, Reardon DA, et al. Updated response assessment criteria for high-grade gliomas: response assessment in neuro-oncology working group. *J Clin Oncol* 2010;28:1963–1972.
8. Byrne MJ, Nowak AK. Modified RECIST criteria for assessment of response in malignant pleural mesothelioma. *Ann Oncol* 2004;15:257–260.
9. Wolchok JD, Hoos A, O'Day S, et al. Guidelines for the evaluation of immune therapy activity in solid tumors: immune-related response criteria. *Clin Cancer Res* 2009;15:7412–7420.
10. Quant EC, Wen PY. Response assessment in neuro-oncology. *Curr Oncol Rep* 2011;13:50–56.
11. Hawkins-Daarud A, Rockne RC, Anderson AR, et al. Modeling tumor-associated edema in gliomas during anti-angiogenic therapy and its impact on imageable tumor. *Front Oncol* 2013;3:66.
12. Fink J, Born D, Chamberlain MC. Pseudoprogression: relevance with respect to treatment of high-grade gliomas. *Curr Treat Options Oncol* 2011;12:240–252.
13. Lin NU, Lee EQ, Aoyama H, et al. Challenges relating to solid tumour brain metastases in clinical trials, part 1: patient population, response, and progression. A report from the RANO group. *Lancet Oncol* 2013;14:e396–e406.
14. Mabille M, Vanel D, Albiter M, et al. Follow-up of hepatic and peritoneal metastases of gastrointestinal tumors (GIST) under Imatinib therapy requires different criteria of radiological evaluation (size is not everything!!!). *Eur J Radiol* 2009;69:204–208.
15. Liu L, Wang W, Chen H, et al. EASL- and mRECIST-evaluated responses to combination therapy of sorafenib with transarterial chemoembolization predict survival in patients with hepatocellular carcinoma. *Clin Cancer Res* 2014;20:1623–1631.
16. Cheson BD, Pfistner B, Juweid ME, et al. Revised response criteria for malignant lymphoma. *J Clin Oncol* 2007;25:579–586.
17. Bernhard J, Dietrich D, Scheithauer W, et al. Clinical benefit and quality of life in patients with advanced pancreatic cancer receiving gemcitabine plus capecitabine versus gemcitabine alone: a randomized multicenter phase III clinical trial—SAKK 44/00-CECOG/PAN.1.3.001. *J Clin Oncol* 2008;26:3695–3701.
18. Burris HA, Moore MJ, Andersen J, et al. Improvements in survival and clinical benefit with gemcitabine as first-line therapy for patients with advanced pancreas cancer: a randomized trial. *J Clin Oncol* 1997;15:2403–2413.
19. Mann BS, Johnson JR, He K, et al. Vorinostat for treatment of cutaneous manifestations of advanced primary cutaneous T-cell lymphoma. *Clin Cancer Res* 2007;13:2318–2322.
20. von Minckwitz G, Untch M, Blohmer JU, et al. Definition and impact of pathologic complete response on prognosis after neoadjuvant chemotherapy in various intrinsic breast cancer subtypes. *J Clin Oncol* 2012;30:1796–1804.
21. Cortazar P, Zhang L, Untch M, et al. Pathological complete response and long-term clinical benefit in breast cancer: the CTNeoBC pooled analysis. *Lancet* 2014 [Epub ahead of print].
22. Bardia A, Baselga J. Neoadjuvant therapy as a platform for drug development and approval in breast cancer. *Clin Cancer Res* 2013;19:6360–6370.
23. Choi H, Charnsangavej C, Faria SC, et al. Correlation of computed tomography and positron emission tomography in patients with metastatic gastrointestinal stromal tumor treated at a single institution with imatinib mesylate: proposal of new computed tomography response criteria. *J Clin Oncol* 2007;25:1753–1759.
24. Schramm N, Englhart E, Schlemmer M, et al. Tumor response and clinical outcome in metastatic gastrointestinal stromal tumors under sunitinib therapy: comparison of RECIST, Choi and volumetric criteria. *Eur J Radiol* 2013;82:951–958.
25. Dudeck O, Zeile M, Reichardt P, et al. Comparison of RECIST and Choi criteria for computed tomographic response evaluation in patients with advanced gastrointestinal stromal tumor treated with sunitinib. *Ann Oncol* 2011;22:1828–1833.
26. Ronot M, Bouattour M, Wassermann J, et al. Alternative response criteria (Choi, European Association for the Study of the Liver, and Modified Response Evaluation Criteria in Solid Tumors [RECIST]) versus RECIST 1.1 in patients with advanced hepatocellular carcinoma treated with sorafenib. *Oncologist* 2014. http://prostatecancer.theoncologist.com/article/alternative-response-criteria-choi-european-association-study-liver-and-modified-response.
27. van der Veldt AA, Meijerink MR, van den Eertwegh AJ, et al. Choi response criteria for early prediction of clinical outcome in patients with metastatic renal cell cancer treated with sunitinib. *Br J Cancer* 2010;102:803–809.
28. Wahl RL, Jacene H, Kasamon Y, et al. From RECIST to PERCIST: evolving considerations for PET response criteria in solid tumors. *J Nucl Med* 2009;50:122S–150S.
29. Shankar LK, Hoffman JM, Bacharach S, et al. Consensus recommendations for the use of 18F-FDG PET as an indicator of therapeutic response in patients in National Cancer Institute Trials. *J Nucl Med* 2006;47:1059–1066.
30. Young H, Baum R, Cremerius U, et al. Measurement of clinical and subclinical tumour response using [18F]-fluorodeoxyglucose and positron emission tomography: review and 1999 EORTC recommendations. European Organization for Research and Treatment of Cancer (EORTC) PET Study Group. *Eur J Cancer* 1999;35:1773–1782.
31. Kramer-Marek G, Capala J. Can PET imaging facilitate optimization of cancer therapies? *Curr Pharm Des* 2012;18:2657–2669.
32. Niederkohr RD, Greenspan BS, Prior JO, et al. Reporting guidance for oncologic 18F-FDG PET/CT imaging. *J Nucl Med* 2013;54:756–761.
33. Liu Y, Litière S, de Vries EG, et al. The role of response evaluation criteria in solid tumour in anticancer treatment evaluation: results of a survey in the oncology community. *Eur J Cancer* 2014;50:260–266.
34. Rubin EH, Allen JD, Nowak JA, et al. Developing precision medicine in a global world. *Clin Cancer Res* 2014;20:1419–1427.
35. Parkinson DR, McCormack RT, Keating SM. Evidence of clinical utility: an unmet need in molecular diagnostics for cancer patients. *Clin Cancer Res* 2014;20:1428–1444.
36. Buyse M, Sargent DJ, Grothey A, et al. Biomarkers and surrogate end points—the challenge of statistical validation. *Nat Rev Clin Oncol* 2010;7:309–317.
37. Karam AK, Karlan BY. Ovarian cancer: the duplicity of CA125 measurement. *Nat Rev Clin Oncol* 2010;7:335–339.

38. Rustin GJ, van der Burg ME, Griffin CL, et al. Early versus delayed treatment of relapsed ovarian cancer (MRC OV05/EORTC 55955): a randomised trial. *Lancet* 2010;376:1155–1163.
39. Vergote I, Rustin GJ, Eisenhauer EA, et al. Re: new guidelines to evaluate the response to treatment in solid tumors [ovarian cancer]. Gynecologic Cancer Intergroup. *J Natl Cancer Inst* 2000;92:1534–1535.
40. Guppy AE, Rustin GJ. CA125 response: can it replace the traditional response criteria in ovarian cancer? *Oncologist* 2002;7:437–443.
41. Rustin GJ, Quinn M, Thigpen T, et al. Re: New guidelines to evaluate the response to treatment in solid tumors (ovarian cancer). *J Natl Cancer Inst* 2004; 96:487–488.
42. Rustin GJ, Vergote I, Eisenhauer E, et al. Definitions for response and progression in ovarian cancer clinical trials incorporating RECIST 1.1 and CA 125 agreed by the Gynecological Cancer Intergroup (GCIG). *Int J Gynecol Cancer* 2011;21:419–423.
43. Eisenhauer EA. Optimal assessment of response in ovarian cancer. *Ann Oncol* 2011;22:viii49–viii51.
44. Bubley GJ, Carducci M, Dahut W, et al. Eligibility and response guidelines for phase II clinical trials in androgen-independent prostate cancer: recommendations from the Prostate-Specific Antigen Working Group. *J Clin Oncol* 1999;17:3461–3467.
45. Scher HI, Halabi S, Tannock I, et al. Design and end points of clinical trials for patients with progressive prostate cancer and castrate levels of testosterone: recommendations of the Prostate Cancer Clinical Trials Working Group. *J Clin Oncol* 2008;26:1148–1159.
46. Mazumdar M, Bajorin DF, Bacik J, et al. Predicting outcome to chemotherapy in patients with germ cell tumors: the value of the rate of decline of human chorionic gonadotrophin and alpha-fetoprotein during therapy. *J Clin Oncol* 2001;19:2534–2541.
47. Fizazi K, Culine S, Kramar A, et al. Early predicted time to normalization of tumor markers predicts outcome in poor-prognosis nonseminomatous germ cell tumors. *J Clin Oncol* 2004;22:3868–3876.
48. Toner GC. Early identification of therapeutic failure in nonseminomatous germ cell tumors by assessing serum tumor marker decline during chemotherapy: still not ready for routine clinical use. *J Clin Oncol* 2004;22:3842–3845.
49. Gilligan TD, Seidenfeld J, Basch EM, et al. American Society of Clinical Oncology Clinical Practice Guideline on uses of serum tumor markers in adult males with germ cell tumors. *J Clin Oncol* 2010;28:3388–3404.
50. Albers P, Albrecht W, Algaba F, et al. EAU guidelines on testicular cancer: 2011 update. *Eur Urol* 2011;60:304–319.
51. Yap T, Lorente D, Omlin A, et al. Circulating tumor cells: a multifunctional biomarker. *Clin Cancer Res* 2014;20:2553–2568.
52. Dawson SJ, Tsui DW, Murtaza M, et al. Analysis of circulating tumor DNA to monitor metastatic breast cancer. *N Engl J Med* 2013;368:1199–1209.
53. Punnoose EA, Atwal S, Liu W, et al. Evaluation of circulating tumor cells and circulating tumor DNA in non-small cell lung cancer: association with clinical endpoints in a phase II clinical trial of pertuzumab and erlotinib. *Clin Cancer Res* 2012; 18:2391–2401.
54. Bettegowda C, Sausen M, Leary RJ, et al. Detection of circulating tumor DNA in early- and late-stage human malignancies. *Sci Transl Med* 2014;6:224ra24.
55. Pazdur R. Endpoints for assessing drug activity in clinical trials. *Oncologist* 2008;13:19–21.
56. Buyse M, Thirion P, Carlson RW, et al. Relation between tumour response to first-line chemotherapy and survival in advanced colorectal cancer: a meta-analysis. Meta-Analysis Group in Cancer. *Lancet* 2000;356:373–378.
57. Bruzzi P, Del Mastro L, Sormani MP, et al. Objective response to chemotherapy as a potential surrogate end point of survival in metastatic breast cancer patients. *J Clin Oncol* 2005;23:5117–5125.
58. Vidaurre T, Wilkerson J, Simon R, et al. Stable disease is not preferentially observed with targeted therapies and as currently defined has limited value in drug development. *Cancer J* 2009;15:366–373.
59. McKee AE, Farrell AT, Pazdur R, et al. The role of the U.S. Food and Drug Administration review process: clinical trial endpoints in oncology. *Oncologist* 2010;15:13–18.
60. Ohorodnyk P, Eisenhauer EA, Booth CM. Clinical benefit in oncology trials: is this a patient-centred or tumour-centred end-point? *Eur J Cancer* 2009; 45:2249–2252.
61. Buyse M. Use of meta-analysis for the validation of surrogate endpoints and biomarkers in cancer trials. *Cancer J* 2009;15:421–425.
62. Wilkerson J, Fojo T. Progression-free survival is simply a measure of a drug's effect while administered and is not a surrogate for overall survival. *Cancer J* 2009;15:379–385.
63. Reck M, von Pawel J, Zatloukal P, et al. Overall survival with cisplatin-gemcitabine and bevacizumab or placebo as first-line therapy for nonsquamous non-small-cell lung cancer: results from a randomised phase III trial (AVAiL). *Ann Oncol* 2010;21:1804–1809.
64. Hortobagyi GN, Gomez HL, Li RK, et al. Analysis of overall survival from a phase III study of ixabepilone plus capecitabine versus capecitabine in patients with MBC resistant to anthracyclines and taxanes. *Breast Cancer Res Treat* 2010; 122:409–418.
65. Hennekens C, Buring J. *Epidemiology in Medicine*. 1st ed. Boston: Little, Brown and Co.; 1987.
66. Cuzick J. Forest plots and the interpretation of subgroups. *Lancet* 2005;365:1308.
67. Huang H, Menefee M, Edgerly M, et al. A phase II clinical trial of ixabepilone (Ixempra; BMS-247550; NSC 710428), an epothilone B analog, in patients with metastatic renal cell carcinoma. *Clin Cancer Res* 2010;16:1634–1641.
68. Stein WD, Gulley JL, Schlom J, et al. Tumor regression and growth rates determined in five intramural NCI prostate cancer trials: the growth rate constant as an indicator of therapeutic efficacy. *Clin Cancer Res* 2011;17:907–917.
69. Stein WD, Wilkerson J, Kim ST, et al. Analyzing the pivotal trial that compared sunitinib and IFN-α in renal cell carcinoma, using a method that assesses tumor regression and growth. *Clin Cancer Res* 2012;18:2374–2381.
70. Maitland ML, Wu K, Sharma MR, et al. Estimation of renal cell carcinoma treatment effects from disease progression modeling. *Clin Pharmacol Ther* 2013;93:345–351.
71. Claret L, Girard P, Hoff PM, et al. Model-based prediction of phase III overall survival in colorectal cancer on the basis of phase II tumor dynamics. *J Clin Oncol* 2009;27:4103–4108.
72. Claret L, Gupta M, Han K, et al. Evaluation of tumor-size response metrics to predict overall survival in Western and Chinese patients with first-line metastatic colorectal cancer. *J Clin Oncol* 2013;31:2110–2114.
73. Wang Y, Sung C, Dartois C, et al. Elucidation of relationship between tumor size and survival in non-small-cell lung cancer patients can aid early decision making in clinical drug development. *Clin Pharmacol Ther* 2009;86:167–174.
74. Oxnard GR, Morris MJ, Hodi FS, et al. When progressive disease does not mean treatment failure: reconsidering the criteria for progression. *J Natl Cancer Inst* 2012;104:1534–1541.
75. Team RDC. R: A language and environment for statistical computing. R Foundation for Statistical Computing. Vienna, Austria: R Foundation for Statistical Computing, 2010. http://www.r-project.org.

PART IV

Cancer Prevention and Screening

31 Tobacco Use and the Cancer Patient

Graham W. Warren, Benjamin A. Toll, Irene M. Tamí-Maury, and Ellen R. Gritz

INTRODUCTION

Tobacco is commonly described as the largest preventable cause of cancer. Over 50 years ago, tobacco was increasingly recognized as the primary cause of lung cancer, with definitive recognition for tobacco use as a causative factor in the seminal 1964 U.S. Surgeon General's Report (SGR) on Smoking and Health.[1] Recent editions of the SGR have described the widespread adverse health effects of tobacco on a spectrum of diseases, including as a causative agent for a spectrum of cancers.[2,3] Tobacco use is an addiction usually initiated in youth prior to the age of 18 and is driven by the highly addictive drug, nicotine.[4] As related to the cancer patient, considerable work has been conducted to associate tobacco use with the risk of developing cancer and how tobacco cessation can substantially reduce cancer risks. However, there is a relative paucity of effort that has been put forth to identify the effects of smoking on outcomes for cancer patients or to establish methods to help cancer patients quit smoking. Fortunately, in recent years, the importance of tobacco use by the cancer patient has been increasingly recognized as an important health behavior, including a National Cancer Institute (NCI)–sponsored conference on tobacco use in 2010, a joint sponsored NCI–American Association of Cancer Research (AACR)–sponsored workshop at the Institute of Medicine in 2012, and recent recommendations by the AACR and the American Society of Clinical Oncology (ASCO) to address tobacco use in cancer patients.[5,6] The recently released 2014 SGR now provides substantial evidence behind the effects of smoking by cancer patients with the following conclusions[7]:

1. In cancer patients and survivors, the evidence is sufficient to infer a causal relationship between cigarette smoking and adverse health outcomes. Quitting smoking improves the prognosis of cancer patients.
2. In cancer patients and survivors, the evidence is sufficient to infer a causal relationship between cigarette smoking and increased all-cause mortality and cancer-specific mortality.
3. In cancer patients and survivors, the evidence is sufficient to infer a causal relationship between cigarette smoking and increased risk for second primary cancers known to be caused by cigarette smoking, such as lung cancer.
4. In cancer patients and survivors, the evidence is suggestive but not sufficient to infer a causal relationship between cigarette smoking and the risk of recurrence, poorer response to treatment, and increased treatment-related toxicity.

The overall objective of this chapter is to discuss tobacco use by cancer patients, the clinical effects of smoking in cancer patients, methods to address tobacco use by cancer patients, and areas of needed research.

NEUROBIOLOGY OF TOBACCO DEPENDENCE

Nicotine is the primary addictive component of tobacco that increases extracellular concentrations of dopamine in the nucleus accumbens and stimulates the mesolimbic dopaminergic system,[8,9] resulting in nicotine's rewarding effect experienced by tobacco users.[10–12] Dopaminergic neurotransmission may also be involved in the assignment of incentive salience, or stimulus for a pleasure based reward, to tobacco use–related environmental cues[13,14] that may become conditioned reinforcers of tobacco use behaviors. For example, an individual who smokes while drinking their morning coffee may associate coffee, or even holding a coffee cup in their hand, with the reward from smoking. Thus, cigarette smoking is directly linked to external nontobacco-based behavioral stimuli. Activation of the nucleus accumbens has further been implicated in drug reinstatement or relapse.[15,16] Individuals who have quit tobacco use for years have restarted a tobacco habit simply by sitting next to a smoker and being exposed to secondhand smoke. Substantial work has been conducted on the addictive nature of tobacco and nicotine, and readers are referred to several comprehensive reviews on this topic.[9,12,17]

TOBACCO USE PREVALENCE AND THE EVOLUTION OF TOBACCO PRODUCTS

Much of the discussion on tobacco use epidemiology and carcinogenesis is presented in Chapter 4. In brief, the prevalence of cigarette smoking among adults in the United States decreased to 19.0% as compared with 22.8% in 2001, but it did not meet the *Healthy People 2010* objective to reduce smoking prevalence to 12%.[18,19] There have been substantial changes in the landscape of tobacco use over time as a direct consequence of cigarette-centered policies and regulations aiming to reduce the harmful effects and number of deaths caused by smoking.[20–22] Under this new landscape, novel and reemergent noncigarette tobacco products such as cigars, cigarillos, snuff, chewing tobacco, water pipes (hookahs), and other forms of tobacco consumption have been growing in demand as a consequence of aggressive and sophisticated marketing by the tobacco industry.[23] Consumption patterns have also changed due to efforts by the tobacco industry to make cigarettes appear safer, such as low tar or filtered cigarettes, and the inclusion of flavoring (menthol, vanilla, fruits, etc.).[24] Although these efforts may have changed consumption patterns, they have not reduced cancer risk. Large patient cohorts demonstrate that the introduction of low tar and filtered cigarettes actually increased risk by promoting deeper inhalation and higher rates of addiction with no reductions in cancer risk,[24,25] resulting in subsequent changes in lung cancer from centrally located squamous cell cancers to peripherally located nonsquamous cell cancers.

The relatively recent introduction of electronic cigarettes (i.e., e-cigarettes, e-cigs, nicotine vaporizers, or electronic nicotine delivery systems [ENDS]) is noteworthy. These electronic or battery-powered devices activate a heating element that vaporizes a liquid solution contained in a cartridge, and then the user inhales this vapor. Levels of nicotine as well as other chemical additives and flavors in the cartridge are uncertain and vary according to the brand.[26] Although there are no research studies that have evaluated the potential harmful effects of the use of e-cigarettes for cancer patients,[27] organizations such as the World Health Organization have already expressed concerns about the safety of these increasingly popular products.[28,29] To date, e-cigarettes have not been approved by the U.S. Food and Drug Administration (FDA) as therapeutic devices to aid in quitting smoking.[26] Readers are referred to a recent editorial on the use of e-cigarettes by cancer patients[27]; however, it will likely be several years before evidence-based health information is available.

TOBACCO USE BY THE CANCER PATIENT

The prevalence of current smoking among long-term adult cancer survivors appears to have declined in the past decade,[30] but data suggest higher rates of smoking among cancer survivors than in the general population.[30–32] These data are often biased by the fact that assessments in cancer patients may not include cancer patients who were current smokers at the time of death. As a result, estimates of smoking rates in cancer survivors may be misleading and may underestimate true tobacco use patterns for cancer patients. Furthermore, alternative tobacco products are often not assessed in cancer patients. Data from the Childhood Cancer Survivor Study and the 2009 Behavioral Risk Factor Surveillance System indicate that approximately 3% to 8% of cancer survivors use smokeless tobacco products.[33,34] Patients may be attracted to these alternative products due to less social stigma and the nonevidence-based perception that these products are healthier alternatives compared to cigarette smoking.

Continued tobacco use by cancer patients often represents a combined failure by the patient to recognize the need to stop smoking even after a cancer diagnosis and the effort by health-care providers to address tobacco use with evidence-based assessments and tobacco cessation support. Approximately 30% of all cancer patients use tobacco at the time of cancer diagnosis with higher rates in traditionally tobacco-related disease sites, such as head and neck or lung cancers, and lower rates in traditionally nontobacco-related disease sites, such as breast or prostate cancers.[35–44] However, findings from several studies indicate that cancer patients are receptive to smoking cessation interventions even as they continue to smoke.[35,38,45–50]

A cancer diagnosis can be used as a window of opportunity, or *teachable moment*, to intervene and provide assistance in the quitting process.[51] A recent study in 12,000 cancer patients, including 2,700 patients who smoked, capitalized on the teachable moment and demonstrated that less than 3% of patients who were contacted by the cessation program rejected tobacco cessation assistance.[45] However, only 1.2% of patients who received a mailed invitation participated in the program. This highlights the idea that patients may be interested in quitting, but methods such as mailed tobacco cessation information may not yield effective participation by cancer patients. Once enrolled, patients and clinicians must realize that although relapses in the general population usually occur within 1 week of cessation, relapses in cancer patients may be delayed due to cancer treatment–related variables such as surgical or other posttreatment healing.[52] Consequently, it is important to continue offering tobacco assessments and cessation support for cancer survivorship efforts.

Defining Tobacco Use by the Cancer Patient

In dealing with tobacco use by cancer patients, it is important to note that virtually all of the evidence associating tobacco with cancer treatment outcomes deals with smoking. Few studies report associations between other forms of tobacco use (e.g., smokeless, cigars, cigarillos) and outcomes in cancer patients. Furthermore, the definition of smoking across published studies varies substantially.[53] In studies of cancer patients, smoking has been defined as current (e.g., smoking after diagnosis, at diagnosis, in the weeks before diagnosis, within the 12 months prior to diagnosis, after diagnosis, within the past 10 years), former (e.g., recent, intermediate-, or long-term quit for 1 month, 3 month, 6 month, 12 month, 2 years, 5 years, 10 years), never, quitting after diagnosis, and according to exposure (e.g., multiple pack year cutoffs, Brinkman index, years of smoking, years of smoking within a predefined period of time such as 5 years prior to diagnosis). Though the nonstandard method of addressing tobacco use in cancer patients has been observed in several reports,[54–57] there are no current standard recommendations for the definition of tobacco use by any national organization. There are four primary categories for smoking status:

1. **Never smoking** is typically defined as having smoked less than 100 cigarettes in a person's lifetime and no current cigarette use. These patients are generally considered as a reference group in many studies. Categories 2 through 4 require that a person has smoked at least 100 cigarettes in their lifetime.
2. **Former smoking** is typically defined as no current cigarette use, usually within the past year.
3. **Recent smoking** (or recent quit) is generally defined as having stopped smoking within the recent past, typically for a period of 1 week to 1 year.
4. **Current smoking** is typically defined as smoking one or more cigarettes per day every day or some days.

Ever smoking is a combination of categories 2 through 4 (i.e., former, recent, and current smokers) that has been used to report negative associations between smoking and cancer outcomes in a number of studies.[58–70] Defining smoking according to *ever* smoking status limits the ability to interpret the effects of current smoking on a clinical outcome, and nothing can be done to address a prior tobacco use history. However, defining exposure according to *current* smoking status allows for the analysis of potentially reversible effects as well as for the potential implementation of smoking cessation to prevent the adverse outcomes of smoking on cancer patients. The primary focus for the remainder of this chapter will be on *current* smoking and will include a discussion of methods to address tobacco use with the cancer patient through accurate assessments and structured tobacco cessation support.

THE CLINICAL EFFECTS OF SMOKING ON THE CANCER PATIENT

Cancer treatment is generally defined according to disease site, stage, treatment type (e.g., surgery, chemotherapy [CT], radiotherapy [RT], or biologic therapy), and primary treatment objective, such as cure or palliation. A comprehensive discussion of the effects of smoking on cancer patients is beyond the scope of a single chapter, but the 2014 SGR provides an excellent evidence base, concluding that "the evidence is sufficient to infer a causal relationship between cigarette smoking and adverse health outcomes."[7] Overall, approximately 75% to 80% of studies in the SGR demonstrated a negative association between smoking and outcome, with approximately 65% to 70% of studies demonstrating statistically significant negative associations. This chapter will provide an illustrative review of studies that demonstrate the adverse effects of tobacco across disease sites and treatment modalities (e.g., surgery, CT, RT), and effects will be discussed across the categories of *mortality*, *recurrence and cancer-related mortality*, *toxicity*, and *risk of a second primary cancer*. Evidence for the benefits of smoking cessation will also be presented within each section.

The Effect of Smoking on Overall Mortality

Substantial evidence demonstrates that current smoking by cancer patients increases the risk of overall mortality across virtually all cancer disease sites and for all treatment modalities. Currently smoking significantly increased the risk of overall mortality by between 17% to 38% as compared with never, former, and recent quit smokers in a large cohort of patients across 13 disease sites.[71] Similar but larger observations were noted in elderly current smokers from a separate cohort (hazard ratio [HR], 1.72, 95% confidence interval [CI], 1.23 to 2.42).[72] A large analysis of over 20,000 patients treated with surgery demonstrated that current smoking increased mortality by 62% in gastrointestinal cancer patients and by 50% in thoracic cancer patients with a nonsignificant trend in urologic cancer patients.[73] Several larger studies with at least 500 patients demonstrated that current smoking increases mortality in head and neck cancer,[74–77] breast cancer,[78–81] gastrointestinal cancers,[82,83] prostate cancer,[84–87] renal cancer,[88] gynecologic cancers,[89,90] and lung cancer.[91–102] Smaller studies demonstrate similar effects for hematolymphoid cancers such as leukemia and lymphoma.[103,104] Studies suggest that the effects of current smoking on mortality may be dose and time dependent, with higher risks in heavier smokers[105,106] and lesser risks in patients whose time since quitting was longer.[105]

Whereas many reports rely on retrospective chart reviews, several prospective studies demonstrate that current smoking increases mortality.[71] Browman et al.[107] was one of the first prospective studies to demonstrate that current smoking increased mortality by 2.3-fold in patients who continued to smoke during RT as compared with nonsmokers. Results from Radiation Therapy Oncology Group (RTOG) 9003 and 0129 cooperative group trials demonstrated that current smoking increased mortality in advanced head and neck cancer patients treated with RT or concurrent chemoradiotherapy (CRT),[108] with a similar effect noted in 165 cervical cancer patients treated with CRT.[109] In the randomized retinoid chemoprevention trial of 1,190 early stage head and neck cancer patients, current smoking increased mortality by 2.5-fold.[110]

Numerous studies have demonstrated that current smoking increases overall mortality as compared with former and never smokers combined.[72,75,76,101,102,107,108] The adverse effects of smoking compared with former and never smokers not only reflect the negative effects of smoking on mortality as a whole, but also demonstrate that the effects of smoking are reversible. Current smoking increased mortality risk as compared with patients who quit within the year[71] or 1 to 3 months prior to diagnosis.[111,112] Furthermore, in 284 limited-stage small-cell lung cancer patients, patients who quit smoking at or following a cancer diagnosis had a 45% reduction in mortality as compared with current smokers.[113] These studies suggest that the effects of smoking on mortality are reversible.

Collectively, these studies provide significant data associating current smoking with increased overall mortality across most disease sites, tumor stages, treatment modalities, and in both traditionally tobacco-related as well as nontobacco-related cancers. The potential significance of smoking is perhaps best exemplified by Bittner et al.,[114] who analyzed causes of death in prostate cancer patients and demonstrated that more than 90% died of causes other than prostate cancer, but that current smoking increased the risks of non–prostate cancer deaths between 3- and 5.5-fold. As a result, tobacco use and cessation may be of paramount importance to cancers with high cure rates, such as prostate cancer or breast cancer, simply because patients may be at the most risk of death from noncancer-related causes such as heart disease, pulmonary disease, or other diseases related to smoking and tobacco use.

The Effect of Smoking on Cancer Recurrence and Cancer-Related Mortality

The primary objective of cancer therapy is to cure cancer and prevent recurrence. However, smoking has been shown to increase cancer recurrence and cancer-related mortality. Across a broad spectrum of cancer patients, current smoking increased cancer mortality as compared with former and never smokers.[71] Current smoking has been shown to increase cancer mortality in patients with head and neck cancer,[108,115–118] breast cancer,[78,119] gastrointestinal cancers,[82,120,121] prostate cancer,[41,84,122] gynecologic cancers,[89,90,106,123–125] and lung cancer.[126] Cancer recurrence, whether local or metastatic, is a key driver behind cancer-related mortality. Several studies demonstrate that current smoking increases the risk of recurrence and decreases response across multiple disease sites.[76,84,107,127,128] The effects of smoking on increasing recurrence or cancer-related mortality have also been reported in several relatively rare cancers.[120,129] In a remarkable report of patients with recurrent head and neck cancers treated with salvage surgery, continued smoking after salvage treatment continued to increase the risk of yet another recurrence by 42%.[130] The striking nature of this last study highlights the continued risks even in recurrent cancer patients and the resilience with which some cancer patients will continue to smoke.

The effects of smoking are also noted in premalignant lesions. In patients with high-grade vulvar intraepithelial neoplasia, current smoking increased the risk of persistent disease after therapy by 30-fold.[131] In a prospective trial of progesterone to treat cervical intraepithelial neoplasia (CIN), current smoking increased the risk of progression as compared with former and never smokers combined.[132] A prospective trial of 516 low-grade cervical intraepithelial neoplasia patients demonstrated that current smoking decreased response by 36%, although a similar effect was also noted in former smokers.[133]

As noted with overall mortality, several studies demonstrated that the effects of current smoking are worse than the effects of former smoking[76,86,89,109,127,134–136,137] and that the effects of smoking may be acutely reversible. Several studies also demonstrate that current smoking increases recurrence or cancer mortality, whereas former smoking has no significant effect.[41,78,82,84,85,119,122–124,138] The acutely reversible effects of smoking were shown by Browman et al.[139] who demonstrated that continued smoking increased the risk of cancer-related mortality by 23% as compared with patients who quit within 12 weeks of starting RT. In 284 colorectal cancer patients, smoking at the first postoperative visit increased the risk of cancer mortality by 2.5-fold as compared with all other patients suggesting that smoking after treatment significantly predict for adverse outcome.[121] In a notable study of over 1,400 prostate cancer patients treated with surgery, continued smoking 1 year after treatment increased the risk of recurrence 2.3-fold, but quitting smoking 1 year after treatment did not confer an increased risk of recurrence.[128] Chen et al.[138] demonstrate that patients who continue to smoke before and following a bladder cancer diagnosis have an increased risk of recurrence as compared with patients who quit in the year prior to diagnosis or within the first 3 months after diagnosis. The reversible effects of smoking on recurrence and mortality are consistent with observations on overall mortality and continue to emphasize the benefit of tobacco cessation for cancer patients who smoke at diagnosis.

The Effect of Smoking on Cancer Treatment Toxicity

Discussion of the effects of smoking on cancer treatment toxicity is highly dependent upon disease site, treatment modality (e.g., surgery, CT, RT), and timing of toxicity. Across disease sites and treatments, current smoking has been shown to increase complications from surgery,[140–149] pulmonary complications,[150,151] toxicity from RT,[117,152–156] mucositis,[157] hospitalization,[158] and vasomotor symptoms.[159] One of the largest recent studies in over 20,000 gastrointestinal, pulmonary, and urologic patients demonstrates that former or current smoking increased the risk of surgical site infection, pulmonary complications, or 30-day mortality in a site-specific manner.[73] The effects of current smoking were most significant for pulmonary complications where former smoking had a lesser or nonsignificant effect. In 13,469 lung cancer patients treated with surgery, current smoking increased the risk of postoperative death with no increased risk in former smokers.[160] Current smoking increased the risk of complications, morbidity, or reoperation following esophagectomy, pancreatectomy, or colorectal surgery.[161–163] A study of 836 prostate cancer patients treated with RT demonstrated that current smoking increased abdominal cramps, rectal urgency, diarrhea, incomplete emptying, and sudden emptying between two- and nine-fold,[164] with similar effects noted in 3,489 cervical cancer patients who smoked more than 1 pack per day (PPD).[156]

Several studies have demonstrated that the effects of smoking on cancer treatment toxicity are reversible. Stopping smoking within 3 weeks of surgery reduced wound healing complications in esophageal cancer patients treated with surgery and reconstruction.[165] In 393 T1 laryngeal cancer patients treated with RT, quitting smoking after diagnosis reduced laryngeal complications as compared with continued smoking.[152] In a large study of 7,990 lung cancer patients from the Society of Thoracic Surgeons Database, current smoking increased the risk of pulmonary complications by 80% and hospital mortality 3.5-fold.[151] However, smoking cessation for 2 weeks eliminated the risks for pulmonary complications, and cessation for 1 month eliminated risks for hospital mortality. Vaporciyan et al.[166] also showed that current smoking increased the risk of pulmonary complications 2.7-fold as compared with smoking cessation for at least 1 month prior to surgery. In a striking example of the potentially reversible effects of smoking in 205 head and neck cancer patients treated with RT,[167] 43% of smoking patients treated in the morning experienced Grade 3+ mucositis compared with 72% of smokers treated in the afternoon ($p = 0.04$). These data suggest that reducing smoking overnight may yield a clinical benefit in reduced toxicity. Whereas all toxicity may not be acutely reversed, these encouraging data show that patients can make clinically meaningful improvements in their health and or cancer treatment within a short time frame by quitting smoking.

The Effect of Smoking on Risk of Second Primary Cancer

Several studies have reported the effects of smoking on the risk of developing a second primary cancer. Park et al.[168] reported on over 14,000 male cancer patients and demonstrated that current smoking increased the risk of developing a second tobacco-related primary cancer twofold, with no increased risk in former smokers. A higher risk was observed in in head and neck cancer patients who smoked more than 10 cigarettes per day, with no increased risk in lighter smokers.[169] Kinoshita et al.[170] showed an 82% increased risk of developing a second primary in gastric cancer patients who are current smokers with no increased risk in former smokers. In the phase III randomized trial of isotretinoin for the prevention of a second primary tumor in 1,190 head and neck cancer patients, current smoking increased the risk of a second primary by 2.2-fold with a nonsignificant trend of 1.6-fold in former smokers.[110] Notably, 39% of patients who reported quitting within the previous year were biochemically confirmed smokers.[171] As a result, these data collectively suggest that some of the increased risk may be biased by continued smoking in patients who deny smoking by self-report.

The effects of smoking on the risk of a second primary cancer are also noted in nontobacco-related cancers and in long-term survivors. In 835 breast cancer patients, smoking increased the risk for the development of lung metastases after breast cancer by more than threefold.[172] Ford et al.[173] demonstrated that breast cancer patients who were former smokers had a threefold increased risk of developing lung cancer, but that current smokers had a 13-fold increased risk. In nearly 1,100 estrogen receptor (ER)-positive breast cancer patients, current smokers had a 1.8-fold increased risk of developing a second contralateral breast cancer, and current smokers at most recent follow-up had a 2.2-fold increased risk, but former smoking at the diagnosis or most recent follow-up had no increased risk.[174] In 2,700 5-year survivors of testicular cancer, current smokers had a 1.8-fold increased risk of developing a second primary as compared with all other survivors.[175]

There are some studies suggesting that smoking, combined with cytotoxic therapy, may have an additive or synergistic effect on the risk of developing a second primary cancer. In 9,780 prostate cancer patients from the Cancer of the Prostate Strategic Urologic Research Endeavor (CaPSURE) study, RT increased the risk of bladder cancer by 1.6-fold, smoking increased the risk by 2.1-fold, and smoking combined with RT increased risk by 3.7-fold.[176] In ER-positive breast cancer patients, treatment with RT had no significant effect on the risk of developing a contralateral breast cancer, but RT combined with current smoking increased the risk of contralateral cancer by ninefold.[173] In a detailed analysis of Hodgkin lymphoma patients, nonheavy smokers (defined as never, former, and less than one PPD) had a second primary relative risk of between fourfold and sevenfold when treated with CT or RT as compared with patients who received no RT or CT.[177] However, heavy smokers had a sixfold increased risk in the absence of RT and CT and a 17- to 49-fold increased risk when combined with RT and/or CT. These observations suggest that smoking combined with cytotoxic cancer therapy may complement the risk of developing a second primary cancer perhaps through the promotion of mutations induced by CT and/or RT in the presence of tobacco smoke. The potential mechanisms of this effect have not been tested or defined at this time, but the mechanism of tobacco-induced carcinogenesis in prior reports[3] supports these observations.

Human Papilloma Virus, Epidermal Growth Factor Receptor, Anaplastic Lymphoma Kinase, Programmed Cell Death Protein 1, and Smoking

Data over the past decade has shown that head and neck cancers that are human papilloma virus (HPV) positive are known to have an improved prognosis as compared with HPV-negative tumors.[178] Patients who have HPV-positive tumors typically have increased p16 expression and often respond better to conventional cancer therapy, including RT and CT. Many HPV-positive patients are never smokers or have a lighter smoking history. However, smoking was an independent adverse risk factor for both overall and cancer-related mortality with a 1% increase in risk per pack-year smoked.[178] Current smoking increased cancer mortality approximately fivefold even in p16-positive patients treated with surgery.[115] Smoking also increased the risk of developing second primary cancer in both HPV-positive and HPV-negative patients.[179] As a consequence, the presence of HPV does not appear to negate the adverse effects of smoking.

A similar effect is noted in lung cancer patients with epidermal growth factor receptor (EGFR)-mutated or anaplastic lymphoma kinase (ALK)-mutated tumors. As with HPV-positive head and neck cancer patients, lung cancer patients who are light or never smokers have a higher rate of EGFR-positive tumors that may respond to biologic therapy using EGFR tyrosine–kinase inhibitors. At this time, most information regarding EGFR-based therapy for lung cancer reports on the effects of ever smoking demonstrating that ever smokers have a decreased response to EGFR therapy. Early, large, randomized trials demonstrate that Tarceva (erlotinib) and Iressa (gefitinib) provide survival and tumor control benefits specifically in never smokers.[180,181] A very similar pattern is noted for ALK-positive patients with a much higher incidence in never smokers and high response rate to the ALK kinase inhibitor crizotinib.[182] Paik et al.[183] have described the importance of driver mutations in EGFR, ALK, and KRAS demonstrating that smokers have a higher preponderance for K-ras drivers, whereas nonsmokers tend to have EGFR or ALK driver mutations. In general, patients who are smokers may be best served with conventional cancer treatments rather than these biologic therapies, but randomized controlled trials confirming this suggestion are lacking at this time.

Although there are essentially no biologic therapies that have shown to have a better response in smokers, there are exciting data presented at the 2013 European CanCer Organization (ECCO) annual conference, suggesting that anti–programmed cell death protein 1 (PD-1)–based therapies may have a better response rate in smokers.[184] These very preliminary data have yet to be replicated or expanded into randomized trials, but if expanded trials prove effective, they may represent one of the only cancer treatments that may specifically benefit smokers.

Summarizing the Clinical Effects of Smoking on the Cancer Patient

Smoking by cancer patients increases mortality, toxicity, recurrence, and the risk of a second primary cancer. There are four important conclusions, and a fifth implied conclusion, to the evidence previously presented:

1. One or more adverse effects of smoking affect all cancer disease sites.
2. One or more adverse effects of smoking affect all treatment modalities.
3. The effects of current smoking are distinct from an ever or former smoking history.
4. Several lines of evidence demonstrate that many of the effects of smoking are reversible.

Although substantial data demonstrate that smoking by cancer patients increases the risk for one or more outcomes, the largest limitations are the lack of standard tobacco use definitions, the lack of assessing tobacco use in cancer patients at follow-up, and the lack of structured tobacco cessation for cancer patients. Importantly, patients may further misrepresent tobacco use. Several studies suggest that approximately 30% of cancer patients who smoke deny tobacco use.[171,185,186] Marin et al.[187] exemplify the importance of an accurate assessment, demonstrating that patients who self-reported smoking had no significant risk associated with surgical complications; however, biochemical confirmation of smoking significantly increased the risk of surgical wound complications. This highlights the potential discrepancy between the effects of smoking based on subjective versus biochemically confirmed assessments. Due to this discrepancy, the *fifth implied conclusion* is that the adverse effects of smoking and the benefits of cessation may be more pronounced than currently reported in the literature.

ADDRESSING TOBACCO USE BY THE CANCER PATIENT

National Oncology Association Statements and Clinical Practice Guidelines

Professional societies are taking leadership roles in recognizing the need to assess patients' tobacco use and to examine the effects of tobacco use in medical treatment, including the important role of tobacco cessation. The American Medical Association (AMA) passed a resolution supporting documentation of smoking behavior in clinical trials, from trial registration through treatment, follow-up, and to end of the study or death.[188] The Oncology Nursing Society (ONS) has also advocated for assessment and cessation.[189,190] Both the AACR[5,191] and ASCO[6,192] have issued policy statements specifically addressing tobacco use in cancer patients, detailing that clinicians have a responsibility to address tobacco use, that all patients should be screened, that all patients who use tobacco should receive evidence-based tobacco cessation support, and that tobacco use should be included in clinical practice and research. These provide strong counsel to address tobacco use in the general population as well as in cancer patients.

Smoking Cessation Guidelines

Overall, the approach to tobacco cessation for the cancer patient is very similar to the approach for the general population. However, there are a few specific details that are important to consider when approaching the cancer patient who smokes. It is important to recognize that virtually all newly diagnosed cancer patients are faced with a life-changing diagnosis that will require intensive treatment approaches. Treatments, toxicity, and outcomes differ according to disease site and treatment modality. Whereas some cancer patients may have a curable cancer, others may have incurable cancer. Smoking in cancer patients is also often associated with comorbid psychiatric diseases, such as depression, that may affect dependence.[193] The urgency of cessation is also important to consider. If smoking decreases the efficacy of cancer treatment, then every effort should be made to stop tobacco use as soon as possible rather than choosing a quit date several weeks or months after a cancer diagnosis. Patients may also be burdened with a "stigma" associated with certain tobacco-related cancers,[193–197] where they may be viewed by others, or themselves, as causing their cancer due to tobacco use. As a result, the rationale and motivation for quitting tobacco use likely differs among cancer patients, but there is a consistent theme that exists. (1) All patients should be asked about tobacco use with structured assessments; (2) all patients who use tobacco or are at risk for relapse should be offered evidence-based cessation support; and 3) tobacco assessment and cessation support should occur at the time of diagnosis, during treatment, and during follow-up for all cancer patients.

Empiric treatment of tobacco use by cancer patients is fundamentally supported by Public Health Service (PHS) Guidelines that are based on evidence from tobacco cessation efforts in noncancer patients. Originally issued in 1996 and renewed in 2008, *The Clinical Practice Guideline: Treating Tobacco Use and Dependence* is a PHS-sponsored, evidence-based guideline designed to assist health-care providers in delivering and supporting effective smoking cessation treatment.[198,199] The basic recommendation states that clinicians should consistently identify, document, and treat every tobacco user seen in a health-care setting. Details of cessation support range from brief to intensive intervention, but emphasize that consistent repeated cessation support and even brief counseling are effective methods to assist patients with stopping tobacco use. It is important to note that physician-delivered interventions significantly increase long-term abstinence rates.[199] Included are newer effective medication options and strong support for counseling and the use of quit lines as effective intervention strategies. As described in the PHS Guidelines, the principal steps in conducting effective smoking cessation interventions are referred to as The 5 A's:

1. *Ask* about tobacco use for every patient.
2. *Advise* every tobacco user to quit.
3. *Assess* the willingness of patients to quit.
4. *Assist* patients with quitting through counseling and pharmacotherapy.
5. *Arrange* follow-up cessation support, preferably within the first week after the quit date.

There is a strong evidence base for these interventions as documented in the clinical practice guideline.[199]

Implementing Smoking Cessation Into Clinical Practice

An algorithm is provided to guide clinicians in implementing the five A's into clinical cancer care (Fig. 31.1).[5,45,194,199] Included in the algorithm are suggested questions that are useful to accurately assess tobacco use by cancer patients where patients can generally be divided into *current, former,* or *never* smokers. The first step (ASK) is to inquire about and document tobacco use behaviors for every

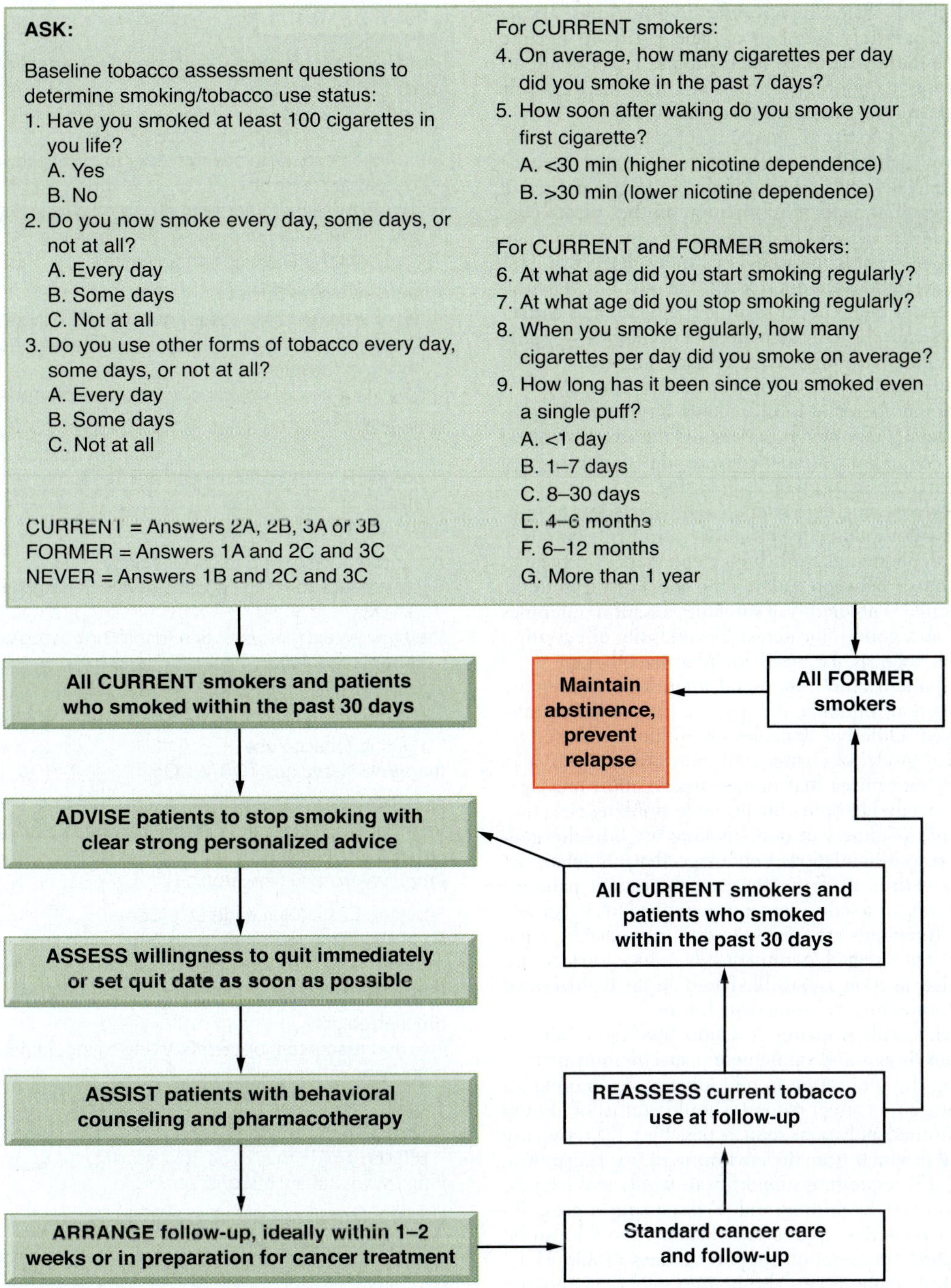

Figure 31.1 This 5 A's screening and smoking cessation treatment schema for cancer patients may be integrated into clinical oncology practice.

patient at every visit including follow-up visits. Whereas a more comprehensive evaluation is necessary at the first consult, only updates to current tobacco use are needed at follow-up. Including smoking status assessments as a "vital sign" for all patients significantly increases the identification and treatment for patients.[200] Tobacco-use status stickers on paper charts or an automated reminder system for electronic records can increase compliance with tobacco assessments.[45] With the recent Meaningful Use standards that were implemented in 2011, hospitals using an electronic medical record (EMR) are essentially required to document tobacco use.[201] A recent report utilized the EMR to implement mandatory tobacco assessments in cancer patients demonstrating that just a few questions at the initial evaluation and at follow-up could yield high referral. Less than 1% of referrals were delayed when assessments were repeated on a monthly basis rather than at every clinic visit.[45] These findings reduce the clinical burden and patient fatigue associated with repeated assessments as frequently as every day such as in patients who are treated with daily RT or CT.

At the time of this chapter release, there were no national guidelines for implementation of specific questions to assess tobacco use in cancer patients. However, Figure 31.1 provides effective questions for assessing tobacco use in cancer patients based on advice from published reports.[5,45,194,199] Current, former, and never smokers are identified in a structured manner. Patients who use tobacco within the past 30 days should have structured support to quit tobacco use, maintain abstinence, and prevent relapse.

Although not explicitly stated by any specific guidelines, asking about tobacco use in family members of cancer patients may be important because family members often support cancer patients during and following treatment, but continued smoking by family members can make quitting much more difficult.[202–204]

Advising is the second step in promoting effective tobacco cessation that involves giving clear, strong, and personalized advice to stop tobacco use. This advice should include the importance of quitting smoking, such as explicit information on the risks of continued smoking and the benefits of cessation for cancer treatment outcomes and overall health regardless of cancer diagnosis. This includes a discussion of how it is not "too late" to quit and that quitting will in fact benefit their cancer treatment efficacy and cancer outcome.[5] Patients can also consider the cost savings of stopping a smoking habit. Clinicians must be particularly sensitive to avoid contributing to any perceived blame for the patient's illness.[195–197,205] Clinicians must remember that most patients started smoking in adolescence and did not completely understand the risks associated with tobacco use. At the same time, the severe addiction associated with chronic tobacco use makes it difficult to stop.

The next step is *assessing* dependence and willingness to quit. Asking "How soon after waking do you smoke your first cigarette?" assesses nicotine dependence, with high dependence associated with a shorter interval between waking and the first cigarette.[206] Nicotine dependence is predictive of smoking cessation outcomes and can be used as a good indicator of the intensity of cessation treatment needed, such as the need for pharmacotherapy.[207,208] Determining the patient's motivation and interest in quitting are critical parameters that influence the types of intervention strategies to be employed. Different strategies for quitting are based on the transtheoretical model of change and motivational interviewing stance, which recognizes that unique intervention messages and strategies are needed to optimally promote smoking cessation based on a patient's readiness to quit smoking.[209,210] In the general population, recommendations encourage that clinicians set a target quit date within 30 days. However, for cancer patients, the reader is encouraged to consider an urgent need to stop smoking immediately. If patients are unable to quit immediately, then patients should be encouraged to immediately reduce tobacco use and to set a quit date as soon as possible based on the typical need to start cancer treatment in the immediate future.

Assisting patients with smoking cessation involves clinicians helping the patient design and implement a specific quit plan or broadly enhancing the motivation to quit tobacco. Promoting an effective quit strategy for cancer patients should consist of (1) setting a quit date (immediately or as soon as possible), (2) removing all tobacco-related products from the environment (e.g., cigarettes, ashtrays, lighters), (3) requesting support from family and friends, (4) discussing challenges to quitting, and (5) discussing or prescribing pharmacotherapy where appropriate. Patients should also be provided information on cessation support services (Table 31.1). In the cancer setting, patients can also be informed that smoking cessation is a critical component of cancer care over which they have complete control, thereby conferring some personal control over their cancer care.

Patients who are unwilling to quit should continue to receive repeated assessments and counseling to help motivate patients to quit smoking. These patients should be encouraged to make immediate reductions in tobacco use and work toward abstinence as soon as possible. Clinician education, reassurance, and gentle encouragement can help them to consider changing their smoking behaviors. Specific strategies include discussing the personal relevance of smoking and benefits to cessation, providing support and acknowledging the difficulty of quitting, educating patients about the positive consequences of quitting smoking, and discussing available pharmacologic methods to assist with quitting.[211] The emphasis should be placed on patient autonomy to quit. Motivational strategies for patients unwilling to quit can be employed (e.g., asking open-ended questions, providing affirmations, reflective listening, summarizing).[198,210,212,213] Table 31.2 provides suggested methods to help clinicians promote tobacco cessation.

The final step in a clinician-delivered smoking cessation intervention involves *arranging* a follow-up contact with the patient. Ideally, cancer patients will follow an immediate quit strategy and follow-up should occur preferably within 1 to 2 weeks. However, a short-term follow-up may also benefit patients who are reluctant to quit smoking. The clinician must remember that a new cancer diagnosis is stressful and patients may rely on continued smoking to

TABLE 31.1

Additional Tobacco Cessation Resources for Patients and Clinicians[a]

American Association for Cancer Research Information about the adverse effects of tobacco and advocacy for tobacco control (http://www.aacr.org/home/public--media/science-policy--government-affairs/science-policy--government-affairs-committee/tobacco-and-cancer.aspx)
American Cancer Society A national cancer organization providing brochures and fact sheets on the health effects of tobacco and resources for smoking cessation (http://www.cancer.org/cancer/cancercauses/tobaccocancer/)
American Legacy Foundation A national independent public health foundation offering programs to help people quit and resources about the health effects of tobacco use (http://www.legacyforhealth.org/)
American Society of Clinical Oncology Resources for tobacco cessation with an emphasis on cancer patients (http://www.asco.org/practice-research/tobacco-cessation-and-control-resources)
Centers for Disease Control and Prevention A collection of online resources, information, and materials about quitting tobacco use (http://www.cdc.gov/TOBACCO/)
North American Quitline Consortium Information on local and national cessation quitlines, 1-800-QUIT-NOW (http://www.naquitline.org/)
Smoking Cessation Leadership Center A collaborative dedicated to disseminating knowledge about the health effects of tobacco and assistance in cessation (http://smokingcessationleadership.ucsf.edu/)
Smokefree.gov Tips and resources for people trying to stop smoking (http://smokefree.gov/)
Tobacco Free Nurses An organization aimed at engaging nurses in tobacco cessation efforts (http://www.tobaccofreenurses.org/)
U.S. Department of Health & Human Services, Surgeon General.gov Tobacco use and cessation information from the Surgeon General (http://www.surgeongeneral.gov/initiatives/tobacco/index.html)
World Health Organization An international organization tasked with implementing and monitoring public health with a focus on tobacco control (http://www.who.int/topics/tobacco/en/)

[a] Current as of December 2013.

TABLE 31.2

Select Treatment Strategies Used for Tobacco Cessation Treatments

Provide and monitor the use of nicotine replacement or other pharmacotherapy.
Provide education regarding the health effects of tobacco use and its addictive and relapsing nature.
Identify and change environmental and psychological cues for tobacco use.
Generate alternative behaviors for tobacco use.
Assist in optimization of social support for cessation efforts and address tobacco use in family members.
Prevent relapse including the identification of future high-risk situations and plans for specific behaviors in those situations.
Provide motivational interventions as needed throughout treatment.
Identify relaxation techniques such as guided imagery and progressive muscle relaxation.
Provide behavioral strategies to address depressed mood (e.g., increasing pleasurable activities).
Provide crisis intervention including appropriate referrals and emergency intervention if indicated.
Recognize and congratulate patients on success with reducing and/or quitting smoking.

relieve stress, but after absorbing the psychological effects of a new cancer diagnosis, patients may be more receptive to smoking cessation. During follow-up, clinicians should congratulate patients on successful cessation efforts, discuss accomplishments and setbacks, and assess pharmacotherapy use and problems. Patients should not be criticized for returning to smoking; rather, it is critical to create a supportive environment for patients to communicate progress, failure, and personal needs. Framing relapses as a learning experience can be helpful, and patients should be encouraged to set another quit date. Referrals to a psychologist or professionally trained smoking cessation counselor should be considered for patients with numerous unsuccessful quit attempts, comorbid depression, anxiety, additional substance abuse disorders, or inadequate social support.

Clinicians who are not well versed in tobacco cessation should realize that smoking is an extremely difficult addiction to overcome and should recognize the clinical pattern associated with cessation. As patients stop smoking, many will experience symptoms of withdrawal, including dry or sore throat, constipation, cravings to smoke, irritability, anxiety, trouble concentrating, restlessness, increased appetite, depression, and insomnia. In the first few weeks, patients may also report an increase in mucous secretions from the airways, a cough, and other upper respiratory tract symptoms. Patients and clinicians should realize that tobacco cessation requires a concerted effort, may require repeated attempts, and symptoms will not resolve immediately. Clinicians should counsel patients on a repeated basis, recognize success, and provide repeated assistance if patients relapse.

Pharmacologic Treatment for Smoking Cessation

The principles of pharmacotherapy to help patients quit smoking are fundamentally based on reducing the craving associated with nicotine withdrawal. Nicotine replacement therapy (NRT), in the form of patches, lozenges, inhalers, sprays, and gum, varenicline (Chantix), and bupropion (Zyban) are the three principal first-line pharmacotherapies recommended for use either alone or in combination according to PHS Guidelines.[199] Table 31.3 presents information on these first-line agents. Nicotine is the primary addictive substance in tobacco and NRT facilitates smoking cessation by reducing craving and withdrawal that smokers experience during abstinence. NRT also weans smokers off nicotine by providing a lower level and, in some cases, slower infusion of nicotine than smoking.[214] Strong evidence from over 100 randomized clinical trials support the use of NRT to increase the odds of quitting approximately twofold as compared with placebo.[215] Pooled analyses demonstrate that 17% of smokers receiving NRT were able to quit versus 10% with placebo after at least 6 months. Recent evidence further shows that combination therapy, or dual NRT (such as a nicotine patch and lozenge), is a very effective smoking cessation therapy that produces high quit rates.[216,217] Data suggest that activation of the nicotinic acetylcholine receptor (nAChR) may promote tumor development,[218] but evidence suggests that the negative aspects of smoking outweigh these concerns.[219,220] Furthermore, there are no clinical trials reporting negative outcomes for NRT in cancer patients as related to mortality or recurrence. Studies also demonstrate that NRT is not associated with an increased risk of carcinogenesis in the general population.[221,222] As a result, NRT should be used as a clinically proven method to help cancer patients stop smoking.

Antidepressants have been studied as non-nicotine–based pharmacotherapy in part due to depression and psychiatric disease being comorbid conditions in smokers.[223] Bupropion (Zyban) is currently the only FDA-approved antidepressant for the treatment of tobacco dependence.[199] Bupropion inhibits the reuptake of both dopamine and norepinephrine, thereby increasing dopamine and norepinephrine concentrations in the mesolimbic systems.[12,224] Bupropion also antagonizes the nAChR, thereby lowering the rewarding effects of nicotine.[225] Should an abstinent smoker relapse, bupropion may function to reduce the pleasure of cigarette smoking experienced by the smoker[226] and help to prevent further relapse. A meta-analysis found that smokers who received bupropion were twice as likely as those who received placebo to have achieved long-term abstinence at either a 6- or 12-month follow-up.[227]

Varenicline (Chantix) is a $\alpha 4\beta 2$ nAChR partial agonist that produces sustained dopamine release in the mesolimbic system that received FDA approval for treating tobacco dependence in 2006. Sustained dopamine release maintains a normal systemic level of the neurotransmitter, which helps to reduce craving and withdrawal during abstinence.[228] Varenicline also antagonizes the rewarding effects of nicotine. Because varenicline attenuates the pleasure smokers experience from smoking, it may decrease motivation to smoke and protect them from relapse. One of the initially reported randomized clinical trials that compared varenicline (2 mg), bupropion (300 mg), and placebo showed that varenicline was superior to bupropion and placebo, with overall continuous abstinence rates between 10% to 23%.[229] A meta-analysis demonstrated that the 1-mg daily dose approximately doubled, whereas the 2-mg daily dose approximately tripled the likelihood of long-term abstinence at 6 months as compared to placebo.[199] As a result, the 1-mg daily dose can be considered as an alternative should the patient experience significant dose-related side effects. Several meta-analyses have shown that varenicline is superior to bupropion and placebo in the general population.[230–233]

In July 2009, the FDA issued a warning after reports that some patients attempting to quit smoking while using varenicline or bupropion experienced unusual changes in behavior, depressed mood, worsening of depression, or had thoughts of suicide. This has prompted recommendations that health-care providers elicit information about a patient's psychiatric history prior to prescribing varenicline or bupropion to closely monitor changes in mood and behavior during the course of treatment. However,

TABLE 31.3

First-Line Pharmacotherapy Agents for the Treatment of Nicotine Depedence

Agent	Dose	Mechanism	Use
Nicotine Replacement			
Transdermal (patches)	16 h or 24 h 7, 14, or 21 mg 1 patch/d	Steady state NRT to reduce craving and withdrawal	6–10 CPD: 14 mg daily × 8 wks then 7 mg daily × 2 wks >10 CPD: 21 mg daily × 6 wks, then 14 mg × 2 wks, then 7 mg × 2 wks
Gum	2 or 4 mg Max: 24 pieces/d	Short-term NRT to reduce craving and withdrawal	First cigarette >30 min after waking: 2 mg PO q1–2 hr First cigarette <30 min after waking: 4 mg PO q1–2 hr
Lozenge	2 or 4 mg Max: 20 lozenges/d	Short-term NRT to reduce craving and withdrawal	1st cigarette >30 min after waking: 2 mg PO q1–2 hr 1st cigarette <30 min after waking: 4 mg PO q1–2 hr
Nasal spray	0.5 mg/spray Max:10 sprays/hr or 80 sprays/d	Short-term NRT to reduce craving and withdrawal	1 spray/nostril q1–5 hr
Inhaler	4 mg/cartridge Max: 16 cartridges/d	Short-term NRT to reduce craving and withdrawal	1 cartridge inhaled over 20 min q1.5–6 hr
Bupropion (Zyban)	150 mg	Block nicotinic receptors and reduces reward	1 tablet daily × 3 d, then 1 tablet twice daily for 7–12 wks
Varenicline (Chantix)	0.5 or 1 mg	Dopaminergic reward and partial nicotinic receptor antagonist	0.5 mg daily × 3 d, then 0.5 mg twice daily × 3 d, then 1 mg twice daily

CPD, cigarettes per day; PO, by mouth; NRT, nicotine replacement therapy.

updated recent safety studies examining very large databases (one database of N = 119,546, one database of N = 35,800) regarding safety have shown no difference in neuropsychiatric side effects between varenicline or bupropion as compared to NRT and no increased risk of depression.[234,235] Another prospective study showed no adverse events when treating participants with current or past major depression and also showed higher abstinence rates for the varenicline group as compared to placebo at weeks 9 to 52 (20.3% versus 10.4%, $p < 0.001$).[236] Varenicline should be considered a viable cessation pharmacotherapy for cancer patients.

The clinical practice guideline also identifies two non-nicotine–based medications—clonidine and nortriptyline—as second-line pharmacotherapies for tobacco dependence. A second-line agent is used when a smoker cannot use first-line medications due to either contraindications or lack of effectiveness. Both clonidine, an antihypertensive, and nortriptyline, a tricyclic antidepressant, have been shown to effectively assist smokers achieve abstinence.[227,237] Unfortunately, many patients who quit will eventually relapse, and rates of long-term abstinence remain low. Because smoking poses enormous health risks to individuals and their families, even a modest reduction in smoking may translate into a significant impact on public health. Clinicians should continue to encourage recalcitrant smokers to stop tobacco use and use pharmacotherapy where appropriate with repeated quit attempts.

Empirically Tested Cessation Interventions with Cancer Patients

The overwhelming majority of cessation research has been performed in the general population, but there are several studies that have been performed in cancer patients. Gritz et al.[238] conducted the first physician- or dentist-delivered randomized cessation intervention comparison in 186 newly diagnosed head and neck cancer patients. Patients were treated with either minimal advice or an enhanced intervention with trained clinicians consisting of strong personalized advice to stop smoking, a contracted quit date, tailored written materials, and booster advice sessions. No significant differences were found between treatments, but a 70.2% continuous abstinence rate was found at 12-month follow-up regardless of treatment condition, suggesting that many cancer patients can benefit from brief physician-delivered advice. A later study by Schnoll et al.,[239] comparing cognitive behavioral treatment with standardized health education advice, also failed to find significant differences in quit rates. All patients received NRT, and quit rates in both groups approached 50% at 1-month follow-up and 40% at 3-month follow-up.

Additional studies, ranging from 15 to 80 patients, examined nurse-delivered cessation interventions for a variety of cancer patients. The lowest cessation rates were found with a single session intervention: a 21% cessation rate in the intervention group versus 14% in the usual care group 6 weeks' postintervention.[240] Higher cessation rates were associated with a more intensive intervention consisting of three inpatient visits, supplementary materials, and five postdischarge follow-up contacts. Additional studies demonstrate higher cessation rates with more intensive intervention (40% to 75%) as compared with usual care (43% to 50%), suggesting more intensive interventions may yield higher cessation rates.[241–243] In general, more intense interventions appear to be more efficacious, but even brief advice is important to achieve tobacco cessation.

In a randomized trial of 432 cancer patients coordinated by the Eastern Cooperative Oncology Group (ECOG) with a physician-delivered intervention (comprised of cessation advice, optional NRT, and written materials) or usual care (unstructured advice from physicians), there were no significant intervention effects and generally low abstinence rates (12% to 15%

at 6 to 12 months).[244] However, patients with head and neck or lung cancer were significantly more likely to have quit smoking compared to patients with tumors that were not smoking related. Analyses of outcomes from the Mayo Clinic Nicotine Dependence Center found that although lung cancer patients were more likely to achieve 6-month tobacco abstinence than controls (22% versus 14%), no significant differences were observed after adjusting for covariates.[245] Garces et al.[246] also found no significant differences in abstinence rates between head and neck cancer patients and controls (33% versus 26%). However, higher abstinence rates were found for both head and neck and lung cancer patients treated within 3 months of diagnosis compared to those treated for more than 3 months after the diagnosis, emphasizing the potential importance of the *teachable moment* at the time of the cancer diagnosis.

The potential importance of addressing smoking combined with considering comorbid disease has been noted in a few studies. In a randomized head and neck cancer patients of usual care versus 9 to 11 sessions of a nurse-administered intervention consisting of cognitive-behavioral therapy and medications, targeting comorbid smoking, drinking, and depression significantly increased quit rates at 6-month follow-up for the intervention group compared to the usual control group (47% versus 31%, $p < 0.05$).[247] In a randomized trial of 246 cancer patients treated with 9 weeks of NRT with or without bupropion, there was no significant difference with the addition of bupropion to NRT, but in patients with depressive symptoms, bupropion increased abstinence rates, lowered withdrawal, and improved quality of life.[248] Patients without depression symptoms did equally well when treated with bupropion versus transdermal nicotine and counseling alone.

Patient recruitment has been a problem noted by some studies, including 5.5 years to accrue 246 patients with telephone screening of over 7,500 potential patients.[249] A pilot trial of varenicline in thoracic oncology patients required screening 1,130 patients to accrue 49 participants randomized to a 12-week course of either varenicline or placebo paired with a behavioral counseling platform of seven sessions.[250] A randomized trial of 185 smoking cancer patients comparing the efficacy of a hospital-based standard care smoking cessation model versus standard care augmented by a behavioral tapering regimen via a handheld device before inpatient hospitalization for cancer surgery demonstrated no difference in quit rates (both 32%,).[251] However, over 29,000 patients were screened to conduct a randomized clinical trial with a smoking cancer patient population. These studies highlight the potential difficulty recruiting participants who smoke, including considerations for the importance of medical comorbidity in guiding smoking cessation treatment, patient mix (multiple tumor sites), treatment status (awaiting treatment to completed treatment), variation in stage of disease, and considering how psychiatric conditions such as depression reflect the difficulty of conducting research in the oncology setting and the importance of these variables in future studies.

Although accruing patients to intervention trials may seem discouraging, several studies demonstrate the benefit of counseling over self-help. Emmons et al.[252] conducted a randomized controlled trial in 796 young adult survivors of pediatric cancer that included six calls, tailored and targeted written materials, and optional NRT as compared with self-help. Significantly higher quit rates were found in the counseling group compared to the self-help group at all reported follow-up time points, including 12 months (15% versus 9%; $p < 0.01$). A randomized trial of a motivational interviewing-based smoking cessation intervention in a south Australian hospital was delivered over a 3-month period, consisted of multiple contacts with a trained counselor, and provided supplementary material tailored to cancer patients with NRT.[253] The control group received brief advice to quit and generic supplementary material. Quit rates did not differ by treatment group (5% to 6% at 3-month follow-up), but the intervention group was significantly more likely to report attempts to quit smoking.

Current Tobacco Assessment and Cessation Support by Oncologists

Access to cessation support is critical to address tobacco use by cancer patients. A recent survey of 58 NCI-designated cancer centers indicated that about 80% reported a tobacco use program available to their patients and about 60% routinely offered educational materials, but less than 50% had a designated individual who provided services.[254] A recent survey of over 1,500 members of the International Association for the Study of Lung Cancer (IASLC)[255] and a parallel study of 1,197 ASCO members[256] observed that approximately 90% of physicians believe that tobacco affects outcomes, tobacco cessation should be a standard part of cancer care, and approximately 80% regularly advise patients to stop using tobacco, but only approximately 40% discuss medications or assist with quitting. Dominant perceived barriers to cessation support were patient resistance to treatment, an inability to get patients to quit, a lack of cessation resources, and a lack of clinician education. These data showed that even motivated clinicians are not regularly providing tobacco cessation support. A recent survey of 155 actively accruing cooperative group clinical trials further demonstrated that only 29% of active trials collected any tobacco use information, 4.5% collected any tobacco use information at follow-up, and none addressed tobacco cessation.[55] Few oncology meetings offer educational workshops or talks, and they are often poorly attended when they are offered.[257] Collectively, these data demonstrate that oncologists are not regularly providing cessation support and that we are not capturing tobacco use information that may be critical to understanding the effects of tobacco on cancer treatment outcomes.

More in-person talks as well as written and Web-based training should be made available, as well as new approaches that move from the traditional 5 A's model delivered by a single professional to referral systems that efficiently connect tobacco users to multiple resources for tobacco cessation.[258–260] The ASCO *Prevention Curriculum* has a chapter devoted to educating oncology healthcare professionals on the evaluation and treatment of tobacco use.[213] Innovative curricula, such as the Texas Tobacco Outreach Education Program (TOEP), are available and can facilitate program development in other states.[261] However, specialty programs in tobacco cessation treatment that are based in cancer centers and other medical centers are valuable resources that need to be further developed.

Addressing tobacco use in cancer patients may be approached in a systematic and efficient manner. A recent report highlighted the potential utility of automated tobacco assessment and smoking cessation using structured assessments in the EMR where all patients were automatically referred to a dedicated cessation program consisting of phone-based cessation support.[45] In 2,700 patients referred for cessation support, half received only a mailing and only 1% contacted the cessation program. However, in the arm with at least five phone call attempts made by the cessation service, 81% of patients were successfully contacted and only 3% refused cessation support. Furthermore, assessments implemented every 4 weeks, rather than more frequent assessments every 2 weeks, resulted in delayed cessation referrals in less than 1% of smokers. This is the first report to try and identify clinically efficient mechanisms of addressing tobacco use that may be useful in clinical practice or research that may be an effective method of increasing patient participation in cessation support, but substantial work is needed to assess who may benefit from low versus high intensity support in such a program.

Examples of Model Tobacco Treatment Programs

Several dedicated tobacco treatment programs at cancer centers have been developed. Table 31.4 contrasts the core elements of

TABLE 31.4

Attributes of Prototypical Tobacco Treatment Programs

Attribute	MDACC	RPCI	Yale	MSKCC
Tobacco assessment of all patients (EMR)	Yes	Yes	Yes	Yes
Automatic referral of all patients	Yes	Yes	No	Yes
In-person counseling	Yes	No	Yes	Yes
Telephone counseling	Yes	Yes	No	Yes
Medications prescribed	Yes	No	Yes	Yes
Biochemical confirmation (CO) testing	Yes	No	Yes	No
Free to patient	Yes	Yes	No	Yes
Third-party payment	No	No	Yes	Yes
Research studies of new treatments	Yes	Yes	Yes	Yes

MDACC, M.D. Anderson Cancer Center, Houston, TX; RPCI, Roswell Park Cancer Institute, Buffalo, NY; Yale, Yale University Hospital, Smilow Cancer Center, New Haven, CT; MSKCC, Memorial Sloan Kettering Cancer Center, New York, NY.

four active model programs at the end of 2013 (University of Texas M.D. Anderson Cancer Center, Roswell Park Cancer Institute, Yale Cancer Center, and Memorial Sloan Kettering Cancer Center), each of which employ different methods to help cancer patients quit smoking. All programs follow the evidence-based 5 A's model described previously from PHS Guidelines.[199] All programs were made available to patients at their respective medical centers and are now designed to evaluate and treat all patients who self-report current tobacco use. Importantly, not all cancer centers can treat smoking cessation in the same manner. Financing of a cessation program is critical and may include institutional funds, state funds, research funds, and third-party billing. Notably, given the broad spectrum of adverse health effects associated with smoking, cancer centers should carefully consider the potential health benefits and cost savings associated with tobacco cessation due to reductions in treatment complications and recurrence associated with smoking by cancer patients. There is no one "correct" way to create and sustain a tobacco treatment program at a cancer center, but at the very least and consistent with evidence, rigorous behavioral counseling should be provided and, if possible, medication management as well.

FUTURE CONSIDERATIONS

Research Considerations

The past several years have shown a surge in activities identifying the effects of tobacco in cancer patients and increasing awareness is being developed for cessation support at cancer centers as well as through several national organizations. There are three fundamental areas of research that need to be expanded:

1. *Evaluating the effects of tobacco use and cessation on clinical cancer outcomes.* The 2014 SGR concluded that smoking caused adverse outcomes in cancer patients,[7] but several limitations remain. Tobacco-use definitions should be standardized and implemented at diagnosis, during treatment, and follow-up. Biochemical confirmation with cotinine or exhaled carbon monoxide may improve the accuracy of tobacco assessment in at-risk groups such as current smokers who are trying to quit or patients who reported quitting in the past year.[171,185,186,262] Although smoking is the predominant form of tobacco consumption, all tobacco products should be considered. A further understanding of the effects of tobacco on the efficacy and toxicity of cancer treatment, tumor response, quality of life, survival, recurrence, compliance, second primary, and noncancer-related comorbidity is needed. All cancer disease sites and stages are important to consider.
2. *Understanding the effects of tobacco and cessation on cancer biology.* Although not a primary focus of this chapter, tobacco and tobacco-related products increase tumor growth, angiogenesis, migration, invasion and metastasis and decrease response to conventional cancer treatments such as CT and RT. These and other areas are important to consider, including the potential effects on immune-related therapy and vaccine development. *In vivo* models of exposure and cancer response are not well developed, yet are critical to this research area. Work is also needed to assess the effect of emerging tobacco-related products such as e-cigarettes.
3. *Advance understanding of models to increase access to cessation support and increase efficacy of tobacco cessation methods for cancer patients.* This diverse area includes assessing the timing of intervention, intensity, duration, follow-up, and the potential effects of harm-reduction strategies. Cessation pharmacology requires additional consideration in combination with unique approaches to motivational and behavioral counseling in cancer patients. Significant work is needed to disseminate evidence-based cessation support and to assess the cost-effectiveness of different cessation strategies, particularly with regard to improving the cost of cancer care as a whole. Preventing relapse and evaluating the safety of transition to alternative products such as e-cigarettes is equally important and increasingly complex with the addition of new tobacco-related products. Identifying and addressing barriers to effective cessation support is also needed. As related to the cancer patient, clinicians and cessation specialists should consider how their research relates to cancer care. Taking advantage of new integrated medical management systems presents a significant opportunity to improve cessation support access as well as to develop a more effective tracking of patient outcomes.

Policy Implications and Systematic Issues

Several national and international organizations have emphasized the importance of tobacco assessments and cessation for the general population and for cancer patients that include tools to evaluate tobacco use at diagnosis, during treatment, and follow-up appointments, as well as routine support for smoking cessation.[5,6,188–191] In 2012, ASCO, with the contribution of the American Legacy Foundation, published a Tobacco Cessation Toolkit for the oncology setting.[263] This evidence-based guideline intends to help oncology providers integrate tobacco cessation strategies into their patient care. Utilization of the EMR and standardized, automated systems for more efficacious and efficient access to tobacco cessation support has also been suggested,[45] but requires participation by clinicians, institutions, insurers, and health departments. Not only should providers be aware of the need for tobacco cessation and available interventions, but health-care institutions must also build such treatment into their overall system of care. Thus, the identification of patients who smoke or use any alternative tobacco product, referral or direct treatment by providers, billing and reimbursement for treatment provided, and consistent efforts from professional oncology organizations are critically important.[257] The tremendous public health burden from tobacco-related disability and death has not been countered by a proportional level of funding in tobacco control, cancer treatment research, or public advocacy. Researchers, clinicians, and advocates must come together to persuade policy makers to increase funding in tobacco-related research, treatment, and policy initiatives on behalf of healthy individuals and patients. A united front is critically needed in support of a common agenda that includes both increased tobacco-control efforts and additional funding for disease-related research and treatment. With clinical rationale, guidelines, and advocacy in place, the final steps in effective tobacco control and improving health outcomes are to implement these recommendations into practice.

REFERENCES

1. U.S. Department of Health, Education, and Welfare. *Smoking and Health: Report of the Advisory Committee to the Surgeon General of the Public Health Service*. PHS Publication No. 1103. Washington, D.C.: U.S. Department of Health, Education, and Welfare, Public Health Service, Center for Disease Control; 1964.
2. Office of the Surgeon General, Office on Smoking and Health. *The Health Consequences of Smoking. A Report of the Surgeon General*. Atlanta: Centers for Disease Control and Prevention; 2004.
3. Centers for Disease Control and Prevention, National Center for Chronic Disease Prevention and Health Promotion, Office on Smoking and Health. *How Tobacco Smoke Causes Disease: The Biology and Behavioral Basis for Smoking-Attributable Disease: A Report of the Surgeon General*. Atlanta: Centers for Disease Control and Prevention; 2010.
4. U.S. Department of Health and Human Services. *The Health Consequences of Smoking: Nicotine Addiction. A Report of the Surgeon General*. DHHS Publication No. (CDC) 88-8406. Atlanta: U.S. Department of Health and Human Services, Public Health Service, Centers for Disease Control, National Center for Chronic Disease Prevention and Health Promotion, Office on Smoking and Health; 1988.
5. Toll BA, Brandon TH, Gritz ER, et al. Assessing tobacco use by cancer patients and facilitating cessation: an American Association for Cancer Research policy statement. *Clin Cancer Res* 2013;19:1941–1948.
6. Hanna N, Mulshine J, Wollins DS, et al. Tobacco cessation and control a decade later: American society of clinical oncology policy statement update. *J Clin Oncol* 2013;31:3147–3157.
7. U.S. Department of Health and Human Services. *The Health Consequences of Smoking—50 Years of Progress: A Report of the Surgeon General*. Atlanta: U.S. Department of Health and Human Services, Centers for Disease Control and Prevention, National Center for Chronic Disease Prevention and Health Promotion, Office on Smoking and Health; 2014.
8. Brunzell DH. Preclinical evidence that activation of mesolimbic alpha 6 subunit containing nicotinic acetylcholine receptors supports nicotine addiction phenotype. *Nicotine Tob Res* 2012;14:1258–1269.
9. Benowitz NL. Nicotine addiction. *N Engl J Med.* 2010;362:2295–2303.
10. Nestler EJ. Is there a common molecular pathway for addiction? *Nat Neurosci* 2005;8:1445–1449.
11. Dani JA, De Biasi M. Cellular mechanisms of nicotine addiction. *Pharmacol Biochem Behav* 2001;70:439–446.
12. Balfour DJ. The neurobiology of tobacco dependence: a preclinical perspective on the role of the dopamine projections to the nucleus accumbens. *Nicotine Tob Res* 2004;6:899–912.
13. Berridge KC, Robinson TE. What is the role of dopamine in reward: hedonic impact, reward learning, or incentive salience? *Brain Res Brain Res Rev* 1998;28:309–369.
14. Schultz W. Multiple dopamine functions at different time courses. *Annu Rev Neurosci* 2007;30:259–288.
15. Kalivas PW, McFarland K. Brain circuitry and the reinstatement of cocaine-seeking behavior. *Psychopharmacology* 2003;168:44–56.
16. Dani JA, Balfour DJK. Historical and current perspective on tobacco use and nicotine addiction. *Trends Neurosci* 2011;34:383–439.
17. Di Chiara G. Role of dopamine in the behavioural actions of nicotine related to addiction. *Eur J Pharmacol* 2000;393:295–314.
18. Centers for Disease Control and Prevention. Current cigarette smoking among adults—United States, 2011. *MMWR Morb Mortal Wkly Rep* 2012;61:889–894.
19. Centers for Disease Control and Prevention. Cigarette smoking among adults—United States, 2001. *MMWR Morb Mortal Wkly Rep* 2003;52: 953–956.
20. Smokefree Laws and Policies. American Lung Association Web site. http://www.lungusa2.org/slati/smokefree_laws.php. Accessed November 25, 2013.
21. Tobacco Policy Project/State Legislated Actions on Tobacco Issues (SLATI). American Lung Association Web site. http://www.lungusa2.org/slati. Accessed November 25, 2013.
22. Tobacco Taxes. American Lung Association Web site. http://www.lungusa2.org/slati/tobacco_taxes.php. Accessed November 25, 2013.
23. Tobacco Situation and Outlook Report, U.S. Department of Agriculture, U.S. Census 1880-2005.
24. Warren GW, Cummings KM. Tobacco and lung cancer: risks, trends, and outcomes in patients with cancer. In: *American Society of Clinical Oncology 2013 Educational Book*. 201; 359–364. ASCO University Web site. http://meetinglibrary.asco.org//content/200-132. Accessed November 25, 2013.
25. Thun MJ, Carter BD, Feskanich D, et al. 50-year trends in smoking-related mortality in the United States. *N Engl J Med.* 2013;368:351–364.
26. U.S. Food and Drug Administration. Summary of Results: Laboratory Analysis of Electronic Cigarettes Conducted by FDA. U.S. Food and Drug Administration Web site. http://www.fda.gov/NewsEvents/PublicHealthFocus/ucm173146.htm. Accessed November 25, 2013.
27. Cummings KM, Dresler CM, Field JK, et al. E-cigarettes and cancer patients. *J Thorac Oncol* 2014;9:438–441.
28. Kuschner WG, Reddy S, Mehrotra N, et al. Electronic cigarettes and thirdhand tobacco smoke: two emerging health care challenges for the primary care provider. *Int J Gen Med* 2011;4:115–120.
29. WHO Study Group on Tobacco Product Regulation. WHO Study Group on Tobacco Product Regulation. Report on the scientific basis of tobacco product regulation: third report of a WHO study group. *World Health Organ Tech Rep Ser* 2009;(955):1–41.
30. National Cancer Institute. Cancer Trends Progress Report – 2011/2012 Update. Nation Cancer Institute Web site. http://progressreport.cancer.gov. Published August 2012. Accessed November 25, 2013.
31. Bellizzi KM, Rowland JH, Jeffery DD, et al. Health behaviors of cancer survivors: examining opportunities for cancer control intervention. *J Clin Oncol* 2005;23:8884–8893.
32. Coups EJ, Ostroff JS. A population-based estimate of the prevalence of behavioral risk factors among adult cancer survivors and noncancer controls. *Prev Med* 2005;40:702–711.
33. Klosky JL, Hum AM, Zhang N, et al. Smokeless and dual tobacco use among males surviving childhood cancer: a report from the Childhood Cancer Survivor Study. *Cancer Epidemiol Biomarkers Prev* 2013;22:1025–1029.
34. Underwood JM, Townsend JS, Tai E, et al. Persistent cigarette smoking and other tobacco use after a tobacco-related cancer diagnosis. *J Cancer Surviv* 2012; 6:333–344.
35. Walker MS, Vidrine DJ, Gritz ER, et al. Smoking relapse during the first year after treatment for early-stage non-small-cell lung cancer. *Cancer Epidemiol Biomarkers Prev* 2006;15:2370–2377.
36. Gritz ER. Smoking and smoking cessation in cancer patients. *Br J Addict* 1991;86:549–554.
37. Lippman SM, Lee JJ, Karp DD, et al. Randomized phase III intergroup trial of isotretinoin to prevent second primary tumors in stage I non-small-cell lung cancer. *J Natl Cancer Inst* 2001;93:605–618.
38. Ostroff JS, Jacobsen PB, Moadel AB, et al. Prevalence and predictors of continued tobacco use after treatment of patients with head and neck cancer. *Cancer* 1995;75:569–576.
39. Hickey K, Do KA, Green A. Smoking and prostate cancer. *Epidemiol Rev* 2001;23:115–125.
40. Plaskon LA, Penson DF, Vaughan TL, et al. Cigarette smoking and risk of prostate cancer in middle-aged men. *Cancer Epidemiol Biomarkers Prev* 2003;12:604–609.
41. Watters JL, Park Y, Hollenbeck A, et al. Cigarette smoking and prostate cancer in a prospective US cohort study. *Cancer Epidemiol Biomarkers Prev* 2009;18:2427–2435.
42. Alberg AJ, Singh S, May JW, et al. Epidemiology, prevention, and early detection of breast cancer. *Curr Opin Oncol* 2000;12:515–520.
43. Johnson KC, Miller AB, Collishaw NE, et al. Active smoking and secondhand smoke increase breast cancer risk: the report of the Canadian Expert Panel on Tobacco Smoke and Breast Cancer Risk (2009). *Tob Control* 2011;20:e2.
44. Breast Cancer Family Registry; Kathleen Cuningham Consortium for Research into Familial Breast Cancer (Australasia); Ontario Cancer Genetics Network (Canada). Smoking and risk of breast cancer in carriers of mutations in BRCA1 or BRCA2 aged less than 50 years. *Breast Cancer Res Treat* 2008;109:67–75.
45. Warren GW, Marshall JR, Cummings KM, et al. Automated tobacco assessment and cessation support for cancer patients. *Cancer* 2014;120:562–569.
46. Centers for Disease Control and Prevention. Cigarette smoking among adults—United States, 2004. *MMWR Morb Mortal Wkly Rep* 2005;54:1121–1124.

47. Centers for Disease Control and Prevention. Tobacco use among adults—United States, 2005. *MMWR Morb Mortal Wkly Rep* 2006;55:1145–1148.
48. Gritz ER, Nisenbaum R, Elashoff RE, et al. Smoking behavior following diagnosis in patients with stage I non-small cell lung cancer. *Cancer Causes Control* 1991;2:105–112.
49. Chen AM, Vazquez E, Courquin J, et al. Tobacco use among long-term survivors of head and neck cancer treated with radiation therapy. *Psychooncology* 2014;23:190–194.
50. Ostroff J, Garland J, Moadel A, et al. Cigarette smoking patterns in patients after treatment of bladder cancer. *J Cancer Educ* 2000;15:86–90.
51. McBride CM, Emmons KM, Lipkus IM. Understanding the potential of teachable moments: the case of smoking cessation. *Health Educ Res* 2003;18:156–170.
52. Gritz ER, Schacherer C, Koehly L, et al. Smoking withdrawal and relapse in head and neck cancer patients. *Head Neck* 1999;21:420–427.
53. Warren GW, Marshall JR, Cummings KM. Smoking, cancer treatment, and design of clinical trials. *Proc AACR* 2013:54:594.
54. Parsons A, Daley A, Begh R, et al. Influence of smoking cessation after diagnosis of early stage lung cancer on prognosis: systematic review of observational studies with meta-analysis. *BMJ* 2010;340:b5569.
55. Peters EN, Torres E, Toll BA, et al. Tobacco assessment in actively accruing National Cancer Institute Cooperative Group Program Clinical Trials. *J Clin Oncol* 2012;30:2869–2875.
56. Land SR. Methodologic barriers to addressing critical questions about tobacco and cancer prognosis. *J Clin Oncol* 2012;30:2030–2032.
57. Gritz ER, Dresler C, Sarna L. Smoking, the missing drug interaction in clinical trials: ignoring the obvious. *Cancer Epidemiol Biomarkers Prev* 2005;14:2287–2293.
58. Yu GP, Ostroff JS, Zhang ZF, et al. Smoking history and cancer patient survival: a hospital cancer registry study. *Cancer Detect Prev* 1997;21:497–509.
59. Dahlstrom KR, Calzada G, Hanby JD, et al. An evolution in demographics, treatment, and outcomes of oropharyngeal cancer at a major cancer center: a staging system in need of repair. *Cancer* 2012;119:81–89.
60. Molina MA, Cheung MC, Perez EA, et al. African American and poor patients have a dramatically worse prognosis for head and neck cancer: an examination of 20,915 patients. *Cancer* 2008;113:2797–2806.
61. Dragun AE, Huang B, Tucker TC, et al. Disparities in the application of adjuvant radiotherapy after breast-conserving surgery for early stage breast cancer: impact on overall survival. *Cancer* 2011;117:2590–2598.
62. Bostrom PJ, Alkhateeb S, Trottier G, et al. Sex differences in bladder cancer outcomes among smokers with advanced bladder cancer. *BJU Int* 2011;109:70–76.
63. Kroeger N, Klatte T, Birkhäuser FD, et al. Smoking negatively impacts renal cell carcinoma overall and cancer-specific survival. *Cancer* 2011;118:1795–1802.
64. Marks DI, Ballen K, Logan BR, et al. The effect of smoking on allogeneic transplant outcomes. *Biol Blood Marrow Transplant* 2009;15:1277–1287.
65. Gridelli C, Ciardiello F, Gallo C, et al. First-line erlotinib followed by second-line cisplatin-gemcitabine chemotherapy in advanced non-small-cell lung cancer: the TORCH randomized trial. *J Clin Oncol* 2012;30:3002–3011.
66. Maeda R, Yoshida J, Ishii G, et al. Influence of cigarette smoking on survival and tumor invasiveness in clinical stage IA lung adenocarcinoma. *Ann Thorac Surg* 2012;93:1626–1632.
67. Maeda R, Yoshida J, Ishii G, et al. The prognostic impact of cigarette smoking on patients with non-small cell lung cancer. *J Thorac Oncol* 2011;6:735–742.
68. Janjigian YY, McDonnell K, Kris MG, et al. Pack-years of cigarette smoking as a prognostic factor in patients with stage IIIB/IV nonsmall cell lung cancer. *Cancer* 2010;116:670–675.
69. Toyooka S, Takano T, Kosaka T, et al. Epidermal growth factor receptor mutation, but not sex and smoking, is independently associated with favorable prognosis of gefitinib-treated patients with lung adenocarcinoma. *Cancer Sci* 2008; 99:303–308.
70. Kawai H, Tada A, Kawahara M, et al. Smoking history before surgery and prognosis in patients with stage IA non-small-cell lung cancer—a multicenter study. *Lung Cancer* 2005;49:63–70.
71. Warren GW, Kasza K, Reid M, et al. Smoking at diagnosis and survival in cancer patients. *Int J Cancer* 2013;132:401–410.
72. Kvale E, Ekundayo OJ, Zhang Y, et al. History of cancer and mortality in community-dwelling older adults. *Cancer Epidemiol* 2011;35:30–36.
73. Gajdos C, Hawn MT, Campagna EJ, et al. Adverse effects of smoking on postoperative outcomes in cancer patients. *Ann Surg Oncol* 2012;19: 1430–1438.
74. Duffy SA, Ronis DL, McLean S, et al. Pretreatment health behaviors predict survival among patients with head and neck squamous cell carcinoma. *J Clin Oncol* 2009;27:1969–1975.
75. Farshadpour F, Kranenborg H, Calkoen EV, et al. Survival analysis of head and neck squamous cell carcinoma: influence of smoking and drinking. *Head Neck* 2011;33:817–823.
76. Meyer F, Bairati I, Fortin A, et al. Interaction between antioxidant vitamin supplementation and cigarette smoking during radiation therapy in relation to long-term effects on recurrence and mortality: a randomized trial among head and neck cancer patients. *Int J Cancer* 2008;122:1679–1683.
77. Shen GP, Xu FH, He F, et al. Pretreatment lifestyle behaviors as survival predictors for patients with nasopharyngeal carcinoma. *PLoS One* 2012;7:e36515.
78. Dal Maso L, Zucchetto A, Talamini R, et al. Effect of obesity and other lifestyle factors on mortality in women with breast cancer. *Int J Cancer* 2008;123: 2188–2194.
79. Hellmann SS, Thygesen LC, Tolstrup JS, et al. Modifiable risk factors and survival in women diagnosed with primary breast cancer: results from a prospective cohort study. *Eur J Cancer Prev* 2010;19:366–673.
80. Holmes MD, Murin S, Chen WY, et al. Smoking and survival after breast cancer diagnosis. *Int J Cancer* 2007;120:2672–2677.
81. Sagiv SK, Gaudet MM, Eng SM, et al. Active and passive cigarette smoke and breast cancer survival. *Ann Epidemiol* 2007;17:385–393.
82. Phipps AI, Baron J, Newcomb PA. Prediagnostic smoking history, alcohol consumption, and colorectal cancer survival: the Seattle Colon Cancer Family Registry. *Cancer* 2011;117:4948–4957.
83. Huang XE, Tajima K, Hamajima N, et al. Effects of dietary, drinking, and smoking habits on the prognosis of gastric cancer. *Nutr Cancer* 2000;38:30–36.
84. Kenfield SA, Stampfer MJ, Chan JM, et al. Smoking and prostate cancer survival and recurrence. *JAMA* 2011;305:2548–2555.
85. Merrick GS, Butler WM, Wallner KE, et al. Androgen-deprivation therapy does not impact cause-specific or overall survival after permanent prostate brachytherapy. *Int J Radiat Oncol Biol Phys* 2006;65:669–677.
86. Pickles T, Liu M, Berthelet E, et al. The effect of smoking on outcome following external radiation for localized prostate cancer. *J Urol* 2004;171: 1543–1546.
87. Taira AV, Merrick GS, Butler WM, et al. Long-term outcome for clinically localized prostate cancer treated with permanent interstitial brachytherapy. *Int J Radiat Oncol Biol Phys* 2011;79:1336–1342.
88. Sweeney C, Farrow DC. Differential survival related to smoking among patients with renal cell carcinoma. *Epidemiology* 2000;11:344–346.
89. Coker AL, DeSimone CP, Eggleston KS, et al. Smoking and survival among Kentucky women diagnosed with invasive cervical cancer: 1995–2005. *Gynecol Oncol* 2009;112:365–369.
90. Modesitt SC, Huang B, Shelton BJ, et al. Endometrial cancer in Kentucky: the impact of age, smoking status, and rural residence. *Gynecol Oncol* 2006;103:300–306.
91. Poullis M, McShane J, Shaw M, et al. Smoking status at diagnosis and histology type as determinants of long-term outcomes of lung cancer patients. *Eur J Cardiothorac Surg* 2012;43:919–924.
92. Kawaguchi T, Tamiya A, Tamura A, et al. Chemotherapy is beneficial for elderly patients with advanced non-small-cell lung cancer: analysis of patients aged 70–74, 75–79, and 80 or older in Japan. *Clin Lung Cancer* 2012;13: 442–447.
93. Pirker R, Pereira JR, Szczesna A, et al. Prognostic factors in patients with advanced non-small cell lung cancer: data from the phase III FLEX study. *Lung Cancer* 2012;77:376–382.
94. Ferketich AK, Niland JC, Mamet R, et al. Smoking status and survival in the national comprehensive cancer network non-small cell lung cancer cohort. *Cancer* 2013;119:847–853.
95. Chansky K, Sculier JP, Crowley JJ, et al. The International Association for the Study of Lung Cancer Staging Project: prognostic factors and pathologic TNM stage in surgically managed non-small cell lung cancer. *J Thorac Oncol* 2009;4:792–801.
96. Myrdal G, Lamberg K, Lambe M, et al. Regional differences in treatment and outcome in non-small cell lung cancer: a population-based study (Sweden). *Lung Cancer* 2009;63:16–22.
97. Saito-Nakaya K, Nakaya N, Akechi T, et al. Marital status and non-small cell lung cancer survival: the Lung Cancer Database Project in Japan. *Psychooncology*. 2008;17:869–876.
98. Zhou W, Heist RS, Liu G, et al. Smoking cessation before diagnosis and survival in early stage non-small cell lung cancer patients. *Lung Cancer* 2006;53:375–380.
99. Tsao AS, Liu D, Lee JJ, et al. Smoking affects treatment outcome in patients with advanced nonsmall cell lung cancer. *Cancer* 2006;106:2428–2436.
100. Ebbert JO, Williams BA, Sun Z, et al. Duration of smoking abstinence as a predictor for non-small-cell lung cancer survival in women. *Lung Cancer* 2005;47:165-172.
101. Tammemagi CM, Neslund-Dudas C, Simoff M, et al. Smoking and lung cancer survival: the role of comorbidity and treatment. *Chest* 2004;125:27–37.
102. Nordquist LT, Simon GR, Cantor A, et al. Improved survival in never-smokers vs current smokers with primary adenocarcinoma of the lung. *Chest* 2004;126:347–351.
103. Ehlers SL, Gastineau DA, Patten CA, et al. The impact of smoking on outcomes among patients undergoing hematopoietic SCT for the treatment of acute leukemia. *Bone Marrow Transplant* 2011;46:285–290.
104. Geyer SM, Morton LM, Habermann TM, et al. Smoking, alcohol use, obesity, and overall survival from non-Hodgkin lymphoma: a population-based study. *Cancer* 2010;116:2993–3000.
105. Deleyiannis FW, Thomas DB, Vaughan TL, et al. Alcoholism: independent predictor of survival in patients with head and neck cancer. *J Natl Cancer Inst* 1996;88:542–549.
106. Ngô C, Alran S, Plancher C, et al. Outcome in early cervical cancer following pre-operative low dose rate brachytherapy: a ten-year follow up of 257 patients treated at a single institution. *Gynecol Oncol* 2011;123:248–252.
107. Browman GP, Wong G, Hodson I, et al. Influence of cigarette smoking on the efficacy of radiation therapy in head and neck cancer. *N Engl J Med* 1993;328:159–163.
108. Gillison ML, Zhang Q, Jordan R, et al. Tobacco smoking and increased risk of death and progression for patients with p16-positive and p16-negative oropharyngeal cancer. *J Clin Oncol* 2012;30:2102–2111.
109. Waggoner SE, Darcy KM, Fuhrman B, et al. Association between cigarette smoking and prognosis in locally advanced cervical carcinoma treated with chemoradiation: a Gynecologic Oncology Group study. *Gynecol Oncol* 2006; 103:853–858.

110. Khuri FR, Lee JJ, Lippman SM, et al. Randomized phase III trial of low-dose isotretinoin for prevention of second primary tumors in stage I and II head and neck cancer patients. *J Natl Cancer Inst* 2006;98:441–450.
111. Karvonen-Gutierrez CA, Ronis DL, Fowler KE, et al. Quality of life scores predict survival among patients with head and neck cancer. *J Clin Oncol* 2008;26:2754–2760.
112. Sardari Nia P, Weyler J, Colpaert C, et al. Prognostic value of smoking status in operated non-small cell lung cancer. *Lung Cancer* 2005;47:351–359.
113. Chen J, Jiang R, Garces YI, et al. Prognostic factors for limited-stage small cell lung cancer: a study of 284 patients. *Lung Cancer* 2010;67:221–226.
114. Bittner N, Merrick GS, Galbreath RW, et al. Primary causes of death after permanent prostate brachytherapy. *Int J Radiat Oncol Biol Phys* 2008;72:433–440.
115. Haughey BH, Sinha P. Prognostic factors and survival unique to surgically treated p16+ oropharyngeal cancer. *Laryngoscope* 2012;122:S13– S33.
116. Kawakita D, Hosono S, Ito H, et al. Impact of smoking status on clinical outcome in oral cavity cancer patients. *Oral Oncol* 2012;48:186–191.
117. Chen AM, Chen LM, Vaughan A, et al. Tobacco smoking during radiation therapy for head-and-neck cancer is associated with unfavorable outcome. *Int J Radiat Oncol Biol Phys* 2011;79:414–419.
118. Junor E, Kerr G, Oniscu A, et al. Benefit of chemotherapy as part of treatment for HPV DNA-positive but p16-negative squamous cell carcinoma of the oropharynx. *Br J Cancer* 2012;106:358–365.
119. Manjer J, Andersson I, Berglund G, et al. Survival of women with breast cancer in relation to smoking. *Eur J Surg* 2000;166:852–858.
120. Kountourakis P, Correa AM, Hofstetter WL, et al. Combined modality therapy of cT2N0M0 esophageal cancer: the University of Texas M. D. Anderson Cancer Center experience. *Cancer* 2011;117:925–930.
121. Munro AJ, Bentley AH, Ackland C, et al. Smoking compromises cause-specific survival in patients with operable colorectal cancer. *Clin Oncol (R Coll Radiol)* 2006;18:436–440.
122. Gong Z, Agalliu I, Lin DW, et al. Cigarette smoking and prostate cancer-specific mortality following diagnosis in middle-aged men. *Cancer Causes Control* 2008;19:25–31.
123. Kjaerbye-Thygesen A, Frederiksen K, Hogdall EV, et al. Smoking and overweight: negative prognostic factors in stage III epithelial ovarian cancer. *Cancer Epidemiol Biomarkers Prev* 2006;15:798–803.
124. Nagle CM, Bain CJ, Webb PM. Cigarette smoking and survival after ovarian cancer diagnosis. *Cancer Epidemiol Biomarkers Prev* 2006;15:2557–2560.
125. Wright JD, Li J, Gerhard DS, et al. Human papillomavirus type and tobacco use as predictors of survival in early stage cervical carcinoma. *Gynecol Oncol* 2005;98:84–91.
126. Sardari Nia P, Van Marck E, Weyler J, et al. Prognostic value of a biologic classification of non-small-cell lung cancer into the growth patterns along with other clinical, pathological and immunohistochemical factors. *Eur J Cardiothorac Surg* 2010;38:628–636.
127. Hoff CM, Grau C, Overgaard J. Effect of smoking on oxygen delivery and outcome in patients treated with radiotherapy for head and neck squamous cell carcinoma—a prospective study. *Radiother Oncol* 2012;103:38–44.
128. Joshu CE, Mondul AM, Meinhold CL, et al. Cigarette smoking and prostate cancer recurrence after prostatectomy. *J Natl Cancer Inst* 2011;103:835–838.
129. Mai SK, Welzel G, Haegele V, et al. The influence of smoking and other risk factors on the outcome after radiochemotherapy for anal cancer. *Radiat Oncol* 2007;2:30.
130. Kim AJ, Suh JD, Sercarz JA, et al. Salvage surgery with free flap reconstruction: factors affecting outcome after treatment of recurrent head and neck squamous carcinoma. *Laryngoscope* 2007;117:1019–1023.
131. Khan AM, Freeman-Wang T, Pisal N, et al. Smoking and multicentric vulval intraepithelial neoplasia. *J Obstet Gynaecol* 2009;29:123–125.
132. Hefler L, Grimm C, Tempfer C, et al. Treatment with vaginal progesterone in women with low-grade cervical dysplasia: a phase II trial. *Anticancer Res* 2010;30:1257–1261.
133. Matsumoto K, Oki A, Furuta R, et al. Tobacco smoking and regression of low-grade cervical abnormalities. *Cancer Sci* 2010;101:2065–2073.
134. Fleshner N, Garland J, Moadel A, et al. Influence of smoking status on the disease-related outcomes of patients with tobacco-associated superficial transitional cell carcinoma of the bladder. *Cancer* 1999;86:2337–2345.
135. Ioffe YJ, Elmore RG, Karlan BY, et al. Effect of cigarette smoking on epithelial ovarian cancer survival. *J Reprod Med* 2010;55:346–350.
136. Schlumbrecht MP, Sun CC, Wong KN, et al. Clinicodemographic factors influencing outcomes in patients with low-grade serous ovarian carcinoma. *Cancer* 2011;117:3741–3749.
137. Fortin A, Wang CS, Vigneault E. Influence of smoking and alcohol drinking behaviors on treatment outcomes of patients with squamous cell carcinomas of the head and neck. *Int J Radiat Oncol Biol Phys* 2009;74:1062–1069.
138. Chen CH, Shun CT, Huang KH, et al. Stopping smoking might reduce tumour recurrence in nonmuscle-invasive bladder cancer. *BJU Int* 2007;100:281–286.
139. Browman GP, Mohide EA, Willan A, et al. Association between smoking during radiotherapy and prognosis in head and neck cancer: a follow-up study. *Head Neck* 2002;24:1031–1037.
140. Clark JR, McCluskey SA, Hall F, et al. Predictors of morbidity following free flap reconstruction for cancer of the head and neck. *Head Neck* 2007;29:1090–1101.
141. Little SC, Hughley BB, Park SS. Complications with forehead flaps in nasal reconstruction. *Laryngoscope*. 2009;119:1093–1099.
142. Patel RS, McCluskey SA, Goldstein DP, et al. Clinicopathologic and therapeutic risk factors for perioperative complications and prolonged hospital stay in free flap reconstruction of the head and neck. *Head Neck* 2010;32:1345–1353.
143. Baumann DP, Lin HY, Chevray PM. Perforator number predicts fat necrosis in a prospective analysis of breast reconstruction with free TRAM, DIEP, and SIEA flaps. *Plast Reconstr Surg* 2010;125:1335–1341.
144. Goodwin SJ, McCarthy CM, Pusic AL, et al. Complications in smokers after postmastectomy tissue expander/implant breast reconstruction. *Ann Plast Surg* 2005;55:16–19.
145. Bertelsen CA, Andreasen AH, Jorgensen T, et al. Anastomotic leakage after anterior resection for rectal cancer: risk factors. *Colorectal Dis* 2010;12:37–43.
146. Cooke DT, Lin GC, Lau CL, et al. Analysis of cervical esophagogastric anastomotic leaks after transhiatal esophagectomy: risk factors, presentation, and detection. *Ann Thorac Surg* 2009;88:177–184.
147. Richards CH, Platt JJ, Anderson JH, et al. The impact of perioperative risk, tumor pathology and surgical complications on disease recurrence following potentially curative resection of colorectal cancer. *Ann Surg* 2011;254:83–89.
148. Nickelsen TN, Jorgensen T, Kronborg O. Lifestyle and 30-day complications to surgery for colorectal cancer. *Acta Oncol* 2005;44:218–223.
149. Begum FD, Hogdall E, Christensen IJ, et al. Serum tetranectin as a preoperative indicator for postoperative complications in Danish ovarian cancer patients. *Gynecol Oncol* 2010;117:446–450.
150. Joo YH, Sun DI, Cho JH, et al. Factors that predict postoperative pulmonary complications after supracricoid partial laryngectomy. *Arch Otolaryngol Head Neck Surg* 2009;135:1154–1157.
151. Mason DP, Subramanian S, Nowicki ER, et al. Impact of smoking cessation before resection of lung cancer: a Society of Thoracic Surgeons General Thoracic Surgery Database study. *Ann Thorac Surg* 2009;88:362–370.
152. van der Voet JC, Keus RB, Hart AA, et al. The impact of treatment time and smoking on local control and complications in T1 glottic cancer. *Int J Radiat Oncol Biol Phys* 1998;42:247–255.
153. Wedlake LJ, Thomas K, Lalji A, et al. Predicting late effects of pelvic radiotherapy: is there a better approach? *Int J Radiat Oncol Biol Phys* 2010;78:1163–1170.
154. Hocevar-Boltezar I, Zargi M, Strojan P. Risk factors for voice quality after radiotherapy for early glottic cancer. *Radiother Oncol* 2009;93:524–529.
155. Lilla C, Ambrosone CB, Kropp S, et al. Predictive factors for late normal tissue complications following radiotherapy for breast cancer. *Breast Cancer Res Treat* 2007;106:143–150.
156. Eifel PJ, Jhingran A, Bodurka DC, et al. Correlation of smoking history and other patient characteristics with major complications of pelvic radiation therapy for cervical cancer. *J Clin Oncol* 2002;20:3651–3657.
157. Wuketich S, Hienz SA, Marosi C. Prevalence of clinically relevant oral mucositis in outpatients receiving myelosuppressive chemotherapy for solid tumors. *Support Care Cancer* 2012;20:175–183.
158. Zevallos JP, Mallen MJ, Lam CY, et al. Complications of radiotherapy in laryngopharyngeal cancer: effects of a prospective smoking cessation program. *Cancer* 2009;115:4636–4644.
159. Gold EB, Flatt SW, Pierce JP, et al. Dietary factors and vasomotor symptoms in breast cancer survivors: the WHEL Study. *Menopause* 2006;13:423–433.
160. Cheung MC, Hamilton K, Sherman R, et al. Impact of teaching facility status and high-volume centers on outcomes for lung cancer resection: an examination of 13,469 surgical patients. *Ann Surg Oncol* 2009;16:3–13.
161. Zingg U, Smithers BM, Gotley DC, et al. Factors associated with postoperative pulmonary morbidity after esophagectomy for cancer. *Ann Surg Oncol* 2011;18:1460–1468.
162. Kelly KJ, Greenblatt DY, Wan Y, et al. Risk stratification for distal pancreatectomy utilizing ACS-NSQIP: preoperative factors predict morbidity and mortality. *J Gastrointest Surg* 2011;15:250–259.
163. Merkow RP, Bilimoria KY, Cohen ME, et al. Variability in reoperation rates at 182 hospitals: a potential target for quality improvement. *J Am Coll Surg*. 2009;209:557–564.
164. Alsadius D, Hedelin M, Johansson KA, et al. Tobacco smoking and long-lasting symptoms from the bowel and the anal-sphincter region after radiotherapy for prostate cancer. *Radiother Oncol* 2011;101:495–501.
165. Kuri M, Nakagawa M, Tanaka H, et al. Determination of the duration of preoperative smoking cessation to improve wound healing after head and neck surgery. *Anesthesiology* 2005;102:892–896.
166. Vaporciyan AA, Merriman KW, Ece F, et al. Incidence of major pulmonary morbidity after pneumonectomy: association with timing of smoking cessation. *Ann Thorac Surg* 2002;73:420–425.
167. Bjarnason GA, Mackenzie RG, Nabid A, et al. Comparison of toxicity associated with early morning versus late afternoon radiotherapy in patients with head-and-neck cancer: a prospective randomized trial of the National Cancer Institute of Canada Clinical Trials Group (HN3). *Int J Radiat Oncol Biol Phys* 2009;73:166–172.
168. Park SM, Lim MK, Jung KW, et al. Prediagnosis smoking, obesity, insulin resistance, and second primary cancer risk in male cancer survivors: National Health Insurance Corporation Study. *J Clin Oncol* 2007;25:4835–4843.
169. Leon X, del Prado Venegas M, Orus C, et al. Influence of the persistence of tobacco and alcohol use in the appearance of second neoplasm in patients with a head and neck cancer. A case-control study. *Cancer Causes Control* 2009;20:645–652.
170. Kinoshita Y, Tsukuma H, Ajiki W, et al. The risk for second primaries in gastric cancer patients: adjuvant therapy and habitual smoking and drinking. *J Epidemiol* 2000;10:300–304.
171. Khuri FR, Kim ES, Lee JJ, et al. The impact of smoking status, disease stage, and index tumor site on second primary tumor incidence and tumor recurrence in the head and neck retinoid chemoprevention trial. *Cancer Epidemiol Biomarkers Prev* 2001;10:823–829.

172. Scanlon EF, Suh O, Murthy SM, et al. Influence of smoking on the development of lung metastases from breast cancer. *Cancer* 1995;75:2693–2699.
173. Ford MB, Sigurdson AJ, Petrulis ES, et al. Effects of smoking and radiotherapy on lung carcinoma in breast carcinoma survivors. *Cancer* 2003;98:1457–1464.
174. Li CI, Daling JR, Porter PL, et al. Relationship between potentially modifiable lifestyle factors and risk of second primary contralateral breast cancer among women diagnosed with estrogen receptor-positive invasive breast cancer. *J Clin Oncol* 2009;27:5312–5318.
175. van den Belt-Dusebout AW, de Wit R, Gietema JA, et al. Treatment-specific risks of second malignancies and cardiovascular disease in 5-year survivors of testicular cancer. *J Clin Oncol* 2007;25:4370–4378.
176. Boorjian S, Cowan JE, Konety BR, et al. Cancer of the Prostate Strategic Urologic Research Endeavor Investigators. Bladder cancer incidence and risk factors in men with prostate cancer: results from Cancer of the Prostate Strategic Urologic Research Endeavor. *J Urol* 2007;177:883–887.
177. Travis LB, Gospodarowicz M, Curtis RE, et al. Lung cancer following chemotherapy and radiotherapy for Hodgkin's disease. *J Natl Cancer Inst* 2002;94:182–192.
178. Ang KK, Harris J, Wheeler R, et al. Human papillomavirus and survival of patients with oropharyngeal cancer. *N Engl J Med* 2010;363:24–35.
179. Peck BW, Dahlstrom KR, Gan SJ, et al. Low risk of second primary malignancies among never smokers with human papillomavirus-associated index oropharyngeal cancers. *Head Neck* 2012;35:794–799.
180. Herbst RS, Prager D, Hermann R, et al. TRIBUTE: a phase III trial of erlotinib hydrochloride (OSI-774) combined with carboplatin and paclitaxel chemotherapy in advanced non-small-cell lung cancer. *J Clin Oncol* 2005;23:5892–5899.
181. Thatcher N, Chang A, Parikh P, et al. Gefitinib plus best supportive care in previously treated patients with refractory advanced non-small-cell lung cancer: results from a randomised, placebo-controlled, multicentre study (Iressa Survival Evaluation in Lung Cancer). *Lancet* 2005;366:1527–1537.
182. Kwak EL, Bang YJ, Camidge DR, et al. Anaplastic lymphoma kinase inhibition in non-small-cell lung cancer. *N Engl J Med* 2010;363:1693–1703.
183. Paik PK, Johnson ML, D'Angelo SP, et al. Driver mutations determine survival in smokers and never-smokers with stage IIIB/IV lung adenocarcinomas. *Cancer* 2012;118:5840–5847.
184. Soria JC, Cruz C, Bahleda R, et al. Clinical activity, safety and biomarkers of PD-L1 blockade in non-small cell lung cancer (NSCLC): additional analyses from a clinical study of the engineered antibody MPDL3280A (anti-PDL1). Presented at: 2013 European Cancer Congress 2013; 2013; Amsterdam.
185. Morales N, Romano M, Cummings KM, et al. Accuracy of self-reported tobacco use in newly diagnosed cancer patients. *Cancer Causes Control* 2013;24:1223–1230.
186. Warren GW, Arnold SM, Valentino JP, et al. Accuracy of self-reported tobacco assessments in a head and neck cancer treatment population. *Radiother Oncol* 2012;103:45–48.
187. Marin VP, Pytynia KB, Langstein HN, et al. Serum cotinine concentration and wound complications in head and neck reconstruction. *Plast Reconstr Surg* 2008;121:451–457.
188. American Medical Association. Tobacco use or exposure as a variable in clinical research (Resolution 424, A-06).www.ama-assn.org.ama1/pub/upload/mm/475/bot479i406.pdf.
189. Sarna L, Bialous SA. Nursing and tobacco cessation: setting a research agenda. Reports from a national conference. In: *Nursing Research*. Philadelphia: Lippincott Williams & Wilkins; 2006: 4S.
190. Sarna L, Bialous SA, Chan S, et al. International symposia: global perspectives on nursing involvement in tobacco control. Presented in: Oncology Nursing Society, 28th Annual Congress Syllabus, May 1–4, 2003, Denver, Colorado. Denver: Oncology Nursing Society; 2003: 112.
191. Viswanath K, Herbst RS, Land SR, et al. Tobacco and cancer: an American Association for Cancer research policy statement. *Cancer Res* 2010;70(17):3419–3430.
192. American Society of Clinical Oncology. American Society of Clinical Oncology policy statement update: tobacco control—Reducing cancer incidence and saving lives. 2003. *J Clin Oncol* 2003;21:2777–2786.
193. Gritz ER, Fingeret MC, Vidrine DJ, et al. Successes and failures of the teachable moment: smoking cessation in cancer patients. *Cancer* 2006;106:17–27.
194. Gritz ER, Dresler C, Sarna L. Smoking, the missing drug interaction in clinical trials: ignoring the obvious. *Cancer Epidemiol Biomarkers Prev* 2005;14:2287–2293.
195. Chappel A, Ziebland S, McPherson A, Stigma, shame, and blame experienced by patients with lung cancer: qualitative study. *BMJ* 2004;328:1470.
196. LoConte NK, Else-Quest NM, Eickhoff J, et al. Assessment of guilt and shame in patients with non-small-cell lung cancer compared with patients with breast and prostate cancer. *Clin Lung Cancer* 2008;9:171–178.
197. Wassenaar TR, Eickhoff JC, Jarzemsky DR, et al. Differences in primary care clinicians' approach to non-small cell lung cancer patients compared with breast cancer. *J Thorac Oncol* 2007;2:722–728.
198. Fiore MC, Bailey WC, Cohen SJ, et al. *Quick Reference Guide for Clinicians. Treating Tobacco Use and Dependence.* Rockville, MD: U.S. Department of Health and Human Services, Public Health Services; 2000. http://health.state.tn.us/Downloads/TQL_Quick%20Reference.pdf. Accessed November 25, 2013.
199. Fiore MC, Jaén CR, Baker TB, et al. *Treating Tobacco Use and Dependence: 2008 Update.* Rockville, MD: U.S. Department of Health and Human Services; 2008. http://www.ncbi.nlm.nih.gov/books/NBK63952/. Accessed November 25, 2013.
200. Fiore MC, Jorenby DE, Schensky AE, et al. Smoking status as the new vital sign: effect on assessment and intervention in patients who smoke. *Mayo Clin Proc* 1995;70:209–213.
201. Blumenthal D, Tavenner M. The "meaningful use" regulation for electronic health records. *N Engl J Med* 2010;363:501–504.
202. Couple approaches to smoking cessation. In: Schmaling KB, Sher TG, eds. *The Psychology of Couples and Illness: Theory, Research, & Practice.* Washington, D.C.: American Psychological Association; 2000: 311–336.
203. Homish GG, Leonard KE. Spousal influence on smoking behaviors in a US community sample of newly married couples. *Soc Sci Med* 2005;61:2557–2567.
204. Hemsing N, Greaves L, O'Leary R, et al. Partner support for smoking cessation during pregnancy: a systematic review. *Nicotine Tob Res* 2012;14:767–776.
205. Tod AM, Joanne R. Overcoming delay in the diagnosis of lung cancer: a qualitative study. *Nurs Stan* 2010;24:35–43.
206. Fagerstrom KO, Schneider NG. Measuring nicotine dependence: a review of the Fagerstrom Tolerance Questionnaire. *J Behav Med* 1989;12:159–182.
207. Baker TB, Piper ME, Bolt DM, et al. Time to first cigarette in the morning smoking as an index of ability to quit smoking: implications for nicotine dependence. *Nicotine Tob Res* 2007;9:S555–S570.
208. Ferguson JA, Patten CA, Schroeder DR, et al. Predictors of 6-month tobacco abstinence among 1224 cigarette smokers treated for nicotine dependence. *Addict Behav* 2003;28:1203–1218.
209. Prochaska JO, DiClemente CC. Stages and processes of self-change of smoking: toward an integrative model of change. *J Consult Clin Psychol* 1983;51:390–395.
210. Prokhorov AV, Hudmon KS, Gritz ER. Promoting smoking cessation among cancer patients: a behavioral model. *Oncology (Williston Park)* 1997;11:1807–1813.
211. Toll BA, Rojewski AM, Duncan L, et al. "Quitting smoking will benefit your health": the evolution of clinician messaging to encourage tobacco cessation. *Clin Cancer Res* 2014;20:301–309.
212. Miller WR, Rose GS. Toward a theory of motivational interviewing. *Am Psychol* 2009;64:527–537.
213. Gritz ER, Fingeret MC, Vidrine DJ. Tobacco control in the oncology setting. In: Brawley OW, Khuri FR, Rock CL, eds. *ASCO Cancer Prevention Curriculum.* Alexandria, VA: American Society of Clinical Oncology; 2007.
214. Henningfield JE, Keenan RM. Nicotine delivery kinetics and abuse liability. *J Consult Clin Psychol* 1993;61:743–750.
215. Silagy C, Lancaster T, Stead L, et al. Nicotine replacement therapy for smoking cessation. *Cochrane Database Syst Rev* 2004;(3):CD000146.
216. Piper M, Smith S, Schlam T, et al. A randomized placebo-controlled clinical trial of 5 smoking cessation pharmacotherapies. *Arch Gen Psychiatry* 2009;66:1253–1262.
217. Smith S, McCarthy D, Japuntich S, et al. Comparative effectiveness of 5 smoking cessation pharmacotherapies in primary care clinics. *Arch Intern Med* 2009;169:2148–2155.
218. Warren GW, Singh AK. Nicotine and lung cancer. *J Carcinog* 2013;12:1–8.
219. Myles PS, Iacono GA, Hunt JO, et al. Risk of respiratory complications and wound infection in patients undergoing ambulatory surgery: smokers versus nonsmokers. *Anesthesiology* 2002;97:842–847.
220. Sørensen L, Hørby J, Friis E, et al. Smoking as a risk factor for wound healing and infection in breast cancer surgery. *Eur J Surg Oncol* 2002;28:815–820.
221. Jorgensen ED, Zhao H, Traganos F, et al. DNA damage response induced by exposure of human lung adenocarcinoma cells to smoke from tobacco- and nicotine-free cigarettes. *Cell Cycle* 2010;9:2170–2176.
222. Murray RP, Connett JE, Zapawa LM. Does nicotine replacement therapy cause cancer? Evidence from the Lung Health Study. *Nicotine Tob Res* 2009;11:1076–1082.
223. Hughes JR, Stead LF, Lancaster T. Nortriptyline for smoking cessation: a review. *Nicotine Tob Res* 2005;7:491–499.
224. Ascher JA, Cole JO, Colin JN, et al. Bupropion: a review of its mechanism of antidepressant activity. *J Clin Psychiatry* 1995;56:395–401.
225. Fryer JD, Lukas RJ. Noncompetitive functional inhibition at diverse, human nicotinic acetylcholine receptor subtypes by bupropion, phencyclidine, and ibogaine. *J Pharmacol Exp Ther* 1999;288:88–92.
226. Cryan JF, Bruijnzeel AW, Skjei KL, et al. Bupropion enhances brain reward function and reverses the affective and somatic aspects of nicotine withdrawal in the rat. *Psychopharmacology* 2003;168:347–358.
227. Hughes JR, Stead LF, Lancaster T. Antidepressants for smoking cessation. *Cochrane Database Syst Rev* 2003;(2):CD000031.
228. Coe JW, Brooks PR, Vetelino MG, et al. Varenicline: an alpha4beta2 nicotinic receptor partial agonist for smoking cessation. *J Med Chem* 2005;48:3474–3477.
229. Jorenby DE, Hays JT, Rigotti NA, et al. Efficacy of varenicline, an alpha4beta2 nicotinic acetylcholine receptor partial agonist, vs placebo or sustained-release bupropion for smoking cessation: a randomized controlled trial. *JAMA* 2006;296:56–63.
230. Cahill K, Stead LF, Lancaster T. Nicotine receptor partial agonists for smoking cessation. *Cochrane Database Syst Rev* 2012;4:CD006103.
231. Hoogendoorn M, Welsing P, Rutten-van Mölken MP. Cost-effectiveness of varenicline compared with bupropion, NRT, and nortriptyline for smoking cessation in the Netherlands. *Curr Med Res Opin* 2008;24:51–61.
232. Linden K, Jormanainen V, Linna M, et al. Cost effectiveness of varenicline versus bupropion and unaided cessation for smoking cessation in a cohort of Finnish adult smokers. *Curr Med Res Opin* 2010;26:549–560.
233. Zimovetz EA, Wilson K, Samuel M, et al. A review of cost-effectiveness of varenicline and comparison of cost-effectiveness of treatments for major smoking-related morbidities. *J Eval Clin Pract* 2011;17:288–297.
234. Gibbons RD, Mann JJ. Varenicline, smoking cessation, and neuropsychiatric adverse events. *Am J of Psychiatry* 2013;170:1460–1467.

235. Thomas KH, Martin RM, Davies NM, et al. Smoking cessation treatment and risk of depression, suicide, and self harm in the Clinical Practice Research Datalink: prospective cohort study. *BMJ* 2013;347:f5704.
236. Anthenelli RM, Morris C, Ramey TS, et al. Effects of varenicline on smoking cessation in adults with stably treated current or past major depression: a randomized trial. *Ann Intern Med* 2013;159:390–400.
237. Gourlay SG, Stead LF, Benowitz NL. Clonidine for smoking cessation. *Cochrane Database Syst Rev* 2004;(3):CD000058.
238. Gritz ER, Carr CR, Rapkin D, et al. Predictors of long-term smoking cessation in head and neck cancer patients. *Cancer Epidemiol Biomarkers Prev* 1993;2:261–270.
239. Schnoll RA, Rothman RL, Wielt DB, et al. A randomized pilot study of cognitive-behavioral therapy versus basic health education for smoking cessation among cancer patients. *Ann Behav Med* 2005;30:1–11.
240. Griebel B, Wewers ME, Baker CA. The effectiveness of a nurse-managed minimal smoking-cessation intervention among hospitalized patients with cancer. *Oncol Nurs Forum* 1998;25:897–902.
241. Wewers ME, Bowen JM, Stanislaw AE, et al. A nurse-delivered smoking cessation intervention among hospitalized postoperative patients—influence of a smoking-related diagnosis: a pilot study. *Heart Lung* 1994;23:151–156.
242. Wewers ME, Jenkins L, Mignery T. A nurse-managed smoking cessation intervention during diagnostic testing for lung cancer. *Oncol Nurs Forum* 1997;24:1419–1422.
243. Stanislaw AE, Wewers ME. A smoking cessation intervention with hospitalized surgical cancer patients: a pilot study. *Cancer Nurs* 1994;17:81–86.
244. Schnoll RA, Zhang B, Rue M, et al. Brief physician-initiated quit-smoking strategies for clinical oncology settings: a trial coordinated by the Eastern Cooperative Oncology Group. *J Clin Oncol* 2003;21:355–365.
245. Sanderson Cox L, Patten CA, Ebbert JO, et al. Tobacco use outcomes among patients with lung cancer treated for nicotine dependence. *J Clin Oncol* 2002;20:3461–3469.
246. Garces YI, Schroeder DR, Nirelli LM, et al. Tobacco use outcomes among patients with head and neck carcinoma treated for nicotine dependence: a matched-pair analysis. *Cancer* 2004;101:116–124.
247. Duffy SA, Ronis DL, Valenstein M, et al. A tailored smoking, alcohol, and depression intervention for head and neck cancer patients. *Cancer Epidemiol Biomarkers Prev* 2006;15:2203–2208.
248. Schnoll RA, Martinez E, Tatum KL, et al. A bupropion smoking cessation clinical trial for cancer patients. *Cancer Causes Control* 2010;21:811–820.
249. Martinez E, Tatum KL, Weber DM, et al. Issues related to implementing a smoking cessation clinical trial for cancer patients. *Cancer Causes Control* 2009;20:97–104.
250. Park ER, Japuntich S, Temel J, et al. A smoking cessation intervention for thoracic surgery and oncology clinics: a pilot trial. *J Thorac Oncol* 2011;6:1059–1065.
251. Ostroff JS, Burkhalter JE, Cinciripini PM, et al. Randomized trial of a presurgical scheduled reduced smoking intervention for patients newly diagnosed with cancer. *Health Psychol* 2013 [Epub ahead of print].
252. Emmons KM, Puleo E, Park E, et al. Peer-delivered smoking counseling for childhood cancer survivors increases rate of cessation: the partnership for health study. *J Clin Oncol* 2005;23:6516–6523.
253. Wakefield M, Olver I, Whitford H, et al. Motivational interviewing as a smoking cessation intervention for patients with cancer: randomized controlled trial. *Nurs Res* 2004;53:396–406.
254. Goldstein AO, Ripley-Moffitt CE, Pathman DE, et al. Tobacco use treatment at the U.S. National Cancer Institute's designated Cancer Centers. *Nicotine Tob Res* 2013;15:52–58.
255. Warren GW, Marshall JR, Cummings KM, et al. Practice patterns and perceptions of thoracic oncology providers on tobacco use and cessation in cancer patients. *J Thorac Oncol* 2013;8:543–548.
256. Warren GW, Marshall JR, Cummings KM, et al. Addressing tobacco use in cancer patients: a survey of American Society of Clinical Oncology (ASCO) members. *J Oncol Pract* 2013;9:258–262.
257. Gritz ER, Sarna L, Dresler C, et al. Building a united front: aligning the agendas for tobacco control, lung cancer research, and policy. *Cancer Epidemiol Biomarkers Prev* 2007;16:859–863.
258. Vidrine JI, Shete S, Cao Y, et al. Ask-Advise-Connect: a new approach to smoking treatment delivery in health care settings. *JAMA Intern Med* 2013;173:458–464.
259. Bernstein SL, Jearld S, Prasad D, et al. Rapid implementation of a smokers' quitline fax referral service in an urban area. *J Health Care Poor Underserved* 2009;20:55–63.
260. Sarna L, Bialous SA, Ong MK, et al. Increasing nursing referral to telephone quitlines for smoking cessation using a web-based program. *Nurs Res* 2012;61:433–440.
261. Stancic N, Mullen PD, Prokhorov AV, et al. Continuing medical education: what delivery format do physicians prefer? *J Contin Educ Health Prof* 2003;23:162–167.
262. Society for Research on Nicotine and Tobacco Committee on Biochemical Verification. Biochemical verification of tobacco use and cessation. *Nicotine Tob Res* 2002;4:149–159.
263. American Society of Clinical Oncology. Tobacco Cessation Guide: for Oncology Providers. ASCO Web site. http://www.asco.org/sites/default/files/tobacco_cessation_guide.pdf. Accessed November 25, 2013.

32 Role of Surgery in Cancer Prevention

José G. Guillem, Andrew Berchuck, Jeffrey F. Moley, Jeffrey A. Norton, Sheryl G. A. Gabram-Mendola, and Vanessa W. Hui

INTRODUCTION

Since the heritable component of some cancer predispositions has been linked to mutations in specific genes, clinical interventions have been formulated for mutation carriers within affected families. The primary interventions for mutation carriers for highly penetrant syndromes, such as multiple endocrine neoplasia (MEN), familial adenomatous polyposis (FAP), hereditary nonpolyposis colorectal cancer (CRC), and hereditary breast and ovarian cancer syndromes, are primarily surgical. This chapter is divided into five sections addressing breast (S.G.A.G.), gastric (J.N.), ovarian and endometrial (A.B.), and MENs (J.F.M.) and colorectal (J.G.G., V.W.H.). For each, the clinical and genetic indications and timing of prophylactic surgery and its efficacy, when known, are provided.

Prophylactic surgery in hereditary cancer is a complex process, requiring a clear understanding of the natural history of the disease and variance of penetrance, a realistic appreciation of the potential benefit and consequence of a risk-reducing procedure in an otherwise potentially healthy individual, and the long-term sequelae of such surgical intervention, as well as the individual patient's and family's perception of surgical risk and anticipated benefit.

PATIENTS AT HIGH RISK FOR BREAST CANCER

Identification of Patients at Risk

A detailed family history is the most important tool for identifying individuals at increased risk for hereditary cancers. The US Preventive Services Task Force updated their recommendation for risk assessment, genetic counseling, and genetic testing for asymptomatic women who have not been diagnosed with a *BRCA*-related cancer. In this update, the use of a risk screening tool is highly recommended to identify appropriate patients for referral for genetic counseling.[1] The American Society of Clinical Oncology has also updated the policy on genetic and genomic testing for cancer susceptibility, and this update includes information on genetic tests of uncertain clinical utility and direct-to-consumer marketing, both of which impact the practice of oncology and preventive medicine.[2] Historically, genetic counseling and testing were offered by health-care providers. However, with the advent of direct-to-consumer marketing, individuals may obtain tests and receive results directly from a company. The American Society of Clinical Oncology still endorses pre- and posttest counseling for thorough disclosure of the impact of testing. Before any woman considers risk-reduction surgery such as bilateral mastectomy or salpingo-oophorectomy, referral to a high-risk or genetic screening program is desirable, as women often overestimate their actual breast cancer risk.[3]

The most common cancer syndromes that place women at risk for breast cancer are *BRCA1*[4] and *BRCA2*[5] gene mutations. Other less common syndromes are listed in Table 32.1.[6,7]

Following referral for genetic assessment, three groups of patients emerge.[8] The first consists of those women who have undergone genetic testing and have been found to harbor a mutated gene associated with high penetrance for breast cancer. Given that the possibility of developing breast cancer in this group may be as high as 90%, there is a role for enhanced surveillance or risk-reduction surgery. The American Cancer Society has published guidelines for magnetic resonance imaging (MRI) screening as a method for enhanced surveillance.[9] Women in this first group qualify for such screening, which can be offered annually but scheduled at 6-month intervals with screening mammography to increase the rate of identifying interval cancers. Alternatively, simultaneous screening with MRI and mammography to compare one modality with the other on an annual basis may also be offered. Another choice for this group of women is to pursue bilateral risk-reduction mastectomy with an option for immediate reconstruction. Bilateral salpingo-oophorectomy for *BRCA1* and *BRCA2* mutation carriers may also be considered, as this procedure has been shown to reduce breast cancer risk by almost 50%.[8,10] This is especially true for *BRCA2* mutation carriers, who tend to develop hormone receptor–positive breast cancers.

The second group consists of women with strong family histories suggestive of hereditary breast cancer who test negative for both the *BRCA1* and *BRCA2* mutations as well as the other described syndromes. In this group, there may not have been a family member with cancer who was tested for the mutation. Therefore, a negative test does not necessarily indicate that a woman's risk is equivalent to that of the general population.[7] There may also be an undetected mutation in such a family, indicating the possibility of higher-than-average risk for that particular woman. These women may or may not qualify for enhanced surveillance with MRI screening,[9] and accurate assessment of their risk may require the use of other risk prediction tools,[3] in addition to evaluating for the presence of lobular carcinoma in situ, atypical lobular hyperplasia, or atypical ductal hyperplasia, and determining if a more intensive surveillance regimen is necessary based on heterogeneously or extremely dense breast tissue on mammography.

The third group consists of women with a strong family history of breast cancer, who for various reasons, have chosen not to pursue genetic testing. These individuals may have other health-related problems, psychological concerns, cost issues, or they may fear perceived medical insurance discrimination. Women in all groups can be educated that with passage of the Genetic Information Nondiscrimination Act in 2008, significant advances have occurred that protect patients from discrimination by employers and health insurers.[11]

Women in the second and third groups may still qualify for bilateral risk-reduction mastectomy and immediate reconstruction. Often, women who elect this path are influenced by their family history or by witnessing breast and/or ovarian cancer deaths in close family members, giving them a significant fear of a breast or ovarian cancer diagnosis. For women in all three groups, the decision of whether to pursue risk-reducing surgery is difficult. Often, the expertise of a cancer clinical psychologist or psychiatrist

TABLE 32.1

Hereditary Carcinoma Syndromes Including Breast Cancer

Syndrome	Chromosome/Gene	Primary Carcinoma	Secondary Carcinoma	Breast Cancer Penetrance
Familial breast cancer/ ovarian cancer syndrome	17q21; *BRCA1* Autosomal dominant	Breast cancer, ovarian cancer	Colon, prostate	60%–80%
Familial breast cancer/ ovarian cancer syndrome	13q12; *BRCA2* Autosomal dominant	Breast cancer, ovarian cancer	Male breast cancer, endometrial, prostate, oropharyngeal, pancreatic	60%–80%
Li-Fraumeni syndrome	17p13.1 and 22q12.1; *TP53* and *CHEK2* Autosomal dominant	Soft tissue cancers (including breast)	Soft tissue sarcoma, leukemia, osteosarcoma, melanoma, colon, pancreas, adrenal syndrome, cortex, and brain tumors	50%–85% (for all types of cancers in this syndrome)
PTEN hamartoma syndrome (Cowdon's)	10q23.31; *PTEN* mutation Autosomal dominant	Breast cancer	Thyroid (follicular) and endometrial carcinoma	25%–50%
Peutz-Jeghers syndrome	19p13.3; *STK11* Autosomal dominant	Gastrointestinal cancers	Esophagus, stomach, small intestine, large bowel, pancreas, lung, ovary, endometrial	29%
Diffuse gastric cancer	16q22.1; *CDH1* Autosomal dominant	Diffuse gastric cancer	Colorectal, lobular breast cancer	39% (lobular breast cancer)
Louis-Bar syndrome	11q22.3; *ATM* Autosomal recessive	Leukemia and lymphoma	Ovarian, breast, gastric, melanoma, leiomyomas, sarcomas	38% (for all types of cancers in the syndrome)

PTEN, phosphatase and tensin homolog.
Data from Lux MP, Fasching PA, Beckmann MW. Hereditary breast and ovarian cancer: review and future perspectives. *J Mol Med* 2006;84:16–28; and Shannon KM, Chittenden A. Genetic testing by cancer site: breast. *Cancer J* 2012;18:310–319.

is enlisted, as risk-reduction mastectomy involves an irreversible procedure with body image and sexual implications.[8]

Updated in 2007, the Society of Surgical Oncology published a position statement on the role of prophylactic mastectomy for patients at high risk for breast cancer, as well as those patients recently diagnosed with breast cancer who are considering contralateral prophylactic breast surgery.[12] For women at high risk, indications fall into three broad categories: presence of a mutation in *BRCA* or other susceptible genes, strong family history with no demonstrable mutation, and histologic risk factors (biopsy-proven atypical ductal hyperplasia, atypical lobular hyperplasia, or lobular carcinoma in situ especially in patients with a strong family history of breast cancer). Recommendations for patients with recently diagnosed breast cancer are similar in that they include the indications for high-risk individuals previously noted, as well as future surveillance challenges for the opposite breast (clinically and mammographically dense breast tissue or diffuse, indeterminate microcalcifications in the contralateral breast). Another important consideration is the need for symmetry in patients with large, ptotic, or disproportionately sized contralateral breasts.

Surgical Issues and Technique

In a single institution's 33-year experience,[13] the risk for breast cancer in both moderate- and high-risk groups of women based on family history was reduced by at least 89% for women who underwent bilateral prophylactic mastectomy. From a technical perspective, in this study, women either had a subcutaneous mastectomy (removal of the majority of breast tissue with sparing of the nipple–areola complex) or total mastectomy (removal of the entire breast through the nipple–areola complex). Most of the recurrences occurred in women undergoing a subcutaneous mastectomy. However, this was the most frequent procedure performed at that time and thus may have contributed to the number of increased recurrences.

Another surgical option for high-risk women is bilateral salpingo-oophorectomy. Among a cohort of women with *BRCA1* and *BRCA2* mutations, this procedure has been associated with a lower risk of mortality from both breast and ovarian cancer.[10] As an additional benefit, this procedure also decreases the risk of breast cancer in this patient population, likely through the mechanism of decreasing hormonal exposure at a younger age.

Contemporary surgical procedures for risk-reducing bilateral mastectomy include total mastectomy, skin-sparing mastectomy (preservation of the skin envelope by removal of the entire breast through a circumareolar incision around the nipple–areola complex), subcutaneous mastectomy, areola-sparing mastectomy (removal of the nipple while sparing the areola), and nipple-sparing mastectomy (removal of entire breast and nipple core tissue but preservation of nipple–areolar skin).[14] Given advances in reconstructive nipple–areolar techniques, it appears that total mastectomy with or without skin-sparing methods reduces the risk of breast cancer to the greatest extent with reasonable cosmesis. More limited and long-term follow-up data are available on areola- and nipple-sparing techniques. The potential limitations of these procedures are distortion of the nipple–areola complex and lack of sensitivity after breast tissue has been completely removed.[8]

Immediate reconstruction is offered to patients and performed in the vast majority undergoing bilateral risk-reduction mastectomy. Choices of reconstruction include a bilateral pedicled or free tissue transverse rectus abdominis muscle flap, a free bilateral deep inferior epigastric perforator flap or superficial inferior epigastric artery flap, bilateral latissimus flaps with or without implant or expanders, or bilateral implant or expander placement alone.[14] Although tissue flap transfer gives a more natural appearance and texture to the reconstructed site, individual body contour drives the ultimate plan for reconstruction. The decision about the type of reconstruction should be made by the plastic surgeon with input from the surgical oncologist, especially for the group of women with breast cancer desiring bilateral mastectomies who may require adjuvant radiation for treatment.

Although the risk reduction is dramatic for bilateral mastectomy, residual breast tissue may be left behind, especially with skin-sparing procedures. Patients should be educated that careful chest wall surveillance is recommended after such a procedure. Local recurrences after bilateral implant reconstruction are reliably detected by clinical examination. Recurrences after reconstruction with autologous tissue present most commonly on the skin 50% to 72% of the time and are detectable by physician examination.[15] Nonpalpable deeper recurrences in this setting are less common, and use of mammography image surveillance may be indicated, especially if significant breast tissue was left behind unintentionally during the bilateral mastectomy procedure. At times, an initial "screening" mammogram may be performed, if significant residual breast tissue is suspected; this should occur well after all healing has taken place to delineate the amount of visible breast tissue on imaging. This drives future decisions of whether to follow a patient with imaging. Finally, all patients should be instructed to return for clinical breast examination with the health provider if any change is noted on the reconstructed breasts, regardless of imaging plan.

Although risk-reduction bilateral mastectomy may be exceedingly beneficial for high-risk women, especially for those testing positive for *BRCA1*, *BRCA2*, or other deleterious mutations, or belonging to a family afflicted with a cancer syndrome, they are never emergent procedures. Along with risk-reduction bilateral salpingo-oophorectomy, risk-reduction bilateral mastectomy resides at the far end of the spectrum of an individual's choices.[16] These procedures should be offered only after appropriate genetic counseling and accurate assessment of a woman's actual risk for breast and ovarian cancer. An in-depth consultation with the patient and her family members is necessary prior to proceeding with an operative plan.

HEREDITARY DIFFUSE GASTRIC CANCER

Gastric cancer is the fourth most common cause of cancer worldwide and is the second leading cause of cancer mortality.[17] Although environmental agents, including *Helicobacter pylori* and diet, are the primary risk factors for this disease, approximately 10% of gastric cancers are a result of familial clustering.[18,19] Histologically, gastric cancers may be classified as either intestinal or diffuse types. The intestinal type histopathology is linked to environmental factors and advanced age. The diffuse type occurs in younger patients and is associated with a familial predisposition. Because of a decrease in intestinal-type gastric cancers, the overall incidence of gastric cancer has declined significantly in the past 50 years. However, the incidence of diffuse gastric cancer (DGC), which is also called signet ring cell or linitis plastica, has remained stable and, by some reports, may be increasing.

Hereditary DGC (HDGC) is a genetic cancer susceptibility syndrome defined by one of the following: (1) two or more documented cases of DGC in first- or second-degree relatives, with at least one diagnosed before the age of 50; or (2) three or more cases of documented DGC in first- or second-degree relatives, independent of age of onset. The average age of onset of HDGC is 38, and the pattern of inheritance is autosomal dominant.[20] Figure 32.1 shows a pedigree with HDGC.

In 1998, inactivating germline mutations in the E-cadherin gene *CDH1* were identified in three Maori families, each with multiple cases of poorly differentiated DGC.[21] The *CDH1* mutations in these families were inherited in an autosomal dominant pattern, with incomplete but high penetrance. Onset of clinically apparent cancer was early, with the youngest affected individual dying of DGC at the age of 14.[21] Since then, germline mutations of *CDH1* have been identified in 30% to 50% of all patients with HDGC.[19,22] More than 50 mutations have been recognized across diverse ethnic backgrounds, including European, African American, Pakistani, Japanese, Korean, and others.[19] In addition to gastric cancers, germline *CDH1* mutations are associated with increased risk of lobular carcinoma of the breast, and this was the first manifestation of a *CDH1* mutation in one series.[23] *CDH1* is, to date, the only gene implicated in HDGC. Penetrance of DGC in patients carrying a *CDH1* mutation is estimated at 70% to 80%, but may be higher. The need for a systematic study of specimens is supported by recent work by Gaya et al.[24] in which initial total gastrectomy specimens were reported as negative, but detailed sectioning and analysis showed invasive carcinoma.

CDH1 is localized on chromosome 16q22.1 and encodes the calcium-dependent cell adhesion glycoprotein E-cadherin. Functionally, E-cadherin impacts maintenance of normal tissue morphology and cellular differentiation. It is hypothesized that *CDH1* acts as a tumor suppressor gene in HDGC, with loss of function leading to loss of cell adhesion and subsequently to proliferation, invasion, and metastases. Figure 32.2 shows the *CDH1* mutation for the pedigree depicted in Figure 32.1.

The germline *CDH1* mutation is most frequently a truncating mutation. Germline missense mutations are causative in a few HDGC kindreds, but are more often clinically insignificant. In vitro assays for cellular invasion and aggregation may predict the functional impact of missense mutations to aid in this distinction.[22] Within the gastric mucosa, the "second hit" leading to complete loss of E-cadherin function results from *CDH1* promoter methylation, as has been described in sporadic gastric cancer.[25]

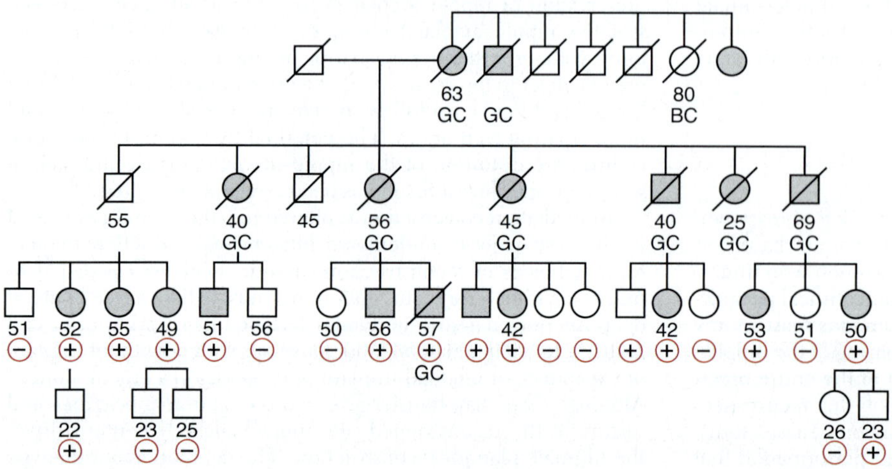

Figure 32.1 A family pedigree showing autosomal dominant inheritance of gastric cancer. Individual mutation testing results for the codon 1003 CDH1 mutation are indicated by + or −. Individuals affected with gastric cancer are *shaded*. (From Norton JA, Ham CM, Van Dam J, et al. CDH1 truncating mutations in the E-cadherin gene: an indication for total gastrectomy to treat hereditary diffuse gastric cancer. *Ann Surg* 2007;245:873.)

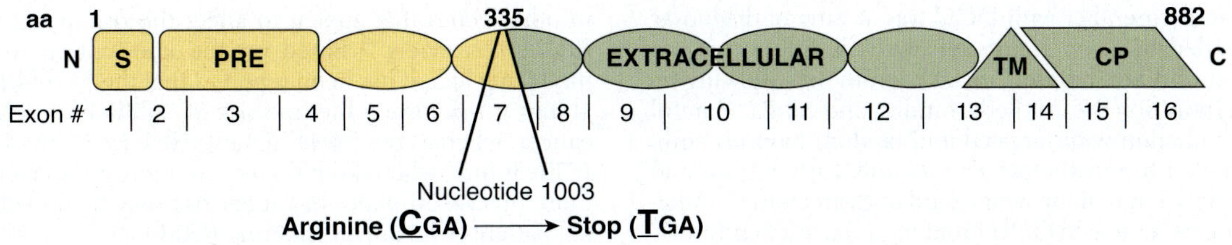

Figure 32.2 The mutation in this kindred is located in the central region of the E-cadherin gene that codes for the extracellular cadherin domains of the protein containing calcium-binding motifs important in the adhesion process. The C →T transition in exon 7 of nucleotide 1003 results in a premature stop codon (R335X), producing truncated peptides that lack the transmembrane and cytoplasmic β-catenin–binding domains essential for tight cell-cell adhesion. *Black* area indicates truncated portion of peptide. N, N-terminus; C, C-terminus; S, signal peptide; PRE, precursor sequence; TM, transmembrane domain; CP, cytoplasmic domain. (From Norton JA, Ham CM, Van Dam J, et al. CDH1 truncating mutations in the E-cadherin gene: an indication for total gastrectomy to treat hereditary diffuse gastric cancer. *Ann Surg* 2007;245:873.)

It remains unclear whether specific *CDH1* mutations are associated with distinctive phenotypic characteristics or rates of penetrance, although this may become apparent as more recurrent mutations are recognized. To date, most mutations identified have been novel and distributed throughout *CDH1*. Recognition of recurrent mutations has usually resulted from independent events; however, there is evidence for the role of founder effects in certain kindreds.[22] At present, it is also unclear whether patients with HDGC without detectable *CDH1* mutations have mutation of a different gene or merely a *CDH1* mutation that has gone unrecognized.

New recommended screening criteria for *CDH1* mutations are as follows:

1. Families with one or more cases of DGC
2. Individuals with DGC before the age of 40 years without a family history
3. Families or individuals with cases of DGC (one case below the age of 50 years) and lobular breast cancer
4. Cases where pathologists detect in situ signet ring cells or pagetoid spread of signet ring cells adjacent to diffuse type gastric cancer[18,26]

As in other familial cancer syndromes, genetic counseling should take place prior to genetic testing so that the family understands the potential impact of the results. After obtaining informed consent, a team comprising a geneticist, gastroenterologist, surgeon, and oncologist should discuss the possible outcomes of testing and the management options associated with each. Genetic testing should first be performed on a family member with HDGC or on a tissue sample if no affected relative is living. In addition to direct sequencing, multiplex ligation-dependent probe amplification is recommended to test for large genomic rearrangements. If a *CDH1* mutation is identified, asymptomatic family members may proceed with genetic testing, preferably by the age of 20.[19] If no mutation is identified in the family member with DGC, the value of testing asymptomatic relatives is low.

Among individuals found to carry a germline *CDH1* mutation, clinical screening is problematic. Histologically, DGC is characterized by multiple infiltrates of malignant signet ring cells, which may underlie normal mucosa.[27] Because these malignant foci are small in size and widely distributed, they are difficult to identify via random endoscopic biopsy. Chromoendoscopy and positron emission tomography have reportedly been used, but the clinical utility of these tools in early detection remains unproven. Lack of a sensitive screening test for HDGC makes early diagnosis extremely challenging. By the time patients are symptomatic and present for treatment, many have diffuse involvement of the stomach or linitis plastica, and rates of mortality are high. Published case reports describe patients who have presented with extensive DGC despite recent normal endoscopy and negative biopsies.[28] The 5-year survival rate for individuals who develop clinically apparent DGC is only 10%, with the majority dying before age 40.

Because of high cancer penetrance, poor outcome, and inadequacy of clinical screening tools for HDGC, prophylactic total gastrectomy is recommended as a management option for asymptomatic carriers of *CDH1* mutations.[18] Although total gastrectomy is performed with prophylactic intent in these cases, most specimens have been found to contain foci of diffuse signet ring cell cancer.[19,28,29] Foci of DGC have been identified even in patients who have undergone extensive negative screening, including high-resolution computed tomography, positron emission tomography scan, chromoendoscopy-guided biopsies, and endoscopic ultrasonography.[19] However, HGDC in asymptomatic *CDH1* carriers is usually completely resected by prophylactic gastrectomy, as pathologic analyses of resected specimens have shown only T1N0 disease.

Because these signet ring cell cancers are multifocal and distributed throughout the entire stomach, especially in the cardia,[30] prophylactic gastrectomy should include the entire stomach, and the surgeon must transect the esophagus and not the proximal stomach. Furthermore, it should be performed by a surgeon experienced in the technical aspects of the procedure and familiar with HDGC. In asymptomatic patients, lymph node metastases have not been observed; therefore, D2 lymph node resection is not necessary. The optimal timing of prophylactic gastrectomy in individuals with *CDH1* mutations is unknown, but recent consensus recommendations indicate that age 20 is reasonable.[18]

Although it is a potentially lifesaving procedure, prophylactic gastrectomy for *CDH1* mutation carries significant risks that must be considered. Overall mortality for total gastrectomy is estimated to be as high as 2% to 4%, although it is estimated to be 1% when performed prophylactically. Patients must also be aware that there is a nearly 100% risk of long-term morbidity associated with this procedure, including diarrhea, dumping, weight loss, and difficulty eating.[19] A recent study of the effects of prophylactic gastrectomy for *CDH1* mutation demonstrated that physical and mental function were normal at 12 months, but specific digestive issues were recognized. Overall, 70% had diarrhea, 63% fatigue, 81% eating discomfort, 63% reflux, 45% eating restrictions, and 44% had altered body image, suggesting that this operation impacted negatively on quality of life.[31] Because of these complications and the fact that lymph node spread has not been observed, some recommend vagus-preserving gastrectomy done either open or laparoscopically. In addition, because the penetrance of *CDH1* mutations is incomplete, some patients who undergo prophylactic gastrectomy would never have gone on to develop clinically significant gastric cancer. Prophylactic gastrectomy has, in fact, been performed on several patients reported to show no evidence of gastric cancer on pathology.[29]

Some individuals with *CDH1* mutations choose not to pursue prophylactic gastrectomy. These individuals should undergo careful surveillance, including biannual chromoendoscopy with biopsies, beginning when they are at least 10 years younger than the youngest family member with DGC was at time of diagnosis. It is recommended that any endoscopically visible lesion is targeted and that six random biopsies are taken from the following regions: antrum, transitional zone, body, fundus, and cardia. Careful white-light examination with targeted and random biopsies combined with detailed histopathology can identify early lesions and help to inform decision making with regard to gastrectomy.[32] Additionally, because women with *CDH1* mutations have a nearly 40% lifetime risk of developing lobular breast carcinoma, they should be carefully screened with annual mammography and breast MRI starting at age 35.[23] They should also do monthly self-examinations and have a breast examination by a physician every 6 months. The same surveillance recommendations are probably appropriate for HDGC families without identifiable *CDH1* mutations, although no current guidelines for this exist.

The emergence of gene-directed gastrectomy as a treatment strategy for patients with HDGC represents the culmination of a successful collaboration between molecular biologists, geneticists, oncologists, gastroenterologists, and surgeons. It is anticipated that the recognition of similar molecular markers in other familial cancer syndromes will transform the approach to the early diagnosis and treatment of a variety of tumors.

SURGICAL PROPHYLAXIS OF HEREDITARY OVARIAN AND ENDOMETRIAL CANCER

Hereditary Ovarian Cancer (*BRCA1, BRCA2*)

Inherited mutations in *BRCA1* and *BRCA2* strongly predispose women to breast cancer and to high-grade serous cancers of the ovary, fallopian tube, and peritoneum.[33,34] About two-thirds are due to *BRCA1* mutations and one-third *BRCA2* mutations, and these account for about 15% to 20% of high-grade serous cases. The lifetime risk of these gynecologic cancers increases from a baseline of 1.5% to about 15% to 25% in *BRCA2* carriers and 30% to 60% in *BRCA1* carriers.[33,34] *BRCA1/2* mutations are rare in most populations (<1 in 500 individuals); one notable exception is the Ashkenazi Jewish population, in which the carrier frequency is 1 in 40.[35] *BRCA1*-associated cases peak in the 50s and *BRCA2*-associated cancers in the 60s.[36] In addition to *BRCA1/2* mutations, germline mutations in a number of other genes in the homologous recombination DNA repair pathway confer high penetrance susceptibility to ovarian cancer (e.g., *RAD51C, RAD51D, BRIP1, PALB2*).[37] This has led to the development of more comprehensive cancer genetic testing panels that are increasingly being used to identify women who are candidates for risk-reducing salpingo-oophorectomy (RRSO).

Genetic testing for inherited high-penetrance mutations in *BRCA1/2* and other genes should be discussed with women who have a significant family history of early onset breast cancer and/or cancers of the ovary, fallopian tube, or peritoneum. Involvement of a genetic counselor prior to testing is helpful, as they have expertise in managing the inherent clinical and social issues. Most *BRCA1/2* mutations involve base deletions or insertions in the coding sequence or splice sites that encode truncated protein products that are clearly dysfunctional. Less frequently, disease-causing mutations may occur that alter a single amino acid, though most of these missense variants represent innocent polymorphisms. The clinical significance of missense mutations can sometimes be elucidated by determining whether they segregate with cancer in other family members. In addition, genomic rearrangements may occur that inactivate *BRCA1* or *BRCA2*, and identification of such alterations requires molecular testing beyond sequencing.

Penetrance of ovarian cancer is not 100% in those with clearly deleterious *BRCA1/2* mutations, but presently it is not possible to provide more precise personalized risk estimates to guide the use of RRSO. However, common variants have been discovered in other genes that appear to affect the risk of ovarian cancer in *BRCA1/2* carriers.[38] Based on the known ovarian cancer risk–modifying loci, it has been reported that the 5% of *BRCA1* carriers at lowest risk have a lifetime risk of ≤28% of developing ovarian cancer, whereas the 5% at highest risk have a ≥63% lifetime risk. In the future, when modifier loci are more completely catalogued, more precise estimates of cancer risk may be provided to individual patients who are considering RRSO.

As about 20% of women with high-grade serous ovarian cancers have *BRCA1/2* mutations, it has been suggested that all of these women undergo genetic testing regardless of family history.[39] Mutational analysis in women with these cancers may increasingly become standard practice as the cost of genetic testing declines. Testing may also be driven by the availability of poly(ADP-ribose) polymerase inhibitor therapy for women whose cancers have germline or sporadic mutations in genes such as *BRCA1/2* and others that are involved in homologous recombination DNA repair.

RRSO is strongly recommended in women who carry *BRCA1/2* mutations because of the high mortality rate of ovarian cancer and the lack of effective screening and prevention approaches. Although screening with pelvic ultrasound and serum CA125 is generally recommended for *BRCA1/2* carriers during their 20s and 30s, it is not proven to reduce ovarian cancer mortality because even early stage high-grade cancers have a very high mortality. Oral contraceptives reduce the risk of ovarian cancer in the general population and appear to have a similar effect in *BRCA1/2* carriers, but this must be balanced against concerns regarding increased breast cancer risks.

The past practice of performing RRSO based solely on family history has been replaced by reliance on genetic testing. Clinical management of women with a strong family history in whom a deleterious germline mutation is not found, or those with variants of uncertain significance, should be resolved on a case-by-case basis. RRSO may be deemed appropriate in some cases, despite the absence of a clearly deleterious mutation. Fortunately, the risk of hereditary ovarian cancer does not rise dramatically until the mid-30s in women with *BRCA1* mutations and the 40s for women with *BRCA2* mutations.[36] As a result, most women are able to complete childbearing prior to undergoing RRSO. It is advisable for *BRCA1* carriers to undergo RRSO around age 35, as there is a 4% risk of ovarian cancer being discovered clinically or at the time of RRSO by age 40.[10] *BRCA2* carriers may choose to delay surgery into their 40s due to their lower risk of ovarian cancer, but this could diminish the protection against breast cancer that is afforded by RRSO. If a mutation carrier, particularly a *BRCA1* carrier, chooses to pursue fertility into her 40s, then she should be counseled that she is at considerable risk of developing a life-threatening cancer that is largely preventable.

Several studies have provided evidence of the efficacy of RRSO. In one early study of *BRCA1/2* carriers, RRSO reduced the rate of breast and ovarian cancer by 75% over several years of follow-up.[40] A separate study in 2002 examined outcome in 551 *BRCA1/2* carriers from various registries.[41] Among 259 women who had undergone RRSO, 6 (2.3%) were found to have stage I ovarian cancer at the time of the procedure and 2 (0.8%) subsequently developed serous peritoneal carcinoma. Among the controls, 58 (20%) women developed ovarian cancer after a mean follow-up of 8.8 years. With the exclusion of the six women whose cancers were diagnosed at surgery, RRSO reduced ovarian cancer risk by 96%. More recently, in 2014, an international registry study of over 5,783 subjects with median follow-up of 5.6 years found that RRSO reduced ovarian, tubal, and peritoneal cancer risk by 80%.[36] There was an estimated lifetime risk of primary peritoneal cancer after RRSO of about 4% for *BRCA1* carriers and 2% for *BRCA2* carriers.[36] The risk of death from all causes was reduced by 77%. A prospective cohort study noted that RRSO was associated with reduction in breast cancer–specific (hazard ratio [HR] = 0.44; 95% confidence interval [CI] = 0.26 to 0.76), ovarian cancer–specific (HR = 0.21; 95% CI = 0.06 to 0.80), and all-cause mortality (HR = 0.40; 95% CI = 0.26 to 0.61).[10]

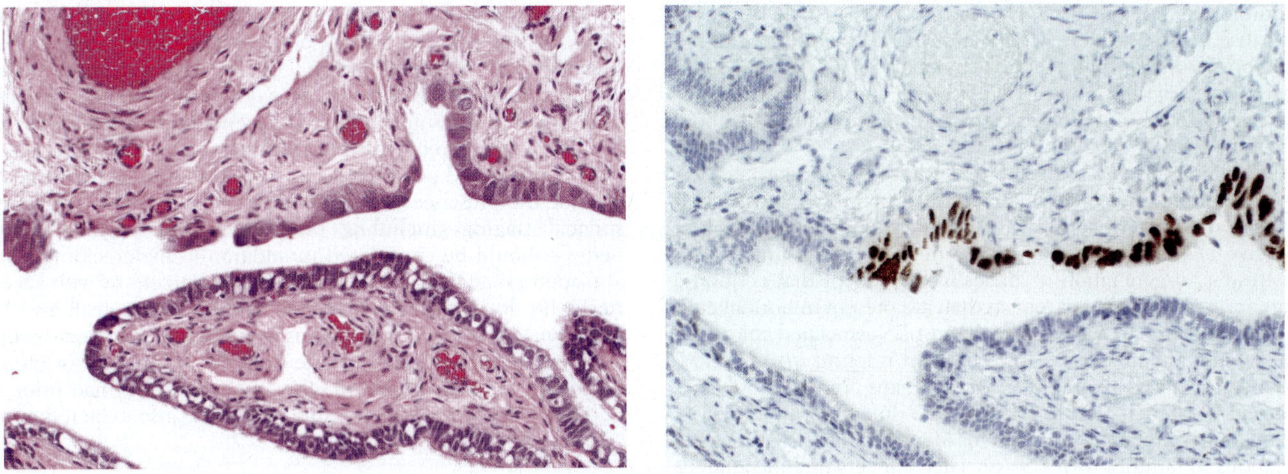

A B

Figure 32.3 Hematoxylin and eosin **(A)** and immunohistochemical staining **(B)** demonstrating overexpression of mutant *TP53* in serous carcinoma in situ of the fallopian tube from a *BRCA1* mutation carrier who underwent risk-reducing bilateral salpingo-oophorectomy.

Removal of the ovaries, as internal organs, usually has little effect on body image and self-esteem, and most *BRCA1/2* mutation carriers elect to undergo RRSO. Insurance payers will almost always pay for RRSO in proven mutation carriers.

RRSO can be performed laparoscopically in most women, with discharge to home the same day. If a laparoscopic approach is problematic due to obesity or adhesions, the surgery can be performed through a small lower abdominal incision. Morbidity including bleeding, infection, and damage to the urinary or gastrointestinal tracts can occur, but the incidence of serious complications is very low. As the fallopian tubes and ovaries are small discrete organs, they are relatively easy to remove completely. Attention should be paid to transecting the ovarian artery and vein proximal to the ovary and tube so that remnants are not left behind. This involves opening the pelvic sidewall peritoneum, visualizing the ureter, and then isolating the ovarian blood supply. If there are adhesions between the adnexa and adjacent structures, careful dissection should be performed to ensure complete removal of the ovaries and fallopian tubes. If the uterus is not removed, care should be taken to remove the entire fallopian tube. A small portion of the tube inevitably will be left in the cornu of the uterus, but the risk of fallopian tube cancer developing in such remnants appears to be negligible.

Though there is not strong evidence that *BRCA1/2* mutations increase uterine cancer risk, many women elect to have the uterus removed as part of the surgical procedure because they have completed their family or have other gynecologic indications. Although the addition of a hysterectomy may increase operative time, blood loss, surgical complications, and hospital stay, it usually can be performed laparoscopically and serious adverse outcomes are infrequent. Furthermore, the likelihood of future exposure to tamoxifen in the context of breast cancer prevention or treatment, which increases endometrial cancer risk two- to three-fold, also argues for concomitant hysterectomy. Women who receive hormone replacement therapy after surgery will require a progestin along with estrogen to protect against the development of endometrial cancer if the uterus is not removed.

In younger women, surgical menopause after RRSO is associated with vasomotor symptoms, vaginal atrophy, decreased libido, and an accelerated onset and incidence of osteoporosis and cardiovascular disease. In premenopausal women who do not have a personal history of breast cancer, estrogen replacement can be administered to ameliorate many of the deleterious effects of premature menopause. Systemic estrogen levels are lower in oophorectomized premenopausal women taking hormone replacement than if the ovaries had been left in place. The therapeutic benefit of oophorectomy in women with breast cancer has long been appreciated, and more recent studies support the contention that RRSO reduces the risk of breast cancer by about half in *BRCA1/2* carriers.[42] However, a meta-analysis showed that while RRSO was strongly protective against estrogen receptor–positive breast cancer (HR = 0.22), there was no protection against estrogen receptor–negative breast cancer.[42] Many carriers are identified after developing early onset breast cancer, and this group represents the most difficult in which to balance the potential risks and benefits of estrogen replacement therapy.

Early stage high-grade serous cancers and in situ lesions with *TP53* mutations have been identified in the fallopian tubes of some RRSO specimens (Fig. 32.3). This has led to a paradigm shift in which it is now thought that most high-grade serous cancers found in the ovary, fallopian tube, and peritoneum are derived from cells that originate in the tubal fimbria.[43] The frequency of occult malignancies has varied between reports, but appears to be about 3%.[43] In view of this, the pelvis and peritoneal cavity should be examined carefully. Malignant cells also have been found in peritoneal cytologic specimens, and washings of the pelvis should be obtained when performing RRSO. The pathologist should be informed of the indication for surgery and serial sections of the fallopian tubes should be performed to look for the presence of early lesions. Patients found to have occult invasive high-grade serous cancers should be treated with chemotherapy after surgery. Those with in situ lesions appear to have a good outcome without chemotherapy.[44]

Cases of peritoneal serous carcinoma indistinguishable from ovarian cancer have been observed years after RRSO, but the origin of these cancers is unclear. Some may represent recurrences of occult ovarian or tubal cancers. In this regard, retrospective examination of the ovaries and fallopian tubes sometimes has revealed primary cancers that were not originally recognized. In contrast, some of these cancers likely arise directly from fallopian tube cells that have implanted in the peritoneum and subsequently become malignant. Patients who undergo RRSO should be made aware of their residual risk of peritoneal cancer, but there is no evidence that continued surveillance using CA125 and/or ultrasound is beneficial.

HEREDITARY ENDOMETRIAL CANCER (LYNCH SYNDROME)

Although Lynch syndrome (LS, also known as hereditary nonpolyposis CRC syndrome) typically manifests as familial clustering of early onset CRC, there is also an increased incidence of several other types of cancers—most notably endometrial cancer in women.[45] About 3% of endometrial cancers are attributable to inherited mutations in the DNA mismatch repair (MMR) genes that cause LS. Most often, *MSH2* and *MLH1* are implicated, but mutations in *MSH6* and *PMS2* also occur.[45] The risk of ovarian cancer is also significantly increased in LS, but to a lesser degree than in *BRCA1/2* mutation carriers, and accounts for only about 1% of all ovarian cancers.

Cells in which one of the LS genes have been inactivated exhibit a phenomenon called microsatellite instability (MSI).[46] This occurs as DNA mismatches cause shortening or lengthening of repetitive DNA sequences and these mismatches go unrepaired. This results in generation of alleles in the cancer that contain a greater or lesser number of repeats than are present in normal cells from that individual. MSI occurs in most LS-associated colorectal and endometrial cancers.[46] However, MSI is found in about 20% of sporadic cancers that arise in these organs, and in most cases is caused by silencing of the *MLH1* gene due to promoter hypermethylation. Screening strategies for identification of MMR gene alterations in families with LS-associated cancers include analysis of tumor tissue for MSI and/or loss of DNA MMR gene expression using immunohistochemistry (IHC).[46] In cancers with MSI or loss of expression of one of the MMR genes, or in families with pedigrees suggestive of LS, these genes can be sequenced to identify disease-causing mutations, most of which cause truncated protein products.[47] Although it has been suggested that it may be cost-effective to do these tests on all endometrial cancers, this approach has not been widely adopted.[47]

The risk of a woman who carries a LS mutation developing endometrial cancer ranges from 20% to 60% in various reports.[45,48] The risk of ovarian cancer is increased to about 5% to 12%. Whereas the mean age of women with sporadic endometrial cancers is in the early 60s, cancers that arise in association with LS are often diagnosed before menopause, with the average age in the 40s. The clinical features of these endometrial cancers are similar to those of most sporadic cases (well-differentiated, endometrioid histology, early stage), and survival is about 90%. The mean age of onset of ovarian cancer in LS is in the early 40s, and the clinical features of these cancers are generally more favorable than in sporadic cases. They usually are identified at an early stage, are well- or moderately differentiated, have favorable survival, and some occur in the setting of a synchronous endometrial cancer.

Recommendations for screening and risk-reducing surgery in LS are better established for CRC than for extracolonic malignancies.[49] Transvaginal ultrasound has been proposed as a screening test for endometrial cancer (and ovarian cancer), but its efficacy is unproven.[50] Endometrial biopsy is the most sensitive means of diagnosing endometrial cancer, and it has been suggested that this should be employed periodically beginning around age 30 to 35. However, there are no published studies demonstrating that this approach prevents endometrial cancer deaths compared to simply performing a biopsy if abnormal uterine bleeding occurs.

Most experts believe that risk-reducing hysterectomy has a role in the management of some women with LS because of the high incidence of endometrial cancer. The risk of endometrial cancer is low during the prime reproductive years, and the uterus does not serve a vital function once childbearing has been completed. In view of the increased risk of ovarian cancer in LS, concomitant bilateral salpingo-oophorectomy should also be considered. One study demonstrated that there were no cases of endometrial or ovarian cancer in 61 LS carriers who underwent risk-reducing hysterectomy and bilateral salpingo-oophorectomy, while endometrial cancer occurred in 33% and ovarian cancer in 5% who retained their uterus and ovaries.[51] Despite the low risk of death from gynecologic cancers in LS, cost-effectiveness analyses of various approaches suggest that risk-reducing hysterectomy and salpingo-oophorectomy leads to both the lowest cost and the greatest increase in quality-adjusted life-years.[52] Estrogen replacement after removal of the ovaries in premenopausal women with LS is not contraindicated, as there is no evidence that this adversely affects the incidence of other cancers.

Many women with LS elect to undergo risk-reducing colectomy, which provides an opportunity to perform concomitant hysterectomy. Hysterectomy in concert with colectomy, either via laparoscopy or laparotomy, does not greatly increase operative time or surgical complications. If an endometrial biopsy has not been performed preoperatively, an intraoperative inspection of the uterine cavity and possibly frozen section should be performed to exclude the presence of cancer. If cancer is found in the uterus, surgical staging—including sampling of the regional lymph nodes—should be considered in addition to hysterectomy.[53] It is also appropriate to discuss risk-reducing hysterectomy with LS carriers who do not elect to undergo prophylactic colectomy. The operative approach (vaginal versus laparotomy versus laparoscopy) can be determined based on the presence or absence of uterine pathology (e.g., myomas), whether the patient has had prior abdominal surgery, and whether the ovaries are also to be removed.

GYNECOLOGIC CANCER RISK IN VERY RARE HEREDITARY CANCER SYNDROMES

Several very rare hereditary cancer syndromes also increase the risk of gynecologic cancers, and some of these women could potentially benefit from risk-reducing surgery to remove the ovaries and/or uterus. Peutz-Jeghers syndrome is characterized by intestinal polyps and an increased risk of colorectal and breast cancers. This rare syndrome is due to inherited mutations in the *STK11* gene. Affected women also have an increased risk of ovarian sex cord–stromal tumors with annular tubules and adenoma malignum of the cervix. Li-Fraumeni syndrome is caused by inherited mutations in the *TP53* gene, and carriers are predisposed to a number of types of cancers including sarcomas and breast cancer. The risk of ovarian cancer is increased as well, but is not a major cause of cancer in these families. Cowden syndrome is due to germline *PTEN* mutations and increases the risk of several malignancies including breast, thyroid, mucocutaneous, and endometrial cancers. Finally, small cell carcinoma of the ovary, hypercalcemic type, is due to mutations in the *SMARCA4* gene. These highly lethal ovarian cancers occur at a very young age (median 24 years) and present difficult challenges related to timing of RRSO. There are no well-accepted evidence-based guidelines for early detection and prevention of gynecologic cancers in these very rare hereditary cancer syndromes. An awareness of the risk and natural history of gynecologic cancers in these families provides a basis for counseling individual patients.

MULTIPLE ENDOCRINE NEOPLASIA TYPE 2

Gene Carriers

The MEN type 2 syndromes include MEN 2A, MEN 2B, and familial (non-MEN) medullary thyroid carcinoma (FMTC).[54–56] These are autosomal dominant inherited syndromes caused by germline mutations in the *RET* proto-oncogene. Their hallmark is the development of multifocal bilateral medullary thyroid carcinoma (MTC) associated with C-cell hyperplasia. MTCs arise from the thyroid C-cells, also called parafollicular cells. C-cells secrete the hormone calcitonin, a specific tumor marker for MTC. A slow-growing tumor in most cases, MTC causes significant morbidity and death in patients with uncontrolled local or metastatic spread. Large tumor burden is associated with diarrhea and flushing. In the MEN 2 syndromes, there is almost complete penetrance of MTC. Other features are variably expressed, with incomplete penetrance (summarized in Table 32.2).

In MEN 2A, all patients develop MTC. Approximately 42% of affected patients also develop pheochromocytomas, associated with adrenal medullary hyperplasia. Hyperparathyroidism develops in

TABLE 32.2

Clinical Features of Sporadic Medullay Thyroid Carcinoma, Multiple Endocrine Neoplasia 2A, Multiple Endocrine Neoplasia 2B, and Familial Medullay Thyroid Carcinoma

Clinical Setting	Features of MTC	Inheritance Pattern	Associated Abnormalities	Genetic Defect
Sporadic MTC	Unifocal	None	None	Somatic *RET* mutations in >20% of tumors
MEN 2A	Multifocal, bilateral	Autosomal dominant	Pheochromocytomas, hyperparathyroidism, cutaneous lichen amyloidosis, Hirshprung's disease	Germline missense mutations in extracellular cysteine codons of *RET*
MEN 2B	Multifocal, bilateral	Autosomal dominant	Pheochromocytomas, mucosal neuromas, megacolon, skeletal abnormalities	Germline missense mutation in tyrosine kinase domain of *RET*
FMTC	Multifocal, bilateral	Autosomal dominant	None	Germline missense mutations in extracellular or intracellular cysteine codons of *RET*

MTC, medullary thyroid carcinoma; MEN, multiple endocrine neoplasia; FMTC, familial medullary thyroid carcinoma.

10% to 35%. Cutaneous lichen amyloidosis and Hirschsprung's disease are infrequently associated with MEN 2A.[57–60]

MEN 2B appears to be the most aggressive form of hereditary MTC. In MEN 2B, MTC develops in all patients at a very young age (infancy). All affected individuals develop neural gangliomas, particularly in the mucosa of the digestive tract, conjunctiva, lips, and tongue; 40% to 50% develop pheochromocytomas. Patients with MEN 2B may also have megacolon, skeletal abnormalities, and markedly enlarged peripheral nerves. They do not develop hyperparathyroidism.

FMTC is characterized by development of MTC in the absence of any other endocrinopathies. MTC in these patients has a more indolent clinical course. Some individuals with FMTC may never manifest clinical evidence (i.e., symptoms or a lump in the neck), although biochemical testing and histologic evaluation of the thyroid demonstrates MTC.[55,56]

RET Genotype-Phenotype Correlations

Mutations in the *RET* proto-oncogene are responsible for MEN 2A, MEN 2B, and FMTC.[61–64] This gene encodes a transmembrane tyrosine kinase protein.[57,65] The mutations that cause the MEN 2 syndromes are activating gain-of-function mutations affecting constitutive activation of the protein. This is unusual among hereditary cancer syndromes, which are usually caused by loss-of-function mutations in the predisposition gene (e.g., familial polyposis, *BRCA1* and 2, von Hippel-Lindau, and MEN 1). More than 30 missense mutations have been described in patients affected by the MEN 2 syndromes (Fig. 32.4).

There is a relationship between the type of inherited *RET* mutation and presentation of MTC. The most virulent form is seen in patients with MEN 2B. These patients most commonly have a germline mutation in codon 918 of *RET* (ATG->ACG), although other mutations have been described (codon 883 and 922). As noted previously, MTC in MEN 2B has an extremely early age of onset (infancy). Despite its distinctive clinical appearance and associated gastrointestinal difficulties, the disease is often not detected until the patient develops a neck mass. Metastatic spread is usually present at the time of initial treatment, and calcitonin levels often remain elevated postoperatively.

MTC has a variable course in patients with MEN 2A, similar to that of sporadic MTC. Codon 634 and 618 mutations are the most common *RET* mutations associated with MEN 2A, although mutations at other codons are also observed (see Fig. 32.4). Some patients do extremely well for many years, even with distant metastases, while others develop inanition, symptomatic liver, lung or skeletal metastases, as well as disabling diarrhea. Recurrence in the central neck, with invasion of the airway or great vessels, may cause death.

In patients with FMTC, MTC is usually indolent. These individuals most commonly have mutations of codons 609, 611, 618, 620, 768, 804, or 891, although mutations of other codons have been identified (see Fig. 32.4). Many patients with FMTC are cured by thyroidectomy alone, and even those with persistent elevation of calcitonin levels do well for many years. Occasionally, patients with FMTC survive into the seventh or eighth decade without clinical signs of disease, although pathologic examination of the thyroid will reveal MTC or C-cell hyperplasia.[66]

Risk-Reducing Thyroidectomy in *RET* Mutation Carriers

Genetic counseling and informed consent should be obtained prior to genetic testing. Specific issues that should be covered in genetic counseling sessions include explaining the patterns of heritability, likelihood of expression of different tumors, their prevention and treatment, insurability, nonpaternity, survivor guilt, and others.

It has been shown that *RET* mutation carriers may harbor foci of MTC in the thyroid gland, even when calcitonin levels are normal.[67] While the age of onset and rate of disease progression may differ, the lifetime penetrance of MTC is near 100% in carriers of *RET* mutations associated with MEN 2 syndromes. At-risk individuals who are found to have inherited a *RET* gene mutation are therefore candidates for thyroidectomy, regardless of their plasma calcitonin levels.

The best option for prevention of MTC in *RET* mutation carriers is complete surgical resection prior to malignant transformation. Prophylactic thyroidectomy prior to the development of MTC is the goal in these patients. A number of studies have demonstrated improved biochemical cure rates and/or decreased recurrence rates from early thyroidectomy, performed after positive screening by calcitonin testing or *RET* mutation testing.[68–70]

MEN 2B mutations are the highest risk level, designated level III (see Fig. 32.4).[55,71] Patients with MEN 2B have the most aggressive form of MTC, with invasive disease reported in patients <1 year of age. These patients should have preventative surgery

Codon	Risk Level	MEN 2B	MEN 2A MTC	MEN 2A Pheo	MEN 2A HPT	FMTC	HSCR
533	I		×	×		×	
9-bp ins	I*					×	
606	I*		×				
609	II*		×	×	×	×	×
611	II		×	×	×	×	×
618	II		×	×	×	×	×
620	II		×	×		×	×
630	II*		×		×	×	
631	I*		×	×		×	
634	II		×	×	×	×	
768	I		×	×		×	
777	I*					×	
790	I		×	×		×	
791	I		×	×	×	×	
804	I		×	×	×	×	
804 +806	III*	×					
883	III	×					
891	I		×	×		×	
912	I*					×	
918	III	×					

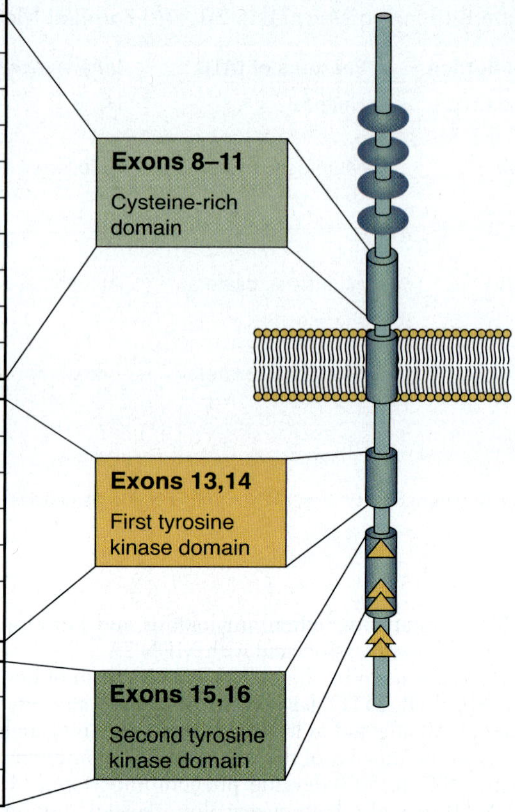

Figure 32.4 *RET* mutation sites associated with multiple endocrine neoplasia (MEN) 2 syndromes. Codons previously reported in association with MEN-2 syndromes are listed by structural domain within the RET protein. Risk level is based on consensus guidelines or more recent clinical reports. Previously reported phenotypes for each codon are shown. MTC, medullary thyroid carcinoma; Pheo, pheochromocytoma; HPT, hyperparathyroidism; FMTC, familial medullary thyroid carcinoma; HSCR, Hirschsprung's disease. *Asterisk* indicates risk level based on recent clinical reports not available at publication of the consensus guidelines. (From Traugott AL, Moley JF. The RET protooncogene. *Cancer Treat Res* 2010;153:303–319.)

early in the first year of life, if possible. Identification and preservation of parathyroid glands can be extremely difficult in these infants, due to their small size, translucent appearance, and the presence of exuberant thymic and perithyroidal nodal tissue. These procedures should be performed by surgeons experienced in parathyroid and/or pediatric thyroid operations.

Patients with MEN 2A with mutations in codons 634, 620, 618, and 611 are also considered high risk (level II).[55,71] Patients with level II mutations should undergo a total thyroidectomy at 5 to 6 years of age. There is evidence that the risk of lymph node metastasis is very low in patients with MEN 2A under the age of 8, with normal calcitonin levels. Central lymph node dissection is associated with higher risk of hypoparathyroidism, and recurrent laryngeal nerve injury and should be reserved for patients with elevated calcitonin levels.

A larger subset of *RET* mutations, associated with MEN 2A and/or FMTC, is considered the lowest risk (level I).[55,71] These include mutations at codons 768, 790, 791, 804, and 891. For patients with low-risk level I mutations, total thyroidectomy is recommended before age 5 to 10 years. This decision, however, regarding ideal age at preventative thyroidectomy in low-risk mutation carriers, is currently being reviewed, and may be driven by additional clinical data such as the basal or stimulated serum calcitonin level.[72,73] There are no guidelines at present that address the issue of timing of surgery based on calcitonin level, and at present, pentagastrin (the primary calcitonin secretagogue used in testing) is not available in the United States. It is anticipated that within a decade, there will be enough published data to direct timing of interventions based upon this information. As with the level II mutations, the need for central lymph node dissection should be guided by calcitonin levels and clinical features of the patient and kindred.

Until recently, some groups recommended total thyroidectomy with central neck lymph node dissection and total parathyroidectomy with autotransplantation for all *RET* mutation carriers. Recent studies and personal experience, however, have demonstrated an extremely low likelihood of nodal metastases in patients with MEN 2A or FMTC younger than 8 years of age, and in patients with a normal calcitonin level.[70] Our current strategy is to leave the parathyroid in situ in these patients, if possible.[74] Often, however, the desired complete removal of thyroid tissue results in compromise of parathyroid blood supply. In these situations, autotransplantation of devascularized parathyroid is required. We routinely remove and autotransplant the parathyroid if a central node dissection is done. In parathyroid autotransplantation, parathyroid glands are sliced into 1 mm × 3 mm fragments and autotransplanted into individual muscle pockets in the muscle of the nondominant forearm in patients with MEN 2A, or in the sternocleidomastoid muscle in patients with FMTC or MEN 2B. Patients are maintained on calcium and vitamin D supplementation for 4 to 8 weeks postoperatively.

In a recent series of thyroidectomies performed in 50 individuals with MEN 2A (identified by genetic screening), total thyroidectomy and central node dissection with parathyroidectomy and parathyroid autografting were performed in all patients (Fig. 32.5).[70]

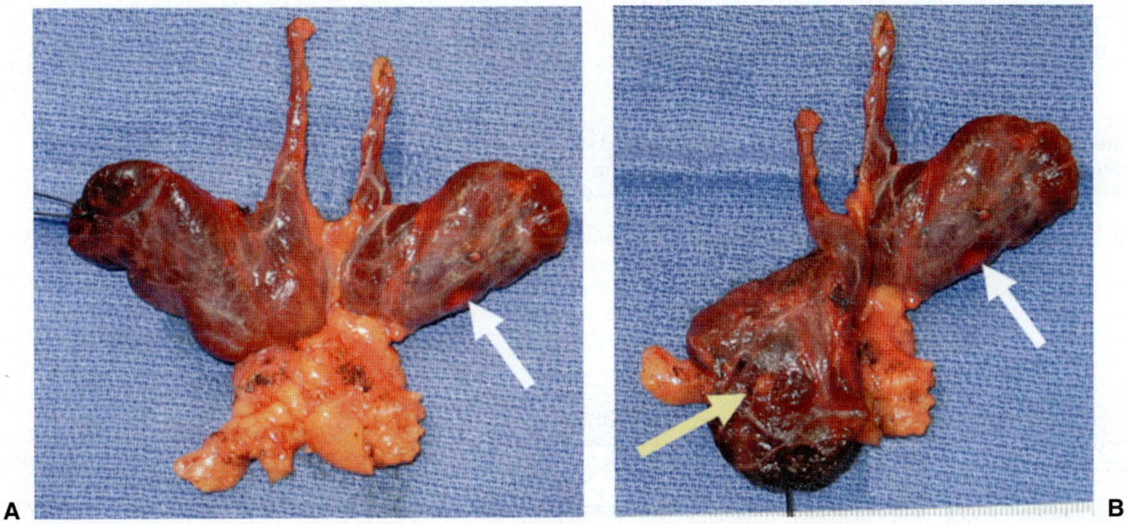

Figure 32.5 Total thyroidectomy specimen with attached central nodes from a patient with germline *RET* mutation and elevated calcitonin levels. Note small visible foci of medullary thyroid carcinoma (*arrows*).

All autografts functioned, but three patients required supplemental calcium. The percentage of individuals requiring calcium supplementation following parathyroidectomy with parathyroid autografting reportedly ranges from 0% to 18%. Parathyroidectomy should be performed in all patients showing gross parathyroid enlargement or biochemical evidence of parathyroid disease at time of surgery. The operating surgeon should have expertise in preservation of parathyroid function. It is important that the surgeon performing an operative procedure for MTC be familiar with the techniques described here. If not, the patient should be referred to a center where these procedures are routinely performed.

Some patients with MEN 2 will be found to have elevated calcitonin levels prior to thyroidectomy. This is usually associated with medullary thyroid carcinoma or C-cell hyperplasia in the gland, and may be associated with lymph node metastases. Much has been written about the correlation between preoperative calcitonin levels and extent of nodal involvement. It has been suggested that preoperative calcitonin level may guide the extent of node dissection. In a study of 300 European patients with MTC, node metastases were not identified when the preoperative basal calcitonin level was <20 pg/ml.[75] Involvement of nodal groups was correlated with basal calcitonin level as follows: ipsilateral central and lateral neck nodes (basal calcitonin >20 pg/ml), contralateral central nodes (basal calcitonin >50 pg/ml), contralateral lateral neck nodes (basal calcitonin >200 pg/ml), and mediastinal nodes (basal calcitonin >500 pg/ml). Based upon these findings, this group (who also wrote the European guidelines) recommends thyroidectomy only if basal calcitonin is <20 pg/ml, ipsilateral central and lateral neck dissection if the calcitonin is 20 to 50 pg/ml, and contralateral central neck dissection if the basal calcitonin is 50 to 200 pg/ml, with the addition of contralateral lateral neck dissection if the calcitonin is 200 to 500 pg/ml. Most experts agree that sternotomy with mediastinal neck dissection should be reserved for patients with image evidence of mediastinal disease. In contrast, most North American surgeons rely heavily upon preoperative ultrasound imaging to map the extent of nodal involvement and determine extent of surgery based upon calcitonin and imaging results.[55,74,76]

Follow-up

Following thyroidectomy, thyroid hormone replacement is required for life. Patients may need several weeks of oral calcium and vitamin D until parathyroid function recovers. Intermittent calcitonin testing may be done to monitor for persistent or recurrent MTC. The importance of regular monitoring of patients' compliance with thyroid medication following thyroidectomy should not be underestimated. Children and teenagers are frequently noncompliant, and this can be determined by routine measurement of thyroid-stimulating hormone levels. Continued noncompliance can result in growth problems. Occasionally, local human services agencies may need to be involved in particularly difficult cases.

The term "biochemical cure" is used to refer to patients with normal calcitonin levels after surgery for MTC. Complete postoperative normalization of calcitonin has been associated with decreased long-term risk of MTC recurrence, though the evidence is less clear for a survival benefit. A persistent or recurrent elevation in calcitonin indicates residual or recurrent MTC and warrants additional investigation by imaging. However, as most MTC has a fairly indolent course, patients with biochemical evidence of recurrent disease may not have corollary imaging findings for some time.

Conclusions

Identification of *RET* gene mutations in individuals at risk for developing hereditary forms of MTC has simplified management, expanding the scope of indications for surgical intervention. Patients who carry this mutation can be offered operative treatment at a very young age, hopefully before the cancer has developed or spread, and those identified as not having the mutation are spared further genetic and biochemical screening. This achievement marks a new paradigm in surgery: the indication that an operation be performed based on the results of a genetic test. As in the decision to perform any surgical procedure, meticulous preparation and detailed discussion with patient and family must precede the final recommendation. It is also important that the patient and family be involved in preoperative discussions with genetic counselors. Postoperative follow-up for compliance with thyroid medication is important, especially in children and teenagers who are still growing and developing into adults.

FAMILIAL ADENOMATOUS POLYPOSIS, *MYH*-ASSOCIATED POLUPOSIS, AND LYNCH SYNDROME

Inherited CRC syndromes with multiple adenomatous polyps include FAP, *MYH*-associated polyposis (MAP), and LS. In some cases, the diagnosis is suspected because of a striking family history

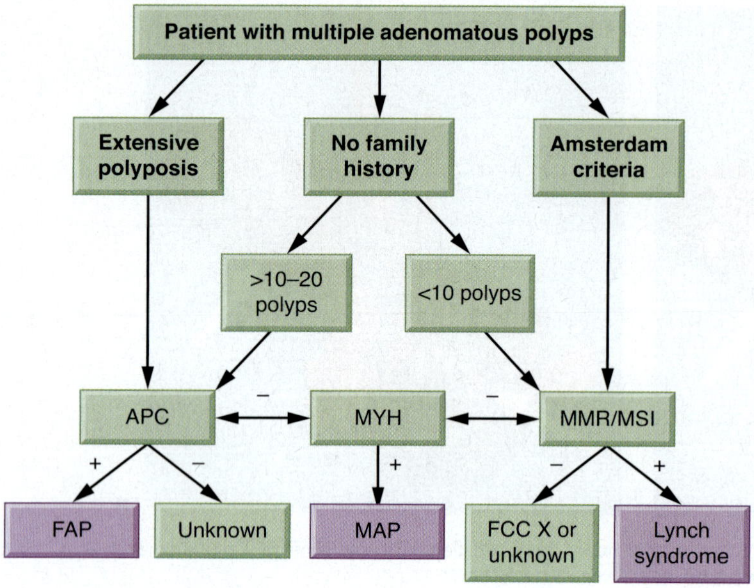

Figure 32.6 Schematic demonstrating the potential genetic workup for a patient with multiple adenomatous colorectal polyps and suspected of having an inherited colorectal cancer syndrome. APC, adenomatous polyposis coli; MMR, mismatch repair; MSI, microsatellite instability; FAP, familial adenomatous polyposis; MAP, *MYH*-associated polyposis; FCC X, familial colorectal cancer syndrome X.

of CRC, while in others, suspicion arises from a very young onset of CRC or florid polyposis.

Although adenomatous polyp burden and family history may suggest one syndrome over another, an initial negative genetic test result should be followed by further evaluation for other syndromes. For example, in clinical practice, a negative adenomatous polyposis coli (*APC*) gene test in a patient with a suspected CRC syndrome is followed by reflex testing for MAP and LS, as shown in Figure 32.6.

FAP is an autosomal dominant syndrome that accounts for <1% of the annual CRC burden, is caused by mutations in the tumor-suppressor *APC* gene. It is characterized by the presence of ≥100 adenomatous polyps in the colorectum, nearly 100% penetrance, and an inevitable risk of CRC if prophylactic colectomy is not performed.[8,77] Patients with a less severe form known as attenuated FAP (AFAP) usually present with <100 colorectal adenomas that tend to be proximally located. MAP is an autosomal recessive syndrome that often presents phenotypically as attenuated polyposis. While an estimated 2% of the general population are monoallelic carriers of a mutated base-excision-repair *MUTYH* (*MYH*) gene, biallelic germline mutations may account for 9% to 18% of patients with FAP or AFAP phenotypes who have no demonstrable *APC* mutation.[78–80]

LS accounts for 1% to 4% of all newly diagnosed CRC and is attributable to a germline mutation in one of the DNA MMR genes (*MLH1*, *MSH2*, *MSH6*, and *PMS2*).[81–83] Epigenetic silencing of the *MSH2* gene via a 3′-end deletion in *EPCAM* (*TACSTD1*), a neighbor of *MSH2* that plays a role in cell adhesion, also accounts for 20% to 25% of all suspected *MSH2* cases and 1% to 6% of LS cases overall.[84–86] LS is characterized by early age-of-onset CRC, predominance of lesions proximal to the splenic flexure, an increased rate of metachronous CRC, and a unique spectrum of benign and malignant extracolonic tumors. Lifetime risk of CRC in patients with LS may be as high as 80%.[83,87] MSI reflects a deficiency in DNA repair secondary to MMR gene mutation and is a hallmark feature of LS-associated tumors.

Variability in penetrance, phenotypic expression, and certainty of disease development mandate distinctly different surgical approaches in these three syndromes, including the type and timing of risk-reducing colon and rectal surgery.[88]

Familial Adenomatous Polyposis

Surveillance of at-risk family members should begin around age 10 to 15 years with an annual colonoscopy or flexible sigmoidoscopy.[89] At-risk individuals who belong to families with an AFAP phenotype should undergo colonoscopic screening every 2 to 3 years starting in their late teens. Informative genetic testing is possible in families with a demonstrated *APC* mutation, and mutations are detected in most pedigrees. However, approximately 25% of patients with FAP will have a de novo *APC* mutation.[87] Severity of polyposis should be established during colonoscopy, as the timing of surgery and the risk of developing colorectal is dependent on the extent of polyp burden. Patients with mild polyposis and a correspondingly lower CRC risk can undergo surgery in their late teens. Patients with severe polyposis, a high degree of dysplasia, multiple adenomas >5 mm in size, and symptoms (bleeding, persistent diarrhea, anemia, failure to thrive, psychosocial stress, etc.) should undergo risk-reducing colorectal surgery as soon as is practical after diagnosis.[90,91] However, in carefully selected, fully asymptomatic patients who have small adenomas but a strong family history of aggressive abdominal desmoid disease, consideration can be given to delaying prophylactic colectomy, as the risk of desmoid-related complication may be greater than the risk of CRC development.

The three current surgical options for patients with FAP are total proctocolectomy (TPC) with permanent ileostomy, total colectomy with ileorectal anastomosis (IRA), and proctocolectomy with ileal pouch-anal anastomosis (IPAA). IPAA can be a double-stapled, end-of-pouch-to-anus anastomosis, which may leave behind approximately 1 cm of anal transition zone. An alternative approach, which is preferred when there is carpeting of the anal transition zone with adenomas, is to perform a mucosal stripping of the anal transition zone down to the dentate line followed by a hand-sewn per anal anastomosis of pouch to the dentate line. Selection of the optimal procedure for an individual patient is based on several factors, including characteristics of the FAP syndrome within the patient and family, differences in likely postoperative functional outcome, preoperative anal sphincter status, and patient preference.[8]

TPC with permanent ileostomy, although rarely chosen as a primary procedure, is used in patients with invasive cancer involving the sphincters or levator complex, or patients for whom an IPAA is not technically feasible (secondary to desmoid disease and foreshortening of the small bowel mesentery, making it surgically impossible to bring the ileal pouch to the anus) nor likely to lead to good function such as massive obesity or weak anal sphincters. However, TPC is occasionally chosen as a primary procedure by patients who perceive that their lifestyle would be compromised by the frequent bowel movements (five to six per day) sometimes associated with the IPAA procedure.

In addition to these issues, the key in deciding between an IPAA and an IRA is based primarily on the risk of rectal cancer development if the rectum is left in situ. The risk of rectal cancer following IRA may range from 3% to 10% at 10 years, while the risk for a secondary proctectomy for uncontrolled rectal polyposis ranges from 10% to 61% at 20 years following initial colectomy with IRA.[92–94] The magnitude of risk in an individual patient is, however, related to the overall extent of colorectal polyposis. IRA may be considered for patients with <1,000 colorectal polyps (including those with attenuated FAP) and <20 rectal adenomas, as these individuals have a relatively low risk of developing rectal cancer.[88,93] Patients with severe rectal (>20 adenomas) or colonic (>1,000 adenomas) polyposis, an adenoma >3 cm, or an adenoma with severe dysplasia should ideally undergo a risk-reducing procedure that will include a proctectomy.[90,91,93]

The risk of secondary rectal excision, due to uncontrollable rectal polyposis or rectal cancer, may be estimated by identifying the specific location of the causative *APC* mutation. Patients with mutations located between codons 1250 and 1464 have been shown to have a six-fold increased risk of developing rectal cancer, compared to those with mutations prior to codon 1250 or after codon 1464 (mean number of rectal polyps 42 versus 22, respectively).[8,92] Although the use of the genotype-phenotype relationship to guide patient management may be appealing,[92] it is important to recognize the variability of phenotypic expression that exists even among members of the same family. This suggests that at the current time, the choice between an IRA and an IPAA should be based primarily on clinical (rather than genetic) grounds.[90]

The risk of polyp and cancer development following primary surgery is not limited to patients undergoing IRA. In patients undergoing IPAA, neoplasia may occur at the site of ileal pouch anastomosis; the frequency appears to be greater after stapled anastomosis (28% to 31%) than after mucosectomy and hand-sewn anastomosis (10% to 14%).[95] In the case of neoplasia developing at the anal transition zone after a stapled anastomosis, transanal mucosectomy may be performed, followed by advancement of the pouch to the dentate line. Of additional concern is the development of adenomatous polyps in the ileal pouch, which occurs in approximately 45% of patients by 10-year follow-up.[96] Consequently, depending on polyp burden, lifetime endoscopic surveillance of the rectal remnant (after IRA) every 6 to 12 months or the ileal pouch (after IPAA) every 1 to 3 years is required following either procedure.[89]

Another important consideration in choosing between IPAA and IRA is postoperative bowel function and quality of life. Some studies have associated IPAA with higher frequency of both daytime and nocturnal bowel movements, higher incidence of passive incontinence and incidental soiling, and greater postoperative morbidity.[97] However, long-term follow-up demonstrates a comparable quality of life following IPAA for FAP relative to the patient's preoperative baseline.[98] Therefore, although the choice of procedure must be carefully individualized, because of the risk of rectal cancer associated with IRA, the authors favor IPAA for most patients with FAP whenever feasible. However, an IRA should be considered in specific circumstances, such as when there is mild rectal polyposis (as in AFAP), or a young patient with rectal sparing who is not interested in undergoing the multiple procedures that accompany an IPAA and diverting loop ileostomy, or a young woman interested in having children and trying to avoid the decreased fecundity associated with an IPAA procedure.[99] The use of minimally invasive techniques such as laparoscopy may reduce the risk of infertility associated with IPAA.[100,101] Though a diverting loop ileostomy should be performed in all IPAA procedures, it is not always feasible due to a number of anatomic factors such as body habitus.

Endoscopic surveillance of the rectal segment at 6- to 12-month intervals after the index surgery is recommended, with subsequent surveillance frequencies dependent on the number and size of adenomas observed.[89] Although small (<5 mm) scattered adenomas can be safely observed or removed with biopsy forceps, polyps >5 mm should be removed by snare. However, repeated fulguration and polypectomy over many years can lead to difficulty with subsequent polypectomy, reduced rectal compliance, and difficulty identifying flat cancers in the background of scar tissue. The development of severe dysplasia and/or villous adenomas not amenable to endoscopic removal is indication for proctectomy.

Long-Term Considerations from Extracolonic Manifestations

Despite the reduced risk of CRC-related death following prophylactic colectomy, patients with FAP are still at increased risk of mortality from both rectal cancer and other causes relative to the general population. The three main causes of death following IRA are progression of desmoid disease, stomach and duodenal cancer, and perioperative mortality. Additional FAP-related extraintestinal manifestations include epidermoid cysts, supernumerary teeth, osteomas of the jaw and/or skull, congenital hypertrophy of the retinal pigment epithelium, cancers of the hepatopancreatobiliary tract and genitourinary tract, and thyroid cancer.[102–104]

Desmoids

Desmoids may occur in 10% to 25% of patients with FAP.[105,106] Unlike those found in the general population, FAP-associated desmoids tend to be intra-abdominal and arise following abdominal surgery.[106,107] Although conflicting reports exist, it appears that female patients, those with extracolonic manifestations of FAP, a positive family history of desmoids, and *APC* mutations located at 3′ of codon 1440 are at increased risk of developing desmoids.[106,108,109] These tumors often involve the small bowel mesentery as well as the retroperitoneum and are often life-threatening due to invasion or compression of adjacent viscera. Further, recurrence and morbidity rates are high following attempted resection, with recurrent disease often more aggressive than the initial desmoid. Estimated 5-year overall survival for patients with intra-abdominal desmoids causing severe symptoms such as significant pain and septic fistula/abscess, diameter >20 cm or rapidly growing, and/or need for parenteral nutrition is only 53%.[107] Therefore, desmoid resection is evaluated on an individualized case-by-case basis with surgery reserved for highly select cases.

Desmoids that involve the small bowel mesentery may preclude the formation of an IPAA secondary to foreshortening of the small bowel mesentery, especially in patients undergoing proctectomy after an initial IRA.[110] Surgery for intra-abdominal and abdominal wall desmoids should be reserved for limited disease where the likelihood of clear margins is high.

In symptomatic cases where resection of an intra-abdominal desmoid may not be feasible, intestinal bypass or ureteral stenting may be necessary to alleviate bowel or urinary obstruction secondary to mass effect. In addition to surgical intervention, several medical options with variable efficacy are available for the management of desmoid disease and include nonsteroidal anti-inflammatory drugs (e.g., sulindac), selective estrogen receptor modulators (e.g., tamoxifen), immunomodulators (e.g., imatinib, sorafenib, interferon), doxorubin-based cytotoxic chemotherapy, and radiation.

MYH-Associated Polyposis

MAP should be suspected in patients with >10 colorectal adenomas, a weak history of CRC, and no family history of FAP. The diagnosis is confirmed by *MUTYH* (*MYH*) gene testing.[80,88]

Depending on the polyp burden, the management of the colon and rectum of a patient with a biallelic *MYH* mutation can be endoscopic or surgical. If the polyp burden is limited and an endoscopic approach is pursued, colonoscopy should be performed every 1 to 3 years.[87,89] If the polyp burden is not amenable to an endoscopic approach at the time of diagnosis, then a resection is indicated. In most cases in which surgery is deemed necessary, an IRA is sufficient. However, if rectal polyposis is severe, an IPAA may be indicated. Indications for surgery following an endoscopic surveillance program include increasing polyp size or number, or worsening histology.

Extracolonic manifestations of MAP are similar to FAP and include osteomas, desmoids, congenital hypertrophy of the retinal pigment epithelium, as well as cancers of the thyroid, ovary, bladder, sebaceous gland, and breast. In addition, patients with MAP are also at a 4% lifetime risk of developing duodenal cancer and require upper endoscopies every 1 to 3 years beginning as early as ages 18 to 20 years and starting no later than ages 30 to 35 years.[87,89,111]

Lynch Syndrome

Due to the discordance associated with the term hereditary nonpolyposis colorectal cancer, the use of this term has largely been abandoned with reversion back to the eponym LS, which refers to individuals with a predisposition to CRC and other malignancies as a result of a germline MMR mutation.[112] Overall, CRC occurs in up to 80% of patients with LS by their mid-40s.[8,82] Endometrial cancer occurs in 40% to 60%, gastric cancer in 11% to 19%, urinary tract cancer in 5% to 18%, and ovarian cancer in 9% to 15% of affected individuals.[8,82,87]

The Amsterdam criteria and revised Bethesda guidelines[113] (Table 32.3) are used in clinical practice to identify patients at risk for LS who require further genetic evaluation. The Amsterdam criteria, which led to the identification of the LS-causing MMR gene mutations require that there be:

- Three relatives (one a first-degree relative of the other two) with colorectal, endometrial, stomach, ovary, small bowel, ureteral/renal pelvis, brain, hepatobiliary, and/or sebaceous cancer;
- In two or more successive generations;
- With at least one case of cancer diagnosed before the age of 50;
- And that FAP as a diagnosis is excluded.[114]

Though the Amsterdam criteria can be used clinically to identify potential patients with LS, using it alone will result in identification of only 42% of LS mutation carriers.[115] Families meeting Amsterdam criteria but lacking an MMR mutation are referred to as having "familial colorectal cancer type X" and appear to have a lower incidence of colorectal and extracolonic cancers than those with a LS germline MMR mutation (see Fig. 32.6). Of note, they have an increased incidence of left-sided and nonmucinous microsatellite stable tumors.[77,88]

Patients with CRC who belong to pedigrees suspicious for LS should be offered screening by IHC for loss of MMR protein expression or by MSI analysis. As the sensitivity of IHC testing for loss of MMR protein expression is comparable to MSI testing, either approach can be pursued.[112] However, IHC testing is less expensive and can also identify a specific MMR protein loss, which can help target subsequent germline testing. Routine IHC testing for loss of MMR protein in individuals younger than 50 years at the time of CRC diagnosis is feasible and has led to the identification of patients with LS who might otherwise have been missed.[116,117] Patients with MSI-high tumors should undergo testing for germline MMR mutations in *MSH2*, *MLH1*, *MSH6*, and *PMS2*. Reflex IHC and/or MSI testing on all newly diagnosed CRC has been advocated by some expert groups and has been successfully implemented at some institutions.[83,112,118] However, a majority of cancer programs nationwide currently do not have a protocol for reflex testing for LS, citing lack of institutional protocols as well as fear of nonreimbursement.[119] As such, a unified move toward universal testing remains some time away. In families for which tumor tissue is not available, initial germline testing may be considered though the financial burden is not insignificant, with the cost of finding a single LS carrier measuring approximately $58,000 (compared to the $5,000 spent in finding a single LS carrier using IHC screening).[120] As in FAP, a mutation in an affected individual must be established for testing in at-risk individuals to be conclusive.

In lieu of universal testing, several predictive models such as the MMRpredict, MMRpro, and PREMM$_{1,2,6}$ have been devised in order to assess an individual's likelihood of harboring LS.[115,121,122] These models quantify an individual's risk for carrying an *MLH1*, *MSH2*, *or MSH6* germline mutation by using clinical characteristics such as age at onset of CRC and/or other LS-associated cancers, location of CRC, family history, history of synchronous or metachronous CRC, among others. A study of these predictive models demonstrated that they all performed better than the revised Bethesda guidelines in terms of identifying patients with germline mutations for LS.[123] The MMRpredict model appeared to have to be the best predictor, with a sensitivity and specificity for LS of 94% and 91%, respectively. Other validation studies, however, have not demonstrated the superiority of MMRpredict compared to the other aforementioned models.[124,125] It appears that the use of clinical characteristics in combination with MSI or MMR protein expression status in predictive models may potentially improve our ability to establish LS diagnoses in patients with CRC. However, the practicality and applicability of these tools in a clinical setting requires further assessment.

Although development of CRC in LS is not a certainty, the 80% lifetime risk, the 16% to 30% risk of metachronous CRC, and the possibly accelerated adenoma-to-carcinoma sequence mandate consideration of prophylactic surgical options.[82,87,126–129] Patients with LS who have a CRC or more than one advanced adenoma should be offered the options of prophylactic total colectomy with IRA or segmental colectomy with annual postoperative surveillance colonoscopy. Careful surveillance is also necessary after total colectomy and IRA, as the risk of high-risk adenomas and cancer in the retained rectum at a median of 104 months are 11% and 8%, respectively.[126] Although there has been no study demonstrating an improved survival for patients with LS undergoing total colectomy and IRA versus segmental colectomy, mathematical models suggest a slight survival benefit for total colectomy and IRA, especially for individuals under the age of 30.[130,131] In addition, because of increased rates of metachronous CRC development and the risk of multiple abdominal surgeries

TABLE 32.3

The Revised Bethesda Guidelines for Testing Colorectal Tumors for Microsatellite Instability

Tumors from individuals should be tested for MSI in the following situations:

1. Colorectal cancer diagnosed in a patient who is <50 y of age.
2. Presence of synchronous, metachronous colorectal, or other HNPCC-associated tumors,[a] regardless of age.
3. Colorectal cancer with the MSI-H[b] histology[c] diagnosed in a patient who is <60 y of age.[d]
4. Colorectal cancer diagnosed in one or more first-degree relatives with an HNPCC-related tumor, with one of the cancers being diagnosed under age 50 years.
5. Colorectal cancer diagnosed in two or more first- or second-degree relatives with HNPCC-related tumors, regardless of age.

MSI, microsatellite instability; HNPCC, hereditary nonpolyposis colorectal cancer; MSI-H, microsatellite instability–high.

[a] HNPCC-related tumors include colorectal, endometrial, stomach, ovarian, pancreas, ureter and renal pelvis, biliary tract, and brain (usually glioblastoma as seen in Turcot syndrome) tumors, sebaceous gland adenomas and keratoacanthomas in Muir-Torre syndrome, and carcinoma of the small bowel.

[b] MSI-H in tumors refers to changes in two or more of the five National Cancer Institute–recommended panels of microsatellite markers.

[c] Presence of tumor-infiltrating lymphocytes, Crohn's-like lymphocytic reaction, mucinous/signet ring differentiation, or medullary growth pattern.

[d] There was no consensus among the workshop participants on whether to include the age criteria in guideline 3; participants voted to keep <60 years of age in the guidelines.

From Umar A, Boland CR, Terdiman JP, et al. Revised Bethesda Guidelines for hereditary nonpolyposis colorectal cancer (Lynch syndrome) and microsatellite instability. *J Natl Cancer Inst* 2004;96:261–268.

in those undergoing a segmental resection, a total colectomy and IRA has emerged as the procedure of choice for the index cancer, with consideration for TPC in cases where a high risk of metachronous rectal cancer can be predicted.[126–128] Targeted genetic testing approaches—such as the single amplicon MSH2 A636P mutation test in Ashkenazi Jewish patients with CRC—have demonstrated how a rapid and inexpensive preoperative genetic test can help direct the extent of colon resection.[132]

LS mutation carriers with a normal colon and without a history of CRC may also be offered prophylactic colectomy in highly select situations. One rationale for this approach is the similarity of lifetime cancer risk between patients with *APC* and MMR gene mutations, and the fact that total abdominal colectomy with IRA produces less functional disturbance than the prophylactic procedure recommended for FAP (TPC with IPAA). However, an alternate strategy for these individuals is surveillance by colonoscopy, which is cost-effective and greatly reduces the rate of CRC development and overall mortality.[133] There is a risk of CRC development in the interval between colonoscopies, though most interval cancers tend to be early stage.[134,135] As such, given that metachronous CRC may develop in as short a duration as a median of 11.3 months,[136] the recommended interval for surveillance colonoscopies is now every 1 to 2 years.[89] While prophylactic colectomy is not routinely recommended, it may be indicated in highly select patients for whom colonoscopic surveillance is not technically possible or in those who refuse to undergo regular surveillance. A decision analysis model suggests that prophylactic subtotal colectomy at age 25 may offer a survival benefit of 1.8 years, compared with surveillance colonoscopy. The benefit of prophylactic colectomy decreases when surgery is delayed until later in life and is negligible when performed at the time of cancer development.[137] Thus, the decision between prophylactic surgery and surveillance for a gene-positive unaffected individual is based on many factors including penetrance of disease in the family, early age-of-onset in affected family members, functional and quality-of-life considerations, and likelihood of compliance with surveillance. Table 32.4 lists some of the pros and cons of a prophylactic colectomy for germline mutation carriers for LS without a history of CRC. Patients with LS and an index rectal cancer should be offered the options of TPC with IPAA or anterior proctosigmoidectomy with primary reconstruction.[128,138] The rationale for TPC is the 10% to 15% associated risk of metachronous colon cancer in the remaining colon following the index rectal cancer. Choosing between the two procedures depends, in part, on the patient's willingness to undergo intensive surveillance of the retained proximal colon, as well as issues regarding quality of life and bowel function.

TABLE 32.4

Prophylactic Total Abdominal Colectomy and Ileorectal Anastomosis for Lynch Syndrome Patients without Cancer

Pros
- Elimination of colon cancer risk
- Elimination of need for surveillance colonoscopy
- Alleviating patient anxiety over the prospect of colon cancer development

Cons
- Persistence of risk of rectal cancer development
- Rectum still requires flexible endoscopic surveillance
- Patient anxiety of prospect of rectal cancer persists
- Possible altered bowel function
- Risk of surgery and possible associated complications

REFERENCES

1. Moyer VA, US Preventive Services Task Force. Risk Assessment, Genetic Counseling, and Genetic Testing for BRCA-Related Cancer in Women: U.S. Preventive Services Task Force Recommendation Statement. *Ann Intern Med* 2014;160.
2. Robson ME, Storm CD, Weitzel J, et al. American Society of Clinical Oncology policy statement update: genetic and genomic testing for cancer susceptibility. *J Clin Oncol* 2010;28:893–901.
3. Amir E, Freedman OC, Seruga B, et al. Assessing women at high risk of breast cancer: a review of risk assessment models. *J Natl Cancer Inst* 2010;102:680–691.
4. Miki Y, Swensen J, Shattuck-Eidens D, et al. A strong candidate for the breast and ovarian cancer susceptibility gene BRCA1. *Science* 1994;266:66–71.
5. Wooster R, Neuhausen SL, Mangion J, et al. Localization of a breast cancer susceptibility gene, BRCA2, to chromosome 13q12-13. *Science* 1994;265:2088–2090.
6. Lux MP, Fasching PA, Beckmann MW. Hereditary breast and ovarian cancer: review and future perspectives. *J Mol Med* 2006;84:16–28.
7. Shannon KM, Chittenden A. Genetic testing by cancer site: breast. *Cancer J* 2012;18:310–319.
8. Guillem JG, Wood WC, Moley JF, et al. ASCO/SSO review of current role of risk-reducing surgery in common hereditary cancer syndromes. *J Clin Oncol* 2006; 24:4642–4660.
9. Saslow D, Boetes C, Burke W, et al. American Cancer Society guidelines for breast screening with MRI as an adjunct to mammography. *CA Cancer J Clin* 2007;57:75–89.
10. Domchek SM, Friebel TM, Singer CF, et al. Association of risk-reducing surgery in BRCA1 or BRCA2 mutation carriers with cancer risk and mortality. *JAMA* 2010;304:967–975.
11. US Equal Employment Opportunity Commission. Genetic information discrimination. http://www.eeoc.gov/laws/types/genetic.cfm. Accessed January 2, 2014.
12. Society of Surgical Oncology. Position statement on prophylactic mastectomy. http://www.surgonc.org/practice-policy/practice-management/consensus-statements/position-statement-on-prophylactic-mastectomy. Accessed February 1, 2014.
13. Hartmann LC, Schaid DJ, Woods JE, et al. Efficacy of bilateral prophylactic mastectomy in women with a family history of breast cancer. *N Engl J Med* 1999;340:77–84.
14. Eldor L, Spiegel A. Breast reconstruction after bilateral prophylactic mastectomy in women at high risk for breast cancer. *Breast J* 2009;15:S81–S89.
15. Zakhireh J, Fowble B, Esserman LJ. Application of screening principles to the reconstructed breast. *J Clin Oncol* 2010;28:173–180.
16. Gabram SG, Dougherty T, Albain KS, et al. Assessing breast cancer risk and providing treatment recommendations: immediate impact of an educational session. *Breast J* 2009;15:S39–S45.
17. Nadauld LD, Ford JM. Molecular profiling of gastric cancer: toward personalized cancer medicine. *J Clin Oncol* 2013;31:838–839.
18. Bardram L, Hansen TV, Gerdes AM, et al. Prophylactic total gastrectomy in hereditary diffuse gastric cancer: identification of two novel CDH1 gene mutations-a clinical observational study. *Fam Cancer* 2014;13:231–242.
19. Norton JA, Ham CM, Van Dam J, et al. CDH1 truncating mutations in the E-cadherin gene: an indication for total gastrectomy to treat hereditary diffuse gastric cancer. *Ann Surg* 2007;245:873–879.
20. Lynch HT, Grady W, Suriano G, et al. Gastric cancer: new genetic developments. *J Surg Oncol* 2005;90:114–133, discussion 133.
21. Guilford P, Hopkins J, Harraway J, et al. E-cadherin germline mutations in familial gastric cancer. *Nature* 1998;392:402–405.
22. Kaurah P, MacMillan A, Boyd N, et al. Founder and recurrent CDH1 mutations in families with hereditary diffuse gastric cancer. *JAMA* 2007;297:2360–2372.
23. Benusiglio PR, Malka D, Rouleau E, et al. CDH1 germline mutations and the hereditary diffuse gastric and lobular breast cancer syndrome: a multicentre study. *J Med Genet* 2013;50:486–489.
24. Gaya DR, Stuart RC, Going JJ, et al. Hereditary diffuse gastric cancer associated with E-cadherin mutation: penetrance after all. *Eur J Gastroenterol Hepatol* 2008;20:1249–1251.
25. Lee KH, Hwang D, Kang KY, et al. Frequent promoter methylation of CDH1 in non-neoplastic mucosa of sporadic diffuse gastric cancer. *Anticancer Res* 2013;33:3765–3774.
26. Oliveira C, Sousa S, Pinheiro H, et al. Quantification of epigenetic and genetic 2nd hits in CDH1 during hereditary diffuse gastric cancer syndrome progression. *Gastroenterology* 2009;136:2137–2148.
27. Carneiro F, Huntsman DG, Smyrk TC, et al. Model of the early development of diffuse gastric cancer in E-cadherin mutation carriers and its implications for patient screening. *J Pathol* 2004;203:681–687.
28. Huntsman DG, Carneiro F, Lewis FR, et al. Early gastric cancer in young, asymptomatic carriers of germ-line E-cadherin mutations. *N Engl J Med* 2001; 344:1904–1909.
29. Suriano G, Yew S, Ferreira P, et al. Characterization of a recurrent germ line mutation of the E-cadherin gene: implications for genetic testing and clinical management. *Clin Cancer Res* 2005;11:5401–5409.

30. Rogers WM, Dobo E, Norton JA, et al. Risk-reducing total gastrectomy for germline mutations in E-cadherin (CDH1): pathologic findings with clinical implications. *Am J Surg Pathol* 2008;32:799–809.
31. Worster E, Liu X, Richardson S, et al. The impact of prophylactic total gastrectomy on health-related quality of life: a prospective cohort study. *Ann Surg* 2014;260:87–93.
32. Lim YC, di Pietro M, O'Donovan M, et al. Prospective cohort study assessing outcomes of patients from families fulfilling criteria for hereditary diffuse gastric cancer undergoing endoscopic surveillance. *Gastrointest Endosc* 2014;80:78–87.
33. Mavaddat N, Peock S, Frost D, et al. Cancer risks for BRCA1 and BRCA2 mutation carriers: results from prospective analysis of EMBRACE. *J Natl Cancer Inst* 2013;105:812–822.
34. Risch HA, McLaughlin JR, Cole DE, et al. Prevalence and penetrance of germline BRCA1 and BRCA2 mutations in a population series of 649 women with ovarian cancer. *Am J Hum Genet* 2001;68:700–710.
35. Struewing JP, Hartge P, Wacholder S, et al. The risk of cancer associated with specific mutations of BRCA1 and BRCA2 among Ashkenazi Jews. *N Engl J Med* 1997;336:1401–1408.
36. Finch AP, Lubinski J, Moller P, et al. Impact of oophorectomy on cancer incidence and mortality in women with a BRCA1 or BRCA2 mutation. *J Clin Oncol* 2014;32:1547–1553.
37. Walsh T, Casadei S, Lee MK, et al. Mutations in 12 genes for inherited ovarian, fallopian tube, and peritoneal carcinoma identified by massively parallel sequencing. *Proc Natl Acad Sci U S A* 2011;108:18032–18037.
38. Couch FJ, Wang X, McGuffog L, et al. Genome-wide association study in BRCA1 mutation carriers identifies novel loci associated with breast and ovarian cancer risk. *PLoS Genet* 2013;9:e1003212.
39. Schrader KA, Hurlburt J, Kalloger SE, et al. Germline BRCA1 and BRCA2 mutations in ovarian cancer: utility of a histology-based referral strategy. *Obstet Gynecol* 2012;120:235–240.
40. Kauff ND, Satagopan JM, Robson ME, et al. Risk-reducing salpingo-oophorectomy in women with a BRCA1 or BRCA2 mutation. *N Engl J Med* 2002;346:1609–1615.
41. Rebbeck TR, Lynch HT, Neuhausen SL, et al. Prophylactic oophorectomy in carriers of BRCA1 or BRCA2 mutations. *N Engl J Med* 2002;346:1616–1622.
42. Kauff ND, Domchek SM, Friebel TM, et al. Risk-reducing salpingo-oophorectomy for the prevention of BRCA1- and BRCA2-associated breast and gynecologic cancer: a multicenter, prospective study. *J Clin Oncol* 2008; 26:1331–1337.
43. Folkins AK, Jarboe EA, Roh MH, et al. Precursors to pelvic serous carcinoma and their clinical implications. *Gynecol Oncol* 2009;113:391–396.
44. Wethington SL, Park KJ, Soslow RA, et al. Clinical outcome of isolated serous tubal intraepithelial carcinomas (STIC). *Int J Gynecol Cancer* 2013; 23:1603–1611.
45. Bonadona V, Bonaiti B, Olschwang S, et al. Cancer risks associated with germline mutations in MLH1, MSH2, and MSH6 genes in Lynch syndrome. *JAMA* 2011;305:2304–2310.
46. Leenen CH, van Lier MG, van Doorn HC, et al. Prospective evaluation of molecular screening for Lynch syndrome in patients with endometrial cancer ≤70 years. *Gynecol Oncol* 2012;125:414–420.
47. Resnick K, Straughn JM Jr, Backes F, et al. Lynch syndrome screening strategies among newly diagnosed endometrial cancer patients. *Obstet Gynecol* 2009;114:530–536.
48. Watson P, Vasen HF, Mecklin JP, et al. The risk of endometrial cancer in hereditary nonpolyposis colorectal cancer. *Am J Med* 1994;96:516–520.
49. Koornstra JJ, Mourits MJ, Sijmons RH, et al. Management of extracolonic tumours in patients with Lynch syndrome. *Lancet Oncol* 2009;10:400–408.
50. Dove-Edwin I, Boks D, Goff S, et al. The outcome of endometrial carcinoma surveillance by ultrasound scan in women at risk of hereditary nonpolyposis colorectal carcinoma and familial colorectal carcinoma. *Cancer* 2002;94:1708–1712.
51. Schmeler KM, Lynch HT, Chen LM, et al. Prophylactic surgery to reduce the risk of gynecologic cancers in the Lynch syndrome. *N Engl J Med* 2006;354: 261–269.
52. Yang KY, Caughey AB, Little SE, et al. A cost-effectiveness analysis of prophylactic surgery versus gynecologic surveillance for women from hereditary nonpolyposis colorectal cancer (HNPCC) Families. *Fam Cancer* 2011;10:535–543.
53. Pistorius S, Kruger S, Hohl R, et al. Occult endometrial cancer and decision making for prophylactic hysterectomy in hereditary nonpolyposis colorectal cancer patients. *Gynecol Oncol* 2006;102:189–194.
54. Traugott AL, Moley JF. Multiple endocrine neoplasia type 2: clinical manifestations and management. *Cancer Treat Res* 2009;153:321–337.
55. American Thyroid Association Guidelines Task Force, Kloos RT, Eng C, et al. Medullary thyroid cancer: management guidelines of the American Thyroid Association. *Thyroid* 2009;19:565–612.
56. Wells SA Jr, Pacini F, Robinson BG, et al. Multiple endocrine neoplasia type 2 and familial medullary thyroid carcinoma: an update. *J Clin Endocrinol Metab* 2013;98:3149–3164.
57. Eng C, Clayton D, Schuffenecker I, et al. The relationship between specific RET proto-oncogene mutations and disease phenotype in multiple endocrine neoplasia type 2. International RET mutation consortium analysis. *JAMA* 1996;276:1575–1579.
58. Howe JR, Norton JA, Wells SA Jr. Prevalence of pheochromocytoma and hyperparathyroidism in multiple endocrine neoplasia type 2A: results of long-term follow-up. *Surgery* 1993;114:1070–1077.
59. Machens A, Niccoli-Sire P, Hoegel J, et al. Early malignant progression of hereditary medullary thyroid cancer. *N Engl J Med* 2003;349:1517–1525.
60. Gagel RF, Levy ML, Donovan DT, et al. Multiple endocrine neoplasia type 2A associated with cutaneous lichen amyloidosis. *Ann Intern Med* 1989; 111:802–806.
61. Santoro M, Carlomagno F, Romano A, et al. Activation of RET as a dominant transforming gene by germline mutations of MEN2A and MEN2B. *Science* 1995;267:381–383.
62. Mulligan LM, Ponder BA. Genetic basis of endocrine disease: multiple endocrine neoplasia type 2. *J Clin Endocrinol Metab* 1995;80:1989–1995.
63. Mulligan L, Kwok J, Healy C. Germ-line mutations of the RET protooncogene in multiple endocrine neoplasia type 2A (MEN 2A). *Nature* 1993; 363:458–460.
64. Donis-Keller H, Dou S, Chi D, et al. Mutations in the RET proto-oncogene are associated with MEN 2A and FMTC. *Hum Mol Genet* 1993;2:851–856.
65. Traugott AL, Moley JF. The RET Protooncogene. *Cancer Treat Res* 2010; 153:303–319.
66. Quayle FJ, Benveniste R, DeBenedetti MK, et al. Hereditary medullary thyroid carcinoma in patients greater than 50 years old. *Surgery* 2004;136:1116–1121.
67. Lips CJ, Landsvater RM, Hoppener JW, et al. Clinical screening as compared with DNA analysis in families with multiple endocrine neoplasia type 2A. *N Engl J Med* 1994;331:828–835.
68. Niccoli-Sire P, Murat A, Baudin E, et al. Early or prophylactic thyroidectomy in MEN 2/FMTC gene carriers: results in 71 thyroidectomized patients. The French Calcitonin Tumours Study Group (GETC). *Eur J Endocrinol* 1999;141:468–474.
69. Rodriguez GJ, Balsalobre MD, Pomares F, et al. Prophylactic thyroidectomy in MEN 2A syndrome: experience in a single center. *J Am Coll Surg* 2002;195: 159–166.
70. Skinner MA, Moley JA, Dilley WG, et al. Prophylactic thyroidectomy in multiple endocrine neoplasia type 2A. *N Engl J Med* 2005;353:1105–1113.
71. Brandi ML, Gagel RF, Angeli A, et al. Guidelines for diagnosis and therapy of MEN type 1 and type 2. *J Clin Endocrinol Metab* 2001;86:5658–5671.
72. Elisei R, Romei C, Renzini G, et al. The timing of total thyroidectomy in RET gene mutation carriers could be personalized and safely planned on the basis of serum calcitonin: 18 years experience at one single center. *J Clin Endocrinol Metab* 2012;97:426–435.
73. Waguespack SG, Rich TA, Perrier ND, et al. Management of medullary thyroid carcinoma and MEN2 syndromes in childhood. *Nat Rev Endocrinol* 2011;7:596–607.
74. Moley JF. Medullary thyroid carcinoma: management of lymph node metastases. *J Natl Compr Canc Netw* 2010;8:549–556.
75. Machens A, Dralle H. Biomarker-based risk stratification for previously untreated medullary thyroid cancer. *J Clin Endocrinol Metab* 2010;95:2655–2663.
76. Solorzano CC, Evans DB. Same-day ultrasound guidance in reoperations for locally recurrent papillary thyroid cancer. *Surgery* 2007;142:973–975.
77. Patel SG, Ahnen DJ. Familial colon cancer syndromes: an update of a rapidly evolving field. *Curr Gastroenterol Rep* 2012;14:428–438.
78. Aretz S, Uhlhaas S, Goergens H, et al. MUTYH-associated polyposis: 70 of 71 patients with biallelic mutations present with an attenuated or atypical phenotype. *Int J Cancer* 2006;119:807–814.
79. Russell AM, Zhang J, Luz J, et al. Prevalence of MYH germline mutations in Swiss APC mutation-negative polyposis patients. *Int J Cancer* 2006; 118:1937–1940.
80. Jasperson KW. Genetic testing by cancer site: colon (polyposis syndromes). *Cancer J* 2012;18:328–333.
81. Hampel H, Frankel WL, Martin E, et al. Screening for the Lynch syndrome (hereditary nonpolyposis colorectal cancer). *N Engl J Med* 2005;352: 1851–1860.
82. Lynch HT, Lynch PM, Lanspa SJ, et al. Review of the Lynch syndrome: history, molecular genetics, screening, differential diagnosis, and medicolegal ramifications. *Clin Genet* 2009;76:1–18.
83. Vasen HF, Blanco I, Aktan-Collan K, et al. Revised guidelines for the clinical management of Lynch syndrome (HNPCC): recommendations by a group of European experts. *Gut* 2013;62:812–823.
84. Niessen RC, Hofstra RM, Westers H, et al. Germline hypermethylation of MLH1 and EPCAM deletions are a frequent cause of Lynch syndrome. *Genes Chromosomes Cancer* 2009;48:737–744.
85. Kuiper RP, Vissers LE, Venkatachalam R, et al. Recurrence and variability of germline EPCAM deletions in Lynch syndrome. *Hum Mutat* 2011;32: 407–414.
86. Rumilla K, Schowalter KV, Lindor NM, et al. Frequency of deletions of EPCAM (TACSTD1) in MSH2-associated Lynch syndrome cases. *J Mol Diagn* 2011;13:93–99.
87. Jasperson KW, Tuohy TM, Neklason DW, et al. Hereditary and familial colon cancer. *Gastroenterology* 2010;138:2044–2058.
88. Steinhagen E, Markowitz AJ, Guillem JG. How to manage a patient with multiple adenomatous polyps. *Surg Oncol Clin N Am* 2010;19:711–723.
89. National Comprehensive Cancer Network. *NCCN Clinical Practice Guidelines in Oncology: Colorectal Cancer Screening.* http://www.nccn.org/professionals/physician_gls/pdf/colorectal_screening.pdf. Accessed February 19, 2014.
90. Vasen HF, Moslein G, Alonso A, et al. Guidelines for the clinical management of familial adenomatous polyposis (FAP). *Gut* 2008;57:704–713.
91. Church J. Familial adenomatous polyposis. *Surg Oncol Clin N Am* 2009; 18:585–598.
92. Nieuwenhuis MH, Bulow S, Bjork J, et al. Genotype predicting phenotype in familial adenomatous polyposis: a practical application to the choice of surgery. *Dis Colon Rectum* 2009;52:1259–1263.

93. Sinha A, Tekkis PP, Rashid S, et al. Risk factors for secondary proctectomy in patients with familial adenomatous polyposis. *Br J Surg* 2010;97:1710–1715.
94. Koskenvuo L, Renkonen-Sinisalo L, Jarvinen HJ, et al. Risk of cancer and secondary proctectomy after colectomy and ileorectal anastomosis in familial adenomatous polyposis. *Int J Colorectal Dis* 2014;29:225–230.
95. Remzi FH, Church JM, Bast J, et al. Mucosectomy vs. stapled ileal pouch-anal anastomosis in patients with familial adenomatous polyposis: functional outcome and neoplasia control. *Dis Colon Rectum* 2001;44:1590–1596.
96. Friederich P, de Jong AE, Mathus-Vliegen LM, et al. Risk of developing adenomas and carcinomas in the ileal pouch in patients with familial adenomatous polyposis. *Clin Gastroenterol Hepatol* 2008;6:1237–1242.
97. Aziz O, Athanasiou T, Fazio VW, et al. Meta-analysis of observational studies of ileorectal versus ileal pouch-anal anastomosis for familial adenomatous polyposis. *Br J Surg* 2006;93:407–417.
98. Fazio VW, Kiran RP, Remzi FH, et al. Ileal pouch anal anastomosis: analysis of outcome and quality of life in 3707 patients. *Ann Surg* 2013;257:679–685.
99. Rajaratnam SG, Eglinton TW, Hider P, et al. Impact of ileal pouch-anal anastomosis on female fertility: meta-analysis and systematic review. *Int J Colorectal Dis* 2011;26:1365–1374.
100. Bartels SA, D'Hoore A, Cuesta MA, et al. Significantly increased pregnancy rates after laparoscopic restorative proctocolectomy: a cross-sectional study. *Ann Surg* 2012;256:1045–1048.
101. Beyer-Berjot L, Maggiori L, Birnbaum D, et al. A total laparoscopic approach reduces the infertility rate after ileal pouch-anal anastomosis: a 2-center study. *Ann Surg* 2013;258:275–282.
102. Steinhagen E, Guillem JG, Chang G, et al. The prevalence of thyroid cancer and benign thyroid disease in patients with familial adenomatous polyposis may be higher than previously recognized. *Clin Colorectal Cancer* 2012;11:304–308.
103. Steinhagen E, Hui VW, Levy RA, et al. Results of a prospective thyroid ultrasound screening program in adenomatous polyposis patients. *Am J Surg* [ePub ahead of print].
104. Jarrar AM, Milas M, Mitchell J, et al. Screening for thyroid cancer in patients with familial adenomatous polyposis. *Ann Surg* 2011;253:515–521.
105. Giardiello FM, Burt RW, Jarvinen H, et al. Familial adenomatous polyposis. In: Bosman FT, Carneiro F, Hruban RH, et al, eds. *Classification of Tumours of the Digestive System*. Lyon: IARC Press; 2010:147–151.
106. Nieuwenhuis MH, Lefevre JH, Bulow S, et al. Family history, surgery, and APC mutation are risk factors for desmoid tumors in familial adenomatous polyposis: an international cohort study. *Dis Colon Rectum* 2011;54:1229–1234.
107. Quintini C, Ward G, Shatnawei A, et al. Mortality of intra-abdominal desmoid tumors in patients with familial adenomatous polyposis: a single center review of 154 patients. *Ann Surg* 2012;255:511–516.
108. Sinha A, Gibbons DC, Phillips RK, et al. Surgical prophylaxis in familial adenomatous polyposis: do pre-existing desmoids outside the abdominal cavity matter? *Fam Cancer* 2010;9:407–411.
109. Schiessling S, Kihm M, Ganschow P, et al. Desmoid tumour biology in patients with familial adenomatous polyposis coli. *Br J Surg* 2013;100:694–703.
110. von Roon AC, Tekkis PP, Lovegrove RE, et al. Comparison of outcomes of ileal pouch-anal anastomosis for familial adenomatous polyposis with and without previous ileorectal anastomosis. *Br J Surg* 2008;95:494–498.
111. Nieuwenhuis MH, Vogt S, Jones N, et al. Evidence for accelerated colorectal adenoma—carcinoma progression in MUTYH-associated polyposis? *Gut* 2012;61:734–738.
112. Palomaki GE, McClain MR, Melillo S, et al. EGAPP supplementary evidence review: DNA testing strategies aimed at reducing morbidity and mortality from Lynch syndrome. *Genet Med* 2009;11:42–65.
113. Umar A, Boland CR, Terdiman JP, et al. Revised Bethesda Guidelines for hereditary nonpolyposis colorectal cancer (Lynch syndrome) and microsatellite instability. *J Natl Cancer Inst* 2004;96:261–268.
114. Vasen HF, Watson P, Mecklin JP, et al. New clinical criteria for hereditary nonpolyposis colorectal cancer (HNPCC, Lynch syndrome) proposed by the International Collaborative group on HNPCC. *Gastroenterology* 1999;116:1453–1456.
115. Barnetson RA, Tenesa A, Farrington SM, et al. Identification and survival of carriers of mutations in DNA mismatch-repair genes in colon cancer. *N Engl J Med* 2006;354:2751–2763.
116. Lee-Kong SA, Markowitz AJ, Glogowski E, et al. Prospective immunohistochemical analysis of primary colorectal cancers for loss of mismatch repair protein expression. *Clin Colorectal Cancer* 2010;9:255–259.
117. Steinhagen E, Shia J, Markowitz AJ, et al. Systematic immunohistochemistry screening for Lynch syndrome in early age-of-onset colorectal cancer patients undergoing surgical resection. *J Am Coll Surg* 2012;214:61–67.
118. Heald B, Plesec T, Liu X, et al. Implementation of universal microsatellite instability and immunohistochemistry screening for diagnosing lynch syndrome in a large academic medical center. *J Clin Oncol* 2013;31:1336–1340.
119. Beamer LC, Grant ML, Espenschied CR, et al. Reflex immunohistochemistry and microsatellite instability testing of colorectal tumors for Lynch syndrome among US cancer programs and follow-up of abnormal results. *J Clin Oncol* 2012;30:1058–1063.
120. Mvundura M, Grosse SD, Hampel H, et al. The cost-effectiveness of genetic testing strategies for Lynch syndrome among newly diagnosed patients with colorectal cancer. *Genet Med* 2010;12:93–104.
121. Chen S, Wang W, Lee S, et al. Prediction of germline mutations and cancer risk in the Lynch syndrome. *JAMA* 2006;296:1479–1487.
122. Kastrinos F, Steyerberg EW, Mercado R, et al. The PREMM(1,2,6) model predicts risk of MLH1, MSH2, and MSH6 germline mutations based on cancer history. *Gastroenterology* 2011;140:73–81.
123. Green RC, Parfrey PS, Woods MO, et al. Prediction of Lynch syndrome in consecutive patients with colorectal cancer. *J Natl Cancer Inst* 2009;101:331–340.
124. Khan O, Blanco A, Conrad P, et al. Performance of Lynch syndrome predictive models in a multi-center US referral population. *Am J Gastroenterol* 2011;106:1822–1827, quiz 1828.
125. Tresallet C, Brouquet A, Julie C, et al. Evaluation of predictive models in daily practice for the identification of patients with Lynch syndrome. *Int J Cancer* 2012;130:1367–1377.
126. Kalady MF, McGannon E, Vogel JD, et al. Risk of colorectal adenoma and carcinoma after colectomy for colorectal cancer in patients meeting Amsterdam criteria. *Ann Surg* 2010;252:507–511, discussion 511–513.
127. Parry S, Win AK, Parry B, et al. Metachronous colorectal cancer risk for mismatch repair gene mutation carriers: the advantage of more extensive colon surgery. *Gut* 2011;60:950–957.
128. Kalady MF, Lipman J, McGannon E, et al. Risk of colonic neoplasia after proctectomy for rectal cancer in hereditary nonpolyposis colorectal cancer. *Ann Surg* 2012;255:1121–1125.
129. Cirillo L, Urso ED, Parrinello G, et al. High risk of rectal cancer and of metachronous colorectal cancer in probands of families fulfilling the Amsterdam criteria. *Ann Surg* 2013;257:900–904.
130. Stupart DA, Goldberg PA, Baigrie RJ, et al. Surgery for colonic cancer in HNPCC: total vs segmental colectomy. *Colorectal Dis* 2011;13:1395–1399.
131. Maeda T, Cannom RR, Beart RW Jr, et al. Decision model of segmental compared with total abdominal colectomy for colon cancer in hereditary nonpolyposis colorectal cancer. *J Clin Oncol* 2010;28:1175–1180.
132. Guillem JG, Glogowski E, Moore HG, et al. Single-amplicon MSH2 A636P mutation testing in Ashkenazi Jewish patients with colorectal cancer: role in presurgical management. *Ann Surg* 2007;245:560–565.
133. Barrow P, Khan M, Lalloo F, et al. Systematic review of the impact of registration and screening on colorectal cancer incidence and mortality in familial adenomatous polyposis and Lynch syndrome. *Br J Surg* 2013;100:1719–1731.
134. Vasen HF, Abdirahman M, Brohet R, et al. One to 2-year surveillance intervals reduce risk of colorectal cancer in families with Lynch syndrome. *Gastroenterology* 2010;138:2300–2306.
135. Stuckless S, Green JS, Morgenstern M, et al. Impact of colonoscopic screening in male and female Lynch syndrome carriers with an MSH2 mutation. *Clin Genet* 2012;82:439–445.
136. Engel C, Rahner N, Schulmann K, et al. Efficacy of annual colonoscopic surveillance in individuals with hereditary nonpolyposis colorectal cancer. *Clin Gastroenterol Hepatol* 2010;8:174–182.
137. Syngal S, Weeks JC, Schrag D, et al. Benefits of colonoscopic surveillance and prophylactic colectomy in patients with hereditary nonpolyposis colorectal cancer mutations. *Ann Intern Med* 1998;129:787–796.
138. Giardiello FM, Allen JI, Axilbund JE, et al. Guidelines on genetic evaluation and management of Lynch syndrome: a consensus statement by the US Multi-Society Task Force on Colorectal Cancer. *Dis Colon Rectum* 2014;57(8):1025–1048.

33 Cancer Risk–Reducing Agents

Dean E. Brenner, Scott M. Lippman, and Susan T. Mayne

WHY CANCER PREVENTION AS A CLINICAL ONCOLOGY DISCIPLINE

Until recently, clinical oncology has been defined as a medical specialty that attempts to intervene in order to slow or reverse the final stage of the cancer process—the clonally derived, genomically damaged, invasive cell mass. Cancer is a long process, a stepwise carcinogenic progression that encompasses critical molecular events that culminate in the loss of key cellular control homeostatic functions (e.g., control of proliferation, apoptosis, invasion, angiogenesis).[1] These events occur prior to and during the morphologic changes that have historically defined neoplasia. Morphologic changes, such as subtle increases in cellular proliferation that progress to early and late precancerous lesions containing dysplastic cells, characterize the carcinogenesis process (Fig. 33.1).[1–3] Opportunities for intervention in this process can include diverse, nonpharmacologic approaches (e.g., obesity management via diet/lifestyle interventions) or pharmacologic interventions (e.g., drugs or nutrients/nonnutrient substances used as drugs) aimed at delaying or reversing the carcinogenesis process prior to or following the appearance of early morphologic changes. Cancer screening and early detection strategies (e.g., surveillance endoscopy, fecal occult blood testing, mammography) identify not only those individuals with early stage, curable malignant transformations, but also those individuals with noninvasive neoplasias who are at risk for progression to transformed invasive malignancies.

Recognizing that cancer is a continuum, oncologists are increasingly expected to be knowledgeable about a diverse array of cancer-related topics including lifestyle behaviors such as diet and exercise, risk assessment, screening, other preventive interventions, in addition to current treatments for advanced malignancy. The understanding, use, and management of interventions designed to delay or reverse the carcinogenesis process have become integral components of the this role.[4]

DEFINING CANCER RISK–REDUCING AGENTS (CHEMOPREVENTION)

Cancer risk reduction, commonly referred to as chemoprevention, is the use of a range of interventions from drugs to isolated dietary components to whole-diet modulation to block, reverse, or prevent the development of invasive cancer.[5,6] Human cancer risk reduction asserts that one can intervene at many steps in the carcinogenic process, which occurs over many years. This prolonged latency provides opportunities to intervene at many time points and at multiple events in the carcinogenic process. Successful deployment of cancer risk–reducing agent interventions requires evidence of reduced cancer-associated incidence and/or mortality.

The concept of field carcinogenesis was first described in the early 1950s as *field cancerization* in squamous cell carcinomas of the head and neck, and subsequently ascribed to many epithelial sites. The field carcinogenesis concept is that patients have a wide surface area of precancerous or cancerous tissue change that can be detected at the gross (oral premalignant lesions, polyps), microscopic (metaplasia, dysplasia), and/or molecular (gene loss or amplification) levels. Recent molecular studies detecting profound genetic alterations in histologically normal tissue from high-risk individuals have provided strong support for the field carcinogenesis concept. The implication of the field effect is that multifocal, genetically distinct, and clonally related premalignant lesions can progress over a broad tissue region.[1] The essence of cancer risk reduction, then, is intervention within the multistep carcinogenic process and throughout a wide field.

IDENTIFYING POTENTIAL CANCER RISK–REDUCING AGENTS

Cancer risk–reducing agent identification results from the synthesis of data from population, basic, translational, and clinical sciences. Findings from all of these disciplines are combined to contribute to the identification of agents with the potential to delay or reverse the carcinogenesis process (see Fig. 33.1).

The Hanahan and Weinberg hallmarks of malignant transformation—self-sufficiency in growth signals, insensitivity to growth-inhibitory signals, evasion of apoptosis, limitless replication potential, sustained angiogenesis, and tissue invasion and metastasis[7]—reflect the loss of cellular signaling control. The molecular damage that results in transformation is triggered by a large array of genetic and environmental stressors such as chronic inflammation, oxidation, inherited genetic mutations, and exogenous environmental exposures. Many such signaling intermediates have common functions in multiple organ sites (see Fig. 33.1). The complexity and overlap of signal transduction pathways suggests that single molecular therapeutic/preventive targets may have limited effectiveness. Interventions aimed at preventing the occurrence of or overcoming the effects of molecular defects in multiple pathways or targets may be required to arrest or reverse carcinogenesis. Using the Hanahan and Weinberg hallmarks, examples of possible targets are shown in Table 33.1.

PRECLINICAL DEVELOPMENT OF CANCER RISK–REDUCING AGENTS

Similar to the development of therapeutic interventions, the assessment of efficacy and toxicity of single chemically synthesized entities, agents designed *in silico*, botanicals, nutrients/nonnutrient substances used as drugs for cancer risk–reducing agent efficacy proceeds through a translational paradigm that identifies efficacy in cell culture models, in live animal models, and in humans. Preclinical models that simulate the carcinogenesis process in target epithelia identify molecular biomarkers for modulation by interventions. These models can be used to identify potential toxicity of interventions and to assess the effect of interventions on the development and progression of preneoplasia/neoplasia.[8]

The U.S. National Cancer Institute's (NCI) PREVENT Cancer Preclinical Drug Development Program is a prime example of a

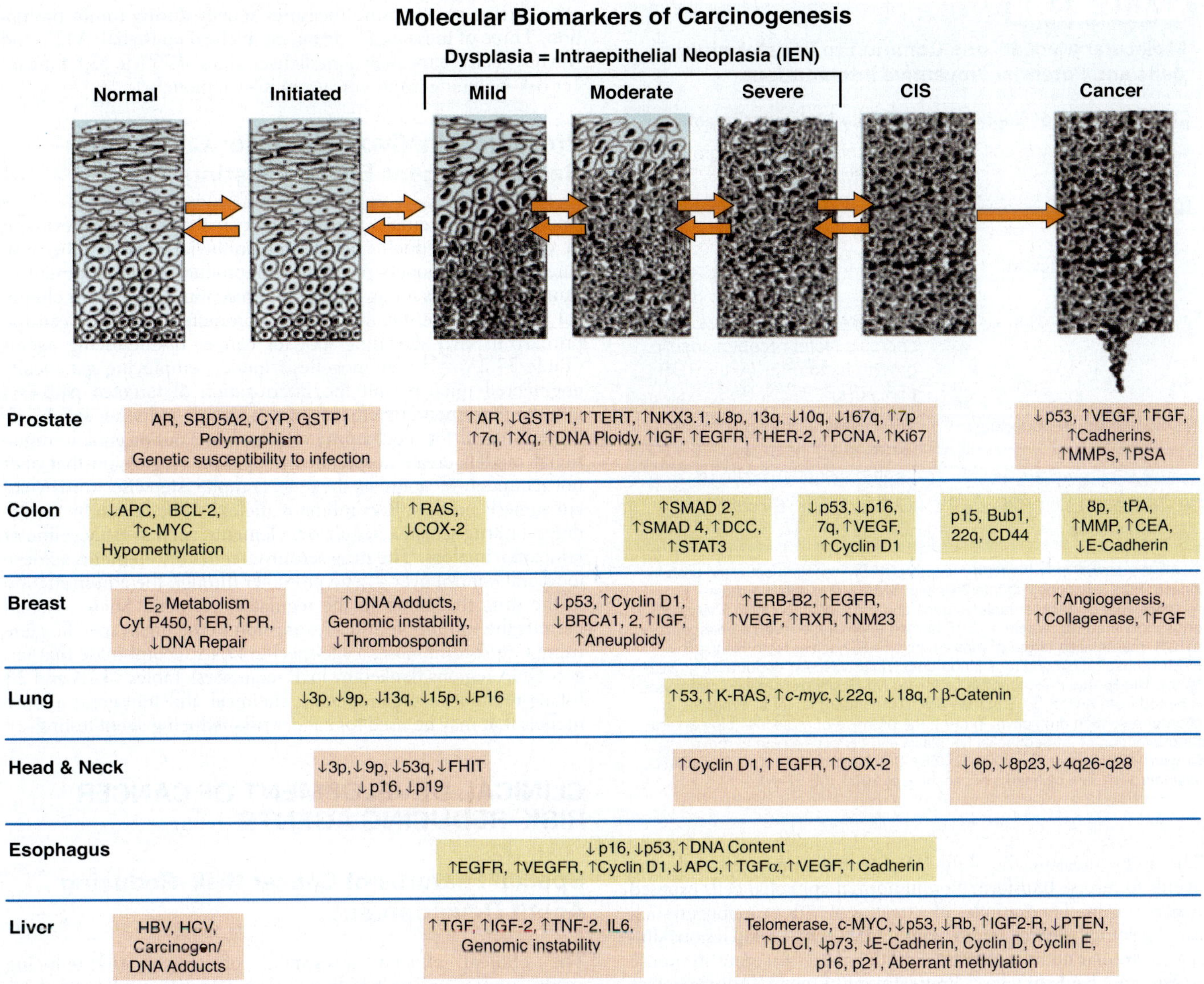

Figure 33.1 Genetic progression in major cancers. Carcinogenesis is driven by genetic progression. This progression is marked by the appearance of molecular biomarkers in distinctive patterns representing accumulating changes in gene expression and correlating with changes in histologic phenotype as cells move from normal through the early stages of clonal expansion to dysplasia and finally to early invasive, locally advanced, and metastatic cancer. The figure[257] shows candidate molecular biomarkers of genetic progression in seven target organs: the prostate,[300–302] the colon,[2] the breast,[303,304] the lung,[305–307] the head and neck,[308–311] the esophagus,[312,313] and the liver.[314] CIS, carcinoma in situ; AR, androgen receptor; CYP, cytochrome P-450; GSTP1, glutathione S transferase P1; TERT, telomerase reverse transcriptase; NKX3.1, NK 3 transcription factor related, locus 1 (prostate specific, androgren regulated); IGF, insulin-like growth factor; EGFR, epidermal growth factor receptor; HER-2, human epidermal growth factor receptor-2; PCNA, proliferating cell nuclear antigen; VEGF, vascular endothelial growth factor; FGF, fibroblast growth factor; MMP, matrix metalloproteinase; PSA, prostate-specific antigen; APC, adenomatous polyposis coli; BCL-2, B cell lymphoma 2 gene, apoptosis control; c-MYC, v-myc avian myelocytomatosis viral oncogene homolog; COX-2, cyclooxygenase-2; SMAD, homolog of mothers against decapentaplegic + *C. Elegans* SMA protein; DCC, deleted in colon cancer gene; CEA, carcinoembryonic antigen; ER, estrogen receptor; PR, progesterone receptor; ERB-B2, Receptor tyrosine-protein kinase erbB-2, same as HER-2; RXR, retinoid X receptor; NM23, Nucleoside disphosphate kinase A; K-RAS, Kirsten rat sarcoma viral oncogene homolog; FHIT, fragile histidine triad protein; TGFα, tumor growth factor alpha; HBV, hepatitis B virus; HCV, hepatitis C virus; TNF-2, tumor necrosis factor 2; IL6, interleukin 6; PTEN, phosphatase and tensin homolog. (Figure and revised caption from Kelloff GJ, Lippman SM, Dannenberg AJ, et al. Progress in chemoprevention drug development: the promise of molecular biomarkers for prevention of intraepithelial neoplasia and cancer—a plan to move forward. *Clin Cancer Res* 2006;12:3661–3697, published with permission from the American Association for Cancer Research.)

rational strategy to select promising agents for clinical trials through a stepwise approach of preclinical in vitro testing followed by *in vivo* screening.[8–10] This system involves several phases: biochemical prescreening assays, in vitro efficacy models, in vivo short-term screening, animal efficacy testing, and preclinical toxicology testing.

Biochemical Prescreening Assays

Prescreening assays are a series of short-term, mechanistic assays developed to evaluate the ability of a test compound to modulate biochemical events presumed to be mechanistically linked to carcinogenesis.[8] These in vitro assays are rapidly completed for potential cancer risk–reducing agents. Examples of such assays include carcinogen-DNA binding, prostaglandin synthesis inhibition, glutathione–S-transferase inhibition, and ornithine decarboxylase inhibition.

In Vitro Efficacy Models

In vitro assays test the cancer risk–reducing activity of a screened compound in four epithelial cell systems (primary rat tracheal epithelial cells, human lung tumor [A427] cells, mouse mammary organ cultures [MMOC], and human foreskin epithelial cells).

TABLE 33.1

Molecular Mechanisms Common to Transforming Cells and Potential Preventive Interventions

Characteristics of Neoplasia	Possible Molecular Targets
■ Self-sufficiency in cell growth	EGFR, platelet-derived growth factor, MAPK, PI3K
■ Insensitivity to antigrowth signals	SMADs, pRb, cyclin-dependent kinases, MYC
■ Limitless replicative potential	hTERT, pRb, p53
■ Evading apoptosis	Bcl-2, BAX, caspases, Fas, tumor necrosis factor receptor, insulin growth factor/PI3K/Akt, mTOR, p53, NF-κB, PTEN, RAS
■ Sustained angiogenesis	VEGF, basic fibroblast growth factor, integrins ($\alpha_v\beta_3$), thrombospondin-1, HIF-1α
■ Tissue invasion and metastases	MMPs, MAPK, E-cadherin

EGFR, epidermal growth factor receptor; MAPK, mitogen-activated protein kinase; PI3K, phosphoinositide 3-kinase; SMAD, drosophila protein, mothers against decapentaplegic gene and the *Elegans* protein SMA; pRb, phosphorylated Rb protein; hTERT, human telomerase reverse transcriptase; mTOR, mammalian target of rapamycin; NF-κB, nuclear factor kappa B; PTEN, phosphatase and tensin homolog; VEGF, vascular endothelial growth factor; HIF-1α, hypoxia-inducible factor-1α; MMP, Matrix metalloproteinases. Adapted from Kelloff GJ, Lippman SM, Dannenberg AJ, et al. Progress in chemoprevention drug development: the promise of molecular biomarkers for prevention of intraepithelial neoplasia and cancer—a plan to move forward. *Clin Cancer Res* 2006;12:3661–3697 and derived from Hanahan D, Weinberg RA. The hallmarks of cancer. *Cell* 2000;100:57–70.

The assays measure the ability of potential cancer risk–reducing agents to reverse transformation in normal epithelial cells exposed to carcinogens. For example, after treatment with a carcinogen such as 7,12-demethylbenz(a)anthracene, MMOCs develop lesions similar to alveolar nodules that are considered precancerous in mouse mammary glands in vivo.[11] Pretreatment of organ cultures before carcinogen exposure measures the effect of cancer risk–reducing agents in the initiation stage of carcinogenesis, whereas treatment after carcinogen exposure measures activity during tumor promotion. Three of these assays (using rat tracheal epithelial, A427, and MMOC cells) have shown predictive values of 76% to 83% for cancer risk–reducing agent efficacy in in vivo models.[8]

Preclinical In Vivo Models for Cancer Risk–Reducing Agent Efficacy Testing

Animal models remain a crucial link in the efficacy assessment of cancer risk–reducing agents for epithelial cancer. Chemical carcinogenesis models provide the reproducible development of tumors in animals following the administration of a known chemical initiator or combination initiator/promoter and have been the primary in vivo screening tool for cancer risk–reducing agents (Table 33.2A).[12,13] Carcinogenesis models employing genetically engineered mice permit the interrogation of targeted pathways and the corresponding efficacy of cancer risk–reducing agents. Although useful for mechanistic studies, knockout or genetic mutational models create accelerated neoplastic progression that does not accurately recapitulate the more complex, stepwise, human carcinogenesis process. Recombinant alleles can be driven by the addition of drug-sensitive regulatory elements, such as tetracycline or tamoxifen analogs. The drug-sensitive regulatory elements achieve temporal control over a gene promoter through the administration of the drug that binds to the regulatory element. Such a system permits the inhibition or overexpression of the organ-specific gene using Cre recombinase, a site-specific DNA recombinase that targets DNA regions flanked by loxP sequences. Tables 33.2A and 2B list representative organ-specific chemical and transgenic mouse models that may be used for cancer risk–reducing agent testing.

CLINICAL DEVELOPMENT OF CANCER RISK–REDUCING AGENTS

Special Features of Cancer Risk–Reducing Agent Development

The clinical efficacy assessment of cancer risk–reducing agents employs phased testing (phase I to III) models used for development of drugs[14] but with crucial differences in study design and end points. Special features for the clinical development of

TABLE 33.2A

Chemical Carcinogenesis Models Used for Screening of Cancer Risk–Reducing Agents for Common Epithelial Neoplasms in Animals

Organ Site	Species	Carcinogen	End Point
Colon	Rat, mouse	Azoxymethane (AOM)	Aberrant crypts, adenomas, adenocarcinomas
Lung	Mouse	N—butyl-N-(4-hydroxylbutyl)nitrosamine (NNK); benzo[a]pyrene; cigarette smoke	Adenomas, adenocarcinomas
	Hamster	Methylnitrosourea (MNU)	Squamous cell carcinomas
	Mouse	N-nitroso-tris-chloroethylurea	Squamous cell carcinomas
Breast	Rat	Dimethylbenz[a]anthracene (DMBA); MNU	Adenocarcinomas, adenomas
Prostate	Rat	MNU + testosterone	Adenocarcinomas
Bladder	Rat, mouse	N-butyl-N-(4-hydroxybutyl)nitrosamine (OH-BBN)	Transitional cell carcinoma
Pancreas	Hamster	N-nitrobis-(2-oxopropyl)amine (BOP)	Ductal carcinomas
Head and neck	Rat	4-nitroquinoline-1-oxide (4-NQO)	Tongue squamous cell carcinomas
	Mouse	DMBA	Squamous cell carcinomas
Esophagus	Rat	Dimethyalbenz[a]anthracene	Squamous cell carcinomas
	Rat	Esophagogastroduodenal anastomosis + iron	Adenocarcinomas

Adapted from Steele VE, Lubet RA. The use of animal models for cancer chemoprevention drug development. *Semin Oncol* 2010;37:327–338.

TABLE 33.2B

Selected Transgenic Animal Models for Carcinogenesis Evaluation

Organ Site	Genes Targeted	End Point	References
Colon	*Apc, Lrig1, gp130, Stat3, Smad3, Wnt-β-catenin, villin, TGFBR2, Kras, Ink4a*	Adenomas and adenocarcinomas	(258, 259)
Lung	*KrasG12D, KrasG12Vgeo, PTEN, BrafV600E, cRaf, Egfr* L858R±T790M, *PIK3CA*, EMLA4-ALK fusion	Adenomas and adenocarcinomas	(260)
	Rb. P53	Small cell	
Breast	Mouse mammary tumor virus long terminal repeat promoter (MMTV) driven *BRCA1, p53, ERα,* aromatase, *TGFα, Her2/neu, wnt,* PELP-1, AIB-1	DCIS, adenocarcinomas	(261)
Prostate	Probasin promotor driving SV40 large T antigen (*TRAMP/LADY*), *c-Myc, TMPRSS-ERG, Akt, Wnt-β-catenin,* androgen receptor	Prostate intraepithelial neoplasia, neuroendocrine tumors (TRAMP); adenocarcinomas (*c-Myc, TMPRESS-ERG, Akt, Wnt,* androgen receptor)	(262)
	Nkx3.1, FGFR1, TGF, PTEN	Adenocarcinomas	
Pancreas	*KrasG12D* alone, *LSL-Kras, PDX-1, R26Notch, Tif1γ* Combined *PDX-1, LSL-Kras, LSL-Trp53*; combined *PDX-1, Brca2, LSL-Kras Trp53; KrasG12D* on *Mist1* locus; *PDX-1, KrasG12D+ Ink4a/Arf* or *Smad4*; *Ptf1a, KrasG12D, TGFBR2*	Pancreatic intraepithelial neoplasia Pancreatic adenocarcinoma	(263)

Note: Most models are mouse models. Such models will permit efficacy testing of specific pathway targets using single agent interventions, combinations, or multimechanism-based natural products.

cancer risk–reducing agents create the following challenges to be overcome: (1) the need for large therapeutic index (doses associated with potential toxicity of an intervention need to substantially exceed doses aimed at delaying or reversing transformation) for use in individuals who are asymptomatic yet may benefit from an extended (years) treatment course; (2) the long latency to malignant transformation (an assessment of effectiveness based on the reduction in cancer incidence requires studies lasting for years and involving thousands of participants); (3) adherence (once-daily dosing regimens using interventions that have sufficiently long half-lives may minimize the impact of a missed dose yet maintain the biologic impact on the physiologic target; minimal toxicity and strong psychological commitment to preventive goals also enhance adherence[15]); and (4) complex risk assessment for cancer (individuals with highly penetrant but infrequent, germ-line genetic susceptibility to breast and colon cancers[16,17] are excellent candidates for cancer risk–reducing agents and are likely to accept some toxicity for reduced cancer risk). For individuals at more modestly increased risk (e.g., long-term, current smokers; persons with a family history of cancer; women with mammographically dense breasts), quantitative risk assessment algorithms may be useful in the future to identify optimal cancer risk–reducing agents. The refinement of cancer risk calculators for breast,[18] colon,[19] and prostate cancer[20] promises to appropriately select high-risk individuals for cancer risk–reducing agents such that anticipated benefits exceed potential risks.

Biomarkers as Cancer Risk–Reducing Agent Targets and Efficacy End Points

A biomarker is a characteristic that is measured and evaluated as an indicator of normal biologic processes, pathogenic processes, or pharmacologic responses to therapeutic interventions.[21] A surrogate end point for cancer prevention assumes that a measured biologic feature will predict the presence or future development of a cancer outcome.[22] Biomarkers enable a reduction in the size and duration of an intervention trial by replacing a rare or distal end point with a more frequent, proximate end point.[23] Intraepithelial neoplasia has served and continues to serve as a biomarker for invasive malignancy (Table 33.3). Although many advocate the use of intraepithelial neoplasia-based biomarkers as regulatory surrogate end points, others caution that intraepithelial neoplasias may not serve as sufficiently robust surrogate biomarkers for cancer incidence or mortality.[24]

In order to be useful as end points for cancer risk–reducing agent efficacy testing as regulatory end points, any biomarker must have statistical accuracy, precision, and effectiveness of results[24] that demonstrate prediction of a *hard* disease end point—cancer incidence or mortality. An independent validation data set must address defined standards of validation that minimize bias in the study design and the populations studied.[25] The biomarker must be generalizable to the specific clinical or screening population (Table 33.4).

Phases of Cancer Risk–Reducing Agent Development

Phase I cancer risk–reducing agent trials define an optimal cancer risk–reducing agent dose. An optimal cancer risk–reducing agent dose is one that is usually nontoxic, scheduled once daily, and modulates a tissue, cellular, or serum biomarker of drug activity (e.g., the dose of aspirin that inhibits prostaglandin production in a target tissue site). The definition of a maximum tolerated dose is not an essential end point of a phase I cancer risk–reducing agent trial. Higher, yet nontoxic doses may lower cancer risk–reducing agent efficacy. For example, β-carotene at high doses has pro-oxidant activity and may enhance the carcinogenesis process, whereas at low doses, it is a potent antioxidant and differentiating agent.[26]

Phase II cancer risk–reducing agent trials begin to define cancer risk–reduction efficacy. These short-term (6 months to 1 year) treatment periods gather evidence of risk reduction by assessing drug effects on tissue, cellular, or blood surrogate markers of carcinogenesis. Phase IIa trials are nonrandomized, biomarker modulation trials. Phase IIb trials are randomized, placebo-controlled trials of several hundred subjects testing, for example, whether a risk-reducing agent reduces recurrence of a previously resected intraepithelial neoplastic lesion as the primary end point. Cellular dynamic

TABLE 33.3

Common Intraepithelial Neoplasias

Epithelium	Intraepithelial Neoplasia	References
Colon and rectum	Adenoma	(264)
Lower esophagus	Barrett esophagus	(265)
Upper esophagus	Squamous dysplasia	(266, 267)
Skin: Squamous/ basal cell	Actinic keratosis	(268)
Skin: Pigmented	Dysplastic nevus	(269)
Cervix	Cervical intraepithelial neoplasia	(270)
Head and neck	Leukoplakia/oral epithelial dysplasia	(271)
Prostate	Prostate intraepithelial neoplasia (PIN), intraductal carcinoma of the prostate	(272)
Lung	Bronchial dysplasia	(273)
Pancreas	Pancreatic intraepithelial neoplasia	(274)

(e.g., proliferation, apoptotic index), biochemical, or molecular (e.g., p53, cyclin D) end points may be used as secondary end points. Preoperative or *window of opportunity trials* enroll subjects for brief study periods prior to obtaining tissue by a planned resection of an invasive neoplasm. Such designs permit the exploration of biomarker modulation in the invasive neoplasm and in contiguous epithelial fields proximal and distal to the invasive neoplasm.[27]

Phase III cancer risk–reducing agent trials define reduction in a hard cancer end point such as cancer incidence or mortality. Such trials, using large, higher risk populations in a randomized, double-blinded intervention, are designed to identify a standard of preventive care for a given risk population. For example, trials of tamoxifen for the reduction of breast cancer incidence,[28,29] finasteride for the reduction of prostate cancer incidence,[30] and β-carotene for the reduction of lung cancer incidence[31] serve as examples of well-conducted, definitive phase III cancer risk–reducing agent clinical trials.

Some investigators consider randomized, controlled clinical trials with an end point sufficient for regulatory review as phase III.

TABLE 33.4

Characteristics of Biomarkers for Use as End Points in Cancer Risk–Reducing Agent Efficacy Assessment

- Variability of expression between phases of the carcinogenesis process
- Detected early in the carcinogenesis process
- Genetic progression or protein pathway based
- Target of modulation by preventive interventions
- Changes in biomarker linked to reduction in incident cancer of epithelial target
- Changes in biomarker linked to clinical benefit
- Can be quantified directly or via closely related activity such as a downstream target or upstream kinase
- Measurable in an accessible biosample (preferably urine, serum, saliva, stool, or breath)
- High throughput, technically feasible, analytical procedure with strong quality assurance/quality control procedures
- Cost-effective

Using such a definition, a clinical trial with an end point of reduction in adenoma recurrence is considered a phase III trial. Other investigators define phase III cancer risk–reducing agent trials as randomized, controlled clinical trials with a cancer incidence or mortality end point. This controversy causes confusion in the literature. For the purpose of clarity in this textbook, the latter definition of phase III trial is used—a prospective, randomized, controlled clinical trial with a cancer incidence or mortality end point. Randomized, controlled clinical trials with a surrogate biomarker end point such as an intraepithelial neoplasia (e.g., adenoma) are defined as phase IIb cancer risk–reducing agent trials.

MICRONUTRIENTS

Definition

Micronutrients comprise a large, diverse group of molecules typically ingested as part of the diet that play roles in normal human biology. This group of compounds has been investigated extensively as cancer risk–reducing agents in purified forms (i.e., supplements), as components of multiagent cocktails, and occasionally, as components of food extracts/other mixtures. Although retinoids are not micronutrients per se, they are related to retinol (vitamin A) and share certain properties with carotenoids, which are diet derived and, therefore, included along with micronutrients.

Retinoids, Carotenoids, and Antioxidant Nutrients

Overview and Mechanisms

Retinoids are the natural derivatives and synthetic analogs of vitamin A.[32] Cancer risk–reduction intervention studies have evaluated the parent compound (retinol, typically given as retinyl acetate or palmitate), naturally occurring retinoids such as all-trans–retinoic acid (ATRA) and 13-cis-retinoic acid (13cRA), and also synthetic retinoids such as etretinate and fenretinide (4-hydroxy[phenyl]retinamide [4HPR]). These agents have been of interest for cancer risk reduction for decades. Mechanistically, retinoids have been shown to modulate cellular growth and differentiation, as well as apoptosis.[32] A large body of research indicates that retinoids have activity in the promotion and progression phases of carcinogenesis, including extensive evidence of efficacy in the setting of premalignant lesions, leading to their evaluation in human Phase III trials. Nuclear retinoic acid receptors mediate many of the retinoid-signaling effects; however, retinoids interact with other signaling pathways, such as estrogen signaling in breast cancer.[33]

Carotenoids are a group of naturally occurring plant pigments, only some of which are found in appreciable levels in the human diet and human tissues, including beta-carotene, alpha-carotene, lycopene, lutein, and β-cryptoxanthin.[34] Of these, the most widely studied carotenoids for cancer risk reduction are beta-carotene and lycopene. Beta-carotene has the highest pro–vitamin A activity of the carotenoids, but alpha-carotene and β-cryptoxanthin also possess pro–vitamin A activity. Other carotenoids, such as lycopene, do not possess vitamin A activity but are known to have potent antioxidant activity, particularly with regard to singlet oxygen quenching.[35] Furthermore, eccentric cleavage products of beta-carotene,[36] as well as other non-pro–vitamin A carotenoids such as lycopene (e.g., apocarotenals, apocarotenoic acids) appear to be biologically active and may also act via retinoid-signaling pathways.[37]

Because of the known antioxidant function of carotenoids, they are often studied for risk-reducing efficacy in combination with other antioxidant nutrients, especially vitamins E and C and selenium (sometimes as a cocktail, versus placebo). Thus, we will consider this group of nutrients first, followed by other micronutrients that are thought to act via different mechanisms and/or pathways.

Epidemiology

A large body of literature indicates that people who consume greater amounts of carotenoids from foods (primarily fruits and vegetables) and people with higher serum or plasma levels of various carotenoids have a lower risk for various cancers.[38] In particular, according to the systematic review of the literature conducted by the World Cancer Research Fund/American Institute for Cancer Research,[38] foods containing carotenoids are "probably" associated with lower risks of cancers of the mouth/pharynx/larynx and lung; foods containing beta-carotene are "probably" associated with lower risks of cancers of the esophagus; and foods containing lycopene are "probably" associated with lower risks of prostate cancer. Preformed retinol intake is inconsistently associated with risks of various cancers but that, in part, likely reflects confounding, because dietary sources of preformed retinol primarily include foods of animal origin (e.g., liver, eggs, milk). Vitamin C in the diet comes primarily from the consumption of fruits and vegetables; therefore, vitamin C and carotenoids often trend together in epidemiologic findings. Vitamin E, in contrast, is found in different foods, especially nuts, seeds, and vegetable oils; intake and blood concentrations are somewhat inconsistently associated with cancer risk.[39] Selenium, being a trace mineral, is difficult to measure in the diet, but higher selenium status has been associated with a lower risk of certain cancers, although the results are not entirely consistent.[39]

Preclinical In Vivo Models

In preclinical models, retinoids induce differentiation as well as arrest proliferation[33] of various cancers, making them attractive agents for cancer risk reduction.[40] The International Agency for Research on Cancer reviewed the preclinical research involving beta-carotene, concluding that there was "sufficient" evidence of cancer preventive activity, particularly involving mouse skin tumor models and the hamster buccal pouch model.[41] Notably, there was inconsistent evidence of efficacy in respiratory tract models. Lycopene has been evaluated in numerous cell culture systems and in a variety of models of prostate carcinogenesis, including chemically induced, orthotopic implantation, transgenic, and xenotransplantation, with mixed evidence of efficacy.[42] Evidence, primarily from cell culture studies, suggests that lycopene metabolites may be at least partially responsible for anticarcinogenic activity.[37]

Clinical Trials: Retinoids, Carotenoids, and Antioxidant Nutrients

Retinoids, carotenoids, and antioxidant nutrients have been evaluated in the setting of preneoplasia/neoplasia in many different organ sites, as will be discussed. Of the many clinical trials of retinoids and carotenoids/other antioxidant nutrients, key trials with cancer incidence/recurrence as primary outcomes are tabulated (see Tables 33.5 and 33.6) and reviewed.

Clinical Efficacy in the Upper Airway

Many trials of cancer risk–reducing agents have been done in the setting of squamous cell carcinomas of the head and neck, in large part because of the substantial clinical problem of relatively high rates of recurrences and second primary tumors in curatively treated cancer patients. Early work demonstrated that high-dose 13cRA (50 to 100 mg/m^2 per day) produced no significant differences in disease recurrence (local, regional, or distant) but significantly lowered the rate of second primary invasive neoplasms,[43] with the benefits persisting for at least 5 years.[44] Substantial retinoid toxicity, however, including skin dryness and peeling, cheilitis, conjunctivitis, and hypertriglyceridemia, was evident in a large proportion of patients. Subsequent trials thus used lower doses of retinoids (13cRA or a synthetic retinoid, etretinate), but failed to show efficacy in reducing second primary tumor formation (Table 33.5).[45,46]

Supplemental beta-carotene has also been studied as a single agent and in combination with other agents for the prevention of second primary cancers of the mouth and throat (Table 33.6). One trial of beta-carotene alone observed no harm or benefit[47]; another observed nonsignificantly fewer second head and neck cancers but more lung cancers[48]; and a third gave beta-carotene with α-tocopherol (400 IU per day).[49] In the third trial, beta-carotene was discontinued early due to adverse findings from lung cancer prevention trials (see the following); however, after a median follow-up of 6.5 years, all-cause mortality was increased, which the authors attributed to the supplemental α-tocopherol. As will be discussed later, adverse effects of antioxidant nutrients are not limited to head and neck cancer patients; potential mechanisms for adverse effects are discussed further.

Clinical Efficacy in the Lung (Lower Airway)

Reversal of Metaplasia or Dysplasia. Active smokers and recent quitters have multiple preinvasive metaplastic and dysplastic lesions in the pulmonary tree. Most of these lesions resolve upon smoking cessation, but some remain and progress to invasive neoplasms. Unfortunately, micronutrient or retinoid interventions have not demonstrated preventive efficacy in most rigorous trials in patients with early lesions. For example, a US trial randomized 755 asbestos workers to receive beta-carotene (50 mg per day) and retinol (25,000 IU every other day) versus placebo; sputum atypia was not reduced after 5 years.[50] As another example, eligible smokers with lung metaplasia or dysplasia were randomized to 6 months of 13cRA or placebo. The extent of metaplasia decreased similarly (in approximately 50% of subjects) in both study arms.[51] Only smoking cessation was associated with a significant reduction in the metaplasia index during the 6-month intervention.

Prevention of Invasive Neoplasms. Large, phase III efficacy trials of beta-carotene plus other micronutrients for primary prevention of lung cancer have been completed, as summarized in Table 33.6. The Alpha-Tocopherol, Beta-carotene (ATBC) Trial involved 29,133 men from Finland who were heavy cigarette smokers at entry.[52] In a two-by-two factorial design, participants were randomized to receive either supplemental α-tocopherol, beta-carotene, the combination, or placebo. Unexpectedly, participants receiving beta-carotene (alone or in combination with α-tocopherol) had a statistically significant 18% increase in lung cancer incidence and an 8% increase in total mortality relative to participants receiving placebo. α-Tocopherol had no effect.

The finding of an increased incidence of lung cancer in the beta-carotene–supplemented smokers was replicated in the Carotene and Retinol Efficacy Trial (CARET), a large randomized trial of supplemental beta-carotene plus retinol versus placebo in asbestos workers and smokers.[53] This trial was terminated early, but, at the time of termination, overall lung cancer incidence was increased by 28% in the supplemented subjects and total mortality was also increased by 17%. In contrast, the Physicians' Health Study (PHS) of supplemental beta-carotene versus placebo in 22,071 male US physicians reported no significant effect—positive or negative—of 12 years of supplementation of beta-carotene on total cancer, lung cancer, or cardiovascular disease (see Table 33.6).[54] Two other trials involving supplemental beta-carotene alone (the Women's Health Study[55]) or with other antioxidant nutrients (the Medical Research Council/British Heart Foundation Heart Protection Study[56]) on overall cancer incidence also failed to observe efficacy.

Prevention of Second Primary Invasive Neoplasms. EUROSCAN was a multicenter trial employing a two-by-two factorial design to test retinyl palmitate and N-acetylcysteine (also a compound with known antioxidant activity) in preventing second primary invasive neoplasms in patients with early stage cancers

TABLE 33.5

Larger, Randomized Trials of Retinoids in Human Cancer Risk Reduction with Cancer Outcomes[a,b]

Population	Drug (Dose)	End Point	Outcomes	References
United States, prior HNSCC	13cRA (50–100 mg/m^2/d)	Second primary tumor	Significant reduction in second primary tumors at 32 and 55 mos; however, substantial toxicity	(43, 44)
France, prior HNSCC	Etretinate (50/25 mg/d)	Second primary tumor	No difference	(46)
United States, prior HNSCC	13cRA (30 mg/d)	Second primary tumor	No difference	(45)
Europe, prior HNSCC, NSCLC	Vitamin A (300,000/150,000 IU/d) +/− N-acetylcysteine	Second primary tumor	No difference	(57)
United States, Prior NSCLC	13cRA (30 mg/d)	Second primary tumor	No difference, but second primary tumors were lower in nonsmokers on drug but higher in smokers on drug	(58)
Italy, prior breast cancer	4HPR (200 mg/d) No treatment	Contralateral breast cancer	Nonsignificant reduction; premenopausal women did better but opposite in postmenopausal women	(60)
United States, prior BCC	13cRA (10 mg/d)	Second basal cell carcinoma	No difference	(65)
United States, prior actinic keratosis	Retinol (25,000 IU/d)	Skin cancer incidence	Reduction in squamous cell carcinomas but not basal cell carcinomas	(67)
United States, prior BCC/ SCC of the skin	13cRA (5–10 mg/d) Retinol (25,000 IU/d)	Second skin cancer	No significant difference for either agent	(66)
Netherlands, renal transplant patients	Acitretin (30 mg/d)	Skin cancer	Significant reduction	(64)
United States, aggressive SCC of the skin	13cRA (1 mg/kg/d) + interferon alpha	Second primary tumors and tumor recurrences	No effect	(275)
United States, prior bladder TCC	Megadose vitamins (40,000 IU retinol/d) versus RDA vitamins	Recurrence	Significant reduction in recurrence	(73)
United States, prior bladder TCC	4HPR (200 mg/d)	Recurrence	No difference	(72)

[a]Trials of retinoids that also included beta-carotene are listed under Table 33.2 only.
[b]Versus placebo unless otherwise indicated.
HNSCC, head and neck squamous cell carcinoma; NSLC, non–small-cell lung cancer; BCC, basal cell carcinoma; TCC, transitional cell carcinoma; RDA, recommended dietary allowance.

of the head and neck or lung. None of the interventions reduced second airway primary invasive neoplasms.[57] The Lung Intergroup Trial randomized patients with surgically resected lung cancer to 13cRA versus placebo and found no significant differences between the two arms in second primary tumors.[58] Notably, smoking status modified the effect of the 13cRA intervention, which was harmful in current smokers yet beneficial in former smokers.

Thus, phase III trials of both carotenoids/antioxidants and retinoids indicate that these agents overall do not reduce the risk of developing invasive lung cancers, nor do they prevent the development of second primary invasive neoplasms. However, the finding that former smokers seemed to benefit from both 13cRA[58] and beta-carotene[53] is intriguing. Mechanistic work suggests this interaction is real rather than chance (see the following), suggesting that (1) risk-reduction in smokers is especially challenging,[59] and (2) trials in former smokers may merit consideration.

Clinical Efficacy in the Breast

Moon et al.[40] first showed that fenretinide was a promising cancer risk–reducing agent for the breast, having a high therapeutic index and synergistic interaction with tamoxifen in mammary carcinogenesis model studies. This laboratory work led to a large-scale randomized trial of fenretinide (versus no treatment) for 5 years to prevent contralateral breast cancer in women aged 30 to 70 years with a history of resected early breast cancer and no prior adjuvant therapy.[60] The intervention produced no significant overall effect, although fenretinide reduced contralateral and ipsilateral breast cancer rates in premenopausal women, with an opposite (adverse) trend observed in postmenopausal women. The reduced incidence of second breast cancer in premenopausal patients persisted with longer follow-up.[61]

Retinoid X receptor (RXR)–selective retinoids are also being evaluated in preclinical and clinical studies. Ongoing work suggests that combination treatment may represent a promising new strategy to suppress both estrogen receptor–negative and estrogen receptor–positive breast tumors, and the combination of retinoids with antiestrogens may be particularly effective.[62]

Clinical Efficacy in the Skin

Retinoids have been widely studied for cancer risk–reducing efficacy in skin. Early work was done in patients who have substantial skin cancer risk either due to xeroderma pigmentosum or medication-induced immunosuppression for transplants. For example, 13cRA reduced skin cancer by 63% in patients with

TABLE 33.6

Randomized Trials of Antioxidant Nutrients in Human Cancer Risk Reduction with Cancer Outcomes[a]

Population	Drug (Dose)	End Point	Outcomes	References
United States, prior head/neck cancer	Beta-carotene (50 mg/d)	Second primary head and neck cancers	Nonsignificant reduction in second head and neck cancer, increase in lung cancer	(48)
Italy, prior head/neck cancer	Beta-carotene (75 mg/d) for 3 mos with 1 mo off	Second primary head and neck cancers	No effect on second primary tumors, nonsignificant decrease in death	(47)
Canada, prior head/neck cancer	30 mg beta-carotene/d + 400 IU vitamin E/d	Deaths	Beta-carotene discontinued, mortality increased at end of trial	(49)
Finland, male smokers	20 mg beta-carotene/d +/− 50 mg vitamin E/d	Lung cancer	Lung cancer increased with beta-carotene, no effect vitamin E	(52)
United States, smokers and asbestos workers	Beta-carotene (30 mg/d) + retinol (25,000 IU/d)	Lung cancer	Lung cancer increased with beta-carotene + vitamin A	(53)
United States, resected stage I non–small-cell lung cancer	Selenized yeast, 200 μg/d versus placebo	Second primary cancer	No effect	(276)
United States, male physicians	Beta-carotene (50 mg every other day)	Total cancer	No effect	(54)
United States, female health professionals	Beta-carotene (50 mg/every other day)	All cancers	No effect	(55)
United Kingdom, adults at risk for coronary heart disease	20 mg beta-carotene/d + 600 mg vitamin E/d + 250 mg vitamin C/d	Total cancers	No effect	(56)
United States, prior skin cancer	50 mg beta-carotene/d	Second skin cancer	No effect	(68)
Australia	Beta-carotene (30 mg/d)	Incident squamous cell skin cancer incident basal cell skin cancer	No effect	(69)
United States, prior skin cancer	200 μg selenium/d	Second skin cancer	No effect, with longer follow-up became adverse	(70)
Linxian County, China, general population	15 mg beta-carotene/d + 30 mg vitamin E/d + 50 μg selenium/d	Stomach cancer death Esophageal cancer death	Significant decrease in stomach cancer death; no effect on esophageal cancer death	(75)
Linxian County, China, esophageal dysplasia	Multivitamin/multimineral + 15 mg beta-carotene/d	Stomach cancer death Esophageal cancer death	No effect	(78)
United States, males	200 μg selenium/d +/− 400 IU vitamin E/d	Prostate cancer incidence	No effect; with longer follow-up vitamin E became adverse	(84)
United States, male physicians II	500 mg vitamin C/d + 400 IU vitamin E every other day	Prostate cancer incidence, total cancer incidence	No effect	(86)

[a] All versus placebo.

CANCER PREVENTION AND SCREENING

xeroderma pigmentosum; however, severe, acute mucocutaneous toxicity with the 13cRA occurred.[63] Also, the preventive effect of the retinoid was lost after stopping retinoid therapy. In renal transplant patients, acitretin (30 mg per day) reduced the numbers of premalignant lesions, the number of patients with skin cancer, and the cumulative number of skin cancers.[64]

In lower risk populations, low-dose 13cRA (10 mg per day)[65] and retinol or 13cRA alone did not reduce the recurrence of basal or squamous cell skin cancers,[66] although retinol alone reduced squamous but not basal cell carcinomas in patients with prior actinic keratoses.[67]

Beta-carotene (50 mg per day), in a randomized trial did not reduce the recurrence of nonmelanoma skin cancers.[68] Consistent with findings in the lung, the risk was increased by 44% in current smokers randomized to beta-carotene but not in never smokers randomized to beta-carotene as compared with placebo. Supplemental beta-carotene (30 mg per day) also did not prevent basal cell carcinoma or squamous cell carcinoma of the skin in an Australian trial.[69]

Clark et al.[70] randomized patients with a history of nonmelanoma skin cancer to 200 μg per day selenium or placebo.[70] Selenium did not reduce the incidence of second skin cancers; a further report of this trial with longer follow-up[71] indicated that there was instead a significant increase in total nonmelanoma skin cancer (hazard ratio [HR] = 1.17; 95% confidence interval [CI], 1.02 to 1.34) and squamous cell skin cancer (HR = 1.25; 95% CI, 1.03 to 1.51).

Clinical Efficacy in the Bladder

A trial of fenretinide (200 mg per day orally for 12 months) versus placebo was conducted for preventing tumor recurrence in patients with nonmuscle-invasive bladder transitional cell carcinoma after transurethral resection with or without adjuvant intravesical bacillus Calmette-Guérin; recurrence rates were similar in both groups.[72] Another trial randomized 65 patients with biopsy-confirmed transitional cell carcinoma of the bladder to a multivitamin (recommended dietary allowance [RDA] levels) alone or supplemented with 40,000 IU retinol, 100 mg pyridoxine, 2,000 mg ascorbic acid, 400 U of α-tocopherol, and 90 mg zinc.[73] The 5-year estimate of tumor recurrence was 91% in the RDA arm versus 41% in the higher-dose nutrient arm ($p = 0.0014$).

Clinical Efficacy in the Cervix

Randomized trials include four with beta-carotene (alone or with other antioxidant nutrients), and five with retinoids. Only one of these trials, involving ATRA,[74] found a significant treatment effect. This trial administered a 0.372% ATRA solution by collagen sponge in a cervical cap delivery system. There was a higher complete response rate in the ATRA group (43%) than the placebo group (27%; $p = 0.041$) among the 141 patients with moderate dysplasia; no significant differences in dysplasia regression rates between the two study arms were detected in patients with severe dysplasia. The investigators experienced substantial losses to follow-up in this patient population.

Clinical Efficacy in the Esophagus and Stomach

Certain regions of China (Huixian and Linxian) have strikingly high incidence rates of esophageal and gastric cancers. Two trials were done in Linxian County; one was a general population trial that tested the efficacy of four different nutrient combinations at inhibiting the development of esophageal and gastric cancers.[75] Those who were given the combination of beta-carotene, vitamin E, and selenium had a 13% reduction in total cancer deaths, a 4% reduction in esophageal cancer deaths, and a 21% reduction in gastric cancer deaths (see Table 33.6). None of the other nutrient combinations reduced gastric or esophageal cancer deaths significantly in this trial. The treatment benefit has been shown to persist for 10 years postintervention, with greater efficacy seen in participants under age 55 years.[76] This finding stands in contrast to most other antioxidant nutrient supplement intervention trials, suggesting that the applicability of these results for populations with adequate nutritional status and for other tumor sites may be limited.[77]

The other Linxian trial evaluated a multivitamin/multimineral preparation plus beta-carotene (15 mg per day) in residents with esophageal dysplasia.[78] There was no clear evidence of efficacy, although confidence intervals were wide.

Clinical Efficacy in the Colon/Rectum

Of the randomized trials aimed at the prevention of recurrent colorectal adenomas with micronutrients that have been completed, some used beta-carotene alone[79] or with other nonmicronutrient interventions.[80] Others evaluated beta-carotene with and without supplemental vitamins C and E.[81] None of the trials observed benefit with supplementation. A subsequent report from one trial noted that alcohol intake and cigarette smoking modified the efficacy of beta-carotene.[82] Among nonsmokers and nondrinkers, beta-carotene was associated with a significant decrease in the risk of one or more recurrent adenomas (relative risk [RR] = 0.56). Among persons who smoked and also drank more than one alcoholic drink per day, beta-carotene significantly increased the risk of recurrent adenoma (RR = 2.07).

Clinical Efficacy in the Prostate

Because oxidative stress may play a role in the etiology of prostate cancer, several antioxidant nutrients, including vitamin E, selenium, and lycopene, have been of interest for preventing prostate cancer. The largest trial to date of these nutrients is the Selenium and Vitamin E Cancer Prevention Trial (SELECT), which tested selenium and vitamin E in a two-by-two factorial design for the primary prevention of prostate cancer. Despite preliminary indications of prostate cancer risk–reducing efficacy for selenium (from a trial of selenium for skin cancer[70]) and vitamin E (from a trial of vitamin E to prevent lung cancer[83]), there was no evidence of efficacy.[84] With extended follow-up, the nonsignificant adverse effect of vitamin E became significantly adverse.[85] Negative/neutral findings also were reported for vitamins E and C and prostate and total cancer in the PHS II randomized controlled trial.[86]

The carotenoid lycopene has generated much interest with regard to prostate cancer risk, and several intervention trials have been conducted based on lycopene supplements. These studies have been small, short term, based on intermediate end points, and often lack adequate control groups. The use of a tomato sauce–based intervention is arguably a better approach to evaluate, based on animal data indicating that tomato powder (which includes lycopene along with other phytochemicals), but not lycopene alone, was effective at inhibiting prostate carcinogenesis.[87]

Mechanisms for Ineffective Retinoid and Carotenoid Cancer Risk–Reducing Activity

There are now a number of trials demonstrating that supplemental beta-carotene/retinoids given to current smokers can produce increases rather than reductions in cancer incidence. In tobacco users, beta-carotene and other carotenoids may produce oxidative carotenoid breakdown products that alter retinoid metabolism and signaling pathways, along with pro-oxidation.[88] For retinoids such as 13cRA, smoking may induce genetic and epigenetic changes in the lung that affect retinoid activity; for example, tobacco smoking can affect RAR-β expression.[58] The adverse effects of supplemental nutrients are not limited to smokers; α-tocopherol increased rather than reduced prostate cancer in SELECT (which had relatively few smokers) and selenium increased prostate cancer among men without a baseline selenium deficiency.[89] This may be a consequence of the relatively high doses used in SELECT,[77] but certainly calls into question the notion that reducing oxidative stress is a pivotal cancer risk–reduction strategy, even in nonsmokers.

It has become clear that reactive oxygen species (ROS), such as hydrogen peroxide, can act as important physiologic regulators of intracellular signaling pathways.[90,91] Data in mouse models have shown that vitamin E accelerates lung tumor growth by disrupting the ROS–p53 axis, potentially by removing oxidative damage to DNA, which can serve as a potent stimulus for p53 activation.[92] Although some of the large cancer risk–reducing trials may have failed in their primary objective, they may indirectly contribute to a clearer understanding of cancer biology, leading to the recognition that the role of oxidative stress and ROS in human disease is much more nuanced than originally hypothesized.[93]

As for the retinoids, these agents are generally too toxic to be used as single agents for risk-reducing efficacy; however, a major area of ongoing research is examining retinoids (low doses) given in combination with other agents, especially those that regulate the epigenome, such histone deacetylase (HDAC) inhibitors.[33]

Folic Acid and Other B Vitamins

Overview and Mechanisms. Folate is a water-soluble B vitamin found in foods, whereas folic acid is the synthetic form found in supplements and fortified foods. Adequate folate is critical for DNA methylation, repair, and synthesis.[94,95] The methylation status of genes can play a key role in gene silencing and gene expression, lending plausibility to the idea that folate could be a key nutrient in regulating cell growth and proliferation.

Epidemiology. Epidemiologic studies have linked low folate intake with higher risk of several cancers, most notably colorectal cancer.[96] Long-term use of multivitamin supplements, which are a major source of folate and other B vitamins, has been associated with a reduction in the risk of colon cancer in some studies, including recent (postfortification) findings.[97–99] Supporting an anticancer role of folate is that genotypes for methylene tetrahydrofolate reductase, an enzyme known to be involved in folate metabolism, predict the risk of colon cancer dependent on folate intake or status.[100] Vitamin B_6 has been less studied in relation to cancer than folate, but some epidemiologic studies suggest that vitamin B_6 may be important for colorectal cancer.[101,102] A higher risk of cancer related to deficiencies of these vitamins has been suggested for alcohol drinkers.[103]

Clinical Trials: Folic Acid and B Vitamins. Risk-reducing efficacy for supplemental folic acid has been primarily evaluated in the setting of prevention of recurrent colorectal adenomas (i.e., in patients with prior adenomas). Of six randomized trials of folic acid, two small trials reported suggestions of benefit of folic acid supplementation.[104,105] However, benefits were not observed in two much larger trials, the Aspirin/Folate Polyp Prevention Study (AFPPS) (dose: 1 mg of folic acid daily)[106] and the United Kingdom Colorectal Adenoma Prevention (ukCAP) trial (dose: 500 μg of folic acid daily).[107] AFPPS found indications of an increased risk for advanced lesions and multiple adenomas with prolonged treatment and follow-up. A third large trial, the Nurses Health Study/Health Professionals Follow-up Study (NHS/HPFS) folic acid polyp prevention trial, showed no overall risk reduction.[108] The most recent trial, done in a Chinese population >50 years of age,[109] reported that 1 mg folic acid per day reduced sporadic colorectal adenomas when compared to no intervention (not a placebo-controlled study). One possible explanation for the discrepancy of the Chinese trial versus North American and European trials is the baseline plasma folate status. In the Chinese trial, the mean baseline folate concentration of 5 ng/mL[109] was half of the reported 10 ng/mL in a United States trial,[106] where folate fortification of the food supply occurs.

Calcium and Vitamin D

Overview and Mechanisms. There are two major forms of vitamin D: ergocalciferol (D_2) and cholecalciferol (D_3). Vitamin D_2 is absorbed through dietary sources such as fortified milk products, and D_3 is synthesized via ultraviolet (UV) B light isomerization of 7-dehydrocholestrol in the epidermis.[110] Vitamin D_3 is converted to calcitriol (1, 25-[OH]$_2$ D_3) in a two-step process requiring both hepatic and renal hydroxylation. Calcitriol binds to the vitamin D receptor, which translocates to the nucleus and binds to multiple gene promoter sites. Through this mechanism, vitamin D regulates cytoplasmic signaling pathways that impact cellular differentiation and growth through proteins such as Ras and mitogen-activated protein kinase (MAPK), protein lipase A, prostaglandins, cyclic adenosine monophosphate (AMP), protein kinase A, and phosphatidyl inositol 3 kinase.[110] 1,25(OH)$_2$D$_3$ regulates cellular proliferation and apoptosis. For example, 1,25(OH)$_2$D$_3$ can induce cleavage of caspase 3, poly (ADP-ribose) polymerase (PARP), and MAPK, leading to apoptosis. 1,25(OH)$_2$D$_3$ inhibits the expression and phosphorylation of Akt, a key regulator of cellular proliferation. The differentiation properties of 1,25(OH)$_2$D$_3$ are mediated through transcriptional activation of the CDK inhibitor p21. The effects of vitamin D on multiple signal transduction pathways operational in cancer cells are reviewed by Deeb et al.[111]

Epidemiology. Observational epidemiologic studies have shown a relatively consistent inverse association between low calcium intake, including that from supplements, and increased colorectal and colon cancer risk.[112,113] Vitamin D exposure is typically assessed by measuring 25(OH)vitamin D in plasma because exposure is derived not only from diet and supplements, but also from cutaneous synthesis following dermal exposure to UV radiation. A large number of observational studies have evaluated the association between vitamin D status and cancer risk, as systematically reviewed by the Agency for Healthcare Research and Quality (AHRQ).[114] The evidence is inconsistent for most cancer sites, with the exception of studies showing that individuals with lower blood vitamin D levels have a higher risk of colorectal cancer or adenoma. Although some observational studies have reported that higher serum vitamin D is associated with lower breast cancer risk, the association is inconsistent.[114,115] Also, there are some studies suggesting high serum vitamin D is associated with increases in certain cancers, particularly pancreatic cancer.[116]

Clinical Trials: Calcium and Vitamin D

Clinical Efficacy in the Colon. Baron et al.[117] randomized subjects with a recent history of colorectal adenomas to either calcium carbonate (1,200 mg per day of elemental calcium) or placebo. Results showed significant benefit for the calcium arm (adjusted RR = 0.81; 95% CI, 0.67 to 0.99; $p = 0.04$). In a smaller, similar study of calcium gluconolactate and carbonate (2 g elemental calcium daily), the adjusted odds ratio (OR) for adenoma recurrence was 0.66 (95% CI, 0.38 to 1.17; $p = 0.16$) for calcium treatment,[118] and while not statistically significant, it was similar to the data of Baron et al.[117]

In the largest trial of calcium and vitamin D with primary cancer end points (e.g., colon, breast), the US Women's Health Initiative (WHI) evaluated the combination of 400 IU of vitamin D per day plus 1,000 mg of calcium per day in 36,282 postmenopausal women. For colon cancer, there was no benefit observed,[119] although the mean baseline intake of calcium was already very high (more than 1,151 mg per day). With regard to vitamin D as a single agent, there was also no suggestion of benefit for colon cancer incidence in a 5-year British trial of vitamin D (100,000 IU every 4 months) that reported colon cancer incidence,[120] although this was not a primary end point.

Clinical Efficacy in the Breast. Vitamin D has received considerable attention for a possible role in the prevention of breast cancer,[121] although no trials have yet investigated vitamin D as a single agent for breast cancer risk reduction. The large WHI trial gave a combination of calcium and vitamin D, as noted previously, and there was no significant effect of this combination on breast cancer risk (HR, 0.96; 95% CI, 0.85 to 1.09).[122] Lappe et al.[123] conducted a trial that examined the relation between calcium plus vitamin D (1,100 IU per day) supplementation (versus calcium alone or placebo) in 1,179 healthy postmenopausal women in Nebraska.[123] Although fracture was the primary outcome of the trial, total cancer incidence was reportedly lower in the calcium plus vitamin D group, although the number of end points was very small (n = 50 total cancers observed during the follow-up). An ongoing randomized trial of vitamin D and omega-3 fatty acids (the **VIT**amin D and Omeg**A**-3 Tria**L** [VITAL]) among 20,000 participants is expected to provide more definitive data on a possible role of vitamin D in the prevention of breast and other cancers.[124]

Summary and Conclusion: Micronutrients

Certain agents, including the retinoids, beta-carotene, folic acid, calcium plus vitamin D, vitamin E, and selenium, have received substantial attention for a possible role in reducing the risk of cancer in humans. As reviewed herein, some of the trials have observed statistically significant reductions in the risk of the primary end point (e.g., retinoids in skin carcinogenesis models, calcium in colorectal adenomas, antioxidant nutrients in Linxian, China, for gastric cancer prevention), whereas others have observed statistically significant increases in the risk of the primary end points (beta-carotene and retinoid lung cancer prevention trials in smokers, vitamin E and prostate cancer, selenium and nonmelanoma skin cancer). Considering the completed trials, there is clear evidence against the general use of nutrient *supplements* for cancer prevention, which is the conclusion also reached by the World Cancer Research Fund/American Institute for Cancer Research.[38] Note that there is no evidence that food sources of these nutrients increase risk.

Having noted that, there are other key themes emerging from this growing body of research. One such theme is that nutrient supplementation may be of benefit to some but not all. One such population that may benefit includes persons who are low in the nutrient of interest at baseline.[77] This was initially suggested in the Linxian Country trial (done in a micronutrient-deficient population), with growing support from subgroup analyses of several completed trials.[77] However, the hypothesis that nutrient supplementation can reduce cancer risk in subgroups selected based on inadequate nutritional status has, to date, not been formally evaluated in intervention trials.

Another consistent theme is that lifestyle factors (e.g., smoking) and genetics (polymorphisms) may determine who is most likely to benefit from supplementation. Trial data will likely be increasingly mined to identify genetic profiles associated with both better outcomes (risk prediction) and response to intervention.[125,126] Ultimately, a more personalized approach to cancer risk reduction may emerge, consistent with the movement toward a more personalized approach for cancer treatment.

Finally, nearly all of these trials initiate intervention with older adults (who are more likely to develop cancer end points during the follow-up); but, animal models suggest that the timing of exposure may likely be quite relevant. For example, folic acid may protect against initiation, but may also promote the proliferation of existing neoplasms.[127] Thus, the dose, form (food versus supplement), timing, and nutritional and lifestyle characteristics may all be relevant in affecting the efficacy of risk-reducing interventions involving nutrients and related substances. Further research, drawing upon newer tools now available through the field of nutritional genomics, will be needed to gain greater clarity on the heterogeneous biologic effects observed in nutrient-based risk reduction.

ANTI-INFLAMMATORY DRUGS

Mechanism

Nonsteroidal anti-inflammatory drugs (NSAIDs) represent a class of drugs that reduce cellular inflammation through multiple mechanisms, the most prominent of them being the modulation of eicosanoid metabolism.[128] Eicosanoids are metabolites of dietary fatty acids, primarily linoleic acid. Linoleic acid is metabolized to arachidonic acid, which is stored in the lipid membrane and, once mobilized from the membrane, further metabolized by prostaglandin-H synthases (PGHS) 1 and 2 to PGD_2, PGE_2, $PGF_{2\alpha}$, PGI_2, or thromboxane A_2 (TxA_2) by specific synthases. Leukotriene pathways involve the conversion of arachidonic acid to leukotriene A_4 by 5-lipoxygenase and subsequent hydrolysis of leukotriene A_4 to other downstream leukotrienes. Newly formed prostaglandins function primarily through binding to prostaglandin receptors (EP receptors), releasing coupled G-proteins to elicit responses in the same or neighboring cells.[129]

Prostaglandins (PG) play crucial roles in controlling cellular proliferation, apoptosis, cellular invasiveness, and angiogenesis and in modulating immunosuppression.[129] Because PGE_2 is the most abundant PG in tumors, reducing local concentrations of PGE_2 may be a pivotal cancer preventive strategy.[129]

PGHS-independent mechanisms of NSAID action may, at least in part, explain NSAID preventive efficacy.[130] A diverse group of NSAIDs inhibit apoptosis via multiple mechanisms. Among the more prominent of these mechanisms is the inhibition of cyclic guanosine monophosphate (cGMP) phosphodiesterase activity, attenuation of beta-catenin mRNA through suppressing transcription of the *CTNNB1* gene, and activation of c-Jun N-terminal kinase 1.[130] NSAIDs activate peroxisome proliferator–activated receptor (PPAR)γ, leading to increased E-cadherin expression and reduced colony formation in vitro, while reducing PPARδ, leading to reduced resistance to apoptosis.[130] Selective cyclooxygenase 2 (COX-2) inhibitors inhibit Akt signaling and induce apoptosis of human colorectal and prostate cancer cells in vitro in a COX-2–independent manner via the inhibition of phosphoinositide-dependent kinase-1 (PDK-1). NSAIDs inhibit nuclear factor kappa B (NF-κB) at pharmacologic concentrations and key cellular proliferation signaling intermediates such as activator protein 1 (AP-1) and other intermediates of the MAPK pathway.[130] The impact of NSAIDs on carcinogenic events driven by these upstream pathways in humans as opposed to preliminary in vitro or in vivo models remains unclear.

Epidemiology

Pooled analyses of 34 controlled trials of aspirin 75 mg to 100 mg daily (69,224 participants), conducted primarily for cardiovascular disease reduction, observed reduced cancer deaths (OR, 0.63; 95% CI, 0.49 to 0.82). Most of the benefit occurred after 5 years follow-up.[131] In a pooled analysis of 150 case control and 45 cohort studies, in addition to a reduced risk of death from colorectal cancer (OR, 0.58; 95% CI, 0.44 to 0.78), chronic and frequent (once daily or more) use of aspirin also reduced the risk of death from esophageal (OR, 0.58; 95% CI, 0.44 to 0.76), gastric (OR, 0.61; 95% CI, 0.40 to 0.93), and breast (OR, 0.81; 95% CI, 0.72 to 0.93) cancers.[132] An analysis of 662,624 men and women enrolled in the American Cancer Society's Cancer Prevention Study II found that aspirin taken at least 16 times per month over a 6-year period conferred a 40% reduced risk of colorectal cancer mortality.[133] Both the 46,363 male patients of the Health Professional Study[134] and the 82,911 patients of the Nurse's Health Study[135] suggest that prolonged use (>10 years) of 325 mg of aspirin twice weekly or more reduces colorectal cancer risk (RR, 0.77; 95% CI, 0.67 to 0.88, from the Nurse's Health Study). Daily NSAID intake is associated with a 40% reduction (OR, 0.56; 95% CI, 0.43 to 0.73) in the risk of esophageal adenocarcinoma.[136]

Evidence in Preclinical In Vivo Carcinogenesis Models

NSAIDs, including aspirin, indomethacin, piroxicam, sulindac, ibuprofen, and ketoprofen, suppress colonic tumorigenesis induced chemically (1,2-dimethylhydrazine or its metabolites) or transgenically (Min^+).[137,138] The selective COX-2 inhibitors were the most efficacious colon tumorigenesis inhibitors in both chemical and transgenic rodent models.[139,140] In preclinical models, NSAIDs affect the onset and progression of cancers in the stomach, skin, breast, lung, prostate, and urinary bladder, although the evidence is more limited than for colon cancers.[141]

Clinical Trials

Key clinical trials of NSAIDs for the prevention of colorectal cancer are summarized in Table 33.7. Sulindac reduced the size and number of preexisting adenomas in patients with familial adenomatous polyposis but did not suppress the development of new adenomas,[142] whereas the selective COX-2 inhibitor, celecoxib, suppressed the development of new adenomatous polyps in patients with familial adenomatous polyposis.[143] Although these results are promising, reports of invasive neoplasms developing in familial adenomatous polyposis patients being treated with sulindac[144] raise the question of whether NSAIDs preferentially alter the formation or regression of those adenomas less likely to progress to invasive adenocarcinomas, as compared to those more likely to progress.

Randomized, double-blinded placebo controlled trials of NSAIDs as cancer risk–reducing agents for colorectal adenocarcinoma (see Table 33.7) have confirmed that aspirin suppresses

TABLE 33.7

Summary of Clinical Trials of Nonsteroidal Anti-Inflammatory Drugs as Colorectal Cancer Risk–Reducing Agents

Population	Drug (Dose), Duration	Phase	Endpoint	Outcome	References
Gene Associated					
Familial adenomatous polyposis (FAP)	Sulindac (300–400 mg/d, divided doses)	IIb	Polyp regression	Colorectal and duodenal polyps regressed in ~50%	(277, 278) (279)
Hereditary nonpolyposis colon cancer (Lynch syndrome)	Aspirin 600 mg/d, resistant starch	III	Cancer	≥2 yr, hazard ratio (HR) colon cancer 0.41; 95% CI, 0.19–0.86; all cancers Incidence rate ratio 0.37; 95% CI, 0.18–0.78; no effect of starch	(280, 281)
Sporadic Risk					
Previous adenomatous polyps, healthy subjects	Aspirin (40, 81, 325, 650 mg once per day)	I, IIa	Dose-biomarker	Aspirin dose of 81 mg daily sufficient to suppress colorectal mucosal prostaglandin E_2	(282–284)
Previous adenomatous polyps	Sulindac (300 mg), 4 mos	IIb	Polyp regression	Sulindac did not significantly decrease the number or size of polyps	(146)
Previous adenomatous polyps	Piroxicam (7.5 mg), 2 yr	IIb	Polyp recurrence	Colorectal mucosal PGE_2 reduced in piroxicam treated arm, unacceptable toxicity	(145)
Prior colorectal cancer	Aspirin (325 mg once per day), 3 yr	IIb	Polyp recurrence	Aspirin use associated with delayed development of adenomatous polyps	(285)
Previous adenomatous polyps	Aspirin (81 mg once per day or 325 mg once per day) and/or folate, 3 yr	IIb	Polyp recurrence	Low-dose aspirin reduced the recurrence of adenomatous polyps	(286)
Previous adenomatous polyps	Celecoxib and rofecoxib	IIb	Polyp recurrence	Celecoxib and rofecoxib reduced the recurrence of adenomatous polyps, unacceptable toxicity	(148–150)

adenoma recurrence in patients previously treated for adenomas or for cancer. Neither sulindac nor piroxicam alone suppressed adenoma formation in high-risk, sporadic populations at tolerable doses.[145,146] Sulindac, in combination with difluoromethylornithine, has potent colorectal anticarcinogenesis effects.[147] Selective COX-2 inhibitors (celecoxib, rofecoxib) reduce the recurrence of adenomas by one-third in all patients previously treated for adenomas and by one-half in patients with previously resected large (≥1 cm) adenomas,[148–150] but they are too toxic as cancer risk–reducing agents due to their cardiovascular toxicity.[151,152] Although most NSAIDs (piroxicam, indomethacin) have sufficient gastrointestinal (GI) toxicity to reduce their acceptability as cancer risk–reducing agents,[153,154] the long-term administration of low-dose aspirin in vascular prevention trials demonstrates acceptable GI toxicity.[155]

Up to 40% of individuals screened for colorectal neoplasms will have an adenomatous polyp detected and removed, yet only 10% of these lesions will progress to invasive neoplasms. To date, prospective NSAID trials of only 2 to 3 years cannot substitute for cancer incidence or mortality end points. Given the 10-year latency between adenoma formation and a cancer event, prospective trials sufficiently powered to detect colorectal cancer incidence end points are unlikely in the future.[156] Alternatively, a follow-up of patients randomized on trials of aspirin in the prevention of vascular events in the 1980s and 1990s offers secondary analysis opportunities. In a pooled analysis of three prospective vascular end point cohort studies, 20-year low-dose aspirin treatments reduced cancer deaths from all solid tumors (OR, 0.69; CI, 0.54 to 0.88) and from lung and esophageal adenocarcinomas (OR, 0.66; CI, 0.56 to 0.77).[155] Despite this, the U.S. Preventive Services Task Force (USPSTF) does not recommend the use of aspirin or NSAIDs as cancer risk–reducing agents for normal risk populations, preferring adherence to colorectal cancer screening recommendations (fecal occult blood testing and endoscopy).[153,154,157]

Minimal prospective cancer risk reduction data are available at other epithelial organ sites. Ketorolac, given as a 1% rinse solution, did not reduce the size or histology of leukoplakia lesions.[158] Celecoxib reduces the Ki67 labeling index and increases the expression of nuclear survivin without significantly changing the cytoplasmic survivin in bronchial biopsies of smokers.[159] Cancer prevention trials of aspirin as interventions for delaying progression from intraepithelial neoplasias in other epithelial sites remain ongoing for the lower esophagus.[136] No prospective, randomized trials or data are available for breast, prostate, or gynecologic cancer prevention.

EPIGENETIC TARGETING AGENTS (SELECTIVE ESTROGEN RECEPTOR MODULATORS, 5α-STEROID REDUCTASE INHIBITORS, POLYAMINE INHIBITORS)

Posttranslational pathway targets remain a fertile source of chemopreventive strategies. Phase III data support cancer risk–reduction agent efficacy of selective estrogen receptor modulators (SERM) and 5α-steroid reductase inhibitors for breast and prostate cancer prevention, respectively. Inhibitors of the polyamine pathway may be useful preventives for colorectal cancer.

Selective Estrogen Receptor Modulators

Mechanism

SERMs function as estrogen receptor (ER) agonists and antagonists depending on the SERM structure and target tissue. Predominant ERα receptors occur in the human uterus, cortical bone, and the liver; whereas predominant ERβ receptors occur in blood vessels, cancellous bone, the whole brain, and immune cells.[160,161] During carcinogenesis, the amount of ERα increases while the amount of ERβ decreases in breast tissues.[162] Ideally, a desirable SERM for cancer prevention will function as an antiestrogen in the breast and uterus, but a partial estrogen agonist in skeletal, cardiovascular, central nervous system (CNS), GI tract, and vaginal tissues. In addition, an ideal SERM will not have procoagulant effects and will not cause perimenopausal symptoms such as hot flashes.[162]

Tamoxifen. Tamoxifen is a triphenylethylene compound developed for the treatment of ER-positive breast cancer in the 1960s and 1970s.[163,164] Tamoxifen inhibits the initiation and promotion phases of breast carcinogenesis in the dimethylbenzanthracene chemical carcinogenesis model.[164,165] When tamoxifen binds to ERβ, which then binds to an AP-1 type gene promoter, it functions as an estrogen agonist. When bound to ERα, which binds to an estrogen response element (ERE) target gene promoter, tamoxifen functions as an estrogen antagonist.[162,166] Tamoxifen has estrogen antagonist effects in the human breast; partial estrogen agonist effects in bone, the cardiovascular system, and CNS; and predominant estrogen agonist effects in the uterus, liver, and vagina. The estrogen agonist effects in the liver and uterus result in tamoxifen's toxicities of thromboembolism and endometrial cancer, respectively. The clinical finding that tamoxifen reduces the incidence of contralateral second primary breast cancers during adjuvant treatment regimens catalyzed the push for its development as a cancer risk–reduction agent.[167,168]

Raloxifene. The benzothiophene structure of raloxifene confers a different tissue-specific ER-binding profile than the triphenylethylene tamoxifen. Raloxifene has greater estrogen agonist activity in bone but reduced estrogen agonist activity in the uterus. Raloxifene was studied for the treatment and prevention of osteoporosis in a large, pivotal trial (the Multiple Outcomes of Raloxifene Evaluation [MORE]) and was found to reduce the rate of vertebral fracture as compared to placebo in postmenopausal women.[169]

Lasofoxifene and Arzoxifene. Lasofoxifene and arzoxifene are third-generation SERMs developed as more potent blockers of bone resorption with the goal of reducing the risk of fractures, breast cancer, and heart disease while minimizing the SERM-induced risk of endometrial hyperplasia in postmenopausal women. Both agents proved potent in vitro and in preliminary clinical trials for bone fracture prevention.[170–173]

Selective Estrogen Receptor Modulators as Risk-Reducing Agents for Breast Cancer Prevention

Efficacy. Table 33.8 summarizes the phase III data for SERM-based breast cancer–risk reduction. In a systematic review of MEDLINE and Cochrane databases through December, 2012, the USPSTF identified seven trials of tamoxifen or raloxifene that showed a reduced incidence of invasive breast cancer by 7 to 9 cases in 1,000 women over 5 years compared to placebo.[174] Tamoxifen is more effective than raloxifene; it reduces breast cancer incidence more than raloxifene by 5 cases in 1,000 women. Both drugs reduce the incidence of ER-positive breast cancer, but neither reduces the risk of ER-negative breast cancer. Neither drug reduced breast cancer–specific or all cause mortality rates. Based on benefit–risk models, women with estimated 5-year risks of breast cancer of 3% or greater are likely to benefit from treatment.[175] Using similar

TABLE 33.8

Phase III, Randomized, Controlled Clinical Trials of SERMs for the Prevention of Breast Cancer

Study	Drug and Daily Dose	N =	Treatment Duration (Years)	Entry Criteria	Overall Outcome HR (95% CI)	References
NSABP P-1	Tamoxifen 20 mg Placebo	13,388	5	Gail model: 5 yr predicted risk of ≥1.66%	0.52 (0.42–0.64)	(28,287)
IBIS-I	Tamoxifen 20 mg Placebo	7,139	5	>Twofold relative risk	0.72 (0.58–0.90)	(288)
Marsden	Tamoxifen 20 mg Placebo	2,471	8	Family history	0.87 (0.63–1.21)	(289)
Italian	Tamoxifen 20 mg Placebo	5,408	5	Normal risk, hysterectomy	0.67 (0.59–0.76)	(290)
NSABP P-2 (STAR)	Raloxifene 60 mg Tamoxifen 20 mg	19,747	5	Gail model: 5 yr predicted risk of ≥1.66%	RR Raloxifene versus tamoxifen 1.02 (0.81–1.28)	(29)
MORE/CORE	Raloxifene 60 mg Placebo Raloxifene 120 mg Placebo	7,705 6,511	5	Normal risk, postmenopausal with osteoporosis	0.42 (0.29–0.60)	(291,292)
RUTH	Raloxifene 60 mg Placebo	10,101	5	Normal risk, postmenopausal with risk of coronary heart disease	0.67(0.47–0.96)	(179)
PEARL	Lasofoxifene 0.5 mg Lasofoxifene 0.25 mg Placebo	8,856	5	Normal risk, postmenopausal, with osteoporosis	0.25 mg: 0.82 (0.45–1.49) 0.5 mg: 0.21 (0.05–0.55)	(170)
GENERATIONS	Arzoxifene 20 mg Placebo	9,354	4	Normal risk, postmenopausal, with osteoporosis	0.42 (0.25–0.68)	(172)

Table and data adapted from Cuzick J, Sestak I, Bonanni B, et al. Selective oestrogen receptor modulators in prevention of breast cancer: an updated meta-analysis of individual participant data. *Lancet* 2013;381:1827–1834.

analysis methods as the USPSTF, the American Society of Clinical Oncology recommends the use of tamoxifen (20 mg per day orally for 5 years) or raloxifene (60 mg per day orally for 5 years) "in premenopausal women who are age ≥35 years with a 5-year projected absolute breast cancer risk ≥1.66% according to the NCI Breast Cancer Risk Assessment Tool (or equivalent measures), or with lobular carcinoma in situ."[176] Tamoxifen reduces the risk of in situ (preinvasive) breast neoplasms (lobular carcinoma in situ, ductal carcinoma in situ) by 50%.[177,178] The reduction during treatment persists for at least 5 years after treatment.[177,178] Raloxifene does not reduce the risk of in situ breast neoplasms.

Data from two trials designed to evaluate the safety and efficacy of lasofoxifene (PEARL)[170,171] and arzoxifene (GENERATIONS)[172,173] as bone fracture preventives have been analyzed for breast cancer–risk reduction. Their effect at reducing breast cancer incidence was captured in secondary analyses (see Table 33.8). Neither lasofoxifene nor arzoxifene have been evaluated in phase III randomized controlled breast cancer prevention trials. Arzoxifene development has been discontinued in the United States.

Toxicity Profiles. Tamoxifen causes a twofold increase in the risk of endometrial adenocarcinoma (RR, 2.13; 95% CI, 1.36 to 3.32) and is related to more benign gynecologic conditions, uterine bleeding, and surgical procedures than the placebo controls, whereas raloxifene did not increase the risk for endometrial cancer or uterine bleeding.[174] Tamoxifen causes a twofold increase in thromboembolic events (RR, 1.93; 95% CI, 1.41 to 2.64), whereas raloxifene causes a 60% increase in risk of venous thromboembolism (RR, 1.60; 95% CI, 1.15 to 2.23).[174] Raloxifene does not differ from tamoxifen in risk of fractures, other cancers, or cardiovascular events.[177] Raloxifene's lower risk of endometrial adenocarcinomas compared to tamoxifen needs to be weighed against the increased risk of stroke seen in in the MORE/CORE trials (see Table 33.8).[179] Raloxifene's effectiveness in the community may also be compromised by its poor bioavailability (2%) due to rapid phase II enzyme metabolism in the gut and liver,[180] whereas tamoxifen is more bioavailable and has active metabolites that permit a prolonged drug effect. Missed raloxifene doses may potentially compromise efficacy and prevention outcomes in widespread, community use.

Aromatase Inhibitors. In adjuvant clinical trials for breast cancer, aromatase inhibitors (anastrozole, exemestane, letrozole) given after 5 years of tamoxifen enhance the reduction of breast cancer recurrence in the contralateral breast compared to tamoxifen alone.[181] In a phase I cancer risk–reducing agent trial, letrozole reduced the Ki-67 proliferation index of breast epithelial cells aspirated from high-risk women.[182] Exemestane reduced the overall risk of ER-positive invasive breast cancer (Table 33.9). It did not reduce the risk of noninvasive breast neoplasms or ER-negative breast cancer.[183] Exemestane has no increased risk of venous thromboembolism, endometrial cancer, fracture, or cataract,[183] but losses in bone mineral density and cortical thickness of the distal tibia and radius occurred after 2 years of treatment despite calcium and vitamin D supplementation.[184] The results of the International Breast Cancer Intervention Study II (IBIS-II), comparing anastrozole with placebo, are similar to those reported for exemestane.[185] Compared to exemestane, anastrozole decreases the incidence of ductal carcinoma in situ (DCIS), whereas exemestane does not. Neither aromatase inhibitor increased survival compared to placebo controls. The American Society of Clinical Oncology recommends exemestane for breast cancer prevention in addition to tamoxifen and raloxifene.

Use Counseling. Despite the widespread evidence of breast cancer preventive efficacy for tamoxifen and raloxifene, only 3% to 20% of eligible high-risk women agree to take tamoxifen for primary prevention.[186] The low willingness of eligible women to take tamoxifen for 5 years demonstrates the issue of risk benefit for cancer risk–reducing agents. Women with high short-term risk (5 year Gail risk of >3%)—for example, those with ER-positive atypical hyperplasia, lobular carcinoma in situ, and the majority of non–high-grade ductal carcinoma in situ lesions—have an acceptable risk to benefit ratio and are the most likely to benefit from a 5-year cancer risk–reducing agent intervention with a SERM.[175,176] The toxicity profile of aromatase inhibitors differs from SERMs. Although aromatase inhibitors may have a more favorable risk to benefit profile than SERMs, long-term outcomes and toxicity experience for aromatase inhibitor risk-reducing agent intervention are not available to date. In the National Surgical Adjuvant Breast and Bowel Project, tamoxifen-treated women with a *BRCA2* mutation but not a *BRCA1* mutation had reduced cancer incidence,[187] but subsequent data from another group have found reduced cancer risk in women with both BRCA mutations.[188] Data remain insufficient to recommend the use of SERMs for risk reduction in women with BRCA mutations.

5α-Steroid Reductase Inhibitors

Mechanism

Prostate cancers require androgens to proliferate and evade apoptosis. The primary nuclear androgen responsible for the maintenance of epithelial function is dihydrotestosterone. The testes and adrenal gland synthesize dihydrotestosterone by the conversion of testosterone by 5α-steroid reductase types 1 and 2 isozymes. Dihydrotestosterone binds to intracellular androgen receptors to form a complex that binds to DNA hormone response elements controlling cellular proliferation and apoptosis. Finasteride, a selective, competitive inhibitor of type 2 5α-steroid reductase,[189] inhibits proliferation in the transformed prostate cell. In the 3,2′-dimethyl-4-aminobiphenyl (DMAB), methylnitrosourea (MNU), and testosterone chemical carcinogenesis models in rats, finasteride reduces prostate tumor incidence by close to six-fold. Finasteride appears to be more effective in the promotion phase of prostate carcinogenesis.[190] Dutasteride inhibits both 5α-steroid reductase inhibitor[190] types 1 and 2 isoforms and has similar anticarcinogenesis activity in preclinical models to finasteride.

TABLE 33.9

Phase III, Randomized, Controlled Clinical Trials of Aromatase Inhibitors for the Prevention of Breast Cancer

Study	Drug and Daily Dose	N =	Treatment Duration (Years)	Entry Criteria	Overall Outcome HR (95% CI)	References
MAP.3	Exemestane 25 mg Placebo	4,560	5	Gail model 5 yr predicted risk of ≥2.3%	0.35 (0.18–0.70)	(183)
IBIS-II	Anastrozole 1 mg Placebo	3,851	5	RR twofold higher than general population or Tyrer-Cuzick 10-yr risk >5%	0.47 (0.32–0.68)	(185)

TABLE 33.10

Phase III, Randomized, Controlled Clinical Trials of 5α-Steroid Reductase Inhibitors for the Prevention of Prostate Cancer

Study	Drug and Daily Dose	N =	Treatment Duration (Years)	Entry Criteria	Overall Outcome HR (95% CI)	References
PCPT	Finasteride 5 mg Placebo	18,880	7	Age ≥55 y, PSA ≤3 ng/mL	0.70 (0.65–0.76)	(30, 193)
REDUCE	Dutaseride 0.5 mg Placebo	6,729	4	Age 50–75 y, PSA 2.5–10.0 ng/mL, core biopsies within 6 mos	RR = 0.77 (0.70–0.85)	(192)

PSA, prostate specific antigen.

Cancer Risk–Reducing Agent Activity

Randomized, placebo-controlled cancer incidence end point risk-reducing agent clinical trials demonstrated that finasteride and dutasteride reduced the incidence of prostate cancer by approximately 22% (Table 33.10).[30,191,192] Patients who are treated with either drug yet progress to transformed neoplasms develop more tumors of a high Gleason grade (7 to 10) compared to the placebo arm (22%). After 18 years of follow-up, no significant differences in overall survival or survival after prostate cancer diagnosis were found in the finasteride-treated group compared to the placebo-treated group.[193] Sexual function side effects (e.g., erectile dysfunction, loss of libido, gynecomastia) were more common in the finasteride- or dutasteride-treated groups.[30,192]

The 5α-steroid reductase inhibitors, finasteride and dutasteride, prevent or delay carcinogenesis progression in the prostate, yet progression of high-grade lesions is unaffected. Use of finasteride for a period of 7 years reduced the incidence of prostate cancer but did not significantly affect mortality.[193] Increasing the diagnosis of low-grade prostate cancer through prostate-specific antigen (PSA) testing or intervention with a drug with a minimal toxicity profile without reducing mortality is of no benefit and "all forms of therapy cause considerable burden to the patient and to society."[193]

SIGNAL TRANSDUCTION MODIFIERS

Both cancer therapy and cancer prevention have investigated drugs that modify specific targets in signal transduction pathways. Although the emphasis in drug development has focused on cancer treatment, interventions aimed at modulating signal transduction pathways promise new approaches to interventions in the carcinogenic process. Because of the complexity of signaling systems, the inhibition of single targets may not be effective or may cause unacceptable toxicity.

Difluoromethylornithine

Mechanism

Polyamines (spermidine, spermine, and the diamine, putrescine) are required to maintain cellular growth and function.[194] In mammalian cells, polyamine inhibition by genetic mutation or pharmaceutical agents is associated with virtual cessation in cellular growth. Difluoromethylornithine (DFMO) is an enzyme-activated irreversible inhibitor of ornithine decarboxylase (which is transactivated by the *c-MYC* oncogene and cooperates with the *RAS* oncogene in malignant transformation).[195]

Evidence in Preclinical In Vivo Carcinogenesis Models

Extensive preclinical data has found that DFMO prevents tumor promotion in a variety of systems, including skin, mammary, colon, cervical, and bladder carcinogenesis models.[194] Synergistic or additive activity with retinoids, butylated hydroxyanisole, tamoxifen, piroxicam, and fish oil has been demonstrated with low concentrations of DFMO.[194]

Clinical Trials

In phase I prevention trials, DFMO at a dose of 0.5 mg/m^2 per day reduced tissue polyamines in the colon and skin[196,197] and causes regression of cervical intraepithelial neoplasia when used topically,[198] but does not reduce tissue polyamines or other biomarkers of cellular proliferation in the human breast.[199] As a single agent, DFMO has anticarcinogenic activity for nonmelanoma skin cancers, primarily basal cell carcinoma. In combination with an NSAID (sulindac), DFMO reduced adenoma recurrences, suggesting a synergistic reduction of colorectal cancer risk (Table 33.11). Preliminary data suggest some cancer risk–reducing agent activity for the lower esophagus and the prostate (see Table 33.11).[200]

Statins

Mechanism

Statins are hydroxyl-3-methylglutaryl coenzyme A (HMG-CoA) reductase inhibitors that inhibit the conversion of HMG-CoA to mevalonate, a cholesterol precursor. The statins are a class of medications with similar structures but with variable moieties that can result in hydrophilic forms (e.g., pravastatin, rosuvastatin) and lipophilic forms (e.g., lovastatin, simvastatin, fluvastatin, atorvastatin).[201] Statins decrease the risk of cancer in preclinical studies by inhibiting *RAS*- and *RHO*-mediated cell proliferation, upregulating cell cycle inhibitors (e.g., p21 and p27), and inducing apoptosis of transformed cells and the inhibition of angiogenesis.[202]

Evidence in Preclinical In Vivo Carcinogenesis Models

Lipophilic statins delay progression of pancreatic intraepithelial neoplasias and the growth of pancreatic carcinoma xenografts. Atorvastatin alone and in combination with NSAIDs reduced colonic adenoma and adenocarcinoma incidence and multiplicity by half in rodent transgenic and chemical carcinogenesis models. Lovastatin reduced lung adenoma multiplicity but not incidence.[201]

Clinical Trials

Although several large trials of pravastatin or simvastatin on cardiovascular disease risk with cancer as secondary end points have shown no benefit for reducing cancer risk with follow-ups between 18 months to 4 years, these trials were not adequately powered to examine cancer end points.[201] Several case control studies evaluating statin effects have shown a significant association with lower risk of colorectal adenocarcinoma with odds ratios ranging from 0.53 to 0.91 for arzoxifene. A secondary analysis of a celecoxib prevention trial demonstrated no statin protection against colorectal

TABLE 33.11

Summary of Clinical Trials of Difluoromethylornithine as a Cancer Risk–Reducing Agent

Population	Dose per Day, Duration	Phase	Endpoint	Outcome	References
Low risk bladder cancer (Ta. T1. Grades 1 or 2)	1 gm versus placebo × 1 year	III	Bladder cancer recurrence	Did not prevent or delay recurrence	(293)
Prostate risk: men with family history prostate cancer, age 35–70 yr	500 mg versus placebo × 1 yr	IIb	Prostate volume, polyamines, PSA	10-fold reduction of prostate size increase over 1 yr compared to placebo, PSA reduction not significant	(294)
Nonmelanoma skin cancer	500 mg/m^2 versus placebo × 4–5 y	III	New nonmelanoma skin cancers	Lower rate of basal cell carcinomas per year (0.28 versus 0.40); persistent reduction in nonmelanoma skin cancers, not statistically significant	(295, 296)
Colon adenomas	DFMO: 500 mg Sulindac: 150 mg versus placebo × 3 y	IIb	Adenoma recurrence	RR for adenoma recurrence for DFMO/sulindac treatment 5 0.30 (0.18–0.49)	(147)

PSA, prostate specific antigen.

neoplasms.[203] The Women's Health Initiative (prospective longitudinal cohort of 159,319 women) found that lovastatin was associated with a lower risk of developing colorectal cancer (HR = 0.62; 95% CI, 0.39 to 0.99).[204] Prospective longitudinal studies have shown mixed results. The PHS reported statin use was inversely associated with prostate cancer (adjusted RR, 0.51),[205] whereas the Nurse's Health Study showed no association with risk of breast cancer.[206] Interventional trials to determine statin preventive efficacy for colon and breast cancer are ongoing.[201] Statins may be effective risk-reducing agents in individuals with the A/A variant of the predominant T/T genotype of rs12654264 of the HMG-CoA reductase gene.[207]

Bisphosphonates

Mechanism

Bisphosphonates are pyrophosphate analogs with a central phosphorus-carbon-phosphorus bond that resists bone degradation preventing bone loss and fractures. Second- and third-generation amino bisphosphonates (pamidronic, alendronic, risedronic, ibandronic, and zoledronic acids) inhibit farnesyl diphosphate synthase downstream of HMG-CoA reductase, leading to decreased post-translational prenylation of GTP-binding proteins such as RAS and Rho. Amino bisphosphonates inhibit cell proliferation, angiogenesis, and cell cycle arrest while inducing apoptosis.[201]

Evidence in In Vivo Preclinical and Clinical Models

HER2-transgenic mice treated with zoledronic acid had increased tumor-free survival and overall survival. Zoledronic acid suppressed bone, lung, and liver metastases when treated prior to an injection of breast cancer cells.[201] The short-term use of bisphosphonates is associated with reduced breast cancer incidence in case control studies[208,209] and prospective cohort studies (HR = 0.68; 95% CI, 0.52 to 0.88 in a prospective cohort study).[210] Randomized trials of amino-bisphosphonates in postmenopausal women with breast cancer treated for 1 year have found a reduction of breast cancer risk in the contralateral breast (HR = 0.39; 95% CI, 0.18 to 0.88).[211] Case control data suggesting a bisphosphonate-associated reduction in colorectal cancer risk have not been confirmed by prospective cohort studies (i.e., Women's Health Initiative, Nurse's Health Study).[201]

Metformin

Mechanism

Metformin, an oral antidiabetic drug in the biguanide class, is the first-line drug of choice for the treatment of type 2 diabetes.[212] Cancers are more common in diabetics and obese individuals than their normal weight and normoglycemic counterparts, leading to the hypothesis that elevated serum insulin concentrations promote cancer risk.[213,214] Insulin and insulin-like growth factors (IGF1 and 2) stimulate cellular DNA synthesis, proliferation, and tumor growth through phosphoinositide-3 kinase (PI3K), mammalian target of rapamycin (mTOR), and the RAS-MAPK signaling pathways.[213] Metformin activates the adenosine monophosphate-activated protein kinase (AMPK) via LKB1, a protein-threonine kinase that has tumor-suppressor activity.[201] Metformin anticarcinogenesis activity appears to be broad and includes downregulation of erbB-2 and epidermal growth factor receptor (EGFR) expression, inhibiting the phosphorylation of erbB family members, IGF1R, Akt, mTOR, and STAT3 in vivo. Low doses of metformin inhibit the self-renewal/proliferation of cancer stem cells in breast, colon, and pancreatic models.[215,216]

Evidence in Preclinical In Vivo Carcinogenesis Models

Metformin reduces tobacco carcinogen–induced tumors in mice, and pancreatic premalignant and malignant tumors in hamsters.[201] However, metformin's anticarcinogenic activity appears dependent on the dose and the induced carcinogenesis process. Metformin promoted carcinogenesis in MNU-induced rat breast cancers, MMTV-Neu ER-negative breast cancers, OH-BBN induced bladder cancer, and Min$^+$ mouse intestinal tumors using nonobese rodents.[217] Metformin cancer risk–reducing agent effects may be limited to obesity- and diabetes-associated carcinogenesis mechanisms.

Clinical Trials

Two large retrospective cohort studies have shown that metformin therapy is associated with a reduced risk of solid tumors by 25% to 30%.[201] The Women's Health Imitative observed a lower incidence of invasive breast cancer in metformin-treated women with type 2 diabetes mellitus.[218] Phase II window of opportunity randomized trials have shown reduced proliferation and increased apoptosis in resected tissue of breast cancer patients.[201]

Diet-Derived Natural Products

Mechanism

Polyphenolic phytochemicals, such as curcumin, resveratrol, epigallocatechin gallate (EGCG), genistein, and ginger, are attractive as cancer risk–reducing agents for their low toxicity and multimechanism anticarcinogenic properties. They have anti-inflammatory activity, in part through scavenging of ROS, modulation of protein kinase signal transduction pathways (e.g., STAT-3, HER2/neu, MAPK, and Akt), and downstream inhibition of eicosanoid synthesis potentially due to upstream inhibition of NF-κB and PPAR or direct blockade or inhibition of eicosanoid-metabolizing enzymes.[219–221] Curcumin, and presumably other polyphenolics, downregulate stem cell driver signaling systems Wnt, Hedgehog, and Notch with subsequent reductions of breast, pancreatic, and colonic stem cell self-renewal.[222,223]

Omega-3 fatty acids (derived from marine products) compete with omega-6 fatty acid substrates for eicosanoid-metabolizing enzymes with subsequent tissue reduction of these inflammatory mediators.[224,225] These fatty acids have other diverse anticarcinogenic mechanisms (e.g., G-protein inhibition, changes in membrane physical characteristics that alter transmembrane signaling protein dynamics) that make them attractive as cancer risk–reducing agents.[226,227]

Whole berries, black raspberries, and strawberries contain mixtures of multiple anticarcinogenic compounds such as ellagic acid, anthocyanins, and tocopherols.[228] Research-grade berries are grown in a standardized cultivation environment and assayed for key components to ensure year-to-year reproducibility despite yearly climatologic variation. Berries have potent stabilization of methylation properties in addition to the expected anti-inflammatory and antioxidative properties associated with the prominent components.[229,230]

Preclinical and Clinical Anticarcinogenesis Efficacy. Diverse diet-derived natural products have moderate-to-strong anticarcinogenic effects in both chemical and transgenic rodent carcinogenesis models (Table 33.12). Phase I clinical trials of curcumin detected little parent compound in plasma or tissues, raising the possibility of biologically active conjugates or deconjugation at the target site.[231–233] Resveratrol's plasma bioavailability exceeds that of curcumin and ginger, and partitions into human colon tissue at 10-fold concentrations compared to plasma.[219,234,235] No natural products have been studied in large prospective, cancer incidence risk–reduction trials. Using intraepithelial biomarker end points in human phase II trials, berry formulations reduce esophageal dysplasia and oral leukoplakia.[236,237] Curcumin reduces the number of colon aberrant crypt foci in human smokers.[238]

ANTI-INFECTIVES

Many infectious agents are known causes of human cancers, including the human hepatitis viruses, hepatitis B virus (HBV) and hepatitis C virus (HCV) for hepatocellular carcinoma[239]; *Helicobacter pylori* for gastric adenocarcinoma[240]; human papilloma viruses (HPV) for cervical, anal, vulva, penis, and oral cavity and pharynx carcinomas[241]; herpes virus-8 for Kaposi sarcoma[242]; Epstein-Barr virus for Burkitt and other lymphomas[243]; liver flukes for cholangiocarcinoma[244]; and schistosomes for bladder carcinoma.[245] The success of the HPV vaccine at reducing the incidence of intraepithelial neoplasia of the cervix is one example that demonstrates the potential of immunochemoprevention for epithelial targets for which an etio logic agent can be identified.

Helicobacter pylori

Intestinal-type gastric adenocarcinoma arises through a multistep process that begins with chronic gastritis initiated by *H. pylori*, progressing through gastric mucosal atrophy, intestinal metaplasia to dysplasia, and ultimately, to adenocarcinoma.[246] *H. pylori* infects 50% of the world's population.[240] Infection occurs early in life, remains quiescent, and may be associated with chronic gastritis of variable intensity but with minimal symptoms. Although the majority of *H. pylori* organisms remain in the gastric mucous layer, 10% adhere to the gastric mucosa through adhesion *BabA*, an outer membrane protein that binds to the Lewis-B histo-blood group antigen.[240] Progression to atrophic gastritis and peptic ulcer disease (occurs in 10% to 15% of infected individuals) requires other bacterial and host cofactors.[245,246] Infection with *H. pylori* is associated with an OR of 2.7 to 6.0 for gastric cancer; *CagA* increases this risk by 20- to 40-fold. The risk of developing gastric adenocarcinoma with an *H. pylori* infection is estimated to be 1% to 3%.[245,246]

The eradication of *H. pylori* with antibiotics and anti-inflammatory agents—for example, amoxicillin, metronidazole, and bismuth subsalicylate—increases the rate of regression of nonmetaplastic gastric atrophy and intestinal metaplasia in geographically diverse regions.[247,248] A combination of a 2-week course of a proton pump inhibitor (omeprazole) and an antibiotic (amoxicillin) reduced the risk of gastric cancer in a high-risk population in China (OR = 0.61; (95% CI, 0.36 to 0.96) for 14.7 years after the treatment.[249] The sequence of giving proton pump inhibitors and antibiotic therapy does not alter the treatment outcome. In addition to contributing to gastric cancer risk, *H. pylori* infections may also contribute to pancreatic cancer risk.[250] Because *H. pylori* infections are so widespread, mass eradication campaigns in high-risk regions are being considered.[251] However, complicating this is that *H. pylori* infections have also been associated with a reduced risk of both esophageal adenocarcinoma and gastric cardia carcinoma.[252]

MULTIAGENT APPROACHES TO CANCER RISK REDUCTION

In the transition to molecularly targeted interventions, combinations of targets that logically address critical carcinogenic pathways may have greater efficacy than single agents. For example, previously demonstrated interactive signaling of EGFRs and COX-2 experiments in Min^+ mice[253] demonstrates cancer preventive synergism. Combining atorvastatin with selective or nonselective COX inhibitors enhanced the inhibition of azoxymethane-induced colon carcinogenesis in F344 rats and reduced the dose of the combined drugs required to achieve a reduction of colon carcinogenesis.[254]

DFMO plus sulindac inhibited adenoma formation in a phase IIb trial of 375 patients with a prior history of adenomas followed for 36 months (see Table 33.11).[147] Cardiovascular-adverse outcomes were higher in DFMO/sulindac-treated patients who had preexisting high baseline cardiovascular risk; however, the cardiovascular-adverse events were similar to placebo in moderate or low cardiovascular risk patients.[255] Using IGF-1 as a biomarker, Guerrieri-Gonzaga et al.[256] showed that the combination of low-dose tamoxifen with low-dose fenretinide is safe but not synergistic. As more data accumulate from in vivo models, combined drugs aimed at specific targets in coordinated signaling pathways will enter clinical biomarker-based trials. Optimal doses, toxicity, and biomarker modulation data will select those combinations useful for risk reduction trials and, ultimately, generalized use in at-risk populations.

TABLE 33.12

Selected Diet-Derived Natural Products with Cancer Risk–Reducing Activity

Nutritional Extract	Source	Mechanisms	In Vivo Anticarcinogenesis Efficacy	Human Trials	References
Curcumin ([1E,6E]-1,7-bis-[4-hydroxy-3-methoxyphenyl]-1,6-heptadiene-3,5-dione/ diferuloylmethane)	Turmeric, rhizome of *Curcuma longa*	Inhibits: PGE_2 synthesis via direct binding to COX-2 and through inhibition of NF-κB; angiogenesis. ErbB2 transduction; PI3K-Akt transduction; Inhibits stem cell self renewal Agonist: vitamin D receptor	Colon, breast, skin	Phase I: Poor bioavailability due to biotransformation in gut, enterohepatic cycling of metabolites; Phase IIa: reduced aberrant crypt foci	(219, 238)
Resveratrol (3,5,4′-trihydroxy-trans-stilbene)	Grapes, mulberries, peanuts, and *Cassia quinquangulata* plants	Inhibits: Carcinogen activation via inhibition of phase I isozyme, eicosanoids via direct binding; NF-κB; Nrf2. Acts as a caloric restriction mimetic, activates the histone deacetylase SIRT1 and AMPK	Colorectal, breast, pancreas, skin, and prostate	Phase I: 1 g dose generated peak concentration ~2 μM, conjugates 10-fold higher; resveratrol tissue concentrations 10-fold higher than plasma; Phase IIa: Small reduction in IGF-1 and IGFBP-1	(220, 234)
Ginger (gingerols, paradols, shagaols)	Rhizome of *Zingiber officinale*	Induces apoptosis via caspase-3 mechanisms; Inhibits NF-κB activation and downstream COX-2 expression; reduces iNOS expression and ornithine decarboxylase activity	Colon, breast, skin, oral cavity, liver	Phase I: 2 g dose nontoxic; Phase IIa: Small reductions in PGE_2, increased Bax in upper colon crypt	(235, 297, 298)
Green tea (epigallocatechin gallate, other catechins)	Green tea extract	Inhibits: PI3K-Akt transduction, IGF-1, IGFBP-3; NK-κB; catenin reduces methylation via inhibition of DNA methyltransferase 1	Lung, prostate, skin, colorectal	Phase IIa: 500–1,000 mg/m^2 × 12 wk reduced oral premalignant lesions in 50%; Phase IIb: 2.5 g × 1 yr reduced colorectal adenoma recurrence by 50%	(221)
Omega-3 fatty acids (eicosapentaenoic acid; docosahexaenoic acid)	Fish oil	Reduction of inflammation via eicosanoid reduction; direct binding to G receptor proteins; PPAR activation; induction of anti-inflammatory lipid mediators (resolvins, protectins, maresins)	Colon, breast, prostate	Phase II: 4–7 mg/d reduced colon adenomas in familial adenomatous polyposis; ongoing trials for sporadic; extensive case control studies	(226, 299)
Berries	Black raspberries, strawberries	Reduction of methylation via inhibition of methyltransferases, re-regulated Wnt; inhibits NF-κB; inhibits cyclooxygenases; inhibits proliferation	Esophageal squamous cell, colon, skin	Phase IIb: Freeze dried strawberries reduced esophageal dysplasia; Phase IIa: Blackberry gel reduced leukoplakia	(228, 229, 236, 237)

IGFBP-1, insulin growth factor binding protein-1; iNOS, inducible isoform of nitric oxide synthase.

REFERENCES

1. Vogelstein B, Papadopoulos N, Velculescu VE, et al. Cancer genome landscapes. *Science* 2013;339:1546–1558.
2. Fearon ER, Vogelstein B. A genetic model for colorectal tumorigenesis. *Cell* 1990;61:759–767.
3. Sidransky D. Emerging molecular markers of cancer. *Nat Rev Cancer* 2002; 2:210–219.
4. Lippman SM, Levin B, Brenner DE, et al. Cancer prevention and the American Society of Clinical Oncology. *J Clin Oncol* 2004;22:3848–3851.
5. Wattenberg L. Chemoprevention of cancer. *Cancer Res* 1985;45:1–8.
6. Greenwald P, Kelloff G. The role of chemoprevention in cancer control. *IARC Scientific Publications (Lyon)* 1996;139:13–22.
7. Hanahan D, Weinberg RA. The hallmarks of cancer. *Cell* 2000;100:57–70.
8. Steele VE, Boone CW, Lubet RA, et al. Preclinical drug development paradigms for chemopreventives. *Hematol Oncol Clin North Am* 1998;12:943–961.
9. Perloff M, Steele VE. Early-phase development of cancer prevention agents: challenges and opportunities. *Cancer Prev Res (Phila)* 2013;6:379–383.
10. National Cancer Institute. PREVENT Cancer Preclinical Drug Development Program. National Cancer Institute Web site. http://prevention.cancer.gov/programs-resources/programs/prevent. Accessed December 7, 2013.
11. Mehta RG, Naithani R, Huma L, et al. Efficacy of chemopreventive agents in mouse mammary gland organ culture (MMOC) model: a comprehensive review. *Curr Med Chem*. 2008;15:2785–2825.
12. Hoenerhoff MJ, Hong HH, Ton TV, et al. A review of the molecular mechanisms of chemically induced neoplasia in rat and mouse models in National Toxicology Program bioassays and their relevance to human cancer. *Toxicol Pathol* 2009;37:835–848.
13. Steele VE, Lubet RA. The use of animal models for cancer chemoprevention drug development. *Semin Oncol* 2010;37:327–338.
14. Shureiqi I, Reddy P, Brenner DE. Chemoprevention: general perspective. *Crit Rev Oncol Hematol* 2000;33:157–167.
15. Becker M. Adherence to prescribed therapies. *Med Care* 1985;23:539–554.
16. Miki Y, Swensen J, Shattuck-Eidens D, et al. A strong candidate for the breast and ovarian cancer susceptibility gene BRCA1. *Science* 1994;266:66–71.
17. Powell SM, Petersen GM, Krush AJ, et al. Molecular diagnosis of familial adenomatous polyposis. *N Engl J Med* 1993;329:1982–1987.
18. Meads C, Ahmed I, Riley RD. A systematic review of breast cancer incidence risk prediction models with meta-analysis of their performance. *Breast Cancer Res Treat* 2012;132:365–377.
19. Kastrinos F, Steyerberg EW, Balmana J, et al. Comparison of the clinical prediction model PREMM(1,2,6) and molecular testing for the systematic identification of Lynch syndrome in colorectal cancer. *Gut* 2013;62:272–279.
20. Ankerst DP, Boeck A, Freedland SJ, et al. Evaluating the PCPT risk calculator in ten international biopsy cohorts: results from the Prostate Biopsy Collaborative Group. *World J Urol* 2012;30:181–187.
21. National Institutes of Health, U.S. Food and Drug Administration. *Biomarkers and Surrogate Endpoints: Advancing Clinical Research and Applications*. Bethesda, MD: National Insitutes of Health; 1999.
22. Schatzkin A, Freedman LS, Schiffman MH, et al. Validation of intermediate end points in cancer research. *J Natl Cancer Inst* 1990;82:1746–1752.
23. Prentice R. Surrogate endpoints in clinical trials: definition and operational criteria. *Statistics Med* 1989;8:431–440.
24. Ransohoff DF. Rules of evidence for cancer molecular-marker discovery and validation. *Nat Rev Cancer* 2004;4:309–314.
25. Pepe MS, Feng Z, Janes H, et al. Pivotal evaluation of the accuracy of a biomarker used for classification or prediction: standards for study design. *J Natl Cancer Inst* 2008;100:1432–1438.
26. Pryor WA, Stahl W, Rock CL. Beta carotene: from biochemistry to clinical trials. *Nutr Rev* 2000;58:39–53.
27. Brenner DE, Hawk E. Trials and tribulations of interrogating biomarkers to define efficacy of cancer risk reductive interventions. *Cancer Prev Res (Phila)* 2013;6:71–73.
28. Fisher B, Costantino J, Wickerham D, et al. Tamoxifen for prevention of breast cancer: report of the National Surgical Adjuvant Breast and Bowel Project P-1 study. *J Natl Cancer Inst* 1998;90:1371–1388.
29. Vogel VG, Costantino JP, Wickerham DL, et al. Update of the National Surgical Adjuvant Breast and Bowel Project Study of Tamoxifen and Raloxifene (STAR) P-2 Trial: Preventing breast cancer. *Cancer Prev Res (Phila)* 2010;3:696–706.
30. Thompson IM, Goodman PJ, Tangen CM, et al. The influence of finasteride on the development of prostate cancer. *N Engl J Med* 2003;349:215–224.
31. Omenn G, Goodman G, Thornquist M, et al. Effects of a combination of beta carotene and vitamin A on lung cancer and cardiovascular disease. *N Engl J Med* 1996;334:1150–1155.
32. Lotan R. Retinoids in cancer chemoprevention. *Faseb J* 1996;10:1031–1039.
33. Tang X-H, Gudas LJ. Retinoids, retinoic acid receptors, and cancer. *Annu Rev Pathol* 2011;6:345–364.
34. Khachik F, Beecher, G, Smith JC Jr. Lutein, lycopene, and their oxidative metabolites in chemoprevention of cancer. *J Cell Biochem* 1995;22:236–246.
35. Di Mascio P, Kaiser S, Sies H. Lycopene as the most efficient biological carotenoid singlet oxygen quencher. *Arch Biochem Biophys* 1989;274:532–538.
36. Eroglu A, Hruszkewycz DP, dela Sena C, et al. Naturally occurring eccentric cleavage products of provitamin A beta-carotene function as antagonists of retinoic acid receptors. *J Biol Chem* 2012;287:15886–15895.
37. Ford NA, Erdman JW Jr. Are lycopene metabolites metabolically active? *Acta Biochim Pol* 2012;59:1–4.
38. World Cancer Research Fund, American Institute for Cancer Research. *Food, Nutrition, Physical Activity, and the Prevention of Cancer: A Global Perspective*. Washington, DC: AICR; 2007.
39. Panel on Dietary Antioxidants and Related Compounds, Subcommittees on Upper Reference Levels of Nutrients and Interpretation and Uses of DRIs, Standing Committee on the Scientific Evaluation of Dietary Reference Intakes, Food and Nutrition Board, Institute of Medicine. *Dietary Reference Intakes for Vitamin C, Vitamin E, Selenium, and Carotenoids*. Washington, DC: National Academy Press; 2000.
40. Moon RC, Mehta RG, Rao KVN. Retinoids and cancer in experimental animals. In: Sporn MB, Roberts AB, Goodman DS, eds., *The Retinoids*. 2nd ed. New York: Raven Press; 1994: 573–595.
41. International Agency for Research on Cancer World Health Organization. *Carotenoids*. Lyon: International Agency for Research on Cancer; 1998.
42. Holzapfel NP, Holzapfel BM, Champ S, et al. The potential role of lycopene for the prevention and therapy of prostate cancer: from molecular mechanisms to clinical evidence. *Int J Mol Sci* 2013;14:14620–14646.
43. Hong WK, Lippman SM, Itri LM, et al. Prevention of second primary tumors with 13cRA in squamous-cell carcinoma of the head and neck. *N Engl J Med* 1990;323:795–801.
44. Benner SE, Pajak TF, Lippman SM, et al. Prevention of second primary tumors with isotretinoin in patients with squamous cell carcinoma of the head and neck: long term follow-up. *J Natl Cancer Inst* 1994;86:140–141.
45. Khuri FR, Lee JJ, Lippman SM, et al. Randomized phase III trial of low-dose isotretinoin for prevention of second primary tumors in stage I and II head and neck cancer patients. *J Natl Cancer Inst* 2006;98:441–450.
46. Bolla M, Lefur R, Ton Van J, et al. Prevention of second primary tumours with etretinate in squamous cell carcinoma of the oral cavity and oropharynx. Results of a multicentric double-blind randomised study. *Eur J Cancer* 1994;30A: 767–772.
47. Toma S, Bonelli L, Sartoris A, et al. beta-carotene supplementation in patients radically treated for stage I-II head and neck cancer: results of a randomized trial. *Oncol Rep* 2003;10:1895–1901.
48. Mayne ST, Cartmel B, Baum M, et al. Randomized trial of supplemental beta-carotene to prevent second head and neck cancer. *Cancer Res* 2001;61:1457–1463.
49. Bairati I, Meyer F, Jobin E, et al. Antioxidant vitamins supplementation and mortality: a randomized trial in head and neck cancer patients. *Int J Cancer* 2006;119:2221–2224.
50. McLarty JW, Holiday DB, Girard WM, et al. Beta-carotene, vitamin A and lung cancer chemoprevention: results of an intermediate endpoint study. *Am J Clin Nutr* 1995;62:1431S–1438S.
51. Lee JS, Lippman SM, Benner SE, et al. Randomized placebo-controlled trial of isotretinoin in chemoprevention of bronchial squamous metaplasia. *J Clin Oncol* 1994;12:937–945.
52. The Alpha-Tocopherol Beta Carotene Cancer Prevention Study Group. The effect of vitamin E and beta carotene on the incidence of lung cancer and other cancers in male smokers. *N Engl J Med* 1994;330:1029–1035.
53. Omenn GS, Goodman G, Thornquist M, et al. Chemoprevention of lung cancer: the beta-Carotene and Retinol Efficacy Trial (CARET) in high-risk smokers and asbestos-exposed workers. *IARC Sci Publ* 1996;67–85.
54. Hennekens CH, Buring JE, Manson JE, et al. Lack of effect of long-term supplementation with beta carotene on the incidence of malignant neoplasms and cardiovascular disease. *N Engl J Med* 1996;334:1145–1149.
55. Lee IM, Cook NR, Manson JE, et al. Beta-carotene supplementation and incidence of cancer and cardiovascular disease: the Women's Health Study. *J Natl Cancer Inst* 1999;91:2102–2106.
56. Heart Protection Study Collaborative Group. MRC/BHF Heart Protection Study of antioxidant vitamin supplementation in 20,536 high-risk individuals: a randomised placebo-controlled trial. *Lancet* 2002;360:23–33.
57. van Zandwijk N, Dalesio O, Pastorino U, et al. EUROSCAN, a randomized trial of vitamin A and N-acetylcysteine in patients with head and neck cancer or lung cancer. For the European Organization for Research and Treatment of Cancer Head and Neck and Lung Cancer Cooperative Groups. *J Natl Cancer Inst* 2000;92:977–986.
58. Lippman SM, Lee JJ, Karp DD, et al. Randomized phase III intergroup trial of isotretinoin to prevent second primary tumors in stage I non-small-cell lung cancer. *J Natl Cancer Inst* 2001;93:605–618.
59. Mayne ST, Lippman SM. Cigarettes: a smoking gun in cancer chemoprevention. *J Natl Cancer Inst* 2005;97:1319–1321.
60. Veronesi U, De Palo G, Marubini E, et al. Randomized trial of fenretinide to prevent second breast malignancy in women with early breast cancer. *J Natl Cancer Inst* 1999;91:1847–1856.
61. De Palo G, Mariani L, Camerini T, et al. Effect of fenretinide on ovarian carcinoma occurrence. *Gynecol Oncol* 2002;86:24–27.
62. Uray IP, Brown PH. Chemoprevention of hormone receptor-negative breast cancer: new approaches needed. *Recent Results Cancer Res* 2011;188:147–162.
63. Kraemer KH, DiGiovanna JJ, Moshell AN, et al. Prevention of skin cancer in xeroderma pigmentosum with the use of oral isotretinoin. *N Engl J Med* 1988;318:1633–1637.
64. Bouwes Bavinck JN, Tieben LM, Van Der Woude FJ, et al. Prevention of skin cancer and reduction of keratotic skin lesions during acitretin therapy in renal

transplant recipients: a double-blind, placebo-controlled study. *J Clin Oncol* 1995;13:1933–1938.
65. Tangrea JA, Edwards BK, Taylor PR, et al. Long-term therapy with low-dose isotretinoin for prevention of basal cell carcinoma: a multicenter clinical trial Isotretinoin-Basal Cell Carcinoma Study Group. *J Natl Cancer Inst* 1992;84:328–332.
66. Levine N, Moon TE, Cartmel B, et al. Trial of retinol and isotretinoin in skin cancer prevention: a randomized, double-blind, controlled trial. Southwest Skin Cancer Prevention Study Group. *Cancer Epidemiol Biomarkers Prev* 1997;6:957–961.
67. Moon TE, Levine N, Cartmel B, et al. Effect of retinol in preventing squamous cell skin cancer in moderate-risk subjects: a randomized, double-blind, controlled trial. Southwest Skin Cancer Prevention Study Group. *Cancer Epidemiol Biomarkers Prev* 1997;6:949–956.
68. Greenberg ER, Baron JA, Stukel TA, et al. A clinical trial of beta carotene to prevent basal-cell and squamous-cell cancers of the skin. The Skin Cancer Prevention Study Group. *N Engl J Med* 1990;323:789–895.
69. Green A, Williams G, Neale R, et al. Daily sunscreen application and beta-carotene supplementation in prevention of basal-cell and squamous-cell carcinomas of the skin: a randomised controlled trial. *Lancet* 1999;354:723–729.
70. Clark LC, Combs GF Jr, Turnbull BW, et al. Effects of selenium supplementation for cancer prevention in patients with carcinoma of the skin. A randomized controlled trial. Nutritional Prevention of Cancer Study Group. *JAMA* 1996;276:1957–1963.
71. Duffield-Lillico AJ, Slate EH, Reid ME, et al. Nutritional Prevention of Cancer Study Group. Selenium supplementation and secondary prevention of nonmelanoma skin cancer in a randomized trial. *J Natl Cancer Inst* 2003;95:1477–1481.
72. Sabichi AL, Lerner SP, Atkinson EN, et al. Phase III prevention trial of fenretinide in patients with resected non-muscle-invasive bladder cancer. *Clin Cancer Res* 2008;14:224–229.
73. Lamm DL, Riggs DR, Shriver JS, et al. Megadose vitamins in bladder cancer: a double-blind clinical trial. *J Urol* 1994;151:21–26.
74. Meyskens FL Jr, Surwit E, Moon TE, et al. Enhancement of regression of cervical intraepithelial neoplasia II (moderate dysplasia) with topically applied all-trans-retinoic acid: a randomized trial. *J Natl Cancer Inst* 1994; 86:539–543.
75. Blot WJ, Li JY, Taylor PR, et al. Nutrition intervention trials in Linxian, China: supplementation with specific vitamin/mineral combinations, cancer incidence, and disease-specific mortality in the general population. *J Natl Cancer Inst* 1993;85:1483–1492.
76. Qiao YL, Dawsey SM, Kamangar F, et al. Total and cancer mortality after supplementation with vitamins and minerals: follow-up of the Linxian General Population Nutrition Intervention Trial. *J Natl Cancer Inst* 2009;101:507–518.
77. Mayne ST, Ferrucci LM, Cartmel B. Lessons learned from randomized clinical trials of micronutrient supplementation for cancer prevention. *Annu Rev Nutr* 2012;32:369–390.
78. Li JY, Taylor PR, Li B, et al. Nutrition intervention trials in Linxian, China: multiple vitamin/mineral supplementation, cancer incidence, and disease-specific mortality among adults with esophageal dysplasia. *J Natl Cancer Inst* 1993;85:1492–1498.
79. Kikendall JW, Mobarhan S, Nelson R, et al. Oral beta carotene does not reduce the recurrence of colorectal adenomas [Abstract]. *Am J Gastroenterol* 1991;36:1356.
80. MacLennan R, Macrae F, Bain C, et al. Randomized trial of intake of fat, fiber, and beta carotene to prevent colorectal adenomas. *J Natl Cancer Inst* 1995;87:1760–1766.
81. Greenberg ER, Baron JA, Tosteson TD, et al. A clinical trial of antioxidant vitamins to prevent colorectal adenoma. Polyp Prevention Study Group. *N Engl J Med* 1994;331:141–147.
82. Baron JA, Cole BF, Mott L, et al. Neoplastic and antineoplastic effects of beta-carotene on colorectal adenoma recurrence: results of a randomized trial. *J Natl Cancer Inst* 2003;95:717–722.
83. Heinonen OP, Albanes D, Virtamo J, et al. Prostate cancer and supplementation with alpha-tocopherol and beta-carotene: incidence and mortality in a controlled trial. *J Natl Cancer Inst* 1998;90:440–446.
84. Lippman SM, Klein EA, Goodman PJ, et al. Effect of selenium and vitamin E on risk of prostate cancer and other cancers: the Selenium and Vitamin E Cancer Prevention Trial (SELECT). *JAMA* 2009;301:39–51.
85. Klein EA, Thompson IM Jr, Tangen CM, et al. Vitamin E and the risk of prostate cancer: the Selenium and Vitamin E Cancer Prevention Trial (SELECT). *JAMA* 2011;306:1549–1556.
86. Gaziano JM, Glynn RJ, Christen WG, et al. Vitamins E and C in the prevention of prostate and total cancer in men: the Physicians' Health Study II randomized controlled trial. *JAMA* 2009;301:52–62.
87. Boileau TW, Liao Z, Kim S, et al. Prostate carcinogenesis in N-methyl-N-nitrosourea (NMU)-testosterone-treated rats fed tomato powder, lycopene, or energy-restricted diets. *J Natl Cancer Inst* 2003;95:1578–1586.
88. Goralczyk R. Beta-carotene and lung cancer in smokers: review of hypotheses and status of research. *Nutr Cancer* 2009;61:767–774.
89. Kristal AR, Darke AK, Morris JS, et al. Baseline Selenium Status and Effects of Selenium and Vitamin E Supplementation on Prostate Cancer Risk. *J Natl Cancer Inst* 2014:106:djt456.
90. Stone JR, Yang S. Hydrogen peroxide: a signaling messenger. *Antioxid Redox Signal* 2006;8:243–270.
91. Finkel T. Signal transduction by reactive oxygen species. *J Cell Biol* 2011; 194:7–15.
92. Sayin V, Ibrahim M, Larsson E, et al. Antioxidants accelerate lung cancer progression in mice. *Sci Transl Med* 2014;6:ra15.
93. Mayne ST. Oxidative stress, dietary antioxidant supplements, and health: is the glass half full or half empty? *Cancer Epidemiol Biomarkers Prev* 2013; 22:2145–2147.
94. Duthie SJ, Narayanan S, Blum S, et al. Folate deficiency in vitro induces uracil misincorporation and DNA hypomethylation and inhibits DNA excision repair in immortalized normal human colon epithelial cells. *Nutr Cancer* 2000;37:245–251.
95. Blount BC, Mack MM, Wehr CM, et al. Folate deficiency causes uracil misincorporation into human DNA and chromosome breakage: implications for cancer and neuronal damage. *Proc Natl Acad Sci U S A* 1997;94:3290–3295.
96. Giovannucci E. Epidemiologic studies of folate and colorectal neoplasia: a review. *J Nutr* 2002;132:2350S–2355S.
97. White E, Shannon JS, Patterson RE. Relationship between vitamin and calcium supplement use and colon cancer. *Cancer Epidemiol Biomarkers Prev* 1997;6:769–774.
98. Jacobs EJ, Connell CJ, Patel AV, et al. Multivitamin use and colon cancer mortality in the Cancer Prevention Study II cohort (United States). *Cancer Causes Control* 2001;12:927–934.
99. Gibson TM, Weinstein SJ, Pfeiffer RM, et al. Pre- and postfortification intake of folate and risk of colorectal cancer in a large prospective cohort study in the United States. *Am J Clin Nutr* 2011;94:1053–1062.
100. Chen J, Giovannucci E, Kelsey, K, et al. A methylenetetrahydrofolate reductase polymorphism and the risk of colorectal cancer. *Cancer Res* 1996;56:4862–4864.
101. Larsson S, Giovannucci, E, Wolk A. Vitamin B6 intake, alcohol consumption, and colorectal cancer: a longitudinal population-based cohort of women. *Gastroenterology* 2005;128:1830–1837.
102. Wei E, Giovannucci E, Selhub J, et al. Plasma vitamin B6 and the risk of colorectal cancer and adenoma in women. *J Natl Cancer Inst* 2005;97:684–692.
103. Giovannucci E, Rimm EB, Ascherio A, et al. Alcohol, low-methionine-low-folate diets, and risk of colon cancer in men. *J Natl Cancer Inst* 1995;87:265–273.
104. Jaszewski R, Misra S, Tobi M, et al. Folic acid supplementation inhibits recurrence of colorectal adenomas: a randomized chemoprevention trial. *World J Gastroenterol* 2008;14:4492–4498.
105. Paspatis GA, Karamanolis DG. Folate supplementation and adenomatous colonic polyps. *Dis Colon Rectum* 1994;37:1340–1341.
106. Cole BF, Baron JA, Sandler RS, et al. Folic acid for the prevention of colorectal adenomas: a randomized clinical trial. *JAMA* 2007;297:2351–2359.
107. Logan RF, Grainge MJ, Shepherd VC, et al. Aspirin and folic acid for the prevention of recurrent colorectal adenomas. *Gastroenterology* 2008;134:29–38.
108. Wu K, Platz EA, Willett WC, et al. A randomized trial on folic acid supplementation and risk of recurrent colorectal adenoma. *Am J Clin Nutr* 2009;90: 1623–1631.
109. Gao Q-Y, Chen H-M, Chen Y-X, et al. Folic acid prevents the initial occurrence of sporadic colorectal adenoma in Chinese older than 50 years of age: a randomized clinical trial. *Cancer prevention research (Phila)* 2013;6:744–752.
110. Ramnath N, Kim S, Christensen PJ. Vitamin D and lung cancer. *Expert Rev Respir Med* 2011;5:305–309.
111. Deeb KK, Trump DL, Johnson CS. Vitamin D signalling pathways in cancer: potential for anticancer therapeutics. *Nat Rev Cancer* 2007;7:684–700.
112. McCullough M, Robertson AS, Rodriguez C, et al. Calcium, vitamin D, dairy products, and risk of colorectal cancer in the cancer prevention study II nutrition cohort (United States). *Cancer Causes Control* 2003;14:1–12.
113. Wu K, Willett WC, Fuchs CS, et al. Calcium intake and risk of colon cancer in women and men. *J Natl Cancer Inst* 2002;94:437–446.
114. Chung M, Balk EM, Brendel M, et al. *Vitamin D and Calcium: A Systematic Review of Health Outcomes*. Evidence Report No. 183 (Prepared by the Tufts Evidence-based Practice Center). Rockville, MD: Agency for Healthcare Research and Quality; 2009.
115. World Health Organization, International Agency for Research on Cancer. Vitamin D and Cancer. Working Group Reports, Volume 5. Lyon, France: IARC; 2008.
116. Stolzenberg-Solomon RZ, Jacobs EJ, Arslan AA, et al. Circulating 25-hydroxyvitamin D and risk of pancreatic cancer: Cohort Consortium Vitamin D Pooling Project of Rarer Cancers. *Am J Epidemiol* 2010;172:81–93.
117. Baron J, Beach M, Mandel JS, et al. Calcium supplements for the prevention of colorectal adenomas. The Calcium Polyp Prevention Study Group. *N Engl J Med* 1999;340:101–107.
118. Bonithon-Kopp C, Kronborg O, Giacosa A, et al. Calcium and fibre supplementation in prevention of colorectal adenoma recurrence: a randomized intervention trial. *Lancet* 2000;356:1300–1306.
119. Wactawski-Wende J, Kotchen JM, Anderson CL, et al. Calcium plus vitamin D supplementation and the risk of colorectal cancer. *N Engl J Med* 2006; 354:684–696.
120. Trivedi DP, Doll R, Khaw KT. Effect of four monthly oral vitamin D3 (cholecalciferol) supplementation on fractures and mortality in men and women living in the community: randomised double blind controlled trial. *BMJ* 2003; 326:469.
121. Cui Y, Rohan TE. Vitamin D, calcium, and breast cancer risk: a review. *Cancer Epidemiol Biomarkers Prev* 2006;15:1427–1437.
122. Chlebowski RT, Johnson KC, Kooperberg C, et al. Calcium plus vitamin D supplementation and the risk of breast cancer. *J Natl Cancer Inst* 2008;100: 1581–1591.
123. Lappe JM, Travers-Gustafson D, Davies KM, et al. Vitamin D and calcium supplementation reduces cancer risk: results of a randomized trial. *Am J Clin Nutr* 2007;85:1586–1591.

124. Manson JE, Bassuk SS, Lee IM, et al. The VITamin D and OmegA-3 TriaL (VITAL): rationale and design of a large randomized controlled trial of vitamin D and marine omega-3 fatty acid supplements for the primary prevention of cancer and cardiovascular disease. *Contemp Clin Trials* 2012;33:159–171.
125. Wu X, Spitz MR, Lee JJ, et al. Novel susceptibility loci for second primary tumors/recurrence in head and neck cancer patients: large-scale evaluation of genetic variants. *Cancer Prev Res (Phila)* 2009;2:617–624.
126. Platz EA. Is prostate cancer prevention with selenium all in the genes? *Cancer Prev Res (Phila)* 2010;3:576–578.
127. Miller JW, Ulrich CM. Folic acid and cancer—where are we today? *Lancet* 2013;381:974–976.
128. Thun MJ, Henley SJ, Patrono C. Nonsteroidal anti-inflammatory drugs as anticancer agents: mechanistic, pharmacologic, and clinical issues. *J Natl Cancer Inst* 2002;94:252–266.
129. Wang D, Mann JR, DuBois RN. The role of prostaglandins and other eicosanoids in the gastrointestinal tract. *Gastroenterology* 2005;128:1445–1461.
130. Gurpinar E, Grizzle WE, Piazza GA. COX-Independent Mechanisms of Cancer Chemoprevention by Anti-Inflammatory Drugs. *Front Oncol* 2013;3:181.
131. Rothwell PM, Wilson M, Price JF, et al. Effect of daily aspirin on risk of cancer metastasis: a study of incident cancers during randomised controlled trials. *Lancet* 2012;379:1591–1601.
132. Rothwell PM, Price JF, Fowkes FG, et al. Short-term effects of daily aspirin on cancer incidence, mortality, and non-vascular death: analysis of the time course of risks and benefits in 51 randomised controlled trials. *Lancet* 2012;379:1602–1612.
133. Thun MJ, Namboodiri MM, Heath C Jr. Aspirin use and reduced risk of fatal colon cancer. *N Engl J Med* 1991;325:1593–1596.
134. Chan AT, Giovannucci EL, Meyerhardt JA, et al. Aspirin dose and duration of use and risk of colorectal cancer in men. *Gastroenterology* 2008;134:21–28.
135. Chan AT, Giovannucci EL, Meyerhardt JA, et al. Long-term use of aspirin and nonsteroidal anti-inflammatory drugs and risk of colorectal cancer. *JAMA* 2005;294:914–923.
136. Liao LM, Vaughan TL, Corley DA, et al. Nonsteroidal anti-inflammatory drug use reduces risk of adenocarcinomas of the esophagus and esophagogastric junction in a pooled analysis. *Gastroenterology* 2012;142:442–452.
137. Pollard M, Luckert PH. Effect of indomethacin on intestinal tumor induced in rats by the acetate derivative of dimethylnitrosamine. *Science* 1981;214:558–559.
138. Jacoby RF, Marshall DJ, Newton MA, et al. Chemoprevention of spontaneous intestinal adenomas in the Apc Min mouse model by the nonsteroidal anti-inflammatory drug piroxicam. *Cancer Res* 1996;56:710–714.
139. Kawamori T, Rao C, Seibert K, et al. Chemopreventive effect of celecoxib, a specific cyclooxygenase-2 inhibitor on colon carcinogenesis. *Cancer Res* 1998;58:409–412.
140. Oshima M, Dinchuk JE, Kargman SL. Suppression of intestinal polyposis in Apc delta 716 knockout ice by inhibition of cyclooxygenase 2 (COX-2). *Cell* 1996;87:803–809.
141. Anderson WF, Umar A, Viner JL, et al. The role of cyclooxygenase inhibitors in cancer prevention. *Curr Pharm Des* 2002;8:1035–1062.
142. Giardiello FM, Yang VW, Hylind LM, et al. Primary chemoprevention of familial adenomatous polyposis with sulindac. *N Engl J Med* 2002;346:1054–1059.
143. Steinbach G, Lynch PM, Phillips RK. The effect of celecoxib, a cyclooxygenase-2 inhibitor, in familial adenomatous polyposis. *N Engl J Med* 2000;342:1946–1952.
144. Thorson AG, Lynch HT, Smyrk TC. Rectal cancer in FAP patient after sulindac. *Lancet* 1994;343:180.
145. Calaluce R, Earnest DL, Heddens D, et al. Effects of piroxicam on prostaglandin E2 levels in rectal mucosa of adenomatous polyp patients: a randomized phase IIb trial. *Cancer Epidemiol Biomarkers Prev* 2000;9:1287–1292.
146. Ladenheim J, Garcia G, Titzer D, et al. Effects of sulindac on sporadic colonic polyps. *Gastroenterology* 1995;108:1083–1087.
147. Meyskens FL Jr, McLaren CE, Pelot D, et al. Difluoromethylornithine plus sulindac for the prevention of sporadic colorectal adenomas: a randomized placebo-controlled, double-blind trial. *Cancer Prev Res (Phila)* 2008;1:32–38.
148. Arber N, Eagle CJ, Spicak J, et al. Celecoxib for the prevention of colorectal adenomatous polyps. *N Engl J Med* 2006;355:885–895.
149. Bertagnolli MM, Eagle CJ, Zauber AG, et al. Celecoxib for the prevention of sporadic colorectal adenomas. *N Engl J Med* 2006;355:873–884.
150. Baron JA, Sandler RS, Bresalier RS, et al. A randomized trial of rofecoxib for the chemoprevention of colorectal adenomas. *Gastroenterology* 2006;131:1674–1682.
151. Bresalier RS, Sandler RS, Quan H, et al. Cardiovascular events associated with rofecoxib in a colorectal adenoma chemoprevention trial. *N Engl J Med* 2005;352:1092–1102.
152. Solomon SD, McMurray JJ, Pfeffer MA, et al. Cardiovascular risk associated with celecoxib in a clinical trial for colorectal adenoma prevention. *N Engl J Med* 2005;352:1071–1080.
153. Rostom A, Dube C, Lewin G, et al. Nonsteroidal anti-inflammatory drugs and cyclooxygenase-2 inhibitors for primary prevention of colorectal cancer: a systematic review prepared for the U.S. Preventive Services Task Force. *Ann Intern Med* 2007;146:376–389.
154. Dube C, Rostom A, Lewin G, et al. The use of aspirin for primary prevention of colorectal cancer: a systematic review prepared for the U.S. Preventive Services Task Force. *Ann Intern Med* 2007;146:365–375.
155. Rothwell PM, Fowkes FG, Belch JF, et al. Effect of daily aspirin on long-term risk of death due to cancer: analysis of individual patient data from randomised trials. *Lancet* 2011;377:31–41.
156. Rothwell PM. Aspirin in prevention of sporadic colorectal cancer: current clinical evidence and overall balance of risks and benefits. *Recent Results Cancer Res* 2013;191:121–142.
157. U.S. Preventive Services Task Force. Routine aspirin or nonsteroidal anti-inflammatory drugs for the primary prevention of colorectal cancer: U.S. Preventive Services Task Force recommendation statement. *Ann Intern Med* 2007;146:361–364.
158. Mulshine JL, Atkinson JC, Greer RO, et al. Randomized, double-blind, placebo-controlled phase IIb trial of the cyclooxygenase inhibitor ketorolac as an oral rinse in oropharyngeal leukoplakia. *Clin Cancer Res* 2004;10:1565–1573.
159. Mao JT, Fishbein MC, Adams B, et al. Celecoxib decreases Ki-67 proliferative index in active smokers. *Clin Cancer Res* 2006;12:314–320.
160. Bord S, Horner A, Beavan S, et al. Estrogen receptors alpha and beta are differentially expressed in developing human bone. *J Clin Endocrinol Metab* 2001;86:2309–2314.
161. Kuiper GG, Carlsson B, Grandien K, et al. Comparison of the ligand binding specificity and transcript tissue distribution of estrogen receptors alpha and beta. *Endocrinology* 1997;138:863–870.
162. Fabian CJ, Kimler BF. Selective estrogen-receptor modulators for primary prevention of breast cancer. *J Clin Oncol* 2005;23:1644–1655.
163. Jordan VC. SERMs: meeting the promise of multifunctional medicines. *J Natl Cancer Inst* 2007;99:350–356.
164. Jordan VC. Tamoxifen (ICI46,474) as a targeted therapy to treat and prevent breast cancer. *Br J Pharmacol* 2006;147:S269–S276.
165. Jordan VC. Effect of tamoxifen (ICI 46,474) on initiation and growth of DMBA-induced rat mammary carcinomata. *Eur J Cancer* 1976;12:419–424.
166. Jordan VC. Chemoprevention of breast cancer with selective oestrogen-receptor modulators. *Nat Rev Cancer* 2007;7:46–53.
167. Cuzick J, Baum M. Tamoxifen and contralateral breast cancer. *Lancet* 1985;2:282.
168. Fisher B, Redmond C. New perspective on cancer of the contralateral breast: a marker for assessing tamoxifen as a preventive agent. *J Natl Cancer Inst* 1991;83:1278–1280.
169. Ettinger B, Black DM, Mitlak BH, et al. Reduction of vertebral fracture risk in postmenopausal women with osteoporosis treated with raloxifene: results from a 3-year randomized clinical trial. Multiple Outcomes of Raloxifene Evaluation (MORE) Investigators. *JAMA* 1999;282:637–645.
170. LaCroix AZ, Powles T, Osborne CK, et al. Breast cancer incidence in the randomized PEARL trial of lasofoxifene in postmenopausal osteoporotic women. *J Natl Cancer Inst* 2010;102:1706–1715.
171. Cummings SR, Ensrud K, Delmas PD, et al. Lasofoxifene in postmenopausal women with osteoporosis. *N Engl J Med* 2010;362:686–696.
172. Cummings SR, McClung M, Reginster JY, et al. Arzoxifene for prevention of fractures and invasive breast cancer in postmenopausal women. *J Bone Miner Res* 2011;26:397–404.
173. Powles TJ, Diem SJ, Fabian CJ, et al. Breast cancer incidence in postmenopausal women with osteoporosis or low bone mass using arzoxifene. *Breast Cancer Res Treat* 2012;134:299–306.
174. Nelson HD, Smith ME, Griffin JC, et al. Use of medications to reduce risk for primary breast cancer: a systematic review for the U.S. Preventive Services Task Force. *Ann Intern Med* 2013;158:604–614.
175. Moyer VA. Medications for risk reduction of primary breast cancer in women: U.S. Preventive Services Task Force recommendation statement. *Ann Intern Med* 2013;159:698-708.
176. Visvanathan K, Hurley P, Bantug E, et al. Use of pharmacologic interventions for breast cancer risk reduction: American Society of Clinical Oncology clinical practice guideline. *J Clin Oncol* 2013;31:2942–2962.
177. Vogel VG, Costantino JP, Wickerham DL, et al. Carcinoma in situ outcomes in National Surgical Adjuvant Breast and Bowel Project Breast Cancer Chemoprevention Trials. *J Natl Cancer Inst Monogr* 2010;2010:181–186.
178. Cuzick J, Sestak I, Bonanni B, et al. Selective oestrogen receptor modulators in prevention of breast cancer: an updated meta-analysis of individual participant data. *Lancet* 2013;381:1827–1834.
179. Barrett-Connor E, Mosca L, Collins P, et al. Effects of raloxifene on cardiovascular events and breast cancer in postmenopausal women. *N Engl J Med* 2006;355:125–137.
180. Snyder KR, Sparano N, Malinowski JM. Raloxifene hydrochloride. *Am J Health Syst Pharm* 2000;57:1669–1675.
181. Goss PE, Ingle JN, Martino S, et al. A randomized trial of letrozole in postmenopausal women after five years of tamoxifen therapy for early-stage breast cancer. *N Engl J Med* 2003;349:1793–1802.
182. Fabian CJ, Kimler BF, Zalles CM, et al. Reduction in proliferation with six months of letrozole in women on hormone replacement therapy. *Breast Cancer Res Treat* 2007;106:75–84.
183. Goss PE, Ingle JN, Ales-Martinez JE, et al. Exemestane for breast-cancer prevention in postmenopausal women. *N Engl J Med* 2011;364:2381–2391.
184. Cheung AM, Tile L, Cardew S, et al. Bone density and structure in healthy postmenopausal women treated with exemestane for the primary prevention of breast cancer: a nested substudy of the MAP.3 randomised controlled trial. *Lancet Oncol* 2012;13:275–284.
185. Cuzick J, Sestak I, Forbes JF, et al. Anastrozole for prevention of breast cancer in high-risk postmenopausal women (IBIS-II): an international, double-blind, randomised placebo-controlled trial. *Lancet* 2014;383:1041–1048.
186. Waters EA, McNeel TS, Stevens WM, et al. Use of tamoxifen and raloxifene for breast cancer chemoprevention in 2010. *Breast Cancer Res Treat* 2012;134:875–880.

187. King MC, Wieand S, Hale K, et al. Tamoxifen and breast cancer incidence among women with inherited mutations in BRCA1 and BRCA2: National Surgical Adjuvant Breast and Bowel Project (NSABP-P1) Breast Cancer Prevention Trial. *JAMA* 2001;286:2251–2256.
188. Gronwald J, Tung N, Foulkes WD, et al. Tamoxifen and contralateral breast cancer in BRCA1 and BRCA2 carriers: an update. *Int J Cancer* 2006; 118:2281–2284.
189. Hess-Wilson JK, Knudsen KE. Endocrine disrupting compounds and prostate cancer. *Cancer Lett* 2006;241:1–12.
190. Andriole G, Bostwick D, Civantos F, et al. The effects of 5alpha-reductase inhibitors on the natural history, detection and grading of prostate cancer: current state of knowledge. *J Urol* 2005;174:2098–2104.
191. Thompson IM, Tangen CM, Goodman PJ, et al. Chemoprevention of prostate cancer. *J Urol* 2009;182:499–507.
192. Andriole GL, Bostwick DG, Brawley OW, et al. Effect of dutasteride on the risk of prostate cancer. *N Engl J Med* 2010;362:1192–1202.
193. Thompson IM Jr, Goodman PJ, Tangen CM, et al. Long-term survival of participants in the prostate cancer prevention trial. *N Engl J Med* 2013;369: 603–610.
194. Gerner EW, Meyskens FL Jr. Polyamines and cancer: old molecules, new understanding. *Nat Rev Cancer* 2004;4:781–792.
195. Meyskens FL Jr, Gerner EW. Development of difluoromethylornithine (DFMO) as a chemoprevention agent. *Clin Cancer Res* 1999;5:945–951.
196. Love R, Carbone P, Verma A, et al. Randomized phase I chemoprevention dose seeking study of alpha-difluoromethylornithine. *J Natl Cancer Inst* 1993;85: 732–737.
197. Alberts DS, Dorr RT, Einspahr JG, et al. Chemoprevention of human actinic keratoses by topical 2-(difluoromethyl)-dl-ornithine. *Cancer Epidemiol Biomarkers Prev* 2000;9:1281–1286.
198. Meyskens FL Jr, Surwit E, Moon TE, et al. Enhancement of regression of cervical intraepithelial neoplasia II (moderate dysplasia) with topically applied all-trans-retinoic acid: randomized trial. *J Natl Cancer Inst* 1994;86: 539–543.
199. Fabian CJ, Kimler BF, Brady DA, et al. A phase II breast cancer chemoprevention trial of oral alpha-difluoromethylornithine: breast tissue, imaging, and serum and urine biomarkers. *Clin Cancer Res* 2002;8:3105–3117.
200. Jeter JM, Alberts DS. Difluoromethylornithine: the proof is in the polyamines. *Cancer Prev Res (Phila)* 2012;5:1341–1344.
201. Gronich N, Rennert G. Beyond aspirin-cancer prevention with statins, metformin and bisphosphonates. *Nat Rev Clin Oncol* 2013;10:625–642.
202. Moyad MA. Why a statin and/or another proven heart healthy agent should be utilized in the next major cancer chemoprevention trial: part II. *Urologic Oncol* 2004;22:472–477.
203. Bertagnolli MM, Hsu M, Hawk ET, et al. Statin use and colorectal adenoma risk: results from the adenoma prevention with celecoxib trial. *Cancer Prev Res (Phila)* 2010;3:588–596.
204. Simon MS, Rosenberg CA, Rodabough RJ, et al. Prospective analysis of association between use of statins or other lipid-lowering agents and colorectal cancer risk. *Ann Epidemiol* 2012;22:17–27.
205. Platz EA, Leitzmann MF, Visvanathan K, et al. Statin drugs and risk of advanced prostate cancer. *J Natl Cancer Inst* 2006;98:1819–1825.
206. Eliassen AH, Colditz GA, Rosner B, et al. Serum lipids, lipid-lowering drugs, and the risk of breast cancer. *Arch Intern Med* 2005;165:2264–2271.
207. Lipkin SM, Chao EC, Moreno V, et al. Genetic variation in 3-hydroxy-3-methylglutaryl CoA reductase modifies the chemopreventive activity of statins for colorectal cancer. *Cancer Prev Res (Phila)* 2010;3:597–603.
208. Rennert G. Bisphosphonates: beyond prevention of bone metastases. *J Natl Cancer Inst* 2011;103:1728–1729.
209. Rennert G, Pinchev M, Rennert HS. Use of bisphosphonates and risk of postmenopausal breast cancer. *J Clin Oncol* 2010;28:3577–3581.
210. Chlebowski RT, Chen Z, Cauley JA, et al. Oral bisphosphonate use and breast cancer incidence in postmenopausal women. *J Clin Oncol* 2010;28: 3582–3590.
211. Monsees GM, Malone KE, Tang MT, et al. Bisphosphonate use after estrogen receptor-positive breast cancer and risk of contralateral breast cancer. *J Natl Cancer Inst* 2011;103:1752–1760.
212. Kirpichnikov D, McFarlane SI, Sowers JR. Metformin: an update. *Ann Intern Med* 2002;137:25–33.
213. Pollack MN. Insulin, insulin-like growth factors, insulin resistance, and neoplasia. *Am J Clin Nutr* 2007;86:s820–s822.
214. Evans JM, Donnelly LA, Emslie-Smith AM, et al. Metformin and reduced risk of cancer in diabetic patients. *BMJ* 2005;330:1304–1305.
215. Zhu P, Davis M, Blackwelder A, et al. Metformin selectively targets tumor initiating cells in erbB-2 overexpressing breast cancer models. *Cancer Prev Res (Phila)* 2014;7:199–210.
216. Lonardo E, Cioffi M, Sancho P, et al. Metformin targets the metabolic achilles heel of human pancreatic cancer stem cells. *PLoS One* 2013;8:e76518.
217. Grubbs C, Clapper M, Reid J, et al. *Metformin Promotes Tumorigenesis in Animal Models of Cancer Prevention.* Washington, DC: American Association for Cancer Research; 2013.
218. Chlebowski RT, McTiernan A, Wactawski-Wende J, et al. Diabetes, metformin, and breast cancer in postmenopausal women. *J Clin Oncol* 2012;30: 2844–2852.
219. Heger M, van Golen RF, Broekgaarden M, et al. The molecular basis for the pharmacokinetics and pharmacodynamics of curcumin and its metabolites in relation to cancer. *Pharmacol Rev* 2014;66:222–307.
220. Whitlock NC, Baek SJ. The anticancer effects of resveratrol: modulation of transcription factors. *Nutr Cancer* 2012;64:493–502.
221. Lambert JD. Does tea prevent cancer? Evidence from laboratory and human intervention studies. *Am J Clin Nutr* 2013;98:1667S–1675S.
222. Kakarala M, Brenner DE, Korkaya H, et al. Targeting breast stem cells with the cancer preventive compounds curcumin and piperine. *Breast Cancer Res Treat* 2010;122:777–785.
223. Norris L, Karmokar A, Howells L, et al. The role of cancer stem cells in the anti-carcinogenicity of curcumin. *Mol Nutr Food Res* 2013;57:1630–1637.
224. Zou H, Yuan C, Dong L, et al. Human cyclooxygenase-1 activity and its responses to COX inhibitors are allosterically regulated by nonsubstrate fatty acids. *J Lipid Res* 2012;53:1336–1347.
225. Wada M, Delong CJ, Hong YH, et al. Enzymes and receptors of prostaglandin pathways with arachidonic acid- vs. eicosapentaenoic acid-derived substrates and products. *J Biol Chem* 2007;282:22254–22266.
226. Laviano A, Rianda S, Molfino A, et al. Omega-3 fatty acids in cancer. *Curr Opin Clin Nutr Metab Care* 2013;16:156–161.
227. Cockbain AJ, Toogood GJ, Hull MA. Omega-3 polyunsaturated fatty acids for the treatment and prevention of colorectal cancer. *Gut* 2012;61:135–149.
228. Stoner GD, Wang LS, Casto BC. Laboratory and clinical studies of cancer chemoprevention by antioxidants in berries. *Carcinogenesis* 2008;29:1665–1674.
229. Wang LS, Dombkowski AA, Seguin C, et al. Mechanistic basis for the chemopreventive effects of black raspberries at a late stage of rat esophageal carcinogenesis. *Mol Carcinog* 2011;50:291–300.
230. Wang LS, Kuo CT, Stoner K, et al. Dietary black raspberries modulate DNA methylation in dextran sodium sulfate (DSS)-induced ulcerative colitis. *Carcinogenesis* 2013;34:2842–2850.
231. Ireson C, Orr S, Jones DJ, et al. Characterization of metabolites of the chemopreventive agent curcumin in human and rat hepatocytes and in the rat in vivo, and evaluation of their ability to inhibit phorbol ester-induced prostaglandin E2 production. *Cancer Res* 2001;61:1058–1064.
232. Ireson CR, Jones DJ, Orr S, et al. Metabolism of the cancer chemopreventive agent curcumin in human and rat intestine. *Cancer Epidemiol Biomarkers Prev* 2002;11:105–111.
233. Vareed SK, Kakarala M, Ruffin MT, et al. Pharmacokinetics of curcumin conjugate metabolites in healthy human subjects. *Cancer Epidemiol Biomarkers Prev* 2008;17:1411–1417.
234. Gescher A, Steward WP, Brown K. Resveratrol in the management of human cancer: how strong is the clinical evidence? *Ann N Y Acad Sci* 2013;1290:12–20.
235. Stoner GD. Ginger: is it ready for prime time? *Cancer Prev Res (Phila)* 2013;6:257–262.
236. Stoner GD, Wang LS. Chemoprevention of esophageal squamous cell carcinoma with berries. *Top Curr Chem* 2013;329:1–20.
237. Mallery SR, Zwick JC, Pei P, et al. Topical application of a bioadhesive black raspberry gel modulates gene expression and reduces cyclooxygenase 2 protein in human premalignant oral lesions. *Cancer Res* 2008;68:4945–4957.
238. Carroll RE, Benya RV, Turgeon DK, et al. Phase IIa clinical trial of curcumin for the prevention of colorectal neoplasia. *Cancer Prev Res (Phila)* 2011;4: 354–364.
239. Seeff LB, Hoofnagle JH. Epidemiology of hepatocellular carcinoma in areas of low hepatitis B and hepatitis C endemicity. *Oncogene* 2006;25:3771–3777.
240. Fox JG, Wang TC. Inflammation, atrophy, and gastric cancer. *J Clin Invest* 2007;117:60–69.
241. Saslow D, Castle PE, Cox JT, et al. American Cancer Society Guideline for human papillomavirus (HPV) vaccine use to prevent cervical cancer and its precursors. *CA Cancer J Clin* 2007;57:7–28.
242. Mohanna S, Maco V, Bravo F, et al. Epidemiology and clinical characteristics of classic Kaposi's sarcoma, seroprevalence, and variants of human herpesvirus 8 in South America: a critical review of an old disease. *Int J Infect Dis* 2005;9:239–250.
243. Castillo JJ, Reagan JL, Bishop KD, et al. Viral lymphomagenesis: from pathophysiology to the rationale for novel therapies. *Br J Haematol* 2014;165: 300–315.
244. Al-Bahrani R, Abuetabh Y, Zeitouni N, et al. Cholangiocarcinoma: risk factors, environmental influences and oncogenesis. *Ann Clin Lab Sci* 2013;43: 195–210.
245. Mostafa MH, Sheweita SA, O'Connor PJ. Relationship between schistosomiasis and bladder cancer. *Clin Microbiol Rev* 1999;12:97–111.
246. Zivny J, Wang TC, Yantiss R, et al. Role of therapy or monitoring in preventing progression to gastric cancer. *J Clin Gastroenterol* 2003;36:S50–S60.
247. Correa P, Fontham ET, Bravo JC, et al. Chemoprevention of gastric dysplasia: randomized trial of antioxidant supplements and anti-helicobacter pylori therapy. *J Natl Cancer Inst* 2000;92:1881–1888.
248. Wong BC, Zhang L, Ma JL, et al. Effects of selective COX-2 inhibitor and Helicobacter pylori eradication on precancerous gastric lesions. *Gut* 2012;61:812–818.
249. Ma JL, Zhang L, Brown LM, et al. Fifteen-year effects of Helicobacter pylori, garlic, and vitamin treatments on gastric cancer incidence and mortality. *J Natl Cancer Inst* 2012;104:488–492.
250. Risch HA, Lu L, Kidd MS, et al. Helicobacter pylori seropositivities and risk of pancreatic carcinoma. *Cancer Epidemiol Biomarkers Prev* 2014;23: 172–178.
251. Mazzoleni LE, Francesconi CF, Sander GB. Mass eradication of *Helicobacter pylori*: feasible and advisable? *Lancet* 2011;378:462–464.
252. Whiteman DC, Parmar P, Fahey P, et al. Association of Helicobacter pylori infection with reduced risk for esophageal cancer is independent of environmental and genetic modifiers. *Gastroenterology* 2010;139:73–83.

CANCER PREVENTION AND SCREENING

253. Torrance CJ, Jackson PE, Montgomery E, et al. Combinatorial chemoprevention of intestinal neoplasia. *Nat Med* 2000;6:1024–1028.
254. Reddy BS, Wang CX, Kong AN, et al. Prevention of azoxymethane-induced colon cancer by combination of low doses of atorvastatin, aspirin, and celecoxib in F 344 rats. *Cancer Res* 2006;66:4542–4546.
255. Zell JA, Pelot D, Chen WP, et al. Risk of cardiovascular events in a randomized placebo-controlled, double-blind trial of difluoromethylornithine plus sulindac for the prevention of sporadic colorectal adenomas. *Cancer Prev Res (Phila)* 2009;2:209–212.
256. Guerrieri-Gonzaga A, Robertson C, Bonanni B, et al. Preliminary results on safety and activity of a randomized, double-blind, 2 x 2 trial of low-dose tamoxifen and fenretinide for breast cancer prevention in premenopausal women. *J Clin Oncol* 2006;24:129–135.
257. Kelloff GJ, Lippman SM, Dannenberg AJ, et al. Progress in chemoprevention drug development: the promise of molecular biomarkers for prevention of intraepithelial neoplasia and cancer—a plan to move forward. *Clin Cancer Res* 2006;12:3661–3697.
258. Washington MK, Powell AE, Sullivan R, et al. Pathology of rodent models of intestinal cancer: progress report and recommendations. *Gastroenterology* 2013;144:705–717.
259. Nandan MO, Yang VW. Genetic and chemical models of colorectal cancer in mice. *Curr Colorectal Cancer Rep* 2010;6:51–59.
260. Kwon MC, Berns A. Mouse models for lung cancer. *Mol Oncol* 2013;7: 165–177.
261. Kirma NB, Tekmal RR. Transgenic mouse models of hormonal mammary carcinogenesis: advantages and limitations. *J Steroid Biochem Mol Biol* 2012;131:76–82.
262. Irshad S, Abate-Shen C. Modeling prostate cancer in mice: something old, something new, something premalignant, something metastatic. *Cancer Metastasis Rev* 2013;32:109–122.
263. Herreros-Villanueva M, Hijona E, Cosme A, et al. Mouse models of pancreatic cancer. *World J Gastroenterol* 2012;18:1286–1294.
264. Winawer SJ, Zauber AG, Ho MN, et al. Prevention of colorectal cancer by colonoscopic polypectomy. The National Polyp Study Workgroup. *N Engl J Med* 1993;329:1977–1981.
265. Spechler S. Barrett's esophagus. *Semin Oncol* 1994;21:431–437.
266. Shen O, Liu S, Dawsey S, et al. Cytologic screening for esophageal cancer: results from 12,877 subjects from a high risk population in China. *Int J Cancer* 1993;54:185–188.
267. Taylor P, Li B, Dawsey S, et al. Prevention of esophageal cancer: the nutrition intervention trials in Linxian, China. Linxian Nutrition Intervention Trials Study Group. *Cancer Res* 1994;54:2029s–2031s.
268. Sober A, Burstein J. Precursors to skin cancer. *Cancer* 1995;75:645–650.
269. Tucker M, Halpern A, Holly E, et al. Clinically recognized dysplastic nevi. A central risk factor for cutaneous melanoma. *JAMA* 1997;277:1439–1444.
270. Gustafsson L, Adami H-O. Natural history of cervical neoplasia:consistent results obtained by an identification technique. *Br J Cancer* 1989;60:132–137.
271. Cawson R. Premalignant lesions in the mouth. *Br Med Bull* 1975;31:164–180.
272. Zhou M. Intraductal carcinoma of the prostate: the whole story. *Pathology* 2013; 45:533–539.
273. Saccomanno G, Archer VE, Auerbach O, et al. Development of carcinoma of the lung as reflected in exfoliated cells. *Cancer* 1974;33:256–270.
274. Cooper CL, O'Toole SA, Kench JG. Classification, morphology and molecular pathology of premalignant lesions of the pancreas. *Pathology* 2013;45:286–304.
275. Brewster AM, Lee JJ, Clayman GL, et al. Randomized trial of adjuvant 13-cis-retinoic acid and interferon alfa for patients with aggressive skin squamous cell carcinoma. *J Clin Oncol* 2007;25:1974–1978.
276. Karp DD, Lee SJ, Keller SM, et al. Randomized, double-blind, placebo-controlled, phase III chemoprevention trial of selenium supplementation in patients with resected stage I non-small-cell lung cancer: ECOG 5597. *J Clin Oncol* 2013;31:4179–4187.
277. Labayle D, Fischer D, Vielh P. Sulindac causes regression of rectal polyps in familial adenomatous polyposis. *Gastroenterology* 1991;101:635–639.
278. Giardiello FM, Hamilton SR, Krush AJ, et al. Treatment of colonic and rectal adenomas with sulindac in familial adenomatous polyposis. *N Engl J Med* 1993;328:1313–1316.
279. Nugent KP, Farmer KC, Sipgelman AD, et al. Randomized controlled trial of the effect of sulindac on duodenal and rectal polyposis and cell proliferation in patients with familial adenomatous polyposis. *Br J Surg* 1993;80: 1618–1619.
280. Mathers JC, Movahedi M, Macrae F, et al. Long-term effect of resistant starch on cancer risk in carriers of hereditary colorectal cancer: an analysis from the CAPP2 randomised controlled trial. *Lancet Oncol* 2012;13:1242–1249.
281. Burn J, Gerdes AM, Macrae F, et al. Long-term effect of aspirin on cancer risk in carriers of hereditary colorectal cancer: an analysis from the CAPP2 randomised controlled trial. *Lancet* 2011;378:2081–2087.
282. Ruffin MT, Krishnan K, Rock CL, et al. Suppression of human colorectal mucosal prostaglandins: determining the lowest effective aspirin dose. *J Natl Cancer Inst* 1997;89:1152–1160.
283. Krishnan K, Ruffin MT, Normolle D, et al. Colonic mucosal prostaglandin E2 and cyclooxygenase expression before and after low aspirin doses in subjects at high risk or at normal risk for colorectal cancer. *Cancer Epidemiol Biomarkers Prev* 2001;10:447–453.
284. Sample D, Wargovich M, Fischer SM, et al. A dose-finding study of aspirin for chemoprevention utilizing rectal mucosal prostaglandin E(2) levels as a biomarker. *Cancer Epidemiol Biomarkers Prev* 2002;11:275–279.
285. Sandler RS, Halabi S, Baron JA, et al. A randomized trial of aspirin to prevent colorectal adenomas in patients with previous colorectal cancer. *N Engl J Med* 2003;348:883–890.
286. Baron JA, Cole BF, Sandler RS, et al. A randomized trial of aspirin to prevent colorectal adenomas. *N Engl J Med* 2003;348:891–899.
287. Fisher B, Costantino JP, Wickerham DL, et al. Tamoxifen for the prevention of breast cancer: current status of the National Surgical Adjuvant Breast and Bowel Project P-1 study. *J Natl Cancer Inst* 2005;97:1652–1662.
288. Cuzick J, Forbes JF, Sestak I, et al. Long-term results of tamoxifen prophylaxis for breast cancer—96-month follow-up of the randomized IBIS-I trial. *J Natl Cancer Inst* 2007;99:272–282.
289. Powles TJ, Ashley S, Tidy A, et al. Twenty-year follow-up of the Royal Marsden randomized, double-blinded tamoxifen breast cancer prevention trial. *J Natl Cancer Inst* 2007;99:283–290.
290. Veronesi U, Maisonneuve P, Rotmensz N, et al. Tamoxifen for the prevention of breast cancer: Late results of the Italian randomzied tamoxifen prevention trial among women with hysterectomy. *J Natl Cancer Inst* 2007;99:727–737.
291. Cauley JA, Norton L, Lippman ME, et al. Continued breast cancer risk reduction in postmenopausal women treated with raloxifene: 4-year results from the MORE trial. Multiple outcomes of raloxifene evaluation. *Breast Cancer Res Treat* 2001;65:125–134.
292. Martino S, Cauley JA, Barrett-Connor E, et al. Continuing outcomes relevant to Evista: breast cancer incidence in postmenopausal osteoporotic women in a randomized trial of raloxifene. *J Natl Cancer Inst* 2004;96: 1751–1761.
293. Messing E, Kim KM, Sharkey F, et al. Randomized prospective phase III trial of difluoromethylornithine vs placebo in preventing recurrence of completely resected low risk superficial bladder cancer. *J Urol* 2006;176:500–504.
294. Simoneau AR, Gerner EW, Nagle R, et al. The effect of difluoromethylornithine on decreasing prostate size and polyamines in men: results of a year-long phase IIb randomized placebo-controlled chemoprevention trial. *Cancer Epidemiol Biomarkers Prev* 2008;17:292–299.
295. Bailey HH, Kim K, Verma AK, et al. A randomized, double-blind, placebo-controlled phase 3 skin cancer prevention study of {alpha}-difluoromethylornithine in subjects with previous history of skin cancer. *Cancer Prev Res (Phila)* 2010;3:35–47.
296. Kreul SM, Havighurst T, Kim K, et al. A phase III skin cancer chemoprevention study of DFMO: long-term follow-up of skin cancer events and toxicity. *Cancer Prev Res (Phila)* 2012;5:1368–1374.
297. Zick SM, Ruffin MT, Djuric Z, et al. Quantitation of 6-, 8- and 10-gingerols and 6-shogaol in human plasma by high-performance liquid chromatography with electrochemical detection. *Int J Biomed Sci* 2010;6:233–240.
298. Zick SM, Turgeon DK, Vareed SK, et al. Phase II study of the effects of ginger root extract on eicosanoids in colon mucosa in people at normal risk for colorectal cancer. *Cancer Prev Res (Phila)* 2011;4:1929–1937.
299. Hull MA. Nutritional agents with anti-inflammatory properties in chemoprevention of colorectal neoplasia. *Recent Results Cancer Res* 2013;191:143–156.
300. Nelson WG, De Marzo AM, Isaacs WB. Prostate cancer. *N Engl J Med* 2003;349:366–381.
301. von Knobloch R, Konrad L, Barth PJ, et al. Genetic pathways and new progression markers for prostate cancer suggested by microsatellite allelotyping. *Clin Cancer Res* 2004;10:1064–1073.
302. Palapattu GS, Sutcliffe S, Bastian PJ, et al. Prostate carcinogenesis and inflammation: emerging insights. *Carcinogenesis* 2005;26:1170–1181.
303. Dontu G, Liu S, Wicha MS. Stem cells in mammary development and carcinogenesis: implications for prevention and treatment. *Stem Cell Rev* 2005;1: 207–213.
304. Liu S, Dontu G, Mantle ID, et al. Hedgehog signaling and Bmi-1 regulate self-renewal of normal and malignant human mammary stem cells. *Cancer Res* 2006;66:6063–6071.
305. Wistuba II, Lam S, Behrens C, et al. Molecular damage in the bronchial epithelium of current and former smokers. *J Natl Cancer Inst* 1997;89: 1366–1373.
306. Massion PP, Carbone DP. The molecular basis of lung cancer: molecular abnormalities and therapeutic implications. *Respir Res* 2003;4:12.
307. Mao C, Koutsky LA, Ault KA, et al. Efficacy of human papillomavirus-16 vaccine to prevent cervical intraepithelial neoplasia: a randomized controlled trial. *Obstet Gynecol* 2006;107:18–27.
308. Califano J, van der Riet P, Westra W, et al. Genetic progression model for head and neck cancer: implications for field cancerization. *Cancer Res* 1996;56: 2488–2492.
309. Califano J, Westra WH, Meininger G, et al. Genetic progression and clonal relationship of recurrent premalignant head and neck lesions. *Clin Cancer Res* 2000;6:347–352.
310. Braakhuis BJ, Tabor MP, Kummer JA, et al. A genetic explanation of Slaughter's concept of field cancerization: evidence and clinical implications. *Cancer Res* 2003;63:1727–1730.
311. Ha PK, Benoit NE, Yochem R, et al. A transcriptional progression model for head and neck cancer. *Clin Cancer Res* 2003;9:3058–3064.
312. Barrett MT, Sanchez CA, Prevo LJ, et al. Evolution of neoplastic cell lineages in Barrett oesophagus. *Nat Genet* 1999;22:106–109.
313. Reid BJ, Levine DS, Longton G, et al. Predictors of progression to cancer in Barrett's esophagus: baseline histology and flow cytometry identify low- and high-risk patient subsets. *Am J Gastroenterol* 2000;95:1669–1676.
314. Thorgeirsson SS, Grisham JW. Molecular pathogenesis of human hepatocellular carcinoma. *Nat Genet* 2002;31:339–346.

34 Cancer Screening

Otis W. Brawley and Howard L. Parnes

INTRODUCTION

Cancer screening refers to a test or examination performed on an asymptomatic individual. The goal is not simply to find cancer at an early stage, nor is it to diagnose as many patients with cancer as possible. The goal of cancer screening is to prevent death and suffering from the disease in question through early therapeutic intervention.

The assumption that early detection improves outcomes can be traced back to the concept that cancer inexorably progresses from a small, localized, primary tumor to local–regional spread, to distant metastases and death. This linear model of disease progression predicts that early intervention would reduce cancer mortality.

Cancer screening was an element of the "periodic physical examination," as espoused by the American Medical Association in the 1920s.[1] It consisted of palpation to find a mass or enlarged lymph nodes and auscultation to find a rub or abnormal sound. Today, screening has grown to include radiologic testing, the measurement of serum markers of disease, and even molecular testing. A positive screening test leads to further diagnostic testing, which might lead to a cancer diagnosis.

The intuitive appeal of early detection accounts for the emphasis that has long been placed on screening. However, it is not widely understood that screening tests are always associated with some harm (e.g., anxiety, financial costs) and may actually cause substantial harm (e.g., invasive follow-up diagnostic or therapeutic procedures). Because screening is, by definition, done in healthy people, all early detection tests should be carefully studied and their risk–benefit ratio determined before they are adopted for widespread usage.

Screening is a public health intervention. However, some draw a distinction between screening an individual within the doctor–patient relationship and mass screening, a program aimed at screening a large population. The latter may involve advertising campaigns to encourage people to be screened for a particular cancer at a shopping mall or at a community event, such as state fair.

Screening may be either *opportunistic* (i.e., a patient sees a health-care provider who chooses to screen or not to screen) or *programmatic*. Programmatic refers to a standardized approach with algorithms for screening and follow-up as well as recall of patients for regular routine screening with quality control measures. Programmatic screening is usually more effective.

PERFORMANCE CHARACTERISTICS

The degree to which a screening test can discriminate between individuals with and without a particular disease is described by its performance characteristics. These include the a test's sensitivity, specificity, positive predictive value (PPV), and negative predictive value (NPV) (Table 34.1). It should be noted that these measures relate to the accuracy of a screening test; they do not provide any information regarding a test's efficacy or effectiveness.

- Sensitivity is the proportion of persons designated positive by the screening test among all individuals who have the disease: true positive (TP)/(TP + false negative [FN]).
- Specificity is the proportion of persons designated negative by the screening test among all individuals who do not have the disease: true negative TN/(TN + false positive [FP]).
- Positive predictive value is the proportion of individuals with a positive screening test who have the disease: (TP)/(TP + FP).
- Negative predictive value is the proportion of individuals with a negative screening test who do not have the disease: (TN)/(TN + false negative [FN]).[2]

For a given screening test, sensitivity and specificity are inversely related. For example, as one lowers the threshold for considering a serum prostate-specific antigen (PSA) level to represent a *positive* screen, the sensitivity of the test increases and more cancers will be detected. This increased sensitivity comes at the cost of decreased specificity (i.e., more men without cancer will have *positive* screenings tests and, therefore, will be subjected to unnecessary diagnostic procedures).

Some screening tests, such as mammograms, are more subjective and operator dependent than others. For this reason, the sensitivity and specificity of screening mammography varies among radiologists. For a given radiologist, the lower his or her threshold for considering a mammogram to be suspicious, the higher the sensitivity and lower the specificity will be for them. However, mammography can have both a higher sensitivity and higher specificity in the hands of a more experienced versus a less experienced radiologist.

As opposed to sensitivity and specificity, the PPV and NPV of a screening test are dependent on disease prevalence. PPV is also highly responsive to small increases in specificity. As shown in Table 34.2, given a disease prevalence of 5 cases per 1,000 (0.005), the PPV of a hypothetical screening test increases dramatically as specificity goes from 95% to 99.9%, but only marginally as sensitivity goes from 80% to 95%. Given a disease prevalence of only 1 per 10,000 (0.0001), the PPV of the same test is poor even at high sensitivity and specificity. The positive association between breast cancer prevalence and age is the major reason why screening mammography is a better test (higher PPV) for women aged 50 to 59 than for women 40 to 49 years of age.

ASSESSING SCREENING TESTS AND OUTCOMES

Screening Test Results

Lead time bias occurs whenever screening results in an earlier diagnosis than would have occurred in the absence of screening.

TABLE 34.1

Performance Characteristics of a Screening Test

Sensitivity is the proportion designated positive by the screening test among all individuals who have the disease.

$$\frac{TP}{TP + FN}$$

Specificity is the proportion designated negative by the screening test among all those who do not have the disease.

$$\frac{TN}{TN + FP}$$

Positive predictive value is the proportion of individuals with a positive test who have the disease.

$$\frac{TP}{TP + FP}$$

Negative predictive value is the proportion of individuals with a negative test negative who do not have the disease.

$$\frac{TN}{TN + FN}$$

TP, true positive, the condition present and the test is positive; FN, false negative, the condition is present and the test is negative; FP, false positive, the condition is absent and the test is positive; TN, true negative, the condition is absent and test is negative.

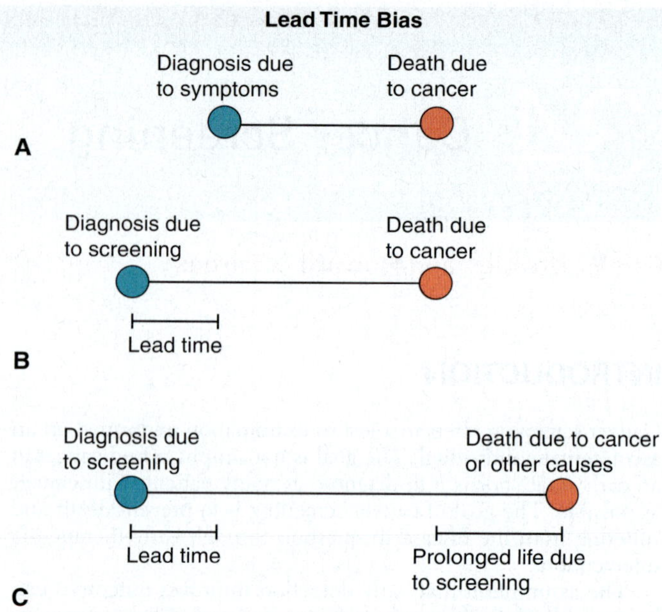

Figure 34.1 Survival is the time from cancer diagnosis to death. **(A)** Lead time bias occurs when screening results in an earlier diagnosis. Without screening, a patient is diagnosed with cancer due to symptoms. **(B)** With screening, the patient is often diagnosed earlier. When screening and treatment do not prolong life, the screened patient can have a longer survival solely due to the earlier diagnosis. The survival increase is pure lead time bias. **(C)** When screening and treatment are beneficial, the patient is diagnosed before the onset of symptoms and the patient lives beyond the point in which death would have occurred without screening.

Because survival is measured *from the time of diagnosis*, an earlier diagnosis, by definition, increases survival. Unless an effective intervention is available, lead time bias has no impact on the natural history of a disease and death will occur at the same time it would have in the absence of early detection (Fig. 34.1).

Length bias is a function of the biologic behavior of a cancer. Slower growing, less aggressive cancers are more likely to be detected by a screening test than faster growing cancers, which are more likely to be diagnosed due to the onset of symptoms between scheduled screenings (interval cancers). Length bias has an even greater effect on survival statistics than lead time bias (Fig. 34.2).

Overdiagnosis is an extreme form of length bias and represents pure harm. It refers to the detection of tumors, often through highly sensitive modern imaging modalities and other diagnostic tests, that fulfill the histologic criteria for malignancy but are not biologically destined to harm the patient (see Fig. 34.2).

There are two categories of overdiagnosis: the detection of histologically defined *cancers* not destined to metastasize or harm the patient, and the detection of cancers not destined to metastasize or cause harm *in the life span of the specific patient*. The importance of this second category is illustrated by the widespread practice in the United States of screening elderly patients with limited life expectancies, who are thus unlikely to benefit from early cancer diagnosis.

Overdiagnosis occurs with many malignancies, including lung, breast, prostate, renal cell, melanoma, and thyroid cancers.[3] Neuroblastoma provides one of the most striking examples of overdiagnosis.[4] Urine vanillylmandelic acid (VMA) testing is a highly sensitive screening test for the detection of this pediatric disease. After screening programs in Germany, Japan, and Canada showed marked increases in the incidence of this disease without a concomitant decline in mortality, it was noticed that nearby areas that did not screen had similar death rates with lower incidence.[4,5] It is now appreciated that screen-detected neuroblastomas have a very good prognosis with minimal or no treatment. Many actually regress spontaneously.

Stage shift—i.e., a cancer diagnosis at an earlier stage than would have occurred in the absence of screening—is necessary, but not sufficient, for a screening test to be effective in terms of reducing mortality. Both lead time bias and length bias contribute to this phenomenon. Although it is tempting to speculate that diagnosis at an earlier stage must confer benefit, this is not necessarily the case. For example, a substantial proportion of men treated with radical prostatectomy for what appears to be a localized prostate cancer relapse after undergoing surgery. Conversely, some men who are treated with definitive therapy would never have gone on to develop metastatic disease in the absence of treatment.

TABLE 34.2

Positive Predictive Value Given Varying Sensitivity and Specificity and Prevalence

Prevalence 0.005		Sensitivity %		
		80	90	95
Specificity %	95	7	8	9
	99	29	31	32
	99.9	80	82	83
Prevalence 0.0001		**Sensitivity %**		
		80	90	95
Specificity %	95	0.2	0.2	2.0
	99	0.8	0.9	0.9
	99.9	0.7	8.0	9.0

PPV improves dramatically in response to small changes in specificity. Changes in specificity influence PPV much more than changes in sensitivity. Note the influence of prevalence on PPV. Screening tests do not perform as well in populations with a low prevalence of disease.

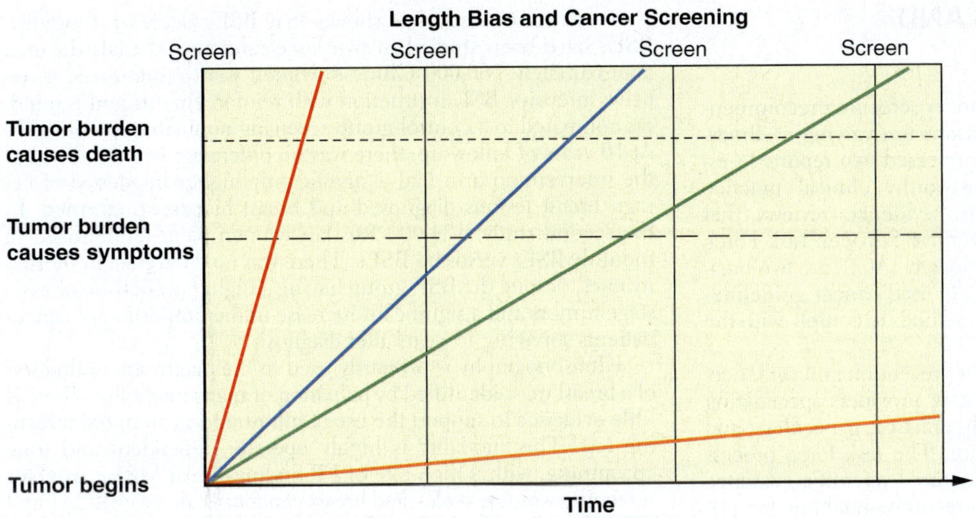

Figure 34.2 Length bias and cancer screening. The *red line* is indicative of a fast-growing tumor that is not amenable to regular screening. The *blue line* is indicative of a fast-growing tumor that can be diagnosed by screening or later by symptoms; death may possibly be prevented by treatment. The *green line* is a slower growing but potentially deadly cancer that can be detected by symptoms or several screenings and treated, possibly preventing death. The *orange line* is indicative of a very slow growing tumor that would never cause death and would never need treatment despite being screen detected. This is classic overdiagnosis.

Selection bias occurs when enrollees in a clinical study differ from the general population. In fact, people who voluntarily participate in clinical trials tend to be healthier than the general population, perhaps due to a greater interest in health and healthcare research. Screening studies tend to enroll individuals healthier than the general population. This so-called *healthy volunteer effect*[6,7] can introduce a powerful bias if not adequately controlled for by randomization procedures.

Assessing Screening Outcomes

The usual primary goal of cancer screening is to reduce mortality from the disease in question (a reduction in disease-specific mortality). Screening studies generally do not have sufficient statistical power to assess the impact of screening for a specific malignancy on overall mortality. (Lung cancer screening provides an exception to this rule; see the following.) As discussed previously, the fact that a screening test increases the percentage of people diagnosed with early stage cancer and decreases that of late stage cancer (stage shift) is not equivalent to proof of mortality reduction. Further, due to the healthy volunteer effect, case control and cohort studies cannot provide definitive evidence of mortality benefit. Prospective, randomized clinical trials are required to address this issue. In such trials, volunteers are randomized to be screened or not and are then followed longitudinally to determine if there is a difference in disease-specific or overall mortality.

A reduction in mortality rates or in the risk of death is often stated in terms of relative risk. However, this method of reporting may be misleading. It is preferable to report both the relative and absolute reduction in mortality. For example, the European Randomized Study of Screening for Prostate Cancer (ERSPC) showed that screening reduced the risk of prostate cancer death by 20%. However, this translates into only 1 prostate cancer death averted per 1,000 men screened (5 prostate cancer deaths per 1,000 men not screened versus 4 prostate cancer deaths per 1,000 men screened) and a relatively modest lifetime reduction in the absolute risk of prostate cancer death of only 0.6%, from 3.0% to 2.4%.[8]

PROBLEMS WITH RANDOMIZED TRIALS

It is important to acknowledge that even prospective, randomized trials can have serious methodologic shortcomings. For example, imbalances caused by flaws in the randomization scheme can prejudice the outcome of a trial. Other flaws include so-called *drop-in* or *contamination*, in which some participants on the control arm get the intervention. Patients on the intervention arm may also *drop out* of the study. Both drop-ins and drop-outs reduce the statistical power of a clinical trial.

In the United States, it is now considered standard to obtain informed consent before randomization takes place. However, there have been several published studies that randomized participants from rosters of eligible subjects such as census lists. In these trials, informed consent was obtained after randomization and only among those randomized to the screening arm of the study. Those randomized to the control arm were not contacted, and indeed, did not know they were in a clinical trial. They were followed through national death registries. Although the study was analyzed on an intent-to-screen basis, this method can still introduce biases. For example, only patients on the intervention arm had access to the screening facility and staff for counseling and treatment if diagnosed; those in the control group were more likely to be treated in the community as opposed to high-volume centers of excellence and were less likely to be treated with surgery and more likely to be treated with hormones alone than those on the screened arm. The study arms would also tend to differ in their knowledge of the disease, which may contribute to an overestimate of the benefits of a screening test.[9]

Virtually every screening test is a balance between known harms and potential benefits. The most important risk of screening is the detection and subsequent treatment of a cancer that would never have come to clinical detection or harmed the patient in the absence of screening (i.e., overdiagnosis and overtreatment). Treatment can cause emotional and physical morbidity and even death.[10] Even when screening has a net mortality benefit, there can be considerable harm. For example, in the recent randomized trial of spiral lung computed tomography (CT) scan, approximately 27,000 current smokers and former smokers were given three annual low-dose CT scans. More than 20% had a *positive* screening CT scan, necessitating further testing. About 1,000 subsequently underwent invasive diagnostic procedures and 16 deaths were reported within 60 days of the procedure.[11] It is not known how many of these deaths were directly related to the screening.

It can be dangerous to extrapolate estimates of benefit from one population to another. In particular, studies showing that a radiographic test is beneficial to average risk individuals may not mean that it is beneficial to a population at high risk, and vice versa. For example, women at high risk for breast cancer due to an inherited mutation of a DNA repair gene may be at higher risk for radiation-induced cancer from mammographies compared to the general population; a screening test (e.g., spiral lung CT scan), shown to be efficacious in a high-risk population of heavy smokers may result in net harm if applied to a low or average risk population.

SCREENING GUIDELINES AND RECOMMENDATIONS

A number of organizations develop cancer screening recommendations or guidelines. These organizations use varying methods. The Institute of Medicine (IOM) has released two reports to establish standards for developing trustworthy clinical practice guidelines and conducting systematic evidence reviews that serve as their basis.[12,13] The U.S. Preventive Services Task Force (USPSTF) and the American Cancer Society (ACS) are two organizations that issue respected and widely used cancer guidelines (Table 34.3). Both have changed their methods to comply with the IOM standards.

The USPSTF is a panel of experts in prevention and evidence-based medicine.[14] They are primary care providers specializing in internal medicine, pediatrics, family practice, gynecology and obstetrics, nursing, and health behavior. The task force process begins by conducting an extensive structured scientific evidence review. The task force then develops recommendations for primary care clinicians and health-care systems. They adhere to some of the highest standards for recommending a screening test. They are very much concerned with the question, "Does the evidence supporting a screening test demonstrate that the benefits outweigh its harms?"

The ACS guidelines date back to the 1970s. The current process for making guidelines involves commissioning academics to do an independent systematic evidence review. A single generalist group digests the evidence review, listens to public input, and writes the guidelines. The ACS panel tries to clearly articulate the benefits, limitations, and harms associated with a screening test.[15]

BREAST CANCER

Mammographies, clinical breast examinations (CBE) by a health-care provider, and breast self-examinations (BSE) have long been advocated[16] for the early detection of breast cancer. In recent years, ultrasound, magnetic resonance imaging (MRI), and other technologies have been added to the list of proposed screening modalities.

Mammographic screening was first advocated in the 1950s. The Health Insurance Plan (HIP) Study was the first prospective, randomized clinical trial to formally assess its value in reducing death from breast cancer. In this study, started in 1963, about 61,000 women were randomized to three annual mammograms with clinical breast examination versus no screening, which was the standard practice at that time. HIP first reported that mammography reduced breast cancer mortality by 30% at about 10 years after study entry. With 18 years of follow-up, those in the screening arm had a 25% lower breast cancer mortality rate.[16]

Nine additional prospective randomized studies have been published. These studies provide the basis for the current consensus that screening women 40 to 75 years of age does reduce the relative risk of breast cancer death by 10% to 25%. The 10 studies demonstrate that the risk–benefit ratio is more favorable for women over 50 years of age. Mammography has also been shown to be operator dependent, with better performance characteristics (higher sensitivity and specificity and lower FP rates) reported by high-volume centers (Table 34.4).

It is important to note that every one of these studies has some flaws and limitations. They vary in the questions asked and their findings. The Canadian screening trial suggests mammographies and clinical breast examinations do not decrease risk of death for woman aged 40 to 49 and that mammographies add nothing to CBEs for women age 50 to 59 years.[17] On the other extreme, the Kopparberg Sweden study suggests that mammographies are associated with a 32% reduction in the risk of death for women aged 40 to 74 years.[18]

To date, no study has shown that BSEs decrease mortality. BSEs have been studied in two large randomized trials. In one, approximately 266,000 Chinese women were randomized to receive intensive BSE instruction with reinforcements and reminders compared to a control group receiving no instruction on BSE. At 10 years of follow-up, there was no difference in mortality, but the intervention arm had a significantly higher incidence of benign breast lesions diagnosed and breast biopsies preformed. In the second study, 124,000 Russian women were randomized to monthly BSEs versus no BSEs. There was no difference in mortality rates, despite the BSE group having a higher proportion of early stage tumors and a significant increase in the proportion of cancer patients surviving 15 years after diagnosis.

Ultrasonography is primarily used in the diagnostic evaluation of a breast mass identified by palpation or mammography. There is little evidence to support the use of ultrasound as an initial screening test. This modality is highly operator dependent and time consuming, with a high rate of FP findings.[19] An MRI is used for screening women at elevated breast cancer risk due to BRCA1 and BRCA2 mutations, Li-Fraumeni syndrome, Cowden disease, or a very strong family history. MRI is more sensitive but less specific than mammography, leading to a high FP rate and more unnecessary biopsies, especially among young women.[20] The impact of MRI breast screening on breast cancer mortality has not yet been determined.

Thermography, an infrared imaging technology, has some advocates as a breast cancer screening modality despite a lack of evidence from several small cohort studies.[21] Nipple aspirate cytology and ductal lavage have also been suggested as possible screening methods. Both should be considered experimental at this time.[22]

Effectiveness of Breast Cancer Screening

Breast cancer screening has been associated with a dramatic rise in breast cancer incidence. At the same time, there has been a dramatic decrease in breast cancer mortality rates. However, in the United States and Europe, incidence-by-stage data show a dramatic increase in the proportion of early stage cancers without a concomitant decrease in the incidence of regional and metastatic cancers.[23] These findings are at odds with the clinical trials data and raise questions regarding the extent to which early diagnosis is responsible for declining breast cancer mortality rates.

From 1976 to 2008, the incidence of early-stage breast cancer for American women aged 40 and older increased from 112 to 234 per 100,000. This is a rise of 122 cases per 100,000, whereas the absolute decrease in late-stage cancers was only 8 cases per 100,000 (from 102 to 94 cases per 100,000). These data raise questions regarding the magnitude of benefit, as well as the potential risks, of breast cancer screening. The discrepancy between the magnitude of the increase of early disease and the decrease of late-stage cancer and cancer mortality suggests that a proportion of invasive breast cancers diagnosed by screening represents overdiagnosis. These data suggest that overdiagnosis accounts for up to 31% of all breast cancers diagnosed by screening.[24] Others have estimated that up to 50% of breast cancers detected by screening mammography are overdiagnosed cancers. In an exhaustive review of the screening literature, a panel of experts concluded that overdiagnosis does exist and estimated it to be 11% to 19% of breast cancers diagnosed by screening.[25]

A confounding factor with regard to the mortality benefits of breast cancer screening is the improvement that has occurred in breast cancer treatment over this period of time. The effects of the advances in therapy are supported by cancer modeling studies. Indeed, the Cancer Intervention and Surveillance Modeling Network (CISNET), supported by the U.S. National Cancer Institute (NCI), has estimated that two-thirds of the observed breast cancer mortality reduction is attributable to modern therapy, rather than to screening.[26]

TABLE 34.3

Screening Recommendations for Normal-Risk Asymptomatic Subjects

Cancer Type	Test or Procedure	American Cancer Society	U.S. Preventive Services Task Force
Breast	Self-examination	Women ≥20 years: Breast self-exam is an option	"D"
	Clinical examination	Women 20–39 years: Perform every 3 years Women ≥40 years: Perform annually	Women ≥40 years: "I" (as a stand alone without mammography)
	Mammography	Women ≥40 years: Screen annually for as long as the woman is in good health	Women 40–49 years: The decision should be an individual one, and take patient context/values into account ("C") Women 50–74 years: Every 2 years ("B") Women ≥75 years: "I"
	MRI	Women >20% lifetime risk of breast cancer: Screen with MRI plus mammography annually Women 15%–20% lifetime risk of breast cancer: Discuss option of MRI plus mammography annually Women <15% lifetime risk of breast cancer: Do not screen annually with MRI	"I"
Cervical	Pap test (cytology)	Women ages 21–29 years: Screen every 3 years Women 30–65 years: Acceptable approach to screen with cytology every 3 years (see HPV test) Women <21 years: No screening Women >65 years: No screening following adequate negative prior screening Women after total hysterectomy for noncancerous causes: Do not screen	Women ages 21–65 years: Screen every 3 years ("A") Women <21 years: "D" Women >65 years, with adequate, normal prior Pap screenings: "D" Women after total hysterectomy for noncancerous causes: "D"
	HPV test	Women <30 years: Do not use HPV testing Women ages 30–65 years: Preferred approach to screen with HPV and cytology cotesting every 5 years (see Pap test) Women >65 years: No screening following adequate negative prior screening Women after total hysterectomy for noncancerous causes: Do not screen	Women ages 30–65 years: Screen in combination with cytology every 5 years if woman desires to lengthen the screening interval (see Pap test) ("A") Women <30 years: "D" Women >65 years, with adequate, normal prior Pap screenings: "D" Women after total hysterectomy for noncancerous causes: "D"
Colorectal	Sigmoidoscopy	Adults ≥50 years: Screen every 5 years Note: For all CRC screening tests, stop screening when benefits are unlikely due to life-limiting comorbidity.	Adults 50–75 years: Every 5 years in combination with high-sensitivity fecal occult blood testing (FOBT) every 3 years ("A")[a] Adults 76–85 years: "C" Adults ≥85 years: "D"
	Fecal occult blood testing (FOBT)	Adults ≥50 years: Screen every year with high sensitivity guaiac based FOBT or fecal immunochemical test (FIT) only	Adults 50–75 years: Annually, for high-sensitivity FOBT ("A") Adults 76–85 years: "C" Adults ≥85 years: "D"
	Colonoscopy	Adults ≥50 years: Screen every 10 years	Adults 50–75 years: every 10 years ("A") Adults 76–85 years: "C" Adults ≥85 years: "D"
	Fecal DNA testing	Adults ≥50 years: Screen, but interval uncertain	"I"
	Fecal immunochemical testing (FIT)	Adults ≥50 years: Screen every year	"I"
	CT colonography	Adults ≥50 years: Screen every 5 years	"I"
Lung	Complete skin examination by clinician or patient	Men and women, 55–74 years, with ≥30 pack-year smoking history, still smoking or have quit within past 15 years: Discuss benefits, limitations, and potential harms of screening. Only perform screening in facilities with the right type of CT scanner and with high expertise/specialists.	"I" ("B" draft recommendation issued for public comment in July 2013)

(continued)

TABLE 34.3

Screening Recommendations for Normal-Risk Asymptomatic Subjects *(continued)*

Cancer Type	Test or Procedure	American Cancer Society	U.S. Preventive Services Task Force
Ovary	CA-125 Transvaginal ultrasound	There is no sufficiently accurate test proven effective in the early detection of ovarian cancer. For women at high risk of ovarian cancer and/or who have unexplained, persistent symptoms, the combination of CA-125 and transvaginal ultrasound with pelvic exam may be offered.	"D" "D"
Prostate	Prostate-specific antigen (PSA)	Starting at age 50, men should talk to a doctor about the pros and cons of testing so they can decide if testing is the right choice for them. If African American or have a father or brother who had prostate cancer before age 65, men should have this talk starting at age 45. How often they are tested will depend on their PSA level.	Men, all ages: "D"
	Digital rectal examination (DRE)	As for PSA; if men decide to be tested, they should have the PSA blood test with or without a rectal exam.	No individual recommendation
Skin	Complete skin examination by clinician or patient	Self-examination monthly; clinical exam as part of routine cancer-related checkup	"I"

Note: Summary of the screening procedures recommended for the general population by the American Cancer Society and the U.S. Preventive Services Task Force. These recommendations refer to asymptomatic persons who have no risk factors for the cancer, other than age or gender.
[a] USPSTF lettered recommendations are defined as follows:
"A": The USPSTF recommends the service, because there is high certainty that the net benefit is substantial.
"B": The USPSTF recommends the service, because there is high certainty that the net benefit is moderate or moderate certainty that the net benefit is moderate to substantial.
"C": The USPSTF recommends selectively offering or providing this service to individual patients based on professional judgment and patient preferences. There is at least moderate certainty that the net benefit is small.
"D": The USPSTF recommends against the service, because there is moderate or high certainty that the service has no net benefit or that the harms outweigh the benefits.
"I": The USPSTF concludes that the current evidence is insufficient to assess the balance of benefits and harms of the service.

Questions have also been raised regarding the quality of the randomized screening trials that demonstrated the mortality benefits of mammography and clinical breast examination because these trials suffered from a variety of design flaws. In some, randomization methods were suboptimal, others reported varying numbers of participants over the years, and still others had substantial contamination (drop-ins). Perhaps more importantly, most trials were started and concluded before the widespread use of more advanced mammographic technology, before the modern era of adjuvant therapy, and before the advent of targeted therapy.

Although randomized control trials (RCT) remain the gold standard for assessing the benefits of a clinical intervention, they cannot take into account improvements in both treatment and patient awareness that occurred over time. For this reason, observational and modeling studies can provide important, complementary information.

One systematic review of 17 published population-based and cohort studies compared breast cancer mortality in groups of women aged 50 to 69 years who started breast cancer screening at different times. Although these studies are subject to methodologic limitations, only four suggested that breast cancer screening reduced the relative risk of breast cancer mortality by 33% or more and five suggested no benefit from screening. The review concluded that breast cancer screening likely reduces the risk of breast cancer death by no more than 10%.[27]

Even with these limitations, a systematic review of the data sponsored by the USPSTF concluded that regular mammography reduces breast cancer mortality in women aged 40 to 74 years.[28] The task force also concluded that the benefits of mammography are most significant in women aged 50 to 74 years.

Screening Women Age 40 to 49

Experts disagree about the utility of screening women in their forties. In the HIP Randomized Control Trial, women who entered at age 40 to 49 years had a mortality benefit at 18 years of follow-up. However, to a large extent, the mortality benefit among those aged 45 to 49 years at entry was driven by breast cancers diagnosed after they reached age 50 years.[16]

Mammography, like all screening tests, is more efficient (higher PPV) for the detection of disease in populations with higher disease prevalence (see Table 34.2). Mammography is, therefore, a better test in women age 50 to 59 years than it is among women age 40 to 49 years because the risk of breast cancer increases with age. Mammography is also less optimal in women age 40 to 49 years compared to women 50 to 59 years of age for the following reasons:

- A larger proportion have increased breast density, which can obscure lesions (lower sensitivity).
- Younger women are more likely to develop aggressive, fast-growing breast cancers that are diagnosed between regular screening visits. By definition, these *interval cancers* are not screen detected.[29]

The USPSTF meta-analysis of eight large randomized trials suggested a 15% relative reduction in mortality (relative risk [RR], 0.85; 95% confidence interval [CI], 0.75 to 0.96) from mammography screening for women aged 40 to 49 years after 11 to 20 years of follow-up. This is equivalent to a needing to invite 1,904 women to screenings over 10 years to prevent one breast cancer death. Studies, however, show that more than half of women aged 40 to 49 years screened annually over a 10-year period will have an FP mammogram necessitating further evaluation, often including biopsy. In addition, estimates of overdiagnosis in this group range from 10% to 40% of diagnosed invasive cancers.[30]

In an effort to decrease FP rates, some have suggested screening every 2 years rather than yearly. Comparing biennial with annual screening, the CISNET Model consistently shows that biennial screening of women ages 40 to 70 only marginally decreases the number of lives saved while halving the false positive rate.[29] Notably, the Swedish two-county trial, which had a planned 24-month screening interval (the actual interval was 33 months) reported one

TABLE 34.4

Randomized Controlled Trials

Study	Randomization	Sample Size	Intervention and Age at Entry	Follow-up	Finding
Health Insurance Plan, United States 1963[a,b]	Individual	60,565–60,857	MMG and CBE for 3 years Age 40–64 years	18 years	RR 0.77 (95% CI: 0.61–0.97)
Malmo, Sweden 1976[c,d]	Individual	42,283	Two-view MMG every 18–24 months × 5 Age 45–69 years	12 years	RR 0.81 (95% CI: 0.62–1.07)
Ostergotland (County E of Two-County Trial) Sweden 1977[e–g]	Geographic cluster	38,405–39,034 study 37,145–37,936 control	Three single-view MMG every 2 years women, Age 40–50 years Every 33 months women, Age 50–74	12 years	RR 0.82 (95% CI: 0.64–1.05)
Kopparberg (County W of Two-County Trial) Sweden 1977[e–g]	Geographic cluster	38,562–39,051 intervention 18,478–18,846 control	Three single-view MMG every 2 years women, Age 40–50 years Every 33 months women, Age 50–74 years	12 years	RR 0.68 (95% CI: 0.52–0.89)
Edinburgh, United Kingdom[h]	Cluster by physician practice	23,266 study 21,904 control	Initially, two-view MMG and CBE Then annual CBE with single-view MMG years 3, 5, and 7, Age 45–64 years	10 years	RR 0.84 (95% CI: 0.63–1.12)
NBSS-1, Canada 1980[i,j]	Individual	25,214 study (100% screened after entry CBE) 25,216 control	Annual two-view MMG and CBE for 4–5 years, Age 40–49 years	13 years	RR 0.97 (95% CI: 0.74–1.27)
NBSS-2, Canada 1980[i,j]	Individual	19,711 study (100% screened after entry CBE) 19,694 control	Annual two-view MMG and CBE versus CBE, Age 50–59 years	11–16 years (mean 13 years)	RR 1.02 (95% CI: 0.78–1.33)
Stockholm, Sweden 1981[k]	Cluster by birth date	40,318–38,525 intervention group 19,943–20,978 control group	Single view MMG every 28 months × 2 Age 40–64 years	8 years	RR 0.80 (95%) CI: 0.53–1.22)
Gothenberg, Sweden 1982[d]	Complex	21,650 invited 29,961 control	Initial two-view MMG, then single-view MMG every 18 months × 4 Single read first three rounds, then double-read, Age 39–59 years	12–14 years	RR 0.79 (95% CI 0.58–1.08) In the evaluation phase RR 0.77 (95% CI 0.60–1.00) In follow-up phase
Age Trial[l]	Individual	160,921 (53,884 invited; 106,956 not invited)	Invited group aged 48 and younger offered annual screening by MMG (double-view first screen, then single mediolateral oblique view thereafter); 68% accepted screening on the first screen an 69% and 70% were reinvited (81% attended at least one screen) Age 39–41 years	10.7 years	RR 0.83 (95% CI: 0.66–1.04)

[a] Shapiro S, Venet W, Strax P, et al. Ten- to fourteen-year effect of screening on breast cancer mortality. *J Natl Cancer Inst* 1982;69:349–355.
[b] Shapiro S. Periodic screening for breast cancer: the HIP Randomized Controlled Trial. Health Insurance Plan. *J Natl Cancer Inst Monogr* 1997:27–30.
[c] Andersson I, Aspegren K, Janzon L, et al. Mammographic screening and mortality from breast cancer: the Malmo mammographic screening trial. *BMJ* 1988;297:943–948.
[d] Nystrom L, Rutqvist LE, Wall S, et al. Breast cancer screening with mammography: overview of Swedish randomised trials. *Lancet* 1993;341:973–978.
[e] Tabar L, Fagerberg CJ, Gad A, et al. Reduction in mortality from breast cancer after mass screening with mammography. Randomised trial from the Breast Cancer Screening Working Group of the Swedish National Board of Health and Welfare. *Lancet* 1985;1:829–832.
[f] Tabar L, Fagerberg G, Duffy SW, Day NE. The Swedish two county trial of mammographic screening for breast cancer: recent results and calculation of benefit. *J Epidemiol Community Health* 1989;43:107–114.
[g] Tabar L, Fagerberg G, Duffy SW, et al. Update of the Swedish two-county program of mammographic screening for breast cancer. *Radiol Clin North Am* 1992;30:187–210.
[h] Roberts MM, Alexander FE, Anderson TJ, et al. Edinburgh trial of screening for breast cancer: mortality at seven years. *Lancet* 1990;335:241–246.
[i] Miller AB, To T, Baines CJ, Wall C. The Canadian National Breast Screening Study-1: breast cancer mortality after 11 to 16 years of follow-up. A randomized screening trial of mammography in women age 40 to 49 years. *Ann Intern Med* 2002;137:305–312.
[j] Miller AB, Wall C, Baines CJ, et al. Twenty five year follow-up for breast cancer incidence and mortality of the Canadian National Breast Screening Study: randomised screening trial. *BMJ* 2014;348–366.
[k] Frisell J, Eklund G, Hellstrom L, et al. Randomized study of mammography screening—preliminary report on mortality in the Stockholm trial. *Breast Cancer Res Treat* 1991;18:49–56.
[l] Moss SM, Cuckle H, Evans A, et al. Effect of mammographic screening from age 40 years on breast cancer mortality at 10 years' follow-up: a randomised controlled trial. *Lancet* 2006;368:2053–2060.

of the greatest reductions in breast cancer mortality among the RCTs conducted to date.

Screening Women at High Risk

There is interest in creating risk profiles as a way of reducing the inconveniences and harms of screening. It might be possible to identify women who are at greater risk of breast cancer and refocus screening efforts on those most likely to benefit.

Risk factors for breast cancer include the following:

- Extremely dense breasts on mammography or a first-degree relative with breast cancer are each associated with at least a twofold increase in breast cancer risk
- Prior benign breast biopsy, second-degree relatives with breast cancer, or heterogeneously dense breasts each increase risk 1.5- to twofold
- Current oral contraceptive use, nulliparity, and age at first birth 30 years and older increase risk 1- to 1.5-fold.[31]

Importantly, these are risk factors for breast cancer diagnosis, not breast cancer mortality. Few studies have assessed the association between these factors and death from breast cancer; however, reproductive factors and breast density have been shown to have limited influence on breast cancer mortality.[32,33]

Genetic testing for *BRCA1* and *BRCA2* mutations and other markers of breast cancer risk has identified a group of women at high risk for breast cancer. Unfortunately, when to begin and the optimal frequency of screening have not been defined. Mammography is less sensitive at detecting breast cancers in women carrying *BRCA1* and *BRCA2* mutations, possibly because such cancers occur in younger women in whom mammography is known to be less sensitive.

MRI screening may be more sensitive than mammography in women at high risk, but specificity is lower. MRIs are associated with both an increase in FP and an increase in the detection of smaller cancers, which are more likely to be biologically indolent. The impact of MRIs on breast cancer mortality with or without concomitant use of mammographies has not been evaluated in a randomized controlled trial.

Breast Density

It is well established that mammogram sensitivity is lower in women with heterogeneously dense or very dense breasts.[29,32] However, at this time, there are no clear guidelines regarding whether or how screening algorithms should take breast density into account.

In the American College of Radiology's Imaging Network (ACRIN)/NCI 666 Trial, breast ultrasound was offered to women with increased mammographic breast density and, if either test was positive, they were referred for a breast biopsy.[34] The radiologists performing the ultrasounds were not aware of the mammographic findings. Mammography detected 7.6 cancers per 1,000 women screened; ultrasound increased the cancer detection rate to 11.8 per 1,000. However, the PPV for mammography alone was 22.6%, whereas the PPV for mammography with ultrasound was only 11.2%.

It has yet to be determined whether supplemental imaging reduces breast cancer mortality in women with increased breast density. Although it continues to be strongly advocated by some, systematic reviews have concluded that the evidence is currently insufficient to recommend for or against this approach.[35] There are also a number of barriers to supplemental imaging, including inconsistent insurance coverage, lack of availability in many communities, concerns about cost-effectiveness (particularly with regard to MRI), and the increased FP rate associated with supplemental imaging leading to unnecessary biopsies.[36]

Newer technologies may improve screening accuracy for women with dense breasts. Compared to conventional mammography, full field digital mammography (FFDM) appears to have less FPs. This could reduce the number of women needing supplemental imaging and biopsies.[37] Digital breast tomosynthesis (DBT) uses x-rays and a digital detector to generate cross-sectional images of the breasts. Data are limited, but compared to mammograms, DBT appears to offer increased sensitivity and a reduction in the recall rates.[38] Another potential supplementary imaging modality currently under investigation is three-dimensional (3-D) automated breast ultrasound, and having screening ultrasounds performed by technologists rather than radiologists.

Ductal Carcinoma In Situ

The incidence of noninvasive ductal carcinoma in situ (DCIS) has increased more than fivefold since 1970 as a direct consequence of widespread screening mammographies.[39] DCIS is a heterogeneous condition with low- and intermediate-grade lesions taking a decade or more to progress. Nevertheless, women with this diagnosis are uniformly subjected to treatment. A better understanding of this entity and an increased ability to predict its biologic behavior may enable more judicious, personalized treatment of DCIS.

There is little evidence that the early detection and aggressive treatment of low- and intermediate-grade DCIS reduces breast cancer mortality. The standard of care for all grades of DCIS is lumpectomy with radiation or mastectomy, followed by tamoxifen for 5 years. Interestingly, patterns of care studies indicate that mastectomy rates are increasing,[40] and that women are more often choosing double mastectomies for the treatment of DCIS.[41] Genomic characterization will hopefully lead to the identification of a subset of noninvasive cancers that can be treated less aggressively or even observed.

Harms

The harms and disadvantages of mammography screening include overdiagnosis, FP tests, FN tests, and the possibility of radiation-induced breast cancer.

The fact that mammography screening has increased the incidence of localized disease without a significant change in metastatic disease at the time of diagnosis suggests that there is some degree of overdiagnosis. The risk of overdiagnosis is greatest at the first screening[3] and varies with patient age, tumor type, and grade of disease.

FP screening tests lead to substantial inconvenience and anxiety in addition to unnecessary invasive biopsies with their attendant complications. In the United States, about 10% of all women screened for breast cancer are called back for additional testing, and less than half of them will be diagnosed with breast cancer.[39] The risk of a FP mammogram is greater for women under the age of 50.[37]

FN tests delay diagnosis and provide false reassurance. They are more common in younger women and in women with dense breasts.[42,43] Certain histologic subtypes are also more difficult to see on mammogram. Mucinous and lobular tumors and rapidly growing tumors tend to blend in with normal breast architecture.[44]

A typical screening mammogram provides approximately 4 mSv of radiation. It has been estimated that annual mammographies will cause up to 1 case of breast cancer per 1,000 women screened from age 40 to age 80 years. Radiation exposure at younger ages causes a greater risk of breast cancer.[45] There is also concern that ionizing radiation from mammographies might disproportionately increase the breast cancer risk for women with certain *BRCA1* or *BRCA2* mutations, because these genes are related to DNA repair.[46]

Recommendations

Women at Average Risk

The ACS and most other medical groups recommend that average risk women undergo a CBE every 3 years starting at age 20 and that women 40 years of age and over should undergo CBEs and screening mammograms annually. Women should be informed of the benefits, limitations, and harms associated with breast cancer screening. A mammography will not detect all breast cancers, and some breast cancers detected with mammographies may still have a poor prognosis. The harms associated with breast cancer screening also include the potential for FP results, causing substantial anxiety. When abnormal findings cannot be resolved with additional imaging, a biopsy is required to rule out the possibility of breast cancer. A majority of biopsies are benign. Finally, some breast cancers detected by a mammography may be biologically indolent, meaning they would not have caused a problem or have been detected in a woman's lifetime had she not undergone a mammography.

The USPSTF, the American College of Physicians, and the Canadian Task Force on the Periodic Health Examination recommend routine screening beginning at age 50 years.[30,47,48] For women aged 40 to 49 years of age, these groups advise physicians to enter into a discussion with the patient. The physician and patient should take into account individual risks and concerns before deciding to screen.[47]

An Advisory Committee on Cancer Prevention in the European Union recommends that women between the ages of 50 and 69 years be offered mammogram screening in an organized screening program with quality assurance.[49] This committee says women aged 40 to 49 years should be advised of the potential harms of screening and, if mammographic screening is offered, it should be performed with strict quality standards and double reading.

Women at High Risk

The ACS has issued guidelines for women who were known or likely carriers of a *BRCA* mutation and other rarer high-risk genetic syndromes, or at high risk for other reasons.[50] Annual screening mammographies and MRIs starting at age 30 is recommended for women:

- With a known *BRCA* mutation
- Who are untested but have a first-degree relative with a *BRCA* mutation
- Who had been treated with radiation to the chest for Hodgkin disease
- Who have an approximately 20% to 25% or greater lifetime risk of breast cancer based on specialized breast cancer risk estimation models.

COLON CANCER SCREENING

Colorectal cancer screening with the rigid sigmoidoscope dates back to the late 1960s. The desire to examine the entire colon led to the use of a barium enema and the development of fecal occult blood tests. With the development of fiber optics, flexible sigmoidoscopies and, later, colonoscopies were employed. Today, fecal occult blood testing (FOBT), stool DNA testing, flexible sigmoidoscopies, colonoscopies, and CT colonographies and, occasionally, barium enemas are all used in colorectal cancer screening. MRI colonoscopy is in development.

Screening examinations of the colon and rectum can find cancer early, but also find precancerous polyps. Randomized trials have demonstrated that endoscopic polypectomies reduce the incidence of colorectal cancer by about 20%.[51–53]

FOBT was the first colorectal screening test studied in a prospective randomized clinical trial. The Minnesota Colon Cancer Control Study randomized 46,551 adults to one of three arms: annual FOBTs, biennial screening, or usual care. A rehydrated guaiac test was used. With 13 years of follow-up, the annual screened arm had a 33% relative reduction in colorectal cancer mortality compared to the usual care group.[54] At 18 years of follow-up, the biennially screened group had a 21% reduction in colorectal cancer mortality.[55] This study would subsequently show that stool blood testing was associated with a 20% reduction in colon cancer incidence.[51] These results were confirmed by two other randomized trials.[56,57] A reduction in colon cancer–specific mortality persisted in the Minnesota trial through 30 years of follow-up. Overall mortality was not affected.

Rehydration increases the sensitivity of FOBT at the expense of lowering specificity.[58] Indeed, rehydrated specimens have a very high FP rate. Overall, 1% to 5% of FOBTs are positive, but only 2% to 10% of those with a positive FOBT have cancer.

Fecal immunochemical tests (FIT) are stool tests that do not react to hemoglobin in dietary products. They appear to have higher sensitivity and specificity for colorectal cancer when compared to nonrehydrated FOBT tests.[59]

Fecal DNA testing is an emerging modality. These tests look for DNA sequences specific to colorectal polyps and colorectal cancer. They may have increased sensitivity and specificity compared to FOBT. Although fecal DNA tests appear to find cancer, the body of evidence on their ability to reduce colorectal cancer mortality is limited due to a lack of study. This test has been intermittently available.

Flexible sigmoidoscopies are, of course, limited to an examination of the rectum and sigmoid colon. A prospective randomized trial of once-only flexible sigmoidoscopies demonstrated a 23% reduction in colorectal cancer incidence and a 31% reduction in colorectal cancer mortality after a median 11.2 years of follow-up.[60] In the NCI's Prostate, Lung, Colorectal, and Ovarian Cancer Screening Trial (PLCO), there was a 21% reduction in colorectal cancer incidence and a 26% reduction in colorectal cancer mortality with two sigmoidoscopies done 3 to 5 years apart compared with the usual care group after a median follow-up of 11.9 years.[53] In both studies, there was no effect on proximal lesions (i.e., right and transverse colon) due to the limited reach of the scope. It is estimated that flexible sigmoidoscopies can find 60% to 80% of cancers and polyps found by colonoscopies.[61]

In two meta-analyses of five randomized controlled trials of sigmoidoscopies, there was an 18% relative reduction in colorectal cancer incidence and a 28% relative reduction in colorectal cancer mortality.[62,63] Participants ranged in age from 50 to 74 years. Follow-up ranged from 6 to 13 years.

The *colonoscopy* has become the preferred screening method of many, although there have been no prospective, randomized trials of colonoscopy screening. A positive FOBT, FIT, fecal DNA test, or sigmoidoscopy warrants a follow-up diagnostic colonoscopy. Perhaps the best support for colonoscopy screening is indirect evidence from the Minnesota Colon Cancer Control Study, which required that all participants with a positive stool blood test have diagnostic imaging of the entire colon. In the Minnesota study, more than 40% of those screened annually eventually received a colonoscopy. One can also make the argument that the sigmoidoscopy studies indirectly support the efficacy of colonoscopy screening, although it can be argued that embryologic and epidemiologic evidence indicate that the right and left colon are biologically distinct and, therefore, the mortality benefits from sigmoidoscopies do not constitute proof that a colonoscopy would similarly reduce mortality from proximal colon lesions.

In studies involving repeat colonoscopies by a second physician, 21% of all adenomas were missed, including 26% of 1 to 5 mm adenomas and 2% of adenomas 10 mm or more in length.[64] Other limitations of colonoscopies include the inconvenience of the bowel preparation and the risk of bowel perforation (about 3 out of 1,000 procedures, overall, with nearly all of the risk among patients who undergo colonoscopic polypectomies). The cost of the procedure and the limited number of physicians who can do the procedure are also of concern.

A *CT colonography* or *virtual* colonoscopy allows a physician to visually reproduce the endoscopic examination on a computer screen. A CT colonography involves the same prep as a colonoscopy, but is less invasive. It might have a higher compliance rate.

In experienced hands, the sensitivity of a CT colonography for the detection of polyps ≥6 mm appears to be comparable to that of a colonoscopy. In a meta-analysis of 30 studies, 2-D and 3-D CT colonographies performed equally well.[65]

The disadvantages of a CT colonography include the fact that it requires a colonic prep and a finding on CT requires a follow-up diagnostic colonoscopy. The rate of extracolonic findings of uncertain significance is high (~15% to 30%), and each one must be evaluated, thereby contributing to additional expense and potential morbidity. The long-term, cumulative radiation risk of repeated colonography screenings is also a concern.

Current Recommendations

The ACS, the American College of Gastroenterology, the American Gastroenterological Association, the American Society for Gastrointestinal Endoscopy, and the American College of Radiology have issued joint colorectal cancer guidelines. These groups consider FOBT, FIT, rigid and flexible sigmoidoscopies, colonoscopies, and CT colonographies to all be reasonable screening methodologies.

They recommend the following: (1) Screening modalities be chosen based on personal preference and access, and (2) average risk adults should begin colorectal cancer screening at age 50 years with *one* of the following options:

1. Annual high sensitivity FOBT or FIT
2. A flexible sigmoidoscopy every 5 years
3. A colonoscopy every 10 years
4. A double contrast barium enema every 5 years
5. A CT colonography every 5 years

No test is of unequivocal superiority. Patient preferences should be incorporated into screening in order to increase compliance. The guidelines also stress that a single screening examination is far from optimal and that patients should be in a program of regular screening.

Although some colorectal cancers are diagnosed in persons under the age of 50 years, screening persons age 40 to 49 years has low yield.[66] The guidelines also state that patients with less than a 10-year life expectancy should not be screened.

The USPSTF issued colorectal cancer screening guidelines in 2008.[67] The guidelines were based on a systematic literature review and decision models. The task force concluded that three screening strategies appear to be equivalent for adults age 50 to 75 years:

1. An annual FOBT with a sensitive test
2. A flexible sigmoidoscopy every 5 years, with a sensitive FOBT every 3 years
3. A colonoscopy every 10 years

The task force recommends that patients age 76 to 85 years be evaluated individually for screening. They found "insufficient evidence" to recommend CT colonographies or fecal DNA testing.

Patients at Increased Risk of Colorectal Cancer

Patients can have higher than average risk of colorectal cancer due to familial or hereditary factors and clinical conditions such as inflammatory bowel disease. These patients technically undergo surveillance and not screening. Nevertheless, there are few clinical studies to guide recommendations. Guidelines have been created based on professional opinion and an understanding of the biology of colorectal cancer (Table 34.5).[68]

OTHER CANCERS OF THE GASTROINTESTINAL TRACT

There are no widely accepted screening guidelines for cancers of the esophagus, stomach, pancreas, and liver. However, surveillance is advocated for some patients at high risk.

Esophageal Cancer Screening

Esophageal cancer screening has centered on endoscopic examinations for those at high risk due to chronic, severe gastroesophageal reflux disease.[69] Some physicians advocate routine endoscopic surveillance of patients with Barrett esophagus. At this time, there is no evidence that such surveillance is effective at reducing cancer mortality.

TABLE 34.5

Colon Cancer Screening Recommendations for People with Familial or Inherited Risk

Familial Risk Category	Screening Recommendation
First-degree relative[a] affected with *colorectal cancer* or an *adenomatous polyp* at age ≥60 years, or two second-degree relatives[b] affected with colorectal *cancer*	Same as average risk but starting at age 40 years
Two or more first-degree relatives with *colon cancer*, or a single first-degree relative with *colon cancer* or *adenomatous polyps* diagnosed at an age <60 years	Colonoscopy every 5 years, beginning at age 40 years or 10 years younger than the earliest diagnosis in the family, whichever comes first
One second-degree or any third-degree relative[b,c] with *colorectal cancer*	Same as average risk
Gene *carrier* or *at risk* for familial adenomatous polyposis[d]	Sigmoidoscopy annually, beginning at age 10–12 years[e]
Gene carrier or at risk for HNPCC	Colonoscopy, every 1–2 years, beginning at age 20–25 years or 10 years younger than the earliest case in the family, whichever comes first

[a] First-degree relatives include patients, siblings, and children.
[b] Second-degree relatives include grandparents, aunts, and uncles.
[c] Third-degree relatives include great-grandparents and cousins.
[d] Includes the subcategories of familial adenomatous polyposis, Gardner syndrome, some Turcot syndrome families, and attenuated adenomatous polyposis coli (AAPC).
[e] In AAPC, colonoscopy should be used instead of sigmoidoscopy because of the preponderance of proximal colonic adenomas. Colonoscopy screening in AAPC should probably begin in the late teens or early 20s.
HNPCC, hereditary nonpolyposis colon cancer.
From Winawer S, Fletcher R, Rex D, et al. Colorectal cancer screening and surveillance: clinical guidelines and rationale: update based on new evidence. *Gastroenterology* 2003;124:544–560, with permission.

Gastric Cancer Screening

Barium-meal photofluorography, serum pepsinogen, and gastric endoscopy have been proposed as screening methods for the early detection of gastric cancer. There are no randomized trials evaluating the impact of these modalities on gastric cancer mortality. Indeed, screening with barium-meal photofluorography has been studied in high-risk populations for more than 40 years without clear evidence of benefit.

Time-trend analysis and case control studies of gastric endoscopy have suggested a decrease in gastric cancer mortality among those at high risk in screened versus unscreened individuals; however, a large observational study in a high-risk population failed to demonstrate a benefit.[70,71]

Although widespread gastric screenings cannot be advocated, there may be justification for endoscopic screenings of high-risk populations. Candidates for screening might include elderly individuals with atrophic gastritis or pernicious anemia, patients who have had partial gastrectomy,[72] those with a history of sporadic adenomas, and patients with familial adenomatous polyposis or hereditary nonpolyposis colon cancer.

Pancreatic Cancer Screening

At this time, there are no data from prospective clinical trials to support a role for pancreatic cancer screening. Some patients with an extensive family history have undergone periodic CT scanning of the abdomen, but this approach has not been shown to reduce pancreatic cancer mortality. There is an ongoing search for screening biomarkers. There is a need to follow large cohorts prospectively after collecting and storing biologic samples to identify biomarkers of risk.[73]

Liver Cancer Screening

Screening for liver cancer or hepatocellular carcinoma (HCC) has focused on very high-risk individuals, such as those with cirrhosis.[54] To date, trial results are unreliable due to small study sizes and a lack of randomization.

Serum alpha-fetoprotein (AFP), a fetal-specific glycoprotein antigen, is an HCC tumor marker used in screening. It is not specific to HCC because it may be elevated in hepatitis, pregnancy, and some germ cell tumors. AFP has variable sensitivity and has not been tested in any randomized clinical trial with a mortality end point.

In one prospective, 16-year, population-based observational study, screening was done on 1,487 Alaska natives with chronic hepatis B virus (HBV) infection. The survival of those with screen-detected HCC was compared with a historical group of clinically diagnosed HCC patients.[74] With a target of AFP determination every 6 months, there was a 97% sensitivity and 95% specificity for HCC. Such high sensitivity and specificity have not been found in other studies. It is not known if AFP screening decreases HCC mortality.[75]

Hepatic ultrasound has been used as an additional method for detection of HCC. This procedure is operator dependent with variable sensitivity and specificity. Ultrasound screening is commonly used in patients with hepatitis and cirrhosis.[76,77]

Interest in CT scanning has grown due to the limitations of AFP and ultrasound. CT scans may be a more sensitive test for HCC than ultrasound or AFP.[75]

GYNECOLOGIC CANCER

Cervical Cancer Screening

Dr. George Papanicolaou first introduced the Pap smear or Pap test in the early 1940s. The test was widely adopted based on its ability to identify squamous premalignancies and malignancies (from the ectodermal cervix) and glandular dysplasia and adenocarcinomas (from the endocervix). It is, however, more sensitive at detecting squamous lesions.

The Pap test was introduced before the advent of the prospective, randomized clinical trial and, therefore, has never been so tested. However, a number of observational studies over the past 60 years support the effectiveness of this screening test.[78,79] Multiple ecologic studies have shown an inverse correlation between the introduction of Pap testing in a given country and reductions in both cervical cancer incidence and mortality.[80] Importantly, mortality reductions in these studies have been proportional to the intensity of screening. In one series, more than half of women diagnosed with cervical cancer either had never had a Pap test or had not been screened within 5 years of diagnosis.[80]

Cervical cytology has evolved over the years. The original Pap smear used an ectocervical spatula to apply a specimen ("smear") to glass slides. It later included an endocervical brush. The smear was fixed, stained, and manually examined under a microscope. That method is still used today, but a liquid-based/thin-layer system capable of being analyzed by computer is gaining in popularity.[81]

Human papillomavirus (HPV) 16 and 18 are the cause of more than 70% of cervical cancers. Thirteen other HPV subtypes are known to be associated with cervical cancer. With increasing understanding of the role of HPV in cervical disease, interest in developing tests to determine the presence of HPV DNA and RNA has grown. HPV screening can be used along with cytology (*cotesting*), in response to an abnormal cytologic test (*reflexive testing*), or as a stand-alone test. One advantage of the liquid-based/thin-layer tests over the older smears is that it makes reflexive testing easier to perform. An abnormal cytology screen can be objectively verified by testing for the presence of the HPV virus without calling the patient back.

HPV testing is especially useful because of its negative predictive value. Although a positive test for HPV infection is not diagnostic of cervical disease, a negative HPV test strongly suggests that the abnormal Pap does not represent a premalignant condition.

The utility of the HPV test is limited in younger women because one-third or more of women in their 20s have active cervical infections at any given time. The overwhelming majority of these infections and resultant dysplasia will regress and resolve within 8 to 24 months. For women over the age of 30, screening for the presence of HPV DNA or RNA appears to be superior to cytology in identifying women at risk for cervical dysplasia and cancer.[82] An HPV infection in women over the age of 30 is more likely to be persistent and clinically significant.[83] The risk of cervical cancer also increases with age, and most cervical cancer deaths occur in women over 50 years of age.

Cytologic Terminology

The terminology of the Pap smear has changed over time. The traditional cytologic categories were mild, moderate, and severe dysplasia and carcinoma in situ. *Mild* correlated with cervical intraepithelial neoplasia (CIN)1 histology on biopsy; *moderate* usually indicated CIN2; and *severe* dysplasia indicated CIN3 or carcinoma in situ.

There was some subjectivity and some overlap, especially in the area of mild and moderate dysplasia. The NCI sponsored the development of the Bethesda system in 1988. This system provides an assessment of the adequacy of the cervical specimen and a way of categorizing and describing the Pap smear findings. It more effectively and uniformly communicates cytology results from the laboratory to the patient caregiver. The Bethesda system was modified in 1991 and again in 2001.[84] Today, more than 40 international professional societies have endorsed the Bethesda system.

The Bethesda system recognizes both squamous and glandular cytologic abnormalities.

Squamous cell abnormalities include:

- Atypical squamous cells (ASC), which are categorized as either:
  - Of undetermined significance (ASC-US)
  - Cannot exclude high-grade squamous intraepithelial lesions (ASC-H)
- Low-grade squamous intraepithelial lesion (LSIL), which correlates with histologic CIN1
- High-grade squamous intraepithelial lesion (HSIL), which correlates with histologic CIN2, CIN3, and carcinoma in situ

Glandular cell abnormalities (features suggestive of adenocarcinoma) include:

- Atypical glandular cells (AGC): endocervical, endometrial, or not otherwise specified
- AGCs, favor neoplastic
- Endocervical or not otherwise specified
- Endocervical adenocarcinoma in situ (AIS)
- Adenocarcinoma

ASCs differ from normal cells but do not meet criteria for LSIL or HSIL. A small proportion of ASC-US smears are from CIN1 lesions; a smaller proportion are from CIN2 or 3. LSILs are usually due to a transient HPV infection. HSILs are more likely to be due to a persistent HPV infection and are more likely to progress to cervical cancer than LSILs.

The Lower Anogenital Squamous Terminology (LAST) project of the College of American Pathology and the American Society for Colposcopy and Cervical Pathology has proposed that histologic cervical findings be described using the same terminology as cytologic findings.[85]

Women under the age of 30 who have not received the HPV vaccine have a high incidence of HPV infection[86] and the highest prevalence of CIN. However, the overwhelming majority of these HPV infections and associated CIN will spontaneously regress.[87,88] Due to the high regression rates, cervical screening and treatment in women aged 20 to 24 years appear to have little or no impact on the incidence of invasive cervical cancer. It is estimated that about 6% of CIN1 lesions progress to CIN3, and 10% to 20% of CIN3 lesions progress to invasive cancer.[89]

The Atypical Squamous Cells of Undetermined Significance (ASCUS)-LSIL Triage Study (ALTS) evaluated women with abnormal Pap smears.[90] The investigators concluded that women with ASC-US should be tested for HPV. Those who are HPV positive should receive a colposcopy. In addition, because most women with LSIL or HSIL had an HPV infection, an immediate colposcopy and a biopsy of lesions was recommended.[91] HPV DNA testing is very sensitive for identifying CIN2 or worse pathology. Among women 30 to 69 years of age, the sensitivity of the Pap test with HPV testing was 95% compared with 55% for the Pap test alone.[92]

Performance Characteristics of Cervical Cytology

The sensitivity of cytology varies and is a function of the adequacy of the cervical specimen. It is also affected by the age of the woman and the experience of the cytologist. The addition of HPV testing increases the number of women referred for a colposcopy. Not surprisingly, sensitivity is improved by serial examinations over time versus a single screen.

Screening Recommendations

Cervical screening, like other screening tests, is associated with some degree of overdiagnosis as evidenced by the phenomenon of spontaneous regression (see previous) and, therefore, potential harm from overtreatment, such as cervical incompetence, which may reduce fertility and the ability to carry a pregnancy to term. Because dysplasia takes years to progress to cervical cancer, increasing the screening interval can reduce overdiagnosis and excessive treatment without decreasing screening efficacy.

In 2012, the ACS, the American Society for Colposcopy and Cervical Pathology (ASCCP), and the American Society for Clinical Pathology (ASCP) issued joint screening guidelines.[93] These guidelines recommend different surveillance strategies and options based on a woman's age, screening history, risk factors, and choice of screening tests. The following are the recommendations for a woman at average risk.

- Screening for cervical cancer should begin at 21 years of age. Women aged 21 to 29 years should receive cytology screening (with either conventional cervical cytology smears or liquid-based cytology) every 3 years. HPV testing should not be performed in this age group (although it can be used to follow-up a diagnosis of ASC-US). Women under 21 years of age should not be screened regardless of their age of sexual initiation.
- For women aged 30 to 65 years, the preferred approach is to be screened every 5 years with both HPV testing and cytology (*cotesting*). It is also acceptable to continue screening every 3 years with cytology alone.
- Women should discontinue screening after age 65 years if they have had three consecutive negative cytology tests or two consecutive negative HPV test results within the 10-year period before ceasing screening, with the most recent test occurring within the last 5 years.
- Women who have undergone a hysterectomy for noncancerous conditions do not need to undergo cervical cancer screening.
- Women, regardless of age, should NOT be screened annually by any screening method.
- Women who have received HPV vaccinations should still be screened according to the previously listed schedule.

Screening in Low Resource Countries

Cytology and HPV testing is not widely available in much of the world. Cervical cancer remains a leading cause of death in many of these areas. Visual inspection of the cervix is a low-tech method of screening that is now recognized as having the potential to save thousands of lives per year. A clustered, randomized trial in India compared one-time cervical visual inspection and immediate colposcopy, biopsy, and/or cryotherapy (where indicated) versus counseling on cervical cancer deaths in women aged 30 to 59 years. After 7 years of follow-up, the age-standardized rate of death due to cervical cancer was 39.6 per 100,000 person-years in the intervention group versus 56.7 per 100,000 person-years in unscreened controls.[94,95] This was the first prospective randomized clinical trial to evaluate cervical cancer screening.

Ovarian Cancer Screening

Modalities proposed for ovarian cancer screening include the bimanual pelvic examination, serum CA-125 antigen measurement, and transvaginal ultrasound (TVU). The bimanual pelvic examination is subjective and not very reproducible, but serum CA-125 can be objectively measured. Unfortunately, CA-125 is neither sensitive nor specific. It is elevated in only about half of women with ovarian cancer and may be elevated in a number of nonmalignant diseases (e.g., diverticulosis, endometriosis, cirrhosis, normal menstruation, pregnancy, uterine fibroids).[96–98] TVU has shown poor performance in the detection of ovarian cancer in average and high-risk women.[99] There is interest in the analysis of serum proteomic patterns, but this should be considered experimental.[100,101]

The combination of CA-125 and TVU has been assessed in two large, prospective randomized trials. The U.S. trial, the Prostate Lung Colorectal and Ovarian trial (PLCO), enrolled

78,216 women of average risk age 55 to 74 years.[102,103] Participants were randomized to receive annual examinations with CA-125 (at entry and then annually for 5 years) and TVU (at entry and then annually for 3 years) (n = 39,105), or usual care (n = 39,111). Participants were followed for a maximum of 13 years, with mortality from ovarian cancer as the main study outcome. At the conclusion of the study, the number of deaths from ovarian cancer was similar in each group. There were 3.1 ovarian cancer deaths per 10,000 women years in the screened group versus 2.6 deaths per 10,000 women years in the control group (RR = 1.18; 95% CI, 0.82 to 1.71).[103]

The U.K. Collaborative Trial of Ovarian Cancer Screening (UKCTOCS) is a randomized trial assessing the efficacy of CA-125 and TVU in more than 200,000 postmenopausal women. In this trial, CA-125 is being used as a first-line test and TVU as a follow-up test using a risk of ovarian cancer algorithm (ROCA).[104] The ROCA measures changes in CA-125 over time rather than using a predefined cut point.[105] ROCA is believed to improve sensitivity for smaller tumors without measurably increasing the FP rate. A mortality assessment is expected in 2015.[106]

No organization currently recommends screening average risk women for ovarian cancer. In 2012, the USPSTF recommended against screening for ovarian cancer, concluding that there was "adequate evidence" that (1) annual screening with TVU and CA-125 does not reduce ovarian cancer mortality and (2) screening for ovarian cancer can lead to important harms, mainly surgical interventions in women without ovarian cancer.[107]

Women at High Risk for Ovarian Cancer

Although no study has shown a mortality benefit for ovarian cancer screening of high-risk individuals, a National Institutes of Health (NIH) consensus panel concluded that it was prudent for women with a known hereditary ovarian cancer syndrome, such as *BRCA1/2* mutations or HNPCC, to have annual rectovaginal pelvic examinations, CA-125 determinations, and TVU until childbearing is completed or at least until age 35 years, at which time a prophylactic bilateral oophorectomy is recommended.[108]

Endometrial Cancer Screening

There is insufficient evidence to recommend endometrial cancer screening either for women at average risk or for those at increased risk due to a history of unopposed estrogen therapy, tamoxifen therapy, late menopause, nulliparity, infertility or failure to ovulate, obesity, diabetes, or hypertension.[109] The ACS recommends that women be informed about the symptoms of endometrial cancer—in particular, vaginal bleeding and spotting—after the onset of menopause. Women should be encouraged to immediately report these symptoms to their physician.

Women at High Risk for Endometrial Cancer

Women with a suspected autosomal-dominant predisposition to colon cancer (e.g. Lynch syndrome), should consider undergoing an annual endometrial biopsy to evaluate endometrial histology, beginning at age 35 years.[110,111] This is based only on *expert opinion*, given the paucity of clinical trial data. Women should be informed about the potential benefits, harms, and limitations of testing for early endometrial cancer.

LUNG CANCER SCREENING

Lung cancer screening programs using chest radiographs (CXR) and sputum cytology began in the late 1940s.[112] An evaluation of these programs showed that screening led to the diagnosis of an increased number of cancers, an increased proportion of early stage cancers, and a larger proportion of screen-diagnosed patients surviving more than 5 years.

These findings led many to advocate for mass lung cancer screening, whereas others called for a prospective, randomized trial with a lung cancer mortality endpoint.[113] The Mayo Lung Project (MLP), which began in 1971, was such a trial. More than 9,200 male smokers were enrolled and randomized to either have sputum cytology collected and CXRs done every 4 months for 6 years or to have these same tests performed annually.

At 13 years of follow-up, there were more early stage cancers in the intensively screened arm (n = 99) than in the control arm (n = 51), but the number of advanced tumors was nearly identical (107 versus 109, respectively).[114] Despite an increase in 5-year survival (35% versus 15%) intensive screening was not associated with a reduction in lung cancer mortality (3.2 versus 3.0 deaths per 1,000 person-years, respectively).[115]

The impact of screening on cancer incidence persisted through nearly 20 years of follow-up. There were 585 lung cancers diagnosed on the intensive screening arm versus 500 on the control arm (p = 0.009) and intensive screening continued to be associated with a significant increase in disease-specific survival. However, a concomitant decrease in lung-cancer mortality did not emerge with long-term follow-up (4.4 lung cancer deaths per 1,000 person-years in the intensively screened arm versus 3.9 per 1,000 person-years in the control arm).[116] This suggests that some lung cancers diagnosed by screening would not have resulted in death had they not been detected (i.e., overdiagnosis).[116]

Two other large, randomized studies of CXR and sputum cytology were conducted in the United States during the same time period. All three studies evaluated different screening schedules rather than screening versus no screening. Paradoxically, a meta-analysis of the three studies found that more frequent screening was associated with an increase (albeit not statistically significant), rather than a decrease, in lung cancer mortality when compared with less frequent screening.[117] A study conducted in Czechoslovakia in the 1980s also failed to show a reduction in lung cancer mortality with CXR screening.[118]

More recently, the NCI conducted the PLCO trial at 10 sites across the United States. This was a prospective, randomized trial of nearly 155,000 men and women, aged 55 to 74 years. Participants were randomized to receive annual, single-view, posteroanterior CXRs for 4 years versus routine care. With 13 years of follow-up, no significant difference in lung cancer mortality was observed. A total of 1,213 lung cancer deaths occurred on the intervention arm versus 1,230 in the control group (RR, 0.99; 95% CI, 0.87 to 1.22).[119]

Low-dose computerized tomography (LDCT) is an appealing technology for lung cancer screening. It uses an average of 1.5 mSv of radiation to perform a lung scan in 15 seconds. A conventional CT scan uses 8 mSv of radiation and takes several minutes. The LDCT image is not as sharp as the conventional image, but sensitivity and specificity for the detection of lung lesions are similar.

As in the early chest radiograph trials, a number of single-arm LDCT studies reported a substantial increase in the number of early stage lung cancers diagnosed. These studies also demonstrated that 5-year survival rates were increased in screened compared to unscreened populations.

These findings led to the conduct of several randomized trials of LDCT for the early detection of lung cancer. The largest, longest, and first to report a mortality end point is the National Lung Screening Trial (NLST). In this trial, approximately 53,000 persons were randomized to receive three annual LDCT scans or single-view posteroanterior CXRs. Eligible participants were current and former smokers between 55 and 74 years of age at the time of randomization with at least a 30 pack-year smoking history; former smokers were eligible if they had quit smoking within the previous 15 years.

With a median follow-up of 6.5 years, 13% more lung cancers were diagnosed and a 20% (95% CI, 6.8 to 26.7; p = 0.004)

CANCER PREVENTION AND SCREENING

relative reduction in lung cancer mortality was observed in the LDCT arm compared to the CXR arm.[11] This corresponds to rates of death from lung cancer of 247 and 309 per 100,000 person-years, respectively.[11] Another important finding from the NLST was a 6.7% (95% CI, 1.2 to 13.6; $p = 0.02$) decrease in death from any cause in the LDCT group.

NLST participants were at high risk for developing lung cancer based on their smoking history. Indeed, 25% of all participant deaths were due to lung cancer. A further analysis of the NLST shows that screening prevented the greatest number of lung cancer deaths among participants who were at the highest risk but prevented very few deaths among those at the lowest risk. These findings provide empirical support for risk-based screening.[120]

LDCT screening is clearly promising, but there are some notable caveats. The risk of a FP finding in the first screen was 21%. Overall, after three CT scans, 39.1% of participants had at least one positive screening result. Of those who screened positive, the FP rate was 96.4% in the LDCT group.[11] Positive results require additional workup, which can include conventional CT scans, a needle biopsy, bronchoscopy, mediastinoscopy, or thoracotomy. These diagnostic procedures are associated with anxiety, expense, and complications (e.g., pneumo- or hemothorax after a lung biopsy). In the LDCT study arm, there were 16 deaths within 60 days of an invasive diagnostic procedure. Of the 16 deaths, 6 ultimately did not have cancer. Although it is not known whether these deaths were directly caused by the invasive procedure, such findings do give pause. Although the radiation dose from LDCT is low, the possibility that this screening test could cause radiation-induced cancers is at least a theoretical concern. The possibility of this long-term phenomenon will have to be assessed in future analyses.

The CXR lung screening studies suggested that there is a reservoir of biologically indolent lung cancer and that a percentage of screen-detected lung cancers represent overdiagnosis. The estimated rate of overdiagnosis in the long-term follow-up of the Mayo Lung Study and the other CXR studies was 17 to 18.5%.[121] Similarly, it is estimated that 18.5% of the cancers diagnosed on the LDCT arm of the NLST represented overdiagnosis.[122]

There are estimates that widespread, high-quality screening has the potential to prevent 12,000 lung cancer deaths per year in the United States.[123] However, the NLST was performed at 33 centers specifically chosen for their expertise in the screening, diagnosis, and treatment of lung cancer. It is not known whether the widespread adoption of LDCT lung cancer screening will result in higher complication rates and a less favorable risk–benefit ratio.

Although LDCT lung cancer screening should clearly be considered for those at high risk of the disease, those at lower risk are equally likely to suffer the harms associated with screening but less likely to reap the benefits.

Following the announcement of the NLST results, the ACS, the American College of Chest Physicians (AACP), the American Society of Clinical Oncology (ASCO), and the National Comprehensive Cancer Network (NCCN) recommended that clinicians should initiate a discussion about lung cancer screening with patients who would have qualified for the trial. That is:

- Age 55 to 74 years
- At least a 30 pack-year smoking history
- Currently smoke or have quit within the past 15 years
- Relatively good health

Core elements of this discussion should include the benefits, uncertainties, and harms associated with screening for lung cancer with LDCT. Adults who choose to be screened should enter an organized screening program at an institution with expertise in LDCT screening, with access to a multidisciplinary team skilled in the evaluation, diagnosis, and treatment of abnormal lung lesions. If such a program is not available, the risks of harm due to screening may be greater than the benefits.[124,125] The guidelines recommend an annual LDCT screening with the caveat that participants in NLST had only three annual screens.

The USPSTF guidelines give LDCT a grade B recommendation, concluding that there is moderate certainty that annual screening for lung cancer with LDCT is of moderate net benefit in asymptomatic persons at high risk for lung cancer based on age, total cumulative exposure to tobacco smoke, and years since quitting.

PROSTATE CANCER SCREENING

Hugh Hampton Young first advocated the early detection of prostate cancer with a careful digital rectal examination (DRE) in 1903. Screening for prostate cancer with the DRE and serum PSA was first advocated in the mid 1980s and became commonplace by 1992. PSA screening is directly responsible for prostate cancer becoming the most common nonskin cancer in American men.

PSA is a glycoprotein produced almost exclusively by the epithelial component of the prostate gland. This protein was discovered in the late 1970s, and a serum test to measure circulating levels was developed in the early 1980s. Although PSA is prostate specific, it is not prostate cancer specific and may be elevated in a variety of conditions (e.g., benign prostatic hyperplasia, inflammation and following trauma to the gland, the presence of prostate cancer).

The PSA test has been widely advocated for prostate cancer screening because it is objective, easily measured, reproducible, noninvasive, and inexpensive. Although PSA screening increases the detection of potentially curable disease, there is substantial debate about the overall utility of the test. This is because PSA screening introduces substantial lead time and length bias as well as being associated with a high FN and FP rates and having a low positive predictive value. The prostate cancer conundrum was best summarized by the distinguished urologist, Willet Whitmore when he said, "Is cure necessary for those in whom it is possible? Is cure possible for those in whom it is necessary?"[126]

Observational studies suggest that the problem of prostate cancer overdiagnosis precedes the PSA era. In a landmark analysis with 20-year follow-up, only a small proportion of 767 men, diagnosed with localized prostate cancer in the 1970s and early 1980s and followed expectantly, died from prostate cancer: 4% to 7% of those with Gleason 2 to 4 tumors, 6% to 11% of those with Gleason 5 disease, and 18% to 30% of men with Gleason 6 cancer.[127]

Although obviously present in the pre-PSA era, overdiagnosis increased substantially after the introduction of PSA screening. This is illustrated by an examination of the prostate cancer incidence and mortality rates in Washington state and Connecticut. Due to the earlier uptake of PSA screening, the incidence of prostate cancer in Washington increased to twice that of Connecticut during the 1990s. However, mortality rates remained similar throughout the decade and, in fact, have remained similar to this day. The Surveillance, Epidemiology, and End Results (SEER) cancer registries show that, over the last 2 decades, a larger proportion of men living in western Washington have been diagnosed with prostate cancer and definitively treated, without a concomitant reduction in prostate cancer mortality compared to that of men living in Connecticut.[128]

Additional evidence of the potential for overdiagnosis comes from the unexpectedly large number of men diagnosed with prostate cancer in the Prostate Cancer Prevention Trial (PCPT). The PCPT was a prospective, randomized, placebo-controlled trial of finasteride for prostate cancer prevention. Men were screened annually during this trial, and those who had not been diagnosed with prostate cancer after 7 years on-study were asked to undergo an end-of-study prostate biopsy. Of 4,692 men on the placebo arm whose prostate cancer status had been determined by biopsy or transurethral resection (TURP), 24.4% were diagnosed with prostate cancer. Given that the lifetime risk of prostate cancer mortality in the United States is less than 3%, it is clear that many men harbor indolent prostate cancer and, therefore, are at risk of being overdiagnosed.

The unexpectantly high rate of positive end-of-study biopsies in men with PSA levels less than or equal to 4.0 ng/mL provided a more accurate assessment of disease prevalence and thus a more accurate assessment of PSA sensitivity than was previously possible. Of the 2,950 men on the placebo arm of the PCPT with PSA levels consistently less than or equal to 4 ng/mL who underwent end-of-study biopsies, 449 (15.2%) were diagnosed with prostate cancer. Accordingly, a PSA level <4.0 ng/mL is more likely to be a *false* negative. Because Sensitivity = True Positives / (True Positives + False Negatives), a higher FN rate means a lower sensitivity at any given PSA threshold. This has prompted some to advocate using a lower PSA threshold for recommending biopsies. However, although lowering the PSA threshold from 4.0 to 2.5 ng/mL increases the sensitivity from 24% to 42.8%, it reduces specificity from 92.7% to an unacceptably low 80%.[129]

In the PCPT, cancer was found on end-of-study biopsies at all PSA levels (e.g., including 10% of biopsies in men with PSA levels between 0.6 and 1.0 ng/mL and 6% of biopsies in men with PSA levels between 0 and 0.6 were positive), suggesting a continuum of prostate cancer risk and no cut point with simultaneously high sensitivity and high specificity. High-grade disease was also documented at all PSA levels, albeit at an overall frequency of only 2.3% of men with PSAs <4 ng/mL.[130,131]

Does Prostate Cancer Treatment Prevent Deaths?

In order for screening to work, treatment has to work. The first prospective, randomized studies showing that any prostate cancer treatment saves lives were published in the late 1990s. These studies demonstrated an overall survival benefit for the addition of long-term androgen deprivation to radiation therapy in men with locally advanced, high-risk prostate cancer.[132]

The value of surgery for localized disease was assessed by the Scandinavian Prostate Cancer Group 4 study (SPCG-4). In this trial, 695 men with clinically localized prostate cancer were prospectively randomized to receive radical prostatectomy (RP) or watchful waiting (WW). In the expectant management group, hormonal therapy was given at the time of symptomatic metastases. About 60% of those enrolled had low-grade, 23% had moderate-grade, 5% had high-grade tumors, and 12% had tumors of unknown grade. At a median follow-up of 12.8 years, the RP group had significantly lower overall (RR 0.75; p = 0.007) and prostate cancer–specific mortality (RR 0.62; p = 0.01), with 14.6% of the PR group and 20.7% of the WW group having died of prostate cancer. The number needed to treat or prevent one prostate cancer death was 15. The survival benefit associated with RP was similar before and after 9 years of follow-up and for men with low and high-risk disease. However, a subset analysis suggested that the mortality benefit of surgery was limited to men less than 65 years of age. An important limitation of this trial is that 75% of the study participants had palpable disease, only 12% had nonpalpable disease, and only 5% of the cancers had been screen detected. It is, therefore, difficult to apply these data to the US prostate cancer population, which is dominated by nonpalpable, screen-detected disease.[133]

In contrast to the SPCG-4, the Prostate Intervention versus Observation Trial (PIVOT) was conducted in the United States during the early PSA era. In this study, 731 men with screen-detected prostate cancer were randomized to receive RP or WW. Of the participants, 50% had nonpalpable disease and, using established criteria for PSA levels, grade, and tumor stage, 43% of men had low-risk, 36% had intermediate-risk, and 21% had high-risk prostate cancer. With a median follow-up of 12 years, during which time 48.4% (354 of 731) of the study participants had died, RP was associated with statistically insignificant 2.9% and 2.6% absolute reductions in overall and prostate cancer–specific mortality, respectively. Subgroup analyses suggested mortality benefits for men with PSA values greater than 10 ng/mL and for those with intermediate- and high-risk disease.[134]

The Prospective Randomized Screening Trials

The PLCO Cancer Screening Trial was a multicenter, phase III trial conducted in the United States by the NCI. In this trial, nearly 77,000 men age 55 to 74 years were randomized to receive annual PSA testing for 6 years or usual care. At 13 years of follow-up, a nonsignificant increase in cumulative prostate cancer mortality was observed among men randomized to annual screening (RR, 1.09; 95% CI, 0.87 to 1.36).[135] The most important limitation of this trial was the high rate of PSA testing among men randomized to the control arm. This *drop-in* or *contamination* served to reduce the statistical power of the study to detect differences in outcome between the two arms. It has also been argued that, due to the high rate of PSA screening on the control arm, PLCO effectively compared regular prostate cancer screening to opportunistic screening rather than comparing screening to no screening.

The ERSPC is a multicenter trial initiated in 1991 in the Netherlands and Belgium; five additional European countries joined between 1994 and 1998.[136,137] The frequency of PSA testing was every 4 years in all countries except Sweden, in which it was every 2 years. The study results were initially reported in 2009 and updated in 2012.[136,137] Although the overall analysis of 182,160 men, aged 50 to 74, did not show a reduction in prostate cancer–specific mortality, screening was associated with a significant decrease in prostate cancer mortality in the prespecified core age group, 55 to 69 years, which included 162,243 men. After a median follow-up of 11 years, a 21% relative reduction of prostate cancer death (RR, 0.79; 95% CI, 0.68 to 0.91) was observed in this group. In absolute terms, prostate cancer mortality was reduced from 5 to 4 men per 1,000 screened and 37 men had to be diagnosed to avert one prostate cancer death. It remains to be seen whether the benefits of screening will increase with continued follow-up.

The recruitment and randomization procedures of the ERSPC differed among countries. Notably, potential participants in Finland, Sweden, and Italy were identified from population registries and underwent randomization *before* written informed consent was obtained. In some trials, men on the control arm were not aware they were in the study. Therefore, men on the intervention arm in these countries were more likely to be cared for at high-volume referral centers. This may have contributed to the higher proportion of men on the screening arm, with clinically localized cancer being treated with RPs.[138]

In a separate report on 20,000 men randomized to screening or a control group in Göteborg, Sweden, there was a 40% (95% CI, 1.50 to 1.80) risk reduction at 14 years of follow-up.[139] They reported 293 (95% CI, 177 to 799) needed to be screened and 12 needed to be diagnosed in order to prevent one prostate cancer death. Three-fourths of the men in this report and 89% of the prostate cancer deaths were included in the published ERSPC analysis. Given this, these data do not constitute independent evidence of the efficacy of prostate cancer screening.

The other site to report separately was in Finland. A total of 80,144 men were randomized to a screening or usual care arm. At 12 years after randomization, there was no statistical difference in risk of prostate cancer death (hazard ratio [HR] = 0.85; 95% CI, 0.69 to 1.04).[140] Possible explanations as to why Sweden and Finland would have such different outcomes include differences in the frequency of screening (every 2 years versus every 4 years, respectively) and the higher background rate of death from prostate cancer in the control group in the Goteborg cohort. Given that the mortality data from these two cohorts have been largely included in the ERSPC analyses, they do not provide independent evidence of the efficacy of prostate cancer screening.

The decline in prostate cancer mortality in the United States since the introduction of PSA screening 2 decades ago is often offered as evidence supporting a mortality benefit for prostate cancer screening. However, prostate cancer mortality rates have also declined in many countries that have not widely adopted screening.[141] Thus, it is likely that improvements in treatment have contributed, at least in part, to the observed decline in prostate cancer mortality. Another possible contributing factor may be the World Health Organization (WHO) algorithm for adjudicating cause of death. A change occurred just as mortality rates began to go up in the late 1970s, and WHO changed back to the older algorithm in 1991 when prostate cancer mortality began declining in many countries.[142] All of these factors, including a beneficial effect from screening, may be contributing to the declining prostate cancer mortality rates in the United States.

Screening Recommendations

The topic of prostate cancer screening tends to evoke strong emotional reactions. Although the intuitive appeal of early detection is undeniable and screening may save some lives, the magnitude of the mortality reduction is relatively small, whereas the harms associated with screening can be substantial. Whether the potential benefits outweigh the known harms is a question that each man must answer for himself based on his individual preferences.

Several professional organizations in the United States, Europe, and Canada have recently reviewed the screening data and issued screening guidelines. All acknowledge that legitimate concerns remain regarding the risk–benefit ratio of prostate cancer screening. There is also general agreement that prostate cancer screening should only be done in the context of fully informed consent and that men should know that experts do not agree as to whether the benefits of screening for this disease outweigh the harms. Most recommend against mass screening in public meeting places, malls, churches, etc.

In 2009, the American Urological Association (AUA) PSA Best Practice Statement was published, which stated, "Given the uncertainty that PSA testing results in more benefit than harm, a thoughtful and broad approach to PSA is critical. Patients need to be informed of the risks and the benefits of testing before it is undertaken. The risks of over-detection and over-treatment should be included in this discussion."[143]

In 2010, the ACS updated their guidelines, stating that the balance of benefits and harms related to prostate cancer early detection are uncertain and the existing evidence is insufficient to support a recommendation for or against the routine use of PSA screening.[144] The ACS called for discussion and shared decision making within the physician–patient relationship.

The most recent 2012 USPSTF guidelines recommend against the use of PSA screening on the basis that there is moderate certainty that the harms of PSA testing outweigh the benefits and, on that basis, recommended against PSA-based screening for all men.[14] The task force did acknowledge that some men will continue to request screening and some physicians will continue to offer it. Like the ACS and AUA, they state that screening under such circumstances should respect patient preferences.

In 2013, the AUA conducted a systematic review of over 300 studies. They recommended against screening men younger than 40 years of age, and against screening average-risk men age 40 to 54 years, most men over 70 years of age, and men with a life expectancy of less than 10 to 15 years. They recommend that screening decisions be individualized for higher risk men ages 40 to 54 years and men over 70 years of age who are in excellent health. They placed primacy on shared decision making versus physician judgments about the balance of benefits and harms at the population level.[145] Even for men aged 55 to 69 years, the AUA concluded that the quality of evidence for benefits associated with screening was moderate, whereas the quality of the evidence for harm was high. They recommended shared decision making for this group, in whom they have concluded the benefits may outweigh the harm.

SKIN CANCER SCREENING

Assessments of skin cancer screening have focused on melanoma end points with very little attention to screening for nonmelanoma skin cancer. A systematic review of skin cancer screening studies examining the available evidence through mid 2005 concluded that direct evidence of improved health outcomes associated with skin cancer screening is lacking.[146]

No randomized, clinical trial of skin cancer screening has been attempted. However, several observational studies have suggested that melanoma screening might reduce mortality. For example, a decrease in melanoma mortality did occur after a Scottish campaign to promote awareness of the signs of suspicious skin lesions and encourage early self-referral. However, uncontrolled, ecologic studies such as this provide a relatively low level of evidence, because it is not possible to determine whether the observed mortality reduction was due to screening or other factors.

More recently, the Skin Cancer Research to Provide Evidence for Effectiveness of Screening project, or SCREEN project, compared a region of Germany in which intensive skin cancer screening was performed to areas of Germany without intensive screening. Approximately 360,000 residents of the Schleswig-Holstein region aged 20 years and older participated. They chose either to be screened by a nondermatologist physician trained in skin examinations or by a dermatologist. Almost 16,000 biopsies were performed and 585 melanomas were diagnosed. Overall, 1 in 23 participants had an excisional skin biopsy and 620 persons needed to be screened to detect one melanoma. This screening effort led to a 16% and 38% increase in melanoma incidence among men and women, respectively, compared to 2 years earlier. The melanoma incidence rate returned to preprogram levels after the program ended. Of the screen-detected melanomas, 90% were less than 1 mm thick. Screening was performed in 2003 to 2004, and melanoma mortality in this region subsequently declined. In 2008, it was nearly 50% lower in both men and women compared to the rest of Germany.[147,148]

Recommendations of Experts

Skin cancer screening recommendations are based on *expert opinion*, given the absence of a randomized clinical trial data and limited observational studies. The ACS recommends monthly skin self-examinations and a yearly clinical skin examination as part of a routine cancer-related checkup.[149] The USPSTF finds insufficient evidence to recommend for or against either routine skin cancer screening of the general population by primary care providers or counseling patients to perform periodic skin self-examinations. The task force does recommend that clinicians "remain alert" for skin lesions with malignant features when performing a physical examination for other purposes, particularly in high-risk individuals. The American Academy of Dermatology recommends that persons at highest risk (i.e., those with a strong family history of melanoma and multiple atypical nevi), perform frequent self-examination and seek a professional evaluation of the skin at least once per year.[150]

High-risk individuals are persons with multiple nevi or atypical moles. There is consensus they should be educated about the need for frequent surveillance by a trained health-care provider beginning at an early age. In the United States, Australia, and Western Europe, Caucasian men age 50 years and over account for nearly half of all melanoma cases. There is some discussion that melanoma early detection efforts should be focused on this population.

REFERENCES

1. Collen MF, Dales LG, Friedman GD, et al. Multiphasic checkup evaluation study. 4. Preliminary cost benefit analysis for middle-aged men. *Prev Med* 1973; 2:236–246.
2. Prorok PC, Kramer BS, Gohagan JK. Screening theory and study design: the basics. In: Kramer B, Prorok P, eds. *Cancer Screening*. New York: Marcel Dekker; 1999: 29–53.
3. Welch HG, Black WC. Overdiagnosis in cancer. *J Natl Cancer Inst* 2010; 102:605–613.
4. Yamamoto K, Hayashi Y, Hanada R, et al. Mass screening and age-specific incidence of neuroblastoma in Saitama Prefecture, Japan. *J Clin Oncol* 1995;13:2033–2038.
5. Woods WG, Gao RN, Shuster JJ, et al. Screening of infants and mortality due to neuroblastoma. *N Engl J Med* 2002;346:1041–1046.
6. Friedman GD, Collen MF, Fireman BH. Multiphasic Health Checkup Evaluation: a 16-year follow-up. *J Chronic Dis* 1986;39:453–463.
7. Pinsky PF, Miller A, Kramer BS, et al. Evidence of a healthy volunteer effect in the prostate, lung, colorectal, and ovarian cancer screening trial. *Am J Epidemiol* 2007;165:874–881.
8. Boyle P, Brawley OW. Prostate cancer: current evidence weighs against population screening. *CA Cancer J Clin* 2009;59:220–224.
9. Autier P, Boyle P, Buyse M, et al. Is FOB screening really the answer for lowering mortality in colorectal cancer? *Recent Results Cancer Res* 2003;163: 254–263.
10. de Boer AG, Taskila T, Ojajarvi A, et al. Cancer survivors and unemployment: a meta-analysis and meta-regression. *JAMA* 2009;301:753–762.
11. Aberle DR, Adams AM, Berg CD, et al. Reduced lung-cancer mortality with low-dose computed tomographic screening. *N Engl J Med* 2011;365: 395–409.
12. Eden J, Levit L, Berg A, et al., eds. *Finding What Works in Health Care: Standards for Systematic Reviews*. Washington DC: The National Academies Press; 2011.
13. Graham R, Mancher M, Wolman DM, et al. Medicine CoSfDTCPGIo. Washington, DC: The National Academies; 2011.
14. Moyer VA. Screening for prostate cancer: U.S. Preventive Services Task Force recommendation statement. *Ann Intern Med* 2012;157:120–134.
15. Brawley O, Byers T, Chen A, et al. New American Cancer Society process for creating trustworthy cancer screening guidelines. *JAMA* 2011;306:2495–2499.
16. Shapiro S. Periodic screening for breast cancer: the HIP Randomized Controlled Trial. Health Insurance Plan. *J Natl Cancer Inst Monogr* 1997:27–30.
17. Miller AB, Wall C, Baines CJ, et al. Twenty five year follow-up for breast cancer incidence and mortality of the Canadian National Breast Screening Study: randomised screening trial. *BMJ* 2014;348:g366.
18. Tabar L, Fagerberg G, Duffy SW, et al. Update of the Swedish two-county program of mammographic screening for breast cancer. *Radiol Clin North Am* 1992;30: 187–210.
19. Moy L, Slanetz PJ, Moore R, et al. Specificity of mammography and US in the evaluation of a palpable abnormality: retrospective review. *Radiology* 2002;225:176–181.
20. Lord SJ, Lei W, Craft P, et al. A systematic review of the effectiveness of magnetic resonance imaging (MRI) as an addition to mammography and ultrasound in screening young women at high risk of breast cancer. *Eur J Cancer* 2007;43:1905–1917.
21. Wishart GC, Campisi M, Boswell M, et al. The accuracy of digital infrared imaging for breast cancer detection in women undergoing breast biopsy. *Eur J Surg Oncol* 2010;36:535–540.
22. Dooley WC, Ljung BM, Veronesi U, et al. Ductal lavage for detection of cellular atypia in women at high risk for breast cancer. *J Natl Cancer Inst* 2001;93:1624–1632.
23. Autier P, Boniol M, Middleton R, et al. Advanced breast cancer incidence following population-based mammographic screening. *Ann Oncol* 2011;22:1726–1735.
24. Bleyer A, Welch HG. Effect of three decades of screening mammography on breast-cancer incidence. *N Engl J Med* 2012;367:1998–2005.
25. Marmot MG, Altman DG, Cameron DA, et al. The benefits and harms of breast cancer screening: an independent review. *Br J Cancer* 2013;108:2205–2240.
26. Berry DA, Cronin KA, Plevritis SK, et al. Effect of screening and adjuvant therapy on mortality from breast cancer. *N Engl J Med* 2005;353:1784–1792.
27. Harris R, Yeatts J, Kinsinger L. Breast cancer screening for women ages 50 to 69 years a systematic review of observational evidence. *Prev Med* 2011;53: 108–114.
28. Nelson HD, Tyne K, Naik A, et al. Screening for breast cancer: an update for the U.S. Preventive Services Task Force. *Ann Intern Med* 2009;151:727–737.
29. Mandelblatt JS, Cronin KA, Bailey S, et al. Effects of mammography screening under different screening schedules: model estimates of potential benefits and harms. *Ann Intern Med* 2009;151:738–747.
30. U.S. Preventive Services Task Force. Screening for breast cancer: U.S. Preventive Services Task Force recommendation statement. *Ann Intern Med* 2009;151:716–726.
31. Nelson HD, Zakher B, Cantor A, et al. Risk factors for breast cancer for women aged 40 to 49 years: a systematic review and meta-analysis. *Ann Intern Med* 2012;156:635–648.
32. Barnett GC, Shah M, Redman K, et al. Risk factors for the incidence of breast cancer: do they affect survival from the disease? *J Clin Oncol* 2008;26: 3310–3316.
33. Gierach GL, Ichikawa L, Kerlikowske K, et al. Relationship between mammographic density and breast cancer death in the Breast Cancer Surveillance Consortium. *J Natl Cancer Inst* 2012;104:1218–1227.
34. Berg WA, Blume JD, Cormack JB, et al. Combined screening with ultrasound and mammography vs mammography alone in women at elevated risk of breast cancer. *JAMA* 2008;299:2151–2163.
35. Gartlehner G, Thaler K, Chapman A, et al. Mammography in combination with breast ultrasonography versus mammography for breast cancer screening in women at average risk. *Cochrane Database Syst Rev* 2013;4:CD009632.
36. Tice JA, O'Meara ES, Weaver DL, et al. Benign breast disease, mammographic breast density, and the risk of breast cancer. *J Natl Cancer Inst* 2013;105: 1043–1049.
37. Kerlikowske K, Hubbard RA, Miglioretti DL, et al. Comparative effectiveness of digital versus film-screen mammography in community practice in the United States: a cohort study. *Ann Intern Med* 2011;155:493–502.
38. Haas BM, Kalra V, Geisel J, et al. Comparison of tomosynthesis plus digital mammography and digital mammography alone for breast cancer screening. *Radiology* 2013;269:694–700.
39. Rosenberg RD, Yankaskas BC, Abraham LA, et al. Performance benchmarks for screening mammography. *Radiology* 2006;241:55–66.
40. Gomez SL, Lichtensztajn D, Kurian AW, et al. Increasing mastectomy rates for early-stage breast cancer? Population-based trends from California. *J Clin Oncol* 2010;28:e155–e157.
41. Tuttle TM, Jarosek S, Habermann EB, et al. Increasing rates of contralateral prophylactic mastectomy among patients with ductal carcinoma in situ. *J Clin Oncol* 2009;27:1362–1367.
42. Rosenberg RD, Hunt WC, Williamson MR, et al. Effects of age, breast density, ethnicity, and estrogen replacement therapy on screening mammographic sensitivity and cancer stage at diagnosis: review of 183,134 screening mammograms in Albuquerque, New Mexico. *Radiology* 1998;209:511–518.
43. Kerlikowske K, Grady D, Barclay J, et al. Effect of age, breast density, and family history on the sensitivity of first screening mammography. *JAMA* 1996;276: 33–38.
44. Porter PL, El-Bastawissi AY, Mandelson MT, et al. Breast tumor characteristics as predictors of mammographic detection: comparison of interval- and screen-detected cancers. *J Natl Cancer Inst* 1999;91:2020–2028.
45. Ronckers CM, Erdmann CA, Land CE. Radiation and breast cancer: a review of current evidence. *Breast Cancer Res* 2005;7:21–32.
46. Pijpe A, Andrieu N, Easton DF, et al. Exposure to diagnostic radiation and risk of breast cancer among carriers of BRCA1/2 mutations: retrospective cohort study (GENE-RAD-RISK). *BMJ* 2012;345:e5660.
47. Qaseem A, Snow V, Sherif K, et al. Screening mammography for women 40 to 49 years of age: a clinical practice guideline from the American College of Physicians. *Ann Intern Med* 2007;146:511–515.
48. Tonelli M, Connor Gorber S, Joffres M, et al. Recommendations on screening for breast cancer in average-risk women aged 40-74 years. *CMAJ* 2011;183: 1991–2001.
49. Recommendations on cancer screening in the European Union. Advisory Committee on Cancer Prevention. *Eur J Cancer* 2000;36:1473–1478.
50. Saslow D, Boetes C, Burke W, et al. American Cancer Society guidelines for breast screening with MRI as an adjunct to mammography. *CA Cancer J Clin* 2007;57:75–89.
51. Mandel JS, Church TR, Bond JH, et al. The effect of fecal occult-blood screening on the incidence of colorectal cancer. *N Engl J Med* 2000;343: 1603 1607.
52. Nishihara R, Wu K, Lochhead P, et al. Long-term colorectal-cancer incidence and mortality after lower endoscopy. *N Engl J Med* 2013;369: 1095–1105.
53. Schoen RE, Pinsky PF, Weissfeld JL, et al. Colorectal-cancer incidence and mortality with screening flexible sigmoidoscopy. *N Engl J Med* 2012;366: 2345–2357.
54. Mandel JS, Bond JH, Church TR, et al. Reducing mortality from colorectal cancer by screening for fecal occult blood. Minnesota Colon Cancer Control Study. *N Engl J Med* 1993;328:1365–1371.
55. Mandel JS, Church TR, Ederer F, et al. Colorectal cancer mortality: effectiveness of biennial screening for fecal occult blood. *J Natl Cancer Inst* 1999;91:434–437.
56. Hardcastle JD, Chamberlain JO, Robinson MH, et al. Randomised controlled trial of faecal occult blood screening for colorectal cancer. *Lancet* 1996;348: 1472–1477.
57. Kronborg O, Fenger C, Olsen J, et al. Randomised study of screening for colorectal cancer with faecal-occult-blood test. *Lancet* 1996;348:1467–1471.
58. Ahlquist DA, Wieand HS, Moertel CG, et al. Accuracy of fecal occult blood screening for colorectal neoplasia. A prospective study using Hemoccult and HemoQuant tests. *JAMA* 1993;269:1262–1267.
59. Levin B, Brooks D, Smith RA, et al. Emerging technologies in screening for colorectal cancer: CT colonography, immunochemical fecal occult blood tests, and stool screening using molecular markers. *CA Cancer J Clin* 2003;53:44–55.
60. Atkin WS, Edwards R, Kralj-Hans I, et al. Once-only flexible sigmoidoscopy screening in prevention of colorectal cancer: a multicentre randomised controlled trial. *Lancet* 2010;375:1624–1633.
61. Levin TR. Flexible sigmoidoscopy for colorectal cancer screening: valid approach or short-sighted? *Gastroenterol Clin North Am* 2002;31:1015–1029.

62. Littlejohn C, Hilton S, Macfarlane GJ, et al. Systematic review and meta-analysis of the evidence for flexible sigmoidoscopy as a screening method for the prevention of colorectal cancer. *Br J Surg* 2012;99:1488–1500.
63. Elmunzer BJ, Hayward RA, Schoenfeld PS, et al. Effect of flexible sigmoidoscopy-based screening on incidence and mortality of colorectal cancer: a systematic review and meta-analysis of randomized controlled trials. *PLoS Med* 2012;9:e1001352.
64. van Rijn JC, Reitsma JB, Stoker J, et al. Polyp miss rate determined by tandem colonoscopy: a systematic review. *Am J Gastroenterol* 2006;101:343–350.
65. Rosman AS, Korsten MA. Meta-analysis comparing CT colonography, air contrast barium enema, and colonoscopy. *Am J Med* 2007;120:203–210.
66. Imperiale TF, Wagner DR, Lin CY, et al. Using risk for advanced proximal colonic neoplasia to tailor endoscopic screening for colorectal cancer. *Ann Intern Med* 2003;139:959–965.
67. U.S. Preventive Services Task Force. Screening for colorectal cancer: U.S. Preventive Services Task Force recommendation statement. *Ann Intern Med* 2008;149:627–637.
68. Winawer S, Fletcher R, Rex D, et al. Colorectal cancer screening and surveillance: clinical guidelines and rationale-Update based on new evidence. *Gastroenterology* 2003;124:544–560.
69. Quintero E, Castells A, Bujanda L, et al. Colonoscopy versus fecal immunochemical testing in colorectal-cancer screening. *N Engl J Med* 2012;366: 697–706.
70. Murakami R, Tsukuma H, Ubukata T, et al. Estimation of validity of mass screening program for gastric cancer in Osaka, Japan. *Cancer* 1990;65:1255–1260.
71. Kampschoer GH, Fujii A, Masuda Y. Gastric cancer detected by mass survey. Comparison between mass survey and outpatient detection. *Scand J Gastroenterol* 1989;24:813–817.
72. Stael von Holstein C, Eriksson S, Huldt B, et al. Endoscopic screening during 17 years for gastric stump carcinoma. A prospective clinical trial. *Scand J Gastroenterol* 1991;26:1020–1026.
73. Shaukat A, Mongin SJ, Geisser MS, et al. Long-term mortality after screening for colorectal cancer. *N Engl J Med* 2013;369:1106–1114.
74. McMahon BJ, Bulkow L, Harpster A, et al. Screening for hepatocellular carcinoma in Alaska natives infected with chronic hepatitis B: a 16-year population-based study. *Hepatology* 2000;32:842–846.
75. Chalasani N, Horlander JC Sr, Said A, et al. Screening for hepatocellular carcinoma in patients with advanced cirrhosis. *Am J Gastroenterol* 1999;94: 2988–2993.
76. Sherman M, Peltekian KM, Lee C. Screening for hepatocellular carcinoma in chronic carriers of hepatitis B virus: incidence and prevalence of hepatocellular carcinoma in a North American urban population. *Hepatology* 1995;22:432–438.
77. Dodd GD 3rd, Miller WJ, Baron RL, et al. Detection of malignant tumors in end-stage cirrhotic livers: efficacy of sonography as a screening technique. *AJR Am J Roentgenol* 1992;159:727–733.
78. Laara E, Day NE, Hakama M. Trends in mortality from cervical cancer in the Nordic countries: association with organised screening programmes. *Lancet* 1987;1:1247–1249.
79. Christopherson WM, Lundin FE Jr, Mendez WM, et al. Cervical cancer control: a study of morbidity and mortality trends over a twenty-one-year period. *Cancer* 1976;38:1357–1366.
80. Janerich DT, Hadjimichael O, Schwartz PE, et al. The screening histories of women with invasive cervical cancer, Connecticut. *Am J Public Health* 1995;85:791–794.
81. Sawaya GF, McConnell KJ, Kulasingam SL, et al. Risk of cervical cancer associated with extending the interval between cervical-cancer screenings. *N Engl J Med* 2003;349:1501–1509.
82. Sankaranarayanan R, Nene BM, Shastri SS, et al. HPV screening for cervical cancer in rural India. *N Engl J Med* 2009;360:1385–1394.
83. Vesco KK, Whitlock EP, Eder M, et al. In: *Screening for Cervical Cancer: A Systematic Evidence Review for the US Preventive Services Task Force*. Rockville, MD: Agency for Healthcare Research and Quality; 2011.
84. Solomon D, Davey D, Kurman R, et al. The 2001 Bethesda System: terminology for reporting results of cervical cytology. *JAMA* 2002;287:2114–2119.
85. Darragh TM, Colgan TJ, Thomas Cox J, et al. The Lower Anogenital Squamous Terminology Standardization project for HPV-associated lesions: background and consensus recommendations from the College of American Pathologists and the American Society for Colposcopy and Cervical Pathology. *Int J Gynecol Pathol* 2013;32:76–115.
86. Ho GY, Bierman R, Beardsley L, et al. Natural history of cervicovaginal papillomavirus infection in young women. *N Engl J Med* 1998;338:423–428.
87. Holowaty P, Miller AB, Rohan T, et al. Natural history of dysplasia of the uterine cervix. *J Natl Cancer Inst* 1999;91:252–258.
88. Richardson H, Kelsall G, Tellier P, et al. The natural history of type-specific human papillomavirus infections in female university students. *Cancer Epidemiol Biomarkers Prev* 2003;12:485–490.
89. Melnikow J, Nuovo J, Willan AR, et al. Natural history of cervical squamous intraepithelial lesions: a meta-analysis. *Obstet Gynecol* 1998;92:727–735.
90. Cox JT, Schiffman M, Solomon D. Prospective follow-up suggests similar risk of subsequent cervical intraepithelial neoplasia grade 2 or 3 among women with cervical intraepithelial neoplasia grade 1 or negative colposcopy and directed biopsy. *Am J Obstet Gynecol* 2003;188:1406–1412.
91. Guido R, Schiffman M, Solomon D, et al. Postcolposcopy management strategies for women referred with low-grade squamous intraepithelial lesions or human papillomavirus DNA-positive atypical squamous cells of undetermined significance: a two-year prospective study. *Am J Obstet Gynecol* 2003;188:1401–1405.
92. Mayrand MH, Duarte-Franco E, Rodrigues I, et al. Human papillomavirus DNA versus Papanicolaou screening tests for cervical cancer. *N Engl J Med* 2007;357:1579–1588.
93. Saslow D, Solomon D, Lawson HW, et al. American Cancer Society, American Society for Colposcopy and Cervical Pathology, and American Society for Clinical Pathology screening guidelines for the prevention and early detection of cervical cancer. *CA Cancer J Clin* 2012;62:147–172.
94. Sankaranarayanan R, Esmy PO, Rajkumar R, et al. Effect of visual screening on cervical cancer incidence and mortality in Tamil Nadu, India: a cluster-randomised trial. *Lancet* 2007;370:398–406.
95. Szarewski A. Cervical screening by visual inspection with acetic acid. *Lancet* 2007;370:365–366.
96. Johnson CC, Kessel B, Riley TL, et al. The epidemiology of CA-125 in women without evidence of ovarian cancer in the Prostate, Lung, Colorectal and Ovarian Cancer (PLCO) Screening Trial. *Gynecol Oncol* 2008;110:383–389.
97. Duffy MJ, Bonfrer JM, Kulpa J, et al. CA125 in ovarian cancer: European Group on Tumor Markers guidelines for clinical use. *Int J Gynecol Cancer* 2005;15:679–691.
98. Moss EL, Hollingworth J, Reynolds TM. The role of CA125 in clinical practice. *J Clin Pathol* 2005;58:308–312.
99. Fishman DA, Cohen L, Blank SV, et al. The role of ultrasound evaluation in the detection of early-stage epithelial ovarian cancer. *Am J Obstet Gynecol* 2005;192:1214–1221.
100. Kobayashi E, Ueda Y, Matsuzaki S, et al. Biomarkers for screening, diagnosis, and monitoring of ovarian cancer. *Cancer Epidemiol Biomarkers Prev* 2012;21:1902–1912.
101. Ren J, Cai H, Li Y, et al. Tumor markers for early detection of ovarian cancer. *Expert Rev Mol Diagn* 2010;10:787–798.
102. Prorok PC, Andriole GL, Bresalier RS, et al. Design of the Prostate, Lung, Colorectal and Ovarian (PLCO) Cancer Screening Trial. *Control Clin Trials* 2000;21:273S–309S.
103. Buys SS, Partridge E, Black A, et al. Effect of screening on ovarian cancer mortality: the Prostate, Lung, Colorectal and Ovarian (PLCO) Cancer Screening Randomized Controlled Trial. *JAMA* 2011;305:2295–2303.
104. Menon U, Gentry-Maharaj A, Hallett R, et al. Sensitivity and specificity of multimodal and ultrasound screening for ovarian cancer, and stage distribution of detected cancers: results of the prevalence screen of the UK Collaborative Trial of Ovarian Cancer Screening (UKCTOCS). *Lancet Oncol* 2009;10:327–340.
105. Drescher CW, Shah C, Thorpe J, et al. Longitudinal screening algorithm that incorporates change over time in CA125 levels identifies ovarian cancer earlier than a single-threshold rule. *J Clin Oncol* 2013;31:387–392.
106. Sharma A, Apostolidou S, Burnell M, et al. Risk of epithelial ovarian cancer in asymptomatic women with ultrasound-detected ovarian masses: a prospective cohort study within the UK collaborative trial of ovarian cancer screening (UKCTOCS). *Ultrasound Obstet Gynecol* 2012;40:338–344.
107. Moyer VA. Screening for ovarian cancer: U.S. Preventive Services Task Force reaffirmation recommendation statement. *Ann Intern Med* 2012;157:900–904.
108. NIH consensus conference. Ovarian cancer. Screening, treatment, and follow-up. NIH Consensus Development Panel on Ovarian Cancer. *JAMA* 1995;273:491–497.
109. Smith RA, von Eschenbach AC, Wender R, et al. American Cancer Society guidelines for the early detection of cancer: update of early detection guidelines for prostate, colorectal, and endometrial cancers. Also: update 2001—testing for early lung cancer detection. *CA Cancer J Clin* 2001;51:38–75.
110. Burke W, Petersen G, Lynch P, et al. Recommendations for follow-up care of individuals with an inherited predisposition to cancer. I. Hereditary nonpolyposis colon cancer. Cancer Genetics Studies Consortium. *JAMA* 1997; 277:915–919.
111. Gull B, Karlsson B, Milsom I, et al. Can ultrasound replace dilation and curettage? A longitudinal evaluation of postmenopausal bleeding and transvaginal sonographic measurement of the endometrium as predictors of endometrial cancer. *Am J Obstet Gynecol* 2003;188:401–408.
112. Scamman CL. Follow-up study of lung cancer suspects in a mass chest X-ray survey. *N Engl J Med* 1951;244:541–544.
113. Croswell JM, Ransohoff DF, Kramer BS. Principles of cancer screening: lessons from history and study design issues. *Semin Oncol* 2010;37:202–215.
114. Fontana RS, Sanderson DR, Taylor WF, et al. Early lung cancer detection: results of the initial (prevalence) radiologic and cytologic screening in the Mayo Clinic study. *Am Rev Respir Dis* 1984;130:561–565.
115. Fontana RS, Sanderson DR, Woolner LB, et al. Screening for lung cancer. A critique of the Mayo Lung Project. *Cancer* 1991;67:1155–1164.
116. Marcus PM, Bergstralh EJ, Zweig MH, et al. Extended lung cancer incidence follow-up in the Mayo Lung Project and overdiagnosis. *J Natl Cancer Inst* 2006;98:748–756.
117. Manser R, Wright G, Hart D, et al. Surgery for early stage non-small cell lung cancer. *Cochrane Database Syst Rev* 2005:CD004699.
118. Kubik A, Parkin DM, Khlat M, et al. Lack of benefit from semi-annual screening for cancer of the lung: follow-up report of a randomized controlled trial on a population of high-risk males in Czechoslovakia. *Int J Cancer* 1990; 45:26–33.
119. Oken MM, Hocking WG, Kvale PA, et al. Screening by chest radiograph and lung cancer mortality: the Prostate, Lung, Colorectal, and Ovarian (PLCO) randomized trial. *JAMA* 2011;306:1865–1873.
120. Kovalchik SA, Tammemagi M, Berg CD, et al. Targeting of low-dose CT screening according to the risk of lung-cancer death. *N Engl J Med* 2013; 369:245–254.

121. Kubik AK, Parkin DM, Zatloukal P. Czech Study on Lung Cancer Screening: post-trial follow-up of lung cancer deaths up to year 15 since enrollment. *Cancer* 2000;89:2363–2368.
122. Patz EF Jr, Pinsky P, Gatsonis C, et al. Overdiagnosis in low-dose computed tomography screening for lung cancer. *JAMA Intern Med* 2014;174:269–274.
123. Ma J, Ward EM, Smith R, et al. Annual number of lung cancer deaths potentially avertable by screening in the United States. *Cancer* 2013;119: 1381–1385.
124. Wender R, Fontham ET, Barrera E Jr, et al. American Cancer Society lung cancer screening guidelines. *CA Cancer J Clin* 2013;63:107–117.
125. Bach PB, Mirkin JN, Oliver TK, et al. Benefits and harms of CT screening for lung cancer: a systematic review. *JAMA* 2012;307:2418–2429.
126. Montie JE, Smith JA. Whitmoreisms: memorable quotes from Willet F. Whitmore, Jr, M.D. *Urology* 2004;63:207–209.
127. Albertsen PC, Hanley JA, Fine J. 20-year outcomes following conservative management of clinically localized prostate cancer. *JAMA* 2005;293:2095–2101.
128. Lu-Yao G, Albertsen PC, Stanford JL, et al. Screening, treatment, and prostate cancer mortality in the Seattle area and Connecticut: fifteen-year follow-up. *J Gen Intern Med* 2008;23:1809–1814.
129. Thompson IM, Chi C, Ankerst DP, et al. Effect of finasteride on the sensitivity of PSA for detecting prostate cancer. *J Natl Cancer Inst* 2006;98:1128–1133.
130. Thompson IM, Pauler DK, Goodman PJ, et al. Prevalence of prostate cancer among men with a prostate-specific antigen level < or =4.0 ng per milliliter. *N Engl J Med* 2004;350:2239–2246.
131. Thompson IM, Ankerst DP, Chi C, et al. Operating characteristics of prostate-specific antigen in men with an initial PSA level of 3.0 ng/ml or lower. *JAMA* 2005;294:66–70.
132. Widmark A, Klepp O, Solberg A, et al. Endocrine treatment, with or without radiotherapy, in locally advanced prostate cancer (SPCG-7/SFUO-3): an open randomised phase III trial. *Lancet* 2009;373:301–308.
133. Bill-Axelson A, Holmberg L, Ruutu M, et al. Radical prostatectomy versus watchful waiting in early prostate cancer. *N Engl J Med* 2011;364: 1708–1717.
134. Wilt TJ, Brawer MK, Jones KM, et al. Radical prostatectomy versus observation for localized prostate cancer. *N Engl J Med* 2012;367:203–213.
135. Andriole GL, Crawford ED, Grubb RL 3rd, et al. Prostate cancer screening in the randomized Prostate, Lung, Colorectal, and Ovarian Cancer Screening Trial: mortality results after 13 years of follow-up. *J Natl Cancer Inst* 2012;104:125–132.
136. Schroder FH, Hugosson J, Roobol MJ, et al. Screening and prostate-cancer mortality in a randomized European study. *N Engl J Med* 2009;360:1320–1328.
137. Schroder FH, Hugosson J, Roobol MJ, et al. Prostate-cancer mortality at 11 years of follow-up. *N Engl J Med* 2012;366:981–990.
138. Wolters T, Roobol MJ, Steyerberg EW, et al. The effect of study arm on prostate cancer treatment in the large screening trial ERSPC. *Int J Cancer* 2010;126:2387–2393.
139. Hugosson J, Carlsson S, Aus G, et al. Mortality results from the Goteborg randomised population-based prostate-cancer screening trial. *Lancet Oncol* 2010;11: 725–732.
140. Kilpelainen TP, Tammela TL, Malila N, et al. Prostate cancer mortality in the Finnish randomized screening trial. *J Natl Cancer Inst* 2013;105: 719–725.
141. Center MM, Jemal A, Lortet-Tieulent J, et al. International variation in prostate cancer incidence and mortality rates. *Eur Urol* 2012;61:1079–1092.
142. Boyle P. Screening for prostate cancer: have you had your cholesterol measured? *BJU Int* 2003;92:191–199.
143. Greene KL, Albertsen PC, Babaian RJ, et al. Prostate specific antigen best practice statement: 2009 update. *J Urol* 2009;182:2232–2241.
144. Wolf AM, Wender RC, Etzioni RB, et al. American Cancer Society guideline for the early detection of prostate cancer: update 2010. *CA Cancer J Clin* 2010;60:70–98.
145. Carter HB. American Urological Association (AUA) guideline on prostate cancer detection: process and rationale. *BJU Int* 2013;112:543–547.
146. Wolff T, Tai E, Miller T. Screening for skin cancer: an update of the evidence for the U.S. Preventive Services Task Force. *Ann Intern Med* 2009;150: 194–198.
147. Katalinic A, Waldmann A, Weinstock MA, et al. Does skin cancer screening save lives?: an observational study comparing trends in melanoma mortality in regions with and without screening. *Cancer* 2012;118:5395–5402.
148. Breitbart EW, Waldmann A, Nolte S, et al. Systematic skin cancer screening in Northern Germany. *J Am Acad Dermatol* 2012;66:201–211.
149. Smith RA, Brooks D, Cokkinides V, et al. Cancer screening in the United States, 2013: a review of current American Cancer Society guidelines, current issues in cancer screening, and new guidance on cervical cancer screening and lung cancer screening. *CA Cancer J Clin* 2013;63:88–105.
150. U.S. Preventive Services Task Force. Screening for skin cancer: U.S. Preventive Services Task Force recommendation statement. *Ann Intern Med* 2009;150: 188–193.

35 Genetic Counseling

Ellen T. Matloff and Danielle C. Bonadies

INTRODUCTION

Clinically based genetic testing has evolved from an uncommon analysis ordered for the rare hereditary cancer family to a widely available tool ordered on a routine basis to assist in surgical and radiation decision making, chemoprevention, and surveillance of the patient with cancer, as well as management of the entire family. The evolution of this field has created a need for accurate cancer genetic counseling and risk assessment. Extensive coverage of this topic by the media, including Angelina Jolie's public disclosure of her *BRCA1+* status in May 2013, and widespread advertising by commercial testing laboratories have further fueled the demand for counseling and testing.

Cancer genetic counseling is a communication process between a health-care professional and an individual concerning cancer occurrence and risk in his or her family.[1] The process, which may include the entire family through a blend of genetic, medical, and psychosocial assessments and interventions, has been described as a bridge between the fields of traditional oncology and genetic counseling.[1]

The goals of this process include providing the client with an assessment of individual cancer risk, while offering the emotional support needed to understand and cope with this information. It also involves deciphering whether the cancers in a family are likely to be caused by a mutation in a cancer gene and, if so, *which one*. There are >30 hereditary cancer syndromes, many of which can be caused by mutations in different genes. Therefore, testing for these syndromes can be complicated. Advertisements by genetic testing companies bill genetic testing as a simple process that can be carried out by health-care professionals with no training in this area; however, there are many genes involved in cancer, the interpretation of the test results is often complicated, the risk of result misinterpretation is great and associated with potential liability, and the emotional and psychological ramifications for the patient and family can be powerful.[2,3] A few hours of training by a company generating a profit from the sale of these tests does not adequately prepare providers to offer their own genetic counseling and testing services.[4] Furthermore, the delegation of genetic testing responsibilities to office staff and, recently, mammography technicians, is alarming and likely presents a huge liability for these ordering physicians, their practices, and their institutions.[5,6] *Providers should proceed with caution before taking on the role of primary genetic counselor for their patients.*

Counseling about hereditary cancers differs from *traditional* genetic counseling in several ways. Clients seeking cancer genetic counseling are rarely concerned with reproductive decisions, which are often the primary focus in traditional genetic counseling, but are instead seeking information about their own and other relatives' chances of developing cancer.[1] Additionally, the risks given are not absolute but change over time as the family and personal history changes and the patient ages. The risk reduction options available are often radical (e.g., chemoprevention or prophylactic surgery), and are not appropriate for every patient at every age. The surveillance and management plan must be tailored to the patient's age, childbearing status, menopausal status, risk category, ease of screening, and personal preferences and will likely change over time with the patient. The ultimate goal of cancer genetic counseling is to help the patient reach the decision best suited to her personal situation, needs, and circumstances.

There are now a significant number of referral centers across the country specializing in cancer genetic counseling, and the numbers are growing. However, some experts insist that the only way to keep up with the overwhelming demand for counseling will be to educate more physicians and nurses in cancer genetics. The feasibility of adding another specialized and time-consuming task to the clinical burden of these professionals is questionable, particularly with average patient encounters of 19.5 and 21.6 minutes for general practitioners and gynecologists, respectively.[7,8] A more practical goal is to better educate clinicians in the area of risk assessment so that they can screen their patient populations for individuals at high risk for hereditary cancer and refer them on to comprehensive counseling and testing programs. Access to genetic counseling is no longer an issue because there are now internet, phone, and satellite-based telemedicine services available (Table 35.1), with most major health insurance companies now covering these services[9–11] and several requiring them.[12]

WHO IS A CANDIDATE FOR CANCER GENETIC COUNSELING?

Only 5% to 10% of most cancer is thought to be caused by single mutations within autosomal-dominant inherited cancer susceptibility genes.[13] The key for clinicians is to determine which patients are at greatest risk to carry a hereditary mutation. There are seven critical risk factors in hereditary cancer (Table 35.2). The first is early age of cancer onset. This risk factor, *even in the absence of a family history*, has been shown to be associated with an increased frequency of germline mutations in many types of cancers.[14] The second risk factor is the presence of the same cancer in multiple affected relatives on the same side of the pedigree. These cancers do not need to be of similar histologic type in order to be caused by a single mutation. The third risk factor is the clustering of cancers known to be caused by a single gene mutation in one family (e.g., breast/ovarian/pancreatic cancer or colon/uterine/ovarian cancers). The fourth risk factor is the occurrence of multiple primary cancers in one individual. This includes multiple primary breast or colon cancers as well as a single individual with separate cancers known to be caused by a single gene mutation (e.g., breast and ovarian cancer in a single individual). Ethnicity also plays a role in determining who is at greatest risk to carry a hereditary cancer mutation. Individuals of Jewish ancestry are at increased risk to carry three specific *BRCA1/2* mutations.[15] The presence of a cancer that presents unusually—in this case, breast cancer in a male—represents a sixth risk factor and is important even when it is the only risk factor present. Finally, the last risk factor is pathology. Certain types of cancer are overrepresented in hereditary cancer families. For example, medullary and triple negative breast

TABLE 35.1

How to Find a Genetic Counselor for Your Patient

American Board of Genetic Counselors
https://abgcmember.goamp.com/Net/ABGCWcm/Find_Counselor/ABGCWcm/PublicDir.aspx?hkey=0ad511c0-d9e9-4714-bd4b-0d73a59ee175
http://bit.ly/1kzTbk9
Directory of board-certified genetic counselors

InformedDNA
www.informeddna.com
(800) 975-4819
A nationwide network of independent genetic counselors that use telephone and internet technology to bring genetic counseling to patients and providers. Covered by many insurance companies.

National Society of Genetic Counselors
www.nsgc.org (click "Find a Counselor" button)
(312) 321-6834
For a listing of genetic counselors in your area who specialize in cancer.

National Cancer Institute Cancer Genetics Services Directory
www.cancer.gov/cancertopics/genetics/directory
(800) 4-CANCER
A free service designed to locate providers of cancer risk counseling and testing services.

cancers (where the estrogen, progesterone and Her2 receptors are all negative, often abbreviated ER-/PR-/Her2) are overrepresented in *BRCA1* families,[16,17] and the National Comprehensive Cancer Network (NCCN) BRCA testing guidelines now include individuals diagnosed with a triple negative breast cancer <age 60 years.[18] However, breast cancer patients without these pathologic findings are *not* necessarily at lower risk to carry a mutation. In contrast, patients with a borderline or mucinous ovarian carcinoma are at lower risk to carry a *BRCA1* or *BRCA2* mutation[19] and may instead carry a mutation in a different gene. It is already well-established that medullary thyroid carcinoma, sebaceous adenoma or carcinoma, adrenocortical carcinoma before the age of 25 years, and multiple adenomatous, hamartomatous, or juvenile colon polyps are indicative of other rare hereditary cancer syndromes.[11,20] These risk factors should be viewed in the context of the entire family history, and must be weighed in proportion to the number of individuals who have not developed cancer. The risk assessment is often limited in families that are small or have few female relatives; in such families, a single risk factor may carry more weight.

A less common, but extremely important, finding is the presence of unusual physical findings or birth defects that are known to be associated with rare hereditary cancer syndromes. Examples include benign skin findings, autism, large head circumference[20,21] and thyroid disorders in Cowden syndrome, odontogenic keratocysts in Gorlin syndrome,[22] and desmoid tumors or dental abnormalities in familial adenomatous polyposis (FAP).[23] These and other findings should prompt further investigation of the patient's family history and consideration of a referral to genetic counseling.

In this chapter, the breast/ovarian cancer counseling session with a female patient will serve as a paradigm by which all other sessions may follow broadly.

TABLE 35.2

Risk Factors that Warrant Genetic Counseling for Hereditary Cancer Syndromes

1. Early age of onset (e.g., <50 years for breast, colon, and uterine cancer)
2. Multiple family members on the same side of the pedigree with the same cancer
3. Clustering of cancers in the family known to be caused by a single gene mutation (e.g., breast/ovarian/pancreatic; colon/uterine/ovarian; colon cancer/polyps/desmoid tumors/osteomas)
4. Multiple primary cancers in one individual (e.g., breast/ovarian cancer; colon/uterine; synchronous/metachronous colon cancers; <15 gastrointestinal polyps; <5 hamartomatous or juvenile polyps)
5. Ethnicity (e.g., Jewish ancestry for breast/ovarian cancer syndrome)
6. Unusual presentation of cancer/tumor (e.g., breast cancer in a male; medullary thyroid cancer; retinoblastoma; even one sebaceous carcinoma or adenoma)
7. Pathology (e.g., triple negative [ER/PR/Her-2] breast cancer <60; medullary breast cancers are overrepresented in women with hereditary breast and ovarian cancer; a colon tumor with an abnormal microsatellite instability (MSI) or immunohistochemistry (IHC) result increases the risk for a hereditary colon cancer syndrome)

COMPONENTS OF THE CANCER GENETIC COUNSELING SESSION

Precounseling Information

Before coming in for genetic counseling, the counselee should be informed about what to expect at each visit, and what information he/she should collect ahead of time. The counselee can then begin to collect medical and family history information and pathology reports that will be essential for the genetic counseling session.

Family History

An accurate family history is undoubtedly one of the most essential components of the cancer genetic counseling session. Optimally, a family history should include at least three generations; however, patients do not always have this information. For each individual affected with cancer, it is important to document the exact diagnosis, age at diagnosis, treatment strategies, and environmental exposures (i.e., occupational exposures, cigarettes, other agents).[24] The current age of the individual, laterality, and occurrence of any other cancers must also be documented. Cancer diagnoses should be confirmed with pathology reports whenever possible. A study by Love et al.[25] revealed that individuals accurately reported the primary site of cancer only 83% of the time in their first degree relatives with cancer, and 67% and 60% of the time in second and third degree relatives, respectively. It is common for patients to report a uterine cancer as an ovarian cancer, or a colon polyp as an invasive colorectal cancer. These differences, although seemingly subtle to the patient, can make a tremendous difference in risk assessment. Individuals should be asked if there are any consanguineous (inbred) relationships in the family, if any relatives were born with birth defects or mental retardation, and whether other genetic diseases run in the family (e.g., Fanconi anemia, Cowden syndrome), because these pieces of information could prove to be important in reaching a diagnosis.

The most common misconception in family history taking is that somehow a maternal family history of breast, ovarian, or uterine cancer is more significant than a paternal history. Conversely, many still believe that a paternal history of prostate cancer is more significant than a maternal history. Few cancer genes discovered thus far are located on the sex chromosomes and, therefore, both maternal and paternal history are significant and must be explored thoroughly. It has also become necessary to elicit the spouse's personal and family history of cancer. This has bearing on the cancer status of common children, but may also determine if children are at increased risk for a serious recessive genetic disease such as Fanconi anemia.[26] Children who inherit two copies of a *BRCA2* mutation (one from each parent) are now known to have this serious disorder characterized by defective DNA repair and high rates of birth defects, aplastic anemia, leukemia, and solid tumors.[26] Patients should be encouraged to report changes in their family history over time (e.g., new cancer diagnoses, genetic testing results in relatives), because this may change their risk assessment and counseling.

A detailed family history should also include genetic diseases, birth defects, mental retardation, multiple miscarriages, and infant deaths. A history of certain recessive genetic diseases (e.g., ataxia telangiectasia, Fanconi anemia) can indicate that healthy family members who carry just one copy of the genetic mutation may be at increased risk to develop cancer.[26,27] Other genetic disorders, such as hereditary hemorrhagic telangiectasia, can be associated with a hereditary cancer syndrome caused by a mutation in the same gene—in this case, juvenile polyposis.[28]

Dysmorphology Screening

Congenital anomalies, benign tumors, and unusual dermatologic features occur in a large number of hereditary cancer predisposition syndromes. Examples include osteomas of the jaw in FAP, palmar pits in Gorlin syndrome, and papillomas of the lips and mucous membranes in Cowden syndrome. Obtaining an accurate past medical history of benign lesions and birth defects, and screening for such dysmorphology can greatly impact diagnosis, counseling, and testing. For example, *BRCA1/2* testing is inappropriate in a patient with breast cancer who has a family history of thyroid cancer and the orocutaneous manifestations of Cowden syndrome.

Risk Assessment

Risk assessment is one of the most complicated components of the genetic counseling session. It is crucial to remember that risk assessment changes over time as the person ages and as the health statuses of their family members change. Risk assessment can be broken down into three separate components.

- What is the chance that the counselee will develop the cancer observed in his/her family (or a genetically related cancer such as ovarian cancer due to a family history of breast cancer)?
- What is the chance that the cancers in this family are caused by a single gene mutation?
- What is the chance that we can identify the gene mutation in this family with our current knowledge and laboratory techniques?

Cancer clustering in a family may be due to genetic and/or environmental factors, or may be coincidental because some cancers are very common in the general population.[29] Although inherited factors may be the primary cause of cancers in some families, in others, cancer may develop because an inherited factor increases the individual's susceptibility to environmental carcinogens. It is also possible that members of the same family may be exposed to similar environmental exposures due to shared geography or patterns in behavior and diet that may increase the risk of cancer.[30] Therefore, it is important to distinguish the difference between a familial pattern of cancer (due to environmental factors or chance) and a hereditary pattern of cancer (due to a shared genetic mutation). Emerging research is also evaluating the role and clinical utility of more common low-penetrance susceptibility genes and single nucleotide polymorphisms (SNP) that may account for a proportion of familial cancers.[31]

Several models are available to calculate the chance that a woman will develop breast cancer, including the Gail and Claus models.[32,33] Computer-based models are also available to help determine the chance that a *BRCA* mutation will be found in a family.[34] At first glance, many of these models appear simple and easy to use, and it may be tempting to exclusively rely on these models to assess cancer risk. However, each model has its strengths and weaknesses, and the counselor needs to understand the limitations well and know which are validated, which are considered problematic, when a model will not work on a particular patient, or when another genetic syndrome should be considered. For example, none of the existing models are able to factor in other risks that may be essential in hereditary risk calculation (e.g., a sister who was diagnosed with breast cancer after radiation treatment for Hodgkin disease).

The risk of a detectable mutation will also vary based on cancer history and the degree of relationship to an affected family member. For example, family members with early-onset breast cancer have a higher likelihood of testing positive than unaffected family members. Therefore, the risk assessment process should include a discussion of which family member is the best candidate for testing.

DNA Testing

DNA testing is now available for a variety of hereditary cancer syndromes. However, despite misrepresentation by the media, testing is feasible for only a small percentage of individuals with cancer. DNA testing offers the important advantage of presenting clients with *actual risks* instead of the empiric risks derived from risk calculation models. DNA testing can be very expensive; full sequencing and rearrangement testing of the *BRCA1/2* genes currently averages $2,500, and full panel testing costs up to $7,000 per patient. Importantly, testing should begin in an affected family member whenever possible to maximize scientific accuracy. Most insurance companies now cover cancer genetic testing in families where the test is medically indicated.

One of the most crucial aspects of DNA testing is accurate result ordering and interpretation. Unfortunately, errors in ordering and interpretation are the greatest risk of genetic testing and are very common.[35] Emerging data reveal that between 30% to 50% of genetic tests are ordered inappropriately, which is problematic for patients, clinicians, and insurers.[36–38] Recent data demonstrate that many medical providers have difficulty interpreting even basic pedigrees and genetic test results.[33–35] Additional studies have demonstrated that an inaccurate interpretation of genetic testing has been shown to result in inappropriate medical management recommendations, unnecessary prophylactic surgeries, a massive waste of health-care dollars, psychosocial distress, and false reassurance for patients.[2,3]

Interpretations are becoming increasingly complicated as more tests and gene panels become available. For example, one study demonstrated that approximately 25% of high-risk families that were *BRCA1* and *BRCA2* negative by commercially available sequencing were found to carry a deletion or duplication in one of these genes, or a mutation in another gene.[39]

This is particularly concerning in an era in which testing companies are canvassing physicians, and now mammography technicians, and encouraging them to perform their own counseling and testing. The potential impact of test results on the patient and his/her family is great and, therefore, accurate interpretation of the results is paramount. Professional groups have recognized this and have adopted standards encouraging clinicians to refer patients to genetics experts to ensure proper ordering and interpretation of genetic tests. The U.S. Preventive Services Task Force recommends that women whose family history is suggestive of a *BRCA* mutation be referred for genetic counseling before being offered genetic testing.[40] The American College of Surgeons' Commission on Cancer standards include "cancer risk assessment, genetic counseling and testing services provided to patients either on site or by referral, by a qualified genetics professional."[4] In an effort to reduce errors, some insurance companies are requiring genetic counseling by a certified genetic counselor before testing for hereditary breast or colon cancer syndromes.[12]

Results can fall into a few broad categories. It is important to note that a negative test result can actually be interpreted in three different ways, detailed in #2, #3, and #4, which follows.

1. Deleterious mutation "positive." When a deleterious mutation in a well-known cancer gene is discovered, the cancer risks for the patient and her family are relatively straightforward. However, with the development of multigene panels and the inclusion of many lesser known genes, the risks of detecting a mutation within a gene whose cancer risks are ill defined and medical management options unknown is much greater. Even for well-known genes, the risks are not precise and should be presented to patients as a risk range.[41,42] When a true mutation is found, it is critical to test both parents (whenever possible) to determine from which side of the family the mutation is originating, even when the answer appears obvious.
2. True negative. An individual does not carry the deleterious mutation found in her family, which ideally, has been proven to segregate with the cancer family history. In this case, the patient's cancer risks are usually reduced to the population risks.
3. Negative. A mutation was not detected, and the cancers in the family are not likely to be hereditary based on the personal and family history assessment. For example, a patient is diagnosed with breast cancer at age 38 years and comes from a large family with no other cancer diagnoses and relatives who died at old ages of other causes.
4. Uninformative. A mutation cannot be found in affected family members of a family in which the cancer pattern appears to be hereditary; there is likely an undetectable mutation within the gene, or the family carries a mutation in a different gene. If, for example, the patient developed breast cancer at age 38 years, has a father with breast cancer, and has a paternal aunt who developed breast and ovarian cancers before age 50 years, a negative test result would be almost meaningless. It would simply mean that the family has a mutation that could not be identified with our current testing methods or a mutation in another cancer gene. The entire family would be followed as high risk.
5. Variant of uncertain significance. A genetic change is identified, the significance of which is unknown. It is possible that this change is deleterious or completely benign. It may be helpful to test other *affected* family members to see if the mutation segregates with disease in the family. If it does not segregate, the variant is less likely to be significant. If it does, the variant is more likely to be significant. Other tools, including a splice site predictor, in conjunction with data on species conservation and amino acid difference scores, can also be helpful in determining the likelihood that a variant is significant. It is rarely helpful (and can be detrimental) to test *unaffected* family members for such variants. The rates of variants of uncertain significance vary greatly depending on the reporting protocols of the lab and the genes analyzed. Creation of open databases through a nationwide movement called Free the Data will likely improve variant reporting for all laboratories.

In order to pinpoint the mutation in a family, an affected individual most likely to carry the mutation should be tested first whenever possible. This is most often a person affected with the cancer in question at the earliest age. Test subjects should be selected with care, because it is possible for a person to develop sporadic cancer in a hereditary cancer family. For example, in an early-onset breast cancer family, it would not be ideal to first test a woman diagnosed with breast cancer at age 65 years because she may represent a sporadic case.

If a mutation is detected in an affected relative, other family members can be tested for the same mutation with a great degree of accuracy. Family members who do not carry the mutation found in their family are deemed true negative. Those who are found to carry the mutation in their family will have more definitive information about their risks to develop cancer. This information can be crucial in assisting patients in decision making regarding surveillance and risk reduction.

If a mutation is not identified in the affected relative, it usually means that either the cancers in the family are (1) not hereditary, or (2) caused by an undetectable mutation or a mutation in a different gene. A careful review of the family history and the risk factors will help to decipher whether interpretation 1 or 2 is more likely. Additional genetic testing may need to be ordered at this point. In cases in which the cancers appear hereditary and no mutation is found, DNA banking should be offered to the proband for a time in the future when improved testing may become available. A letter indicating exactly who in the family has access to the DNA should accompany the banked sample.

The genetic counseling result disclosure session should also include a detailed discussion of which other family members would benefit from genetic counseling and testing and referral information. This can apply not only to families who have been found to carry a deleterious mutation, but may also prove useful in other families (e.g., test a higher risk relative or determine segregation of a variant within a family).

The penetrance of mutations in cancer susceptibility genes is also difficult to interpret. Initial estimates derived from high-risk families provided very high cancer risks for *BRCA1* and *BRCA2* mutation carriers.[43] More recent studies done on populations that were not selected for family history have revealed lower penetrances.[44] Because exact penetrance rates cannot be determined for individual families at this time, and because precise genotype/phenotype correlations remain unclear, it is prudent to provide patients with a range of cancer risk and to explain that their risk probably falls somewhere within this spectrum. This can prove challenging for genes that lack published long-term data on cancer associations and risks.

Female carriers of *BRCA1* and *BRCA2* mutations have a 50% to 85% lifetime risk to develop breast cancer and between a 15% to 60% lifetime risk to develop ovarian cancer.[15,42,43] It is important to note that the classification "ovarian cancer" also includes cancer of the fallopian tubes and primary peritoneal carcinoma.[44,45] *BRCA2* carriers also have an increased lifetime risk of male breast cancer, pancreatic cancer, and possibly, melanoma.[46,47]

Options for Surveillance, Risk Reduction, and Tailored Treatment

The cancer risk counseling session is a forum to provide counselees with information, support, options, and hope. Mutation carriers can be offered: earlier and more aggressive surveillance, chemoprevention, and/or prophylactic surgery. Detailed management options for *BRCA* carriers are discussed in this chapter.

Surveillance recommendations are evolving with newer techniques and additional data. At this time, it is recommended that individuals at increased risk for breast cancer, particularly those who carry a *BRCA* mutation, have annual mammograms beginning at age 25 years, with a clinical breast exam by a breast specialist, a yearly breast magnetic resonance imaging (MRI) with a clinical breast exam by a breast specialist, and a yearly clinical breast exam by a gynecologist.[48,49] It is suggested that the mammogram and MRI be spaced out around the calendar year so that some intervention is planned every 6 months. Recent data suggest that MRI may be safer and more effective in *BRCA* carriers <40 years of age and may someday replace mammograms in this population.[50]

BRCA carriers may take a selective estrogen-receptor modulator (SERM) or aromatase inhibitor in hopes of reducing their risks of developing breast cancer. These medications have been proven effective in women at increased risk due to a positive family history

CANCER PREVENTION AND SCREENING

of breast cancer.[51–53] There are limited data on the effectiveness of such medications in unaffected *BRCA* carriers[54–56]; however, there are some data to suggest that *BRCA* carriers taking tamoxifen as treatment for a breast cancer reduce their risk of a contralateral breast cancer.[57] Additionally, the majority of *BRCA2* carriers who develop breast cancer develop an estrogen-positive form of the disease,[58] and it is hoped that this population will respond especially well to chemoprevention. Further studies in this area are necessary before drawing conclusions about the efficacy of chemoprevention in this population. Prophylactic bilateral mastectomy reduces the risk of breast cancer by >90% in women at high-risk for the disease.[59] Before genetic testing was available, it was not uncommon for entire generations of cancer families to have at-risk tissues removed without knowing if they were *personally* at increased risk for their familial cancer. Fifty percent of unaffected individuals in hereditary cancer families will *not* carry the inherited predisposition gene and can be spared prophylactic surgery or invasive high-risk surveillance regimens. Therefore, it is clearly not appropriate to offer prophylactic surgery until a patient is referred for genetic counseling and, if possible, testing.[60]

Women who carry *BRCA1/2* mutations are also at increased risk to develop second contralateral and ipsilateral primaries of the breast.[61] These data bring into question the option of breast conserving surgery in women at high risk to develop a second primary within the same breast. For this reason, the *BRCA1/2* carrier status can have a profound impact on surgical decision making,[62] and many patients have genetic counseling and testing immediately after diagnosis and before surgery or radiation therapy. Those patients who test positive and opt for prophylactic mastectomy can often be spared radiation and the resulting side effects that can complicate reconstruction. Approximately 30% to 60% of previously irradiated patients who later opt for mastectomy with reconstruction report significant complications or unfavorable cosmetic results.[62,63]

Women who carry *BRCA1/2* mutations are also at increased risk to develop ovarian, fallopian tube, and primary peritoneal cancer, even if no one in their family has developed these cancers. Surveillance for ovarian cancer includes transvaginal ultrasounds and CA-125 testing; however, the effectiveness of such surveillance in detecting ovarian cancers at early, more treatable stages has not been proven in any population. Oral contraceptives reduce the risk of ovarian cancer in all women, including *BRCA* carriers.[64] Recent data indicate that the impact of this intervention on increasing breast cancer risk, if any, is low.[56,65] Given the difficulties in screening and in the treatment of ovarian cancer, the risk/benefit analysis likely favors the use of oral contraceptives in young carriers of *BRCA1/2* mutations[30] who are not yet ready to have their ovaries removed. Prophylactic bilateral salpingo-oophorectomy (BSO) is currently the most effective means to reduce the risk of ovarian cancer and is recommended to *BRCA1/2* carriers by the age of 35 to 40 or when childbearing is complete.[66] Specific operative and pathologic protocols have been developed for this prophylactic surgery.[67] In *BRCA1/2* carriers whose pathologies come back normal, this surgery is highly effective at reducing the subsequent risk of ovarian cancer.[68] A decision analysis, comparing various surveillance and risk-reducing options available to *BRCA* carriers, has shown an increase in life expectancy if BSO is pursued by age 40.[69] Emerging data indicate that most ovarian cancers begin in the fallopian tube, and that salpingectomy may someday be sufficient in reducing ovarian cancer risk in young women; however, more data are needed before this option is offered to patients outside of clinical trials.[70] A relatively small percentage of women who pursue BSO may develop primary peritoneal carcinoma.[44,71] There has been some debate about whether *BRCA1/2* carriers should also opt for total abdominal hysterectomy (TAH) due to the fact that small stumps of the fallopian tubes remain after BSO alone. The question of whether *BRCA* carriers are at increased risk for uterine serous papillary carcinoma (USPC) has also been raised.[72–74] If a relationship does exist between *BRCA* mutations and uterine cancer, the risk appears to be low and not elevated over that of the general population.[75] Removing the uterus may make it possible for a *BRCA* carrier to take unopposed estrogen or tamoxifen in the future without the risk of uterine cancer, but this surgery is associated with a longer recovery time and has more side effects than does BSO alone. Each patient should be counseled about the pros and cons of each procedure and the risks associated with premature menopause before having surgery.[76]

A secondary, but important, reason for female *BRCA* carriers to consider prophylactic oophorectomy is that it also significantly reduces the risk of a subsequent breast cancer, particularly if they have this surgery before menopause.[77,78] The reduction in breast cancer risk remains even if a healthy premenopausal carrier elects to take low-dose hormone-replacement therapy (HRT) after this surgery[79]. Early data suggest that tamoxifen, in addition to premenopausal oophorectomy, in *BRCA* carriers may have little additional benefit in terms of breast cancer risk reduction.[80] Research is needed in balancing quality of life issues secondary to estrogen deprivation with cancer risk reduction in these young female *BRCA1/2* carriers.

New developments are also emerging in the treatment and, possibly, the prevention of *BRCA*-related cancers. Early data revealed that breast and ovarian cancers in *BRCA* carriers were particularly sensitive to treatment with poly adenosine diphosphate (ADP)-ribose polymerases (PARP) inhibitors in combination with chemotherapy.[81,82] New trials are focusing on which chemotherapeutic regimens are most effective in mutation carriers. More data are needed on larger cohorts of patients and are currently being studies in multiple clinical trials.

Genetic counseling and testing is also available for dozens of cancer syndromes, including Lynch syndrome, von Hippel-Lindau syndrome, multiple endocrine neoplasias, and familial adenomatous polyposis. Surveillance and risk reduction for patients who are known mutation carriers for such conditions may decrease the associated morbidity and mortality of these syndromes.

Follow-up

A follow-up letter to the patient is a concrete means of documenting the information conveyed in the sessions so that the patient and his/her family members can review it over time. This letter should be sent to the patient and health-care professionals to whom the patient has granted access to this information. A follow-up phone call and/or counseling session may also be helpful, particularly in the case of a positive test result. Some programs provide patients with an annual or biannual newsletter updating them on new information in the field of cancer genetics or patient support groups. It is now recommended that patients return for follow-up counseling sessions months, or even years, after their initial consult to discuss advances in genetic testing and changes in surveillance and risk reduction options. This can be beneficial for individuals who have been found to carry a hereditary predisposition, for those in whom a syndrome/mutation is suspected but yet unidentified, and for those who are ready to move forward with genetic testing. Follow-up counseling is also recommended for patients whose life circumstances have changed (e.g., preconception, after childbearing is complete), who are preparing for prophylactic surgery, or who are ready to discuss the family genetics with their children.

ISSUES IN CANCER GENETIC COUNSELING

Psychosocial Issues

The psychosocial impact of cancer genetic counseling cannot be underestimated. Just the process of scheduling a cancer risk counseling session may be quite difficult for some individuals with a family history who are not only frightened about their own cancer risk, but also are reliving painful experiences associated with the cancer of their loved ones.[13] Counselees may be faced with an onslaught of emotions, including anger, fear of developing cancer, fear of disfigurement and dying, grief, lack of control, negative body image, and a sense of isolation.[24] Some counselees wrestle with the fear that insurance companies, employers, family members, and even future partners will react negatively to their cancer risks. For many, it is a double-edged sword as they balance their fears and apprehensions about dredging up these issues with the possibility of obtaining reassuring news and much needed information.

A person's perceived cancer risk is often dependent on many "nonmedical" variables. They may estimate that their risk is higher if they look like an affected individual, or share some of their personality traits.[24] Their perceived risks will vary depending on if their relatives were cancer survivors or died painful deaths from the disease. Many people wonder not *if* they are going to get cancer, but *when*.

The counseling session is an opportunity for individuals to express why they believe they have developed cancer, or why their family members have cancer. Some explanations may revolve around family folklore, and it is important to listen to and address these explanations rather than dismiss them.[24] In doing this, the counselor will allow the clients to alleviate their greatest fears and to give more credibility to the medical theory. Understanding a patient's perceived cancer risk is important, because that fear may *decrease* surveillance and preventive health-care behaviors.[83] For patients and families who are moving forward with DNA testing, a referral to a mental health-care professional is often very helpful. Genetic testing has an impact not only on the patient, but also on his/her children, siblings, parents, and extended relatives. This can be overwhelming for an individual and the family, and should be discussed in detail prior to testing.

To date, studies conducted in the setting of pre- and post-genetic counseling have revealed that, at least in the short term, most patients do not experience adverse psychological outcomes after receiving their test results.[84,85] In fact, preliminary data have revealed that individuals in families with known mutations who seek testing seem to fare better psychologically at 6 months than those who avoid testing.[84] Among individuals who learn they are *BRCA* mutation carriers, anxiety and distress levels appear to increase slightly after receiving their test results but returned to pretest levels in several weeks.[86] Although these data are reassuring, it is important to recognize that genetic testing is an individual decision and will not be right for every patient or every family.

Presymptomatic Testing in Children

Presymptomatic testing in children has been widely discussed, and most concur that it is appropriate only when the onset of the condition regularly occurs in childhood or if there are useful interventions that can be applied.[87] For example, genetic testing for mutations in the *BRCA* genes and other adult-onset diseases is generally limited to individuals who are >18 years of age. The American College of Medical Genetics states that if the "medical or psychosocial benefits of a genetic test will not accrue until adulthood . . . genetic testing generally should be deferred."[88] In contrast, the DNA-based diagnosis of children and young adults at risk for hereditary medullary thyroid carcinoma (MTC) is appropriate and has improved the management of these patients.[89] DNA-based testing for MTC is virtually 100% accurate and allows at-risk family members to make informed decisions about prophylactic thyroidectomy. FAP is a disorder that occurs in childhood and in which mortality can be reduced if detection is presymptomatic.[90] Testing is clearly indicated in these instances.

Questions have been raised about the parents' right to demand testing for adult-onset diseases, and this is now happening regularly with direct-to-consumer tests and whole exome testing of children.[91] The risks of such testing to the child, and the child's right *not* to be tested must be considered. Whenever childhood testing is not medically indicated, it is preferable that testing decisions are postponed until the children are adults and can decide for themselves whether to be tested.

Confidentiality

The level of confidentiality surrounding cancer genetic testing is paramount due to concerns of genetic discrimination. Careful consideration should be given to the confidentially of family history information, pedigrees, genetic test results, pathology reports, and the carrier status of other family members as most hospitals and clinicians transition to electronic medical records systems. The goal of electronic records is to share information about the patient with his/her entire health-care team. However, genetics is a unique specialty that involves the whole family. Patient's charts often contain Health Insurance Portability and Accountability Act (HIPAA)–protected health information and genetic test results for many other family members. This information may not be appropriate to enter into an electronic record. The unique issues of genetics services need to be considered when designing electronic medical record standards.

Confidentiality of test results *within* a family can also be of issue, because genetic counseling and testing often reveals the risk statuses of family members other than the patient. Under confidentiality codes, the patient needs to grant permission before at-risk family members can be contacted. For this reason, many programs have built in a "share information with family members" clause to their informed consent documents. It has been questioned whether or not a family member could sue a health-care professional for negligence if they were identified at high risk yet not informed.[92] Most recommendations have stated that the burden of confidentiality lies between the provider and the patient. However, more recent recommendations state that confidentiality *should* be violated if the potential harm of not notifying other family members outweighs the harm of breaking a confidence to the patient.[93] There is no patent solution for this difficult dilemma, and situations must be considered on a case-by-case basis with the assistance of the in-house legal department and ethics committee.

Insurance and Discrimination Issues

When genetic testing for cancer predisposition first became widely available, the fear of health insurance discrimination by both patients and providers was one of the most common concerns.[94,95] It appears that the risks of health insurance discrimination were overstated and that almost no discrimination by health insurers has been reported.[96] HIPAA banned the use of genetic information as a preexisting condition.[97,98] In May of 2008, Congress passed the Genetic Information Nondiscrimination Act (GINA, HR 493), which provides broad protection of an individual's genetic information against health insurance and employment discrimination.[99] In addition, the Heath Care and Education Reconciliation Act of 2010 (HR 4872) prohibits group health plans from denying insurance based on preexisting conditions and from increasing premiums based on health status.[100] Health-care providers can now more confidently reassure their patients that genetic counseling and testing will not put them at risk of losing group or individual health insurance.

More and more patients are choosing to submit their genetic counseling and/or testing charges to their health insurance companies. In the past few years, more insurance companies have agreed to pay for counseling and/or testing,[101] perhaps in light of data that show these services reduce errors related to ordering and interpreting genetic testing and that decision analyses have revealed subsequent prophylactic surgeries to be cost effective.[102] The risk of life or disability insurance discrimination, however, is more realistic. Patients should be counseled about such risks before they pursue genetic testing.

Reproductive Issues

Reproductive technology in the form of preimplantation genetic diagnosis, prenatal testing, or sperm sorting are options[103] for men and women with a hereditary cancer syndrome, but are requested by few patients for adult-onset conditions in which there are viable options for surveillance and risk reduction. Importantly, if a *BRCA2* carrier is considering having a child, it is important to assess the spouse's risk of also carrying a *BRCA2* mutation. If the spouse is of Jewish ancestry or has a personal or family history of breast, ovarian, or pancreatic cancer, *BRCA* testing should be considered and a discussion of the risk of Fanconi anemia in a child with two *BRCA2* mutations should take place.[104]

RECENT ADVANCES AND FUTURE DIRECTIONS

Cancer genetic counseling and testing were thrust into the national spotlight in the spring of 2013 when Hollywood icon Angelina Jolie publically disclosed that she was a *BRCA1* carrier. One month later the Supreme Court unanimously ruled against gene patents. Referrals for genetic testing spiked across the country and have not returned to baseline levels at most centers. Within hours of the ruling, other labs began offering less expensive and more comprehensive *BRCA* testing, dramatically changing the marketplace of genetic testing for hereditary breast cancer.

All laboratories that have entered the *BRCA* marketplace have done so by including *BRCA1* and *BRCA2* in gene panels. These panels simultaneously analyze groups of genes that contribute to increased risk for breast, colon, ovarian, uterine, and other cancers. The cost of this technology continues to decrease with some multigene panels costing just a few hundred dollars *less* than traditional *BRCA* testing (~$4,000). Some panels include only well-known genes (e.g., *p53, APC, MLH1*), although many include lesser known genes (e.g., *BRIP1, NBN, MRE11A*) for which cancer risks are ill defined and medical management options are unknown. Because testing for these genes is new to the clinical setting, it is expected to take several years to compile accurate cancer risk estimates and appropriate recommendations for surveillance and risk reduction. Furthermore, the rate of *variants of uncertain significance* will likely be more common in the lesser known genes. These changes have increased the complexity of genetic testing exponentially. In response, several state and one national insurance company have mandated genetic counseling by certified providers before they will cover cancer genetic testing. In a surprising response, the American Society of Clinical Oncology (ASCO) opposed this insurer's decision, despite more than a decade's worth of data demonstrating that the majority of physicians do not have the time or expertise to offer genetic counseling and testing([38,105-108]). The AMA will decide whether to back the ASCO resolution in June 2014.

Some companies are now offering direct-to-consumer (DTC) genetic testing via websites. The accuracy of some of these DTC genetic tests are in question, and the leading company, 23andMe, has recently come under fire by the U.S. Food and Drug Administration.[105]

Maintaining high standards for thorough genetic counseling, informed consent, and accurate result interpretation will be paramount in reducing potential risks and maximizing the benefits of genetic technology in the next century.

REFERENCES

1. Peters J. Breast cancer genetics: relevance to oncology practice. *Cancer Control* 1995;2:195–208.
2. Brierley KL, Campfield D, Ducaine W, et al. Errors in delivery of cancer genetics services: implications for practice. *Conn Med* 2010;74:413–423.
3. Brierley KL, Blouch E, Cogswell W, et al. Adverse events in cancer genetic testing: medical, ethical, legal, andt financial implications. *Cancer J* 2012;18: 303–309.
4. American College of Surgeons, Commission on Cancer: Cancer Program Standards 2012: Ensuring Patient-Centered Care. http://www.facs.org/cancer/coc/programstandards2012.html Accessed on December 3, 2012.
5. Yale Cancer Genetic Counseling Program. Mammography techs ordering their own genetic testing? It appears our suspicion was correct. yalecancer geneticcounseling.blogspot.com October 2, 2013. http://yalecancergenetic counseling.blogspot.com/2013/10/mammography-techs-ordering-their -own.html
6. Lubin IM, Caggana M, Constantin C, et al. Ordering molecular genetic tests and reporting results: practices in laboratory and clinical settings. *J Mol Diagn* 2008;10:459–468.
7. Weeks WB, Wallace AE. Time and money: a retrospective evaluation of the inputs, outputs, efficiency, and incomes of physicians. *Arch Intern Med* 2003;163(8):944–948.
8. Doksum T, Bernhardt BA, Holtzman NA. Does knowledge about the genetics of breast cancer differ between nongeneticist physicians who do or do not discuss or order BRCA testing? *Genet Med* 2003;5:99–105.
9. Rosenthal ET. Shortage of genetics counselors may be anecdotal, but need is real. *Oncology Times* 2007;29:34–36.
10. Informed Medical Decisions. Adult Genetics: Genetic counseling for your health concerns. Available at: http://www.informeddna.com/index.php/patients/adult-genetics.html. Accessed August 24, 2009.
11. Informed Medical Decisions. News: Aetna Press Release: Aetna to offer access to confidential telephonic cancer genetic counseling to health plan members. Available at: http://www.informeddna.com/images/stories/news_articles/aetna%20press%20release%20bw.pdf. Accessed August 24, 2009.
12. Schneider, ME. Cigna to require counseling for some genetic tests. Internal Medicine News Digital Network. July 26, 2013. http://www.internalmedicine news.com/single-view/cigna-to-require-counseling-for-some-genetic-tests /efd4f421df8b46ba2208da423adf198d.html
13. Claus E, Schildkraut J, Thompson W, et al. The genetic attributable risks of breast and ovarian cancer. *Cancer* 1996;77:2318–2324.
14. Loman N, Johannsson O, Kristoffersson U. Family history of breast and ovarian cancers and BRCA1 and BRCA2 mutations in a population-based series of early-onset breast cancer. *J Natl Cancer Inst* 2001;93:1215.
15. Struewing J, Hartge P, Wacholder S. The risk of cancer associated with specific mutations of BRCA1 and BRCA2 among Ashkenazi Jews. *N Engl J Med* 1997;336:1401–1408.
16. Eisinger F, Jacquemier J, Charpin C, et al. Mutations at BRCA1: the medullary breast carcinoma revisited. *Cancer Res* 1998;58:1588–1592.
17. Kandel M, Stadler Z, Masciari S, et al. Prevalence of BRCA1 mutations in triple negative breast cancer. Paper presented at: 2006 42nd Annual ASCO Meeting; 2006; Atlanta, GA.
18. National Comprehensive Cancer Network Clinical Guidelines in Oncology: Genetics/Familial High-Risk Assessment - Breast and Ovarian Cancer. http://www.nccn.org/professionals/physician_gls/f_guidelines.asp#detection Accessed November 2, 2012.
19. Risch H, McLaughlin J, Cole D, et al. Population BRCA1 and BRCA2 mutation frequencies and cancer penetrances: a kin-cohort study in Ontario, Canada. *JNCI* 2006;98:1694–706.
20. Matloff E, Brierley K, Chimera C. A clinician's guide to hereditary colon cancer. *Cancer J* 2004;10(5):280–287.
21. Pilarski R. Cowden syndrome: a critical review of the clinical literature. *J Genet Couns* 2009 Feb;18:13–27.
22. Varga EA, Pastore M, Prior T, et al. The prevalence of PTEN mutations in a clinical pediatric cohort with autism spectrum disorders, developmental delay, and macrocephaly. *Genet Med* 2009;11:111–117.
23. Gorlin R. Nevoid basal-cell carcinoma syndrome. *Medicine* 1987;66(2): 98–113.
24. Schneider K. *Counseling About Cancer: Strategies for Genetic Counseling*. 2nd ed. Wiley-Liss; 2001.
25. Love R, Evan A, Josten D. The accuracy of patient reports of a family history. *J Chronic Dis* 1985;38(4):289–293.
26. Alter B, Rosenberg P, Brody L. Clinical and molecular features associated with biallelic mutations in FANCD1/BRCA2. *J Med Genet* 2007;44:1–9.
27. Thompson D, Duedal S, Kirner J, et al. Cancer risks and mortality in heterozygous ATM mutation carriers. *J Natl Cancer Inst* 2005;97:813–822.
28. Korzenik J, Chung D, Digumarthy S, at al. Case 33-2005: a 43 year-old man with lower gastrointestinal bleeding. *N Engl J Med* 2005;353:1836–1844.
29. American Cancer Society. *Cancer Facts and Figures 2009*. Atlanta, GA: American Cancer Society; 2009.

30. Olopade O, Weber B. Breast cancer genetics: toward molecular characterization of individuals at increased risk for breast cancer. Part II. PPO Updates 1998;12:1–8.
31. Stratton MR, Rahman N. The emerging landscape of breast cancer susceptibility. *Nat Genet* 2008;40:17–22.
32. Gail M, Brinton L, Byar D. Projecting individualized probabilities of developing breast cancer for white females who are being examined annually. *J Natl Cancer Inst* 1989;81:1879–1886.
33. Claus E, Risch N, Thompson W. Autosomal dominant inheritance of early-onset breast cancer. *Cancer* 1994;73:643.
34. Parmigiani G, Berry D, Agiular O. Determining carrier probabilities for breast cancer susceptibility genes BRCA1 and BRCA2. *Am J Hum Genet* 1998;62:145–158.
35. Friedman S. *Thoughts from FORCE: Comments Submitted to the Secretary's Advisory Committee on Genetics Health and Society.* http://facingourrisk.wordpress.com/2008/12/03/comments-submitted-to-the-secretarys-advisory-committee-on-genetics-health-and-society/. Accessed April 6, 2010.
36. UnitedHealth. *Personalized Medicine: Trends and Prospects for the New Science of Genetic Testing and Molecular Diagnostics.* Working Paper 7. Minnetonka, MN: UnitedHealth Center for Health Reform & Modernization; March 2012.
37. ARUP Laboratories. *Value of Genetic Counselors in the Laboratory.* Salt Lake City: ARUP Laboratories; March 2011.
38. Plon SE, Cooper HP, Parks B, et al. Genetic testing and cancer risk management recommendations by physicians for at-risk relatives. *Genet Med* 2011;13:148–154.
39. Walsh T. *More Than 25% of Breast Cancer Families with Wild-Type Results from Commercial Genetic Testing of BRCA1 and BRCA2 Are Resolved by BROCA Sequencing of All Known Breast Cancer Genes.* Paper presented at: 2013 American Society of Human Genetics Meeting Session #19; 2013; Boston, MA.
40. U.S. Preventive Services Task Force. *Genetic Risk Assessment and BRCA Mutation Testing for Breast and Ovarian Cancer Susceptibility.* Rockville, MD: Agency for Healthcare Research and Quality; 2013. http://www.uspreventiveservicestaskforce.org/uspstf12/brcatest/brcatestfinalrs.htm. Accessed June 2, 2014.
41. King MC, Marks JH, Mandell JB, et al. Breast and ovarian cancer risks due to inherited mutations in BRCA1 and BRCA2. *Science* 2003;302:643–646.
42. Antoniou A, Pharoah PD, Narod S, et al. Average risks of breast and ovarian cancer associated with BRCA1 or BRCA2 mutations detected in case Series unselected for family history: a combined analysis of 22 studies. *Am J Hum Genet* 2003;72:1117–1130.
43. Ford D, Easton D, Bishop D, et al. Risks of cancer in BRCA1 mutation carriers. *Lancet* 1994;343:692–695.
44. Piver M, Jishi M, Tsukada Y. Primary peritoneal carcinoma after prophylactic ooophorectomy in women with a family history of ovarian cancer. *Cancer* 1993;71:2751–2755.
45. Aziz S, Kuperstein G, Rosen B. A genetic epidemiological study of carcincoma of the fallopian tube. *Gynecol Oncol* 2001;80:341–345.
46. van Asperen C, Brohet R, Meijers-Heijboer, et al. Cancer risks in BRCA2 families: estimates for sites other than breast and ovary. *J Med Genet* 2005;42: 711–719.
47. Breast Cancer Linkage Consortium. Cancer risks in BRCA2 mutation carriers. *J Natl Cancer Inst* 1999;91:1310–1316.
48. Warner E, Plewes D, Hill K, et al. Surveillance of BRCA1 and BRCA2 mutation carriers with magnetic resonance imaging, ultrasound, mammography, and clinical breast examination. *JAMA* 2004;202:1317–1325.
49. Kriege M, Brekelmans CT, Boetes C, et al. Efficacy of MRI and mammography for breast-cancer screening in women with a familial or genetic predisposition. *N Engl J Med* 2004;29:351:427–437.
50. Kuhl C, Weigel S, Schrading S, et al. Prospective multicenter cohort study to refine management recommendations for women at elevated familial risk of breast cancer: the EVA Trial. *J Clin Oncol* 2010:1450–1457.
51. Powles T, Ashley S, Tidy A, et al. Twenty-year follow-up of the Royal Marsden randomized, double-blinded tamoxifen breast cancer prevention trial. *J Natl Cancer Inst* 2007;99:283–290.
52. Cuzick J, Forbes J, Sestak I, et al. Long-term results of tamoxifen prophylaxis for breast cancer: 96 month follow-up of the randomized IBIS-I trial. *J Natl Cancer Inst* 2007;99:272–282.
53. Goss PE, Ingle JN, Alés-Martínez JE, et al. Exemestane for breast-cancer prevention in postmenopausal women. *N Engl J Med* 2011;364:2381.
54. Fisher B, Constantino J, Wickerman D. Tamoxifen for the prevention of breast cancer: report of the National Surgical Adjuvant Breast and Bowel Project P-1 Study. *J Natl Cancer Inst* 1998;90:1371–1388.
55. King M, Wieand S, Hale K. Tamoxifen and breast cancer incidence among women with inherited mutations in BRCA1 and BRCA2. *JAMA* 2001;286:2251–2256.
56. Narod S, Brunet J, Ghadirian P. Tamoxifen and risk of contralateral breast cancer in BRCA1 and BRCA2 mutation carriers: a case-control study. *Lancet* 2000;356:1876–1881.
57. Phillips KA, Milne RL, Rookus MA, et al. Tamoxifen and risk of contralateral breast cancer for BRCA1 and BRCA2 mutation carriers. *J Clin Oncol* 2013;31:3091–3099.
58. Lakhani S, van de Vijver M, Jacquemier J, et al. The pathology of familial breast cancer: predictive value of immunohistochemical markers estrogen receptor, progesterone receptor, HER-2, and p53 in patients with mutations in BRCA1 and BRCA2. *J Clin Oncol* 2002;20:2310–2318.
59. Hartmann L, Schaid D, Woods J. Efficacy of bilateral prophylactic mastectomy in women with a family history of breast cancer. *N Engl J Med* 1999;340:77–84.
60. Matloff E. The breast surgeon's role in BRCA1 and BRCA2 testing. *Am J Surg* 2000; 180:294–298.
61. Turner B, Harold E, Matloff E, et al. BRCA1/BRCA2 germline mutations in locally recurrent breast cancer patients after lumpectomy and radiation therapy: Implications for breast-conserving management in patients with BRCA1/BRCA2 mutations. *J Clin Oncol* 1999;17:3017–3024.
62. Contant CM, et al. Clinical experience of prophylactic mastectomy followed by immediate breast reconstruction in women at hereditary risk of breast cancer (HBOC) or a proven BRCA1 or BRCA2 germ-line mutation. *Eur J Surg Oncol* 2002;28:627–632.
63. Forman DL, Chiu J, Restifo RJ, et al. Breast reconstruction in previously irradiated patients using tissue expanders and implants: a potentially unfavorable result. *Ann Plast Surg* 1998;40:360–363.
64. McLaughlin J, Risch H, Lubinski J, et al. Reproductive risk factors for ovarian cancer in carriers of BRCA1 or BRCA2 mutations: a case-control study. *Lancet* 2007;8:26–34.
65. Milne R, Knight J, John E, et al. Oral contraceptive use and risk of early-onset breast cancer in carriers and noncarriers of BRCA1 and BRCA2 mutations. *Cancer Epidemiol Biomarkers Prev* 2005;14:350–356.
66. Domchek S, Friebel T, Neuhausen S, et al. Mortality reduction after risk-reducing bilateral salpingo-oophorectomy in a prospective cohort of BRCA1 and BRCA2 mutation carriers. *Lancet Oncol* 2006;7:223–229.
67. Powel CB, Kenley E, Chen LM, et al. Risk-reducing salpingo-oophorectomy in BRCA mutation carriers: role of serial sectioning in the detection of occult malignancy. *J Clin Oncol* 2005;23:127–132.
68. Finch A, Beiner M, Lubinski J, et al. Salpingo-oophorectomy and the risk of ovarian, fallopian tube, and peritoneal cancers in women with a BRCA1 or BRCA2 mutation. *JAMA* 2006;296:185–192.
69. Kurian AW, Sigal BM, Plevritis SK. Survival analysis of cancer risk reduction strategies for BRCA1/2 mutation carriers. *J Clin Oncol* 2010;10;28:222–231.
70. Kwon JS, Tinker A, Pansegrau G, et al. Prophylactic salpingectomy and delayed oophorectomy as an alternative for BRCA mutation carriers. *Obstet Gynecol* 2013;121:14–24.
71. American College of Obstetricians and Gynecologists. ACOG committee opinion. Breast–ovarian cancer screening. Number 176, October 1996. Committee on Genetics. The American College of Obstetricians and Gynecologists. *Int J Gynaecol Obstet* 1997;56:82–83.
72. Hornreich G, Beller U, Lavie O. Is uterine serous papillary carcinoma a BRCA1 related disease? Case report and review of the literature. *Gynecol Oncol* 1999;75(2):300–304.
73. Levine D, Lin P, Barakat R. Risk of endometrial carcinoma associated with BRCA mutation. *Gynecol Oncol* 2001;80(3):395–398.
74. Goshen R, Chu W, Elit L. Is uterine papillary serous adenocarcinoma a manifestation of the hereditary breast-ovarian cancer syndrome? *Gynecol Oncol* 2000;79(3):477–481.
75. Boyd J. The breast, ovarian, and other cancer genes. *Gynecol Oncol* 2001; 80(3):337–340.
76. Campfield Bonadies D, Moyer A, Matloff ET. What I wish I'd known before surgery: BRCA carriers' perspectives after bilateral salipingo-oophorectomy. *Fam Cancer* 2011;10:79–85.
77. Rebbeck T, Lynch H, Neuhausen S, et al. Prophylactic oophorectomy in carriers of BRCA1 or BRCA2 mutations. *N Engl J Med* 2002;346:1616–1622.
78. Kauff N, Satagopan J, Robson M, et al. Risk-reducing salpingo-oophorectomy in women with a BRCA1 or BRCA2 mutation. *N Engl J Med* 2002;346: 1609–1615.
79. Rebbeck T, Friebel T, Wagner T, et al. Effect of short-term hormone replacement therapy on breast cancer risk reduction after bilateral prophylactic oophorectomy in BRCA1 and BRCA2 mutation carriers: the PROSE study group. *J Clin Oncol* 2005;23:7804–7810.
80. Gronwald J, Tung N, Foulkes W, et al. Tamoxifen and contralateral breast cancer in BRCA1 and BRCA2 carriers: an update. *Int J Cancer* 2006;118: 2281–2284.
81. Fong PC, Boss DS, Yap TA, et al. Inhibition of Poly (ADPRibose) Polymerase in Tumors from BRCA Mutation Carriers. *N Engl J Med* 2009;361:1–12.
82. Inglhart JD, Silver DP. Synthetic lethality – a new direction in cancer-drug development. *N Engl J Med* 2009;361:1–3.
83. Kash K, Holland J, Halper M, et al. Psychological distress and surveillance behaviors of women with a family history of breast cancer. *J Natl Cancer Inst* 1992;84:24–30.
84. Lerman C, Hughes C, Lemon S. What you don't know can hurt you: adverse psychologic effects in members of BRCA1-linked and BRCA2-linked families who decline genetic testing. *J Clin Oncol* 1998;16:1650–1654
85. Croyle R, Smith K, Botkin J. Psychological responses to BRCA1 mutation testing: preliminary findings. *Health Psychol* 1997;16:63–72.
86. Hamilton JG, Lobel M, Moyer A. Emotional distress following genetic testing for hereditary breast and ovarian cancer: a meta-analytic review. *Health Psychol* 2009;28:510–518.
87. Clayton E. Removing the shadow of the law from the debate about genetic testing of children. *Am J Med Genet* 1995;57:630–634.
88. ASHG/ACMG. Points to consider: ethical, legal, and psychosocial implications of genetic testing in children and adolescents. American Society of Human Genetics Board of Directors, American College of Medical Genetics Board of Directors. *Am J Hum Genet* 1995;57:1233–1241.
89. Ledger G, Khosia S, Lindor N, et al. Genetic testing in the diagnosis and management of multiple endocrine neoplasia type II. *Ann Intern Med* 1995; 122:118–124.

90. Rhodes M, Bradburn D. Overview of screening and management of familial adenomatous polyposis. *Br J Surg* 1992;33:125–123.
91. Howard HC, Avard D, Borry P. Are the kids really all right? Direct-to-consumer genetic testing in children: are company policies clashing with professional norms? *Eur J Hum Genet* 2011;19:1122–1126.
92. Tsoucalas C. Legal aspects of cancer genetics - screening, counseling, and registers. In: Lynch H, Kullander S, eds. *Cancer Genetics in Women*. Vol I. Boca Raton, FL: CRC Press, Inc.; 1987:9.
93. American Society of Human Genetics. ASHG Statement: professional disclosure of familial genetic information. *Am J Hum Genet* 1998;62:474–483.
94. Bluman L, Rimer B, Berry D. Attitudes, knowledge, and risk perceptions of women with breast and/or ovarian cancer considering testing for BRCA1 and BRCA2. *J Clin Oncol* 1999; 17:1040–1046.
95. Matloff E, Shappell H, Brierley K, et al. What would you do? Specialists' perspectives on cancer genetic testing, prophylactic surgery and insurance discrimination. *J Clin Oncol* 2000;18:2484–2492.
96. Hall MA, Rich SS. Patients' fear of genetic discrimination by health insurers: the impact of legal protections *Genet Med* 2000:2:214–221.
97. Leib JR, Hoodfar E, Larsen Haidle J, Nagy R. The new genetic privacy law. *Community Oncol* 2008;5:351–354.
98. Hudson KL, Holohan JD, Collins FS. Keeping pace with the times — the Genetic Information Nondiscrimination Act of 2008. *N Engl J Med* 2008;358:2661–2663.
99. The Genetic Information Nondiscrimination Act of 2008 (H.R. 493). Library of Congress Web site. http://beta.congress.gov/bill/110th-congress/house-bill/493. Accessed June 2, 2014.
100. The Health Care and Education Affordability Reconciliation Act of 2010 (H.R. 4872). Library of Congress Web site. http://beta.congress.gov/bill/111th-congress/house-bill/4872: Accessed June 2, 2014.
101. Manley S, Pennell R, Frank T. Insurance coverage of BRCA1 and BRCA2 sequence analysis. *J Genet Couns* 1998;7:A462.
102. Grann V, Whang W, Jabcobson J, et al. Benefits and costs of screening Ashkenazi Jewish women for BRCA1 and BRCA2. *J Clin Oncol* 1999;17: 494–500.
103. Offit K, Kohut K, Clagett B, et al. Cancer genetic testing and assisted reproduction. *J Clin Oncol* 2006;24:4775–4782.
104. Offit K, Levran O, Mullaney B, et al. Shared genetic susceptibility to breast cancer, brain tumors, and Fanconi anemia. *J Natl Cancer Inst* 2003;95(20): 1548–1551.
105. Greendale K, Pyeritz RE. Empowering primary care health professionals in medical genetics: How soon? How fast? How far? *Am J Med Genet* 2001;106:223–232.
106. Wilkins-Haug L, Hill LD, Power ML, et al. Gynecologists' training, knowledge, and experiences in genetics: a survey. *Obstet Gynecol* 2000;95:421–424.
107. Wood ME, Stockdale A, Flynn BS. Interviews with primary care physicians regarding taking and interpreting the cancer family history. *Fam Pract* 2008; 25:334–340.
108. Bellcross CA, Kolor K, Goddard K, et al. Awareness and utilization of BRCA1/2 testing among U.S. primary care physicians. *Am J Prev* Med 2011;40:61–66.
109. Pollack A. F.D.A. Orders genetic testing firm to stop selling DNA analysis service. *New York Times.* November 25, 2013. http://www.nytimes.com/2013/11/26/business/fda-demands-a-halt-to-a-dna-test-kits-marketing.html?_r=0

PART V

Cancer of the Thoracic Cavity

36 Molecular Biology of Lung Cancer

Leora Horn, Luiz Henrique de Lima Araujo, Patrick Nana-Sinkam, Gregory A. Otterson, Terence M. Williams, and David P. Carbone

INTRODUCTION

Lung cancer tumorigenesis is a multistep process of transformation from normal bronchial epithelium to overt lung cancer. Various molecular events resulting in gain or loss of function cause dysregulation of key genetic pathways involved in cellular proliferation, differentiation, apoptosis, migration, invasion, and other processes characteristic of the malignant phenotype. Mutations, including single nucleotide substitution or deletion, and translocation, deletion, or amplification of larger portions of genetic material may result from environmental factors, inherited susceptibility, or random events. Many genes are involved in tumorigenesis of both small cell lung cancer (SCLC) and non–small-cell lung cancer (NSCLC) (Table 36.1 and Fig. 36.1), but there are also unique genetic aberrations associated with each tumor type. The identification of the nature and frequency of these molecular abnormalities is necessary to determine their clinical implications (e.g., associations with smoking, histologic type, stage, survival, response to therapy), and define their clinical utility for the prevention and early diagnosis of lung cancer, and the development of therapeutic targets.

SUSCEPTIBILITY TO LUNG CANCER: GENETIC SUSCEPTIBILITY AND CARCINOGENS IN TOBACCO SMOKE

Tobacco use is the most important environmental factor associated with the development of lung cancer. Approximately 85% of lung cancer occurs in current or former smokers. Cigarette smoke contains more than 60 known carcinogens, 20 of which have been convincingly shown to cause lung tumors in laboratory animals or humans.[1] Of these, polycyclic aromatic hydrocarbons, such as benzo(a)pyrene, tobacco-specific nitrosamines, such as 4-(methylnitrosamino)-1-(3-pyridyl)-1-butanone (NNK), and aromatic amines, such as 4-aminobiphenyl, appear to have an important role in cancer causation. Nitrosamines such as NNK induce lung tumors in mice independent of the route of administration. Among the polycyclic aromatic hydrocarbons, benzo(a)pyrene is the most extensively tested and the first to be detected in tobacco smoke. Its role in cancer tumorigenesis is well described, and its diol epoxide metabolite has been implicated as a cause of mutations in the TP53 gene.[2] One of the carcinogenic effects of tobacco smoke in the lung is the formation of DNA adducts, leading to errors in DNA replication and resulting in mutations. DNA adducts have been identified in the bronchial tissue of patients with lung cancer. In current smokers, adduct levels correlate with the amount of tobacco smoke exposure.[3,4] In addition, in former smokers, the age at smoking initiation has been inversely associated with levels of DNA adducts, suggesting that the prevention of smoking in adolescence is of utmost importance in decreasing lung cancer risks.

Although tobacco use can account for the majority of lung cancers, most chronic smokers still do not develop lung cancer. Differences in inherent susceptibility may be related to variations in carcinogen metabolizing enzymes, DNA repair mechanisms, chromosome fragility, and other homeostatic mechanisms. Among genes for carcinogen-metabolizing enzymes, polymorphisms in the cytochrome P-450 genes, CYP1A1, CYP2D6, and CYP2E1, and in mu-class glutathione S-transferase (GSTM1) have received the most attention. In addition to inherent susceptibility to the carcinogenic effects of tobacco smoke, large genomewide association studies have identified lung cancer susceptibility loci at 15q25, 5p15, and 6p21.[5,6] In particular, polymorphisms in and around nicotinic cholinergic receptors at chromosome 15q25 appear to correlate with mRNA and protein expression of these receptors as well as functional changes in the calcium ion channel of the A5 nicotine receptor; these differences confer susceptibility to smoking behaviors.[7]

Researchers are optimistic that molecular epidemiology will help identify individuals at the highest risk of developing lung cancer. Such information, in addition to the smoking history, will be of great value in new lung cancer screening trials and in chemoprevention trials to identify persons at the highest risk of developing lung cancer.

MOLECULAR CHANGES IN PRENEOPLASIA

Before lung cancer is clinically recognizable, a series of morphologically distinct changes (hyperplasia, metaplasia, dysplasia, and carcinoma in situ) are thought to occur. It is believed that dysplasia and carcinoma in situ represent true preneoplastic changes. It is evident that preneoplastic cells contain several genetic abnormalities identical to some of the abnormalities found in overt lung cancer cells. For squamous cell carcinomas (SQCC), an immunohistochemical analysis has confirmed the abnormal expression of proto-oncogenes (cyclin D1) and TSGs (p53).[8] Allelotyping of precisely microdissected, preneoplastic foci of cells shows that 3p allele loss is currently the earliest known change, suggesting that one or more 3p TSGs may act as gatekeepers for lung cancer pathogenesis.[9] This is followed by 9p, 8p, and 17p allele loss and p53 mutation. Similarly, atypical alveolar hyperplasia, the potential precursor lesion of adenocarcinomas, can harbor KRAS mutations and allele losses of 3p, 9p, and 17p.[10] Other genetic alterations, such as inactivation of LKB1, whose germline mutations cause Peutz-Jeghers syndrome, have also been implicated in the development of adenocarcinoma. These observations are consistent with the multistep model of carcinogenesis and a field cancerization process, whereby the whole tissue region is repeatedly exposed to carcinogenic damage and is at risk for the development of multiple, separate foci of neoplasia.[11] Although all types of lung cancers

TABLE 36.1

Most Frequently Acquired Molecular Abnormalities in Lung Cancer

Abnormalities	Small Cell Lung Cancer	Non–Small-Cell Lung Cancer
Microsatellite instabilities	~35%	~22%
Autocrine loops	GRP/GRP receptor; SCF/KIT	TGF-α/EGFR; heregulin/HER2/neu; HGF/MET
RAS point mutation	<1%	15%–20%
EGFR mutation	<1%	<10% (West), ~40% (Asia)
EML4-ALK	0%	3%–7%
ROS1	0%	1%
RET	0%	1%
ERBB2	0%	2%–4%
PIK3CA	0%	1%–3%
FGFR	0%	20%
MYC family overexpression	15%–30%	5%–10%
P53 inactivation	~90%	~50%
RB inactivation	~90%	15%–30%
$p16^{INK4A}$ inactivation	0%–10%	30%–70%
LKB1 inactivation	~40%–60% (IHC)	20%–40%
Frequent allelic loss	3p, 4p, 4q, 5q, 8p, 10q, 13q, 17p, 22q	3p, 6q, 8p, 9p, 13p, 17p, 19q
Telomerase activity	~100%	80%–85%
BCL2 expression	75%–95%	10%–35%

GRP, gastrin-releasing peptide; SCF, stem cell factor; TGF-α, transforming growth factor-α; EGFR, epidermal growth factor receptor; HER2, human epidermal growth factor receptor 2; HGF, hepatocyte growth factor; RB, retinoblastoma protein; IHC, immunohistochemistry.

have associated molecular abnormalities in their normal and preneoplastic lung epithelium, SCLC patients in particular appear to have multiple genetic alterations occurring in their histologically normal-appearing respiratory epithelium.

Molecular changes have been found not only in the lungs of patients with lung cancer, but also in the lungs of current and former smokers without lung cancer. These molecular alterations are thus important targets for use in the early detection of lung cancer and for use as surrogate biomarkers in following the efficacy of lung cancer chemoprevention. The challenge is to identify not only the prevalence and temporal sequence of molecular lesions in lung preneoplasia, but also to determine which are rate

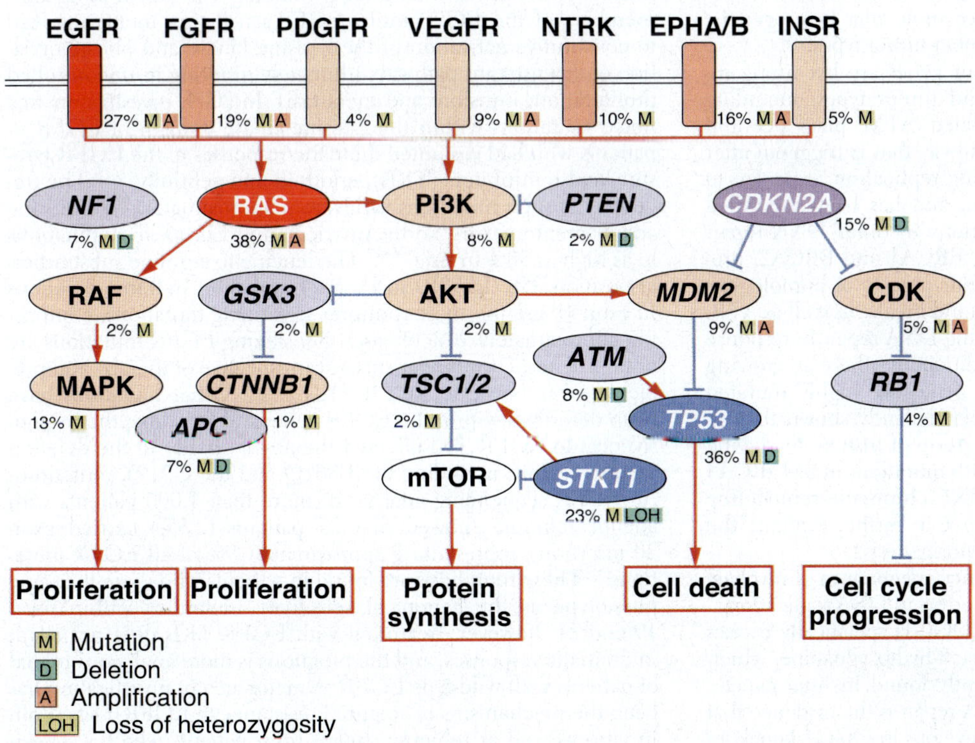

Figure 36.1 Significantly mutated pathways in lung adenocarcinomas. Genetic alterations in lung adenocarcinoma frequently occur in genes of the MAPK signaling, p53 signaling, Wnt signaling, cell cycle, and mammalian target of rapamycin (mTOR) pathways. Oncoproteins are indicated in *pink* to *red* and tumor suppressor proteins are shown in *light* to *dark blue*. The darkness of the colors is positively correlated to the percentage of tumors with genetic alterations. Frequency of genetic alterations for each of these pathway members in 188 tumors is indicated. (Reprinted by permission from Macmillan Publishers Ltd: Nature. Ding L, Getz G, Wheeler DA, et al. Somatic mutations affect key pathways in lung adenocarcinoma. *Nature* 2008;455:1069–1075. Copyright 2007.)

limiting and indispensable and thus represent potential candidates for intermediate biomarker monitoring and therapeutic efforts.

GENETIC AND EPIGENETIC ALTERATIONS IN LUNG CANCERS

Genomic Instability and DNA Repair Genes

Similar to other epithelial tumors, lung cancer cells typically display chromosomal instability—both numeric abnormalities (aneuploidy) of chromosomes and structural cytogenetic abnormalities.[12] Allele loss on chromosome 3p is thought to be the among the earliest genetic change occurring in both NSCLC and SCLC.[13] In addition, nonreciprocal translocations and recurrent losses involving 1p, 4p, 4q, 5q, 6p 6q, 8p, 9p, 11p, 13q, 17p, 18q, and 22q may occur, representing changes in known and potential tumor suppressor genes (TSGs).[14] Polysomes or regions of gene amplifications also occur and often involve proto-oncogenes, such as epidermal growth factor receptor (*EGFR*) and myelocytomatosis viral oncogene homolog (*MYC*).[15,16] Simple reciprocal translocations are uncommonly observed in lung cancer, although translocations that give rise to BRD4-NUT, CRCT1-MAML2, SLC34A2–ROS1, and EML4-ALK fusion proteins have been recently reported.[17–19] ALK and ROS1 translocations have been shown to drive the development and proliferation of tumors, and targeted therapy has resulted in clinical responses in patients with these abnormalities (see the following). In addition, alterations in microsatellite polymorphic repeat sequences are found in 35% of SCLC and 22% of NSCLC.[20] Most recently, a comprehensive genomic analysis of lung squamous cell cancers has revealed a high-frequency selective amplification of chromosome 3q compared to lung adenocarcinomas.[21] Furthermore, large-scale genomic profiling has established that there is a higher rate of copy number alterations, somatic rearrangements, and mutations found in squamous and adenocarcinoma lung cancers compared to other tumors.[22] For example, squamous cell lung cancers exhibit 8.1 somatic mutations per megabase (Mb) compared to other cancers where the frequency ranges from 1.0 to 3.2 mutations per megabase. These studies highlight the increased genetic complexity, genomic instability, higher mutation rate, and thus more extensive molecular heterogeneity that typifies lung cancer compared to other tumor types.

Recurring mutations in DNA repair genes are becoming increasingly recognized in multiple solid tumor types, including lung cancer. Ataxia telangiectasia mutated (ATM) plays a central role in the DNA damage response pathway that is triggered after genomic insults, including errors during replication, exposure to genotoxic drugs, or ionizing radiation, and has been identified in lung adenocarcinomas.[22–24] Alterations in other DNA repair genes have been identified, including BRCA1 and BRCA2, proteins that are both involved in the repair process of homologous recombination especially for double-strand breaks, as well as ATR, which functions in sensing and activating DNA repair in response to single-stranded DNA breaks.[22] Additionally, there is growing evidence that chromatin remodeling genes are highly mutated in lung cancer. Specifically, it has been recently shown that alterations in MLL2, MLL3, MLL4 (a group of histone-modifying genes) cluster in lung cancers, along with mutations in SMARCA4 and ARID1A (members of the SWI/SNF chromatin-remodeling complex).[21–24] Ongoing studies will serve to further evaluate the role of these putative TSGs in lung tumorigenesis.

The most powerful tumor surveillance mechanism is involved in DNA damage response and repair of errors in DNA replication.[25] The DNA glycosylase 8-oxo guanine (OGG1) specifically excises the oxidatively damaged mutagenic base 8-hydroxyguanine, which causes G:C→T:A transversions frequently found in lung cancer. Proof that OGG1 is central to this DNA repair is the evidence that lung adenocarcinoma spontaneously develops in OGG1 knockout mice and 8-hydroxyguanine accumulates in their genomes.[26,27] Individuals with low OGG activity have a greatly increased risk of developing lung cancer. Polymorphisms in other DNA repair genes including *ERCC1*, *XRCC1*, *ERCC5/XPG*, and *MGMT/AGT* have been correlated with a reduction of polyaromatic hydrocarbon DNA adduct formation as well as with lower lung cancer risks in case-control studies. Furthermore, high expression of ERCC1 is associated with decreased response to platinum-based chemotherapy, and overexpression of ERCC1 correlates with better overall prognosis in NSCLC,[28] reflecting improved repair of lethal DNA damage by platinum on the one hand, and greater DNA stability with less aggressive disease course on the other. More recent studies, however, have called into question the predictive ability of ERCC1 expression alone to predict cisplatin response, at least by immunohistochemical detection.[29] Similarly, ribonucleotide reductase M1 (RRM1) overexpression correlates with better de novo prognosis but resistance to gemcitabine.[30,31] High levels of the mismatch repair protein MSH2 have also been shown to be associated with poor survival with cisplatin, and may enhance the predictive significance of ERCC1 expression.[32] Prospective clinical trials investigating ERCC1 and RRM1 biomarker-guided therapy are currently underway.

PROTOONCOGENES, GROWTH FACTOR SIGNALING, AND GROWTH FACTOR–TARGETED THERAPIES

Advances in the understanding of lung carcinogenesis have yielded to a rapid discovery of novel driver oncogenes activated by mutations, translocations, or gene amplification. These alterations occur in genes that encode receptors or intracellular proteins crucial for cellular growth, proliferation, and survival, driving tumor formation and maintenance.

Receptor Tyrosine Kinases

EGFR is one of the most commonly mutated proto-oncogenes in lung adenocarcinoma. It is a transmembrane receptor-tyrosine kinase that is normally activated by binding with one of its ligands, members of the EGF family. EGFR-sensitizing mutations lead to constitutive activation of the tyrosine kinase and phosphorylation of downstream pathways ultimately resulting in uncontrolled proliferation, invasion, and metastasis. In 2004, investigators first noted mutations within the tyrosine-kinase domain of *EGFR* in patients who had sustained dramatic responses to the EGFR tyrosine-kinase inhibitors (TKIs), erlotinib and gefitinib.[33–35] The frequency of such mutations varies from approximately 10% of lung adenocarcinomas in North American and European populations to as high as 50% in Asia.[36–39] The leucine to arginine substitution at position 858 (L858R) in exon 21 and short in-frame deletions in exon 19 are the most common sensitizing mutations, comprising approximately 90% of cases. Sensitizing *EGFR* mutations are both prognostic for longer survival irrespective of therapy and predictive of response to EGFR TKIs.[35,39–47] Other mutations have been described within the *EGFR* gene, and for some, the responsiveness to EGFR TKI-directed therapy is similar to the deletion 19 and L858R, including the L861Q and the G719X mutations. An *EGFR* sequencing analysis of more than 1,000 patients with adenocarcinoma showed that 27 patients (2.5%) carried exon 20 insertions, representing approximately 9% of all *EGFR* mutations.[48] These mutations are found in patients who share the same phenotype as the canonical sensitivity mutations within exon 19 and 21; however, treatment with EGFR TKIs does not result in dramatic responses, and the prognosis is more analogous to that of patients with wild-type *EGFR*. A major area of investigation has been the mechanisms of acquired resistance to EGFR TKIs. Both in vitro as well as rebiopsy studies from patients who have been treated and subsequently progressed on treatment have shown two broad resistance mechanisms, secondary *EGFR* alterations and non-*EGFR bypass* mechanisms.[49] Approximately 50% of EGFR TKI resistance is due to a second site mutation, the T790M mutation occurring within exon 20.[50,51] Other, non-EGFR mechanisms of TKI resistance include *MET* amplification, *PIK3CA* mutations, and change in histology to a small cell appearance.[49] The T790M mutation is also found to be present at a very low prevalence in the germ line and appears to increase lung cancer risk independent of smoking.[52]

ERBB2 (formerly human epidermal growth factor receptor 2 [HER2]/neu) is a member of the erbB receptor family, along with *EGFR*. It is overexpressed in about 20% of NSCLCs, and amplified in 2% to 4% of cases.[53] *ERBB2* mutations have been identified in approximately 2% of NSCLCs, comprising in-frame insertions of 3 to 12 base pairs into exon 20, usually around the codon 776.[34,38,54] A meta-analysis suggested that ERBB2 overexpression is an indicator of poor survival in lung adenocarcinoma,[55] but amplification or mutations do not seem to be prognostic.[55,56] Early trials examining targeted therapies selected patients on the basis of ERBB2 overexpression and were mostly unsuccessful.[57] However, recent data suggest that trastuzumab, a recombinant humanized monoclonal antibody against ERBB2, may be active in *ERBB2*-mutant lung adenocarcinomas.[34] In addition, irreversible TKIs targeting ERBB2 are in early clinical trials.

Hepatocyte growth factor receptor (HGFR) is a receptor tyrosine kinase encoded by *MET*. *MET* amplification has been reported in about 2% of NSCLCs, and has been implicated in up to 20% of cases with acquired resistance to EGFR TKIs.[58] Several therapeutic strategies, including antibodies that target HGFR and anti-HGFR TKIs are under clinical evaluation in NSCLC patients, mostly aiming to prevent or overcome EGFR TKI resistance.[59–61]

Three other receptors have been nominated as potential druggable targets, especially in lung SQCC.[62,63] Insulin-like growth factor receptor 1 (IGFR1) is a tyrosine kinase receptor that activates the MAPK and PI3K/AKT/mTOR pathways, playing an important role in cancer growth and progression.[64] IGFR1 expression is higher in lung SQCC, and gene copy number has been associated with survival.[65] Despite an initial promise, phase III studies of some anti-IGFR1 agents has halted due to excess toxicities, including treatment-related deaths in the experimental arm. Fibroblast growth factor receptor 1 (FGFR1) is a member of the family of fibroblast growth factor (FGF) receptors that are dysregulated in a variety of cancers. *FGFR1* amplification has been described in approximately 20% of lung SQCCs and has been associated with cigarette smoking and worse survival.[66,67] In vitro studies showed activity with anti-FGFR inhibitors in cell lines harboring this feature, and pan-FGFR and multikinase inhibitors are in early phases of clinical investigation. Discoidin death receptor 2 (*DDR2*) is a member of the DDR family of transmembrane receptors that signals through SRC and STAT pathways. Mutations in the kinase domain have been reported in nearly 4% of lung SQCCs and were shown to yield malignant transformation in vitro.[68] Interestingly, some FDA-approved agents for chronic myelogenous leukemia seem to be active against the DDR family, including dasatinib, nilotinib, and imatinib.[69]

Translocated Genes in Lung Cancer

The anaplastic lymphoma kinase (ALK) fusion protein is an activating oncogenic driver of lung adenocarcinomas occurring in 3% to 7% of all NSCLCs.[70,71] Multiple ALK variants have been identified in lung cancer, and different ALK partners like kinesin family member 5B (KIF5B) have been described.[70,72,73] Similar to *EGFR* mutations, ALK fusions occur almost exclusively in adenocarcinomas, specifically with acinar histology, in never or former light smokers.[70,74–76] ALK fusions are not found in tumors with mutations in *EGFR* or *KRAS*, and patients appear to be of younger age compared to those with *EGFR* mutant tumors.[76] The gold standard test for *ALK* translocations is fluorescence in situ hybridization (FISH), but a variety of methods have been proposed, including immunohistochemistry, reverse transcription polymerase chain reaction (RT-PCR), and next-generation sequencing (NGS). The clinical activity of crizotinib—an oral inhibitor against c-MET, ALK, and ROS1—was impressive in early trials involving patients with the EML4-ALK translocation.[71] In a randomized phase III trial, crizotinib significantly improved progression-free survival (PFS), response rate (RR), and quality of life in comparison to second-line chemotherapy among patients with metastatic NSCLC harboring ALK translocations.[77] In a fashion analogous to that seen with EGFR TKI resistance, initial reports of resistance mechanisms include both *ALK* dependent (e.g., secondary mutations within *ALK* or amplification of the mutant *ALK* allele) and bypass tracks (e.g., the development of secondary *KRAS* and *EGFR* mutations have been described).[78–81] Importantly, several second-generation inhibitors are under clinical investigation and have shown promising activity in patients with acquired resistance to crizotinib.[82,83]

More recently, fusions involving the receptor tyrosine kinases ROS1 and RET have been described in NSCLC, each with oncogenic activity and potential utility as clinical biomarkers. ROS1 belongs to the insulin receptor family and is not normally expressed in the human lung tissue.[84] It has been demonstrated that ROS1 fusions induce autophosphorylation and downstream activation of common growth and survival pathways like mitogen-activated protein kinase (MAPK), STAT3, and PI3K/AKT. *ROS1* rearrangements occur in approximately 1% to 2% of NSCLC patients, mostly in adenocarcinoma histology, younger patients, and never smokers.[85] It has been shown that selective ALK inhibitors are also active in tumors harboring *ROS1* translocations, both in vitro and in vivo.[86] *RET* rearrangements were only described in NSCLC in 2011, involving KIF5B as a partner.[87,88] Subsequently, CCD6, NCOA4, and TRIM33 have been described as alternative RET fusion partners.[89,90] Similar to *ALK* translocations, RET partners contain a coiled-coil domain that functions as a dimerization unit, leading to ligand-independent homodimerization of the fused protein and constitutive activation of the RET kinase activity mediated by autophosphorylation. Like ALK and ROS1, RET fusions are associated with a lack of smoking history and adenocarcinoma histology, with a frequency slightly higher than 1% in all comers.[91] Agents including cabozantinib,[90] sorafenib, sunitinib, vandetanib, and ponatinib are being evaluated in this patient population.

Intracellular Signaling

Because downstream effectors are required for intracellular transduction of incoming growth factors or receptor signals, it is not surprising that proteins important in cytoplasmic signal transduction cascades are also implicated in carcinogenesis. The *RAS* gene family—in particular, *KRAS*—can be activated by point mutations at codons 12 or 13 in exon 2 in approximately 20% to 30% of NSCLCs. *KRAS* mutations more commonly occur in patients with significant smoking history and adenocarcinoma histology.[92] Approximately 70% are G→T transversions, with the substitution of glycine by either cysteine or valine. Similar G→T transversions are observed in the mutated p53 gene, representing similar DNA damage as a result of bulky DNA adducts caused by the polycyclic hydrocarbons and nitrosamines in tobacco smoke. In a meta-analysis of 3,779 lung cancer patients, mutant *KRAS* was correlated to a worse prognosis in adenocarcinoma histology, but this link was not confirmed in a prospective study.[93] The poor prognosis has been proposed to be related to the fact that KRAS mutations rarely occur with EGFR mutations, and EGFR mutant tumors have a better prognosis than EGFR wild type. Thus, if KRAS mutations are evaluated only in EGFR wild-type tumors, the adverse prognostic effect of KRAS disappears.[94] Although the oncogenicity of aberrant *KRAS* is well established, effective agents that inhibit KRAS have not reached the clinic. Another strategy has been to target downstream effectors of RAS, like the RAF family proteins and MEK. For instance, sorafenib—a broad-spectrum kinase inhibitor including the RAF family—led to a disease control rate of 79% in the BATTLE trial[95] among patients with either *KRAS* or *BRAF* mutations. However, these findings were not confirmed in a large phase III trial.[96] The addition of selumetinib (AZD6244), a MEK1/2 inhibitor, to docetaxel significantly improved RR and PFS in a randomized, phase II trial.[97] A phase III study evaluating this combination in patients with KRAS-mutant NSCLC is ongoing. Another MEK inhibitor, trametinib (GSK1120212), also showed promising results in combination with chemotherapy in early phase I/Ib studies.[98,99] However, it is not clear whether these agents have a differential effectiveness according to the *KRAS* status, because similar responses have been observed in *KRAS* wild-type tumors.

The RAF proteins are serine/threonine kinases downstream of RAS, represented by three isoforms in mammals (ARAF, BRAF, and RAF1 [also known as CRAF]). *BRAF* is a known oncogene in lung adenocarcinoma, being mutated in approximately 3% of cases.[100] In contrast to melanoma, where the majority of *BRAF* mutations occur at valine 600 (V600E) within exon 15, V600E comprises only half of cases in lung adenocarcinoma. Interestingly, *BRAF* mutations are more likely to occur in former/current smokers. Dabrafenib (BRF113928)—a specific V600E BRAF inhibitor—demonstrated a promising RR of 40% in a phase II trial involving patients with lung adenocarcinoma harboring this mutation.[101] Dramatic responses have also been reported with vemurafenib, another specific inhibitor that is U.S. Food and Drug Administration (FDA)-approved for the treatment of melanoma.[102] Apart from *BRAF*, recurrent mutations at *ARAF* and *RAF1* inhibitory sites were recently described in lung adenocarcinoma. Importantly, these mutations seem to be oncogenic in vitro, and may predict a response to targeted therapies, including sorafenib and MEK inhibitors.[103]

MAP2K1 (also known as MEK1) is a serine/threonine kinase downstream of RAF. In NSCLC, point mutations have been identified in 1% of cases, comprising three major nucleotide substitutions (Q56P, K57N, and D67N).[104] These mutations tend to be nonoverlapping with other drivers and induce constitutive extracellular signal-regulated kinase (ERK) phosphorylation and cell proliferation in vitro. It is still unknown if these mutations will predict clinical benefit from anti-MEK therapies.

Another frequently altered intracellular pathway in lung cancer is PI3K–AKT–mammalian target of rapamycin (mTOR). Phosphatidylinositol 3-kinases (PI3Ks) are lipid kinases that participate in regulating cell growth, proliferation, and survival. They comprise heterodimers formed by an 85-kDa regulatory subunit and a 110-kDa catalytic subunit, the latter being encoded by *PIK3CA*. *PIK3CA* mutations have been reported in several cancer types, including a frequency of 1% to 4% in lung adenocarcinoma.[105,106] However, a higher frequency of 16% was reported in the lung squamous section of The Cancer Genome Atlas (TCGA),[107] suggesting a predominance in this histologic subtype. The most common hotspots are at codons E542 and E545 in exon 9 (helical domain) and at codon H1047 in exon 20 (kinase domain). As opposed to other drivers, *PIK3CA* mutations often coexist with other oncogenic mutations in the case of lung adenocarcinoma and are not associated with smoking status.[108] *PIK3CA* mutations were shown to induce constitutive pathway activation and cell transformation in vitro[109] and have been associated with poor clinical prognosis.[110] The best strategy to target PI3K and the population to be selected is still a matter of debate.

AKT1 is downstream of PI3K and is a member of a family of serine-threonine kinases. Recurrent mutations within the plekstrin homology/lipid binding domain of *AKT1* at E17K have been described in up to 1% of patients with lung adenocarcinoma.[111] This mutation causes constitutive activation of AKT and leads to cellular transformation in vitro and in vivo.[112]

Phosphatase and tensin homolog (PTEN) is a lipid/protein phosphatase that is integral to cellular processes and acts as a TSG gene by inhibiting the activity of the PI3K pathway. While germline mutations in *PTEN* lead to Cowden syndrome, somatic mutations have been found in patients with lung cancer, as well as epigenetic inactivation. *PTEN* mutations may be more common in smokers and those with squamous cancer, and are also seen in patients with SCLC.[113]

THE TECHNOLOGY OF GENOMIC ANALYSES OF LUNG CANCER

In recent years, technologic advances have enabled the comprehensive analyses of gene expression, copy number alterations, mutations, and other genetic perturbations across a large number of tumors.[114] In the lung cancer setting, such global approaches have led to the understanding of cancer biology and the molecular mechanisms underlying key cancer phenotypes at an unprecedented scope. More importantly, this knowledge has leveraged the identification of subsets of tumors whose biology may be affected by interventions targeted against key dysregulated genes or pathways.[115] These efforts have been increasingly applied in individual institutions or collaborative groups as will be described.

Although direct dideoxynucleotide (ddNTP) sequencing (or Sanger sequencing) has traditionally been the gold standard for the detection of recurrent point mutations in NSCLC (like EGFR), newer methodologies have been developed that are not only less dependent on the tumor fraction in the sample, but also simultaneously determine the mutational status of many genes in a single reaction. Multiplex genotyping comprises methods such as Sequenom (Sequenom, San Diego, CA) and SNaPShot (Applied Biosystems, Foster City, CA).[116,117] In an early report using these techniques from the Massachusetts General Hospital in 2009, at least one alteration was evident in 51% of 552 cases, and no overlap was observed among the main driver oncogenes.[118] More recently, the Lung Cancer Mutation Consortium (LCMC)—a collaborative group that genotyped 1,000 lung adenocarcinomas in the United States—detected genetic alterations in 54% of cases, and 97% were mutually exclusive.[119]

NGS platforms, also known as massively parallel sequencing, offer a wide range of opportunities to characterize the cancer genome for DNA, mRNA, transcription factor binding sites, microRNA (miRNA), and DNA methylation patterns.[120,121] In TCGA, 230 lung adenocarcinomas and adjacent samples were analyzed using various NGS platforms.[122] A whole-exome approach was used in all cases, whereas whole-genome sequencing was performed in 34 samples. The authors found a very high mutation rate (median 4.56 mutations per megabase), consistent with a median of 159 mutations per tumor (range, 13 to 1,339). As demonstrated in prior experiences, this was among the highest rates in TCGA projects, only behind lung SQCC and melanoma. Somatic mutations were found in known oncogenes, like *KRAS*, *EGFR*, and *BRAF*, as well as chromatin modifiers as *ARID1A*, *SMARCA4*, and *SETD2*. A number of recurrent noncanonical mutations were documented, including a *MET* Y1003* mutation. Lung SQCC was also explored in TCGA, including 178 pairs of tumor/normal samples from patients with stages I through IV disease.[107] A total of 48,690 nonsilent mutations were identified through whole-exome sequencing, with a mean of 360 total exonic mutations per tumor (median, 8.4 per megabase). Ten genes were considered to harbor significant mutations, including *TP53*, *CDKN2A*, *PTEN*, *PIK3CA*, *KEAP1*, *MLL2*, *HLA-A*, *NFE2L2*, *NOTCH1*, and *RB1*. Frequent alterations were present in the following pathways: CDKN2A/RB1 (cell cycle control), NFE2L2/KEAP1/CUL3 (response to oxidative stress), PI3K/AKT (apoptotic signaling), and SOX2/TP63/NOTCH1 (squamous differentiation). In addition, whole-transcriptome sequencing and microarray expression was carried out. The mRNA expression data clustered in four distinct subtypes named classical, basal, secretory, and primitive, which correlate with miRNA, methylation, somatic copy number alterations, and mutation spectrum.

As a more comprehensive insight into the lung cancer genome emerges, it becomes clear that its complex biology will require continuous efforts and more integrative analyses. For instance, it is somewhat disappointing that approximately half of lung adenocarcinomas still lack a plausible target for drug development. It comes without saying that many alterations are detected in TSGs, for which no targeted therapies are available. These observations may also serve to argue that a fraction of driver mechanisms may be mediated by epigenetic or other regulatory mechanisms, as opposed to structural genomic alterations. One approach to fill this gap is the coordinated analysis of multiple types of data from large cohorts like TCGA. For example, integrating mutational data to gene expression, miRNA, or methylation profiling could potentially determine associations with particular sets of genes. Such gene sets could be subjected to computational analyses and biochemical studies to discover the biologic and clinical significance, as well as proposing alternative therapeutic strategies. The Clinical Proteomic Tumor Analysis Consortium (CPTAC) is an ongoing program that exemplifies the integration of high-throughput cancer genomics and proteomics using samples from TCGA, as well as cell lines and xenograft models.[123]

It is also intriguing that current genomic studies rely primarily on computational approaches to identify *driver* events and distinguish them from the background of *passenger* mutations. Such analyses may be flawed not only by the relatively low sample size, but also by the filtering method on its own.[124,125] Indeed, most comprehensive genomic studies (as previously described) included a few more than a hundred samples and are not empowered to detect rare mutations. Larger efforts will be essential to achieve a larger number of cases per cancer type, as exemplified by TCGA and the International Cancer Genome Consortium. In addition, continuously improving the accuracy of analytical methods will be key to avoid false discoveries and to avoid overlooking potential targetable alterations.

EPIGENETICS/EPIGENOME

Over the last 20 years, it has become apparent that epigenetics dysregulation is nearly universal in cancers, and specifically in lung cancer. Indeed, a recent study showed that the determination of the methylation status of a four gene panel (CDKN2A, CDH13, RASSF1A, and APC) is predictive of lymph node recurrence in stage I cancers.[126] A separate study confirmed the prognostic impact of a separate panel of methylated genes.[127] Unfortunately, despite the near universal finding of hypermethylation of tumor-relevant genes and the prognostic impact of transcriptional silencing of these genes, attempts at interfering with this epigenetic program by using hypomethylating agents (usually in conjunction with histone deacetylase inhibitors) has failed to have a dramatic impact on typical tumor response criteria, although each of these trials showed tantalizing evidence of biologic effect.[128–130]

More recently, mutations within epigenetic modifying genes have been discovered in a variety of thoracic tumors. These include mutations within the SWI/SNF complex proteins SMARCA4/BRG1 and ARID1A.[24] The SWI/SNF complex is an important chromatin modeling complex that is essential in yeast and is thought to function as a tumor suppressor in many human tumors, including lung cancers. Other mutations or overexpression of other epigenetic modifiers, including histone methyltransferases, histone acetyltransferase coactivators and the histone lysine demethylase KDM2A, have been described as well.[21,131,132] Whether these mutations or overexpression of genes act as *drivers* of oncogenesis or act as passenger mutations/alterations has not yet been clarified. Furthermore, if these findings will serve as useful predictors of response to epigenetic therapy will depend on the development of well-designed prospective biomarker-driven and/or stratified trials.

TUMOR SUPPRESSOR GENES AND GROWTH SUPPRESSION

A number of TSGs have been identified that inhibit lung tumorigenesis or suppress key phenotypes in developed lung carcinomas. Many classical tumor suppressors have been identified by decades of work examining genes involved in human-inherited cancer syndromes and elucidating their role in sporadic cancers. Germ-line mutations in some TSGs, such as LKB1/STK11, *p53*, and *RB1*, give rise to inherited tumor syndromes; however, a somatic loss of TSGs within sporadic cancers is more commonly seen, including p53, PTEN, CDKN2A (encoding both $p16^{INK4A}$ and $p14^{ARF}$), ATM, NF1, RB1, and APC. These have all been found to be mutated or lost in lung cancer through multiple mechanisms, such as inactivating mutations, chromosomal loss, methylation, or overexpression of other proteins that inhibit the suppressive gene's expression or activity.[23,24] We discuss several of the most frequently lost TSGs in the following paragraphs.

p53 Pathway

The *p53* gene, located at chromosome 17p13, is crucial for maintaining genomic integrity in the face of cellular stress from DNA damage through gamma and ultraviolet irradiation, carcinogens, and chemotherapy. It is the most frequently mutated TSG in human malignancies, and mutations affect approximately 90% of SCLCs and >50% of NSCLCs. In NSCLCs, p53 alterations occur more frequently in SQCC (81%) than adenocarcinomas (~50%).[21,22,24] *p53* mutations have been linked to poorer prognosis retrospectively and in the TCGA Pan-Cancer analysis; however, they have not been shown to correlate with survival in a prospective randomized clinical trial.[133,134] Most p53 mutations are G→T transversions, which correlate with cigarette smoking.[2] The Li-Fraumeni syndrome of inherited germline *p53* mutation may also lead to increased susceptibility to lung cancer in adults; this risk is magnified by tobacco smoking, because carriers who smoked had a 3.16-fold higher risk for lung cancer than nonsmokers.[135] The majority of missense mutations occur in the DNA-binding domain of the protein, and five of the six most prevalently mutated sites are arginine residues that are involved with electrostatic interactions with DNA strands.[136] Missense mutations prolong the half-life of the p53 protein, leading to increased protein levels detectable with immunohistochemistry. Also, because p53 exerts its cellular actions as a tetramer, mutant forms of the protein appear to exert dominant negative effects on wild-type p53 and have also been shown to inhibit the function of p63 and p73 family members.[137]

In addition to mutational or deletional loss of p53, other regulatory components of the p53 pathway are altered in lung cancer, including the *ATM* gene, the p53 binding protein MDM2, and the $p14^{ARF}$ tumor suppressor. *ATM* and the related protein ATR are tumor-suppressive serine/threonine kinases that activate cell cycle checkpoints in response to DNA damage and, ultimately, activate and stabilize p53.[138] Although ATR and the downstream checkpoint kinases (CHEK) are mutated in less than 1% of lung adenocarcinomas, ATM has been found to have deleterious mutations in 7% of lung adenocarcinomas. These mutations were largely mutually exclusive with p53 mutations, likely indicating that mutations in both genes would have redundant effects, especially because it has been shown that gain-of-function mutations in p53 can inactivate ATM.[139,140] Conversely, the MDM2 E3 ubiquitin ligase negatively regulates p53 by binding its transcriptional activation domain, inducing its nuclear export, and by polyubiquitinating p53, marking it for proteasomal degradation.[141] Abnormal overexpression of MDM2 is found in NSCLC, where it is amplified in a significant number of tumors. MDM2 activity is inhibited by other tumor suppressor genes in the p53 pathway, including ATM and also the $p14^{ARF}$ tumor suppressor gene.[142]

When p53 is functional, it is activated by phosphorylation in response to cellular stress (e.g., DNA damage). Once activated, p53 strongly induces the expression of other tumor suppressor genes that control cell cycle checkpoints (e.g., $p21^{WAF1/CIP1}$), apoptosis (*BAX*), DNA repair (*GADD45*), and angiogenesis (thrombospondin).[143] p53 activation has also been found to alter miRNA expression and maturation.[144,145] The high frequency of p53 loss across

CANCER OF THE THORACIC CAVITY

the entire spectrum of human tumors is a strong testament to its importance in inhibiting tumor development and growth. Restoring p53 activity in tumors is effective at halting their growth and could represent an effective therapy, although development of this strategy is challenging.[146] Several gene therapy clinical trials have been reported in which lung cancers are treated by an intratumoral injection introducing a wild-type *p53* gene using retroviral or adenoviral vectors.[147] Other strategies have been developed to restore p53 activity without attempting to reintroduce the entire gene into tumor cells.[148,149] The vaccination of patients with advanced cancer with a custom vaccine corresponding to their tumor's mutation in *p53* or *RAS* has demonstrated the generation of mutant oncogene–specific immune responses associated with prolonged survival.[150] A trial of p53 vaccination in SCLCs produced measurable increases in tumor-specific immune response that was associated with improved outcome and response to therapy in some patients.[151,152]

CYCLINS AND CELL CYCLE REGULATORY PATHWAYS

$p16^{INK4A}$ is a cyclin-dependent kinase (CDK) inhibitor important for the integrity of the G1 checkpoint. Loss of $p16^{INK4A}$ frees CDKs from inhibition, permitting constitutive phosphorylation of retinoblastoma (RB) protein and inactivation of its growth suppressive function. Approximately 40% of primary NSCLCs lose $p16^{INK4A}$, located on chromosome 9p21, making it the most common component of the $p16^{INK4A}$–cyclin D1–CDK4–RB pathway to be inactivated in NSCLC. Other CDK inhibitors are also lost at a lower prevalence in NSCLC, and the RB gene is mutated or lost in a significant minority of cases.[153] In contrast, a strikingly different pattern of pathway dysregulation is observed in SCLCs, in which abnormalities in p16 are rarely observed, but RB itself is nearly always abnormal. Although $p16^{INK4A}$ point mutations in NSCLCs were observed in only 14% of tumors, homozygous deletions or aberrant promoter methylation are common mechanisms for $p16^{INK4A}$ inactivation.[20] Indeed, aberrant $p16^{INK4A}$ methylation is a frequent, early preneoplastic event in the pathogenesis of SQCC.[154] Furthermore, $p16^{INK4A}$ and $p14^{ARF}$ are alternative splice forms of RNA transcripts from the same DNA locus. $p14^{ARF}$ is also a tumor suppressor gene and functions to stabilize p53. Thus, alteration at the $p16^{INK4A}$ locus may not only abrogate $p16^{INK4A}$ function but also disrupt p53 pathway through $p14^{ARF}$.[155]

In the absence of inhibitory regulation by the CDK inhibitors, cyclins, and their catalytic partners, the CDKs phosphorylate the retinoblastoma protein, a growth-suppressive nuclear phosphoprotein located on chromosomal region 13q14. When in its active, unphosphorylated form, RB binds and inactivates proteins such as transcription factor E2F-1, preventing G1/S transition. The RB protein is absent or structurally abnormal in more than 90% of SCLCs and 15% to 30% of NSCLCs. Lung-targeted, conditional deletion of RB and p53 in mice leads to the development of SCLC that recapitulate that observed in humans.[156] Although the p16 and RB tumor-suppressive components of this pathway are frequently lost in lung cancer, the growth promoting cyclin and CDK components of the pathway are often overexpressed, and cyclin D1, cyclin E1, and CDK4 have each been shown to be amplified in a subset of lung cancers[157] and are overexpressed by immunohistochemical evaluation.

LKB1, AMPK, AND MTOR PATHWAY

LKB1 is a serine/threonine kinase that serves as a *master regulator* of several key intracellular pathways through phosphorylation of downstream regulatory kinases. Its tumor-suppressive role became apparent when it was discovered that inherited mutations in LKB1 gave rise to a rare autosomal-dominant polyposis/cancer susceptibility disease, Peutz-Jeghers syndrome.[158,159] Subsequent to this discovery it was found that LKB1 is somatically mutated and deleted in a range of other carcinomas, most prevalently in NSCLC, where approximately 20% to 30% of adenocarcinomas exhibit LKB1 loss.[160–162] SQCCs and large cell lung carcinomas also exhibit LKB1 loss but at a lower frequency, and an immunohistochemical analysis revealed absent LKB1 expression in two-thirds of SCLCs.[163] In a mouse model, tumors rapidly develop when conditional LKB1 knockout was combined with conditional expression of oncogenic KRAS using inhaled adenovirus-expressing Cre recombinase. Additionally, whereas most other mouse models of lung tumorigenesis (e.g., oncogenic KRAS with conditional p53 deletion) cause only lung adenocarcinomas, more than half of the tumors resulting from KRAS with conditional LKB1 deletion showed squamous or mixed histology, and large cell histology was also observed.[161] LKB1 regulates a key metabolic checkpoint through its phosphorylation of the AMP-activated protein kinase AMPK. Phosphorylation of AMPK results in the suppression of tumor growth and metabolic activity by direct phosphorylation of metabolic enzymes and by activation of the tuberous sclerosis complex tumor suppressors, which block activation of the mTOR pathway.[164] In tumors that have lost LKB1, this growth-suppressive checkpoint is inactivated.[165,166] Metformin, an oral hypoglycemic drug commonly used in diabetics, activates AMPK and has been found to inhibit proliferation and colony formation in vitro.[167] Retrospective analyses demonstrate reduced incidence of cancer among diabetics treated with metformin.[168–170] In addition, metformin treatment of diabetics is associated with higher rates of complete response among neoadjuvantly treated breast cancer patients.[171] Although metformin appears to require functional LKB1 in order to effect AMPK activation, other compounds have been identified that circumvent this requirement. Thus, direct pharmacologic reactivation of the downstream tumor-suppressive functions of AMPK may be a viable therapeutic strategy for LKB1-deficient tumors. In addition to its role in regulating the AMPK metabolic checkpoint, LKB1 has many other distinct roles dependent on other downstream effector kinases, such as salt-inducible kinase, NUAK, and microtubule-affinity regulating kinase. These actions play a role in regulating a variety of cellular phenotypes important to cancer, such as cellular motility and transcriptional regulation, and LKB1 has been shown to exert profound effects in maintaining cellular polarity.[172,173] However, the relative importance of these various phenotypes in the biology of LKB1-deficient lung cancers is poorly understood.

OTHER PUTATIVE TUMOR SUPPRESSORS

Several other genes that are less well characterized than the tumor suppressor genes detailed previously have been identified as targets of recurrent mutational inactivation, chromosomal loss, and epigenetic repression in lung cancer. These candidate suppressor genes are often identified as regions of copy number loss or loss of heterozygosity (LOH) that occur in multiple tumors in large, genomewide studies of chromosomal architecture in lung cancer. Further experimentation is required to elucidate which molecular pathways and cellular phenotypes are affected and to define the functional importance of these candidates. Common regions of genomic loss surround the chromosomal regions of classical tumor suppressors CDKN2A, CDKN2B, LKB1, and RB1 (in small cell lung cancer). Other areas of recurrent loss in NSCLC occur at 9p23, 3p14.2, 3p21.3 16q23.1, 2q21.2, 4q35, 5q12.1, and 13q12.11.[157] Many of these regions are also altered in SCLC, although there are fewer data available for this tumor type. Determining the functional roles of each individual gene can be challenging. Of genes included in the regions listed previously, missense mutations have been identified in PTPRD (9p23), LRP1B (2q21.2), BLU (3p21.3), and WWOX (16q23.1).[174,175] Experimental reexpression of candidate genes has been shown to inhibit proliferation in tumor cell lines for many of these putative tumor suppressors, including PTPRD, LRP1B, WWOX (16q23.1), FHIT (3p14.2), SMARCA4 (19p13.2), PTEN (10q23), and RASSF1, FUS1, BLU, and SEMA3B (3p21.3).[176,177] However, for most of these candidates, the biologic implications of gene loss in a tumor is uncertain.

Immune Checkpoint Inhibitors

Immune checkpoint inhibitors have recently demonstrated promising results in lung cancer patients. In particular, inhibitors to cytotoxic T-lymphocyte–associated antigen 4 (CTLA-4) and programmed death 1 (PD-1) and programmed death receptor ligand 1 (PD-L1) are currently in clinical trials in both small cell and non–small-cell lung cancer patients. CTLA-4 is expressed on T cells and suppresses T-cell signaling.[178] Ipilimumab is a monoclonal antibody that inhibits CTLA-4 and is FDA approved for the treatment of melanoma. Randomized phase II trials in small cell and non–small-cell lung cancer patients demonstrated promising results when ipilimumab was combined with chemotherapy.[179,180] Randomized phase III trials in SCLCs and NSCLCs are ongoing. Antibodies that block PD-1 include nivolumab (BMS-936558) and MK3475. These agents inhibit binding of PD-1 to both its ligands, PD-L1 and PD-L2. Antibodies that block PD-L1 include MPDL3280A and MEDI-4736. These agents inhibit binding of the ligand to its receptor PD-1 and B7.1. A large phase I trial of nivolumab included 129 NSCLC patients and reported a 17.1% response rate, 1-year survival of 42%, and 2-year survival of 24%.[181,182] Based on this promising data, two randomized phase III trials in squamous and nonsquamous NSCLC patients and a single-arm phase II trial in squamous NSCLC patients have been completed with results anticipated. In patients with tumor samples available for assessment, PD-L1 expression by immunohistochemistry was associated with a response to therapy, whereas no response was observed in patients with tumors that were PD-L1 negative.[181] A phase I trial that included 85 NSCLC patients treated with MPDL3280A reported a response rate of 23%.[183] Preliminary data reported that the response rate was higher in tumors that were IHC3 positive (83%), defined as 10% of tumors staining positive for the expression of PD-L1, and in smokers. Although anti-CTLA-4 antibodies are being employed with chemotherapy in lung cancer patients, single agent data with anti-PD-1 and PD-L1 antibodies appears promising, and it is unclear if these agents should be used alone or in combination with chemotherapy or targeted therapy in lung cancer patients.

OTHER BIOLOGIC ABNORMALITIES IN LUNG CANCER

Cellular Immortality Resulting from Increased Telomerase Activity

Cellular senescence is mainly regulated by telomerase, a ribonucleoprotein enzyme responsible for maintaining telomere length by de novo synthesis of telomeres and elongation of existing telomeres. The human telomerase reverse transcriptase (hTERT) catalytic subunit is the major determinant of telomerase activity in vitro and in vivo. During normal cell division, telomere shortening leads to cell senescence and thus governs normal cell mortality. TERT maintains telomere ends via the synthesis of TTAGG nucleotide repeats. Telomerase activation is considered mandatory for tumor cells to escape senescence and contributes to immortalization and cancer pathogenesis. For example, immortalization of primary human airway epithelial cells can be achieved by the successive introduction of the simian virus SV40 early region and *hTERT*.[184] Malignant transformation is seen when these immortalized cells are transfected by an activated *RAS* oncogene. Approximately 100% of SCLCs and 80% to 85% of NSCLCs have been demonstrated to express high levels of telomerase activity. Furthermore, hTERT gene amplification occurs in 57% of NSCLCs, suggesting that this pathway is commonly targeted in lung cancer.[185] The prognostic significance of hTERT expression or activity remains controversial, although a recent study demonstrated that the copy number of serum *hTERT* mRNA was independently correlated with tumor size, tumor number, presence of metastasis, likelihood of recurrence, and smoking.[186] Furthermore, elevated telomerase activity and hTERT levels have been associated with worse DFS and overall survival in patients with stage I NSCLC.[187] In preneoplastic lesions, telomerase activity or expression of its RNA component, or both, are observed in situ in lesions with the expression proportional to the severity of histology grade, supporting a temporal role for telomerase activation during lung preneoplasia.[188] Thus, telomerase activity or expression can be used as a potential biomarker to detect premalignant as well as tumor cells. For these reasons, there is much interest in developing antitelomerase drugs as new therapeutics.[189,190]

Deregulation of Apoptosis

Loss of normal apoptosis commonly occurs in many cancer types and is associated with the expansion of viable cells and the development of resistance to chemotherapy and radiation therapy. Many members of both the mitochondrial (intrinsic) and the death receptor (extrinsic) apoptotic signaling pathways are found to be abnormal in lung cancer. A member of the intrinsic pathway, the antiapoptotic gene *BCL2* originally described in follicular lymphomas, is abnormally overexpressed in SCLCs (75% to 95%) and some NSCLCs (25% of SQCC and approximately 10% of adenocarcinoma) and is the prototypical member of the antiapoptotic Bcl2 family proteins.[191–193] BCL-2 expression is associated with good prognosis in NSCLCs.[194] Cytotoxicity of many chemotherapeutic agents is induced through the Bcl-2 apoptotic pathway; overexpression of Bcl-2 is associated with increased resistance to these agents.[195,196] Other prosurvival Bcl-2 family members include Bcl-xL, Bcl-w, and Mcl-1. Conversely, a number of Bcl-2 family members have proapoptotic functions, including Bim, Bak, Bax, Bad, and Puma. Given the role of Bcl-2 and other members of this family in suppressing apoptosis and in reducing the efficacy of chemotherapy and radiotherapy, considerable effort is being made to develop Bcl-2 family targeted therapeutics in combination with chemotherapy.

In the extrinsic apoptotic pathway, death receptors are members of the tumor necrosis factor (TNF)/TRAIL receptor gene superfamily that consists of more than 20 proteins with a broad range of biologic functions, including regulation of cell death and survival, differentiation, or immune regulation. The best-characterized death receptor, Fas (CD95), and its ligand, FasL, have also been implicated in lung cancer. In general, lung cancers express FasL but not the receptor. However, as T cells express Fas, one model that may help explain the resistance of lung cancer cells to immune surveillance involves the clonal deletion of immune T cells that would otherwise be directed against lung cancer antigens by this Fas–FasL interaction. Both caspase-8 and caspase-10 expression appears to be decreased in lung cancer. Homozygous deletion or methylation of the *CASP8* gene has been observed in SCLC cell lines, with 79% demonstrating loss of expression, suggesting that therapies that utilize the TNF/TRAIL receptor pathway of apoptotic activation may not achieve success in SCLC due to the impaired formation of the death-inducing signaling complex (DISC).[197] Of note, TRAIL-induced apoptosis is independent of *p53* gene status. Conversely, because NSCLC has high rates of p53 inactivation (but predominantly intact caspase 8 pathways) and high levels of TRAIL receptor expression, this mode of therapy may prove beneficial. Polymorphisms in the promoter region of caspase-9 have been shown to contribute to risk of lung cancer development.[198]

Another family of proteins that promote tumor survival are the inhibitors of apoptosis (IAP), which bind to and block caspase function, especially caspase-3 and -7. IAPs also inhibit apoptosis via the modulation of the transcription of nuclear factor κ B (NF-κB). In addition to X-linked inhibitor of apoptosis protein (XIAP), one of the best-known members of this class of protein is survivin. Its expression is high in the tumor but nearly nonexistent in adult normal tissue, and higher expression has been correlated with poor outcomes in NSCLCs.[199,200] The suppression of survivin has been shown to sensitize lung cancer cells to radiation, suggesting that it can be a potential target for intervention.[201] During the activation of apoptosis, another class of proteins called Smac proteins are released from the mitochondria and neutralize IAPs, by competing with caspases for the binding of IAPs. Bcl-2 family inhibitors, TRAIL receptor agonists, Smac mimetics, and IAP inhibitors are currently undergoing clinical testing as agents that sensitize lung tumor cells to chemotherapy and radiation in order to promote apoptosis.[202]

microRNAS IN LUNG CANCER DIAGNOSTICS AND THERAPY

Approximately 2 decades ago, investigators made the startling discovery that components of the human genome, previously considered to be nonfunctional, actually harbored noncoding RNAs (ncRNAs) with gene regulatory properties.[203,204] Termed microRNAs (miRNAs or miRs), these 22 nucleotide ncRNAs are now known to be highly conserved, are often localized within fragile chromosomal regions and have the capacity for gene regulation through either mRNA degradation or the inhibition of translation.[205] Given their relative short length and redundancy, it is estimated that miRNAs may regulate up to 60% of the human genome. miRNAs have been implicated as regulators of biologic processes fundamental to both the initiation and progression of cancer (differentiation, proliferation, angiogenesis).[206,207] The mechanisms of change in miRNA expression in cancers are multifactorial. First, miRNAs tend to be localized to fragile chromosomal regions. Such chromosomal regions harbor amplifications, deletions, and translocations, many of which have been described in lung cancers.[208] Thus, in some cases, patterns of miRNA deregulation may be linked to chromosomal aberrations. Changes in miRNA expression and function may also be driven by epigenetic changes, miRNA or target polymorphisms, environmental stimuli (e.g., cigarette smoke), and either tumor suppressors or oncogenes (e.g., p53).[209,210] Although the function of many miRNAs remains largely unknown, research suggests that miRNA function is both disease and cell specific.

microRNA Biogenesis

The process of miRNA biogenesis is a complex one and investigators continue to explore the mechanisms that drive miRNA production (Fig. 36.2). Initially, a long primary transcript (pri)-miRNA transcript undergoes transcription by RNA polymerase II.[211] The pri-miRNAs are then bound to the double-stranded RNA-binding domain (dsRBD) protein known as DiGeorge syndrome critical region gene 8 (DGCR8) for vertebrates.[212] Subsequently, the RNase III endonuclease termed RNASEN/Drosha converts the pri-miRNA to a smaller stem-loop ~70 nucleotide (nt) precursor miRNA (pre-miRNA). These pre-miRNAs are then transported from the nucleus to the cytoplasm using the dsRBD, Exportin 5.[213] Once in the cytoplasm, the pre-miRNA is cleaved to a mature 18 to 25 nucleotide miRNA using Dicer. The mature miRNA sequence is then loaded into the RNA-induced silencing complex (RISC) complex after which it may then form complementarity to either the 3′ or 5′ untranslated region (UTR) of a target gene to induce either RNA degradation of the inhibition of translation. It is important to recognize that investigators have now identified

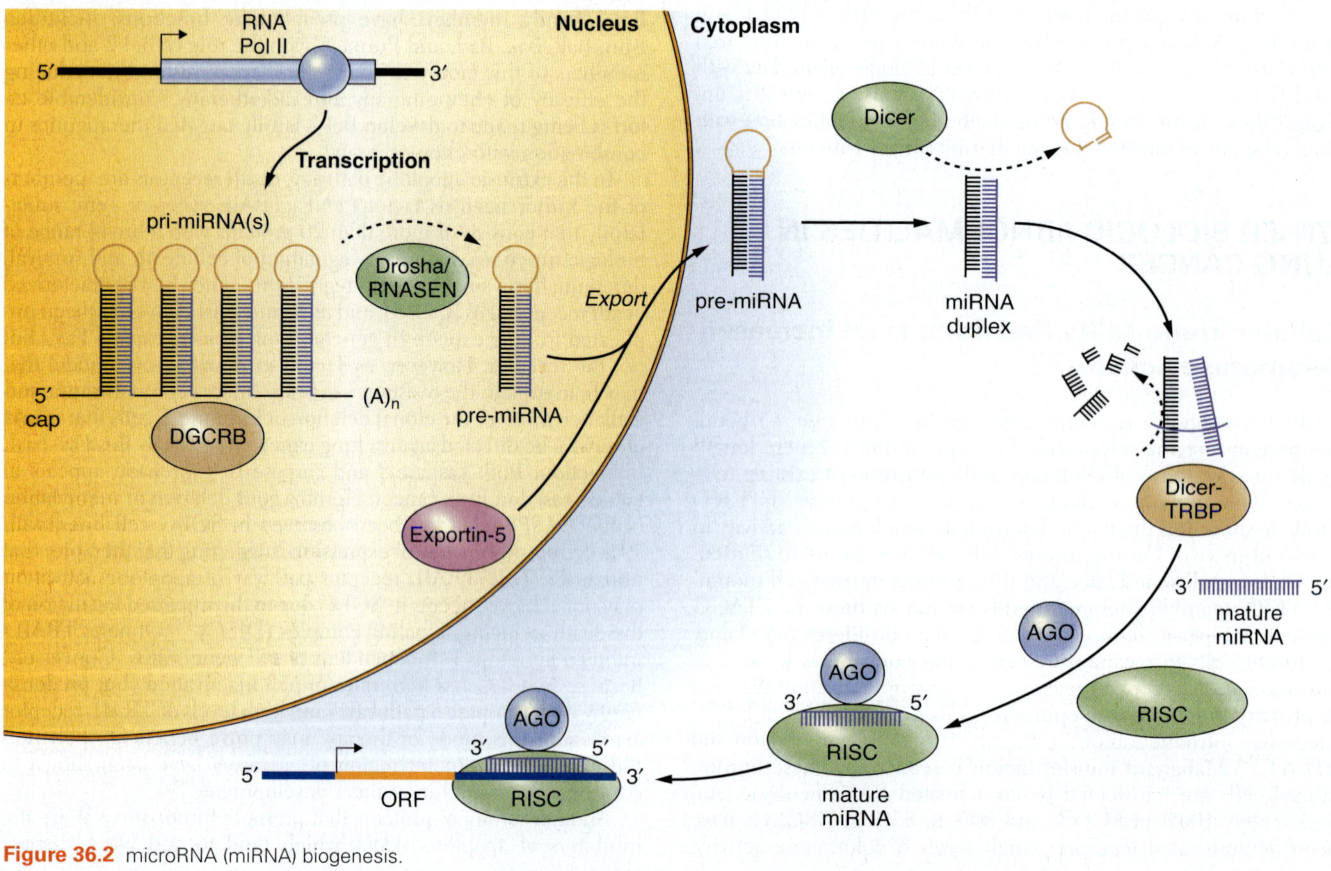

Figure 36.2 microRNA (miRNA) biogenesis.

additional mechanisms for miRNA biogenesis, suggesting that we are just beginning to understand the complexities of this process.

miRNA PROFILING IN LUNG CANCER

Early investigations in lung cancer have focused on applying high throughput platforms as a means for linking patterns of miRNA deregulation to clinical parameters. Of note, targeted the disruption of miRNA processing through the targeting of Dicer can promote lung tumorigenesis and has been associated with clinical outcome.[214] Yanaihara and colleagues[215] conducted high throughput profiling of cases of stage I adenocarcinoma of the lung. They identified over 40 miRNAs that distinguished lung tumors from adjacent uninvolved lung.[215] Of these miRNAs, decreased Let-7a-2 and increased miR-155 appeared to correlate with patient outcome. Because of that initial study, investigators have conducted multiple similar studies with the primary goals of identifying a prognostic miRNA signature[216–218] and potentially actionable miRNAs.[218]

Despite the multitude of miRNA profiling studies, investigators have yet to reach a consensus on which miRNAs confer the most accurate prognostic information. A primary reason for the lack of reproducibility is that, similar to other high throughput platforms, miRNA profiling studies are susceptible certain biases including small cohort sizes, varying platforms (array, sequencing, RT-PCR), and variability in data interpretation. In addition, most platforms are based on previously identified miRNAs. A recent study by Keller and colleagues[219] sought to use NGS to identify both previously unknown and novel mature forms of miRNAs. The authors conducted NGS on peripheral whole blood obtained from 10 patients with NSCLCs (stages 1A through IIIA) and 10 healthy control patients. They identified 32 known and 7 novel miRNAs that were significantly altered in patients with lung cancer. In addition, they identified 41 novel mature forms of previously identified precursors and 76 novel miRNAs, thus suggesting that we have yet to identify all miRNAs that may be of potential clinical and biologic relevance.

miRNAs and Mutational Status in Lung Cancer

The identification of actionable somatic mutations such as EGFR and ALK has markedly altered clinical practice in lung cancer. Few studies have correlated lung tumor mutational status with miRNA deregulation. Dacic and colleagues[220] examined EGFR-mutated, KRAS-mutated, and double-negative lung tumors for miRNA expression and identified few mutation-specific miRNAs. miR-155 was upregulated in double negative lung tumors, whereas miR-495 was upregulated only in KRAS-positive tumors and miR-25 was upregulated only in EGFR-mutated tumors. miRNAs have been implicated as drivers of both EGFR sensitivity and resistance. For example, Garofalo and colleagues[221] demonstrated that deregulation of select miRNAs miR-30b, miR-30c, miR-221/222, miR103, and miR-203 contributed to both in vitro and in vivo sensitivity of NSCLC to gefitinib.[221] Several miRNAs, including miR-128b, miR-7, and miR-145, have been validated as directly targeting EGFR.[222–224] In the case of miR-7, investigators determined both in vitro and in vivo that EGFR signaling was mediated in part by miR-7 induction in a Ras/ERK/Myc dependent manner.[225] Conversely, liposomal-mediated delivery of miR-7 has been shown to overcome EGFR resistance in T790M-mutated lung cancer cell lines.[226]

Integrating miRNAs into Clinical Decision Making in Lung Cancer

Although significant progress has been made in miRNA discovery, few miRNAs have reached clinical application in human disease; however, two recent discoveries have led to the application of miRNAs as directed therapeutics. The first involves the directed targeting of miR-122 as a therapeutic in hepatitis C, whereas the other study, which is much earlier in development, involves supplemental replacement of the tumor suppressor miRNA miR-34 in the setting of hepatocellular carcinoma or solid malignancies that have metastasized to the liver.[227,228] No such studies have reached clinical application in lung cancer; however, ongoing investigation suggests that miRNA signatures may be of value in both diagnostic and therapeutic decision making. In particular, investigators are exploring the potential for miRNA signatures in the settings of indeterminate lung nodules and early detection, histologic classification, and chemotherapeutic response, each of which can present clinical challenges. Schembri and colleagues[229] demonstrated that the human airway epithelium was susceptible to changes in miRNA expression following cigarette smoke exposure. They identified 28 miRNAs that were differentially expressed in airway epithelium from current and never smokers. One particular miRNA was miR-218, which was downregulated in smokers. Since that initial finding, studies have demonstrated downregulation of miR-218 in SQCC of the lung.[230] Few studies to date have identified a miRNA signature for solitary lung nodules.[231] The concept of integrating miRNA profiling in lung cancer early detection is an intriguing one. Using cohorts drawn from a longitudinal lung cancer screening trial, Boeri and colleagues[232] tested and identified plasma-based miRNA signatures that could predict the risk for the development of lung cancer, diagnosis, and prognosis.

Another potential area for integration for miRNA biology into the clinic is in the setting of determining chemotherapeutic response. Several studies have been conducted using miRNAs to distinguish chemosensitive from chemoresistent tumors.[34,221,233,234]

Noninvasive miRNA Detection

There have been numerous studies exploring potential noninvasive biomarkers in lung cancer. These biomarkers have included circulating DNA, transcripts, select proteins, cytokines, and angiogenic factors. Despite such exciting studies, a lack of reproducibility and a lack absence of mechanistic insight have limited the clinical impact. Recently, investigators demonstrated the utility of sputum miRNA in the early detection of lung cancer. Using a training set of 154 patients (66 with lung cancer and 68 controls) and a test set of 64 lung cancer patients and 73 smoking controls, Shen and colleagues[235] showed that sputum levels of miR-31 and miR-210 had a sensitivity of 65.2% and a specificity of 89.7% in diagnosing lung cancer. Interestingly, when combined with a computed tomography (CT) scan, the resultant specificity was higher than with a CT scan alone.[235] An independent study identified sputum miR-205, miR-210, and miR-708 as potential diagnostic biomarkers in early stage lung cancer.[236]

Investigators recognize that components of the lung tumor microenvironment, including endothelial cells, macrophages, and fibroblasts to name a few, each harbor distinct biologic programs that drive cross-talk with the primary tumor, thus fostering tumor progression. Although several mechanisms that underlie this exchange of information have been proposed and explored, there are likely to be many others. Although multiple gain of function and silencing studies have shed light on the multitude of intracellular physiologic functions of miRNAs, few have truly explored the manner by which miRNAs may carry genetic information and programming between cells and their environment. Recently, investigators have demonstrated that miRNAs may circulate both freely attached to select proteins (e.g., Ago) or lipids and packaged within extracellular vesicles (EV), including exosomes, apoptotic bodies, and microvesicles (Fig. 36.3). The concept of *packaged* miRNAs is particularly intriguing as a mechanism for the intercellular transfer of genetic material.[237] These paradigm-shifting discoveries have led to an intense investigation for novel mechanisms by which circulating miRNA may serve as mediators of intercellular communication. However, several unanswered questions remain, including defining the distribution and mechanism by which miRNAs are processed

CANCER OF THE THORACIC CAVITY

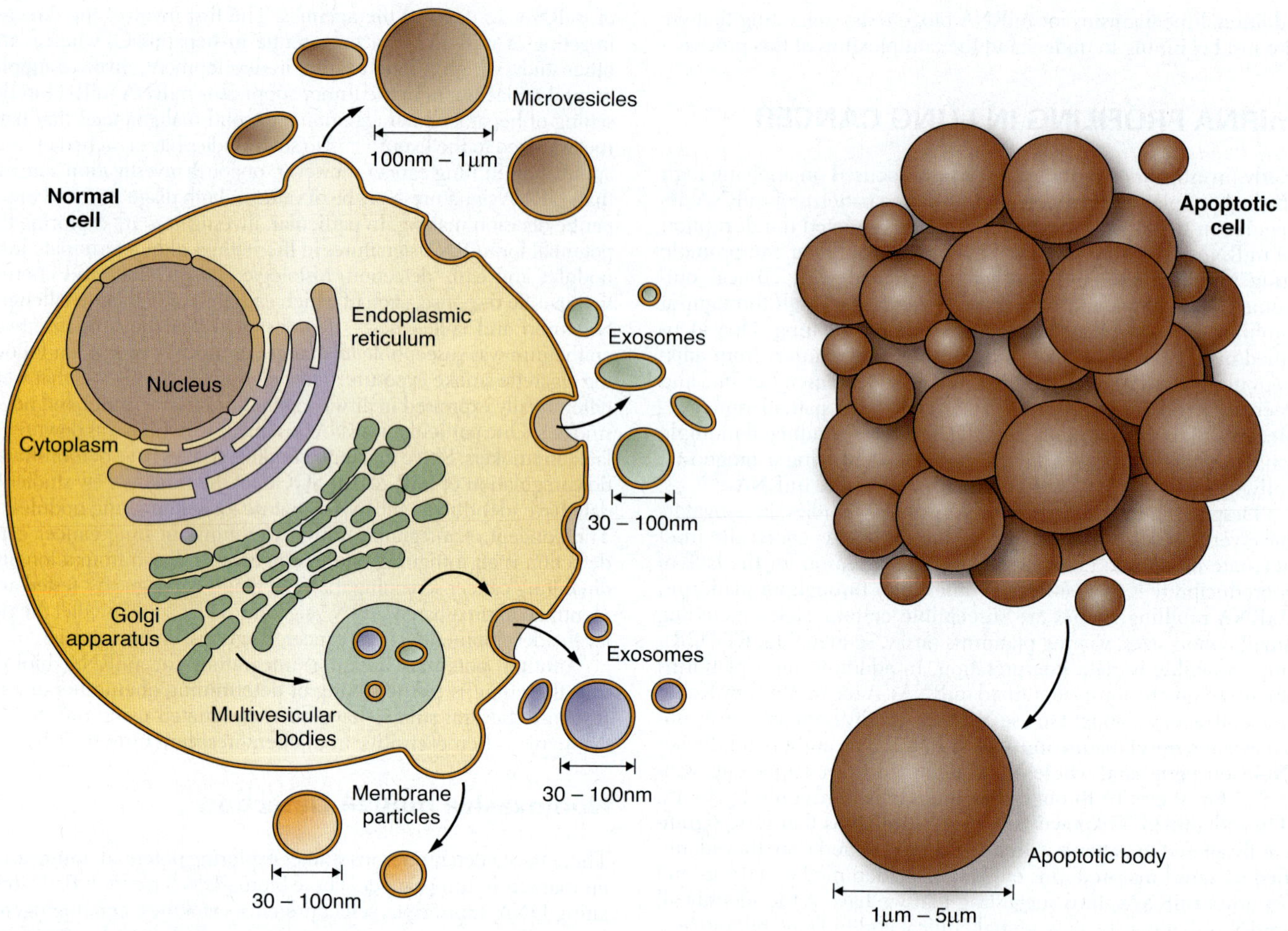

Figure 36.3 Extracellular vesicles.

for cellular release, how they are packaged into EVs versus being bound to molecules, and ultimately, their biologic function in circulation. To date, some studies suggest that the majority of circulating miRNAs are not associated with exosomes but rather are bound to select proteins.[238] Surprisingly, very few studies have examined the clinical and biologic role for extracellular miRNAs in lung cancer. Although the majority of studies to date have focused on linking global expression patterns of miRNAs in blood or other bodily fluids to clinical parameters, the reproducibility of signatures has been limited by variability in the compartment analyzed (whole blood, peripheral blood mononuclear cells [PBMC], serum, or plasma) and low cohort numbers. Identifying the *lung cancer signature* within these compartments is a major challenge.

Very few studies to date have examined the presence of miRNAs in the circulation as either diagnostic or prognostic biomarkers in lung cancer. The earliest studies to examine miRNAs in the circulation were focused on merely providing scientific feasibility for the presence of miRNAs in the circulation. Studies have targeted whole blood, peripheral mononuclear cells, and plasma with no clearly reproducible signature.[147,148,150]

INVASION, METASTASIS, AND ANGIOGENESIS

An investigation of the molecular mechanisms of invasion and metastasis has yielded a variety of candidate genes, including cell adhesion molecules such as the cadherins, integrins, and CD44. The E-cadherin–catenin complex is critical for intercellular adhesiveness and the maintenance of normal and malignant tissue architecture. Epigenetically reduced expression of this complex in malignant disease is associated with tumor invasion, metastasis, and unfavorable prognosis in lung cancer. Another family of adhesion molecules are the integrins. α_3 Integrin has been shown to be important for normal lung development, and diminished expression correlated with a poor prognosis for patients with lung adenocarcinoma. Specific isoforms of CD44 may also be associated with lung cancer metastasis. Matrix metalloproteinases (MMP) are zinc-dependent proteases that belong to a family of endopeptidases, which degrade the extracellular matrix and basement membrane, necessary first steps in angiogenesis. The increased expression of MMPs has been strongly implicated in tumor growth, invasion, and metastasis. MMP2 and MMP9 have been associated with poorer prognosis. However, despite its established role in invasion and metastasis, many randomized phase III trials of MMP inhibitors have failed to demonstrate a survival benefit in patients with advanced lung cancer.[239] This is perhaps related to the lack of specificity of these inhibitors and recent findings that some MMPs actually inhibit tumor growth.[240] The stimuli that regulate tumor cell invasiveness are often generated or influenced by surrounding stromal or inflammatory cells and, as such, the invasive phenotype seems to be quite plastic, complex, and highly dependent on the context of the tumor microenvironment.[241]

Angiogenesis, the formation of new blood capillaries, is necessary for a tumor mass to grow beyond a few millimeters in size. The angiogenic switch results from perturbation in the balance between inducers and inhibitors, both of which are produced by tumor and host cells. Vascular endothelial growth factor (VEGF), basic fibroblast growth factor (bFGF), and angiogenic cytokines, such as interleukin-8, have all been implicated in lung cancer.[242]

Furthermore, high microvessel density (MVD) and VEGF overexpression are predictive of poor outcome. Thus, tumor angiogenesis has become a major new therapeutic target for lung cancer.[243] Clinical trials in NSCLC with bevacizumab, the humanized monoclonal antibody to VEGF, to chemotherapy prolongs PFS in phase III clinical trials, although improvements in overall survival were not always observed.[244–246]

CANCER STEM CELL HYPOTHESIS

The cancer stem cell hypothesis proposes that a self-renewing undifferentiated stem cell population comprising a small fraction of the total tumor burden gives rise to more numerous and more differentiated progeny that populate the tumor.[247] Among the characteristics reported to distinguish stemlike cells from cells constituting the bulk of tumors include the potential for supporting the continued growth of the local tumor mass, for seeding metastases throughout the body, and a resistance to cytotoxic therapies allowing the residual viable stem cells to repopulate the tumor after treatment. Because of their resistance to treatment and the potential for seeding distant metastatic disease, the study of cancer stem cells and the development of strategies effectively to eradicate all residual stem cells is of critical importance in cancer treatment.

Cancer stemlike cells can be isolated from a variety of tumor types using antibodies to unique cell surface proteins. They are capable of forming xenograft tumors at a high frequency after injection into immunocompromised mice. Empirically selected surface markers have been used to isolate putative stem cells from human breast cancer, glioblastoma multiforme, colon cancer, and other carcinomas, and these cells have a demonstrably greater potential for xenograft formation than do unselected tumor cells. The resulting tumors recapitulate the histologic appearance of the primary tumor as well as the heterogeneous expression of various surface and intracellular molecular markers.[247]

Putative lung progenitor cells have been described as cells residing at the bronchoalveolar duct junction that express both clara cell and pneumocyte markers or as lung resident cells of hematopoietic origin that express CD133.[248,249] These cells have not been conclusively shown to be lung adult stem cell populations but are intriguing and have been shown to be involved in the repair of lung tissue after injury and may be involved in cancer development. In lung tumors, CD133[250–253] and other commonly used markers of stemlike tumor cells (Hoechst dye efflux and aldehyde dehydrogenase activity)[254] have been shown to identify subsets of tumor cells that display characteristics consistent with the cancer stem cell hypothesis. CD133 has been shown to segregate with template DNA in lung cells undergoing asymmetric cell division.[255] However, conflicting reports suggest that CD133 may not define a specific subset of cells, because interconversion between CD133+ and CD133− populations is observed and CD133 expression may be associated with specific stages of cell cycle progression[256]; furthermore, some studies show no association between CD133 expression and propensity to initiate tumors.[257] The cancer stem cell hypothesis has other important grey areas as well. It is not yet certain whether a consistent developmental hierarchy would exist for every individual tumor or only in certain cases, whether lineage differentiation in a tumor can be reversible, and which basic properties should be required to define a stemlike phenotype in a given population of cells. A highly increased propensity for xenograft formation is one of the most convincing features that can be demonstrated experimentally for proposed cancer stemlike cells. However, even the reliability of this evidence is called into question by the observation that a much higher rate of tumor formation is observed when mouse tumor lines are propagated in isogenic immunocompetent mice, which raises the possibility that the xenograft initiation phenotype may be related to the ability to adapt to the tissue environment of an immunocompromised mouse, rather than a general property of enhanced tumor formation.[258]

Nevertheless, the balance of evidence from diverse tumor types favors the hypothesis that stemlike cells are present within tumors and may play a key role in certain aspects of tumor biology. Furthermore, developmental pathways that are proposed to be important in governing cancer stem cell biology may be important oncogenic drivers of proliferation and invasion for unselected tumor cell populations in certain subsets of tumors, and are important avenues of research in their own right. For instance, the activity of particular genes—achaete-scute complex homolog 1[253] and OCT4 transcription factors[251]—have been implicated in regulating this subset of lung tumor cells.

Recent studies have defined aldehyde dehydrogenase (ALDH) activity as a robust marker for lung adenocarcinoma stemlike cells.[259] ALDH-positive cells are highly tumorigenic and clonogenic as well as capable of self-renewal compared to the ALDH subpopulation. This subset and its behavior was shown to be dependent on Notch activity, specifically NOTCH3. The expression of ALDH7A1 was associated with increased risk of recurrence after surgical resection.[260]

Given the far-reaching implications of the cancer stem cell hypothesis and especially the concept that targeting developmental pathways cancer stem cells or, in particular, subsets of cancer could represent an important therapeutic strategy, these complex and exciting areas warrant further study in lung cancer.

MOLECULAR TOOLS IN THE LUNG CANCER CLINIC

Our understanding of the molecular genetic changes in lung cancer pathogenesis is advancing rapidly. Many genetic abnormalities identified in lung cancer are common to other human cancers, whereas others appear more specific to lung cancer, perhaps because of characteristics of the cells of origin and the unique nature of carcinogen exposure. Where their biochemical function is known, the proteins rendered abnormal appear to fall into several growth regulatory pathways.[261] Thus, our understanding of the fundamental workings and diverse molecular drivers of lung cancer is becoming clearer. A substantial effort has been made to translate the current scientific knowledge of these abnormalities from the bench to the bedside in order to improve patient outcomes. These approaches fall into three general categories:

- Development of early detection tools to identify primary and recurrent disease to enable effective early treatment. Because lung cancer eventually develops in only 1 of 10 cigarette smokers, the identification of persons with a genetic susceptibility to lung cancer should allow for targeting and the intensification of smoking cessation, early detection, and chemoprevention efforts. The National Lung Cancer Screening Trial (NLST)[262] randomized patients at high risk for developing lung cancer, defined as individuals between 55 and 74 years of age with a =30 pack-years history of cigarette smoking; former smokers must have quit within the previous 15 years. There was a 20% reduction in lung cancer mortality in the LDCT screened population (95% confidence interval [CI], 6.8% to 26.7%; $p = 0.001$). Based on this data, the U.S. Preventive Services Task Force has recommended annual CT screening for these high-risk patients. The high false-positive rate and the fact that many lung cancers arise in patients who do not meet these eligibility criteria stress the need for developing diagnostic biomarkers to aid in defining an appropriate management of CT-detected nodules and biomarkers of risk for better defining the population who would benefit from screening, including, potentially, germ line T790M.
- Development of new cancer-specific therapies based on knowledge of genetic abnormalities. These may include replacing or pharmacologically reactivating mutant tumor suppressor genes, developing new drugs targeting activated proto-oncogenes,

CANCER OF THE THORACIC CAVITY

interfering with autocrine or paracrine growth stimulatory loops, and inhibiting angiogenesis, metastasis, and antiapoptosis. Some new therapies may be highly effective as single agents in some patients. However, it is likely that for many patients, combinations of two or more targeted or cytotoxic agents will be required to maximize clinical benefit, and determining the optimal combination of therapy for a given patient will be an additional challenge in the field.

- Identification of prognostic and predictive biomarkers, such as the EGFR mutation and ALK-EML4, ROS1, and RET fusion previously described that are both direct targets and predict the response and outcomes to specific therapies. Such tools will play an increasingly important role in selecting optimal treatment strategies as the number of molecularly targeted therapies expands.

These are exciting times in the molecular biology field of lung cancer, in which the science directly informs patient care and vice versa. Improved outcomes are surely to be the result, and patients can be given a degree of hope never before possible.

REFERENCES

1. Hecht SS. Tobacco smoke carcinogens and lung cancer. *J Natl Cancer Inst* 1999;91:1194–1210.
2. Denissenko MF, Pao A, Tang M, et al. Preferential formation of benzo[a]pyrene adducts at lung cancer mutational hotspots in P53. *Science* 1996;274:430–432.
3. Wiencke JK, Thurston SW, Kelsey KT, et al. Early age at smoking initiation and tobacco carcinogen DNA damage in the lung. *J Natl Cancer Inst* 1999;91:614–619.
4. Phillips DH, Hewer A, Martin CN, et al. Correlation of DNA adduct levels in human lung with cigarette smoking. *Nature* 1988;336:790–792.
5. Landi MT, Chatterjee N, Yu K, et al. A genome-wide association study of lung cancer identifies a region of chromosome 5p15 associated with risk for adenocarcinoma. *Am J Hum Genet* 2009;85:679–691.
6. Truong T, Hung RJ, Amos CI, et al. Replication of lung cancer susceptibility loci at chromosomes 15q25, 5p15, and 6p21: a pooled analysis from the International Lung Cancer Consortium. *J Natl Cancer Inst* 2010;102:959–971.
7. Sherva R, Wilhelmsen K, Pomerleau CS, et al. Association of a single nucleotide polymorphism in neuronal acetylcholine receptor subunit alpha 5 (CHRNA5) with smoking status and with 'pleasurable buzz' during early experimentation with smoking. *Addiction* 2008;103:1544–1552.
8. Lonardo F, Rusch V, Langenfeld J, et al. Overexpression of cyclins D1 and E is frequent in bronchial preneoplasia and precedes squamous cell carcinoma development. *Cancer Res* 1999;59:2470–2476.
9. Wistuba II, Behrens C, Virmani AK, et al. High resolution chromosome 3p allelotyping of human lung cancer and preneoplastic/preinvasive bronchial epithelium reveals multiple, discontinuous sites of 3p allele loss and three regions of frequent breakpoints. *Cancer Res* 2000;60:1949–1960.
10. Westra WH. Early glandular neoplasia of the lung. *Respir Res* 2000;1:163–169.
11. Braakhuis BJ, Tabor MP, Kummer JA, et al. A genetic explanation of Slaughter's concept of field cancerization: evidence and clinical implications. *Cancer Res* 2003;63:1727–1730.
12. Balsara BR, Testa JR. Chromosomal imbalances in human lung cancer. *Oncogene* 2002;21:6877–6883.
13. Braithwaite KL, Rabbitts PH. Multi-step evolution of lung cancer. *Sem Cancer Biol* 1999;9:255–265.
14. Virmani AK, Gazdar AF. Tumor suppressor genes in lung cancer. *Methods Mol Biol* 2003;222:97–115.
15. Miura I, Graziano SL, Cheng JQ, et al. Chromosome alterations in human small cell lung cancer: frequent involvement of 5q. *Cancer Res* 1992;52:1322–1328.
16. Testa JR, Siegfried JM. Chromosome abnormalities in human non-small cell lung cancer. *Cancer Res* 1992;52:2702s–2706s.
17. Rikova K, Guo A, Zeng Q, et al. Global survey of phosphotyrosine signaling identifies oncogenic kinases in lung cancer. *Cell* 2007;131:1190–1203.
18. Haruki N, Kawaguchi KS, Eichenberger S, et al. Cloned fusion product from a rare t(15;19)(q13.2;p13.1) inhibit S phase in vitro. *J Med Genet* 2005;42:558–564.
19. Soda M, Choi YL, Enomoto M, et al. Identification of the transforming EML4-ALK fusion gene in non–small-cell lung cancer. *Nature* 2007;448:561–566.
20. Sekido Y, Fong KM, Minna JD. Molecular genetics of lung cancer. *Ann Rev Med* 2003;54:73–87.
21. Cancer Genome Atlas Research Network. Comprehensive genomic characterization of squamous cell lung cancers. *Nature* 2012;489:519–525.
22. Kandoth C, McLellan MD, Vandin F, et al. Mutational landscape and significance across 12 major cancer types. *Nature* 2013;502:333–339.
23. Ding L, Getz G, Wheeler DA, et al. Somatic mutations affect key pathways in lung adenocarcinoma. *Nature* 2008;455:1069–1075.
24. Imielinski M, Berger AH, Hammerman PS, et al. Mapping the hallmarks of lung adenocarcinoma with massively parallel sequencing. *Cell* 2012;150:1107–1120.
25. Klein G, Klein E. Surveillance against tumors—is it mainly immunological? *Immunol Lett* 2005;100:29–33.
26. Sakumi K, Tominaga Y, Furuichi M, et al. Ogg1 knockout-associated lung tumorigenesis and its suppression by Mth1 gene disruption. *Cancer Res* 2003;63:902–905.
27. Zienolddiny S, Campa D, Lind H, et al. Polymorphisms of DNA repair genes and risk of non-small cell lung cancer. *Carcinogenesis* 2006;27:560–567.
28. Olaussen KA, Dunant A, Fouret P, et al. DNA repair by ERCC1 in non–small-cell lung cancer and cisplatin-based adjuvant chemotherapy. *N Engl J Med* 2006;355:983–991.
29. Friboulet L, Olaussen KA, Pignon JP, et al. ERCC1 isoform expression and DNA repair in non–small-cell lung cancer. *N Engl J Med* 2013;368:1101–1110.
30. Zheng Z, Chen T, Li X, et al. DNA synthesis and repair genes RRM1 and ERCC1 in lung cancer. *N Engl J Med* 2007;356:800–808.
31. Bepler G, Kusmartseva I, Sharma S, et al. RRM1 modulated in vitro and in vivo efficacy of gemcitabine and platinum in non–small-cell lung cancer. *J Clin Oncol* 2006;24:4731–4737.
32. Kamal NS, Soria JC, Mendiboure J, et al. MutS homologue 2 and the long-term benefit of adjuvant chemotherapy in lung cancer. *Clin Cancer Res* 2010;16:1206–1215.
33. Lynch TJ, Bell DW, Sordella R, et al. Activating mutations in the epidermal growth factor receptor underlying responsiveness of non–small-cell lung cancer to gefitinib. *N Engl J Med* 2004;350:2129–2139.
34. Gao W, Lu X, Liu L, et al. MiRNA-21: a biomarker predictive for platinum-based adjuvant chemotherapy response in patients with non-small cell lung cancer. *Cancer Biol Ther* 2012;13:330–340.
35. Pao W, Miller V, Zakowski M, et al. EGF receptor gene mutations are common in lung cancers from "never smokers" and are associated with sensitivity of tumors to gefitinib and erlotinib. *Proc Natl Acad Sci U S A* 2004;101:13306–13311.
36. Jänne PA, Engelman JA, Johnson BE. Epidermal growth factor receptor mutations in non–small-cell lung cancer: implications for treatment and tumor biology. *J Clin Oncol* 2005;23:3227–3234.
37. Cappuzzo F, Hirsch FR, Rossi E, et al. Epidermal growth factor receptor gene and protein and gefitinib sensitivity in non–small-cell lung cancer. *J Natl Cancer Inst* 2005;97:643–655.
38. Shigematsu H, Takahashi T, Nomura M, et al. Somatic mutations of the HER2 kinase domain in lung adenocarcinomas. *Cancer Res* 2005;65:1642–1646.
39. Tsao MS, Sakurada A, Cutz JC, et al. Erlotinib in lung cancer—molecular and clinical predictors of outcome. *N Engl J Med* 2005;353:133–144.
40. Thatcher N, Chang A, Parikh P, et al. Gefitinib plus best supportive care in previously treated patients with refractory advanced non–small-cell lung cancer: results from a randomised, placebo-controlled, multicentre study (Iressa Survival Evaluation in Lung Cancer). *Lancet* 2005;366:1527–1537.
41. Tamura K, Okamoto I, Kashii T, et al. Multicentre prospective phase II trial of gefitinib for advanced non-small cell lung cancer with epidermal growth factor receptor mutations: results of the West Japan Thoracic Oncology Group trial (WJTOG0403). *Br J Cancer* 2008;98:907–914.
42. Mok TS, Wu YL, Thongprasert S, et al. Gefitinib or carboplatin-paclitaxel in pulmonary adenocarcinoma. *N Engl J Med* 2009;361:947–957.
43. Sequist LV, Yang JC, Yamamoto N, et al. Phase III study of afatinib or cisplatin plus pemetrexed in patients with metastatic lung adenocarcinoma with EGFR mutations. *J Clin Oncol* 2013;31:3327–3334.
44. Yang JC, Shih JY, Su WC, et al. Afatinib for patients with lung adenocarcinoma and epidermal growth factor receptor mutations (LUX-Lung 2): a phase 2 trial. *Lancet Oncol* 2012;13:539–548.
45. Maemondo M, Inoue A, Kobayashi K, et al. Gefitinib or chemotherapy for non–small-cell lung cancer with mutated EGFR. *N Engl J Med* 2010;362:2380–2388.
46. Mitsudomi T, Morita S, Yatabe Y, et al. Gefitinib versus cisplatin plus docetaxel in patients with non–small-cell lung cancer harbouring mutations of the epidermal growth factor receptor (WJTOG3405): an open label, randomised phase 3 trial. *Lancet Oncol* 2010;11:121–128.
47. Zhou C, Wu YL, Chen G, et al. Erlotinib versus chemotherapy as first-line treatment for patients with advanced EGFR mutation-positive non–small-cell lung cancer (OPTIMAL, CTONG-0802): a multicentre, open-label, randomised, phase 3 study. *Lancet Oncol* 2011;12:735–742.
48. Oxnard GR, Lo PC, Nishino M, et al. Natural history and molecular characteristics of lung cancers harboring EGFR exon 20 insertions. *J Thorac Oncol* 2013;8:179–184.
49. Sequist LV, Waltman BA, Dias-Santagata D, et al. Genotypic and histological evolution of lung cancers acquiring resistance to EGFR inhibitors. *Sci Transl Med* 2011;3:75ra26.

50. Kobayashi S, Boggon TJ, Dayaram T, et al. EGFR mutation and resistance of non–small-cell lung cancer to gefitinib. *N Engl J Med* 2005;352:786–792.
51. Pao W, Miller VA, Politi KA, et al. Acquired resistance of lung adenocarcinomas to gefitinib or erlotinib is associated with a second mutation in the EGFR kinase domain. *PLoS Med* 2005;2:e73.
52. Bell DW, Gore I, Okimoto RA, et al. Inherited susceptibility to lung cancer may be associated with the T790M drug resistance mutation in EGFR. *Nat Genet* 2005;37:1315–1316.
53. Hirsch FR, Varella-Garcia M, McCoy J, et al. Increased epidermal growth factor receptor gene copy number detected by fluorescence in situ hybridization associates with increased sensitivity to gefitinib in patients with bronchioloalveolar carcinoma subtypes: a Southwest Oncology Group Study. *J Clin Oncol* 2005;23:6838–6845.
54. Arcila ME, Chaft JE, Nafa K, et al. Prevalence, clinicopathologic associations, and molecular spectrum of ERBB2 (HER2) tyrosine kinase mutations in lung adenocarcinomas. *Clin Cancer Res* 2012;18:4910–4918.
55. Liu L, Shao X, Gao W, et al. The role of human epidermal growth factor receptor 2 as a prognostic factor in lung cancer: a meta-analysis of published data. *J Thorac Oncol* 2010;5:1922–1932.
56. Tomizawa K, Suda K, Onozato R, et al. Prognostic and predictive implications of HER2/ERBB2/neu gene mutations in lung cancers. *Lung Cancer* 2011;74:139–144.
57. Gatzemeier U, Groth G, Butts C, et al. Randomized phase II trial of gemcitabine-cisplatin with or without trastuzumab in HER2-positive non–small-cell lung cancer. *Ann Oncol* 2004;15:19–27.
58. Nguyen KS, Kobayashi S, Costa DB. Acquired resistance to epidermal growth factor receptor tyrosine kinase inhibitors in non–small-cell lung cancers dependent on the epidermal growth factor receptor pathway. *Clin Lung Cancer* 2009;10:281–289.
59. Sadiq AA, Salgia R. MET as a possible target for non–small-cell lung cancer. *J Clin Oncol* 2013;31:1089–1096.
60. Spigel DR, Ervin TJ, Ramlau RA, et al. Randomized phase II trial of onartuzumab in combination with erlotinib in patients with advanced non–small-cell lung cancer. *J Clin Oncol* 2013;31:4105–4114.
61. Sequist LV, von Pawel J, Garmey EG, et al. Randomized phase II study of erlotinib plus tivantinib versus erlotinib plus placebo in previously treated non–small-cell lung cancer. *J Clin Oncol* 2011;29:3307–3315.
62. Drilon A, Rekhtman N, Ladanyi M, et al. Squamous-cell carcinomas of the lung: emerging biology, controversies, and the promise of targeted therapy. *Lancet Oncol* 2012;13:e418–e426.
63. Rooney M, Devarakonda S, Govindan R. Genomics of squamous cell lung cancer. *Oncologist* 2013;18:707–716.
64. Pollak MN. Insulin-like growth factors and neoplasia. *Novartis Found Symp* 2004;262:84–98.
65. Dziadziuszko R, Merrick DT, Witta SE, et al. Insulin-like growth factor receptor 1 (IGF1R) gene copy number is associated with survival in operable non–small-cell lung cancer: a comparison between IGF1R fluorescent in situ hybridization, protein expression, and mRNA expression. *J Clin Oncol* 2010;28:2174–2180.
66. Weiss J, Sos ML, Seidel D, et al. Frequent and focal FGFR1 amplification associates with therapeutically tractable FGFR1 dependency in squamous cell lung cancer. *Sci Transl Med* 2010;2:62ra93.
67. Dutt A, Ramos AH, Hammerman PS, et al. Inhibitor-sensitive FGFR1 amplification in human non-small cell lung cancer. *PLoS One* 2011;6:e20351.
68. Hammerman PS, Sos ML, Ramos AH, et al. Mutations in the DDR2 kinase gene identify a novel therapeutic target in squamous cell lung cancer. *Cancer Discov* 2011;1:78–89.
69. Day E, Waters B, Spiegel K, et al. Inhibition of collagen-induced discoidin domain receptor 1 and 2 activation by imatinib, nilotinib and dasatinib. *Eur J Pharmacol* 2008;599:44–53.
70. Koivunen JP, Mermel C, Zejnullahu K, et al. EML4-ALK fusion gene and efficacy of an ALK kinase inhibitor in lung cancer. *Clin Cancer Res* 2008;14:4275–4283.
71. Kwak EL, Bang YJ, Camidge DR, et al. Anaplastic lymphoma kinase inhibition in non–small-cell lung cancer. *N Engl J Med* 2010;363:1693–1703.
72. Choi YL, Takeuchi K, Soda M, et al. Identification of novel isoforms of the EML4-ALK transforming gene in non-small cell lung cancer. *Cancer Res* 2008;68:4971–4976.
73. Wong DW, Leung EL, So KK, et al. The EML4-ALK fusion gene is involved in various histologic types of lung cancers from nonsmokers with wild-type EGFR and KRAS. *Cancer* 2009;115:1723–1733.
74. Inamura K, Takeuchi K, Togashi Y, et al. EML4-ALK lung cancers are characterized by rare other mutations, a TTF-1 cell lineage, an acinar histology, and young onset. *Mod Pathol* 2009;22:508–515.
75. Inamura K, Takeuchi K, Togashi Y, et al. EML4-ALK fusion is linked to histological characteristics in a subset of lung cancers. *J Thorac Oncol* 2008;3:13–17.
76. Shaw AT, Yeap BY, Mino-Kenudson M, et al. Clinical features and outcome of patients with non–small-cell lung cancer who harbor EML4-ALK. *J Clin Oncol* 2009;27:4247–4253.
77. Shaw AT, Kim DW, Nakagawa K, et al. Crizotinib versus chemotherapy in advanced ALK-positive lung cancer. *N Engl J Med* 2013;368:2385–2394.
78. Doebele RC, Pilling AB, Aisner DL, et al. Mechanisms of resistance to crizotinib in patients with ALK gene rearranged non-small cell lung cancer. *Clin Cancer Res* 2012;18:1472–1482.
79. Katayama R, Khan TM, Benes C, et al. Therapeutic strategies to overcome crizotinib resistance in non-small cell lung cancers harboring the fusion oncogene EML4-ALK. *Proc Natl Acad Sci U S A* 2011;108:7535–7540.
80. Qi J, McTigue MA, Rogers A, et al. Multiple mutations and bypass mechanisms can contribute to development of acquired resistance to MET inhibitors. *Cancer Res* 2011;71:1081–1091.
81. Choi YL, Soda M, Yamashita Y, et al. EML4-ALK mutations in lung cancer that confer resistance to ALK inhibitors. *N Engl J Med* 2010;363:1734–1749.
82. Shaw AT, Mehra R, Kim D-W, et al. Clinical activity of the ALK inhibitor LDK378 in advanced, ALK-positive NSCLC. *J Clin Oncol* 2013;31:abstr 8010.
83. Nakagawa K, Kiura K, Nishio M, et al. A phase I/II study with a highly selective ALK inhibitor CH5424802 in ALK-positive non-small cell lung cancer (NSCLC) patients: updated safety and efficacy results from AF-001 JP. *J Clin Oncol* 2013;31:abstr 8033.
84. Acquaviva J, Wong R, Charest A. The multifaceted roles of the receptor tyrosine kinase ROS in development and cancer. *Biochim Biophys Acta* 2009;1795:37–52.
85. Bergethon K, Shaw AT, Ou SH, et al. ROS1 rearrangements define a unique molecular class of lung cancers. *J Clin Oncol* 2012;30:863–870.
86. Shaw AT, Camidge D, Engelman JA, et al. Clinical activity of crizotinib in advanced non-small cell lung cancer (NSCLC) harboring ROS1 gene rearrangement. *J Clin Oncol* 2012;30:abstr 7508.
87. Ju YS, Lee WC, Shin JY, et al. A transforming KIF5B and RET gene fusion in lung adenocarcinoma revealed from whole-genome and transcriptome sequencing. *Genome Res* 2012;22:436–445.
88. Kohno T, Ichikawa H, Totoki Y, et al. KIF5B-RET fusions in lung adenocarcinoma. *Nat Med* 2012;18:375–377.
89. Takeuchi K, Soda M, Togashi Y, et al. RET, ROS1 and ALK fusions in lung cancer. *Nat Med* 2012;18:378–381.
90. Drilon A, Wang L, Hasanovic A, et al. Response to Cabozantinib in patients with RET fusion-positive lung adenocarcinomas. *Cancer Discov* 2013;3:630–635.
91. Wang R, Hu H, Pan Y, et al. RET fusions define a unique molecular and clinicopathologic subtype of non–small-cell lung cancer. *J Clin Oncol* 2012;30:4352–4359.
92. Ahrendt SA, Decker PA, Alawi EA, et al. Cigarette smoking is strongly associated with mutation of the K-ras gene in patients with primary adenocarcinoma of the lung. *Cancer* 2001;92:1525–1530.
93. Mascaux C, Iannino N, Martin B, et al. The role of RAS oncogene in survival of patients with lung cancer: a systematic review of the literature with meta-analysis. *Br J Cancer* 2005;92:131–139.
94. Shepherd FA, Domerg C, Hainaut P, et al. Pooled analysis of the prognostic and predictive effects of KRAS mutation status and KRAS mutation subtype in early-stage resected non–small-cell lung cancer in four trials of adjuvant chemotherapy. *J Clin Oncol* 2013;31:2173–2181.
95. Kim ES, Herbst RS, Wistuba II, et al. The BATTLE trial: personalizing therapy for lung cancer. *Cancer Discov* 2011;1:44–53.
96. Mok TSK, Paz-Ares L, Wu Y-L, et al. Association between tumor EGFR and KRAS mutation status and clinical outcomes in NSCLC patients randomized to sorafenib plus best supportive care (BSC) or BSC alone: subanalysis of the phase III MISSION trial [abstract]. *Ann Oncol* 2013;23:Abstract LBA9_PR.
97. Jänne PA, Shaw AT, Pereira JR, et al. Selumetinib plus docetaxel for KRAS-mutant advanced non–small-cell lung cancer: a randomised, multicentre, placebo-controlled, phase 2 study. *Lancet Oncol* 2013;14:38–47.
98. Kelly K, Mazieres J, Leighl NB, et al. Oral MEK1/MEK2 inhibitor trametinib (GSK1120212) in combination with pemetrexed for KRAS-mutant and wild-type (WT) advanced non-small cell lung cancer (NSCLC): A phase I/Ib trial. *J Clin Oncol* 2013;31:abstr 8027.
99. Gandara DR, Hiret S, Blumenschein GR, et al. Oral MEK1/MEK2 inhibitor trametinib (GSK1120212) in combination with docetaxel in KRAS-mutant and wild-type (WT) advanced non-small cell lung cancer (NSCLC): A phase I/Ib trial. *J Clin Oncol* 2013;31:abstr 8028.
100. Paik PK, Arcila ME, Fara M, et al. Clinical characteristics of patients with lung adenocarcinomas harboring BRAF mutations. *J Clin Oncol* 2011;29:2046–2051.
101. Planchard D, Mazieres J, Riely GJ, et al. Interim results of phase II study BRF113928 of dabrafenib in BRAF V600E mutation–positive non-small cell lung cancer (NSCLC) patients. *J Clin Oncol* 2013;31:abstr 8009.
102. Peters S, Michielin O, Zimmermann S. Dramatic response induced by vemurafenib in a BRAF V600E-mutated lung adenocarcinoma. *J Clin Oncol* 2013;31:e341–e344.
103. Imielinski M, Greulich H, Kaplan B, et al. Oncogenic and sorafenib-sensitive ARAF mutations in lung adenocarcinomas. *J Clin Invest* 2014;124:1582–1586.
104. Marks JL, Gong Y, Chitale D, et al. Novel MEK1 mutation identified by mutational analysis of epidermal growth factor receptor signaling pathway genes in lung adenocarcinoma. *Cancer Res* 2008;68:5524–5528.
105. Samuels Y, Wang Z, Bardelli A, et al. High frequency of mutations of the PIK3CA gene in human cancers. *Science* 2004;304:554.
106. Kawano O, Sasaki H, Endo K, et al. PIK3CA mutation status in Japanese lung cancer patients. *Lung Cancer* 2006;54:209–215.
107. Cancer Genome Atlas Research Network. Comprehensive genomic characterization of squamous cell lung cancers. *Nature* 2012;489:519–525.
108. Chaft JE, Arcila ME, Paik PK, et al. Coexistence of PIK3CA and other oncogene mutations in lung adenocarcinoma-rationale for comprehensive mutation profiling. *Mol Cancer Ther* 2012;11:485–491.
109. Kang S, Bader AG, Vogt PK. Phosphatidylinositol 3-kinase mutations identified in human cancer are oncogenic. *Proc Natl Acad Sci U S A* 2005;102:802–807.
110. Zhang L, Shi L, Zhao X, et al. PIK3CA gene mutation associated with poor prognosis of lung adenocarcinoma. *Onco Targets Ther* 2013;6:497–502.

111. Bleeker FE, Felicioni L, Buttitta F, et al. AKT1(E17K) in human solid tumours. *Oncogene* 2008;27:5648–5650.
112. Carpten JD, Faber AL, Horn C, et al. A transforming mutation in the pleckstrin homology domain of AKT1 in cancer. *Nature* 2007;448:439–444.
113. Jin G, Kim MJ, Jeon HS, et al. PTEN mutations and relationship to EGFR, ERBB2, KRAS, and TP53 mutations in non-small cell lung cancers. *Lung Cancer* 2010;69:279–283.
114. Tran B, Dancey JE, Kamel-Reid S, et al. Cancer genomics: technology, discovery, and translation. *J Clin Oncol* 2012;30:647–660.
115. Buettner R, Wolf J, Thomas RK. Lessons learned from lung cancer genomics: the emerging concept of individualized diagnostics and treatment. *J Clin Oncol* 2013;31:1858–1865.
116. Dias-Santagata D, Akhavanfard S, David SS, et al. Rapid targeted mutational analysis of human tumours: a clinical platform to guide personalized cancer medicine. *EMBO Mol Med* 2010;2:146–158.
117. MacConaill LE, Campbell CD, Kehoe SM, et al. Profiling critical cancer gene mutations in clinical tumor samples. *PLoS One* 2009;4:e7887.
118. Sequist LV, Heist RS, Shaw AT, et al. Implementing multiplexed genotyping of non–small-cell lung cancers into routine clinical practice. *Ann Oncol* 2011;22:2616–2624.
119. Kris MG, Johnson BE, Kwiatkowski DJ, et al. Identification of driver mutations in tumor specimens from 1,000 patients with lung adenocarcinoma: The NCI's Lung cancer Mutation Consortium (LCMC). *J Clin Oncol* 2011;29:abstr CRA7506.
120. Rothberg JM, Hinz W, Rearick TM, et al. An integrated semiconductor device enabling non-optical genome sequencing. *Nature* 2011;475:348–352.
121. Loman NJ, Misra RV, Dallman TJ, et al. Performance comparison of benchtop high-throughput sequencing platforms. *Nat Biotechnol* 2012;30:434–439.
122. Chmielecki J, Rosenberg M, Imielinski M, et al. Whole exome and whole genome sequence analysis of lung adenocarcinoma. *Am Assoc Cancer Res* 2013:abstract 1112.
123. Ellis MJ, Gillette M, Carr SA, et al. Connecting genomic alterations to cancer biology with proteomics: The NCI Clinical Proteomic Tumor Analysis Consortium. *Cancer Discov* 2013;3:1108–1112.
124. Macconaill LE, Garraway LA. Clinical implications of the cancer genome. *J Clin Oncol* 2010;28:5219–5228.
125. Lawrence MS, Stojanov P, Polak P, et al. Mutational heterogeneity in cancer and the search for new cancer-associated genes. *Nature* 2013;499:214–218.
126. Brock MV, Hooker CM, Ota-Machida E, et al. DNA methylation markers and early recurrence in stage I lung cancer. *N Engl J Med* 2008;358:1118–1128.
127. Sandoval J, Mendez-Gonzalez J, Nadal E, et al. A prognostic DNA methylation signature for stage I non–small-cell lung cancer. *J Clin Oncol* 2013;31:4140–4147.
128. Juergens RA, Wrangle J, Vendetti FP, et al. Combination epigenetic therapy has efficacy in patients with refractory advanced non-small cell lung cancer. *Cancer Discov* 2011;1:598–607.
129. Chu BF, Karpenko MJ, Liu Z, et al. Phase I study of 5-aza-2'-deoxycytidine in combination with valproic acid in non–small-cell lung cancer. *Cancer Chemother Pharmacol* 2013;71:115–121.
130. Schrump DS, Fischette MR, Nguyen DM, et al. Phase I study of decitabine-mediated gene expression in patients with cancers involving the lungs, esophagus, or pleura. *Clin Cancer Res* 2006;12:5777–5785.
131. Behrens C, Solis LM, Lin H, et al. EZH2 protein expression associates with the early pathogenesis, tumor progression, and prognosis of non-small cell lung carcinoma. *Clin Cancer Res* 2013;19:6556–6565.
132. Wagner KW, Alam H, Dhar SS, et al. KDM2A promotes lung tumorigenesis by epigenetically enhancing ERK1/2 signaling. *J Clin Invest* 2013;123:5231–5246.
133. Mitsudomi T, Oyama T, Kusano T, et al. Mutations of the p53 gene as a predictor of poor prognosis in patients with non–small-cell lung cancer. *J Natl Cancer Inst* 1993;85:2018–2023.
134. Kosaka T, Yatabe Y, Onozato R, et al. Prognostic implication of EGFR, KRAS, and TP53 gene mutations in a large cohort of Japanese patients with surgically treated lung adenocarcinoma. *J Thorac Oncol* 2009;4:22–29.
135. Hwang SJ, Cheng LS, Lozano G, et al. Lung cancer risk in germline p53 mutation carriers: association between an inherited cancer predisposition, cigarette smoking, and cancer risk. *Hum Genet* 2003;113:238–243.
136. Joerger AC, Fersht AR. Structural biology of the tumor suppressor p53. *Annu Rev Biochem* 2008;77:557–582.
137. Lang GA, Iwakuma T, Suh YA, et al. Gain of function of a p53 hot spot mutation in a mouse model of Li-Fraumeni syndrome. *Cell* 2004;119:861–872.
138. Cheng Q, Chen J. Mechanism of p53 stabilization by ATM after DNA damage. *Cell Cycle* 2010;9:472–478.
139. Song H, Hollstein M, Xu Y. p53 gain-of-function cancer mutants induce genetic instability by inactivating ATM. *Nat Cell Biol* 2007;9:573–580.
140. Weir BA, Woo MS, Getz G, et al. Characterizing the cancer genome in lung adenocarcinoma. *Nature* 2007;450:893–898.
141. Klein C, Vassilev LT. Targeting the p53-MDM2 interaction to treat cancer. *Br J Cancer* 2004;91:1415–1419.
142. Eymin B, Gazzeri S, Brambilla C, et al. Mdm2 overexpression and p14(ARF) inactivation are two mutually exclusive events in primary human lung tumors. *Oncogene* 2002;21:2750–2761.
143. Menendez D, Inga A, Resnick MA. The expanding universe of p53 targets. *Nat Rev Cancer* 2009;9:724–737.
144. Tarasov V, Jung P, Verdoodt B, et al. Differential regulation of microRNAs by p53 revealed by massively parallel sequencing: miR-34a is a p53 target that induces apoptosis and G1-arrest. *Cell Cycle* 2007;6:1586–1593.
145. Raver-Shapira N, Marciano E, Meiri E, et al. Transcriptional activation of miR-34a contributes to p53-mediated apoptosis. *Mol Cell* 2007;26:731–743.
146. Wang W, El-Deiry WS. Restoration of p53 to limit tumor growth. *Curr Opin Oncol* 2008;20:90–96.
147. Rabinowits G, Gercel-Taylor C, Day JM, et al. Exosomal microRNA: a diagnostic marker for lung cancer. *Clin Lung Cancer* 2009;10:42–46.
148. Cazzoli R, Buttitta F, Di Nicola M, et al. microRNAs derived from circulating exosomes as noninvasive biomarkers for screening and diagnosing lung cancer. *J Thorac Oncol* 2013;8:1156–1162.
149. Al-Nedawi K, Meehan B, Kerbel RS, et al. Endothelial expression of autocrine VEGF upon the uptake of tumor-derived microvesicles containing oncogenic EGFR. *Proc Natl Acad Sci U S A* 2009;106:3794–3799.
150. Aushev VN, Zborovskaya IB, Laktionov KK, et al. Comparisons of microRNA patterns in plasma before and after tumor removal reveal new biomarkers of lung squamous cell carcinoma. *PloS One* 2013;8:e78649.
151. Antonia SJ, Mirza N, Fricke I, et al. Combination of p53 cancer vaccine with chemotherapy in patients with extensive stage small cell lung cancer. *Clin Cancer Res* 2006;12:878–887.
152. Baylin SB, Jones PA. A decade of exploring the cancer epigenome - biological and translational implications. *Nat Rev Cancer* 2011;11:726–734.
153. Weir BA, Woo MS, Getz G, et al. Characterizing the cancer genome in lung adenocarcinoma. *Nature* 2007;450:893–898.
154. Belinsky SA, Nikula KJ, Palmisano WA, et al. Aberrant methylation of p16(INK4a) is an early event in lung cancer and a potential biomarker for early diagnosis. *Proc Natl Acad Sci U S A* 1998;95:11891–11896.
155. Zhang Y, Xiong Y, Yarbrough WG. ARF promotes MDM2 degradation and stabilizes p53: ARF-INK4a locus deletion impairs both the Rb and p53 tumor suppression pathways. *Cell* 1998;92:725–734.
156. Meuwissen R, Linn SC, Linnoila RI, et al. Induction of small cell lung cancer by somatic inactivation of both Trp53 and Rb1 in a conditional mouse model. *Cancer Cell* 2003;4:181–189.
157. Beroukhim R, Mermel CH, Porter D, et al. The landscape of somatic copy-number alteration across human cancers. *Nature* 2010;463:899–905.
158. Hearle N, Schumacher V, Menko FH, et al. Frequency and spectrum of cancers in the Peutz-Jeghers syndrome. *Clin Cancer Res* 2006;12:3209–3215.
159. Jansen M, Ten Klooster JP, Offerhaus GJ, et al. LKB1 and AMPK family signaling: the intimate link between cell polarity and energy metabolism. *Physiol Rev* 2009;89:777–798.
160. Carretero J, Medina PP, Pio R, et al. Novel and natural knockout lung cancer cell lines for the LKB1/STK11 tumor suppressor gene. *Oncogene* 2004;23:4037–4040.
161. Ji H, Ramsey MR, Hayes DN, et al. LKB1 modulates lung cancer differentiation and metastasis. *Nature* 2007;448:807–810.
162. Matsumoto S, Iwakawa R, Takahashi K, et al. Prevalence and specificity of LKB1 genetic alterations in lung cancers. *Oncogene* 2007;26:5911–5918.
163. Amin RMS, Hiroshima K, Iyoda A, et al. LKB1 protein expression in neuroendocrine tumors of the lung. *Pathol Int* 2008;58:84–88.
164. Gwinn D, Shackelford D, Egan D, et al. AMPK phosphorylation of raptor mediates a metabolic checkpoint. *Mol Cell* 2008;30:214–226.
165. Mahoney CL, Choudhury B, Davies H, et al. LKB1/KRAS mutant lung cancers constitute a genetic subset of NSCLC with increased sensitivity to MAPK and mTOR signalling inhibition. *Br J Cancer* 2009;100:370–375.
166. Robinson J, Lai C, Martin A, et al. Oral rapamycin reduces tumour burden and vascularization in Lkb1(+/−) mice. *J Pathol* 2009;219:35–40.
167. Liu B, Fan Z, Edgerton SM, et al. Metformin induces unique biological and molecular responses in triple negative breast cancer cells. *Cell Cycle* 2009;8:2031–2040.
168. Bowker SL, Majumdar SR, Veugelers P, et al. Increased cancer-related mortality for patients with type 2 diabetes who use sulfonylureas or insulin: Response to Farooki and Schneider. *Diabetes Care* 2006;29:1990–1991.
169. Evans JM, Donnelly LA, Emslie-Smith AM, et al. Metformin and reduced risk of cancer in diabetic patients. *BMJ* 2005;330:1304–1305.
170. Libby G, Donnelly L, Donnan P, et al. New users of metformin are at low risk of incident cancer: A cohort study among people with type 2 diabetes. *Diabetes Care* 2009;32:1620–1625.
171. Jiralerspong S, Palla SL, Giordano SH, et al. Metformin and pathologic complete responses to neoadjuvant chemotherapy in diabetic patients with breast cancer. *J Clin Oncol* 2009;27:3297–3302.
172. Baas AF, Kuipers J, van der Wel NN, et al. Complete polarization of single intestinal epithelial cells upon activation of LKB1 by STRAD. *Cell* 2004;116:457–466.
173. Shackelford DB, Shaw RJ. The LKB1–AMPK pathway: metabolism and growth control in tumour suppression. *Nat Rev Cancer* 2009;9:563–575.
174. Baykara O, Demirkaya A, Kaynak K, et al. WWOX gene may contribute to progression of non–small-cell lung cancer (NSCLC). *Tumour Biol* 2010;31:315–320.
175. Ding L, Getz G, Wheeler DA, et al. Somatic mutations affect key pathways in lung adenocarcinoma. *Nature* 2008;455:1069–1075.
176. Hesson LB, Cooper WN, Latif F. Evaluation of the 3p21.3 tumour-suppressor gene cluster. *Oncogene* 2007;26:7283–7301.
177. Lerman MI, Minna JD. The 630-kb lung cancer homozygous deletion region on human chromosome 3p21.3: identification and evaluation of the resident candidate tumor suppressor genes. The International Lung Cancer Chromosome 3p21.3 Tumor Suppressor Gene Consortium. *Cancer Res* 2000;60:6116–6133.
178. Brunet JF, Denizot F, Luciani MF, et al. A new member of the immunoglobulin superfamily—CTLA-4. *Nature* 1987;328:267–270.

179. Lynch TJ, Bondarenko I, Luft A, et al. Ipilimumab in combination with paclitaxel and carboplatin as first-line treatment in stage IIIB/IV non–small-cell lung cancer: results from a randomized, double-blind, multicenter phase II study. *J Clin Oncol* 2012;30:2046–2054.
180. Reck M, Bondarenko I, Luft A, et al. Ipilimumab in combination with paclitaxel and carboplatin as first-line therapy in extensive-disease-small-cell lung cancer: results from a randomized, double-blind, multicenter phase 2 trial. *Ann Oncol* 2013;24:75–83.
181. Topalian SL, Hodi FS, Brahmer JR, et al. Safety, activity, and immune correlates of anti-PD-1 antibody in cancer. *N Engl J Med* 2012;366:2443–2454.
182. Brahmer J, Horn L, Antonia S, et al. Nivolumab (anti-PD-1; BMS-936558; ONO-4538) in patients with non-small cell lung cancer (NSCLC): overall survival and long-term safety in a phase I trial. Abstract presented at: 2013 World Conference on Lung Cancer; 2013; Sydney, Australia.
183. Soria JC, Cruz C, Bahleda R, et al. Clinical activity, safety, and biomarkers of PD-L1 blockade in non-small cell lung cancer; additional analyses from a clinical study of the engineered antibody MPDL2380A (Anti-PD-L1). Abstract presented at: 2013 European Cancer Congress; 2013; Amsterdam.
184. Lundberg AS, Randell SH, Stewart SA, et al. Immortalization and transformation of primary human airway epithelial cells by gene transfer. *Oncogene* 2002;21:4577–4586.
185. Zhu CQ, Cutz JC, Liu N, et al. Amplification of telomerase (hTERT) gene is a poor prognostic marker in non–small-cell lung cancer. *Br J Cancer* 2006;94:1452–1459.
186. Miura N, Nakamura H, Sato R, et al. Clinical usefulness of serum telomerase reverse transcriptase (hTERT) mRNA and epidermal growth factor receptor (EGFR) mRNA as a novel tumor marker for lung cancer. *Cancer Sci* 2006;97:1366–1373.
187. Marchetti A, Pellegrini C, Buttitta F, et al. Prediction of survival in stage I lung carcinoma patients by telomerase function evaluation. *Lab Invest* 2002;82:729–736.
188. Shibuya K, Fujisawa T, Hoshino H, et al. Increased telomerase activity and elevated hTERT mRNA expression during multistage carcinogenesis of squamous cell carcinoma of the lung. *Cancer* 2001;92:849–855.
189. Brunsvig PF, Kyte JA, Kersten C, et al. Telomerase peptide vaccination in NSCLC: a phase II trial in stage III patients vaccinated after chemoradiotherapy and an 8-year update on a phase I/II trial. *Clin Cancer Res* 2011;17:6847–6857.
190. Georgoulias V, Douillard JY, Khayat D, et al. A multicenter randomized phase IIb efficacy study of Vx-001, a peptide-based cancer vaccine as maintenance treatment in advanced non–small-cell lung cancer: treatment rationale and protocol dynamics. *Clin Lung Cancer* 2013;14:461–465.
191. Adams JM, Cory S. The Bcl-2 apoptotic switch in cancer development and therapy. *Oncogene* 2007;26:1324–1337.
192. Pezzella F, Turley H, Kuzu I, et al. bcl-2 protein in non–small-cell lung carcinoma. *N Engl J Med* 1993;329:690–694.
193. Ikegaki N, Katsumata M, Minna J, et al. Expression of bcl-2 in small cell lung carcinoma cells. *Cancer Res* 1994;54:6–8.
194. Martin B, Paesmans M, Berghmans T, et al. Role of Bcl-2 as a prognostic factor for survival in lung cancer: a systematic review of the literature with meta-analysis. *Br J Cancer* 2003;89:55–64.
195. Campos L, Rouault JP, Sabido O, et al. High expression of bcl-2 protein in acute myeloid leukemia cells is associated with poor response to chemotherapy. *Blood* 1993;81:3091–3096.
196. Mortenson MM, Schlieman MG, Virudachalam S, et al. Reduction in BCL-2 levels by 26S proteasome inhibition with bortezomib is associated with induction of apoptosis in small cell lung cancer. *Lung Cancer* 2005;49:163–170.
197. Shivapurkar N, Reddy J, Matta H, et al. Loss of expression of death-inducing signaling complex (DISC) components in lung cancer cell lines and the influence of MYC amplification. *Oncogene* 2002;21:8510–8514.
198. Park JY, Park JM, Jang JS, et al. Caspase 9 promoter polymorphisms and risk of primary lung cancer. *Hum Mol Genet* 2006;15:1963–1971.
199. Huang LN, Wang DS, Chen YQ, et al. Expression of survivin and patients survival in non-small cell lung cancer: a meta-analysis of the published studies. *Mol Biol Rep* 2013;40:917–924.
200. Zhang LQ, Wang J, Jiang F, et al. Prognostic value of survivin in patients with non-small cell lung carcinoma: a systematic review with meta-analysis. *PLoS One* 2012;7:e34100.
201. Lu B, Mu Y, Cao C, et al. Survivin as a therapeutic target for radiation sensitization in lung cancer. *Cancer Res* 2004;64:2840–2845.
202. Pore MM, Hiltermann TJ, Kruyt FA. Targeting apoptosis pathways in lung cancer. *Cancer Lett* 2013;332:359–368.
203. Ambros V. The functions of animal microRNAs. *Nature* 2004;431:350–355.
204. Lagos-Quintana M, Rauhut R, Lendeckel W, et al. Identification of novel genes coding for small expressed RNAs. *Science* 2001;294:853–858.
205. Croce CM. Causes and consequences of microRNA dysregulation in cancer. *Nat Rev Genet* 2009;10:704–714.
206. Calin GA, Cimmino A, Fabbri M, et al. MiR-15a and miR-16-1 cluster functions in human leukemia. *Proc Natl Acad Sci U S A* 2008;105:5166–5171.
207. Dews M, Homayouni A, Yu D, et al. Augmentation of tumor angiogenesis by a Myc-activated microRNA cluster. *Nat Genet* 2006;38:1060–1065.
208. Calin GA, Croce CM. MicroRNA signatures in human cancers. *Nat Rev Cancer* 2006;6:857–866.
209. Bommer GT, Gerin I, Feng Y, et al. p53-mediated activation of miRNA34 candidate tumor-suppressor genes. *Curr Biol* 2007;17:1298–1307.
210. Izzotti A, Calin GA, Arrigo P, et al. Downregulation of microRNA expression in the lungs of rats exposed to cigarette smoke. *FASEB J* 2009;23:806–812.
211. Gregory RI, Yan KP, Amuthan G, et al. The Microprocessor complex mediates the genesis of microRNAs. *Nature* 2004;432:235–240.
212. Han J, Lee Y, Yeom KH, et al. The Drosha-DGCR8 complex in primary microRNA processing. *Genes Dev* 2004;18:3016–3027.
213. Bohnsack MT, Czaplinski K, Gorlich D. Exportin 5 is a RanGTP-dependent dsRNA-binding protein that mediates nuclear export of pre-miRNAs. *RNA* 2004;10:185–191.
214. Karube Y, Tanaka H, Osada H, et al. Reduced expression of Dicer associated with poor prognosis in lung cancer patients. *Cancer Sci* 2005;96:111–115.
215. Yanaihara N, Caplen N, Bowman E, et al. Unique microRNA molecular profiles in lung cancer diagnosis and prognosis. *Cancer Cell* 2006;9:189–198.
216. Lu Y, Govindan R, Wang L, et al. MicroRNA profiling and prediction of recurrence/relapse-free survival in stage I lung cancer. *Carcinogenesis* 2012;33:1046–1054.
217. Nadal E, Chen G, Gallegos M, et al. Epigenetic Inactivation of microRNA-34b/c Predicts Poor Disease-Free Survival in Early-Stage Lung Adenocarcinoma. *Clin Cancer Res* 2013;19:6842–6852.
218. Akagi I, Okayama H, Schetter AJ, et al. Combination of protein coding and noncoding gene expression as a robust prognostic classifier in stage I lung adenocarcinoma. *Cancer Res* 2013;73:3821–3832.
219. Keller A, Backes C, Leidinger P, et al. Next-generation sequencing identifies novel microRNAs in peripheral blood of lung cancer patients. *Mol Biosyst* 2011;7:3187–3199.
220. Dacic S, Kelly L, Shuai Y, et al. miRNA expression profiling of lung adenocarcinomas: correlation with mutational status. *Mod Pathol* 2010;23:1577–1582.
221. Garofalo M, Romano G, Di Leva G, et al. EGFR and MET receptor tyrosine kinase-altered microRNA expression induces tumorigenesis and gefitinib resistance in lung cancers. *Nat Med* 2012;18:74–82.
222. Weiss GJ, Bemis LT, Nakajima E, et al. EGFR regulation by microRNA in lung cancer: correlation with clinical response and survival to gefitinib and EGFR expression in cell lines. *Ann Oncol* 2008;19:1053–1059.
223. Webster RJ, Giles KM, Price KJ, et al. Regulation of epidermal growth factor receptor signaling in human cancer cells by microRNA-7. *J Biol Chem* 2009;284:5731–5741.
224. Cho WC, Chow AS, Au JS. MiR-145 inhibits cell proliferation of human lung adenocarcinoma by targeting EGFR and NUDT1. *RNA Biol* 2011;8:125–131.
225. Chou YT, Lin HH, Lien YC, et al. EGFR promotes lung tumorigenesis by activating miR-7 through a Ras/ERK/Myc pathway that targets the Ets2 transcriptional repressor ERF. *Cancer Res* 2010;70:8822–8831.
226. Rai K, Takigawa N, Ito S, et al. Liposomal delivery of MicroRNA-7-expressing plasmid overcomes epidermal growth factor receptor tyrosine kinase inhibitor-resistance in lung cancer cells. *Mol Cancer Ther* 2011;10:1720–1727.
227. Janssen HL, Reesink HW, Lawitz EJ, et al. Treatment of HCV infection by targeting microRNA. *N Engl J Med* 2013;368:1685–1694.
228. Mirna Therapeutics, Inc. A Multicenter Phase I Study of MRX34, MicroRNA miR-RX34 Liposome Injectable Suspension. Clinical Trials.gov Web site. http://clinicaltrials.gov/ct2/show/NCT01829971.
229. Schembri F, Sridhar S, Perdomo C, et al. MicroRNAs as modulators of smoking-induced gene expression changes in human airway epithelium. *Proc Natl Acad Sci U S A* 2009;106:2319–2324.
230. Davidson MR, Larsen JE, Yang IA, et al. MicroRNA-218 is deleted and downregulated in lung squamous cell carcinoma. *PloS One* 2010;5:e12560.
231. Shen J, Liu Z, Todd NW, et al. Diagnosis of lung cancer in individuals with solitary pulmonary nodules by plasma microRNA biomarkers. *BMC Cancer* 2011;11:374.
232. Boeri M, Verri C, Conte D, et al. MicroRNA signatures in tissues and plasma predict development and prognosis of computed tomography detected lung cancer. *Proc Natl Acad Sci U S A* 2011;108:3713–3718.
233. Lei L, Huang Y, Gong W. miR-205 promotes the growth, metastasis and chemoresistance of NSCLC cells by targeting PTEN. *Oncol Rep* 2013;30:2897–2902.
234. Romano G, Acunzo M, Garofalo M, et al. MiR-494 is regulated by ERK1/2 and modulates TRAIL-induced apoptosis in non–small-cell lung cancer through BIM down-regulation. *Proc Natl Acad Sci U S A* 2012;109:16570–16575.
235. Shen J, Liao J, Guarnera MA, et al. Analysis of microRNAs in sputum to improve computed tomography for lung cancer diagnosis. *J Thorac Oncol* 2014;9:33–40.
236. Xing L, Todd NW, Yu L, et al. Early detection of squamous cell lung cancer in sputum by a panel of microRNA markers. *Mod Pathol* 2010;23:1157–1164.
237. Kosaka N, Iguchi H, Yoshioka Y, et al. Secretory mechanisms and intercellular transfer of microRNAs in living cells. *J Biol Chem* 2010;285:17442–17452.
238. Turchinovich A, Weiz L, Langheinz A, et al. Characterization of extracellular circulating microRNA. *Nucleic Acids Res* 2011;39:7223–7233.
239. Isobe T, Herbst RS, Onn A. Current management of advanced non-small cell lung cancer: targeted therapy. *Semin Oncol* 2005;32:315–328.
240. Acuff HB, Sinnamon M, Fingleton B, et al. Analysis of host- and tumor-derived proteinases using a custom dual species microarray reveals a protective role for stromal matrix metalloproteinase-12 in non-small cell lung cancer. *Cancer Res* 2006;66:7968–7975.
241. Gibbons DL, Lin W, Creighton CJ, et al. Contextual extracellular cues promote tumor cell EMT and metastasis by regulating miR-200 family expression. *Genes Dev* 2009;23:2140–2151.
242. Sandler AB. Targeting angiogenesis in lung cancer. *Semin Oncol* 2005;32:S16–S22.

243. Mineo TC, Ambrogi V, Baldi A, et al. Prognostic impact of VEGF, CD31, CD34, and CD105 expression and tumour vessel invasion after radical surgery for IB-IIA non-small cell lung cancer. *J Clin Pathol* 2004;57:591–597.
244. Reck M, von Pawel J, Zatloukal P, et al. Phase III trial of cisplatin plus gemcitabine with either placebo or bevacizumab as first-line therapy for nonsquamous non–small-cell lung cancer: AVAil. *J Clin Oncol* 2009;27:1227–1234.
245. Reck M, von Pawel J, Zatloukal P, et al. Overall survival with cisplatin-gemcitabine and bevacizumab or placebo as first-line therapy for nonsquamous non–small-cell lung cancer: results from a randomised phase III trial (AVAiL). *Ann Oncol* 2010;21:1804–1809.
246. Sandler A, Gray R, Perry MC, et al. Paclitaxel-carboplatin alone or with bevacizumab for non–small-cell lung cancer. *N Engl J Med* 2006;355:2542–2550.
247. Jordan CT, Guzman ML, Noble M. Cancer stem cells. *N Engl J Med* 2006;355:1253–1261.
248. Germano D, Blyszczuk P, Valaperti A, et al. Prominin-1/CD133+ lung epithelial progenitors protect from bleomycin-induced pulmonary fibrosis. *Am J Respir Crit Care Med* 2009;179:939–949.
249. Kim CFB, Jackson EL, Woolfenden AE, et al. Identification of bronchioalveolar stem cells in normal lung and lung cancer. *Cell* 2005;121:823–835.
250. Bertolini G, Roz L, Perego P, et al. Highly tumorigenic lung cancer CD133+ cells display stem-like features and are spared by cisplatin treatment. *Proc Natl Acad Sci U S A* 2009;106:16281–16286.
251. Chen Y-C, Hsu H-S, Chen Y-W, et al. Oct-4 expression maintained cancer stem-like properties in lung cancer-derived CD133-positive cells. *PLoS One* 2008;3:e2637.
252. Eramo A, Lotti F, Sette G, et al. Identification and expansion of the tumorigenic lung cancer stem cell population. *Cell Death Differ* 2008;15:504–514.
253. Jiang T, Collins BJ, Jin N, et al. Achaete-scute complex homologue 1 regulates tumor-initiating capacity in human small cell lung cancer. *Cancer Res* 2009;69:845–854.
254. Jiang F, Qiu Q, Khanna A, et al. Aldehyde dehydrogenase 1 is a tumor stem cell-associated marker in lung cancer. *Mol Cancer Res* 2009;7:330-338.
255. Pine SR, Ryan BM, Varticovski L, et al. Microenvironmental modulation of asymmetric cell division in human lung cancer cells. *Proc Natl Acad Sci U S A* 2010;107:2195–2200.
256. Jaksch M, Múnera J, Bajpai R, et al. Cell cycle-dependent variation of a CD133 epitope in human embryonic stem cell, colon cancer, and melanoma cell lines. *Cancer Res* 2008;68:7882–7886.
257. Shmelkov SV, Butler JM, Hooper AT, et al. CD133 expression is not restricted to stem cells, and both CD133+ and CD133− metastatic colon cancer cells initiate tumors. *J Clin Invest* 2008;118:2111–2120.
258. Kelly PN, Dakic A, Adams JM, et al. Tumor growth need not be driven by rare cancer stem cells. *Science* 2007;317:337.
259. Sullivan JP, Spinola M, Dodge M, et al. Aldehyde dehydrogenase activity selects for lung adenocarcinoma stem cells dependent on notch signaling. *Cancer Res* 2010;70:9937–9948.
260. Giacalone NJ, Den RB, Eisenberg R, et al. ALDH7A1 expression is associated with recurrence in patients with surgically resected non–small-cell lung carcinoma. *Future Oncol* 2013;9:737–745.
261. Bild AH, Yao G, Chang JT, et al. Oncogenic pathway signatures in human cancers as a guide to targeted therapies. *Nature* 2006;439:353–357.
262. Aberle DR, Adams AM, Berg CD, et al. Reduced lung-cancer mortality with low-dose computed tomographic screening. *N Engl J Med* 2011;365:395–409.

37 Non-Small Cell Lung Cancer

Frank C. Detterbeck, Roy H. Decker, Lynn Tanoue, and Rogerio C. Lilenbaum

INCIDENCE AND ETIOLOGY

Lung cancer is the most common cause of cancer death worldwide. The World Health Organization International Agency for Research on Cancer reported the global incidence of lung cancer at approximately 1.8 million new cases in 2012.[1] The overall ratio of mortality to incidence is high, with the 5-year survival rate in the United States still only 17%.[2] Consequently, the mortality burden is staggering, with lung cancer causing an estimated 1.59 million deaths per year around the world. Lung cancer accounts for nearly one-third of all cancer deaths in the United States and causes as many cancer deaths as the next four leading causes of cancer deaths combined (breast, colon, prostate, and pancreas).[2]

A relatively unique aspect of lung cancer is the strong association with a potentially avoidable risk factor, namely smoking. This has far-reaching psychological, social, political, and societal implications. An attitude of blame has contributed to low prioritization of lung cancer research and a lack of activism among people affected by the disease. Furthermore, this attitude and the relatively poor outcomes have promoted nihilism in both the medical and patient community about both treatment of the disease and attempts to make advances.

It is important to look beyond the simple association of lung cancer and smoking. Over half of those diagnosed with lung cancer in the United States are either never-smokers or people who quit smoking many years earlier.[3–5] Furthermore, lung cancer occurring in never-smokers is relatively common, occurring in about 20,000 individuals in the United States; this puts deaths from lung cancer in never-smokers among the top 10 causes of cancer deaths in the United States (e.g., more than cancer of the ovaries, uterus, or lymphomas).[2] This underscores that the etiology of lung cancer is complex and not well understood.

Major advances have been made in all aspects of lung cancer, from screening, to surgical, chemotherapy and radiotherapy (RT) treatment, methods of palliation, as well as the understanding of fundamental aspects of the biology of the disease. Lung cancer has become a vibrant and dynamic field, with a vast and growing literature describing advances in every facet of this disease. This makes it an impossible task to summarize the state of the art in one short chapter; it is inevitable that some areas will be missed or covered superficially, and new advances will have emerged during the course of publication. Nevertheless, this chapter is an attempt to cover the most important clinical aspects of lung cancer, which represents a major source of suffering and mortality throughout the world.

The highest incidence and mortality rates from lung cancer are observed in men in Central and Eastern Europe, Southern Europe, Eastern Asia, Micronesia, and Northern America, and in women in Northern America, Northern Europe, Australia/New Zealand, and Micronesia (Fig. 37.1). The highest estimated age-standardized lung cancer incidence rates occur in more developed regions of the world, where smoking is more prevalent (Fig. 37.2). Globally, lung cancer is still more common in men than in women, reflecting different historical and temporal exposure to tobacco smoking. The evidence does not suggest that women are either more or less susceptible than men to the carcinogenic effects of tobacco. On a hopeful note, the incidence rates in men appear to be falling or at least stabilizing in all regions, likely reflecting the impact of successful national initiatives focused on tobacco control (Fig. 37.3). In contrast, incidence rates in women appear to be increasing in most regions or at best stabilizing in a few.

Smoking

At the turn of the 20th century, lung cancer was a rare malignancy. In an extensive autopsy review in the United States and Western Europe in 1916, Adler found that lung cancers represented <0.5% of all cancer cases.[6] Over the next several decades, a substantive increase in the incidence of lung cancer was noted; at the same time, observations of the adverse health effects of smoking were made. In 1941, Ochsner and DeBakey stated, "it is our definite conviction that the increase in the incidence of pulmonary carcinoma is due largely to the increase in smoking, particularly cigaret *(sic)* smoking."[7] Two landmark case-control studies published in 1950 by Doll and Hill[8] in the United Kingdom and Wynder and Graham[9] in the United States established a causal link between cigarette smoking and bronchogenic carcinoma. The Royal College of Physicians in the United Kingdom in 1962[10] and the Surgeon General of the United States in 1964[11] endorsed the conclusion that cigarette smoking is the major cause of lung cancer. Population trends of lung cancer incidence mirror smoking behavior, with a typical lag time of approximately 20 years (see Figs. 37.1 and 37.2). Both the number of cigarettes smoked per day and the duration of smoking correlate with lung cancer risk, with longer duration in particular being associated with a much higher risk.[12]

Cigarette smoke is a complex aerosol, with nicotine being the primary determinant of addiction and tar being the particulate residue left when nicotine and water are removed from tobacco smoke. More than 50 carcinogens in tobacco smoke have been identified, including N-nitrosoamines formed by nitrosation of nicotine during smoking, and polycyclic aromatic hydrocarbines.[13–15] The N-nitrosoamine 4-(methylnitrosamino)-1(3-pyridyl)-1-butanone is associated with DNA adduct formation and DNA mutations that result in the activation of *KRAS* oncogenes.[16,17] Both N-nitrosoamines and polycyclic aromatic hydrocarbines may be metabolically activated to become carcinogenic, or alternatively may be metabolically detoxified; the balance of these processes will determine exposure. Other carcinogens in tobacco smoke carcinogens do not require activation (e.g., benzene, vinyl chloride, or radon). The dose of carcinogen(s) received from smoking will vary with the composition of the cigarette itself, including whether a filter is present, and the intensity of inhalation. Because of regulatory mandates, cigarettes contain less nicotine and tar than in years past. However, smokers may compensate by smoking more intensively (more puffs per minute and deeper, longer inhalations) to satisfy nicotine addiction. Mentholation of cigarettes may also facilitate

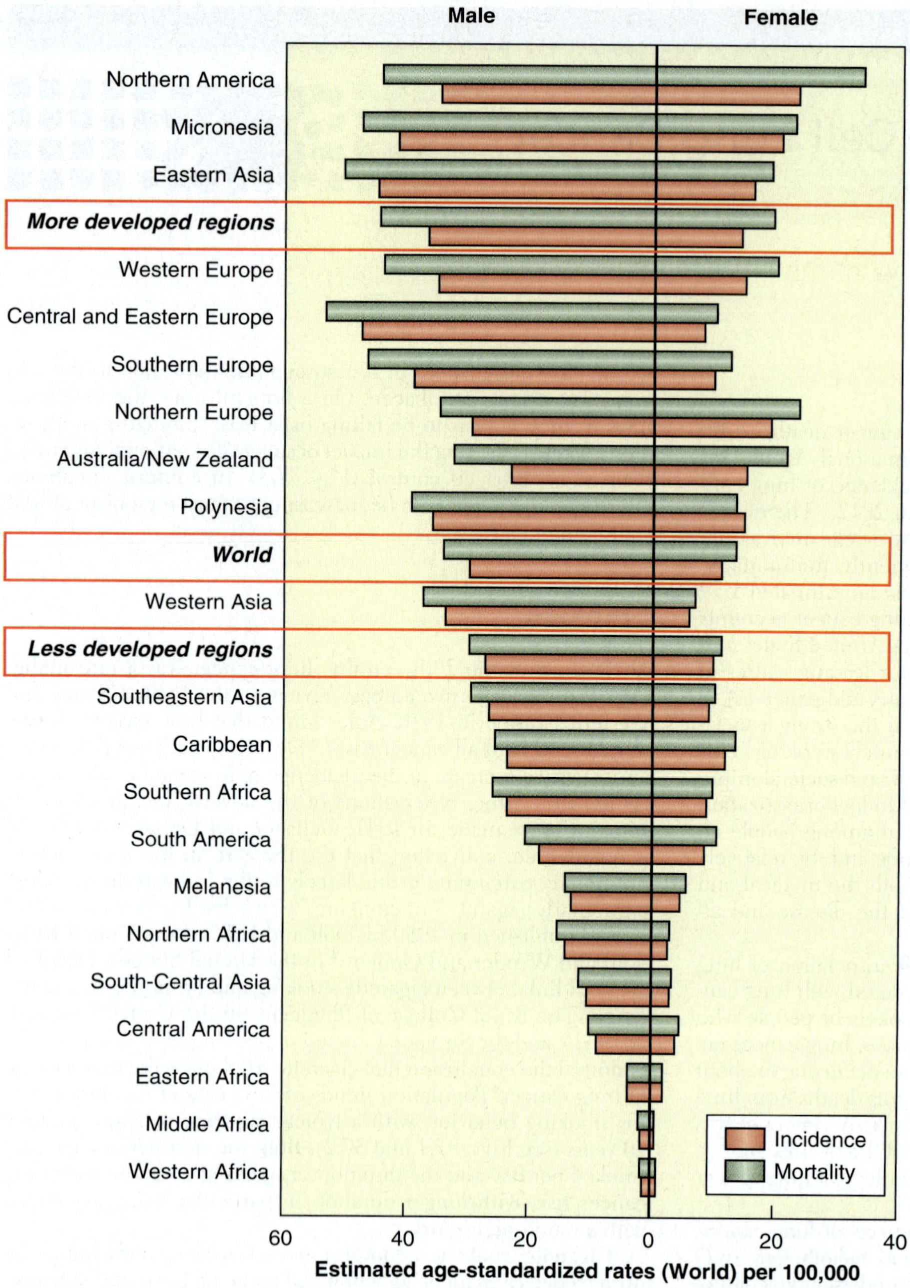

Figure 37.1 Estimated age-standardized rates of lung cancer per 100,000 population by region of the world. (Reproduced from GLOBOCAN 2012, International Agency for Research on Cancer, World Health Organization.)

more intense smoking, as it changes the aroma of the smoke and decreases the irritant effect of the smoke, thereby facilitating more intense inhalation.[18,19]

Genetic Predisposition

The cumulative lifetime risk for lifelong smokers in their eighth decade of life is approximately 16%.[20] The host factors that confer "protection" from lung cancer in the majority of individuals who smoke and never develop lung cancer, or determine increased susceptibility in those individuals who do, are not clear. An estimated 300,000 lung cancer deaths occur in nonsmokers annually in the world; in many of these cases, no specific risk or exposure can be identified.[21,22] It is widely accepted that genetic (inherited) factors as well as epigenetic (acquired) DNA changes contribute to the development of malignancy. The association of lung cancer with rare Mendelian cancer syndromes or in family aggregates supports the contribution of high-penetrance, low-frequency genes.[23,24] Mutations in low-penetrance, high-frequency genes that encode enzymes involved in activation or detoxification of carcinogens, or enzymes involved in DNA repair, also influence lung cancer susceptibility.[25–27]

A large European case control study and meta-analysis of 41 studies demonstrated that the risk of lung cancer increased if there was a first-degree family member with lung cancer (odds ratio = 1.63) and increased further if two or more family members had lung cancer (odds ratio = 3.6).[28] The Liverpool Lung Project reported that a family history of early onset lung cancer (age <60 years) was associated with an odds ratio for lung cancer of 2.02.[29] While some polymorphisms in a few candidate genes have been identified, the broad field of host genetic factors determining lung cancer susceptibility is still poorly understood and is an area of intense investigation. We do not yet have the tools to identify which individuals might be intrinsically more likely to develop lung cancer or more vulnerable to the carcinogenic effects of cigarettes. Such knowledge eventually may help define specific populations who should be targeted for lung cancer screening.

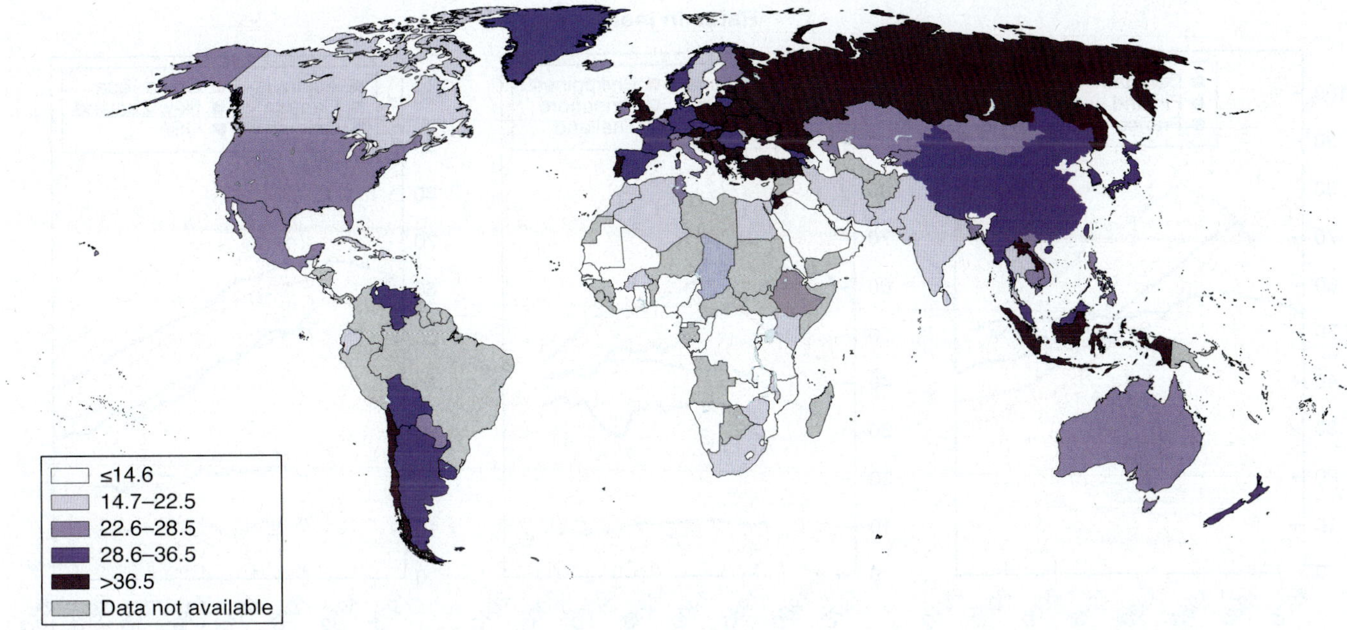

Figure 37.2 Percentage of tobacco use among adults by country in 2005. (Reproduced from GLOBOCAN 2012, International Agency for Research on Cancer, World Health Organization.)

Occupational/Environmental

Though smoking is clearly the most important modifiable risk factor, many other factors influence the development of lung cancer. It is estimated that approximately 10% of lung cancer cases are at least in part related to occupational exposures.[30] Many workplace materials have been identified as carcinogens, including, among others, arsenic, asbestos, beryllium, cadmium, chromium, nickel, radon, and vinyl chloride. Of these, asbestos is the most common, having been used widely for its insulating properties and recognized as a lung carcinogen as early as the 1940s.[31] There has been controversy as to whether asbestos exposure per se confers lung cancer risk or whether asbestosis, the associated interstitial lung disease, is required. A recent long-term follow-up of a large group of North American insulators originally studied in the early 1980s provided further data on asbestos exposure, asbestosis, and cigarette smoking.[32] In the nonsmoking cohort, lung cancer risk was increased with asbestos exposure alone, and further increased if asbestosis was also present. In the smoking cohort, there was an additive risk of smoking and asbestos exposure, with a supra-additive increase in risk if both smoking and asbestosis were present. Thus it appears that while asbestosis clearly increases lung cancer risk, particularly in smokers, asbestos exposure alone also increases risk, albeit to a lesser degree.

Radon gas was first implicated as increasing lung cancer risk in workers in underground uranium mines. The awareness of radon as a carcinogen has focused attention on domestic radon gas as a common indoor pollutant.[33–36] Radon is felt to contribute to an estimated 15,000 to 20,000 lung cancer deaths in the United States annually.[36] Other indoor air pollutant carcinogens include environmental tobacco smoke and byproducts of biomass fuels used for heating and cooking. Outdoor air pollution contains carcinogens generated by fossil fuel combustion and diesel exhaust, which can be adsorbed to fine particulates small enough to be inhaled into the airways. These exposures are of particular concern in countries such as China, where indoor domestic use of coal and wood, intense urban outdoor pollution, and an epidemic of tobacco smoking are likely all contributing to an alarming rise in lung cancer incidence.

Cancer risk related to medical imaging has been an area of increasing public health concern, particularly with the escalation of use of high technology studies such as computed tomography (CT) and positron emission tomography (PET). Radiation exposure acquired in this way is cumulative, with risk extrapolated on a linear model based on known cancer risk in survivors of the atomic bomb in Japan, and after therapeutic radiation given in the past for medical diseases including tuberculosis and ankylosing spondylitis.[37–40] Based on this model, even lower cumulative doses incur some risk. Recognition of the potential harms of radiation from medical imaging makes more urgent the need to utilize these tests judiciously, develop methods to track cumulative radiation exposure to specific organs, and improve technologies that will minimize patient exposure. This need is particularly cogent anticipating implementation of lung cancer screening with low-dose chest CT scanning.

Lung cancer is typically a disease of older individuals; ironically, as overall health status improves in developing countries and those populations acquire longer life expectancy, their lung cancer risk may increase. Whether gender is a factor has been a topic of considerable debate. At present, the body of evidence does not support any significant sex-related difference in susceptibility to smoking-associated lung cancer.[41] African Americans have consistently been observed to have higher lung cancer rates as well as worse 5-year survival than Caucasian Americans.[2] In developed nations, socioeconomic factors including education and income are inversely associated with risk. Lifestyle factors, including diet and physical activity, likely influence risk. An inverse association of diets higher in fruit and vegetable (cruciferous and carotenoid-rich) consumption with lung cancer risk has been consistently described.[42,43] The evidence for physical activity is less clear, though higher levels of activity have been described as associated with lower cancer risk.[44]

The presence of underlying pulmonary disease is increasingly recognized to influence lung cancer risk. Cigarette smoking is the major etiologic factor in both lung cancer and chronic obstructive pulmonary disease (COPD). COPD per se is an independent risk factor after controlling for smoking.[45,46] The mechanism(s) by which fixed airways disease may etiologically be implicated in carcinogenesis are not defined, but potentially include mutagenesis through activation of the NF-kappaB inflammatory pathway, protease-antiprotease imbalance, or chronic inflammation itself.[47–49] The presence of interstitial lung disease has also been associated

CANCER OF THE THORACIC CAVITY

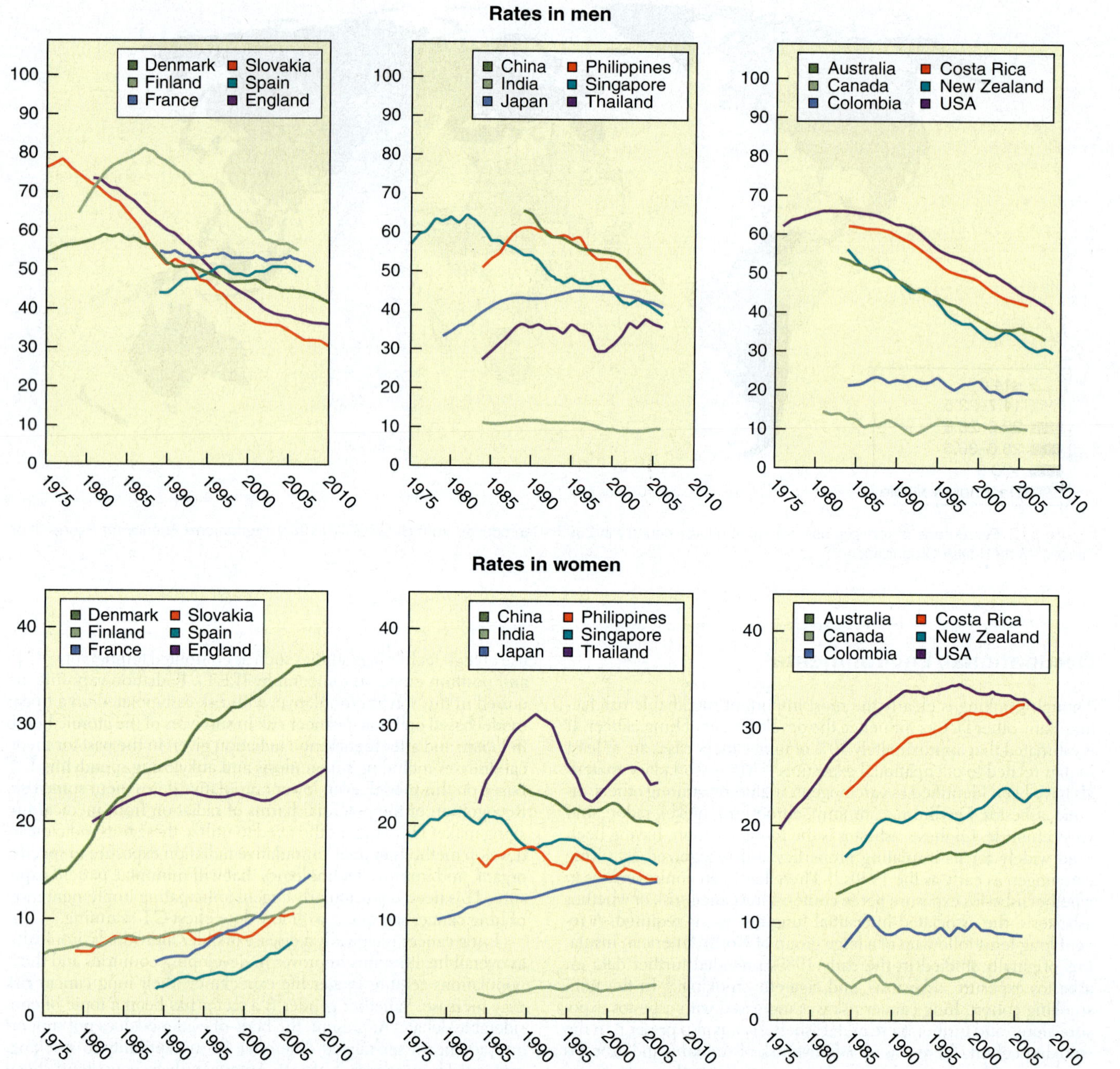

Figure 37.3 Trends in mortality from lung cancer showing the age-standardized mortality rate from lung cancer per 100,000 men (*top row*) and women (*bottom row*) in selected countries. (Reproduced from GLOBOCAN 2012. International Agency for Research on Cancer, World Health Organization.)

with an increase in lung cancer risk. In particular, patients with idiopathic pulmonary fibrosis have been reported to have an odds ratio for lung cancer of 8.25 compared to controls.[50,51] In contrast to COPD, cigarette smoking is usually not etiologically implicated in interstitial diseases, although chronic inflammation typically is felt to contribute to the pathologic process.

ANATOMY AND PATHOLOGY

Stage Classification

The stage classification for non–small-cell lung cancer (NSCLC) follows the tumor, node, metastasis (TNM) paradigm used for most solid tumors. Staging ensures a uniform standardized nomenclature to describe the anatomic extent of disease, namely the primary tumor site (T component) as well as cancer spread to nodes (N component) or distant metastatic sites (M component). The most recent (seventh edition) of the lung cancer stage classification is based on an unprecedented effort directed by the International Association for the Study of Lung Cancer (IASLC).[52–55] This involved an international database of over 100,000 patients, identified over the period 1990 to 2000 from 46 sources in 19 countries in North America, Asia, Australia, and Europe, and a sophisticated statistical analysis with extensive internal and external validation.[56] This stage classification applies to small cell and NSCLCs as well as carcinoid tumors.[57,58]

Several characteristics of the IASLC database are important to recognize in order to appropriately interpret some of the results. This was a retrospective database, with limitations in the level of details available. For example, some of the definitions of the TNM descriptors contained too few patients to allow statistical analysis of the impact of that tumor characteristic. Because the database consisted of patients diagnosed between 1990 and 2000, advances in technology (e.g., PET imaging) and treatment modalities that are routine today are not reflected. The analysis did not account for what treatment (if any) was given. In fact, there was a great deal of variation in outcomes depending on the type of source data and the geographic region. Thus, while the outcomes created a phenomenal tool to define where to draw distinctions between TNM categories and groupings, the outcomes themselves represent a global cross-section from the past with less clear relevance to specific patients today.

The definitions of the T, N, and M categories for both NSCLC and small-cell lung cancer (SCLC) are outlined in detail in Table 37.1.[59] The T, N, and M categories are then grouped to define particular stages of lung cancer (both NSCLC and SCLC), as outlined in Fig. 37.4. While ideally each stage would represent a homogeneous group of patients, this is not necessarily the case, as is evident in the range of T, N, and M combinations that comprise stage IIB or IIIA, for example. Nevertheless, the system provides a practical way of managing the complexity of a large number of T, N and M categories into a more limited number of stage groups.

TABLE 37.1

Stage Classification: T, N, M Descriptors

Category	Descriptor Definition	Subgroup[a]
T (Primary Tumor)		
T0	No primary tumor	
T1	Tumor ≤3 cm,[b] surrounded by lung or visceral pleura, not more proximal than the lobar bronchus	
T1a	Tumor ≤2 cm[b]	*T1a*
T1b	Tumor >2 but ≤3 cm[b]	*T1b*
T2	Tumor >3 but ≤7 cm[b] or tumor with any of the following[c]: Invades visceral pleura, involves main bronchus ≥2 cm distal to the carina, atelectasis/obstructive pneumonia extending to hilum but not involving the entire lung	
T2a	Tumor >3 but ≤5 cm[b]	*T2a*
T2b	Tumor >5 but ≤7 cm[b]	*T2b*
T3	Tumor >7 cm[a]	$T3_{>7}$
	or directly invading chest wall, diaphragm, phrenic nerve, mediastinal pleura, parietal pericardium,	$T3_{Inv}$
	or tumor in the main bronchus <2 cm distal to the carina,[d]	$T3_{Centr}$
	or atelectasis/obstructive pneumonitis of entire lung,	
	or separate tumor nodule(s) in the same lobe	$T3_{Satell}$
T4	Tumor of any size with invasion of heart, great vessels, trachea, recurrent laryngeal nerve, esophagus, vertebral body, or carina;	$T4_{Inv}$
	or separate tumor nodule(s) in a different ipsilateral lobe	$T4_{Ipsi\ Nod}$
N (Regional Lymph Nodes)		
N0	No regional node metastasis	
N1	Metastasis in ipsilateral peribronchial and/or perihilar lymph nodes and intrapulmonary nodes, including involvement by direct extension	
N2	Metastasis in ipsilateral mediastinal and/or subcarinal lymph node(s)	
N3	Metastasis in contralateral mediastinal, contralateral hilar, ipsilateral, or contralateral scalene or supraclavicular lymph node(s)	
M (Distant Metastasis)		
M0	No distant metastasis	
M1a	Separate tumor nodule(s) in a contralateral lobe;	$M1a_{Contr\ Nod}$
	or tumor with pleural nodules or malignant pleural dissemination[e]	$M1a_{Pl\ Dissem}$
M1b	Distant metastasis	*M1b*
Special Situations		
TX, NX, MX	T, N, or M status not able to be assessed	
T*is*	Focus of in situ cancer	*Tis*
T1[d]	Superficial spreading tumor of any size but confined to the wall of the trachea or mainstem bronchus	$T1_{SS}$

[a]These subgroup labels are not defined in the International Association for the Study of Lung Cancer publications (see Goldstraw P, Crowley J, Chansky K, et al. The IASLC Lung Cancer Staging Project: proposals for the revision of the TNM stage groupings in the forthcoming [seventh] edition of the TNM Classification of malignant tumours. *J Thorac Oncol* 2007;2:706–714; Rami-Porta R, Ball D, Crowley J, et al. The IASLC Lung Cancer Staging Project: proposals for the revision of the T descriptors in the forthcoming (seventh) edition of the TNM classification for lung cancer. *J Thorac Oncol* 2007,2.593–602; Rusch VW, Crowley J, Giroux DJ, et al. The IASLC Lung Cancer Staging Project: proposals for the revision of the N descriptors in the forthcoming seventh edition of the TNM classification for lung cancer. *J Thorac Oncol* 2007;2:603–612; Postmus PE, Brambilla E, Chansky K, et al. The IASLC Lung Cancer Staging Project: proposals for revision of the M descriptors in the forthcoming [seventh] edition of the TNM classification of lung cancer. *J Thorac Oncol* 2007;2:686–693) but are added here to facilitate a clear discussion.

[b]In greatest dimension.

[c]T2 tumors with these features are classified as T2a if ≤5 cm.

[d]The uncommon superficial spreading tumor in central airways is classified as T1.

[e]Pleural effusions are excluded that are cytologically negative, nonbloody, transudative, and clinically judged not to be due to cancer.

Reproduced with permission from the American College of Chest Physicians from Detterbeck F, Tanoue L, Boffa DJ. The new lung cancer staging system. *Chest* 2009;136:260–271.

T/M	Subgroup	N0	N1	N2	N3
T1	T1a	Ia	IIa	IIIa	IIIb
	T1b	Ia	IIa	IIIa	IIIb
T2	T2a	Ib	IIa	IIIa	IIIb
	T2b	IIa	IIb	IIIa	IIIb
T3	T3 $_{>7}$	IIb	IIIa	IIIa	IIIb
	T2 $_{Inv}$	IIb	IIIa	IIIa	IIIb
	T3 $_{Satell}$	IIb	IIIa	IIIa	IIIb
T4	T4 $_{Inv}$	IIIa	IIIa	IIIb	IIIb
	T4 $_{Ipsi\ Nod}$	IIIa	IIIa	IIIb	IIIb
M1	M1a $_{Contra\ Nod}$	IV	IV	IV	IV
	M1a $_{Pl\ Disem}$	IV	IV	IV	IV
	M1b	IV	IV	IV	IV

Figure 37.4 Stage classification: Stage groups. Inv, invasion; Satell, satellite; Ipsi Nod, ipsilateral nodule; Contra Nod, contralateral nodule; Pl Disem, pleural dissemination. (Reproduced with permission from Detterbeck F, Tanoue L, Boffa DJ. The new lung cancer staging system. *Chest* 2009;136:262.)

It is worth emphasizing what the stage classification system does and cannot accomplish. It is designed to be a consistent, stable nomenclature for the anatomic extent of disease. Although this is a major component in a patient's prognosis, the prognosis depends on many other factors, including age, comorbidities, environmental factors, and treatment factors. Particular tumor or patient factors (e.g., genetic mutations, central/peripheral lung location) may have a major impact in certain settings (e.g., a particular treatment strategy) but not in others, and at certain times during the course of the disease. Therefore, stage classification is not sufficient to capture the complexity of prognostic prediction for specific patients in specific clinical settings. Furthermore, although the anatomic extent of disease is an important component of selecting a treatment approach, this is also determined by other factors (e.g., histologic type, molecular information, patient-specific factors such as comorbidities). In addition, stage classification must remain relatively static and consistent to be useful, while treatment should continually evolve and improve. Thus, treatment must be determined by the results of clinical trials and cannot be determined merely by a stage classification nomenclature.

Histologic Classification

The histologic spectrum of lung cancer has clearly changed over the past several decades. SCLC has decreased from about 25% to <15% of all lung cancers.[60] Adenocarcinoma is now the most dominant histologic type, replacing squamous carcinoma. With the advent of more frequent CT imaging, an increased proportion of more indolent small tumors is being recognized.[61]

The histologic classification of lung cancer has become much more nuanced. In the past, the major NSCLC histologic types (adenocarcinoma, squamous cell carcinoma, and large cell carcinoma) were simply lumped together. It is critical to differentiate these because they respond differently to certain chemotherapeutic agents. Immunohistochemical stains and genetic characterization can facilitate the distinction between subtypes.[62,63] It is recognized that the vast majority of adenocarcinomas are mixed subtypes; these are now classified according to the predominant subtype with the percent of each noted in 10% increments.[63] Furthermore, the adenocarcinoma subtypes have been defined according to preinvasive, minimally invasive, and invasive groups (Table 37.2),[63] reflecting the increasingly recognized spectrum of aggressiveness of lung cancers encountered in the Western world today. Finally, bronchopulmonary carcinoid and salivary gland tumors are less common types that are also included among lung cancers.[64]

TABLE 37.2

International Association for the Study of Lung Cancer/American Thoracic Society/ European Respiratory Society Classification of Lung Adenocarcinoma in Resection Specimens

- Preinvasive lesions
  - Atypical adenomatous hyperplasia
  - Adenocarcinoma in situ (≤3 cm, formerly BAC)
    - Nonmucinous
    - Mucinous
    - Mixed mucinous/nonmucinous
- Minimally invasive adenocarcinoma (≤3 cm lepidic predominant tumor with >5 mm invasion)
  - Nonmucinous
  - Mucinous
  - Mixed mucinous/nonmucinous
- Invasive adenocarcinoma
  - Lepidic predominant (formerly nonmucinous BAC pattern, with >5 mm invasion)
  - Acinar predominant
  - Papillary predominant
  - Micropapillary predominant
  - Solid predominant with mucin production
- Variants of invasive adenocarcinoma
  - Invasive mucinous adenocarcinoma (formerly mucinous BAC)
  - Colloid
  - Fetal (low and high grade)
  - Enteric

BAC, bronchioloalveolar carcinoma.
Reproduced with permission from Travis WD, Brambilla E, Noguchi M, et al. International Association for the Study of Lung Cancer/American Thoracic Society/European Respiratory Society international multidisciplinary classification of lung adenocarcinoma. *J Thorac Oncol* 2011;6:244.

Genetic Characterization

A fairly detailed understanding of cellular and genetic characteristics of cancer has emerged. A way to organize this is the concept of "hallmarks of cancer." Initially 6 hallmarks were defined; by 2011, this had increased to 10 (resisting cell death, sustaining proliferative signaling, evading growth suppressors, enabling replicative immortality, activating invasion and metastasis, inducing angiogenesis, deregulating cellular energetics, avoiding immune destruction, genome instability and mutation, tumor-promoting inflammation).[65,66] A potential 11th hallmark has recently been suggested (epigenetic or RNA deregulation).[67] The ability to identify mutations in genes that play a role in various of these mechanisms has substantiated the importance of these hallmarks as being fundamental to malignant behavior.

Genetic characterization allows better classification of lung cancers. A systematic characterization of genetic alterations in 1,255 patients with lung cancer reveals that most histologic types have a characteristic pattern of genetic alteration.[62] Large-cell lung cancer is the exception, exhibiting alterations associated with each of the other major histologic types. Using genetic characterization, the vast majority of cases initially classified simply as large-cell lung cancer could be assigned to another histologic group (e.g., adenocarcinoma, squamous carcinoma, SCLC), which was corroborated by prognostic and other similarities among the genetically grouped cohorts.[62]

Particular mutations have sparked a great deal of attention, primarily because they have led to dramatic therapeutic breakthroughs (Table 37.3). Mostly these involve driver mutations for sustained proliferative signaling. Mutations in the epidermal growth factor receptor (EGFR) gene are the best-known examples. Such driver mutations have received much attention because targeted treatment can yield dramatic results, although the overall proportion of patients with these mutations may be quite small. Particularly because identification of these genetic alterations drives the choice of treatment, some have suggested that classification based on targetable mutations may be a better way to classify lung cancers than by histologic features.

Classification by genetic alterations is thwarted by the complexity of these changes. Whole genome and whole exome sequencing of 183 lung adenocarcinomas revealed greater complexity in genetic alterations than what is seen in most other cancers.[67] Although many mutated genes were found, 15% did not have a single hallmark alteration, and almost 40% have fewer than four hallmark alterations.[67] Focusing on mutations in which a targeted therapy is available or being developed may be practical, but belies the complexity of cancer biology. Even in those instances where dramatic responses have been achieved, in most cases resistance eventually develops. Furthermore, while driver mutations can sometimes clearly play a major role in cancer growth, alterations in many of the other hallmarks of cancer are less amenable to treatment, at least at this time. Finally, the well-documented finding that some EGFR-mutated adenocarcinomas that have become resistant to treatment with a tyrosine kinase inhibitor (TKI) have been transformed into a SCLC underscores that our understanding of the fundamental nature of lung cancer is still rudimentary.

Prognostic Factors

Prediction of prognosis is fervently desired, but remains an elusive goal. Developing a system to do this is complex and must solve a number of inherent conflicts. Hence the state of affairs is that we have identified a few factors that have prognostic value (at least in some clinical settings), but it is spotty and explains only a small amount of the actual observed outcomes.

Prediction of prognosis is inherently complex.[68] There are many factors that contribute; these can be grouped roughly into environmental factors, tumor-related factors, and patient-related factors (Fig. 37.5). The prognosis is inherently linked to a specific clinical scenario and to the outcome of interest. The scenario includes treatment-related factors and timing (e.g., the prognostic significance of an EGFR mutation is different if the patient is to undergo treatment with an EGFR inhibitor, regular chemotherapy, or neither, and different prior to treatment than upon developing resistance).

There are inherent conflicts in prognostication.[68,69] We derive our knowledge from studying groups of patients with a particular characteristic, but we seek individualized prognostic prediction, tailored to a particular person. The ability to individualize is limited because we do not have sufficient detail of all of the other factors of the group to assess how well the group fits with the individual. Even if we had more and more detail, the more specific we get, the more limited the dataset available to derive the prediction becomes, and thus the greater the uncertainty about the prediction. Finally, the data we base the prediction on is inherently based on past observation, yet the prediction is for the future, and thus cannot take into account new developments that inevitably occur.

Prognostic prediction is inherently different than stage classification.[69] Stage classification is a nomenclature to describe the anatomic extent of disease. It must remain relatively static and be used in a consistent uniform manner; the classification we assign to a particular extent of tumor today must be the same as what we assign to the same extent next year or else it is a useless nomenclature. However, prognostication is inherently fluid and constantly changing as advances occur and the setting changes. Stage classification must be consistent and definitive while prognostic prediction is inherently speculative and uncertain.

CANCER OF THE THORACIC CAVITY

TABLE 37.3

Genetic Alterations in Non–Small-Cell Lung Cancer

Genetic Alteration	Frequency	Test	Targeted Agents[a]
Nonsquamous			
KRAS mutation	25%	Sequence	None
EGFR mutation	15%	Sequence	Gefitinib, erlotinib, afatinib
ALK rearrangement	5%–7%	FISH	Crizotinib, ceritinib
ROS1 rearrangement	1%–2%	FISH	Crizotinib
HER2 (mutation only)	2%–4%	Sequence	Traztuzumab, pertuzumab, lapatinib, afatinib
BRAF mutation	2%–3%	Sequence	Vemurafenib, dabrafenib
RET rearrangement	1%–2%	FISH	Carbozantinib
MET (mutation only)	1%–2%	Sequence	None
MEK1 mutation	<1%	Sequence	None
PIK3CA mutation	1%–2%	Sequence	None
Squamous			
FGFR1 amplification	20%–25%	FISH	None
FGFR1 mutation	5%	Sequence	None
PIK3CA mutation	5%–10%	Sequence	None
DDR2 mutation	3%–5%	Sequence	Dasatinib
PTEN mutation/deletion	15%–20%	Sequence	None

FISH, fluorescence in situ hybridization.
[a] Agents listed do not all have proof of efficacy and are not all approved.

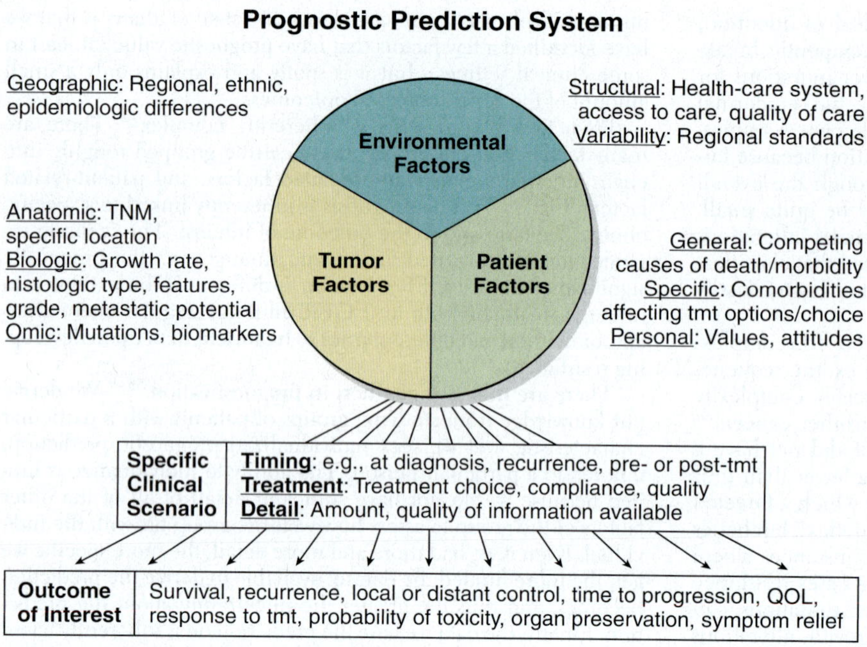

Figure 37.5 Schematic of a prognostic prediction system, taking into account environmental, patient-related, and tumor-related factors. The prediction must be specific to the clinical scenario and the outcome of interest. TNM, tumor, node, metastases; QOL, quality of life; tmt, treatment.

As part of the stage classification project, the international staging committee undertook a review of data on prognostic factors in lung cancer among surgically treated patients in the worldwide IASLC database.[70] Pathologic TNM class was most important, but age and gender also had independent prognostic significance. Histologic cell type (particularly bronchioloalveolar carcinoma [BAC]) may have some prognostic value; however, this is linked to other variables and is probably best understood when we can take into account the newer subclassification of adenocarcinoma, which was not available at the time of the analysis.[63] Many other potential factors, such as genetic features or PET intensity, were also not available for analysis. In sum, development of a prognostic model is very complex, situation specific, and constantly changing. We have only a rudimentary understanding at this point, and no overarching system of how to develop a universal prognostic prediction model.

PREVENTION AND SCREENING

Prevention

Tobacco Control

The global epidemic of lung cancer is linked most strongly to population engagement in cigarette smoking. While other modifiable risk factors (e.g., exposure to occupational or domestic carcinogens) are clearly identifiable, it is tobacco smoking that has driven the steep rises in lung cancer incidence and mortality witnessed over the last century in developed and developing nations. Primary prevention has the greatest overall potential to minimize lung cancer risk, and smoking cessation is still the most powerful intervention to diminish lung cancer risk in persons who smoke. Smoking cessation even into the seventh decade of life results in a decrease in lung cancer incidence, and so it is never too late to quit.[20,71] While smoking rates have decreased dramatically since the publication of the first surgeon general's report on the health consequences of smoking in 1964, approximately 20% of adult Americans still habitually smoke.

Important public health interventions have included stricter control of tobacco products by government regulatory agencies, limitations on cigarette advertising, particularly those geared toward children, the use of text and graphic warnings on cigarette packaging, and global initiatives to inform the public of the health hazards of smoking.[72–75]

Smoking Cessation

There are many physiologic and psychological factors that contribute to make smoking a difficult addiction to overcome. However, there have been major advances in understanding these, and solid scientific data regarding which interventions work best and in which individuals. Nicotine acts in an area of the brain associated with a sense of "safety" and "survival functions."[76] This appears to explain the paradox of difficulty in giving up smoking even when faced with a life-threatening disease that is a consequence of smoking. This struggle and the illogical nature of it, combined with the stigmatism associated with smoking, lead to feelings of shame, helplessness, and depression that further aggravate the problem.[76] It is easy to succumb to a fatalistic defense that "it is too late anyhow." However, data clearly shows that patients with lung cancer who continue to smoke approximately double their risk of dying.[76] Quitting smoking is associated with better response to treatment, better quality of life (QOL), better long-term survival, and a lower risk of second primary cancers.[76–79] Furthermore, data shows that a diagnosis of lung cancer represents a particularly opportune moment to intervene.[76]

Smoking cessation intervention should be included in the health care of any individual smoking cigarettes. It is important to use a sophisticated, evidence-based approach and an organized smoking cessation program to achieve the best results.[76] A simple recommendation to stop smoking or provision of self-help materials is largely ineffective. Several points are important. Tobacco dependence is best managed in a chronic disease model with repeated intervention over time. Intensive behavioral therapy and counseling (e.g., weekly) is of significant benefit in several randomized controlled trials (RCT). In addition, seven first-line medications reliably increase long-term smoking abstinence rates (bupropion, varenicline, nicotine patch, gum, lozenges, inhaler, and nasal spray).[76] These increase effectiveness two- or three-fold and result in abstinence rates of ~25%. Often, combinations of these may be more effective than a single intervention. These medications have been shown to be safe in most patients, including those who are about to undergo either surgery, RT, or chemotherapy. It is best to initiate the cessation interventions at the outset. Specifically, it is safe (and beneficial) for patients to stop smoking even a short time (e.g., 1 to

2 weeks) before undergoing surgery; pharmacologic interventions are safe to continue in the perioperative period as well.[76] A well-organized thoracic oncology program, therefore, should include an evidence-based smoking cessation program that is fully integrated with the diagnostic and treatment components of patient care.

Chemoprevention

The concept of chemoprevention is based on the data that lung cancer is the end result of a multistep accumulation of carcinogen-driven genetic and epigenetic changes. In theory, chemical agents might prevent these changes by a variety of proposed mechanisms, such as detoxifying carcinogens and modifying pathways that influence cell growth and behavior. Epidemiologic and animal studies had suggested that derivatives of the antioxidant vitamins A and E might be protective against lung cancer. However, large clinical trials of alpha-tocopherol and beta carotene in subjects at risk of developing lung cancer failed to demonstrate any benefit, and two studies suggested that beta carotene was actually associated with an increased incidence of lung cancer as well as cardiovascular disease.[80–83] To date, no chemopreventative intervention has been demonstrated to be of benefit for lung cancer. The focus has shifted from large RCTs to studies to better define the underlying biology and appropriate surrogate end points.[84]

Screening

At present, the majority of patients with lung cancer have advanced disease at the time of diagnosis. This preponderance of advanced disease, where prognosis is poor even with treatment, is a major contributor to the dismal overall 5-year survival rate of 18%; this contrasts starkly with breast, colon, and prostate cancers, the next three leading causes of cancer death, whose 5-year survival rates over the past several decades have increased to 90%, 65%, and nearly 100%, respectively.[2] These improved survival rates are arguably attributable at least in part to early detection resulting from widely available and broadly accepted, albeit still controversial, screening interventions.

An effective screening tool for early detection of lung cancer has been an elusive goal for decades. Several large randomized trials performed during the 1960s and 1970s evaluating lung cancer screening with chest radiography with or without sputum analysis at varying time intervals failed to demonstrate any mortality benefit,[85–89] and a Cochrane meta-analysis[90] concluded that there was no evidence to support the use of chest radiography or sputum cytology as a lung cancer screening modality. More recently, chest radiography was re-examined as a lung cancer screening tool in the Prostate, Lung, Colorectal and Ovarian trial, which enrolled 154,901 participants aged 55 to 74 years from 1993 to 2001.[91] No difference in lung cancer mortality was seen between those randomized to screening with annual chest radiography versus no screening, regardless of the degree of smoking. Together, these studies clearly demonstrate that there is no mortality benefit associated with serial chest radiography as a screening tool.

In the 1990s, intense interest was generated by the results of a number of observational studies evaluating low-dose CT (LDCT) as a lung cancer screening modality. Eventually, a number of RCTs were performed in various sites around the world. The largest of the RCTs was the National Lung Screening Trial (NLST), which included 53,454 subjects, ages 55 to 74 with at least 30 pack-years of cigarette smoking, who were either currently smoking or had quit smoking within the prior 15 years.[92] NLST subjects underwent three rounds of annual screening, randomized to either chest radiograph or LDCT. Approximately 1% of subjects had lung cancer over the duration of the trials. At a median follow-up of 6.5 years, there was a 20% relative reduction in lung cancer mortality observed in the LDCT arm (Fig. 37.6).[92] None of the other RCTs evaluating lung cancer screening with LDCT is of the scale of the NLST; in the trials in which the data has become available, the mortality benefit has been nonsignificant, and without a trend toward a benefit.[93–95] The subjects in all of these studies had smoked and were of middle to older age. A multisociety systematic review of lung cancer screening with LDCT analyzed the evidence from 8 RCTs and 13 prospective cohort studies.[96] This review found a composite significant benefit for LSCT screening, with few ensuing harms, when LDCT screening was conducted in the setting of an organized, structured program. Consistent with this, many organizations (American College of Chest Physicians [ACCP], American Cancer Society, Society of Thoracic Surgeons, American Association of Thoracic Surgery, National Comprehensive Cancer Network [NCCN], US Preventative Services Task Force) have recommended that healthy smokers or former smokers (quit <15 years ago, ≥30 pack years of smoking) age 55 to 74 years or 80 years be considered for LDCT screening.[96–101]

Teasing out further details on who to consider for screening will rely heavily on modeling studies as the effort needed for further RCTs is too great. To explore this, the Cancer Intervention and Surveillance Modeling Network developed five independent models based on a US cohort born in 1950.[102] All five models included dose-response information relating to cigarette exposure; 26 scenarios varying in age, screening frequency, and smoking exposure were modeled with respect to the percentage of cancers detected at an early stage, the number of lung cancer deaths prevented, and life-years gained were balanced against outcome measurements of harm, including the number of CT screenings

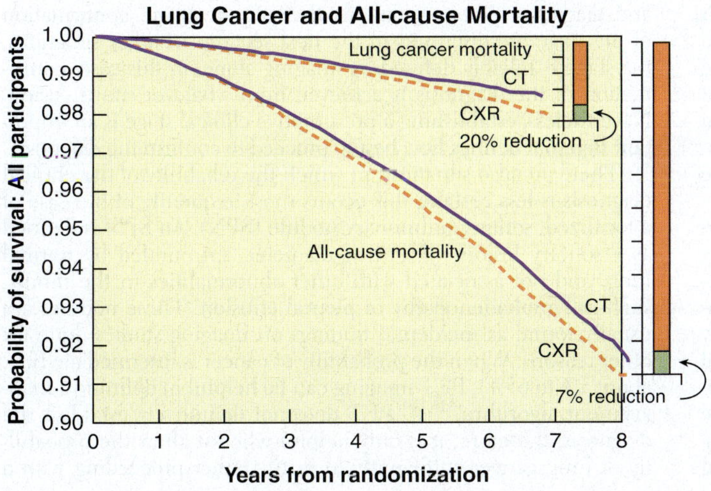

Figure 37.6 Lung cancer mortality and overall mortality reduction by computed tomography (CT) screening in the National Lung Screening Trial. CXR, chest X-ray. Data taken from Aberle D, Adams A, Berg C, et al. Reduced lung-cancer mortality with low-dose computed tomographic screening. *N Eng J Med* 2011;365:395–409.

required, the number of follow-up imaging exams, the number of overdiagnosed lung cancers, and radiation-related lung cancer deaths. Based on the models, a range of different screening scenarios are arguably valid, with different balances of benefits and harms, with the most efficient screening projected in a population similar to the NLST. On the basis of the Cancer Intervention and Surveillance Modeling Network analysis, the US Preventative Services Task Force now recommends "annual screening for lung cancer with low-dose computed tomography in adults ages 55 to 80 years who have a 30 pack-year smoking history and currently smoke or have quit within the past 15 years."[101]

There are potential downsides to screening with LDCT that must be considered in the decision to pursue screening for any population or for a given patient. The most obvious of these is the high rate (20% to 50%) of finding small nodules, which are benign and inconsequential in about 97%.[96] These findings can create unnecessary anxiety, lead to further more intense imaging with significant radiation exposure, and sometimes invasive biopsies with potential complications. In the highly organized LDCT screening studies, only 1.2% to 5.6% of subjects underwent a surgical biopsy or procedure, about 25% of these were for what turned out to be benign nodules.[97] Finally, it is clear that screening detects a higher proportion of slow-growing, less aggressive cancer, some of which may even be inconsequential.[103,104] Appropriate management of these issues that are inextricably linked to screening is essential in order to minimize harms and achieve the greatest benefits.

The complexities of the identification of the "right" population or individuals to screen, combined with the potential harms associated with LDCT screening, argue strongly that screening for lung cancer is a multifaceted process, involving much more than the simple ordering of a scan. The process for most individuals should include an individualized risk assessment for lung cancer[29,105–108]; a discussion about the potential harms of screening, including false-positive results; the potential for cumulative diagnostic radiation; and the possibility of invasive evaluation to diagnose nonmalignant disease. Smoking cessation intervention should be an integral part of this process for individuals still smoking or at risk for relapse. This process should be performed in a multidisciplinary setting. There is data to suggest that if lung cancer screening is done in an unstructured way, the ratio of benefits to harms may be significantly altered. Because implementation of lung screening is just beginning, careful consideration and monitoring is needed to see if the benefit seen in the NLST can be achieved with broader application.

DIAGNOSIS

Clinical Presentation

Approximately a quarter of patients with lung cancer are diagnosed at early stage. These patients are typically free of symptoms; their cancers are identified incidentally during evaluation of unrelated issues. While the proportion of asymptomatic early stage lung cancers may increase with the implementation of screening, at present more than half of patients have advanced lung cancer at the time of diagnosis. These patients typically come to attention because of symptoms related to the primary tumor, metastasis to distant sites, or paraneoplastic syndromes.[109]

The most common pulmonary symptoms are cough, hemoptysis, and dyspnea.[109] Cough may represent the effects of the primary tumor on the airways, with endobronchial or extrinsic airway obstruction, postobstructive atelectasis or infection, or airway inflammation with secretions. Hemoptysis may also result from airway inflammation or necrosis, but may also be related to parenchymal tumor necrosis and cavitation. Dyspnea may arise from a wide variety of tumor-related issues, including mechanical compromise of the airways, lymphangitic spread, pleural effusion, hypercoagulability with pulmonary thromboembolism, or even pericardial effusion. Direct extension of the primary tumor to adjacent structures may cause pain from invasion of the chest wall or brachial plexus, hoarseness from impingement of the recurrent laryngeal nerve, superior vena cava (SVC) syndrome, Horner syndrome (ptosis, miosis, anhidrosis) from invasion of the sympathetic chain and stellate ganglion, or pericardial tamponade.[109]

Symptoms related to metastatic disease may be constitutional or organ related. The most common sites of NSCLC metastases are the brain, bone, liver, adrenals, and lung, though any organ can be affected. Focal neurologic symptoms, persistent headache, bony pain, or unexplained weight loss, anorexia, or fatigue should raise the suspicion for metastatic disease. Likewise, laboratory abnormalities such as anemia, liver function test abnormalities, or hypercalcemia should raise concern for distant spread.[109]

Paraneoplastic syndromes are well described with lung cancer; it is important to recognize that these syndromes are unrelated to metastatic disease and do not preclude curative intent therapy. Hyponatremia related to syndrome of inappropriate secretion of antidiuretic hormone is seen most commonly with SCLC but can occur with other malignant or benign lung processes. Hypercalcemia related to ectopic production of parathyroid hormone–related peptide is more common than hypercalcemia related to bony metastases and is most commonly associated with squamous cell carcinomas. Ectopic corticotrophin (Cushing syndrome) is usually associated with SCLC or early stage carcinoid tumors. Hypertrophic pulmonary osteoarthropathy typically manifests as symmetric and painful arthropathy of the limbs associated with characteristic findings of new periosteal bone formation of the long bones. Neurologic syndromes are less common but include the Lambert-Eaton myasthenic syndrome and encephalomyelitis-subacute sensory neuropathy, both of which are typically associated with SCLC.[109]

Diagnostic Approach

In most patients, an experienced clinician can make a clinical diagnosis of lung cancer with a high degree of reliability (>95%).[110] The main factors that contribute to this are the risk factors for development of lung cancer (e.g., age, smoking history, family history, presence of significant COPD), the clinical presentation, and the radiographic appearance of the lesion on CT (e.g., spiculated, upper lobe, node enlargement). If needed, algorithms are available that can predict the likelihood of lung cancer,[108,112–115] but the judgment of experienced clinicians is just as good.[112]

If the probability of lung cancer is high (e.g., >80%), it is generally more efficient to proceed with evaluation of the stage than confirmation of the diagnosis.[110,116,117] Frequently, this will identify a necessary procedure that will serve both to confirm the stage as well as the diagnosis. For example, biopsy of a potential solitary metastasis or of a suspicious mediastinal node can confirm both the stage and diagnosis. Those situations that require tissue confirmation of the stage are discussed in the next section. In other situations, the stage is reliably defined by imaging alone; in this case, confirmation of the diagnosis is achieved from whatever site is easiest. Nevertheless, establishing a presumptive clinical stage is an important step that defines how best to proceed to confirm the diagnosis.

There are also situations in which the reliability of the clinical diagnosis is less certain; this occurs most frequently in the case of a localized, solitary pulmonary nodule (SPN). An SPN is defined as a solitary lesion <3 cm in diameter, surrounded by normal lung, and not associated with other abnormalities in the thorax, such as lymphadenopathy or pleural effusion. These nodules are usually found as incidental findings on imaging studies done for other reasons. When the probability of cancer is intermediate (i.e., about 5% to 65%), PET imaging can be helpful in defining a management algorithm.[118,119] PET does not definitively establish the diagnosis; therefore, it is only helpful when it alters the probability of lung cancer sufficiently to justify either proceeding with a

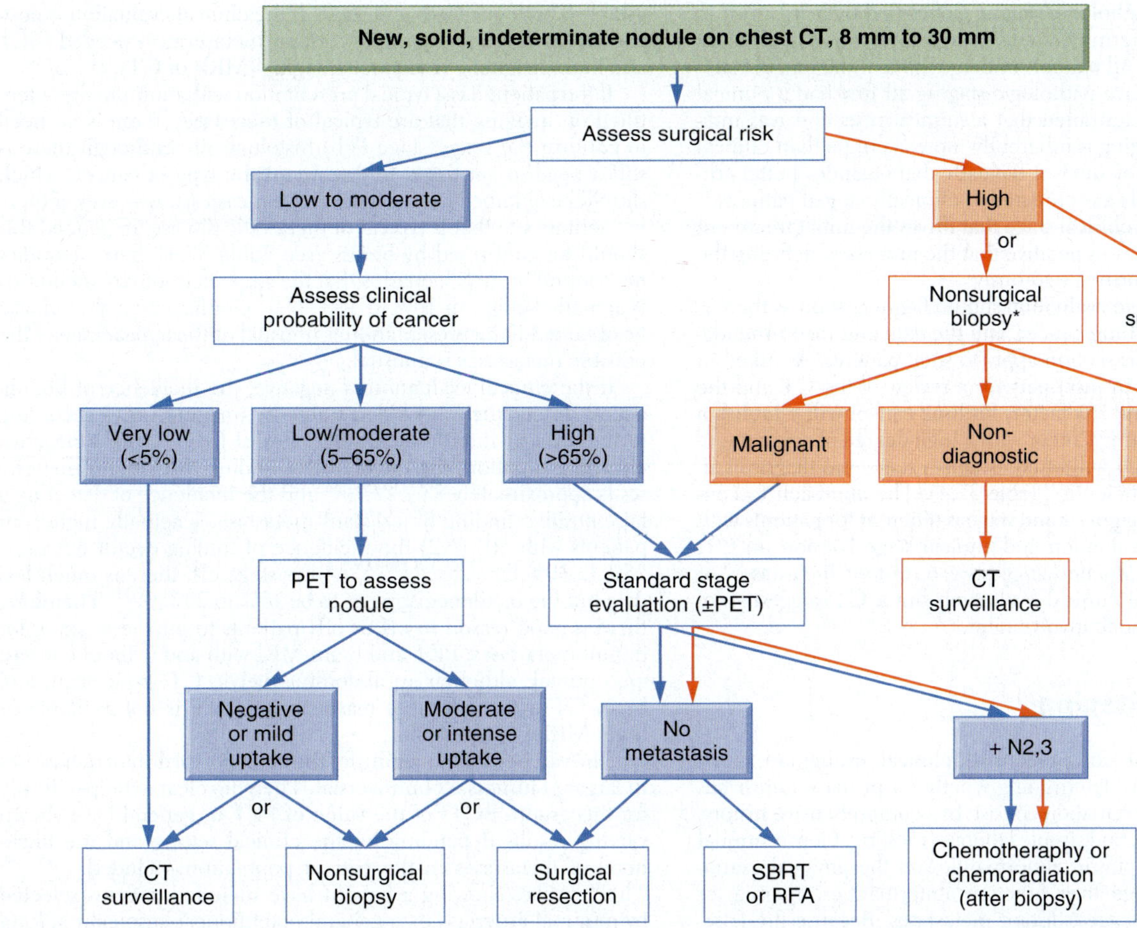

Figure 37.7 Management algorithm for individuals with solid pulmonary nodules 8 to 30 mm in diameter. *Branches* indicate steps in the algorithm following nonsurgical biopsy. *Among individuals at high risk for surgical complications, we recommend either computed tomography (CT) scan surveillance (when the clinical probability of malignancy is low to moderate) or nonsurgical biopsy (when the clinical probability of malignancy is moderate to high). PET, positron emission tomography; SBRT, stereotactic body radiotherapy; RFA, radiofrequency ablation. (Reproduced with permission from the American College of Chest Physicians Lung Cancer Guidelines, Gould MK, Donington J, Lynch W, et al. Evaluation of individuals with pulmonary nodules: when is it lung cancer? *Chest* 2013;143:e93S–120S.)

biopsy or observation. False-positive PET results may occur with any inflammatory or infectious process: tuberculosis, fungal infections, rheumatoid nodules, and sarcoidosis—when such a process is suspected, PET is generally not helpful (it does not differentiate between such a process and cancer). PET also carries a high false-negative rate with ground glass opacities (GGO), carcinoid tumors, or small lesions; in these situations, PET should also generally be avoided. Specifically, the false-negative rate of PET in a GGO is approximately 90%.[118] The false-negative rate in solid lesions <1.5 cm is ~15% and in lesions <1 cm ~30% to 50%.[118] Although the "resolution" of modern PET scanners is ~6 mm, this is a technical and not a clinical term—a lesion must have a diameter of *four times the resolution* in order to detect >90% of the 18-fluorodeoxyglucose activity that is present. This fact also explains why the detected standard uptake value of a lesion falls linearly for lesions smaller than ~2 cm, even if the actual amount of 18-fluorodeoxyglucose activity remains the same.[118,120]

A nonsurgical biopsy can be accomplished by transthoracic needle aspiration (usually guided by CT) or via bronchoscopy. This is most useful when a benign diagnosis is suspected, but this is rather uncommon.[121] In patients with a high suspicion of lung cancer, a biopsy can confirm the diagnosis, but in this situation the false-negative rate of a nonspecific diagnosis is ~20%[116]; therefore, a surgical biopsy should be pursued unless the patient is too high risk.[119] When doing a tissue biopsy, it is crucial to obtain enough tissue for histologic and molecular characterization.[116]

To summarize, PET is most useful when there is an intermediate probability of lung cancer; PET should not be used for lesions that are <1 cm or for a GGO. A biopsy can be important in certain instances when there is doubt about the diagnosis. With a high probability of cancer, it is best to complete the stage evaluation and obtain tissue in a manner that is suited to confirm the stage as well. A detailed management approach for SPN is available for the ACCP lung cancer guidelines, as summarized in Fig. 37.7.[119]

STAGE EVALUATION

General Approach

Staging is a critical aspect of the evaluation of all patients known or suspected of having lung cancer. Clinical stage (identified by a "c" prior to the stage group) is determined by all information available before any definitive treatment. This may involve merely a simple history and physical examination, may include imaging studies, or may involve invasive biopsies or surgical procedures with sampling the primary tumor, intrathoracic lymph nodes, pleural fluid, or extrathoracic sites. Pathologic staging (identified by a "p" prior to the stage group) is determined only if surgical resection with intent to cure is performed. All patients undergo clinical staging; the subset of patients who have pathologic staging all first had a clinical stage defined that determined that a surgical resection was indicated. Pathologic staging is inherently more accurate than clinical staging; comparison of survival typically demonstrates better survival for pathologically as compared to clinically staged patients.[52] Nonetheless, it is the clinical stage that drives the initial treatment decisions, and thus it is imperative that the process of defining the clinical stage be performed rigorously.

The process of stage evaluation should begin as soon as there is a strong suspicion of lung cancer, and the data and recommendations in the rest of this section apply to such patients. As noted in the previous section, in most patients a review of the CT and the patient's symptoms and risk factors for lung cancer will establish a clinical diagnosis of lung cancer with a high degree of accuracy.[110] A thoughtful approach will often establish stage and diagnosis simultaneously and efficiently (Table 37.4). The approach to confirming the clinical diagnosis and stage is different for patients with a negative clinical evaluation and clinical stage I lesion on CT, a positive clinical evaluation suggestive of distant metastases, or those with a negative clinical evaluation but a CT suggestive of hilar or mediastinal node involvement.[110]

Extrathoracic Staging

As noted, the initial comprehensive clinical evaluation is an important first step in determining whether a primary tumor has spread. The clinical evaluation consists of a comprehensive history, physical examination, and simple laboratory testing. Constitutional symptoms, focal symptoms, abnormalities on the physical examination, or unexplained liver function abnormalities, anemia, or hypercalcemia may suggest distant metastases. Because the false-positive rate of this evaluation is around 50%, this suspicion must be confirmed. If the clinical evaluation points strongly to a particular site, further imaging or biopsy should be targeted to the observed abnormalities. For example, needle aspiration of enlarged supraclavicular nodes identified on physical examination may efficiently establish both diagnosis and stage. If the clinical evaluation is positive but less focal, imaging for distant metastases is needed (PET and brain magnetic resonance imaging [MRI] or CT).[122]

If the patient has a typical presentation with multiple sites identified on imaging that are typical of metastases, there is no need to confirm the stage (stage IVb) histologically (although there is still a need to get tissue to document the type of cancer, which should be obtained from whatever site is easiest). However, if there is a solitary site that is typical of metastatic disease, in general this should be confirmed by biopsy (see Table 37.4). Several studies have found in such scenarios that the suspected solitary metastasis is actually benign in 10% to 50%.[123,124] Confirmation should also be obtained if the presentation is unusual or the appearance of the possible metastases is unusual.

If the clinical evaluation is negative, the incidence of finding occult distant metastases detectable by imaging varies according to the clinical intrathoracic stage. For cI by CT with a negative clinical evaluation, the incidence of finding true distant metastases is approximately 5%,[110,124–132] and the incidence of detecting a false-positive finding of a distant metastasis is actually higher. In patients with cIII (N2) the incidence of finding occult disease is 25% to 30%.[110,125,127,128,130,133–136] For stage cII, there is much less data but the incidence appears to be 15% to 20%.[110,128] Therefore, there is good reason in cII or cIII patients to pursue imaging for distant metastases: PET and brain MRI with and without contrast are optimal, although an abdominal/pelvic CT, bone scan, and brain CT with contrast is reasonable if PET is not available or brain MRI is not possible.

The value of PET imaging for the detection of distant metastases in larger cI tumors is controversial. There no clear data specifically for this group. RCTs of the value of PET in general have shown varying results depending on the clinical setting and the likelihood of metastases in the patient population included.[131,137–140] Those studies showing a benefit have included patients selected by minimal criteria (i.e., a general practitioner's suspicion of lung cancer based on a chest X-ray alone) or patients with clinical findings suggestive of metastases and little conventional imaging,[138,139] whereas those that have found no difference involved patients that had a low suspicion of metastases based on the clinical evaluation by a lung cancer specialist and who had already undergone

TABLE 37.4

Approach Diagnosis and Staging of Patients with Probable Lung Cancer

Clinical Scenario	Result of Clinical Evaluation	Confirmation of Extrathoracic Stage	Confirmation of Intrathoracic Stage	Confirmation of Diagnosis
NSCLC				
Peripheral cI	Neg (FN 5%)	Not needed	CT alone (FN <10%)	Surgical resection
cII, central cI	Neg (FN 5%–15%)[a]	PET	Mediastinoscopy vs. EBUS[b]	Surgical resection
cIII, discrete N2,3 enlargement	Neg (FN 30%)	PET, brain MRI	EBUS vs. mediastinoscopy[b]	Mediastinal node biopsy
cIII, diffuse infiltration	Neg (FN 30%)	PET, brain MRI	CT alone is sufficient	Easiest site[c]
cIV	Pos (FP 50%)	PET, brain MRI	not needed	Easiest site if multiple typical metastases[c] Biopsy of suspected site if solitary potential metastasis
SCLC				
Any	Any	PET, brain MRI	CT	Easiest site[c]

NSCLC, Non-small cell lung cancer; cI, clinical stage I; Neg, negative; FN, false negative; CT, computed tomography; cII, clinical stage II; PET, positron emission tomography; EBUS, endobronchial ultrasound; cIII, clinical stage III; MRI, magnetic resonance imaging; cIV, clinical stage IV; Pos, positive; FP, false positive; SCLC, small-cell lung cancer;

[a] Rate not specifically defined for stage II (defined for stage I and II combined). FN rate may be up to 15%.

[b] Fine needle aspiration carries FN rate of about 30% in most series.

[c] For example, sputum, bronchoscopy, fine needle aspiration of supraclavicular node, transthoracic needle aspiration.

conventional imaging.[131,137] The ACCP and NCCN guidelines are relatively generic in recommending PET in essentially all patients with a suspected or diagnosed lung cancer, without accounting for details of the clinical stage before PET or the clinical setting (only cIa and GGO lesions are excluded from the PET recommendation by the ACCP).[110,141]

Mediastinal Staging

If there are no distant metastases, the status of the mediastinal nodes becomes critical in determining the right treatment strategy. Much information is already available from the CT scan. However, while there are situations in which it is reliable, there are also many in which it is notoriously unreliable. One can distinguish four groups of patients based on the CT findings: (A) tumors with mediastinal infiltration, meaning that discrete lymph nodes can no longer be distinguished or measured; (B) tumors with enlargement of discrete mediastinal node(s) (≥1 cm in short axis diameter on an axial image); (C) normal mediastinal nodes but either N1 node enlargement or a central (hilar) tumor; and (D) peripheral tumors with no evidence of N1 or N2,3 node enlargement.[110]

In group A, clinical experience shows the false-positive rate is essentially 0; thus, invasive biopsy is not needed to confirm mediastinal involvement (Fig. 37.8). The rate of a false positive of discrete node enlargement in category B is ~40%, making invasive staging necessary. For central tumors (category C), the false-negative rate of the lack of N2,3 enlargement is ~25%, again making invasive biopsy important. In category D (peripheral tumor with no N1-3 enlargement), the false-negative rate of CT is ~10% (<10% for T1 and ~12% for T2); thus, many feel that invasive confirmation of a lack of N2,3 involvement is not needed (especially if PET is also negative; see the following), whereas some feel this rate is high enough to justify invasive biopsy.[110]

PET scanning adds information, but does not alter the indications for invasive staging significantly.[110] A positive PET in an enlarged node (group B) carries a 15% to 20% false-positive rate, whereas a negative PET in an enlarged node carries a 20% false-negative rate, making invasive biopsy necessary either way.[110] For central tumors (group C), a negative PET still has a 20% false-negative rate, and a positive PET in the mediastinum has a 20% chance of being a false positive. For a peripheral tumor with no node enlargement, a negative PET has a false-negative rate of ~3% (but a positive PET may be false positive). This data makes it clear that in groups A and D imaging can generally be considered adequate, but in groups B and C invasive biopsy is needed regardless of the PET results (unless compelling data for distant metastases is present).[110]

There are multiple techniques to invasively confirm the presence or absence of N2,3 involvement. These include traditional mediastinoscopy, video-mediastinoscopy, so-called super mediastinoscopies that involve a complete mediastinal lymphadenectomy performed as an outpatient via a cervical incision, endobronchial ultrasound (EBUS) and needle aspiration, esophageal ultrasound and needle aspiration, simple "blind" transbronchial needle aspiration, video-assisted thoracic surgery (VATS), and rarely CT-guided transthoracic needle aspiration. There are differences in which nodes are accessible, whether these procedures are applicable to multiple node sampling, and how feasible they are for sampling normal sized versus enlarged nodes (Table 37.5). The technique and thoroughness of how the procedure is done probably has a major impact on the reliability of the results.[110,142]

The choice of which invasive staging technique to use is probably best tailored to specifics of the institution and the patient. In trained hands, all can be performed with low morbidity and mortality. There is RCT data to suggest that if good quality EBUS is available, this may be the best first step in most patients.[110,143] However, the institutional availability of expertise is an important factor. In many reports, the false-negative rate of EBUS has been ~20%, although in expert hands this appears to be lower (particularly if lymphocytes are obtained). Similarly, a video-assisted lymphadenectomy via mediastinoscopy has a false-negative rate of ~2%, but is not available in most institutions. What is critical is an interest in thorough staging and experience with at least some of the various techniques available.

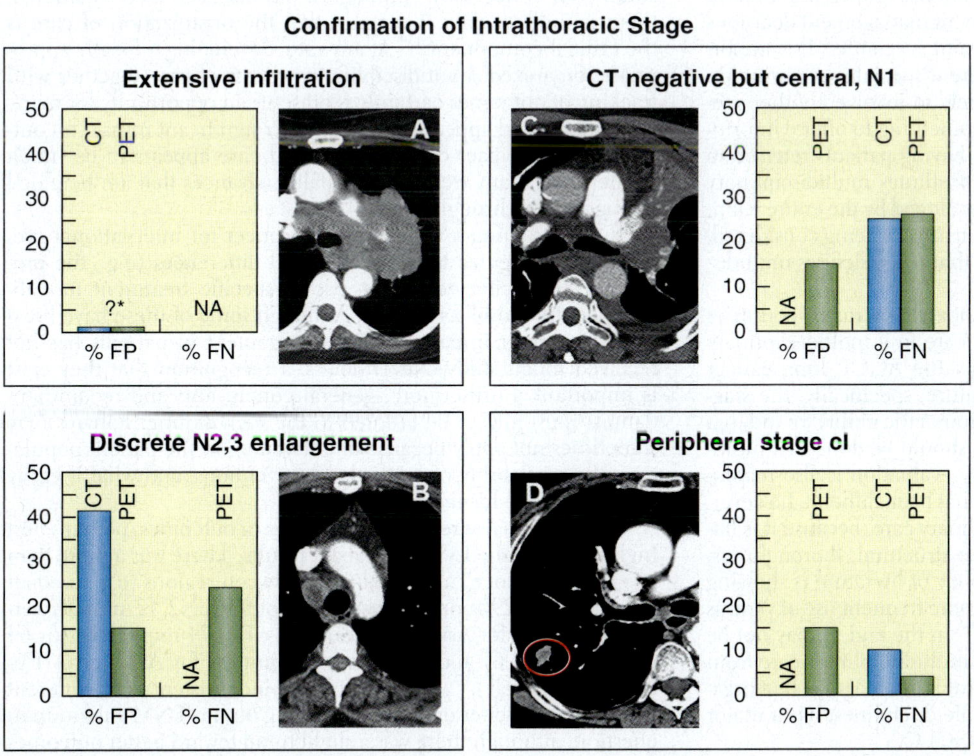

Figure 37.8 False-positive and false-negative rates for computed tomography (CT) and positron emission tomography (PET) assessment of mediastinal nodes by the American College of Chest Physicians intrathoracic radiographic (CT) classification categories. ?*, estimated, no actual data available; NA, not applicable; % FP, percent of positive test results that are false positive (= 100 − positive predictive value%); % FN, percent of negative test results that are false negative (= 100 − negative predictive value %). (Reproduced with permission from the American College of Chest Physicians Lung Cancer Guidelines, Silvestri GA, Gonazalez AV, Jantz M, et al. Methods of staging for non-small cell lung cancer: diagnosis and management of lung cancer, 3rd ed: American College of Chest Physicians evidence-based clinical practice guidelines. *Chest* 2013; 143:e211S–e250S.)

TABLE 37.5

Accessibility of Node Stations to Various Invasive Mediastinal Staging Techniques

Invasive Mediastinal Staging Technique	Accessible Lymph Node Stations
Traditional Mediastinoscopy	1, 2R, 2L, 3, 4R, 4L, anterior 7
Videomediastinoscopy	1, 2R, 2L, 3, 4R, 4L, 5, 7, 8, 10R
Anterior mediastinotomy (Chamberlain)	5, 6
Video-assisted thoracic surgery	Right-sided: R2, R4, 7, 10, 11
	Left-sided: L2, L4, 5, 6, 7, 10, 11
Transthoracic needle aspiration or biopsy	Variable; restricted to enlarged nodes
Transbronchial needle aspiration	2R, 2L, 3, 4R, 4L, 7, 10, 11
Endoscopic ultrasound with needle aspiration	4L, 5, 7, 8, 9
Endobronchial ultrasound with needle aspiration	2R, 2L, 3, 4R, 4L, 7, 10, 11, 12

MANAGEMENT BY STAGE

Overview of Lung Cancer Treatment Modalities

Structural Aspects of Patient Care

The field of lung cancer has grown to encompass a huge body of knowledge, more than what any one person can stay abreast of. Furthermore, it has become complex, with many different specialties that contribute to the evaluation and management of the patient. This makes it important to provide care in a multidisciplinary manner. The key aspect is to have a system of care delivery that is developed together with all relevant disciplines, and to have a forum for discussion so that major patient management decisions can be made with involvement of relevant specialties. It is important to provide an opportunity for different specialties to bring up points that one is unaware of, not merely to involve another specialty when one knows that they have something to offer. Unfortunately, many people think that simply having patients referred to another specialty from time to time constitutes multidisciplinary care; however, it is the system of care developed by the entire team, the ability to introduce salient points that are not being considered, and the collaborative decision making that really defines multidisciplinary care.

It is recommended and even mandated in many countries that patients with lung cancer receive care in a multidisciplinary fashion.[109,144] This is recommended by the ACCP lung cancer guidelines, based on a review of literature; specifically, the staging evaluation, the physiologic evaluation of the ability to undergo treatment, and the treatment planning should be done in a multidisciplinary setting.[144] Multidisciplinary evaluation is also recommended by the NCCN guidelines.[141] It has been difficult, however, to quantitate the impact of multidisciplinary care, because it is difficult to separate this aspect from other structural, thoroughness, and quality of care issues. A growing body of literature is showing benefits in terms of timeliness of care, more frequent use of various treatment modalities, and survival.[109,144] In the end, it may not be important to disentangle the impact of multidisciplinary care from other quality of care issues. The key point is to recognize that organization of care, which involves multiple disciplines, has a major impact on outcomes of patients with NSCLC.

There is extensive data that the care for a large proportion of patients with lung cancer is suboptimal. A study of the US National Cancer Database revealed that the proportion of patients with NSCLC and *no comorbidities* that received suboptimal care (defined as deviating from guidelines that were in place at the time) was approximately 33% for stage I, 40% for stage II, 46% for stage III, and 47% for stage IV.[145] Other studies show that there are major regional differences (more than three-fold) in the United States in the frequency of use of different treatment modalities, implying that these are not related to patient factors or what is appropriate, but likely related to regional differences in the quality of care delivery.[146,147] Several studies have shown that despite the existence of clinical guidelines for many years recommending careful mediastinal staging with biopsy confirmation, the large majority of patients are staged using CT alone (which is notoriously inaccurate).[148–150] Furthermore, such limited clinical staging was associated with dramatically worse outcomes, stage for stage (adjusted hazard ratio [HR] for death of ~1.7 to 2.3 for overall and cancer-specific survival).[148]

There is extensive evidence that structural aspects of care (e.g., case volume, specialization) have a marked effect on outcomes.[151,152] A comprehensive literature review on effect of volume/specialization in quality of cancer care concluded that "An extensive, consistent literature that supports a volume-outcome relationship was found for cancers treated with technologically-complex surgical procedures. . . . Across studies, the benefit from care at high-volume centers exceeds the benefits from breakthrough treatments."[153] In lung cancer, most of these studies have focused on surgical treatment. With very few exceptions, these studies have found lower perioperative mortality and better long-term survival in high-volume versus low-volume centers, teaching versus nonteaching facilities, and when treatment is delivered by thoracic versus general surgeons (Fig. 37.9).[151,152]

However, the relationship between volume and outcomes is not consistent on an individual institution level; there are low-volume institutions with excellent outcomes and vice versa. This suggests that volume is only a marker for other aspects of care. It is possible that low-volume centers have less availability of expertise or cutting-edge treatment interventions. However, it is much more likely that it is a marker for how organized the care delivery is. In most high-volume institutions, care will become more organized simply out of necessity. Although it has not been directly studied, there is indirect data to support that the organization of care is the critical component.[154] At any rate, developing a locally appropriate, organized, multidisciplinary process of care together with tracking of outcomes certainly represents an opportunity for many institutions, and appears likely to have a significant impact on outcomes. The impact of such organized care appears to be much greater than many treatment modality advances that are heralded as major breakthroughs.[148,155,156]

In constructing a review of lung cancer for international use, one must recognize there are regional differences (e.g., the proportion of specific cell types, use of specific treatment modalities, penetration of screening). Although some of these have been identified, their impact on the management of patients has not received much study. Nevertheless, a recognition that they exist is important. Furthermore, general conclusions and recommendations must always be tailored to the local setting. Policies may sometimes not apply because of differences in the patient population, the availability of particular interventions, and what is easily accepted in the local culture.

There are major regional differences in outcomes, perhaps best highlighted by the IASLC database results. There was a more than two-fold difference in survival rates between regions (e.g., median survival cN0 29 months versus 70 months; cN2 12 months versus 20 months for Asia versus Europe; cT1a 74 months versus 64 months, cT1b 67 months versus 46 months for Asia versus Europe, respectively).[157] The results were inconsistent, with different regions being better or worse depending on the TNM subgroup in question, although there was a slight trend toward better outcomes

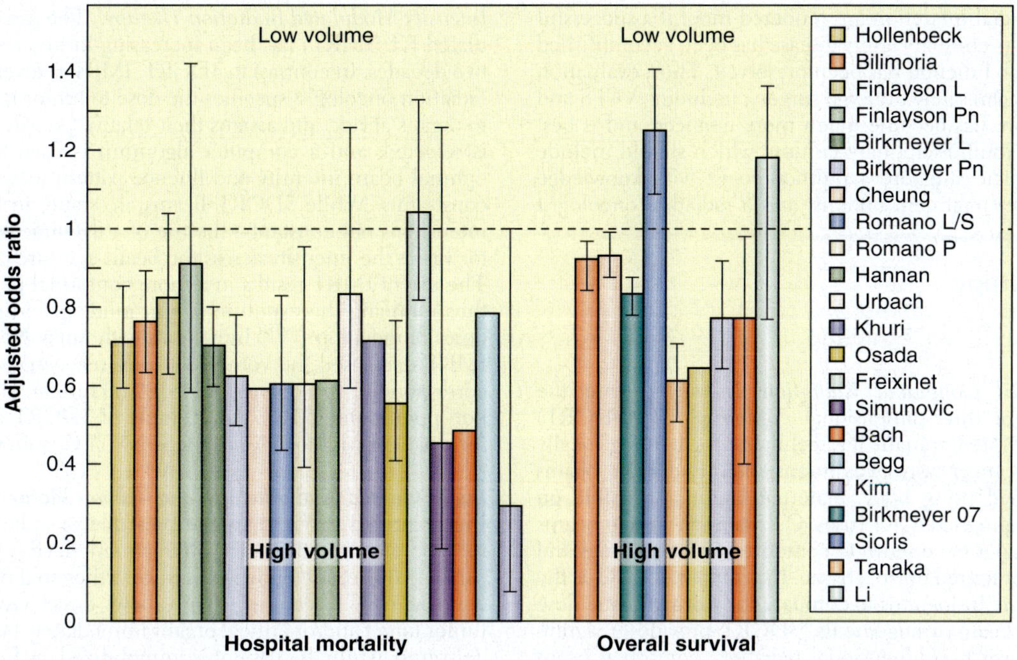

Figure 37.9 Surgical outcomes according to case volume. Perioperative mortality and long-term survival according to institutional case volume of patients undergoing surgical resection for lung cancer. (Data taken from Howington J, Blum M, Chang A, et al. Treatment of stage I and II non-small cell lung cancer: Diagnosis and management of lung cancer, 3rd ed: American College of Chest Physicians evidence-based clinical practice guidelines. *Chest* 2013;143:e278S–313S.)

in Asia.[158] It is not clear what the reasons for these differences are. It is well known that the incidence of EGFR mutation is higher in the Asian lung cancer population. There are differences in the proportion of subtypes of NSCLC. There are societal differences regarding how aggressive and which treatment modalities are generally accepted. There are differences in the availability of various technologies and treatment methods (e.g., EBUS, PET, VATS, four-dimensional RT, stereotactic body RT [SBRT], genetic testing). The impact of these differences is not clear, but it does emphasize that general recommendations need to be thoughtfully considered in light of differences as compared with the population and setting in which the data was derived.

Surgery

There have been major advances in surgical treatment of lung cancer in the past two decades, just as there have been in RT and chemotherapy. Most prominent is perhaps the use of minimally invasive resection (VATS), which makes a lung cancer resection a very different experience for the patient. The perioperative morbidity is cut in half, the hospital stay reduced to 3 to 4 days in the United States, and the return to normal functioning is dramatically quicker. This is well documented in several meta-analyses,[159–165] large-scale outcomes studies,[166–170] propensity matched studies,[168,171–182] and small randomized studies.[183–185]

While the data makes VATS the recommended treatment in the ACCP lung cancer guidelines,[151] it is used variably in different centers. Those that have embraced it perform about 80% of resections by VATS, but there remain many institutions that are not comfortable and use VATS relatively sparingly. It is likely this will change, given the amount of data supporting the VATS approach. Furthermore, robotic-assisted thoracic surgery is now being practiced at some centers. It is clear this is also a safe and effective approach. Whether there are benefits for the patient with respect to perioperative or long-term outcomes for robotic versus VATS resections is unclear.

Even open thoracotomy has changed. Smaller, muscle-sparing incisions are now commonly used. There are many newer ways of pain management that allow greater patient mobility and avoidance of complications. The management of postoperative air leaks has changed; quantitation using digital devices allows earlier chest tube removal and earlier hospital discharge.[186] Such postoperative management approaches have changed the experience for patients undergoing thoracotomy from what it typically was 20 years ago.

The value of care delivered by dedicated thoracic surgeons, who have a focused interest in noncardiac thoracic surgery and lung cancer in particular, is increasingly recognized. The ACCP lung cancer guidelines recommend that surgical care be delivered by such an individual, on the basis of a review of the literature that demonstrates better outcomes.[151] Intraoperative lymph node staging was previously often spotty; there is now a much better appreciation for the necessity to do this for both the surgeon and pathologist, and acceptance of substandard intraoperative staging is diminishing.[151]

There has also been a major advance in the ability to safely carry out extensive resections, for example involving cancers invading the thoracic inlet, vertebral column, and SVC. This makes it feasible to consider surgery as part of the treatment approach for tumors that appear to be only locally invasive. In the past, many of these tumors were simply considered unresectable; however, the modern techniques and ways of reducing morbidity make surgery a reasonable option.

The advances in surgical therapy have changed patient selection for surgery. The improved perioperative outcomes allow older and more frail patients to undergo surgery (e.g., a VATS resection or a segmentectomy).[151,166,187] Patient selection is also altered by the recognition that previous criteria had been very conservative. These had primarily defined thresholds above which there was little concern; however, they ignored the fact that risk is a continuous variable and that many patients below previous thresholds could undergo resection with quite acceptable low risk of perioperative mortality. Other previous contraindications for surgery such as a history of myocardial infarction are rendered moot if a successful intervention for the coronary artery disease has been accomplished and overall cardiac function has been preserved. Thus, evaluation of which patients can safely undergo surgery, including VATS and sublobar resection, has become much more nuanced and is best approached in a multidisciplinary fashion, which should include a dedicated thoracic surgeon, a pulmonologist with knowledge about lung cancer treatment options, and a radiation oncologist as well.

Radiation Therapy

Advances in Radiation Technique

Three-Dimensional Conformal Radiation Therapy. Before the widespread use of three-dimensional conformal RT (3DCRT) in the 1990s, the predominant RT technique for treating locally advanced lung cancer was two-dimensional. Radiation beams would be designed using bony anatomic landmarks visible on fluoroscopic imaging. 3DCRT uses CT datasets, using beams from multiple angles to conform to contoured target volumes and similarly avoid contoured normal tissue. Inherent in 3DCRT is the use of dose-volume histograms to compare the normal tissue dose among different beam arrangements. 3DCRT provides a significant advantage over two-dimensional radiation: conformal beam design and the ability to manipulate beam geometry and weighting through the planning process improves coverage of the tumor target, and decreases the dose to normal tissue. The use of CT datasets in RT planning also enables the fusion of complementary imaging modalities, such as PET or MRI.

Intensity-Modulated Radiation Therapy. The use of intensity-modulated RT (IMRT) has been increasing in frequency over the past two decades. In contrast to 3DCRT, IMRT is inverse planned. The radiation oncologist specifies the dose to tumor targets, dose limits to organs at risk, and assigns their relative priority. Beam geometry is selected, and a computer algorithm is used to determine the optimal beam intensity and fluence pattern to meet the planning constraints. While 3DCRT beams are static, in IMRT the beam intensity is not constant—the use of a dynamic multileaf collimator varies the intensity across the beam aperture during treatment. The use of IMRT results in a more conformal plan than 3DCRT, thus reducing the exposure of surrounding normal tissue to high doses of radiation.[188,189] In patients with bulky NSCLC, the use of IMRT decreased the volume of lung receiving >20 Gy by 10%, corresponding to a decrease of >10% in the calculated risk of radiation pneumonitis (RP). An example of 3DCRT and IMRT plans for a patient with locally advanced NSCLC is shown in Fig. 37.10.

Image-Guided Radiotherapy and Tumor Motion Considerations. Image-guided RT implies the presence of radiographic imaging incorporated into the radiation treatment device. Commonly used imaging devices include kilovoltage orthogonal planar imaging or cone-beam CT scanning. This allows direct visualization of the tumor target and/or critical organs immediately before treatment is delivered, while the patient is immobilized, as frequently as every treatment fraction. The use of image-guided RT allows the reduction of the expansion margin around the clinical target volume, since interfraction variations in patient positioning are reduced.[190] This can, in turn, reduce the exposure of the surrounding normal lung tissue.

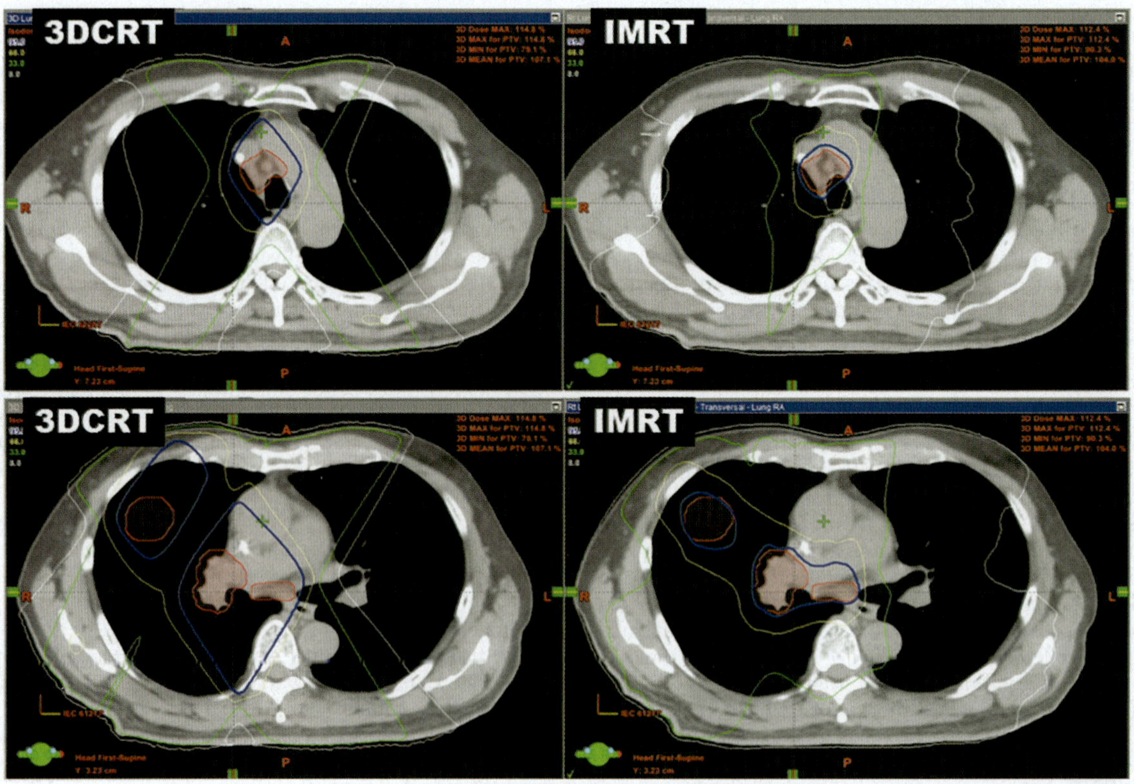

Figure 37.10. Radiation treatment plans: Comparison of two methods. A 64-year-old former smoker presented with stage IIIA non–small-cell lung cancer, with disease in the right lower lobe, hilum, and mediastinal station R4. Concurrent chemoradiation was recommended. Radiation plans were generated using three-dimensional conformal radiotherapy (3DCRT) and intensity-modulated radiotherapy (IMRT). Representative axial slices from the two plans are shown: the *top panels* compare 3DCRT (*left*) to IMRT (*right*) at the level of the aortic arch, the *bottom panels* are similarly presented for an axial level below the carina. The planning target volume is shown in *red*, isodose lines are demonstrated for 60 Gy (*dark blue*), 40 Gy (*yellow*), 20 Gy (*green*) and 5 Gy (*white*). The use of IMRT decreased the mean lung dose (16 Gy versus 13 Gy) and V20 (32% versus 23%), but increased the volume of lung receiving 5 Gy. The esophageal dose was also lower with IMRT; V30 was reduced from 41% to 23%.

A large component of the expansion margin for lung cancer is designed to allow for positional uncertainty of the tumor that corresponds with the respiratory excursion of the diaphragm. Allowing for intrafraction respiratory motion is a required part of radiation treatment planning for lung cancer, and can be accomplished in several ways. The use of four-dimensional CT scans in treatment planning allows the accurate measurement of tumor motion for an individual patient,[191] and the correlation of tumor position with an external fiducial. After the acquisition of a four-dimensional CT scan, various motion management techniques can be employed: expansion of the intended treatment volume based on the measured motion, gated treatment in which the patient is only treated during a portion of the respiratory cycle, or abdominal compression where the diaphragmatic motion is damped using external compression devices. Tumor tracking, where the radiation aperture follows tumor while it moves, is an area of growing interest.

Proton Therapy. The use of charged particle therapy such as protons is an area of active investigation in lung cancer. Protons have distinct physical characteristics that suggest they can be used to deliver thoracic radiation with a lower risk of side effects, when compared to standard photon therapy. The deposition of proton energy in tissue can be modulated by changing the beam energy, leading to much lower entry doses than photons, and an even more significant in the drop-off of the exit dose. Proton radiation beam arrangements do not need to enter and exit through lung tissue to avoid critical structures such as the spinal cord, which should decrease the risk of RP and radiation fibrosis.[192] Phase 2 trials of fractionated proton therapy with concurrent chemotherapy in locally advanced lung cancer have demonstrated excellent median survival, with relatively low toxicity.[193,194] A large cooperative group randomized trial is ongoing.

Radiation Toxicity. The risk and severity of radiation toxicity are related to the dose and volume of normal tissue that are exposed, to the presence or absence of underlying comorbidities, as well as the functional organization of the particular organ at risk. Emami et al.[195] published a comprehensive review of partial-volume organ tolerances for normal tissue that served for more than a decade as the standard source for radiation dose limits, and risk of toxicity. These parameters were based predominantly on clinical data from older, two-dimensional RT planning. Recently, a large multidisciplinary effort was undertaken, the Quantitative Analysis of Normal Tissue Effects in the Clinic, to summarize the published three-dimensional dose-volume/toxicity data in the literature, review normal tissue complication probability modeling, and provide practical guidance for organ dose limits.[196]

Radiation Pneumonitis and Pulmonary Fibrosis. Clinically significant pneumonitis occurs in somewhere between 5% and 50% of patients receiving definitive fractionated radiation for locally advanced lung cancer, and is often the dose-limiting factor in radiation planning. RP may occur during fractionated treatment or up to 18 months afterward, with a peak incidence at approximately 2 months. The most common clinical presentation is a persistent, nonproductive cough; dyspnea; low-grade fever; and fatigue. Chest X-ray or CT scan may be normal, or depending on the time course there may be GGO (within 2 to 6 months), patchy consolidation (4 to 12 months), or fibrosis (≥10 months). The earliest radiographic changes occur within the medium- to high-dose radiation volumes, though later changes may extend into unirradiated lung. Pulmonary function testing shows reduced lung volumes, tidal volumes, and diffusion capacity. A variety of dose-volume models have been evaluated as predictive metrics of RP, including threshold volumes (i.e., V_{dose}), mean lung dose (MLD), and normal tissue complication probability models. Accumulated data from the Quantitative Analysis of Normal Tissue Effects in the Clinic effort suggest that while there is gradually increasing risk with increasing exposure, with no safe threshold dose below which the risk of RP is zero,[196] the risk of grade 2 or greater RP was <20% when the MLD was held to <20 Gy during conventional radiation fractionation. Commonly used thresholds include a V_{20} <30% to 35%, or V_5 <60%, corresponding to a risk of RP of <20%.

RP occurs less commonly after SBRT in comparison to conventionally fractionated radiation.[197] The risk of symptomatic RP does seem to follow a similar relationship to dose and volume irradiated as seen in conventionally fractionated treatment,[198] though specific dose thresholds are evolving as experience with SBRT grows. Takeda et al.[199] retrospectively examined 265 patients, and with a median follow-up of 19 months the incidence of grade 2 to 5 pneumonitis was 18.5%, 4.5%, 0%, and 0.4%, respectively. Predictors of grade 2 or higher RP on multivariate analysis included V_{20}. A large series from Indiana University examined dosimetric predictors of pneumonitis[200] in a group of 143 patients treated with SBRT. RP (grade 2 to 4) occurred in 9.4% of cases. Pneumonitis was noted in 4.3% of patients with a MLD of ≤4 Gy, compared with 17.6% of patients with MLD of >4 Gy ($p = 0.02$), and in 4.3% of patients with a V_{20} ≤4% compared with 16.4% of patients with V_{20} of ≥4% ($p = 0.03$).

RT-induced dyspnea may have several contributing causes, including not only RP but also RT to other thoracic organs at risk. Emerging evidence suggests an interaction between cardiac dose and RP,[201] and there may be additive dyspnea due to pleural and pericardial effusions, cardiomyopathy, and bronchial stenosis or bronchiectasis. Bronchial fibrosis and stenosis has been reported with radiation dose escalation beyond 70 Gy.[202]

Several patient- and treatment-related factors also impact the risk of RP, independent of dose and volume. In a large dataset derived from patients treated on Radiation Therapy Oncology Group (RTOG) trials, the risk of RP was significantly higher for tumors in the lower lung fields.[203] Older age may increase the risk of RP, and patients who continue to smoke through treatment may be at decreased risk.[196] Several chemotherapy agents that are commonly administered to patients with lung cancer concurrently are associated with an increased risk of RP, including docetaxel, gemcitabine, and particularly the commonly used carboplatin and paclitaxel combination.[204]

Glucocorticoids are commonly used to treat RP in patients who have moderate to severe symptoms, although the efficacy and appropriate starting dose and tapering schedule have not been defined in a prospective fashion. Prophylactic antibiotics or anticoagulants do not appear to effect the development of RP, although they are frequently given. Pulmonary parenchymal fibrosis is the underlying cause of long-term dyspnea after thoracic radiation, likely the result of chronic treatment-induced inflammation. No standard clinical approach has been definitively demonstrated to reverse or even slow the progression of pulmonary fibrosis, though several therapies have shown signs of activity, including pentoxifylline.[205] Amifostine is a radioprotector that has been tested in several randomized trials, with mixed results.[206,207] Captopril is an angiotensin-converting enzyme inhibitor that has been shown to reduce the development of radiation-induced fibrosis in animal models.[208]

Esophagitis and Esophageal Stenosis. Acute esophagitis is typically the dose-limiting side effect during fractionated RT for thoracic malignancies. Grade 3 or greater acute symptoms (i.e., severely altered eating/swallowing, tube feeding, parenteral nutrition, or hospitalization indicated) occurred 18% of the time, in a series of >1,000 patients undergoing chemoradiation.[204] Acute esophagitis may coexist with, and be exacerbated by, comorbid conditions such as candidiasis or reflux disease. Other factors identified as increasing the risk or severity of acute esophagitis include the use of accelerated fractionation and older patient age.[209] The use of concurrent chemotherapy is associated with an increased risk.[210] The use of concurrent bevacizumab with RT has led to case reports of fistulae.[211,212] Clinically significant late toxicity, such as stenosis or fistula formation, is less common after conventionally fractionated radiation, occurring in <5% of patients.[213,214]

Treatment of acute esophagitis is primarily supportive, frequently requiring topical agents, dietary changes, and narcotic pain medication. It is often prudent to either evaluate or treat empirically for viral or candida esophagitis. Patients may benefit from proton pump inhibitors for comorbid reflux disease, and topical agents for mucosal irritation such as sucralfate or local anesthetic agents. The ability of the radioprotectant amifostine to reduce the risk and severity of acute esophagitis has been evaluated in several prospective trials, but no benefit was noted in a large randomized, cooperative group study.[207]

Heart. For thoracic malignancies, the dose and volume of radiation to the heart and great vessels varies considerably, depending upon the anatomic distribution of the target and the treatment technique. The overall excess risk of cardiac mortality after thoracic RT is low,[215] but moderate toxicities have been reported more commonly. Acutely, this can include pericarditis, which can develop during treatment or within several months afterward. Months after radiation, there can be pericardial effusion, and over years progressive fibrosis may rarely lead to constrictive pericarditis. Ischemic changes in the cardiac muscle can manifest with a long latency and may lead clinically to congestive heart failure or ultimately a higher cardiac mortality.[216] Valvular abnormalities have been reported, presumably due to late fibrotic changes. In the great vessels, there can accelerated atherosclerosis that worsens over years to decades, leading to an increased risk of structural damage such as aneurysm. Comorbid clinical conditions may increase the risk of RT-induced cardiac toxicity,[217] including hypertension, diabetes, obesity, and genetic predisposition. The risk of cardiac mortality from RT has been specifically demonstrated to be increased in patients over 60 years old, and by tobacco use.[218,219] There are reports that concurrent paclitaxel may also increase this risk.[220,221]

Brachial Plexus. Radiation brachial plexopathy is a rare but serious complication of fractionated radiation to conventional doses. There are case reports of early, transient neuropathy that may occur during or shortly after radiation, and may resolve spontaneously.[222] Late radiation plexopathy is more clinically significant; it manifests years after radiation to the supraclavicular area and may manifest as hypesthesia, paresthesia, and weakness of the affected arm and shoulder. It may progress to total paralysis of the affected arm, and severe pain. The dose tolerance of the brachial plexus is less defined than other thoracic organs, partly due to the difficulty in defining the plexus radiographically during radiation treatment planning. A contouring atlas has been adopted, so that more robust clinical data can be collected.[223] Late plexopathy is rare in patients who receive conventional doses of fractionated radiation.[224] For SBRT, brachial plexopathy is a more significant concern, because the biologically effective dose prescribed to the target exceeds the tolerance of the plexus.

Chemotherapy

There has been a long evolution in the treatment of NSCLC since the early editions of this textbook. It was not until the late 1980s that the benefits of chemotherapy with respect of overall survival (OS) and QOL versus supportive care were appreciated in patients with advanced disease.[225–227] In the early 1990s, a new generation of chemotherapeutic agents, used in combination with platinum analogs, consolidated the benefits of treatment and established chemotherapy.

In the mid to late 1990s, the combination of chemotherapy and RT in patients with stage III disease showed superior outcomes compared to single modality and created a new paradigm of combined modality therapy, still considered the standard to this date.[225] During the 2000s, chemotherapy was tested in the adjuvant setting and became a new standard of care by improving the cure rates in selected patients with stage IB through IIIA disease.[228] Remarkably, over the course of two decades, or five editions of this textbook, chemotherapy has become an established treatment modality for the majority of patients with NSCLC.

The discovery of somatic mutations in a subset of lung tumors is the most significant paradigm shift in the treatment of lung cancer in the last decade. Since the initial report on EGFR,[229] the understanding that specific molecular alterations serve as oncogenic drivers, and that blockade of these pathways by specific agents can lead to robust and prolonged responses, has revolutionized the approach to patients with lung cancer. This discovery has launched the era of personalized medicine, in which patients are managed based on specific characteristics of their tumors.

The evolution of chemotherapeutic management of NSCLC has ushered in many more fundamental changes in how we think about stage IV NSCLC. At one time, it was questionable whether the treatment was worse than the disease, now this is a vibrant, successful, fast-paced field with new discoveries that challenge the ability to keep pace. There are many effective cytotoxic agents, targeted therapy, and immunotherapy, and which are used in first-, second-, and third-line settings. The treatments can be dramatically effective, and it is no longer surprising when a patient with incurable NSCLC can be successfully managed over many years. We are clearly moving toward management of stage IV NSCLC as a chronic disease.

The management of stage IV NSCLC is complex. It is not merely a question of which drug to use, but which sequence, how to plan the first course of therapy taking into account later options, and when to initiate a new treatment. Treatment is viewed less as a defined course of therapy and more as a continuum over time. The lines between treatment courses are blurred: when does a course of therapy become maintenance, when is maintenance therapy early institution of second-line treatment? More aggressive palliation of specific symptoms or conditions (brain, spine, bone metastases, airway obstruction, etc.) has far-reaching effects, including a better QOL and a more positive attitude, but also a better ability to tolerate active treatment.

The evolution of chemotherapy treatment of NSCLC has led to different end points in clinical trials. OS, once considered a hard end point, has become problematic. Because OS reflects the entire continuum of management and a combination of interventions, it is often difficult to discern what effect a particular portion of the treatment strategy has on OS. Progression-free survival (PFS) has become more prominent as it can assess a specific portion of the continuum of treatment. However, it is controversial whether and under what circumstances it is an appropriate measure.[230] More subtle measures such as toxicity and QOL are also used as primary end points. Thus, end points of clinical research have become more difficult to measure and attribute to a particular intervention. At the same time, the standards of what is considered clinically relevant and sufficient to call a trial positive has decreased.[231] The combination of these trends raises issues for clinical research moving forward.

The treatment has become much more specific; having evolved from a one-size-fits-all NSCLC approach to being histology based, and even more specifically directed to small cohorts identified by particular genetic mutations. These markers have an impact not only on response but also on susceptibility to toxicity in some cases. This radically changes the economics of treatment, research, and drug development. The specific cohorts are smaller and more difficult to identify. The need to screen a larger population to identify a few individuals can be costly and inefficient. Cost is determined not just by the cost of therapy but also cost of and ability to find the right cohort.[232–234] The dramatic response that can be seen with such targeted therapy can lead to approval of a therapy based on nonrandomized data alone, reducing the costs of drug development. However, the more limited cohort for whom it is applicable also limits the potential return. The pace of new discoveries in specific tumor subgroups creates challenges in how to conduct appropriate clinical research in a timely enough manner. New approaches to trial design, such as an adaptive Bayesian structure, may offer innovative, more flexible options than the traditional phase 1, 2, and 3 research schema.[235] There are many forces in play in the dynamic, rapidly changing field.

Preinvasive and Minimally Invasive Disease (Bronchial Intraepithelial Neoplasia, Adenocarcinoma in Situ, Ground Glass Nodules)

Bronchial intraepithelial neoplasia appears to be a precursor to central airway squamous cell carcinomas. These lesions are infrequently encountered, usually in patients with abnormal sputum cytology or during surveillance of the central airways. Although techniques have been developed (autofluorescence bronchoscopy, narrow-band imaging) that are more sensitive in detecting such lesions, it is unclear how these should be implemented.[236] Among high-risk patients who participated in a screening program, about 30% of high-grade dysplasia and 50% of carcinoma in situ lesions were observed to progress; however, the rates were highly variable among studies (with follow-up periods of ~1 to 10 years).[236] A substantial proportion of lesions regresses during follow-up. One of the problems is that there is moderate interobserver variability in the classification of such biopsies. Photodynamic therapy seems to be fairly effective at treating lesions deemed worthy of intervention, but it is not well established which lesions need intervention, as many do not progress.[236]

In 2011, a new subclassification of adenocarcinoma was introduced, covering a spectrum from atypical adenomatous hyperplasia (AAH), adenocarcinoma in situ (AIS), minimally invasive adenocarcinoma (MIA), lepidic predominant adenocarcinoma, and various types of invasive adenocarcinoma (acinar, papillary, micropapillary, etc.).[63] Although not conclusively established, this carries the implication that the earlier lesions (e.g., AAH, AIS) may be precursors to invasive adenocarcinoma. It must be emphasized that these entities can only be classified after resection (not on the basis of a limited biopsy).[63] However, there is a strong correlation between the histologic classification and the radiographic appearance, although this has not been quantitatively defined. AAH and AIS lesions generally appear as pure ground glass nodules (GGN) on CT, and MIA and lepidic predominant adenocarcinoma are often part-solid GGNs, while other types of adenocarcinoma are generally mostly solid-appearing lesions on CT. The increased use of CT has led to more frequent recognition of these lesions and creates a need to define how to manage them.

Pure GGNs are focal lesions seen incidentally on a chest CT; this is distinct from more diffuse or patchy ground glass appearance of the lung, which generally signifies benign interstitial or inflammatory lung disease. A number of studies have reported outcomes of such lesions during a period of observation of 1 to 3 years.[237] It is difficult to be precise because of slight differences in definitions and inclusion criteria and duration of follow-up. Approximately 10% to 20% of pure GGNs disappear, usually within 3 months. About 10% decrease in size, but it should be noted that approximately 20% of adenocarcinomas that were eventually resected after a period of observation were observed to have decreased in size.[237] Most remain stable, around 20% increase in size, and ~10% (range, 0% to 30%) develop a solid component.[237]

Other papers have focused on diagnoses made during observation of a GGN, which may skew the data toward the more suspicious lesions that motivated intervention. These studies have found that approximately 75% of pure GGNs are benign (and still followed), ~10% are AAH, 10% to 20% are BAC, and ~5% are adenocarcinoma.[237] It is hard to translate the older terms BAC and adenocarcinoma used in these studies into the new subclassification of adenocarcinoma. Among studies that focused on lesions that were actually resected, ~30% of pure GGNs were benign (including AAH), the majority was BAC, and ~10% were diagnosed as adenocarcinoma. The incidence of adenocarcinoma was <5% in pure GGNs <10 mm in size, and ~25% if >10 mm.[237]

The rate of invasive cancer is substantially higher in part-solid GGNs (although these are by definition still >50% ground glass). A diagnosis of adenocarcinoma is made in ~10% during a period of observation. Of those coming to actual resection, ~30% are adenocarcinoma and most of the rest were classified as BAC; ~10% were adenocarcinoma among part-solid GGN <10 mm versus ~40% if >10 mm.[237]

Triggers for intervention are still evolving. There is a growing impression that pure GGNs may be simply observed, while a part-solid GGN usually warrants intervention, especially if the solid component has recently developed. The rate of growth should also be factored in—a lesion that has grown 2 mm in 5 years may not warrant intervention. Significant growth over the course of a year or development of a solid component should generally trigger resection.[119,237,238] Exact definition of recommendations and specific documentation of results is hampered by the short periods of follow-up in studies so far, the loose correlation between radiographic appearance and histologic results, the inability to establish a diagnosis of a preinvasive lesion before resection, and the uncertainty about the malignant potential of AAH, AIS, MIA, and even lepidic predominant adenocarcinoma.

Multiple studies suggest that a limited resection of a pure or >50% GGN results in excellent outcomes (5-year survival >95% with no recurrences).[237] One can question whether all of these lesions actually need to be resected in the first place. Nevertheless, one prospective carefully done study of limited resection found no recurrence at 5 years, but by 10 years 13% developed a staple line recurrence of a genetically apparently identical tumor, despite a reasonably wide negative margin originally.[239] The ACCP lung cancer guidelines suggest a sublobar resection for a pure GGN <2 cm with careful attention to achieving an adequate margin.[151]

Patients with GGNs often have several lesions. These lesions should be approached conceptually as independent lesions. Each lesion should be managed individually, intervening when necessary and observing other when there is no change and a low suspicion of invasive cancer.[119,237,238] There is no reason to give chemotherapy to these patients if these are independent early cancers or preinvasive lesions; chemotherapy has no role as a chemopreventative agent.

Stage I (T1,2 N0)

The standard of care for healthy patients with a clinical stage I NSCLC is surgical resection.[141,151] This is based on decades of experience showing good long-term survival rates with few recurrences after resection. Examination of the 2010-11 US National Cancer Database shows that surgery was the dominant treatment strategy (surgery in 66%, RT in 23%, and no treatment in 9%). In the US Surveillance Epidemiology and End Results (SEER)-Medicare database (i.e., patients age >65 years), the treatment given to stage cI patients in 2007 was surgery in 67%, RT in 16%, and no treatment in 18%.[240] The ACCP Lung Cancer Guideline recommends that patients with stage I NSCLC being considered for curative therapy be evaluated by a thoracic surgeon or a multidisciplinary team (even if nonsurgical therapy is being considered). Those undergoing surgery should be treated by a thoracic surgeon with a demonstrated focus on lung cancer (grade 1B).[151] There is a growing body of literature that demonstrates that outcomes are demonstrably better with specialty training and at higher volume centers (HR = 0.7 for perioperative mortality and 0.9 for long-term outcome in high-volume centers in a recent meta-analysis).[152]

Across the world, for NSCLC cases diagnosed between 1990 and 2000, staged and treated according to the local routines at the time the survival as reported by the huge IASLC database is 50% for cIa and 43% for cIb, and 73% for pIa and 58% for pIb.[52] More recent Japanese national cancer statistics demonstrate 5-year survival rates of 77% and 60% for cIa and cIb, and 84% and 66% for pIa and pIb.[241] It is important to note that only about half of the deaths within 5 years in stage I NSCLC are due to recurrences; the 5-year recurrence rate is only about 20%.[242–244] The majority (60%) of recurrences are identified within the first 2 years.[244,245] Late recurrences beyond 5 years are seen in 10% to 20% of patients, but it is unclear how many of these "recurrences" are actually new primary cancers.[246,247]

The ACCP Lung Cancer Guideline suggests that a minimally invasive (e.g., thoracoscopic [VATS] or robotically assisted) resection is preferred over an open thoracotomy for stage I NSCLC (grade 2C).[151] This is based on consistent data from small RCTs, matched case-control studies, propensity matched cohort studies, meta-analyses, and large outcomes studies, which demonstrate lower perioperative mortality, fewer complications, and shorter hospitalization as well as at least equivalent long-term stage-matched survival.[151,159,160,168,171,176,248–250] The penetration of VATS for major lung resection has been growing annually at US academic medical centers, but is performed almost exclusively by thoracic surgeons (not cardiac, general, or oncology surgeons).[251] RCTs and large database outcome studies show no difference in the ability to biopsy or resect mediastinal nodes by VATS,[159,176,183,184,252,253] although there may be a less thorough assessment of N1 nodes.[252] The ability of patients to receive adjuvant chemotherapy is improved following VATS lobectomy.[254,255]

A lobectomy remains the treatment of choice for good-risk patients with stage I NSCLC in general (ACCP Lung Cancer Guideline grade 1B).[151] This is a general conclusion, which is a different issue than asking whether an alternative resection is acceptable in patients that cannot tolerate a lobectomy, or whether there are particular cohorts for which the general statement does not apply. The recommendation for lobectomy over a more limited resection is based on better survival and lower local recurrence rates after lobectomy. Unfortunately, the data is not of high quality. This result is demonstrated by a RCT with only minor flaws,[256,257] but because it stems from the late 1980s, the relevance to the current era can be questioned. Other uncontrolled comparative studies corroborate these results, but the patients undergoing sublobar resection were clearly not the same (often not able to tolerate lobectomy or with smaller tumors). Furthermore, the sublobar resections often involved a mixture of segmentectomy and wedge resection, although segmentectomy generally results in better survival and less local recurrence than a wedge.

Specific groups that have been considered to be potentially suitable for a sublobar resection include patients with tumors <2 cm, <1 cm, pure GGO lesions, and elderly patients. For solid smaller lesions and older patients, the data is unclear; comparisons have yielded conflicting results, probably because of the inability to account for selection and confounding factors. Comparisons involving primarily wedge resection tend to show worse results, whereas those involving segmentectomy are more similar to lobectomy.[151] Two RCTs are under way to address the value of segmentectomy for solid tumors <2 cm. Increased perioperative mortality or competing causes of death such as might be present in older patients are reasonable to consider; however, clear guidance on when this tips the balance away from lobectomy is not possible from the currently available data.[151] On the other hand, there is fairly extensive data that patients with predominantly GGO lesions <2 cm consistently experience excellent 5-year outcomes after sublobar resection (predominantly segmentectomy), with the implication that it would be difficult for lobectomy to yield even better results. This led the ACCP guideline committee to recommend sublobar resection for predominantly GGO lesions <2 cm (grade 2C).[151] However, it is important to have an adequate margin, and there is data from a carefully done prospective study that segmentectomy may be associated with late recurrences (between 5 and 10 years).[239]

At the time of surgical resection, at least a systematic lymph node sampling should be performed. This involves systematically looking for and sampling a representative node from N1 and ipsilateral mediastinal node stations. Data supports that this results in more accurate staging than selective sampling.[258–261] However, there appears to be no survival benefit to a complete lymph node dissection in RCTs, at least not in clinical stage I patients.[151,260–262]

Adjuvant chemotherapy or RT is not indicated after complete resection of stage I NSCLC. Although the majority of recurrences after resection of stage I NSCLC are distant, multiple RCTs that have included stage I patients have suggested that there is no benefit to adjuvant chemotherapy.[263–265] A meta-analysis that addressed stage-specific subgroups did not find a benefit for either stage Ia or Ib.[155] An unplanned subgroup analysis in one study suggested that there may be a benefit for tumors ≥4 cm,[266] but this has not been borne out by further follow-up or other analyses. Other negative prognostic factors have been suggested (i.e., tumor differentiation, vascular invasion, histologic features), but the argument that chemotherapy will have an impact is purely speculative. The ACCP NSCLC guideline, which is more evidence based, takes the position that adjuvant chemotherapy should not be given for stage Ia or Ib with the stance that speculative arguments should not overpower RCT data.[151] The NCCN guideline, however, which is primarily consensus based, suggests considering adjuvant chemotherapy for high-risk stage Ib patients, by taking into account potential negative prognostic factors.[141] On the other hand, tegafur (an oral 5-fluorouracil agent available in Japan) has been found to improve survival in two RCTs when given orally for 2 years.[267,268]

Adjuvant RT is also not indicated after complete resection of a stage I NSCLC; in fact, the RCT data suggest it is likely to be harmful.[151,269] A more recent RCT and an outcomes analysis of the SEER database confirm this result.[270,271]

While lobectomy remains the standard of care for stage I NSCLC, there are patients who are considered poor candidates for this approach. However, poor risk for lobectomy is difficult to define. VATS resection has decreased the perioperative mortality,[272,273] data shows that lung function is reduced much less or even improved in patients with severe COPD,[272,274–276] and the majority of data mixes lobectomy and various forms of sublobar resection together (often including good-risk patients with low-risk tumors together with poor-risk patients with high-risk tumors). Furthermore, data suggest that limited pulmonary reserve correlates primarily with perioperative mortality, whereas long-term functional limitations are often due to random unpredictable events. The ACCP guideline recommends caution about undertaking lobectomy if the predicted postoperative FEV1 or predicted postoperative DLCO is <30% or <22 m on a stairclimbing test.[272] Such patients should undergo a formal exercise test and a careful multidisciplinary evaluation. While lobectomy may still be found to be appropriate, other options such as a segmentectomy, wedge, SBRT, or radiofrequency ablation (RFA) should also be considered.[272] The multidisciplinary decision making is crucial, because there are many aspects that must be taken into account (e.g., how functional the portion of lung is that contains the cancer, technical issues with doing either surgery, SBRT or RFA, and issues related to confirming the stage of the patient).

Sublobar resection undertaken as a compromise due to poor pulmonary reserve cannot be compared to sublobar resection undertaken electively because of favorable tumor characteristics. Furthermore, the outcomes for a segmentectomy cannot be compared to a wedge resection, although frequently these are combined. The available studies show that the perioperative mortality for a sublobar resection in compromised patients is around 5%, even when the resection involves a thoracotomy (not VATS).[151] The issue is one of long-term results. In the ACCP guideline review, 5-year survival after segmentectomy/wedge for stage I NSCLC in compromised patients ranged from 40% to 70%; there was a trend to worse outcomes than for lobectomy in case-matched comparisons, although the differences were not statistically significant in most studies.

The recurrence rate after sublobar resection was 0% to 18%.[151] In one of the few series to specifically compare (retrospectively) compromised patients undergoing segmentectomy versus wedge, the 5-year survival was better for segmentectomy (80% versus 48%; $p = 0.005$) and the recurrence rate was lower (16% versus 55%; $p = 0.001$).[277] In conclusion, when surgery (usually open thoracotomy) was judged to be reasonable in compromised patients, a sublobar resection could be accomplished quite safely (mortality ~5%) and the long-term outcomes were encouraging, especially for segmentectomy, which appears to be better than a wedge resection.

Nonsurgical treatment options have also emerged for compromised patients. SBRT has received the most attention. In contrast to conventionally fractionated radiation therapy, which uses small daily fractions over the course of 6 or more weeks, an SBRT treatment plan typically delivers a much higher biologically effective dose over three to five treatment visits. This requires a high degree of precision to avoid delivering the increased dose to the surrounding tissue. For lung cancer, this means highly reproducible immobilization, management of respiratory motion, and accurate localization during treatment delivery. The result is markedly higher rate of local control and survival and markedly lower toxicity when compared to conventional RT.

Because SBRT is well tolerated, does not require general anesthesia, and results in minimal damage to surrounding lung, it has been used primarily in the management of early stage lung cancers in patients who could not tolerate surgical resection of any type. In general, these appear to have been rather severely compromised patients in reported studies. The diagnosis of lung cancer was confirmed in about 75% of patients (range, 30% to 100%). In many of the studies, the cases not confirmed by biopsy were clinically diagnosed as lung cancer by a multidisciplinary tumor board on the basis of growth and/or PET activity. The lesions treated appear to have been primarily solid typical lung cancers, not indolent, ground glass tumors or screening detected cancers. The median tumor size has generally been 2 to 3 cm.

Many of the studies involving SBRT for NSCLC have reported 2-year outcomes. Survival is approximately 60% at 2 years (45% to 79%) and 40% at 5 years (24% to 50%).[151] Cancer-specific survival is approximately 75% at 2 years (50% to 90%) and 60% at 5 years (31% to 73%).[151] Disease control at the primary tumor site is approximately 90% at 2 years (83% to 100%).

Early prospective trials suggested that SBRT is associated with a higher risk of moderate to severe adverse events in a central or perihilar tumors. However, there are several published examples of safe SBRT schedules for such patients, all delivering a somewhat lower biologically effective radiation dose than that described in the RTOG 0236.[278–281] Taken together, the cumulative experience in SBRT for central lung tumors suggests that the use of more protracted fractionation, lower dose, and prioritizing normal tissue dose constraints over target volume coverage appear to reduce the risk, but there is a suggestion that this comes at the cost of somewhat lower local control. The RTOG 0813 was a phase 1/2 dose escalation study of SBRT in central tumors that has completed accrual, and the results will inform treatment of these tumors.

There is much less data for RFA, but reported OS is approximately 80% at 2 years and 30% at 5 years (20% to 61%), with a control at the primary tumor site being achieved in approximately 60% (58% to 92%). It is very difficult to compare outcomes of patients treated surgically to those treated with SBRT or RFA—the degree of comorbidity is different, the confirmation of stage and diagnosis is different, and the definition of local control outcomes are different. Randomized studies have not been able to be conducted.

In summary, it can be said that surgical resection remains the standard for stage cI NSCLC. This should involve a lobectomy with at least a systematic mediastinal node sampling and should be performed by VATS in an experienced center. Tumors that are amenable to a sublobar resection (with attention to adequate margins!) are primarily GGO lesions <2 cm; the data for small solid tumors or in elderly patients is not clear. In patients with limited pulmonary reserve who are considered poor risk for lobectomy, segmentectomy can be accomplished safely in selected patients with good long-term outcomes. A wedge resection is probably oncologically similar to nonsurgical treatment. Although survival results appear slightly better for wedge resection than SBRT, any comparison is confounded because the patients, tumors, and workup are quite different. However, the results of such interventions appear to be good enough to justify their use and appear to be better than that of completely untreated, conventionally detected stage I NSCLC.

Stage II (T1,2 N1)

The recommended treatment for clinical stage II NSCLC without major comorbidities is surgical resection followed by adjuvant chemotherapy.[141,151] Surgery has been the mainstay of treatment for many decades; an additional benefit to adjuvant chemotherapy has been demonstrated more recently (discussed subsequently). The ACCP recommends that patients be evaluated by a thoracic surgeon with a focus on lung cancer and be discussed in a multidisciplinary forum (grade Ib).[151] This is the standard in many European countries as well.

In the IASLC database, the 5-year survival was 36% for cIIa and 25% for cIIb (representing frequent stage misclassification). Survival was 46% for pIIa and 36% for pIIb.[52] These patients were diagnosed and treated between 1990 and 2000, mostly without the availability of PET scanning and likely mostly by surgery alone. In the Japanese national database, the 5-year survival rates in 2004 were 54% and 44% for cIIa and cIIb, and 61% and 47% for pIIa and pIIb, respectively.[241] In the Lung Adjuvant Cisplatin Evaluation meta-analysis of patients receiving resection plus adjuvant chemotherapy, the 5-year survival was estimated to be 45% for stage II NSCLC.[282] In stage II NSCLC, approximately 75% of deaths are due to recurrence.[283,284]

At the time of resection, the ACCP suggests that a formal mediastinal node dissection be performed (grade 2B), because there is some data suggesting that survival may be improved.[151] Selective sampling of only abnormal-appearing nodes is clearly substandard, and does not accurately define the pathologic stage. There is no difference in the accuracy of stage definition between a systematic mediastinal node sampling and a complete mediastinal node dissection.[151,258,260] However, there is a suggestion that survival and recurrence is better after a complete node dissection from randomized and nonrandomized studies.[151,258,260,285,286] Although substandard node assessment at the time of resection has been common, it should no longer be accepted given the data and value of adjuvant chemotherapy.

Stage II NSCLC involves either hilar (N1) nodes or a central (hilar) primary tumor. Whenever possible, a sleeve resection should be performed as opposed to a pneumonectomy.[151] A sleeve resection involves resection of a portion of the bronchus to the lung with an end-to-end anastomosis of the main bronchus to that of the uninvolved lobes of the lung. The same can be done for the pulmonary artery. Although the data is retrospective and subject to potential confounding by other factors, several reviews have found lower operative mortality and complications for sleeve resection versus pneumonectomy, equivalent or better long-term survival, lower recurrence rates, and better QOL.[151,287,288]

Adjuvant chemotherapy is clearly indicated after complete resection of stage IIa,b (N1) NSCLC, and adjuvant platinum-based chemotherapy is recommended by the ACCP and NCCN clinical guidelines.[141,151] This is based on the results of several randomized trials and meta-analyses.[155] There is data suggesting that cisplatin-vinorelbine may offer the best efficacy compared with other doublets.[155,289] While a few RCTs have not been positive, they have generally had significant flaws.[151]

The benefit of adjuvant therapy rests in the use of cisplatin-based combinations.[155] Carboplatin was used in one randomized

CANCER OF THE THORACIC CAVITY

trial, exclusive to patients with stage IB disease, which did not show a statistically improvement in survival, save for a subset of patients, identified in a post hoc analysis, with tumors ≥4 cm in greatest diameter.[266] Although carboplatin may be considered an alternative for patients with an absolute contraindication to cisplatin, the majority of candidates for adjuvant chemotherapy should receive cisplatin in combination with vinorelbine, docetaxel, gemcitabine, or with pemetrexed in patients with nonsquamous histology. While the bulk of the adjuvant data is based on cisplatin-vinorelbine, other regimens have been endorsed by the National Cancer Institute. It is assumed, though not yet demonstrated, that these regimens have comparable efficacy in this setting as in more advanced stages. Four cycles of adjuvant chemotherapy are typically recommended.

There are a number of nuances to mention. While the survival benefit of adjuvant therapy is sustained in late follow-up, it is diminished and there are late intracranial failures.[263,290] The lack of benefit in some RCTs suggests that factors such as the quality of surgery, the choice of chemotherapy, and the use of RT may play an important role. Whether adjuvant chemotherapy should be used for larger primary tumors (>5 cm) without local lymph node metastasis (T2bN0M0) is unclear. The ACCP guideline does not recommend this (based on equivalent survival in JBR10 and Cancer and Leukemia Group B [CALGB] 9633),[151] but the NCCN guideline suggests this can be considered.[141]

Postoperative RT (PORT) is not recommended for completely resected NSCLC.[141,151] The PORT meta-analysis found a nonsignificant survival detriment for PORT in N1 patients.[269] However, techniques of RT have advanced from what was used in many studies included in the PORT meta-analysis, and there are nuances that may be important. A SEER analysis found slightly worse survival for stage II patients receiving adjuvant RT.[271] A subset analysis of stage II patients in the ANITA study demonstrated a 12% survival advantage of PORT in the no adjuvant chemotherapy arm, but a 16% survival disadvantage in the arm receiving adjuvant chemotherapy.[291] In the setting of a positive bronchial margin, PORT is recommended by the ACCP and NCCN, although there is very little available data addressing this.[141,151] In summary, adjuvant RT should not be used after complete resection of stage II NSCLC; while modern techniques may change this recommendation in the future, it is also possible that better adjuvant chemotherapy obviates the benefit of RT.

Preoperative chemotherapy is not recommended. This has been addressed by one RCT involving stage I-II NSCLC, although about two-thirds of the patients were stage Ib; 624 patients were randomized to either surgery alone, preoperative chemotherapy, or surgery and adjuvant chemotherapy (three cycles of paclitaxel/carboplatin).[292] There was no difference in OS or disease-free survival between any of the arms. A subgroup analysis of stage II (T3 or N1) patients found a nonsignificant trend in disease-free survival favoring preoperative chemotherapy versus surgery alone (HR = 0.88; 95% confidence interval = 0.69 to 1.12; 5-year disease-free survival 41% versus 35%; $p = 0.31$). There was no benefit to adjuvant chemotherapy versus surgery alone in this subgroup analysis (HR = 1.01; 5-year disease-free survival 37% versus 35%; $p = 0.97$). However, given the limited number of patients, no suggestive conclusions can be drawn from this experience.[292]

Locally Invasive Tumors (T3,4 N0,1)

Certain tumors are characterized by local invasiveness (or size). Although they are classified as stage IIb, IIIa or IIIb, they may be biologically different than tumors distinguished primarily by nodal involvement.

T3N0,1

T3N0M0 tumors are classified as stage IIb, whereas T3N1M0 tumors are stage IIIa.[293,294] Most commonly, this involves tumors that are locally invasive into adjacent structures, with the chest wall being the most common site. The presence or absence of pain is probably the best indicator of chest wall involvement. In patients with cT3N0M0 tumors, the ACCP and NCCN guidelines suggest imaging for potential distant metastases and invasive mediastinal staging to detect possible occult N2,3 involvement, although data defining the incidence of such involvement is not available.[141,295]

Surgical resection is the recommended therapy for T3N0,1M0 NSCLC involving the chest wall.[141,295] The 5-year survival after an en bloc complete resection is consistently 50% to 60% for T3N0M0 tumors, whereas it is <5% with no resection or an incomplete resection (even with adjuvant RT).[295] Because a discontinuous (versus en bloc) resection is associated with worse outcomes, there should be a low threshold to chest wall resection whenever there is suspicion of involvement. Several retrospective studies of completely resected patients found no difference in OS or recurrence with or without PORT[296,297] with one exception.[298] Currently, postoperative chemotherapy or RT for completely resected T3 chest wall tumors is not recommended, although the data is limited.[295]

The 5-year survival for other resected T3N0 tumors (i.e., involving the mainstem bronchus or other central T3 structures) appears to be slightly lower at about 25% to 30%.[299,300] Careful stage evaluation followed by resection is the recommended approach. There is no data that defines the role of adjuvant therapy after complete resection. Nevertheless, the NCCN guidelines recommend adjuvant chemotherapy for all T3N0,1 tumors after an R0 resection, without providing any data or details.[141] The ACCP guidelines do not address this question.

The seventh edition of the stage classification classifies tumors ≥7 cm as T3, even without invasion into adjacent structures. A few studies of large cancer databases have investigated the impact of size.[301–303] Among $T3_{\geq 7}N0$ tumors, the use of preoperative therapy was not associated with significantly better survival; negative prognostic factors were age and a size of >10 cm.[302] For $T3_{\geq 7}N1$ tumors, the best outcomes were seen after a combination of surgical resection and adjuvant chemotherapy; negative prognostic factors by multivariate analysis included a size of >10 cm and the need for pneumonectomy.[303]

Pancoast Tumors

Pancoast tumors are lung cancers that invade the structures of the thoracic inlet (i.e., the first rib, brachial plexus, subclavian vessels, or upper thoracic spine).[295,304] These tumors typically present with shoulder or arm pain; however, pain down the arm or a Horner syndrome is not required to classify a tumor as a Pancoast tumor. The key feature is the involvement of structures in a complex area that raises challenges for local treatment. There is no direct data, but given the treatment challenges it is recommended that imaging for distal metastases and invasive mediastinal staging be done routinely.[295]

The standard treatment is concurrent chemoradiation followed by resection for localized tumors.[295,305] This is based on several phase II studies that have shown better complete resection rates and lower local recurrence when compared with historical series using preoperative RT alone.[295] The chemotherapy regimen typically involves a platinum doublet (e.g., cisplatin, etoposide), and usually 45 Gy of RT is given although some recommend more.[295]

Surgical resection of Pancoast tumors has advanced, with a better understanding of the anatomy of the anterior, middle, and posterior portions of the thoracic inlet, and the advent of different surgical approaches addressing particular problems each situation presents.[304] Furthermore, techniques allowing extended resections have developed. In specialized institutions, resection and reconstruction of subclavian vessels or vertebral bodies can be accomplished safely. The long-term survival of such resections is encouraging (20% to 40%); this is usually combined with pre- or postoperative additional chemotherapy or RT.[306–311] Resection should involve a lobectomy and all involved structures; it is crucial to achieve a complete resection, and surgery should only be undertaken in an institution with the ability to carry out resection of whatever is encountered.

The outcomes of neoadjuvant chemoradiotherapy followed by resection have found an R0 resection rate of ~90% and a pathologic complete response rate of ~50%.[295] The average 5-year survival was approximately 55% (range, 37% to 84%), and the average local recurrence rate was 6%. However, it must be noted that approximately 20% of patients enrolled in these studies dropped out for various reasons, and are not included in the outcomes reported. Approximately one-third of the enrolled patients had T4 tumors, and only a few had N2,3 nodal involvement.[295] In contrast, 5-year survival of patients treated with preoperative RT and resection is ~25%, with about one-third having an incomplete resection and about two-thirds experiencing a local recurrence.

If resection cannot be accomplished, curative intent treatment with chemoradiotherapy should be considered, as suggested by ACCP and NCCN guidelines.[141,295] If palliation is the goal, RT is suggested, which is effective in relieving pain in about 75% of patients.[295]

T4N0,1

Most patients with involvement of T4 structures have involvement of N2,3 nodes; these patients should be treated with chemoradiotherapy just like patients with infiltrative stage IIIa,b (N2,3) NSCLC. However, there are a small number of patients with tumors that are locally invasive but without significant nodal involvement (T4N0,1M0). Surgical techniques have advanced significantly so that T4 structures such as the carina, SVC, aorta, and vertebral column can be resected and reconstructed relatively safely. Resection appears reasonable even when cardiopulmonary bypass is needed: in a review of all reported cases, the perioperative mortality rate was 0% and the 5-year survival was 37%.[312] However, these remain major surgical interventions and should be reserved for specialized centers. Reports from such centers demonstrate perioperative mortality rates of ~10% (lower in more recent reports), with 5-year survival rates of approximately 30%.[295] These long-term outcomes appear to be better than what is reported in series of T4 patients treated with definitive chemoradiotherapy, but this observation must be made with recognition that the resected patients are probably more highly selected.

In patients with cT4N0,1M0 tumors, a careful search for distant metastases and invasive mediastinal staging is suggested.[295] The incidence of occult N2,3 node involvement is not well documented, but many series include a substantial proportion of patients who were found to be pN2. The presence of N2,3 disease is a negative prognostic factor in many (but not all) studies.[295]

The role of preoperative chemotherapy or chemoradiotherapy is not well defined, but limited data suggest it may be of benefit.[313–315] The data generally demonstrate high rates of complete resection and good long-term survival rates after preoperative therapy. While this data cannot disentangle the effect of selection from that of treatment, it does suggest that preoperative therapy should be considered when combined with the more robust data for stage IIIa (N2) patients. demonstrating that preoperative therapy is better than primary surgical resection.[316]

Stage III (N2,3)

Stage III encompasses a large group of patients; discussion of management of these patients is aided by division into several subgroups. Although there are many ways to divide this, we find that the method used by the ACCP is simple and practical, and lends itself to clinical application.[317] We distinguish patients with "incidental N2" disease, meaning there was no reason to suspect N2 involvement preoperatively but it is nevertheless found intra- or postoperatively. The next group is patients with discrete N2,3 node involvement. Such nodes can be individually distinguished and measured, and are suspicious either due to enlargement, PET activity, or because of a central primary tumor or N1 involvement (which correlates with a ~25% chance of occult N2,3 involvement).[110] These patients are distinguished from those with infiltrative stage IIIa,b disease, in which matted nodes or tumor infiltration makes distinction/measurement of individual nodes difficult. This division can be reasonably easily defined clinically and provides a structure for discussion.

Incidental Stage IIIa (N2)

Patients in whom N2 disease is not suspected but nevertheless found post- or intraoperatively are classified as incidental N2.[317,318] It is assumed that appropriate staging for distant or mediastinal nodes has been done. If N2 is discovered intraoperatively in a patient with clinical signs pointing to possible N2 involvement (enlarged or PET-positive N1-3 nodes)—in other words an inadequately preoperatively staged patient—the ACCP suggests it is better to abort the resection and proceed first with appropriate staging.[316] The data and recommendations in the following sections only apply to patients who are incidental N2 despite appropriate preoperative stage evaluation.

Postoperative Chemotherapy. The Non-Small Cell Lung Cancer Collaborative Group[225] conducted a meta-analysis in 1995 evaluating the effect of adjuvant chemotherapy in stage I-IIIa NSCLC, including 14 trials and 4,357 patients. Five trials used alkylating agents, eight used cisplatin combinations, and three used tegafur or tegafur-uracil. There was a significant decrease in survival after treatment with alkylating agents ($p = 0.005$), no change in survival with 5-fluorouracil alone or in combination, and platinum-based chemotherapy produced an improvement in survival of 5% at 5 years ($p = 0.08$). A number of randomized trials conducted in Europe and North America since the 1995 meta-analysis have examined the efficacy of platinum-based chemotherapy after surgery. Three trials showed no significant benefit,[265,319,320] but several others showed improvement in recurrence-free survival or OS.[266,290,321–323] The Lung Adjuvant Cisplatin Evaluation meta-analysis[155] included 4,584 patients treated on the five largest platinum-based adjuvant trials (ALPI, ANITA, BLT, IALT, and JBR-10), and revealed an absolute 5-year OS benefit of 5.4%. Four of the studies included stage III disease; there were a total of 760 patients with N2 lymph nodes. Although there was no improvement in survival in stage I disease, there was a significant survival benefit in patients with stage II and III disease. There appeared to be no difference between vinorelbine, etoposide, vinca alkaloids, or other agents when combined with cisplatin.

Both the ACCP and NCCN guidelines recommend adjuvant chemotherapy for completely resected stage IIIa (N2) disease.[141,316]

Postoperative Radiotherapy. Despite appropriate preoperative staging, at times a patient will undergo surgical resection as primary therapy for presumed stage I or II disease, and mediastinal sampling at the time of surgery will be positive. For select patients, there may be a role for PORT. While the role of adjuvant chemotherapy has been relatively well defined in multiple prospective randomized trials, the indications for and benefit of PORT are subject to debate. Considerations include both the T and N stage, the status of surgical margins, and consideration of the extent and type of surgery. The variability in the extent of both surgical resection and surgical staging, both independent indicators of outcome, presents a challenge to identifying patients who might benefit from adjuvant RT.

A large retrospective SEER analysis[271] included a subset analysis of resected stage III (N2) patients (data on the margin status was not available). In this group, PORT was associated with a significant improvement in OS (27% versus 20% at 5 years). Although this retrospective analysis suffers from a lack of information about

CANCER OF THE THORACIC CAVITY

patient characteristics, how the treatment approach was selected, or details of the treatment given, it suggested lower toxicity associated with better radiation treatment techniques may have decrease the toxicity of PORT and allowed a survival benefit to emerge. A follow-up SEER study supported that treatment-related morbidity was declining as radiation techniques improved.[324] Specifically, PORT was associated with increased cardiac mortality in patients with stage II or III NSCLC between 1983 and 1988 (HR = 1.49), but not in patients treated between 1989 and 1993 (HR = 1.08; p = not significant). Similarly, a recent work stratified the randomized PORT trials by the use or nonuse of linear accelerators.[325] PORT decreased local recurrence, whether patients were treated with linear accelerators or cobalt machines. There was a survival benefit associated with PORT (an absolute increase of 13% at 5 years) when delivered with linear accelerators, but not when delivered with older cobalt units. These studies support the hypothesis that PORT delivered using modern radiation technology may be associated with a lower risk of treatment-related death than was noted in older, randomized studies, and therefore radiation-related morbidity and mortality is less likely to detract from a potential survival benefit in the modern era.

The ACCP suggests adjuvant RT when the concern about local recurrence is high.[316] The NCCN suggests that adjuvant RT sequentially after adjuvant chemotherapy may be an option, but does not specify further how to make this decision.[141]

Postoperative Chemoradiotherapy. The PORT meta-analysis and the majority of the retrospective and population-based studies of PORT examined patients that were treated before the benefit of adjuvant chemotherapy was established. In the modern era, most patients with N2 disease receive adjuvant cisplatin-based chemotherapy. The additional benefit of PORT in the setting of adjuvant chemotherapy was examined in a post hoc subset analysis of the Adjuvant Navelbine International Trialist Association (ANITA) study.[291] The trial randomized patients with stage IB to IIIA NSCLC to adjuvant cisplatin and vinorelbine, or observation. PORT was recommended, but not required or randomized, for patients with node-positive disease. Out of 840 patients, 232 received PORT. On multivariate analysis, PORT improved survival in patients with N2 disease, in both the chemotherapy and no-chemotherapy arms. Shen et al.[326] conducted a trial in completely resected stage IIIA, N2 NSCLC randomized to paclitaxel and cisplatin with or without RT. There was an improvement in local and distant relapse in the RT group, and in the subgroup of patients with two or more lymph nodes positive, there was an improvement in OS.

Single-arm prospective studies have established the efficacy and safety of PORT with concurrent chemotherapy,[327,328] and several randomized studies have evaluated PORT with or without chemotherapy. The addition of concurrent chemotherapy to PORT, compared to PORT alone, does not appear to improve local control, disease-free survival, or OS.[329–331] A comparison of sequential to concurrent chemotherapy with PORT showed increased toxicity, without an increase in OS, with concurrent therapy.[332] Together, the data suggest that when PORT and chemotherapy are recommended adjuvantly, sequential therapy provides the same benefit as concurrent with less toxicity. For patients at the highest risk of local/regional recurrence (e.g., a positive surgical margin), the value of concurrent therapy can only be extrapolated from studies demonstrating a benefit to concurrent chemoradiotherapy in patients with gross unresectable disease.

Adjuvant chemotherapy for completely resected stage IIIa (N2) disease is not recommended by either the ACCP or NCCN guidelines.[141,316]

Discrete N2 Node Involvement

Discrete N2/N3 involvement defines patients in whom individual mediastinal nodes can be identified and measured on a CT. These nodes may be enlarged on CT or normal sized but suspected by PET uptake or by other characteristics such as a central tumor or N1 node involvement.[316] The terms “resectable” and “unresectable” are specifically avoided because they are notoriously subjective and inaccurate; for example, it is consistently shown that 25% to 35% of stage IIIa (N2) patients who are selected for surgery end up with an incomplete resection.[316,317]

Such patients should undergo invasive mediastinal staging to confirm N2 or N3 involvement (the false-positive rate for discrete node enlargement on CT is ~40%, and for PET positivity it is ~15% to 20%).[110] Furthermore, such patients should undergo a careful evaluation for distant metastases, which are found in about 25% despite a negative clinical evaluation.[110] The subsequent discussion assumes that appropriate staging evaluation has been carried out; it is not acceptable to proceed to resection without thorough invasive mediastinal staging or imaging for distant metastases in patients in whom there is reasonable suspicion of N2 node involvement.[110,317] The results reported in this chapter do not apply to patients that are mismanaged (i.e., in whom clinical standards for stage evaluation prior to treatment have been ignored).

In evaluating treatment approaches for patients with discrete N2 involvement, it is best to focus on RCTs or on intent-to-treat analyses. However, the literature is replete with reported outcomes of particular cohorts of patients; these cohorts are often selected by characteristics that can only be defined in retrospect. While these studies provide data on these specific cohorts, it must be recognized that the outcomes represent not only a treatment effect but probably most predominantly the effect of selection. A common mistake is to attribute the outcomes entirely to the treatment and forget that the effect of treatment cannot be disentangled from that of selection. Another common mistake is to assume that the outcomes of patients who complete a treatment approach apply to all patients who start on this approach. The extent of attrition and its effect on outcomes is perhaps best illustrated in a comprehensive analysis of 402 preoperatively identified patients with N2 involvement who were selected for preoperative chemotherapy with planned subsequent surgery (Fig. 37.11).[333] While the 5-year survival of the patients who completed the planned approach was ~50%, this represented only about one-quarter of the original group; the 5-year survival of all patients selected for the treatment plan was only 13%. Finally, it must be emphasized that selection of a treatment approach must be based on factors that can be identified as pretreatment; the outcomes of patients according to factors that are available only in retrospect are useless to identify how to select patients for treatment.

Several RCTs have compared initial surgical resection for proven N2 versus preoperative chemotherapy.[316] These have generally found better survival in patients given preoperative therapy (average 2-year survival 40% versus 29%, 5-year survival 24% versus 17%).[316] However, most of these studies were underpowered and did not show a statistically significant difference. A 2007 Cochrane meta-analysis of stage III patients found a trend to better survival for preoperative platinum-based chemotherapy versus surgery alone (HR = 0.73; 95% confidence interval = 0.51 to 1.07; $p = 0.1$).[334]

Some groups have advocated that initial surgical resection is appropriate for some patients with N2 involvement. This argument is generally made citing good outcomes for cN0,1 patients with incidental N2 after resection[335]—this is not applicable to patients with N2 disease confirmed or suspected preoperatively. A few centers have published their results of preoperatively confirmed N2 patients that were selected for primary surgery; the average 5-year survival for all patients selected was 13%.[316,336–338]

In summary, the data suggests that selection of patients with good outcomes after primary surgery has not been demonstrated, and limited data suggests that outcomes are better after preoperative therapy. Neither the ACCP nor the NCCN guidelines recommend primary surgery for confirmed N2 involvement.[141,316]

However, it must be recognized that some of the data is relatively old. Techniques of mediastinal evaluation have progressed, at least in some institutions. The results of a microscopic deposit of cancer in an N2 node identified via video-assisted mediastinal

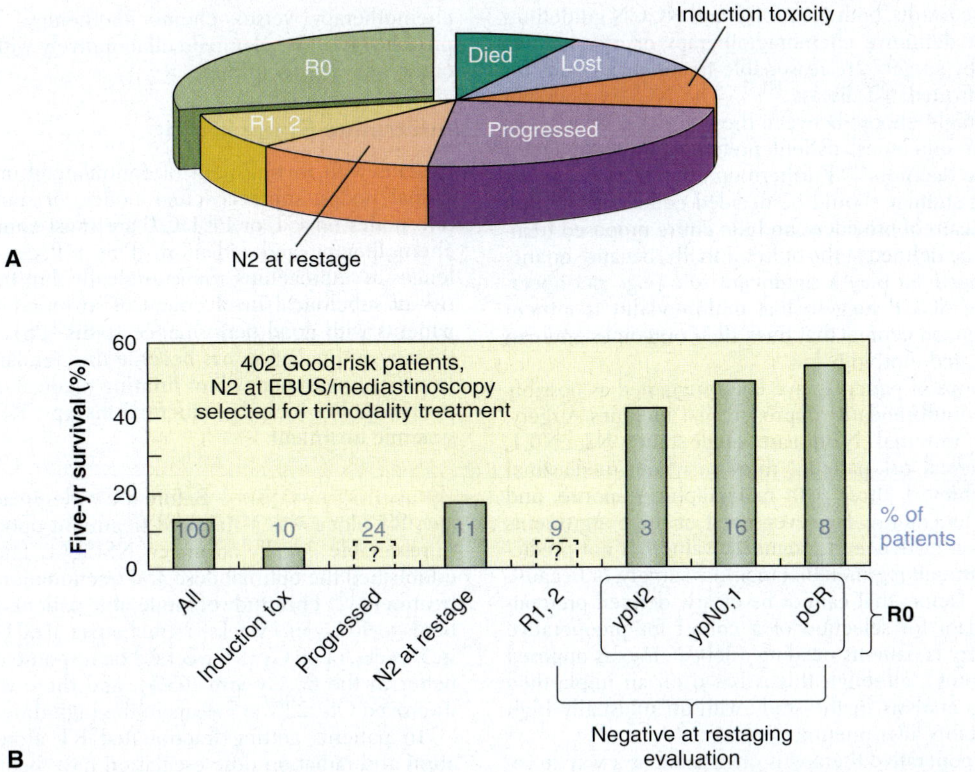

Figure 37.11 Fate of stage IIIa(N2) patients selected for neoadjuvant therapy and resection. Analysis of the fate of 402 good-risk patients, identified as having histologically proven but limited N2 involvement, who were selected as good candidates for preoperative chemotherapy followed by planned subsequent surgery. **(A)** Fate of all patients selected for this treatment approach. **(B)** Five-year survival of subgroups of patients based on subsequent outcomes and events during the planned treatment. EBUS, endobronchial ultrasound. (Data taken from Cerfolio RJ, Maniscalco L, Bryant AS. The treatment of patients with stage IIIA non-small cell lung cancer from N2 disease: who returns to the surgical arena and who survives. *Ann Thorac Surg* 2008;86:912–920.)

lymphadenectomy may not be the same as that derived from older literature. Furthermore, there appear to be regional differences, with survival being better for cN2 patients in Asia than North America or Europe.[157] However, no studies have defined how these factors can lead to appropriate selection of patients for primary surgery.

Several RCTs have compared preoperative therapy followed by surgery versus chemoradiotherapy alone.[316,339–342] These have found no significant difference, even in adequately powered studies, between these approaches, although arguably one can interpret there might be a slight trend to better survival in the surgical arms. In one larger study, a suggestion of better outcomes after treatment was completed was offset by higher treatment-related mortality in the surgical arm, particularly after pneumonectomy (Fig. 37.12).[339] However, the perioperative mortality in this study appears to have been significantly higher than in other studies.[343]

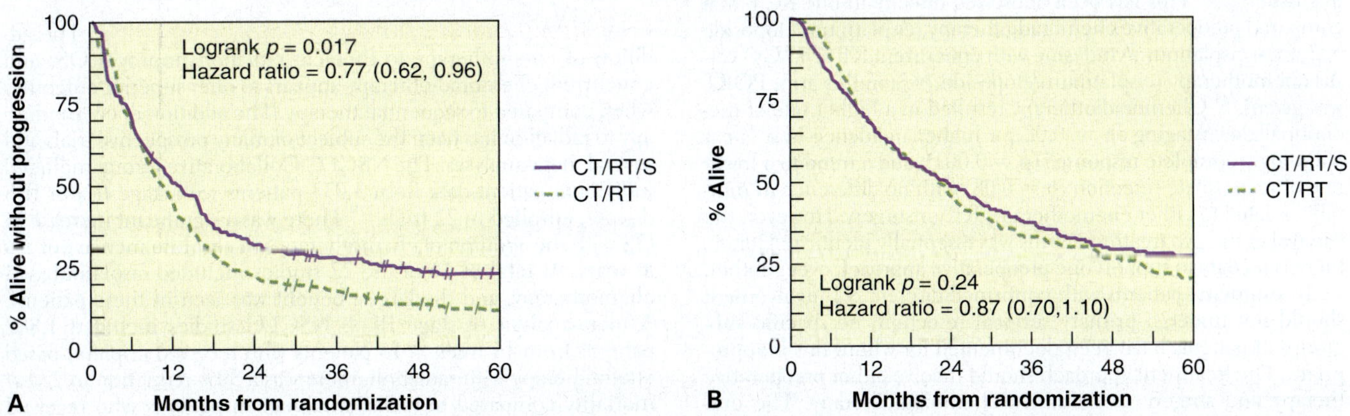

Figure 37.12 Trimodality versus bimodality treatment of stage IIIa(N2) lung cancer. Survival of patients with stage IIIA (N2) non–small-cell lung cancer treated with trimodality (CT/RT/S) versus bimodality (CT/RT) therapy from the North American Intergroup Study 0139. The initial steeper slope of the trimodality arm demonstrates the importance of the perioperative mortality rate on the overall results of trimodality therapy. **(A)** Progreesion-free survival. **(B)** Overall survival. CT/RT/S, chemotherapy and radiotherapy followed by surgery; CT/RT, chemotherapy and radiotherapy. (Reproduced with permission from Albain KS, Swann RS, Rusch VW, et al. Radiotherapy plus chemotherapy with or without surgical resection for stage III non-small-cell lung cancer: a phase III randomised controlled trial. *Lancet* 2009;374:379–386.)

Reflecting these results, both the ACCP and NCCN guidelines suggest that either definitive chemoradiotherapy or preoperative therapy followed by surgery are reasonable treatment options for patients with confirmed N2 disease.[141,316] The NCCN does not suggest how one might choose between these; the ACCP suggests that, given similar outcomes, patient preferences should factor significantly in the decision.[316] Furthermore, the ACCP suggests that the treatment strategy should be decided collectively by the multidisciplinary team of providers, and the entire proposed treatment plan should be defined at the outset. Finally, because quality of care aspects appear to play a significant role (e.g., perioperative mortality), the ACCP suggests that multimodality treatment be done at experienced centers that track their outcomes and can keep treatment-related morbidity low.

Various subgroups of patients have been suggested as possibly benefiting from a multimodality approach that includes surgery, such as those with "minimal" N2 disease, single station N2, cN0,1, younger, good surgical risk patients, those in whom mediastinal downstaging is achieved, those with radiographic response, and those requiring a lobectomy. However, most of these arguments are flawed, based on evidence of prognostic value but not predictive value for a treatment regimen that includes surgery, or because they are based on factors that cannot be clearly defined pretreatment. The best data for selection of a cohort for preoperative therapy with surgery is patients needing a lobectomy (as opposed to a pneumonectomy), although this is based on an unplanned matched-subgroup analysis in the study with an unusually high perioperative mortality after pneumonectomy.[339]

Response to preoperative therapy is often cited as a way to select patients who will benefit from resection. While this is prognostic (responders do better), there is no data that demonstrates that the better prognosis is affected whether resection is undertaken or not.[316] Furthermore, arguments that outcomes are poor in those who are not downstaged are confounded because most of the nondownstaged patients are not resected. Those that are resected despite ypN2 involvement have a 5-year survival of about 15%.[316] Finally, radiographic response by CT is notoriously inaccurate to define downstaging, and invasive methods other than a first-time mediastinoscopy are associated with high false-negative rates.[344] The data regarding survival of downstaged patients relates to the postoperative stage. Therefore, the ACCP concludes that identification of patients that are more likely to benefit from surgical resection is not possible at this time based on pretreatment characteristics.

There is also debate about the choice of preoperative therapy (chemotherapy versus chemoradiotherapy). The NCCN suggests either approach is acceptable; the ACCP does not address this issue.[141,316] This has been addressed directly in one RCT that compared preoperative chemoradiotherapy (cisplatinum/etoposide × 3, then cisplatinum/vindesine with concurrent RT of 45 Gy) versus chemotherapy (cisplatinum/etoposide × 3; in this arm, PORT was given).[345] Chemoradiotherapy resulted in a higher rate of mediastinal downstaging ($p = 0.02$), a higher incidence of a "near pathologic complete response" ($p = 0.001$), and a trend to a lower rate of incomplete resection ($p = 0.08$) with no difference in mortality related to either chemotherapy, RT, or surgery. However, the survival of the two treatment arms was essentially identical. Hence, there is no data to support one preoperative approach over another.

In summary, patients with confirmed discrete N2 involvement should not undergo primary surgical resection; no specific subgroups of patients have been documented for whom this is appropriate. The treatment approach should involve either preoperative therapy and surgery or definitive chemoradiotherapy. The outcomes of these two strategies appear to be similar, and factors such a patient preferences as well as local expertise and minimization of morbidity and mortality should play a major role in deciding upon a treatment approach. Definition of subgroups that are more likely to benefit from the inclusion of surgery is not possible from the available data; there is also no difference between preoperative chemotherapy versus chemoradiotherapy. The treatment approach should be planned collaboratively with involvement of all of the relevant disciplines.

Infiltrative Stage III a,b

Patients with involvement of contralateral or multistation mediastinal nodes, supraclavicular nodes, or multiple clinically visible nodes on CT or PET/CT are most commonly treated with chemotherapy and radiation. This reflects not only the challenges in approaching these surgically, but the inherently higher risk of subclinical involvement of surrounding regional sites. In patients with good performance status (PS), concurrent chemotherapy and radiation has become the standard of care approach. In patients with poor PS or limiting medical comorbidities, therapeutic options include sequential therapy, RT alone, or palliative systemic treatment.

Radiotherapy Alone. Before the widespread use of chemotherapy, RT alone was a standard treatment option for patients with unresectable, locally advanced NSCLC. The RTOG 7301 trial established the optimal dose and fractionation for single-modality treatment.[346] This study of inoperable patients randomized 375 patients to 40 Gy in 4 weeks, a split course of 40 Gy in 6 weeks, 50 Gy in 5 weeks, or 60 Gy in 6 weeks. The response rate was significantly better in the 60 Gy arm (63%), and there was parallel trend in improved OS (22% at 3 years in the high-dose arm).

In patients getting fractionated RT alone, altered fractionation and radiation dose escalation have been investigated in an effort to improve the relatively poor response and survival that is seen after standard 60 Gy. A dose escalation study conducted at the University of Michigan included 106 patients with stage I to III NSCLC, using doses from 63 to 103 Gy in daily fractions.[347] Patients were allocated to dose based on the tumor volume and risk of pneumonitis, so no optimal dose was identified, but higher dose was associated with improved control and survival. The RTOG 8311 included 840 patients in a dose escalation trial, from 60 Gy to 79.2 Gy delivered in twice-daily 1.2 Gy fractions.[348] The best OS, 29% at 2 years, was associated with 69.6 Gy twice daily. Similarly, the European Organisation for Research and Treatment of Cancer conducted a randomized phase II/III study of standard RT (60 Gy in 6 weeks) versus continuous hyperfractionated accelerated RT (CHART).[349] CHART is given in 1.5 Gy fractions, three times daily, 7 days per week, to a total dose of 54 Gy. The use of CHART was associated with improved OS (20% versus 13%), but also a higher rate of severe acute dysphagia (49% versus 19%).

Concurrent and Sequential Chemoradiotherapy. The addition of chemotherapy to thoracic radiation improves OS, and concurrent chemoradiotherapy appears to offer superior outcomes when compared to sequential therapy. The addition of chemotherapy to radiation has been the subject of many prospective trials and several meta-analyses. The NSCLC Collaborative Group included individual patient data from 3,033 patients with stage IIIa or IIIb disease, enrolled in 22 trials.[225] There was a significant increase in OS with the addition of chemotherapy, an absolute increase of 2% at years. At total of 11 of the 22 studies included cisplatin-based chemotherapy, and the largest benefit was seen in these patients. A meta-analysis of stage IIIa,b NSCLC studies included 1,887 patients from 14 trials.[350] In patients who received cisplatin-based chemotherapy with radiation, there was a 30% reduction in 2-year mortality compared to radiation alone. In patients who received other chemotherapy, there was an 18% reduction. The preference for cisplatin-based chemotherapy was confirmed in a more recent meta-analysis, which was limited to studies that combined radiation with either cisplatin- or carboplatin-based chemotherapy.[351] They analyzed 1,764 patients from nine trials, and found an absolute improvement in OS of 4% at 2 years.

The use of concurrent, rather than sequential, chemotherapy with thoracic RT appears to improve OS, at the cost of increased acute toxicity. The RTOG 9410 was a three-arm trial: cisplatin and vindesine followed by RT (63 Gy once daily), cisplatin and vindesine with concurrent RT (63 Gy once daily), or cisplatin and etoposide concurrently with RT (69.6 Gy twice daily).[352] The median OS was significantly better in the concurrent arm with daily radiation, compared to sequential therapy (17 months versus 14.6 months), as was local control (66% versus 59%). Acute grade ≥3 toxicity was similarly higher with concurrent therapy; 48% versus 30% nonhematologic. Serious late toxicity was significantly different. The survival in the concurrent chemotherapy and twice-daily RT arm was 15.6 months, not significantly better than the control arm. This was confirmed in a trial by the West Japan Lung Cancer Group, in which patients were randomized to receive either sequential or concurrent chemotherapy.[353] The chemotherapy was cisplatin, mitomycin, and vindesine in both arms. Sequential RT was 56 Gy in 5.5 weeks; the concurrent RT was 56 Gy in 7.5 weeks with a 2-week break midcourse. The median survival was better in the concurrent arm (17 months versus 13 months). There was no difference in esophageal toxicity.

Cisplatin- and carboplatin-based are the most common chemotherapy combinations delivered concurrently with thoracic radiation, extrapolated from the superiority of such combinations in the meta-analyses of sequential treatment. The best specific combination has not yet been clearly defined. In a three-arm noninferiority trial conducted by the West Japan Lung Cancer Group, the use of concurrent weekly carboplatin (40 mg/m^2) and paclitaxel (area under the curve = 2) (CP) had comparable survival to mitomycin, vindesine, and cisplatin, and to irinotecan and carboplatin, with lower toxicity.[354] A small randomized study compared weekly carboplatin (45 mg/m^2 and area under the curve = 2, respectively) to cisplatin and etoposide (CE) delivered every 3 weeks (cisplatin 50 mg/m^2 on day 1, etoposide 50 mg/m^2 on days 1 to 5).[355] Both arms received concurrent thoracic RT to 60 Gy. The survival was superior in the CE arm (33% versus 13%). Neutropenia was more common with CE, and RP more common with carboplatin. A larger, phase 2/3 randomized study from the Chinese Academy of Medical Sciences (NCT01494558) comparing carboplatin to CE has completed enrollment and may answer this question. The use of pemetrexed in combination with platinum compounds is equally effective, and less toxic, than other combinations in patients with nonsquamous histology. The use of this combination, carboplatin (area under the curve = 5) and pemetrexed (500 mg/m^2) with thoracic RT (70 Gy), has been shown to be both safe and effective in a phase 2 study from the CALGB.[356] A large international randomized study comparing pemetrexed and cisplatin to etoposide and cisplatin with RT has been conducted but not yet reported. Attempts have been made to add targeted agents to standard chemoradiotherapy platforms in the setting of stage III disease, in an effort incorporate chemo- and radiosensitizing agents. The addition of antiangiogenics has not improved outcomes: a randomized trial adding antiangiogenic AE-941 to carboplatin and radiation failed to show an improvement in OS.[357] Similarly, a randomized trial conducted by the Eastern Cooperative Oncology Group added thalidomide to concurrent or sequential chemoradiation did not show any benefit. Bevacizumab, the monoclonal antibody to the vascular endothelial growth factor receptor has been added to chemoradiation in a phase 2 study that also incorporated an EGFR TKI and escalated radiation dose.[212] There was no improvement over standard therapy. Several phase 2 studies have incorporated the monoclonal EGFR antibody cetuximab. A randomized phase 2 study, the CALGB 30407,[356] suggested no benefit. Consistent with this, a phase 3 trial, the RTOG 0617, randomized patients getting carboplatin and thoracic RT to the addition of cetuximab. The preliminary results suggest no incremental benefit. The addition of EGFR TKIs to chemoradiation in unselected patients has been similarly disappointing; the Southwest Oncology Group S0023 randomized patients with stage III NSCLC to gefitinib or placebo after CE and RT.[358] OS was worse with gefitinib. Effort to incorporate TKIs into the treatment of stage III patients, in selected patients based on molecular profiling, are ongoing.

Induction or Adjuvant Chemotherapy with Chemoradiation. The role of adjuvant chemotherapy after definitive concurrent chemoradiation is not entirely defined and is likely dependent on the choice of concurrent systemic therapy. There are no published, randomized trials that support this specific approach with high-level evidence. The phase 3 Hoosier Oncology Group study enrolled patients receiving concurrent radiation and CE randomized to three cycles of docetaxel versus no further therapy.[359] Enrollment stopped when futility analysis determined that there would be no chance of observing a benefit; the median survival was 21.2 months after adjuvant chemotherapy and 23.3 months for observation. The continued interest in adjuvant therapy likely stems from the desire to administer more than two cycles of full-dose chemotherapy in the setting of stage III disease, consistent with that given adjuvantly after surgery. This is relevant for concurrent regimens that include two cycles of concurrent chemotherapy, but of particular interest when the concurrent regimen is weekly carboplatin, as opposed to combinations that can be delivered concurrently with radiation at full systemic dose, such as cisplatin and etoposide or cisplatin and vinorelbine.

In the induction setting, the CALGB 39081 randomized patients to two cycles of carboplatin followed by RT and weekly carboplatin, or immediate treatment with RT and weekly carboplatin.[360] In 366 enrolled patients, survival was not improved by the addition of two cycles of carboplatin before concurrent therapy. Induction therapy is not routinely employed before definitive chemoradiation but instead reserved for those patients where circumstances or disease volume precludes immediate chemoradiation.

Radiation Dose and Fractionation for Concurrent Treatment. The RTOG 7301 established 60 Gy in 6 weeks as the standard radiation for single modality therapy, and this regimen was adopted as one possible standard when combined with sequential or concurrent chemoradiotherapy. But the risk of local, in-field relapse among patients receiving definitive chemoradiation is high, between 30% and 50% depending on the length and manner of follow-up. A number of radiation dose escalation trials suggest that increasing radiation dose may improve local control and can be accomplished in at least a subset of patients. The RTOG 9311 was the first large dose escalation trial conduced with three-dimensional conformal radiation techniques. In an effort to increase the dose to the gross tumor and involved nodes, nodal regions without confirmed macroscopic or microscopic disease were not electively included. Either radiation alone or sequential chemoradiation were allowed.[327] For each patient, the lung V20 was calculated, and the maximum dose cohort was based on their predicted risk of pneumonitis. Patients were treated from 70.9 Gy to 90.3 Gy in daily 2.15-Gy fractions. Dose escalation was well tolerated up to 83.8 Gy in the lowest-risk group and 77.4 Gy in the intermediate-risk group. The follow-up study, the RTOG 0117, escalated dose in the setting of concurrent cisplatin and docetaxel.[361] The study started at 75.25 Gy in 2.15 Gy fractions and was designed to escalate by increasing the dose per fraction (and decreasing the overall treatment duration). After excess toxicity was observed at the starting dose, dose de-escalation was done, reducing to 74 Gy in 2-Gy fractions. A total of 55 patients were treated at this dose, with a median survival of 21.6 months for stage III patients. A similar, small dose escalation study in 15 stage III patients receiving weekly chemotherapy also concluded that the maximum tolerated dose was 74 Gy in two fractions[362]; the median survival was 37 months.

A series of prospective studies conducted at the University of North Carolina also evaluated escalating radiation dose from 60 Gy to 74 Gy in 2-Gy fractions, with an expansion at 74 Gy. Patients received induction and concurrent carboplatin.[363] With a median follow-up of 5 years for 62 patients, the OS at 5 years was 27%. A follow-up phase 2 study with chemoradiation to 74 Gy and erlotinib included 48 patients. The median survival was 18 months, with a 29% rate of grade 3 or 4 toxicity. The CALGB 30105 was a randomized phase 2 study that also incorporated 74 Gy into two different induction and concurrent chemotherapy schedules. The median survival was 24 months in 69 patients in the superior chemotherapy arm.[364]

Finally, the RTOG 0617 sought to determine the absolute benefit of 74 Gy, versus standard 60 Gy, with concurrent weekly carboplatin. This was a two-by-two factorial design, where patients were randomized to standard or high dose, and to standard chemotherapy or chemotherapy and cetuximab concurrently with radiation. The 74-Gy arm was closed early when futility analysis determined that there would be no benefit over 60 Gy. The result of this randomization was presented; high-dose radiation was associated with worse OS compared to standard radiation (median survival 19.5 months versus 28.7 months). There were more treatment-related deaths in the high dose arm, and a higher rate of grade 3 or greater esophagitis. Oddly, local control was worse in the high-dose arm.[365]

Altered Fractionation with Chemotherapy. The use of standard, daily radiation fractionation is designed to balance the delivery of definitive dose to the tumor, while allowing daily repair of the surrounding normal tissue. Altered fractionation schedules take advantage of radiobiologic principles: hyperfractionation (increased number of fractions) should result in increased opportunity for normal tissue repair and a lower risk of late side effects. Accelerated radiation (shorter treatment duration) should improve local control by allowing less tumor repopulation. Hypofractionation (higher dose per fraction) is one method to achieve acceleration, typically at the cost of increased acute toxicity. SBRT is extreme hypofractionation, combined with precision targeting to reduce exposure of normal tissue. Because both hypofractionation and accelerated hyperfractionation may increase the acute side effects of radiation therapy, combining these regimens with concurrent radiosensitizing chemotherapy remains investigational.

The RTOG 9410 was a three-arm randomized trial: sequential chemoradiotherapy with 60 Gy once daily, concurrent chemoradiotherapy with 60 Gy once daily, and concurrent chemotherapy with 69.6 Gy twice daily (hyperfractionation). While the addition of concurrent chemotherapy improved survival, the hyperfractionated radiation arm was no better than daily treatment.[352] Schild et al.[366] conducted a similar phase 3 trial, comparing concurrent CE with either daily RT to 60 Gy, or twice daily RT to 60 Gy in 6 weeks. There was no difference in local control or OS.

The use of CHART improved OS when compared to daily treatment, when radiation was the sole modality, but the advantage of hyperfractionation with concurrent chemotherapy has not been similarly demonstrated. The Eastern Cooperative Oncology Group 2597 examined hyperfractionated accelerated radiation therapy with sequential chemotherapy. Patients were randomized after two cycles of carboplatin to daily radiation (64 Gy in 32 fractions) versus hyperfractionated accelerated radiation therapy (57.6 Gy three times daily over 2.5 weeks).[367] The study was closed early, partially because of the difficult logistic of three times daily treatment. Overall, 141 patients were randomized, and there was no significant difference in median survival (20.3 months versus 14.9 months favoring hyperfractionated accelerated radiation therapy).

The European Organisation for Research and Treatment of Cancer tested the use of hypofractionated RT in inoperable NSCLC.[368] Overall, 158 patients were randomized to either gemcitabine and cisplatin before RT, or low-dose daily cisplatin (6 mg/m^2) concurrent with RT. The radiation was delivered in 24 fractions of 2.75 Gy in 32 days (total 66 Gy). The combination of sequential or concurrent chemotherapy with hypofractionated radiation was well tolerated, with grade 3 esophagitis in 14% of patients in the concurrent arm. Similarly, a phase 2 trial in 49 patients with stage III disease used 60 Gy in 5 weeks with carboplatin, with a median survival of 28 months[369]; 29 of 49 patients had grade 2 or greater toxicity, and two patients died of bleeding complications.

Choice of Chemotherapy. In the setting of stage III disease, either prior to surgical intervention (neoadjuvant therapy), or when used concurrently with RT (combined modality therapy), cisplatin-based combinations are preferred. Combinations with etoposide, vinorelbine, paclitaxel, docetaxel, and pemetrexed have all been tested in this setting. Gemcitabine is generally avoided in this context due to its potent radiosensitizing properties and potential severe complications.[370] However, unlike in adjuvant therapy, the use of carboplatin in the context of combined modality therapy for stage III disease is better documented. In particular, the use of carboplatin, administered on a weekly schedule and administered concurrently with standard thoracic RT, yielded roughly the same survival results as trials using cisplatin-based combinations.[365] In stage III disease, neither induction nor consolidation chemotherapy appears to add to concurrent treatment.[359,371] However, practitioners in the United States have been reluctant to limit treatment to two cycles of chemotherapy and tend to recommend an additional two cycles for total of four cycles.

Stage IV

Selection for Treatment

Patients with advanced NSCLC are often symptomatic and require prompt intervention. A "watch and wait" approach is generally not recommended.[372] A few selected patients who are asymptomatic at the time of the diagnosis and wish to forgo immediate treatment must be followed closely by clinical and radiographic criteria. In some circumstances, it is appropriate to administer local therapy prior to systemic therapy, such as symptomatic central nervous system disease, cord compression, painful skeletal metastases, or uncontrolled hemoptysis (discussed in more detail in the section "Specific Symptom Management"). However, chemotherapy is also an effective palliative tool and individualized judgment is recommended.

Chemotherapy is the mainstay of treatment for patients who present with stage IV disease at diagnosis or who experience recurrent disease that is not amenable to local therapy. In the 1990s and early 2000s, multiple RCTs clearly established that treatment of patients with stage IV NSCLC and good PS prolongs survival compared with basic supportive care alone.[373,374] Because this question is considered to have been clearly answered, further trials addressing this have not been conducted in the last decade.

Patients are frequently more focused on QOL and express concern that treatment with chemotherapy will negatively impact this. Multiple RCTs have evaluated this and consistently shown that treatment with chemotherapy improves QOL compared to best supportive care in good PS patients.[373,374] Chemotherapy for stage IV NSCLC is given as an outpatient; significant toxicity (grade ≥3) is uncommon. Nevertheless, QOL continues to be an important end point in studies comparing one regimen to another.

Therefore, both the ACCP and NCCN guidelines recommend that patients with stage IV NSCLC and a PS of 0,1 be treated with chemotherapy (based on level 1 evidence or a unanimous consensus, respectively).[141,374] Patients with a PS of 2 may also benefit from chemotherapy, and this is recommended by the ACCP and NCCN guidelines, but in a nuanced fashion. This patient population is addressed specifically in a subsequent section.

Recent studies have demonstrated a median survival of approximately 10 to 12 months for patients with nonsquamous histology, and 9 to 10 months for squamous carcinoma (Table 37.6).[375] The respective 1-year survival rates are 20% to 25% and 15% to 20%. These estimates are lower for patients with PS 2, regardless

TABLE 37.6

Efficacy of Chemotherapy in Advanced Non–Small-Cell Lung Cancer[a]

	ORR	PFS	MST	1-y OS
Nonsquamous				
Doublet	15%–25%	4 mo	8–10 mo	40%
Doublet + bevacizumab	25%–35%	5–6 mo	10–12mo	50%
Doublet + maintenance		5–6 mo	12–14 mo	55%–60%
Squamous				
Doublet	15%–25%	4 mo	8–10 mo	35%

ORR, objective response rate; PFS, progression-free survival; MST, median survival time; OS overall survival.
[a] Results apply to patients with performance status 0-1 and wild-type tumors.

of histology.[376] Patients with sensitizing mutations treated with targeted therapy have a more favorable outcome, as detailed in the following.

First-Line Therapy

The approach is based on the patient's histologic subtype and PS (Fig. 37.13). Patients with nonsquamous histology, regardless of PS, should have the tumor submitted for molecular analysis and, in the presence of an actionable mutation, be treated with the appropriate targeted agent. For patients with nonsquamous cancers without a mutation and for patients with squamous histology, combination chemotherapy is the standard of care for patients with PS 0-1.[141,374] Platinum-based regimens are the standard. An extensive literature has attempted to determine the "optimal platinum analog," cisplatin or carboplatin, in advanced disease. There is a general consensus that while cisplatin may be slightly more active, particularly with respect to response rate, the impact on OS is minimal, if any, and toxicity, especially nonhematologic, is worse.[377] Carboplatin tends to be widely used in the United States, while cisplatin is still frequently utilized in Europe and Latin America. Agents that are typically combined with a platinum analog include pemetrexed (except in squamous carcinoma), paclitaxel, docetaxel, nab-paclitaxel, gemcitabine, vinorelbine, irinotecan, and etoposide (see Table 37.6). Studies have failed to demonstrate superiority of one regimen over another, and decisions regarding which agent to use are based on the toxicity profile, ease and convenience of administration, and cost.[378]

The choice of regimens tends to differ between the histologic types. Pemetrexed has no efficacy in squamous cell carcinomas and should not be used in these patients.[379] Bevacizumab, an antiangiogenesis inhibitor, has a high rate of bleeding complications in squamous cell carcinomas and should not be used in these patients.[156,380] The addition of a third cytotoxic agent does not improve outcomes and is not recommended.[381] The use of nonplatinum doublets in first-line therapy is not encouraged but may be an alternative to occasional patients who have contraindications to both platinum analogs.[382]

The general standard is to administer four to six cycles of chemotherapy unless progression or toxicity prevents this.[141,374] This is administered either alone or in combination with a biologic agent (bevacizumab). The biologic agent is typically continued until disease progression (see subsequent section). In addition, administration of maintenance chemotherapy should be considered (also as discussed in a later section).

PS 2 patients have a poorer prognosis and tend to benefit less from chemotherapy.[383] However, new data have demonstrated a survival benefit for combination chemotherapy over single agent in patients with PS 2 despite higher toxicity rates.[384] This trial demonstrated a significant improvement in survival for carboplatin and pemetrexed compared to pemetrexed alone. Benefits with respect

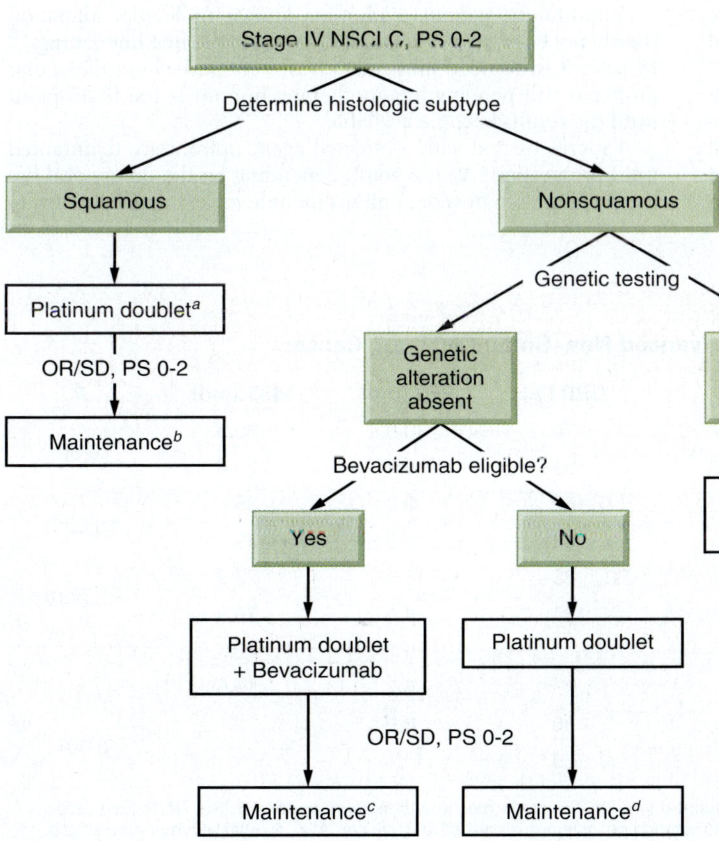

Figure 37.13 Algorithm for first-line chemotherapy management of patients with stage IV non–small-cell lung cancer (NSCLC). OR, objective response; SD, stable disease; PS, performance status.
[a] Avoid Pemetrexed
[b] Switch maintenance with Erlotinib
[c] Bevacizumab maintenance or Pemetrexed maintenance (either switch or continuation) or switch maintenance with Erlotinib
[d] Pemetrexed maintenance (either switch or continuation) or switch maintenance with Erlotinib

to symptom reduction and QOL have also been reported in PS 2 patients.[385] Patients with PS 3 or lower are typically not candidates for chemotherapy.

Age alone is not a restriction to chemotherapy. In the past, patients aged ≥70 years were felt to be at high risk for complications and many were treated with single-agent therapy or denied active treatment altogether.[386] A robust literature published in the past decade has demonstrated that elderly patients benefit from standard combination chemotherapy compared to single agent, including a pivotal clinical trial in which the combination of carboplatin, administered weekly, was superior to single-agent therapy.[387] Toxicity, as in PS 2 patients, tends to be more severe. Carboplatin is easier to tolerate, and the use of cisplatin is discouraged in these patients. Octogenarians have been poorly represented in clinical trials, and caution is advised when applying these data to this age subset.[388]

Monoclonal Antibodies

Guidelines recommend the addition of bevacizumab, a monoclonal antibody directed against the vascular endothelial growth factor ligand, in addition to combination chemotherapy.[141,374] Bevacizumab should be continued until disease progression. This is based largely on a US RCT in which bevacizumab in combination with carboplatin led to a significant improvement in survival in patients with nonsquamous cell histology with PS 0-1.[156] However, toxicity in general and treatment-related deaths in particular were significantly higher in the bevacizumab arm, including rates of pulmonary hemorrhage, thromboembolic phenomena, and neutropenia and thrombocytopenia. A similar study conducted in Europe, using two different doses of bevacizumab in combination with cisplatin and gemcitabine, showed a significant improvement in PFS (the primary end point) but not in OS.[389]

A recent study (Pointbreak trial) compared the two most frequently used bevacizumab-containing regimens: the original carboplatin-paclitaxel-bevacizumab versus carboplatin-pemetrexed-bevacizumab developed by investigators in Chicago.[390] Both combinations were administered for four cycles followed by maintenance bevacizumab alone in the paclitaxel arm, and both pemetrexed and bevacizumab in the other arm. There was no significant difference in survival. Toxicity, while slightly different between the arms, did not seem statistically different.

These data demonstrate that bevacizumab can be used in eligible patients with advanced NSCLC in combination with chemotherapy. The benefit is modest, and toxicity can be significant. Patients with squamous cell carcinoma and hemoptysis should not receive bevacizumab, while patients on anticoagulation and with previously treated brain metastases are eligible.[391] Patients with PS 2 do not typically receive bevacizumab.

Cetuximab, a monoclonal antibody directed against the EGFR, also demonstrated a significant improvement in survival when added to cisplatin and vinorelbine in a single randomized trial.[392] However, the clinical significance of the results has been questioned and, along with other negative trials in the first- and second-line setting,[393,394] has not led to the approval of cetuximab in NSCLC. The ACCP guidelines do not recommend the addition of cetuximab to standard chemotherapy, but the NCCN guidelines suggest this is an option.[141,374] Preliminary results of a new monoclonal antibody, necitumumab, have been positive in patients with squamous cell histology, while negative in patients with adenocarcinoma.

First-Line Therapy with Targeted Agents

For patients whose tumors harbor an actionable molecular alteration, in particular EGFR-sensitizing mutations and anaplastic lymphoma kinase (ALK) rearrangement, first-line therapy with the corresponding targeted agent should be considered. Several trials have demonstrated that in patients with EGFR-mutated cancers, gefitinib, erlotinib, or afatinib yield superior response rates and longer PFS compared to standard chemotherapy, with a more favorable toxicity profile (Table 37.7).[395–399] Similarly, in patients with ALK-rearranged tumors, RCTs have confirmed the superiority of crizotinib over conventional chemotherapy.[400] However, none of the trials demonstrated a significant improvement in OS for the targeted agent compared to chemotherapy. Although this is often attributed to crossover upon progression, other explanations such as acquired resistance may also play a role.

Other trials have tested whether a combination of chemotherapy and a targeted agent is superior to either chemotherapy or the targeted agent alone in patients selected based on clinical characteristics without mutational testing.[401,402] None of these trials has demonstrated an advantage over the targeted agent, and the concurrent administration of chemotherapy and a TKI in first-line therapy is not recommended.

Importantly, patients without a known molecular alteration should not be treated with targeted agents in the first-line setting.[403] In patients who need immediate treatment and whose molecular profile is still pending, chemotherapy upfront is the best option until the results become available.

Patients treated with a targeted agent upfront are maintained until progression. At that point, depending on the nature and the tempo of the progression, options include local/ablative therapy to

TABLE 37.7

Chemotherapy Versus Targeted Therapy in First-Line Advanced Non–Small-Cell Lung Cancer

Target	Trial	N	Regimen	ORR (%)	PFS (mo)	MST (mo)	*P*
EGFR	NEJSG	228	Gefitinib	74	10.8	30.5	<0.001
			Carboplatin-paclitaxel	31	5.4	23.6	
	WJTOG	177	Gefitinib	62	9.2	36	<0.0001
			Cisplatin-docetaxel	32	6.3	39	
	Optimal	154	Erlotinib	83	13.1	22.7	<0.0001
			Carboplatin-gemcitibine	36	4.6	28.9	
	EURTAC		Erlotinib		9.7	19.3	
			Chemotherapy		5.2	19.5	
ALK	LUX Lung 3	345	Afatinib	56	6.9		0.001
			Cisplatin-pemetrexed	23	11.1		

ORR, objective response rate; PFS, progression-free survival; MST, median survival time; EGFR, epidermal growth factor receptor; NEJSG, North East Japan Study Group; WJTOG, West Japan Thoracic Oncology Group; EURTAC, EGFR mutation-positive non-small-cell lung cancer; ALK, anaplastic lymphoma kinase.

site(s) of oligoprogression and continuation of the targeted agent; change to a second generation inhibitor; and institution of chemotherapy, which can be done with or without continuation of the targeted agent.[404,405] Patients with EGFR-mutated tumors should be carefully monitored once the TKI is discontinued due to the risk of "flare," which can be severe and at times fatal.[406] It is recommended that once a change in therapy is decided, the washout period be limited to a minimum. Interestingly, patients later rechallenged with the same EGFR inhibitor often have prolonged periods of stabilization.

Maintenance Therapy

The continuation of the same combination chemotherapy regimen beyond four to six cycles yields no discernible benefit.[407–409] Assuming no evidence of progression, options at that juncture include close observation with treatment at progression or maintenance therapy. Continuation maintenance means that the nonplatinum agent used in the initial regimen is continued until disease progression. Another strategy is switch maintenance in which a new agent, one not used in the initial regimen, is initiated after the initial regimen. Both maintenance strategies have been shown to improve survival.

Continuation pemetrexed has led to an improvement in OS after four cycles of cisplatin-pemetrexed (Table 37.8).[410] A French trial also demonstrated an improvement in progression-free survival when gemcitabine was continued after four cycles of cisplatin-gemcitabine.[411] Continuation maintenance is also frequently used with bevacizumab based on the pivotal trial previously discussed,[156] despite the lack of randomized data demonstrating a benefit for maintenance versus no maintenance.

Switch maintenance therapy trials have shown a benefit for pemetrexed and erlotinib after four cycles of a platinum-based doublet (see Table 37.8).[412,413] A prior trial with docetaxel showed a progression-free survival advantage but the difference in OS, while clinically meaningful, did not reach statistical significance.[414] One criticism of these trials is that a relatively small percentage of patients randomized to the nonmaintenance arm actually received the same agent upon relapse.[415] In fact, in the Fidias trial,[414] a post hoc analysis of the patients who received this agent at the time of progression showed similar survival to those who received it as switch maintenance. This has led many thought leaders to interpret that switch maintenance is akin to early institution of second-line therapy.

Maintenance therapy must be discussed as an option rather than a universal recommendation. Several patients can be safely watched and benefit from a treatment break. On the other hand, a number of patients recur with devastating complications and miss the "window of opportunity" for second-line therapy. As of now, there are no clinical, radiographic, or biologic markers that predict outcome after first-line therapy. The ACCP and NCCN guidelines suggest maintenance pemetrexed in nonsquamous NSCLC, either as continuation maintenance if the patient is on a pemetrexed regimen, or switch maintenance if they are not.[141,374] Consideration of switch maintenance erlotinib is also suggested by both guidelines. The NCCN suggests continuation maintenance gemcitibine (category 2b), but the ACCP guideline recommends against it. However, it is clear that many factors must be considered in the decision, and clinical judgment is needed.

Second-Line Therapy

Multiple randomized trials have demonstrated that second-line therapy, with a noncross-resistant agent, leads to an improvement in survival compared to supportive care.[374] In addition, consistent improvement in QOL has been documented.[416,417] Cytotoxic agents used in this setting include docetaxel and pemetrexed.[379,418] Gemcitabine is also used in previously treated patients despite the lack of randomized data. Efficacy is similar among the chemotherapy agents, but toxicity profiles are somewhat different. EGFR TKIs have also shown benefit in this setting.[419] Erlotinib received its original approval for previously treated patients, unselected by molecular criteria, and still is used in this setting.

Recently trials have addressed whether conventional chemotherapy is preferable to erlotinib (or gefitinib where applicable) for EGFR wild-type patients in the second-line setting.[420–422] While only one trial showed an advantage with respect to OS, all trials showed a consistent trend toward better outcomes with chemotherapy. Based on these data, second-line chemotherapy is preferred for EGFR wild-type patients; erlotinib or gefitinib is usually used in these patients only after two lines of chemotherapy.

For patients whose tumors carry an EGFR mutation and who are treated with an inhibitor in the first-line setting, options at progression depend on the mechanism of resistance. The majority

CANCER OF THE THORACIC CAVITY

TABLE 37.8

Maintenance Chemotherapy

	Trial	Induction	Randomization	N	PFS	MST
Switch	Fidias	Cisplatin-gemcitabine	Immediate docetaxel	153	5.7	12.3
			Delayed docetaxel	156	2.7	9.7
	Ciuleanu[a]	Platinum doublet	Pemetrexed	441	4.5	15.5
			Placebo	222	2.6	10.3
	Capuzzo	Platinum doublet	Erlotinib	438	2.8	12
			Placebo	451	2.6	11
	Perol[b]	Cisplatin-gemcitabine	Erlotinib	155	2.9	11.4
			Observation	155	1.9	10.8
Continuation	Paz-Ares	Cisplatin-pemetrexed	Pemetrexed	539	4.1	13.9
			Placebo		2.8	11
	Perol[b]	Cisplatin-gemcitabine	Gemcitabine	154	3.8	12.1
			Observation	155	1.9	10.8

PFS, progression-free survival; MST, median survival time.
[a] Squamous subset.
[b] Three-arm trial: observation versus erlotinib versus gemcitabine.

of these patients have a secondary mutation, T790M, in exon 20, which shifts the affinity of the receptor preferentially to adenosine triphosphate.[423] Several new agents that target T790M are in development.[424] Other known mechanisms include conversion to a small-cell histology (usually responsive to platinum-etoposide combinations) and Her2 amplification.[405] A repeat biopsy at the time of progression is therefore advised to better guide the second-line therapy options. In addition, some patients with EGFR-mutated disease have an indolent or limited progression, including central nervous system involvement, which can be managed with local/ablative techniques, without discontinuation of the systemic therapy.[425]

Patients with ALK rearrangement also have multiple mechanisms of resistance, including de novo mutations.[426] While the same management principles apply to these patients, particularly those with indolent progression, the emergence of more specific second-generation ALK inhibitors, such as LDK 378, has become an appealing option.[427]

Third-Line Therapy

Contrary to second-line therapy, no randomized trial has shown a survival benefit for third-line therapy compared to placebo. The only agent approved for third-line therapy in the United States is erlotinib based on the same trial that led to the approval in second-line.[419] Candidates for third-line therapy were randomized to erlotinib or placebo, and those treated with the former experienced a survival benefit as well as improvement in symptom control of the same magnitude seen in second-line patients. Although no standard chemotherapy agent is formally approved for this indication, patients who have progressed on two prior lines and still maintain an acceptable PS are often treated in clinical practice with additional chemotherapy. The ACCP and NCCN guidelines recommend third-line treatment with erlotinib over basic supportive care in good PS patients.[141,374]

SPECIAL CLINICAL SITUATIONS

Oligometastases

In general, the presence of distant metastases indicates incurable disease that must be treated palliatively, usually by chemotherapy. However, a small subset of patients presents with a limited number (e.g., one to three) number of metastatic sites. This is called oligometastatic disease, and there is ample evidence that a curative intent treatment approach can be successful.

The greatest amount of data comes from patients with NSCLC and isolated brain metastases. Definitive treatment of brain metastases can be an important component of palliative-intent treatment, but in this section we focus on eradication of all known disease with intent to cure. The ACCP and NCCN guidelines recommend this be considered in NSCLC patients with isolated brain metastases.[141,295] A careful search (PET, brain MRI/CT) should be conducted to find evidence of more diffuse metastases. The number of brain metastases is not crucial as long as they can each be treated definitively.[295] Invasive mediastinal staging should be done; involvement of N2,3 nodes is considered a contraindication for curative-intent therapy.[141,295]

Treatment of patients with isolated brain metastases (T1-3N0-1M1b) generally begins with stereotactic radiosurgery or surgical resection of the brain metastases because of the devastating consequences of untreated brain lesions. Stereotactic radiosurgery and surgery for the brain metastases are complementary approaches with equivalent effectiveness; surgery is generally used with larger lesions that produce more mass effect and if the morbidity of a surgical approach is low. Curative resection of the primary lung tumor should follow the same principles dictated by the primary tumor regardless of the brain metastasis. Adjuvant chemotherapy is then recommended, although based only on indirect data of a benefit in earlier stage patients.[141,295] There is no data regarding the sequence (i.e., after treatment of the brain metastasis, whether to resect the lung lesion followed by chemotherapy or to administer chemotherapy and then later resect the lung primary). However, given the rapid recovery in general from modern (usually VATS) lung resection, it is probably best to get this accomplished before chemotherapy in general. Both the ACCP and NCCN recommend adjuvant whole-brain RT (WBRT) as well to decrease the chance of a brain recurrence; however, the data for the benefit of WBRT (for either survival or the rate of brain recurrences) is conflicting and indirect (not specific to oligometastatic tumors and curative-intent treatment).

Outcomes of curative-intent treatment of NSCLC with isolated brain oligometastases are reasonable. The surgical mortality from both resection of the brain lesion and the lung primary is about 2% in a recent systematic review.[295] The 5-year survival is about 15% on average.[295] The outcomes are the same whether patients present with a synchronous brain metastases or a metachronous brain metastasis that is found after a previous resection of an early stage NSCLC. Prognostic factors are poorly defined; outcomes may be slightly better in patients that are younger, have good PS, and have a lower T stage of the primary tumor.

There is data supporting a similar treatment approach for patients with isolated adrenal metastases.[141,295] The staging approach and treatment strategy is similar, although the urgency of treatment of the brain metastasis missing. Usually, the adrenal metastasis is treated by surgical resection (often laparoscopic) followed in about 2 weeks by lung resection (often by VATS). Both the ACCP and NCCN recommend adjuvant chemotherapy, but this is based on extrapolation from patients with other disease stages.[141,295]

A systematic review of outcomes found an average 5-year survival of 27% with curative-intent treatment of patients with NSCLC and isolated adrenal metastases.[295] Prognostic factors have not been defined. The outcomes appear to be similar for synchronous and metachronous presentations.

Limited data is available regarding curative-intent treatment of oligometastatic disease in other distant sites. However, reported outcomes are quite good (5-year survival of 32% to 86%).[295] The observation that outcomes are better for adrenal and other sites compared with brain oligometastatic disease probably simply reflects that clinicians have been more selective in choosing patients for curative-intent treatment involving nonbrain oligometastases. A prospective trial of aggressive curative-intent treatment for nonbrain oligometastatic disease found a median survival of only 11 months; however, this trial was not very selective and included many patients with N2 disease.[428]

Second Primary Lung Cancers, Additional Nodules, and Multifocal Lung Cancer

Patients with a lung cancer and additional nodules or lesions are challenging to manage. The additional lesion may be benign, may be a synchronous second primary lung cancer, one manifestation of systemic metastases, an additional nodule of cancer, or multifocal lung cancer. Appropriate categorization is difficult because the terms and definitions are ambiguous and the usage varies over time and between centers. The ACCP lung cancer guidelines have proposed a definition of terms and a structure for classification.[158,295] This structure is based on the clinical presentation rather than pathology, which makes it applicable at the time of clinical decision making. Table 37.9 provides a summary of the approach to patients with additional lesions according to the clinical presentation. The NCCN guidelines also address these patients, but without any clarity about how to classify them.[141]

A critical step for most of these patients is evaluation by a multidisciplinary team. One must be careful; often, there is tendency

TABLE 37.9

Approach to Patients with Additional Nodule(s)

Presentation	Data Summary	Initial Evaluation	Assessment	Categorization	Management
Typical solid cancer, additional nodule on CT, no clinical signs of distant disease[a]	Large majority are benign	Multidisciplinary team[b] discussion	Judged very likely benign	Benign lesion	Treatment of primary lung cancer, observation of nodule per Fleischner guidelines
Locally advanced NSCLC, nodule(s), and clinical signs of distant disease[a]	No formal data	PET and brain MRI/ CT Multidisciplinary team[b] discussion	Judged very likely stage IV	Stage IV	Stage IV treatment (i.e., chemotherapy)
			Judged unclear	Suspicious for Stage IV	Biopsy of nodule and other potential sites (N2,3 or M1b)
Typical solid cancer[c] and additional typical solid cancer[c]	~1.5% incidence	Thorough workup to rule out N2,3 or M1b Multidisciplinary team[b] discussion	Meets criteria for synchronous primaries if evaluation negative	Synchronous primaries	Manage each primary accordingly, and as patient will tolerate physiologically
Typical solid cancer and additional solid nodule	IASLC DB, but patients poorly defined, survival after resection better than for solitary M1b	Thorough workup to rule out N2,3 or M1b Multidisciplinary team[b] discussion	Judged unlikely to be synchronous second primary, but lesion suspected (or proven) malignant with same histology	Lung cancer with additional cancer nodule	Manage aggressively if T3 or T4 (consider resection), unclear if M1a (contralateral lung)
Lung cancer with GGO component and additional GGO (or semisolid) lesions	Indirect data, patients poorly defined	Multidisciplinary team[b] discussion	Fits pattern of multifocal disease	Multifocal lung cancer	Manage primary accordingly, and manage additional lesions according to guidelines for GGO

CT, computed tomography; NSCLC, non-small cell lung cancer; PET, positron emission tomography; MRI, magnetic resonance imaging; IASLC DB, International Association for the Study of Lung Cancer database; GGO, ground glass opacity.
[a] Fatigue, weight loss, anorexia, bone pain, neurologic symptoms.
[b] Team should include a chest radiologist, pulmonologist, and thoracic surgeon.
[c] Spiculated solid lesion.
Table modified from the Kozower B, Larner JM, Detterbeck FC, et al. Special treatment issues in non-small cell lung cancer: diagnosis and management of lung cancer, 3rd ed: American College of Chest Physicians evidence-based clinical practice guidelines *Chest* 2013;143:e369S–e399S.

to be swayed by the stage classification of additional nodules (e.g., $T3_{satell}$, $T4_{ipsi\ nod}$, or $M1a_{contra\ nod}$) and forget that many if not most patients belong in other categories. The classification of $T3_{satell}$, $T4_{ipsi\ nod}$, or $M1a_{contra\ nod}$ is explicitly contraindicated when dealing with a second primary lung cancer or patients with distant metastases from lung cancer.[55] It is particularly important to remember that, in patients with a clinical and radiographic presentation consistent with early stage lung cancer and an additional subcentimeter nodule on CT, the large majority of these nodules are benign.[295,429–431] Furthermore, identification of second primary lung cancers on clinical grounds has been quite accurate (as evidenced by survival outcomes), and these have most often been of the *same* cell type. Thus, it is clinical recognition and not necessarily a biopsy result that is critical to define second primary lung cancers. Because of these and other factors, the judgment of a multidisciplinary team is important in the evaluation of patients found to have additional lesions by CT.

Second primary lung cancers occur in about 5% of resected cases (either synchronous or metachronous presentation) and at a rate of about 1.5% per patient per year after curative treatment of a NSCLC. Approximately two-thirds of second primary lung cancers have been of the same histologic type; quite consistently the outcomes of tumors classified as second primary lung cancer based on different histology versus based on other features have been the same.[295] It is reasonable to consider the radiographic appearances in making a clinical determination of a second primary lung cancer. It has also been suggested to use molecular markers or the percentage of different subtypes of adenocarcinoma in making this determination, but this has not been extensively evaluated. All of the data available should be considered (clinical, radiographic, and pathologic) in making the determination whether a second focus of cancer is a second primary lung cancer or not.

When a synchronous second primary lung cancer is suspected, a careful search should be made for distant or mediastinal metastases as recommended by the ACCP and NCCN.[141,295] If this evaluation is negative, each primary cancer should be treated in the usual fashion for early stage cancer, provided the patient has adequate reserve. SBRT offers another treatment option. The vast majority of reported synchronous second primary lung cancers have been resected (often a limited resection); the 5-year survival after resection is approximately 25% for all and 40% if both tumors are stage pI (range, 0% to 79%).

A metachronous second primary lung cancer is best defined as a cancer with either a different histology or an interval of >4 years—in these situations, one can be fairly certain it is not a recurrence. A site of cancer of the same histologic type appearing within 2 years is most likely a metastasis, and between 2 and 4 years is a gray zone.[295] Once ~2 years have evolved, the stage of the initial NSCLC does not appear to affect the likelihood of recurrence versus new primary cancer. The judgment of a multidisciplinary team, taking all factors into account, is important in classifying the situation as a second primary lung cancer versus a recurrence.

The staging evaluation of a metachronous second primary lung cancer should generally proceed as dictated by the characteristics of the second primary tumor alone.[295] Most metachronous second primary cancers that are reported have been resected (often a limited resection); the 5-year survival after resection is approximately 30% for all and 40% for stage pI (range, 20% to 70%). No data is available regarding outcomes of unresected patients.[295]

Attention has been drawn to additional nodules ($T3_{satell}$, $T4_{ipsi\ nod}$, or $M1a_{contra\ nod}$) by the seventh edition of the lung cancer staging system.[293,294] The patients with additional nodules in the IASLC database were poorly defined, but specifically excluded those with second primary lung cancers or with distant metastases.[55] The additional nodules were probably recognized clinically in most cases (either pre- or intraoperatively) and proven pathologically to be of the same histologic type. The ACCP suggests that the additional nodule designations should be used for patients with a dominant "classic" lung cancer (i.e., solid, spiculated) and an additional solid nodule identified clinically or on pathologic examination.[158] It should be noted that most reports of patients with additional nodules of cancer have specifically excluded BAC because BAC is recognized to often present as multifocal disease. The ACCP clinically based definition effectively also excludes what was formerly called BAC pathologically from the cohort of patients classified as having additional nodules.

No additional diagnostic workup is recommended by the ACCP in patients with a secondary lesion in the same lobe ($T3_{satell}$). The data does not suggest a higher rate of occult distant or mediastinal metastases from what is predicted based on the dominant cancer, and the treatment recommendation is the same with or without an additional nodule in the same lobe (i.e., lobectomy).[295] The 5-year survival appears to be about 10% to 15% worse, stage for stage, with an additional nodule compared to the same dominant cancer without an additional nodule.[295,432] There does not appear to be a difference in survival whether there is one or several additional nodules.[295]

For additional nodules of cancer in a different lobe, the ACCP suggests a thorough search for distant disease (i.e., PET, brain MRI/CT) and invasive mediastinal staging, although direct data to support this stance is not available.[295] If there is no N2,3 or M1b disease, resection of both the dominant cancer and an ipsilateral, different lobe nodule is recommended. The reported 5-year survival for resection of such patients with ipsilateral, different lobe, additional nodules is ~20%.[295] The outcomes do appear to be better than if resection was not done. Much of the reported data comes from Asia, although there is no evidence of a geographic difference in outcomes in this cohort in the IASLC database. The survival appears to be worse if there is more than one additional ipsilateral, different lobe nodule, or with lymph node involvement.[295]

The ACCP also suggests resection of a contralateral additional nodule if thorough staging reveals no N2,3 or M1b involvement.[295] Very limited data is available on resected patients; in the IASLC database, 98% of patients were not resected, and survival was poor (5-year survival = 3%). This has been corroborated by other registry reports.[295]

Multifocal BAC was a well-recognized entity. The term BAC has been abandoned because it was used loosely in many different settings.[63] In the context of multifocal BAC, this was probably most often what would now be called a lepidic predominant invasive adenocarcinoma. The combination of abandonment of the term BAC and the seventh edition of the stage classification has left a void in how to classify multifocal lung cancer, which is still an entity that is regularly encountered. The ACCP has proposed a definition of multifocal lung cancer as multiple lesions arising from GGOs, which may develop a solid component.[158,295] This is a clinically focused definition, rather than one focused on particular pathologic findings; some of these lesions may be AAH, AIS, or MIA, but most are lepidic predominant invasive adenocarcinoma. A diffuse infiltrative pattern of disease (also called "pneumonic type" of adenocarcinoma) is also included in the ACCP definition. For stage classification, the ACCP recommends that the T(m) designation should be used for patients with multifocal lung cancer (a designation that has been used rarely in lung cancer although it has been part of the stage classification system for more than a decade).[158,293,294]

Multifocal lung cancer appears to have a decreased propensity for nodal or systemic spread and an increased propensity for additional pulmonary foci. The ACCP lung cancer guidelines therefore suggest that for multifocal lung cancer a search for distant or mediastinal metastases (i.e., PET, invasive mediastinal staging) is not necessary unless there is clinical suspicion.[295] Additionally, the rate of recurrence after resection, which has often been a limited resection, is low. Therefore, the ACCP guidelines suggest that a limited resection be performed of any multifocal lesions that are thought to be invasive cancer.[295] Lesions that are thought not to be invasive cancer (i.e., pure GGO) should generally be followed, because most of these appear to remain stable, at least for many years.[119,151,295] Adjuvant therapy for R0 resected patients without nodal involvement is not recommended.

The published outcomes for resected patients with multifocal disease have been quite good (5-year survival of approximately 90%; range, 64% to 100%).[295]

PALLIATIVE CARE

Role of Palliative Care

A large number of patients with lung cancer will develop symptoms related to their disease. Metastases to the brain and spinal column may threaten significant neurologic compromise; airway obstruction or SVC syndrome may present urgently or with milder symptoms that progress to become severe if left untreated. And more common, less acutely severe, symptoms such as pain, dyspnea, cough, anorexia, or fatigue can significantly impact QOL, and may preclude cancer-directed therapy.[433] The importance of palliative efforts in lung cancer care was highlighted in an RCT involving 151 patients with metastatic NSCLC who received standard oncologic treatment and were randomized to receive early palliative care or not.[434] In patients who received early palliative care, there was a significant improvement in QOL and fewer depressive symptoms. Because the care mode resulted in better documentation of end-of-life preferences, patients receiving early palliative care were less likely to have aggressive resuscitation efforts and less likely to receive chemotherapy in favor of hospice care. Despite this, the authors also observed significantly improved OS (median, 11.6 months versus 8.9 months). While unexpected, this finding is consistent with prior studies that demonstrated shorter survival in patients with more severe depressed mood and worse QOL.[435] These results suggest a model for improving patient mood and QOL during cancer care, and validate the importance of the early initiation of such efforts.

Specific Symptom Management

Airway obstruction is common in patients with lung cancer, as a result of tumor mass effect, bleeding, or mucous production.[433] Therapeutic bronchoscopy is appropriate for evaluation, with interventions including mechanical disimpaction, brachytherapy, ablation, or stenting. Hemoptysis responds well to ablation with laser or electrocautery, and brachytherapy or external beam radiation may also be considered. A cough can be the direct result of malignancy, or due to secondary infection, or chemotherapy- or RT-induced pneumonitis. Evaluation and treatment for the latter etiologies should be considered, and otherwise cough suppression with opioids is appropriate. Malignant effusions, if symptomatic, respond to tunneled pleural catheters when the lung can be re-expanded. Pleurodeisis can be pursued for recurrent effusions, via talc slurry or poudrage.[433]

Pain, whether due to bone or soft tissue disease, is one of the most common symptoms of lung cancer. Nonsteroidal anti-inflammatory drugs should be prescribed to all patients, unless contraindicated, and, for those who require chronic medication, appropriate gastrointestinal prophylaxis (i.e., misprostol, H2 antagonists, or proton pump inhibitors) should be added. For those patients who have a neuropathic component to their pain, the addition of an anticonvulsant or tricycylic antidepressant improves pain control. For moderate to severe pain, morphine or an alternative narcotic is recommended.[433]

Bony metastases without pathologic fracture or significant structural weakness can be managed with short-course RT and bisphosphonates. Patients with pathologic fractures, or with focal lytic lesions that involve >50% of the cortex of weight-bearing bones, should undergo surgical fixation to prevent debilitating injury, followed by RT. Vertebral compression fractures with instability can be stabilized surgically or through augmentation procedures.

Epidural spinal cord compression (ESCC) is one of the most serious complications of metastatic cancer. The most common presenting symptom is local pain, with or without radicular component.[439,437] A bony metastatic lesion arising in the vertebral body can extend directly into the epidural space, impinging upon the spinal cord or cauda equina, or an induced vertebral compression fracture may retropulse bony fragments into the same space. Progressive pressure on the cord or nerve roots can lead to edema, ischemia, and irreversible neurologic compromise. MRI is the primary diagnostic intervention, although CT myelography may also demonstrate the characteristic impingement on the thecal sac. Additional plain films or CT imaging may be required to differentiate soft tissue extension from bony retropulsion. Corticosteroids should be administered as early as feasible. A small, single-blind randomized study of corticosteroids showed that the addition of dexamethasone to RT improved ambulation, an effect that was durable to 6 months (59% versus 33% remained ambulatory), without an effect on survival.[438] The doses administered were higher than are typically used in the modern era, 96 mg intravenously followed by 96 mg/day and tapered over 10 days. Lower doses are typically used in an effort to avoid steroid-related complications.

Surgical or augmentation procedures are indicated for ESCC when there is spinal instability or the cause of the cord impingement is bony in nature. For symptoms caused by direct tumor compression, either surgical intervention or local RT may be appropriate. Evidence suggests that neurologic compromise of short duration is more apt to be meaningfully reversed by surgery than symptoms that have been present for longer duration.[439] Patchell et al.[439] conducted a randomized trial of surgery versus RT (30 Gy in 10 fractions) in 101 patients with symptomatic ESCC, all with neurologic symptoms of <2 days duration. Patients who underwent surgery were more likely to have symptomatic relief (62% versus 19%), more likely to ambulate (84% versus 57%), and had better OS (median, 126 days versus 100 days), clearly indicating that surgery should be strongly considered in patients with ESCC, particularly those with neurologic signs and symptoms of relatively acute onset. RT as primary treatment offers reasonable palliation of pain, but is highly unlikely to restore ambulation or otherwise reverse neurologic compromise.

Lung cancer accounts for approximately half of all brain metastases. Historically, survival after diagnosis of brain metastases is poor; a median of 6 months in the most robust candidates (i.e., those of young age, good PS, and brain-only disease).[440] In patients with NSCLC, significant prognostic factors for survival in patients with brain metastases include age, PS, the presence of extracranial metastases, and the number of brain metastases.[441] The increased availability of active systemic therapy and targeted agents options has resulted in a subset of patients with brain metastases whose survival is significantly longer, increasing the importance of selecting the appropriate brain-directed therapy to maximize control and minimize potential long-term morbidity.

Brain metastases are often accompanied by significant surrounding cerebral edema, and the latter is the most common cause of symptoms such as headache, nausea, vomiting, and ataxia. Steroids with predominant glucocorticoid activity, such as dexamethasone, are commonly used to address symptomatic patients, and can partially or completely relieve symptoms in otherwise untreated patients for several weeks. There is no evidence to suggest that steroid treatment of asymptomatic patients confers any benefit. For patients with severe symptoms due to mass effect or edema that are not amenable to steroid treatment, consideration should be given to surgical decompression. Noninvasive therapies such as radiosurgery or WBRT are unlikely to acutely improve symptoms.

WBRT was the standard-of-care approach to most patients with brain metastases for several decades, since a randomized trial demonstrated a 40% improvement in OS when compared to steroid treatment and supportive care alone.[442] Because WBRT can lead to significant fatigue and somnolence in the short term, and permanent neurocognitive deficits in the late term, patients with less bulky disease or those with an expectation of more prolonged survival are frequently treated with surgery or radiosurgery in place of whole-brain treatment.

For patients with a single brain metastasis, surgery or radiosurgery, either with our without WBRT, has become the standard-of-care approach. A landmark pair of studies by Patchell et al.[443,444] established the separate roles of resection and WBRT in this setting. In the first trial, 84 patients with a solitary brain metastasis were randomized to surgical resection followed by WBRT or WBRT alone.[443] The OS was significantly longer in the surgical arm (45 weeks versus 40 weeks), reflecting the marked benefit of local therapy for patients with good PS. The use of radiosurgery in place of surgery in patients with a solitary lesion also improves OS when given in addition to WBRT in a parallel fashion.[445] The companion study from Patchell et al addressed the role of WBRT.[444] In this trial, 95 patients with a solitary metastatic lesion underwent surgery, and then were randomized to WBRT or no further therapy. The addition of WBRT significantly improved local control of the resected lesion, reduced "elsewhere" failures in the brain, but did not improve OS.[444] The significant reduction in brain recurrence seen in this study has been cited to support the routine use of WBRT after surgery or radiosurgery to a solitary brain metastasis, but the lack of any survival benefit has also been cited to suggest that active surveillance after local therapy is a reasonable approach.

Patients with one to three brain metastases may be treated with radiosurgery alone, WBRT, or both in combination. The value of radiosurgery in this population was established in the RTOG 9508,[445] in which 333 patients with one to three metastases were randomized to either WBRT alone or WBRT followed by radiosurgery. In the subset of patients with a single metastasis, the addition of radiosurgery improved OS, consistent with the Patchell trial of surgical resection in the setting of WBRT. Patients with two or three lesions who received radiosurgery in addition to WBRT had better PS at 6 months posttreatment, but no incremental survival benefit. Withholding WBRT in these patients and treating them with radiosurgery alone is predicated on avoiding the neurocognitive sequelae of WBRT. In a small randomized trial, Chang et al.[446] answered the question of whether WBRT could be avoided, randomizing patients with one to three brain metastases to either radiosurgery alone or radiosurgery and WBRT. The trial was stopped early when an interim analysis demonstrated an OS benefit to withholding WBRT. This finding was not consistent with prior surgical data and could be due to the increased opportunity to deliver subsequent chemotherapy in patients who did not have WBRT, or could be simply an anomalous finding in a relatively small study population. The clear and consistent result was that neurocognitive function was significantly better when WBRT was withheld.

In patients with poor PS or extensive extracranial disease, WBRT is appropriately the treatment of choice. In patients with more than five brain metastases, good PS, and limited extracranial disease, the role of WBRT versus stereotactic radiosurgery is ill-defined.[447] Several efforts are currently under way to determine the optimal treatment for this population.

SVC syndrome may have various neoplastic and nonneoplastic causes. Bronchogenic carcinoma is the most common cause of SVC syndrome, underlying approximately 80% of cases at diagnosis.[448] When the SVC becomes obstructed, blood returns to the heart through collateral vessels via the azygous vein or inferior vena cava. Venous collaterals dilate over weeks, compensating for the loss of SVC patency. Upper body venous pressure and resulting edema of the arm and face decrease over time, so that symptoms with sudden onset, from acute obstruction, can diminish over several weeks even without intervention. The severity of the symptoms is due not only to the degree of SVC narrowing, but also to the rapidity with which it develops. The characteristic signs include cyanosis, plethora, distention of subcutaneous veins, and edema of the head, neck, and arm. Patients may develop dyspnea and cough. In rare cases, severe and acute obstruction can result in cerebral edema or laryngeal stridor. The specific cause of SVC syndrome in a patient with known malignancy may be extrinsic compression from tumor mass or due to thrombus in the setting of hypercoagulability. Even in the case of malignant, extrinsic compression, the clinical course may be complicated by the subsequent development of a thrombus in the SVC or brachiocephalic vein, or the simultaneous tumor mass effect on the bronchi or heart.

Traditionally, SVC syndrome was viewed as a medical emergency, but accumulating experience demonstrates that the course of SVC is rarely life-threatening. In a review of 107 patients in whom intervention was withheld during evaluation, there were no serious consequences to deferring treatment until diagnosis and staging was completed.[449] The symptoms often improve without active intervention, as collateral vessels dilate.[450] Immediate intervention is warranted when symptoms are life threatening (e.g., cerebral edema leading to altered mental status, stridor, or clinically significant hemodynamic compromise). When urgent intervention is indicated, intravascular stenting provides the most immediate relief. In the absence of life-threatening symptoms, the patient should be appropriately staged, biopsied, and the underlying malignancy treated in a manner appropriate for its stage and presentation. Patients with metastatic SCLC and SVC syndrome will likely respond to systemic therapy, which may be more appropriate than the initiation of urgent radiation. Patients with limited-stage SCLC and SVC syndrome should respond rapidly to chemoradiotherapy, or induction chemotherapy if that can be started more promptly. Patients with NSCLC and SVC syndrome are less likely to respond quickly to either chemotherapy or radiation, and so the threshold for placing an endovascular stent is somewhat lower. SVC syndrome is a poor prognostic factor in NSCLC, with a median survival from presentation of 5 months.[451]

CONCLUSION

Lung still remains by far the leading cause of cancer deaths. The blame, guilt, and nihilism that stems from the relationship of smoking to lung cancer continues to be an issue, despite a better understanding of smoking as an addiction and the fact that most patients diagnosed will have quit smoking many years earlier. However, lung cancer has become a dynamic and vibrant field. Screening is able to reduce the rate of lung cancer deaths by decreasing the proportion that is diagnosed with advanced disease. Major improvements have been made in all treatment modalities: minimally invasive surgery, better RT targeting and delivery, and a diverse array of chemotherapeutic agents and methods of palliation of many symptoms. There have also been advances in epidemiology (focusing on more than simply smoking), in imaging, in accurate definition of the stage, and on understanding some of the biologic and genetic alterations encountered. Many questions remain, but there is no question that lung cancer is a dynamic, challenging, and exciting area in which much progress is being made.

REFERENCES

1. GLOBOCAN 2012: Estimated Cancer Incidence, Mortality and Prevalence Worldwide in 2012. Lung Cancer [database on the Internet]. International Agency for Research on Cancer, World Health Organization. 2013 [cited January 8, 2014]. http://globocan.iarc.fr/Pages/fact_sheets_cancer.aspx.
2. Siegel R, Naishadham D, Jemal A. Cancer statistics, 2013. *CA Cancer J Clin* 2013;63:11–30.
3. Tong L, Spitz MR, Fueger JJ, et al. Lung carcinoma in former smokers. *Cancer* 1996;78:1004–1010.
4. Garces YI, Yang P, Parkinson J, et al. The relationship between cigarette smoking and quality of life after lung cancer diagnosis. *Chest* 2004;126:1733–1741.
5. Visbal AL, Williams BA, Nichols FC 3rd, et al. Gender differences in non-small-cell lung cancer survival: an analysis of 4,618 patients diagnosed between 1997 and 2002. *Ann Thorac Surg* 2004;78:209–215, discussion 215.
6. Adler I. *Primary Malignant Growth of the Lung and Bronchi*. New York, NY: Longman, Green Company; 1912.
7. Ochsner A, DeBakey M. Carcinoma of the lung. *Arch Surg* 1941;42:209–258.
8. Doll R, Hill AB. Smoking and carcinoma of the lung; preliminary report. *Br Med J* 1950;2:739–748.
9. Wynder EL, Graham EA. Tobacco smoking as a possible etiologic factor in bronchiogenic carcinoma; a study of 684 proved cases. *JAMA* 1950;143:329–336.
10. *Smoking and Health: Summary of a Report of the Royal College of Physicians of London on Smoking in Relation to Cancer of the Lung and Other Diseases*. London, UK: Pitman Medical Publishing; 1962.
11. US Public Health Service. *Smoking and Health. Report of the Advisory Committee to the Surgeon General for the Public Health Service*. Publication No. 1103. Washington, DC: US Department of Health, Education, and Welfare, Public Health Service; 1964.
12. Burns DM, Anderson CM, Gray N. Has the lung cancer risk from smoking increased over the last fifty years? *Cancer Causes Control* 2011;22:389–397.
13. Rodgman A, Smith CJ, Perfetti TA. The composition of cigarette smoke: a retrospective, with emphasis on polycyclic components. *Hum Exp Toxicol* 2000;19:573–595.
14. Smith CJ, Perfetti TA, Mullens MA, et al. "IARC group 2B Carcinogens" reported in cigarette mainstream smoke. *Food Chem Toxicol* 2000;38:825–848.
15. Smith CJ, Perfetti TA, Rumple MA, et al. "IARC group 2A Carcinogens" reported in cigarette mainstream smoke. *Food Chem Toxicol* 2000;38:371–383.
16. Hoffmann D, Djordjevic MV, Rivenson A, et al. A study of tobacco carcinogenesis. LI. Relative potencies of tobacco-specific N-nitrosamines as inducers of lung tumours in A/J mice. *Cancer Lett* 1993;71:25–30.
17. Belinsky SA, Devereux TR, Maronpot RR, et al. Relationship between the formation of promutagenic adducts and the activation of the K-ras protooncogene in lung tumors from A/J mice treated with nitrosamines. *Cancer Res* 1989;49:5305–5311.
18. Eccles R. Menthol and related cooling compounds. *J Pharm Pharmacol* 1994; 46:618–630.
19. Brooks DR, Palmer JR, Strom BL, et al. Menthol cigarettes and risk of lung cancer. *Am J Epidemiol* 2003;158:609–616, discussion 617–620.
20. Peto R, Darby S, Deo H, et al. Smoking, smoking cessation, and lung cancer in the UK since 1950: combination of national statistics with two case-control studies. *BMJ* 2000;321:323–329.
21. Samet JM, Avila-Tang E, Boffetta P, et al. Lung cancer in never smokers: clinical epidemiology and environmental risk factors. *Clin Cancer Res* 2009;15: 5626–2645.
22. Sun S, Schiller JH, Gazdar AF. Lung cancer in never smokers—a different disease. *Nat Rev Cancer* 2007;7:778–790.
23. Takemiya M, Shiraishi S, Teramoto T, et al. Bloom's syndrome with porokeratosis of Mibelli and multiple cancers of the skin, lung and colon. *Clin Genet* 1987;31:35–44.
24. Bailey-Wilson JE, Amos CI, Pinney SM, et al. A major lung cancer susceptibility locus maps to chromosome 6q23-25. *Am J Hum Genet* 2004;75:460–474.
25. Spitz MR, Wei Q, Dong Q, et al. Genetic susceptibility to lung cancer: the role of DNA damage and repair. *Cancer Epidemiol Biomarkers Prev* 2003;12:689–698.
26. Zhou W, Liu G, Thurston SW, et al. Genetic polymorphisms in N-acetyltransferase-2 and microsomal epoxide hydrolase, cumulative cigarette smoking, and lung cancer. *Cancer Epidemiol Biomarkers Prev* 2002;11:15–21.

27. Ye Z, Song H, Higgins JP, et al. Five glutathione s-transferase gene variants in 23,452 cases of lung cancer and 30,397 controls: meta-analysis of 130 studies. *PLoS Med* 2006;3(4):e91.
28. Lissowska J, Foretova L, Dabek J, et al. Family history and lung cancer risk: international multicentre case-control study in Eastern and Central Europe and meta-analyses. *Cancer Causes Control* 2010;21:1091–1104.
29. Cassidy A, Myles JP, van Tongeren M, et al. The LLP risk model: an individual risk prediction model for lung cancer. *Br J Cancer* 2008;98:270–276.
30. De Matteis S, Consonni D, Bertazzi PA. Exposure to occupational carcinogens and lung cancer risk. Evolution of epidemiological estimates of attributable fraction. *Acta Biomed* 2008;79:34–42.
31. Doll R. Mortality from lung cancer in asbestos workers. *Br J Ind Med* 1955; 12:81–86.
32. Markowitz SB, Levin SM, Miller A, et al. Asbestos, asbestosis, smoking, and lung cancer. New findings from the North American insulator cohort. *Am J Respir Crit Care Med* 2013;188:90–96.
33. Lubin JH, Boice JD Jr, Edling C, et al. Lung cancer in radon-exposed miners and estimation of risk from indoor exposure. *J Natl Cancer Inst* 1995;87: 817–827.
34. Krewski D, Lubin JH, Zielinski JM, et al. Residential radon and risk of lung cancer: a combined analysis of 7 North American case-control studies. *Epidemiology* 2005;16:137–145.
35. Darby S, Hill D, Auvinen A, et al. Radon in homes and risk of lung cancer: collaborative analysis of individual data from 13 European case-control studies. *BMJ* 2005;330:223.
36. US Environmental Protection Agency. *Technical Support Document for the 1992 Citizen's Guide to Radon*. Washington, DC: US Environmental Protection Agency; 1992.
37. Shimizu Y, Kato H, Schull WJ. Studies of the mortality of A-bomb survivors. 9. Mortality, 1950-1985: Part 2. Cancer mortality based on the recently revised doses (DS86). *Radiat Res* 1990;121:120–141.
38. Darby SC, Doll R, Gill SK, et al. Long term mortality after a single treatment course with X-rays in patients treated for ankylosing spondylitis. *Br J Cancer* 1987;55:179–190.
39. Davis FG, Boice JD Jr, Hrubec Z, et al. Cancer mortality in a radiation-exposed cohort of Massachusetts tuberculosis patients. *Cancer Res* 1989;49:6130–6136.
40. Epstein DM, Gefter WB, Miller WT. Lobar bronchioloalveolar cell carcinoma. *Am J Radiol* 1982;139:463–466.
41. Bain C, Feskanich D, Speizer FE, et al. Lung cancer rates in men and women with comparable histories of smoking. *J Natl Cancer Inst* 2004;96: 826–834.
42. Gallicchio L, Boyd K, Matanoski G, et al. Carotenoids and the risk of developing lung cancer: a systematic review. *Am J Clin Nutr* 2008;88:372–383.
43. Lam TK, Gallicchio L, Lindsley K, et al. Cruciferous vegetable consumption and lung cancer risk: a systematic review. *Cancer Epidemiol Biomarkers Prev* 2009;18:184–195.
44. Tardon A, Lee WJ, Delgado-Rodriguez M, et al. Leisure-time physical activity and lung cancer: a meta-analysis. *Cancer Causes Control* 2005;16:389–397.
45. Mannino DM, Aguayo SM, Petty TL, et al. Low lung function and incident lung cancer in the United States: data from the First National Health and Nutrition Examination Survey follow-up. *Arch Intern Med* 2003;163:1475–1480.
46. Turner MC, Chen Y, Krewski D, et al. Chronic obstructive pulmonary disease is associated with lung cancer mortality in a prospective study of never smokers. *Am J Respir Crit Care Med* 2007;176:285–290.
47. Siemes C, Visser LE, Coebergh JW, et al. C-reactive protein levels, variation in the C-reactive protein gene, and cancer risk: the Rotterdam Study. *J Clin Oncol* 2006;24:5216–5222.
48. Yang SR, Chida AS, Bauter MR, et al. Cigarette smoke induces proinflammatory cytokine release by activation of NF-kappaB and posttranslational modifications of histone deacetylase in macrophages. *Am J Physiol Lung Cell Mol Physiol* 2006;291:L46–L57.
49. Yang P, Sun Z, Krowka MJ, et al. Alpha1-antitrypsin deficiency carriers, tobacco smoke, chronic obstructive pulmonary disease, and lung cancer risk. *Arch Intern Med* 2008;168:1097–1103.
50. Hubbard R, Venn A, Lewis S, et al. Lung cancer and cryptogenic fibrosing alveolitis. A population-based cohort study. *Am J Respir Crit Care Med* 2000;161:5–8.
51. Le Jeune I, Gribbin J, West J, et al. The incidence of cancer in patients with idiopathic pulmonary fibrosis and sarcoidosis in the UK. *Respir Med* 2007;101:2534–2540.
52. Goldstraw P, Crowley J, Chansky K, et al. The IASLC Lung Cancer Staging Project: proposals for the revision of the TNM stage groupings in the forthcoming (seventh) edition of the TNM Classification of malignant tumours. *J Thorac Oncol* 2007;2:706–714.
53. Rami-Porta R, Ball D, Crowley J, et al. The IASLC Lung Cancer Staging Project: proposals for the revision of the T descriptors in the forthcoming (seventh) edition of the TNM classification for lung cancer. *J Thorac Oncol* 2007;2:593–602.
54. Rusch VW, Crowley J, Giroux DJ, et al. The IASLC Lung Cancer Staging Project: proposals for the revision of the N descriptors in the forthcoming seventh edition of the TNM classification for lung cancer. *J Thorac Oncol* 2007;2:603–612.
55. Postmus PE, Brambilla E, Chansky K, et al. The IASLC Lung Cancer Staging Project: proposals for revision of the M descriptors in the forthcoming (seventh) edition of the TNM classification of lung cancer. *J Thorac Oncol* 2007;2:686–693.
56. Goldstraw P, Crowley J. The International Association for the Study of Lung Cancer International Staging Project on Lung Cancer. *J Thorac Oncol* 2006;1:281–286.
57. Shepherd FA, Crowley J, Van Houtte P, et al. The International Association for the Study of Lung Cancer lung cancer staging project: proposals regarding the clinical staging of small cell lung cancer in the forthcoming (seventh) edition of the tumor, node, metastasis classification for lung cancer. *J Thorac Oncol* 2007;2:1067–1077.
58. Travis WD, Giroux DJ, Chansky K, et al. The IASLC Lung Cancer Staging Project: proposals for the inclusion of broncho-pulmonary carcinoid tumors in the forthcoming (seventh) edition of the TNM Classification for Lung Cancer. *J Thorac Oncol* 2008;3:1213–1223.
59. Detterbeck F, Tanoue L, Boffa DJ. The new lung cancer staging system. *Chest* 2009;136:260–271.
60. Govindan R, Page N, Morgensztern D, et al. Changing epidemiology of small-cell lung cancer in the United States over the last 30 years: analysis of the surveillance, epidemiologic, and end results database. *J Clin Oncol* 2006;24:4539–4544.
61. Detterbeck FC. Maintaining aim at a moving target. *J Thor Oncol* 2011;6: 417–422.
62. Clinical Lung Cancer Genome Project (CLCGP), Network Genomic Medicine (NGM). A genomics-based classification of human lung tumors. *Sci Transl Med* 2013;5:209ra153.
63. Travis WD, Brambilla E, Noguchi M, et al. International Association for the Study of Lung Cancer/American Thoracic Society/European Respiratory Society: international multidisciplinary classification of lung adenocarcinoma. *J Thorac Oncol* 2011;6:244–285.
64. Travis WD, Brambilla E, Muller-Hernlink HD, et al., eds. *Pathology and Genetics of Tumours of the Lung, Pleura, Thymus and Heart*. Lyon, France: IARC Press; 2004.
65. Hanahan D, Weinberg RA. Hallmarks of cancer: the next generation. *Cell* 2011;144:646–674.
66. Hanahan D, Weinberg RA. The hallmarks of cancer. *Cell* 2000;100:57–70.
67. Imielinski M, Berger AH, Hammerman PS, et al. Mapping the hallmarks of lung adenocarcinoma with massively parallel sequencing. *Cell* 2012;150: 1107–1120.
68. Detterbeck FC. Stage classification and prognosis: an intersection of medicine, quantum physics and religion? *Thorax* 2011;66:1016–1017.
69. Detterbeck FC. Stage classification and prediction of prognosis: difference between accountants and speculators. *J Thor Oncol* 2013;8:820–822.
70. Chansky K, Sculier J, Crowley J, et al. The International Association for the Study of Lung Cancer Staging Project: prognostic factors and pathologic TNM stage in surgically managed non-small cell lung cancer. *J Thorac Oncol* 2009;4:792–801.
71. Brennan P, Crispo A, Zaridze D, et al. High cumulative risk of lung cancer death among smokers and nonsmokers in Central and Eastern Europe. *Am J Epidemiol* 2006;164:1233–1241.
72. World Health Organization. *WHO Framework Convention on Tobacco Control*. Geneva, Switzerland: World Health Organization; 2007.
73. Hammond D, Fong GT, Borland R, et al. Text and graphic warnings on cigarette packages: findings from the international tobacco control four country study. *Am J Prev Med* 2007;32:202–209.
74. Wright AA, Katz IT. Tobacco tightrope—balancing disease prevention and economic development in China. *N Engl J Med* 2007;356:1493–1496.
75. Public Law 111-31 June 22, 2009. Family Smoking Prevention and Tobacco Control Act.
76. Leone F, Evers-Casey S, Toll B, et al. Treatment of tobacco use in lung cancer: diagnosis and management of lung cancer, 3rd ed: American College of Chest Physicians evidence-based clinical practice guidelines. *Chest* 2013;143: e61S–e77S.
77. Trousse D, Barlesi F, Loundou A, et al. Synchronous multiple primary lung cancer: an increasing clinical occurrence requiring multidisciplinary management. *J Thorac Cardiovasc Surg* 2007;133:1193–1200.
78. Tucker MA, Murray N, Shaw EG, et al. Second primary cancers related to smoking and treatment of small-cell lung cancer. *J Natl Cancer Inst* 1997;89:1782–1788.
79. Johnson BE. Second lung cancers in patients after treatment for an initial lung cancer. *J Natl Cancer Inst* 1998;90:1335–1345.
80. Omenn GS, Goodman GE, Thornquist MD, et al. Effects of a combination of beta carotene and vitamin A on lung cancer and cardiovascular disease. *N Engl J Med* 1996;334:1150–1155.
81. The effect of vitamin E and beta carotene on the incidence of lung cancer and other cancers in male smokers. The Alpha-Tocopherol, Beta Carotene Cancer Prevention Study Group. *N Engl J Med* 1994;330:1029–1035.
82. Virtamo J, Pietinen P, Huttunen JK, et al. Incidence of cancer and mortality following alpha-tocopherol and beta-carotene supplementation: a postintervention follow-up. *JAMA* 2003;290:476–485.
83. Hennekens CH, Buring JE, Manson JE, et al. Lack of effect of long-term supplementation with beta carotene on the incidence of malignant neoplasms and cardiovascular disease. *N Engl J Med* 1996;334:1145–1149.
84. Szabo E, Mao JT, Lam S, et al. Chemoprevention of lung cancer: diagnosis and management of lung cancer, 3rd ed: American College of Chest Physicians evidence-based clinical practice guidelines. *Chest* 2013;143:e40S–e60S.
85. Marcus PM, Bergstralh EJ, Zweig MH, et al. Extended lung cancer incidence follow-up in the Mayo Lung Project and overdiagnosis. *J Natl Cancer Inst* 2006;98:748–756.

86. Doria-Rose VP, Marcus PM, Szabo E, et al. Randomized controlled trials of the efficacy of lung cancer screening by sputum cytology revisited: a combined mortality analysis from the Johns Hopkins Lung Project and the Memorial Sloan-Kettering Lung Study. *Cancer* 2009;115:5007–5017.
87. Melamed MR, Flehinger BJ, Zaman MB, et al. Screening for early lung cancer. Results of the Memorial Sloan-Kettering study in New York. *Chest* 1984;86:44–53.
88. Fontana RS, Sanderson DR, Woolner LB, et al. Screening for lung cancer. A critique of the Mayo Lung Project. *Cancer* 1991;67:1155–1164.
89. Kubik A, Parkin DM, Khlat M, et al. Lack of benefit from semi-annual screening for cancer of the lung: follow-up report of a randomized controlled trial on a population of high-risk males in Czechoslovakia. *Int J Cancer* 1990;45:26–33.
90. Manser RL, Irving LB, Stone C, et al. Screening for lung cancer. *Cochrane Database Syst Rev* 2004;(1):CD001991.
91. Oken MM, Hocking WG, Kvale PA, et al. Screening by chest radiograph and lung cancer mortality: the Prostate, Lung, Colorectal, and Ovarian (PLCO) randomized trial. *JAMA* 2011;306:1865–1873.
92. Aberle D, Adams A, Berg C, et al. Reduced lung-cancer mortality with low-dose computed romographic screening. *N Eng J Med* 2011;365:395–409.
93. Infante M, Cavuto S, Lutman FR, et al. A randomized study of lung cancer screening with spiral computed tomography. *Am J Respir Crit Care Med* 2009;180:445–453.
94. Saghir Z, Dirksen A, Ashraf H, et al. CT screening for lung cancer brings forward early disease. The randomised Danish Lung Cancer Screening Trial: status after five annual screening rounds with low-dose CT. *Thorax* 2012;67: 296–301.
95. Pastorino U, Rossi M, Rosato V, et al. Annual or biennial CT screening versus observation in heavy smokers: 5-year results of the MILD trial. *Eur J Cancer Prev* 2012;21:308–315.
96. Bach PB, Mirkin JN, Oliver TK, et al. Benefits and harms of CT screening for lung cancer: a systematic review. *JAMA* 2012;307:2418–2429.
97. Detterbeck FC, Mazzone PJ, Naidich DP, et al. Screening for lung cancer: diagnosis and management of lung cancer, 3rd ed: American College of Chest Physicians evidence-based clinical practice guidelines. *Chest* 2013;143: e78S–e92S.
98. Jaklitsch MT, Jacobson FL, Austin JH, et al. The American Association for Thoracic Surgery guidelines for lung cancer screening using low-dose computed tomography scans for lung cancer survivors and other high-risk groups. *J Thorac Cardiovasc Surg* 2012;144:33–38.
99. Rocco G, Allen M, Altorki N, et al. Clinical statement on the role of the surgeon and surgical issues relating to CT screening programs for lung cancer: Report from The Society of Thoracic Surgeons CT Screening for Lung Cancer Task Force. *Ann Thorac Surg* 2013;96:357–360.
100. Wood D, Eapen G, Ettinger D, et al. Lung cancer screening. *J Natl Compr Canc Netw* 2011;10:240–265.
101. Moyer V, U.S. Preventive Services Task Force. Screening for lung cancer: U.S. Preventive Services Task Force recommendation statement. *Ann Intern Med* 2014;160:330–338.
102. de Koning H, Meza R, Plevritis S, et al. *Benefits and Harms of Computed Tomography Lung Cancer Screening Programs for High-Risk Populations*. AHRQ Publication No. 13-05196-EF-2. Rockville, MD: Agency for Healthcare Research and Quality; 2013.
103. Detterbeck F, Gibson C. Turning gray: the natural history of lung cancer over time. *J Thorac Oncol* 2008;3:781–792.
104. Detterbeck FC. Cancer, concepts, cohorts and complexity: avoiding oversimplification of overdiagnosis. *Thorax* 2012;67:842–845.
105. Bach PB, Gould MK. When the average applies to no one: personalized decision making about potential benefits of lung cancer screening. *Ann Intern Med* 2012;157:571–573.
106. Tammemagi MC, Katki HA, Hocking WG, et al. Selection criteria for lung-cancer screening. *N Engl J Med* 2013;368:728–736.
107. Spitz MR, Hong WK, Amos CI, et al. A risk model for prediction of lung cancer. *J Natl Cancer Inst* 2007;99:715–726.
108. Bach PB, Kattan MW, Thornquist MD, et al. Variations in lung cancer risk among smokers. *J Natl Cancer Inst* 2003;95:470–478.
109. Ost D, Yeung S, Tanoue L, et al. Clinical and organizational factors in the initial evaluation of patients with lung cancer: Diagnosis and management of lung cancer, 3rd ed: American College of Chest Physicians evidence-based clinical practice guidelines. *Chest* 2013;143:e121S.
110. Silvestri GA, Gonazalez AV, Jantz M, et al. Methods of staging for non-small cell lung cancer: diagnosis and management of lung cancer, 3rd ed: American College of Chest Physicians evidence-based clinical practice guidelines. *Chest* 2013;143:e211S–e250S.
111. Swensen SJ, Silverstein MD, Ilstrup DM, et al. The probability of malignancy in solitary pulmonary nodules: application to small radiologically indeterminate nodules. *Arch Intern Med* 1997;157:849–855.
112. Swensen SJ, Silverstein MD, Edell ES, et al. Solitary pulmonary nodules: Clinical prediction model versus physicians. *Mayo Clin Proc* 1999;74:319–329.
113. Cummings S, Lillington G, Richard R. Estimating the probability of malignancy in solitary pulmonary nodules: a Bayesian approach. *Am Rev Respir Dis* 1986;134:449–452.
114. Tammemagi C, Pinsky P, Caporaso N, et al. Lung cancer risk prediction: prostate, lung, colorectal and ovarian cancer screening trial models and validation. *J Natl Cancer Inst* 2011;103:1058–1068.
115. McWilliams A, Tammemagi MC, Mayo JR, et al. Probability of cancer in pulmonary nodules detected on first screening CT. *N Engl J Med* 2013;369:910–919.
116. Rivera M, Mehta AC, Wahidi MM. Establishing the diagnosis of lung cancer: diagnosis and management of lung cancer, 3rd ed: American College of Chest Physicians evidence-based clinical practice guidelines. *Chest* 2013;143: e142S–e165S.
117. Ost DE, Niu J, S Elting L, et al. Quality gaps and comparative effectiveness in lung cancer staging and diagnosis. *Chest* 2014;145:331–345.
118. Detterbeck F, Khandani AH. The role of PET imaging in solitary pulmonary nodules. *Clin Pulm Med* 2009;16:81–88.
119. Gould MK, Donington J, Lynch W, et al. Evaluation of individuals with pulmonary nodules: when is it lung cancer? *Chest* 2013;143:e93S–e120S.
120. Vesselle H, Schmidt RA, Pugsley JM, et al. Lung cancer proliferation correlates with [F-18]fluorodeoxyglucose uptake by positron emission tomography. *Clin Cancer Res* 2000;6:3837–3844.
121. Rolston KV, Rodriguez S, Dholakia N, et al. Pulmonary infections mimicking cancer: a retrospective, three-year review. *Support Care Cancer* 1997;5:90–93.
122. Silvestri GA, Littenberg B, Colice GL. The clinical evaluation for detecting metastatic lung cancer. A meta-analysis. *Am J Respir Crit Care Med* 1995;152: 225–230.
123. Patchell RA, Tibbs PA, Walsh JW, et al. A randomized trial of surgery in the treatment of single metastases to the brain. *N Engl J Med* 1990;322:494–500.
124. Reed C, Harpole D, Posther K, et al. Results of the American College of Surgeons Oncology Group Z0050 Trial: the utility of positron emission tomography in staging potentially operable non-small cell lung cancer. *J Thorac Cardiovasc Surg* 2003;126:1943–1951.
125. Grant D, Edwards D, Goldstraw P. Computed tomography of the brain, chest, and abdomen in the postoperative assessment of non-small cell lung cancer. *Thorax* 1988;43:883–886.
126. Ichinose Y, Hara N, Ohta M, et al. Preoperative examination to detect distant metastasis is not advocated for asymptomatic patients with stages 1 and 2 non-small cell lung cancer: preoperative examination for lung cancer. *Chest* 1989;96:1104–1109.
127. Salvatierra A, Baamonde C, Llamas JM, et al. Extrathoracic staging of bronchogenic carcinoma. *Chest* 1990;97:1052–1058.
128. MacManus MP, Hicks RJ, Matthews JP, et al. High rate of detection of unsuspected distant metastases by PET in apparent stage III non-small-cell lung cancer: implications for radical radiation therapy. *Int J Radiation Oncology Biol Phys* 2001;50:287–293.
129. Sazon DA, Santiago SM, Hoo GW, et al. Fluorodeoxyglucose—positron emission tomography in the detection and staging of lung cancer. *Am J Respir Crit Care Med* 1996;153:417–421.
130. Weder W, Schmid RA, Bruchhaus H, et al. Detection of extrathoracic metastases by positron emission tomography in lung cancer. *Ann Thorac Surg* 1998;66:886–893.
131. Viney RC, Boyer MJ, King MT, et al. Randomized controlled trial of the role of positron emission tomography in the management of stage I and II non-small-cell lung cancer. *J Clin Oncol* 2004;22:2357–2362.
132. Farrell MA, McAdams HP, Herndon JE, et al. Non-small cell lung cancer: FDG PET for nodal staging in patients with stage I disease. *Radiology* 2000;215:886–890.
133. Eschmann SM, Friedel G, Paulsen F, et al. FDG PET for staging of advanced non-small cell lung cancer prior to neoadjuvant radio-chemotherapy. *Eur J Nucl Med Mol Imaging* 2002;29:804–808.
134. Michel F, Soler M, Imhof E, et al. Initial staging of non-small cell lung cancer: value of routine radioisotope bone scanning. *Thorax* 1991;40:409–413.
135. Modini C, Passariello R, Iascone C, et al. TNM staging in lung cancer: role of computed tomography. *J Thorac Cardiovasc Surg* 1982;84:569–574.
136. Quinn DL, Ostrow LB, Porter DK, et al. Staging of non-small cell bronchogenic carcinoma: relationship of the clinical evaluation to organ scans. *Chest* 1986;89:270–275.
137. Maziak DE, Darling GE, Inculet RI, et al. Positron emission tomography in staging early lung cancer. *Ann Intern Med* 2009;151:221–228.
138. Fischer B, Lassen U, Mortensen J, et al. Preoperative staging of lung cancer with combined PET-CT. *N Engl J Med* 2009;361:32–39.
139. van Tinteren H, Hoekstra OS, Smit EF, et al. Effectiveness of positron emission tomography in the preoperative assessment of patients with suspected non-small-cell lung cancer: the PLUS multicentre randomised trial. *Lancet* 2002;359:1388–1392.
140. Herder GJ, Kramer H, Hoekstra OS, et al. Traditional versus up-front [18F] fluorodeoxyglucose-positron emission tomography staging of non-small-cell lung cancer: a Dutch cooperative randomized study. *J Clin Oncol* 2006;24: 1800–1806.
141. National Comprehensive Cancer Network. Non-Small Cell Lung Cancer Version 2.2014.
142. Detterbeck F, Puchalski J, Rubinowitz A, et al. Classification of the thoroughness of mediastinal staging of lung cancer. *Chest* 2010;137:436–442.
143. Annema JT, van Meerbeeck JP, Rintoul RC, et al. Mediastinoscopy vs endosonography for mediastinal nodal staging of lung cancer. *JAMA* 2010;304: 2245–2252.
144. Detterbeck FC, Lewis S, Diekemper R, et al. Executive summary: diagnosis and management of lung cancer, 3rd ed: American College of Chest Physicians evidence-based clinical practice guidelines. *Chest* 2013;143:7S–37S.
145. Little AG, Gay EG, Gaspar LE, et al. National survey of non-small cell lung cancer in the United States: epidemiology, pathology and patterns of care. *Lung Cancer* 2007;57:253–260.
146. Earle CC, Venditti LN, Neumann PJ, et al. Who gets chemotherapy for metastatic lung cancer? *Chest* 2000;117:1239–1246.

147. Potosky AL, Saxman S, Wallace RB, et al. Population variations in the initial treatment of non-small-cell lung cancer. *J Clin Oncol* 2004;22:3261–3268.
148. Farjah F, Flum D, Ramsey S, et al. Multi-modality mediastinal staging for lung cancer among Medicare beneficiaries. *J Thorac Oncol* 2009;4:355–363.
149. Little AG, Rusch VW, Bonner JA, et al. Patterns of surgical care of lung cancer patients. *Ann Thorac Surg* 2005;80:2051–2056.
150. Vest M, Tanoue L, Soulos P, et al. Thoroughness of mediastinal staging in stage IIIA non-small cell lung cancer. *J Thor Oncol* 2012;7:188–195.
151. Howington J, Blum M, Chang A, et al. Treatment of stage I and II non-small cell lung cancer. *Chest* 2013;432:e278S–e313S.
152. von Meyenfeldt E, Gooiker G, van Gijn W, et al. The relationship between volume or surgeon specialty and outcome in the surgical treatment of lung cancer: a systematic review and meta-analysis. *J Thorac Oncol* 2012;7:1170–1178.
153. Hillner BE, Smith TJ, Desch CE. Hospital and physician volume or specialization and outcomes in cancer treatment: importance in quality of cancer care. *J Clin Oncol* 2000;18:2327–2340.
154. Ghaferi AA, Birkmeyer JD, Dimick JB. Variation in hospital mortality associated with inpatient surgery. *N Engl J Med* 2009;361:1368–1375.
155. Pignon JP, Tribodet H, Scagliotti GV, et al. Lung adjuvant cisplatin evaluation: a pooled analysis by the LACE Collaborative Group. *J Clin Oncol* 2008;26: 3552–3559.
156. Sandler A, Gray R, Perry MC, et al. Paclitaxel-carboplatin alone or with bevacizumab for non-small-cell lung cancer. *N Engl J Med* 2006;355:2542–2550.
157. Groome PA, Bolejack V, Crowley J, et al. The IASLC Lung Cancer Staging Project: validation of the proposals for revision of the T, N, and M descriptors and consequent stage groupings in the forthcoming (seventh) edition of the TNM classification of malignant tumours. *J Thorac Oncol* 2007;2:694–705.
158. Detterbeck FC, Postmus PE, Tanoue L. The stage classification of lung cancer: diagnosis and management of lung cancer, 3rd ed: American College of Chest Physicians evidence-based clinical practice guidelines. *Chest* 2013;143: e191s–e210s.
159. Cheng D, Downey RJ, Kernstine K, et al. Video-assisted thoracic surgery in lung cancer resection: a meta-analysis and systematic review of controlled trials. *Innovations* 2007;2:261–292.
160. Yan TD, Black D, Bannon PG, et al. Systematic review and meta-analysis of randomized and nonrandomized trials on safety and efficacy of video-assisted thoracic surgery lobectomy for early-stage non-small-cell lung cancer. *J Clin Oncol* 2009;27:2553–2562.
161. Chen FF, Zhang D, Wang YL, et al. Video-assisted thoracoscopic surgery lobectomy versus open lobectomy in patients with clinical stage non-small cell lung cancer: a meta-analysis. *Eur J Surg Oncol* 2013;39:957–963.
162. Zhang Z, Zhang Y, Feng H, et al. Is video-assisted thoracic surgery lobectomy better than thoracotomy for early-stage non-small-cell lung cancer? A systematic review and meta-analysis. *Eur J Cardiothorac Surg* 2013;44:407–414.
163. Taioli E, Lee DS, Lesser M, et al. Long-term survival in video-assisted thoracoscopic lobectomy vs open lobectomy in lung-cancer patients: a meta-analysis. *Eur J Cardiothorac Surg* 2013;44:591–597.
164. Cai Y, Fu X, Xu Q, et al. Thoracoscopic lobectomy versus open lobectomy in Stage I non small cell lung cancer: a meta-analysis. *PLoS One* 2013;8:e82366.
165. Li Z, Liu H, Li L. Video-assisted thoracoscopic surgery versus open lobectomy for stage I lung cancer: A meta-analysis of long-term outcomes. *Exp Ther Med* 2012;3:886–892.
166. Ceppa D, Kosinski A, Berry M, et al. Thoracoscopic lobectomy has increasing benefit in patients with poor pulmonary function: a Society of Thoracic Surgeons database analysis. *Ann Surg* 2012;256:487–493.
167. Farjah F, Wood DE, Mulligan MS, et al. Safety and efficacy of video-assisted versus conventional lung resection for lung cancer. *J Thorac Cardiovasc Surg* 2009;137:1415–1421.
168. Park H, Detterbeck F, Boffa D, et al. Impact of hospital volume of thoracoscopic lobectomy on primary lung cancer outcomes. *Ann Thorac Surg* 2012;93: 372–379.
169. Swanson SJ, Meyers BF, Gunnarsson CL, et al. Video-assisted thoracoscopic lobectomy is less costly and morbid than open lobectomy: a retrospective multiinstitutional database analysis. *Ann Thorac Surg* 2012;93:1027–1032.
170. Licht PB, Jørgensen OD, Ladegaard L, et al. A national study of nodal upstaging after thoracoscopic versus open lobectomy for clinical stage I lung cancer. *Ann Thorac Surg* 2013;96:943–950.
171. Paul S, Altorki NK, Sheng S, et al. Thoracoscopic lobectomy is associated with lower morbidity than open lobectomy: a propensity-matched analysis from the STS database. *J Thorac Cardiovasc Surg* 2010;139:366–378.
172. Paul S, Sedrakyan A, Chiu YL, et al. Outcomes after lobectomy using thoracoscopy vs thoracotomy: a comparative effectiveness analysis utilizing the Nationwide Inpatient Sample database. *Eur J Cardiothorac Surg* 2013;43:813–817.
173. Cao C, Manganas C, Ang SC, et al. Video-assisted thoracic surgery versus open thoracotomy for non-small cell lung cancer: a meta-analysis of propensity score-matched patients. *Interact CardioVasc Thorac Surg* 2013;16:244–249.
174. Cao C, Zhu ZH, Yan TD, et al. Video-assisted thoracic surgery versus open thoracotomy for non-small-cell lung cancer: a propensity score analysis based on a multi-institutional registry. *Eur J Cardiothorac Surg* 2013;44:849–854.
175. Su S, Scott WJ, Allen MS, et al. Patterns of survival and recurrence after surgical treatment of early stage non–small cell lung carcinoma in the ACOSOG Z0030 (ALLIANCE) trial. *J Thorac Cardiovasc Surg* 2014;147:747–753.
176. Scott WJ, Allen MS, Darling G, et al. Video-assisted thoracic surgery versus open lobectomy for lung cancer: a secondary analysis of data from the American College of Surgeons Oncology Group Z0030 randomized clinical trial. *J Thorac Cardiovasc Surg* 2010;139:976–983.
177. Flores RM, Park BJ, Dycoco J, et al. Lobectomy by video-assisted thoracic surgery (VATS) versus thoracotomy for lung cancer. *J Thorac Cardiovasc Surg* 2009;138:11–18.
178. Villamizar NR, Darrabie MD, Burfeind WR, et al. Thoracoscopic lobectomy is associated with lower morbidity compared with thoracotomy. *J Thorac Cardiovasc Surg* 2009;138:419–425.
179. Lee PC, Nasar A, Port JL, et al. Long-term survival after lobectomy for non-small cell lung cancer by video-assisted thoracic surgery versus thoracotomy. *Ann Thorac Surg* 2013;96:951–961.
180. Ilonen IK, Räsänen JV, Knuuttila A, et al. Anatomic thoracoscopic lung resection for non-small cell lung cancer in stage I is associated with less morbidity and shorter hospitalization than thoracotomy. *Acta Oncol* 2011;50:1126–1132.
181. Jeon JH, Kang CH, Kim HS, et al. Video-assisted thoracoscopic lobectomy in non-small-cell lung cancer patients with chronic obstructive pulmonary disease is associated with lower pulmonary complications than open lobectomy: a propensity score-matched analysis. *Eur J Cardiothorac Surg* 2014;45:640–645.
182. Scott W, Matteotti R, Egleston B, et al. A comparison of perioperative outcomes of Video-Assisted Thoracic Surgical (VATS) Lobectomy with open thoracotomy and lobectomy: results of an analysis using propensity score based weighting. *Ann Surg Innov Res* 2010;4:1.
183. Kirby TJ, Mack MJ, Landreneau RJ, et al. Lobectomy—video-assisted thoracic surgery versus muscle-sparing thoracotomy: a randomized trial. *J Thorac Cardiovasc Surg* 1995;109:997–1002.
184. Sugi K, Kaneda Y, Esato K. Video-assisted thoracoscopic lobectomy achieves a satisfactory long-term prognosis in patients with clinical stage IA lung cancer. *World J Surg* 2000;24:27–31.
185. Craig SR, Leaver HA, Yap PL, et al. Acute phase responses following minimal access and conventional thoracic surgery. *Eur J Cardiothorac Surg* 2001;20: 455–463.
186. Pompili C, Detterbeck F, Papagiannopoulos K, et al. Multicenter international randomized comparison of objective and subjective outcomes between electronic and traditional chest drainage systems. *Ann Thorac Surg* 2014;98: 490–497.
187. Cattaneo SM, Park BJ, Wilton AS, et al. Use of video-assisted thoracic surgery for lobectomy in the elderly results in fewer complications. *Ann Thorac Surg* 2008;85:231–236.
188. Grills IS, Yan D, Martinez AA, et al. Potential for reduced toxicity and dose escalation in the treatment of inoperable non-small-cell lung cancer: a comparison of intensity-modulated radiation therapy (IMRT), 3D conformal radiation, and elective nodal irradiation. *Int J Radiat Oncol Biol Phys* 2003;57:875–890.
189. Liu HH, Wang X, Dong L, et al. Feasibility of sparing lung and other thoracic structures with intensity-modulated radiotherapy for non-small-cell lung cancer. *Int J Radiat Oncol Biol Phys* 2004;58:1268–1279.
190. Grills IS, Hugo G, Kestin LL, et al. Image-guided radiotherapy via daily online cone-beam CT substantially reduces margin requirements for stereotactic lung radiotherapy. *Int J Radiat Oncol Biol Phys* 2008;70:1045–1056.
191. Keall P. 4-dimensional computed tomography imaging and treatment planning. *Semin Radiat Oncol* 2004;14:81–90.
192. Chang JM, Lee HJ, Goo JM, et al. False positive and false negative FDG-PET scans in various thoracic diseases. *Korean J Radiol* 2006;7:57–69.
193. Chang JY, Komaki R, Lu C, et al. Phase 2 study of high-dose proton therapy with concurrent chemotherapy for unresectable stage III nonsmall cell lung cancer. *Cancer* 2011;117:4707–4713.
194. Oshiro Y, Mizumoto M, Okumura T, et al. Results of proton beam therapy without concurrent chemotherapy for patients with unresectable stage III non-small cell lung cancer. *J Thorac Oncol* 2012;7:370–375.
195. Emami B, Lyman J, Brown A, et al. Tolerance of normal tissue to therapeutic irradiation. *Int J Radiat Oncol Biol Phys* 1991;21:109–122.
196. Marks LB, Bentzen SM, Deasy JO, et al. Radiation dose-volume effects in the lung. *Int J Radiat Oncol Biol Phys* 2010;76:S70–S76.
197. Timmerman R, McGarry R, Yiannoutsos C, et al. Excessive toxicity when treating central tumors in a phase II study of stereotactic body radiation therapy for medically inoperable early-stage lung cancer. *J Clin Oncol* 2006;24:4833–4839.
198. Borst GR, Ishikawa M, Nijkamp J, et al. Radiation pneumonitis after hypofractionated radiotherapy: evaluation of the LQ(L) model and different dose parameters. *Int J Radiat Oncol Biol Phys* 2010;77:1596–1603.
199. Takeda A, Kunieda E, Ohashi T, et al. Severe COPD is correlated with mild radiation pneumonitis following stereotactic body radiotherapy. *Chest* 2012;141:858–866.
200. Barriger RB, Forquer JA, Brabham JG, et al. A dose-volume analysis of radiation pneumonitis in non-small cell lung cancer patients treated with stereotactic body radiation therapy. *Int J Radiat Oncol Biol Phys* 2012;82:457–462.
201. Huang EX, Hope AJ, Lindsay PE, et al. Heart irradiation as a risk factor for radiation pneumonitis. *Acta Oncol* 2011;50:51–60.
202. Miller KL, Shafman TD, Anscher MS, et al. Bronchial stenosis: an underreported complication of high-dose external beam radiotherapy for lung cancer? *Int J Radiat Oncol Biol Phys* 2005;61:64–69.
203. Bradley JD, Hope A, El Naga I, et al. A nomogram to predict radiation pneumonitis, derived from a combined analysis of RTOG 9311 and institutional data. *Int J Radiat Oncol Biol Phys* 2007;69:985–992.
204. Palma DA, Senan S, Oberije C, et al. Predicting esophagitis after chemoradiation therapy for non-small cell lung cancer: an individual patient data meta-analysis. *Int J Radiat Oncol Biol Phys* 2013;87:690–696.
205. Ozturk B, Egehan I, Atavci S, et al. Pentoxifylline in prevention of radiation-induced lung toxicity in patients with breast and lung cancer: a double-blind randomized trial. *Int J Radiat Oncol Biol Phys* 2004;58:213–219.

206. Antonadou D, Coliarakis N, Synodinou M, et al. Randomized phase III trial of radiation treatment +/− amifostine in patients with advanced-stage lung cancer. *Int J Radiat Oncol Biol Phys* 2001;51:915–922.
207. Movsas B, Scott C, Langer C, et al. Randomized trial of amifostine in locally advanced non-small-cell lung cancer patients receiving chemotherapy and hyperfractionated radiation: radiation therapy oncology group trial 98-01. *J Clin Oncol* 2005;23:2145–2154.
208. Ward WF, Molteni A, Kim YT, et al. Structure-function analysis of angiotensin-converting enzyme inhibitors as modifiers of radiation-induced pulmonary endothelial dysfunction in rats. *Br J Radiol* 1989;62:348–354.
209. Turrisi AT 3rd, Kim K, Blum R, et al. Twice-daily compared with once-daily thoracic radiotherapy in limited small-cell lung cancer treated concurrently with cisplatin and etoposide. *N Engl J Med* 1999;340:265–271.
210. O'Rourke N, Roque IFM, Farre Bernado N, et al. Concurrent chemoradiotherapy in non-small cell lung cancer. *Cochrane Database Syst Rev* 2010;(6): CD002140.
211. Spigel DR, Hainsworth JD, Yardley DA, et al. Tracheoesophageal fistula formation in patients with lung cancer treated with chemoradiation and bevacizumab. *J Clin Oncol* 2010;28:43–48.
212. Socinski MA, Stinchcombe TE, Moore DT, et al. Incorporating bevacizumab and erlotinib in the combined-modality treatment of stage III non-small-cell lung cancer: results of a phase I/II trial. *J Clin Oncol* 2012;30:3953–3959.
213. Singh AK, Lockett MA, Bradley JD. Predictors of radiation-induced esophageal toxicity in patients with non-small-cell lung cancer treated with three-dimensional conformal radiotherapy. *Int J Radiat Oncol Biol Phys* 2003;55:337–341.
214. Qiao WB, Zhao YH, Zhao YB, et al. Clinical and dosimetric factors of radiation-induced esophageal injury: radiation-induced esophageal toxicity. *World J Gastroenterol* 2005;11:2626–2629.
215. Gagliardi G, Constine LS, Moiseenko V, et al. Radiation dose-volume effects in the heart. *Int J Radiat Oncol Biol Phys* 2010;76:S77–S85.
216. Schytte T, Hansen O, Stolberg-Rohr T, et al. Cardiac toxicity and radiation dose to the heart in definitive treated non-small cell lung cancer. *Acta Oncol* 2010;49:1058–1060.
217. King V, Constine LS, Clark D, et al. Symptomatic coronary artery disease after mantle irradiation for Hodgkin's disease. *Int J Radiat Oncol Biol Phys* 1996;36: 881–889.
218. Harris EE, Correa C, Hwang WT, et al. Late cardiac mortality and morbidity in early-stage breast cancer patients after breast-conservation treatment. *J Clin Oncol* 2006;24:4100–4106.
219. Hooning MJ, Botma A, Aleman BM, et al. Long-term risk of cardiovascular disease in 10-year survivors of breast cancer. *J Natl Cancer Inst* 2007;99:365–375.
220. Doyle JJ, Neugut AI, Jacobson JS, et al. Chemotherapy and cardiotoxicity in older breast cancer patients: a population-based study. *J Clin Oncol* 2005;23: 8597–8605.
221. Gianni L, Dombernowsky P, Sledge G, et al. Cardiac function following combination therapy with paclitaxel and doxorubicin: an analysis of 657 women with advanced breast cancer. *Ann Oncol* 2001;12:1067–1073.
222. Churn M, Clough V, Slater A. Early onset of bilateral brachial plexopathy during mantle radiotherapy for Hodgkin's disease. *Clin Oncol (R Coll Radiol)* 2000;12:289–291.
223. Kong FM, Ritter T, Quint DJ, et al. Consideration of dose limits for organs at risk of thoracic radiotherapy: atlas for lung, proximal bronchial tree, esophagus, spinal cord, ribs, and brachial plexus. *Int J Radiat Oncol Biol Phys* 2011;81:1442–1457.
224. Eblan MJ, Corradetti MN, Lukens JN, et al. Brachial plexopathy in apical non-small cell lung cancer treated with definitive radiation: dosimetric analysis and clinical implications. *Int J Radiat Oncol Biol Phys* 2013;85:175–181.
225. The Non-small Cell Lung Cancer Collaborative Group. Chemotherapy in non-small cell lung cancer: a meta-analysis using updated data on individual patients from 52 randomised clinical trials. *Br Med J* 1995;311:899–909.
226. Ellis PA, Smith IE, Hardy JR, et al. Symptom relief with MVP (mitomycin C, vinblastine and cisplatin) chemotherapy in advanced non-small-cell lung cancer. *Br J Cancer* 1995;71:366–370.
227. Thatcher N, Anderson H, Betticher DC, et al. Symptomatic benefit from gemcitabine and other chemotherapy in advanced non-small cell lung cancer: changes in performance status and tumour-related symptoms. *Anticancer Drugs* 1995;6:39–48.
228. Pignon J, Tribodet H, Scagliotti G, et al. Lung Adjuvant Cisplatin Evaluation (LACE): a pooled analysis of five randomized clinical trials including 4,584 patients. *J Clin Oncol* 2007;24:7008.
229. Lynch TJ, Bell DW, Sordella R, et al. Activating mutations in the epidermal growth factor receptor underlying responsiveness of non-small-cell lung cancer to gefitinib. *N Engl J Med* 2004;350:2129–2139.
230. Johnson DH. Setting the bar for therapeutic trials in non–small-cell lung cancer: how low can we go? *J Clin Oncol* 2014;32:1389–1391.
231. Sacher AG, Le LW, Leighl NB. Shifting patterns in the interpretation of phase III clinical trial outcomes in advanced non–small-cell lung cancer: the bar is dropping. *J Clin Oncol* 2014;32:1407–1411.
232. Atherly AJ, Camidge DR. The cost-effectiveness of screening lung cancer patients for targeted drug sensitivity markers. *Br J Cancer* 2012;106:1100–1106.
233. Djalalov S, Beca J, Hoch JS, et al. Cost effectiveness of EML4-ALK fusion testing and first-line crizotinib treatment for patients with advanced ALK-positive non–small-cell lung cancer. *J Clin Oncol* 2014;32:1012–1019.
234. Kelley MJ, McCrory DC. Prevention of lung cancer: summary of published evidence. *Chest* 2003;123:50S–59S.
235. Kim ES, Herbst RS, Wistuba II, et al. The BATTLE trial: personalizing therapy for lung cancer. *Cancer Discov* 2011;1:44–53.
236. Wisnievesky J, Yung RC, Mathur PN, et al. Diagnosis and treatment of bronchial intraepithelial neoplasia and early lung cancer of the central airways: diagnosis and management of lung cancer, 3rd ed: American College of Chest Physicians evidence-based clinical practice guidelines. *Chest* 2013;143: e263S–e277S.
237. Detterbeck FC, Homer RJ. Approach to the ground-glass nodule. *Clin Chest Med* 2011;32:799–810.
238. Naidich DP, Bankier AA, MacMahon H, et al. Recommendations for the management of subsolid pulmonary nodules detected at CT: a statement from the Fleischner Society. *Radiology* 2013;266:304–317.
239. Yoshida J, Ishii G, Yokose T, et al. Possible delayed cut-end recurrence after limited resection for ground-glass opacity adenocarcinoma, intraoperatively diagnosed as Noguchi Type B, in three patients. *J Thor Oncol* 2010;5:546–550.
240. Vest M, Herrin J, Soulos P, et al. Use of new treatment modalities for non-small cell lung cancer care in the Medicare population. *Chest* 2013;143:429–435.
241. Asamura H, Goya T, Koshiishi Y, et al. A Japanese Lung Cancer Registry study: prognosis of 13,010 resected lung cancers. *J Thorac Oncol* 2008;3:46–52.
242. Harpole DH Jr, Herndon JE II, Young WG Jr, et al. Stage I nonsmall cell lung cancer: a multivariate analysis of treatment methods and patterns of recurrence. *Cancer* 1995;76:787–796.
243. Jones DR, Detterbeck FC. Surgery for stage I non-small cell lung cancer. In: Detterbeck FC, Rivera MP, Socinski MA, et al., eds. *Diagnosis and Treatment of Lung Cancer: An Evidence-Based Guide for the Practicing Clinician*. Philadelphia, PA: W. B. Saunders; 2001:177–190.
244. Martini N, Bains MS, Burt ME, et al. Incidence of local recurrence and second primary tumors in resected stage I lung cancer. *J Thorac Cardiovasc Surg* 1995;109:120–129.
245. Cangemi A, Volpino P, D'Andrea N, et al. Local and/or distant recurrences in T1-2/N0-1 non-small cell lung cancer. *Eur J Cardiothorac Surg* 1995;9: 473–478.
246. Hubbard MO, Fu P, Margevicius S, et al. Five-year survival does not equal cure in non-small cell lung cancer: a surveillance, epidemiology, and end results-based analysis of variables affecting 10- to 18-year survival. *J Thorac Cardiovasc Surg* 2012;143:1307–1313.
247. Maeda R, Yoshida J, Hishida T, et al. Late recurrence of non-small cell lung cancer more than 5 years after complete resection: incidence and clinical implications in patient follow-up. *Chest* 2010;138:145–150.
248. West D, Rashid S, Dunning J. Does video-assisted thoracoscopic lobectomy produce equal cancer clearance compared to open lobectomy for non-small cell carcinoma of the lung? *Interact Cardiovasc Thorac Surg* 2007;6:110–116.
249. Whitson BA, Groth SS, Duval SJ, et al. Surgery for early-stage non-small cell lung cancer: a systematic review of the video-assisted thoracoscopic surgery versus thoracotomy approaches to lobectomy. *Ann Thorac Surg* 2008;86:2008–2018.
250. Phillips JD, Merkow RP, Sherman KL, et al. Factors affecting selection of operative approach and subsequent short-term outcomes after anatomic resection for lung cancer. *J Am Coll Surg* 2012;215:206–215.
251. Cooke D, Wisner D. Who performs complex noncardiac thoracic surgery in United States academic medical centers? *Ann Thorac Surg* 2012;94:1060–1064.
252. Boffa DJ, Kosinski A, Paul S, et al. Lymph node evaluation by open or video assisted approaches in 11,500 anatomic lung cancer resections. *Ann Thorac Surg* 2012;94:347–353.
253. Palade E, Passlick B, Osei-Agyemang T, et al. Video-assisted vs open mediastinal lymphadenectomy for Stage I non-small-cell lung cancer: results of a prospective randomized trial. *Eur J Cardiothorac Surg* 2013;44:244–249.
254. Petersen RP, Pham D, Burfeind WR, et al. Thoracoscopic lobectomy facilitates the delivery of chemotherapy after resection for lung cancer. *Ann Thorac Surg* 2007;83:1245–1250.
255. Jiang G, Yang F, Li X, et al. Video-assisted thoracoscopic surgery is more favorable than thoracotomy for administration of adjuvant chemotherapy after lobectomy for non-small cell lung cancer. *World J Surg Oncol* 2011;21:170.
256. Ginsberg RJ, Rubinstein LV. Randomized trial of lobectomy versus limited resection for T1 N0 non-small cell lung cancer. Lung Cancer Study Group. *Ann Thorac Surg* 1995;60:615–622, discussion 623.
257. Lederle FA. Lobectomy versus limited resection in T1 N0 lung cancer (Letter). *Ann Thorac Surg* 1996;62:1249–1250.
258. Kim AW, Detterbeck F. Mediastinal lymph node dissection. In: Franco K, Thourani V, eds. *Cardiothoracic Surgery Review*. Philadelphia, PA: Lippincott Williams & Wilkins; 2012:1019–1022.
259. Darling GE, Allen MS, Decker PA, et al. Number of lymph nodes harvested from a mediastinal lymphadenectomy: results of the randomized, prospective ACOSOG Z0030 trial. *Chest* 2011;139:1124–1129.
260. Izbicki JR, Passlick B, Pantel K, et al. Effectiveness of radical systematic mediastinal lymphadenectomy in patients with resectable non-small cell lung cancer. *Ann Surg* 1998;227:138–144.
261. Sugi K, Nawata K, Fujita N, et al. Systematic lymph node dissection for clinically diagnosed peripheral non-small-cell lung cancer less than 2 cm in diameter. *World J Surg* 1998;22:290–294.
262. Allen MS, Darling GE, Pechet TT, et al. Morbidity and mortality of major pulmonary resections in patients with early-stage lung cancer: initial results of the randomized, prospective ACOSOG Z0030 trial. *Ann Thorac Surg* 2006;81:1013–1020.
263. Arriagada R, Dunant A, Pignon JP, et al. Long-term results of the international adjuvant lung cancer trial evaluating adjuvant cisplatin-based chemotherapy in resected lung cancer. *J Clin Oncol* 2010;28:35–42.
264. Scagliotti GV. The ALPI trial: the Italian/European experience with adjuvant chemotherapy in resectable non–small lung cancer. *Clin Cancer Res* 2005;11:5011s–5016s.

265. Waller D, Peake MD, Stephens RJ, et al. Chemotherapy for patients with non-small cell lung cancer: the surgical setting of the Big Lung Trial. *Eur J Cardiothorac Surg* 2004;26:173–182.
266. Strauss GM, Herndon JE II, Maddaus MA, et al. Adjuvant paclitaxel plus carboplatin compared with observation in stage IB non-small-cell lung cancer: CALGB 9633 with the Cancer and Leukemia Group B, Radiation Therapy Oncology Group, and North Central Cancer Treatment Group study groups. *J Clin Oncol* 2008;26:5043–5051.
267. Hamada C, Tanaka, F, Ohta, M, et al. Meta-analysis of postoperative adjuvant chemotherapy with tegafur-uracil in non-small-cell lung cancer. *J Clin Oncol* 2005;23:4999.
268. Wada H, Hitomi S, Teramatsu T. Adjuvant chemotherapy after complete resection in non-small-cell lung cancer. West Japan Study Group for Lung Cancer Surgery. *J Clin Oncol* 1996;14:1048–1054.
269. PORT Meta-analysis Trialists Group. Postoperative radiotherapy in non-small-cell lung cancer: systemic review and meta-analysis of individual patient data from nine randomised controlled trials. *Lancet* 1998;352:257–263.
270. Trodella L, Granone P, Valente S, et al. Adjuvant radiotherapy in non-small cell lung cancer with pathological stage I: definitive results of a phase III randomized trial. *Radiother Oncol* 2002;62:11–19.
271. Lally BE, Zelterman D, Colasanto JM, et al. Postoperative radiotherapy for stage II or III non-small-cell lung cancer using the surveillance, epidemiology, and end results database. *J Clin Oncol* 2006;24:2998–3006.
272. Brunelli A, Kim AW, Berger K, et al. Physiologic evaluation of the patient with lung cancer being considered for resectional surgery: diagnosis and management of lung cancer, 3rd ed: American College of Chest Physicians evidence-based clinical practice guidelines. *Chest* 2013;143:e166S–e190S.
273. Lau KK, Martin-Ucar AE, Nakas A, et al. Lung cancer surgery in the breathless patient—the benefits of avoiding the gold standard. *Eur J Cardiothorac Surg* 2010;38:6–13.
274. Brunelli A, Socci L, Refai M, et al. Quality of life before and after major lung resection for lung cancer: a prospective follow-up analysis. *Ann Thorac Surg* 2007;84:410–416.
275. Bobbio A, Chetta A, Carbognani P, et al. Changes in pulmonary function test and cardio-pulmonary exercise capacity in COPD patients after lobar pulmonary resection. *Eur J Cardiothorac Surg* 2005;28:754–758.
276. Endoh H, Tanaka S, Yajima T, et al. Pulmonary function after pulmonary resection by posterior thoracotomy, anterior thoracotomy or video-assisted surgery. *Eur J Cardiothorac Surg* 2010;37:1209–1214.
277. Sienel W, Dango S, Kirschbaum A, et al. Sublobar resections in stage IA non-small cell lung cancer: segmentectomies result in significantly better cancer-related survival than wedge resections. *Eur J Cardiothorac Surg* 2008;33:728–734.
278. Chang JY, Balter PA, Dong L, et al. Stereotactic body radiation therapy in centrally and superiorly located stage I or isolated recurrent non-small-cell lung cancer. *Int J Radiat Oncol Biol Phys* 2008;72:967–971.
279. Rowe BP, Boffa DJ, Wilson LD, et al. Stereotactic body radiotherapy for central lung tumors. *J Thorac Oncol* 2012;7:1394–1399.
280. Nuyttens JJ, van der Voort van Zyp NC, Praag J, et al. Outcome of four-dimensional stereotactic radiotherapy for centrally located lung tumors. *Radiother Oncol* 2012;102:383–387.
281. Palma DA, Senan S, Haasbeek CJ, et al. Radiological and clinical pneumonitis after stereotactic lung radiotherapy: a matched analysis of three-dimensional conformal and volumetric-modulated arc therapy techniques. *Int J Radiat Oncol Biol Phys* 2011;80:506–513.
282. NSCLC Meta-analyses Collaborative Group, Arriagada R, Auperin A, et al. Adjuvant chemotherapy, with or without postoperative radiotherapy, in operable non-small-cell lung cancer: two meta-analyses of individual patient data. *Lancet* 2010;375:1267–1277.
283. Martini N, Burt ME, Bains MS, et al. Survival after resection of stage II non-small cell lung cancer. *Ann Thorac Surg* 1992;54:460–466.
284. van Velzen E, Snijder RJ, de la Riviere AB, et al. Type of lymph node involvement influences survival rates in T1N1M0 non-small cell lung carcinoma. *Chest* 1996;110:1469–1473.
285. Lardinois D, Suter H, Hakki H, et al. Morbidity, survival, and site of recurrence after mediastinal lymph-node dissection versus systematic sampling after cpmplete resection for non-small cell lung cancer. *Ann Thorac Surg* 2005;80:268–275.
286. Wu Y, Huang ZF, Wang SY, et al. A randomized trial of systematic nodal dissection in resectable non-small cell lung cancer. *Lung Cancer* 2002;36:1–6.
287. Ferguson MK, Lehman AG. Sleeve lobectomy or pneumonectomy: optimal management strategy using decision analysis techniques. *Ann Thorac Surg* 2003;76:1782–1788.
288. Ma Z, Dong A, Fan J, et al. Does sleeve lobectomy concomitant with or without pulmonary artery reconstruction (double sleeve) have favorable results for non-small cell lung cancer compared with pneumonectomy? A meta-analysis. *Eur J Cardiothorac Surg* 2007;32:20–28.
289. Douillard J, Tribodet H, Aubert D, et al. Adjuvant cisplatin and vinorelbine for completely resected non-small cell lung cancer: subgroup analysis of the Lung Adjuvant Cisplatin Evaluation. *J Thorac Oncol* 2010;5:220–228.
290. Butts CA, Ding K, Seymour L, et al. Randomized phase III trial of vinorelbine plus cisplatin compared with observation in completely resected stage IB and II non-small-cell lung cancer: updated survival analysis of JBR-10. *J Clin Oncol* 2010;28:29–34.
291. Douillard JY, Rosell R, De Lena M, et al. Impact of postoperative radiation therapy on survival in patients with complete resection and stage I, II, or IIIA non-small-cell lung cancer treated with adjuvant chemotherapy: the Adjuvant Navelbine International Trialist Association (ANITA) randomized trial. *Int J Radiat Oncol Biol Phy* 2008;72:695–701.
292. Felip E, Rosell R, Maestre JA, et al. Preoperative chemotherapy plus surgery versus surgery plus adjuvant chemotherapy versus surgery alone in early-stage non-small-cell lung cancer. *J Clin Oncol* 2010;28:3138–3145.
293. American Joint Committee on Cancer. *AJCC Cancer Staging Manual*. 7th ed. New York, NY: Springer; 2009.
294. International Union for Cancer Control. *TNM Classification of Malignant Tumors*. 7th ed. Hoboken, NJ: Wiley-Blackwell; 2009.
295. Kozower B, Larner JM, Detterbeck FC, et al. Special treatment issues in non-small cell lung cancer: diagnosis and management of lung cancer, 3rd ed: American College of Chest Physicians evidence-based clinical practice guidelines. *Chest* 2013;143:e369S–e399S.
296. Piehler JM, Pairolero PC, Weiland LH, et al. Bronchogenic carcinoma with chest wall invasion: factors affecting survival following en bloc resection. *Ann Thorac Surg* 1982;34:684–691.
297. Gould PM, Bonner JA, Sawyer TE, et al. Patterns of failure and overall survival in patients with completely resected T3 N0 M0 non-small cell lung cancer. *Int J Radiat Oncol Biol Phys* 1999;45:91–95.
298. Patterson GA, Ilves R, Ginsberg RJ, et al. The value of adjuvant radiotherapy in pulmonary and chest wall resection for bronchogenic carcinoma. *Ann Thorac Surg* 1982;34:692–697.
299. Detterbeck FC, Socinski MA. IIB or not IIB: the current question in staging non-small cell lung cancer. *Chest* 1997;112:229–234.
300. Detterbeck FC, Kiser AC. T3 non-small cell lung cancer (stage IIb-IIIa). In: Detterbeck FC, Rivera MP, Socinski MA, et al., eds. *Diagnosis and Treatment of Lung Cancer: An Evidence-Based Guide for the Practicing Clinician*. Philadelphia, PA: W. B. Saunders; 2001:223–232.
301. Morgensztern D, Waqar S, Subramanian J, et al. Prognostic significance of tumor size in patients with stage III non-small-cell lung cancer: a surveillance, epidemiology, and end results (SEER) survey from 1998 to 2003. *J Thorac Oncol* 2012;7:1479–1484.
302. Moreno A, Morgensztern D, Yu J, et al. Impact of preoperative radiation on survival of patients with T3N)>7-cm non-small cell lung cancers treated with anatomic resection using the Surveillance, Epidemiology, and End Results database. *J Surg Res* 2013;184:10–18.
303. Moreno A, Morgensztern D, Boffa D, et al. Treating stage IIIA-N1 disease: an analysis of very large, hilar lymph node positive non-small cell lung cancer using the National Cancer Data Base. *Ann Thorac Surg* 2014;97:1149–1155.
304. Detterbeck FC. Changes in the treatment of Pancoast tumors. *Ann Thorac Surg* 2003;75:1990–1997.
305. Foroulis CN, Zarogoulidis P, Darwiche K, et al. Superior sulcus (Pancoast) tumors: current evidence on diagnosis and radical treatment. *J Thorac Dis* 2013;5:S342–S358.
306. Anraku M, Waddell TK, de Perrot M, et al. Induction chemoradiotherapy facilitates radical resection of T4 non-small cell lung cancer invading the spine. *J Thorac Cardiovasc Surg* 2009;137:441–447.e1.
307. Bilsky MH, Vitaz TW, Boland PJ, et al. Surgical treatment of superior sulcus tumors with spinal and brachial plexus involvement. *J Neurosurg Spine* 2009;97:301–309.
308. Bolton WD, Rice DC, Goodyear A, et al. Superior sulcus tumors with vertebral body involvement: a multimodality approach. *J Thorac Cardiovasc Surg* 2009;137:1379–1387.
309. Fadel E, Missenard G, Chapelier A, et al. En bloc resection of non-small cell lung cancer invading the thoracic inlet and intervertebral foramina. *J Thorac Cardiovasc Surg* 2002;123:676–685.
310. Gandhi S, Walsh GL, Komaki R, et al. A multidisciplinary surgical approach to superior sulcus tumors with vertebral invasion. *Ann Thorac Surg* 1999;68:1778–1785.
311. Grunenwald DH, Mazel C, Girard P, et al. Radical en bloc resection for lung cancer invading the spine. *J Thorac Cardiovasc Surg* 2002;123:271–279.
312. Muralidaran A, Detterbeck FC, Boffa DJ, et al. Long-term survival after lung resection for NSCLC with circulatory bypass: a systematic review. *J Thorac Cardiovasc Surg* 2011;142:1137–1142.
313. Kim AW, Detterbeck FC. Surgery for T4 and N3 non-small cell lung cancer, additional pulmonary nodules and isolated distant metastases. In: Kernstine K, Reckamp K, Thomas CJ, eds. *Lung Cancer: A Multidisciplinary Approach to Diagnosis and Management*. New York, NY: Demos Medical Publishing; 2011:161–182.
314. Rendina EA, Venuta F, De Giacomo T, et al. Induction chemotherapy for T4 centrally located non-small cell lung cancer. *J Thorac Cardiovasc Surg* 1999;117:225–233.
315. Rusch VW, Giroux DJ, Kraut MJ, et al. Induction chemoradiation and surgical resection for superior sulcus non-small-cell lung carcinomas: long-term results of Southwest Oncology Group Trial 9416 (Intergroup Trial 0160). *J Clin Oncol* 2007;25:313–318.
316. Ramnath N, Dilling T, Harris L, et al. Treatment of stage III non-small cell lung cancer: diagnosis and management of lung cancer, 3rd ed: American College of Chest Physicians evidence-based clinical practice guidelines. *Chest* 2013;143:e314S–e340S.
317. Detterbeck F. What to do with surprise N2: intraoperative management of patients with non-small cell lung cancer. *J Thorac Oncol* 2008;3:289–302.
318. Detterbeck FC. N2 disease discovered at thoracotomy: resect or abort? In: Ferguson MK, ed. *Difficult Decisions in Thoracic Surgery: An Evidence-Based Approach*. 2nd ed. London, UK: Springer-Verlag; 2011:89–103.
319. Tada H, Tsuchiya R, Ichinose Y, et al. A randomized trial comparing adjuvant chemotherapy versus surgery alone for completely resected pN2 non-small cell lung cancer (JCOG9304). *Lung Cancer* 2004;43:167–173.

320. Scagliotti GV, Fossati R, Torri V, et al. Randomized study of adjuvant chemotherapy for completely resected stage I, II, or IIIA non-small-cell Lung cancer. *J Natl Cancer Inst* 2003;95:1453–1461.
321. Arriagada R, Bergman B, Dunant A, et al. Cisplatin-based adjuvant chemotherapy in patients with completely resected non-small-cell lung cancer. *N Engl J Med* 2004;350:351–360.
322. Winton T, Livingston R, Johnson D, et al. Vinorelbine plus cisplatin vs. observation in resected non-small-cell lung cancer. *N Engl J Med* 2005;352: 2589–2597.
323. Douillard JY, Rosell R, De Lena M, et al. Adjuvant vinorelbine plus cisplatin versus observation in patients with completely resected stage IB-IIIA non-small-cell lung cancer (Adjuvant Navelbine International Trialist Association [ANITA]): a randomised controlled trial. *Lancet Oncol* 2006;7:719–727.
324. Lally BE, Detterbeck FC, Geiger AM, et al. The risk of death from heart disease in patients with nonsmall cell lung cancer who receive postoperative radiotherapy: analysis of the Surveillance, Epidemiology, and End Results database. *Cancer* 2007;110:911–917.
325. Billiet C, Decaluwe H, Peeters S, et al. Modern post-operative radiotherapy for stage III non-small cell lung cancer may improve local control and survival: a meta-analysis. *Radiother Oncol* 2014;110:3–8.
326. Shen WY, Ji J, Zuo YS, et al. Comparison of efficacy for postoperative chemotherapy and concurrent radiochemotherapy in patients with IIIA-pN2 non-small cell lung cancer: an early closed randomized controlled trial. *Radiother Oncol* 2014;110:120–125.
327. Bradley J, Graham MV, Winter K, et al. Toxicity and outcome results of RTOG 9311: a phase I-II dose-escalation study using three-dimensional conformal radiotherapy in patients with inoperable non-small-cell lung carcinoma. *Int J Radiat Oncol Biol Phys* 2005;61:318–328.
328. Feigenberg SJ, Hanlon AL, Langer C, et al. A phase II study of concurrent carboplatin and paclitaxel and thoracic radiotherapy for completely resected stage II and IIIA non-small cell lung cancer. *J Thorac Oncol* 2007;2:287–292.
329. The benefit of adjuvant treatment for resected locally advanced non-small-cell lung cancer. The Lung Cancer Study Group. *J Clin Oncol* 1988;6:9–17.
330. Pisters KM, Le Chevalier T. Adjuvant chemotherapy in completely resected non-small-cell lung cancer. *J Clin Oncol* 2005;23:3270–3278.
331. Keller SM, Adak S, Wagner H, et al. A randomized trial of postoperative adjuvant therapy in patients with completely resected stage II or IIIA non-small-cell lung cancer. Eastern Cooperative Oncology Group. *N Engl J Med* 2000;343: 1217–1222.
332. Dautzenberg B, Chastang C, Arriagada R, et al. Adjuvant radiotherapy versus combined sequential chemotherapy followed by radiotherapy in the treatment of resected nonsmall cell lung carcinoma. A randomized trial of 267 patients. GETCB (Groupe d'Etude et de Traitement des Cancers Bronchiques). *Cancer* 1995;76:779–786.
333. Cerfolio RJ, Maniscalco L, Bryant AS. The treatment of patients with stage IIIA non-small cell lung cancer from N2 disease: who returns to the surgical arena and who survives. *Ann Thorac Surg* 2008;86:912–920.
334. Burdett S, Stewart L, Rydzewska L. Chemotherapy and surgery versus surgery alone in non-small cell lung cancer. *Cochrane Database Syst Rev* 2007;(3):CD006157.
335. Andre F, Grunenwald D, Pignon JP, et al. Survival of patients with resected N2 non–small-cell lung cancer: evidence for a subclassification and implications. *J Clin Oncol* 2000;18:2981–2989.
336. Coughlin M, Deslauriers J, Beaulieu M, et al. Role of mediastinoscopy in pretreatment staging of patients with primary lung cancer. *Ann Thorac Surg* 1985;40:556–560.
337. Pearson FG, DeLarue NC, Ilves R, et al. Significance of positive superior mediastinal nodes identified at mediastinoscopy in patients with resectable cancer of the lung. *J Thorac Cardiovasc Surg* 1982;83:1–11.
338. Vansteenkiste JF, De Leyn PR, Deneffe GJ, et al. Clinical prognostic factors in surgically treated stage IIIA-N2 non-small cell lung cancer: analysis of the literature. *Lung Cancer* 1998;19:3–13.
339. Albain KS, Swann RS, Rusch VW, et al. Radiotherapy plus chemotherapy with or without surgical resection for stage III non-small-cell lung cancer: a phase III randomised controlled trial. *Lancet* 2009;374:379–386.
340. Johnstone DW, Byhardt RW, Ettinger D, et al. Phase III study comparing chemotherapy and radiotherapy with preoperative chemotherapy and surgical resection in patients with non-small-cell lung cancer with spread to mediastinal lymph nodes (N2); final report of RTOG 89-01. Radiation Therapy Oncology Group. *Int J Radiat Oncol Biol Phys* 2002;54:365–369.
341. Stephens R, Girling D, Hopwood P, et al. A randomised controlled trial of preoperative chemotherapy followed, if feasible, by resection versus radiotherapy in patients with inoperable stage T3, N1, M0 or T1-3, N2, M0 non-small cell lung cancer. *Lung Cancer* 2005;49:395–400.
342. Van Meerbeeck JP, Kramer GW, Van Schil PE, et al. Randomized controlled trial of resection versus radiotherapy after induction chemotherapy in stage IIIA-N2 non-small-cell lung cancer. *J Natl Cancer Inst* 2007;99:442–450.
343. Kim AW, Faber LP, Warren WH, et al. Pneumonectomy after chemoradiation therapy for non-small cell lung cancer: does "side" really matter? *Ann Thorac Surg* 2009;88:937–944.
344. de Cabanyes Candela S, Detterbeck F. A systematic review of restaging after induction therapy for stage IIIa lung cancer: prediction of pathologic stage. *J Thorac Oncol* 2010;5:389–398.
345. Thomas M, Rübe C, Hoffknecht P, et al. Effect of preoperative chemoradiation in addition to preoperative chemotherapy: a randomised trial in stage III non-small-cell lung cancer. *Lancet Oncol* 2008;9:636–648.
346. Perez CA, Stanley K, Rubin P, et al. A prospective randomized study of various irradiation doses and fractionation schedules in the treatment of inoperable non-oat-cell carcinoma of the lung. Preliminary report by the Radiation Therapy Oncology Group. *Cancer* 1980;45:2744–2753.
347. Kong FM, Hayman JA, Griffith KA, et al. Final toxicity results of a radiation-dose escalation study in patients with non-small-cell lung cancer (NSCLC): predictors for radiation pneumonitis and fibrosis. *Int J Radiat Oncol Biol Phys* 2006;65:1075–1086.
348. Cox JD, Azarnia N, Byhardt RW, et al. A randomized phase I/II trial of hyperfractionated radiation therapy with total doses of 60.0 Gy to 79.2 Gy: possible survival benefit with greater than or equal to 69.6 Gy in favorable patients with Radiation Therapy Oncology Group stage III non-small-cell lung carcinoma: report of Radiation Therapy Oncology Group 83-11. *J Clin Oncol* 1990;8:1543–1555.
349. Saunders M, Dische S, Barrett A, et al. Continuous, hyperfractionated, accelerated radiotherapy (CHART) versus conventional radiotherapy in non-small cell lung cancer: mature data from the randomised multicentre trial. CHART Steering committee. *Radiother Oncol* 1999;52:137–148.
350. Marino P, Preatoni A, Cantoni A. Randomized trials of radiotherapy alone versus combined chemotherapy and radiotherapy in stages IIIa and IIIb nonsmall cell lung cancer. A meta-analysis. *Cancer* 1995;76:593–601.
351. Auperin A, Le Pechoux C, Pignon JP, et al. Concomitant radio-chemotherapy based on platin compounds in patients with locally advanced non-small cell lung cancer (NSCLC): a meta-analysis of individual data from 1764 patients. *Ann Oncol* 2006;17:473–483.
352. Curran WJ Jr, Paulus R, Langer CJ, et al. Sequential vs. concurrent chemoradiation for stage III non-small cell lung cancer: randomized phase III trial RTOG 9410. *J Natl Cancer Inst* 2011;103:1452–1460.
353. Furuse K, Fukuoka M, Kawahara M, et al. Phase III study of concurrent versus sequential thoracic radiotherapy in combination with mitomycin, vindesine, and cisplatin in unresectable stage III non-small-cell lung cancer. *J Clin Oncol* 1999;17:2692–2699.
354. Yamamoto N, Nakagawa K, Nishimura Y, et al. Phase III study comparing second- and third-generation regimens with concurrent thoracic radiotherapy in patients with unresectable stage III non-small-cell lung cancer: West Japan Thoracic Oncology Group WJTOG0105. *J Clin Oncol* 2010;28:3739–3745.
355. Wang L, Wu S, Ou G, et al. Randomized phase II study of concurrent cisplatin/etoposide or paclitaxel/carboplatin and thoracic radiotherapy in patients with stage III non-small cell lung cancer. *Lung Cancer* 2012;77:89–96.
356. Govindan R, Bogart J, Stinchcombe T, et al. Randomized phase II study of pemetrexed, carboplatin, and thoracic radiation with or without cetuximab in patients with locally advanced unresectable non-small-cell lung cancer: Cancer and Leukemia Group B trial 30407. *J Clin Oncol* 2011;29:3120–3125.
357. Lu C, Lee JJ, Komaki R, et al. Chemoradiotherapy with or without AE-941 in stage III non-small cell lung cancer: a randomized phase III trial. *J Natl Cancer Inst* 2010;102:859–865.
358. Kelly K, Chansky K, Gaspar LE, et al. Phase III trial of maintenance gefitinib or placebo after concurrent chemoradiotherapy and docetaxel consolidation in inoperable stage III non-small-cell lung cancer: SWOG S0023. *J Clin Oncol* 2008;26:2450–2456.
359. Hanna N, Neubauer M, Yiannoutsos C, et al. Phase III study of cisplatin, etoposide, and concurrent chest radiation with or without consolidation docetaxel in patients with inoperable stage III non-small-cell lung cancer: the Hoosier Oncology Group and U.S. Oncology. *J Clin Oncol* 2008;26:5755–5760.
360. Vokes EE, Herndon JE 2nd, Kelley MJ, et al. Induction chemotherapy followed by chemoradiotherapy compared with chemoradiotherapy alone for regionally advanced unresectable stage III Non-small-cell lung cancer: Cancer and Leukemia Group B. *J Clin Oncol* 2007;25:1698–1704.
361. Bradley JD, Bae K, Graham MV, et al. Primary analysis of the phase II component of a phase I/II dose intensification study using three-dimensional conformal radiation therapy and concurrent chemotherapy for patients with inoperable non-small-cell lung cancer: RTOG 0117. *J Clin Oncol* 2010;28: 2475–2480.
362. Schild SE, McGinnis WL, Graham D, et al. Results of a Phase I trial of concurrent chemotherapy and escalating doses of radiation for unresectable non-small-cell lung cancer. *Int J Radiat Oncol Biol Phys* 2006;65:1106–1111.
363. Stinchcombe TE, Lee CB, Moore DT, et al. Long-term follow-up of a phase I/II trial of dose escalating three-dimensional conformal thoracic radiation therapy with induction and concurrent carboplatin and paclitaxel in unresectable stage IIIA/B non-small cell lung cancer. *J Thorac Oncol* 2008;3:1279–1285.
364. Socinski MA, Blackstock AW, Bogart JA, et al. Randomized phase II trial of induction chemotherapy followed by concurrent chemotherapy and dose-escalated thoracic conformal radiotherapy (74 Gy) in stage III non-small-cell lung cancer: CALGB 30105. *J Clin Oncol* 2008;26:2457–2463.
365. Bradley JD, Paulus R, Komaki R, et al. A randomized phase III comparison of standard-dose (60 Gy) versus high-dose (74 Gy) conformal chemoradiotherapy with or without cetuximab for stage III non-small cell lung cancer: results on radiation dose in RTOG 0617. *J Clin Oncol* 2013;31:Abstr 7501.
366. Schild SE, Stella PJ, Geyer SM, et al. Phase III trial comparing chemotherapy plus once-daily or twice-daily radiotherapy in Stage III non-small-cell lung cancer. *Int J Radiat Oncol Biol Phys* 2002;54:370–378.
367. Belani CP, Wang W, Johnson DH, et al. Phase III study of the Eastern Cooperative Oncology Group (ECOG 2597): induction chemotherapy followed by either standard thoracic radiotherapy or hyperfractionated accelerated radiotherapy for patients with unresectable stage IIIA and B non-small-cell lung cancer. *J Clin Oncol* 2005;23:3760–3767.

368. Belderbos J, Uitterhoeve L, van Zandwijk N, et al. Randomised trial of sequential versus concurrent chemo-radiotherapy in patients with inoperable non-small cell lung cancer (EORTC 08972-22973). *Eur J Cancer* 2007;43:114–121.
369. Cho KH, Ahn SJ, Pyo HR, et al. A Phase II study of synchronous three-dimensional conformal boost to the gross tumor volume for patients with unresectable Stage III non-small-cell lung cancer: results of Korean Radiation Oncology Group 0301 study. *Int J Radiat Oncol Biol Phys* 2009;74:1397–1404.
370. Arrieta O, Gallardo-Rincon D, Villarreal-Garza C, et al. High frequency of radiation pnemonitis in patients with locally advanced non-small cell lung cancer treated with concurrent radiotherapy and gemcitabine after induction with gemcitabine and carboplating. *J Thorac Oncol* 2009;4:845–852.
371. Vokes EE, Herndon JE, Kelley MJ, et al. Induction chemotherapy followed by chemoradiotherapy compared wtih chemoradiotherapy alone for regionally advanced unresectable stage III Non-small-cell lung cancer: Cancer and Leukemia Group B. *J Clin Oncol* 2007;25:1698–1704.
372. Noonan K, Laskin J, Tong K, et al. Evaluation of a "Watch and Wait" approach for patients with newly diagnosed advanced NSCLC in a diverse community population. *J Thorac Oncol* 2013;8:Abstr 015.01.
373. Socinski MA, Crowell R, Hensing TE, et al. Treatment of non-small cell lung cancer, stage IV: ACCP evidence-based clinical practice guidelines (2nd Edition). *Chest* 2007;132:277S–289S.
374. Socinski MA, Evans T, Gettinger S, et al. Treatment of stage IV non-small cell lung cancer: diagnosis and management of lung cancer, 3rd ed: American College of Chest Physicians evidence-based clinical practice guidelines. *Chest* 2013;143:e341S–e368S.
375. Ellis LM, Bernstein DS, Voest EE, et al. American Society of Clinical Oncology perspective: raising the bar for clinical trials by defining clinically meaningful outcomes. *J Clin Oncol* 2014;32:1277–1280.
376. Lilenbaum RC, Herndon JE 2nd, List MA, et al. Single-agent versus combination chemotherapy in advanced non-small-cell lung cancer: the cancer and leukemia group B (study 9730). *J Clin Oncol* 2005;23:190–196.
377. Ardizzoni A, Boni L, Tiseo M, et al. Cisplatin- versus carboplatin-based chemotherapy in first-line treatment of advanced non–small-cell lung cancer: an individual patient data meta-analysis. *J Natl Cancer Inst* 2007;99:847–857.
378. Schiller JH, Harrington D, Belani CP, et al. Comparison of four chemotherapy regimens for advanced non-small-cell lung cancer. *N Engl J Med* 2002;346:92–98.
379. Hanna N, Shepherd FA, Fossella FV, et al. Randomized phase III trial of pemetrexed versus docetaxel in patients with non-small-cell lung cancer previously treated with chemotherapy. *J Clin Oncol* 2004;22:1589–1597.
380. Johnson DH, Fehrenbacher L, Novotny WF, et al. Randomized phase II trial comparing bevacizumab plus carboplatin and paclitaxel with carboplatin and paclitaxel alone in previously untreated locally advanced or metastatic non-small-cell lung cancer. *J Clin Oncol* 2004;22:2184–2191.
381. Delbaldo C, Michiels S, Syz N, et al. Benefits of adding a drug to a single-agent or a 2-agent chemotherapy regimen in advanced non-small-cell lung cancer: a meta-analysis. *JAMA* 2004;292:470–484.
382. D'Addario G, Pintilie M, Leighl NB, et al. Platinum-based versus non-platinum-based chemotherapy in advanced non-small-cell lung cancer: a meta-analysis of the published literature. *J Clin Oncol* 2005;23:2926–2936.
383. Sweeney CJ, Zhu J, Sandler AB, et al. Outcome of patients with a performance status of 2 in Eastern Cooperative Oncology Group Study E1594: a Phase II trial in patients with metastatic nonsmall cell lung carcinoma. *Cancer* 2001;92:2639–2647.
384. Zukin M, Barrios CH, Rodrigues Pereira J, et al. Randomized phase III trial of single-agent pemetrexed versus carboplatin and pemetrexed in patients with advanced non–small-cell lung cancer and Eastern Cooperative Oncology Group performance status of 2. *J Clin Oncol* 2013;31:2849–2853.
385. Hikish TF, Smith IE, O'Brien ME, et al. Clinical benefit from palliative chemotherapy in non-small-cell lung cancer extends to the elderly and those with poor prognostic factors. *Br J Cancer* 1998;78:28–33.
386. Pallis AG, Gridelli C, van Meerbeeck JP, et al. EORTC Elderly Task Force and Lung Cancer Group and International Society for Geriatric Oncology (SIOG) experts' opinion for the treatment of non-small-cell lung cancer in an elderly population. *Ann Oncol* 2010;21:692–706.
387. Quoix E, Zalcman G, Oster JP, et al. Carboplatin and weekly paclitaxel doublet chemotherapy compared with monotherapy in elderly patients with advanced non-small-cell lung cancer: IFCT-0501 randomised, phase 3 trial. *Lancet* 2011;378:1079–1088.
388. Hesketh PJ, Lilenbaum R, Chansky K, et al. Chemotherapy in patients > or = 80 with advanced non-small cell lung cancer: combined results from SWOG 0027 and LUN 6. *J Thor Oncol* 2007;2:494–498.
389. Reck M, von Pawel J, Zatloukal P, et al. Phase III trial of cisplatin plus gemcitabine with either placebo or bevacizumab as first-line therapy for nonsquamous non-small-cell lung cancer: AVAiL. *J Clin Oncol* 2009;27:1227–1234.
390. Patel JD, Socinski MA, Garon EB, et al. PointBreak: a randomized phase III study of pemetrexed plus carboplatin and bevacizumab followed by maintenance pemetrexed and bevacizumab versus paclitaxel plus carboplatin and bevacizumab followed by maintenance bevacizumab in patients with stage IIIB or IV nonsquamous non-small-cell lung cancer. *J Clin Oncol* 2013;31:4349–4357.
391. Crinò L, Dansin E, Garrido P, et al. Safety and efficacy of first-line bevacizumab-based therapy in advanced non-squamous non-small-cell lung cancer (SAiL, MO19390): a phase 4 study. *Lancet Oncol* 2010;11:733–740.
392. Pirker R, Pereira JR, Szczesna A, et al. Cetuximab plus chemotherapy in patients with advanced non-small-cell lung cancer (FLEX): an open-label randomised phase III trial. *Lancet* 2009;373:1525–1531.
393. Lynch TJ, Patel T, Dreisbach L, et al. Cetuximab and first-line taxane/carboplatin chemotherapy in advanced non-small-cell lung cancer: results of the randomized multicenter phase III trial BMS099. *J Clin Oncol* 2010;28:911–917.
394. Kim ES, Neubauer M, Cohn A, et al. Docetaxel or pemetrexed with or without cetuximab in recurrent or progressive non-small-cell lung cancer after platinum-based therapy: a phase 3, open-label, randomised trial. *Lancet Oncol* 2013;14:1326–1336.
395. Sequist LV, Yang JC-H, Yamamoto N, et al. Phase III study of afatinib or cisplatin plus pemetrexed in patients with metastatic lung adenocarcinoma with EGFR mutations. *J Clin Oncol* 2013;31:3327–3334.
396. Maemondo M, Inoue A, Kobayashi K, et al. Gefitinib or chemotherapy for non-small-cell lung cancer with mutated EGFR. *N Engl J Med* 2010;362:2380–2388.
397. Mitsudomi T, Morita S, Yatabe Y, et al. Gefitinib versus cisplatin plus docetaxel in patients with non-small-cell lung cancer harbouring mutations of the epidermal growth factor receptor (WJTOG3405): an open label, randomised phase 3 trial. *Lancet Oncol* 2010;11:121–128.
398. Zhou C, Wu Y, Liu X, et al. Overall survival (OS) results from OPTIMAL (CTONG0802), a phase III trial of erlotinib (E) versus carboplatin plus gemcitabine (GC) as first-line treatment for Chinese patients with EGFR mutation-positive advanced non-small cell lung cancer (NSCLC) [abstract 7520]. *J Clin Oncol* 2012;30:30.
399. Rosell R, Carcereny E, Gervais R, et al. Erlotinib versus standard chemotherapy as first-line treatment for European patients with advanced EGFR mutation-positive non-small-cell lung cancer (EURTAC): a multicentre, open-label, randomised phase 3 trial. *Lancet Oncol* 2012;13:239–246.
400. Shaw AT, Kim DW, Nakagawa K, et al. Crizotinib versus chemotherapy in advanced ALK-positive lung cancer. *N Engl J Med* 2013;368:2385–2394.
401. Jänne PA, Wang X, Socinski MA, et al. Randomized phase II trial of erlotinib alone or with carboplatin and paclitaxel in patients who were never or light former smokers with advanced lung adenocarcinoma: CALGB 30406 trial. *J Clin Oncol* 2012;30:2063–2069.
402. Wu YL, Lee JS, Thongprasert S, et al. Intercalated combination of chemotherapy and erlotinib for patients with advanced stage non-small-cell lung cancer (FASTACT-2): a randomised, double-blind trial. *Lancet Oncol* 2013;14:777–786.
403. Mok TS, Wu YL, Thongprasert S, et al. Gefitinib or carboplatin-paclitaxel in pulmonary adenocarcinoma. *N Engl J Med* 2009;361:947–957.
404. Oxnard G, Arcila M, Chmielecki J, et al. New strategies in overcoming acquired resistance to epidermal growth factor receptor tyrosine kinase inhibitors in lung cancer. *Clin Cancer Res* 2011;17:5530–5537.
405. Sequist LV, Waltman BA, Dias-Santagata D, et al. Genotypic and histological evolution of lung cancers acquiring resistance to EGFR inhibitors. *Sci Transl Med* 2011;3:75ra26.
406. Chaft J, Oxnard G, Sima CS, et al. Disease flare after tyrosine kinase inhibitor discontinuation in patients with EGFR-mutant lung cancer and acquired resistance to erlotinib or gefitinib: implications for clinical trial design. *Clin Cancer Res* 2011;17:6298–6303.
407. Socinski MA, Schell MJ, Peterman A, et al. Phase III trial comparing a defined duration of therapy versus continuous therapy followed by second-line therapy in advanced-stage IIIB/IV non-small-cell lung cancer. *J Clin Oncol* 2002;20:1335–1343.
408. Smith IE, O'Brien MER, Talbot DC, et al. Duration of chemotherapy in advanced non-small-cell lung cancer: a randomized trial of three versus six courses of mitomycin, vinblastine, and cisplatin. *J Clin Oncol* 2001;19:1336–1343.
409. Park JO, Kim SW, Ahn JS, et al. Phase III trial of two versus four additional cycles in patients who are nonprogressive after two cycles of platinum-based chemotherapy in non small-cell lung cancer. *J Clin Oncol* 2007;25:5233–5239.
410. Paz-Ares LG, de Marinis F, Dediu M, et al. PARAMOUNT: Final overall survival results of the phase III study of maintenance pemetrexed versus placebo immediately after induction treatment with pemetrexed plus cisplatin for advanced nonsquamous non-small-cell lung cancer. *J Clin Oncol* 2013;31:2895–2902.
411. Pérol M, Chouaid C, Pérol D, et al. Randomized, phase III study of gemcitabine or erlotinib maintenance therapy versus observation, with predefined second-line treatment, after cisplatin-gemcitabine induction chemotherapy in advanced non-small-cell lung cancer. *J Clin Oncol* 2012;30:3516–3524.
412. Ciuleanu T, Brodowicz T, Zielinski C, et al. Maintenance pemetrexed plus best supportive care versus placebo plus best supportive care for non-small-cell lung cancer: a randomised, double-blind, phase 3 study. *Lancet* 2009;374:1432–1440.
413. Cappuzzo F, Ciuleanu T, Stelmakh L, et al. Erlotinib as maintenance treatment in advanced non-small-cell lung cancer: a multicentre, randomised, placebo-controlled phase 3 study. *Lancet Oncol* 2010;11:521–529.
414. Fidias PM, Dakhil SR, Lyss AP, et al. Phase III study of immediate compared with delayed docetaxel after front-line therapy with gemcitabine plus carboplatin in advanced non-small-cell lung cancer. *J Clin Oncol* 2009;27:591–598.
415. Edelman M, Le Chevalier T, Soria J. Maintenance therapy and advanced non-small-cell lung cancer: a skeptic's view. *J Thor Oncol* 2012;7:1331–1336.
416. Bezjak A, Tu D, Seymour L, et al. Symptom improvement in lung cancer patients treated with erlotinib: quality of life analysis of the National Cancer Institute of Canada Clinical Trials Group Study BR.21. *J Clin Oncol* 2006;24:3831–3837.
417. Dancey J, Shepherd FA, Gralla RJ, et al. Quality of life assessment of second-line docetaxel versus best supportive care in patients with non-small-cell lung cancer previously treated with platinum-based chemotherapy: results of a prospective, randomized phase III trial. *Lung Cancer* 2004;43:183–194.

418. Shepherd FA, Dancey J, Ramlau R, et al. Prospective randomized trial of docetaxel versus best supportive care in patients with non-small-cell lung cancer previously treated with platinum-based chemotherapy. *J Clin Oncol* 2000;18:2095–2103.
419. Shepherd FA, Rodrigues Pereira J, Ciuleanu T, et al. Erlotinib in previously treated non-small-cell lung cancer. *N Engl J Med* 2005;353:123–132.
420. Ciuleanu T, Stelmakh L, Cicenas S, et al. Efficacy and safety of erlotinib versus chemotherapy in second-line treatment of patients with advanced, non-small-cell lung cancer with poor prognosis (TITAN): a randomised multicentre, open-label, phase 3 study. *Lancet Oncol* 2012;13:300–308.
421. Kim E, Hirsh V, Mok T, et al. Gefitinib versus docetaxel in previously treated non-small-cell lung cancer (INTEREST): a randomised phase III trial. *Lancet* 2008;372:1809–1818.
422. Garassino MC, Martelli O, Bettini A, et al. TAILOR: A phase III trial comparing erlotinib with docetaxel as the second-line treatment of NSCLC patients with wild-type (wt) EGFR. *J Clin Oncol* 2012;30:Abstr LBA7501.
423. Yun CH, Mengwasser KE, Toms AV, et al. The T790M mutation in EGFR kinase causes drug resistance by increasing the affinity for ATP. *Proc Natl Acad Sci U S A* 2008;105:2070–2075.
424. Janne P, Ramalingam S, Yang J, et al. Clinical activity of the mutant-selective EGFR inhibitor AZD9291 in patients (pts) with EGFR inhibitor-resistant non-small cell lung cancer (NSCLC). *J Clin Oncol* 2014;32:Abstr 8009.
425. Yu H, Sima C, Huang J, et al. Local therapy with continued EGFR tyrosine kinase inhibitor therapy as a treatment strategy in EGFR-mutant advanced lung cancers that have developed acquired resistance to EGFR tyrosine kinase inhibitors. *J Thorac Oncol* 2013;8:346–351.
426. Gainor JF, Shaw AT. Emerging paradigms in the development of resistance to tyrosine kinase inhibitors in lung cancer. *J Clin Oncol* 2013;31:3987–3996.
427. Shaw AT, Kim DW, Mehra R, et al. Ceritinib in ALK-rearranged non–small-cell lung cancer. *N Engl J Med* 2014;370:1189–1197.
428. Downey RJ, Ng KK, Kris MG, et al. A phase II trial of chemotherapy and surgery for non-small cell lung cancer patients with a synchronous solitary metastasis. *Lung Cancer* 2002;38:193–197.
429. Cerfolio RJ, Bryant AS. Is palpation of the nonresected pulmonary lobe(s) required for patients with non-small cell lung cancer? A prospective study. *J Thorac Cardiovasc Surg* 2008;135:261–268.
430. Keogan MT, Tung KT, Kaplan DK, et al. The significance of pulmonary nodules detected on CT staging for lung cancer. *Clin Radiol* 1993;48:94–96.
431. Kunitoh H, Eguchi K, Yamada K, et al. Intrapulmonary sublesions detected before surgery in patients with lung cancer. *Cancer* 1992;70:1876–1879.
432. Port JL, Korst RJ, Lee PC, et al. Surgical resection for multifocal (T4) non-small cell lung cancer: is the T4 designation valid? *Ann Thorac Surg* 2007;83:397–400.
433. Simoff MJ, Lally B, Slade MG, et al. Symptom management in patients with lung cancer: diagnosis and management of lung cancer, 3rd ed: American College of Chest Physicians evidence-based clinical practice guidelines. *Chest* 2013;143:e455S–e497S.
434. Temel JS, Greer JA, Muzikansky A, et al. Early palliative care for patients with metastatic non-small-cell lung cancer. *N Engl J Med* 2010;363:733–742.
435. Movsas B, Moughan J, Sarna L, et al. Quality of life supersedes the classic prognosticators for long-term survival in locally advanced non-small-cell lung cancer: an analysis of RTOG 9801. *J Clin Oncol* 2009;27:5816–5822.
436. Perrin RG. Metastatic tumors of the axial spine. *Curr Opin Oncol* 1992;4:525–532.
437. Sundaresan N, Galicich JH, Lane JM, et al. Treatment of neoplastic epidural cord compression by vertebral body resection and stabilization. *J Neurosurg* 1985;63:676–684.
438. Sorensen S, Helweg-Larsen S, Mouridsen H, et al. Effect of high-dose dexamethasone in carcinomatous metastatic spinal cord compression treated with radiotherapy: a randomised trial. *Eur J Cancer* 1994;30a:22–27.
439. Patchell RA, Tibbs PA, Regine WF, et al. Direct decompressive surgical resection in the treatment of spinal cord compression caused by metastatic cancer: a randomised trial. *Lancet* 2005;366:643–648.
440. Gaspar LE, Scott C, Murray K, et al. Validation of the RTOG recursive partitioning analysis (RPA) classification for brain metastases. *Int J Radiat Oncol Biol Phys* 2000;47:1001–1006.
441. Sperduto PW, Kased N, Roberge D, et al. Effect of tumor subtype on survival and the graded prognostic assessment for patients with breast cancer and brain metastases. *Int J Radiat Oncol Biol Phys* 2012;82:2111–2117.
442. Horton J, Baxter DH, Olson KB. The management of metastases to the brain by irradiation and corticosteroids. *Am J Roentgenol Radium Ther Nucl Med* 1971;111:334–336.
443. Patchell RA, Tibbs PA, Walsh JW, et al. A randomized trial of surgery in the treatment of single metastases to the brain. *N Engl J Med* 1990;322:494–500.
444. Patchell RA, Tibbs PA, Regine WF, et al. Postoperative radiotherapy in the treatment of single metastases to the brain: a randomized trial. *JAMA* 1998;280:1485–1489.
445. Andrews DW, Scott CB, Sperduto PW, et al. Whole brain radiation therapy with or without stereotactic radiosurgery boost for patients with one to three brain metastases: phase III results of the RTOG 9508 randomised trial. *Lancet* 2004;363:1665–1672.
446. Chang EL, Wefel JS, Hess KR, et al. Neurocognition in patients with brain metastases treated with radiosurgery or radiosurgery plus whole-brain irradiation: a randomised controlled trial. *Lancet Oncol* 2009;10:1037–1044.
447. Tsao MN, Rades D, Wirth A, et al. Radiotherapeutic and surgical management for newly diagnosed brain metastasis(es): an American Society for Radiation Oncology evidence-based guideline. *Pract Radiat Oncol* 2012;2:210–225.
448. Wilson LD, Detterbeck FC, Yahalom J. Clinical practice. Superior vena cava syndrome with malignant causes. *N Engl J Med* 2007;356:1862–1869.
449. Schraufnagel DE, Hill R, Leech JA, et al. Superior vena caval obstruction. Is it a medical emergency? *Am J Med* 1981;70:1169–1174.
450. Yu JB, Wilson LD, Detterbeck FC. Superior vena cava syndrome—a proposed classification system and algorithm for management. *J Thorac Oncol* 2008;3:811–814.
451. Martins SJ, Pereira JR. Clinical factors and prognosis in non-small cell lung cancer. *Am J Clin Oncol* 1999;22:453–457.

38 Small Cell and Neuroendocrine Tumors of the Lung

M. Catherine Pietanza, Lee M. Krug, Abraham J. Wu, Mark G. Kris, Charles M. Rudin, and William D. Travis

SMALL CELL LUNG CANCER

Incidence and Etiology

Although the incidence of small cell lung cancer (SCLC) is declining, it remains a worldwide public health problem. The Surveillance, Epidemiologic, and End Results (SEER) database reports the proportion of SCLC cases among all lung cancers in the United States decreased from 17% to 13% in the past 30 years (Fig. 38.1),[1] whereas the age-adjusted rates per 100,000 decreased from 10.65 in 1990 to 6.74 in 2010.[2] Among the predicted 228,190 lung cancer cases in the United States in 2013,[3] an estimated 29,665 cases of SCLC were diagnosed.

Only 2% to 3% of patients with this malignancy are never smokers[4,5]; thus, as tobacco exposure causes SCLC in over 97% of cases, its incidence rates mirror smoking patterns. Peak cigarette consumption occurred in the 1960s, but declined following the Surgeon General's report linking smoking to cancer and the subsequent ban on tobacco advertising on television.[6] The percentage of men who smoke decreased from 50% in 1965 to 21.6% in 2011, which is a much greater proportional reduction than in women, who went from a rate of 32% to 16.5% during the same time period.[6,7] Correspondingly, the incidence of SCLC in men peaked in 1984 and since has been trending steadily down, whereas in women, the incidence peaked later and only has declined slightly.[8] The gender gap has narrowed such that currently about half of the patients diagnosed with SCLC are women (see Fig. 38.1).

Anatomy and Pathology

Neuroendocrine tumors of the lung encompass a spectrum of tumors, including low-grade typical carcinoid, intermediate-grade atypical carcinoid, high-grade large cell neuroendocrine carcinoma (LCNEC), and SCLC.[9] Because of their shared neuroendocrine properties, these tumors have common morphologic, ultrastructural, immunohistochemical, and molecular features. Despite this, there are also important differences in clinical, epidemiologic, histologic, and molecular characteristics.

SCLC is readily diagnosed on small specimens such as bronchoscopic biopsies, fine-needle aspirates, core biopsies, and cytology. The diagnosis of SCLC is based primarily on light microscopy (Fig. 38.2A): dense sheets of small cells with scant cytoplasm, finely granular nuclear chromatin, inconspicuous or absent nucleoli, and frequent mitoses. Necrosis is common and frequently shows large areas. The tumor cells usually measure less than the diameter of three small resting lymphocytes. They are round to be fusiform in shape and have scant cytoplasm. The nuclear chromatin is finely granular and nucleoli are inconspicuous or absent.[9–11] The mitotic rate is characteristically high, averaging 60 to 80 per 2 mm^2. Crush artifact is a frequent finding in small transbronchial or mediastinal biopsy specimens and can make pathologic interpretation difficult. The tumor cells of SCLC also have a tendency to show a streaming artifact. This can also occur with non–small-cell lung cancer (NSCLC), lymphoma, and chronic inflammation. In surgically resected specimens where the tumor cells achieve better fixation, the cells of SCLC appear larger than in small biopsies.[10,12] When a component of NSCLC, including adenocarcinoma, squamous cell carcinoma, large cell carcinoma, spindle cell carcinoma, and giant cell carcinoma, is present, the term *combined SCLC* is used with mention of the specific histology of the non–small-cell component.[9,10] In resected specimens, combined SCLC may occur in up to 28% of cases.[10] To diagnose combined SCLC and large cell carcinoma, the large cell carcinoma component must comprise at least 10% of the overall tumor.[9,10]

The following immunohistochemical stains are helpful in difficult cases. A pancytokeratin antibody such as AE1/AE3 is useful to confirm if the tumor is a carcinoma. Neuroendocrine differentiation can be demonstrated using a panel of markers such as CD56, chromogranin, and synaptophysin. However, up to 10% of SCLCs may be negative for all neuroendocrine markers.[13] A high proliferation rate of 80% to 100% should be seen with Ki-67. Thyroid transcription factor-1 (TTF-1) is positive in 70% to 80% of small cell carcinomas.[14–16] Notably, TTF-1 can be positive in extrapulmonary small cell carcinomas, so it is not useful in determining the primary site of small cell carcinomas.[17]

Genetics

SCLC has been characterized by frequent inactivating mutations in the critical tumor suppressor genes *TP53* (75% to 90%)[18] and *RB1* (60% to 90%).[19,20] A mouse model with conditional inactivation of these two tumor suppressors in the lung generates lung tumors histologically and biologically similar to human SCLC.[21]

Recent reports including exome, transcriptome, and limited whole genome sequencing have provided insights into the fuller landscape of genetic alterations in SCLC.[22,23] In addition to confirming *TP53* and *RB1* inactivation, these studies define other alterations of interest in SCLC, with potential therapeutic implications. One consistent finding from both reports was an exceptionally high degree of genomic alteration in this tumor type, including mutations, insertions, deletions, large scale copy number alterations, and gross inter- and intrachromosomal rearrangements. *MYC* family member alterations, including gene amplification of *MYC*, *MYCN*, and *MYCL1*, as well as a recurrent gene fusion involving *MYCL1*, are frequent in SCLC and may represent important drivers of SCLC oncogenesis. The tumor suppressor phosphatase and tensin homolog (*PTEN*) appears to be inactivated in approximately 10% of SCLC, and mutations of other factors in the same signaling pathway were also identified. Other alterations implicated as potential drivers in subsets of SCLC include amplification of the tyrosine kinase *FGFR1* (in 6% of cases) and of the developmental regulator and transcription factor *SOX2* (in up to 27% of cases). The therapeutic implications of the large majority of

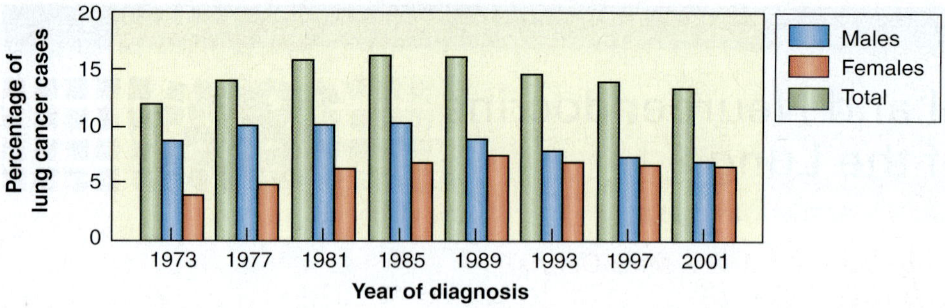

Figure 38.1 Patients diagnosed with small cell lung cancer as a percentage of all lung cancer cases and the breakdown by gender.

the genetic alterations documented to date in SCLC have not been defined.

Several reports have described the rare phenomenon of transformation to SCLC as a mechanism of acquired resistance to epidermal growth factor receptor (EGFR) tyrosine-kinase inhibitors (TKI) in patients initially treated for *EGFR*-mutant lung adenocarcinomas.[4] Of those cases with acquired resistance to EGFR TKIs, 3% to 14% will undergo SCLC transformation. Importantly, pure SCLC lack *EGFR* mutations and *ALK* rearrangements, even in those patients with this malignancy who are never smokers.[4,24] However, in the rare cases of SCLC transformation as a mechanism of acquired resistance to EGFR TKIs, there is persistence of the original *EGFR* mutation in the tumors confirmed on biopsy. In all cases where SCLC has been documented as a mechanism of acquired resistance to EGFR TKIs, the original tumor was a pure adenocarcinoma prior to EGFR TKI treatment, and the transformation was validated by histologic examination and confirmed by expression of neuroendocrine markers.

Screening

Screening computed tomography (CT) scans detect NSCLCs at an earlier stage compared to chest x-ray (CXR), or no screening, and can decrease lung cancer–specific mortality in heavy smokers.[25] However, the natural history of SCLC is characterized by rapid tumor growth and early metastatic spread. As such, the diagnosis of SCLC in an asymptomatic patient is rare.

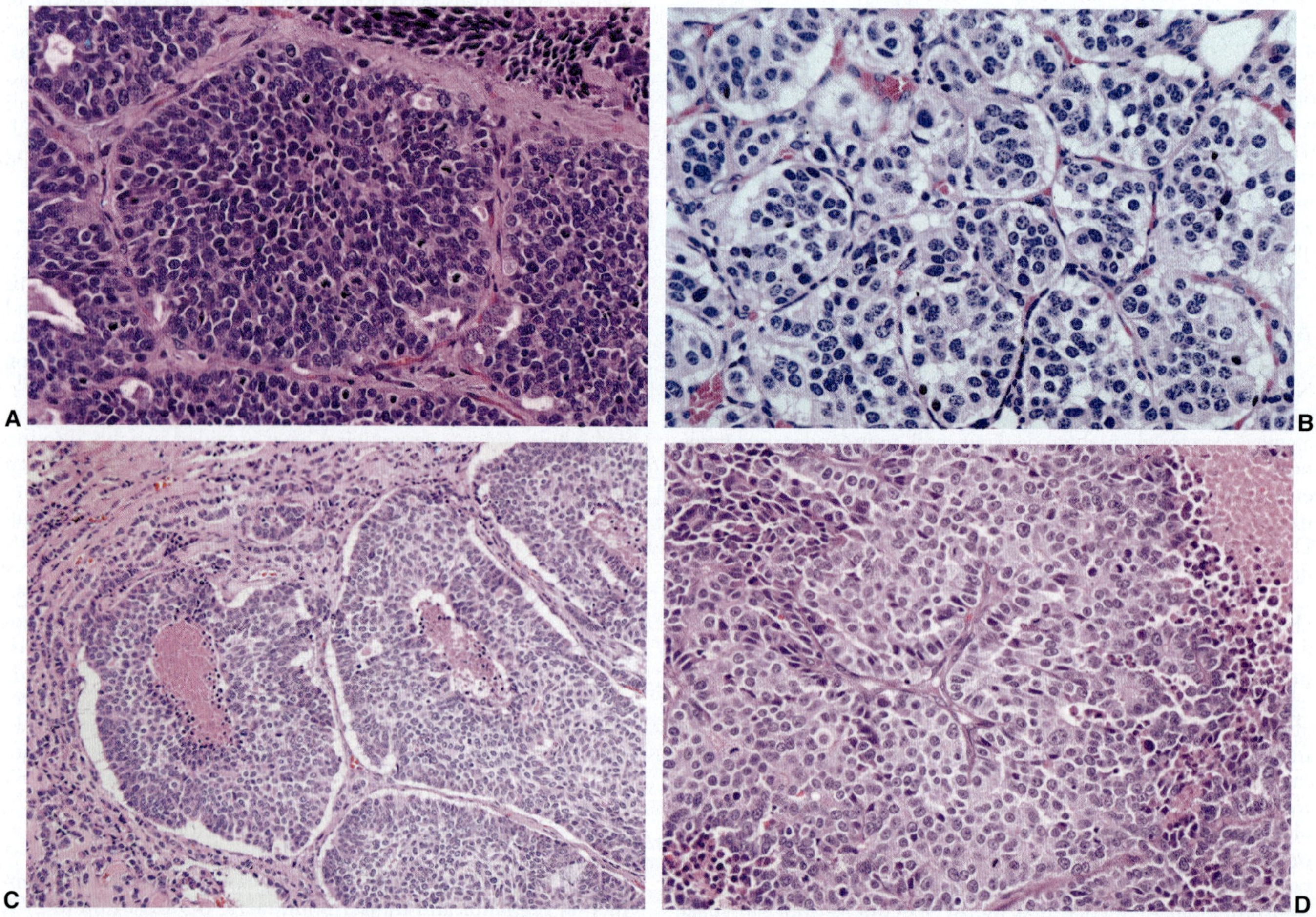

Figure 38.2 Histologic appearance of neuroendocrine carcinomas. **(A)** Small cell carcinoma. **(B)** Typical carcinoid. **(C)** Atypical carcinoid. **(D)** Large cell neuroendocrine carcinoma.

The National Lung Screening Trial (NLST) enrolled 53,454 Americans age 55 to 74 years with a history of at least 30 pack-years of cigarette smoking, and randomly assigned them to undergo three annual screenings with either low-dose CT scans (LDCT) or standard CXR. LDCT screening identified a preponderance of adenocarcinomas, including many with bronchioloalveolar subtype. SCLCs were not detected at early stages by either LDCT or CXR in the NLST. Although the study demonstrated a reduction in lung-cancer specific mortality compared to CXR, the similar rates and patterns of detection of SCLC make it unlikely that LDCT screening will reduce mortality specific to SCLC. Therefore, screening for SCLC by any method is not recommended.[25]

Diagnosis

Presenting symptoms in patients with SCLC can be constitutional, pulmonary, the result of extrathoracic spread, or due to paraneoplastic disorders.[26,27] In one series in which patient-reported symptoms were recorded using the Lung Cancer Symptom Scale, fatigue was the most common, symptom with decreased physical activity, cough, dyspnea, decreased appetite, weight loss, and pain occurring sometime in the course of the illness in the majority of patients.[27] Hemoptysis was noted in 14% in the same series.[27] The primary tumor often presents as a large central mass invading or compressing the mediastinum. Superior vena cava obstruction is present at diagnosis in 10% of patients with SCLC (Fig. 38.3),[28] and in these cases, the symptoms are often worsened by associated thrombosis in the compromised blood vessel. Chest imaging typically shows hilar and mediastinal adenopathy. Rarely, SCLC presents as a solitary pulmonary nodule.[29,30] No more than 2% of SCLC present as a superior sulcus tumor.[31]

Most patients with SCLC have metastases at diagnosis. Bone involvement is usually characterized by osteolytic lesions, often in the absence of bone pain, or elevations in the serum alkaline phosphatase.[32] Osteoblastic bone metastases do occur in some patients. Hepatic and adrenal lesions are typically asymptomatic. Brain metastases can be detected in at least 18% of patients at diagnosis,[33] which are often asymptomatic.

Paraneoplastic syndromes are common in SCLC and differ from those observed with NSCLC. SCLC accounts for approximately 75% of the tumors associated with the syndrome of inappropriate antidiuretic hormone (SIADH). Although serum concentrations of antidiuretic hormone are elevated in the majority of those with SCLC, only approximately 10% of patients fulfill the criteria of SIADH, and symptoms are present in no more than 5%. In some cases, ectopic production of atrial natriuretic factor contributes to the disorder in sodium homeostasis. The primary treatment for hyponatremia in SCLC patients is chemotherapy aimed at treating the disease. Additional management strategies include fluid restriction in mild cases or intravenous hypertonic saline in severe, symptomatic cases. Older pharmacologic interventions that have been used in SIADH, include demeclocycline and lithium, both of which induce nephrogenic diabetes insipidus.[34] More recently, tolvaptan, an oral vasopressin V2-receptor antagonist, has been shown to significantly improve serum sodium in patients with SIADH over a 4- and 30-day period.[35] Tolvaptan therapy should be initiated while patients are in the hospital to allow monitoring of the therapeutic response. Increased serum levels of adrenocorticotropic hormone can be detected in up to 50% of patients with lung cancer, but Cushing syndrome develops in only 5% of patients with SCLC. Low serum sodium is an adverse prognostic factor,[36] and patients with Cushing syndrome have a very limited survival.[37] The primary treatment of Cushing syndrome in SCLC patients is chemotherapy, although agents such as ketoconazole and mitotane have been used.[38] Hypercalcemia is rare in SCLC.

Paraneoplastic neurologic disorders seen in patients with SCLC include sensory, sensorimotor, and autoimmune neuropathies and encephalomyelitis.[39] These syndromes are thought to occur through autoimmune mechanisms, and antinuclear antibodies that bind to SCLC and to neuronal tissues have been identified. Symptoms may precede the diagnosis by many months and are often the presenting complaint. They may also be the initial sign of relapse from remission. An aggressive search may be required to discover small tumor nodules causing profound neurologic syndromes. Subacute peripheral sensory neuropathy associated with the anti-Hu antibody may be the most frequent paraneoplastic neurologic disorder seen in those with SCLC. Less common is the Lambert-Eaton syndrome, characterized by proximal muscle weakness that improves with continued use, hyporeflexia, and dysautonomia. Classic electromyographic findings confirm the diagnosis. The cause is related to autoantibody impairment of voltage-gated calcium channels. Rarer neurologic disorders seen in patients with SCLC include cerebellar degeneration or retinopathy. Two studies conflicted when evaluating whether the presence of paraneoplastic antibodies have prognostic implications[40,41]; the utilization of different techniques to measure antibody levels may account for the discrepant results.[42]

In contrast to the endocrine syndromes, for which successful treatment of the tumor effectively controls the symptoms, the occurrence and severity of the neurologic symptoms is unrelated to tumor bulk and usually does not resolve with antineoplastic therapy. Various therapies such as plasma exchange and immunosuppressive therapy with agents such as corticosteroids, cyclophosphamide, and tacrolimus have been tried, but generally offer little benefit. In patients with Lambert-Eaton syndrome, two randomized placebo-controlled trials of 3,4 diaminopyridine, which blocks potassium channel efflux from nerve terminals, demonstrated that treatment with this agent increases compound muscle action potentials and significantly improves muscle strength.[43] In a randomized trial with a crossover design, intravenous immunoglobulin also improved limb strength as measured by myometry over placebo in 10 patients with Lambert-Eaton syndrome.[43] However, the benefit was short lived and began to dissipate after just 8 weeks.

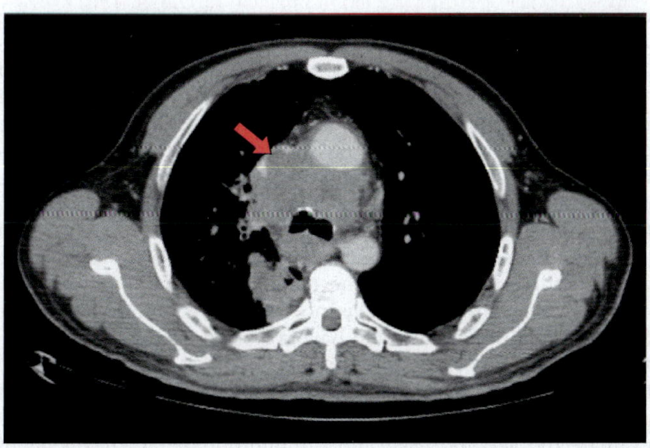

Figure 38.3 Computed tomography scan showing small cell lung cancer with an infiltrative mediastinal mass causing compression of the superior vena cava (*arrow*).

Staging

A simple two-stage system, introduced by the Veterans' Administration Lung Study Group (VALSG), has historically been utilized instead of the tumor, node, metastasis (TNM) system employed for most other cancer types.[44] In the VALSG system, limited stage is defined as disease confined to one hemithorax that can be "encompassed" in a "tolerable" radiation field. These patients currently are treated with a combined modality approach. All other patients are considered to have extensive-stage disease. At presentation, approximately two-thirds of patients with SCLC have extensive disease and one-third have limited-stage disease.[1]

In the VALSG staging system, the appropriate classification of ipsilateral pleural effusion, supraclavicular lymphadenopathy (ipsilateral or contralateral), or contralateral mediastinal lymphadenopathy as either limited or extensive stage remains controversial. Some large series have not found a survival difference between patients with an isolated ipsilateral pleural effusion and other patients with limited SCLC.[45] However, analyses of two large cooperative group databases, which included over 4,000 patients, showed that the survival of individuals with an isolated effusion was similar to that of patients with extensive disease.[46,47] In clinical practice, it is assumed that an effusion is malignant unless three criteria are met: the fluid is transudative, nonhemorrhagic, and cytologically negative on repeated examinations. Patients with a malignant effusion are appropriate to exclude from a combined modality treatment because hemithoracic radiotherapy to encompass the entirety of the pleura is impractical.

The presence of supraclavicular lymphadenopathy commonly is associated with extensive disease but, when encountered in patients with otherwise limited disease (5% of cases), carries a trend toward poorer survival.[47] Contralateral mediastinal involvement also is usually classified as limited-stage disease. However, two studies that evaluated twice-a-day radiation regimens excluded patients with contralateral hilar disease to reduce the normal lung volume irradiated and the risk for toxicity.[48,49]

For patients who appear to have limited-stage SCLC, some additional tests may be appropriate to confirm this assessment. Unilateral iliac crest bone marrow aspiration and biopsy are still a routine part of staging for many oncologists and should be performed in limited-stage patients with elevations of serum lactate dehydrogenase (LDH)[50,51] and evidence of myelophthisis (nucleated red blood cells, leukopenia, or thrombocytopenia) on the peripheral blood smear. If there is evidence of a pleural effusion, a thoracentesis or thoracoscopy may help confirm that the effusion is nonbloody, transudative, and cytologically negative. Effusions too small to permit image-guided sampling should not be considered in staging.[52] Osseous abnormalities seen on positron-emission tomography (PET) or bone scan require confirmation with magnetic resonance imaging (MRI), CT scan, or biopsy if they represent the only disease site that makes a patient extensive stage.

For the American Joint Committee on Cancer (AJCC) seventh edition, the use of a TNM staging system for SCLC has been revisited. To establish the accuracy of outcomes based on stage, cases of completely resected SCLC were staged using the same definitions as used for NSCLC.[53] The use of pathologic stage was necessary to accurately stage the patients used for this analysis. More favorable outcomes of patients have been reported in patients previously classified as *very limited* disease (i.e., no evidence of mediastinal metastases by CT or mediastinoscopy) treated with chemotherapy and radiation, as compared with other patients with limited-stage disease.[54–56] The use of the TNM system is best applied for cases of early stage disease and may have less relevance for the majority of patients presenting with metastatic disease.

Clinical and Serologic Predictive and Prognostic Factors

Multivariable analyses suggest that performance status is a strong and reproducible predictive and prognostic factor.[47,57,58] Poorer performance status can additionally identify individuals at higher risk for treatment-related complications. Several other clinical parameters have been proposed. Female gender has been associated with improved response and survival in patients with SCLC.[47,57,58] Older age (variably defined) has not been identified as an adverse prognostic factor in patients with SCLC in most[59–62] but not all[36,46,47] series. Older age has been associated with decreased performance status and more comorbid illnesses and often results in compromised chemotherapy dose intensity,[63,64] which may partially explain its prognostic implications. Certain metastatic sites, such as the liver,[65–67] the brain,[66,68] bone marrow,[67] and bone,[68] as well as the total number of metastatic sites involved,[47] have been found to be of prognostic significance for patients with extensive-stage disease. Paraneoplastic Cushing syndrome has been correlated with a poor response to therapy and short survival.[37] Continued use of tobacco during combined modality therapy was identified as an adverse prognostic factor in a group of 186 patients with limited disease.[69] Elevation of serum LDH is found in 33% to 57% of all patients with SCLC and up to 85% of patients with extensive-stage disease and is a strong prognostic and predictive factor.[46,57,65,66,68,70–72] Serum LDH elevation is associated with the presence of bone marrow involvement.[50] Although many other serum markers have been proposed to have prognostic significance, including neuron-specific enolase,[61,66] chromogranin, and precursors of gastrin-releasing peptide,[73,74] none have been strong and reliable enough to warrant general use. Carcinoembryonic antigen (CEA) has been found to predict outcome in SCLC in multiple series.[57,75,76]

Management by Stage

General Recommendations for Initial Management

Once the pathologic diagnosis of SCLC is confirmed, a complete history and physical examination is the next step. Special attention should be paid to the cigarette smoking history. If a patient is a current smoker, he or she should be advised to quit immediately in the strongest terms and offered the most aggressive smoking cessation intervention available.[69] If the patient is a never smoker, the pathologic diagnosis of SCLC should be reviewed as only 2% to 3% of never smokers develop SCLC.[4,5] The National Comprehensive Cancer Network (NCCN) has compiled consensus guidelines for the initial evaluation of individuals with SCLC.[52] A complete blood cell count (CBC) with platelet count, electrolytes, calcium, creatinine, blood urea nitrogen (BUN), liver function tests, and LDH are recommended. All patients should undergo a contrast-enhanced CT scan of the chest, a gadolinium-enhanced MRI of the head, and whole-body PET or a bone scan. A PET scan can identify sites of metastases undetected by other modalities[77–79] and can replace the bone scan.[80]

All fit patients (Karnofsky performance status greater than 60% or Eastern Cooperative Oncology Group [ECOG] performance status 0, 1, or 2) should initially receive combination chemotherapy with etoposide plus either cisplatin or carboplatin for four to six cycles (Fig. 38.4).[52] Supportive data, specifics of chemotherapy regimens, duration of therapy, and alternatives for patients with contraindications or special needs are discussed in the sections that follow. Patients with limited-stage disease should receive the chemotherapy concurrently with twice-daily thoracic irradiation beginning with the first, second, or third cycle.[49,81,82] Patients who achieve a response to chemotherapy should receive prophylactic whole-brain radiotherapy at the conclusion of chemotherapy or chemoradiotherapy.[83] There is no routine recommendation for the treatment of patients who have a Karnofsky performance status of 50% or less or ECOG performance status 3 or 4. Because the toxicity of all treatment worsens and effectiveness lessens in patients with a low performance status, clinicians must carefully evaluate the agent(s) used and the appropriateness and goals of therapy individually. For many patients in this low performance status group, supportive care only and referral to hospice are the best options.

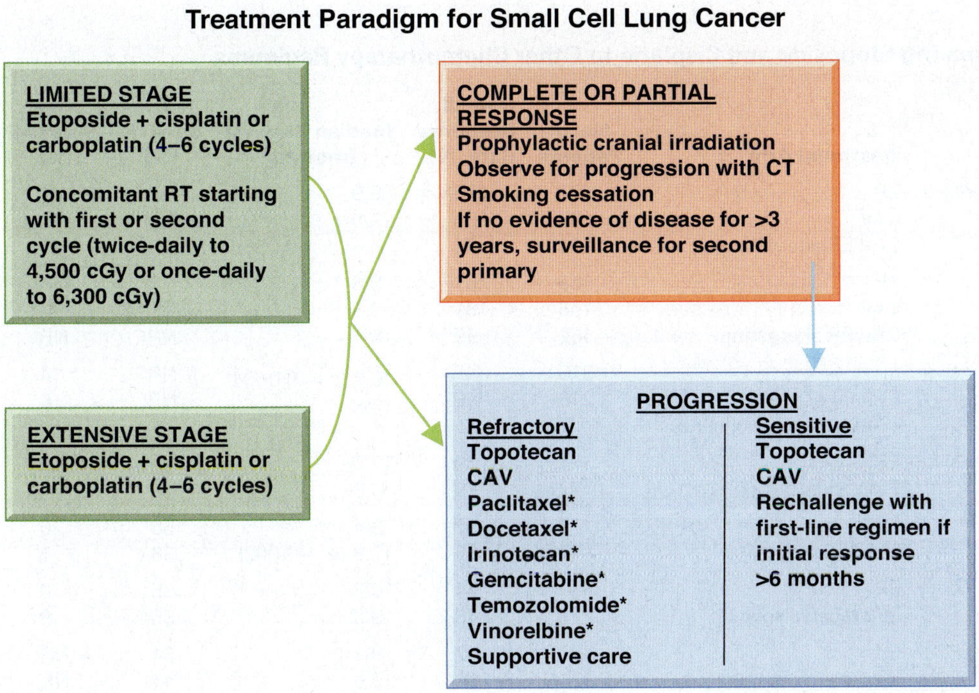

Figure 38.4 General treatment paradigm for small cell lung cancer. *Single agents evaluated in phase II trials with activity in SCLC.

Chemotherapy

Evolution of Chemotherapy Regimens. The sensitivity of SCLC to chemotherapy agents was recognized about 50 years ago, and the primary role of systemic treatment in SCLC was established early on. Alkylating agents, anthracyclines, vinca alkaloids, and antifolates all showed single-agent efficacy. In the 1980s, the epipodophyllotoxin, etoposide, and the platinum analogs, cisplatin and carboplatin, were introduced, and their activity ranged from 40% to 60% in previously untreated patients.[84] Since then, numerous other chemotherapeutic agents have demonstrated activity in SCLC, but aside from the camptothecins, the drugs identified in the 1970s and 1980s remain the backbone of therapy. Ultimately, randomized trials of combinations demonstrated superior activity to single agents.[85,86]

Livingston et al.[87] developed the cyclophosphamide, doxorubicin, vincristine (CAV) combination, and reported on 358 patients who received this combination followed sequentially by thoracic and brain irradiation. For patients with extensive disease, the complete response rate was 14%, the overall response rate was 57%, and the median survival was 26 weeks. For patients with limited disease, the rates were 41%, 75%, and 52 weeks, respectively. With these data, CAV became the standard chemotherapy regimen.

With the identification of etoposide as perhaps the most active agent, several modifications of the CAV regimen that included etoposide were tested. A randomized trial showed greater response duration and survival with cyclophosphamide, doxorubicin, and etoposide (CAE) compared with CAV.[88] Hong et al.[89] compared intensive cyclophosphamide and vincristine (CV) (with the dose of cyclophosphamide increased from 1,000 to 2,000 mg/m^2) to CAV and to cyclophosphamide, etoposide, and vincristine (CEV) and reported that patients treated with CV had a shorter survival and experienced more myelosuppression than those treated on the other two arms. Five randomized trials have evaluated the addition of etoposide (CAVE) to the CAV regimen.[90–94] In the three studies in which the doses of CAV were equivalent in each arm,[90–92] a better response rate was evident in the arm that contained etoposide, in at least some patient subsets, with increased hematologic toxicity, although a nonstatistical improvement in survival was seen in only one study.[90] Two studies intensified components of this regimen in the CAV arm compared to the CAVE arm,[93] leading to equivalent myelotoxicity, response rates, and survival.

The etoposide/cisplatin (EP) regimen was tested in SCLC cases because this combination produced synergistic activity in preclinical systems. In addition, both agents could be given at full doses because of less myelosuppression with cisplatin. The first report by Sierocki et al.[95] at Memorial Sloan-Kettering Cancer Center in 1979 demonstrated the activity of this combination in SCLC. Subsequent studies by Evans et al.[96,97] reported response rates of 55% in patients previously treated with CAV and 86% in newly diagnosed patients. Einhorn et al.[98] reported that two cycles of consolidation with EP, when added to the treatment of patients with limited disease who were responding to six cycles of CAV, produced longer survival than with CAV only. Three randomized trials have compared EP to cyclophosphamide, vincristine, and an anthracycline.[99–101] Less myelosuppression occurred with EP, and, if given with radiation, patients experienced less esophagitis and interstitial pneumonitis. Furthermore, the largest trial showed that EP produced a better median (15 months versus 10 months) and 5-year (10% versus 3%) survival for patients with limited disease.[101] Retrospective analyses and meta-analyses also support the superiority of cisplatin- or carboplatin-containing chemotherapy for SCLC.[102–104] As a result, EP is now the standard first-line chemotherapy regimen for SCLC (Table 38.1).

Carboplatin has been substituted for cisplatin in SCLC chemotherapy regimens in an effort to decrease nonhematologic toxicities. Randomized trials comparing cisplatin and carboplatin suggest that they may have similar efficacy. The Hellenic Cooperative Oncology Group randomized 147 patients with either limited or extensive disease to receive etoposide 100 mg/m^2 days 1 to 3, and cisplatin 100 mg/m^2 or carboplatin 300 mg/m^2.[105] Concurrent radiation also was administered to responding patients starting with the third cycle. Response and survival were similar in the two arms. Nausea, vomiting, nephrotoxicity, and neurotoxicity were significantly lower in the patients who received carboplatin, as was grade 4 leukopenia. However, the sample size of this study is inadequate to confirm equivalent efficacy. A meta-analysis that evaluated individual subject data from four randomized trials with a total of 663 patients found that median overall survival (OS), median progression-free survival (PFS), and response rates were similar in the cisplatin and carboplatin arms. Although hematologic toxicities were higher in those patients that receive carboplatin, nonhematologic toxicities were increased in those that receive cisplatin.[106] Based on these data, etoposide and carboplatin can

TABLE 38.1

Randomized Clinical Trials Comparing Etoposide and Cisplatin to Other Chemotherapy Regimens

Study (Ref.)	Stage	Treatment Arm	No. of Patients	Overall Response Rate (%)	Median Survival (months)	1-Year Survival (%)	2-Year Survival (%)
Fukuoka, et al.[99]	Limited and extensive	EP	97	78	9.9	NR	12
		CAV	97	55	9.9	NR	10
		CAV/EP alternating	94	76	11.8 ($p = 0.056$)	NR	21
Roth, et al.[100]	Extensive	EP	159	61	8.6	NR	NR
		CAV	156	51	8.3	NR	NR
		CAV/EP alternating	162	59	8.1	NR	NR
Sundstrom, et al.[101]	Limited and extensive	EP	218	NR	10.2 ($p = 0.0004$)	NR	14
		Cyclophosphate, epirubicin, vincristine	218	NR	7.8	NR	6
Skarlos, et al.[105]	Limited and extensive	EP	71	69	12.5	NR	NR
		Etoposide/carboplatin	72	78	11.8	NR	NR
Noda, et al.[108]	Extensive	EP	77	52	9.4	58	20
		Irinotecan/cisplatin	77	65	12.8 ($p = 0.002$)	38	5
Hanna, et al.[425]	Extensive	EP	110	44	10.2	35	8
		Irinotecan/cisplatin	221	48	9.3	35	8
Lara, et al.[109]	Extensive	EP	327	57	9.1	34	NR
		Irinotecan/cisplatin	324	60	9.9	41	NR
Eckardt, et al.[115]	Extensive	EP	395	69	9.4	31	NR
		Oral topotecan/cisplatin	389	63	9.2	31	NR
Miyamoto, et al.[130]	Limited and extensive	EP	45	78	12.8	53	15
		Ifosfamide with EP	47	74	13.0	62	17
Loehrer, et al.[131]	Extensive	EP	84	67	7.3	27	5
		Ifosfamide with EP	87	73	9.1 ($p = 0.045$)	36	13
Mavroudis, et al.[135]	Limited and extensive	EP	71	48	10.5	37	NR
		Paclitaxel with EP	62	50	9.5	38	NR
Niell, et al.[136]	Extensive	EP	282	68	9.9	37	8
		Paclitaxel with EP	283	75	10.6	38	11

EP, etoposide and cisplatin; CAV, cyclophosphamide, doxorubicin, and vincristine; NR, not reported.

be considered an appropriate first-line regimen, particularly in patients who cannot tolerate cisplatin.

More recently, platinum combinations with topotecan and irinotecan have emerged as potential regimens for initial therapy. Irinotecan was shown to have single-agent efficacy in Japanese studies.[107] The Japan Clinical Oncology Group compared cisplatin and irinotecan to EP as initial treatment in extensive disease.[108] The study was terminated after 154 of the planned 230 patients were enrolled because median (12.8 months versus 9.4 months) and 2-year (19.5% versus 5.2%) survival were significantly better in the group treated with cisplatin and irinotecan. Significant diarrhea occurred only in the irinotecan group, and myelosuppression was the most common toxicity in both groups and more frequent with EP. Two confirmatory studies were subsequently launched in the United States. In the first trial, the irinotecan/cisplatin schedule was modified in an effort to decrease toxicity, leading to equivalent response rates (48% for irinotecan/cisplatin versus 44% for EP), median time to progression (4 versus 5 months), and median OS (9 versus 10 months).[425] The Southwest Oncology Group (SWOG) compared these two regimens with the same dose and schedule used in the Japanese trial and also showed, in a well-powered study, that outcomes are equivalent with the two regimens in Caucasian patients.[109] High response rates have been reported in several trials using irinotecan and carboplatin with varied dosing schedules.[110,111] A phase III trial comparing that regimen with etoposide/cisplatin showed improved survival, but the median survival of 7 months in the control arm, which used oral etoposide, was lower than expected.[112] Many hypothesize that population-based polymorphisms in uridine 5′-diphospho (UDP)-glucuronosyltransferase (UGT1A1), the enzyme responsible for detoxifying SN-38, the active metabolite of irinotecan, may account for differences in toxicity and efficacy between Japanese and Americans.[113] The regimen of topotecan plus cisplatin also has undergone phase II and III testing.[114,115] Eckardt et al.[115] reported the results of a randomized trial including 784 patients in which patients received oral topotecan (1.7 mg/m^2 per day for 5 days) plus cisplatin, or standard etoposide and cisplatin. The response rates, median survival, and 1-year survival were identical. Severe neutropenia occurred more often with EP, but oral topotecan and cisplatin caused more anemia and thrombocytopenia.

Strategies to Improve Outcomes with Chemotherapy Regimens

Alternating Cycles of Combination Chemotherapy Regimens. The recognition of clonal heterogeneity within a tumor and the intolerability of treatment regimens that included more than four drugs due to overlapping toxicity led to trials of alternating chemotherapy combinations. The somatic mutation model developed by Goldie et al.[116] predicted that the best probability of cure was achieved by the earliest possible introduction and the most rapid alternation of all active agents. If two equally effective non–cross-resistant regimens were available, the model predicted that alternating between regimens every other cycle would be more effective than alternating after every three cycles or giving one regimen continuously for five cycles before switching to the second regimen.

Many randomized clinical trials have tested the concept of alternating multidrug combinations.[100,117–121] The fact that the EP regimen was effective in patients who had progressed after cyclophosphamide-based chemotherapy suggested that these drug combinations were non–cross-resistant.[122] With this in mind, the National Cancer Institute of Canada conducted a study in which 289 patients were randomized to CAV or CAV alternating with EP.[119] Chemotherapy was given for a total of six cycles. The response rate (65% versus 47%), PFS, and median survival time (10 months versus 8 months) favored the patients who had received alternating therapy. The authors postulated that these findings could be the result of the inclusion of a more active regimen (i.e., EP) within the alternating arm, an advantage due to greater drug diversity with five effective drugs rather than three, or support of the Goldie et al. concept. A Japanese study compared CAV to EP to alternating CAV/EP in 288 patients with limited or extensive stage disease.[99] Patients with limited disease received four cycles of chemotherapy followed by thoracic irradiation and were found to have improved survival with the alternating regimen compared with CAV ($p = 0.058$) or EP ($p = 0.032$). No differences in survival were noted in the patients with extensive disease. Roth et al.[100] evaluated 437 patients with extensive disease in a randomized trial comparing EP for four cycles, CAV for six cycles, or CAV alternating with EP for a total of six cycles. Although a slight improvement occurred in PFS ($p = 0.052$) with the alternating regimen, there was no difference in response rate or OS among the treatment arms. The patients whose tumors did not respond to CAV and were crossed over to EP were twice as likely to benefit as individuals who initially received EP and were crossed over to CAV, although these differences were not significant (28% versus 14% for induction responders who relapsed and 15% versus 8% for patients with primary resistance). The modest activity seen when refractory patients were crossed over from one of these regimens to the other suggests that the CAV and EP combinations are not entirely cross-resistant, which works against a primary assumption of the Goldie et al. hypothesis. Taking all of these studies together, alternating regimens appears to have slight or no benefit over initial treatment with EP alone.

Additional studies have evaluated alternating chemotherapy introduced after achieving a response to an induction regimen.[123–125] The National Cancer Institute of Canada designed a randomized trial in which 300 patients with limited disease received either CAV for three cycles followed by EP for three cycles or CAV alternating with EP for a total of six cycles.[126] Response rates, time to treatment failure, or survival did not differ. Wolf et al.[123] randomized 321 patients to treatment with ifosfamide plus etoposide given until a response plateau, followed by CAV or ifosfamide plus etoposide alternating with CAV. A total of six cycles of chemotherapy were delivered in each arm. No difference in outcome was noted.

Studies also have evaluated alternating more intensive regimens. For example, a German multicenter trial demonstrated that an alternating eight-drug regimen was superior to CAV.[127] Two other European trials testing three drugs regimens alternating with four drug regimens found no survival advantage to that approach.[120,128] Again, the median survival times observed in these studies were no different from those that used EP alone.[99,100]

Addition of a Third Chemotherapeutic Agent to Etoposide Plus Cisplatin. All efforts to add a third drug to the standard EP regimen have resulted in more toxicity with little or no improvement in survival. The three-drug regimen of etoposide, ifosfamide, and cisplatin (VIP), developed initially for refractory germ cell tumors, also has been evaluated in SCLC.[129] In randomized trials comparing VIP to EP, one study, which included patients with limited and extensive disease, found no difference in survival between the two treatment groups,[130] whereas another, which was larger and enrolled only patients with extensive disease, identified a significant difference in median survival (9 months versus 7 months) and 2-year survival rates (13% versus 5%).[131] In both studies, myelosuppression was more severe in the ifosfamide-containing arm. Single-arm studies substituting carboplatin for cisplatin in ifosfamide, carboplatin, and etoposide (ICE) have shown impressive response rates, yet cumulative myelosuppression.[132,133] A large trial comparing ICE plus a midcycle dose of vincristine to other standard therapy demonstrated an improvement in the median and 1-year survival rates.[134] However, an increased rate of septicemia was noted with ifosfamide, carboplatin, and etoposide-vincristine (ICE-V) (15% versus 7% in the control arm).

Studies that added paclitaxel to EP reach the same conclusion: enhanced toxicity with similar efficacy. Two studies that compared EP to EP plus paclitaxel showed that the addition of the third drug increased toxicity, as well as treatment-related mortality, without improving survival.[135,136] A German study that added paclitaxel to etoposide and carboplatin demonstrated a significantly better median survival (13 months versus 12 months) and 3-year survival (17% versus 9%) only in patients with limited disease as compared to treatment with etoposide, carboplatin, and vincristine.[137]

Maintenance Therapy. A large number of randomized studies have examined whether maintenance chemotherapy prolongs survival in SCLC.[117,138–148] Three studies that randomized patients in complete remission after induction therapy to maintenance treatment or observation identified improved survival with the prolonged treatment program in some patient groups.[117,141,144] The Cancer and Leukemia Group B (CALGB) randomized 258 patients to one of four chemotherapy regimens, and 57 patients in complete remission underwent a second randomization to maintenance therapy or observation. Among the 46 patients with limited disease who proceeded to the second randomization, the median survival was improved with maintenance chemotherapy (17 months versus 7 months).[144] However, the initial regimens used in this study might be considered inferior to currently used treatments. In a second study, patients treated with six cycles of CAV and in complete remission were randomized to six additional cycles of the same chemotherapy or observation.[111] For the patients with extensive disease, the median survival was improved by approximately 4 months with maintenance treatment. In an ECOG trial, patients were randomized to CAV alternating with another three-drug combination or CAV alone and, subsequently, those in complete remission after six to eight cycles of induction underwent a second randomization to maintenance treatment or observation.[117] Patients assigned to CAV and maintenance therapy had a longer PFS and OS ($p = 0.09$) than patients who received only CAV with no maintenance. In contrast, for the patients who received the six-drug regimen, those who were given no maintenance survived longer than the patients who received maintenance treatment. These studies suggest that there may be patients—perhaps those with particularly chemotherapy-sensitive disease—who derive a benefit from maintenance. In unselected patients, however, clinical trials that have evaluated treatment programs that extend beyond six cycles of chemotherapy have not demonstrated an advantage in survival.

The Medical Research Council randomized 265 patients who had responded to six cycles of induction chemotherapy to an additional six cycles of maintenance or observation.[138] Overall, there was no difference in survival between patients treated with 6 or 12 cycles of chemotherapy, although for patients in complete remission at the time of randomization, a subset analysis suggested that maintenance provides a survival benefit. Three other large studies that randomized patients responding to 5 or 6 cycles of induction to a total of 12 cycles of chemotherapy or observation found no difference in outcome.[142,143,146] Another study that randomized patients with limited disease from the start of chemotherapy to a total of 6 or 12 cycles identified inferior survival in the arm treated with the longer course of therapy.[140]

Other studies have evaluated whether four cycles of chemotherapy are adequate.[139,145,149] Spiro et al.[149] designed a study that included a double randomization at diagnosis. Patients received four or eight cycles of CEV and on relapse were given additional chemotherapy or supportive care. Of the four treatment arms, patients who received four cycles of chemotherapy and only supportive care at relapse had a significantly inferior median survival of 30 weeks. Four cycles of treatment were found to be adequate, provided that chemotherapy was offered to patients appropriate for additional therapy at relapse. Two additional studies evaluated four cycles of induction with longer treatment programs. A European trial randomized patients with limited and extensive disease who responded to four cycles of EP to CAV for up to 10 additional cycles or to observation with no survival differences, although the study had limited power due to small sample size.[139] ECOG enrolled 402 eligible patients with extensive-stage disease into a trial that delivered four cycles of EP followed by a randomization of patients with at least stable disease to four additional cycles of topotecan or to observation.[145] Although maintenance therapy increased the time before documentation of disease progression, there was no difference in OS.

Two recent meta-analyses have been conducted evaluating maintenance chemotherapy showing small improvements in survival and an increase in toxicity.[150,151] Bozcuk and colleagues[150] reported an improved 1- and 2-year survival by 9% and 4%, respectively. Although Rossi et al.[151] showed a significant OS benefit (hazard ratio [HR], 0.89, 95% confidence interval [CI], 0.81 to 0.92; $p = 0.02$) for maintenance treatment, this improvement was projected to an additional 2 weeks.[151] Further, there was a high heterogeneity among the included trials.

In summary, four to six cycles of chemotherapy appear to be optimal in the management of limited and extensive SCLC. After the completion of this initial treatment, patients should be monitored closely and then offered further chemotherapy at the time of progression. Both the NCCN and the European Society of Medical Oncology Guidelines support this approach.[52,152]

Dose Intensification. In experimental models, numerous chemotherapy drugs display log-linear or near linear dose-response curves,[153] and high-dose chemotherapy has proven effective at treating hematologic diseases. It seemed reasonable to test the hypothesis that more intensive chemotherapy could improve outcomes in SCLC. Methods used have included the use of higher chemotherapy doses without or with hematopoietic growth factor support, shortened cycle length, or extreme dose intensification with marrow or peripheral blood stem cell support.

Several investigators evaluated whether increasing the dose of drugs beyond the usual dose improves survival.[154–159] Three randomized trials comparing standard versus high-dose CAV[156,158] or EP[157] found no difference in response rates or median survival. No hematopoietic growth factors were used in these three trials, and, as such, myelosuppression and infections were significantly more severe in the high-dose arms. A randomized trial that did utilize granulocyte-macrophage colony-stimulating factor (GM-CSF) with dose escalation found that excess toxicity actually resulted in lower drug delivery and poorer response and survival rates in the dose-intense arm.[159] Only a French study with 105 limited-stage patients demonstrated improvements in PFS at 2 years (28% versus 8%) and OS (43% versus 26%) with the administration of higher drug doses.[154] Few oncologists have embraced this approach.

A number of studies have evaluated whether shortening the interval between chemotherapy cycles improves survival. A multicenter study randomized 300 patients, mostly with limited-stage disease, to six cycles of ICE-V delivered every 4 weeks or every 3 weeks.[160] In a second randomization, patients were given GM-CSF or placebo after each chemotherapy cycle. The delivered dose intensity was increased by 26% in the group receiving chemotherapy every 3 weeks compared to those treated every 4 weeks. The median survival (443 days versus 351 days) and the 2-year survival rate (33% versus 18%) were better in the intensified arm ($p = 0.0014$). GM-CSF did not reduce the incidence or the duration of febrile neutropenia, and there was no difference in survival between the patients who received GM-CSF or placebo. In a subsequent study, ICE given every 4 weeks was compared to ICE given every 2 weeks with support of GM-CSF, and autologous blood collected before the cycle was reinfused 24 hours after the chemotherapy.[161] Although the median delivered dose intensity was increased by 82% without significant increased toxicity, no survival benefit was identified. Two studies compared treatment with cyclophosphamide, doxorubicin, and etoposide given either every 3 weeks, or every 2 weeks with GM-CSF support.[162,163] The larger trial,[163] which also included a higher percentage of limited-stage patients, showed an improvement in complete response rate and OS, but the other trial did not. No fewer than four randomized trials have shown that intensive multidrug weekly regimens are no better, yet significantly more toxic than standard regimens.[164–167]

Numerous reports cite the use of high-dose chemotherapy with autologous bone marrow or stem cell rescue for treating SCLC.[168–186] These studies have included small numbers of highly selected patients.[161,182,183,187–189] Survival has not been shown to be better than conventional treatment. As in other chemosensitive solid tumors like breast cancer, high-dose chemotherapy with stem cell support does not appear to have a role in SCLC.

Treatment After Relapse Following Initial Therapy. The strongest predictor of outcome for patients with relapsed SCLC is the duration of remission. As such, patients are distinguished as having *sensitive* or *refractory* disease. The term *sensitive* implies an appropriate response to initial therapy that is maintained for 3 months or more. These patients have a higher likelihood of response to any additional chemotherapy; although, at best, it is approximately half that expected in the first-line setting. Survival from the start of a second regimen averages around 6 months. Patients with *refractory* disease either had no response to initial therapy or progressed within 3 months after completing treatment. Their chance of response to additional therapy is less than 10%, and their median survival from the start of a second regimen is 4 months.

The only approved agent in relapsed disease is topotecan. Ardizzoni et al.[190] reported a phase II trial in which topotecan, administered at a dose of 1.5 mg/m^2 daily for 5 days, yielded a response rate of 38% in sensitive patients and 6% in refractory patients. Median survival from the start of second-line therapy was 7 and 5 months, respectively. A randomized trial compared topotecan, administered at that same dose and schedule, to CAV in patients who relapsed at least 2 months after initial therapy.[191] The response rates for topotecan (24%) and for CAV (18%) were similar. The median survival was 6 months in both arms. Symptom improvement was better with topotecan for four of the eight symptoms queried, and as such, the U.S. Food and Drug Administration approved intravenous topotecan for sensitive relapsed SCLC. Oral topotecan has also undergone extensive testing in patients with relapsed SCLC. In a randomized phase II study, oral topotecan at a dose of 2.3 mg/m^2 daily for 5 days was comparable to intravenous topotecan 1.5 mg/m^2 daily for 5 days with regard to response rate (23% versus 15%), median survival (32 weeks versus 25 weeks), and symptom control.[192] Subsequently, the Medical Research Council showed that oral topotecan improved survival in relapsed sensitive and refractory SCLC over best supportive care alone (26 versus 14 weeks, respectively).[193] Oral topotecan led to a response rate of 7%, with a slower deterioration of quality of life and symptomatology. Another phase III study randomized 309 SCLC patients who had relapsed ≥90 days after first-line therapy to receive oral topotecan or intravenous topotecan.[194] The overall response rate and median survival time were 18.3% and 33 weeks, respectively, for patients who received oral topotecan compared to 21.9% and 35 weeks, respectively, for those who received intravenous topotecan. Although oral topotecan was associated with a lower incidence of grade 4 neutropenia, diarrhea occurred more often in this group of patients. Oral topotecan also has received regulatory approval for second-line therapy of SCLC.

Amrubicin, a third-generation synthetic 9-amino-anthracycline with diverse molecular effects including DNA intercalation, inhibition of topoisomerase II, and stabilization of topoisomerase IIa cleavable complexes, has been studied extensively and has received approval in Japan for SCLC treatment.[195] A randomized phase II trial conducted there showed higher response rates and PFS compared with topotecan.[196] Two North American phase II trials of amrubicin showed encouraging results.[197,198] In patients with refractory SCLC, the overall response rate for single-agent amrubicin was found to be 21%, with median PFS and OS of 3.2 and 6 months, respectively. Subsequently, 76 patients with sensitive SCLC were randomized in a 2:1 fashion to receive amrubicin or topotecan. Amrubicin treatment resulted in a significantly higher response rate than topotecan (44% versus 15%, $p = 0.021$), which led to improved PFS (4.5 versus 3.3 months) and OS (9.2 versus 7.6 months).[198] Despite phase II activity, preliminary results of the phase III study, which compared amrubicin to topotecan, were disappointing.[199] Although the activity of amrubicin was apparent, there was no statistically significant difference in OS observed between the two arms. The trend favored amrubicin (HR, 0.82; 95% CI, 0.68 to 0.99; $p = 0.036$), especially in the subgroup of patients with primary refractory disease (HR, 0.77; 95% CI, 0.59 to 1.0; $p = 0.047$). Although lower hematologic adverse events were noted in the amrubicin arm, these patients had a higher incidence of infections. The role of amrubicin for the treatment of patients with relapsed SCLC remains to be defined.

Temozolomide is an oral alkylating agent that crosses the blood–brain barrier. A phase II clinical trial of temozolomide in 64 patients with relapsed sensitive or refractory SCLC has been performed.[200] Temozolomide therapy was well tolerated and associated with an overall response rate of 20% in this patient population, with a 23% response rate in the sensitive group ($n = 48$) and a 13% response rate in the refractory cohort ($n = 16$). Responses also were noted in patients receiving temozolomide as third-line treatment and in those with brain metastases.[200] There is an ongoing multicenter phase II study comparing temozolomide and veliparib (a poly [ADP-ribose] polymerase [PARP] inhibitor) versus temozolomide and placebo in patients with relapsed sensitive and refractory SCLC (ClinicalTrials.gov identifier: NCT01638546).

Multiple trials have been conducted using other agents in this patient population. A list of single agents and their activity in relapsed SCLC is found in Table 38.2, many of which also have been tested in combination studies. In summary, the optimal drug or combination of drugs in relapsed SCLC has not been established. Single-agent topotecan or CAV are appropriate for patients with sensitive relapse. These regimens also could be used for patients with refractory SCLC, although the response rates are lower. Agents evaluated in phase II trials with activity in SCLC can be considered. For patients with relapse 6 months or more after initial therapy, rechallenging with the same regimen as used in first-line treatment is also a consideration.[52]

Immunotherapy and Other Targeted Therapies

In light of the therapeutic plateau achieved with current chemotherapy, investigators have studied a wide range of novel therapies in the hopes of improving outcomes (Table 38.3).

Receptor Tyrosine Kinases and Growth Factors. Small molecule kinase inhibitors are now established therapies for several diseases, but as yet, have not proven efficacious in SCLC. c-Kit protein expression has been reported in 28% to 93% of SCLC tumors.[201] In vitro studies support the role of c-kit and its ligand, stem cell factor (SCF), on SCLC autocrine and paracrine growth stimulation,[202] and imatinib has demonstrated growth inhibition of multiple SCLC cell lines.[203] Nonetheless, three phase II studies in SCLC failed to demonstrate a single radiologic response to imatinib, even when enrollment was restricted to patients with tumors expressing c-kit protein by immunohistochemistry.[201,204,205]

The PI3K/AKT/mammalian target of rapamycin (mTOR) signal pathway is defective in SCLC: SCLC cells possess a constitutively active PI3K[206] and harbor PI3K and PTEN mutations[22,23,207]; phosphorylated AKT is present in 70% of tumors in SCLC patients[208]; and protein expression of mTOR, S6K1, and phosphorylated 4EBP1 are elevated in SCLC cells compared to type II epithelial cells.[209] Such alterations lead to growth, survival, and chemotherapy resistance in SCLC. Temsirolimus—the small molecule inhibitor of mTOR—was evaluated in an ECOG trial in which patients were randomized after initial chemotherapy to maintenance therapy with either high-dose or low-dose temsirolimus.[210] Although the PFS (1.8 months versus 2.5 months) and OS were better for the high dose arm (6.5 months versus 9.0 months), these results were no better than those observed in the previous ECOG trial of topotecan maintenance therapy,[145] suggesting no added benefit from temsirolimus. Similarly, a phase II trial of everolimus in relapsed SCLC did not demonstrate antitumor activity for this agent.[211]

The insulinlike growth factor receptor (IGF-1R), a member of the insulin receptor subclass of receptor tyrosine kinase, is activated by the ligands IGF-1 and IGF-2 and signals mitogenic and antiapoptotic signaling pathways contributing to cellular transformation and malignant growth.[208] IGF-1R and its ligand, IGF-1, are expressed at increased levels in SCLC.[208] The IGF-1R activates the PI3K-AKT pathway in SCLC, playing a role in the development and growth of the disease, as well as resistance to chemotherapy.[208] Therefore, targeted inhibition of IGF-1R represents an attractive approach to enhancing chemotherapeutic efficacy and inhibiting tumor recurrence in patients with SCLC. Yet, the ECOG 1508 phase II study evaluating the monoclonal antibody, cixutumumab, together with cisplatin and etoposide in a randomized trial, failed to show an improvement in PFS with IGF-1R inhibition.[212]

Developmental Pathways: The Hedgehog Pathway. The Hedgehog pathway is essential in early lung development and has a role in regulating stem cell maintenance and differentiation.[213] Hedgehog signaling may play a significant role in the development and proliferation of SCLC, which is a relatively undifferentiated airway epithelial tumor that may recapitulate aspects of early lung development.[214,215] In vitro and in vivo studies have demonstrated that Hedgehog antagonists can inhibit SCLC and, when administered following chemotherapy, such inhibition may delay or prevent the recurrence of residual disease.[215] The ECOG 1508 phase II randomized trial in patients with extensive stage disease included an arm evaluating the addition of vismodegib, a Hedgehog inhibitor, to cisplatin and etoposide, which unfortunately, did not lead to an improvement in PFS.[212]

Nonreceptor Oncogenes: Bcl-2 Genes. The antiapoptotic gene product, bcl-2 protein, is expressed in 80% to 90% of SCLC tumor samples and, as such, is a potential therapeutic target.[216,217] Oblimersen (G3139) is an antisense oligonucleotide that suppresses bcl-2 expression. The CALGB conducted a series of studies with oblimersen in combination with chemotherapy for SCLC.[218,219] In a randomized phase II study of etoposide/carboplatin with or without oblimersen, survival was inferior in the patients receiving oblimersen (HR for OS, 2.13; $p = 0.02$).[220] Insufficient suppression of bcl-2 by this agent may explain its lack of efficacy. Navitoclax, a selective high-affinity small molecule inhibitor of bcl-2 and bcl-x_L (another antiapoptotic protein of the Bcl-2 family), resulted in dramatic tumor responses in SCLC cell line xenograft tumors as a single agent and enhanced the efficacy of standard cytotoxic agents against SCLC models.[221–227] Yet, a recent phase II study of navitoclax demonstrated limited activity in patients

TABLE 38.2

Activity of Single Agent Chemotherapy in Relapsed Small Cell Lung Cancer

Drug (Ref.)	Dose/Schedule	N	Sensitive/Refractory	Response Rate (%)	Median Survival (mo)
Topotecan (IV)[190]	1.5 mg/m^2 daily × 5 days	45 47	Sensitive Refractory	38 6	6.9 4.7
Topotecan (IV)[191]	1.5 mg/m^2 daily × 5 days	107	Sensitive (60 days)	24	6.0
Topotecan (IV)[192]	1.5 mg/m^2 daily × 5 days	54	Sensitive	15	5.8
Topotecan (oral)[192]	2.3 mg/m^2 daily × 5 days	52	Sensitive	23	7.5
Topotecan (oral)[193]	2.3 mg/m^2 daily × 5 days	71 30 41	Sensitive + refractory Sensitive Refractory	7 3 10	6.0
Topotecan (IV)[194]	1.5mg/m^2 daily × 5 days	151	Sensitive	22	8.8
Topotecan (oral)[194]	2.3 mg/m^2 daily × 5 days	153	Sensitive	18	8.0
Irinotecan[107]	100 mg/m^2 weekly	16	Sensitive[a]	47	6.2
Paclitaxel[426]	175 mg/m^2 every 3 wks	24	Refractory	29	3.0
Docetaxel[427]	100 mg/m^2 every 3 wks	34	Not specified[b]	25	NR
Gemcitabine[428]	1,000 mg/m^2 d1, 8, 15 every 4 wks	46	Both	12	7.1
Gemcitabine[429]	1,250 mg/m^2 d1, 8 every 3 wks	27	Both	0	6.4
Gemcitabine[430]	1,000 mg/m^2 d1, 8, 15 every 4 wks	38	Refractory	13	4.0
Vinorelbine[431]	25 mg/m^2 weekly	24	Both	13	5.0
Vinorelbine[432]	30 mg/m^2 weekly	26	Sensitive	16	NR
Amrubicin[433]	40 mg/m^2 daily × 3 every 3 wks	44 16	Sensitive Refractory	52 50	10.3 11.6
Amrubicin[434]	40 mg/m^2 daily × 3 every 3 wks	75	Refractory	21	6.0
Amrubicin[198]	40 mg/m^2 daily × 3 every 3 wks	50	Sensitive	44%	9.2
Amrubicin[199]	40 mg/m^2 daily × 3 every 3 wks	225 199	Sensitive Refractory	31% (both sensitive & refractory)	9.2 6.2
Picoplatin[435]	120–150 mg/m^2 every 3 wks	24 13	Sensitive Refractory	8 15	8.1 6.2
Picoplatin[436]	150 mg/m^2 every 3 wks	6 27 44	Sensitive Resistant[c] Refractory[d]	4 (all three groups)	6.1 (all three groups)
Picoplatin[437]	150 mg/m^2 every 3 wks	268	Relapsed disease[e]	4	4.7
Temozolomide[200]	75 mg/m^2 daily for 21 out of 28 days	48 16	Sensitive Refractory	23 13	6.0 5.6

[a] All but one patient had a chemotherapy-free interval of >90 days.
[b] Previously untreated patients also included.
[c] Defined as patients that relapsed within 90 days of the end of first-line platinum-containing chemotherapy.
[d] Defined as patients that did not have a response to first-line platinum-containing chemotherapy.
[e] Defined as those patients with relapse <6 months of completing first-line platinum-based chemotherapy.
IV, intravenous; NR, not reported; N, number of patients.

with recurrent and progressive SCLC.[228] Results of a completed phase I trial of navitoclax with first-line combination chemotherapy for SCLC are not yet available (ClinicalTrials.gov identifier: NCT00878449). A third agent, obatoclax mesylate, which is a small-molecule BH3-mimetic that exhibits binding affinity for a range of bcl-2 family members, has been evaluated in various clinical scenarios. A phase II trial of obatoclax mesylate added to topotecan did not exceed the historic response rate seen in topotecan alone in patients with relapsed SCLC.[229] The phase II randomized study of carboplatin and etoposide with or without obatoclax followed by maintenance obatoclax in patients with newly diagnosed extensive stage SCLC failed to meet its primary endpoint of improved response rate for those receiving obatoclax, although there was a trend for improved PFS (6 versus 5.4 months, $p = 0.084$) and OS (10.6 versus 9.9 months, $p = 0.052$).[230]

Angiogenesis Inhibitors. Angiogenesis inhibitors have entered into standard clinical practice for numerous malignancies, and they are being tested in SCLC as well. Two phase III trials that tested thalidomide as maintenance therapy after first-line chemotherapy showed no significant effect on OS.[231,232] Likewise, vandetanib, an oral TKI of vascular endothelial growth factor receptor 2 (VEGFR-2) and EGFR, failed to improve PFS in a randomized phase II maintenance trial.[233] In all of these cases, toxicity was significantly greater in the treatment arms. Similarly, sorafenib (inhibitor of RAF; VEGFR-2,-3; platelet-derived growth factor receptor alpha [PDGFRα]) and cediranib (inhibitor of VEGFR-1, -2, -3; PDGFRβ; c-KIT) showed minimal activity for relapsed disease when evaluated as single agents, although cediranib demonstrated a promising PFS of 8 months when administered with cisplatin and etoposide in a phase I study.[234–236]

TABLE 38.3

Immunotherapies and Other Targeted Agents That Have Undergone Testing in Small Cell Lung Cancer

Agent (Ref.)	Mechanism of Action	Study Design	Result
Interferon-alfa[438–441]	Immunomodulator	Phase III (multiple)	Two studies with improved survival in limited-stage patients, two studies with no survival benefit
Interferon-gamma[442, 443]	Immunomodulator	Phase III (multiple)	No improvement in survival
Interleukin-2[444]	Immunomodulator	Phase II	21% response rate but excessive toxicity
Warfarin[445,446]	Anticoagulant	Randomized phase II Randomized phase III	Significant improvement in PFS and OS Warfarin added to chemotherapy significantly improved response rates, and nonsignificant improvement in PFS and OS
Aspirin (1 g/d)[447]	Anticoagulant	Randomized phase II	Aspirin added to chemotherapy did not improve survival
Subcutaneous unfractionated heparin[448]	Anticoagulant	Randomized phase II	Heparin added to chemotherapy during first 5 weeks of treatment led to significantly improved response rates and PFS, as well as OS in limited stage disease
Ipilimumab[245]	Humanized anti-CTLA4 antibody	Randomized phase II	Improved immune-related PFS when administered with carboplatin/paclitaxel in phased dosing schedule in chemo-naïve extensive stage SCLC
Marimastat[449]	Matrix metalloproteinase inhibitor	Phase III	No improvement in PFS or OS
Tanomastat[450]	Matrix metalloproteinase inhibitor	Phase III	No improvement in PFS or OS
Imatinib[201,204,205]	c-Kit tyrosine kinase inhibitor	Phase II (multiple)	No responses
Temsirolimus[210]	mTOR inhibitor	Randomized phase II	Improved survival at higher dose but no improvement in outcome compared with prior trials
Everolimus[211]	mTOR inhibitor	Phase II	Limited antitumor activity in relapsed SCLC
Tipifarnib[451]	Farnesyl transferase inhibitor	Phase II	No responses
Cixutumumab[212]	Monoclonal IGF-1R antibody	Randomized phase II	No improvement in PFS when added to cisplatin/etoposide in chemo-naïve extensive stage SCLC
Vismodegib[212]	Hedgehog pathway inhibitor	Randomized phase II	No improvement in PFS when added to cisplatin/etoposide in chemo-naïve extensive stage SCLC
Oblimersen[220]	Bcl-2 antisense	Randomized phase II	No improvement in response rate
Navitoclax[220]	Bcl-2 and bcl-x_L inhibitor	Phase II	Limited activity in recurrent and progressive disease
Obatoclax mesylate[229,230]	BH3-mimetic exhibits binding affinity for bcl-2 family members, including bcl-2, bcl-XL, and mcl-1	Phase II Randomized phase II	No increased response rate when added to topotecan in relapsed SCLC Trend toward improved response rate, PFS and OS in chemo-naïve extensive stage SCLC
Bortezomib[452]	Proteosome inhibitor	Phase II	One response in refractory patient (2% overall response rate)
BEC-2 + Bacille Calmette-Guerin (BCG) adjuvant[453]	Ganglioside (GD3) anti-idiotype vaccine	Phase III	No improvement in PFS or OS
Thalidomide[231,232]	Multiple immunomodulatory effects, also inhibits VEGF	Phase III Phase III	Improved survival from 8.7 to 11.7 months but not significant (HR, 0.74; $p = 0.16$) No improvement in any parameters
Vandetanib[233]	Tyrosine kinase inhibitor of VEGFR-2 and EGFR	Randomized phase II	No improvement in PFS
Sorafenib[234]	RAF, VEGFR-2, VEGFR-3, PDGFRα inhibitor	Phase II	5% response rate in relapsed disease

(continued)

TABLE 38.3

Immunotherapies and Other Targeted Agents That Have Undergone Testing in Small Cell Lung Cancer *(continued)*

Agent (Ref.)	Mechanism of Action	Study Design	Result
Cediranib[235,236]	VEGFR-1, VEGFR-2, VEGFR-3, PDGFRβ, c-KIT inhibitor	Phase II	Minimal activity as a single agent in relapsed disease
		Phase I	8-month PFS with cisplatin and etoposide
Bevacizumab[238–241]	Monoclonal antibody to VEGF	Phase II (multiple)	No increased risk of hemorrhage Favorable survival compared with historical control
		Randomized phase II	Improved PFS for bevacizumab, but not in OS

PFS, progression-free survival; OS, overall survival; mTOR, mammalian target of rapamycin; VEGF, vascular endothelial growth factor; PDGFR, platelet-derived growth factor receptor.

Sunitinib, which is known to inhibit VEGFR-1, -2, -3; PDGFRα; PDGFRβ; c-KIT; and FLT3, was evaluated in a phase II trial as maintenance treatment after chemotherapy in patients with untreated extensive-stage SCLC (CALGB 30504).[237] After receiving four to six cycles of etoposide with cisplatin or carboplatin, patients were randomized to sunitinib or placebo until progression of disease. Patients in the placebo arm could cross over to receive sunitinib at the time of progression. The study met its primary endpoint of PFS after chemotherapy from the time of randomization (3.77 versus 2.3 months for sunitinib and placebo, respectively; HR, 1.53; 90% CI, 1.03 to 2.27; $p = 0.037$). Further, there was evidence of single-agent activity for sunitinib as maintenance therapy and at crossover, as well as a trend toward improvement in survival.[237]

Multiple phase II studies adding the VEGF monoclonal antibody, bevacizumab, to chemotherapy have not shown any increased risk of pulmonary hemorrhage in this cohort of patients who commonly have central tumors and have yielded favorable survival rates when compared to historical controls.[238–240] A randomized phase II study evaluated cisplatin or carboplatin plus etoposide with or without bevacizumab, for four cycles followed by single-agent bevacizumab or placebo until progression or unacceptable toxicity in patients with untreated extensive stage SCLC.[241] Median PFS was higher in the bevacizumab group than in the placebo group (5.5 versus 4.4 months; HR, 0.53; 95% CI, 0.32 to 0.86); however, there was no difference observed in OS, but a trend that favored placebo was noted (9.4 versus 10.9 months for bevacizumab and placebo groups, respectively; HR, 1.16; 95% CI, 0.66 to 2.04). Although no new or unexpected safety signals for bevacizumab were observed, the trend toward worse OS calls future prospects of bevacizumab into question unless a biomarker for benefit is discovered to select patients for this therapy.

Antigen-Independent Immunotherapy: Ipilimumab. Ipilimumab, a humanized immunoglobulin (Ig)G1 monoclonal antibody against cytotoxic T-lymphocyte antigen-4 (CTLA-4), has been approved for the treatment of patients with metastatic melanoma.[242] By blocking the inhibitory signal provided by CTLA-4, this class of antibodies can prolong the activation and proliferation of tumor-directed cytotoxic T cells, thus promoting an antitumor immune response.[243] A randomized, double-blind, three arm phase II trial in patients with untreated stage IIIB/IV NSCLC or extensive stage SCLC was performed to evaluate the efficacy and safety of paclitaxel and carboplatin with or without ipilimumab given on two dosing schedules.[244] Among the 130 patients with SCLC, the phased dosing schedule, in which ipilimumab was started in cycle three of paclitaxel and carboplatin, appeared to improve immune-related PFS (median 6.4 months for the phased ipilimumab arm versus 5.3 months for the control arm ($p = 0.03$)), immune-related best overall response rate (71% [95% CI, 55 to 84] versus 53% [95% CI, 38 to 68]) and OS (median 12.9 months versus 9.9 months [$p = 0.13$]), compared to paclitaxel and carboplatin, whereas the concurrent regimen did not lead to improved outcomes.[245] Ipilimumab did not potentiate the toxicities of the chemotherapy, but was associated with moderate immune-related adverse events.[245] Given these favorable results, a randomized, multicenter, double-blind phase III trial comparing the efficacy of platinum/etoposide with or without ipilimumab in patients with newly diagnosed extensive stage disease SCLC, with OS as the primary endpoint, has been conducted and the results are forthcoming. (ClinicalTrials.gov identifier: NCT01450761).

As seen previously, distinct pathways contribute to the pathogenesis of SCLC, leading to its unique biology and clinical features. The therapeutic strategies employed previously to target the basic molecular and cellular changes in SCLC have not led to significant changes in the management and outcomes of the disease, thus far. However, continued, rational, target-based approaches ultimately should lead to improved survival of patients with SCLC.

Radiation

Role of Radiotherapy in Limited Disease. Despite being exquisitely chemo- and radioresponsive, neither modality alone controls all aspects of disease. The CALGB trial of the late 1980s demonstrated that 90% of patients treated with chemotherapy alone failed locally.[246] The meta-analysis of Pignon and Arriagada[247] provided more data to mandate thoracic radiotherapy, but a number of treatment issues remained to be determined, including sequencing of radiation with chemotherapy, early versus late radiotherapy, altered fractionation, and prophylactic cranial irradiation.

Concurrent combined modality therapy is the standard treatment for SCLC patients with limited-stage disease.[52] It requires close coordination between medical and radiation oncologists. A combined modality treatment approach requires patients with an excellent performance status. Single-modality therapy may be appropriate for those who are debilitated or have serious comorbidities. If the patient's condition improves sufficiently after the initial chemotherapy or radiotherapy, subsequent treatment with the other modality may be considered. Although gains in radiotherapy delivery and integration with PET imaging have been made, disease failure in local, distant, and sanctuary sites continue to be substantial clinical challenges.

Sequencing of Radiation with Chemotherapy. Concurrent therapy is the delivery of chemotherapy and radiation therapy throughout the same time period. Sequential therapy is the delivery of one modality only after the completion of the other, often requiring a delay to allow for adequate recovery from the initial modality. A 1992 meta-analysis evaluated trials in which more than 2,100 patients with limited-stage SCLC were randomized to receive chemotherapy alone or with chest irradiation.[248] Patients given combined modality therapy had a 14% reduction in death rate and an absolute 5.4% improvement in 3-year survival compared with those who received chemotherapy alone. Both differences were highly significant. A second and independent meta-analysis reached similar conclusions.[249]

The trials included in the meta-analysis used cyclophosphamide- and doxorubicin-based chemotherapy, which is excessively toxic when given with concurrent thoracic radiotherapy. Therefore, individual trials used strategies such as sequential or interdigitated chemoradiation and used different chemotherapy regimens during the concurrent phases. However, the current standard chemotherapy regimen of cisplatin and etoposide can be used safely with concurrent radiotherapy.

Thoracic Radiation Dose and Fractionation. Due to the radioresponsiveness of SCLC, modest doses of radiation from 45 to 50 Gy have been used. However, with modest-dose radiation therapy there is a high rate of local failure. For example, in the Intergroup trial, the control arm of 45 Gy given once daily had a 75% rate of intrathoracic relapse.[250] Therefore, higher radiation doses or intensification (i.e., acceleration) appear necessary to improve local control. A retrospective review from Massachusetts General Hospital suggested that there may be continued dose response beyond 50 Gy.[251] The maximum tolerated dose of concurrent thoracic chemoradiation seems to be 45 to 51 Gy with a twice-daily approach and 70 Gy daily.[252] However, the advent of highly conformal radiotherapy techniques, such as intensity-modulated radiation therapy (IMRT) and the shift away from targeting clinically uninvolved nodal stations, may lead to tolerance of higher radiation doses, as discussed in the following paragraphs.

CALGB-39808 determined that 70 Gy delivered with daily fractions of 2 Gy with concurrent chemotherapy is feasible in the cooperative group setting and was associated with a median survival of 22.4 months and acceptable rates of esophagitis and pneumonitis.[253] Other CALGB trials also have used 70 Gy of thoracic irradiation with concurrent chemotherapy.[254] Once-daily fractionation is more familiar for radiation oncologists and typically is more convenient for patients, although it should be noted that some patients prefer the decreased overall treatment duration with a twice-daily schedule.

SCLC appears to be an ideal neoplasm for twice-daily treatment in that it has a high growth fraction, short cell cycle time, and small-to-absent shoulder on the in vitro cell survival curve, which may allow for a reduction in long-term pulmonary toxicity while maintaining antitumor efficacy.[255] Pilot studies in the late 1980s combining etoposide and platinum with twice-daily chest radiation were promising, with median survivals greater than 2 years and, in most series, low rates of pneumonitis.[250,256,257] An Intergroup study randomized 417 patients with limited-stage SCLC receiving 45 Gy in either daily fractions of 1.8 Gy or twice-daily fractions of 1.5 Gy, both given concurrently with the first of four cycles of EP.[49] Although fractionation is the obvious variable, the overall duration of radiotherapy varied as well (3 weeks versus 5 weeks), and longer treatment times may exert selective pressure on the emergence of resistant clones. The target volume included the primary tumor, bilateral mediastinal nodes, and the ipsilateral hilum, excluding uninvolved supraclavicular nodes. Local failure was reduced from 52% to 36% with the twice-daily schedule ($p = 0.06$). Of interest, only 6% of patients with twice-daily radiation failed in both local and distant sites, compared to 23% with daily treatment ($p = 0.01$). More importantly, although statistically significant differences in survival were not seen at 2 years,[257] by 5 years the survival was 16% with once-daily treatment, compared to 26% with a twice-daily schedule ($p = 0.04$).[49] All patients who achieved less than complete response were scored as local failures, but some of those treated with the accelerated scheme who achieved only a partial response survived, as well as those with a complete response, implying that the local failure rate was overestimated by imaging on that arm. There was a higher frequency of grade 3 esophagitis with twice-daily treatment, but overall long-term morbidities were not significantly different between the two arms.

A North Central Cancer Treatment Group trial attempted to reduce morbidity of twice-daily radiation by inserting a 2.5-week pause between two courses of 24 Gy each (therefore, the overall course was longer than the standard duration).[48,258] After three cycles of induction chemotherapy, fit and responding patients were randomized to receive either the 48 Gy split-course regimen, or 54 Gy in a once daily regimen in 6 weeks.[258] The 20% rate of 5-year survival was less than the benchmark 26% from the Intergroup trial. However, a follow-up trial used a higher dose of twice-daily radiation (total 60 Gy) with a 2-week treatment break and reported a favorable 5-year survival of 24%.[259]

A phase I trial conducted by the Radiation Therapy and Oncology Group (RTOG) and CALGB evaluated the use of 70 Gy delivered in daily fractionation or 45 Gy given in twice-a-day fractionation.[260] Although it was intended to establish the maximum-tolerated doses (MTD) of irinotecan given with cisplatin and thoracic radiation, it also was the first trial to evaluate 70 Gy delivered at cycle one. Of the 15 patients treated to 70 Gy, 2 had dose-limiting toxicities (diarrhea, esophagitis, and cardiovascular complications).

RTOG-9712 was a phase I trial to establish the MTD of radiation therapy with delayed accelerated hyperfractionation.[261] With this technique, a large field encompassing the gross tumor and mediastinum was treated to 45 Gy. A smaller field that encompassed only the gross tumor was treated as a second daily 1.8 Gy treatment for the last 3 to 11 days. The MTD was found to be 61.2 Gy with this regimen, which subsequently was evaluated in RTOG-0239, a phase II trial.[262] It reported a 2-year OS of 37%, short of the predicted survival of 60%. However, the regimen demonstrated an excellent local control of 73%.

Currently, a randomized phase III trial is being conducted by the RTOG and CALGB to evaluate three fractionation schemes: 45 Gy in 1.5-Gy twice-daily fractions (standard), 70 Gy in 2-Gy fractions (Arm B), and 61.2 Gy with delayed accelerated hyperfractionation (Arm C). In the first part of this trial, toxicity was to be assessed and the less toxic of Arms B and C was to be compared head to head with the standard arm. Although no clear difference in toxicity was observed between Arms B and C, the delayed accelerated hyperfractionation arm has been dropped due to slow accrual, and the study is continuing as a two-arm trial. A separate Phase III randomized trial is also evaluating once versus twice-daily radiotherapy with concurrent chemoradiotherapy in Europe, comparing 66 Gy in daily 2-Gy fractions against the same control arm of 45 Gy in twice-daily 1.5-Gy fractions. Until results from these trials are available, twice-daily fractionation as established by the Intergroup trial remains the reference regimen for fit patients. However, it should be noted that the logistical and toxicity obstacles with twice-daily treatment apparently are substantial, because a recent survey of practice patterns indicated that fewer than a quarter of limited-stage SCLC patients receive twice-daily treatment in the United States.[263]

Early Versus Late Radiotherapy. Randomized trials have yielded conflicting results on whether concurrent irradiation is best given early or late in the chemotherapy program. There have been multiple meta-analyses of the timing of thoracic irradiation.[264–268] One meta-analysis[265] reviewed seven randomized trials with a total of 1,524 patients that addressed the timing of radiotherapy relative to chemotherapy. Early radiation therapy was defined as beginning before 9 weeks after the initiation of chemotherapy and before the third cycle of chemotherapy. Late radiation therapy began 9 weeks or more after the initiation of chemotherapy or after the beginning of the third cycle. They reported a small but statistically significant improvement in 2-year survival for patients receiving early radiation therapy. A greater benefit was observed in patients receiving hyperfractionated radiation. Another meta-analysis[269] evaluated four randomized trials consisting of 1,056 patients to determine whether the time from the start of chemotherapy until the end of radiotherapy (SER) was a predictor of survival. They found that there was a significantly higher 5-year survival rate in the treatment arms with a shorter SER. In addition, a low SER was associated with a higher incidence of severe esophagitis. This suggests that an important factor in the treatment of SCLC involves counteracting accelerated repopulation that occurs after treatment with chemotherapy. However, definitive evidence that early integration of radiotherapy leads to improved survival remains elusive. A recent randomized trial from Korea assigned patients to receive radiotherapy (albeit a nonstandard regimen of 52.5 Gy) with either the first or third cycle of chemotherapy with cisplatin or etoposide. There was no difference in survival or local control, but rather an increase in febrile neutropenia with early radiotherapy, suggesting that later integration of radiotherapy was preferable.[82]

In clinical practice, it is often prudent to initiate chemotherapy immediately in these patients who are typically highly symptomatic and not delay treatment until radiation treatment planning is complete. Starting radiotherapy with the second cycle of chemotherapy is more readily achievable and should preserve the potential gains in efficacy obtained with early integration of radiotherapy with chemotherapy.

Radiation Therapy Treatment Volumes and Technique. An early randomized trial by SWOG showed no difference in recurrence rate whether pre- or postchemotherapy imaging was used to determine radiation therapy treatment fields.[270] Of course, if early radiation therapy is used, then there is no postchemotherapy treatment volume. The Intergroup trial[49] included gross disease, the bilateral mediastinum, and the ipsilateral hilum in the treatment field. The uninvolved supraclavicular area was excluded. RTOG-9712[261] allowed for the treatment of the uninvolved supraclavicular area in the setting of apical tumors. A small phase II trial suggested that there may be increased elective nodal failure in the supraclavicular area if it is excluded from the treatment field.[271] Consultants from the International Atomic Energy Agency reviewed available literature in 2008 and found little evidence to guide the use of elective nodal irradiation.[272] However, a number of prospective and retrospective experiences have since been published and increasingly suggest that involved-field radiation therapy is not associated with an excessive rate of local–regional failure, particularly in an era of routine PET staging. A Dutch phase II trial of concurrent chemoradiation limited radiotherapy (RT) fields to the primary tumor and clinically involved lymph nodes and reported a relatively low local failure rate of 16%.[273]

Utilizing PET to guide the design of limited radiotherapy fields appears to reduce the probability of elective nodal failure due to the improved sensitivity of PET to detect nodal disease compared to CT alone. A follow-up trial from the same group that found a worrisome rate of elective nodal failure when utilizing involved-field RT in CT-staged patients showed that the rate of isolated nodal failure was only 3% with PET staging, compared to 11% without.[274] A retrospective experience from the M.D. Anderson Cancer Center similarly showed a low rate of isolated elective nodal failure in a PET-staged cohort of patients who were treated with IMRT, a technique that gives lower incidental radiation doses to untargeted lymph node regions and, therefore, would theoretically increase the risk of elective nodal failure.[275] Overall, these and other recent publications suggest that with modern staging and treatment techniques, the omission of elective nodal irradiation does not lead to an excessive rate of isolated nodal failure.[276–278] Neither of the ongoing trials of daily versus twice-daily thoracic radiotherapy employ elective nodal irradiation in any of the trial arms (with the exception of mandatory coverage of hilar lymph nodes in the CALGB trial), indicating that the omission of elective nodal irradiation is increasingly considered within the standard of care for PET-staged patients.

In addition to the omission of elective nodal irradiation, another area of investigation in radiation technique is the implementation of more highly conformal delivery methods, such as IMRT or proton therapy. These techniques allow for significantly greater control of the location of radiation dose, particularly of incidental radiation dose outside of the target volume. Although this would seem to be an unequivocal advantage, theoretic concerns have persisted regarding the sensitivity of these techniques to respiratory organ motion, and the possibility that decreasing the incidental dose outside of the target volume might increase rates of regional or nodal failure. Investigators from the M.D. Anderson Cancer Center retrospectively compared outcomes with patients receiving standard three-dimensional (3D)-conformal radiation therapy and IMRT, and found no significant difference in OS or DFS.[279] Proton therapy, which reduces the dose outside of the target volume more fully than is possible with any form of photon radiotherapy, has not yet been widely used in SCLC, with only one small report published so far.[280] However, if the phase III trials demonstrate an advantage to higher dose radiotherapy, then IMRT and photon therapy are likely to gain in importance, because highly conformal techniques are often required to achieve high target doses while respecting dose limits to critical normal structures.

Toxicity of Radiation Therapy. The addition of chest irradiation has increased myelosuppressive, pulmonary, and esophageal complications of treatment, particularly with concurrent cyclophosphamide-based regimens.[281–283] Esophagitis is a difficult toxicity to compare because trials often use unique grading systems. However, most trials with concurrent chemoradiation with a cisplatin-based regimen report a 10% to 25% rate of severe esophagitis.[284] A retrospective review revealed that various radiation dosimetric parameters, such as mean esophageal dose and volume of esophagus receiving 15 Gy, were associated with a higher incidence of grade 3 or worse esophagitis in patients receiving twice-daily radiation.[285] More recently, a large individual patient data meta-analysis of esophagitis after concurrent thoracic chemoradiotherapy indicated that the best predictor of esophagitis was the volume of esophagus receiving greater than or equal to 60 Gy, with the highest risk seen when 17% or more of the esophagus was exposed to such doses.[286]

Radiation pneumonitis (RP) has not been as well studied in SCLC as it has in NSCLC, most likely due to the fact that most trials have used a moderate dose of radiation therapy, below which high rates of RP rarely are seen. Recent trials report a RP rate of approximately 10%.[253,287] This is lower than some of the trials reported in the 1980s and 1990s, probably due to improved radiation therapy techniques and better distinction between pneumonitis and other etiologies of respiratory distress, such as infection or tumor recurrence. The volume of lung receiving 20 Gy (V20) is a standard parameter used to predict lung toxicity in patients with NSCLC. A recent collaborative effort to define consensus dose limits for RP recommended that the V20 be kept below 30% to 35% in order to keep the risk of pneumonitis less than 20%.[288] It has been shown to have value in patients receiving concurrent accelerated hyperfractionated treatment for SCLC as well, with a V20 less than 25% associated with a lower rate of RP.[289]

Role of Chest Irradiation in Extensive Disease. Reviews of the historical literature indicated that the addition of chest irradiation plus chemotherapy for patients who have extensive-stage SCLC may improve local control in the thorax, but without change in survival.[290,291] Successive large studies by the SWOG also confirmed a benefit on local control but not survival.[118,292] Because patients with extensive disease generally achieve complete response rates of only 20% to 25% with current chemotherapy regimens and frequently relapse in distant metastatic sites, it is unsurprising that the routine application of additional local therapy did not have a clear impact on survival. Several clinical trials have randomized patients with extensive disease to chemotherapy alone or in combination with irradiation to the chest disease, as well as to some or all sites of overt distant metastases.[292–295] Although most of these did not show survival advantages with the addition of radiotherapy, it is notable that the most recent trial did.[293] In this trial, patients with at least a partial response to chemotherapy at the primary site and a complete response in distant sites were randomized to receive thoracic radiation with additional chemotherapy, or chemotherapy alone. Thoracic radiotherapy was associated with significantly better survival and a trend toward better local control. A recent, small phase II trial of consolidative thoracic radiation suggested that rates of symptomatic recurrence in the chest were low with this strategy and may, therefore, have an important quality of life benefit irrespective of any survival benefit.[296] Preliminary results from the Dutch phase III trial randomizing extensive stage SCLC patients who have had a response to four to six cycles of chemotherapy to thoracic radiation therapy or no thoracic radiation therapy has found a survival benefit at two years but not at one year, which was the primary endpoint.[297] The RTOG is conducting a randomized trial in which patients with extensive-stage disease and four or fewer metastatic lesions (excluding the central nervous system [CNS]) receive prophylactic cranial irradiation and consolidative RT to the thorax and all metastatic sites, or prophylactic cranial irradiation (PCI) alone. Although the routine use of consolidative thoracic radiation cannot yet be justified, the improved local control, attendant impact on symptomatic progression, and possible survival benefit make it a reasonable consideration in patients with significant responses to initial chemotherapy.

Prophylactic Cranial Irradiation. Brain metastases are detected in at least 18% of SCLC patients at diagnosis[33] and eventually are diagnosed in another 20% to 25%, with an increasing likelihood seen with lengthening survival.[298,299] An actuarial analysis reveals a probability of brain metastases ranging from 50% to 80% in patients who survive 2 years.[298,230] At postmortem examination, they are found in up to 65% of patients.[301] Because these metastases are sometimes the sole site of clinical relapse and are frequently clinically disabling, PCI has been recommended by many,[302] but not all,[303] authorities. The rationale is essentially an extrapolation from original strategies used in acute lymphocytic leukemia of childhood.

A large number of early prospective randomized trials assessed the benefit of PCI given at or within a few months of diagnosis.[144,304–307] When these trials were considered together, PCI reduced the frequency of clinically detectable brain metastases from 24% to 6%. However, no significant impact of PCI on survival was seen in any of those studies. Retrospective analyses suggested that virtually all benefit with PCI was confined to patients who achieved a complete remission from their initial treatment.[300] In an actuarial analysis, partial responders or nonresponders have similar risks of recurrence in the brain regardless of whether PCI was administered. This is not surprising because persistent systemic cancer could readily metastasize to the CNS after the completion of PCI.

In a meta-analysis of almost 1,000 patients in seven trials between 1977 and 1995, patients were evaluated with and without PCI after initially obtaining a complete response.[308] PCI doses ranged from 24 to 40 Gy in most patients. The meta-analysis suggested that a significant gain in survival with PCI, with 3-year survival figures increasing from 15% to almost 21%. PCI significantly decreased the probability of brain metastases and increased the likelihood of disease-free survival. Higher doses appeared to have no impact on survival, although seemed to have an increasing effect of preventing brain metastases. A trend also was seen toward a decreased risk of brain metastases when PCI was administered earlier. The meta-analysis was not able to assess the impact of PCI on cognitive function, because most of the studies did not include thorough neurocognitive assessments. Two studies that assessed baseline neuropsychological function before treatment demonstrated that many patients appear to have abnormalities of cognitive function as initial manifestations of their cancer, even when brain metastases were not detected and before any treatment.[309,310]

An Intergroup trial evaluated standard-dose versus higher dose PCI after complete response for limited-stage disease.[311] Seven hundred twenty patients were randomized to either 25 Gy in 10 fractions or 36 Gy delivered in 18 daily fractions of 2 Gy or 24 twice-daily fractions of 1.5 Gy. There was no significant difference in incidences of brain metastases between the standard-dose group and the high-dose group. The OS was significantly was worse in the higher dose group, although this was due to extracranial disease progression rather than toxicity. The reason for this counterintuitive result remains unclear. This study further established 2,500 cGy in 10 fractions as the standard dose of PCI for limited-stage patients, although some practitioners use a regimen of 3,000 cGy in 15 fractions, which should have similar biologic efficacy.

A recent EORTC randomized trial demonstrated a survival benefit with PCI in patients with extensive-stage SCLC who had had a response to chemotherapy.[83] The use of PCI significantly improved the rate of 1-year freedom from symptomatic brain metastases from 14.6% to 40.4% and the 1-year survival from 13.3% to 27.1% in the 286 randomized patients. Various fractionation schemes were used, but the most common ones were 20 Gy in five fractions and 30 Gy in 10 fractions. A common criticism of this trial is its lack of mandatory pretreatment brain imaging to rule out clinically occult brain metastases, raising the question of whether the observed survival benefit was due to treatment of patients who already had detectable brain metastases. In an era of routine and regular imaging of the brain with sensitive MRI examinations, it has been suggested that the actual rate of developing brain metastases in thoroughly staged extensive-stage patients is relatively low, which may attenuate the potential benefit of routine PCI in this cohort. Nevertheless, the results of the EORTC trial established PCI as a standard consideration for all extensive-stage patients achieving a response to initial therapy.

A major concern with recommending PCI is the significant risk of toxicity associated with it. It is evident that some long-term survivors have neurologic and intellectual impairment as well as abnormalities on CT scan that may be related to PCI.[312,313] In one study, CT scan and CNS abnormalities were significantly more frequent in patients who had received PCI or therapeutic brain irradiation than in those who had not.[314] These findings were especially disturbing because complete responders are at greater risk for possible complications. Many deficits on neuropsychological testing have been unsuspected on casual examination, but a few patients have obvious major impairments. CT scan abnormalities continue to worsen for several years after treatment has ended, although the abnormalities may eventually stabilize.[315] Neurologic abnormalities were most prominent in one series of patients who were given PCI concurrently with high-dose chemotherapy or in individual radiation fractions of 4 Gy.[312] Some authorities suggest that PCI should be administered only in standard fractions of 2 Gy after the completion of chemotherapy.[250]

After PCI, neuropsychological and imaging abnormalities may or may not be due to PCI. Chemotherapy, paraneoplastic syndromes, micrometastases, and chronic cigarette and alcohol abuse may be important contributors. In one study that evaluated cognitive function in patients before and after chemoradiation but before PCI, deficits were discovered in verbal memory, frontal lobe function, and motor coordination within both groups of patients.[118] A similar, more recent study indicated that 47% of SCLC patients had impaired cognitive function before PCI, and that PCI was not associated with persistent declines in cognitive function.[316] The administration of methotrexate, procarbazine, and lomustine has decreased over the past 15 years; these particular agents have been incriminated in neuropsychological dysfunction. One of the studies included in the meta-analysis had almost 300 patients who were randomized to receive PCI after having achieved a complete remission to initial treatment.[304] There were no obvious differences in the neuropsychological function between the two groups, but only 33 patients underwent a complete reassessment at 18 months. Inasmuch as neuropsychological abnormalities possibly due to PCI progress over time, these data are insufficient to exclude radiation-associated cognitive damage, but they are nonetheless relevant.

A recent decision analysis suggests that for patients who have had a complete response to initial therapy, PCI offers a better quality-adjusted life expectancy, even if a mild to moderate neurotoxicity rate was assumed.[317] If PCI is not administered concurrently with chemotherapy, radiation-induced permeability alterations that allow more of the chemotherapeutic agent into the brain parenchyma should be obviated. The authors' guidelines for PCI, after a thorough discussion with the patient of potential risks and benefits, are as follows: (1) PCI is typically recommended as soon as a partial or complete response to induction therapy has been confirmed, and after acute toxicities have resolved, which is typically 2 to 4 weeks after completion of all chemotherapy. Note that in the EORTC trial of PCI for extensive-stage patients, PCI was given 4 to 6 weeks after chemotherapy. (2) The standard fractionation of 2500 cGy in 10 fractions is recommended for all patients in whom PCI is deemed appropriate, with a consideration of 2000 cGy in five fractions for extensive-stage patients for whom, due to borderline performance status or significant logistical impediments, shortening overall treatment time is felt to be important.

Role of Chemotherapy and Radiation Therapy to the Neuraxis. For overt metastatic lesions within the CNS, doses of 3 Gy daily to a dose of 30 Gy typically is used. Overt intracranial metastases appear to be more difficult to sterilize than intrathoracic disease.[318] Due to the propensity for SCLC patients to develop multifocal brain metastases, stereotactic treatment for brain metastases is typically not appropriate because the risk of brain relapse beyond the treated lesion would be unacceptably high. However, in the context of prior whole brain radiation or prophylactic cranial irradiation, stereotactic treatment may be considered as a salvage option.[319]

Chemotherapy also is a therapeutic option for brain metastases, perhaps because the blood–brain barrier is disrupted in the setting of macroscopic metastatic disease. Small series of patients in whom brain metastases were present at diagnosis have been treated with standard chemotherapy regimens without radiation, and the majority have demonstrated clinical and radiographic improvement.[320] Chemotherapy also has been used at the time of relapse, and response rates of 33% to 43% have been reported.[320–322] In previously treated patients, the response to chemotherapy in the brain appears to be comparable to the response rates in other organs, and it is not dissimilar from the activity of irradiation, which in one series produced a partial response rate of 50%; the median survival was 4.7 months in a series of 22 patients.[323] In the phase II trial evaluating temozolomide in patients with relapsed or refractory SCLC, patients with progressive brain metastases that had received prior cranial irradiation demonstrated an intracranial response to the agent.[200] Thus, although brain irradiation remains the standard for patients who have not been previously irradiated, chemotherapy is a reasonable option for those in whom recurrent disease develops after prior brain radiation, particularly if active systemic disease is also present.

Surgery

Even before the advent of combination chemotherapy for SCLC, the poor outcomes in various case series clearly indicated that surgery is not advisable as a sole treatment modality in this disease.[324–327]

Given that SCLC patients generally present with bulky unresectable disease, studies evaluating surgery are limited. In some cases, patients who undergo thoracotomy for an abnormal pulmonary nodule are unexpectedly diagnosed with SCLC.[55] About 4% of solitary pulmonary nodules are diagnosed as SCLC.[29,30] In these cases, a complete surgical resection should be performed and the patient should be referred for adjuvant therapy. Based on current recommendations, patients with N0 disease should then receive adjuvant chemotherapy, whereas patients with nodal involvement should receive chemotherapy and mediastinal radiation.[52]

Nodal status and primary tumor (T) status have significant effects on the survival of patients who have undergone resection. Angeletti et al.[328] and Shepherd et al.[329] reported increased survival of node-negative compared to N1 and N2 patients after surgical resection and postoperative chemotherapy, whereas Macchiarini et al.[330] found a decrease in 5-year survival with increasing T category in surgically resected patients without nodal metastases. Rea et al.[331] reported that 51 stage I or II SCLC patients resected and given chemotherapy after resection had 5-year survival rates of 52% (stage I) and 30% (stage II). In the review by Lucchi et al.,[332] stage I or II resected SCLC patients who underwent postoperative chemotherapy had 5-year survival rates of 47% and 15%, respectively. Stage III patients from this series who underwent surgery followed by adjuvant therapy had a 5-year survival of 14%. The largest experience examining the role of surgery followed by adjuvant therapy in SCLC was a cooperative group trial conducted by the International Society of Chemotherapy Lung Cancer Study Group.[54] Four-year survival rates for completely resected, pathologically staged SCLC patients with N0 (n = 69), N1 (n = 58), and N2 (n = 36) who received postoperative therapy were 60%, 36%, and 33%, respectively. Based on these studies, most authorities believe that surgery may have a role as part of a multimodality approach, but only for patients with stage I disease.[52] A mediastinoscopy should be performed in all patients who are being considered for resection of known SCLCs. In a large series from the University of Toronto, surgery followed by chemotherapy had the same outcome as treatment in the reverse order.[329]

Surgical resection also has been studied as a way of reducing the risk of local recurrence in patients with limited disease after the completion of chemoradiation. Although most patients with SCLC succumb to metastatic disease, local recurrence occurs in 35% to 50%.[49] Furthermore, tumors may have a mixed histology such that residual NSCLC remains after treatment of the more chemosensitive SCLC component. Of 38 cases resected after chemoradiation in a University of Toronto study, 29 had pure SCLC but 4 were pure NSCLC, 2 had a mixed histology, and 3 had no residual tumor.[333] Several groups have reported the feasibility of this approach, although notably in these prospective studies, only about half of the cases were resectable and pneumonectomies were frequently required.[305–307] One randomized trial attempted to address the question of whether surgical resection of persistent local disease adds any benefit to the usual approach of chemoradiation for limited-stage patients.[334] The Lung Cancer Study Group enrolled 328 patients who were first treated with CAV for five cycles. Fit patients with at least a partial response were then randomized to surgical resection or not. All patients were then intended to receive thoracic and prophylactic cranial irradiation. As with the previously reported studies, only a fraction of the patients were eligible for surgery after induction therapy; only 146 patients were randomized, and this diminished the power of the statistical analysis. Nonetheless, no differences in OS or even in local control rates were noted between the two groups. NSCLC or mixed NSCLC/SCLC comprised 11% of the resected specimens. These data suggest that surgical resection of residual disease in limited-stage SCLC does not improve outcomes. The use of surgery for patients with SCLC should be restricted to patients with stage I tumors.

Palliative Care

Survivorship Issues

Although minor advances have transpired over the past 3 decades, there has been no dramatic change in outcomes for SCLC since the introduction of EP chemotherapy in the late 1970s, with median survival improving only by 2 months from 7 to 9 months between 1972 and 1990.[335] Although this therapy significantly changes the natural history of SCLC, and the use of twice-daily concomitant radiotherapy and prophylactic cranial irradiation adds incremental benefit in patients with limited disease, the number of persons cured remains small. Few patients with extensive disease attain long-term survival. Patients are at greatest risk of dying from SCLC during the first 24 months after diagnosis. This risk declines between years 2 and 3 and is further reduced beyond year 3. In the SEER program database, OS at 2, 3, and 5 years was 12%, 7%, and 5%, respectively.[336]

Excessive mortality in long-term survivors is due primarily to the development of second primary tumors, mainly NSCLC, and other illnesses associated with cigarette smoking.[67,337–340] Late relapse can occur in approximately 10% of patients at 5 years.[341] Overall, the relative risk of a second primary tumor in patients who survive beyond 2 years is increased 3.5-fold. The second lung cancer risk is increased 13-fold among those who received chest irradiation.[337] Because most of the second primary tumors are NSCLC or other malignancies of the upper aerodigestive tract, it is likely that field cancerization due to tobacco exposure has occurred.[337,338] The risk of a second primary tumor increases significantly over time and with continued smoking. Treatment with alkylating agents further magnifies this risk.[337] For example, the risk of a second lung cancer in patients who continue to smoke was approximately fourfold more than those who stopped before the diagnosis of SCLC and twofold greater in patients who received chest irradiation compared to nonirradiated patients. The cumulative risk of a second lung cancer was 32% at 12 years and continued to increase beyond that time point. Secondary leukemias have been seen as well.[339,340] Patients successfully treated for SCLC constitute an extraordinarily high-risk group for second malignancies and require close surveillance. The cigarette smoking status of every long-term survivor of SCLC should be assessed at every visit. Aggressive smoking cessation efforts should be marshaled for any patient who expresses an interest in quitting. In addition, this population should be considered for studies evaluating new surveillance technologies and chemoprevention.

Long-term survivors are also at increased risk for non–cancer-related problems, including complications of treatment (e.g., pulmonary fibrosis in patients receiving thoracic irradiation, neurologic impairment both as a consequence of treatment with cranial irradiation and paraneoplastic effects of SCLC, and the acceleration of coronary artery disease following thoracic irradiation) as well as tobacco-related illnesses like heart disease, stroke, and chronic obstructive pulmonary disease. In a French study of patients surviving beyond 30 months, treatment-related sequelae included neurologic impairment in 13% of the patients, pulmonary fibrosis in 18%, and cardiac disorders in 10%.[342] A return to work was possible in 40% of these patients and was not influenced by the presence of late treatment-related complications. In a Danish analysis of patients surviving 5 years or more, there was a sixfold increased risk of death from noncancer causes, particularly cardiovascular and pulmonary diseases.[343] Physicians who care for survivors of SCLC should aggressively implement all strategies to reduce cardiovascular disease. These patients should be considered high risk and managed like any other high-risk individual.

TYPICAL AND ATYPICAL CARCINOID TUMORS

Incidence and Etiology

Although over 60% of carcinoid tumors originate in the gastrointestinal system, about 25% of all carcinoids have a pulmonary origin, representing the second most common involved site.[344] Pulmonary carcinoids comprise about 2% of all primary lung tumors.[345] Over the past 30 years, the age-adjusted incidence rate in pulmonary carcinoids has significantly increased, which may represent the improvement in classification of these tumors, as well as the rise of imaging techniques.[344] There is a higher incidence of pulmonary carcinoids in women compared to men and whites compared to blacks.[346,347]

Atypical carcinoids, which have a higher likelihood of metastatic spread or relapse after surgery, are distinguished from the typical carcinoids, which have a more favorable prognosis. Ten percent to 30% of pulmonary carcinoids are atypical.[348–350] Patients with typical carcinoids are approximately 10 years younger than those with atypical carcinoids, which occur in the 6th decade of life.[347,351] Carcinoids are not clearly caused by smoking like SCLC and LCNEC, although some series suggest that a higher percentage of patients with atypical carcinoid smoke as compared to patients with typical carcinoid tumors.[347,348,352] Pulmonary carcinoids occur rarely in association with multiple endocrine neoplasia type 1 (MEN-1) syndrome. Some sporadic pulmonary carcinoid tumors demonstrate inactivation of the *MEN-1* gene located on chromosome 11q13.[353]

Anatomy and Pathology

All carcinoids are malignant. Typical carcinoids are low grade and atypical carcinoids are intermediate grade. Although carcinoid tumors can be diagnosed by small biopsies or cytology, it is difficult to separate a typical from an atypical carcinoid. This distinction usually requires a surgical biopsy or resection specimen. The histologic appearance of typical and atypical carcinoids is similar with a uniform population of tumor cells arranged in organoid nests with a moderate amount of cytoplasm with an eosinophilic hue (see Fig. 38.2B,C). The finely granular nuclear chromatin frequently has a salt-and-pepper appearance. There are a wide variety of histologic patterns in these tumors, including spindle cell, oncocytic, glandular, follicular, clear cell, and melanocytic. Stromal ossification can occur as well. Atypical carcinoids show increased mitoses (see Fig. 38.2C) with 2 to 10 mitoses per 2 mm^2 or necrosis that is typically punctate.[354] Mitotic activity is the most important way to distinguish typical from atypical carcinoid. The most useful immunohistochemical neuroendocrine markers are chromogranin, synaptophysin, and CD56. If the mitotic count is 11 or more mitoses per 2 mm^2 (10 high power fields), a diagnosis of LCNEC or SCLC is favored over atypical carcinoid.[354,355] In small specimens where mitotic figures are difficult to demonstrate, it may be helpful to use Ki-67 staining because most typical carcinoids show less than 5% staining, atypical carcinoids are usually 10% to 30%, and most LCNECs or SCLCs usually have a very high proliferation index of 80% to 100%.[356]

Nodular neuroendocrine proliferations 0.5 cm or larger are called *carcinoid tumors*. Smaller proliferations are called *tumorlets*, which are separated from carcinoid tumors by size, but with identical morphology of cells. Tumorlets usually are incidental histologic findings of no clinical significance, although they can be seen in interstitial or airway inflammatory and fibrosing conditions. A very rare condition called *diffuse idiopathic pulmonary neuroendocrine cell hyperplasia* (DIPNECH) is regarded as a preinvasive condition for pulmonary carcinoids. Patients with DIPNECH have widespread neuroendocrine cell hyperplasia and tumorlets in their airways and can develop multiple carcinoid tumors.[357]

Screening

Screening for pulmonary carcinoids is not useful. They represent a very small percentage of all lung malignancies and have an indolent natural history. In one study, atypical carcinoid was diagnosed in only 2 of 31,567 (0.006%) asymptomatic patients undergoing baseline lung cancer screening CT scans.[358]

Diagnosis

Two-thirds of carcinoids develop in the major bronchi. As a result, the most common presenting symptoms include obstructive pneumonia, pleuritic pain, atelectasis, dyspnea, and cough.[348,359] Hemoptysis may occur in 10% to 20% of patients. Up to 30% of patients with pulmonary carcinoid tumors are asymptomatic at presentation. In contrast to carcinoids of gastrointestinal origin, carcinoid syndrome (facial flushing, diarrhea, wheezing) is rare in pulmonary carcinoids, occurring in only about 2% of cases.[348,359] Cushing syndrome due to ectopic corticotropin production has been reported in approximately 2% of pulmonary carcinoids.[360] A rare manifestation of pulmonary carcinoids is acromegaly due to the ectopic production of growth hormone–releasing hormone (GHRH), yet these tumors are the most common cause of extrapituitary secretion of GHRH.[361]

The initial workup proceeds in a similar fashion as with other lung tumors, but once a diagnosis of carcinoid is confirmed, more specific radiologic and serologic evaluations for these neuroendocrine tumors may be employed. A biopsy of the central tumors can be easily obtained by bronchoscopy. A biopsy of peripheral lesions by fine needle can be performed, but a definitive diagnosis may be difficult to ascertain in small cytology samples. In addition to routine chest imaging with CT scans, nuclear medicine studies are helpful adjuncts for staging (Fig. 38.5). Due to the overexpression of somatostatin receptors, immunoscintigraphy by somatostatin analogs such as octreotide is widely used. In one series, the sensitivity and specificity was 90% and 83%, respectively.[362] In patients with somatostatin receptor–positive pulmonary carcinoids, octreotide scans have been found to be useful for follow-up and in the detection of recurrent disease, as well as for guiding treatment options.[363] Fluorine-18 (18F) fluorodeoxyglucose (FDG)-PET scanning may be less accurate because these indolent tumors generally have a low standard uptake value (SUV),[364] but some still advocate its potential use.[365] Recent series have shown that 18F-FDG–PET is useful for the assessment of intermediate- and high-grade neuroendocrine tumors and may have prognostic value.[366,367] Elevated chromogranin A levels have been measured in serum or plasma, although they have been found to be lower in pulmonary carcinoids compared to gastroenteropancreatic endocrine tumors.[368,369] In the setting of advanced or metastatic disease, chromogranin A levels can be useful to follow disease activity.[369] Urinary 5-hydroxyindoleacetic acid (5-HIAA) may be elevated in patients with carcinoid syndrome.

Staging

Pulmonary carcinoid tumors are staged according to the TNM classification used for NSCLC in the AJCC seventh edition. The International Association for the Study of Lung Cancer (IASLC) proposed and approved this in 2009 when it was determined that the TNM staging system was helpful in predicting the prognosis for pulmonary carcinoids.[370] Applying this staging system to cases in the National Cancer Institute SEER registry and cases submitted to the IASLC database, it was determined that 5-year OS for patients with stage I was 93%, stage II was 74% to 85%, stage III was 67% to 75%, and stage IV was 57%.[370] Survival is significantly better for

A

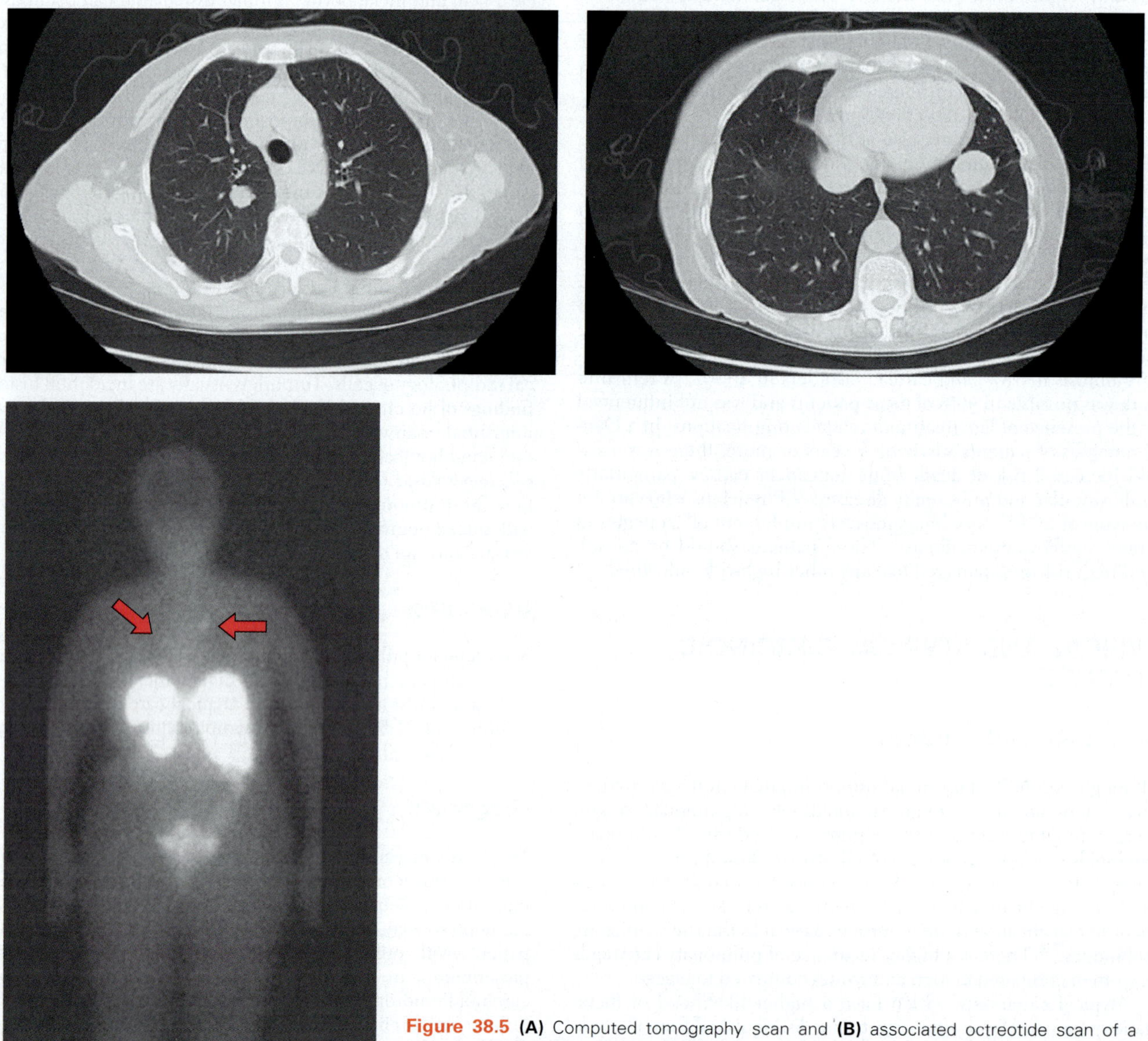

B

Figure 38.5 (A) Computed tomography scan and **(B)** associated octreotide scan of a patient with bilateral typical carcinoid.

typical carcinoid than for atypical carcinoid. Five-year and 10-year survival rates have been reported at 87% and 87%, respectively, for typical carcinoids, whereas they were 56% and 35%, respectively, for atypical carcinoids.[353] Predictors of survival include stage, tumor size, higher mitotic rates (i.e., atypical subtype), and age greater than 60.[347,352,370] Importantly, patients with multiple nodules have a very favorable prognosis, likely reflected by the fact that these individuals tend to have the underlying preinvasive lesion, diffuse idiopathic pulmonary neuroendocrine cell hyperplasia.[370]

Management by Stage

Stages I, II, and III

Surgery is the primary treatment modality and the only curative option for patients with pulmonary carcinoids. Because carcinoids often present centrally, a pneumonectomy or bilobectomy is frequent, but most patients undergo a lobectomy.[345,352] For patients with favorable prognostic features, such as typical histology and the absence of lymph node involvement, a more limited resection has been proposed.[359,371] Patients with atypical carcinoids should be resected using the same principles guiding surgery for NSCLC.[372]

Because mediastinal lymph node metastases occur in patients with pulmonary carcinoids, complete mediastinal lymph node dissection is advocated, with surgical resection of nodal metastases when feasible.[351,373–377] Multiple series have found decreased incidences of local recurrence[351,375] and improved survival when a complete mediastinal lymph node dissection is performed.[350,373]

Adjuvant chemotherapy after surgical resection for patients with typical carcinoid with or without regional lymph node metastases (stages I, II, and III) is not recommended,[378] because the risk of recurrence has been shown to be low: In a series of 291 resected typical carcinoids, only 3% of patients suffered recurrence.[351,379] Similarly, following surgical resection, patients with stage I atypical carcinoid are followed expectantly. However, because systemic recurrence occurs more frequently in patients with atypical carcinoid with N1 or N2 involvement (stages II and III), documented to be as high as 26% in a surgical series,[379] adjuvant chemotherapy after surgical resection has been advocated by some,[378] but it is unknown whether this is beneficial. There is no defined adjuvant regimen for atypical carcinoid, yet due to similarities with SCLC, etoposide with cisplatin or carboplatin is generally used.[378]

The use of radiation therapy for carcinoid tumors is most similar to its pattern of use in NSCLCs. For tumors that are resectable, adjuvant radiation therapy is typically recommended in situations of residual disease (R1 resection) and mediastinal lymphadenopathy (N2 disease). The use of adjuvant radiation therapy for nodal disease is probably of greater utility in the more aggressive atypical carcinoid.[378] In patients with unresectable disease, radiation therapy can be used after induction chemotherapy or concurrently.[380] Doses of 60 Gy are typical. Carcinoid tumors are less responsive to radiation therapy than SCLC.[381]

Stage IV

Data regarding the efficacy of chemotherapy specifically in pulmonary carcinoid (as opposed to gastrointestinal carcinoids) are lacking, because this tumor type has not been studied independently of other neuroendocrine tumors and occasionally has been omitted from such trials. Many of the studies have used older classification systems for carcinoids and different criteria for response. Various chemotherapeutic agents have been used, including doxorubicin, 5-fluorouracil, dacarbazine, cisplatin, carboplatin, etoposide, streptozocin, and interferon-alpha.[368,382] Yet, in general, carcinoid tumors have no significant therapies that consistently induce regression.

Octreotide has been used in the treatment of these tumors. Retrospective reviews, including small numbers of patients with pulmonary carcinoids, have reported on the use of somatostatin analogs with improvement in carcinoid syndrome symptoms, as well as prolonged disease control and survival, with very few individuals achieving a tumor response.[383,384,385] These results are similar to the experience with octreotide in gastrointestinal carcinoids.[386] Notably, the recent PROMID study showed that long-acting–release octreotide acetate significantly prolonged time to tumor progression compared with placebo in patients with newly diagnosed functionally active or inactive well-differentiated midgut neuroendocrine tumors (14.3 versus 6 months; HR, 0.34; 95% CI, 0.20 to 0.59; $p = 0.000072$). However, there was no improvement in OS.[387] Although some studies evaluating peptide receptor radionuclide therapy with radiolabeled somatostatin analogs in patients resistant to octreotide have included bronchial carcinoids, the number of patients with this histology is small thus far to generate any meaningful conclusions. However, such agents have been found to have reasonable response rates and outcomes in patients with pancreatic neuroendocrine tumors and gastrointestinal carcinoids.[388]

Regimens typically used for SCLC often are recommended.[378,389] However, typical carcinoids and atypical carcinoids are clearly less chemosensitive than SCLCs. In two small series that included 26 patients in total treated with chemotherapy (mostly etoposide and cisplatin), the response rate was about 20%.[368,380] EP was administered to 18 patients with foregut-origin carcinoids (lung and thymus) who had progressed after first- or second-line treatment in a prospective study. Radiographic response was noted in 2 of the 5 patients with atypical carcinoid (40%) and in 5 of the 13 with typical carcinoid (39%). The median response duration was 9 months (range, 6 to 30 months).[390] Similarly, etoposide with cisplatin or carboplatin was administered to 17 pulmonary carcinoid patients, with a 23.5% radiologic response (2 patients each with atypical and typical carcinoid) and median PFS of 7 months.[385]

Newer agents are being studied actively in neuroendocrine carcinoma. Temozolomide, a nonclassical oral alkylating agent, has been evaluated either alone or in combination with other agents. Thirteen patients with pulmonary carcinoids (10 typical, 3 atypical) were included in a retrospective study using single-agent temozolomide. Four of these patients (31%) had a partial response to treatment (3 typical, 1 atypical), and 62% derived clinical benefit (response or stable disease) with temozolomide.[391] In a larger retrospective study of 31 patients that included both typical and atypical pulmonary carcinoids, a partial response to treatment was noted in 3 patients (14%), whereas stable disease was observed in 11 patients (52%); median PFS and OS were 5.3 months and 23.2 months, respectively.[392] Eighteen patients with carcinoid and pancreatic neuroendocrine tumors metastatic to the liver that received capecitabine and temozolomide, were evaluated for response and outcome.[393] The overall response rate was 61%, and three of the four carcinoid patients attained clinical benefit (complete response, n = 1; partial response, n = 1, stable disease, n = 1). From the time of liver metastases, median PFS and OS were 14 months (range, 4 to 18 months) and 83 months (range, 18.5 to 140 months) for this combination, respectively. These results suggest that the regimen of capecitabine and temozolomide is active and may prolong survival in this malignancy.[393] In contrast, in two prospective trials that included patients with carcinoid tumors, a 7% response rate was noted using temozolomide with thalidomide and no response was observed using temozolomide and bevacizumab.[394,395] However, because some studies have shown promising results for temozolomide, either alone or in combination with other agents in metastatic pulmonary carcinoids, larger prospective studies should be developed.

The mTOR pathway, which regulates cell growth, proliferation, and metabolism, has been implicated in the pathogenesis of neuroendocrine tumors.[396] To determine if the addition of everolimus improved PFS, the randomized, placebo-controlled phase III study of everolimus plus octreotide long-acting repeatable (LAR) (RADIANT-2) included 429 patients with low-grade or intermediate-grade carcinoids, of which 44 were of pulmonary histology.[396] Median PFS was 16.4 months (95% CI, 13.7 to 21.2 months) for the group receiving the combination of everolimus and octreotide LAR compared to 11.3 months (95% CI, 8.4 to 14.6 months) in the octreotide LAR–only group (HR, 0.77; 95% CI, 0.59 to 1.0, p = 0.026); thus achieving the primary endpoint of the study. For the 44 bronchial carcinoid patients, median PFS was 13.6 and 5.6 months in the everolimus plus octreotide LAR group versus octreotide LAR–only group, respectively.[396] Currently, we are awaiting results from the randomized, double-blind, phase III study of everolimus versus placebo in patients with advanced neuroendocrine tumors of gastrointestinal (GI) or lung origin only (RADIANT-4) (ClinicalTrials.gov identifier: NCT01524783). Well-differentiated carcinoid tumors are highly vascularized and extensively express VEGF, Hypoxia inducible factor 1-alpha, and microvessel density.[397] As such, angiogenesis inhibitors have been investigated in this disease. In a phase II study, in low- to intermediate-grade neuroendocrine tumors, patients were randomized to receive either bevacizumab or pegylated interferon-alfa-2b (IFNα–2b). Only four patients with pulmonary carcinoids were included in this trial, where an 18% partial response rate was observed in the bevacizumab group compared with no responses in the pegylated IFNα–2b arm.[398] Fourteen patients with foregut carcinoids of the lung and stomach were included in a phase II study using sunitinib, a multitargeted oral TKI. The overall response rate for patients with carcinoid tumors was only 2.4% with a median time tumor progression of 10.2 months.[399] In contrast, in pancreatic neuroendocrine carcinoma, the randomized phase III trial of sunitinib versus placebo, demonstrated a significant improvement in PFS (11.4 versus 5.5 months, respectively; HR, 0.42; 95% CI, 0.26 to 0.66; $p < 0.001$).[400]

In patients with liver metastases, hepatic artery embolization, with or without intra-arterial chemotherapy has been associated with responses and improved outcomes in carcinoid patients.[401] Nine patients with pulmonary carcinoids who developed liver metastases underwent hepatic artery chemoembolization in a recently reported single institution retrospective review. Prolonged stable disease lasting up to 19 months was noted in eight of these patients, with three achieving a partial response.[385] A newer embolization method, utilizing injectable particles conjugated to yttrium-90, permits the delivery of internal radiation into hepatic arteries that supply carcinoid liver metastases.[397] Because randomized trials in embolization methods are lacking and some do experience treatment-related toxicities, patients must be selected carefully for these procedures.

In the approach to metastatic carcinoid tumors, many advocate using somatostatin analogs as first-line treatment in patients with well-differentiated tumors with little tumor bulk in the setting of a positive octreotide scan[363,383] and chemotherapy for those with more rapidly progressing tumors or those who have progressed on less toxic treatments.[402,403] Additional prospective, randomized studies are needed for both traditional cytotoxic and molecularly targeted agents in this disease, because early results are promising. Palliative radiation therapy can be used for symptomatic lesions.[381]

LARGE CELL NEUROENDOCRINE CARCINOMA

Incidence and Etiology

LCNEC of the lung was first described in 1991 as a form of high-grade non–small-cell neuroendocrine carcinoma.[404] LCNEC accounts for about 3% of surgically resected lung cancers.[405] In previously reported series, LCNEC patients have a median age of 62 years (range, 33 to 87 years) and the vast majority of patients are male cigarette smokers.[347,405]

Anatomy and Pathology

In the 2004 World Health Organization (WHO) classification, LCNEC is classified as a variant of large cell carcinoma.[9,405,406] There are four ways that neuroendocrine differentiation can be manifest within large cell carcinomas: (1) If both neuroendocrine morphology by light microscopy as well as neuroendocrine differentiation by immunohistochemistry or electron microscopy are seen, the tumor is classified as LCNEC; (2) if there is no neuroendocrine morphology by light microscopy and neuroendocrine differentiation is seen by immunohistochemistry or electron microscopy, the tumor is classified as large cell carcinoma with neuroendocrine differentiation (LCC-NED); (3) if the tumor lacks both neuroendocrine morphology by light microscopy and neuroendocrine differentiation by immunohistochemistry or electron microscopy, it is classified as a classic large cell carcinoma; and (4) if the neuroendocrine morphology (LCNEM) has neuroendocrine morphology but lacks neuroendocrine differentiation by electron microscopy or immunohistochemistry, it is classified as large cell carcinoma.[9,405,406] Little is known about the latter category.

LCNEC are diagnosed based on the following criteria (Fig. 38.2D): (1) neuroendocrine morphology with organoid nesting, palisading, or rosettelike structures; (2) high mitotic rate greater than 10 mitoses per 2 mm^2 (average 60 to 80 mitoses per 2 mm^2); (3) non–small-cell cytologic features, including large cell size, low nuclear or cytoplasmic ratio, nucleoli, or vesicular chromatin; and (4) neuroendocrine differentiation by immunohistochemistry (chromogranin, CD56, or synaptophysin) or electron microscopy.[9,354] The tumor grows in organoid nests with peripheral palisading and rosettelike structures. The tumor cells have abundant cytoplasm, prominent nucleoli, and frequent mitoses.

When LCNEC has components of adenocarcinoma, squamous cell carcinoma, giant cell carcinoma, or spindle cell carcinoma, it is called combined LCNEC and the specific components present should be mentioned.[9,354] Adenocarcinoma is the histologic type found most often in combined LCNEC. When SCLC is combined with LCNEC, the tumor becomes a combined SCLC, and LCNEC and should be regarded as a SCLC.

LCNEC will be positive for pancytokeratin and at least one neuroendocrine marker such as chromogranin, CD56, or synaptophysin. TTF-1 will be positive in 60% to 80% of cases. There is a very high proliferation index with 80% to 100% positive tumor cells.[405,407] When the differential diagnosis of basaloid carcinoma is a consideration, diffuse strong staining for p63 or p40 would favor this diagnosis over LCNEC.[15]

It is difficult to make the diagnosis of LCNEC on small biopsies or cytology because the characteristic neuroendocrine morphologic pattern and neuroendocrine differentiation by immunohistochemistry are difficult to demonstrate in minute pieces of tissue.[405,407] Therefore, in the vast majority of cases, a definite diagnosis of LCNEC will require a surgical biopsy. Separation of LCNEC from SCLC requires consideration of multiple histologic features such as cell size, nucleoli, chromatin pattern, and nuclear to cytoplasmic ratio, rather than a single criterion. Artifacts such as those introduced by frozen sections or poor quality hematoxylin and eosin-stained sections, can distort cellular morphology, resulting in confusion with SCLC.[11,405,407]

Screening

Clinically, LCNEC is characterized by similar behavior to SCLC, with rapid tumor growth and early metastatic spread.[347] Further, LCNEC represents a small percentage of all lung malignancies. In one study, LCNEC was diagnosed in only 15 of 31,567 (0.05%) asymptomatic patients undergoing baseline lung cancer screening CT scans.[358] Therefore, screening for LCNEC is not useful.

Diagnosis

In patients with LCNEC, presenting symptoms mimic those of SCLC and other NSCLC. For example, in one series of 83 patients, the main symptoms were hemoptysis (30%), chest pain (22%), dyspnea (16%), cough (16%), and weight loss (13%); only 4% of patients were asymptomatic.[408] Ectopic hormone production and paraneoplastic syndromes are typically absent.[347]

LCNEC generally present as peripheral tumors. When centrally located, endobronchial growth and obstructive pneumonia can be found.[409] On CT scan, these tumors are often well defined and lobulated, without air bronchograms or calcifications; spiculated margins are less commonly observed.[409,410] Inhomogeneous enhancement is found in larger diameter (33 mm or larger) tumors secondary to necrosis.[409] LCNEC typically have homogenously high FDG uptake on PET scans, which is helpful in locating extrathoracic metastases.[410] A definitive diagnosis may be difficult to determine in small specimens or by cytology, as indicated previously[405,407]; thus, a surgical biopsy is often needed in LCNEC.

Staging

The TNM classification used for NSCLC in the AJCC seventh edition is used for the staging of LCNEC.

Survival for LCNEC is poor and appears to be significantly worse than that of nonneuroendocrine NSCLC.[411] In a series of 335 pathologic stage IA NSCLCs comprising 259 adenocarcinomas, 65 squamous cell carcinomas, and 11 large cell neuroendocrine carcinomas, the histology of LCNEC was found to have a significant adverse prognostic impact and was predictive of poorer overall survival.[411] Asamura et al.[347] found that the survival curve of LCNEC can be superimposed on that for SCLC, with no difference in survival stage for stage between the two, confirming the findings of multiple other series. Reported overall 5-year survival after surgical resection of LCNEC ranges between 15% and 57%,[405] indicating that the recurrence rate after surgery is high. Data from different series reveal that the 5-year survival rate ranges between 33% to 62% in stage I patients, 18% to 75% in stage II patients, 8% to 45% in stage III patients, and 0% in stage IV patients.[347,408,411–413] Factors significantly related to survival among clinicopathologic parameters are tumor stage and size (less than 3 cm versus 3 cm or greater),[406] as well as male gender.[414]

Management by Stage

Patients with LCNEC are managed as if they have NSCLC with the same treatment algorithm stage for stage. The controversy in LCNEC centers on the choice of chemotherapy. Based on the neuroendocrine features, should LCNEC be treated with the same chemotherapy regimens used for SCLC? Certainly the aggressive natural history and propensity to metastasize are similar to SCLC, yet LCNEC clearly does not demonstrate the same chemosensitivity. Published reports about LCNEC are not instructive because essentially all are small, retrospective series with a focus on patients who underwent surgery. Details regarding chemotherapy treatment, such as the agents used or the response rates, are generally not provided.

Stages I, II, and III

For patients with early stage LCNECs, resection is recommended. The modalities of choice are either lobectomy or pneumonectomy, with systematic nodal dissection.[415] After careful mediastinal lymph node sampling, patients without lymph node metastases seem to experience improved survival.[415]

Given the aggressive nature of LCNEC, surgery alone is not sufficient for its treatment. Several small, retrospective studies have attempted to discern the role of neoadjuvant or adjuvant chemotherapy in LCNEC. In this setting, the use of SCLC-based regimens is supported. A Japanese group compiled data on 16 patients who received postoperative chemotherapy and 57 who did not.[413] For all patients, the 5-year survival was 62% for stage I, 18% for stage II, and 17% for stage III. The authors noted that the 5-year survival for the five patients with stage I disease who received adjuvant chemotherapy was 100%, whereas it was 51% for the 23 patients who did not. Postoperative chemotherapy did not affect survival for other stages.[413] In a retrospective review of 100 patients with resected LCNEC evaluating the use of perioperative chemotherapy,[414] there was no association observed between OS and receipt of neoadjuvant (n = 22) or adjuvant (n = 20) platinum-based regimens (OS at 5 years was 50% for no therapy versus 45% for those that received chemotherapy, p adjusted for propensity score = 0.18). However, when the analysis was restricted to patients with completely resected advanced stage IB-IIIA disease, the receipt of platinum-based chemotherapy in either the induction and/or the adjuvant setting was marginally associated with improved median OS: 2 years (95% CI, 1 to 5.3 years) in the no platinum chemotherapy group, compared to 7.4 years (95% CI, 2.5 to not reached) in the platinum chemotherapy group (p adjusted for propensity score = 0.052).[414] In a retrospective analysis of 144 surgical LCNEC cases, Veronesi et al.[412] showed that although perioperative chemotherapy only led to a trend toward improved survival in stage I patients, a statistically significant survival benefit was found across all stages compared to surgery alone (p = 0.04). In a retrospective review of 45 surgically resected patients with LCNEC, patients who did not receive chemotherapy after surgery were more likely to die than patients who underwent surgery plus chemotherapy (n = 23) (HR, 9.472; 95% CI, 1.050 to 85.478; p = 0.0457).[416] An improvement in OS was found in 23 of 63 patients who received perioperative platinum-based chemotherapy compared to those who underwent surgery alone (74.4% versus 32.3%, respectively; p = 0.042).[417] A multivariate analysis utilizing age, gender, pathologic stage, surgical procedure, and perioperative chemotherapy revealed that those patients who underwent surgery with chemotherapy had a significantly better prognosis than those who underwent surgery alone (HR, 0.323; 95% CI, 0.112 to 0.934, p = 0.0371).[417]

As stated, SCLC-based regimens in the adjuvant treatment of LCNEC is supported, in particular. Iyoda et al.[418] performed a prospective analysis on 15 LCNEC patients who received adjuvant chemotherapy with EP and compared outcomes to a historic cohort of LCNEC patients treated without platinum-based adjuvant therapy. Prolonged survival was noted for the patients that received at least two cycles of SCLC-based regimens; the 5-year overall survival rates were 88.9% and 47.4% in the adjuvant chemotherapy group and in the control group, respectively. Further, those receiving platinum-based adjuvant chemotherapy were noted to have a significantly lower rate of tumor recurrence when compared to patients receiving non–platinum-based adjuvant chemotherapy or no adjuvant chemotherapy.[419] Finally, in an Italian retrospective series of 83 LCNEC cases, the 13 patients who received SCLC-based regimens had significantly better survival than the 15 patients who received drug combinations used in NSCLC (median survival, 42 months versus 11 months, respectively, $p < 0.0001$). The best prognosis was noted in stage I LCNEC patients who received SCLC-based adjuvant chemotherapy. In univariate and multivariate analyses, the administration of adjuvant chemotherapy with cisplatin or carboplatin plus etoposide was the most important variable correlating with survival.[408] The interpretation of these reports is limited by their retrospective nature and the small sample size. However, these data, along with the known poor natural history and the routine use of adjuvant chemotherapy for SCLC and NSCLC, suggest that postoperative treatment with etoposide and cisplatin is appropriate in patients with completely resected LCNEC, including patients with stage I disease.

Data regarding the use of radiation therapy in this disease are sparse, but its role in the adjuvant setting is likely similar to that in NSCLC. As per the NCCN guidelines, definitive radiation therapy is recommended for patients who are unable to undergo surgical resection.[420]

Stage IV

The optimal chemotherapeutic regimen in relapsed or stage IV disease is not defined, although treatment with platinum-based regimens is advocated. Several studies have shown that the response rate of LCNEC to cisplatin-based chemotherapy is comparable to SCLC. A retrospective series of 20 patients with advanced LCNEC (stage IIIA, 3; stage IIIB, 6; stage IV, 6; postoperative recurrence, 5) treated with platinum-based therapy showed a response rate of 50% (complete response, 1; partial response, 9).[421] Interestingly, the response rate for chemotherapy-naïve patients (64%) was better than those patients who were previously treated (17%).[421] Rossi et al.[408] showed that in metastatic disease, the 12 patients who received SCLC-based chemotherapy had a significantly better median survival than the 15 patients who received common NSCLC regimens (51 versus 21 months, respectively; $p < 0.001$). Only the patients who received SCLC-based chemotherapy had a complete or partial response. In another retrospective review of 45 patients with pathologically confirmed LCNEC receiving first-line chemotherapy, response rates and outcomes were compared between those that received SCLC (n = 11) and NSCLC (n = 34) regimens. Those treated with SCLC regimens had nonsignificant higher response rates and median PFS and OS compared to patients in the NSCLC chemotherapy group (73% versus 50%, $p = 0.19$; 6.1 versus 4.9 months, respectively, $p = 0.41$; 16.5 versus 9.2 months, respectively, $p = 0.10$).[422]

Two single arm, multicenter phase II studies have been performed in patients with newly diagnosed stage IV LCNEC, each of which had the response rate as the primary endpoint.[423,424] In Japan, 44 patients were enrolled to receive cisplatin and irinotecan every 4 weeks. After careful pathologic review, 30 patients had confirmed LCNEC, whereas 10 actually were reclassified as SCLC. Comparing the two groups, the response rate for this regimen was 47% and 80% for patients with LCNEC and SCLC, respectively ($p = 0.082$). The median PFS and OS were higher in the SCLC group compared to the LCNEC group, 6.2 months versus 5.8 months ($p = 0.382$), and 17.3 months versus 12.6 months ($p = 0.047$), respectively.[423] In the multicenter French study, 42 patients were enrolled to receive EP every 21 days. Here, the LCNEC pathology was confirmed in 29 patients, the response rate of which was 34%. In the analysis confined to the patients with confirmed LCNEC, the median PFS was 5 months and the median OS was 8 months, which was not significantly different than the group with other confirmed diagnoses (SCLC, 9; NSCLC, 1; and atypical carcinoid, 1).[424]

As can be seen, information regarding the treatment of LCNEC has been derived from small studies and suggests that these cancers should be treated as SCLC, although the response rates are lower and outcomes are inferior. Larger, randomized prospective studies are needed to determine the optimal treatment regimen for this disease.

REFERENCES

1. Govindan R, Page N, Morgensztern D, et al. Changing epidemiology of small-cell lung cancer in the United States over the last 30 years: analysis of the surveillance, epidemiologic, and end results database. *J Clin Oncol* 2006;24:4539–4544.
2. Howlader N, Noone AM, Krapcho M, et al. SEER Cancer Statistics Review, 1975–2010. Bethesda, MD: National Cancer Institute; 2013. http://seer.cancer.gov/csr/1975_2011/
3. Siegel R, Naishadham D, Jemal A. Cancer statistics, 2013. *CA Cancer J Clin* 2013;63:11–30.
4. Varghese A, Zakowski MF, Yu HA, et al. Small-cell lung cancers in patients who never smoked cigarettes. *J Thorac Oncol* 2014:9:892–896
5. Ou SH, Ziogas A, Zell JA. Prognostic factors for survival in extensive stage small cell lung cancer (ED-SCLC): the importance of smoking history, socioeconomic and marital statuses, and ethnicity. *J Thorac Oncol* 2009;4:37–43.
6. Garfinkel L. Trends in cigarette smoking in the United States. *Prev Med* 1997;26:447–450.
7. Centers for Disease Control and Prevention (CDC). Current Cigarette Smoking Among Adults – United States, 2011. *MMWR Morb Mort Wkly Rep* 2012;61:889–894.
8. Wingo PA, Ries LA, Giovino GA, et al. Annual report to the nation on the status of cancer, 1973–1996, with a special section on lung cancer and tobacco smoking. *J Natl Cancer Inst* 1999;91:675–690.
9. Travis WD, Brambilla E, Muller-Hermelink HK, et al. *Pathology and Genetics: Tumours of the Lung, Pleura, Thymus and Heart.* Lyon: International Agency for Research on Cancer; 2004.
10. Nicholson SA, Beasley MB, Brambilla E, et al. Small cell lung carcinoma (SCLC): a clinicopathologic study of 100 cases with surgical specimens. *Am J Surg Pathol* 2002;26:1184–1197.
11. Travis WD. Update on small cell carcinoma and its differentiation from squamous cell carcinoma and other non-small cell carcinomas. *Mod Pathol* 2012;25:S18–S30.
12. Vollmer RT. The effect of cell size on the pathologic diagnosis of small and large cell carcinomas of the lung. *Cancer* 1982;50:1380–1383.
13. Hiroshima K, Iyoda A, Shida T, et al. Distinction of pulmonary large cell neuroendocrine carcinoma from small cell lung carcinoma: a morphological, immunohistochemical, and molecular analysis. *Mod Pathol* 2006; 19:1358–1368.
14. Folpe AL, Gown AM, Lamps LW, et al. Thyroid transcription factor-1: immunohistochemical evaluation in pulmonary neuroendocrine tumors. *Mod Pathol* 1999;12:5–8.
15. Sturm N, Lantuejoul S, Laverriere MH, et al. Thyroid transcription factor 1 and cytokeratins 1, 5, 10, 14 (34betaE12) expression in basaloid and large-cell neuroendocrine carcinomas of the lung. *Hum Pathol* 2001;32:918–925.
16. Sturm N, Rossi G, Lantuejoul S, et al. Expression of thyroid transcription factor-1 in the spectrum of neuroendocrine cell lung proliferations with special interest in carcinoids. *Hum Pathol* 2002;33:175–182.
17. Agoff SN, Lamps LW, Philip AT, et al. Thyroid transcription factor-1 is expressed in extrapulmonary small cell carcinomas but not in other extrapulmonary neuroendocrine tumors. *Mod Pathol* 2000;13:238–242.
18. Wistuba II, Gazdar AF, Minna JD. Molecular genetics of small cell lung carcinoma. *Semin Oncol* 2001;28:3–13.
19. Mori N, Yokota J, Akiyama T, et al. Variable mutations of the RB gene in small-cell lung carcinoma. *Oncogene* 1990;5:1713–1717.
20. Arriola E, Canadas I, Arumi M, et al. Genetic changes in small cell lung carcinoma. *Clin Transl Oncol* 2008;10:189–197.
21. Meuwissen R, Linn SC, Linnoila RI, et al. Induction of small cell lung cancer by somatic inactivation of both Trp53 and Rb1 in a conditional mouse model. *Cancer Cell* 2003;4:181–189.
22. Peifer M, Fernandez-Cuesta L, Sos ML, et al. Integrative genome analyses identify key somatic driver mutations of small-cell lung cancer. *Nat Geneti* 2012;44:1104–1110.
23. Rudin CM, Durinck S, Stawiski EW, et al. Comprehensive genomic analysis identifies SOX2 as a frequently amplified gene in small-cell lung cancer. *Nat Genet* 2012;44:1111–1116.
24. Rekhtman N, Marchetti A, Lau C, et al. Analysis of EGFR and KRAS mutations in small cell carcinoma and large cell neuroendocrine carcinoma. Presented at: 2011 14th World Conference on Lung Cancer; July 2011; Amsterdam, The Netherlands.
25. Aberle DR, Adams AM, Berg CD, et al. Reduced lung-cancer mortality with low-dose computed tomographic screening. *N Engl J Med* 2011;365:395–409.
26. Chute CG, Greenberg ER, Baron J, et al. Presenting conditions of 1539 population-based lung cancer patients by cell type and stage in New Hampshire and Vermont. *Cancer* 1985;56:2107–2111.
27. Hollen PJ, Gralla RJ, Kris MG, et al. Quality of life assessment in individuals with lung cancer: testing the Lung Cancer Symptom Scale (LCSS). *Eur J Cancer* 1993;29A:S51–S58.
28. Sculier JP, Evans WK, Feld R, et al. Superior vena caval obstruction syndrome in small cell lung cancer. *Cancer* 1986;57:847–851.
29. Higgins GA, Shields TW, Keehn RJ. The solitary pulmonary nodule. Ten-year follow-up of veterans administration-armed forces cooperative study. *Arch Surg* 1975;110:570–575.
30. Quoix E, Fraser R, Wolkove N, et al. Small cell lung cancer presenting as a solitary pulmonary nodule. *Cancer* 1990;66:577–582.
31. Johnson DH, Hainsworth JD, Greco FA. Pancoast's syndrome and small cell lung cancer. *Chest* 1982;82:602–606.
32. Levitan N, Byrne RE, Bromer RH, et al. The value of the bone scan and bone marrow biopsy staging small cell lung cancer. *Cancer* 1985;56:652–654.
33. Seute T, Leffers P, ten Velde GP, et al. Neurologic disorders in 432 consecutive patients with small cell lung carcinoma. *Cancer* 2004;100:801–806.
34. Castillo JJ, Vincent M, Justice E. Diagnosis and management of hyponatremia in cancer patients. *Oncologist* 2012;17:756–765.
35. Verbalis JG, Adler S, Schrier RW, et al. Efficacy and safety of oral tolvaptan therapy in patients with the syndrome of inappropriate antidiuretic hormone secretion. *Eur J Endocrinol* 2011;164:725–732.
36. Osterlind K, Andersen PK. Prognostic factors in small cell lung cancer: multivariate model based on 778 patients treated with chemotherapy with or without irradiation. *Cancer Res* 1986;46:4189–4194.
37. Shepherd FA, Laskey J, Evans WK, et al. Cushing's syndrome associated with ectopic corticotropin production and small-cell lung cancer. *J Clin Oncol* 1992;10:21–27.

38. Ilias I, Torpy DJ, Pacak K, et al. Cushing's syndrome due to ectopic corticotropin secretion: twenty years' experience at the National Institutes of Health. *J Clin Endocrinol Metab* 2005;90:4955–4962.
39. Darnell RB, Posner JB. Paraneoplastic syndromes involving the nervous system. *N Engl J Med* 2003;349:1543–1554.
40. Graus F, Dalmou J, Rene R, et al. Anti-Hu antibodies in patients with small-cell lung cancer: association with complete response to therapy and improved survival. *J Clin Oncol* 1997;15:2866–2872.
41. Monstad SE, Drivsholm L, Storstein A, et al. Hu and voltage-gated calcium channel (VGCC) antibodies related to the prognosis of small-cell lung cancer. *J Clin Oncol* 2004;22:795–800.
42. Darnell R. Tumor immunity in small-cell lung cancer. *J Clin Oncol* 2004; 22:762–764.
43. Maddison P, Newsom-Davis J. Treatment for Lambert-Eaton myasthenic syndrome. *Cochrane Database Syst Rev* 2005;(2):CD003279.
44. Zelen M. Keynote address on biostatistics and data retrieval. *Cancer Chemother Rep [3]* 1973;4:31–42.
45. Livingston RB, McCracken JD, Trauth CJ, et al. Isolated pleural effusion in small cell lung carcinoma: favorable prognosis. A review of the Southwest Oncology Group experience. *Chest* 1982;81:208–211.
46. Albain KS, Crowley JJ, LeBlanc M, et al. Determinants of improved outcome in small-cell lung cancer: an analysis of the 2,580-patient Southwest Oncology Group data base. *J Clin Oncol* 1990;8:1563–1574.
47. Spiegelman D, Maurer LH, Ware JH, et al. Prognostic factors in small-cell carcinoma of the lung: an analysis of 1,521 patients. *J Clin Oncol* 1989;7:344–354.
48. Bonner JA, Sloan JA, Shanahan TG, et al. Phase III comparison of twice-daily split-course irradiation versus once-daily irradiation for patients with limited stage small-cell lung carcinoma. *J Clin Oncol* 1999;17:2681–2691.
49. Turrisi AT 3rd, Kim K, Blum R, et al. Twice-daily compared with once-daily thoracic radiotherapy in limited small-cell lung cancer treated concurrently with cisplatin and etoposide. *N Engl J Med* 1999;340:265–271.
50. Doll DC. Serum lactate dehydrogenase and bone marrow involvement in small-cell carcinoma of the lung. *N Engl J Med* 1985;312:1262.
51. Van den Brande P, Demedts M. Serum lactate dehydrogenase in small-cell lung cancer. *N Engl J Med* 1989;320:61.
52. Kalemkerian GP, Akerley W, Bogner P, et al. Small cell lung cancer. *J Natl Compr Canc Netw* 2013;11:78–98.
53. Vallieres E, Shepherd FA, Crowley J, et al. The IASLC Lung Cancer Staging Project: proposals regarding the relevance of TNM in the pathologic staging of small cell lung cancer in the forthcoming (seventh) edition of the TNM classification for lung cancer. *J Thorac Oncol* 2009;4:1049–1059.
54. Karrer K, Ulsperger E. Surgery for cure followed by chemotherapy in small cell carcinoma of the lung. For the ISC-Lung Cancer Study Group. *Acta Oncol* 1995;34:899–906.
55. Kreisman H, Wolkove N, Quoix E. Small cell lung cancer presenting as a solitary pulmonary nodule. *Chest* 1992;101:225–231.
56. Shepherd FA, Ginsberg RJ, Haddad R, et al. Importance of clinical staging in limited small-cell lung cancer: a valuable system to separate prognostic subgroups. The University of Toronto Lung Oncology Group. *J Clin Oncol* 1993;11:1592–1597.
57. Gronowitz JS, Bergstrom R, Nou E, et al. Clinical and serologic markers of stage and prognosis in small cell lung cancer. A multivariate analysis. *Cancer* 1990;66:722–32.
58. Paesmans M, Sculier JP, Lecomte J, et al. Prognostic factors for patients with small cell lung carcinoma: analysis of a series of 763 patients included in 4 consecutive prospective trials with a minimum follow-up of 5 years. *Cancer* 2000;89:523–533.
59. Yuen AR, Zou G, Turrisi AT, et al. Similar outcome of elderly patients in intergroup trial 0096: Cisplatin, etoposide, and thoracic radiotherapy administered once or twice daily in limited stage small cell lung carcinoma. *Cancer* 2000;89:1953–1960.
60. Siu LL, Shepherd FA, Murray N, et al. Influence of age on the treatment of limited-stage small-cell lung cancer. *J Clin Oncol* 1996;14:821–828.
61. Jorgensen LG, Osterlind K, Genolla J, et al. Serum neuron-specific enolase (S-NSE) and the prognosis in small-cell lung cancer (SCLC): a combined multivariable analysis on data from nine centres. *Br J Cancer* 1996;74:463–467.
62. Jara C, Gomez-Aldaravi JL, Tirado R, et al. Small-cell lung cancer in the elderly—is age of patient a relevant factor? *Acta Oncol* 1999;38:781–786.
63. Ludbrook JJ, Truong PT, MacNeil MV, et al. Do age and comorbidity impact treatment allocation and outcomes in limited stage small-cell lung cancer? a community-based population analysis. *Int J Radiat Oncol Biol Phys* 2003;55: 1321–1330.
64. Hurria A, Kris MG. Management of lung cancer in older adults. *CA Cancer J Clin* 2003;53:325–341.
65. Dearing MP, Steinberg SM, Phelps R, et al. Outcome of patients with small-cell lung cancer: effect of changes in staging procedures and imaging technology on prognostic factors over 14 years. *J Clin Oncol* 1990;8: 1042–1049.
66. Bremnes RM, Sundstrom S, Aasebo U, et al. The value of prognostic factors in small cell lung cancer: results from a randomised multicenter study with minimum 5 year follow-up. *Lung Cancer* 2003;39:303–313.
67. Lassen U, Osterlind K, Hansen M, et al. Long-term survival in small-cell lung cancer: posttreatment characteristics in patients surviving 5 to 18+ years—an analysis of 1,714 consecutive patients. *J Clin Oncol* 1995;13:1215–1220.
68. Sagman U, Maki E, Evans WK, et al. Small-cell carcinoma of the lung: derivation of a prognostic staging system. *J Clin Oncol* 1991;9:1639–1649.
69. Videtic GM, Stitt LW, Dar AR, et al. Continued cigarette smoking by patients receiving concurrent chemoradiotherapy for limited-stage small-cell lung cancer is associated with decreased survival. *J Clin Oncol* 2003;21:1544–1549.
70. Maestu I, Pastor M, Gomez-Codina J, et al. Pretreatment prognostic factors for survival in small-cell lung cancer: a new prognostic index and validation of three known prognostic indices on 341 patients. *Ann Oncol* 1997;8:547–553.
71. Quoix E, Purohit A, Faller-Beau M, et al. Comparative prognostic value of lactate dehydrogenase and neuron-specific enolase in small-cell lung cancer patients treated with platinum-based chemotherapy. *Lung Cancer* 2000;30: 127–134.
72. Kawahara M, Fukuoka M, Saijo N, et al. Prognostic factors and prognostic staging system for small cell lung cancer. *Jpn J Clin Oncol* 1997;27:158–165.
73. Pujol JL, Quantin X, Jacot W, et al. Neuroendocrine and cytokeratin serum markers as prognostic determinants of small cell lung cancer. *Lung Cancer* 2003;39:131–138.
74. Shingyoji M, Takiguchi Y, Watanabe R, et al. Detection of tumor specific gene expression in bone marrow and peripheral blood from patients with small cell lung carcinoma. *Cancer* 2003;97:1057–1062.
75. Laberge F, Fritsche HA, Umsawasdi T, et al. Use of carcinoembryonic antigen in small cell lung cancer. Prognostic value and relation to the clinical course 1. *Cancer* 1987;59:2047–2052.
76. Sculier JP, Feld R, Evans WK, et al. Carcinoembryonic antigen: a useful prognostic marker in small-cell lung cancer. *J Clin Oncol* 1985;3:1349–1354.
77. Bradley JD, Dehdashti F, Mintun MA, et al. Positron emission tomography in limited-stage small-cell lung cancer: a prospective study. *J Clin Oncol* 2004;22:3248–3254.
78. Chin R Jr, McCain TW, Miller AA, et al. Whole body FDG-PET for the evaluation and staging of small cell lung cancer: a preliminary study. *Lung Cancer* 2002;37:1–6.
79. Pandit N, Gonen M, Krug L, et al. Prognostic value of [18F]FDG-PET imaging in small cell lung cancer. *Eur J Nucl Med Mol Imaging* 2003;30:78–84.
80. Cheran SK, Herndon JE 2nd, Patz EF Jr. Comparison of whole-body FDG-PET to bone scan for detection of bone metastases in patients with a new diagnosis of lung cancer. *Lung Cancer* 2004;44:317–325.
81. Murray N, Coy P, Pater JL, et al. Importance of timing for thoracic irradiation in the combined modality treatment of limited-stage small-cell lung cancer. The National Cancer Institute of Canada Clinical Trials Group. *J Clin Oncol* 1993;11:336–344.
82. Park K, Sun J-M, Kim S-W, et al. Phase III trial of concurrent thoracic radiotherapy with either the first cycle or the third cycle of cisplatin and etoposide chemotherapy to determine the optimal timing of thoracic radiotherapy for limited-disease small cell lung cancer. *J Clin Oncol* 2012;30:abstract 7004.
83. Slotman B, Faivre-Finn C, Kramer G, et al. Prophylactic cranial irradiation in extensive small-cell lung cancer. *N Engl J Med* 2007;357:664–672.
84. Cavalli F, Sonntag RW, Jungi F, et al. VP-16-213 monotherapy for remission induction of small cell lung cancer: a randomized trial using three dosage schedules. *Cancer Treat Rep* 1978;62:473–475.
85. Lowenbraun S, Bartolucci A, Smalley RV, et al. The superiority of combination chemotherapy over single agent chemotherapy in small cell lung carcinoma. *Cancer* 1979;44:406–413.
86. Hansen HH, Dombernowsky P, Hansen M, et al. Chemotherapy of advanced small-cell anaplastic carcinoma. Superiority of a four-drug combination to a three-drug combination. *Ann Intern Med* 1978;89:177–181.
87. Livingston RB, Moore TN, Heilbrun L, et al. Small-cell carcinoma of the lung: combined chemotherapy and radiation: a Southwest Oncology Group study. *Ann Intern Med* 1978;88:194–199.
88. Bunn PA Jr, Greco FA, Einhorn L. Cyclophosphamide, doxorubicin, and etoposide as first-line therapy in the treatment of small-cell lung cancer. *Semin Oncol* 1986;13:45–53.
89. Hong WK, Nicaise C, Lawson R, et al. Etoposide combined with cyclophosphamide plus vincristine compared with doxorubicin plus cyclophosphamide plus vincristine and with high-dose cyclophosphamide plus vincristine in the treatment of small-cell carcinoma of the lung: a randomized trial of the Bristol Lung Cancer Study Group. *J Clin Oncol* 1989;7:450–456.
90. Jackson DV Jr, Case LD, Zekan PJ, et al. Improvement of long-term survival in extensive small-cell lung cancer. *J Clin Oncol* 1988;6:1161–1169.
91. Jackson DV Jr, Zekan PJ, Caldwell RD, et al. VP-16-213 in combination chemotherapy with chest irradiation for small-cell lung cancer: a randomized trial of the Piedmont Oncology Association. *J Clin Oncol* 1984;2: 1343–1351.
92. Jett JR, Everson L, Therneau TM, et al. Treatment of limited-stage small-cell lung cancer with cyclophosphamide, doxorubicin, and vincristine with or without etoposide: a randomized trial of the North Central Cancer Treatment Group. *J Clin Oncol* 1990;8:33–38.
93. Lowenbraun S, Birch R, Buchanan R, et al. Combination chemotherapy in small cell lung carcinoma. A randomized study of two intensive regimens. *Cancer* 1984;54:2344–2350.
94. Messeih AA, Schweitzer JM, Lipton A, et al. Addition of etoposide to cyclophosphamide, doxorubicin, and vincristine for remission induction and survival in patients with small cell lung cancer. *Cancer Treat Rep* 1987;71: 61–66.
95. Sierocki JS, Hilaris BS, Hopfan S, et al. cis-Dichlorodiammineplatinum(II) and VP-16-213: an active induction regimen for small cell carcinoma of the lung. *Cancer Treat Rep* 1979;63:1593–1597.
96. Evans WK, Osoba D, Feld R, et al. Etoposide (VP-16) and cisplatin: an effective treatment for relapse in small-cell lung cancer. *J Clin Oncol* 1985;3:65–71.

97. Evans WK, Shepherd FA, Feld R, et al. VP-16 and cisplatin as first-line therapy for small-cell lung cancer. *J Clin Oncol* 1985;3:1471–1477.
98. Einhorn LH, Crawford J, Birch R, et al. Cisplatin plus etoposide consolidation following cyclophosphamide, doxorubicin, and vincristine in limited small-cell lung cancer. *J Clin Oncol* 1988;6:451–456.
99. Fukuoka M, Furuse K, Saijo N, et al. Randomized trial of cyclophosphamide, doxorubicin, and vincristine versus cisplatin and etoposide versus alternation of these regimens in small-cell lung cancer. *J Natl Cancer Inst* 1991;83:855–861.
100. Roth BJ, Johnson DH, Einhorn LH, et al. Randomized study of cyclophosphamide, doxorubicin, and vincristine versus etoposide and cisplatin versus alternation of these two regimens in extensive small-cell lung cancer: a phase III trial of the Southeastern Cancer Study Group. *J Clin Oncol* 1992;10:282–291.
101. Sundstrom S, Bremnes RM, Kaasa S, et al. Cisplatin and etoposide regimen is superior to cyclophosphamide, epirubicin, and vincristine regimen in small-cell lung cancer: results from a randomized phase III trial with 5 years' follow-up. *J Clin Oncol* 2002;20:4665–4672.
102. Chute JP, Venzon DJ, Hankins L, et al. Outcome of patients with small-cell lung cancer during 20 years of clinical research at the US National Cancer Institute. *Mayo Clin Proc* 1997;72:901–912.
103. Mascaux C, Paesmans M, Berghmans T, et al. A systematic review of the role of etoposide and cisplatin in the chemotherapy of small cell lung cancer with methodology assessment and meta-analysis. *Lung Cancer* 2000;30:23–36.
104. Pujol JL, Carestia L, Daures JP. Is there a case for cisplatin in the treatment of small-cell lung cancer? A meta-analysis of randomized trials of a cisplatin-containing regimen versus a regimen without this alkylating agent. *Br J Cancer* 2000;83:8–15.
105. Skarlos DV, Samantas E, Kosmidis P, et al. Randomized comparison of etoposide-cisplatin vs. etoposide-carboplatin and irradiation in small-cell lung cancer. A Hellenic Co-operative Oncology Group study. *Ann Oncol* 1994;5:601–607.
106. Rossi A, Di Maio M, Chiodini P, et al. Carboplatin- or cisplatin-based chemotherapy in first-line treatment of small-cell lung cancer: the COCIS meta-analysis of individual patient data. *J Clin Oncol* 2012;30:1692–1698.
107. Masuda N, Fukuoka M, Kusunoki Y, et al. CPT-11: a new derivative of camptothecin for the treatment of refractory or relapsed small-cell lung cancer. *J Clin Oncol* 1992;10:1225–1229.
108. Noda K, Nishiwaki Y, Kawahara M, et al. Irinotecan plus cisplatin compared with etoposide plus cisplatin for extensive small-cell lung cancer. *N Engl J Med* 2002;346:85–91.
109. Lara PN Jr, Natale R, Crowley J, et al. Phase III trial of irinotecan/cisplatin compared with etoposide/cisplatin in extensive-stage small-cell lung cancer: clinical and pharmacogenomic results from SWOG S0124. *J Clin Oncol* 2009;27:2530–2535.
110. Naka N, Kawahara M, Okishio K, et al. Phase II study of weekly irinotecan and carboplatin for refractory or relapsed small-cell lung cancer. *Lung Cancer* 2002;37:319–323.
111. Chen G, Huynh M, Fehrenbacher L, et al. Phase II trial of irinotecan and carboplatin for extensive or relapsed small-cell lung cancer. *J Clin Oncol* 2009;27:1401–1404.
112. Hermes A, Bergman B, Bremnes R, et al. Irinotecan plus carboplatin versus oral etoposide plus carboplatin in extensive small-cell lung cancer: a randomized phase III trial. *J Clin Oncol* 2008;26:4261–4267.
113. Ando Y, Saka H, Ando M, et al. Polymorphisms of UDP-glucuronosyltransferase gene and irinotecan toxicity: a pharmacogenetic analysis. *Cancer Res* 2000;60:6921–6926.
114. Ardizzoni A, Manegold C, Debruyne C, et al. European organization for research and treatment of cancer (EORTC) 08957 phase II study of topotecan in combination with cisplatin as second-line treatment of refractory and sensitive small cell lung cancer. *Clin Cancer Res* 2003;9:143–150.
115. Eckardt JR, von Pawel J, Papai Z, et al. Open-label, multicenter, randomized, phase III study comparing oral topotecan/cisplatin versus etoposide/cisplatin as treatment for chemotherapy-naive patients with extensive-disease small-cell lung cancer. *J Clin Oncol* 2006;24:2044–2051.
116. Goldie JH, Coldman AJ, Gudauskas GA. Rationale for the use of alternating non-cross-resistant chemotherapy. *Cancer Treat Rep* 1982;66:439–449.
117. Ettinger DS, Finkelstein DM, Abeloff MD, et al. A randomized comparison of standard chemotherapy versus alternating chemotherapy and maintenance versus no maintenance therapy for extensive-stage small-cell lung cancer: a phase III study of the Eastern Cooperative Oncology Group. *J Clin Oncol* 1990;8:230–240.
118. Livingston RB, Mira JG, Chen TT, et al. Combined modality treatment of extensive small cell lung cancer: a Southwest Oncology Group study. *J Clin Oncol* 1984;2:585–590.
119. Evans WK, Feld R, Murray N, et al. Superiority of alternating non-cross-resistant chemotherapy in extensive small cell lung cancer. A multicenter, randomized clinical trial by the National Cancer Institute of Canada. *Ann Intern Med* 1987;107:451–458.
120. Postmus PE, Scagliotti G, Groen HJ, et al. Standard versus alternating non-cross-resistant chemotherapy in extensive small cell lung cancer: an EORTC Phase III trial. *Eur J Cancer* 1996;32A:1498–1503.
121. Osterlind K, Sorenson S, Hansen HH, et al. Continuous versus alternating combination chemotherapy for advanced small cell carcinoma of the lung. *Cancer Res* 1983;43:6085–6089.
122. Andersen M, Kristjansen PE, Hansen HH. Second-line chemotherapy in small cell lung cancer. *Cancer Treat Rev* 1990;17:427–436.
123. Wolf M, Pritsch M, Drings P, et al. Cyclic-alternating versus response-oriented chemotherapy in small-cell lung cancer: a German multicenter randomized trial of 321 patients. *J Clin Oncol* 1991;9:614–624.
124. Aisner J, Whitacre M, Van Echo DA, et al. Combination chemotherapy for small cell carcinoma of the lung: continuous versus alternating non-cross-resistant combinations. *Cancer Treat Rep* 1982;66:221–230.
125. Ettinger DS, Lagakos S. Phase III study of CCNU, cyclophosphamide, adriamycin, vincristine, and VP-16 in small-cell carcinoma of the lung. *Cancer* 1982;49:1544–1554.
126. Feld R, Evans WK, Coy P, et al. Canadian multicenter randomized trial comparing sequential and alternating administration of two non-cross-resistant chemotherapy combinations in patients with limited small-cell carcinoma of the lung. *J Clin Oncol* 1987;5:1401–1409.
127. Havemann K, Wolf M, Holle R, et al. Alternating versus sequential chemotherapy in small cell lung cancer. A randomized German multicenter trial. *Cancer* 1987;59:1072–1082.
128. Urban T, Baleyte T, Chastang CL, et al. Standard combination versus alternating chemotherapy in small cell lung cancer: a randomised clinical trial including 394 patients. 'Petites Cellules' Group. *Lung Cancer* 1999;25:105–113.
129. Loehrer PJ Sr, Rynard S, Ansari R, et al. Etoposide, ifosfamide, and cisplatin in extensive small cell lung cancer. *Cancer* 1992;69:669–673.
130. Miyamoto H, Nakabayashi T, Isobe H, et al. A phase III comparison of etoposide/cisplatin with or without added ifosfamide in small-cell lung cancer. *Oncology* 1992;49:431–435.
131. Loehrer PJ Sr, Ansari R, Gonin R, et al. Cisplatin plus etoposide with and without ifosfamide in extensive small-cell lung cancer: a Hoosier Oncology Group study. *J Clin Oncol* 1995;13:2594–2599.
132. Thatcher N, Lind M, Stout R, et al. Carboplatin, ifosfamide and etoposide with mid-course vincristine and thoracic radiotherapy for 'limited' stage small cell carcinoma of the bronchus. *Br J Cancer* 1989;60:98–101.
133. Wolff AC, Ettinger DS, Neuberg D, et al. Phase II study of ifosfamide, carboplatin, and oral etoposide chemotherapy for extensive-disease small-cell lung cancer: an Eastern Cooperative Oncology Group pilot study. *J Clin Oncol* 1995;13:1615–1622.
134. Thatcher N, Qian W, Clark PI, et al. Ifosfamide, carboplatin, and etoposide with midcycle vincristine versus standard chemotherapy in patients with small-cell lung cancer and good performance status: clinical and quality-of-life results of the British Medical Research Council multicenter randomized LU21 trial. *J Clin Oncol* 2005;23:8371–8379.
135. Mavroudis D, Papadakis E, Veslemes M, et al. A multicenter randomized clinical trial comparing paclitaxel-cisplatin-etoposide versus cisplatin-etoposide as first-line treatment in patients with small-cell lung cancer. *Ann Oncol* 2001;12:463–470.
136. Niell HB, Herndon JE 2nd, Miller AA, et al. Randomized phase III intergroup trial of etoposide and cisplatin with or without paclitaxel and granulocyte colony-stimulating factor in patients with extensive-stage small-cell lung cancer: Cancer and Leukemia Group B Trial 9732. *J Clin Oncol* 2005;23:3752–3759.
137. Reck M, von Pawel J, Macha HN, et al. Randomized phase III trial of paclitaxel, etoposide, and carboplatin versus carboplatin, etoposide, and vincristine in patients with small-cell lung cancer. *J Natl Cancer Inst* 2003;95:1118–1127.
138. Controlled trial of twelve versus six courses of chemotherapy in the treatment of small-cell lung cancer. Report to the Medical Research Council by its Lung Cancer Working Party. *Br J Cancer* 1989;59:584–590.
139. Beith JM, Clarke SJ, Woods RL, et al. Long-term follow-up of a randomised trial of combined chemoradiotherapy induction treatment, with and without maintenance chemotherapy in patients with small cell carcinoma of the lung. *Eur J Cancer* 1996;32A:438–443.
140. Byrne MJ, van Hazel G, Trotter J, et al. Maintenance chemotherapy in limited small cell lung cancer: a randomised controlled clinical trial. *Br J Cancer* 1989;60:413–418.
141. Cullen M, Morgan D, Gregory W, et al. Maintenance chemotherapy for anaplastic small cell carcinoma of the bronchus: a randomised, controlled trial. *Cancer Chemother Pharmacol* 1986;17:157–160.
142. Giaccone G, Dalesio O, McVie GJ, et al. Maintenance chemotherapy in small-cell lung cancer: long-term results of a randomized trial. European Organization for Research and Treatment of Cancer Lung Cancer Cooperative Group. *J Clin Oncol* 1993;11:1230–1240.
143. Lebeau B, Chastang C, Allard P, et al. Six vs twelve cycles for complete responders to chemotherapy in small cell lung cancer: definitive results of a randomized clinical trial. The "Petites Cellules" Group. *Eur Respir J* 1992;5:286–290.
144. Maurer LH, Tulloh M, Weiss RB, et al. A randomized combined modality trial in small cell carcinoma of the lung: comparison of combination chemotherapy-radiation therapy versus cyclophosphamide-radiation therapy effects of maintenance chemotherapy and prophylactiv whole brain irradiation. *Cancer* 1980;45:30–39.
145. Schiller JH, Adak S, Cella D, et al. Topotecan versus observation after cisplatin plus etoposide in extensive-stage small-cell lung cancer: E7593—a phase III trial of the Eastern Cooperative Oncology Group. *J Clin Oncol* 2001;19:2114–2122.
146. Sculier JP, Paesmans M, Bureau G, et al. Randomized trial comparing induction chemotherapy versus induction chemotherapy followed by maintenance chemotherapy in small-cell lung cancer. European Lung Cancer Working Party. *J Clin Oncol* 1996;14:2337–2344.
147. Bleehen NM, Girling DJ, Machin D, et al. A randomised trial of three or six courses of etoposide cyclophosphamide methotrexate and vincristine or six courses of etoposide and ifosfamide in small cell lung cancer (SCLC). I: Survival and prognostic factors. Medical Research Council Lung Cancer Working Party. *Br J Cancer* 1993;68:1150–1156.
148. Bleehen NM, Girling DJ, Machin D, et al. A randomised trial of three or six courses of etoposide cyclophosphamide methotrexate and vincristine or six

courses of etoposide and ifosfamide in small cell lung cancer (SCLC). II: Quality of life. Medical Research Council Lung Cancer Working Party. *Br J Cancer* 1993;68:1157–1166.

149. Spiro SG, Souhami RL, Geddes DM, et al. Duration of chemotherapy in small cell lung cancer: a Cancer Research Campaign trial. *Br J Cancer* 1989;59: 578–583.
150. Bozcuk H, Artac M, Ozdogan M, et al. Does maintenance/consolidation chemotherapy have a role in the management of small cell lung cancer (SCLC)? A metaanalysis of the published controlled trials. *Cancer* 2005;104:2650–2657.
151. Rossi A, Garassino MC, Cinquini M, et al. Maintenance or consolidation therapy in small-cell lung cancer: a systematic review and meta-analysis. *Lung Cancer* 2010;70:119–128.
152. Fruh M, De Ruysscher D, Popat S, et al. Small-cell lung cancer (SCLC): ESMO Clinical Practice Guidelines for diagnosis, treatment and follow-up. *Ann Oncol* 2013;24:vi99–vi105.
153. Teicher B. Preclinical models for high-dose therapy. In: Armitage J, Antman K, eds. *High-Dose Chemotherapy: Pharmacology, Hematopoietins, Stems cells.* Baltimore: Williams & Wilkins; 1992.
154. Arriagada R, Le Chevalier T, Pignon JP, et al. Initial chemotherapeutic doses and survival in patients with limited small-cell lung cancer. *N Engl J Med* 1993;329:1848–1852.
155. Cohen MH, Creaven PJ, Fossieck BE Jr, et al. Intensive chemotherapy of small cellbronchogenic carcinoma. *Cancer Treat Rep* 1977; 61:349–354.
156. Figueredo AT, Hryniuk WM, Strautmanis I, et al. Co-trimoxazole prophylaxis during high-dose chemotherapy of small-cell lung cancer. *J Clin Oncol* 1985;3:54–64.
157. Ihde DC, Mulshine JL, Kramer BS, et al. Prospective randomized comparison of high-dose and standard-dose etoposide and cisplatin chemotherapy in patients with extensive-stage small-cell lung cancer. *J Clin Oncol* 1994;12:2022–2034.
158. Johnson DH, Einhorn LH, Birch R, et al. A randomized comparison of high-dose versus conventional-dose cyclophosphamide, doxorubicin, and vincristine for extensive-stage small-cell lung cancer: a phase III trial of the Southeastern Cancer Study Group. *J Clin Oncol* 1987;5:1731–1738.
159. Pujol JL, Douillard JY, Riviere A, et al. Dose-intensity of a four-drug chemotherapy regimen with or without recombinant human granulocyte-macrophage colony-stimulating factor in extensive-stage small-cell lung cancer: a multicenter randomized phase III study. *J Clin Oncol* 1997;15:2082–2089.
160. Steward WP, von Pawel J, Gatzemeier U, et al. Effects of granulocyte-macrophage colony-stimulating factor and dose intensification of V-ICE chemotherapy in small-cell lung cancer: a prospective randomized study of 300 patients. *J Clin Oncol* 1998;16:642–650.
161. Lorigan P, Woll PJ, O'Brien ME, et al. Randomized phase III trial of dose-dense chemotherapy supported by whole-blood hematopoietic progenitors in better-prognosis small-cell lung cancer. *J Natl Cancer Inst* 2005;97:666–674.
162. Ardizzoni A, Tjan-Heijnen VC, Postmus PE, et al. Standard versus intensified chemotherapy with granulocyte colony-stimulating factor support in small-cell lung cancer: a prospective European Organization for Research and Treatment of Cancer-Lung Cancer Group Phase III Trial-08923. *J Clin Oncol* 2002;20:3947–3955.
163. Thatcher N, Girling DJ, Hopwood P, et al. Improving survival without reducing quality of life in small-cell lung cancer patients by increasing the dose-intensity of chemotherapy with granulocyte colony-stimulating factor support: results of a British Medical Research Council Multicenter Randomized Trial. Medical Research Council Lung Cancer Working Party. *J Clin Oncol* 2000;18:395–404.
164. Sculier JP, Paesmans M, Bureau G, et al. Multiple-drug weekly chemotherapy versus standard combination regimen in small-cell lung cancer: a phase III randomized study conducted by the European Lung Cancer Working Party. *J Clin Oncol* 1993;11:1858–1865.
165. Souhami RL, Rudd R, Ruiz de Elvira MC, et al. Randomized trial comparing weekly versus 3-week chemotherapy in small-cell lung cancer: a Cancer Research Campaign trial. *J Clin Oncol* 1994;12:1806–1813.
166. Furuse K, Fukuoka M, Nishiwaki Y, et al. Phase III study of intensive weekly chemotherapy with recombinant human granulocyte colony-stimulating factor versus standard chemotherapy in extensive-disease small-cell lung cancer. The Japan Clinical Oncology Group. *J Clin Oncol* 1998;16:2126–2132.
167. Murray N, Livingston RB, Shepherd FA, et al. Randomized study of CODE versus alternating CAV/EP for extensive-stage small-cell lung cancer: an Intergroup Study of the National Cancer Institute of Canada Clinical Trials Group and the Southwest Oncology Group. *J Clin Oncol* 1999;17:2300–2308.
168. Elias A. Dose-intensive therapy in small cell lung cancer. *Chest* 1998;113: 101S–106S.
169. Spitzer G, Dicke KA, Litam J, et al. High-dose combination chemotherapy with autologous bone marrow transplantation in adult solid tumors. *Cancer* 1980;45:3075–3085.
170. Lazarus HM, Spitzer TR, Creger RJ. Phase I trial of high-dose etoposide, high-dose cisplatin, and reinfusion of autologous bone marrow for lung cancer. *Am J Clin Oncol* 1990;13:107–112.
171. Elias AD, Ayash LJ, Wheeler C, et al. Phase I study of high-dose ifosfamide, carboplatin and etoposide with autologous hematopoietic stem cell support. *Bone Marrow Transplant* 1995;15:373–379.
172. Littlewood TJ, Bentley DP, Smith AP. High-dose etoposide with autologous bone marrow transplantation as initial treatment of small cell lung cancer—a negative report. *Eur J Respir Dis* 1986;68:370–374.
173. Souhami RL, Hajichristou HT, Miles DW, et al. Intensive chemotherapy with autologous bone marrow transplantation for small-cell lung cancer. *Cancer Chemother Pharmacol* 1989;24:321–325.
174. Lange A, Kolodziej J, Tomeczko J, et al. Aggressive chemotherapy with autologous bone marrow transplantation in small cell lung carcinoma. *Arch Immunol Ther Exp (Warsz)* 1991;39:431–439.
175. Nomura F, Shimokata K, Saito H, et al. High dose chemotherapy with autologous bone marrow transplantation for limited small cell lung cancer. *Jpn J Clin Oncol* 1990;20:94–98.
176. Stahel RA, Takvorian RW, Skarin AT, et al. Autologous bone marrow transplantation following high-dose chemotherapy with cyclophosphamide, BCNU and VP-16 in small cell carcinoma of the lung and a review of current literature. *Eur J Cancer Clin Oncol* 1984; 20:1233–1238.
177. Klastersky J, Nicaise C, Longeval E, et al. Cisplatin, adriamycin, and etoposide (CAV) for remission induction of small-cell bronchogenic carcinoma. *Cancer* 1982;50:652–658.
178. Banham S, Soukop M, Burnett A, et al. Treatment of small cell carcinoma of lung with late dosage intensification programmes containing cyclophosphamide and mesna. *Cancer Treat Rev* 1983;10:73–77.
179. Cunningham D, Banham SW, Hutcheon AH, et al. High-dose cyclophosphamide and VP 16 as late dosage intensification therapy for small cell carcinoma of lung. *Cancer Chemother Pharmacol* 1985;15:303–306.
180. Sculier JP, Klastersky J, Stryckmans P. Late intensification in small-cell lung cancer: a phase I study of high doses of cyclophosphamide and etoposide with autologous bone marrow transplantation. *J Clin Oncol* 1985;3:184–191.
181. Spitzer G, Farha P, Valdivieso M, et al. High-dose intensification therapy with autologousbone marrow support for limited small-cell bronchogenic carcinoma. *J Clin Oncol* 1986;4:4–13.
182. Ihde DC, Deisseroth AB, Lichter AS, et al. Late intensive combined modality therapy followed by autologous bone marrow infusion in extensive stage small-cell lung cancer. *J Clin Oncol* 1986;4:1443–1454.
183. Humblet Y, Symann M, Bosly A, et al. Late intensification chemotherapy with autologous bone marrow transplantation in selected small-cell carcinoma of the lung: a randomized study. *J Clin Oncol* 1987;5:1864–1873.
184. Wilson C, Pickering D, Stewart S, et al. High dose chemotherapy with autologous bone marrow rescue in small cell lung cancer. *In Vivo* 1988;2:331–334.
185. Goodman GE, Crowley J, Livingston RB, et al. Treatment of limited small-cell lung cancer with concurrent etoposide/cisplatin and radiotherapy followed by intensification with high-dose cyclophosphamide: a Southwest Oncology Group study. *J Clin Oncol* 1991;9:453–457.
186. Elias A, Ibrahim J, Skarin AT, et al. Dose-intensive therapy for limited-stage small-cell lung cancer: long-term outcome. *J Clin Oncol* 1999;17:1175.
187. Elias A. Hematopoietic stem cell transplantation for small cell lung cancer. *Chest* 1999;116:531S–538S.
188. Fetscher S, Brugger W, Engelhardt R, et al. Standard- and high-dose etoposide, ifosfamide, carboplatin, and epirubicin in 100 patients with small-cell lung cancer: a mature follow-up report. *Ann Oncol* 1999;10:561–567.
189. Buchholz E, Manegold C, Pilz L, et al. Standard versus dose-intensified chemotherapy with sequential reinfusion of hematopoietic progenitor cells in small cell lung cancer patients with favorable prognosis. *J Thorac Oncol* 2007; 2:51–58.
190. Ardizzoni A, Hansen H, Dombernowsky P, et al. Topotecan, a new active drug in the second-line treatment of small-cell lung cancer: a phase II study in patients with refractory and sensitive disease. The European Organization for Research and Treatment of Cancer Early Clinical Studies Group and New Drug Development Office, and the Lung Cancer Cooperative Group. *J Clin Oncol* 1997;15:2090–2096.
191. von Pawel J, Schiller JH, Shepherd FA, et al. Topotecan versus cyclophosphamide, doxorubicin, and vincristine for the treatment of recurrent small-cell lung cancer. *J Clin Oncol* 1999;17:658–667.
192. von Pawel J, Gatzemeier U, Pujol JL, et al. Phase II comparator study of oral versus intravenous topotecan in patients with chemosensitive small-cell lung cancer. *J Clin Oncol* 2001;19:1743–1749.
193. O'Brien ME, Ciuleanu TE, Tsekov H, et al. Phase III trial comparing supportive care alone with supportive care with oral topotecan in patients with relapsed small-cell lung cancer. *J Clin Oncol* 2006;24:5441–5447.
194. Eckardt JR, von Pawel J, Pujol JL, et al. Phase III study of oral compared with intravenous topotecan as second-line therapy in small-cell lung cancer. *J Clin Oncol* 2007;25:2086–2092.
195. Ettinger DS. Amrubicin for the treatment of small cell lung cancer: does effectiveness cross the Pacific? *J Thorac Oncol* 2007;2:160–165.
196. Inoue A, Sugawara S, Yamazaki K, et al. Randomized phase II trial comparing amrubicin with topotecan in patients with previously treated small-cell lung cancer: North Japan Lung Cancer Study Group Trial 0402. *J Clin Oncol* 2008;26:5401–5406.
197. Ettinger DS, Jotte R, Lorigan P, et al. Phase II study of amrubicin as second-line therapy in patients with platinum-refractory small-cell lung cancer. *J Clin Oncol* 2010;28:2598–2603.
198. Jotte R, Conkling P, Reynolds C, et al. Randomized phase II trial of single-agent amrubicin or topotecan as second-line treatment in patients with small-cell lung cancer sensitive to first-line platinum-based chemotherapy. *J Clin Oncol* 2011;29:287–293.
199. Jotte R, Von Pawel J, Spigel DR, et al. Randomized phase III trial of amrubicin versus topotecan as second-line treatment for small cell lung cancer. *J Clin Oncol* 2011;29:abstract 7000.
200. Pietanza MC, Kadota K, Huberman K, et al. Phase II trial of temozolomide in patients with relapsed sensitive or refractory small cell lung cancer, with assessment of methylguanine-DNA methyltransferase as a potential biomarker. *Clin Cancer Res* 2012;18:1138–1145.

201. Krug LM, Crapanzano JP, Azzoli CG, et al. Imatinib mesylate lacks activity in small cell lung carcinoma expressing c-kit protein: a phase II clinical trial. *Cancer* 2005;103:2128–2131.
202. Krystal GW, Hines SJ, Organ CP. Autocrine growth of small cell lung cancer mediated by coexpression of c-kit and stem cell factor. *Cancer Res* 1996;56:370–376.
203. Krystal GW, Honsawek S, Litz J, et al. The selective tyrosine kinase inhibitor STI571 inhibits small cell lung cancer growth. *Clin Cancer Res* 2000;6:3319–3326.
204. Dy GK, Miller AA, Mandrekar SJ, et al. A phase II trial of imatinib (ST1571) in patients with c-kit expressing relapsed small-cell lung cancer: a CALGB and NCCTG study. *Ann Oncol* 2005;16:1811–1816.
205. Johnson BE, Fischer T, Fischer B, et al. Phase II study of imatinib in patients with small cell lung cancer. *Clin Cancer Res* 2003;9:5880–5887.
206. Moore SM, Rintoul RC, Walker TR, et al. The presence of a constitutively active phosphoinositide 3-kinase in small cell lung cancer cells mediates anchorage-independent proliferation via a protein kinase B and p70s6k-dependent pathway. *Cancer Res* 1998;58:5239–5247.
207. Krystal GW, Sulanke G, Litz J. Inhibition of phosphatidylinositol 3-kinase-Akt signaling blocks growth, promotes apoptosis, and enhances sensitivity of small cell lung cancer cells to chemotherapy. *Mol Cancer Ther* 2002;1:913–922.
208. Fischer B, Marinov M, Arcaro A. Targeting receptor tyrosine kinase signalling in small cell lung cancer (SCLC): what have we learned so far? *Cancer treatment reviews* 2007;33:391–406.
209. Marinov M, Ziogas A, Pardo OE, et al. AKT/mTOR pathway activation and BCL-2 family proteins modulate the sensitivity of human small cell lung cancer cells to RAD001. *Clin Cancer Res* 2009;15:1277–1287.
210. Pandya KJ, Levy DE, Hidalgo M, et al. A randomized, phase II ECOG trial of two dose levels of temsirolimus (CCI-779) in patients with extensive stage small cell lung cancer in remission after induction chemotherapy. A preliminary report. *J Clin Oncol* 2005;23:abstr 7005.
211. Tarhini A, Kotsakis A, Gooding W, et al. Phase II study of everolimus (RAD001) in previously treated small cell lung cancer. *Clin Cancer Res* 2010;16:5900–5907.
212. Belani CP, Dahlberg SE, Rudin CM, et al. Three-arm randomized phase II study of cisplatin and etoposide versus cisplatine and etoposide with either vismodegib or cixutumumab for patients with extensive stage-small cell lung cancer (ECOG 1508). *J Clin Oncol* 2013;31:abstract 7508.
213. Pepicelli CV, Lewis PM, McMahon AP. Sonic hedgehog regulates branching morphogenesis in the mammalian lung. *Curr Biol* 1998;8:1083–1086.
214. Liu H, Kho AT, Kohane IS, et al. Predicting survival within the lung cancer histopathological hierarchy using a multi-scale genomic model of development. *PLoS Med* 2006;3:e232.
215. Park KS, Martelotto LG, Peifer M, et al. A crucial requirement for Hedgehog signaling in small cell lung cancer. *Nature Med* 2011;17:1504–1508.
216. Jiang SX, Sato Y, Kuwao S, et al. Expression of bcl-2 oncogene protein is prevalent in small cell lung carcinomas. *J Pathol* 1995;177:135–138.
217. Yan JJ, Chen FF, Tsai YC, et al. Immunohistochemical detection of Bcl-2 protein in small cell carcinomas. *Oncology* 1996;53:6–11.
218. Rudin CM, Kozloff M, Hoffman PC, et al. Phase I study of G3139, a bcl-2 antisense oligonucleotide, combined with carboplatin and etoposide in patients with small-cell lung cancer. *J Clin Oncol* 2004;22:1110–1117.
219. Rudin CM, Otterson GA, Mauer AM, et al. A pilot trial of G3139, a bcl-2 antisense oligonucleotide, and paclitaxel in patients with chemorefractory small-cell lung cancer. *Ann Oncol* 2002;13:539–545.
220. Rudin CM, Salgia R, Wang X, et al. Randomized phase II Study of carboplatin and etoposide with or without the bcl-2 antisense oligonucleotide oblimersen for extensive-stage small-cell lung cancer: CALGB 30103. *J Clin Oncol* 2008;26:870–876.
221. Oltersdorf T, Elmore SW, Shoemaker AR, et al. An inhibitor of Bcl-2 family proteins induces regression of solid tumours. *Nature* 2005;435:677–681.
222. Tahir SK, Yang X, Anderson MG, et al. Influence of Bcl-2 family members on the cellular response of small-cell lung cancer cell lines to ABT-737. *Cancer Res* 2007;67:1176–1183.
223. Tse C, Shoemaker AR, Adickes J, et al. ABT-263: a potent and orally bioavailable Bcl-2 family inhibitor. *Cancer Res* 2008;68:3421–3428.
224. Shoemaker AR, Mitten MJ, Adickes J, et al. Activity of the Bcl-2 family inhibitor ABT-263 in a panel of small cell lung cancer xenograft models. *Clin Cancer Res* 2008;14:3268–3277.
225. Shoemaker AR, Oleksijew A, Bauch J, et al. A small-molecule inhibitor of Bcl-XL potentiates the activity of cytotoxic drugs in vitro and in vivo. *Cancer Res* 2006;66:8731–8739.
226. Kim KW, Moretti L, Mitchell LR, et al. Combined Bcl-2/mammalian target of rapamycin inhibition leads to enhanced radiosensitization via induction of apoptosis and autophagy in non-small cell lung tumor xenograft model. *Clin Cancer Res* 2009;15:6096–6105.
227. Tan N, Malek M, Zha J, et al. Navitoclax enhances the efficacy of taxanes in non-small cell lung cancer models. *Clin Cancer Res* 2011;17:1394–1404.
228. Rudin CM, Hann CL, Garon EB, et al. Phase II study of single-agent navitoclax (ABT-263) and biomarker correlates in patients with relapsed small cell lung cancer. *Clin Cancer Res* 2012;18:3163–3169.
229. Paik PK, Rudin CM, Pietanza MC, et al. A phase II study of obatoclax mesylate, a Bcl-2 antagonist, plus topotecan in relapsed small cell lung cancer. *Lung Cancer* 2011;74:481–485.
230. Langer CJ, Albert I, Kovacs P, et al. A randomized phase II study of carboplatin and etoposide with or without pan-BCL-2 antagonist obatoclax in extensive-stage small cell lung cancer. *J Clin Oncol* 2011;29:abstract 7001.
231. Pujol JL, Breton JL, Gervais R, et al. Phase III double-blind, placebo-controlled study of thalidomide in extensive-disease small-cell lung cancer after response to chemotherapy: an intergroup study FNCLCC cleo04 IFCT 00-01. *J Clin Oncol* 2007;25:3945–3951.
232. Lee SM, Woll PJ, Rudd R, et al. Anti-angiogenic therapy using thalidomide combined with chemotherapy in small cell lung cancer: a randomized, double-blind, placebo-controlled trial. *J Natl Cancer Inst* 2009;101:1049–1057.
233. Arnold AM, Seymour L, Smylie M, et al. Phase II study of vandetanib or placebo in small-cell lung cancer patients after complete or partial response to induction chemotherapy with or without radiation therapy: National Cancer Institute of Canada Clinical Trials Group Study BR.20. *J Clin Oncol* 2007;25:4278–4284.
234. Gitlitz BJ, Moon J, Glisson BS, et al. Sorafenib in platinum-treated patients with extensive stage small cell lung cancer: a Southwest Oncology Group (SWOG 0435) phase II trial. *J Thorac Oncol* 2010;5:1835–1840.
235. Ramalingam SS, Belani CP, Mack PC, et al. Phase II study of Cediranib (AZD 2171), an inhibitor of the vascular endothelial growth factor receptor, for second-line therapy of small cell lung cancer (National Cancer Institute #7097). *J Thorac Oncol* 2010;5:1279–1284.
236. Heymach J, Glisson BS, Doebele RC, et al. Phase I open-label study of cediranib plus etoposide and cisplatin as first-line therapy for patients with small cell lung cancer or lung neuroendocrine cancer. *J Clin Oncol* 2010;28:abstract 7050.
237. Ready N, Pang H, Gu L, et al. Chemotherapy with or without maintenance sunitinib for untreated extensive-stage small cell lung cancer: a randomized, placebo controlled phase II study CALGB 30504 (ALLIANCE). *J Clin Oncol* 2013;31:abstract 7506.
238. Horn L, Dahlberg SE, Sandler AB, et al. Phase II study of cisplatin plus etoposide and bevacizumab for previously untreated, extensive-stage small-cell lung cancer: Eastern Cooperative Oncology Group Study E3501. *J Clin Oncol* 2009;27:6006–6011.
239. Ready N, Dudek AZ, Wang XF, et al. CALGB 30306: A phase II study of cisplatin, irinotecan and bevacizumab for untreated extensive stage small cell lung cancer. *J Clin Oncol* 2007;25:Abstr 7563.
240. Spigel DR, Greco FA, Zubkus JD, et al. Phase II trial of irinotecan, carboplatin, and bevacizumab in the treatment of patients with extensive-stage small-cell lung cancer. *J Thorac Oncol* 2009;4:1555–1560.
241. Spigel DR, Townley PM, Waterhouse DM, et al. Randomized phase II study of bevacizumab in combination with chemotherapy in previously untreated extensive-stage small-cell lung cancer: results from the SALUTE trial. *J Clin Oncol* 2011;29:2215–2222.
242. Hodi FS, O'Day SJ, McDermott DF, et al. Improved survival with ipilimumab in patients with metastatic melanoma. *N Engl J Med* 2010;363:711–723.
243. Fong L, Small EJ. Anti-cytotoxic T-lymphocyte antigen-4 antibody: the first in an emerging class of immunomodulatory antibodies for cancer treatment. *J Clin Oncol* 2008;26:5275–5283.
244. Lynch TJ, Bondarenko I, Luft A, et al. Ipilimumab in combination with paclitaxel and carboplatin as first-line treatment in stage IIIB/IV non-small-cell lung cancer: results from a randomized, double-blind, multicenter phase II study. *J Clin Oncol* 2012;30:2046–2054.
245. Reck M, Bondarenko I, Luft A, et al. Ipilimumab in combination with paclitaxel and carboplatin as first-line therapy in extensive-disease-small-cell lung cancer: results from a randomized, double-blind, multicenter phase 2 trial. *Ann Oncol* 2013;24:75–83.
246. Perry MC, Eaton WL, Propert KJ, et al. Chemotherapy with or without radiation therapy in limited small-cell carcinoma of the lung. *N Engl J Med* 1987;316:912–918.
247. Pignon JP, Arriagada R. Role of thoracic radiotherapy in limited-stage small-cell lung cancer: quantitative review based on the literature versus meta-analysis based on individual data. *J Clin Oncol* 1992;10:1819–1820.
248. Pignon JP, Arriagada R, Ihde DC, et al. A meta-analysis of thoracic radiotherapy for small-cell lung cancer. *N Engl J Med* 1992;327:1618–1624.
249. Warde P, Payne D. Does thoracic irradiation improve survival and local control in limited-stage small-cell carcinoma of the lung? A meta-analysis [see comments]. *J Clin Oncol* 1992;10:890.
250. Turrisi AT 3rd, Glover DJ. Thoracic radiotherapy variables: influence on local control in small cell lung cancer limited disease. *Int J Radiat Oncol Biol Phys* 1990;19:1473–1479.
251. Roof KS, Fidias P, Lynch TJ, et al. Radiation dose escalation in limited-stage small-cell lung cancer. *Int J Radiat Oncol Biol Phys* 2003;57:701–708.
252. Choi NC, Herndon JE 2nd, Rosenman J, et al. Phase I study to determine the maximum-tolerated dose of radiation in standard daily and hyperfractionated-accelerated twice-daily radiation schedules with concurrent chemotherapy for limited-stage small-cell lung cancer. *J Clin Oncol* 1998;16:3528–3536.
253. Bogart JA, Herndon JE 2nd, Lyss AP, et al. 70 Gy thoracic radiotherapy is feasible concurrent with chemotherapy for limited-stage small-cell lung cancer: analysis of Cancer and Leukemia Group B study 39808. *Int J Radiat Oncol Biol Phys* 2004;59:460–468.
254. Miller AA, Wang XF, Bogart JA, et al. Phase II trial of paclitaxel-topotecan-etoposide followed by consolidation chemoradiotherapy for limited-stage small cell lung cancer: CALGB 30002. *J Thorac Oncol* 2007;2:645–651.
255. Carney DN, Mitchell JB, Kinsella TJ. In vitro radiation and chemotherapy sensitivity of established cell lines of human small cell lung cancer and its large cell morphological variants. *Cancer Res* 1983;43:2806–2811.
256. Ihde DC, Grayson J, Woods E, et al. Twice daily chest irradiation an adjuvant to etoposide/cisplatin therapy of limited stage small cell lung cancer. In: Salmon S, ed. *Adjuvant Therapy of Cancer*. 6th ed. Philadelphia: WB Saunders; 1990.

257. Turrisi AT 3rd, Glover DJ, Mason BA. A preliminary report: concurrent twice-daily radiotherapy plus platinum-etoposide chemotherapy for limited small cell lung cancer. *Int J Radiat Oncol Biol Phys* 1988;15:183–187.
258. Schild SE, Bonner JA, Shanahan TG, et al. Long-term results of a phase III trial comparing once-daily radiotherapy with twice-daily radiotherapy in limited-stage small-cell lung cancer. *Int J Radiat Oncol Biol Phys* 2004;59:943–951.
259. Schild SE, Bonner JA, Hillman S, et al. Results of a phase II study of high-dose thoracic radiation therapy with concurrent cisplatin and etoposide in limited-stage small-cell lung cancer (NCCTG 95-20-53). *J Clin Oncol* 2007; 25:3124–3129.
260. Langer CJ, Swann S, Werner-Wasik M, et al. Phase i study of irinotecan (ir) and cisplatin (ddp) in combination with thoracic radiotherapy (rt) either twice daily (45 Gy) or once daily (70 Gy), in patients with limited (ltd) small cell lung cancer (sclc): early analysis of rtog 0241. *Proc Am Soc Clin Oncol* 2006;24:1.
261. Komaki R, Swann RS, Ettinger DS, et al. Phase I study of thoracic radiation dose escalation with concurrent chemotherapy for patients with limited small-cell lung cancer: Report of Radiation Therapy Oncology Group (RTOG) protocol 97-12. *Int J Radiat Oncol Biol Phys* 2005;62:342–350.
262. Komaki R, Paulus R, Ettinger DS, et al. Phase II study of accelerated high-dose radiotherapy with concurrent chemotherapy for patients with limited small-cell lung cancer: Radiation Therapy Oncology Group protocol 0239. *Int J Radiat Oncol Biol Phys* 2012;83:e531–e536.
263. Komaki R, Khalid N, Langer CJ, et al. Penetration of recommended procedures for lung cancer staging and management in the United States over 10 years: a quality research in radiation oncology survey. *Int J Radiat Oncol Biol Phys* 2013;85:1082–1099.
264. Spiro SG, James LE, Rudd RM, et al. Early compared with late radiotherapy in combined modality treatment for limited disease small-cell lung cancer: a London Lung Cancer Group multicenter randomized clinical trial and meta-analysis. *J Clin Oncol* 2006;24:3823–3830.
265. Fried DB, Morris DE, Poole C, et al. Systematic review evaluating the timing of thoracic radiation therapy in combined modality therapy for limited-stage small-cell lung cancer. *J Clin Oncol* 2004;22:4837–4845.
266. De Ruysscher D, Pijls-Johannesma M, Vansteenkiste J, et al. Systematic review and meta-analysis of randomised, controlled trials of the timing of chest radiotherapy in patients with limited-stage, small-cell lung cancer. *Ann Oncol* 2006;17:543–552.
267. Pijls-Johannesma MC, De Ruysscher D, Lambin P, et al. Early versus late chest radiotherapy for limited stage small cell lung cancer. *Cochrane Database Syst Rev* 2005;(1):CD004700.
268. Huncharek M, McCarry R. A meta-analysis of the timing of chest irradiation in the combined modality treatment of limited-stage small cell lung cancer. *Oncologist* 2004;9:665–672.
269. De Ruysscher D, Pijls-Johannesma M, Bentzen SM, et al. Time between the first day of chemotherapy and the last day of chest radiation is the most important predictor of survival in limited-disease small-cell lung cancer. *J Clin Oncol* 2006;24:1057–1063.
270. Kies MS, Mira JG, Crowley JJ, et al. Multimodal therapy for limited small-cell lung cancer: a randomized study of induction combination chemotherapy with or without thoracic radiation in complete responders; and with wide-field versus reduced-field radiation in partial responders: a Southwest Oncology Group Study. *J Clin Oncol* 1987;5:592–600.
271. De Ruysscher D, Bremer RH, Koppe F, et al. Omission of elective node irradiation on basis of CT-scans in patients with limited disease small cell lung cancer: a phase II trial. *Radiother Oncol* 2006;80:307–312.
272. Videtic GM, Belderbos JS, Spring Kong FM, et al. Report from the International Atomic Energy Agency (IAEA) consultants' meeting on elective nodal irradiation in lung cancer: small-cell lung cancer (SCLC). *Int J Radiat Oncol Biol Phys* 2008;72:327–334.
273. Baas P, Belderbos JS, Senan S, et al. Concurrent chemotherapy (carboplatin, paclitaxel, etoposide) and involved-field radiotherapy in limited stage small cell lung cancer: a Dutch multicenter phase II study. *Br J Cancer* 2006;94:625–630.
274. van Loon J, De Ruysscher D, Wanders R, et al. Selective nodal irradiation on basis of (18)FDG-PET scans in limited-disease small-cell lung cancer: a prospective study. *Int J Radiat Oncol Biol Phys* 2010;77:329–336.
275. Shirvani SM, Komaki R, Heymach JV, et al. Positron emission tomography/computed tomography-guided intensity-modulated radiotherapy for limited-stage small-cell lung cancer. *Int J Radiat Oncol Biol Phys* 2012;82:e91–e97.
276. Hu X, Bao Y, Zhang L, et al. Omitting elective nodal irradiation and irradiating postinduction versus preinduction chemotherapy tumor extent for limited-stage small cell lung cancer: interim analysis of a prospective randomized non-inferiority trial. *Cancer* 2012;118:278–287.
277. Xia B, Chen GY, Cai XW, et al. Is involved-field radiotherapy based on CT safe for patients with limited-stage small-cell lung cancer? *Radiother Oncol* 2012;102:258–262.
278. Colaco R, Sheikh H, Lorigan P, et al. Omitting elective nodal irradiation during thoracic irradiation in limited-stage small cell lung cancer—evidence from a phase II trial. *Lung Cancer* 2012;76:72–77.
279. Shirvani SM, Juloori A, Allen PK, et al. Comparison of 2 common radiation therapy techniques for definitive treatment of small cell lung cancer. *Int J Radiat Oncol Biol Phys* 2013;87:139–147.
280. Colaco RJ, Huh S, Nichols RC, et al. Dosimetric rationale and early experience at UFPTI of thoracic proton therapy and chemotherapy in limited-stage small cell lung cancer. *Acta Oncol* 2013;52:506–513.
281. Brooks BJ Jr, Seifter EJ, Walsh TE, et al. Pulmonary toxicity with combined modality therapy for limited stage small-cell lung cancer. *J Clin Oncol* 1986;4:200–209.
282. Osterlind K, Hansen HH, Hansen HS, et al. Chemotherapy versus chemotherapy plus irradiation in limited small cell lung cancer. Results of a controlled trial with 5 years follow-up. *Br J Cancer* 1986;54:7–17.
283. Bunn PA Jr, Lichter AS, Makuch RW, et al. Chemotherapy alone or chemotherapy with chest radiation therapy in limited stage small cell lung cancer. A prospective, randomized trial. *Ann Intern Med* 1987;106:655–662.
284. Albain KS, Crowley JJ, Turrisi AT 3rd, et al. Concurrent cisplatin, etoposide, and chest radiotherapy in pathologic stage IIIB non-small-cell lung cancer: a Southwest Oncology Group phase II study, SWOG 9019. *J Clin Oncol* 2002;20: 3454–3460.
285. Watkins JM, Wahlquist AE, Shirai K, et al. Factors associated with severe acute esophagitis from hyperfractionated radiotherapy with concurrent chemotherapy for limited-stage small-cell lung cancer. *Int J Radiat Oncol Biol Phys* 2009;74:1108–1113.
286. Palma DA, Senan S, Oberije C, et al. Predicting esophagitis after chemoradiation therapy for non-small cell lung cancer: an individual patient data meta-analysis. *Int J Radiat Oncol Biol Phys* 2013;87:690–696.
287. Ettinger DS, Berkey BA, Abrams RA, et al. Study of paclitaxel, etoposide, and cisplatin chemotherapy combined with twice-daily thoracic radiotherapy for patients with limited-stage small-cell lung cancer: a Radiation Therapy Oncology Group 9609 phase II study. *J Clin Oncol* 2005;23:4991–4998.
288. Marks LB, Bentzen SM, Deasy JO, et al. Radiation dose-volume effects in the lung. *Int J Radiat Oncol Biol Phys* 2010;76:S70–S76.
289. Tsujino K, Hirota S, Kotani Y, et al. Radiation pneumonitis following concurrent accelerated hyperfractionated radiotherapy and chemotherapy for limited-stage small-cell lung cancer: dose-volume histogram analysis and comparison with conventional chemoradiation. *Int J Radiat Oncol Biol Phys* 2006;64:1100–1105.
290. Lichter AS, Bunn PA, Ihde DC, et al. The role of radiation therapy in the treatment of small cell lung cancer. *Cancer* 1985;55:2163–2175.
291. Seifter EJ, Ihde DC. Therapy of small cell lung cancer: a perspective on two decades of clinical research. *Semin Oncol* 1988;15:278–299.
292. Livingston RB, Schulman S, Mira JG, et al. Combined alkylators and multiple-site irradiation for extensive small cell lung cancer: a Southwest Oncology Group study. *Cancer Treat Rep* 1986;70:1395–1401.
293. Jeremic B, Shibamoto Y, Nikolic N, et al. Role of radiation therapy in the combined-modality treatment of patients with extensive disease small cell lung cancer: a randomized study. *J Clin Oncol* 1999;17:2092–2099.
294. Williams C, Alexander M, Glatstein EJ, et al. The role of radiation therapy in combination with chemotherapy in extensive oat cell cancer of the lung: a randomized study. *Cancer Treat Rep* 1977;61:1427–1431.
295. Wilson HE, Stanley K, Vincent RG, et al. Comparison of chemotherapy alone versus chemotherapy and radiation therapy of extensive small cell carcinoma of the lung. *J Surg Oncol* 1983;23:181–184.
296. Yee D, Butts C, Reiman A, et al. Clinical trial of post-chemotherapy consolidation thoracic radiotherapy for extensive-stage small cell lung cancer. *Radiother Oncol* 2012;102:234–238.
297. Slotman BJ, Faivre-Finn C, van Tinteren H, et al. Randomized trial on thoracic radiotherapy (TRT) in extensive-stage small cell lung cancer. *J Clin Oncol* 2014; 32:5s.
298. Komaki R, Cox JD, Whitson W. Risk of brain metastasis from small cell carcinoma of the lung related to length of survival and prophylactic irradiation. *Cancer Treat Rep* 1981;65:811–814.
299. Nugent JL, Bunn PA Jr, Matthews MJ, et al. CNS metastases in small cell bronchogenic carcinoma: increasing frequency and changing pattern with lengthening survival. *Cancer* 1979;44:1885–1893.
300. Rosen ST, Makuch RW, Lichter AS, et al. Role of prophylactic cranial irradiation in prevention of central nervous system metastases in small cell lung cancer. Potential benefit restricted to patients with complete response. *Am J Med* 1983;74:615–624.
301. Hirsch FR, Paulson OB, Hansen HH, et al. Intracranial metastases in small cell carcinoma of the lung: correlation of clinical and autopsy findings. *Cancer* 1982;50:2433–2437.
302. Glantz MJ, Choy H, Yee L. Prophylactic cranial irradiation in small cell lung cancer: rationale, results, and recommendations. *Semin Oncol* 1997;24:477–483.
303. Einhorn LH 3rd. The case against prophylactic cranial irradiation in limited small cell lung cancer. *Semin Radiat Oncol* 1995;5:57–60.
304. Arriagada R, Le Chevalier T, Borie F, et al. Prophylactic cranial irradiation for patients with small-cell lung cancer in complete remission. *J Natl Cancer Inst* 1995;87:183–190.
305. Cox JD, Petrovich Z, Paig C, et al. Prophylactic cranial irradiation in patients with inoperable carcinoma of the lung. *Cancer* 1978;42:1135–1140.
306. Hansen HH, Dombernowsky P, Hirsch FR, et al. Prophylactic irradiation in bronchogenic small cell anaplastic carcinoma: A comparative trial of localized versus extensive radiotherapy including prophylactic brain irradiation in patients receiving combination chemotherapy. *Cancer* 1980;46:279–384.
307. Seydel HG, Creech R, Pagano M, et al. Prophylactic versus no brain irradiation in regional small cell lung carcinoma. *Am J Clin Oncol* 1985;8:218–223.
308. Auperin A, Arriagada R, Pignon J, et al. Prophylactic cranial irradiation for patients with small-cell lung cancer in complete remission. *N Engl J Med* 1999;341:476–484.
309. Gregor A, Cull A, Stephens RJ, et al. Prophylactic cranial irradiation is indicated following complete response to induction therapy in small cell lung cancer: results of a multicentre randomised trial. United Kingdom Coordinating Committee for Cancer Research (UKCCCR) and the European Organization for Research and Treatment of Cancer (EORTC). *Eur J Cancer* 1997;33:1752–1758.

310. Meyers CA, Byrne KS, Komaki R. Cognitive deficits in patients with small cell lung cancer and after chemotherapy. *Lung Cancer* 1995;12:231–235.
311. Le Pechoux C, Dunant A, Senan S, et al. Standard-dose versus higher-dose prophylactic cranial irradiation (PCI) in patients with limited-stage small-cell lung cancer in complete remission after chemotherapy and thoracic radiotherapy (PCI 99-01, EORTC 22003-08004, RTOG 0212, and IFCT 99-01): a randomised clinical trial. *Lancet Oncol* 2009;10:467–474.
312. Fleck JF, Einhorn LH, Lauer RC, et al. Is prophylactic cranial irradiation indicated in small-cell lung cancer? *J Clin Oncol* 1990;8:209–214.
313. Johnson BE, Becker B, Goff WB, et al. Neurologic, neuropsychologic, and cranial computed tomography scan abnormalities in 2-10 year survivors of small cell lung cancer. *J Clin Oncol* 1985;3:1659–1667.
314. Lee JS, Umsawasdi T, Lee Y, et al. Neurotoxicity in long-term survivors of small cell lung cancer. *In J Radiat Oncol Biol Phys* 1986;12:313–321.
315. Johnson BE, Patronas N, Hayes W, et al. Neurologic, computed cranial tomographic, and magnetic resonance imaging abnormalities in patients with small-cell lung cancer: further follow-up of 6- to 13-year survivors. *J Clin Oncol* 1990;8:48–56.
316. Grosshans DR, Meyers CA, Allen PK, et al. Neurocognitive function in patients with small cell lung cancer: effect of prophylactic cranial irradiation. *Cancer* 2008;112:589–595.
317. Lee JJ, Bekele BN, Zhou X, et al. Decision analysis for prophylactic cranial irradiation for patients with small-cell lung cancer. *J Clin Oncol* 2006;24:3597–603.
318. Carmichael J, Crane JM, Bunn PA, et al. Results of therapeutic cranial irradiation in small cell lung cancer. *In J Radiat Oncol Biol Phys* 1988;14:455–459.
319. Harris S, Chan MD, Lovato JF, et al. Gamma knife stereotactic radiosurgery as salvage therapy after failure of whole-brain radiotherapy in patients with small-cell lung cancer. *Int J Radiat Oncol Biol Phys* 2012;83:e53–e59.
320. Kristensen CA, Kristjansen PE, Hansen HH. Systemic chemotherapy of brain metastases from small-cell lung cancer: a review. *J Clin Oncol* 1992;10:1498–1502.
321. Groen HJ, Smit EF, Haaxma-Reiche H, et al. Carboplatin as second line treatment for recurrent or progressive brain metastases from small cell lung cancer. *Eur J Cancer* 1993;29A:1696–1699.
322. Postmus PE, Smit EF, Haaxma-Reiche H, et al. Teniposide for brain metastases of small-cell lung cancer: a phase II study. European Organization for Research and Treatment of Cancer Lung Cancer Cooperative Group. *J Clin Oncol* 1995;13:660–665.
323. Postmus PE, Haaxma-Reiche H, Gregor A, et al. Brain-only metastases of small cell lung cancer; efficacy of whole brain radiotherapy. An EORTC phase II study. *Radiother Oncol* 1998;46:29–32.
324. Martini N, Wittes RE, Hilaris BS, et al. Oat cell carcinoma of the lung. *Clin Bull* 1975;5:144–148.
325. Mountain CF. Clinical biology of small cell carcinoma: relationship to surgical therapy. *Semin Oncol* 1978;5:272–279.
326. Fox W, Scadding JG. Medical Research Council comparative trial of surgery and radiotherapy for primary treatment of small-celled or oat-celled carcinoma of bronchus. Ten-year follow-up. *Lancet* 1973;2:63–65.
327. Shields TW, Higgins GA Jr, Matthews MJ, et al. Surgical resection in the management of small cell carcinoma of the lung. *J Thorac Cardiovasc Surg* 1982;84:481–488.
328. Angeletti CA, Macchiarini P, Mussi A, et al. Influence of T and N stages on long-term survival in resectable small cell lung cancer. *Eur J Surg Oncol* 1989;15:337–340.
329. Shepherd FA, Ginsberg RJ, Feld R, et al. Surgical treatment for limited small-cell lung cancer. The University of Toronto Lung Oncology Group experience. *J Thorac Cardiovasc Surg* 1991;101:385–393.
330. Macchiarini P, Hardin M, Basolo F, et al. Surgery plus adjuvant chemotherapy for T1-3N0M0 small-cell lung cancer. Rationale for current approach. *Am J Clin Oncol* 1991;14:218–224.
331. Rea F, Callegaro D, Favaretto A, et al. Long term results of surgery and chemotherapy in small cell lung cancer. *Eur J Cardiothorac Surg 1998*;14:398–402
332. Lucchi M, Mussi A, Chella A, et al. Surgery in the management of small cell lung cancer. *Eur J Cardiothorac Surg* 1997;12:689–693.
333. Shepherd FA, Ginsberg RJ, Patterson GA, et al. A prospective study of adjuvant surgical resection after chemotherapy for limited small cell lung cancer. A University of Toronto Lung Oncology Group study. *J Thorac Cardiovasc Surg* 1989;97:177–186.
334. Lad T, Piantadosi S, Thomas P, et al. A prospective randomized trial to determine the benefit of surgical resection of residual disease following response of small cell lung cancer to combination chemotherapy. *Chest* 1994;106:320S–323S.
335. Chute JP, Chen T, Feigal E, et al. Twenty years of phase III trials for patients with extensive-stage small-cell lung cancer: perceptible progress. *J Clin Oncol* 1999;17:1794–801.
336. Merrill RM, Henson DE, Barnes M. Conditional survival among patients with carcinoma of the lung. *Chest* 1999;116:697–703.
337. Tucker MA, Murray N, Shaw EG, et al. Second primary cancers related to smoking and treatment of small-cell lung cancer. Lung Cancer Working Cadre. *J Natl Cancer Inst* 1997;89:1782–1788.
338. Kawahara M, Ushijima S, Kamimori T, et al. Second primary tumours in more than 2-year disease-free survivors of small-cell lung cancer in Japan: the role of smoking cessation. *Br J Cancer* 1998;78:409–412.
339. Heyne KH, Lippman SM, Lee JJ, et al. The incidence of second primary tumors in long-term survivors of small-cell lung cancer. *J Clin Oncol* 1992;10:1519–1524.
340. Sagman U, Lishner M, Maki E, et al. Second primary malignancies following diagnosis of small-cell lung cancer. *J Clin Oncol* 1992;10:1525–1533.
341. Sekine I, Nishiwaki Y, Kakinuma R, et al. Late recurrence of small-cell lung cancer: treatment and outcome. *Oncology* 1996;53:318–321.
342. Jacoulet P, Depierre A, Moro D, et al. Long-term survivors of small-cell lung cancer (SCLC): a French multicenter study. Groupe d'Oncologie de Langue Francaise. *Ann Oncol* 1997;8:1009–1014.
343. Osterlind K, Hansen HH, Hansen M, et al. Long-term disease-free survival in small-cell carcinoma of the lung: a study of clinical determinants. *J Clin Oncol* 1986;4:1307–1313.
344. Modlin IM, Lye KD, Kidd M. A 5-decade analysis of 13,715 carcinoid tumors. *Cancer* 2003;97:934–959.
345. Harpole DH Jr, Feldman JM, Buchanan S, et al. Bronchial carcinoid tumors: a retrospective analysis of 126 patients. *Ann Thorac Surg* 1992;54:50–54.
346. Yao JC, Hassan M, Phan A, et al. One hundred years after "carcinoid": epidemiology of and prognostic factors for neuroendocrine tumors in 35,825 cases in the United States. *J Clin Oncol* 2008;26:3063–3072.
347. Asamura H, Kameya T, Matsuno Y, et al. Neuroendocrine neoplasms of the lung: a prognostic spectrum. *J Clin Oncol* 2006;24:70–76.
348. Fink G, Krelbaum T, Yellin A, et al. Pulmonary carcinoid: presentation, diagnosis, and outcome in 142 cases in Israel and review of 640 cases from the literature. *Chest* 2001;119:1647–51.
349. Kulke MH, Mayer RJ. Carcinoid tumors. *N Engl J Med* 1999;340:858–868.
350. Davini F, Gonfiotti A, Comin C, et al. Typical and atypical carcinoid tumours: 20-year experience with 89 patients. *J Cardiovasc Surg (Torino)* 2009;50:807–811.
351. Thomas CF Jr, Tazelaar HD, Jett JR. Typical and atypical pulmonary carcinoids : outcome in patients presenting with regional lymph node involvement. *Chest* 2001;119:1143–1150.
352. McCaughan BC, Martini N, Bains MS. Bronchial carcinoids. Review of 124 cases. *J Thorac Cardiovasc Surg* 1985;89:8–17.
353. Debelenko LV, Brambilla E, Agarwal SK, et al. Identification of MEN1 gene mutations in sporadic carcinoid tumors of the lung. *Hum Mol Genet* 1997;6:2285–2290.
354. Travis WD, Rush W, Flieder DB, et al. Survival analysis of 200 pulmonary neuroendocrine tumors with clarification of criteria for atypical carcinoid and its separation from typical carcinoid. *Am J Surg Pathol* 1998;22:934–944.
355. Beasley MB, Thunnissen FB, Brambilla E, et al. Pulmonary atypical carcinoid: Predictors of survival in 106 cases. *Hum Pathol* 2000;31:1255–1265.
356. Pelosi G, Rodriguez J, Viale G, et al. Typical and atypical pulmonary carcinoid tumor overdiagnosed as small-cell carcinoma on biopsy specimens: a major pitfall in the management of lung cancer patients. *Am J Surg Pathol* 2005;29:179–187.
357. Davies SJ, Gosney JR, Hansell DM, et al. Diffuse idiopathic pulmonary neuroendocrine cell hyperplasia. An under recognised spectrum of disease. *Thorax* 2007;62:248–252.
358. Henschke CI, Yankelevitz DF, Libby DM, et al. Survival of patients with stage I lung cancer detected on CT screening. *N Engl J Med* 2006;355:1763–1771.
359. Chughtai TS, Morin JE, Sheiner NM, et al. Bronchial carcinoid—twenty years' experience defines a selective surgical approach. *Surgery* 1997;122:801–808.
360. Limper AH, Carpenter PC, Scheithauer B, et al. The Cushing syndrome induced by bronchial carcinoid tumors. *Ann Intern Med* 1992;117:209–214.
361. Athanassiadi K, Exarchos D, Tsagarakis S, et al. Acromegaly caused by ectopic growth hormone-releasing hormone secretion by a carcinoid bronchial tumor: a rare entity. *J Thorac Cardiovasc Surg* 2004;128:631–632.
362. Yellin A, Zwas ST, Rozenman J, et al. Experience with somatostatin receptor scintigraphy in the management of pulmonary carcinoid tumors. *Isr Med Assoc J* 2005;7:712–716.
363. Granberg D, Sundin A, Janson ET, et al. Octreoscan in patients with bronchial carcinoid tumours. *Clin Endocrinol (Oxf)* 2003;59:793–799.
364. Erasmus JJ, McAdams HP, Patz EF Jr, et al. Evaluation of primary pulmonary carcinoid tumors using FDG PET. *AJR Am J Roentgenol* 1998;170:1369–1373.
365. Daniels CE, Lowe VJ, Aubry MC, et al. The utility of fluorodeoxyglucose positron emission tomography in the evaluation of carcinoid tumors presenting as pulmonary nodules. *Chest* 2007;131:255–260.
366. Kayani I, Bomanji JB, Groves A, et al. Functional imaging of neuroendocrine tumors with combined PET/CT using 68Ga-DOTATATE (DOTA-DPhe1,Tyr3-octreotate) and 18F-FDG. *Cancer* 2008;112:2447–2455.
367. Binderup T, Knigge U, Loft A, et al. 18F-fluorodeoxyglucose positron emission tomography predicts survival of patients with neuroendocrine tumors. *Clin Cancer Res* 2010;16:978–985.
368. Granberg D, Eriksson B, Wilander E, et al. Experience in treatment of metastatic pulmonary carcinoid tumors. *Ann Oncol* 2001;12:1383–1391.
369. Campana D, Nori F, Piscitelli L, et al. Chromogranin A: is it a useful marker of neuroendocrine tumors? *J Clin Oncol* 2007;25:1967–1973.
370. Travis WD, Giroux DJ, Chansky K, et al. The IASLC Lung Cancer Staging Project: proposals for the inclusion of broncho-pulmonary carcinoid tumors in the forthcoming (seventh) edition of the TNM Classification for Lung Cancer. *J Thorac Oncol* 2008;3:1213–1223.
371. Yendamuri S, Gold D, Jayaprakash V, et al. Is sublobar resection sufficient for carcinoid tumors? *Ann Thorac Surg* 2011;92:1774–1778.
372. Marty-Ane CH, Costes V, Pujol JL, et al. Carcinoid tumors of the lung: do atypical features require aggressive management? *Ann Thorac Surg* 1995;59:78–83.
373. Garcia-Yuste M, Matilla JM, Cueto A, et al. Typical and atypical carcinoid tumors: analysis of the experience of the Spanish Multi-centric Study of Neuroendocrine Tumors of the Lung. *Eur J Cardiothorac Surg* 2007;31:192–197.
374. Cardillo G, Sera F, Di Martino M, et al. Bronchial carcinoid tumors: nodal status and long-term survival after resection. *Ann Thorac Surg* 2004;77:1781–1785.

375. Mineo TC, Guggino G, Mineo D, et al. Relevance of lymph node micrometastases in radically resected endobronchial carcinoid tumors. *Ann Thorac Surg* 2005;80:428–432.
376. Wurtz A, Benhamed L, Conti M, et al. Results of systematic nodal dissection in typical and atypical carcinoid tumors of the lung. *J Thorac Oncol* 2009;4: 388–394.
377. Ferolla P, Daddi N, Urbani M, et al. Tumorlets, multicentric carcinoids, lymph-nodal metastases, and long-term behavior in bronchial carcinoids. *J Thorac Oncol* 2009;4:383–387.
378. Kalemkerian GP, Akerley W, Blum MG, et al. Practice Guidelines: Small Cell Lung Cancer. 2010 (accessed May 8, 2010).
379. Lou F, Sarkaria I, Pietanza C, et al. Recurrence of pulmonary carcinoid tumors after resection: implications for postoperative surveillance. *Ann Thorac Surg* 2013;96:1156–1162.
380. Wirth LJ, Carter MR, Janne PA, et al. Outcome of patients with pulmonary carcinoid tumors receiving chemotherapy or chemoradiotherapy. *Lung Cancer* 2004;44:213–220.
381. Mackley HB, Videtic GM. Primary carcinoid tumors of the lung: a role for radiotherapy. *Oncology (Williston Park)* 2006;20:1537–1543.
382. Moertel CG, Hanley JA. Combination chemotherapy trials in metastatic carcinoid tumor and the malignant carcinoid syndrome. *Cancer Clin Trials* 1979;2:327–334.
383. Filosso PL, Ruffini E, Oliaro A, et al. Long-term survival of atypical bronchial carcinoids with liver metastases, treated with octreotide. *Eur J Cardiothorac Surg* 2002;21:913–917.
384. Srirajaskanthan R, Toumpanakis C, Karpathakis A, et al. Surgical management and palliative treatment in bronchial neuroendocrine tumours: a clinical study of 45 patients. *Lung Cancer* 2009;65:68–73.
385. Forde PM, Hooker CM, Boikos SA, et al. Systemic therapy, clinical outcomes, and overall survival in locally advanced or metastatic pulmonary carcinoid: a brief report. *J Thorac Oncol* 2014;9:414–418.
386. Modlin IM, Kidd M, Latich I, et al. Current status of gastrointestinal carcinoids. *Gastroenterology* 2005;128:1717–1751.
387. Rinke A, Muller HH, Schade-Brittinger C, et al. Placebo-controlled, double-blind, prospective, randomized study on the effect of octreotide LAR in the control of tumor growth in patients with metastatic neuroendocrine midgut tumors: a report from the PROMID Study Group. *J Clin Oncol* 2009;27:4656–4663.
388. Gridelli C, Rossi A, Airoma G, et al. Treatment of pulmonary neuroendocrine tumours: state of the art and future developments. *Cancer Treat Rev* 2013;39: 466–472.
389. Detterbeck FC. Management of carcinoid tumors. *Ann Thorac Surg* 2010;89: 998–1005.
390. Fjallskog ML, Granberg DP, Welin SL, et al. Treatment with cisplatin and etoposide in patients with neuroendocrine tumors. *Cancer* 2001;92:1101–1107.
391. Ekeblad S, Sundin A, Janson ET, et al. Temozolomide as monotherapy is effective in treatment of advanced malignant neuroendocrine tumors. *Clin Cancer Res* 2007;13:2986–2991.
392. Saranga-Perry V, Morse B, Centeno B, et al. Treatment of metastatic neuroendocrine tumors of the thymus with capecitabine and temozolomide: a case series. *Neuroendocrinology* 2013;97:318–321.
393. Fine RL, Gulati AP, Krantz BA, et al. Capecitabine and temozolomide (CAPTEM) for metastatic, well-differentiated neuroendocrine cancers: The Pancreas Center at Columbia University experience. *Cancer Chemother Pharmacol* 2013;71:663–670.
394. Kulke MH, Stuart K, Enzinger PC, et al. Phase II study of temozolomide and thalidomide in patients with metastatic neuroendocrine tumors. *J Clin Oncol* 2006;24:401–406.
395. Kulke MH, Stuart K, Earle CC, et al. A phase II study of temozolomide and bevacizumab in patients with advanced neuroendocrine tumors. *J Clin Oncol* 2006;24:4044.
396. Pavel ME, Hainsworth JD, Baudin E, et al. Everolimus plus octreotide long-acting repeatable for the treatment of advanced neuroendocrine tumours associated with carcinoid syndrome (RADIANT-2): a randomised, placebo-controlled, phase 3 study. *Lancet* 2011;378:2005–2012.
397. Reidy-Lagunes D, Thornton R. Pancreatic neuroendocrine and carcinoid tumors: what's new, what's old, and what's different? *Curr Oncol Rep* 2012;14: 249–256.
398. Yao JC, Phan A, Hoff PM, et al. Targeting vascular endothelial growth factor in advanced carcinoid tumor: a random assignment phase II study of depot octreotide with bevacizumab and pegylated interferon alpha-2b. *J Clin Oncol* 2008;26:1316–1323.
399. Kulke MH, Lenz HJ, Meropol NJ, et al. Activity of sunitinib in patients with advanced neuroendocrine tumors. *J Clin Oncol* 2008;26:3403–3410.
400. Raymond E, Dahan L, Raoul JL, et al. Sunitinib malate for the treatment of pancreatic neuroendocrine tumors. *N Engl J Med* 2011;364:501–513.
401. Gupta S, Johnson MM, Murthy R, et al. Hepatic arterial embolization and chemoembolization for the treatment of patients with metastatic neuroendocrine tumors: variables affecting response rates and survival. *Cancer* 2005;104: 1590–1602.
402. Moertel CG, Kvols LK, O'Connell MJ, et al. Treatment of neuroendocrine carcinomas with combined etoposide and cisplatin. Evidence of major therapeutic activity in the anaplastic variants of these neoplasms. *Cancer* 1991;68:227–232.
403. Sun W, Lipsitz S, Catalano P, et al. Phase II/III study of doxorubicin with fluorouracil compared with streptozocin with fluorouracil or dacarbazine in the treatment of advanced carcinoid tumors: Eastern Cooperative Oncology Group Study E1281. *J Clin Oncol* 2005;23:4897–4904.
404. Travis WD, Linnoila RI, Tsokos MG, et al. Neuroendocrine tumors of the lung with proposed criteria for large-cell neuroendocrine carcinoma. An ultrastructural, immunohistochemical, and flow cytometric study of 35 cases. *Am J Surg Pathol* 1991;15:529–553.
405. Travis WD, Krug LM, Rusch V, et al. Large Cell Neuroendocrine Carcinoma. *Textbook of Uncommon Cancer.* Chichester, England: John Wiley & Sons, Ltd.; 2006: 298–306.
406. Chen LC, Travis WD, Krug LM. Pulmonary neuroendocrine tumors: What (little) do we know? *J Natl Compr Canc Netw* 2006;4:623–630.
407. Travis WD. Neuroendocrine lung tumors. *Path Case Reviews* 2006;11:235–242.
408. Rossi G, Cavazza A, Marchioni A, et al. Role of chemotherapy and the receptor tyrosine kinases KIT, PDGFRalpha, PDGFRbeta, and Met in large-cell neuroendocrine carcinoma of the lung. *J Clin Oncol* 2005;23:8774–8785.
409. Oshiro Y, Kusumoto M, Matsuno Y, et al. CT findings of surgically resected large cell neuroendocrine carcinoma of the lung in 38 patients. *AJR Am J Roentgenol* 2004;182:87–91.
410. Chong S, Lee KS, Kim BT, et al. Integrated PET/CT of pulmonary neuroendocrine tumors: diagnostic and prognostic implications. *AJR Am J Roentgenol* 2007;188:1223–1231.
411. Takei H, Asamura H, Maeshima A, et al. Large cell neuroendocrine carcinoma of the lung: a clinicopathologic study of eighty-seven cases. *J Thorac Cardiovasc Surg* 2002;124:285–292.
412. Veronesi G, Morandi U, Alloisio M, et al. Large cell neuroendocrine carcinoma of the lung: a retrospective analysis of 144 surgical cases. *Lung Cancer* 2006;53:111–115.
413. Iyoda A, Hiroshima K, Toyozaki T, et al. Adjuvant chemotherapy for large cell carcinoma with neuroendocrine features. *Cancer* 2001;92:1108–1112.
414. Sarkaria IS, Iyoda A, Roh MS, et al. Neoadjuvant and adjuvant chemotherapy in resected pulmonary large cell neuroendocrine carcinomas: a single institution experience. *Ann Thorac Surg* 2011;92:1180–1186.
415. Zacharias J, Nicholson AG, Ladas GP, et al. Large cell neuroendocrine carcinoma and large cell carcinomas with neuroendocrine morphology of the lung: prognosis after complete resection and systematic nodal dissection. *Ann Thorac Surg* 2003;75:348–352.
416. Saji H, Tsuboi M, Matsubayashi J, et al. Clinical response of large cell neuroendocrine carcinoma of the lung to perioperative adjuvant chemotherapy. *Anticancer Drugs* 2010;21:89–93.
417. Tanaka Y, Ogawa H, Uchino K, et al. Immunohistochemical studies of pulmonary large cell neuroendocrine carcinoma: a possible association between staining patterns with neuroendocrine markers and tumor response to chemotherapy. *J Thorac Cardiovasc Surg* 2013;145:839–846.
418. Iyoda A, Hiroshima K, Moriya Y, et al. Prospective study of adjuvant chemotherapy for pulmonary large cell neuroendocrine carcinoma. *Ann Thorac Surg* 2006;82:1802–1807.
419. Iyoda A, Hiroshima K, Moriya Y, et al. Postoperative recurrence and the role of adjuvant chemotherapy in patients with pulmonary large-cell neuroendocrine carcinoma. *J Thorac Cardiovasc Surg* 2009;138:446–453.
420. Ettinger DS, Akerley W, Borghaei H, et al. Non-small cell lung cancer, version 2. *J Natl Compr Canc Netw*. 2013;11:645–653, quiz 653.
421. Yamazaki S, Sekine I, Matsuno Y, et al. Clinical responses of large cell neuroendocrine carcinoma of the lung to cisplatin-based chemotherapy. *Lung Cancer* 2005;49:217–223.
422. Sun JM, Ahn MJ, Ahn JS, et al. Chemotherapy for pulmonary large cell neuroendocrine carcinoma: similar to that for small cell lung cancer or non-small cell lung cancer? *Lung Cancer* 2012;77:365–370.
423. Niho S, Kenmotsu H, Sekine I, et al. Combination chemotherapy with irinotecan and cisplatin for large-cell neuroendocrine carcinoma of the lung: a multicenter phase II study. *J Thorac Oncol* 2013;8:980–984.
424. Le Treut J, Sault MC, Lena H, et al. Multicentre phase II study of cisplatin-etoposide chemotherapy for advanced large-cell neuroendocrine lung carcinoma: the GFPC 0302 study. *Ann Oncol* 2013;24:1548–1552.
425. Hanna N, Bunn PA Jr, Langer C, et al. Randomized phase III trial comparing irinotecan/cisplatin with etoposide/cisplatin in patients with previously untreated extensive-stage disease small-cell lung cancer. *J Clin Oncol* 2006;24: 2038–2043.
426. Smit EF, Fokkema E, Biesma B, et al. A phase II study of paclitaxel in heavily pretreated patients with small-cell lung cancer. *Br J Cancer* 1998;77:347–351.
427. Smyth JF, Smith IE, Sessa C, et al. Activity of docetaxel (Taxotere) in small cell lung cancer. The Early Clinical Trials Group of the EORTC. *Eur J Cancer* 1994;30A:1058–1060.
428. Masters GA, Declerck L, Blanke C, et al. Phase II trial of gemcitabine in refractory or relapsed small-cell lung cancer: Eastern Cooperative Oncology Group Trial 1597. *J Clin Oncol* 2003;21:1550–1555.
429. Hoang T, Kim K, Jaslowski A, et al. Phase II study of second-line gemcitabine in sensitive or refractory small cell lung cancer. *Lung Cancer* 2003;42:97–102.
430. van der Lee I, Smit EF, van Putten JW, et al. Single-agent gemcitabine in patients with resistant small-cell lung cancer. *Ann Oncol* 2001;12:557–561.
431. Furuse K, Kubota K, Kawahara M, et al. Phase II study of vinorelbine in heavily previously treated small cell lung cancer. Japan Lung Cancer Vinorelbine Study Group. *Oncology* 1996;53:169–172.
432. Jassem J, Karnicka-Mlodkowska H, van Pottelsberghe C, et al. Phase II study of vinorelbine (Navelbine) in previously treated small cell lung cancer patients. EORTC Lung Cancer Cooperative Group. *Eur J Cancer* 1993;29A:1720–1722.
433. Onoda S, Masuda N, Seto T, et al. Phase II trial of amrubicin for treatment of refractory or relapsed small-cell lung cancer: Thoracic Oncology Research Group Study 0301. *J Clin Oncol* 2006;24:5448–5453.

434. Ettinger DS, Jotte R, Lorigan P, et al. Phase II study of amrubicin as second-line therapy in patients with platinum-refractory small-cell lung cancer. *J Clin Oncol* 2010;28:2598–2603.
435. Treat J, Schiller J, Quoix E, et al. ZD0473 treatment in lung cancer: an overview of the clinical trial results. *Eur J Cancer* 2002;38:S13–S18.
436. Eckardt JR, Bentsion DL, Lipatov ON, et al. Phase II study of picoplatin as second-line therapy for patients with small-cell lung cancer. *J Clin Oncol* 2009;27:2046–2051.
437. Ciuleanu T, Samarzjia M, Demidchik Y, et al. Randomized phase III study (SPEAR) of picoplatin plus best supportive care or best supportive care alone in patients with SCLC refractory or progressive within 6 months after first-line platinum-based chemotherapy. *J Clin Oncol* 2010;28:abstract 7002.
438. Mattson K, Niiranen A, Pyrhonen S, et al. Natural interferon alfa as maintenance therapy for small cell lung cancer. *Eur J Cancer* 1992;28A:1387–1391.
439. Prior C, Oroszy S, Oberaigner W, et al. Adjunctive interferon-alpha-2c in stage IIIB/IV small-cell lung cancer: a phase III trial. *Eur Respir J* 1997;10:392–396.
440. Ruotsalainen TM, Halme M, Tamminen K, et al. Concomitant chemotherapy and IFN-alpha for small cell lung cancer: a randomized multicenter phase III study. *J Interferon Cytokine Res* 1999;19:253–259.
441. Kelly K, Crowley JJ, Bunn PA Jr, et al. Role of recombinant interferon alfa-2a maintenance in patients with limited-stage small-cell lung cancer responding to concurrent chemoradiation: a Southwest Oncology Group study. *J Clin Oncol* 1995;13:2924–2930.
442. Jett JR, Maksymiuk AW, Su JQ, et al. Phase III trial of recombinant interferon gamma in complete responders with small-cell lung cancer. *J Clin Oncol* 1994;12:2321–2326.
443. van Zandwijk N, Groen HJ, Postmus PE, et al. Role of recombinant interferon-gamma maintenance in responding patients with small cell lung cancer. A randomised phase III study of the EORTC Lung Cancer Cooperative Group. *Eur J Cancer* 1997;33:1759–1766.
444. Clamon G, Herndon J, Perry MC, et al. Interleukin-2 activity in patients with extensive small-cell lung cancer: a phase II trial of Cancer and Leukemia Group B. *J Natl Cancer Inst* 1993;85:316–320.
445. Zacharski LR, Henderson WG, Rickles FR, et al. Effect of warfarin on survival in small cell carcinoma of the lung. Veterans Administration Study No. 75. *JAMA* 1981;245:831–835.
446. Chahinian AP, Propert KJ, Ware JH, et al. A randomized trial of anticoagulation with warfarin and of alternating chemotherapy in extensive small-cell lung cancer by the Cancer and Leukemia Group B. *J Clin Oncol* 1989;7:993–1002.
447. Lebeau B, Chastang C, Muir JF, et al. No effect of an antiaggregant treatment with aspirin in small cell lung cancer treated with CCAVP16 chemotherapy. Results from a randomized clinical trial of 303 patients. The "Petites Cellules" Group. *Cancer* 1993;71:1741–1745.
448. Lebeau B, Chastang C, Brechot JM, et al. Subcutaneous heparin treatment increases survival in small cell lung cancer. "Petites Cellules" Group. *Cancer* 1994;74:38–45.
449. Shepherd FA, Giaccone G, Seymour L, et al. Prospective, randomized, double-blind, placebo-controlled trial of marimastat after response to first-line chemotherapy in patients with small-cell lung cancer: a trial of the National Cancer Institute of Canada-Clinical Trials Group and the European Organization for Research and Treatment of Cancer. *J Clin Oncol* 2002;20:4434–4439.
450. Rigas JR, Denham CA, Rinaldi DA, et al. Randomized placebo-controlled trials of the matrix metalloproteinase inhibitor BAY12-9566 as adjuvant therapy for patients with small cell and non-small cell lung cancer. *Proc Am Soc Clin Oncol* 2003;22:Abstr 2525.
451. Heymach JV, Johnson DH, Khuri FR, et al. Phase II study of the farnesyl transferase inhibitor R115777 in patients with sensitive relapse small-cell lung cancer. *Ann Oncol* 2004;15:1187–1193.
452. Lara PN Jr, Chansky K, Davies AM, et al. Bortezomib (PS-341) in relapsed or refractory extensive stage small cell lung cancer: a Southwest Oncology Group phase II trial (S0327). *J Thorac Oncol* 2006;1:996–1001.
453. Giaccone G, Debruyne C, Felip E, et al. Phase III study of adjuvant vaccination with Bec2/bacille Calmette-Guerin in responding patients with limited-disease small-cell lung cancer (European Organisation for Research and Treatment of Cancer 08971-08971B; Silva Study). *J Clin Oncol* 2005;23:6854–6864.

39 Neoplasms of the Mediastinum

Robert B. Cameron, Patrick J. Loehrer, and Percy P. Lee

THYMIC NEOPLASMS

Incidence and Etiology

Thymic neoplasms, predominantly thymomas, constitute 30% and 15% of anterior mediastinal masses in adults and children, respectively. Surveillance, Epidemiology, and End Results (SEER) data suggest that 15 thymomas occur in every 100,000 person-years, are more common in males and Pacific Islanders, and increase in frequency into the 8th decade of life.[1] Other studies document an incidence as low as 0.15 to 0.32 per 100,000 persons. No specific etiology or risk factors are known, but a well-known association with myasthenia gravis (MG) does exist. Thymic carcinoma is a rare, aggressive thymic neoplasm that has a particularly poor prognosis and infrequently is associated with MG or other paraneoplastic syndromes.[2] Like thymoma, it is an epithelial tumor, but unlike thymoma it exhibits malignant cytologic features. Although it is unclear if thymoma and thymic carcinoma share a common cell of origin because molecular markers are unique for each, both most often are located in the anterior mediastinum, although other sites have been reported.[3] Suster and Rosai[4] reported on 60 patients with thymic carcinoma ranging in age from 10 to 76 years and with a slight male predominance. Nearly 70% of patients had symptoms of cough, chest pain, or superior vena cava syndrome. Extensive local invasion and distant metastases are more common than in thymomas.

Anatomy and Pathology

The thymus is an incompletely understood lymphatic organ functioning in T-lymphocyte maturation. It is composed of thymocytes, lymphocytes, and an epithelial stroma. Although lymphomas, carcinoid tumors, and germ-cell tumors all may arise within the thymus, only thymomas, thymic carcinomas, and thymolipomas arise from true thymic elements.[5,6] The thymus develops from a paired epithelial anlage in the ventral portion of the third pharyngeal pouch and is closely associated with the developing parathyroid glands.[7] The thymic epithelial stromal cells are likely derived from both ectodermal and endodermal components.[8] During weeks 7 and 8 of development, the thymus elongates and descends caudally and ventromedially into the anterior mediastinum. Lymphoid cells arrive during week 9 and are separated from the perivascular spaces by a flat epithelial cell layer that creates the blood–thymus barrier. Maturation and differentiation occurs in this antigen-free environment and, during the 4th fetal month, lymphocytes begin to circulate to peripheral lymphoid tissue.[8] Six subtypes of epithelial cells have been identified in the mature thymus.[8] Four exist primarily in the cortical region and two in the medullary region. Type 6 cells form Hassall corpuscles that are characteristic of the thymus. These cells have an ectodermal origin and are displaced into the thymic medulla, where they hypertrophy, form tonofilaments, and finally appear as concentric cells without nuclei.[7,8]

At maturity, the thymus gland is an irregular, lobulated organ. It attains its greatest relative weight at birth, but its absolute weight increases to 30 to 40 g by puberty. During adulthood, it slowly involutes and is replaced by adipose tissue. Ectopic thymic tissue has been found to be widely distributed throughout the mediastinum and neck, particularly the aortopulmonary window and retrocarinal area, and often is indistinguishable from mediastinal fat.[9] This ectopic tissue is the likely explanation for thymomas outside the anterior mediastinum and possibly for failure in some cases of a simple thymectomy to improve MG.

THYMOMA

Ninety percent of thymomas occur in the anterior mediastinum and the remainder arise in the neck or other areas of the mediastinum, including, rarely, the heart.[10] The normal contour of the thymus is biconcave or flat. The diseased thymus gland displays a more convex margin. Thymomas grossly are lobulated, firm, tan-pink to gray tumors that may contain cystic spaces, calcification, or hemorrhage. They may be encapsulated, adherent to surrounding structures, or frankly invasive. Microscopically, thymomas arise from thymic epithelial cells, although thymocytes or lymphocytes may predominate histologically. True thymomas contain cytologically bland cells and should be distinguished from thymic carcinomas, which have malignant cytologic characteristics. Originally, in 1976, Rosai and Levine[11] proposed that thymomas be divided into three types: lymphocytic, epithelial, or mixed (lymphoepithelial). In 1985, Marino and Muller-Hermelink[12] proposed a histologic classification system determined by the thymic site of origin—that is, cortical thymomas, medullary thymomas, and mixed thymomas—which were later subdivided further.[13,14] To unify the pathology of thymic neoplasms[15–17] the World Health Organization (WHO) adopted a new classification system for thymic neoplasms (Table 39.1).[17] WHO type A and B2 tumors are more likely to present with locoregional disease, compared with WHO type B3 and C tumors.[18,19]

Although Suster and Moran[20] have proposed a simpler classification schema that separates thymic tumors into three categories of thymic carcinoma: well-differentiated (WHO types A, AB, B1, and B2), moderately differentiated (WHO type B3), and poorly differentiated (WHO type C), the full WHO classification system remains more broadly accepted.

Currently, the terms *noninvasive* and *invasive* thymoma are preferred over *benign* and *malignant* designations. Noninvasive thymomas have an intact capsule, are mobile, and are easily resected, although they can be adherent to adjacent organs. In contrast, invasive thymomas invade surrounding structures and should be removed with en bloc resection of involved structures despite a benign cytologic appearance. Metastatic disease may occur in both noninvasive and invasive thymomas and is most commonly seen as pleural implants or pulmonary nodules. Metastases to extrathoracic sites, such as the liver, brain, bone, and kidney, rarely occur.[21]

In 1981, Masaoka et al.[22] developed a surgical staging system, shown in Table 39.2. An update of this series of 273 patients confirmed that both WHO histology and clinical staging were independently predictive of 20-year survival.[23] The Groupe

TABLE 39.1

World Health Organization Classification System for Thymic Epithelial Tumors

Tumor Type	Cells	Clinicopathologic Classification	Histologic Terminology
A	Spindle or oval	Benign thymoma	Medullary
B B1 B2 B3	Epithelioid or dendritic	Category I malignant thymoma	Cortical; organoid Lymphocyte rich; predominately cortical Cortical Well-differentiated thymic carcinoma
AB		Benign thymoma	Mixed
C		Category II malignant thymoma	Nonorganotypic; thymic carcinoma, epidermoid keratinizing and nonkeratinizing carcinoma, lymphoepitheliomalike carcinoma, sarcomatoid carcinoma, clear-cell carcinoma, basaloid carcinoma, mucoepidermoid carcinoma, undifferentiated carcinoma

From Patterson GA. Thymomas. *Semin Thorac Cardiovasc Surg* 1992;4:39–44 with permission.

d'Etudes des Tumeurs Thymiques (GETT) has another surgically oriented staging system.[24] The Istituto Nazionale Tumori system combines the Masaoka classifications in three distinct stage groupings (locally restricted, locally advanced, and systemic disease) and may better encompass all WHO subtypes.[25] Although the Masaoka staging system[26] and a tumor-node-metastasis (TNM) classification system[27] (Table 39.3) also have been used in staging thymic carcinoma, their utility is largely unproven.

THYMIC CARCINOMA

The histologic classification of thymic carcinoma was proposed by Levine and Rosai[28] and revised by Suster and Rosai.[4] Tumors are classified broadly as low or high grade. Low-grade tumors include squamous cell carcinoma, mucoepidermoid carcinoma, and basaloid carcinoma. High-grade neoplasms include lymphoepithelioma-like carcinoma and small-cell, undifferentiated, sarcomatoid, and clear-cell carcinomas.[4,26,29,30] Although the histologic classification of thymic carcinomas was designed to be descriptive, correlations with prognosis have been made. For instance, low-grade tumors may have a more favorable clinical course (median survival rates of 25.4 months to more than 6.6 years) when compared with higher grade malignancies (median survival of only 11.3 months to 15.0 months).[4,26]

TABLE 39.2

Thymoma Staging System of Masaoka

Stage	Description	5-/10-year Survival (%)
I	Macroscopically completely encapsulated and microscopically no capsular invasion	96/67
II	1. Macroscopic invasion into surrounding fatty tissue or mediastinal pleura, or 2. Microscopic invasion into capsule	86/60
III	Macroscopic invasion into neighboring organs (pericardium, great vessels, lung)	69/58
IV	a. Pleural or pericardial dissemination, or b. Lymphogenous or hematogenous metastasis	50/0

Adapted from Masaoka A, Monden Y, Nakahara K, Tanioka T. Follow-up study of thymomas with special reference to their clinical stages. *Cancer* 1981;48:2485–2492.

Molecular profiling of rare solid tumors, such as thymic neoplasms, has taken place over the past decade.[31] Emerging analyses do suggest that mutations in genes of the epidermal growth factor receptor (EGFR) and KIT pathways have documented a progressive increase in observed genomic aberrations from WHO subtype A thymoma to WHO subtype C thymic carcinoma.[32]

Diagnosis

A meticulous history and physical examination, along with serologic and imaging studies, usually suggests the diagnosis. Although most anterior mediastinal masses are thymic malignancies, other etiologies also exist (Table 39.4). An improved pathologic analysis of image-guided percutaneous core needle biopsy specimens makes surgical biopsy rarely necessary.

Symptoms and Signs

Approximately 40% of mediastinal masses are asymptomatic and discovered incidentally on routine chest imaging.[1] The remaining 60% have symptoms related to either compression or direct invasion of adjacent mediastinal structures or to paraneoplastic syndromes. Asymptomatic patients are more likely to have benign lesions, whereas symptomatic patients more often harbor malignancies. Davis et al.[33] found that 85% of patients with a malignancy were symptomatic, but only 46% of patients with benign neoplasms had identifiable complaints. The most common symptoms are chest pain, cough, and dyspnea. Superior vena cava syndrome, Horner syndrome, hoarseness, and neurologic deficits are less common and often signal a malignancy.[33] Systemic syndromes associated with mediastinal neoplasms are shown in Tables 39.4 and 39.5.

Associated Systemic Syndromes

A myriad of associated systemic disorders may be identified in 71% of patients with thymomas, including autoimmune diseases (MG, systemic lupus erythematosus, polymyositis, myocarditis, Sjögren syndrome, ulcerative colitis, Hashimoto thyroiditis, rheumatoid arthritis, sarcoidosis, and scleroderma), endocrine disorders (hyperthyroidism, hyperparathyroidism, stiff-person syndrome, Addison disease, and panhypopituitarism), blood disorders (red cell aplasia, hypogammaglobulinemia, T-cell deficiency syndrome, erythrocytosis, pancytopenia, megakaryocytopenia, T-cell lymphocytosis, and pernicious anemia), neuromuscular syndromes (myotonic dystrophy,

TABLE 39.3

Istituto Nazionale Tumori Tumor-Node-Metastatis (TNM)–Based Staging System

TNM	Description
T1	No capsular invasion
T2	Microscopic invasion into the capsule, or extracapsular involvement limited to the surrounding fatty tissue or normal thymus
T3	Direct invasion into the mediastinal pleura and/or anterior pericardium
T4	Direct invasion into neighboring organs, such as the sternum, great vessels, and lungs; implants to the mediastinal pleura or pericardium, only if anterior to phrenic nerves
N0	No lymph nodes metastasis
N1	Metastasis to anterior mediastinal lymph nodes
N2	Metastasis to intrathoracic lymph nodes other than anterior mediastinal
N3	Metastasis to prescalene or supraclavicular nodes
M0	No hematogenous metastasis
M1a	Implants to the pericardium or mediastinal pleura beyond the sites defined in the T4 category
M1b	Hematogenous metastasis to other sites, or involvement of lymph nodal stations other than those described in the N categories
Stage Grouping	**Description**
I	Locally restricted disease
	T1–2 N0 M0
II	Locally advanced disease
	T3–4 N0 M0
	Any T N1–2 M0
III	Systemic
	Any T N3 M0
	Any T any N M1
Classification Description of Residual Disease	
R0	No residual tumor
R1	Microscopic residual tumor
R2a	Local macroscopic residual tumor after reductive resection (more than 80% of the tumor)
R2b	Other features of residual tumor

Adapted from Shimizu J, Hayashi Y, Monita K, et al. Primary thymic carcinoma: a clinicopathological and immunohistochemical study. *J Surg Oncol* 1994;56:159–164.

TABLE 39.4

Systemic Syndromes Associated with Mediastinal Neoplasms

Tumor	Syndrome
Thymoma	Acute pericarditis, Addison disease, agranulocytosis, alopecia areata, Cushing syndrome, hemolytic anemia, hypogammaglobulinemia, limbic encephalopathy, myasthenia gravis, myocarditis, nephrotic syndrome, panhypopituitarism, pernicious anemia, polymyositis, pure red cell aplasia, rheumatoid arthritis, sarcoidosis, scleroderma, sensorimotor radiculopathy, stiff-person syndrome, thyroiditis, ulcerative colitis
Hodgkin lymphoma	Alcohol-induced pain, Pel-Ebstein fever
Neurofibroma	von Recklinghausen disease, osteoarthritis
Thymic carcinoid	Multiple endocrine neoplasia
Neuroblastoma	Opsomyoclonus, erythrocyte abnormalities
Neurilemoma	Peptic ulcer

TABLE 39.5

Systemic Manifestations of Hormone Production by Mediastinal Neoplasms

Symptoms	Hormone	Tumor
Hypertension	Catecholamines	Pheochromocytoma, chemodectoma, neuroblastoma, ganglioneuroma
Hypercalcemia	Parathyroid hormone	Parathyroid adenoma
Thyrotoxicosis	Thyroxine	Thyroid
Cushing syndrome	ACTH	Carcinoid tumor
Gynecomastia	HCG	Germ cell tumor
Hypoglycemia	? Insulin	Mesenchymal tumors
Diarrhea	VIP	Ganglioneuroma, neuroblastoma, neurofibroma

ACTH, adrenocorticotropic hormone; HCG, human chorionic gonadotropin; VIP, vasoactive intestinal polypeptide.

myositis, and Eaton-Lambert syndrome), as well as other disorders (hypertrophic osteoarthropathy, nephrotic syndrome, minimal change nephropathy, pemphigus, and chronic mucocutaneous candidiasis).[34] Symptoms of one or more of these disorders may lead to the original discovery of the mediastinal tumor.

Myasthenia Gravis

MG is the most common autoimmune disorder associated with thymoma, occurring in 30% to 50% of patients.[35] Younger women and older men usually are affected, with a female-to-male ratio of 2:1. Myasthenia is a disorder of neuromuscular transmission. The temporal association is variable and a prolonged interval between the diagnosis of MG and the development of a visible thymic tumor can occur.[36] Symptoms (e.g., diplopia, ptosis, dysphagia, fatigue) begin insidiously and result from the production of antibodies to the postsynaptic nicotinic acetylcholine receptor at the myoneural junction. Ocular symptoms are the most frequent initial complaint, eventually progressing to generalized weakness in 80% of cases. The role of the thymus in MG remains unclear, but autosensitization of T lymphocytes to acetylcholine-receptor proteins or an unknown action of thymic hormones remains possible.[37] The altered microenvironment may adversely impact the output of T-regulatory (Treg) cells, thus altering autoimmune homeostasis.[38] Pathologic thymic changes are noted in 70% of MG patients, with lymphoid hyperplasia predominating and thymomas seen only in 15% of patients.[37]

The treatment of MG involves the use of anticholinesterase mimetic agents (i.e., pyridostigmine bromide [Mestinon]). In severe cases, plasmapheresis may be required to remove high antibody titers. Thymectomy has become an increasingly accepted procedure in the treatment of MG, although the indications, timing, and surgical approach remain controversial.[39] Some improvement in MG symptoms frequently occurs after a thymectomy, but complete remission rates vary from 7% to 63%.[39] Patients with thymomas do not respond as well to a thymectomy as MG patients without thymomas. Age 54 years and older and a symptom duration of less than 1 year are associated with poor outcomes[40]; however, MG does not necessarily portend a poor outcome.[41]

Red Cell Aplasia

Pure red cell aplasia, an autoimmune disorder, occurs in 5% of patients with thymomas.[42] Of patients with red cell aplasia, 30% to 50% have associated thymomas. Affected patients are older than 40 years of age in 96% of cases. A bone marrow examination reveals an absence of erythroid precursors and, in 30% of cases, a poorly understood associated decrease in platelet and leukocyte numbers. A thymectomy has produced remission in up to 38% of patients. For patients with recurrent disease, octreotide and prednisone were effective in case reports.[42,43]

Hypogammaglobulinemia

Hypogammaglobulinemia is seen in 5% to 10% of patients with thymoma (Good syndrome), and 10% of patients with hypogammaglobulinemia have been shown to have thymoma. Recurrent sinusitis is a common associated symptom in such patients. Defects in both cellular and humoral immunity have been described, and many patients also have red cell hypoplasia.[44] Thymectomy has not proven beneficial in this disorder.

Radiographic Imaging Studies

Imaging studies initially localize mediastinal neoplasms.[45] The posteroanterior and lateral chest radiographs define the location, size, density, and calcification of a mass, which helps focus the initial diagnostic testing; however, an intravenous contrast-enhanced spiral computed tomography (CT) scan remains the best imaging modality to accurately assess the nature of the lesion (cystic versus solid), detect fat and calcium, determine the relationship to surrounding anatomic structures, and, in some instances, predict invasiveness of the tumors.[46,47]

Recent advances in electrocardiogram-gating and real-time magnetic resonance imaging (MRI) and angiography have dramatically increased the usefulness of this modality in the evaluation of mediastinal masses. Not only is it superior to CT in defining vascular involvement, but an MRI scan can also detect subtle differences in tumor contour, capsule clarity, and intratumoral signal (low), which correlate with the WHO classification of thymomas.[48]

Recently, the usefulness of positron emission tomography (PET) scans in the evaluation of thymic tumors has expanded significantly. In a study of 51 patients, Benveniste et al. suggested that 18-fluorodeoxyglucose (18F-FDG) uptake by PET/CT scans was higher in thymic carcinomas than thymomas. Additionally, higher *focal* 18F-FDG uptake correlated with B3 thymomas, and greater 18F-FDG avid tumor volume predicted higher stage tumors.[49] In a contemporary study of 47 patients, Lococo et al. demonstrated that maximum standardized uptake values (SUV_{max}) and SUV_{max}/tumor size index, as determined by PET/CT, not only distinguished thymomas from thymic carcinomas, but also both parameters correlated with WHO malignancy grade and SUV_{max} predicted Masaoka stage.[50] On serial PET/CT imaging, decreased 18F-FDG uptake in 56 patients with stage III/IV thymic epithelial malignancies treated after only 6 weeks of chemotherapy was shown by Thomas et al.[51] to correlate with longer progression-free survival (11.5 versus 4.6 months; $p = 0.044$) and a trend toward longer overall survival (31.8 versus 18.4 months; $p = 0.14$).

Serology and Chemistry

Many germ-cell neoplasms release chemical markers into the serum that may be measured to confirm a diagnosis, evaluate the response to therapy, and monitor for tumor recurrence. Lactate dehydrogenase, α-fetoprotein (AFP), and human chorionic gonadotropin-β (β-hCG) are common tumor markers that should be obtained in male patients with anterior mediastinal masses. Also, adrenocorticotropic hormone, thyroid hormone, and parathormone may help differentiate certain mediastinal masses (see Table 39.4).

Invasive Diagnostic Tests

An accurate histologic diagnosis is essential for appropriate treatment of nearly all mediastinal neoplasms. Although some patients may still require open surgical biopsies, CT- or ultrasound-guided percutaneous needle biopsy is now standard in the initial evaluation of mediastinal masses.[10] Although fine-needle specimens may distinguish carcinomas from benign pathology, core biopsies are necessary for most mediastinal neoplasms, especially lymphoma and thymoma. Recent series report diagnostic yields for percutaneous needle biopsy in excess of 90%.[52] Complications include simple pneumothorax (25%), hemoptysis (7% to 15%), and pneumothorax, requiring chest tube placement (5%).[52] In some circumstances, fine-needle aspiration of posterior and middle mediastinal tumors can be performed endoscopically using transesophageal ultrasonography.[53]

Surgical procedures occasionally are still required in the diagnosis of mediastinal tumors. A mediastinoscopy is a relatively simple procedure with a diagnostic accuracy of more than 90% for biopsies of the upper middle and, in some surgeons' hands, the anterior and posterior mediastinum.[54] Anterior parasternal mediastinotomy (Chamberlain procedure) yields a diagnosis in 95% of anterior mediastinal masses and may be accomplished under local anesthesia.[54,55] A thoracoscopy is a minimally invasive procedure that provides a diagnostic accuracy of nearly 100% in most areas of the mediastinum.[54] Currently, thoracotomy rarely is necessary solely as a diagnostic procedure.

Management by Stage

Thymomas, albeit slow growing, should be considered potentially malignant neoplasms. Surgery, radiation, and chemotherapy all may play a role in their management.[41,56] Few prospective, well-designed clinical trials in the management of thymomas have been conducted, particularly evaluating the role of surgery and radiotherapy; however, the newly formed International Thymic Malignancy Interest Group is planning cohort studies to help guide diagnostic and therapeutic interventions.[57]

Masaoka Stage I/II Thymoma

Complete surgical resection is the mainstay of therapy for stage I/II thymomas and is the most important predictor of long-term survival.[58–61] Although a median sternotomy with a vertical or submammary skin incision is most commonly used, bilateral anterolateral thoracotomies with transverse sternotomy, or the *clam-shell procedure*, is useful with advanced or laterally displaced large tumors. Recently, the use of minimally invasive surgery in stage I and II thymomas has expanded dramatically. One study comparing 76 thoracoscopic thymectomies to 44 transsternal resections reported a shorter hospital stay with the thoracoscopies.[62] Similarly, two reports of robotic-assisted surgery, including a multicenter European study, were associated with less blood loss, fewer complications, and a shorter hospital stay, as well as similar operative times and short-term outcomes compared to sternotomies.[63,64] Although randomized, prospective clinical trials are still lacking, it is highly likely that minimally invasive surgery in the hands of experienced surgeons can produce identical oncologic outcomes with less morbidity than open surgery, as has been shown in other thoracic tumors, such as lung and esophageal cancers.

During any surgery, a careful assessment of areas of possible invasion and adherence should be made. Extended total thymectomy, including all tissue anterior to the pericardium from the diaphragm to the neck and laterally from one phrenic nerve to the other, including en bloc pericardium, phrenic nerve, chest wall, lung, and diaphragmatic resection (with reconstruction) in up to two-thirds of cases in order to achieve an R0 resection is recommended in all good performance status patients.[41,58–60] Operative mortality is less than 3% in experienced centers.[41]

In the past, ionizing radiation has been used to treat various stages of thymomas. Furthermore, modern imaging, three-dimensional treatment planning, and delivery techniques have allowed thoracic radiotherapy to be prescribed in a safer fashion than noted in the past century. Radiation therapy is delivered in doses ranging from 30 to 60 Gy in 1.8- to 2.0-Gy fractions for 3 to 6 weeks.[58,65,66] There are suggestions of a dose–response relationship with local control in some patients, albeit from retrospective data, although it is not clear that doses exceeding 60 Gy offer any consistent advantage[67,68]; however, completely resected and microscopic residual disease can be well controlled with only 40 to 45 Gy.[61,69] Emerging data suggest that certain histologic subtypes (WHO type B1 and B2) are more likely to respond to radiotherapy compared to others subtypes (WHO type B3), suggesting that the response is limited to the lymphocytic and not the epithelial cell component of the tumors.[41,70–72] Gating techniques to minimize respiratory variation and intensity-modulated radiation therapy are new techniques that can minimize the dose heterogeneity, increase total dose and fraction size, and minimize toxicity.[69,73,75]

Masaoka Stage III/IV Thymoma

The role of subtotal surgical resection, or *debulking* surgery, in stage III and IV disease remains highly controversial.[76] Several studies have documented improved 5-year survival rates after subtotal resection compared to a biopsy alone.[58,61] Another study suggested no survival advantage to *debulking* surgery followed by radiation when compared with radiation alone, and a more recent report reached the opposite conclusion.[76] The use of surgery in recurrent disease remains to be defined.

Radiation therapy may be beneficial in selected patients with locally advanced disease.[61,65,67,77] Large variations in the amount of tumor treated, radiation delivered, and tumor biology, however, make interpretation of these results difficult.[61,67,78,79]

Cytotoxic chemotherapy has been used with increasing frequency in the treatment of invasive thymomas.[80] Both single-agent and combination therapy have demonstrated activity in the adjuvant and neoadjuvant settings. Doxorubicin, cisplatin, ifosfamide, corticosteroids, and cyclophosphamide all have been used as single-agent therapies.[81] The most active agents are cisplatin, doxorubicin, ifosfamide, and corticosteroids; however, only a few single agents, such as cisplatin, ifosfamide, pemetrexed, gefitinib, and imatinib, have undergone formal phase II trials.

A number of molecular targets have been identified in thymic tissue.[83] Overexpression of the EGFR has been found in more than two thirds of patients, mostly WHO B2 and 3 subtypes.[84–86] The overexpression of *c-kit* is common in thymic carcinoma, although *c-kit* mutations are less frequent.[85,87,88]

Thymic Carcinoma

The optimal treatment of thymic carcinoma remains undefined, but currently, a multimodality approach, including surgical resection, postoperative radiation, and chemotherapy, is recommended.[89] Initial surgical resection followed by radiation has been used in most studies.[4,26,27,29,90] Complete resection should be attempted, but often is not possible.[26,91] One analysis noted a 9.5-month median survival after resection and postoperative photon-beam radiation therapy,[90]

CANCER OF THE THORACIC CAVITY

with a trend toward improved survival in other studies.[4,26,29] Chemotherapy with cisplatin-based regimens similar to those used with thymomas have produced variable responses in a small number of patients.[4,26,29] Combinations of doxorubicin, cyclophosphamide, and cisplatin also have generated partial responses, as has the combination of 5-fluorouracil and leucovorin in recurrent disease. Use of neoadjuvant chemotherapy has been reported in a small number of patients.[89,92]

Results of Treatment

Thymoma

In nearly 700 patients in the SEER database treated between 1973 and 1998, advanced disease was associated with decreasing survival.[42] According to various retrospective series, the 5- and 10-year survival rates for stage I, III, and IV tumors are reported to be 89% to 95% and 78% to 90%; 70% to 80% and 21% to 80%; and 50% to 60% and 30% to 40%, respectively.[58,93] Ten-year disease-free survival rates of 74%, 71%, 50%, and 29% also have been reported for stage I, II, III, and IV disease, respectively.[58] Long-term results from an experienced Indiana University group has yielded a 66% 1-year overall survival.[41] Although Maggi et al.[58] reported a 10% overall recurrence rate in 241 patients, less than 5% of noninvasive thymomas and 20% of invasive thymomas were noted to recur. A large Japanese multi-institutional experience with 1,320 patients reported 5-year survival rates of 100%, 98.4%, 88.7%, 70.6%, and 52.8% for Masaoka stages I, II, III, IVa, and IVb, respectively.[59] Although MG once was considered an adverse prognostic factor, this is no longer the case because of improved perioperative care, and in fact, MG actually may be associated with an improved survival owing to earlier tumor detection.[41,94] Complete surgical resection of thymomas is associated with an 82% overall 7-year survival rate, whereas survival with incomplete resection is 71%, and with biopsy is only 26%.[58] Survival after a complete tumor resection has been similar in patients with noninvasive and invasive thymomas in several studies.[59,60] Patients with MG and thymoma have a 56% to 78% 10-year survival rate and a 3% recurrence rate with 4.8% (1.7% since 1980) operative mortality after an extended thymectomy.[61,95] Rarely, a syndrome of myasthenia crisis may occur following surgery and may lead to increased perioperative morbidity.[95]

Although the data on whether outcomes are related to WHO subtype is inconclusive,[41,71,72] it may be that when coupled with other factors such as completeness of resection, the WHO subtype may be prognostic in some patients.[96]

For example, in stage I thymomas, adjuvant radiotherapy has been administered but has not improved on the excellent results with surgery alone (more than 80% 10-year survival rate).[58,61] In stage II and III invasive disease, adjuvant radiation can decrease recurrence rates after complete surgical resection from 28% to 5%.[67] In addition, Pollack et al.[65] reported an increase in 5-year disease-free survival for stage II to IVa from 18% to 62% with the addition of adjuvant radiation, despite a 50% infield relapse rate in patients recurring with prior radiation. Stage II patients with cortical tumors[97,98] and invasion of pleura or the pericardium are most likely to benefit from postoperative radiation.[77] Preoperative radiotherapy for extensive tumors has been reported in limited studies that suggest a decreased tumor burden and potential for tumor seeding at the time of surgery, although multivariate analyses suggested that chemotherapy may have played a role.[58,61] Data suggest that not all Masaoka stage II patients may necessarily require postoperative radiotherapy (PORT).[56,101] Indeed, a review of SEER registry data from 1975 to 2003 demonstrated a worse cancer-specific survival for patients with resected, localized thymoma who received PORT compared to those without (91% versus 98%; $p = 0.03$). For patients with regional disease, PORT had a slight but nonstatistically significant difference (91% versus 86%; $p = 0.12$).[102] The absence of statistically significant therapeutic efficacy for PORT, despite the suggestion of a lower local recurrence rate (i.e., 0% versus 8%) again has been confirmed in two recent studies.[102]

Masaoka Stage III/IV Thymoma

The role of subtotal surgical resection or *debulking* surgery in stage III and IV disease remains highly controversial.[76] Several studies have documented 5-year survival rates from 60% to 75% after subtotal resection and 24% to 40% after biopsy alone.[58,61] Although one study did suggest no survival advantage to debulking followed by radiation when compared with radiation alone, another more recent experience reached the opposite conclusion.[76] The use of surgery in recurrent disease remains to be defined. Maggi et al.[58] reported a 71% 5-year survival rate in 12 surgery patients and a 41% survival rate in 11 patients treated with radiation and chemotherapy alone. Prolonged tumor-free survival also was reported by Kirschner[74] in 23 patients. However, Urgesi et al.[78] noted a 74% 5-year survival rate in 11 patients undergoing surgery and radiation, compared with 65% in 10 patients treated with radiation alone (not statistically different). In 71 patients with thymoma (WHO types A and B3) with stage I to IVA disease, 53 (75.3%) patients are alive and free of disease, with 6 additional patients alive with disease with a mean follow-up of 66 months.[41]

Radiation therapy may be beneficial in selected patients with locally advanced disease.[61,63,65,68,77] Radiotherapy after incomplete surgical resection produces local control rates of 35% to 74% and 5-year survival rates ranging from 50% to 70% for stage III and 20% to 50% for stage IVa tumors.[61,66,67] In addition, Ciernik et al.[67] and others[78] have reported similar survival rates (87% 5-year and 70% 7-year) in patients treated with radiation alone compared with partial surgical resection and adjuvant radiation in small numbers of stage III and IV patients and patients with intrathoracic recurrences. Weksler et al.[105] reviewed SEER data on 322 patients with stage III thymoma who received postoperative adjuvant radiation and found that by multivariate analysis, disease-specific survival was improved ($p = 0.049$) but overall survival was not. However, large variations in the amount of tumor treated, radiation delivered, and tumor biology in particular make interpretation of these results difficult at best.[61,67,78,79]

Cytotoxic chemotherapy has been used with increasing frequency in the treatment of invasive thymomas.[80] Both single-agent and combination therapy have demonstrated activity in the adjuvant and neoadjuvant settings. The most commonly used active agents are cisplatin and doxorubicin; however, only a few single agents, such as cisplatin, ifosfamide, pemetrexed, gefitinib, and imatinib, have undergone formal phase II trials.[80] Cisplatin at doses of 100 mg/m^2 has produced complete responses lasting up to 30 months, but lower doses (50 mg/m^2) have associated response rates of only 10%.[81] In 13 earlier patients, ifosfamide (with mesna) was given at a single dose of 7.5 g/m^2 or as a continuous infusion of 1.5 g/m^2 per day for 5 days every 3 weeks and resulted in five (38.7%) complete and one (7.7%) partial responses.[106] Varying regimens of corticosteroids have shown effectiveness in the treatment of all histologic subtypes of thymoma (with and without myasthenia), with a 77% overall response rate in limited numbers of patients.[82,107,108] Corticosteroids also have been effective for patients unsuccessful with chemotherapy[82]; however, the actual impact may only be on the lymphocytic and not the malignant epithelial component of the tumor.

Combination chemotherapy regimens have shown higher response rates and have been used in both neoadjuvant and metastatic settings in the treatment of advanced invasive, metastatic, and recurrent thymoma. Cisplatin plus doxorubicin-containing regimens appear to be the most active. Fornasiero et al.[93] reported a 43% complete and 91.8% overall response rate with a median survival of 15 months in 37 previously untreated patients with stage III or IV invasive thymoma treated with monthly (median, 5 months) cisplatin, 50 mg/m^2 on day 1; doxorubicin, 40 mg/m^2 on day 1; vincristine, 0.6 mg/m^2 on day 3; and cyclophosphamide, 700 mg/m^2 on day 4. Loehrer et al.[109] documented 10% complete and 50% overall response rates with a median survival of 37.7 months in 29 patients with metastatic or locally progressive recurrent thymoma treated with cisplatin, 50 mg/m^2; doxorubicin, 50 mg/m^2; and cyclophosphamide, 500 mg/m^2, given every 3 weeks for a maximum of eight cycles after radiotherapy. Park et al.[110] retrospectively described 35% complete and 64% overall response rates with a median survival of 67 months in responding and 17 months in nonresponding patients in 17 patients with invasive stage II and IV thymoma initially treated after relapse with cyclophosphamide, doxorubicin, and cisplatin, with or without prednisone. The European Organisation for Research and Treatment of Cancer noted 31% complete and 56% overall response rates with a median survival of 4.3 years in a small study of 16 patients with advanced thymoma treated with cisplatin and etoposide.[111] The addition of ifosfamide to cisplatin and etoposide had a lower than anticipated response rate (approximately 32%) in patients with thymoma and thymic carcinoma in a prospective Eastern Cooperative Oncology Group (ECOG) trial of 28 patients.[90]

ECOG also conducted a prospective trial in patients with thymoma (n = 25) and thymic carcinoma (n = 21) who were treated with carboplatin plus paclitaxel, with a 33% objective response rate for the former group and 24% for the latter.[112] In total, these data suggest higher objective response rates achieved with anthracycline-based regimens.

Combined Modality Approaches

The use of neoadjuvant (induction or preoperative) chemotherapy has been evaluated as part of a multimodality approach to stage III and IV thymoma. Six combined reports document 31% complete and 89% overall response rates in 61 total patients treated with a variety of neoadjuvant chemotherapy regimens (80% cisplatin based).[113] Twenty-two patients (36%) underwent surgery, with 11 (18%) achieving a complete resection (all treated with cisplatin). Nineteen patients were treated with radiotherapy, but only five patients had disease-free survivals exceeding 5 years. Rea et al.[114] reported 43% complete and 100% overall response rates with median and 3-year survival rates of 66 months and 70%, respectively, in 16 stage III and IVa patients treated initially with cisplatin, doxorubicin, vincristine, and cyclophosphamide, followed by surgery. At surgery, 69% were completely resected and the other 31% received postoperative radiation. A recent report from the Amsterdam team noted a 50% objective response rate using the Response Evaluation Criteria in Solid Tumors (RECIST) criteria in 16 patients with locally advanced tumors.[111] Macchiarini et al.[115] reported similar findings. Recently, the Japan Clinical Oncology Group reported a phase II trial (JCOG 9606) that treated 23 patients with unresectable stage III thymoma with 9 weeks of chemotherapy, including cisplatin 25 mg/m^2 on weeks 1 through 9; vincristine 1 mg/m^2 on weeks 1, 2, 4, 6, and 8; and doxorubicin 40 mg/m^2 and etoposide 80 mg/m^2 CODE on days 1 through 3 of weeks 1, 3, 5, 7, and 9.[116] Twelve patients (57%) completed the planned 9-week therapy without mortality. Of 21 eligible patients, zero, 13 (62%), and 7 achieved a complete response, partial response, and stable disease, respectively. Subsequently, 13 (62%) underwent thoracotomies, with 9 (39%) undergoing complete R0 resection and postoperative radiotherapy (48 or 60 Gy in completely or incompletely resected disease, respectively). Progression-free survival at 2 and 5 years was 80% and 43%, respectively, and overall survival at 5 and 8 years was 85% and 69%, respectively. Survival was not improved by surgical resection. Finally, 25% complete (3 patients) and 92% overall response rates (11 patients) with an 83% 7-year disease-free survival rate (10 patients) were reported in only 12 patients at the M.D. Anderson Cancer Center who received cisplatin, doxorubicin, cyclophosphamide, and prednisone induction chemotherapy followed by surgical resection (80% complete) and adjuvant radiotherapy for locally advanced (unresectable) thymoma.[117] The degree of chemotherapy-induced tumor necrosis correlated with Ki-67 expression.

Using two to four cycles of cisplatin, doxorubicin, and cyclophosphamide chemotherapy and sequential radiotherapy (54 Gy), a multi-institutional prospective trial demonstrated a 22% complete and 70% overall response rate. Also noted was a median survival of 93 months and a Kaplan-Meier 5-year failure-free survival rate of 54.3% in 23 patients with stage III (22/23) unresectable thymoma (GETT stage IIIA/IIIB), stage IV (1/23) thymoma, and thymic carcinoma (2/23).[118] Approximately 25% of these patients also had MG. Although these results compare favorably with those obtained with neoadjuvant therapy followed by surgical resection and radiation, further data are required. In summary, postoperative (adjuvant) chemotherapy cannot be recommended based on these data.[41]

Molecularly Targeted Therapy

Molecular profiles of thymic epithelial malignancies have shown some differences between thymoma and thymic carcinoma, but overall, clinically relevant findings are inconsistent.[119] For example, EGFR often is overexpressed in thymic epithelial malignancies, but activating mutations are rare.[119–125] However, with rare case reports of radiographic responses to cetuximab in advanced thymoma,[122,123] a combined-modality phase II trial in locally advanced or recurrent but resectable stage II and IVA patients is now underway (NCT01025089). Other trials with gefitinib as a single agent and erlotinib plus bevacizumab in previously treated patients had minimal activity. Tyrosine–kinase inhibitors also have been investigated. Despite an initial reported brief thymic carcinoma response to imatinib, two subsequent trials in 20 thymic carcinoma patients failed to find any activity.[124] Some antitumor activity has been reported in thymic malignancies with dasatinib, an oral, multitargeted kinase inhibitor of *Bcr-Abl* and *src* kinases; ephrin receptor kinases; platelet-derived growth factor receptor; c-kit; and with sunitinib, another multikinase inhibitor.[125] A phase II sunitinib study in patients with previously treated thymic malignancies is underway (NCT01621568). The histone deacetylase inhibitor, belinostat, has demonstrated a promising 65% control rate (response rate = 5%) in a 41 patient phase II study and currently is being tested in combination with first-line chemotherapy (NCT01100944).[126] Thymus-specific targeted therapy, specifically with somatostatin analogs, has shown promise in small clinical trials.[84] Although the mechanism of action is unclear, inhibition of the insulinlike growth factor or EGFR pathways are possible. Response rates were seen in more than one third (37%) of patients with tumors that were resistant to cytotoxic chemotherapy with octreotide plus prednisone.[84] The median and progression-free survival of 15 months and 14 months, respectively, is encouraging. In thymoma patients with positive radionuclide octreotide scans, 12.5% of the patients demonstrated a partial response to octreotide alone, which increased to 32% with the addition of prednisone.[84]

Thymic Carcinoma

The prognosis of thymic carcinoma is poor because of early metastatic involvement of mediastinal, cervical, and axillary lymph nodes; the pleura; the lungs; the brain; bone; and the liver.[4,92,128] The overall survival rate at 5 years is approximately 35%.[4,26] The recently reported Japanese experience noted a 88.2%, 51.7%, and 37.6% 5-year survival in patients with stages I/II, III, and IV, respectively.[59] Improved survival has been correlated with encapsulated tumors, lobular growth pattern, low mitotic activity, early-stage tumors, low histologic grade, lymphoepitheliomalike histology, and complete surgical resection.[4,87,91,108] Furthermore, in multivariate analysis of SEER data, Masaoka stage and ethnicity emerge as significant determinants of survival in thymic carcinoma patients undergoing complete resection.[108] In addition, patients with stage IVa disease appear to benefit more from treatment than those with more disseminated disease (stage IVb).[88]

THYMIC CARCINOID

Thymic carcinoid tumors are rare, male-predominant tumors that are associated with Cushing syndrome, multiple endocrine neoplasia, and, rarely, carcinoid syndrome.[129–136] Thymic neuroendocrine tumors may be differentiated from similar pulmonary tumors by their different PAX 8 (32% versus 8%) and thyroid transcription factor 1 (TTF-1) (8% versus 76%) staining characteristics.[136] Complete surgical resection with adjuvant radiotherapy for incompletely resected tumors is recommended.[130–133] Chemotherapy rarely has been used.[137,138] Although a 5-year survival rate of 60% has been reported with complete surgical resection,[131] long-term survival is generally poor and is correlated with the extent of disease and the degree of tumor differentiation.[139]

THYMOLIPOMA

Thymolipomas are rare soft, lobulated, and encapsulated benign neoplasms of the anterior mediastinum, which are composed of mature adipose and thymic tissue and account for 1% to 5% of thymic neoplasms.[140] They are also known as *lipothymomas, mediastinal lipomas with thymic remnants*, and *thymolipomatous hamartomas*.[140,141] A review of 27 patients noted an equal gender distribution and a mean age of 27 years.[141] Approximately 50% of patients presented with symptoms of vague chest pain, dyspnea, and tachypnea. Others have reported an association with MG, red cell aplasia, hypogammaglobulinemia, lichen planus, and Graves disease in adult patients, but less often than with thymoma.[140,142–144] They often attain a large size before becoming symptomatic[145] and frequently are found in the anterior–inferior mediastinum "draped along the diaphragm" and connected to the thymus by a small pedicle, conforming to the shape of the cardiac and mediastinal structures.[141] Microscopically, more than 50% consists of adipose tissue with the remainder being thymic tissue, often with calcified Hassall corpuscles.[141] Malignant transformation does not occur. Treatment is a complete resection.[145]

GERM CELL TUMORS

Incidence and Etiology

Mediastinal germ-cell (MGC) neoplasms account for only 2% to 5% of all germinal tumors but constitute 50% to 70% of all extragonadal tumors.[146] Most commonly seen in the anterior mediastinum, they account for 10% to 15% of all primary mediastinal tumors. MGC tumors are most commonly diagnosed in the third decade of life, but patients as old as 60 years of age have been reported. The incidence is equal in all ethnicities. Benign teratomas are the most common MGC tumor, accounting for 70% of the MGC tumors in children and 60% of those in adults. They can occur at any age, but most commonly occur between 20 and 40 years of age. Primary pure mediastinal seminomas account for roughly 35% of malignant MGC tumors and principally arise in men aged 20 to 40 years.[147] Although benign germ-cell tumors have no sex predilection, 90% of adult malignant germ-cell tumors occur in men, with a mean age of 29. Both benign and malignant extragonadal pediatric germ-cell tumors occur with equal sex distribution.

Anatomy and Pathology

Extragonadal germ-cell tumors arise along the body's midline from the cranium (pineal gland) to the presacral area, corresponding to the embryologic urogenital ridge, presumably from aberrantly migrated germ cells.[146] MGC tumors are broadly classified as benign or malignant. Benign tumors include mature teratomas and mixed teratomas with an immature component of less than 50%. Malignant germ-cell tumors are divided into seminomas (dysgerminomas) and nonseminomatous tumors. In addition, MGC tumors have a propensity to develop a component of non–germ-cell malignancy (e.g., rhabdomyosarcoma, adenocarcinoma, permeative neuroectodermal tumor), which can become the predominant histology.

Teratomas

Teratomas contain elements from all three germ-cell layers, with a predominance of the ectodermal component in most tumors, including the skin, hair, sweat glands, sebaceous glands, and teeth. The mesoderm is represented by fat, smooth muscle, bone, and cartilage. Respiratory and intestinal epithelium are often seen as the endodermal component. Teratomas may be solid or cystic in appearance and are often referred to as *dermoid cysts* if unilocular. The majority of mediastinal teratomas are composed of mature ectodermal, mesodermal, and endodermal elements and exhibit a benign course. Immature teratomas, which phenotypically appear as malignant ectodermal, mesodermal, or endodermal tumors, behave aggressively and generally are not responsive to therapy.

Seminomas

Seminomas uncommonly may exist in a pure form, but any elevation of serum AFP levels indicates the presence of at least a small element of nonseminomatous tumor.

Nonseminomatous Tumors

Mediastinal nonseminomatous germ-cell tumors are most commonly found in the anterior mediastinum and appear grossly as invasive, lobulated masses with a thin capsule. Nonseminomatous tumors include embryonal carcinomas, choriocarcinomas, yolk sac tumors, and immature teratomas.[148] They may occur in pure form, but in approximately one third of cases, multiple cell types are present. Other malignant components, including adenocarcinoma, squamous cell carcinoma, small cell undifferentiated carcinoma, neuroblastoma, rhabdomyosarcoma, or other sarcomas, may be present or even predominate, as usually occurs in immature teratomas.[146] Other synchronous hematologic malignancies, such as acute myeloid leukemia, acute nonlymphocytic leukemia, erythroleukemia, myelodysplastic syndrome, malignant histiocytosis, thrombocytosis, and most interestingly, acute megakaryocytic leukemia, also have been reported and may antedate the discovery of the germ-cell tumor. Karyotypic abnormalities, particularly the 47XXY pattern of Klinefelter syndrome, have been found in up to 20% of patients.[149] Of patients, 85% to 95% have systemic disease at the time of diagnosis. Common metastatic sites include the lungs, pleura, lymph nodes, the liver, and, less commonly, bone.[147]

Diagnosis

Many patients with benign tumors, including 50% of teratomas, are asymptomatic; however, 90% to 100% of patients with malignant tumors have symptoms of chest pain, dyspnea, cough, fever, or complaints from compression or invasion of adjacent mediastinal structures.[149,150] Seminomas typically grow slowly and metastasize later than their nonseminomatous counterparts, and they may reach a large size by the time of diagnosis with 20% to 30% remaining asymptomatic until discovered.[147] Symptoms are usually related to their affects on the surrounding mediastinal structures. Pulmonary and other intrathoracic metastases are present in 60% to 70% of patients, whereas extrathoracic metastases usually involve bone.[147]

The determination of serum tumor markers is important in the diagnosis and follow-up of MGC tumors. Immunoassays for serum β-hCG and AFP should be obtained in all patients who have suspicious mediastinal masses. The elevation of β-hCG and AFP confirm a malignant tumor, and AFP (60% to 80%), β-hCG (30% to 50%), or both are elevated in 80% to 85% of nonseminomatous germ-cell tumors.[150] Patients with pure seminoma may have low levels of β-hCG, but AFP is not detected unless a nonseminomatous component also exists. Patients with benign teratomas have normal markers. Isochromosome 12p is diagnostic of undifferentiated germ-cell malignancies even in the absence of elevated serum markers.

MGC tumors typically are detected by standard chest radiographs, which are abnormal in 95% of cases. Most masses are noted in the anterior mediastinum, but 3% to 8% of tumors arise within the posterior mediastinum.[149] Chest CT scans demonstrate large inhomogeneous masses containing areas of hemorrhage and necrosis and also define the extent of disease, the relationship to surrounding structures, and the presence of cystic areas and calcification within the tumor. In teratomas, sonographic patterns may improve the diagnostic accuracy of CT scans alone.[151] Abdominal imaging should be performed to assess for liver metastases. Careful examination of the testes, including a testicular ultrasound, should always be performed; however, a blind testicular biopsy or orchiectomy in patients with normal physical and ultrasound findings is not indicated because an isolated anterior mediastinal mass without retroperitoneal adenopathy is not consistent with a primary testicular tumor.[146] The diagnosis of nonseminomatous germ-cell tumors in young males with anterior mediastinal masses and elevated serum tumor markers (AFP and β-hCG) may be made without a tissue biopsy, and treatment may be initated.[152] If a tissue confirmation is necessary, a core needle biopsy with cytologic staining for tumor markers usually is adequate. Rarely, an open biopsy via an anterior mediastinotomy approach is necessary.[152]

Management by Histology

MGC tumors are not formally staged according to the American Joint Committee on Cancer (AJCC) staging system but can be characterized as localized, locally advanced, and metastatic. Due to the lack of a staging system, these tumors will be discussed by histologic subtype.

Teratoma

Treatment of a mature mediastinal teratoma consists of complete surgical resection, which results in excellent long-term cure rates.[148] The tumor may be adherent to surrounding structures, necessitating resection of the pericardium, pleura, or the lung. Radiotherapy and chemotherapy play no role in the management of this tumor. For teratomas with a malignant component (immature) in patients over 15 years of age, adjuvant cisplatin-based combination chemotherapy (four cycles of cisplatin, etoposide, and bleomycin or vinblastine, ifosfamide, and cisplatin) is recommended. Neoadjuvant chemotherapy may be considered if the tumor is not completely resectable.[148]

Seminoma

The treatment of mediastinal seminoma has evolved since the early 1970s. Seminomas are extremely radiosensitive tumors, and for many years, high-dose mediastinal radiation was used as the definitive therapy, resulting in long-term survival rates of 60% to 80%.[152] Radiation therapy in the extragonadal seminoma, including recommendations for mediastinal and bilateral supraclavicular fields as well as for doses of 35 to 45 Gy was reviewed by Hainsworth.[147]

Mediastinal seminoma, however, often presents as a bulky, extensive, and locally invasive disease, requiring large radiotherapy portals that would result in excessive irradiation of surrounding the normal lung, heart, and other structures. Additionally, 20% to 40% of irradiated patients fail at distant sites.[147] Currently, due to these limitations, only an isolated mediastinal seminoma with minimal disease is managed with radiotherapy alone. Instead, the use of cisplatin-based combination chemotherapy, which was previously used only in advanced gonadal seminoma, is now used as first-line therapy. Lemarie et al.[150] reported that 12 of 13 patients treated experienced complete remission, with only 2 subsequent recurrences. Bokemeyer et al.[153] reported an international analysis of 51 patients with mediastinal seminoma. Chemotherapy was primarily cisplatin based (45, 88%), but carboplatin was also used (3, 5.9%) and had a lower objective response rate (80% versus 93%). In this study, patients were treated with chemotherapy (38, 74.5%), chemotherapy and radiation (10, 19.6%), or radiation alone (3, 5.9%). The progression-free survival and overall survival were 77% and 88%, respectively. Patients with extrathoracic metastases (6, 11.8%) had a worse prognosis. In a collective review of 52 patients by Hainsworth,[147] 14 patients had received prior radiation therapy, but all underwent chemotherapy with cisplatin and various combinations of cyclophosphamide, vinblastine, bleomycin, or etoposide. Complete responses to treatment were noted in 85% of patients, with 83% disease-free long-term survival.

Pure mediastinal seminoma, even with visceral metastases, falls into the intermediate-risk category of the new International Staging System for Germ Cell Tumors, and all patients should be treated with curative intent. Locally advanced and bulky disease should be treated initially with cisplatin-based combination chemotherapy, which is most often four cycles of cisplatin and etoposide with or without supradiaphragmatic radiotherapy. Patients with distant metastases should undergo chemotherapy alone as the initial treatment. Salvage chemotherapy (vinblastine, ifosfamide, and cisplatin) may be required for persistent or recurrent disease.[154]

Despite a recent report of 76.9% long-term survival patients using primary surgical resection followed by adjuvant therapy,[155] most authors believe that surgery does not play a role in the definitive treatment of a seminoma.[152] In addition, surgical debulking of large tumors has not been shown to be of benefit in improving local control or survival.[147]

The management of patients with residual radiographic abnormalities after chemotherapy is controversial. Studies have shown that the residual mass is a dense scirrhous reaction or fibrosis in 85% to 90% of patients, and the presence of a viable seminoma is rare. Others have shown a 25% incidence of residual viable seminoma in these patients treated with chemotherapy followed by resection of residual masses larger than 3 cm.[155] Close observation without surgery is recommended for residual masses after chemotherapy unless the mass enlarges.[147,152] An evaluation with PET scans is superior to CT alone in seminoma patients with a sensitivity and specificity of 80% and 100%, respectively, versus 73% and 73% for CT alone. There were no false-positive scans in lesions larger than 3 cm, and all 11 lesions greater than 3 cm with a residual tumor were PET avid, making this a useful modality to avoid unnecessary surgery and empiric radiation therapy.[147,152]

Nonseminomatous Germ-Cell Tumors

The mainstay of treatment of nonseminomatous germ-cell tumors is cisplatin-based chemotherapy, which is identical to that of gonadal nonseminomatous germ-cell tumors. Overall complete remission rates of 40% to 64% were obtained in most series.[147,148,150,153] In an international review of 287 patients, responses were noted in 178 (64%), and the progression-free and overall survival were 62% and 45%, respectively.[153] Patients with relapsing mediastinal nonseminomatous germ-cell tumors do extraordinarily poorly even with salvage therapy, such as vinblastine, ifosfamide, and cisplatin,[154] with only 9 of 79 patients (11%) becoming disease free in one study.[153] Surgical resection of the residual disease despite persistently elevated tumor markers has been reported by several authors to be beneficial.[155–157]

Prognosis

Immature teratomas are potentially malignant tumors, and their prognosis is influenced by the anatomic site of the tumor, the patient's age, and the fraction of the tumor that is immature.[148] In patients younger than 15 years, immature teratomas behave similarly to their mature counterparts. In older patients, they may behave as highly malignant tumors. Nonseminomatous MGC tumors carry a poorer prognosis than either pure extragonadal seminomas or their gonadal nonseminomatous counterparts. All primary mediastinal nonseminomatous germ-cell tumors fall into the poor-risk category of the International Germ Cell Consensus Classification.[158]

REFERENCES

1. Engels EA, Pfeiffer RM. Malignant thymoma in the United States: demographic patterns in incidence and associations with subsequent malignancies. *Int J Cancer* 2003;105:546–551.
2. Chang C-C, Chang Y-L, Lee Y-C. Thymic carcinoma associated with Sjogren's syndrome and syndrome of inappropriate antidiuretic hormone. *J Thorac Cardiovasc Surg* 2010;139(2):e1–e2.
3. Kadowaki T, Hamada H, Yokoyama A, et al. Thymic carcinoma originating from the mid-posterior mediastinum. *Respirology* 2005;10:689–691.
4. Suster S, Rosai J. Thymic carcinoma: a clinicopathologic study of 60 cases. *Cancer* 1991;67:1025–1032.
5. Tomaszek S, Wigle DA, Keshavjee S, et al. Thymomas: review of current clinical practice. *Ann Thorac Surg* 2009;87:1973–1980.
6. Shimizu K, Yoshida J, Kakegawa S, et al. Primary thymic mucosa-associated lymphoid tissue lymphoma: diagnostic tips. *J Thorac Oncol* 2010;5:117–121.
7. Skandalakis JE, Gray SW, Todd NW. Pharynx and its derivatives. In: Skandalakis JE, Gray SW, eds. *Embryology for Surgeons*, 2nd ed. Baltimore: Williams & Wilkins; 1994.
8. Von Gaudecker B. Functional histology of the human thymus. *Anat Embryol* 1991;183:1–15.
9. Fukai I, Funato Y, Mizuno T, et al. Distribution of thymic tissue in the mediastinal adipose tissue. *J Thorac Cardiovasc Surg* 1991;101:1099–1102.
10. Kazemi S, Kress DC, Gal RA, et al. A rare case of intracardiac thymoma. *Echocardiography* 2006;24:348–349.
11. Tumors of the thymus pathology. In: Hartmann WH (ed) Atlas of Tumor Pathology, Fascicle 13, Series 2. Washington, DC: Armed Forces Institute of Pathology;1976:34–153.
12. Marino M, Muller-Hermelink HK. Thymoma and thymic carcinoma: relation of thymoma epithelial cells to the cortical and medullary differentiation of thymus. *Virchows Arch A Pathol Anat Histopathol* 1985;407:119–149.
13. Kirchner T, Muller-Hermelink H. New approaches to the diagnosis of thymic epithelial tumors. *Prog Surg Pathol* 1989;10:167–189.
14. Quintanilla-Martinez L, Wilkins EW, Choi N, et al. Thymoma: histologic subclassification is an important prognostic factor. *Cancer* 1994;74:606–617.
15. Shimosato Y. Controversies surrounding the subclassification of thymoma. *Cancer* 1994;74:542–544.
16. Suster S, Moran CA. Primary thymic epithelial neoplasms: current concepts and controversies. In: Fechner RE, Rosen PP, eds. *Anatomic Pathology 1997*, Vol 2. Chicago: American Society for Clinical Pathology Press; 1997: 1.
17. Marx A, Muller-Hermelink HK. From basic immunobiology to the upcoming WHO-classification of tumors of the thymus. *Pathol Res Pract* 1999;195:515–533.
18. Rieker RJ, Hoegel J, Morresi-Hauf A, et al. Histologic classification of thymic epithelial tumors: comparison of established classification schemes. *Int J Cancer* 2002;98:900–906.
19. Detterbeck FC. Clinical value of the WHO classification system of thymoma. *Ann Thorac Surg* 2006;81:2328–2334.
20. Suster S, Moran CA. Thymoma classification: current status and future trends. *Am J Clin Pathol* 2006;125:542–554.
21. Patterson GA. Thymomas. *Semin Thorac Cardiovasc Surg* 1992;4:39–44.
22. Masaoka A, Monden Y, Nakahara K, et al. Follow-up study of thymomas with special reference to their clinical stages. *Cancer* 1981;48:2485–2492.
23. Okumura M, Ohta M, Tateyama H, et al. The World Health Organization Histologic Classification System reflects oncologic behavior of thymoma. *Cancer* 2002;94:624–632.
24. Gamondes JP, Balawi A, Greenland T, et al. Seventeen years of surgical treatment of thymoma: factors influencing survival. *Eur J Cardiothorac Surg* 1991;5:124–131.
25. Bedini AV, Andreani SM, Tavecchio L, et al. Proposal of a novel system for the staging of thymic epithelial tumors. *Ann Thorac Surg* 2005;80:1994–2000.
26. Hsu CP, Chan CY, Chen CL, et al. Thymic carcinoma: ten years' experience in twenty patients. *J Thorac Cardiovasc Surg* 1994;107:615–620.
27. Shimizu J, Hayashi Y, Monita K, et al. Primary thymic carcinoma: a clinicopathological and immunohistochemical study. *J Surg Oncol* 1994;56:159–164.
28. Levine GD, Rosai J. Thymic hyperplasia and neoplasia: a review of current concepts. *Hum Pathol* 1978;9:495–515.
29. Weide LG, Ulbright TM, Loehrer PJ, et al. Thymic carcinoma: a distinct clinical entity responsive to chemotherapy. *Cancer* 1993;71:1219–1223.
30. Suster S, Moran CA. Spindle cell thymic carcinoma: clinicopathologic and immunohistochemical study of a distinctive variant of primary thymic epithelial neoplasm. *Am J Surg Pathol* 1999;23:681–700.
31. Marchevsky AM, Gupta R, McKenna RJ, et al. Evidence-based pathology and the pathologic evaluation of thymomas: the World Health Organization classification can be simplified into only 3 categories other than thymic carcinoma. *Cancer* 2008;112:2780–2788.
32. Girard N, Shen R, Guo T, et al. Comprehensive genomic analysis reveals clinically relevant molecular distinctions between thymic carcinomas and thymomas. *Clin Cancer Res* 2009;15:6790–6799.
33. Davis RD, Oldham HN, Sabiston DC. The mediastinum. In: Sabiston DC, Spencer FC, eds. *Surgery of the Chest*. 5th ed. Philadelphia: WB Saunders; 1989.
34. Iwata T, Inoue K, Mizuguchi S, et al. Thymectomy for paraneoplastic stiff-person syndrome associated with invasive thymoma. *J Thorac Cardiovasc Surg* 2006;132:196–197.
35. Rinadi TP, Batocchi AP, Evoli A, et al. Thymic lesions and myasthenia gravis: diagnosis based on mediastinal imaging and pathological findings. *Acta Radiol* 2002;43:380–384.
36. Hengstman GJ, Drost G, Wagenaar M, et al. Persistent increased risk for thymoma in myasthenia gravis associated with myositis. *Muscle Nerve* 2006; 34:251–252.
37. Berrih-Akin S, Morel E, Raimond F, et al. The role of the thymus in myasthenia gravis: immunohistological and immunological studies in 115 cases. *Ann N Y Acad Sci* 1987;505:50–71.
38. Ströbel P, Preisshofen T, Helmreich M, et al. Pathomechanisms of paraneoplastic myasthenia gravis. *Clin Dev Immunol* 2003;10:7–12.
39. Blossom GB, Ernstoff RM, Howells GA, et al. Thymectomy for myasthenia gravis. *Arch Surg* 1993;128:854–862.
40. Lopez-Cano M, Ponseti-Bosch JM, Espin-Basany E, et al. Clinical and pathologic predictors of outcome in thymoma-associated myasthenia gravis. *Ann Thorac Surg* 2003;76:1643–1649.
41. Okereke IC, Kesler KA, Morad MH, et al. Prognostic indicators after surgery for thymoma. *Ann Thorac Surg* 2010;89:1071–1077.
42. Palmieri G, Lastoria S, Cala O, et al. Successful treatment of a patient with a thymoma and pure red cell aplasia with octreotide and prednisone. *N Engl J Med* 1997;336:263–265.
43. Zaucha R, Zaucha JM, Jassem J. Resolution of thymoma-related pure red cell aplasia after octreotide. *Acta Oncologica* 2007;46:864–865.
44. Kelesidis T, Yang O. Good's syndrome remains a mystery after 54 years. A systematic review of the scientific evidence. *Clin Immunol* 2010;135:347–363.
45. Nasseri F, Eftekhari F. Clinical and radiologic review of the normal and abnormal thymus: pearls and pitfalls. *Radiographics* 2010;30:413–428.
46. Bogot NR, Quint LE. Imaging of thymic disorders. *Cancer Imaging* 2005; 5:139–149.
47. Tomiyama H, Muller NL, Ellis SJ, et al. Invasive and noninvasive thymoma: distinctive CT features. *J Comput Assist Tomogr* 2001;25:388–393.
48. Inoue A, Tomiyama N, Fujimoto K, et al. MR imaging of thymic epithelial tumors: correlation with World Health Organization classification. *Radiat Med* 2006;24:171–181.
49. Benveniste MF, Moran CA, Mawlawi O, et al. FDG PET-CT aids in the preoperative assessment of patients with newly diagnosed thymic epithelial malignancies. *J Thorac Oncol* 2013;8:502–510.
50. Lococo F, Cesario A, Okami J, et al. Role of combined (18)F-FDG-PET/CT for predicting theWHO malignancy grade of thymic epithelial tumors: A multicenter analysis. *Lung Cancer* 2013;82:245–251.
51. Thomas A, Mena E, Kurdziel K, et al. 18F-fluorodeoxyglucose positron emission tomography in the management of patients with thymic epithelial tumors. *Clin Cancer Res* 2013;19:1487–1493.
52. Morrissey B, Adams H, Gibbs AR, et al. Percutaneous needle biopsy of the mediastinum: review of 94 procedures. *Thorax* 1993;48:632–637.
53. Bressler EL, Kirkham JA. Mediastinal masses: alternative approaches to CT-guided needle biopsy. *Radiology* 1994;191:391–396.
54. Rendina EA, Venuta F, DeGiacomo T, et al. Comparative merits of thoracoscopy, mediastinoscopy, and mediastinotomy for mediastinal biopsy. *Ann Thorac Surg* 1994;57:992–995.
55. Redina EA, Venuta F, De Giacomo T, et al. Biopsy of anterior mediastinal masses under local anesthesia. *Ann Thorac Surg* 2002;74:1720–1722.
56. Falkson CB, Bezjak A, Darling G, et al. The management of thymoma: a systematic review and practice guideline. *J Thorac Oncol* 2009;4:911–919.
57. Detterbeck F, Giaccone G, Loehrer P, et al. International thymic malignancy interest group. *J Thorac Oncol* 2010;5:1–2.
58. Maggi G, Casadio C, Cavallo A, et al. Thymoma: results of 241 operated cases. *Ann Thorac Surg* 1991;51:152–156.
59. Kondo K, Monden Y. Therapy for thymic epithelial tumors: a clinical study of 1,320 patients from Japan. *Ann Thorac Surg* 2003;76:878–884.
60. Crucitti F, Daghetto GB, Bellantone R, et al. Effects of surgical treatment in thymoma with myasthenia gravis: our experience in 103 patients. *J Surg Oncol* 1992;50:43–46.
61. Cowen D, Mornex RF, Bachelot T, et al. Thymoma: results of a multicentric retrospective series of 149 non-metastatic irradiated patients and review of the literature. *Radiother Oncol* 1995;34:9–16.
62. Liu TJ, Lin MW, Hsieh MS, et al. Video-assisted thoracoscopic surgical thymectomy to treat early thymoma: a comparison with the conventional transsternal approach. *Ann Surg Oncol* 204;21:322–328
63. Marulli G, Rea F, Melfi F, et al. Robot-aided thoracoscopic thymectomy for early-stage thymoma: a multicenter European study. *J Thorac Cardiovasc Surg* 2012;144:1125–1130.
64. Weksler B, Tavares J, Newhook TE, et al. Robot-assisted thymectomy is superior to transsternal thymectomy. *Surg Endosc* 2012;26:261–266.
65. Pollack A, Komaki R, Cox JD, et al. Thymoma: treatment and prognosis. *Int J Radiol Oncol Biol Phys* 1992;23:1037–1043.
66. Latz D, Schraube P, Oppitz U, et al. Invasive thymoma: treatment with postoperative radiation therapy. *Radiology* 1997;204:859–864.
67. Ciernik IF, Meier U, Lutolf UM. Prognostic factors and outcome of incompletely resected invasive thymoma following radiation therapy. *J Clin Oncol* 1994;12:1484–1490.
68. Zhu G, He S, Fu X, et al. Radiotherapy and prognostic factors for thymoma: a retrospective study of 175 patients. *Int J Radiat Oncol Biol Phys* 2004;60:1113–1119.
69. Marks LB. The impact of organ structure on radiation response. *Int J Radiat Oncol Biol Phys* 1996;34:1165–1171.
70. Onuki T, Ishikawa S, Yamamoto T, et al. Pathologic radio response of preoperatively irradiated invasive thymomas. *J Thorac Oncol* 2008;3:270–276.

71. Wright CD, Wain JC, Wong DR, et al. Predictors of recurrence in thymic tumors: importance of invasion, World Health Organization histology, and size. *J Thorac Cardiovasc Surg* 2005;130:1413–1421.
72. D'Angelillo RM, Trodella L, Ramella S, et al. Novel prognostic groups in thymic epithelial tumors: assessment of risk and therapeutic strategy selection. *Int J Radiat Oncol Biol Phys* 2008;71:420–427.
73. Thomas CR Jr, Williams TE, Turrisi AT 3rd. Lung toxicity in the treatment of lung cancer: thoughts at the end of the millennium. In: Meyer J, Karger T, eds. *Radiation Injury: Prevention and Treatment. Frontiers of Radiation Therapy and Oncology*. Basel, Switzerland: Karger Medical and Scientific Publishers; 1999.
74. Kirschner PA. Reoperation for thymoma: report of 23 cases. *Ann Thorac Surg* 1990;49:550–554.
75. Bogart J, Sagerman RH. High-dose hemithorax irradiation in a patient with recurrent thymoma: a study of pulmonary and cardiac radiation tolerance. *Am J Clin Oncol* 1999;22:441–445.
76. Liu H-C, Chen Y-J, Tzen C-Y, et al. Debulking surgery for advanced Thymoma. *Eur J Surg Oncol* 2006;32:1000–1005.
77. Haniuda M, Miyazawa M, Yoshida K, et al. Is postoperative radiotherapy for thymoma effective? *Ann Surg* 1996;224:219–224.
78. Urgesi A, Monetti U, Rossi G, et al. Aggressive treatment of intrathoracic recurrences of thymoma. *Radiother Oncol* 1992;24:221–225.
79. Mornex F, Resbeut M, Richard P, et al. Radiotherapy and chemotherapy for invasive thymomas: a multicentric retrospective review of 90 cases. *Int J Radiat Oncol Biol Phys* 1995;32:651–659.
80. Schmitt J, Loehrer PJ. The role of chemotherapy in advanced thymoma. *J Thorac Oncol* 2010;5:357–360.
81. Bonomi PD, Finkelstein D, Aisner S, et al. EST 2582 Phase II trial of cisplatin in metastatic or recurrent thymoma. *Am J Clin Oncol* 1993;16:342–345.
82. Kobayashi Y, Fujii Y, Yano M, et al. Preoperative steroid pulse therapy for invasive thymoma: clinical experience and mechanism of action. *Cancer* 2006;106:1901–1907.
83. Hammond-Thelin LA, Thomas CR Jr. Systemic therapeutic options in thymic malignancies: a glimmer of hope. *Rev Recent Clin Trials* 2007;2:191–205.
84. Loehrer PJ Sr, Wang W, Johnson DH, et al. Octreotide alone or with prednisone in patients with advanced thymoma and thymic carcinoma: an Eastern Cooperative Oncology Group phase II trial. *J Clin Oncol* 2004;22:293–299.
85. Ionescu DN, Sasatomi E, Ciepley K, et al. Protein expression and gene amplification of epidermal growth factor receptor in thymomas. *Cancer* 2005;103:630–636.
86. Strobel P, Hartmann M, Jakob A, et al. Thymic carcinoma with overexpression of mutated KIT and the response to imatinib. *N Engl J Med* 2004;350:2625–2626.
87. Pan CC, Chen PC, Chiang H. KIT (CD117) is frequently overexpressed in thymic carcinomas but is absent in thymomas. *J Pathol* 2004;202:375–381.
88. Lin J-T, Wei-Shu W, Yen C-C, et al. Stage IV thymic carcinoma: a study of 2-patients. *Am J Med Sci* 2005;330:172–175.
89. Magois E, Guigay J, Blancard PS, et al. Multimodal treatment of thymic carcinoma: report of nine cases. *Lung Cancer* 2008;59:126–132.
90. Loehrer PJ, Jiroutek M, Aisner S, et al. Phase II trial of etoposide (V), ifosfamide (I), plus cisplatin (P) in patients with advanced thymoma (T) or thymic carcinoma (TC): preliminary results from a ECOG coordinated intergroup trial. *Proc Am Soc Clin Oncol* 1998;17:30 (abst 118).
91. Liu H, Hsu W, Chen Y, et al. Primary thymic carcinoma. *Ann Thorac Surg* 2002;73:1076–1081.
92. Yano T, Hara N, Ichinose Y, et al. Treatment and prognosis of primary thymic carcinoma. *J Surg Oncol* 1993;52:255–258.
93. Fornasiero A, Danilele O, Ghiotto C, et al. Chemotherapy for invasive thymoma: a 13 year experience. *Cancer* 1991;68:30–33.
94. Nieto IP, Robledo JP, Pajuelo MC, et al. Prognostic factors for myasthenia gravis treated by thymectomy: review of 61 cases. *Ann Thorac Surg* 1999;67:1568–1571.
95. Fang W, Chen W, Chen G, et al. Surgical management of thymic epithelial tumors: a retrospective review of 204 cases. *Ann Thorac Surg* 2005;80:2002–2007.
96. Kang M-W, Lee E-S, Jo J, et al. Stage III thymic epithelial neoplasms are not homogeneous with regard to clinical, pathological, and prognostic features. *J Thorac Oncol* 2009;4:1561–1567.
97. Quintanilla-Martinez L, Wilkins EW Jr, Ferry JA, et al. Thymoma: morphologic subclassification correlates with invasiveness and immunohistologic features. A study of 122 cases. *Hum Pathol* 1993;24:958–969.
98. Harris N. Classification of thymic epithelial neoplasms. In: Marx A, Muller-Hermelink HK, eds. *Epithelial Tumors of the Thymus. Pathology, Biology, Treatment*. New York: Plenum; 1997:1.
99. Mangi AA, Wain JC, Donahue DM, et al. Adjuvant radiation therapy of stage III thymoma: is it necessary? *Ann Thorac Surg* 2005;79:1834–1839.
100. Utsumi T, Shiono H, Kadota Y, et al. Postoperative radiation therapy after complete resection of thymoma has little impact on survival. *Cancer* 2009;115:5413–5420.
101. Korst RJ, Kansler AL, Christos PJ, et al. Adjuvant radiotherapy for thymic epithelial tumors: a systematic review and meta-analysis. *Ann Thorac Surg* 2009;87:1641–1647.
102. Forquer JA, Rong N, Fakiris AJ, et al. Postoperative radiotherapy after surgical resection of thymoma: differing roles in localized and regional disease. *Int J Radiat Oncol Biol Phys* 2010;76:440–445.
103. Chen YD, Feng QF, Lu HZ, et al. Role of adjuvant radiotherapy for stage II thymoma after complete tumor resection. *Int J Radiat Oncol Biol Phys* 2010;78:1400–1406.
104. Berman AT, Litzky L, Livolsi V, et al. Adjuvant radiotherapy for completely resected stage 2 thymoma. *Cancer* 2011;117:3502–3508.
105. Weksler B, Shende M, Nason KS, et al. The role of adjuvant radiation therapy for resected stage III thymoma: a population-based study. *Ann Thorac Surg* 2012;93:1822–1828.
106. Harper P, Highly M, Rankin E, et al. Treatment of invasive thymoma with single-agent ifosfamide. *J Clin Oncol* 1999;17:2737–2744.
107. Tomiak EM, Evans WK. The role of chemotherapy in invasive thymoma: a review of the literature and considerations for future clinical trials. *Crit Rev Oncol Hematol* 1993;15:113–124.
108. Kirkove C, Berghmans J, Noel H, et al. Dramatic response of recurrent invasive thymoma to high dose corticosteroids. *Clin Oncol (R Coll Radiol)* 1992;4:64–66.
109. Loehrer PJ, Kim KM, Aisner SC, et al. Cisplatin plus doxorubicin plus cyclophosphamide in metastatic or recurrent thymoma: final results of an intergroup trial. *J Clin Oncol* 1994;12:1164–1168.
110. Park HS, Shin DM, Lee JS, et al. Thymoma: a retrospective study of 87 cases. *Cancer* 1994;73:2491.
111. Giaccone G, Ardizzoni A, Kirkpatrick A, et al. Cisplatin and etoposide combination chemotherapy for locally advanced or metastatic thymoma. A phase II study of the European Organization for Research and Treatment of Lung Cancer Cooperative Group. *J Clin Oncol* 1996;14:814–820.
112. Lemma GL, Loehrer PJ, Lee JW, et al. A phase II study of carboplatin plus paclitaxel in advanced thymoma and thymic carcinoma: E1C99. *J Clin Oncol* 2008;26:(abst 8018).
113. Tomiak EM, Evans WK. The role of chemotherapy in invasive thymoma: a review of the literature and considerations for future clinical trials. *Crit Rev Oncol Hematol* 1993;15:113–124.
114. Rea F, Sartori F, Lay M, et al. Chemotherapy and operation for invasive thymoma. *J Cardiovasc Surg* 1993;106:543–549.
115. Macchiarini P, Chella A, Ducci F, et al. Neoadjuvant chemotherapy, surgery and postoperative radiation therapy for invasive thymoma. *Cancer* 1991;68:706–713.
116. Kunitoh H, Tamura T, Shibata T, et al. A phase II trial of dose-dense chemotherapy followed by surgical resection and/or thoracic radiotherapy in locally advanced thymoma: report of a Japan Clinical Oncology Group trial (JCOG 9606). *Br J Cancer* 2010;103:6–11.
117. Shin DM, Walsh GL, Komaki R, et al. A multidisciplinary approach to therapy for unresectable malignant thymoma. *Ann Intern Med* 1998;129:100–104.
118. Papadopoulos KP, Thomas CR Jr. Current chemotherapy options for thymic epithelial neoplasms. *Expert Opinion Pharmacother* 2005;6:1169–1177.
119. Girard N, Shen R, Guo T, et al. Comprehensive genomic analysis reveals clinically relevant molecular distinctions between thymic carcinomas and thymomas. *Clin Cancer Res* 2009;15:6790–6799.
120. Kelly RJ, Petrini I, Rajan A, et al. Thymic malignancies: from clinical management to targeted therapies. *J Clin Oncol* 2011;29:4820–4827.
121. Suzuki E, Sasaki H, Kawano O, et al. Expression and mutation statuses of epidermal growth factor receptor in thymic epithelial tumors. *Jpn J Clin Oncol* 2006;36:351–356.
122. Farina G, Garassino MC, Gambacorta M, et al. Response of thymoma to cetuximab. *Lancet Oncol* 2007;8:449–450.
123. Palmieri G, Marino M, Salvatore M, et al. Cetuximab is an active treatment of metastatic and chemorefractory thymoma. *Front Biosci* 2007;12:757–761.
124. Giaccone G, Rajan A, Ruijfer R, et. al. Imatinib mesylate in patients with WHO B3 thymomas and thymic carcinomas. *J Thorac Oncol* 2009;4:1270–1273.
125. Ströbel P, Bargou R, Wolff A, et al. Sunitinib in metastatic thymic carcinomas: laboratory findings and initial clinical experience. *Br J Cancer* 2010;103:196–200.
126 Giaccone G, Rajan A, Berman A, et al. Phase II study of belinostat in patients with recurrent or refractory advanced thymic epithelial tumors. *J Clin Oncol* 2011;29:2052–2059.
127. Henley JD, Koukoulis GK, Loehrer PJ Sr. Epidermal growth factor receptor expression in invasive thymoma. *J Cancer Res Clin Oncol* 2002;128:167–170.
128. Kong D-S, Lee J-I, Nam DH, et al. Cerebral involvement of metastatic thymic carcinoma. *J Neurooncol* 2005;75:143–147.
129. Rosai J, Higa E. Mediastinal endocrine neoplasm of probable thymic origin related to carcinoid tumors. *Cancer* 1972;29:1061–1074.
130. Wang DY, Chang DB, Kuo SH, et al. Carcinoid tumors of the thymus. *Thorax* 1994;49:357–360.
131. Vietri F, Illuminati R, Guglielmi R, et al. Carcinoid tumor of the thymus gland. *Eur J Surg* 1994;160:645–647.
132. Gibril F, Chen YJ, Schrump DS, et al. Prospective study of thymic carcinoids in patients with multiple endocrine neoplasia type 1. *J Clin Endocrinol Metab* 2003;88:1066–1081.
133. Asbun HJ, Calabria RP, Calmes S, et al. Thymic carcinoid. *Am Surg* 1991;57:442–445.
134. Zeiger MA, Swartz SE, Macgillivary DC, et al. Thymic carcinoid in association with MEN syndromes. *Am Surg* 1992;58:430–434.
135. Chaer R, Massad MG, Evans E, et al. Primary neuroendocrine tumors of the thymus. *Ann Thorac Surg* 2002;74:1733–1740.
136. Weissferdt A, Tang X, Wistuba II, et al. Comparative immunohistochemical analysis of pulmonary and thymic neuroendocrine carcinomas using PAX8 and TTF-1. *Mod Pathol* 2013;26:1554–1560.
137. Tiffet O, Nicholson AG, Landas G, et al. A clinicopathologic study of 12 neuroendocrine tumors arising in the thymus. *Chest* 2003;124:141–146.
138. Ferolla P, Falchetti A, Filooso P, et al. Thymic neuroendocrine carcinoma (carcinoid) in multiple endocrine neoplasia type 1 syndrome: the Italian series. *J Clin Endocrinol Metab* 2005;90:2603–2609.

139. Moran CA, Suster S. Neuroendocrine carcinomas (carcinoid tumor) of the thymus. *Am J Clin Pathol* 2000;114:100–110.
140. McManus KG, Allen MS, Trastek VF, et al. Lipothymoma with red cell aplasia, hypogammaglobulinemia and lichen planus. *Ann Thorac Surg* 1994; 58:1534–1536.
141. Rosado-de-Christenson ML, Pugatch RD, Moran CA, et al. Thymolipoma: analysis of 27 cases. *Radiology* 1994;193:121–126.
142. Litano Y, Yokomari K, Ohkura M, et al. Giant thymolipoma in a child. *J Pediatr Surg* 1993;28:1622–1625.
143. Zambudio AR, Lanzas JT, Roca Calvo MJ, et al. Thymolipomas in association with myasthenia gravis. *J Thorac Cardiovasc Surg* 2001;122:825–826.
144. Kilic D, Giray S, Bolat FA, et al. A rare combination of thymic tumor: radiologically invisible thymolipoma associated with myasthenia gravis. *Neurol India* 2006;54:322–324.
145. Jiang X, Fang Y, Wang G. Images in cardiothoracic surgery. Giant thymolipoma involving both chest cavities. *Ann Thorac Surg* 2009;87:1960.
146. Nichols CR, Fox EP. Extragonadal and pediatric germ cell tumors. *Hematol Oncol Clin North Am* 1991;5:1189–1209.
147. Hainsworth JD, Greco FA. Extragonadal germ cell tumors and unrecognized germ cell tumors. *Semin Oncol* 1992;19:119–127.
148. Dulmet EM, Macchiarini P, Suc B, et al. Germ cell tumors of the mediastinum: a 30-year experience. *Cancer* 1993;72:1894–1901.
149. Luna M, Valenzuela-Tamaritz J. Germ-cell tumors of the mediastinum, postmortem findings. *Am J Clin Pathol* 1976;65:450–454.
150. Lemarié E, Assouline PS, Diot P, et al. Primary mediastinal germ cell tumors. Results of a French retrospective study. *Chest* 1992;102:1477–1483.
151. Wu TT, Wang HC, Chang YC, et al. Mature mediastinal teratoma: sonographic imaging patterns and pathologic correlation. *J Ultrasound Med* 2002; 21:759–765.
152. Ginsberg RJ. Mediastinal germ cell tumors: the role of surgery. *Semin Thorac Cardiovasc Surg* 1992;4:51–54.
153. Bokemeyer C, Nichols CR, Draz J, et al. Extragonadal germ cell tumors of the mediastinum and retroperitoneum: results from an international analysis. *J Clin Onocol* 2002;20:1864–1873.
154. Becherer A, De Santis M, Karanikas G, et al. FDG PET is superior to CT in the prediction of viable tumour in post-chemotherapy seminoma residuals. *Eur J Radiol* 2005;54:284–288.
155. Hartmann JT, Einhorn L, Nichols CR, et al. Second-line chemotherapy in patients with relapsed extragonadal nonseminomatous germ cell tumors: results of an international multicenter analysis. *J Clin Oncol* 2001;19:1641–1648.
156. Nakamura Y, Matsumura A, et al. Cisplatin-based chemotherapy followed by surgery for malignant nonseminomatous germ cell tumor of mediastinum: one institution's experience. *Gen Thorac Cardiovasc Surg* 2009;57:363–368.
157. Kesler KA, Einhorn LH. Multimodality treatment of germ cell tumors of the mediastinum.*Thorac Surg Clin* 2009;19:63–69.
158. International Germ Cell Consensus Classification: a prognostic factor-based staging system for metastatic germ cell cancers. International Germ Cell Cancer Collaborative Group. *J Clin Oncol* 1997;15:594–603.

40 Benign and Malignant Mesothelioma

Harvey I. Pass, Michele Carbone, Lee M. Krug, and Kenneth E. Rosenzweig

INTRODUCTION

Malignant mesotheliomas (MM) are highly aggressive neoplasms that arise primarily from the surface serosal cells of the pleural, peritoneal, and pericardial cavities. The disease is characterized by a long latency from the time of exposure to asbestos to the onset of disease, suggesting that multiple somatic genetic events are required for tumorigenic conversion of a normal mesothelial cell.

MECHANISM OF ASBESTOS CARCINOGENESIS

There are six types of asbestos: amosite, crocidolite, anthophyllite, actinolite, tremolite, and chrysotile.[1] The five types other than chrysotile are termed *amphibole asbestos*. Several nonasbestos minerals (e.g., erionite, wincherite) are very similar to asbestos structurally and chemically and are also capable of causing mesothelioma in humans. The mechanisms responsible for asbestos carcinogenicity are linked to the secretion of tumor necrosis factor (TNF)-alpha by mesothelial cells and macrophages exposed to asbestos that in turn leads to NFκB activation.[2] The activation of the NFκB pathway in mesothelial cells allows them to survive the toxic insult and the genetic damage caused by asbestos, and these damaged but viable cells may proliferate into a mesothelioma.[2]

Animal Models of Asbestos Carcinogenicity

Mesotheliomas and sarcomas are induced in a dose-dependent fashion after intrapleural and intraperitoneal injection of asbestos into animals.[3–5] Chronic inhalational studies are thought to be the best representation of asbestos carcinogenicity. Because of the cost of these experiments, however, very few have been performed.

Asbestos Carcinogenicity in Humans

Although injection and inhalation studies in animals suggest that all forms of asbestos are equally carcinogenic and that there is a clear dose-response relationship between asbestos exposure and mesothelioma risk, epidemiologic studies in humans do not support these observations. The proportion of mesotheliomas that are thought to be associated with asbestos varies in the literature from 16% to 90%.[1] Although this wide range may reflect the distinct populations studied, it is more likely a result of the different methodologies used to determine exposure rates.[1] Most human studies have indicated that amosite and crocidolite exposure carry a much greater risk than exposure to chrysotile.[6,7] Chrysotile, however, is frequently combined with tremolite, an amphibole, that may instead be responsible for mesothelioma development.[8]

In humans, there is no clear dose-response curve to asbestos, and a threshold level below which mesotheliomas do not develop has not been determined, although it is generally accepted in the scientific community that background levels of exposure, such as those found in the lungs of almost all individuals, do not increase the risk of mesothelioma. It is estimated that <5% of asbestos miners exposed to high levels of asbestos develop mesotheliomas[1]; however, wives of some of these workers have developed mesotheliomas after they were presumably exposed to lower levels of asbestos compared to their husbands while washing their clothes.[9,10] Similarly, mesothelioma development commonly occurs in workers in occupations in which asbestos exposure is higher than in the general population, but much lower than in asbestos miners. The carpenters, electricians, and construction workers who have developed mesotheliomas are a reflection of this.[11] These data suggest that high levels of exposure are not necessarily correlated with increased risk of malignancy compared to moderate asbestos exposure, arguing against a classic dose-response relationship.[1]

Mechanism of Asbestos Pathogenicity

It is thought that when fibers reach the alveoli after inhalation, smaller fibers are phagocytized and efficiently removed from the lung. Larger fibers are not easily engulfed and can usually only be removed if solubilized. However, amphiboles are not soluble and thus remain in the lung. These fibers may eventually reach the pleura via the lymphatics or direct extension, where they may lead to pleural plaques, fibrosis, and mesothelioma. In the pleura, asbestos fibers may cause mutagenic changes through hydroxy radical and superoxide anion production during phagocytosis, leading to DNA strand breaks and deletions. Most recently, data implicating necrosis in the genesis of mesothelioma have been reported in which the release of HMGB1 is necessary as a critical initial step in the pathogenesis of asbestos-related disease and provides a mechanistic link between asbestos-induced cell death, chronic inflammation, and mesothelial carcinogenesis.[12] Inflammation due to asbestos deposition contributes to asbestos carcinogenesis.[2,13,14] Phagocytic macrophages at these sites of inflammation internalize asbestos and release mutagenic reactive oxygen species and numerous cytokines including TNF-α and interleukin (IL)-1, which have been linked to asbestos-related carcinogenesis.[2,15] By inducing cell necrosis, asbestos causes the release of HMGB1,[12] a typical damage-associated molecular pattern[16,17] and a key mediator of inflammation.[18] Activation of Nalp3 inflammasome ensues with subsequent IL-1β secretion, a process that is enhanced by asbestos-induced production of reactive oxygen species.[19,20] Additionally, HMGB1 is released by reactive macrophages, other inflammatory cells, and human mesothelial cells (HMC[12]) upon exposure to asbestos. HMGB1 is a critical regulator in the initiation of asbestos-mediated inflammation leading to the release of TNF-α and subsequent NF-κB signaling[12] (Fig. 40.1). During programmed necrosis, HMGB1 translocates from the nucleus to the cytosol and the extracellular space, where it binds several proinflammatory molecules and triggers the inflammatory responses that distinguish this type of cell death from apoptosis. Secreted

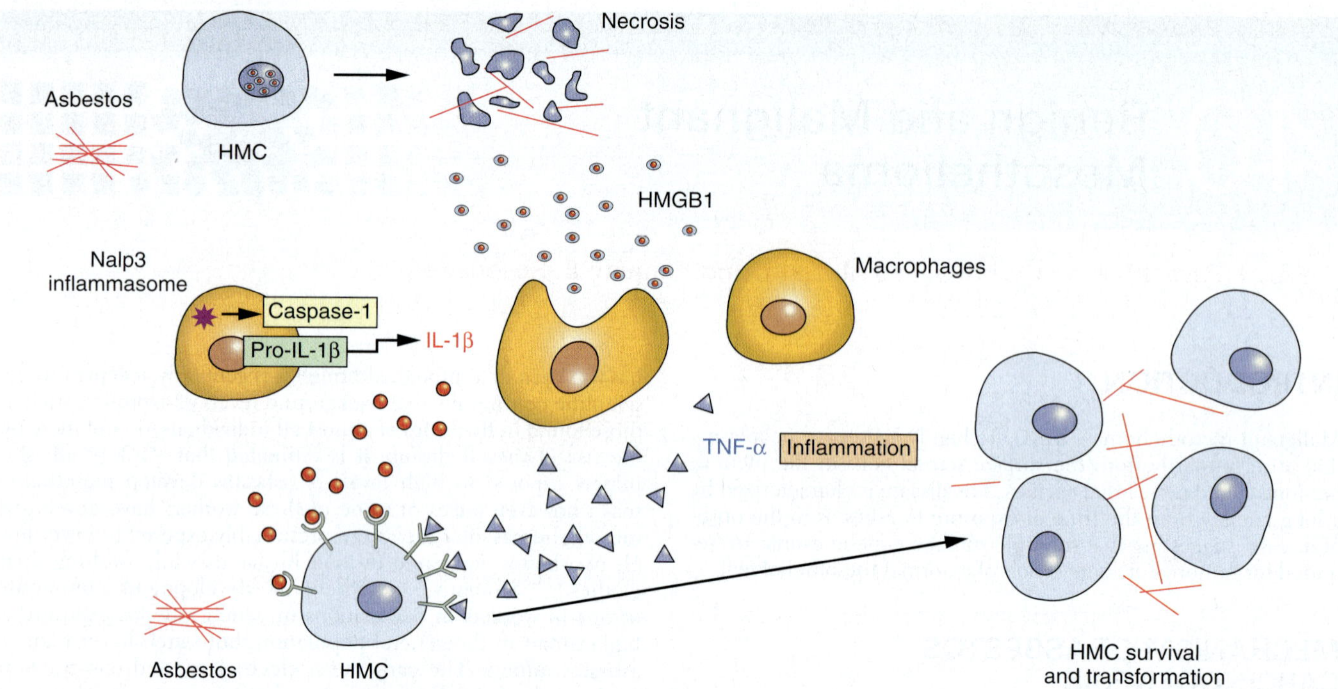

Figure 40.1 Working hypothesis for mesothelioma carcinogenesis. Asbestos causes necrotic human mesothelial cell (*HMC*) death, leading to the release of HMGB1 into the extracellular space. As a typical damage-associated molecular pattern and a key mediator of inflammation, HMGB can induce activation of Nalp3 inflammasome and subsequent interleukin (*IL*)-1β secretion, as well as eliciting macrophage accumulation and triggering the inflammatory response and tumor necrosis factor–α secretion, which increases the survival of asbestos-damaged HMCs. This allows key genetic alterations to accumulate within HMCs that sustain asbestos-induced DNA damage, leading to the initiation of mesothelioma.

HMGB1 stimulates RAGE, TLR2, and TLR4 (the three main HMGB1 receptors) expressed on neighboring inflammatory cells such as macrophages and induces the release of several inflammatory cytokines, including TNF-α and IL-1β. TNF-α–induced NF-κB signaling has been shown to be a critical link between inflammation and carcinogenesis in multiple cancer models, including mesothelioma.[2] Specifically, asbestos-mediated TNF-α signaling induces the activation of NF-κB–dependent mechanisms, promoting the survival of HMCs after asbestos exposure,[2] and thus allowing HMCs with accumulated asbestos-induced genetic damage to survive, divide, and propagate genetic aberrations in premalignant cells that can give rise to a malignant clone. In addition, HMGB1 enhances the activity of NF-κB, which promotes tumor formation, progression, and metastasis.[21] An investigation into the targeting of extracellular HMGB1 as a novel strategy for mesothelioma prevention and/or therapy is currently under way.[22]

It is difficult to reconcile what is known about the carcinogenic actions of asbestos and the long latency period between asbestos exposure and mesothelioma development. Lanphear and Buncher[23] reviewed 21 studies of 1,690 mesotheliomas and found that 96% occurred at least 20 years after exposure; the mean latency was 32 years. Several theories have been postulated to describe what happens during this latency period.[24] It is widely believed that asbestos induces genetic alterations in mesothelial cells over a long period that eventually lead to malignant cells. This may occur if a key regulatory gene, such as the *INK4a/ARF* locus, is deleted or silenced. With loss of key regulatory genes, additional mutations could accumulate rapidly. INK4a/ARF codes for p16 (a cyclin-dependent kinase inhibitor) and for p14ARF, which promotes murine double minute-2 degradation, preventing murine double minute-2 from neutralizing p53. Both p16 and p14ARF are often deleted in MM (see "Alterations of Specific Tumor Suppressor Genes in Mesothelioma"). This process may allow enough mutations to accumulate to lead to malignancy. Cell growth from this point would be rapid, leading to a clinically detectable tumor.[1]

OVERVIEW OF MOLECULAR MECHANISMS IN MESOTHELIOMA

Cytogenetic Assessment of Malignant Mesotheliomas

Deletions of specific chromosomal sites in the short (p) arms of chromosomes 1, 3, and 9, and long (q) arm of 6 are repeatedly observed in these tumors. Using newer molecular platforms including array comparative genomic hybridization and representational oligonucleotide microarray analysis, deletions in chromosomes 22q12.2, 19q13.32, and 17p13.1 appear to be the most frequent events (55% to 74%), followed by deletions in 1p, 9p, 9q, 4p, and 3p, and gains in 5p, 18q, 8q, and 17q (23% to 55%). Increasing numbers of copy number abnormalities in mesothelioma are associated with poor prognosis, especially when associated with deletions in 9p21.3 encompassing CDKN2A/ARF and CDKN2B, as detailed later.[24] Analysis of the minimal common areas of frequent gains and losses has pointed to novel potential tumor suppressor genes (TSG) including OSM (22q12.2), FUS1, PL6 (3p21.3), DNAJA1 (9p21.1), and CDH2 (18q11.2–q12.3).[25]

Alterations of Specific Tumor Suppressor Genes in Mesothelioma

p16

Cheng et al.[26] reported homozygous deletions of one or more of the three *p16* exons in 34 of 40 (85%) malignant mesothelioma cell lines and a point mutation in one cell line. Downregulation of *p16* was observed in four of the remaining cell lines. Homozygous deletions of *p16* were identified in 5 of 23 (22%) malignant mesothelioma tumor samples. Downregulation of *p16* in malignant mesothelioma cells may result from 5′CpG island hypermethylation, as has been demonstrated in other types of cancer. *P16* inactivation by homozygous deletions or methylation is a frequent event in Japanese patients with malignant pleural mesotheliomas (MPM).[27] Homozygous deletion is the major cause of the *P16* inactivation,[28] but methylation also leads to the inactivation of *P16* when the *P16* alleles are retained.[27] Homozygous deletions at this locus can lead to the inactivation of another putative TSG, *p14*ARF, because *p16* and *p14*ARF share exons 2 and 3 although their reading frames differ.[29,30] The prognostic significance of p16/CDKN2A loss in MM has been defined both by immunohistochemistry and fluorescence in situ hybridization (FISH). With the FISH analysis of primary MM tissue samples or MM cells from the pleural effusion, over 70% of cases showed homozygous deletions of the *CDKN2A/ARF* locus. Both loss of p16 protein expression by immunohistochemistry and homozygous deletion of p16 by FISH are associated with an adverse prognosis.[31] Loss of p15 is also associated with codeletion of microRNA (miR)-31.[32] Protein phosphatase (PPP6C), upregulated in MPM, is a target of mir-31, and reintroduction of miR-31 in mesothelioma cells has a suppressive effect on MM cells.[32]

p53

Cell lines derived from murine models of asbestos-induced mesothelioma have reduced or absent expression of p53 messenger RNA (mRNA) compared to the RNA from nontumorigenic cell lines or reactive mesothelial cells.[33] In human cell lines derived from patients with malignant mesothelioma, attention has turned to specific mutations or genetic abnormalities in *p53*. In general, mutational analyses of *p53* in mesothelioma have not revealed reasons for its inactivation.

Wilms Tumor Gene

The detection of Wilms tumor gene (*WT1*) mRNA or protein provides a specific molecular or immunohistochemical marker for differentiation of mesothelioma from other pleural tumors, in particular adenocarcinoma.[34] Vaccination protocols that exploit the selective presence of *WT1* in mesothelioma are under way at selected institutions.[35]

Neurofibromatosis Gene

The tumor suppressor merlin is encoded by the neurofibromatosis type 2 gene (*NF2*), which is located on chromosome 22q12, and mutations in this gene have been found in 40% of mesothelioma and 50% of malignant mesothelioma cell lines.[36,37] Mutations including deletions and insertions lead to truncated and inactivated merlin. Experimental animal models indicate that disruption of the *NF2* signaling pathway, together with a deficiency in *ink4a*, is essential for mesothelioma development.[38]

ALTERATIONS OF ONCOGENES IN MESOTHELIOMA

C-sis (Platelet-Derived Growth Factor)

Malignant mesothelioma cell lines produce numerous growth factors and cytokines, possibly as a consequence of altered oncogene status. One of the more intriguing oncogenes in malignant mesothelioma is C-sis, which codes for one of the two chains (alpha and beta) of platelet-derived growth factor (PDGF). Gerwin et al.[39] were the first to describe elevation of RNA levels for both chains of PDGF in mesothelioma cell lines and correlated the increase with PDGF-like activity secreted by the cells. It is of interest that overexpression of A chain transforms human mesothelial cells to the tumorigenic phenotype in vitro and that the use of antisense ODN to the A chain inhibits growth of mesothelioma cell lines. PDGF-D promotes mesothelioma cell proliferation by targeting ROCK or MAP kinase through autocrine activation of PDGF-beta receptor[40]; however, in general, therapies targeting PDGF in mesothelioma have been unsuccessful.[41]

Transforming Growth Factor

Transforming growth factor-B (TGF-B) is another growth-regulatory and immunomodulatory cytokine, and high levels of TGF-B have been described in several human and mouse malignant mesothelioma cell lines.[42,43] TGF-B may have a potential role in regulation of the differential PDGF receptor expression in malignant mesothelioma and thus have an effect on proliferation as well as other events. TGF-B production by tumors plays a significant role in blocking immune response by preventing T-cell infiltration into tumors, inhibition of T-cell activation/function, and mediation of T regulatory cell–induced immunosuppression. TGF-blockers (soluble receptors/antibodies) and receptor inhibitors have antitumor effects that, in several models, are due primarily to immunologic mechanisms. TGF blockade had antitumor effects that were CD8+ T-cell dependent in a murine malignant mesothelioma model.[44] Recently, it was reported that a combined triple treatment of anti-CD25 monoclonal antibody, anti–cytotoxic T-lymphocyte antigen-4 monoclonal antibody and TGF-beta soluble receptor resulted in long-term clearance of MPM tumors and memory against tumor rechallenge.[45]

Insulin Growth Factor

Insulin growth factor (IGF) is another of the important autocrine loops in mesothelioma.[46] The IGF receptor-1 pathway is a significant regulator of mesothelioma growth acting through downstream kinases such as Akt. In humans, both normal mesothelium and mesothelioma cell lines express IGF-1 and IGF-1R RNAs (by Northern blot or reverse transcriptase polymerase chain reaction), and IGF-1 protein is detected in their conditioned media. These studies suggest that mesothelioma growth, both in human and animal models for the disease, may involve the IGFs, and trials using anti-IGF-1R antibodies or small-molecule IGF blockade are being formulated for mesothelioma.[47] Cixutumumab, a humanized monoclonal antibody to IGF-IR, has been investigated using early passage tumor cells and an in vivo human mesothelioma tumor xenograft model. Cixutumumab induced antibody-dependent cell-mediated toxicity and in vivo, cixutumumab treatment delayed growth of H226 mesothelioma tumor xenografts in mice and improved the overall survival of these mice compared to controls.[48] A phase 2 clinical trial of cixutumumab is currently ongoing for the treatment of patients with mesothelioma.

Angiogenic Mechanisms in Mesothelioma

The most relevant cytokines and growth factors in angiogenic pathways involve the ILs (specifically IL-6 and IL-8), fibroblast growth factors (FGF), vascular endothelial growth factors (VEGF), platelet-derived endothelial growth factors, and IGFs. Moreover, mutational or posttranslational silencing of TSGs or their products, particularly *p53* and *p16*, has also been associated with increased angiogenic mechanisms.

IL-6 levels are elevated in the serum and pleural effusions of patients with mesothelioma, and there have been correlations seen between the IL-6 level and the degree of thrombocytosis in these patients.[49] IL-6 expression is elevated in tissues undergoing angiogenesis, but by itself it has a limited role in proliferation of endothelial cells. IL-6, however, induces angiogenesis by elevating the expression of VEGF, a specific mitogen for vascular endothelial cells. Serum VEGF and IL-6 levels are elevated in patients with mesothelioma, and their levels each correlate with platelet count.[50] IL-8 is also an important angiogenic factor for the development of new capillaries in vivo and has direct growth-potentiating activity in mesothelioma. Pleural fluid from patients with mesothelioma has significantly higher IL-8 levels by enzyme-linked assay compared to patients with other malignant effusions.[51] Mesotheliomas present with a high intratumoral vessel density that also have prognostic relevance,[42,52,53] and immunohistochemically, VEGF, FGF-1 and -2, and TGF-B immunoreactivity are present in 81%, 67%, 92%, and 96%, respectively, of mesotheliomas, and in 20%, 50%, 40%, and 10%, respectively, of samples of the nonneoplastic mesothelium. Depending on the study, high immunohistochemical FGF-2 expression[53] or VEGF expression by reverse transcriptase polymerase chain reaction correlate with more tumor aggressiveness and worse prognosis for mesothelioma.[52,54]

Simian Virus 40

SV40 is a DNA tumor virus that has been associated with the development of malignant mesothelioma.[55] Although this virus is endogenous in rhesus monkeys, epidemiologic studies have shown that it is also widespread among the human population. The mode by which the virus was transferred from monkey to human is uncertain, but the bulk of this transfer may have occurred from 1954 to 1963 through SV40-contaminated polio vaccines administered worldwide. Moreover, polio vaccines produced in the former Union of Soviet Socialist Republics remained contaminated with infectious SV40 at least until 1978.[56]

The association of SV40 with mesothelioma started with the observation that when hamsters were injected with SV40 into the pleural space, all of the animals developed mesotheliomas within 6 months. This finding prompted investigations into the possibility that some mesotheliomas in humans could be attributed to SV40 infection directly or with SV40 acting as a cocarcinogen with asbestos. Mesothelioma samples studied in 1994 showed that 60% of the samples contained SV40 DNA and expressed the SV40 large T antigen. The results were confirmed by numerous laboratories using a variety of techniques such as PCR, FISH, Western blot, immunohistochemistry, and laser dissection/PCR, but the percentage of positive samples varied from 6% to 83%, and a few studies were completely negative. Technical and geographical differences may account for these variances.

Although the epidemiologic data are not available, mechanistic experiments in human mesothelial cells[57,58] and animal experiments[59] strongly support a pathogenic role of SV40 in mesothelioma. It is unlikely, however, that SV40 acts alone in mesothelioma development, as most cancers are multifactorial, and most mesotheliomas occur in asbestos-exposed individuals. SV40 has been shown to be a cocarcinogen in causing mesothelioma in animals and malignant transformation of mesothelial cells in tissue culture.[60,61] It is safe to say that a definitive role for the virus in human mesothelioma has not been unequivocally demonstrated but ongoing debate regarding its role will continue.

Radiation and Mesothelioma

In the literature, there are a few studies reporting mesothelioma development in patients exposed to thorotrast (intravenously) or who had received radiation to the chest and abdomen.[1] In some of these cases, asbestos exposure could not be ruled out, and SV40 status was not investigated. However, in a few cases in which mesotheliomas developed in young adults who received radiotherapy (RT) because of Wilms tumor, radiation was the only likely causative factor. Studies in rats support a role for radiation as a causative factor. Although it appears that radiation may cause mesotheliomas, the number of mesotheliomas for which it is responsible is probably small.

Carbon Nanoparticles

Engineered single-wall carbon nanotubes (SWCNT) are a class of nanoparticles being actively evaluated for myriad industrial and biomedical applications.[62] Preliminary cellular and animal exposure investigations on the toxicity and pathogenicity of SWCNTs have demonstrated biologic interactions, including toxicity, inflammatory reactions, oxidative stress, and fibroproliferative response.[63–65] SWCNTs are biopersistent and have the ability to distribute to subpleural areas after pharyngeal aspiration. Reports have described the induction of mesothelioma in p53+/− mice by multiwall carbon nanotubes.[66,67] These investigations compelled the present studies of potential interactions of SWCNTs with mesothelial cells. Exposure to SWCNTs induced reactive oxygen species generation, increased cell death, enhanced DNA damage and H2AX phosphorylation, and activated poly(adenosine diphosphate-ribose) polymerase, AP-1, NFκB, p38, and Akt in a dose-dependent manner. These events recapitulate some of the key molecular events involved in mesothelioma development associated with asbestos exposure.[68,69] In addition, nickel nanoparticles enhance the in vitro activity of PDGF in regulating chemokine production in rat mesothelial cells through a mechanism involving reactive oxygen species generation and prolonged activation of ERK-1.[70]

Genetic Predisposition to Mesothelioma: Erionite and BAP1

Recent evidence indicates that genetic predisposition plays an important role in determining individual susceptibility to mineral fiber carcinogenesis and to the development of mesothelioma. In the villages of Karain (population ~600), Tuzkoy (population ~1,400), and Sarihidir (this village was abandoned) in Cappadocia, a region in Central Anatolia, Turkey, ≥50% of deaths are caused by malignant mesothelioma.[71] This epidemic has been linked to exposure to a mineral fiber called *erionite*, one of the most potent mineral fibers in causing mesothelioma. However, mesothelioma was more frequent in certain families than others, leading to observations that some families in Turkey were unusually susceptible to erionite carcinogenesis.[71] Erionite is present in many parts of the world, including western American states such as North Dakota,[72,73] but so far the contribution of erionite to the increased incidence of mesothelioma has not been studied except in Turkey.

Similar families have also been identified in other parts of the world[74] and in the United States, where they appear to be unusually susceptible to asbestos carcinogenesis. Recently, BRCA-associated protein 1 (BAP1) has been identified as a novel MPM TSG. BAP1 is located at the 3p21, a region frequently deleted in MM, and encodes for a deubiquitinase enzyme known to target histones and other proteins. BAP1 appears to exert its antitumor activities mainly in a BRCA-independent manner,[75] with regulation of the cell epigenome, via modulation of histone H2A ubiquitination and chromatin accessibility.[76] However, the relevance of BAP1 to the biology of normal and cancer cells remains largely unexplained; in fact, manipulation of BAP1 in cancer cells has often yielded unexpected or even contradictory results. For example, silencing of BAP1 in MM and uveal melanoma cell lines resulted in reduced cell growth.[77,78]

Bott et al.[77] originally described the association of somatic mutations of BAP1 in 23% of mesothelioma samples. In a larger series of patients, the same group confirmed that somatic BAP1 mutations occur in about 20% of pleural MM and reported that the only clinical variable significantly different among those with and without BAP1 mutations was smoking (former or current), with BAP1 mutations more prevalent among smokers (75% versus 42%).[79] A Japanese study reported BAP1 gene alterations (either deletions or sequence-level mutations) in 61% of their 23 MM samples.[80] Whether this discrepancy results from the different methodologies

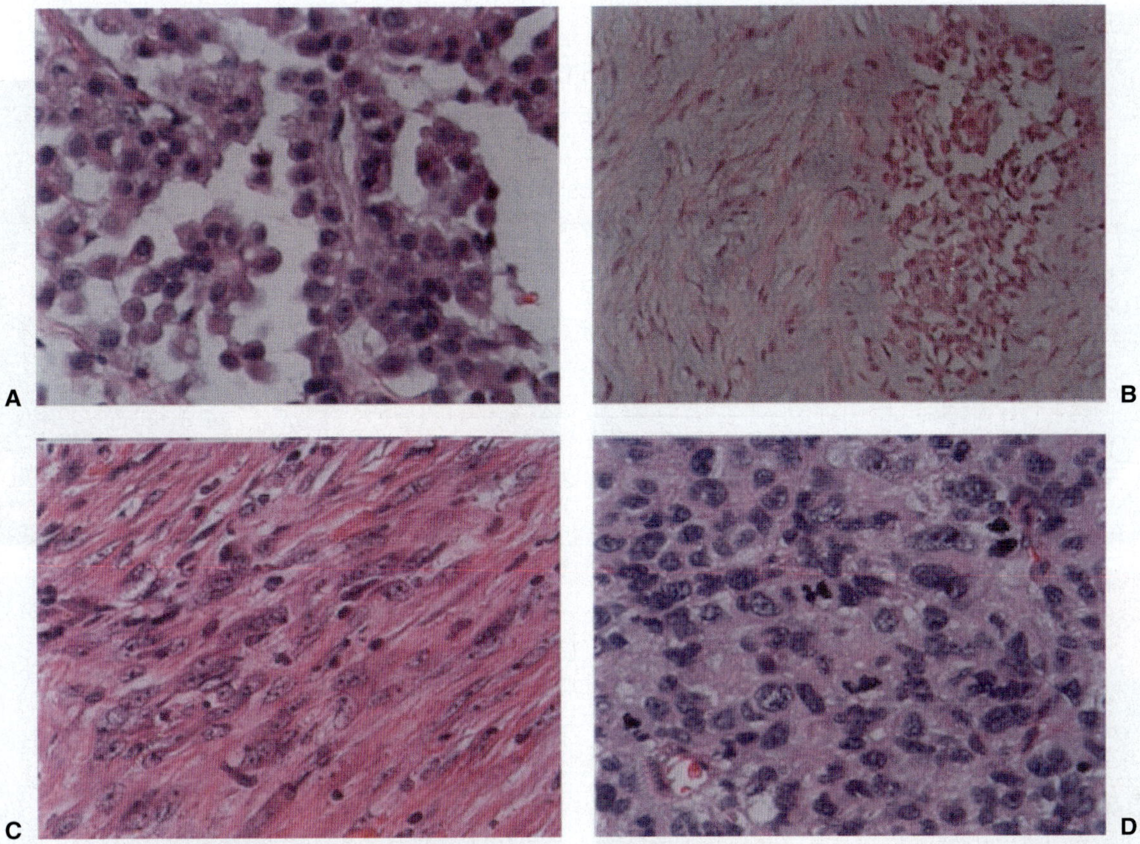

Figure 40.2 Histology of mesothelioma. **(A)** Epithelioid mesothelioma. Note tubular structures and malignant mesothelioma cells showing a hobnail morphology with bland nuclei and abundant cytoplasm. **(B)** Biphasic malignant mesothelioma, showing a nest of mesothelioma cells with epithelial differentiation within the sarcomatoid component. **(C)** Sarcomatoid mesothelioma, positivity for pankeratin, and rare foci of cells suggestive of epithelioid differentiation indicated the diagnosis. **(D)** High-grade sarcoma, a highly aggressive tumor that is vimentin-positive but vimentin-negative over 15 different immunostains for other markers and without distinctive electron microscopic features. In this case, the diagnosis of mesothelioma could not be confirmed. Original magnification: **A**, **C**, and **D**, × 400; **B**, × 200.

in sample preparation and detection of BAP1 mutations or it is an intrinsic difference between the two populations (e.g., due to ethnicity) has still to be determined. A third recent study from Arzt et al.,[81] with a separate cohort of 52 pleural MM, reported absence of BAP1 IHC staining in 60% of pleural MM, confirming previous results. Moreover, there was no correlation between BAP1 expression and asbestos exposure, and it was suggested that expression of BAP1 in tumor samples is inversely correlated to survival.

Germline BAP1 mutations were reported by Testa and Carbone[82] in two US families having a high frequency of MPMs. In the same study, 22% sporadic MM tumors harbored somatic BAP1 mutations. These findings have promoted speculation that BAP1 germline mutations can cause a novel cancer syndrome characterized by a significant excess of both pleural and peritoneal MM, uveal and cutaneous melanoma, and possibly other tumors.

PATHOLOGY OF MESOTHELIOMA

Benign Mesotheliomas

There are a number of benign mesothelial proliferations that must be distinguished from malignant mesothelioma including multicystic mesothelioma (*multilocular peritoneal inclusion cyst*), adenomatoid mesotheliomas, and well-differentiated papillary mesothelioma. Localized mesothelioma, better referred to as *localized fibrous tumor of the pleura* (FTP), is similar to other fibrous tumors found elsewhere in the body. The tumor cells have a benign appearance and are usually immersed in a fibrous and characteristically vascular stroma. FTPs are characteristically negative for cytokeratin (a marker of mesothelial cells) and positive for CD34, which suggests that these cells are not of mesothelial origin. The most important predictive factor in the prognosis of FTP is whether the tumor can be completely resected. Pedunculated tumors have a much better prognosis than tumors that grow over a broad pleural area.[83–85] Surgical resection (Fig. 40.2) is the treatment of choice, with complete resection of the tumor and its pedunculated portion along with the site of origin. Five-year survival rates as high as 97% have been reported. En bloc resection of the lung, chest wall, or diaphragm may be necessary. For recurrences, re-excision is the treatment of choice. Long-term survival with re-excision is possible, but with incomplete resection or malignant transformation the median survival is 24 to 36 months.

Malignant Mesothelioma

Histologically, malignant mesothelioma can show an epithelial morphology (malignant mesothelioma epithelial type), a fibrous morphology (malignant mesothelioma fibrous type, also called sarcomatoid type), or a combination of both (mixed type or biphasic malignant mesothelioma) (Fig. 40.3). Most MM (50% to 60%) are of the epithelial type, approximately 10% are sarcomatoid, and the remainder are biphasic MM.

The diagnosis of malignant mesothelioma is usually straightforward, in contrast to common belief, provided that the pathologist

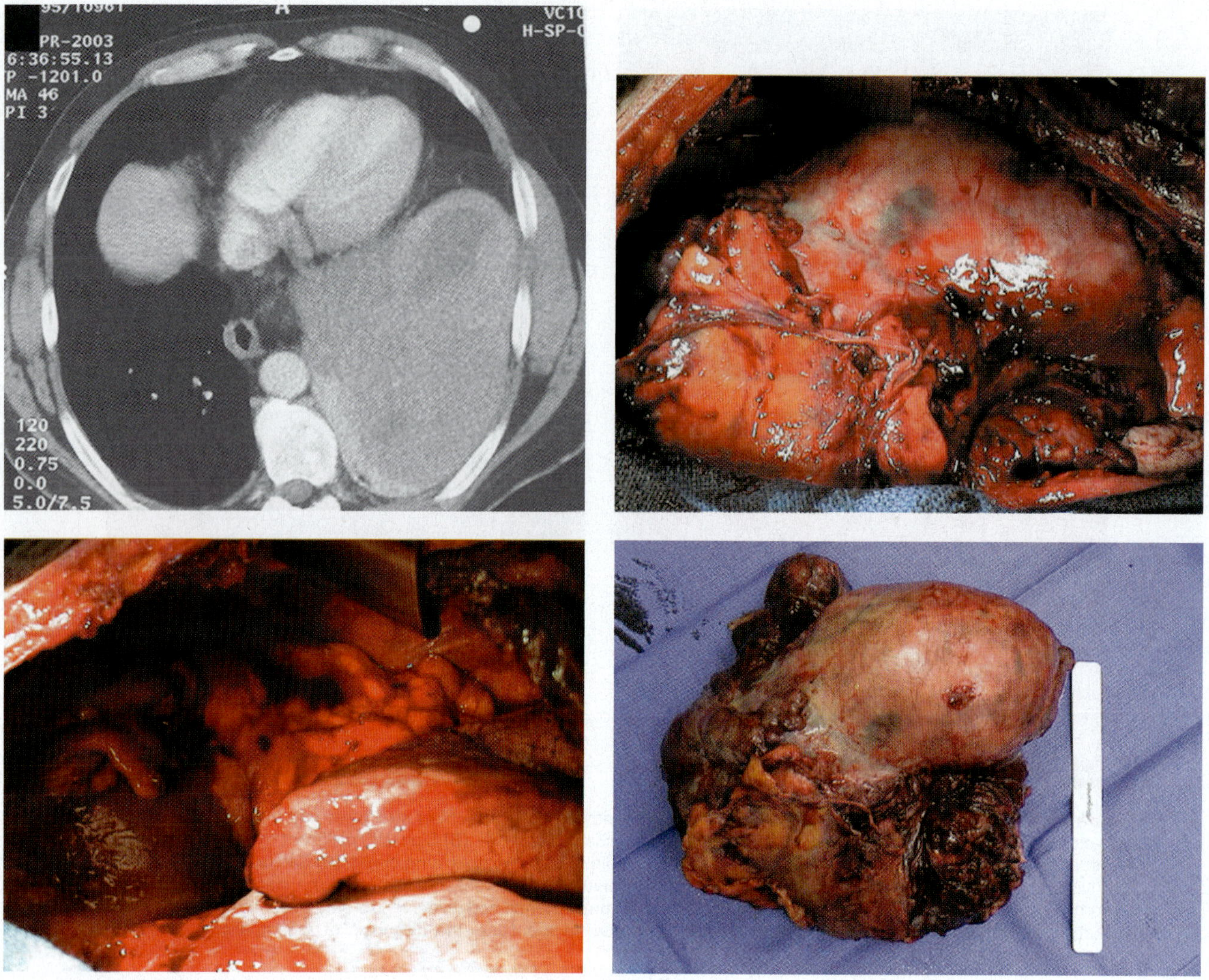

Figure 40.3 Fibrous tumor of pleura. **(A)** Computed tomography reveals a large mass compressing the lower lobe of the lung. **(B)** Intraoperative photograph. Tumor arose from a wide stalk on the diaphragm. **(C)** Intraoperative photograph after resection of the mass revealing expansion of the lung and no other disease. **(D)** Resected specimen.

has extensive experience with this malignancy. Some epithelial mesotheliomas grow forming sheets of epithelioid cells. To rule out mimics of mesothelioma, the diagnosis should be confirmed by immunohistochemistry, which shows that the tumor cells are diffusively positive for pankeratin, keratin 5/6, calretinin, and WT-1, and negative for the epithelial markers such as CEA, CD15, Ber-EP4, Moc-31, TTF-1, and B72.3. For epithelial mesotheliomas, positive stainings for pankeratin and calretinin and negative stainings for three epithelial markers are considered sufficient for diagnosis.

Biphasic mesotheliomas can be distinguished from carcinosarcomas metastasizing from various organs and from biphasic synovial sarcomas by using either electron microscopy or molecular testing for the X;18 translocation that is diagnostic of synovial sarcoma.[86]

Newer methods are under development for distinguishing mesothelioma from adenocarcinoma and include microRNA profiling of the tumors. Gee et al.[87] have described the use of seven miRNAs (miR-200c, miR-141, miR-200b, miR-200a, miR-429, miR-203, and miR-205) to distinguish lung adenocarcinoma from mesothelioma with a 10% misclassification error. Others have described a three microRNA profile (mir-205, mir-193a-3p, and mir-192) for the differential diagnosis of mesothelioma from colon, renal, lung, and breast cancer with a 95% specificity and 96% sensitivity.[88]

EPIDEMIOLOGY AND CLINICAL PRESENTATION

The death rates for mesothelioma parallel the consumption of asbestos by individual countries. When one considers mesothelioma death rates from 2000 to 2004 as a function of asbestos usage in the 1960s, Australia has the highest death rate for the disease in the world.[89] It is predicted that between 2000 and 2049, over 400,000 lives will be lost in those countries from the disease.[90] In the United States, there have been 2,500 deaths per year from the disease since 1999, with workers with industrial exposures in construction and shipbuilding being at highest risk, followed by plumbers, pipe fitters, and steamers. Mesothelioma affects men in their 50s, 60s, and 70s due to the aforementioned 25- to 40-year latency period between occupational asbestos exposure and the development of the tumor.[91] Women and children can have the disease, but the male-to-female ratio is approximately 4.5:1.[92]

Symptoms

As many as 25% of patients with the disease have symptoms for ≥6 months before seeking medical attention. The right side is affected more than the left side (60% versus 40%), most likely because of the right side's greater volume.

Approximately 60% of the patients present with nonpleuritic chest pain that classically is located posterolaterally and low in the thorax. Dyspnea is present in 50% to 70% of the cases, and, indeed, 80% of the patients present with dyspnea and effusion. The presence of a pleural effusion is documented at some time in the course of the disease in 95% of patients with MPM. With the increasing use of positron emission tomography for pretreatment planning, between 5% and 25% of patients are found to have metastatic disease at presentation.[93]

Physical Examination

Physical examination reveals decreased breath sounds, dullness to percussion, or decreased motion of the involved chest wall. Failure to significantly relieve the dyspnea after thoracentesis may indicate that the lung is "trapped." In the late stages of the disease, there is often dramatic cachexia, marked contraction of the involved chest with narrowed interspaces, and hypertrophy of the contralateral hemithorax. A chest wall mass occurs in up to 25% of patients, often at the site(s) of prior thoracentesis, thoracotomy, or thoracoscopy wounds.

Laboratory Examination and Blood Biomarkers

Mesothelioma patients have nonspecific laboratory findings, including hypergammaglobulinemia, eosinophilia, and/or anemia of chronic disease. It has been recently noted that 14% to 15% of patients have elevated homocysteine levels, reflecting folic acid deficiency; 17% have biochemical evidence of vitamin B_{12} deficiency; and 32% have biochemical signs of vitamin B_6 deficiency.[94] The most striking laboratory abnormality is thrombocytosis (>400,000), which is seen in 60% to 90% of patients,[95] and approximately 15% of patients have platelet counts >1,000,000.

Soluble mesothelin-related peptide (SMRP), osteopontin (OPN), and megakaryocyte potentiating factor are presently under investigation as early detection or therapy monitoring markers. Robinson et al.[96] reported that determination of SMRP in serum is a marker of mesothelioma with a sensitivity of 83% and specificity of 95% in the first 48 patients with MPM tested. These data have been validated by other laboratories in the United States[97,98] and internationally.[99] Changes in serum SMRP levels parallel clinical course/tumor size, and SMRP was elevated in 75% of patients at diagnosis.[100] Studies using SMRP in an attempt to diagnose early mesothelioma in high-risk cohorts have so far been disappointing, but follow-up is still short.[101,102]

OPN is a glycoprotein that mediates cell-matrix interactions and is regulated by proteins in cell-signaling pathways that have been associated with asbestos-induced carcinogenesis.[103] In a study that compared serum OPN levels of patients with MPM to those of asbestos-exposed individuals without cancer, serum OPN levels rose with duration of asbestos exposure and degree of radiographic abnormality (plaques and fibrosis versus other lesser findings[104]), and using a cutpoint of 48.3 ng of OPN per milliliter resulted in 77.6% sensitivity and 85.5% specificity when comparing the group exposed to asbestos with the group with mesothelioma. Follow-up studies have demonstrated that serum OPN is not reliable because of the presence of a thrombin cleavage site, which causes degradation of the marker.[105] Plasma OPN,[106] although not specific to mesothelioma, is being evaluated in the disease for both prognosis and early detection utility. A blinded validation of plasma fibulin 3 confirmed excellent discrimination between MPM plasma and all non-MPM cohorts including those with benign or malignant effusions. Pleural effusion fibulin 3 was also discriminatory between MPM effusions and non-MPM effusions.[107]

Radiologic Examination

Malignant mesothelioma can have a diverse radiographic appearance. Many of the early changes are associated with a previous exposure to asbestos, consisting both of pleural and parenchymal changes, including pleural plaques or parenchymal pulmonary fibrosis.

Chest Radiography

The most common chest radiography features associated with mesothelioma progression and symptoms include the presence of a pleural effusion, diffuse pleural thickening, and nodularity. The involved hemithorax can eventually have smooth, lobular pleural masses that infiltrate the pleural space and fissures[108–110] in 45% to 60% of patients with contraction and fixation of the chest (Fig. 40.4). The lung becomes encased, and the mediastinum shifts because of volume loss.

Chest Tomography

Pleural changes on chest tomography (CT) include pleural plaques, diffuse pleural thickening, and pleural effusion. Additional CT features of mesothelioma are localized nodular or plaque-like pleural thickening, possibly associated with pleural effusion. The lobulated pleural encasement frequently causes lower lobe collapse (Fig. 40.5). Intrapulmonary nodules can occur in 60% of patients, and infiltration into fissures along with enlarged hilar and mediastinal lymph nodes may be seen. The CT allows a better view of the involved pericardium, which is irregularly thickened and associated with infiltration to the pericardial fat pad. A clear fat plane between the inferior diaphragmatic surface and the adjacent abdominal organs as well as a smooth inferior diaphragmatic contour may imply resectability.[111] CT may reveal a hemidiaphragm encased by a mass or poor definition between the liver, stomach, and inferior diaphragmatic surface.

Volumetric measurements using CT have recently been studied with regard to their prognostic capability (see "Prognostic Indicators").

Magnetic Resonance Imaging

Studies have suggested that gadolinium contrast enhancement magnetic resonance imaging can improve mesothelioma staging (Fig. 40.6). Detection of diaphragm invasion and invasion of endothoracic fascia or a single chest wall focus may be better with magnetic resonance imaging compared with CT.[111]

Positron Emission Tomography Imaging

There are a number of studies of positron emission tomography (PET) and the radionuclide imaging agent [^{18}F]fluorodeoxyglucose (FDG) in mesothelioma (Fig. 40.7). Early studies reported that FDG-PET was accurate in the diagnosis of pleural malignancies, specifically mesothelioma.[112–116] Recent studies have concentrated on the accuracy of PET in defining nodal and extrathoracic metastases prior to surgical therapy.[93,112] Because of false-positive results in patients with FDG-avid pleural inflammatory/infectious etiologies, all FDG-avid extrathoracic sites should be histologically confirmed in patients with MPM being considered for extrapleural pneumonectomy (EPP).

DIAGNOSTIC APPROACH FOR PRESUMED MESOTHELIOMA

Thoracentesis and Closed Pleural Biopsy

Patients who present with a large, unexplained pleural effusion and minimal or moderate evidence of pleural thickening should have initial thoracentesis and pleural biopsy, especially if a history of asbestos exposure or mesothelioma in a family member is elicited. By preserving a cell block from the pleural fluid and using both histochemical

CANCER OF THE THORACIC CAVITY

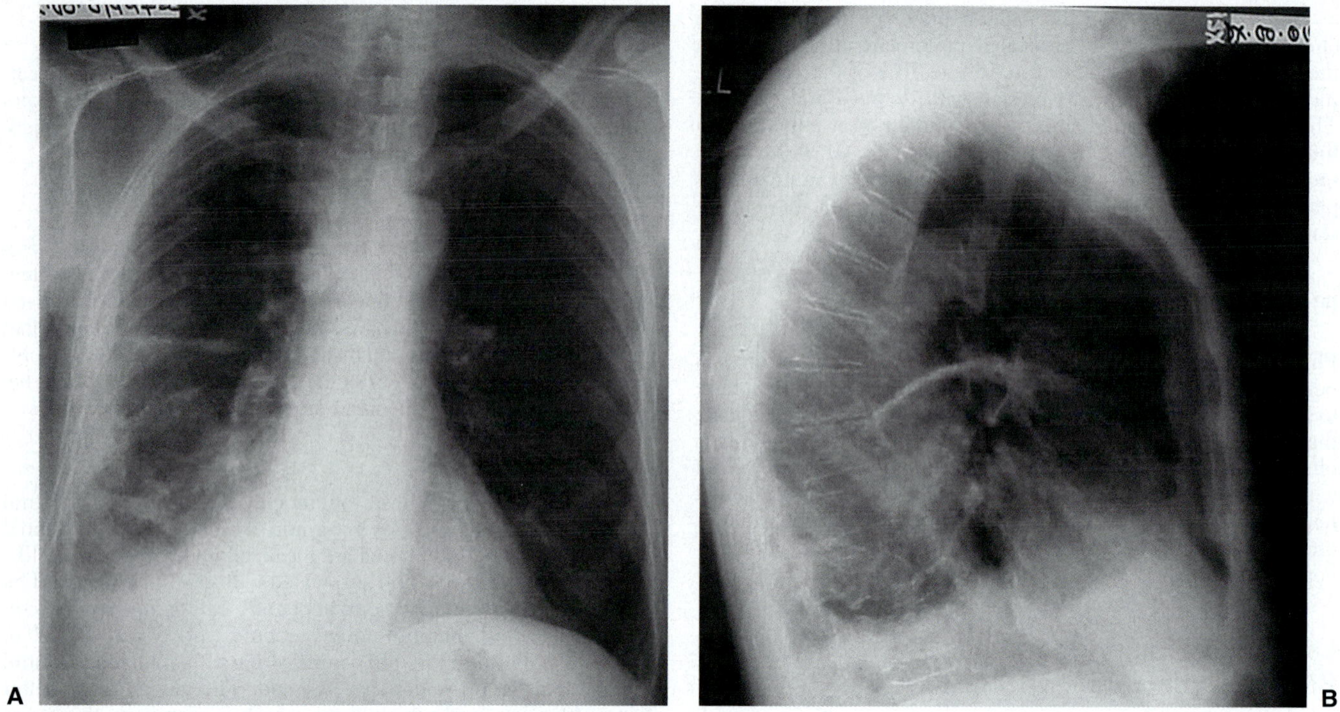

Figure 40.4 Chest radiography of malignant pleural mesothelioma. **(A)** Anteroposterior view reveals a contracted right hemithorax with nodular scalloping of the pleura at the right base. There is fluid or tumor in the fissure, and the diaphragm and right heart border are obscured. **(B)** Lateral view demonstrates fluid or tumor at the right base with thickened pleura and disease in the fissure.

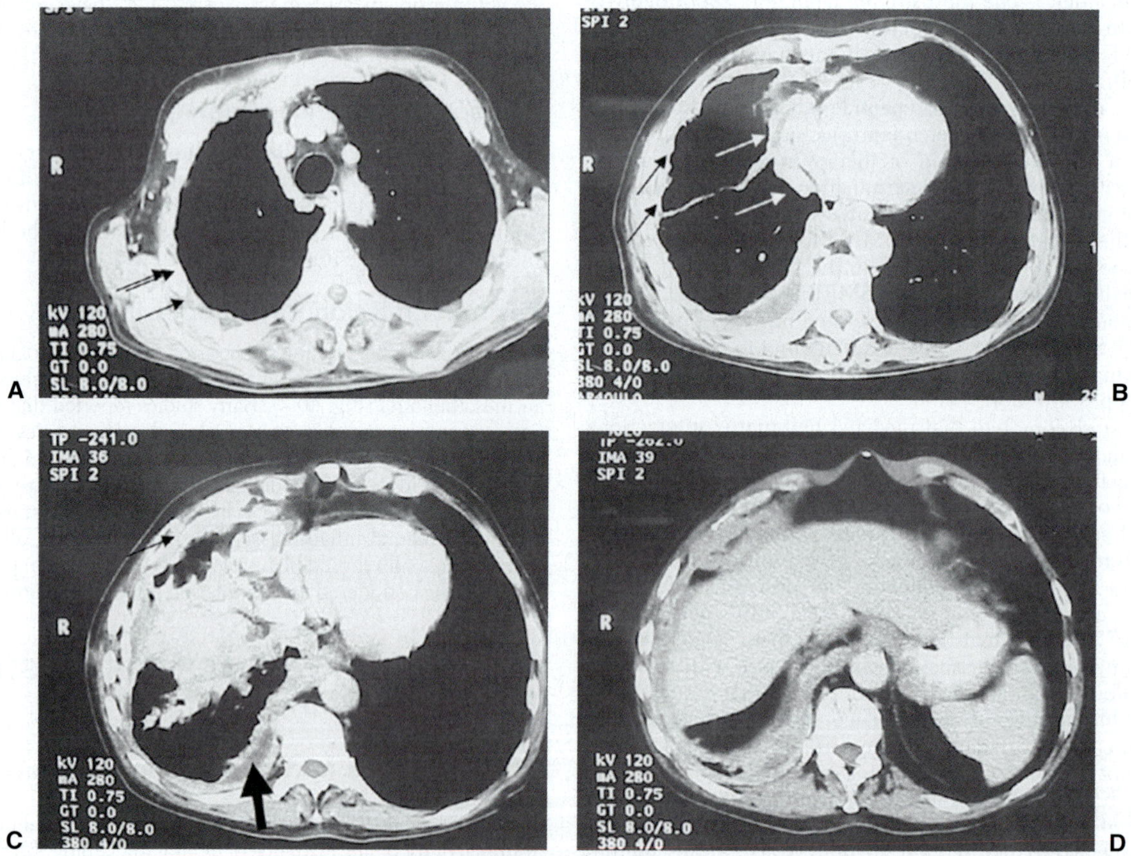

Figure 40.5 Computed tomography of a patient with a right-sided pleural mesothelioma. As one progresses from the apex **(A)** to the diaphragm **(D)**, loculated fluid (*bold black arrow*), thickened pleura (*thin black arrows*) **(B)**, and thickened pericardium (*white arrows*) can be appreciated in panel **C**.

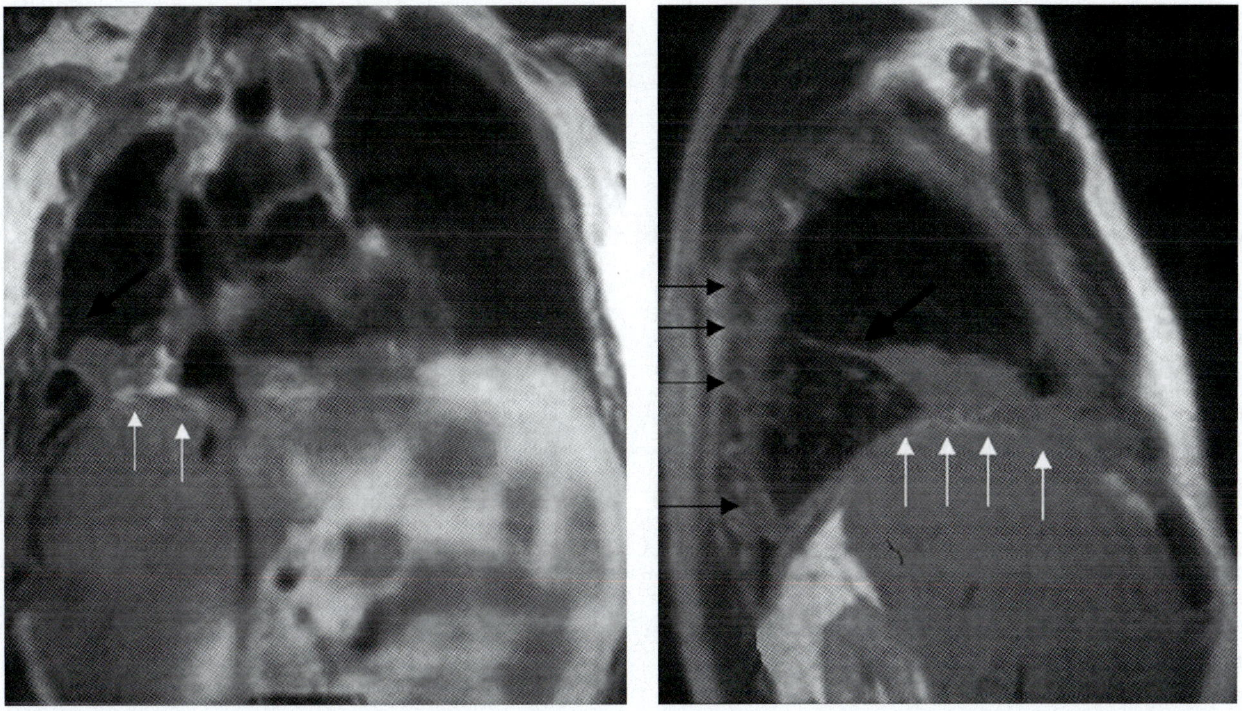

A B

Figure 40.6 Magnetic resonance imaging and mesothelioma. **(A)** Coronal magnetic resonance imaging of a right-sided pleural mesothelioma. *White arrows* indicate diaphragmatic involvement. *Black arrows* delineate fluid in fissure and associated mass. **(B)** Sagittal magnetic resonance image of same patient reveals the thickened pleura (*thin black arrows*), involvement in the fissure (*thick black arrow*), and involvement of the diaphragm (*white arrows*).

and immunohistochemical staining techniques along with electron microscopic analysis, the diagnosis of mesothelioma can be obtained from the pleural effusion in as high as 84% of suspected cases.

Thoracoscopy

A video-assisted thoracoscopy is indicated for patients at risk for mesothelioma who (1) develop a large effusion and who have negative studies on thoracentesis and pleural biopsy, or (2) recur with effusion after initial thoracentesis. Thoracoscopy can be invaluable for estimating extent of disease with regard to the lung, diaphragm, pericardium, chest wall, and nodes.[117,118] Development of chest wall masses from seeding of the biopsy site or surgical scar is an uncommon complication (approximately 10%) of any diagnostic procedure, and the efficacy of radiotherapy to the scar to prevent recurrence is controversial.[119–121]

If there is no free pleural space because of previous treatment of pleural effusion and the bulk of the disease in the hemithorax is

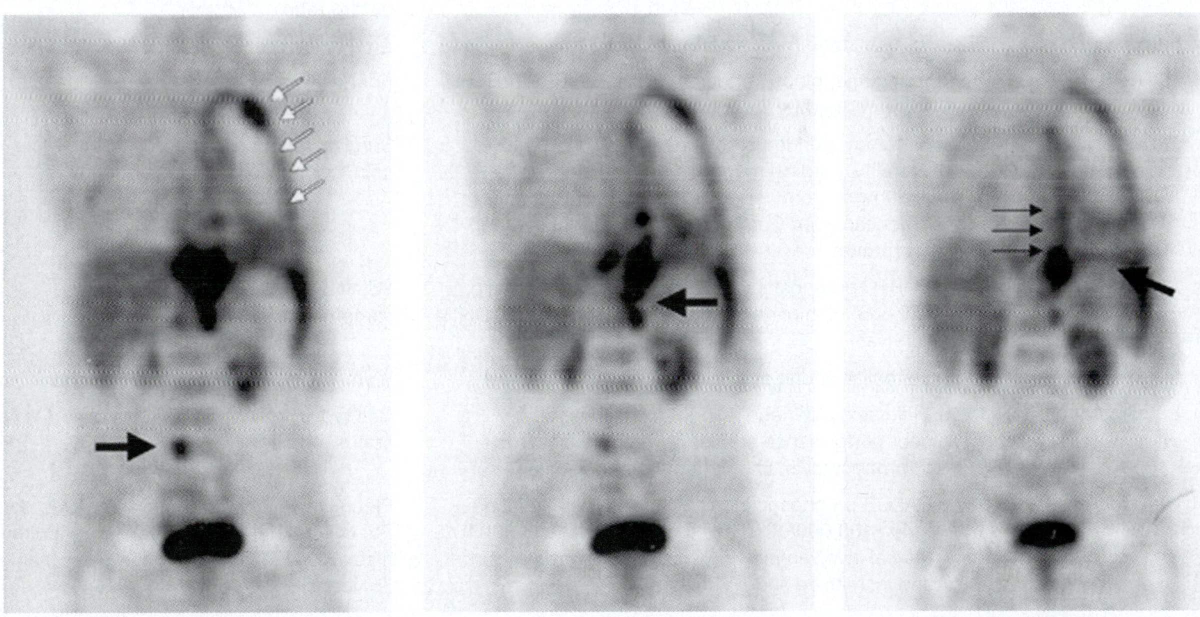

A,B C

Figure 40.7 Positron emission tomography with [^{18}F] fluorodeoxyglucose in a patient with an unresectable stage IV mesothelioma. **(A)** *White arrows* outline the involved pleura, with an area of bulky disease superiorly. *Black arrow* points out an occult metastasis in the abdomen. **(B)** *Black arrow* depicts posterior infracrural mediastinal lymph node disease. **(C)** *Bold black arrow* points out diaphragmatic involvement. *Thin black arrows* depict mesothelioma medially.

solid, open biopsy should be performed such that the scar can be incorporated into the incision at the time of cytoreduction surgery.

NATURAL HISTORY

The majority of patients with treated or untreated pleural mesothelioma die of complications of local disease because of (1) increasing tumor bulk that eventually replaces the pleural effusion and causes progressive respiratory compromise, pneumonia, or myocardial dysfunction with arrhythmias; (2) unrelenting chest wall pain requiring narcotics, which leads to cachexia; and/or (3) dysphagia from tumor compression of the esophagus. Patients generally die of respiratory failure or pneumonia. Small bowel obstruction from direct extension through the diaphragm develops in approximately one-third of patients, and 10% die of pericardial or myocardial involvement.[122] One of the most important clinical predictor of survival in noncytoreduced patients is performance status.[95]

Extrathoracic metastases occur late in the course of disease and are not usually the direct cause of the patient's death. In the largest series of patients with MPM who had autopsy, 54% to 82% had distant metastases, with the most frequently involved organs being the liver, adrenal gland, kidney, and contralateral lung.[123,124] Intracranial metastases are seen in approximately 3% of patients and are predominantly of the sarcomatous type.[124,125]

Prognostic Indicators

The best-known clinical prognostic scoring systems for MPM have originated from European Organisation for Research and Treatment of Cancer (EORTC) and Cancer and Leukemia Group B (CALGB), and use a combination of biologic and clinical factors. Poor performance status, nonepithelioid histology, male gender, low hemoglobin, high platelet count, high white blood cell count, and high lactate dehydrogenase were found to be poor prognostic indicators in mesothelioma.[95,126] The EORTC model was validated at St. Bartholomew's Hospital in sequential chemotherapy trials,[127] and both models were validated by Edwards.[128] Many other studies have explored clinical and pathologic features of MPM as seen in Table 40.1. Most recently, the ratio of absolute neutrophil to lymphocyte ratio was promising in segregation of risk for death[129–131]; however, a recent study found that the aforementioned EORTC and CALGB indices were superior.[132]

The molecular prognostication of mesothelioma has also been explored using gene expression array technology.[133,134] There has, however, been variability in the gene sets and results of these prognostic tests when used in other MPM cohorts.[135]

The presence of a single microRNA, mir-29c*, has been associated with improved time to progression and overall survival but needs further validation.[136] A variety of other tissue-based prognostic markers, including thymidylate synthase,[137] OPN,[138,139] and HAPLN1,[140] have been reported but require validation.

TABLE 40.1

Clinicopathologic Prognostic Studies of Malignant Pleural Mesothelioma[a]

Year	Author	N	Univariate Predictors	Multivariate Predictors
2013	Baud et al.[267]	170	Asbestos exposure, age, ASA class III versus ASA classes I and II, nonepithelioid histology, CRP >3 mg/L, and white cell count >12,000/mm³	Nonepithelioid histology, age, CRP, WBC >12,000/mm³
2011	Nojiri et al.[268]	314	Demographic and laboratory parameters	Age >70, nonepithelial, low PS, high WBC, high CRP
2010	Tanrikulu et al.[269]	363	Glucose <40,CRP >50 ↓ survival	KPS, serum LDH, presence of pleural effusion, pleural thickening >1 cm, and PLT >420 k
2010	Richards et al.[149]	354	Stratification of T and N status, epithelial only	N2b versus N2a nodal status with different hazard ratio
2009	Francart et al.[270]	523	PS >0, stage IV, nonepithelial ↓ PFS	Age, histotype, stage, PS, hgb, WBC
2009	Yan et al.[271]	456	Young age, pleural effusion, epithelial, EPP, PET scan, adjuvant therapy ↑ survival	Epithelial and EPP: ↑ survival
2007	Flores et al.[272]	945	Histology, gender, smoking, asbestos exposure, laterality, surgical resection by extrapleural pneumonectomy or pleurectomy/decortication, American Joint Committee on Cancer stage, and symptoms	Surgical resection, nonsmokers, female, no pain, epithelial, left side: ↑ survival
2005	Steele et al.[273]	145	EORTC prognostic index: PS, nonepithelial, male, low hgb, high platelet count, high WBC, high LDH ↓ survival	PS, WBC, hgb, uncertain diagnosis, sarcomatoid: ↓ survival
2004	Neumann et al.[274]	155	Epithelial, young age, female gender: ↑ survival	Epithelial, young age, female gender: ↑ survival
2000	Edwards et al.[128]	142	Male sex, older age, weight loss, chest pain, poor performance status, low hgb, leukocytosis, thrombocytosis, and nonepithelial cell type ↓ survival	Cell type, hgb, white cell count, performance status, and sex
1998	Herndon et al.[95]	337	CALGB prognostic index: PS, chest pain, dyspnea, PLT >400,000/uL, weight loss, LDH level >500 IU/L, pleural involvement, low hgb level, high WBC count, and increasing age >75 years	Pleural involvement, LDH >500 IU/L, poor PS, chest pain, PLT >400,000, nonepithelial histology, and increasing age older than 75 years

ASA, American Society of Anesthesiologists; CRP, C-reactive protein; WBC, white blood cell; PS, performance status; PFS, progression free survival; KPS, Karnovsky performance status; LDH, lactate dehydrogenase; PLT, platelet count; hgb, hemoglobin; EPP, PET, positron emission tomography; EORTC, European Organisation for Research and Treatment of Cancer; CALGB, Cancer and Leukemia Group B.
[a]Table modified from Pass.[275]

TABLE 40.2

Radiographic Prognostic Studies[a]

Marker	Year	Author	N	Univariate Predictors	Multivariate Predictors
PET-CT	2013	Abakay et al.[276]	177	Male gender, nonepithelial, KPS <60, stage III-IV, hgb <12.3 g/dl, serum ALP >79 u/L, presence of pleural thickening >1 cm, BSC treatment regimen, SUVmax >5	Male gender, KPS <60, BSC, stage III-IV, SUVmax >5
CT volume	2012	Gill et al.[151]	88	Tumor volume predicts survival after EPP	Tumor volume, hgb, adjuvant therapy
PET-CT	2011	Sharif et al.[142]	1,108	SUV >10 associated with decreased survival in best evidence review of 15 papers	NA
PET-CT volume	2010	Lee et al.[143]	13	High metabolic tumor volume decreased survival	Metabolic tumor volume
Quantitative FDG	2010	Nowak et al.[144]	89	High total glycolytic volume decreased survival, histology, weight loss, CT stage, EORTC prognostic score	Total glycolytic volume and weight loss for sarcomatoid histology

PET, positron emission tomograpy; CT, computed tomography; KPS, Karnovsky performance status; hgb, hemoglobin; ALP, alkaline phosphatase; BSC, best supportive care; SUV, standardized uptake value; EPP; extrapleural pneumonectomy; NA, not available; FDG, fluorodeoxyglucose; EORTC, European Organisation for Research and Treatment of Cancer.
[a]Table modified from Pass.[275]

Quantification of the standardized uptake value (SUV) for PET scanning has also been investigated in mesothelioma as a prognostic marker (Table 40.2). Low SUV and epithelial histology predict the best survival, whereas high SUV and nonepithelial histology indicate the worst survival.[112,141–144]

Staging

The original MPM staging system proposed by Butchart et al.[145] relied on pathologic generalizations instead of specific quantitative aspects of the disease and was designed at a time that was well before recognition of different prognostic implications of N1 and N2 nodes. The American Joint Committee on Cancer staging system for mesothelioma (Table 40.3) was adopted from that proposed by the International Mesothelioma Interest Group (IMIG) in 1995[146] and has been validated in a number of surgically based trials. In collaboration with IMIG, the International Staging and Prognostic Factors Committee of the International Association for the Study of Lung Cancer recently formed a Mesothelioma Domain in order to improve the current staging system resulting in the first large, international MPM database, which included over 2,000 staged patients with MPM diagnosed from 1995 to 2008 who had a surgical procedure. As described by Rusch et al.,[147] a set of covariates were identified as predictive of survival in a "core" model for this analysis which included best staging information, age, sex, histology (epithelioid or not), and type of surgical procedure (palliative versus extrapleural pneumonectomy or pleurectomy decortication).[147]

Regrouping of the T and N combinations based on relative hazard and Kaplan-Meier survival analysis of 368 patients having EPP resulted in improved stage distribution (stage I–IV: 8%, 43%, 33%, 16%, respectively) and survival stratification (51 months, 26 months, 15 months, 8 months, respectively).[148,149] A stage-independent model of risk for death in patients having surgical cytoreduction has expanded on the data from Pass et al.,[150] which described the influence of tumor volume and survival in MPM. Gill et al.,[151] in a study of 88 epithelial MPMs having EPP, reported that tumor volume, hemoglobin concentration, platelet count, pathologic TNM (tumor, node, metastasis) category, and administration of adjuvant chemotherapy or RT were associated with survival. In the final multivariate model, tumor volume, hemoglobin concentration, and administration of adjuvant chemotherapy or RT were identified as independently associated with overall survival.[151] Richards et al.[152] recently described a validated model for survival and time to recurrence in cytoreduced MPM using hemoglobin, CT volume, thickness of the fissures, and histologic subtype.

TREATMENT

Overview

For unresectable patients who are candidates for chemotherapy, the well-powered phase 3 trial that showed a 3- to 4-month survival advantage for the two-drug regimen of pemetrexed and cisplatin compared with the one-drug regimen of cisplatin has defined the standard of care[94] (Fig. 40.8). Recommendations for the management of pleural mesothelioma have been made by the European Society for Medical Oncology[153] and the National Comprehensive Cancer Center Network.

Supportive Care

The median survival of patients with MPM who select supportive care ranges only from 4 months[128] to 13 months.[122] This variation is likely due to variations in tumor biology, host response to tumor, detection bias, lead-time bias, and the use of ad hoc or unreported treatments by some patients and physicians.

There are a number of options for the control of pleural effusion, including repeated thoracenteses, talc pleurodesis, or placement of a PleurX (Denver Biomedical, Denver, CO) catheter.[154] Talc pleurodesis is performed by instilling 2 to 5 g of asbestos-free, sterile talc over the lung and the parietal surfaces. Success rates in effusion control with talc, used either via thoracoscopy or via slurry, approach 90%.

The MesoVats trial was a randomization between 2003 and 2012 of 87 video-assisted thoracoscopic pleurectomy or 88 talc pleurodesis. A total of 84% had epithelioid disease, 78% were IMIG stage ¾, and 49% were high risk as per EORTC criteria. Although there was no difference in survival between the two groups, pleural effusion was better controlled with patients who underwent pleurectomy at 1 month and 6 months. Moreover, there was a significant benefit in quality of life at 6 months and 12 months in favor of the pleurectomy group.[155] Failure of these techniques is usually associated with lung trapped by the tumor, a large solid tumor mass, a long history of effusion with multiple thoracenteses leading to loculations, age older than 70 years, or

TABLE 40.3

International Staging System for Diffuse Malignant Pleural Mesothelioma

T: Tumor

T1a
Tumor limited to the ipsilateral parietal ± mediastinal ± diaphragmatic pleura
No involvement of the visceral pleura

T1b
Tumor involving the ipsilateral parietal ± mediastinal ± diaphragmatic pleura
Tumor also involving the visceral pleura

T2
Tumor involving each of the ipsilateral pleural surfaces (parietal, mediastinal, diaphragmatic, and visceral pleura) with at least one of the following features:
Involvement of diaphragmatic muscle
Extension of tumor from visceral pleura into the underlying pulmonary parenchyma

T3
Describes locally advanced but potentially resectable tumor
Tumor involving all of the ipsilateral pleural surfaces (parietal, mediastinal, diaphragmatic, and visceral pleura) with at least one of the following features:
- Involvement of the endothoracic fascia
- Extension into the mediastinal fat
- Solitary, completely resectable focus of tumor extending into the soft tissues of the chest wall
- Nontransmural involvement of the pericardium

T4
Describes locally advanced technically unresectable tumor
Tumor involving all the ipsilateral pleural surfaces (parietal, mediastinal, diaphragmatic, and visceral pleura) with at least one of the following features:
- Diffuse extension or multifocal masses of tumor in the chest wall, with or without associated rib destruction
- Direct transdiaphragmatic extension of tumor to the peritoneum
- Direct extension of tumor to the contralateral pleura
- Direct extension of tumor to mediastinal organs
- Direct extension of tumor into the spine
- Tumor extending through to the internal surface of the pericardium with or without a pericardial effusion; or tumor involving the myocardium

N: Lymph Nodes

NX: Regional lymph nodes cannot be assessed
N0: No regional lymph node metastases
N1: Metastases in the ipsilateral bronchopulmonary or hilar lymph nodes
N2: Metastases in the subcarinal or the ipsilateral mediastinal lymph nodes, including the ipsilateral internal mammary nodes
N3: Metastases in the contralateral mediastinal, contralateral internal mammary, ipsilateral, or contralateral supraclavicular lymph nodes

M: Metastases

MX: Presence of distant metastases cannot be assessed
M0: No distant metastasis
M1: Distant metastasis present

Stage I
Ia: T1aN0 M0
Ib: T1bN0 M0

Stage II
T2 N0 M0

Stage III
Any T3 M0
Any N1 M0
Any N2 M0

Stage IV
Any T4
Any N3
Any M1

Based on Edge SB, Byrd DR, Compton CC, et al. *AJCC Cancer Staging Manual.* 7th ed. New York: Springer, 2010; and Rusch VW. A proposed new international TNM staging system for malignant pleural mesothelioma: from the International Mesothelioma Interest Group. *Chest* 1995;108:1122.

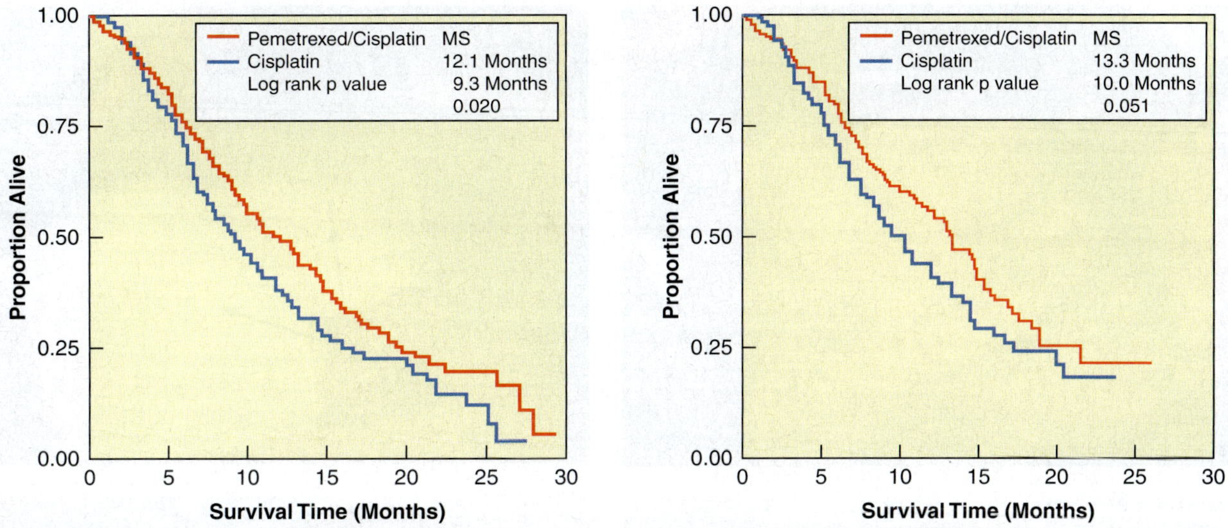

A

Pts at Risk							
Pem/Cls	226	185	111	50	19	7	0
Cls	222	173	91	32	19	3	0

B

Pts at Risk							
Pem/Cls	168	141	86	35	9	1	0
Cls	163	128	89	20	9	0	0

Figure 40.8 Results of the phase 3 trial of pemetrexed (Pem) and cisplatin (Cis) versus cisplatin alone. See text for details. MS, median survival; Pts, patients.

poor performance status. In such cases, the PleurX catheter with its one-way valve can be implanted under local anesthesia into pleural effusion, and patients can drain themselves at home using the available disposable drainage kits.[156]

The chest pain of malignant mesothelioma requires narcotics, and these patients should be seen in consultation by a dedicated pain management team to assist in the optimization of the patient's quality of life. Subcutaneous tunneling of epidural catheters for long-term out-of-hospital use has also been used in selective cases. When only local RT has been delivered solely for chest wall pain or chest wall nodules, the median survival has been reported to be 4 to 5 months.[157,158]

SURGERY FOR PLEURAL MESOTHELIOMA

The Controversy

Surgery for pleural mesothelioma remains a controversial subject not only among medical oncologists, but with thoracic surgeons. Much of the controversy remains as the result of the early trials of EPP with reported mortality rates of 31%,[159] as well as the lack of systemic therapies besides pemetrexed and cisplatinum with response rates >30%, which can complement present surgical therapy with mortality rates of 4%. Despite strict functional criteria for the selection of patients to undergo mesothelioma surgery, there are no reliable prognostic predictors to stratify patients by the biology of the disease in order to determine which patients will recur rapidly after cytoreductive surgery. As discussed in the following, the type of operation to be performed (EPP or some sort of lung sparing pleurectomy with decortication (P/D) is one of the more debatable subjects for the management of the disease, and at present, suffers from the lack of randomized data that defines the present cadre of surgical interventions in a uniform manner. These issues, as well as the interpretation of high profile recently completed trials, have led to geographical variation in physicians' use of surgery as part of the management plan.[160] In a questionnaire answered by 802 thoracic surgeons belonging to The European Association for Cardio-Thoracic Surgery, The European Society of Thoracic Surgeons, or the Society of Thoracic Surgeons, EPP was believed to be more effective than P/D and the addition of adjuvant chemotherapy and multimodality therapy were believed to increase the chance of cure (see the following). American surgeons, however, were twice as likely to believe that EPP alone can cure mesothelioma as those in Europe (45% versus 23%).

The Purpose of Surgery

Operation for malignant pleural mesothelioma can be done simply for *diagnostic* or *palliative purposes*, but in selected patients, it is performed as a maximal cytoreductive procedure in which the persistent disease at the end of the operation is microscopic.

Diagnostic Procedures

In patients with localized or free flowing pleural effusion suspected of having mesothelioma, video thoracoscopy allows for definitive diagnosis. For subtype classification of mesothelioma histology, biopsy by open pleural biopsy or thoracotomy was found to be the most accurate in subtype classification (83%) compared with thoracoscopy (74%) and imaging-guided core or needle biopsy (44%) in a study comparing histologic subtype recorded by pre-EPP diagnostic method to the EPP surgical specimen.[161,162]

Maximal Cytoreductive Procedures

The goal of cytoreductive surgery in MPM should be the removal of all visible or palpable tumor (R0 or R1) or a "macroscopic complete resection" (MCR). MCR should be the goal of cytoreductive surgery, regardless of whether that involves EPP or a lung-preserving operation. The Mesothelioma Domain of the International Association for the Study of Lung Cancer has recommended the following as uniform nomenclature for pleural mesothelioma resections.[163]

EPP: en bloc resection of the parietal and visceral pleura with the ipsilateral lung, pericardium, and diaphragm. In cases where the pericardium and/or diaphragm are not involved by tumor, these structures may be left intact (Fig. 40.9).

Extended P/D: parietal and visceral pleurectomy to remove all gross tumor with resection of the diaphragm and/or pericardium.

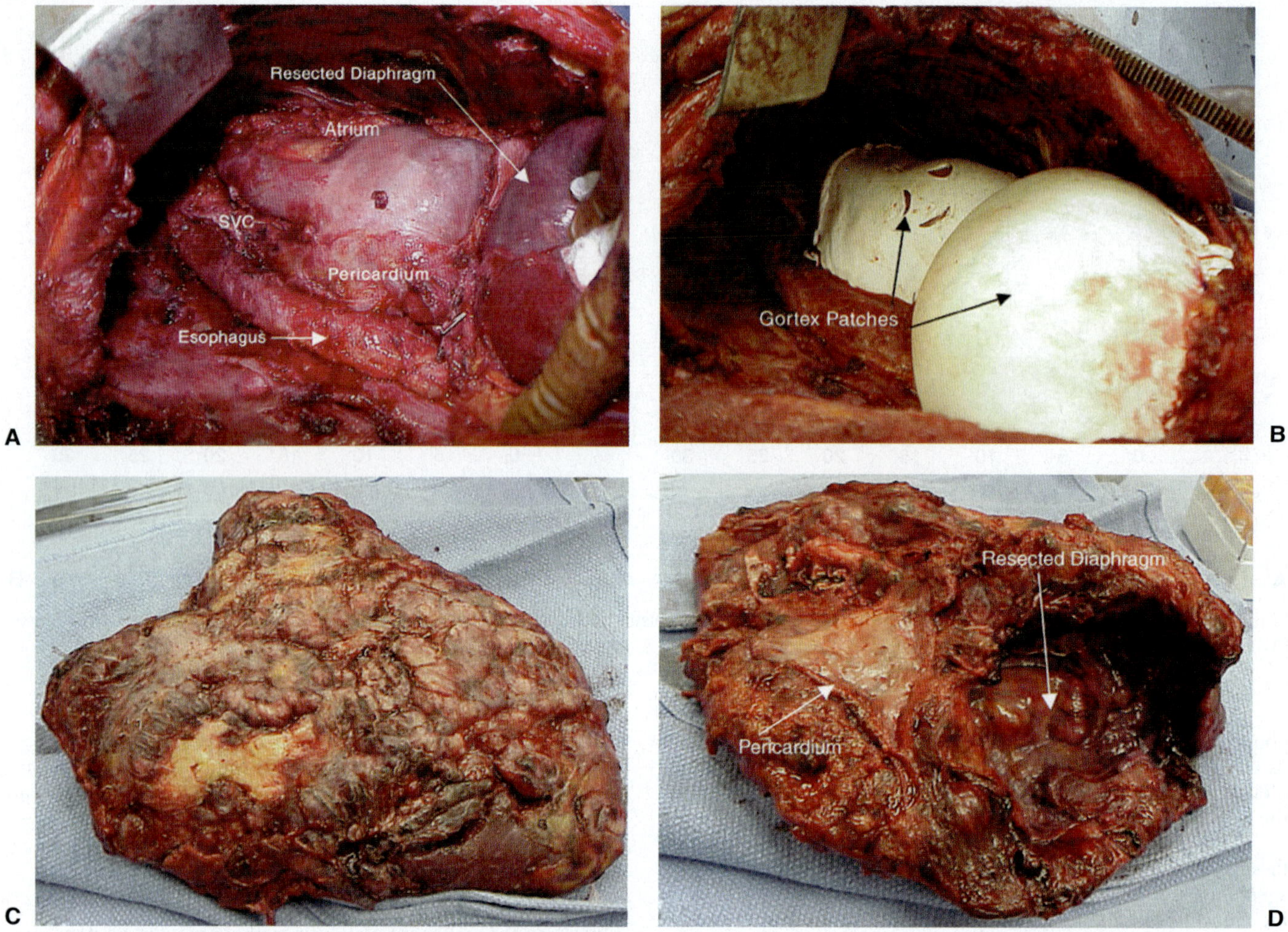

Figure 40.9 Intraoperative and specimen photography. **(A)** Right hemithorax after resection of lung, pleura, diaphragm, pericardium, and lymph nodes. **(B)** Replacement of the diaphragm and pericardium with Gore-Tex material (W.L. Gore & Associates, Inc., Reisterstown, MD). **(C)** View of lateral aspect of specimen, which reveals the entire lung coated with thickened, mesothelioma-involved pleura. **(D)** Medial view of specimen revealing the resected pericardium and diaphragm, hilar structures, and lung. SVC, superior vena cava.

P/D: parietal and visceral pleurectomy to remove all gross tumor without diaphragm or pericardial resection.

Partial pleurectomy: partial removal of parietal and/or visceral pleura for diagnostic or palliative purposes but leaving gross tumor behind.

Palliation or MCR?: Only approximately 20% of patients presenting with pleural MPM will be candidates for an MCR. The decision to actually palliate a patient with mesothelioma begins with palliation of fluid in order to improve dyspnea or cough, as described previously. Patients who have an excellent result from drainage, with partial or full lung expansion, may then be considered candidates for MCR depending on other factors including (1) the experience of the thoracic surgeon, (2) the cardiopulmonary/functional status of the patient, and (3) patient/tumor demographics at presentation. Any preoperative staging radiologic examination that points to disease outside the involved hemithorax eliminates the use of an MCR. Thoracic surgeons at major centers with mesothelioma programs decide not only whether the patient is a candidate for cytoreduction or palliation but also the appropriate cytoreductive procedure. Patients who present with Eastern Cooperative Oncology Group performance status ≥2, or who have limiting cardiac reserve either with nonreversible myocardial ischemia or compromised ventricular function (ejection fraction <50%) are usually not candidates for cytoreductive procedures. Moreover, patients with compromised pulmonary function testing who are not felt to be candidates for pneumonectomy must be carefully evaluated for either extended P/D in that the cytoreduction should not compromise existing lung function but may recruit trapped lung and possibly improve dyspnea.

CONTROVERSY REGARDING PERFORMANCE OF EXTRAPLEURAL PNEUMONECTOMY

Extrapleural Pneumonectomy Results

The use of EPP for MCR has evolved since the first description alluded to previously. As detailed in a systematic review of the use of EPP for MPM,[164] which included survival and perioperative outcomes, the median overall survival varied from 9.4 to 27.5 months, and 1-, 2-, and 5-year survival rates ranged from 36% to 83%, 5% to 59%, and 0% to 24%, respectively. Overall perioperative mortality rates ranged from 0% to 11.8%, and the perioperative morbidity rates ranged from 22% to 82%. In Sugarbaker and Wolf's[165] series, the mortality of EPP is reported at 3.4%, which has been achieved by improving preoperative staging, anesthesia, resection, reconstruction, and perioperative management of procedure-related complications. The chief complication is reversible atrial fibrillation, which occurs in 44.2% of patients and other major causes of morbidity are myocardial infarction (1.5%), epicarditis (2.7%), pulmonary complications (7.9%), thrombosis (6.4%), empyema (2.4%), technical complications (6.1%), and gastrointestinal complications (0.9%).[166] Some of the technical issues include herniation of the heart due to failure of the pericardial patch or herniation of abdominal contents into the pleural space secondary to dehiscence of the diaphragmatic repair, vocal cord dysfunction secondary to recurrent laryngeal nerve injury, bronchopleural fistula, empyema, and prolonged respiratory failure. EPP alone does not appear to prolong survival. In most EPP series, median survival is <2 years, but 10% to 20% of patients are 5-year survivors. Patients with sarcomatoid histology and/or lymph node involvement have an even poorer prognosis and should not be considered as candidates for EPP.[167]

Trimodality Therapy in the Context of an Extrapleural Pneumonectomy

Trimodality therapy (TMT) for MPM began with evidence of a decreasing mortality and standardization of techniques for EPP, as well as the demonstration of increased tumor responses and survival with cisplatinum doublets using either gemcitabine[168] or pemetrexed.[169] TMT consists of induction chemotherapy, followed by EPP, and RT either as hemithorax radiation to the pneumonectomy cavity or as intensity modulated RT.[170] Because of the morbidity and mortality with EPP, patient selection is a critical factor. The ideal patient is younger than 65 years old, has pure epithelial histology, an absence of lymph node involvement, and is physiologically able to tolerate pneumonectomy. Although EPP has been reported thus far as the primary surgical MCR technique in this selected group of patients, it should not be considered the only option, as detailed later. Table 40.4 describes the major TMT trials to date using EPP for MCR, and overall demonstrates a 3.1% mortality for EPP, along with a 27.7-month median survival in the 60% of presenting patients who completed the full package.

Randomized Trials of Surgery for Malignant Pleural Mesothelioma Involving Extrapleural Pneumonectomy

As of 2002, only one randomized trial involving surgery for MPM had been performed,[171] and that trial did not address the issue of the utility of surgery, specifically EPP in MPM. In an attempt to define the efficacy of EPP, Mesothelioma and Radical Surgery (MARS) was originally designed as a randomized trial with 670 patients needed comparing induction chemotherapy, EPP, and postoperative RT to induction therapy but no EPP.[172] When difficulty arose in recruiting patients, an initial feasibility study was performed randomizing 50 patients to EPP or no EPP. The final results of the trial demonstrated that it may be feasible to randomize MPM patients to a surgical or nonsurgical arm; however, the conclusions of the study's authors have caused considerable controversy among surgeons and medical oncologists dealing with MPM. The study as published revealed nonsignificant differences in the 6, 12, 18 months and median survivals comparing the surgery arm to the nonsurgical arm, with a median survival of 14.4 months versus 19.5 months, respectively. Amongst many practitioners, the study has been interpreted not only as a condemnation of EPP in the management of MPM but also as an indictment of surgery as nonefficacious in the disease. One of the main criticisms of the study includes an 18% operative mortality from EPP, which is to be contrasted to the data noted previously for other phase 2 TMT trials (3.1%). Moreover, other flaws included (1) the lack of power of the study, which demanded a sample size of 670 randomized individuals; (2) the fact that the preoperative chemotherapy was not standardized; (3) the crossover of individuals from one arm to the other in six instances; (4) the lack of data on the interval from the end of chemotherapy to surgery; and (5) only one-third of the individuals received the full TMT while, as demonstrated previously, 60% of the individuals in the phase 2 setting completed the TMT and recorded a median overall survival of 27.7 months.[173]

CANCER OF THE THORACIC CAVITY

TABLE 40.4

Trimodality Studies in Pleural Malignant Pleural Mesothelioma Involving Extrapleural Pneumonectomy

Ref	N	RR	EPP Done	Mortality	Completed Trimodal	OS (ITT) Mo	OS: Subsets Mo	PFS Mo
Weder et al.,[277] 2004	19	32%	84%	0%	68%	23	NR	CT + EPP: 16.5
Weder et al.,[278] 2007	61	NR	74%	2.2%	59%	19.8	CT + EPP:23	CT + EPP:13.5
Rea et al.,[279] 2007	21	33%	81%	0%	71%	25.5	27.5	CT + EPP: 16.3
Flores et al.,[280] 2006	21	26%	42%	0%	42%	19	CT + EPP + RT: 33.5	NR
Opitz et al.,[281] 2006	63	32%	—	3.2%	—	NR	NR	NR
Buduhan et al.,[282] 2009	55	NR	84%	4.3%	69%	NR	CT + EPP: 24 TMT: 25	NR
de Perrot et al.,[283] 2009	60	NR	75%	6.7%	50%	14	NR	NR
Krug et al.,[284] 2009	77	32%	70%	4%	52%	16.8	CT + EPP: 21.9 TMT: 29.1	ITT: 10.1 CT + EPP: 18.3
Van Schil et al.,[285] 2010	58	43%	72%	6.5%	65%	18.4	TMT: 33	ITT: 13.9
Pasello,[286] 2012	54	29%	83%	NR	41%	15.5	NR	ITT PFS: 8.6
Bille et al.[287] 2012	25	NR	88%	4%	71%	12.8	NR	NR
Okada,[288] 2012	27	NR	100%	3.7%	63%	13	23 (CT/RT after EPP)	NR

RR, response rate; EPP, extrapleural pneumonectomy; OS, overall survival; ITT, intent to treat; PFS, progression-free survival; NR, not recorded; CT, chemotherapy; RT, radiation therapy; TMT, trimodality therapy.

TABLE 40.5

Pleurectomy/Decortication and Macroscopic Complete Resection of Pleural Mesothelioma

Ref	N	RX	MCR P/D Done	Mortality	Completed Trimodal	OS (ITT) Mo	OS: Subsets Mo	PFS Mo
Neragi-Miandoab, Richards, and Sugarbaker,[289] 2008	64	Palliative P/D	—	3.1	—	9.4	Epith: 21.7 Nonepith: 5.8	—
Nakas et al.,[175] 2008	102	P/D, radical Nonradical	51 51	5.9 R 9.8 NR	65% 26%	15.3 7.1	25.4R Epith 10.2 NR Epith	—
Luckraz et al.[290] 2010	24	P/D CT + RT	24	1.1	24	26	—	—
Shahin et al.,[176] 2011	26	P/D, Radical Nonradical	13 13	—	CT: 54%, RT: 46% CT: 54%, RT: 15%	16.9 6.8	—	—
Bolukbas,[291] 2012	88	P/D, RT, CT	NR	2.3%	84%	26	—	13
Cameron, Olevsky, and Selch,[292] 2012	121	P/D, RT ± CT	100	NR	NR	13.8	19.7 P/D and RT	NR
Friedberg, Culligan, and Mick,[293] 2012	44	P/D, PDT, CT	97%	2.3%	100	~33	Epith: 37–57 Nonepith: 6.8	9.6
Bille, Okiror, and Lang-Lazdunski,[294] 2012	65	P/D, HPov, RT, CT	NR	0	100	5y:33.4	—	9

RX, treatment protocol; MCR, maximal cytoreductive surgery; P/D, pleurectomy decortication; OS, overall survival; ITT, intent to treat; PFS, progression-free survival; epith, epithelial; CT, chemotherapy; RT, radiation therapy; PDT, photodynamic therapy; HPov, hyperthermic povidone.

EVOLUTION OF LUNG SPARING APPROACHES FOR MACROSCOPIC COMPLETE RESECTION

Questions regarding the ability to perform the same degree of MCR and also spare lung parenchyma arose while studies investigating TMT with EPP as well the MARS trial were accruing patients. A retrospective review of 663 consecutive patients (538 men and 125 women with MPM who underwent EPP or P/D at three US mesothelioma centers) reported an operative mortality of 7% for EPP ($n = 27/385$) and 4% for P/D ($n = 13/278$).[174] The cytoreduction for these patients was described as a macroscopic tumor clearance, both pleurae, and as needed resection of the diaphragm and/or pericardium. Besides significant survival advantages seen for earlier stage ($p < 0.001$), epithelioid versus nonepithelioid histology ($p < 0.001$), multimodality therapy versus surgery alone ($p < 0.001$), and female versus male gender ($p < 0.001$), the type of operation, EPP versus P/D ($p < 0.001$), also influenced survival. Multivariate analysis demonstrated a 1.4-fold greater chance for death with EPP ($p < 0.001$) controlling for stage, histology, gender, and multimodality therapy. This study was the first to postulate that patients who underwent P/D could have comparable survival to those who underwent EPP; however, the reasons for such a conclusion were multifactorial and subject to selection bias. Other studies followed as seen in Table 40.5. The studies by Nakas et al.[175] and Shahin et al.[176] highlight the difference in results for P/D performed either for palliation or for MCR, and both revealed a doubling of overall survival if the P/D is performed to remove all macroscopic disease in a compulsive fashion. All of the subsequent studies, most of which involved a postoperative multimodality adjuvant approach with or without intraoperative therapies, demonstrate superior overall survival of P/D to historical studies of palliative P/D, and exceptional survivals especially in pure epithelial MPM.

Nevertheless, short of a randomized trial, the direct comparison of EPP and P/D performed by the same surgeon. The data for four such centers is seen in Table 40.6. Essentially in all studies,

TABLE 40.6

The Most Recent Published Multimodality Data Comparing Pleurectomy Decortication and Extrapleural Pneumonectomy

Ref	Procedure	n	Thirty-d mortality	Morbidity	Median Follow-up Mo	OS Mo	Two Yr	Five Yr
Lang-Lazdunski et al.[295] 2012	P/D (V/P/dgm/peri) EPP	54 22	0 4.5%	28% 68%	15.7 12.9	23 12.8	49% 18.2%	30.1% 9%
Rena and Casadio,[296] 2012	P/D (? extended) EPP	37 40	0 5%	24% 62%	2–45 10–41	25 20	55% 35%	NA NA
Sorensen, Ravn, and Krisetensen,[297] 2012	P/D EPP	34 28	0 0	NR NR		28.4 31.9		27% 16%
Pass,[298] 2012	P/D (all stages, 24 extended) EPP P/D Stage I/II (11 extended) EPP Stage I/II	78 102 38 20	1.3% 4.9% 2% 5%	22% 57% 20% 30%	22 (0–204) 12 (0–118) 35 (0–204) 27.5 (0–105)	23 12 44 25	46% 23% 66% 55%	19% 5% 35% 29%

OS, overall survival; P/D, pleurectomy decortication; V/P, visceral/parietal; dgm, diaphragm; peri, pericardium; EPP, extrapleural pneumonectomy; NR, not reported.

P/D seems to have less mortality, less morbidity, and a comparable overall survival to EPP. The similarity of the data is quite striking and attests to experienced mesothelioma programs with surgical techniques that are comparable. For early stage mesothelioma, the results also seem to be similar if one compares P/D to EPP.

As extended P/D is a less extensive operation with lower morbidity and mortality than EPP, a newly designed MARS-2 trial will attempt to demonstrate whether this type of operation can offer survival and/or quality-of-life benefits to patients with MPM.[177] Recruitment will most likely be improved compared to MARS-1. Patients with MPM registered on MARS-2 will receive two cycles of pemetrexed-platinum chemotherapy. Patients who do not progress on CT scan will then be randomized to up to four further cycles of pemetrexed-platinum chemotherapy or extended P/D followed by up to four further cycles of postoperative pemetrexed-platinum chemotherapy. An EORTC trial will investigate the timing of the chemotherapy in combination with extended P/D.[178] Patients with MPM will be randomly allocated to extended P/D preceded or followed by four cycles of cisplatin/pemetrexed at standard doses. It is hoped that this randomized trial will address the feasibility of the operation in combination with standard (neo) adjuvant chemotherapy and set the experimental arm of an ensuing phase 3 trial exploring the role of surgery in MPM or could be a standard arm for future trials of surgery in MPM.

CHEMOTHERAPY

First-Line Therapy

Over the past three decades, nearly all chemotherapeutic agents have been tested for malignant mesothelioma as single agents or in combination regimens primarily in single-arm uncontrolled trials.[179] Most single-agent studies exhibited poor response rates and short median survival times (with the exception of cisplatin and the antifolates), while combination therapy generally demonstrated greater efficacy. A meta-analysis of 59 trials confirmed greater response rates for platinum-containing versus non–platinum-containing regimens (23.2% versus 11.6%, respectively; $p < 0.001$).[180]

The report that first garnered enthusiasm regarding the possible chemosensitivity of MPM was the phase 2 trial of gemcitabine plus cisplatin from Byrne et al.[181] Forty-seven percent of treated patients (10 of 21) had a ≥30% reduction in the thickness of the pleural rind and improvement in symptoms. A follow-up multicenter trial from Australia using the same regimen in 53 patients reported a lower response rate at 33% and a median survival of 11.2 months.[182] These studies, and other multicenter phase 2 studies using gemcitabine/cisplatin[183] or gemcitabine/carboplatin,[184] ultimately led to its widespread use for a period of time.

A 1998 report from the United Kingdom also encouraged the use of chemotherapy for MPM by showing that an overall improvement in symptoms occurred in 62% of patients treated with a regimen of three agents: mitomycin C, vinblastine, and cisplatin (MVP).[185] Steele et al.[186] reported a similar rate of clinical benefit with the single agent vinorelbine. Based on these data, the Medical Research Council and British Thoracic Society conducted the first, and only, trial to evaluate whether chemotherapy improved survival over supportive care.[187] Patients with MPM were randomized to either (1) active supportive care (ASC) alone, (2) ASC + MVP, or (3) ASC + vinorelbine. ASC was defined as regular follow-up in a specialist clinic, and treatment could include steroids, analgesics, bronchodilators, and palliative radiation. The trial was originally intended to enroll 840 patients, but due to slow accrual, the statistical design was modified such that only 409 patients were enrolled and the results of the two chemotherapy arms were combined. A small, nonsignificant survival benefit was seen for ASC + CT (hazard ratio [HR] = 0.89; 95% confidence interval [CI] = 0.72 to 1.1; p = .029). The median survival for the ASC arm was 7.6 months, and it was 8.5 months for the ASC + CT arm. In an exploratory analysis, treatment with vinorelbine trended toward providing a survival advantage over ASC (HR = 0.80 [0.63 to 1.02]; $p = 0.08$), but this was not observed for MVP. No difference in four predefined quality-of-life measures (physical functioning, pain, dyspnea, and global health status) was observed between the groups in the first 6 months.

The development of antifolates ultimately had the greatest impact on establishing the standard of care chemotherapy regimen for MPM. Pemetrexed inhibits dihydrofolate reductase, thymidylate synthase, and glycinamide ribonucleotide formyltransferase, enzymes involved in purine and pyrimidine synthesis.[188] Pemetrexed enters the cell primarily through the reduced folate carrier and undergoes extensive intracellular polyglutamation by folylpoly-gamma-glutammate synthetase. The polyglutamated forms, retained for long periods within the cell, have >100-fold greater affinity for thymidylate synthase and glycinamide ribonucleotide formyltransferase than the parent drug, pemetrexed monoglutamate. Moreover, malignant mesothelioma cells overexpress the α-folate receptor, and high levels of expression of this receptor may make malignant mesothelioma more susceptible to antifolate drugs.[189]

The potential activity of pemetrexed and cisplatin in MPM was first noted serendipitously in a phase 1 trial of the combination,[190] and it was this observation that led to the randomized phase 3 trial comparing that combination to treatment with cisplatin alone in patients with advanced MPM. Vogelzang et al.[94] randomized a total of 456 patients with malignant mesothelioma; 226 received a combination of pemetrexed with cisplatin and 222 received cisplatin alone. They were treated with pemetrexed 500 mg/m^2 intravenously followed by cisplatin 75 mg/m^2 on day 1 of a 21-day cycle, or with a normal saline infusion (to maintain single blinding) followed by the same dose of cisplatin alone. Median survival time in the pemetrexed/cisplatin arm was 12.1 months versus 9.3 months in the control arm ($p = 0.020$). The HR for death of patients in the pemetrexed/cisplatin arm versus those in the control arm was 0.77. Median time to progression was significantly longer in the pemetrexed/cisplatin arm: 5.7 months versus 3.9 months ($p = 0.001$), and response rates were 41.3% in the pemetrexed/cisplatin arm versus 16.7% in the control arm ($p < 0.0001$). Analysis of various pemetrexed trials conducted up to that time suggested that supplementation with folic acid and vitamin B_{12} could lessen toxicity from pemetrexed, and this, in fact, was noted in the subset of patients who received supplementation once that was implemented midway through the trial. Interestingly, the cisplatin-alone arm also derived some benefit, possibly enabling patients to receive more cycles of chemotherapy. This pivotal trial led to the establishment of pemetrexed and cisplatin as the standard first-line chemotherapy regimen for MPM, and its regulatory approval for that indication.

Another trial with an identical design confirmed the benefits of adding an antifolate to platinum for the treatment of MPM. That study, run by EORTC, utilized raltitrexed, a more specific thymidylate synthase inhibitor.[191] A total of 250 patients with MPM were randomized to raltitrexed in the presence or absence of cisplatin. The combination of raltitrexed with cisplatin improved response rate (23.6% versus 13.6%; $p = 0.056$), median survival (11.4 months versus 8.8 months; 95% CI = 7.8 to 10.8), and 1-year survival (46% versus 40%; $p = 0.048$).

For patients who are unable to tolerate cisplatin due to gastrointestinal, renal, neurologic, or ototoxicities, substitution with carboplatin is a reasonable alternative. In large, single-arm phase 2 trials,[192,193] and also in the Expanded Access Program that provided patients with access to pemetrexed before its commercial availability,[194] pemetrexed and carboplatin was shown to have comparable response and survival rates. For patients who cannot tolerate any platinum or who have a poor performance status, pemetrexed alone can be considered, though the single-agent response rates are clearly lower.[195,196] If pemetrexed is not available, or results in toxicity, the use of cisplatin or carboplatin together with gemcitabine can be considered as another option.

Second-Line Therapy

No standard of care regimen for patients with previously treated malignant mesothelioma exists, and there are no clear data confirming that second-line therapy increases overall survival. Best supportive care, local RT, and pain medications should be given to patients when required, and chemotherapy may also be considered. Only one phase 3 trial has been conducted in this setting, but it included patients who did not receive a pemetrexed-based regimen as first-line therapy.[195,197] In this study, 243 patients were treated with single-agent pemetrexed and supportive care, or supportive care alone. Treatment with pemetrexed increased the response rate (18.7% versus 1.7%; $p <.0001$) and disease control rate (59.3% versus 19.2%; $p <0.0001$), though overall survival was not improved because a significant number of patients in the supportive care arm ended up receiving chemotherapy. Treatment with pemetrexed or pemetrexed plus cisplatin also yielded high disease control rates in previously treated patients in the Expanded Access Trial.[195,198] However, the current widespread use of pemetrexed/cisplatin as first-line therapy makes these findings mostly irrelevant.

Patients who receive pemetrexed combinations as first-line therapy may derive further benefit from being retreated with pemetrexed, particularly if there is a long interval before progression. In a retrospective analysis of second-line therapy, 42 patients who had been pretreated with pemetrexed were rechallenged, and this resulted in a higher disease control rate, longer progression-free survival, and longer overall survival as compared to treatment with a different agent.[199]

The data supporting the use of other second-line therapies is similarly lacking. A multiple regression analysis that adjusted for baseline prognostic factors found that patients enrolled in the phase 3 trial comparing pemetrexed/cisplatin to cisplatin alone had a longer survival if they received poststudy chemotherapy which primarily consisted of either gemcitabine or vinorelbine.[200] As treatment with single-agent vinorelbine trended toward improving survival in the Medical Research Council phase 3 three-arm trial, it seems a reasonable option for second-line therapy. Stebbing et al.[201] conducted a phase 2 trial with vinorelbine given at a dose of 30mg/m^2 weekly and found a 16% response rate and overall survival of 9.6 months. Only a fraction of the patients in that trial were previously treated with pemetrexed and cisplatin, however. In a retrospective analysis including 56 evaluable patients who had mostly received pemetrexed-based first-line therapy and were treated with vinorelbine or gemcitabine as second- or third-line therapy, there was 1 partial response (with gemcitabine) giving a response rate of 2% (95% CI = 0% to 5%). Forty-six percent of patients had stable disease. Median progression free survival was 1.4 months for both vinorelbine and gemcitabine, while overall median survival was 5.4 months and 4.7 months, respectively. Given the unclear benefit of further chemotherapy, these patients should ideally be enrolled in a clinical trial if available.

NOVEL THERAPEUTIC APPROACHES

Angiogenesis Inhibition

Several lines of evidence support angiogenesis inhibition as a potential therapeutic strategy in mesothelioma. VEGF induces proliferation of mesothelial cells in culture, and the addition of VEGF-neutralizing antibodies inhibits this effect.[52,202] Mesothelioma tumor specimens express VEGF and its receptors.[203,204] High levels of VEGF have also been detected in the serum and pleural effusions of patients with mesothelioma and correlate with poorer survival.[203,205]

The VEGF monoclonal antibody bevacizumab has been extensively studied in mesothelioma. In a randomized phase 2 trial, 106 patients received six cycles of gemcitabine and cisplatin combined with bevacizumab or placebo followed by maintenance therapy with bevacizumab or placebo.[206] No improvement in response rate, progression-free survival, or overall survival was seen with the addition of bevacizumab. A subgroup analysis noted that higher baseline plasma VEGF levels were correlated with a shorter progression-free and overall survival, and that patients with VEGF levels less than the median had longer progression-free and overall survival when treated with bevacizumab. Other studies have explored bevacizumab in combination with pemetrexed and cisplatin. In a single-arm, phase 2 trial with this regimen, 53 patients enrolled at four US centers achieved a progression-free survival of 6.9 months, a disease control rate of 75%, and a median overall survival of 14.8 months; these results compare favorably with historical controls.[207] A French Intergroup study is currently testing pemetrexed/cisplatin plus bevacizumab versus placebo in a definitive randomized phase 2/3 design.

Thalidomide, a drug with a checkered past due to its teratogenic effects, but effective and approved for use in multiple myeloma, has a putative mechanism of action of antiangiogenesis. A phase 1/2 study of thalidomide identified a suitable dose of 200 mg daily and demonstrated 28% disease stabilization for >6 months.[208] However, a phase 3 trial conducted in the Netherlands that randomized 222 patients to maintenance thalidomide versus observation after completion of platinum-based chemotherapy did not demonstrate any benefit in progression-free survival (3.6 months versus 3.5 months; HR = 0.95).[209]

A number of VEGF receptor multikinase inhibitors have been tested in mesothelioma, and they demonstrate a consistent low level of activity (Table 40.7). Most of these drugs also inhibit other growth signaling pathways including PDGF receptors and c-KIT which are also relevant in MPM.[210,211] The first agent in this class to be tested was SU5416, which yielded responses in 11% of patients, but clinical development for this drug was subsequently halted.[212] A CALGB study with sorafenib highlights the issues of patient selection when studying novel agents in mesothelioma.[213] In this trial, patients could receive sorafenib as first- or second-line therapy. Patients who had received previous chemotherapy survived for a median of 13.2 months, compared with 5 months for chemonaïve patients, though this large difference was not statistically significant ($p = 0.3$). One-year survival was also greater in the previously treated patients compared with those who were chemonaïve (57% versus 30%). This suggests that the patients treated as first-line may have been poor candidates for standard chemotherapy, while the patients treated as second-line had maintained a good performance status after chemotherapy. Sunitinib malate was tested in two phase 2 trials. In the Australian study,[214] 53 patients received sunitinib as second-line therapy at a dose of 50 mg on an intermittent schedule of 28 out of every 42 days. The confirmed response rate was 12%, but 65% had stable disease including many patients with some degree of tumor shrinkage. That response rate could not be confirmed, however, in a Canadian trial,[215] which noted only one response in an untreated patient and none in the cohort of previously treated patients. Survival rates were generally poor in both studies. The sum of these trials suggests that these agents may have limited activity, but perhaps should optimally be combined with chemotherapy. This concept is being tested in a Southwest Oncology Group randomized phase 2 trial of pemetrexed/cisplatin with or without cederinib.

Histone Deacetylase Inhibitors

In addition to directly regulating transcription through changes in chromatin structure, histone deacetylase inhibitors modulate the acetylation of transcription factors and other nonhistone proteins. This leads to a range of biologic effects that have shown relevance to MPM in preclinical studies.[216] Vorinostat is an oral agent that binds to the catalytic site of histone deacetylase subtypes 1, 2, 3, and 6 thereby inhibiting their activity.[217] In a phase 1 trial of

TABLE 40.7

Phase 2 Studies with Multikinase Inhibitors of Vascular Endothelial Growth Factor Receptor

Agent	Line of Therapy	N	Overall Response Rate (%)	Stable Disease Rate (%)	Progression-Free Survival (mo)	Overall Survival (mo)
SU5416[212]	Second	23	11	38	2	12.4
Cediranib[299]	First or second	51	10	34	1.8	4.4
Cediranib[300]	Second	54	9	34	2.6	9.5
Pazopanib[301]	First or second	34	NR	56	4.4	11.1
Sorafenib[213]	First or second	51	6	54	3.6	9.7
Sunitinib[302]	Second	53	12	65	3.5	6.1
Sunitinib[303]	First or second	35	3	60	2.7	7.5
Vatalanib[41]	First	47	6	72	4.1	10.0

NR, not reported.

vorinostat, two unconfirmed partial responses were observed in the 13 patients with mesothelioma, and several others had prolonged disease stabilization.[218] These data led to the largest phase 3 trial in mesothelioma in which 661 patients previously treated with one or two prior chemotherapy regimens were randomized 1:1 to vorinostat or placebo. However, vorinostat did not impact overall survival; the median overall survival for vorinostat versus placebo was 30.7 weeks versus 27.1 weeks with a HR of 0.98.[219]

Mammalian Target of Rapamycin Inhibitors

The neurofibromatosis-2 (NF2) gene is mutated in 50% to 60% of MM resulting in loss of the protein Merlin. Merlin mediates contact-dependent inhibition of cell proliferation in normal cells, primarily through inhibition of mammalian target of rapamycin (mTOR).[220] In knockout models of Merlin, mTOR activity becomes unregulated, and this leads to increased cell proliferation that can be abrogated by mTOR inhibition. In mesothelioma cell lines, Merlin loss activates mTORC1 signaling, and cells with NF2 mutations are selectively sensitive to drugs targeting mTORC1.[221] These data provide the rationale for studying the mTOR inhibitors in patients with mesothelioma. However, a Southwest Oncology Group phase 2 study with everolimus in previously treated patients failed to reach its predefined 4-month progression-free survival end point.[222] Agents that also block phosphoinositide-3-kinase along with mTOR appear to have greater efficacy in early trials, though. In an expansion cohort of a phase 1 trial with GDC0980, four patients achieved a partial response, including one patient at 50 mg, one patient with the PIK3CA mutation R88Q at 8 mg, and two at the recommended phase 2 dose of 30 mg. Furthermore, 11 (41%) patients remained on study for >6 months, and 2 (7%) remained on study >12 months.[223]

Mesothelin-Directed Therapy

Mesothelin is an immunogenic cell surface antigen[224,225] involved in cell proliferation, cell signaling, adhesion, and metastases.[226–228] In normal tissues, it is expressed only in the pleura, pericardium, and peritoneum at low levels,[225,229] and it is expressed in essentially all MPM tumors.[98,224,230–232] Several therapeutic approaches targeting mesothelin have shown promise. Amatuximab (MORAb-009) is a chimeric IgG1 antibody tested in a single-arm phase 2 trial in combination with standard chemotherapy for patients with advanced MPM. Although progression-free survival did not differ from historical control and thus the trial did not meet its predefined primary end point, 90% of patients had a radiographic response or stable disease, and overall survival was significantly greater than anticipated with a number of patients remaining on maintenance antibody treatment for an extended time. A follow-up randomized trial with that agent is planned. A mesothelin immunoconjugate, SS1P, consisting of antimesothelin Fv fused to Pseudomonas exotoxin A, demonstrated minor activity in phase 1 trials; however, efficacy was hampered by the development of neutralizing antibodies.[229,233] However, when SS1P was administered along with immunosuppressive agents pentostatin and cyclosphosphamide, dramatic tumor regressions were observed in 3 out of 10 patients, and 2 other patients had major responses to chemotherapy following that therapy.[234] The group at the University of Pennsylvania has begun treating patients with genetically engineered T cells targeting mesothelin and have reported on one patient having a minor response after recovery from a severe infusion reaction.

RADIOTHERAPY FOR MESOTHELIOMA

Curative Radiation Therapy as a Single Modality

The limitation of potentially "curative" RT for treatment of MPM is the inability to treat a large volume of disease in the chest with a curative radiation dose (>60 Gy) because of the risks of severe damage to normal tissue. Previous studies from the 1980s administered approximately 50 Gy to the pleural space with most studies demonstrating a median overall survival ranging from 3 to 10 months. Patients who received treatment had an improved outcome than those who did not receive treatment, although this is likely the result of a selection bias, with those fit enough to undergo a full course of radiation likely to have a greater survival regardless of treatment given.[123,235–239] RT as a sole therapy should be used rarely and only in the setting of patients who are unable to tolerate any form of systemic chemotherapy.

Combined Chemotherapy and Definitive Radiotherapy

The poor results reported for definitive RT alone have led to studies evaluating the combination of chemotherapy and radiation. Both Ruffie et al.[236] and Linden et al.[240] have reported that the median survival is increased in patients treated with combined modality therapy compared with RT alone. Some investigators have evaluated the addition of radiation sensitizers to definitive RT. Herscher et al.[241] from the National Cancer Institute studied the use of a 5-day continuous infusion of paclitaxel with radical RT in patients with mesothelioma and non–small-cell lung cancer. In patients with mesothelioma, the hemithoracic radiation was delivered before the chemotherapy. Chen et al.[242] reported a 12% complete response rate and an 88% partial response rate when pulsed paclitaxel was delivered during RT in a phase 1 trial. Although these combination approaches are interesting, it is not likely that the addition of radiation sensitizers to radical RT will be curative, and as such, definitive chemoradiotherapy should be considered experimental for patients with mesothelioma.

Combined Surgical Resection and Definitive Radiotherapy

RT can be used as an adjuvant treatment after EPP or P/D. After an EPP, radical RT can be administered without concern for damage to the underlying ipsilateral lung because it has been removed surgically. However, radical RT after a P/D continues to place the intact ipsilateral lung at risk for substantial loss of function and toxicity.

Rusch et al.[140,243] at Memorial Sloan Kettering Cancer Center completed a phase 2 trial of EPP followed by postoperative radiation in patients with pleural mesothelioma. Eighty-eight patients with biopsy-confirmed mesothelioma were treated. Twenty-one patients were unresectable and taken off the study. The majority of patients ($n = 62$) underwent an EPP followed by 54 Gy delivered through anterior and posterior fields in 30 fractions of 1.8 Gy. Five patients were treated with a pleurectomy (PL), which was followed by intraoperative RT to a dose of 15 Gy using a high-dose iridium applicator. This was followed by 54 Gy to the hemithorax via anterior and posterior fields in the same fractionation schedule as those who underwent EPP. There were seven postoperative deaths, all primarily related to pulmonary complications in patients who had undergone an EPP. A total of 33 patients had some complications, with the most common being atrial arrhythmias (17 patients), respiratory failure (6 patients), pneumonia (5 patients), and empyema (5 patients). Only the patients who underwent EPP were considered for survival analysis. The median survival was 17 months, with an overall survival of 27% at 3 years. Only 13% had locoregional recurrence, with the majority of patients failing to respond and having distant metastases. The authors concluded that their approach of aggressive surgery with EPP followed by high-dose radiation to the entire hemithorax provided a favorable outcome for those patients who were able to complete the therapy when compared to historical data.

Intensity-modulated RT (IMRT) offers the potential for administering higher doses of RT with better target coverage to the hemithorax while minimizing normal tissue toxicities. IMRT is a highly conformal radiation technique that allows more effective sparing of normal tissues, providing an opportunity for safer, less toxic treatments and increased efficacy by enabling higher radiation doses to the tumor. It comes with a much higher level of dosimetric control and certainty leading to better target coverage than conventional techniques.[244] Areas of dose inhomogeneity are readily recognizable and can be corrected. Rice et al.[245] and Forster et al.[246] at the MD Anderson Cancer Center treated patients with MPM with IMRT after EPP. Recent data in 100 patients who underwent EPP, 63 of whom were treated with IMRT, reveal a median survival of 14.2 months and 3-year survival of 20% for patients with IMRT. Recurrences in the irradiated field occurred in only three patients, and distant disease observed in 54% of patients was the major pattern of failure. Liver injury has been documented after hemithoracic IMRT.[247] However, pulmonary toxicity appears to be the most significant late toxicity observed in patients with MPM after IMRT.[248–250] Allen et al.[248] reported fatal pulmonary complications in 6 of 13 patients with MPM treated with IMRT to a dose of 54 Gy to the clinical target volume. The median time from completion of IMRT to the onset of radiation pneumonitis was 30 days (range, 5 to 57 days). Recent data from Kristensen et al.[250] showed fatal pulmonary toxicity in 4 of 26 (15%) of patients with MPM treated with induction chemotherapy, EPP, and postoperative IMRT to a pleural surface dose of 50 Gy. These reports of pulmonary toxicity emphasize that care should be taken when planning and delivering IMRT to the hemithorax. An alternative technique using electrons and IMRT has been reported as an alternative to IMRT alone. However, it appears that better coverage of the target volume is achieved with IMRT.[251,252] If the use of IMRT after EPP is planned, doses of 45 to 50 Gy in 1.8 to 2.0 Gy fractions are typically recommended. In addition to other standard normal tissue constraints, a mean lung dose of $\leq$9 Gy and a V5 (volume of lung receiving $\geq$5 Gy) of $\leq$65% should be used during the planning process.

Gomez et al.[253] retrospectively analyzed 86 patients who underwent hemithoracic IMRT after EPP at MD Anderson Cancer Center. Grade 3 or worse pulmonary toxicity occurred in 11.6% of patients. There were five fatal cases of pulmonary toxicity: three from radiation pneumonitis and two from bronchopleural fistula. At 2 years, the rates of overall survival, local control, and distant control were 32%, 55%, and 40% respectively. Fourteen patients (16%) experienced local failure and only two of these patients had local failure alone. Fifty-one patients (59%) had distant metastases, which included failures in the contralateral hemithorax and the abdomen.

A retrospective review from the University of North Carolina examined 30 patients who received IMRT following EPP.[254] The median dose to the ipsialteral hemithorax was 45 Gy with an 8 to 25 Gy boost in nine patients. Two-year local control, disease-free survival, and overall survival rates were 47%, 34%, and 50%, respectively. Four patients (13%) developed radiation pneumonitis, including one fatality (3%).

Radiation After Lung Sparing

In a retrospective review of patients having P/D at Memorial Sloan Kettering Cancer Center from 1974 to 2003, 123 patients received external-beam RT (median dose, 42.5 Gy; range, 7.2 to 67.8 Gy) to the ipsilateral hemithorax postoperatively. The median and 2-year overall survival for all patients was 13.5 months (range, 1 to 199 months) and 23%, respectively. Multivariate analysis for overall survival revealed a radiation dose <40 Gy ($p = 0.001$), nonepithelioid histology ($p = 0.002$), left-sided disease ($p = 0.01$), and the use of an implant ($p = 0.02$) to be unfavorable. These data reinforce the concept that residual disease cannot be eradicated with external RT with or without brachytherapy and that a more extensive surgery followed by external RT might be required to improve local control and overall survival.[255] Moreover, intraoperative RT for mesothelioma is associated with toxicity and failure to prolong survival.[256]

An experience with pleural IMRT in 36 patients with two intact lungs has recently been reported.[257] All patients were planned with a PET/CT scan to aid target delineation. With a median dose of 46.8 Gy, 1- and 2- year survival was 75% and 53%, respectively, with a median survival of 26 months in patients who underwent P/D. Seven (20%) patients experienced grade 3 or 4 pneumonitis. A typical treatment plan is presented in Figure 40.10.

A prospective study from Aviano, Italy, reported on 28 patients who were treated with helical tomotherapy after P/D or biopsy alone.[258] All patients had FDG-PET scans after surgery for staging and were treated to an intended dose of 50 to 60 Gy. Five patients (18%) had respiratory toxicity, but only two were grade 3 (7%); none were grade 5. The contralateral lung dose was strongly correlated with the risk of pneumonitis.

Prevention of Scar Recurrences

Malignant seeding in approximately 20% to 50% of patients with mesothelioma along thoracentesis tracts, biopsy tracts, chest

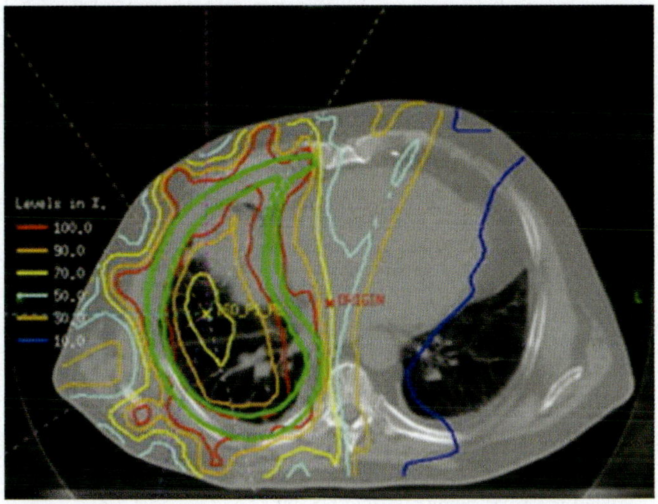

Figure 40.10 Radiation therapy after pleurectomy decortication. Isodense beam distribution showing example of typical isodose distribution using eight angles equally spaced over the 200-degree to 240-degree sector encompassing the ipsilateral lung. Area within *green lines* depicts target volume. (Color version of figure is available online at http://www.semthorcardiovascsurg.com). (Reprinted from Rosenzweig KE, Zauderer MG, Laser B, et al. Pleural intensity-modulated radiotherapy for malignant pleural mesothelioma. *Int J Radiat Oncol Biol Phys* 2012;83:1278–1283, Copyright (2012), with permission from Elsevier.)

tube sites, and surgical incisions is a common complication of procedures in these patients.[119,259] Boutin et al.[119] randomized 40 patients after an invasive diagnostic procedure to either RT (7 Gy × three fractions) or no treatment. No patient in the radiation treatment group developed subcutaneous nodules. Alternatively, 8 of 20 patients in the untreated group developed metastases. Two additional small randomized trials have suggested that the use of short-course RT does not reduce the frequency of cutaneous seeding after invasive procedures.[121,260] These data are inconclusive, and reviews of contemporary practice patterns suggest that radiation is commonly used to prevent scar recurrences.[261,262]

Palliation Using Radiation Therapy

RT is commonly used to palliate pain in patients with advanced mesothelioma,[157] and investigators from the Netherlands have reported using palliative RT to treat painful chest wall metastases in patients with mesothelioma. Ball and Cruickshank[237] reported a 72% rate of symptom improvement using palliative courses of RT. Ruffie et al.[263] and Davis et al.[264] reported the results of palliative RT in patients with mesothelioma. When doses >45 Gy were used, pain relief was attained in >50% of the cases.

More recently, some centers have investigated the use of IMRT for unresectable patients. Treatment techniques prior to the advent of IMRT would have necessitated significant dose inhomogeneity in the setting of intact lung. Palliative RT to the entire hemithorax should only be considered when first-line and second-line chemotherapeutic options have been exhausted.

Proton Beam Radiation

The widespread interest in proton RT has begun to carry over to MPM. To date, two theoretical planning studies have been published that suggest that proton therapy allows better sparing of normal organs at risk while providing better target coverage in patients after EPP.[265,266] However, many uncertainties regarding the feasibility of proton therapy in thoracic RT remain, given the significant impact of respiratory motion and stark tissue density variation in the thorax on accurate proton dosimetry. Clinical validation of proton therapy for MPM remains to be shown.

REFERENCES

1. Carbone M, Kratzke RA, Testa JR. The pathogenesis of mesothelioma. *Semin Oncol* 2002;29:2–17.
2. Yang H, Bocchetta M, Kroczynska B, et al. TNF-alpha inhibits asbestos-induced cytotoxicity via a NF-kappaB-dependent pathway, a possible mechanism for asbestos-induced oncogenesis. *Proc Natl Acad Sci U S A* 2006;103:10397–10402.
3. Altomare DA, Vaslet CA, Skele KL, et al. A mouse model recapitulating molecular features of human mesothelioma. *Cancer Res* 2005;65:8090–8095.
4. Wagner JC, Berry G, Timbrell V. Mesotheliomata in rats after inoculation with asbestos and other materials. *Br J Cancer* 1973;28:173–185.
5. Smith WE. Asbestos, talc and nitrites in relation to gastric cancer. *Am Ind Hyg Assoc J* 1973;34:227–228.
6. Stanton MF, Wrench C. Mechanisms of mesothelioma induction with asbestos and fibrous glass. *J Natl Cancer Inst* 1972;48:797–821.
7. Mossman BT, Bignon J, Corn M, et al. Asbestos: scientific developments and implications for public policy. *Science* 1990;247:294–301.
8. Smith AH, Wright CC. Chrysotile asbestos is the main cause of pleural mesothelioma. *Am J Ind Med* 1996;30:252–266.
9. Vianna NJ, Polan AK. Non-occupational exposure to asbestos and malignant mesothelioma in females. *Lancet* 1978;1:1061–1063.
10. Li FP, Lokich J, Lapey J, et al. Familial mesothelioma after intense asbestos exposure at home. *JAMA* 1978;240:467.
11. Yates DH, Corrin B, Stidolph PN, et al. Malignant mesothelioma in south east England: clinicopathological experience of 272 cases. *Thorax* 1997;52:507–512.
12. Yang H, Rivera Z, Jube S, et al. Programmed necrosis induced by asbestos in human mesothelial cells causes high-mobility group box 1 protein release and resultant inflammation. *Proc Natl Acad Sci U S A* 2010;107:12611–12616.
13. Carbone M, Ly BH, Dodson RF, et al. Malignant mesothelioma: facts, myths, and hypotheses. *J Cell Physiol* 2012;227:44–58.
14. Hillegass JM, Shukla A, Lathrop SA, et al. Inflammation precedes the development of human malignant mesotheliomas in a SCID mouse xenograft model. *Ann N Y Acad Sci* 2010;1203:7–14.
15. Wang Y, Faux SP, Hallden G, et al. Interleukin-1beta and tumour necrosis factor-alpha promote the transformation of human immortalised mesothelial cells by erionite. *Int J Oncol* 2004;25:173–178.
16. Franchi L, Eigenbrod T, Munoz-Planillo R, et al. The inflammasome: a caspase-1-activation platform that regulates immune responses and disease pathogenesis. *Nat Immunol* 2009;10:241–247.
17. Martinon F, Mayor A, Tschopp J. The inflammasomes: guardians of the body. *Annu Rev Immunol* 2009;27:229–265.
18. Bianchi ME. DAMPs, PAMPs and alarmins: all we need to know about danger. *J Leukoc Biol* 2007;81:1–5.
19. Dostert C, Petrilli V, Van Bruggen R, et al. Innate immune activation through Nalp3 inflammasome sensing of asbestos and silica. *Science* 2008;320:674–677.
20. Cassel SL, Eisenbarth SC, Iyer SS, et al. The Nalp3 inflammasome is essential for the development of silicosis. *Proc Natl Acad Sci U S A* 2008;105:9035–9040.
21. Ellerman JE, Brown CK, de Vera M, et al. Masquerader: high mobility group box-1 and cancer. *Clin Cancer Res* 2007;13:2836–2848.
22. Jube S, Rivera ZS, Bianchi ME, et al. Cancer cell secretion of the DAMP protein HMGB1 supports progression in malignant mesothelioma. *Cancer Res* 2012;72:3290–3301.
23. Lanphear BP, Buncher CR. Latent period for malignant mesothelioma of occupational origin. *J Occup Med* 1992;34:718–721.
24. De Rienzo A, Testa JR. Recent advances in the molecular analysis of human malignant mesothelioma. *Clin Ter* 2000;151:433–438.
25. Ivanov SV, Miller J, Lucito R, et al. Genomic events associated with progression of pleural malignant mesothelioma. *Int J Cancer* 2009;124:589–599.
26. Cheng JQ, Jhanwar SC, Klein WM, et al. p16 alterations and deletion mapping of 9p21-p22 in malignant mesothelioma. *Cancer Res* 1994;54:5547–5551.
27. Kobayashi N, Toyooka S, Yanai H, et al. Frequent p16 inactivation by homozygous deletion or methylation is associated with a poor prognosis in Japanese patients with pleural mesothelioma. *Lung Cancer* 2008;62:120–125.
28. Altomare DA, Menges CW, Xu J, et al. Losses of both products of the Cdkn2a/Arf locus contribute to asbestos-induced mesothelioma development and cooperate to accelerate tumorigenesis. *PLoS One* 2011;6:e18828.

29. Yang CT, You L, Uematsu K, et al. p14(ARF) modulates the cytolytic effect of ONYX-015 in mesothelioma cells with wild-type p53. *Cancer Res* 2001;61:5959–5963.
30. Yang CT, You L, Lin YC, et al. A comparison analysis of anti-tumor efficacy of adenoviral gene replacement therapy (p14ARF and p16INK4A) in human mesothelioma cells. *Anticancer Res* 2003;23:33–38.
31. Dacic S, Kothmaier H, Land S, et al. Prognostic significance of p16/cdkn2a loss in pleural malignant mesotheliomas. *Virchows Arch* 2008;453:627–635.
32. Ivanov SV, Goparaju CM, Lopez P, et al. Pro-tumorigenic effects of miR-31 loss in mesothelioma. *J Biol Chem* 2010;285:22809–22817.
33. Marsella JM, Liu BL, Vaslet CA, et al. Susceptibility of p53-deficient mice to induction of mesothelioma by crocidolite asbestos fibers. *Environ Health Perspect* 1997;105:1069–1072.
34. Amin KM, Litzky LA, Smythe WR, et al. Wilms' tumor 1 susceptibility (WT1) gene products are selectively expressed in malignant mesothelioma. *Am J Pathol* 1995;146:344–356.
35. Zauderer MG, Krug LM. Novel therapies in phase II and III trials for malignant pleural mesothelioma. *J Natl Compr Canc Netw* 2012;10:42–47.
36. Cheng JQ, Lee WC, Klein MA, et al. Frequent mutations of NF2 and allelic loss from chromosome band 22q12 in malignant mesothelioma: evidence for a two-hit mechanism of NF2 inactivation. *Genes Chromosomes Cancer* 1999;24:238–242.
37. Thurneysen C, Opitz I, Kurtz S, et al. Functional inactivation of NF2/merlin in human mesothelioma. *Lung Cancer* 2009;64:140–147.
38. Jongsma J, van Montfort E, Vooijs M, et al. A conditional mouse model for malignant mesothelioma. *Cancer Cell* 2008;13:261–271.
39. Gerwin BI, Lechner JF, Reddel RR, et al. Comparison of production of transforming growth factor-beta and platelet-derived growth factor by normal human mesothelial cells and mesothelioma cell lines. *Cancer Res* 1987;47:6180–6184.
40. Honda M, Kanno T, Fujita Y, et al. Mesothelioma cell proliferation through autocrine activation of PDGF-betabeta receptor. *Cell Physiol Biochem* 2012;29:667–674.
41. Jahan T, Gu L, Kratzke R, et al. Vatalanib in malignant mesothelioma: a phase II trial by the Cancer and Leukemia Group B (CALGB 30107). *Lung Cancer* 2012;76:393–396.
42. Kumar-Singh S, Weyler J, Martin MJ, et al. Angiogenic cytokines in mesothelioma: a study of VEGF, FGF-1 and -2, and TGF beta expression. *J Pathol* 1999;189:72–78.
43. Maeda J, Ueki N, Ohkawa T, et al. Transforming growth factor-beta 1 (TGF-beta 1)- and beta 2-like activities in malignant pleural effusions caused by malignant mesothelioma or primary lung cancer. *Clin Exp Immunol* 1994;98:319–322.
44. Kim S, Buchlis G, Fridlender ZG, et al. Systemic blockade of transforming growth factor-beta signaling augments the efficacy of immunogene therapy. *Cancer Res* 2008;68:10247–10256.
45. Kissick HT, Ireland DJ, Krishnan S, et al. Tumour eradication and induction of memory against murine mesothelioma by combined immunotherapy. *Immunol Cell Biol* 2012;90:822–826.
46. Lee TC, Zhang Y, Aston C, et al. Normal human mesothelial cells and mesothelioma cell lines express insulin-like growth factor I and associated molecules. *Cancer Res* 1993;53:2858–2864.
47. Pass HI, Mew DJ, Carbone M, et al. The effect of an antisense expression plasmid to the IGF-1 receptor on hamster mesothelioma proliferation. *Dev Biol Stand* 1998;94:321–328.
48. Kalra N, Zhang J, Yu Y, et al. Efficacy of anti-insulin-like growth factor I receptor monoclonal antibody cixutumumab in mesothelioma is highly correlated with insulin growth factor-I receptor sites/cell. *Int J Cancer* 2012;131:2143–2152.
49. Nakano T, Chahinian AP, Shinjo M, et al. Interleukin 6 and its relationship to clinical parameters in patients with malignant pleural mesothelioma. *Br J Cancer* 1998;77:907–912.
50. Adachi Y, Aoki C, Yoshio-Hoshino N, et al. Interleukin-6 induces both cell growth and VEGF production in malignant mesotheliomas. *Int J Cancer* 2006;119:1303–1311.
51. Antony VB, Hott JW, Godbey SW, et al. Angiogenesis in mesotheliomas. Role of mesothelial cell derived IL-8. *Chest* 1996;109:21S–22S.
52. Ohta Y, Shridhar V, Bright RK, et al. VEGF and VEGF type C play an important role in angiogenesis and lymphangiogenesis in human malignant mesothelioma tumours. *Br J Cancer* 1999;81:54–61.
53. Kumar-Singh S, Vermeulen PB, Weyler J, et al. Evaluation of tumour angiogenesis as a prognostic marker in malignant mesothelioma. *J Pathol* 1997;182:211–216.
54. Ohta Y, Shridhar V, Kalemkerian GP, et al. Thrombospondin-1 expression and clinical implications in malignant pleural mesothelioma. *Cancer* 1999;85:2570–2576.
55. Gazdar AF, Butel JS, Carbone M. SV40 and human tumours: myth, association or causality? *Nat Rev Cancer* 2002;2:957–964.
56. Carbone M, Pass HI. Evolving aspects of mesothelioma carcinogenesis: SV40 and genetic predisposition. *J Thorac Oncol* 2006;1:169–171.
57. Carbone M, Strianese O, Theos K, et al. Mesothelioma. *Hawaii Med J* 2007;66:48–50.
58. Klein G. Simian virus 40 and the human mesothelium. *Proc Natl Acad Sci U S A* 2000;97:9830–9831.
59. Cicala C, Pompetti F, Carbone M. SV40 induces mesotheliomas in hamsters. *Am J Pathol* 1993;142:1524–1533.
60. Kroczynska B, Cutrone R, Bocchetta M, et al. Crocidolite asbestos and SV40 are cocarcinogens in human mesothelial cells and in causing mesothelioma in hamsters. *Proc Natl Acad Sci U S A* 2006;103:14128–14133.
61. Cleaver AL, Bhamidipaty K, Wylie B, et al. Long-term exposure of mesothelial cells to SV40 and asbestos leads to malignant transformation and chemotherapy resistance. *Carcinogenesis* 2014;35:407–414.
62. Dresselhaus MS, Dresselhaus G, Charlier JC, et al. Electronic, thermal and mechanical properties of carbon nanotubes. *Philos Trans A Math Phys Eng Sci* 2004;362:2065–2098.
63. Lam CW, James JT, McCluskey R, et al. Pulmonary toxicity of single-wall carbon nanotubes in mice 7 and 90 days after intratracheal instillation. *Toxicol Sci* 2004;77:126–134.
64. Shvedova AA, Kagan VE, Fadeel B. Close encounters of the small kind: adverse effects of man-made materials interfacing with the nano-cosmos of biological systems. *Annu Rev Pharmacol Toxicol* 2010;50:63–88.
65. Shvedova AA, Kisin E, Murray AR, et al. Inhalation vs. aspiration of single-walled carbon nanotubes in C57BL/6 mice: inflammation, fibrosis, oxidative stress, and mutagenesis. *Am J Physiol Lung Cell Mol Physiol* 2008;295:L552–L565.
66. Takagi A, Hirose A, Futakuchi M, et al. Dose-dependent mesothelioma induction by intraperitoneal administration of multi-wall carbon nanotubes in p53 heterozygous mice. *Cancer Sci* 2012;103:1440–1444.
67. Takagi A, Hirose A, Nishimura T, et al. Induction of mesothelioma in p53+/− mouse by intraperitoneal application of multi-wall carbon nanotube. *J Toxicol Sci* 2008;33:105–116.
68. Pacurari M, Castranova V, Vallyathan V. Single- and multi-wall carbon nanotubes versus asbestos: are the carbon nanotubes a new health risk to humans? *J Toxicol Environ Health A* 2010;73:378–395.
69. Pacurari M, Yin XJ, Zhao J, et al. Raw single-wall carbon nanotubes induce oxidative stress and activate MAPKs, AP-1, NF-kappaB, and Akt in normal and malignant human mesothelial cells. *Environ Health Perspect* 2008;116:1211–1217.
70. Glista-Baker EE, Taylor AJ, Sayers BC, et al. Nickel nanoparticles enhance platelet-derived growth factor-induced chemokine expression by mesothelial cells via prolonged mitogen-activated protein kinase activation. *Am J Respir Cell Mol Biol* 2012;47:552–561.
71. Carbone M, Emri S, Dogan AU, et al. A mesothelioma epidemic in Cappadocia: scientific developments and unexpected social outcomes. *Nat Rev Cancer* 2007;7:147–154.
72. Carbone M, Baris YI, Bertino P, et al. Erionite exposure in North Dakota and Turkish villages with mesothelioma. *Proc Natl Acad Sci U S A* 2011;108:13618–13623.
73. Dogan AU, Dogan M, Hoskins JA. Erionite series minerals: mineralogical and carcinogenic properties. *Environ Geochem Health* 2008;30(4):367–381.
74. Ascoli V, Aalto Y, Carnovale-Scalzo C, et al. DNA copy number changes in familial malignant mesothelioma. *Cancer Genet Cytogenet* 2001;127:80–82.
75. Carbone M, Yang H, Pass HI, et al. BAP1 and cancer. *Nat Rev Cancer* 2013;13:153–159.
76. Dey A, Seshasayee D, Noubade R, et al. Loss of the tumor suppressor BAP1 causes myeloid transformation. *Science* 2012;337:1541–1546.
77. Bott M, Brevet M, Taylor BS, et al. The nuclear deubiquitinase BAP1 is commonly inactivated by somatic mutations and 3p21.1 losses in malignant pleural mesothelioma. *Nat Genet* 2011;43:668–672.
78. Matatall KA, Agapova OA, Onken MD, et al. BAP1 deficiency causes loss of melanocytic cell identity in uveal melanoma. *BMC Cancer* 2013;13:371.
79. Zauderer MG, Bott M, McMillan R, et al. Clinical characteristics of patients with malignant pleural mesothelioma harboring somatic BAP1 mutations. *J Thorac Oncol* 2013;8:1430–1433.
80. Yoshikawa Y, Sato A, Tsujimura T, et al. Frequent inactivation of the BAP1 gene in epithelioid-type malignant mesothelioma. *Cancer Sci* 2012;103:868–874.
81. Arzt L, Quehenberger F, Halbwedl I, et al. BAP1 protein is a progression factor in malignant pleural mesothelioma. *Pathol Oncol Res* 2014;20:145–151.
82. Testa JR, Cheung M, Pei J, et al. Germline BAP1 mutations predispose to malignant mesothelioma. *Nat Genet* 2011;43:1022–1025.
83. Robinson LA. Solitary fibrous tumor of the pleura. *Cancer Control* 2006;13:264–269.
84. Brozzetti S, D'Andrea N, Limiti MR, et al. Clinical behavior of solitary fibrous tumors of the pleura. An immunohistochemical study. *Anticancer Res* 2000;20:4701–4706.
85. Filosso PL, Oliaro A, Rena O, et al. Severe hypoglycaemia associated with a giant solitary fibrous tumor of the pleura. *J Cardiovasc Surg (Torino)* 2002;43:559–561.
86. Carbone M, Rizzo P, Powers A, et al. Molecular analyses, morphology and immunohistochemistry together differentiate pleural synovial sarcomas from mesotheliomas: clinical implications. *Anticancer Res* 2002;22:3443–3448.
87. Gee GV, Koestler DC, Christensen BC, et al. Downregulated microRNAs in the differential diagnosis of malignant pleural mesothelioma. *Int J Cancer* 2010;127:2859–2869.
88. Benjamin H, Lebanony D, Rosenwald S, et al. A diagnostic assay based on microRNA expression accurately identifies malignant pleural mesothelioma. *J Mol Diagn* 2010;12:771–779.
89. Lin RT, Takahashi K, Karjalainen A, et al. Ecological association between asbestos-related diseases and historical asbestos consumption: an international analysis. *Lancet* 2007;369:844–849.
90. Peto J, Decarli A, La Vecchia C, et al. The European mesothelioma epidemic. *Br J Cancer* 1999;79:666–672.
91. Roggli VL, Sharma A, Butnor KJ, et al. Malignant mesothelioma and occupational exposure to asbestos: a clinicopathological correlation of 1445 cases. *Ultrastruct Pathol* 2002;26:55–65.
92. Wolf AS, Richards WG, Tilleman TR, et al. Characteristics of malignant pleural mesothelioma in women. *Ann Thorac Surg* 2010;90:949–956.

93. Erasmus JJ, Truong MT, Smythe WR, et al. Integrated computed tomography-positron emission tomography in patients with potentially resectable malignant pleural mesothelioma: Staging implications. *J Thorac Cardiovasc Surg* 2005;129:1364–1370.
94. Vogelzang NJ, Rusthoven JJ, Symanowski J, et al. Phase III study of pemetrexed in combination with cisplatin versus cisplatin alone in patients with malignant pleural mesothelioma. *J Clin Oncol* 2003;21:2636–2644.
95. Herndon JE, Green MR, Chahinian AP, et al. Factors predictive of survival among 337 patients with mesothelioma treated between 1984 and 1994 by the Cancer and Leukemia Group B. *Chest* 1998;113:723–731.
96. Robinson BW, Creaney J, Lake R, et al. Mesothelin-family proteins and diagnosis of mesothelioma. *Lancet* 2003;362:1612–1616.
97. Beyer HL, Geschwindt RD, Glover CL, et al. MESOMARK: a potential test for malignant pleural mesothelioma. *Clin Chem* 2007;53:666–672.
98. Pass HI, Wali A, Tang N, et al. Soluble mesothelin-related peptide level elevation in mesothelioma serum and pleural effusions. *Ann Thorac Surg* 2008;85: 265–272.
99. Hollevoet K, Reitsma JB, Creaney J, et al. Serum mesothelin for diagnosing malignant pleural mesothelioma: an individual patient data meta-analysis. *J Clin Oncol* 2012;30:1541–1549.
100. Creaney J, Robinson BW. Detection of malignant mesothelioma in asbestos-exposed individuals: the potential role of soluble mesothelin-related protein. *Hematol Oncol Clin North Am* 2005;19:1025–1040, v.
101. Park EK, Sandrini A, Yates DH, et al. Soluble mesothelin-related protein in an asbestos-exposed population: the dust diseases board cohort study. *Am J Respir Crit Care Med* 2008;178:832–837.
102. Imashimizu K, Shiomi K, Maeda M, et al. Feasibility of large-scale screening using N-ERC/mesothelin levels in the blood for the early diagnosis of malignant mesothelioma. *Exp Ther Med* 2011;2:409–411.
103. Sandhu H, Dehnen W, Roller M, et al. mRNA expression patterns in different stages of asbestos-induced carcinogenesis in rats. *Carcinogenesis* 2000;21: 1023–1029.
104. Pass HI, Lott D, Lonardo F, et al. Asbestos exposure, pleural mesothelioma, and serum osteopontin levels. *N Engl J Med* 2005;353:1564–1573.
105. Grigoriu BD, Grigoriu C, Chahine B, et al. Clinical utility of diagnostic markers for malignant pleural mesothelioma. *Monaldi Arch Chest Dis* 2009;71:31–38.
106. Creaney J, Yeoman D, Demelker Y, et al. Comparison of osteopontin, megakaryocyte potentiating factor, and mesothelin proteins as markers in the serum of patients with malignant mesothelioma. *J Thorac Oncol* 2008;3:851–857.
107. Pass HI, Levin SM, Harbut MR, et al. Fibulin-3 as a blood and effusion biomarker for pleural mesothelioma. *N Engl J Med* 2012;367:1417–1427.
108. Wechsler RJ, Rao VM, Steiner RM. The radiology of thoracic malignant mesothelioma. *Crit Rev Diagn Imaging* 1984;20:283–310.
109. Heller RM, Janower ML, Weber AL. The radiological manifestations of malignant pleural mesothelioma. *Am J Roentgenol Radium Ther Nucl Med* 1970;108:53–59.
110. Solomon A. Radiological features of diffuse mesothelioma. *Environ Res* 1970;3:330–338.
111. Patz EF Jr, Shaffer K, Piwnica-Worms DR, et al. Malignant pleural mesothelioma: value of CT and MR imaging in predicting resectability. *AJR Am J Roentgenol* 1992;159:961–966.
112. Flores RM. The role of PET in the surgical management of malignant pleural mesothelioma. *Lung Cancer* 2005;49:S27–S32.
113. Schneider DB, Clary-Macy C, Challa S, et al. Positron emission tomography with f18-fluorodeoxyglucose in the staging and preoperative evaluation of malignant pleural mesothelioma. *J Thorac Cardiovasc Surg* 2000;120:128–133.
114. Benard F, Sterman D, Smith RJ, et al. Prognostic value of FDG PET imaging in malignant pleural mesothelioma. *J Nucl Med* 1999;40:1241–1245.
115. Gerbaudo VH, Mamede M, Trotman-Dickenson B, et al. FDG PET/CT patterns of treatment failure of malignant pleural mesothelioma: relationship to histologic type, treatment algorithm, and survival. *Eur J Nucl Med Mol Imaging* 2011;38:810–821.
116. Gerbaudo VH, Sugarbaker DJ, Britz-Cunningham S, et al. Assessment of malignant pleural mesothelioma with (18)F-FDG dual-head gamma-camera coincidence imaging: comparison with histopathology. *J Nucl Med* 2002;43:1144–1149.
117. Boutin C, Rey F, Gouvernet J, et al. Thoracoscopy in pleural malignant mesothelioma: a prospective study of 188 consecutive patients. Part 2: Prognosis and staging. *Cancer* 1993;72:394–401.
118. Boutin C, Rey F. Thoracoscopy in pleural malignant mesothelioma: a prospective study of 188 consecutive patients. Part 1: Diagnosis. *Cancer* 1993;72:389–393.
119. Boutin C, Rey F, Viallat JR. Prevention of malignant seeding after invasive diagnostic procedures in patients with pleural mesothelioma. A randomized trial of local radiotherapy. *Chest* 1995;108:754–758.
120. Muirhead R, O'Rourke N. Drain site radiotherapy in malignant pleural mesothelioma: a wasted resource. *Eur Respir J* 2007;30:1021–1025.
121. O'Rourke N, Garcia JC, Paul J, et al. A randomised controlled trial of intervention site radiotherapy in malignant pleural mesothelioma. *Radiother Oncol* 2007;84:18–22.
122. Antman KH, Blum RH, Greenberger JS, et al. Multimodality therapy for malignant mesothelioma based on a study of natural history. *Am J Med* 1980;68: 356–362.
123. Law MR, Hodson ME, Heard BE. Malignant mesothelioma of the pleura: relation between histological type and clinical behaviour. *Thorax* 1982;37:810–815.
124. Falconieri G, Grandi G, DiBonito L, et al. Intracranial metastases from malignant pleural mesothelioma. Report of three autopsy cases and review of the literature. *Arch Pathol Lab Med* 1991;115:591–595.
125. Davies MJ, Ahmedzai S, Arsiwala SS, et al. Intracranial metastases from malignant pleural mesothelioma. *Scand J Thorac Cardiovasc Surg* 1995;29:97–99.
126. Curran D, Sahmoud T, Therasse P, et al. Prognostic factors in patients with pleural mesothelioma: the European Organization for Research and Treatment of Cancer experience. *J Clin Oncol* 1998;16:145–152.
127. Fennell DA, Parmar A, Shamash J, et al. Statistical validation of the EORTC prognostic model for malignant pleural mesothelioma based on three consecutive phase II trials. *J Clin Oncol* 2005;23:184–189.
128. Edwards JG, Abrams KR, Leverment JN, et al. Prognostic factors for malignant mesothelioma in 142 patients: validation of CALGB and EORTC prognostic scoring systems. *Thorax* 2000;55:731–735.
129. Kao SC, Vardy J, Chatfield M, et al. Validation of prognostic factors in malignant pleural mesothelioma: a retrospective analysis of data from patients seeking compensation from the New South Wales Dust Diseases Board. *Clin Lung Cancer* 2013;14:70–77.
130. Kao SC, Klebe S, Henderson DW, et al. Low calretinin expression and high neutrophil-to-lymphocyte ratio are poor prognostic factors in patients with malignant mesothelioma undergoing extrapleural pneumonectomy. *J Thorac Oncol* 2011;6:1923–1929.
131. Kao SC, Pavlakis N, Harvie R, et al. High blood neutrophil-to-lymphocyte ratio is an indicator of poor prognosis in malignant mesothelioma patients undergoing systemic therapy. *Clin Cancer Res* 2010;16:5805–5813.
132. Meniawy TM, Creaney J, Lake RA, et al. Existing models, but not neutrophil-to-lymphocyte ratio, are prognostic in malignant mesothelioma. *Br J Cancer* 2013;109:1813–1820.
133. Gordon GJ, Jensen RV, Hsiao LL, et al. Using gene expression ratios to predict outcome among patients with mesothelioma. *J Natl Cancer Inst* 2003;95:598–605.
134. Pass HI, Liu Z, Wali A, et al. Gene expression profiles predict survival and progression of pleural mesothelioma. *Clin Cancer Res* 2004;10:849–859.
135. Lopez-Rios F, Chuai S, Flores R, et al. Global gene expression profiling of pleural mesotheliomas: overexpression of aurora kinases and P16/CDKN2A deletion as prognostic factors and critical evaluation of microarray-based prognostic prediction. *Cancer Res* 2006;66:2970–2979.
136. Pass HI, Goparaju C, Ivanov S, et al. hsa-miR-29c* is linked to the prognosis of malignant pleural mesothelioma. *Cancer Res* 2010;70:1916–1924.
137. Righi L, Papotti MG, Ceppi P, et al. Thymidylate synthase but not excision repair cross-complementation group 1 tumor expression predicts outcome in patients with malignant pleural mesothelioma treated with pemetrexed-based chemotherapy. *J Clin Oncol* 2010;28:1534–1539.
138. Hollevoet K, Nackaerts K, Gosselin R, et al. Soluble mesothelin, megakaryocyte potentiating factor, and osteopontin as markers of patient response and outcome in mesothelioma. *J Thorac Oncol* 2011;6:1930–1937.
139. Cappia S, Righi L, Mirabelli D, et al. Prognostic role of osteopontin expression in malignant pleural mesothelioma. *Am J Clin Pathol* 2008;130:58–64.
140. Ivanova AV, Goparaju CM, Ivanov SV, et al. Protumorigenic role of HAPLN1 and its IgV domain in malignant pleural mesothelioma. *Clin Cancer Res* 2009;15:2602–2611.
141. Gerbaudo VH, Britz-Cunningham S, Sugarbaker DJ, et al. Metabolic significance of the pattern, intensity and kinetics of 18F-FDG uptake in malignant pleural mesothelioma. *Thorax* 2003;58:1077–1082.
142. Sharif S, Zahid I, Routledge T, et al. Does positron emission tomography offer prognostic information in malignant pleural mesothelioma? *Interact Cardiovasc Thorac Surg* 2011;12:806–811.
143. Lee HY, Hyun SH, Lee KS, et al. Volume-based parameter of 18)F-FDG PET/CT in malignant pleural mesothelioma: prediction of therapeutic response and prognostic implications. *Ann Surg Oncol* 2010;17:2787–2794.
144. Nowak AK, Francis RJ, Phillips MJ, et al. A novel prognostic model for malignant mesothelioma incorporating quantitative FDG-PET imaging with clinical parameters. *Clin Cancer Res* 2010;16:2409–2417.
145. Butchart EG, Ashcroft T, Barnsley WC, et al. Pleuropneumonectomy in the management of diffuse malignant mesothelioma of the pleura. Experience with 29 patients. *Thorax* 1976;31:15–24.
146. Rusch VW. A proposed new international TNM staging system for malignant pleural mesothelioma. From the International Mesothelioma Interest Group. *Chest* 1995;108:1122–1128.
147. Rusch VW, Giroux D, Kennedy C, et al. Initial analysis of the international association for the study of lung cancer mesothelioma database. *J Thorac Oncol* 2012;7:1631–1639.
148. Zellos L, Sugarbaker DJ. Current surgical management of malignant pleural mesothelioma. *Curr Oncol Rep* 2002;4:354–360.
149. Richards WG, Godleski JJ, Yeap BY, et al. Proposed adjustments to pathologic staging of epithelial malignant pleural mesothelioma based on analysis of 354 cases. *Cancer* 2010;116:1510–1517.
150. Pass HI, Temeck BK, Kranda K, et al. Preoperative tumor volume is associated with outcome in malignant pleural mesothelioma. *J Thorac Cardiovasc Surg* 1998;115:310–317.
151. Gill RR, Richards WG, Yeap BY, et al. Epithelial malignant pleural mesothelioma after extrapleural pneumonectomy: stratification of survival with CT-derived tumor volume. *AJR Am J Roentgenol* 2012;198:359–363.
152. Richards W, Gill RR, Yeap B, et al. Validation of a stage-independent pre-operative risk assessment algorithm for patients considering surgery for malignant pleural mesothelioma. Presented at the 15th International Association for the Study of Lung Cancer Meeting, October 2013, Sydney, Australia.
153. Stahel RA, Weder W, Felip E. Malignant pleural mesothelioma: ESMO clinical recommendations for diagnosis, treatment and follow-up. *Ann Oncol* 2009;20:73–75.

154. Pilling JE, Dusmet ME, Ladas G, et al. Prognostic factors for survival after surgical palliation of malignant pleural effusion. *J Thorac Oncol* 2010;5:1544–1550.
155. Rintoul RC, Ritchie AJ, Edwards JG, et al. MesoVATS: A multi-centre randomised controlled trial of video assisted thoracoscopic pleurectomy versus talc pleurodesis in malignant pleural mesothelioma (MesoVATS): an open-label, randomised, controlled trial. *Lancet* 2014;14:60418–60419.
156. Pien GW, Gant MJ, Washam CL, et al. Use of an implantable pleural catheter for trapped lung syndrome in patients with malignant pleural effusion. *Chest* 2001;119:1641–1646.
157. de Graaf-Strukowska L, van der Zee J, van Putten W, et al. Factors influencing the outcome of radiotherapy in malignant mesothelioma of the pleura—a single-institution experience with 189 patients. *Int J Radiat Oncol Biol Phys* 1999;43:511–516.
158. Bissett D, Macbeth FR, Cram I. The role of palliative radiotherapy in malignant mesothelioma. *Clin Oncol (R Coll Radiol)* 1991;3:315–317.
159. Butchart EG, Ashcroft T, Barnsley WC, et al. Pleuropneumonectomy in the management of diffuse malignant mesothelioma of the pleura. Experience with 29 patients. *Thorax* 1976;31:15–24.
160. Treasure T, Internullo E, Fiorentino F, et al. A survey of opinions and beliefs concerning surgery for malignant pleural mesothelioma amongst 802 members of the European Association for Cardio-Thoracic Surgery (EACTS), the European Society of Thoracic Surgeons (ESTS) and the Society of Thoracic Surgeons (STS). *Interact Cardiovasc Thorac Surg* 2011;12:341–346.
161. Kao SC, Yan TD, Lee K, et al. Accuracy of diagnostic biopsy for the histological subtype of malignant pleural mesothelioma. *J Thorac Oncol* 2011;6:602–605.
162. Bueno R, Reblando J, Glickman J, et al. Pleural biopsy: a reliable method for determining the diagnosis but not subtype in mesothelioma. *Ann Thorac Surg* 2004;78:1774–1776.
163. Rice D, Rusch V, Pass H, et al. Recommendations for uniform definitions of surgical techniques for malignant pleural mesothelioma: a consensus report of the international association for the study of lung cancer international staging committee and the international mesothelioma interest group. *J Thorac Oncol* 2011;6:1304–1312.
164. Cao CQ, Yan TD, Bannon PG, et al. A systematic review of extrapleural pneumonectomy for malignant pleural mesothelioma. *J Thorac Oncol* 2010; 5:1692–1703.
165. Sugarbaker DJ, Wolf AS. Surgery for malignant pleural mesothelioma. *Expert Rev Respir Med* 2010;4:363–372.
166. Sugarbaker DJ, Jaklitsch MT, Bueno R, et al. Prevention, early detection, and management of complications after 328 consecutive extrapleural pneumonectomies. *J Thorac Cardiovasc Surg* 2004;128:138–146.
167. Balduyck B, Trousse D, Nakas A, et al. Therapeutic surgery for nonepithelioid malignant pleural mesothelioma: is it really worthwhile? *Ann Thorac Surg* 2010;89:907–911.
168. Kindler HL, van Meerbeeck JP. The role of gemcitabine in the treatment of malignant mesothelioma. *Semin Oncol* 2002;29:70–76.
169. Vogelzang NJ, Rusthoven JJ, Symanowski J, et al. Phase III study of pemetrexed in combination with cisplatin versus cisplatin alone in patients with malignant pleural mesothelioma. *J Clin Oncol* 2003;21:2636–2644.
170. Ahamad A, Stevens CW, Smythe WR, et al. Promising early local control of malignant pleural mesothelioma following postoperative intensity modulated radiotherapy (IMRT) to the chest. *Cancer J* 2003;9:476–484.
171. Pass HI, Temeck BK, Kranda K, et al. Phase III randomized trial of surgery with or without intraoperative photodynamic therapy and postoperative immunochemotherapy for malignant pleural mesothelioma. *Ann Surg Oncol* 1997;4:628–633.
172. Treasure T, Lang-Lazdunski L, Waller D, et al. Extra-pleural pneumonectomy versus no extra-pleural pneumonectomy for patients with malignant pleural mesothelioma: clinical outcomes of the Mesothelioma and Radical Surgery (MARS) randomised feasibility study. *Lancet Oncol* 2011;12:763–772.
173. Weder W, Stahel RA, Baas P, et al. The MARS feasibility trial: conclusions not supported by data. *Lancet Oncol* 2011;12:1093–1094.
174. Flores RM, Pass HI, Seshan VE, et al. Extrapleural pneumonectomy versus pleurectomy/decortication in the surgical management of malignant pleural mesothelioma: results in 663 patients. *J Thorac Cardiovasc Surg* 2008;135: 620–626.
175. Nakas A, Trousse DS, Martin-Ucar AE, et al. Open lung-sparing surgery for malignant pleural mesothelioma: the benefits of a radical approach within multimodality therapy. *Eur J Cardiothorac Surg* 2008;34:886–891.
176. Shahin Y, Wellham J, Jappie R, et al. How successful is lung-preserving radical surgery in the mesothelioma and radical surgery-trial environment? A case-controlled analysis. *Eur J Cardiothorac Surg* 2011;39:360–363.
177. Steele JP, Walley T, Edwards J. A randomized trial of extended pleurectomy and decortication with pemetrexed and platinum chemotherapy versus pemetrexed and platinum chemotherapy in patients with malignant pleural mesothelioma. Presented at International Mesothelioma Interest Group Meeting, October 2012, Boston, MA.
178. Lang-Lazdunski L, van Meerbeeck JP. EORTC randomized phase II study of extended pleurectomy/decortication (E-Pd) preceded or followed by chemotherapy in patients with early stage malignant pleural mesothelioma (MPM). Presented at International Mesothelioma Interest Group Meeting, October 2012, Boston, MA.
179. Krug LM. An overview of chemotherapy for mesothelioma. *Hematol Oncol Clin North Am* 2005;19:1117–1136, vii.
180. Berghmans T, Paesmans M, Lalami Y, et al. Activity of chemotherapy and immunotherapy on malignant mesothelioma: a systematic review of the literature with meta-analysis. *Lung Cancer* 2002;38:111–121.
181. Byrne MJ, Davidson JA, Musk AW, et al. Cisplatin and gemcitabine treatment for malignant mesothelioma: a phase II study. *J Clin Oncol* 1999;17:25–30.
182. Nowak AK, Byrne MJ, Williamson R, et al. A multicentre phase II study of cisplatin and gemcitabine for malignant mesothelioma. *Br J Cancer* 2002;87:491–496.
183. van Haarst JM, Baas P, Manegold C, et al. Multicentre phase II study of gemcitabine and cisplatin in malignant pleural mesothelioma. *Br J Cancer* 2002;86:342–345.
184. Favaretto AG, Aversa SM, Paccagnella A, et al. Gemcitabine combined with carboplatin in patients with malignant pleural mesothelioma: a multicentric phase II study. *Cancer* 2003;97:2791–2797.
185. Andreopoulou E, Ross PJ, O'Brien ME, et al. The palliative benefits of MVP (mitomycin C, vinblastine and cisplatin) chemotherapy in patients with malignant mesothelioma. *Ann Oncol* 2004;15:1406–1412.
186. Steele JP, Shamash J, Evans MT, et al. Phase II study of vinorelbine in patients with malignant pleural mesothelioma. *J Clin Oncol* 2000;18:3912–3917.
187. Muers MF, Stephens RJ, Fisher P, et al. Active symptom control with or without chemotherapy in the treatment of patients with malignant pleural mesothelioma (MS01): a multicentre randomised trial. *Lancet* 2008;371:1685–1694.
188. Chattopadhyay S, Moran RG, Goldman ID. Pemetrexed: biochemical and cellular pharmacology, mechanisms, and clinical applications. *Mol Cancer Ther* 2007;6:404–417.
189. Bueno R, Appasani K, Mercer H, et al. The alpha folate receptor is highly activated in malignant pleural mesothelioma. *J Thorac Cardiovasc Surg* 2001;121: 225–233.
190. Thodtmann R, Depenbrock H, Dumez H, et al. Clinical and pharmacokinetic phase I study of multitargeted antifolate (LY231514) in combination with cisplatin. *J Clin Oncol* 1999;17:3009–3016.
191. Van Meerbeeck JP, Gaafar R, Manegold C, et al. Randomized phase III study of cisplatin with or without raltitrexed in patients with malignant pleural mesothelioma: an intergroup study of the European Organisation for Research and Treatment of Cancer Lung Cancer Group and the National Cancer Institute of Canada. *J Clin Oncol* 2005;23:6881–6889.
192. Ceresoli GL, Zucali PA, Favaretto AG, et al. Phase II study of pemetrexed plus carboplatin in malignant pleural mesothelioma. *J Clin Oncol* 2006;24:1443–1448.
193. Castagneto B, Botta M, Aitini E, et al. Phase II study of pemetrexed in combination with carboplatin in patients with malignant pleural mesothelioma (MPM). *Ann Oncol* 2008;19:370–373.
194. Santoro A, O'Brien ME, Stahel RA, et al. Pemetrexed plus cisplatin or pemetrexed plus carboplatin for chemonaive patients with malignant pleural mesothelioma: results of the International Expanded Access Program. *J Thorac Oncol* 2008;3:756–763.
195. Taylor P, Castagneto B, Dark G, et al. Single-agent pemetrexed for chemonaive and pretreated patients with malignant pleural mesothelioma: results of an International Expanded Access Program. *J Thorac Oncol* 2008;3:764–771.
196. Scagliotti GV, Shin DM, Kindler HL, et al. Phase II study of pemetrexed with and without folic acid and vitamin B12 as front-line therapy in malignant pleural mesothelioma. *J Clin Oncol* 2003;21:1556–1561.
197. Jassem J, Ramlau R, Santoro A, et al. Phase III trial of pemetrexed plus best supportive care compared with best supportive care in previously treated patients with advanced malignant pleural mesothelioma. *J Clin Oncol* 2008;26:1698–1704.
198. Janne PA, Wozniak AJ, Belani CP, et al. Pemetrexed alone or in combination with cisplatin in previously treated malignant pleural mesothelioma: outcomes from a phase IIIB expanded access program. *J Thorac Oncol* 2006;1:506–512.
199. Zucali PA, Simonelli M, Michetti G, et al. Second-line chemotherapy in malignant pleural mesothelioma: results of a retrospective multicenter survey. *Lung Cancer* 2012;75:360–367.
200. Manegold C, Symanowski J, Gatzemeier U, et al. Second-line (post-study) chemotherapy received by patients treated in the phase III trial of pemetrexed plus cisplatin versus cisplatin alone in malignant pleural mesothelioma. *Ann Oncol* 2005;16:923–927.
201. Stebbing J, Powles T, McPherson K, et al. The efficacy and safety of weekly vinorelbine in relapsed malignant pleural mesothelioma. *Lung Cancer* 2009;63:94–97.
202. Masood R, Kundra A, Zhu S, et al. Malignant mesothelioma growth inhibition by agents that target the VEGF and VEGF-C autocrine loops. *Int J Cancer* 2003;104:603–610.
203. Strizzi L, Catalano A, Vianale G, et al. Vascular endothelial growth factor is an autocrine growth factor in human malignant mesothelioma. *J Pathol* 2001;193:468–475.
204. Konig J, Tolnay E, Wiethege T, et al. Co-expression of vascular endothelial growth factor and its receptor flt-1 in malignant pleural mesothelioma. *Respiration* 2000;67:36–40.
205. Linder C, Linder S, Munck-Wikland E, et al. Independent expression of serum vascular endothelial growth factor (VEGF) and basic fibroblast growth factor (bFGF) in patients with carcinoma and sarcoma. *Anticancer Res* 1998;18:2063–2068.
206. Kindler HL, Karrison TG, Gandara DR, et al. Multicenter, double-blind, placebo-controlled, randomized phase II trial of gemcitabine/cisplatin plus bevacizumab or placebo in patients with malignant mesothelioma. *J Clin Oncol* 2012;30:2509–2515.
207. Dowell JE, Dunphy FR, Taub RN, et al. A multicenter phase II study of cisplatin, pemetrexed, and bevacizumab in patients with advanced malignant mesothelioma. *Lung Cancer* 2012;77:567–571.
208. Baas P, Boogerd W, Dalesio O, et al. Thalidomide in patients with malignant pleural mesothelioma. *Lung Cancer* 2005;48:291–296.
209. Buikhuisen WA, Burgers JA, Vincent AD, et al. Thalidomide versus active supportive care for maintenance in patients with malignant mesothelioma after

first-line chemotherapy (NVALT 5): an open-label, multicentre, randomised phase 3 study. *Lancet Oncol* 2013;14:543–551.
210. Langerak AW, De Laat PA, Van der Linden-Van Beurden CA, et al. Expression of platelet-derived growth factor (PDGF) and PDGF receptors in human malignant mesothelioma in vitro and in vivo. *J Pathol* 1996;178:151–160.
211. Catalano A, Rodilossi S, Rippo MR, et al. Induction of stem cell factor/c-Kit/slug signal transduction in multidrug-resistant malignant mesothelioma cells. *J Biol Chem* 2004;279:46706–46714.
212. Kindler HL, Vogelzang NJ, Chien K, et al. SU5416 in malignant mesothelioma: A University of Chicago Phase II Consortium Study. *Proc Am Soc Clin Oncol* 2001;20:abstract 1359.
213. Dubey S, Janne PA, Krug L, et al. A phase II study of sorafenib in malignant mesothelioma: results of Cancer and Leukemia Group B 30307. *J Thorac Oncol* 2010;5:1655–1661.
214. Nowak AK, Millward MJ, Creaney J, et al. A phase II study of intermittent sunitib malate as second-line therapy in progressive malignant pleural mesothelioma. *J Thorac Oncol* 2012;7:1449–1456.
215. Laurie SA, Gupta A, Chu Q, et al. Brief report: A phase II study of sunitib in malignant pleural mesothelioma. The NCIC Clinical Trials Group. *J Thorac Oncol* 2011;6:1950–1954.
216. Paik PK, Krug LM. Histone deacetylase inhibitors in malignant pleural mesothelioma: preclinical rationale and clinical trials. *J Thorac Oncol* 2010;5:275–279.
217. Marks PA, Richon VM, Miller T, et al. Histone deacetylase inhibitors. *Adv Cancer Res* 2004;91:137–168.
218. Krug LM, Curley T, Schwartz L, et al. Potential role of histone deacetylase inhibitors in mesothelioma: clinical experience with suberoylanilide hydroxamic acid. *Clin Lung Cancer* 2006;7:257–261.
219. Krug L, Kindler H, Calvert AH. VANTAGE 014: Vorinostat in patients with advanced malignant pleural mesothelioma who have failed prior pemetrexed and etiehr cisplain or carboplatin therapy: a phase III, randomized, double-blind, placebo-controlled trial. *Eur J Cancer* 2011;1:2–3.
220. Okada T, Lopez-Lago M, Giancotti FG. Merlin/NF-2 mediates contact inhibition of growth by suppressing recruitment of Rac to the plasma membrane. *J Cell Biol* 2005;171:361–371.
221. Lopez-Lago MA, Okada T, Murillo MM, et al. Loss of the tumor suppressor gene NF2, encoding merlin, constitutively activates integrin-dependent mTORC1 signaling. *Mol Cell Biol* 2009;29:4235–4249.
222. Garland L, Ou G, Moon J, et al. SWOG 0722: A phase II study of mTOR inhibitor everolimus (RAD001) in malignant pleural mesothelioma (MPM). *J Clin Oncol* 2012;30(Suppl): Abst. 7083.
223. Kindler H, Dolly S, Bendell J, et al. Evaluation of tolerability and antitumor activity of GDC-0980, an oral PI3K/mROT inhibitor, administered to patients with advanced malignant pleural mesothelioma. Paper presented at: 11th International Conference of the International Mesothelioma Interest Group. September 12, 2012. Boston, MA.
224. Hassan R, Ho M. Mesothelin targeted cancer immunotherapy. *Eur J Cancer* 2008;44:46–53.
225. Ho M, Hassan R, Zhang J, et al. Humoral immune response to mesothelin in mesothelioma and ovarian cancer patients. *Clin Cancer Res* 2005;11:3814–3820.
226. Uehara N, Matsuoka Y, Tsubura A. Mesothelin promotes anchorage-independent growth and prevents anoikis via extracellular signal-regulated kinase signaling pathway in human breast cancer cells. *Mol Cancer Res* 2008;6:186–193.
227. Kaneko O, Gong L, Zhang J, et al. A binding domain on mesothelin for CA125/MUC16. *J Biol Chem* 2009;284:3739–3749.
228. Tang Z, Qian M, Ho M. The role of mesothelin in tumor progression and targeted therapy. *Anticancer Agents Med Chem* 2013;13:276–280.
229. Hassan R, Bullock S, Premkumar A, et al. Phase I study of SS1P, a recombinant anti-mesothelin immunotoxin given as a bolus I.V. infusion to patients with mesothelin-expressing mesothelioma, ovarian, and pancreatic cancers. *Clin Cancer Res* 2007;13:5144–5149.
230. Palumbo C, Bei R, Procopio A, et al. Molecular targets and targeted therapies for malignant mesothelioma. *Curr Med Chem* 2008;15:855–867.
231. Roe OD, Creaney J, Lundgren S, et al. Mesothelin-related predictive and prognostic factors in malignant mesothelioma: a nested case-control study. *Lung Cancer* 2008;61:235–243.
232. Rodriguez Portal JA, Rodriguez BE, Rodriguez RD, et al. Serum levels of soluble mesothelin-related peptides in malignant and nonmalignant asbestos-related pleural disease: relation with past asbestos exposure. *Cancer Epidemiol Biomarkers Prev* 2009;18:646–650.
233. Kreitman RJ, Hassan R, FitzGerald DJ, et al. Phase I trial of continuous infusion anti mesothelin recombinant immunotoxin SS1P. *Clin Cancer Res* 2009;15:5274–5279.
234. Hassan R, Miller AC, Sharon E, et al. Major cancer regressions in mesothelioma after treatment with an anti-mesothelin immunotoxin and immune suppression. *Sci Transl Med* 2013;5:208ra147.
235. Law MR, Gregor A, Hodson ME, et al. Malignant mesothelioma of the pleura: a study of 52 treated and 64 untreated patients. *Thorax* 1984;39:255–259.
236. Ruffie P, Feld R, Minkin S, et al. Diffuse malignant mesothelioma of the pleura in Ontario and Quebec: a retrospective study of 332 patients. *J Clin Oncol* 1989;7:1157–1168.
237. Ball DL, Cruickshank DG. The treatment of malignant mesothelioma of the pleura: review of a 5-year experience, with special reference to radiotherapy. *Am J Clin Oncol* 1990;13:4–9.
238. Holsti LR, Pyrhonen S, Kajanti M, et al. Altered fractionation of hemithorax irradiation for pleural mesothelioma and failure patterns after treatment. *Acta Oncol* 1997;36:397–405.
239. Alberts AS, Falkson G, Goedhals L, et al. Malignant pleural mesothelioma: a disease unaffected by current therapeutic maneuvers. *J Clin Oncol* 1988;6:527–535.
240. Linden CJ, Mercke C, Albrechtsson U, et al. Effect of hemithorax irradiation alone or combined with doxorubicin and cyclophosphamide in 47 pleural mesotheliomas: a nonrandomized phase II study. *Eur Respir J* 1996;9:2565–2572.
241. Herscher LL, Hahn SM, Kroog G, et al. Phase I study of paclitaxel as a radiation sensitizer in the treatment of mesothelioma and non-small-cell lung cancer. *J Clin Oncol* 1998;16:635–641.
242. Chen Y, Pandya K, Keng PP, et al. Schedule-dependent pulsed paclitaxel radiosensitization for thoracic malignancy. *Am J Clin Oncol* 2001;24:432–437.
243. Rusch VW, Rosenzweig K, Venkatraman E, et al. A phase II trial of surgical resection and adjuvant high-dose hemithoracic radiation for malignant pleural mesothelioma. *J Thorac Cardiovasc Surg* 2001;122:788–795.
244. Krayenbuehl J, Oertel S, Davis JB, et al. Combined photon and electron three-dimensional conformal versus intensity-modulated radiotherapy with integrated boost for adjuvant treatment of malignant pleural mesothelioma after pleuropneumonectomy. *Int J Radiat Oncol Biol Phys* 2007;69:1593–1599.
245. Rice DC, Smythe WR, Liao Z, et al. Dose-dependent pulmonary toxicity after postoperative intensity-modulated radiotherapy for malignant pleural mesothelioma. *Int J Radiat Oncol Biol Phys* 2007;69:350–357.
246. Forster KM, Smythe WR, Starkschall G, et al. Intensity-modulated radiotherapy following extrapleural pneumonectomy for the treatment of malignant mesothelioma: clinical implementation. *Int J Radiat Oncol Biol Phys* 2003;55:606–616.
247. Munden RF, Erasmus JJ, Smythe WR, et al. Radiation injury to the liver after intensity-modulated radiation therapy in patients with mesothelioma: an unusual CT appearance. *AJR Am J Roentgenol* 2005;184:1091–1095.
248. Allen AM, Czerminska M, Janne PA, et al. Fatal pneumonitis associated with intensity-modulated radiation therapy for mesothelioma. *Int J Radiat Oncol Biol Phys* 2006;65:640–645.
249. Miles EF, Larrier NA, Kelsey CR, et al. Intensity-modulated radiotherapy for resected mesothelioma: the Duke experience. *Int J Radiat Oncol Biol Phys* 2008;71:1143–1150.
250. Kristensen CA, Nottrup TJ, Berthelsen AK, et al. Pulmonary toxicity following IMRT after extrapleural pneumonectomy for malignant pleural mesothelioma. *Radiother Oncol* 2009;92:96–99.
251. Baldini EH. Radiation therapy options for malignant pleural mesothelioma. *Semin Thorac Cardiovasc Surg* 2009;21:159–163.
252. Gupta V, Krug LM, Laser B, et al. Patterns of local and nodal failure in malignant pleural mesothelioma after extrapleural pneumonectomy and photon-electron radiotherapy. *J Thorac Oncol* 2009;4:746–750.
253. Gomez DR, Hong DS, Allen PK, et al. Patterns of failure, toxicity, and survival after extrapleural pneumonectomy and hemithoracic intensity-modulated radiation therapy for malignant pleural mesothelioma. *J Thorac Oncol* 2013;8:238–245.
254. Patel PR, Yoo S, Broadwater G, et al. Effect of increasing experience on dosimetric and clinical outcomes in the management of malignant pleural mesothelioma with intensity-modulated radiation therapy. *Int J Radiat Oncol Biol Phys* 2012;83:362–368.
255. Gupta V, Mychalczak B, Krug L, et al. Hemithoracic radiation therapy after pleurectomy/decortication for malignant pleural mesothelioma. *Int J Radiat Oncol Biol Phys* 2005;63:1045–1052.
256. Rosenzweig KE, Fox JL, Zelefsky MJ, et al. A pilot trial of high-dose-rate intraoperative radiation therapy for malignant pleural mesothelioma. *Brachytherapy* 2005;4:30–33.
257. Rosenzweig KE, Zauderer MG, Laser B, et al. Pleural intensity-modulated radiotherapy for malignant pleural mesothelioma. *Int J Radiat Oncol Biol Phys* 2012;83:1278–1283.
258. Trovo M, Minatel E. Tomotherapy after pleurectomy or decortication or biopsy for malignant pleural mesothelioma. *J Thorac Oncol* 2013;8:e50–e51.
259. Agarwal PP, Seely JM, Matzinger FR, et al. Pleural mesothelioma: sensitivity and incidence of needle track seeding after image-guided biopsy versus surgical biopsy. *Radiology* 2006;241:589–594.
260. Bydder S, Phillips M, Joseph DJ, et al. A randomised trial of single-dose radiotherapy to prevent procedure tract metastasis by malignant mesothelioma. *Br J Cancer* 2004;91:9–10.
261. De Ruysscher D, Slotman B. Treatment of intervention sites of malignant pleural mesothelioma with radiotherapy: a Dutch-Belgian survey. *Radiother Oncol* 2003;68:299–302.
262. Lee C, Bayman N, Swindell R, et al. Prophylactic radiotherapy to intervention sites in mesothelioma: a systematic review and survey of UK practice. *Lung Cancer* 2009;66:150–156.
263. Ruffie P, Lehmann M, Galateau-Salle F, et al. Malignant mesothelioma. *Br J Cancer* 2001;84:49–50.
264. Davis SR, Tan L, Ball DL. Radiotherapy in the treatment of malignant mesothelioma of the pleura, with special reference to its use in palliation. *Australas Radiol* 1994;38:212–214.
265. Krayenbuehl J, Hartmann M, Lomax AJ, et al. Proton therapy for malignant pleural mesothelioma after extrapleural pleuropneumonectomy. *Int J Radiat Oncol Biol Phys* 2010;78:628–634.
266. Lorentini S, Amichetti M, Spiazzi L, et al. Adjuvant intensity-modulated proton therapy in malignant pleural mesothelioma. A comparison with intensity-modulated radiotherapy and a spot size variation assessment. *Strahlenther Onkol* 2012;188:216–225.
267. Baud M, Strano S, Dechartres A, et al. Outcome and prognostic factors of pleural mesothelioma after surgical diagnosis and/or pleurodesis. *J Thorac Cardiovasc Surg* 2013;145:1305–1311.

268. Nojiri S, Gemba K, Aoe K, et al. Survival and prognostic factors in malignant pleural mesothelioma: a retrospective study of 314 patients in the west part of Japan. *Jpn J Clin Oncol* 2011;41:32–39.
269. Tanrikulu AC, Abakay A, Kaplan MA, et al. A clinical, radiographic and laboratory evaluation of prognostic factors in 363 patients with malignant pleural mesothelioma. *Respiration* 2010;80:480–487.
270. Francart J, Vaes E, Henrard S, et al. A prognostic index for progression-free survival in malignant mesothelioma with application to the design of phase II trials: a combined analysis of 10 EORTC trials. *Eur J Cancer* 2009;45:2304–2311.
271. Yan TD, Boyer M, Tin MM, et al. Extrapleural pneumonectomy for malignant pleural mesothelioma: outcomes of treatment and prognostic factors. *J Thorac Cardiovasc Surg* 2009;138:619–624.
272. Flores RM, Zakowski M, Venkatraman E, et al. Prognostic factors in the treatment of malignant pleural mesothelioma at a large tertiary referral center. *J Thorac Oncol* 2007;2:957–965.
273. Steele JP, Klabatsa A, Fennell DA, et al. Prognostic factors in mesothelioma. *Lung Cancer* 2005;49:S49–S52.
274. Neumann V, Rutten A, Scharmach M, et al. Factors influencing long-term survival in mesothelioma patients—results of the German mesothelioma register. *Int Arch Occup Environ Health* 2004;77:191–199.
275. Pass HI. Biomarkers and prognostic factors for mesothelioma. *Ann Cardiothorac Surg* 2012;1:449–456.
276. Abakay A, Komek H, Abakay O, et al. Relationship between 18 FDG PET-CT findings and the survival of 177 patients with malignant pleural mesothelioma. *Eur Rev Med Pharmacol Sci* 2013;17:1233–1241.
277. Weder W, Kestenholz P, Taverna C, et al. Neoadjuvant chemotherapy followed by extrapleural pneumonectomy in malignant pleural mesothelioma. *J Clin Oncol* 2004;22:3451–3457.
278. Weder W, Stahel RA, Bernhard J, et al. Multicenter trial of neo-adjuvant chemotherapy followed by extrapleural pneumonectomy in malignant pleural mesothelioma. *Ann Oncol* 2007;18:1196–1202.
279. Rea F, Marulli G, Bortolotti L, et al. Induction chemotherapy, extrapleural pneumonectomy (EPP) and adjuvant hemi-thoracic radiation in malignant pleural mesothelioma (MPM): Feasibility and results. *Lung Cancer* 2007;57:89–95.
280. Flores RM, Krug LM, Rosenzweig KE, et al. Induction chemotherapy, extrapleural pneumonectomy, and postoperative high-dose radiotherapy for locally advanced malignant pleural mesothelioma: a phase II trial. *J Thorac Oncol* 2006;1:289–295.
281. Opitz I, Kestenholz P, Lardinois D, et al. Incidence and management of complications after neoadjuvant chemotherapy followed by extrapleural pneumonectomy for malignant pleural mesothelioma. *Eur J Cardiothorac Surg* 2006;29:579–584.
282. Buduhan G, Menon S, Aye R, et al. Trimodality therapy for malignant pleural mesothelioma. *Ann Thorac Surg* 2009;88:870–875.
283. de Perrot M, Feld R, Cho BC, et al. Trimodality therapy with induction chemotherapy followed by extrapleural pneumonectomy and adjuvant high-dose hemithoracic radiation for malignant pleural mesothelioma. *J Clin Oncol* 2009;27:1413–1418.
284. Krug LM, Pass HI, Rusch VW, et al. Multicenter phase II trial of neoadjuvant pemetrexed plus cisplatin followed by extrapleural pneumonectomy and radiation for malignant pleural mesothelioma. *J Clin Oncol* 2009;27:3007–3013.
285. Van Schil PE, Baas P, Gaafar R, et al. Trimodality therapy for malignant pleural mesothelioma: results from an EORTC phase II multicentre trial. *Eur Respir J* 2010;36:1362–1369.
286. Pasello G, Marulli G, Polo V, et al. Pemetrexed plus carboplatin or cisplatin as neoadjuvant treatment of operable malignant pleural mesothelioma (MPM). *Anticancer Res* 2012;32:5393–5399.
287. Bille A, Belcher E, Raubenheimer H, et al. Induction chemotherapy, extrapleural pneumonectomy, and adjuvant radiotherapy for malignant pleural mesothelioma: experience of Guy's and St Thomas' hospitals. *Gen Thorac Cardiovasc Surg* 2012;60:289–296.
288. Okada K. Personal communication. Trimodality therapy with extrapleural pneumonectomy, radiation therapy, and chemotherapy for malignant pleural mesothelioma. *11th International Conference of the International Mesothelioma Interest Group*. 2012.
289. Neragi-Miandoab S, Richards WG, Sugarbaker DJ. Morbidity, mortality, mean survival, and the impact of histology on survival after pleurectomy in 64 patients with malignant pleural mesothelioma. *Int J Surg* 2008;6:293–297.
290. Luckraz H, Rahman M, Patel N, et al. Three decades of experience in the surgical multi-modality management of pleural mesothelioma. *Eur J Cardiothorac Surg* 2010;37:552–556.
291. Bolukbas S. Long-term outcome after radical pleurectomy followed by chemoradiation for malignant pleural mesothelioma: a 10-year single center experience. *11th International Conference of the International Mesothelioma Interest Group*. September 12, 2012, Boston, MA.
292. Cameron RB, Olevsky O, Selch M. The timing of chemotherapy in the multimodality therapy of pleural mesothelioma. *11th International Conference of the International Mesothelioma Interest Group*, September 12, 2012, Boston, MA.
293. Friedberg J, Culligan MJ, Mick R. Radical pleurectomy and intraoperative porfimer sodium photodynamic therapy for malignant. *11th International Conference of the International Mesothelioma Interest Group*. September 12, 2012, Abstract.
294. Bille A, Okiror L, Lang-Lazdunski L. Pleurectomy/decortication, hyperthermic pleural lavage with povidone-iodine followed by adjuvant chemotherapy: survival analysis in 65 consecutive patients. *11th International Conference of the International Mesothelioma Interest Group*. September 12, 2012, Boston, MA.
295. Lang-Lazdunski L, Bille A, Lal R, et al. Pleurectomy/decortication is superior to extrapleural pneumonectomy in the multimodality management of patients with malignant pleural mesothelioma. *J Thorac Oncol* 2012;7:737–743.
296. Rena O, Casadio C. Extrapleural pneumonectomy for early stage malignant pleural mesothelioma: a harmful procedure. *Lung Cancer* 2012;77:151–155.
297. Sorensen JB, Ravn J, Krisetensen C. Two simultaneous consecutive non-randomized cohorts of operable patients with MPM receiving induction therapy followed either by EPP and postoperative radiotherapy or pleurectomy decortication alone. Presented at International Mesothelioma Interest Group Meeting, October 2012, Boston, MA.
298. Pass H. Mesothelioma revisited: a multidisciplinary approach. Presented at International Mesothelioma Interest Group Meeting, October 2012, Boston, MA.
299. Campbell NP, Kunnavakkam R, Leighl N, et al. Cediranib in patients with malignant mesothelioma: a phase II trial of the University of Chicago Phase II Consortium. *Lung Cancer* 2012;78:76–80.
300. Garland LL, Chansky K, Wozniak AJ, et al. Phase II study of cediranib in patients with malignant pleural mesothelioma: SWOG S0509. *J Thorac Oncol* 2011;6:1938–1945.
301. Molina JR, Mandrekar S, Ziegler K. A phase II study of the VEGFR inhibitor pazopanib (P) in patients with newly diagnosed or relapsed malignant pleural mesothelioma (MPM): an NCCTG study. *J Thorac Oncol* 2009;4:S456.
302. Nowak AK, Millward MJ, Creaney J, et al. A phase II study of intermittent sunitinib malate as second-line therapy in progressive malignant pleural mesothelioma. *J Thorac Oncol* 2012;7:1449–1456.
303. Laurie SA, Gupta A, Chu Q, et al. Brief report: a phase II study of sunitinib in malignant pleural mesothelioma. The NCIC Clinical Trials Group. *J Thorac Oncol* 2011;6:1950–1954.

41 Peritoneal Metastases and Peritoneal Mesothelioma

Marcello Deraco, Dominique M. Elias, Olivier Glehen, C. William Helm, Paul H. Sugarbaker, and Vic J. Verwaal

INTRODUCTION

Peritoneal carcinomatosis, mesothelioma, and sarcomatosis are included in the group of diseases collectively referred to, in this chapter, as peritoneal metastases. Over the past three decades, there has emerged an increasing optimism concerning an individualized management plan for cancer dissemination within the abdomen and pelvis. The clinical problem was originally defined by several important clinical studies that established the natural history of peritoneal surface malignancy.[1–3]

Concomitant with these manuscripts that identified the dismal prognosis of patients with peritoneal metastases, isolated reports appeared concerning an emerging technology that described a new approach to management. This alternative treatment plan had two essential components. First, cytoreductive surgery (CRS) was used in an attempt to resect all visible implants within the abdomen and pelvis. Peritonectomy along with visceral resections was developed to surgically eradicate cancer on peritoneal surfaces.[4] The second component was local-regional chemotherapy (intraperitoneal chemotherapy) used in the operating room or within the early postoperative period before adhesions develop. Chemotherapy used in the operating room with moderate heat has been referred to as hyperthermic intraperitoneal chemotherapy (HIPEC)[5]; chemotherapy used within the early postoperative period has been referred to as early postoperative intraperitoneal chemotherapy (EPIC).[6] The chemotherapy is used in an attempt to eradicate free cancer cells and minute attached nodules that remain following surgery.[7]

The unique aspect of this new combination of treatments was the perioperative timing of the chemotherapy. Currently, the perioperative chemotherapy may be both intravenous and intraperitoneal, and may be administered in the operating room or in the early postoperative period. HIPEC now abbreviates the term hyperthermic perioperative chemotherapy and includes all perioperative chemotherapy regimens. It is not adjuvant chemotherapy and it is not neoadjuvant chemotherapy; it is chemotherapy used simultaneously with a major cytoreductive surgical procedure. Of course, all efforts to maintain benefits from systemic chemotherapy in patients with peritoneal metastases or mesothelioma must continue. Patients with peritoneal surface malignancy are required to be a focus of the multidisciplinary team (MDT).

NATURAL HISTORY STUDIES DOCUMENT THE IMPORTANCE OF LOCAL-REGIONAL PROGRESSION

A strong rationale for the emergence of CRS and HIPEC as a valid treatment option comes from natural history studies. In a proportion of patients, recurrence of the primary cancer isolated to the surfaces of the abdomen and pelvis is a reality. Primary or recurrent disease at the resection site and on peritoneal surfaces in the absence of hepatic metastases or systemic metastases does occur; these patients are appropriate for treatment by CRS and HIPEC. Isolated peritoneal surface progression of abdominal or pelvic malignancy is not unusual.[8–12]

To fully understand the importance of cancer cells that gain access to the peritoneal space prior to or at the time of a cancer resection, one must appreciate the pathophysiology of disease. Figure 41.1 illustrates the mechanism of local-regional progression. Cancer cells at low density result in peritoneal metastases at a distance from the primary cancer resection. Cancer cells at higher density become trapped within raw tissue surfaces at the resection site. A fusiform layer of cancer that conforms to the anatomic structures within the bed of the primary resection site results from high-density seeding.[13] The progression of cancer implants within the resection site and on peritoneal surfaces in the absence of liver metastases or systemic disease presents a major rationale for comprehensive local-regional treatments.[14]

PATIENT SELECTION USING QUANTITATIVE PROGNOSTIC INDICATORS

A second factor strongly recommending CRS and HIPEC as a valid treatment option comes from well-established selection factors applied to this patient population. With some variations between diseases, the same group of quantitative prognostic indicators operates for all patients with peritoneal surface malignancy. Now, prognostic indicators are used to refine the selection of patients to those most likely to benefit and to exclude those who are unlikely to benefit.[15,16] Histopathology, the peritoneal cancer index (PCI), the completeness of cytoreduction score (CC), radiologic imaging by computed tomography (CT), and TNM (tumor, node, metastasis) stage with peritoneal cytology play a central role in patient selection.

Biologic Aggressiveness as Measured by Histopathology for Epithelial Appendiceal Neoplasms and Peritoneal Mesothelioma

Mucinous appendiceal neoplasms have a broad spectrum of aggressiveness, and the histologic type of the appendiceal neoplasm has a profound effect on survival following treatment by CRS and HIPEC.[17] Patients with adenomucinosis obtain maximal survival benefit, while those with mucinous carcinoma show survivals similar to that for peritoneal metastases of colorectal origin.[18]

Seven different histologic patterns of peritoneal mesothelioma contribute to three distinct histologic groups that have a very different prognosis following treatment with CRS and HIPEC: poor prognosis for sarcomatoid, deciduoid, or biphasic types; intermediate prognosis for papillary and epithelial types; and excellent prognosis for low-grade or multicystic types.[19,20]

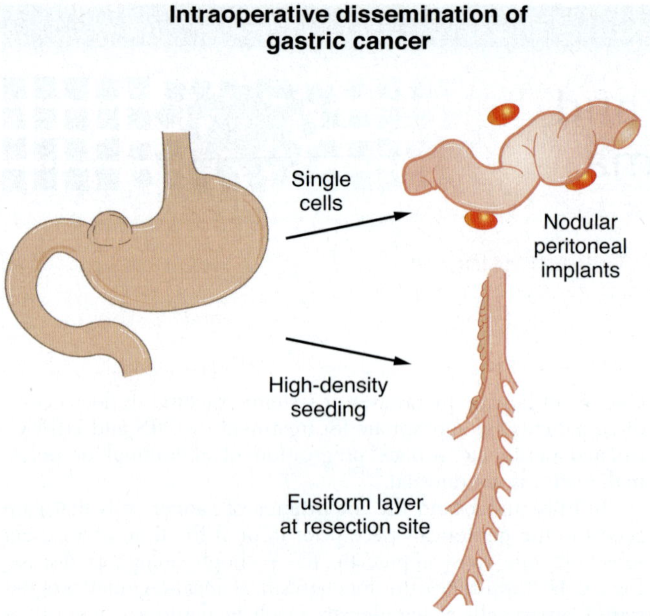

Figure 41.1 Intraoperative dissemination of gastric cancer cells. If cancer cells gain access to the peritoneal space either prior to or at the time of gastrectomy, two patterns of dissemination are observed. Low density of cancer cells into the free peritoneal space results in nodules as peritoneal implants. A high density of cancer cells dropped into the cancer resection site results in a layering of cancer.

Extent of Disease as Measured by the Peritoneal Cancer Index

The PCI is an assessment combining lesion size (0 to 3) with tumor distribution (abdominopelvic regions 0 to 12) to estimate the extent of disease within the abdomen and pelvis as a numerical score (Fig. 41.2).[21] It is calculated from observations obtained at the time of surgical exploration of the abdomen and pelvis, and should be recorded by the surgeon before leaving the operating room. The higher the PCI, the less likely CRS and HIPEC will result in long-term survival for all the peritoneal surface malignancies discussed in this chapter.

The Completeness of Cytoreduction Score Performed after the Resection

The size of residual tumor nodules visually determined after CRS has been completed has a profound effect on outcome. The new definition of complete cytoreduction is no visible evidence of cancer or only minute nodules reliably penetrated by HIPEC, a completeness of cytoreduction score of 0 (CC-0) or CC-1, respectively. With few exceptions, a CC-0 or CC-1 score is necessary for long-term benefit with CRS and HIPEC.[21]

Preoperative Radiologic Imaging by Computed Tomography

CT of the chest, abdomen, and pelvis is an essential tool in the selection of patients for CRS with HIPEC. Systemic metastases and spread to pleural surfaces can be identified. The location and quantity of mucinous carcinoma within the peritoneal cavity can be accurately determined.[22,23] Unfortunately, nonmucinous peritoneal metastases may be greatly underestimated by CT.[24] If the small bowel and its mesentery are layered by tumor or a large mass of cancer occupies the epigastric region, the likelihood of achieving complete cytoreduction is small. The CT should be performed with maximal intravenous and oral contrast in order to identify patients who have small bowel compartmentalization versus diffuse involvement of the small bowel and its mesentery.

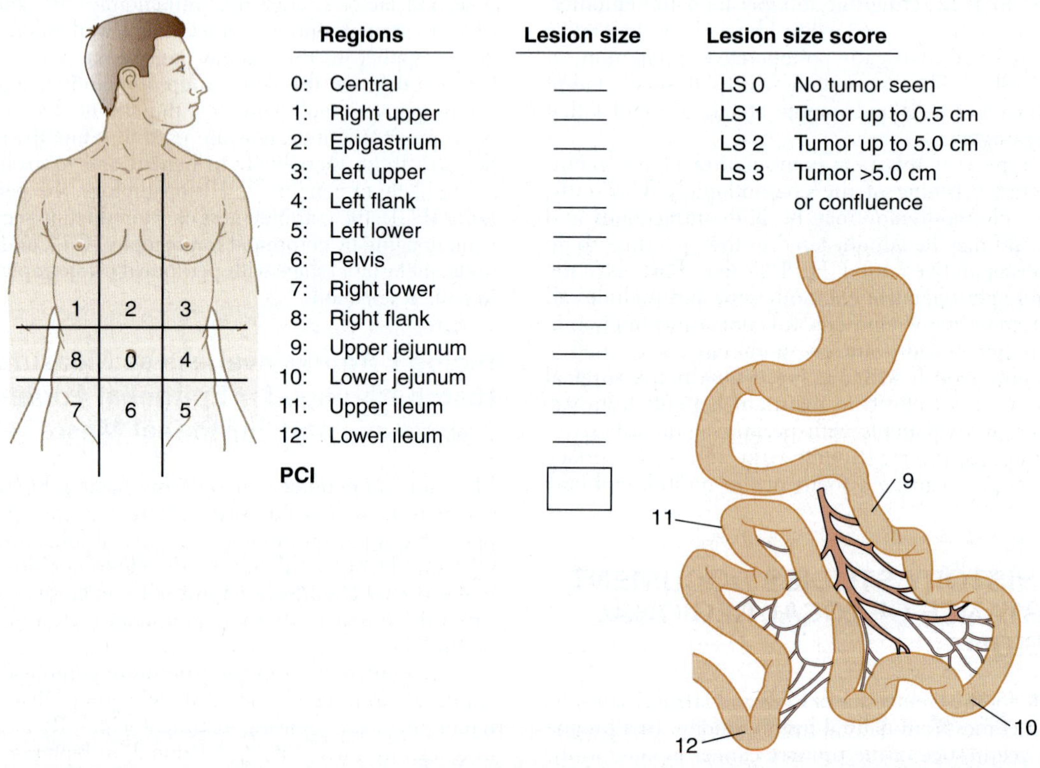

Figure 41.2 The peritoneal cancer index (*PCI*). This index combines a size and a distribution parameter to achieve a numerical score. The lesion size (*LS*) is used to quantitate the size of peritoneal nodules. The distribution of tumor is determined within the 13 abdominopelvic regions.

Tumor, Node, Metastasis Stage, Peritoneal Cytology, and Clinical Features of the Primary Cancer

A careful survey of the peritoneal surfaces at the time of primary gastrointestinal cancer resection combined with a knowledgeable and timely gross and histopathologic assessment of the resected specimen can accurately predict the incidence of peritoneal metastases that will occur in follow-up. Also, in advanced gastrointestinal cancers, peritoneal cytology provides important prognostic information. This information should be used by the MDT to consider proactive treatment with CRS and HIPEC. It is possible to prevent peritoneal metastases in high-risk groups or treat peritoneal metastases by second-look surgery in patients with documented disease.[25–30] The fast pace at which peritoneal metastases progress and the profound effect of extent of disease (PCI) on outcome indicate this approach. Table 41.1 presents the clinical features that should alert the MDT to a high risk for peritoneal metastases.[31,32]

Pharmacokinetic Advantage of Perioperative Chemotherapy

Another argument in favor of CRS and HIPEC as a treatment option for peritoneal surface malignancy is a well-studied pharmacologic rationale. As determined by physical properties, some chemotherapy agents are especially appropriate for hyperthermic use in the peritoneal cavity after CRS has been completed. Other cell cycle–specific chemotherapy agents are more appropriate for EPIC. As experience with different perioperative chemotherapy regimens has accumulated, the use of multiple-agent chemotherapy given both intravenously and intraperitoneally has evolved and promises to be increasingly effective. Heat targeting of both intravenous and intraperitoneal chemotherapy to the peritoneal surface cancer nodule is a goal of treatment.

TABLE 41.1

Tumor, Node, Metastasis Stage, Peritoneal Cytology, and Clinical Features of the Primary Cancer as an Estimate of the Incidence of Subsequent Peritoneal Metastases to Guide Proactive Treatment Strategies

	Incidence of Peritoneal Metastases Observed in Follow-up (%)	
Clinical Feature	**Colorectal Cancer**	**Gastric Cancer**
Peritoneal nodules detected with primary cancer resection	70[a]	100
Ovarian metastases	60[a]	100
Perforation through the primary cancer	50[a]	75[b]
Positive margin of resection (R-1 resection)	70	70
Positive peritoneal cytology before or after resection	40[a]	80
Adjacent organ or structure invasion	20[a]	40
T3	20	60
T4	20	75
T3/T4 mucinous cancer	40[a]	NA
Signet ring histomorphology	20	70
Fistula formation	20	NA
Obstruction of primary cancer	20	60

NA, not applicable.
[a] Data from Honore C, Goere D, Souadka A, et al. Definition of patients presenting a high risk of developing peritoneal carcinomatosis after curative surgery for colorectal cancer: a systematic review. *Ann Surg Oncol* 2013;20:183–192.
[b] Data from Tsujimoto H, Hiraki S, Sakamoto N, et al. Outcome after emergency surgery in patients with a free perforation caused by gastric cancer. *Exp Ther Med* 2010;1:199–203.

Combined Use of Cytoreductive Surgery and Perioperative Chemotherapy as a Standard of Care in Selected Patients

A final argument for use of CRS and HIPEC as a treatment option for peritoneal surface malignancy concerns the well-defined management parameters that are currently in practice at experienced treatment centers. A standardized cytoreductive surgical procedure involves visceral resections and peritonectomy procedures in an attempt to leave the abdomen visibly free of cancer. After the CRS is complete, tubes and drains are positioned to facilitate inflow and outflow of the chemotherapy solution. The chemotherapy solution circulates through roller pumps and a heat exchanger to maintain moderate hyperthermia (42°C/109°F) within the abdomen and pelvis. The skin edges are elevated on a self-retaining retractor (open method) or the skin closed (closed method) in order to create a reservoir for the hyperthermic chemotherapy solution.

The sequence of cancer resection, intraoperative chemotherapy washing, and then intestinal reconstruction may be important to optimize the destruction of small volumes of cancer cells and prevent tumor cell entrapment in adhesions, suture lines, and the abdominal incision. During the peritonectomy and visceral resections, large volumes of cancer are removed; however, residual cancer cells remain and must be eradicated.

A review of the important recent contributions to the literature that critically assesses the benefits of CRS and HIPEC in different disease states constitutes the remainder of this chapter.

APPENDICEAL MALIGNANCY

Natural History

Although similarities exist, there are unique features of appendiceal malignancies as compared to colorectal adenocarcinoma. The first and probably the most obvious difference between the colon and the appendix malignancies is the diameter of the bowel lumen involved. A colon tumor grows as an intraluminal mass in the bowel and will invade through the wall. The intraluminal growth pattern causes the primary cancer to reach the serosa in a late stage. In contrast, the appendix is a small organ, up to 1 cm in diameter, with a thin wall. A tumor may obliterate the appendix lumen in an early stage. This may cause a rupture of the wall of the appendix, allowing a spreading of tumor cells into the abdominal and pelvic cavity. Early in the natural history of the disease, these neoplastic cells implant with a high efficiency throughout the peritoneal cavity and progress as peritoneal metastases.[33,34]

Histologic Classification

The biology of appendiceal malignancies varies from simple mucinous adenoma to solid intestinal type adenocarcinoma. The histology of the peritoneal metastases from the primary tumor itself has a major influence on the outcome of the treatment by CRS and HIPEC. Ronnett et al.[35] and Bruin et al.[36] described three different types in their analyses of appendiceal malignancies. Metastases

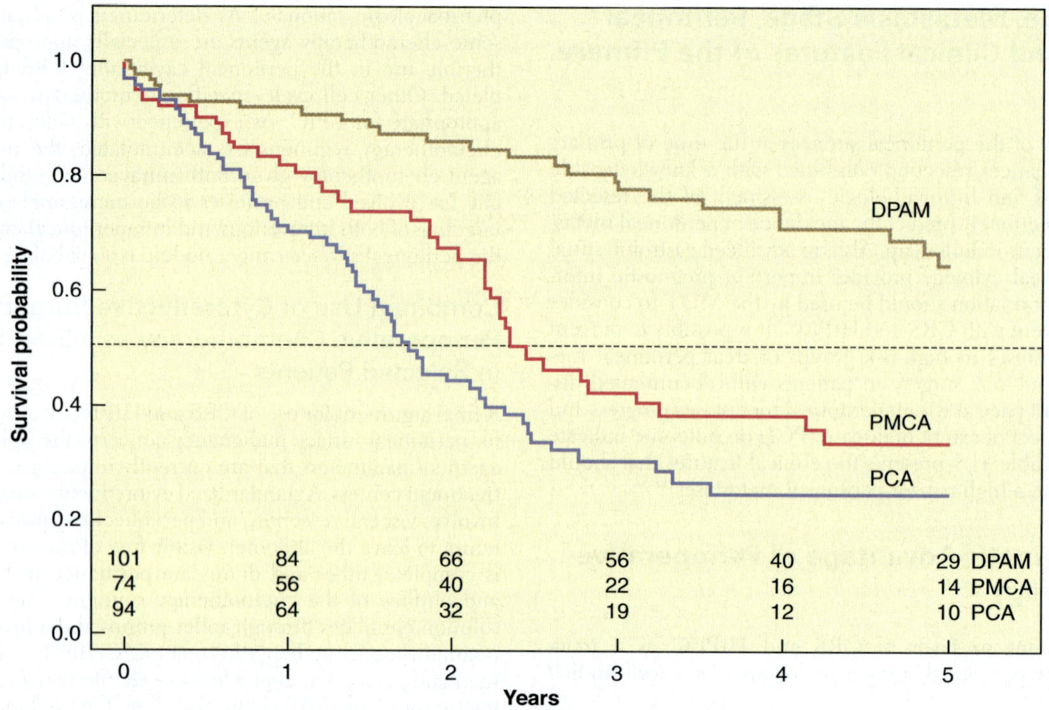

Figure 41.3 Survival of 269 patients with peritoneal metastases of an appendiceal neoplasm by histologic classification. DPAM, disseminated peritoneal adenomucinosis; PMCA, peritoneal mucinous carcinoma; PCA, peritoneal carcinoma. (From Bruin S, Verwaal VJ, Vincent A, et al. A clinicopathologic analysis of peritoneal metastases from colorectal and appendiceal origin. *Ann Surg Oncol* 2010;17:2330–2340.)

with >90% mucus, flat epithelial cells, no atypia, and no mitoses had a good prognosis despite a high PCI. At the other end of the spectrum, peritoneal metastases with much atypia, abundant mitoses, and <50% mucus has a prognosis similar to colorectal carcinomatosis and is referred to as peritoneal carcinoma.

Outcome of Treatment of Peritoneal Dissemination by Cytoreductive Surgery Followed by Hyperthermic Perioperative Chemotherapy

The survival outcome with peritoneal dissemination of appendiceal origin neoplasms is shown in Figure 41.3. The overall survival is shown according to the histologic classification. For the least aggressive form (disseminated peritoneal adenomucinosis), the median survival is not reached within 5 years.[36] Those patients who were affected by peritoneal carcinoma had a much poorer prognosis. The median survival was only 14 months in these patients. These survival data compare with the median survival of peritoneal metastases of colorectal origin treated with cytoreduction followed by HIPEC. Accepting the fact that complete resection is always the goal of CRS, these data document that survival with peritoneal metastases from appendiceal malignancies is highly dependent upon the histopathologic characteristics of the tumor.

Success in the treatment of recurrence after primary treatment with CRS followed by HIPEC is a unique feature of appendiceal peritoneal metastases. Benefit depends largely on the number and location of tumor masses. With a limited number of locations, the first choice is resection; if more diffuse disease is present and CRS is complete, a second HIPEC can be performed.[37,38] In patients in whom the pathology is more aggressive, definitive treatment with systemic chemotherapy, with all it limitations, should be considered by the MDT.

Surgical Learning Curve

Cytoreduction followed by HIPEC is a complex treatment that demonstrates a surgical learning curve.[39,40] The peak of the learning curve in the study of Smeenk et al.[31] was reached after approximately 130 procedures. Surgical skill is undoubtedly the main component of this learning process, but modified treatment strategies for an individual patient and experience in handling complications by the entire medical team has contributed to a decreased morbidity and mortality.[41,42]

COLORECTAL PERITONEAL METASTASES: CURATIVE TREATMENT AND PREVENTION

Stage IV colorectal cancer is a very morbid disease, with a 5-year survival rate of 10% and a median survival of 14.4 months. The prognosis is significantly worse when peritoneal metastases are present, with a median survival of 6.7 months versus 18.1 months without peritoneal metastases (p <0.01).[43] When colorectal peritoneal metastases are diagnosed, the crucial question for the MDT is whether curative (complete CRS with HIPEC) or palliative therapy (systemic chemotherapy) should be the goal of treatment.

Incidence of the Disease and Incidence of Peritoneal Metastases

At the initial diagnosis of colon cancer, the peritoneal surface is involved with tumor in 10% to 15% of patients.[11,44] Besides the liver, the peritoneal surfaces are the most common sites of cancer recurrence after "curative" colorectal cancer resections. Unfortunately, cancer progression occurs in as many as 50% of patients who have an R0 resection. In 10% to 35% of patients with recurrent disease, the anatomic site of treatment failure is confined to the peritoneal surface.[11,44] With recurrent disease, when peritoneal metastases are of limited extent (low PCI), potentially curative treatment options should be considered.

Useful Prognostic Indicators for the Disease

Contraindications for this combined treatment are the presence of metastases at another site (although, up to three easily resectable liver metastases is not an absolute contraindication),[45] a poor general status (the combined treatment is rather aggressive), and extensive peritoneal metastases (PCI >20). Extensive disease is likely to be unresectable in its entirety. Also, even when a complete cytoreduction is possible, the prognosis is poor. Most of the series using complete CRS with HIPEC report a poor survival rate when the PCI is higher than 20.[46,47]

Results of Treatment

Figure 41.4 reports the survival rates according to the completeness of surgery in the 523 patients collected by the Association Française de Chirurgie.[47] Five years after surgery, no patient was alive if the size of the residual tumor nodules exceeded 2.5 mm after surgery, whereas 30% of the patients were alive if complete CRS was possible (p <0.0001). These data are confirmed in the Dutch HIPEC study, which included 960 patients.[48]

A crucial role for hyperthermia for HIPEC is currently unknown for humans. In a randomized trial in rats, those treated with HIPEC survived longer than those treated with intraperitoneal chemotherapy alone or with intraperitoneal hyperthermia alone.[49] A recent retrospective study compared similar patients (all of whom underwent a laparotomy) with resectable peritoneal metastases treated with complete CRS and HIPEC to patients who received standard systemic chemotherapy. Median survival was 63 months in the complete CRS with HIPEC group versus 24 months in the systemic chemotherapy group.[50]

Summary of Important Results from Other Institutions

This combined treatment (complete CRS and HIPEC) is effective. Benefits were definitively demonstrated by the randomized study of the Amsterdam group: 105 patients who presented with colorectal peritoneal metastases were randomized between surgery with HIPEC and systemic chemotherapy versus systemic chemotherapy alone.[51] In this study, close to 50% of the patients in the experimental arm were at presentation not good candidates for HIPEC because their peritoneal metastases could not be completely resected. Despite this bias, the reported median survival was 22 months in the experimental arm versus 13 months in the control group (p = 0.032). At eight years the benefit persisted.[52]

The results obtained with complete CRS with HIPEC in the Association Française de Chirurgie study showed a 5-year overall survival of 30%.[47] This result accepts clinical data over an 18-year interval and includes the learning curves of 28 different centers. It is the least favorable data ever to be reported by the authors' group. The results of experienced centers concerning patients who underwent complete CRS and HIPEC show 5-year overall survival rates close to 40%. It was 32% for the 70 patients in the study by da Silva et al.,[46] 43% for the 59 patients in the Verwaal et al.[51] study, and 48% for the 30 patients treated by Elias et al.[53] Such a survival rate has never been published before for colorectal peritoneal metastases, even if the report includes only selected patients.

Furthermore, these results in the treatment of peritoneal metastases are similar to those obtained with hepatectomy for liver metastases. Selected patients with peritoneal metastases should be treated with this combined therapy just as selected patients with liver metastases should be treated with hepatectomy given that similar results are achieved in terms of survival.[54]

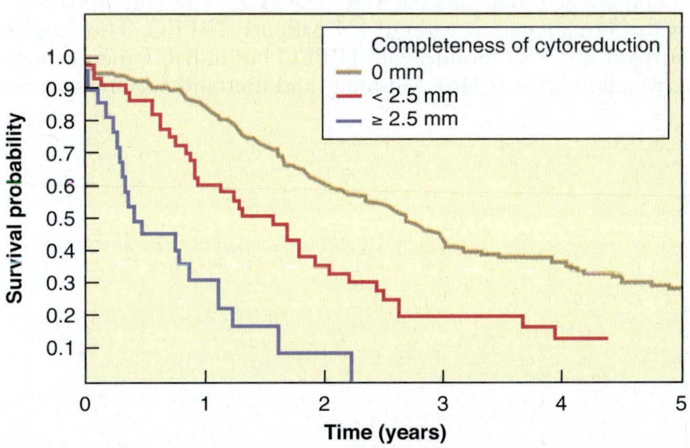

Figure 41.4 Overall survival according to the completeness of cytoreduction after cytoreductive surgery and hyperthermic perioperative chemotherapy for peritoneal metastases. (Elias D, Gilly F, Boutitie F, et al. Peritoneal colorectal carcinomatosis treated with surgery and perioperative intraperitoneal chemotherapy: retrospective analysis of 523 patients from a multicentric French study. *J Clin Oncol* 2010:28:63–68.)

Prevention of Peritoneal Metastases in Patients at High Risk for Progression

Unfortunately, early diagnosis of peritoneal metastases is not possible with radiologic imaging, but only with a laparotomy. This is why the authors proposed second-look surgery plus HIPEC in asymptomatic patients who presented with a primary exhibiting a high risk of developing peritoneal metastases.[28,55] High-risk patients were those who presented with a few (resected) peritoneal implants, ovarian metastases, or perforated tumors. Second-look surgery was performed 6 months after the end of the classic 6 months of systemic adjuvant chemotherapy. Among 47 patients, macroscopic peritoneal metastases was found and treated in 50% of them. In the remaining patients with no macroscopic peritoneal metastases, peritoneal recurrence occurred frequently in those who did not receive HIPEC, but rarely in those who did receive HIPEC (p = 0.02). Finally, only 17% of the patients treated at the time of second-look surgery with HIPEC developed a peritoneal recurrence.[28]

Reports of complete CRS and HIPEC being used to simultaneously treat the primary colorectal cancer and the peritoneal metastases have appeared.[25–27] Also, patients without established peritoneal disease but at high risk for subsequent peritoneal progression are being treated with HIPEC during the same procedure used to resect the primary tumor.[26] The rationale for this proactive approach is three-fold. First, after the primary cancer resection and complete CRS, the PCI was maximally low. Second, reliable radiologic tests to detect the progression of a low volume of peritoneal metastases do not exist. And third, this proactive approach does not require a second-look surgery. With rectal cancer, a second-look approach with CRS and HIPEC may rarely, if ever, be curative.[46,56]

DIFFUSE MALIGNANT PERITONEAL MESOTHELIOMA

Clinical Presentation and Diagnosis

Diffuse malignant peritoneal mesothelioma (DMPM) is characterized by progressive peritoneal seeding, eventually leading to the patient's death due to tumor layering on peritoneal surfaces, bowel obstruction, and intractable malignant ascites. Patients are usually diagnosed with presenting signs and symptoms of advanced disease. In a recently published series of 81 patients with DMPM reported by an Italian group, ascites, abdominal pain, and asthenia were the most frequent symptoms present on 77%, 69%, and 43% of patients, respectively. CT scan shows ascites, peritoneal thickening, abdominal mass, and mesenteric thickening, respectively, on 80%, 63%, 32%, and 29% of cases.[57] CT scan is used as an accurate prognostic radiologic test for patient selection for comprehensive treatment.[23]

Cytologic diagnosis of ascitic fluid is often inconclusive, as cells frequently resemble elements with mesothelial hyperplasia. In the series of the Washington Cancer Institute, diagnosis was made by fluid sampling in 0 of 68 patients. Laparotomy was required in 44% of patients, laparoscopy in 52%, and ultrasound/CT-guided biopsy in 4%.[58] Recently, refined cytological and ultrastructural methods have enhanced the diagnostic accuracy of cytologic assessment.[56]

Treatment and Results with Systemic Chemotherapy

Numerous single-drug and combination regimens have been tested over the past decades with modest results. Preliminary data also suggest a possible survival advantage for a combination of cisplatin and pemetrexed as compared to cisplatin alone. Other cytotoxic agents that have shown to be active in this setting include vinorelbine and gemcitabine, either alone or combined with platinum compounds. In historical case series, standard therapy with palliative surgery and systemic or intraperitoneal chemotherapy is associated with a median survival of about 1 year, ranging from 9 to 15 months.[59,60]

The combined approach consisting of CRS and HIPEC modified the natural history of DMPM with a dramatic improvement in outcomes in multiple single institution studies and in a multi-institutional registry series.[9,19,61–64] Median survival grew from 12 months with a systemic chemotherapy treatment to 53 months with CRS with HIPEC, with 50% 5-year overall survival.[65]

GASTRIC CANCER

Treatment and Prevention of Peritoneal Metastases

Peritoneal dissemination is the most frequent pattern of metastasis and recurrence with gastric cancer. Also, it occurs in 5% to 20% of patients being explored for potentially curative resection.[66] In the past, gastric cancer peritoneal metastases was regarded as a terminal disease, only to be palliated. Over the past two decades, novel therapeutic approaches have emerged, combining gastrectomy and peritonectomy procedures with perioperative chemotherapy.[67] Because of the aggressive nature of gastric cancer, the question regarding the efficiency of this combined procedure remains controversial.

Natural History and Palliative Treatment

The studies that prospectively evaluated patients with peritoneal dissemination of gastric cancer indicated median survival of not more than 6 months.[2] Despite improvements in systemic chemotherapy with encouraging tumor response rates, there has been no improvement in survival.[68] Positive effects of palliative gastric cancer resection have been recently reported in patients with peritoneal metastases but without any long-term survivors.[66]

Curative Treatment: Cytoreductive Surgery and Hyperthermic Perioperative Chemotherapy

The experience of a few single institution phase 2 studies showed encouraging survival results following treatment of peritoneal metastases along with primary gastric cancer.[69–74] Recently, a collaborative effort of French institutions collected data from 159 patients and represents the largest experience with treatment of peritoneal metastases of gastric origin.[72] With a median follow-up of 20.4 months, the overall median survival was only 9.2 months but the 5-year survival rate was 13%, with some long-term survivors. These survival results are less encouraging than those obtained for other peritoneal surface malignancies, reflecting a more aggressive disease process, less response to this combined treatment modality, and the need for more strict patient selection. But the combination of CRS with HIPEC was the only therapeutic strategy that reported survivors at 5 years. In the recent French study, a 5-year survival of 23% and a median survival of 15 months were obtained in patients treated with complete macroscopic resection (Fig. 41.5).[72]

Primary gastric cancer with localized and small peritoneal nodules seems to be the best indication for this combined procedure. In the French study, in patients who had undergone complete CRS, the extent of peritoneal metastases measured by PCI represented the only strong prognostic factor.[72] When the PCI was >12, despite a complete CRS, no patient was alive at 3 years. The institution in which the procedure was performed played an important role in the postoperative course and in survival, suggesting the importance of a learning curve.[41,42,75,76] The high rates of morbidity and mortality reported may reach 60% and 6.5%, respectively.[72] These high rates of morbidity and mortality emphasize the necessity for patient selection using strict criteria regarding physiologic age and general status.

Important data regarding the treatment of peritoneal metastases from gastric cancer was provided by Yang and colleagues.[77] In a randomized trial, patients were treated by cytoreductive surgery with (34 patients) or without (34 patients) HIPEC. The median survival was 11.9 months with HIPEC but only 6.5 months with CRS alone ($p = 0.046$). Morbidity and mortality was the same in

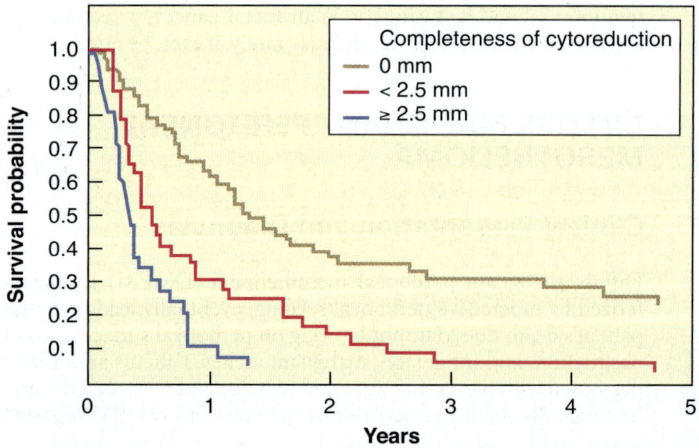

Figure 41.5 Overall survival of 159 patients with peritoneal metastases from gastric cancer treated by cytoreductive surgery and hyperthermic intraperitoneal chemotherapy according to completeness of cytoreduction. (From Glehen O, Gilly FN, Arvieux C, et al. Peritoneal carcinomatosis from gastric cancer: a multi-institutional study of 159 patients treated by cytoreductive surgery combined with perioperative intraperitoneal chemotherapy. *Ann Surg Oncol* 2010;17:2370–2377.)

both groups. Limited but real benefits for HIPEC were demonstrated. Currently, Rau and colleagues in Germany are conducting a similar phase 3 trial, the GASTRIPEC study.[78]

Prevention of Gastric Cancer Peritoneal Metastases

For many Korean and Japanese researchers, HIPEC has been performed in an adjuvant setting in phase 3 trials. Most of them demonstrated the benefit of HIPEC, especially for T3, T4, and lymph node–positive gastric tumors.[79–82] In Western countries, some small experiences also suggested the benefit of using HIPEC as adjuvant treatment for primary gastric cancer presenting with peritoneal metastases.[83,84] Yan and coworkers in a meta-analysis showed that HIPEC with or without EPIC after resection of advanced gastric primary cancer is associated with improved overall survival. However, increased risk of intra-abdominal abscess and neutropenia were also demonstrated.[85] Xu et al., in their meta-analysis, reported similar results.[86] Currently, a prospective randomized trial is being performed in France to test adjuvant HIPEC in gastric cancer.[87]

PERITONEAL METASTASES IN OVARIAN CANCER

Cytoreductive Surgery and Hyperthermic Perioperative Chemotherapy in Epithelial Ovarian Cancer

There is emerging data helping to define the potential role of HIPEC for epithelial ovarian cancer. A registry for patients with ovarian cancer was initiated to collect data from many centers in a format that allowed analysis for factors such as prognostic indicators, variations in technique, and outcomes.[88] Patient eligibility included epithelial ovarian, fallopian tube, or primary peritoneal carcinoma treated with HIPEC at some point in the natural history of the disease. Each participating institution used its own HIPEC technology regarding chemotherapy solutions, duration of perfusion, temperature, and technique of open or closed peritoneal lavage. In the initial report, 141 women were analyzed who had been treated with either frontline (n = 26), at interval debulking (n = 19), for consolidation (n = 12), or for recurrence (n = 83). The median overall survival was 30.3 months. In multivariable analysis, the factors significant for increased survival were sensitivity to platinum response ($p = 0.048$), completeness of cytoreduction score of 1 or 0 ($p = 0.025$), carboplatin alone or combination ($p = 0.011$), and duration of hospital stays of ≤10 days ($p = 0.021$).

Ceelen and coworkers reported on 42 women treated for recurrent heavily pretreated ovarian cancer with extensive CRS and HIPEC.[89] In multivariate analysis, overall survival was influenced by completeness of cytoreduction, type of chemoperfusion drug, nodal status, and tumor grade. In a Cox regression model, only completeness of cytoreduction (hazard ratio = 0.06 to 0.8; $p = 0.022$) and tumor grade (hazard ratio = 1.23 to 12.6; $p = 0.021$) were independent predictors of overall survival.

Bakrin et al.[90] reported a French multicenter prospective study of 246 women with recurrent or persistent ovarian cancer treated by CRS and HIPEC. The effects of PCI, CC score, and platinum sensitivity versus resistance are shown in Figure 41.6. They conclude that salvage therapy combining optimal CRS and HIPEC is feasible and may achieve long-term survival in highly selected patients with recurrent ovarian carcinoma, including those with platinum-resistant disease, with acceptable morbidity. Into their updated experience on 566 patients, they underlined the role of PCI in patient selection because of its major and independent prognostic impact for advanced and recurrent ovarian cancer.[91]

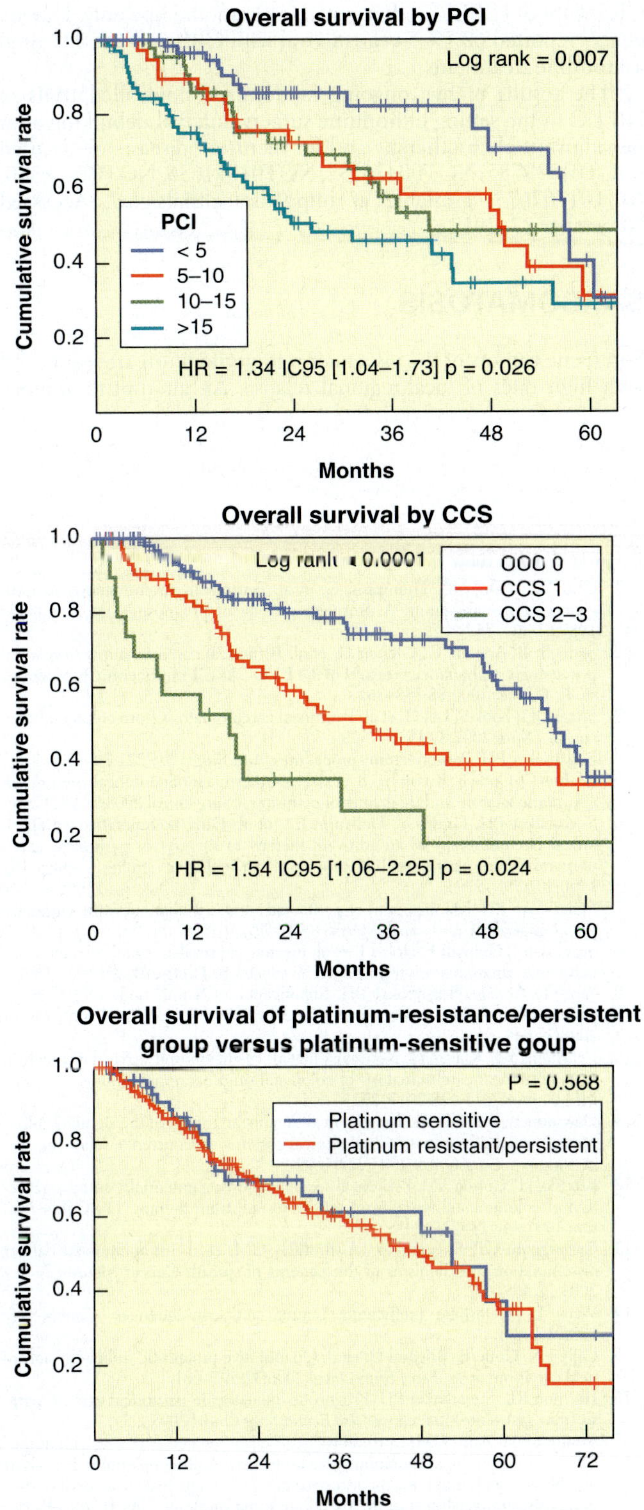

Figure 41.6 Overall survival of 246 patients with recurrent or persistent ovarian cancer by (*top*) peritoneal cancer index (*PCI*), (*middle*) completeness of cytoreduction (*CCS*), (*bottom*) platinum-resistant/persistent group versus platinum-sensitive group. HR, hazard ratio. (From Bakrin N, Cotte E, Golfier F, et al. Cytoreductive surgery and hyperthermic intraperitoneal chemotherapy (HIPEC) for persistent and recurrent advanced ovarian carcinoma: A multicenter, prospective study of 246 patients. *Ann Surg Oncol* 2012;19:4052–4058.)

In a case-control study, Fagotti et al.[92] reported significantly better 5-year survival of 68.4% versus 42.7% ($p = 0.017$) for 30 cases of platinum-sensitive recurrent ovarian cancer undergoing CRS and HIPEC versus 37 control patients who underwent either

CRS without HIPEC and/or systemic chemotherapy only. Deraco et al.[93] reported 60.7% 5-year survival with CRS and HIPEC used as frontline treatments.

The results of five ongoing randomized controlled trials of HIPEC in the setting of frontline surgery, interval debulking after neoadjuvant chemotherapy and for recurrent disease are awaited (NCT01539785, NCT00426257, NCT01091636, NCT01628380, NCT01767675: available at http://clinicaltrials.gov/. Accessed November 27, 2013).

SARCOMATOSIS

Soft tissue tumors of the viscera or retroperitoneum are associated with high rates of local-regional relapse. An attempt to achieve adequate margins of excision may be impossible because of anatomic constraints. Cancer cell seeding into the peritoneal cavity either prior to or at the time of sarcoma resection combined with positive or narrow margins of excision result in this high likelihood of local-regional recurrence.[94] In patients with local-regional disease progression or sarcomatosis, the survival is limited to approximately 2 years.

If CRS is performed in this group of patients and combined with HIPEC, the median survival is extended past 2 years. In four of the five studies referenced, an overall 5-year survival was >30%.[95–99] Unusually large benefits with CRS and HIPEC in patients with uterine sarcomatosis have been reported.[100] The mechanical removal of sarcoma peritoneal metastases that occurs with HIPEC may be as important or even more important than the cytotoxic effects. A consensus statement has been published.[101]

REFERENCES

1. Chu DZ, Lang NP, Thompson C, et al. Peritoneal carcinomatosis in nongynecologic malignancy. A prospective study of prognostic factors. *Cancer* 1989;63:364–367.
2. Sadeghi B, Arvieux C, Glehen O, et al. Peritoneal carcinomatosis from nongynecologic malignancies: results of the EVOCAPE 1 multicentric prospective study. *Cancer* 2000;88:358–363.
3. Jayne DG, Fook S, Loi C, et al. Peritoneal carcinomatosis from colorectal cancer. *Br J Surg* 2002;89:1545–1550.
4. Sugarbaker PH. Peritonectomy procedures. *Ann Surg* 1995;221:29–42.
5. Glehen O, Cotte E, Kusamura S, et al. Hyperthermic intraperitoneal chemotherapy: nomenclature and modalities of perfusion. *J Surg Oncol* 2008;98:242–246.
6. Sugarbaker PH, Graves T, DeBruijn EA, et al. Early postoperative intraperitoneal chemotherapy as an adjuvant therapy to surgery for peritoneal carcinomatosis from gastrointestinal cancer: pharmacological studies. *Cancer Res* 1990;50:5790–5794.
7. Sugarbaker PH. Management of peritoneal surface malignancy: the surgeon's role. *Langenbeck Arch Surg* 1999;384:576–587.
8. Segelman J, Granath F, Holm T, et al. Incidence, prevalence and risk factors for peritoneal carcinomatosis from colorectal cancer. *Br J Surg* 2012;99:699–705.
9. Yan TD, Yoo D, Sugarbaker PH. Significance of lymph node metastasis in patients with diffuse malignant peritoneal mesothelioma. *Eur J Surg Oncol* 2006;32:948–953.
10. Lemmens VE, Klaver YL, Verwaal VJ, et al. Predictors and survival of synchronous peritoneal carcinomatosis of colorectal origin: a population-based study. *Int J Cancer* 2011;128:2717–2725.
11. Dawson LE, Russell AH, Tong D, et al. Adenocarcinoma of the sigmoid colon: sites of initial dissemination and clinical patterns of recurrence following surgery alone. *J Surg Oncol* 1983;22:95–99.
12. Brodsky JT, Cohen AM. Peritoneal seeding following potentially curative resection of colonic carcinoma: implications for adjuvant therapy. *Dis Colon Rectum* 1991;34:723–727.
13. Carmignani CP, Sugarbaker TA, Bromley CM, et al. Intraperitoneal cancer dissemination: mechanisms of the patterns of spread. *Cancer Metastasis Rev* 2003;22:465–472.
14. Weiss L. Metastatic inefficiency: causes and consequences. *Cancer Rev* 1986;3:1–24.
15. Gilly FN, Cotte E, Brigand C, et al. Quantitative prognostic indices in peritoneal carcinomatosis. *Eur J Surg Oncol* 2006;32:597–601.
16. Harmon RL, Sugarbaker PH. Prognostic indicators in peritoneal carcinomatosis from gastrointestinal cancer. *Int Semin Surg Oncol* 2005;2:3.
17. Ronnett BM, Zahn CM, Kurman RJ, et al. Disseminated peritoneal adenomucinosis and peritoneal mucinous carcinomatosis. A clinicopathologic analysis of 109 cases with emphasis on distinguishing pathologic features, site of origin, prognosis, and relationship to "pseudomyxoma peritonei." *Am J Surg Pathol* 1995;19:1390–1408.
18. Sugarbaker PH. Epithelial appendiceal neoplasms. *Cancer J* 2009;15:225–235.
19. Yan TD, Deraco M, Baratti D, et al. Cytoreductive surgery and hyperthermic intraperitoneal chemotherapy for malignant peritoneal mesothelioma: multi-institutional experience. *J Clin Oncol* 2009;27:6237–6242.
20. Cerruto CA, Brun EA, Chang D, et al. Prognostic significance of histomorphologic parameters in diffuse malignant peritoneal mesothelioma. *Arch Pathol Lab Med* 2006;130:1654–1661.
21. Jacquet P, Sugarbaker PH. Current methodologies for clinical assessment of patients with peritoneal carcinomatosis. *J Exp Clin Cancer Res* 1996;15:49–58.
22. Jacquet P, Jelinek JS, Chang D, et al. Abdominal computed tomographic scan in the selection of patients with mucinous peritoneal carcinomatosis for cytoreductive surgery. *J Am Coll Surg* 1995;181:530–538.
23. Yan TD, Haveric N, Carmignani CP, et al. Computed tomographic characterization of malignant peritoneal mesothelioma. *Tumori* 2005;91:394–400.
24. Jacquet P, Jelinek JS, Steves MA, et al. Evaluation of computer tomography in patients with peritoneal carcinomatosis. *Cancer* 1993;72:1631–1636.
25. Pestieau SR, Sugarbaker PH. Treatment of primary colon cancer with peritoneal carcinomatosis: comparison of concomitant vs. delayed management. *Dis Colon Rectum* 2000;43:1341–1346, discussion 1347–1348.
26. Sammartino P, Sibio S, Biacchi D, et al. Prevention of peritoneal metastases from colon cancer in high-risk patients: Preliminary results of surgery plus prophylactic HIPEC. *Gastroenterol Res Pract* 2012;2012:141585.
27. Braam HJ, Boerma D, Wiezer MJ, et al. Hyperthermic perioperative chemotherapy during primary tumour resection limits extent of bowel resection compared to two-stage treatment. *Eur J Surg Oncol* 2013;39:988–993.
28. Elias D, Goere D, Di Pietrantonio D, et al. Results of systematic second-look surgery in patients at high risk of developing colorectal peritoneal carcinomatosis. *Ann Surg* 2008;247:445–450.
29. Sugarbaker PH. Comprehensive management of disseminated colorectal cancer. *Ann Surg Oncol* 2008;15:3327–3330.
30. Delhorme JB, Triki E, Zeca I, et al. Mandatory second-look surgery after surgical treatment of peritoneal carcinomatosis of colonic origin. (personal communication)
31. Honore C, Goere D, Souadka A, et al. Definition of patients presenting a high risk of developing peritoneal carcinomatosis after curative surgery for colorectal cancer: a systematic review. *Ann Surg Oncol* 2013;20:183–192.
32. Tsujimoto H, Hiraki S, Sakamoto N, et al. Outcome after emergency surgery in patients with a free perforation caused by gastric cancer. *Exp Ther Med* 2010;1:199–203.
33. Smeenk RM, van Velthuysen ML, Verwaal VJ, et al. Appendiceal neoplasms and pseudomyxoma peritonei: a population based study. *Eur J Surg Oncol* 2008;34:196–201.
34. Sugarbaker PH. Pseudomyxoma peritonei. A cancer whose biology is characterized by a redistribution phenomenon. *Ann Surg* 1994;219:109–111.
35. Ronnett BM, Shmookler BM, Sugarbaker PH, et al. Pseudomyxoma peritonei: new concepts in diagnosis, origin, nomenclature, and relationship to mucinous borderline (low malignant potential) tumors of the ovary. *Anat Pathol* 1997;2:197–226.
36. Bruin S, Verwaal VJ, Vincent A, et al. A clinicopathologic analysis of peritoneal metastases from colorectal and appendiceal origin. *Ann Surg Oncol* 2010;17:2330–2340.
37. Smeenk RM, Verwaal VJ, Antonini N, et al. Progression of pseudomyxoma peritonei after combined modality treatment: management and outcome. *Ann Surg Oncol* 2007;14:493–499.
38. Yan TD, Bijelic L, Sugarbaker PH. Critical analysis of treatment failure after complete cytoreductive surgery and perioperative intraperitoneal chemotherapy for peritoneal dissemination from appendiceal mucinous neoplasms. *Ann Surg Oncol* 2007;14:2289–2299.
39. Kusamura S, Baratti D, Virzì S, et al. Learning curve for cytoreductive surgery and hyperthermic intraperitoneal chemotherapy in peritoneal surface malignancies: analysis of two centres. *J Surg Oncol* 2013;107:312–319.
40. Verwaal VJ, van Tinteren H, Ruth SV, et al. Toxicity of cytoreductive surgery and hyperthermic intra-peritoneal chemotherapy. *J Surg Oncol* 2004;85:61–67.
41. Moran BJ. Establishment of a peritoneal malignancy treatment centre in the United Kingdom. *Eur J Surg Oncol* 2006;32:614–618.
42. Smeenk RM, Verwaal VJ, Zoetmulder FA. Learning curve of combined modality treatment in peritoneal surface disease. *Br J Surg* 2007;94:1408–1414.
43. Rosen SA, Buell JF, Yohida A, et al. Initial presentation with stage IV colorectal cancer. *Arch Surg* 2000;135:530–534.
44. Russel AH, Tong D, Dawson LE, et al. Adenocarcinoma of the retroperitoneal ascending and descending colon: sites of initial dissemination and clinical patterns of recurrence following surgery alone. *Int Radiat Oncol Biol Phys* 1983;9:361–365.
45. Elias D, Benizri E, Pocard M, et al. Treatment of synchronous peritoneal carcinomatosis and liver metastases from colorectal cancer. *Eur J Surg Oncol* 2006;32:632–636.

46. da Silva RG, Sugarbaker PH. Analysis of prognostic factors in seventy patients having a complete cytoreduction plus perioperative intraperitoneal chemotherapy for carcinomatosis from colorectal cancer. *J Am Coll Surg* 2006;203: 878–886.
47. Elias D, Gilly F, Boutitie F, et al. Peritoneal colorectal carcinomatosis treated with surgery and perioperative intraperitoneal chemotherapy: retrospective analysis of 523 patients from a multicentric French study. *J Clin Oncol* 2010: 28:63–68.
48. Kuijpers AM, Mirck B, Aalbers AG, et al. Cytoreduction and HIPEC in the Netherlands: Nationwide long-term outcome following the Dutch Protocol. *Ann Surg Oncol* 2013;20:4224–4230.
49. Koga S, Hamazoe R, Maeta M, et al. Treatment of implanted peritoneal cancer in rats by continuous hyperthermic peritoneal perfusion in combination with an anticancer drug. *Cancer Res* 1984;44:1840–1842.
50. Elias D, Lefevre JH, Chevalier J, et al. Complete cytoreductive surgery plus intraperitoneal chemohyperthermia with oxaliplatin for peritoneal carcinomatosis of colorectal origin. *J Clin Oncol* 2009;27:681–685.
51. Verwaal VC, van Ruth S, de Bree E, et al. Randomized trial of cytoreduction and hyperthermic intraperitoneal chemotherapy versus systemic chemotherapy and palliative surgery in patients with peritoneal carcinomatosis from colorectal cancer. *J Clin Oncol* 2003;21:3737–3743.
52. Verwaal VJ, van Ruth S, Witkamp A, et al. Long-term survival of peritoneal carcinomatosis of colorectal origin. Ann Surg Oncol 2005;12:65–71.
53. Elias D, Raynard B, Farkhondeh F, et al. Peritoneal carcinomatosis of colorectal origin. *Gastroenterol Clin Biol* 2006;30:1200–1204.
54. Elias D. Peritoneal carcinomatosis or liver metastases from colorectal cancer: similar standards for a curative surgery? *Ann Surg Oncol* 2004;11:122–123.
55. Sugarbaker PH. Second-look surgery for colorectal cancer: revised selection factors and new treatment options for greater success. *Int J Surg Oncol* 2011;2011:915078.
56. Verwaal VJ, van Tinteren H, van Ruth S, et al. Predicting the survival of patients with peritoneal carcinomatosis of colorectal origin treated by aggressive cytoreduction and hyperthermic intraperitoneal chemotherapy. *Br J Surg* 2004;91:739–746.
57. de Pangher Manzini V, Recchia L, Cafferata M, et al. Malignant peritoneal mesothelioma: a multicenter study on 81 cases. *Ann Oncol* 2010;21:348–353.
58. Sugarbaker PH, Welch LS, Mohamed F, et al. A review of peritoneal mesothelioma at the Washington Cancer Institute. *Surg Oncol Clin North Am* 2003;12:605–621, xi.
59. Carteni G, Manegold C, Martin Garcia G, et al. Malignant peritoneal mesothelioma. Results from the International Expanded Access Program using pemetrexed alone or in combination with a platinum agent. *Lung Cancer* 2009;64:211–218.
60. Garcia-Carbonero R, Paz-Ares L. Systemic chemotherapy in the management of malignant peritoneal mesothelioma. *Eur J Surg Oncol* 2006;32:676–681.
61. Feldman AL, Libutti SK, Pingpank JF, et al. Analysis of factors associated with outcome in patients with malignant peritoneal mesothelioma undergoing surgical debulking and intraperitoneal chemotherapy. *J Clin Oncol* 2003;21:4560–4567.
62. Sugarbaker PH, Yan TD, Stuart OA, et al. Comprehensive management of diffuse malignant peritoneal mesothelioma. *Eur J Surg Oncol* 2006;32:686–691.
63. Deraco M, Nonaka D, Baratti D, et al. Prognostic analysis of clinicopathologic factors in 49 patients with diffuse malignant peritoneal mesothelioma treated with cytoreductive surgery and intraperitoneal hyperthermic perfusion. *Ann Surg Oncol* 2006;13:229–237.
64. Deraco M, Baratti D, Zaffaroni N, et al. Advances in clinical research and management of diffuse peritoneal mesothelioma. *Recent Results Cancer Res* 2007;169:137–155.
65. Deraco M, Bartlett D, Kusamura S, et al. Consensus statement on peritoneal mesothelioma. *J Surg Oncol* 2008;98:268–272.
66. Hioki M, Gotohda N, Konishi M, et al. Predictive factors improving survival after gastrectomy in gastric cancer patients with peritoneal carcinomatosis. *World J Surg* 2010;34:555–562.
67. Glehen O, Mohamed F, Gilly FN. Peritoneal carcinomatosis from digestive tract cancer: new management by cytoreductive surgery and intraperitoneal chemohyperthermia. *Lancet Oncol* 2004;5:219–228.
68. Boku N. Gastrointestinal Oncology Study Group of Japan Clinical Oncology Group. Chemotherapy for metastatic disease: review from JCOG trials. *Int J Clin Oncol* 2008;13:196–200.
69. Yonemura Y, Kawamura T, Bandou E, et al. Treatment of peritoneal dissemination from gastric cancer by peritonectomy and chemohyperthermic peritoneal perfusion. *Br J Surg* 2005;92:370–375.
70. Glehen O, Cotte F, Sayag-Beaujard AC, et al. Cytoreductive surgery and intraperitoneal chemohyperthermia for peritoneal carcinomatosis arising from gastric cancer. *Arch Surg* 2004;139:20–26.
71. Fujimoto S, Takahashi M, Mutou T, et al. Improved mortality rate of gastric carcinoma patients with peritoneal carcinomatosis treated with intraperitoneal hyperthermic chemoperfusion combined with surgery. *Cancer* 1997;79:884–891.
72. Glehen O, Gilly FN, Arvieux C, et al. Peritoneal carcinomatosis from gastric cancer: a multi-institutional study of 159 patients treated by cytoreductive surgery combined with perioperative intraperitoneal chemotherapy. *Ann Surg Oncol* 2010;17:2370–2377.
73. Yonemura Y, Fujimura T, Nishimura G, et al. Effects of intraoperative chemohyperthermia in patients with gastric cancer with peritoneal dissemination. *Surgery* 1996;119:437–444.
74. Hall JJ, Loggie BW, Shen P, et al. Cytoreductive surgery with intraperitoneal hyperthermic chemotherapy for advanced gastric cancer. *J Gastrointest Surg* 2004;8:454–463.
75. Mohamed F, Moran BJ. Morbidity and mortality with cytoreductive surgery and intraperitoneal chemotherapy. *Cancer J* 2009;15:196–199.
76. Yan TD, Links M, Fransi S, et al. Learning curve for cytoreductive surgery and perioperative intraperitoneal chemotherapy for peritoneal surface malignancy—a journey to becoming a Nationally Funded Peritonectomy Center. *Ann Surg Oncol* 2007;14:2270–2280.
77. Yang XJ, Huang CQ, Suo T, et al. Cytoreductive surgery and hyperthermic intraperitoneal chemotherapy improves survival of patients with peritoneal carcinomatosis from gastric cancer: final results of a phase III randomized clinical trial. *Ann Surg Oncol* 2011;18:1575–1581.
78. Prospektive multizentrische Phase III-Studie zur zytoreduktiven Chirurgie mit hyperthermer intraperitonealer Chemoperfusion nach präoperativer Chemotherapie beim Magenkarzinom inkl. AEG mit primärer peritonealer Metastasierung (Gastripec I). EudraCT-Number: 2006-006088-22 Phase III-Trial.
79. Yonemura Y, de Aretxabala X, Fujimura T, et al. Intraoperative chemohyperthermic peritoneal perfusion as an adjuvant to gastric cancer: final results of a randomized controlled study. *Hepatogastroenterology* 2001;48:1776–1782.
80. Fujimoto S, Takahashi M, Mutou T, et al. Successful intraperitoneal hyperthermic chemoperfusion for the prevention of postoperative peritoneal recurrence in patients with advanced gastric carcinoma. *Cancer* 1999;85: 529–534.
81. Kim JY, Bae HS. A controlled clinical study of serosa-invasive gastric carcinoma patients who underwent surgery plus intraperitoneal hyperthermo-chemo-perfusion (IHCP). *Gastric Cancer* 2001;4:27–33.
82. Zhu ZG, Tang R, Yan M, et al. Efficacy and safety of intraoperative peritoneal hyperthermic chemotherapy for advanced gastric cancer patients with serosal invasion. A long-term follow-up study. *Dig Surg* 2006;23:93–102.
83. Scaringi S, Kianmanesh R, Sabate JM, et al. Advanced gastric cancer with or without peritoneal carcinomatosis treated with hyperthermic intra-peritoneal-chemotherapy: a single Western center experience. *Eur J Surg Oncol* 2008;34: 1246–1252.
84. De Roover A, Detroz B, Detry O, et al. Adjuvant hyperthermic intraperitoneal preoperative chemotherapy (HIPEC) associated with curative surgery for locally advanced gastric carcinoma. An initial experience. *Acta Chir Belg* 2006;106:297–301.
85. Yan TD, Black D, Sugarbaker PH, et al. A systematic review and meta-analysis of the randomized controlled trials on adjuvant intraperitoneal chemotherapy for resectable gastric cancer. *Ann Surg Oncol* 2007;14:2702–2713.
86. Xu DZ, Zhan YQ, Sun XW, et al. Meta-analysis of intraperitoneal chemotherapy for gastric cancer. *World J Gastroenterol* 2004;10:2727–2730.
87. D2 Resection and HIPEC (Hyperthermic Intraperitoneal Chemoperfusion) in Locally Advanced Gastric Carcinoma (GASTRICHIP). ClinicalTrials.gov Identifier: NCT01882933 (http://clinicaltrials.gov/show/NCT01882933).
88. Helm CW, Richard SD, Pan J, et al. Hyperthermic intraperitoneal chemotherapy in ovarian cancer: first report of the HYPER-O registry. *Int J Gynecol Cancer* 2010;20:61–69.
89. Ceelen WP, Van Nieuwenhove Y, Van Belle S, et al. Cytoreduction and hyperthermic intraperitoneal chemoperfusion in women with heavily pretreated recurrent ovarian cancer. *Ann Surg Oncol* 2012;19:2352–2359.
90. Bakrin N, Cotte E, Golfier F, et al. Cytoreductive surgery and hyperthermic intraperitoneal chemotherapy (HIPEC) for persistent and recurrent advanced ovarian carcinoma: A multicenter, prospective study of 246 patients. *Ann Surg Oncol* 2012;19:4052–4058.
91. Bakrin N, Bereder JM, Decullier E, et al. Peritoneal carcinomatosis treated with cytoreductive surgery and Hyperthermic Intraperitoneal Chemotherapy (HIPEC) for advanced ovarian carcinoma: A French multicentre retrospective cohort study of 566 patients. *Eur J Surg Oncol* 2013;39:1435–1443.
92. Fagotti A, Costantini B, Petrillo M, et al. Cytoreductive surgery plus HIPEC in platinum-sensitive recurrent ovarian cancer patients: a case-control study on survival in patients with two year follow-up. *Gynecol Oncol* 2012;127: 502–505.
93. Deraco M, Kusamura S, Virzì S, et al. Cytoreductive surgery and hyperthermic intraperitoneal chemotherapy as upfront therapy for advanced epithelial ovarian cancer: multi-institutional phase-II trial. *Gynecol Oncol* 2011;122:215–220.
94. Karakousis CP, Kontzoglou K, Driscoll DL. Intraperitoneal chemotherapy in disseminated abdominal sarcoma. *Ann Surg Oncol* 1997;4:496–498.
95. Bilimoria MM, Holtz DJ, Mirza NQ, et al. Tumor volume as a prognostic factor for sarcomatosis. *Cancer* 2002;94:2441–2446.
96. Berthet B, Sugarbaker TA, Chang D, et al. Quantitative methodologies for selection of patients with recurrent abdominopelvic sarcoma for treatment. *Eur J Cancer* 1999;35:413–419.
97. Eilber FC, Rosen G, Forscher C, et al. Surgical resection and intraperitoneal chemotherapy for recurrent abdominal sarcomas. *Ann Surg Oncol* 1999;6:645–650.
98. Rossi CR, Deraco M, De Simone M, et al. Hyperthermic intraperitoneal intraoperative chemotherapy after cytoreductive surgery for the treatment of abdominal sarcomatosis: clinical outcome and prognostic factors in 60 consecutive patients. *Cancer* 2004;100:1943–1950.
99. Bonvalot S, Cavalcanti A, Le Pechoux C, et al. Randomized trial of cytoreduction followed by intraperitoneal chemotherapy versus cytoreduction alone in patients with peritoneal sarcomatosis. *Eur J Surg Oncol* 2005;31:917–923.
100. Baratti D, Pennacchioli E, Kusamura S, et al. Peritoneal sarcomatosis: is there a subset of patients who may benefit from cytoreductive surgery and hyperthermic intraperitoneal chemotherapy? *Ann Surg Oncol* 2010;17:3220–3228.
101. Rossi CR, Casali P, Kusamura S, et al. The consensus statement on the locoregional treatment of abdominal sarcomatosis. *J Surg Oncol* 2008;98:291–294.

INDEX

Note: Page locators followed by *f* and *t* indicate figure and table, respectively.

D

E

N

Q

R

T